The Managed Health Care Handbook

Fourth Edition

Edited by

Peter R. Kongstvedt, MD, FACP

AN ASPEN PUBLICATION®
Aspen Publishers, Inc.
Gaithersburg, Maryland
2001

This publication is designed to provide accurate and authoritative information in regard to the Subject Matter covered. It is sold with the understanding that the publisher is not engaged in rendering legal, accounting, or other professional service. If legal advice or other expert assistance is required, the service of a competent professional person should be sought. (From a Declaration of Principles jointly adopted by a Committee of the American Bar Association and a Committee of Publishers and Associations.)

Library of Congress Cataloging-in-Publication Data

The managed health care handbook/[edited by] Peter R. Kongstvedt.—4th ed.
p. ; cm.
Includes bibliographical references and index.
ISBN 0-8342-1726-0
1. Managed care plans (Medical care)—United States—Management.   I. Kongstvedt,
Peter R. (Peter Reid)
[DNLM: 1. Managed Care Programs—organization & administration—United States.
W 130 AA1 M26 2000]
RA413.M28 2000
362.1'04258—dc21
00-035580

Orders: (800) 638-8437
Customer Service: (800) 234-1660

About Aspen Publishers • For more than 40 years, Aspen has been a leading professional publisher in a variety of disciplines. Aspen's vast information resources are available in both print and electronic formats. We are committed to providing the highest quality information available in the most appropriate format for our customers. Visit Aspen's Internet site for more information resources, directories, articles, and a searchable version of Aspen's full catalog, including the most recent publications: **www.aspenpublishers.com**
Aspen Publishers, Inc. • The hallmark of quality in publishing
Member of the worldwide Wolters Kluwer group.

Editorial Services: Ruth Bloom
Library of Congress Catalog Card Number: 00-035580
ISBN: 0-8342-1726-0

Printed in the United States of America

1   2   3   4   5

This book is dedicated to my family:
my late father, *Gerald Nicholas Kongstvedt*;
my mother, *Elizabeth Pearson Kongstvedt*;
my sister *Chris Lieberman*,
and especially my wife, *Sheryl* and my son *David*.

Table of Contents

About the Editor .... **xxiv**

Contributors .... **xxv**

Preface .... **xxix**

Acknowledgments .... **xxxi**

PART I—INTRODUCTION TO MANAGED CARE **1**

CHAPTER 1—AN OVERVIEW OF MANAGED CARE **3**

Peter D. Fox

Introduction 3
Managed Care: The Early Years (Pre–1970) 4
The Adolescent Years: 1970–1985 5
Managed Care Comes of Age: 1985 to the Present 9
Future Issues Facing Managed Care 13
Conclusion 15

CHAPTER 2—MANAGED CARE'S REGULATORY EVOLUTION:
DRIVING CHANGE IN THE NEW CENTURY **17**

Frederick B. Abbey

Forces Driving Federal Health Policy 17
Major Areas of Policy Development 21
Outlook 25

CHAPTER 3—TYPES OF MANAGED CARE ORGANIZATIONS **28**

Eric R. Wagner

Types of MCOs 30
HMO Models 33
Conclusion 41

CHAPTER 4—INTEGRATED HEALTH CARE DELIVERY SYSTEMS 42

Peter R. Kongstvedt, David W. Plocher, and Jean C. Stanford

Introduction 42
Highly Integrated Delivery Systems 43
Market Characteristics 44
Types of IDSs 45
IPAs 45
PPMCs 47
Consolidated Medical Groups 50
PHOs 52
MSOs 56
Foundations 57
Staff Model 58
Physician Ownership Model 59
PSOs 60
Virtual Integration 62
Global Capitation 62
Acquisition of Physician Practices 64
Legal Pitfalls for IDSs 66
Critical Success Factors for IDSs 68
Conclusion 71

**CHAPTER 5—ELEMENTS OF THE MANAGEMENT CONTROL
AND GOVERNANCE STRUCTURE** 73

Peter R. Kongstvedt

Board of Directors 73
Key Management Positions 76
Committees 78
Management Control Structure 79
Conclusion 80

CHAPTER 6—EXAMINING COMMON ASSERTIONS ABOUT MANAGED CARE 81

Richard I. Smith, Daniel Thornton, and Terry Sollom

Introduction 81
Managed Care Myths 82
Conclusion 88

PART II—THE HEALTH CARE DELIVERY SYSTEM 91

CHAPTER 7—PRIMARY CARE IN MANAGED HEALTH CARE PLANS 93

Peter R. Kongstvedt

Introduction and Definitions 93
Recruiting 94
Nonphysician or Midlevel Practitioners 95
Types of Contracting Situations 97
Credentialing 100
The National Practitioner Data Bank 101
Healthcare Integrity and Protection Data Bank 103
Compensation 105
Orientation 105

Network Maintenance 105
Internet-Based Activities 106
Removing Physicians from the Network 107
Conclusion 108

**CHAPTER 8—COMPENSATION OF PRIMARY CARE PHYSICIANS
IN MANAGED HEALTH CARE** **110**

Peter R. Kongstvedt

Introduction 110
Basic Models of Reimbursement 111
Capitation 113
Withholds and Risk/Bonus Arrangements 118
Capitation Pools for Referral and Institutional Services 118
Full Professional Risk Capitation 124
Reasons To Capitate 125
Problems with Capitation Systems 126
Effect of Benefits Design on Reimbursement 127
Fee for Service 129
A Special Requirement for Reimbursement When Coinsurance Is in Place 131
Out-of-Network Fees 132
Discounts, Negotiated Fee Schedules, Fee Maximums, or Fee Allowances 132
Relative Value Scales 133
Global Fees 134
Problems with FFS in Managed Health Care Plans 137
Legislation and Regulation Applicable to Physician Incentive Programs 138
Civil Liability in Physician Compensation Programs 143
Conclusion 144

**CHAPTER 9—PHYSICIAN COMPENSATION IN MEDICAL GROUPS
AND HEALTH SYSTEMS** **147**

James A. Rodeghero

Background 147
Traditional Concepts in Pay Plan Design 148
Pay Plan Design Issues 150
General Design Alternatives 153
Measurement Issues 156
The Role of Benefits in Total Compensation 157
Compensating Medical Directors and Administrative Physicians 158
Compensating Hospital-Based Practitioners 159
Compensation in Faculty Practice Plans under Managed Care 159
Examples 161
Designing Performance Measures 162
Conclusion 163

**CHAPTER 10—NONUTILIZATION–BASED INCENTIVE
COMPENSATION FOR PHYSICIANS** **166**

Peter R. Kongstvedt

Introduction 166
Problems with Evaluation Systems 167
Categories for Evaluation of Physician Performance 168
Measuring the Categories and Producing a Result 172
Conclusion 174

CHAPTER 11—CONTRACTING AND REIMBURSEMENT OF SPECIALTY PHYSICIANS **175**

Peter R. Kongstvedt

Introduction 175
How Many Specialty Care Physicians? 175
Primary versus Specialty Care Designation 176
Credentialing 177
Types of Reimbursement Arrangements 178
Organizational Models for Capitating Specialty Services 184
Common Problems with Specialty Capitation 186
Other Forms of Specialty Physician Reimbursement 187
Risk and Reward 189
Conclusion 189

CHAPTER 12—NEGOTIATING AND CONTRACTING WITH HOSPITALS AND INSTITUTIONS **191**

Peter R. Kongstvedt

Introduction 191
Hospital Network Development 191
Types of Reimbursement Arrangements 196
Outpatient Procedures 204
Conclusion 205

CHAPTER 13—ACADEMIC HEALTH CENTERS AND MANAGED CARE **206**

Jennifer H. Lofland and David B. Nash

Dimensions of the Problem 207
Strategies for Success 213
A New Role for MCOs 223
Conclusion 225

CHAPTER 14—HEALTH CENTERS AND MANAGED HEALTH CARE **228**

Pamela J. Byrnes, Judith Shea, and Richard J. Jacobsen

Introduction 228
Community Health Centers 230
Public Policy and Support 231
Entry into Managed Care 233
Operational and Strategic Responses to Managed Care 234
Formation of CHC-Sponsored Health Plans 237
The Impact of Managed Care and Challenges for the Future 240
Conclusion 243

CHAPTER 15—COMPLEMENTARY AND ALTERNATIVE MEDICINE INTEGRATION: TRENDS, STRUCTURES, AND CHALLENGES **245**

John Weeks

Introduction 245
Orientation: Stakeholder Activity 245
Models and Challenges: Network Delivered Services 251

Challenges and Models: Hospitals and Health Systems 258
Conclusion: Exploratory Integration for Moving CAM Out of Quarantine 260

PART III—MEDICAL MANAGEMENT 265

CHAPTER 16—CARE MANAGEMENT AND CLINICAL INTEGRATION COMPONENTS 267

David W. Plocher, Wendy L. Wilson, Jacqueline A. Lutz, and Ann Huston

The Context for Advanced Care Management 267
Defining Advanced Care Management 268
Integrating the Components of Care Management 269
The Role of Physicians in Care Management 272
Building an Advanced Care Management System: A Typical Process 273
Defining the Future State of Care Management 278
Conclusion 280
Appendix 16–A—Description of the Components of the Advanced Care
Management System 281

CHAPTER 17—PRIMARY PREVENTION IN MANAGED HEALTH CARE 284

Leif I. Solberg

Introduction 284
Why Should an MCO Do Prevention? 285
Typology of HP/DP Activities 285
A Framework for Action 286
Taking Advantage of the Clinical Setting 287
Health Data Systems 291
Population-Based (Member) Programs 291
Community Outreach Programs 291
Public Policy Initiatives 292
Conclusion 292

CHAPTER 18—MANAGING BASIC MEDICAL-SURGICAL UTILIZATION 294

Peter R. Kongstvedt

Introduction 294
Return on Investment in Management of Medical Costs 294
Demand Management 295
Measurements of Utilization 298
Variations in Utilization 301
The Role of Electronic Commerce 305
Authorization or Denial of Payment for Services 305
Managing Utilization of Specialty Services 306
The Role of the Primary Care Physician in Specialty Services Management 307
Single Visit Authorizations Only 309
Specialty Physicians As Primary Physicians 310
Prohibition of Secondary Referrals and Authorizations 311
Review of Reasons for Referral 311
Institutional Utilization Management 313
Common Methods for Managing Utilization 314
Alternatives to Acute Care Hospitalization 324
Case Management 326
Conclusion 327

CHAPTER 19—CLINICAL SERVICES REQUIRING AUTHORIZATION 331

Peter R. Kongstvedt

Definition of Services Requiring Authorization 331
Definition of Who Can Authorize Services 332
Claims Payment 334
Categories of Authorization 335
Staffing 337
Common Data Elements 338
Methods of Data Capture and Authorization Issuance 339
Authorization System Reports 341
Open Access HMOs 341
Specialty-Physician Based Authorization Systems 342
Non-Physician-Based Authorization Systems 342
Conclusion 343

CHAPTER 20—ANCILLARY DIAGNOSTIC AND THERAPEUTIC SERVICES 344

Peter R. Kongstvedt

Introduction 344
Ancillary Services 344
Physician-Owned Ancillary Services 345
Data Capture 346
Financial Incentives 346
Feedback 346
Control Points 346
Contracting and Reimbursement for Ancillary Services 347
Conclusion 349

CHAPTER 21—THE EMERGENCY DEPARTMENT AND MANAGED CARE 351

Casey Jason and Meera Kanhouwa

Overview 351
Challenges Shared by Managed Care and Emergency Medicine 352
Creating Efficiencies and Improving Productivity 355
Technology Impact 363
Opportunities with Managed Care 366

CHAPTER 22—CASE MANAGEMENT AND MANAGED CARE 371

Catherine M. Mullahy

The Case Manager's Role 371
Patient Profile: Not Every Case Needs a Case Manager 372
On-Site versus Telephone-Based Case Management 374
Case Managers in Managed Care 375
Case Management Work Format and Process 375
Utilization Review: Preadmission and Concurrent Review and Case Management 384
Preadmission and Concurrent Review Case Management Reports 388
Red Flags: Indicators for Case Management 393
Timing Case Management Intervention 393
Beyond the Case Management Basics 397
A Long-Term Solution to a Long-Term Problem 400

**CHAPTER 23—FUNDAMENTALS AND CORE COMPETENCIES OF
DISEASE MANAGEMENT** **402**

David W. Plocher

Definition and Clarification 402
Barriers and Drivers for Disease Management 405
Business Plan 405
Survey of Disease Management Programs 406
Important Linkages 408
Support from Electronic Commerce 409
Conclusion 411

CHAPTER 24—PRESCRIPTION DRUG BENEFITS IN MANAGED CARE **413**

Robert P. Navarro

Financial Basis for Pharmacy Benefit Management 413
Pharmacy Program Cost Components 415
Principles of Pharmacy Benefit Management 417
Managing the Supply and Demand 418
Pharmacy Information Systems and Health Informatics 418
Pharmacy Benefit Management Companies (PBMs) 423
Pharmacy Benefit Management Program Components 426
Physician Provider Network 428
Pharmacy Provider Network 429
Pharmacy Provider Audits 432
Drug Formulary Management 433
Pharmaceutical Manufacturer Discount and Rebate Contracts 438
Prescription Patient Copayments 439
Role of Pharmacy Programs in Disease Management and Quality Improvement
    Programs 444
Quality Improvement in Pharmacy Benefit Management 444
Measuring Pharmacy Benefit Management Program Performance 446
Future Changes in Pharmacy Benefit Management 447
Conclusion 447

**CHAPTER 25—MANAGED BEHAVIORAL HEALTH CARE AND
CHEMICAL DEPENDENCY SERVICES** **451**

*Donald F. Anderson, Jeffrey L. Berlant, Katherine O. Sternbach, Danna Mauch,
    H.G. Whittington, William R. Maloney, and Terri Goens*

Introduction 451
Historical Perspective 452
Key Treatment Principles 456
Benefit Plan Design 461
Utilization Management 463
Channeling Mechanisms 465
Provider Structures for Integrated Delivery Systems To Meet Managed Care Objectives 467
Quality Assurance 469
BH Information Systems 473
Public/Private Systems Integration 476
Emerging Issues 477
Conclusion 478

CHAPTER 26—HOME HEALTH CARE **480**

Peggy H. Rodebush, Laura L. Waltrip, and G. David Baker

Introduction 480
What Is Home Care? 481
History of Home Care 481
Indicators and Predictors of Home Care Demand 482
Home Care Services and Disciplines 486
Home Care Providers 486
Regulations Guiding Home Care 488
Financing Home Care Services 490
Recent Legislation and Regulatory Issues Affecting Home Care 492
Measuring Quality in Home Care Services 493
Examples of Advanced Clinical Practices in Home Care 494

**CHAPTER 27—SUBACUTE CARE WITHIN THE MANAGED
CARE SYSTEM** **496**

Kathleen M. Griffin

Categories 496
Subacute Patients 496
Subacute Providers 497
Subacute Care Sites in the Future 499
Subacute Care within a Continuum of Care 499
Payment for Subacute Care 500
Selecting a Quality Subacute Provider 501
Conclusion 504
Appendix 27–A—NSCA and Joint Commission Definitions of Subacute Care ... 505
Appendix 27–B—Categories of Subacute Care 506

CHAPTER 28—HOSPICE AND END-OF-LIFE CARE **508**

Anne C. Dye, Peggy H. Rodebush, and Geri Hempel

Medical Management and End-of-Life Care 508
The Basics of Hospice Care 510
Financing and Reimbursement 511
Size of the U.S. Hospice Industry 512
Major Policy Issues 513
Service Models 515
Hospice Cost and Staffing 517
Specialty Programs 517
Future Integration and Affiliation Strategies 519

**CHAPTER 29—CLINICAL PATHWAYS: LINKING OUTCOMES FOR
PATIENTS, CLINICIANS, PAYERS, AND EMPLOYERS** **521**

Richard J. Coffey and Sarah S. LeRoy

Introduction 521
Background and Terminology 522
Scopes and Uses 522
Environment 524
Development 525
Application 528

Alternative Formats and Sample Uses 529
Results 533
Conclusion 538

CHAPTER 30—QUALITY MANAGEMENT IN MANAGED CARE **539**

Pamela B. Siren

Introduction 539
Traditional Quality Assurance 539
Components of a Quality Management Program 543
A Process Model for a Modern Quality Management Program 544
Conclusion 554

CHAPTER 31—MEASURING AND MANAGING OF CLINICAL OUTCOMES **556**

Michael Pine

Domains of Clinical Outcomes Measurement 556
Goals of Clinical Outcomes Measurement 556
Measuring Comparative Risk-Adjusted Clinical Outcomes 558
Using Data on Risk-Adjusted Costs To Craft Measures of Clinical Performance 567
Using Adverse Outcome Rates To Reduce Costs 570
Using Control Charts To Get a Dynamic View of Performance 572
Relating Clinical Outcomes to Processes of Care 572
Monitoring Clinical Outcomes of Ambulatory Care 575
Conclusion 578

CHAPTER 32—USING DATA AND PROVIDER PROFILING IN MEDICAL MANAGEMENT **579**

Peter R. Kongstvedt, Norbert I. Goldfield, and David W. Plocher

Introduction 579
Use of Data and Information in Medical Management 580
Patient Data Confidentiality 583
Data Elements and the Application of Reports 586
General Types of Reports 590
Provider Profiling 595
Desired Characteristics of Provider Profiles 597
The Need To Adjust for Severity of Illness 600
Selection of a Profiling Vendor 610
The Future of Data Use 614
Conclusion 615

CHAPTER 33—PHYSICIAN BEHAVIOR CHANGE IN MANAGED HEALTH CARE **618**

Peter R. Kongstvedt

Introduction 618
General Aspects of Physician Practice Behavior 618
General Approaches to Changing Behavior 626
Programmatic Approaches to Changing Physician Behavior 628
Addressing Noncompliance by Individual Physicians 630
Conclusion 633

CHAPTER 34—MEMBER BEHAVIOR CHANGE **637**

Nancy W. Spangler

Introduction 637
They Know Better, So Why Don't They Just Stop? 637
Models for Affecting Patient Behaviors 641
Tools for Enhancing Change 646
From Theory into Practice: Humana's CHIP Program 649
Conclusion 651

PART IV—OPERATIONAL MARKETING AND MANAGEMENT **655**

CHAPTER 35—INFORMATION SYSTEMS IN MANAGED HEALTH CARE PLANS **657**

James S. Slubowski

Introduction 657
Core Managed Care Information System 658
Electronic Data Interchange 662
Privacy and Confidentiality under HIPAA 663
Value-Added Services—The Next Generation 666
HEDIS 670
Information Services Department 673
Conclusion 674

**CHAPTER 36—INFORMATION SYSTEMS AND ELECTRONIC COMMERCE FOR
PROVIDER SYSTEMS IN MANAGED HEALTH CARE** **676**

Robert G. Reese and Rick Majzun

Introduction: Major Issues Facing Health Care Provider Organizations
    in the Year 2000 676
Health Care Is a Business in an Information Economy 676
Health Care Provider Organizations Are Building the Information Infrastructure
    for a New Era in Health Care 677
Pressures on Both the Cost and Revenue Sides of the Equation Are Increasing 677
Information Technology Should Support Business Strategy and Market Need 677
Interconnectivity 678
Data Repositories or Warehouses: The Backbone of the Organization's
    Clinical and Financial Systems 679
Enterprise-Wide Information Systems 680
Use of Information Technology in Managing Care 680
Computerized Medical Records 681
Clinical Decision Support Systems 682
Knowledge Management Systems 683
Data Privacy and Security 684
Electronic Commerce 684
Capital Budgeting for Information Technology 687
Organizational Structure of Information Technology Departments 689
Client Relationships 689
Outsourcing the Information Technology Function 691
Conclusion: Information Technology Will Play a Key Role in Improving the
    Health Care Provider Organization's Ability To Manage Care 692

CHAPTER 37—ELECTRONIC COMMERCE IN MANAGED HEALTH CARE **694**

Britton L. Pim and Sean D. Kenny

E-Commerce in Health Care 694
E-Commerce Technologies 696
E-Commerce Functionality 701
External Impact 703
Internal E-Commerce Opportunities 705
Challenges 707
Critical Success Factors 708
Conclusion 709

CHAPTER 38—CLAIMS AND BENEFITS ADMINISTRATION **710**

Robin L. McElfatrick and Robert S. Eichler

Introduction 710
Claims: Positioning, Purpose, and Opportunities 711
Organizational Structure and Staffing 713
Claims Operations Management 718
Productivity 729
Turn Around Time 731
Staff Training and Development 732
Quality 735
Policy and Procedure 737
Coordination with Other Departments/Functions 739
Systems Support 739
Claims Business Functions 743
Other Issues 751
Conclusion 754

**CHAPTER 39—OTHER PARTY LIABILITY AND COORDINATION OF
BENEFITS** **755**

Barry S. Scheur, Robin L. McElfatrick, and Robert S. Eichler

Definitions 756
Contractual Support/Requirements 758
Legal Issues Based on Case Law 760
Organizational Placement (with Dedicated Staff) 761
COB: Basic Procedure Defined 761
Subrogation: Basic Procedure Defined 763
Accounting for OPL 763
OPL Policy Issues 766
OPL in a Capitated Environment 766
Outsourcing OPL 768
Conclusion 769

CHAPTER 40—MEMBER SERVICES AND CONSUMER AFFAIRS **771**

Peter R. Kongstvedt

Provision of General Information 772
Conclusion 797

CHAPTER 41—SALES AND MARKETING IN MANAGED HEALTH CARE PLANS: THE PROCESS OF DISTRIBUTION **798**

Gail Marcus and John C. Thomson

What Managed Care Organizations Deliver 798
Challenges Facing MCOs 800
An Overview of the Managed Care Market 804
Key Decision Makers and Influencers in the Managed Care Distribution Process 804
The Managed Care Sales Process 809
How the Managed Care Team Delivers 812
The Management of Sales and Marketing Professionals 815
Conclusion 816

CHAPTER 42—THE EMPLOYER'S VIEW OF MANAGED HEALTH CARE: SHOW ME THE VALUE **817**

Michael J. Taylor

Recent Managed Care Trends Affecting Employers 817
How These Trends Impact Employers Both Large and Small 818
The Large Group Employer: 5,000 Lives Plus 818
The Moderate Group Employer: 500–5,000 Lives 819
The Medium Group Employer: 50–500 Lives 819
The Small Group Employer: 0–50 Lives 820
How Employers Purchase Value (1988–1998) 820
Looking for Value: 2000 and Beyond 822
Future Trends 824
Conclusion 825

CHAPTER 43—THE IMPACT OF CONSUMERISM ON MANAGED HEALTH CARE **828**

Jacqueline A. Lutz and Hindy J. Shaman

Why Is Consumerism a Significant Trend? 828
Who Is the New Health Care Consumer? 835
What Are the Implications of Consumerism? 836
How Can Organizations Develop a Consumer Strategy? 845
What Consumerism Means for the Managed Care Industry 846
Conclusion 846

CHAPTER 44—ACCREDITATION AND PERFORMANCE MEASUREMENT PROGRAMS FOR MANAGED CARE ORGANIZATIONS **849**

Margaret E. O'Kane

Introduction 849
Oversight by Type of Organization 850
National Committee for Quality Assurance 851
The Utilization Review Accreditation Commission 861
Joint Commission on Accreditation of Healthcare Organizations 865
Conclusion 869

CHAPTER 45—RISK MANAGEMENT IN MANAGED CARE **871**

Barbara J. Youngberg

Introduction 871
Changes in the Health Care Organization Related to Managed Care 873
Operational Risks under Managed Care 875

Managing Corporate Negligence 876
Clinical Decision Making 879
Utilization Management Issues 879
Emerging Case Law 879
Reducing Utilization Management Exposure 880
Externally Imposed Practice Guidelines or Standards of Care 881
Multi-Site Challenges 881
The Convergence of Financial and Risk Management 882
Using the Risk Management Process To Control the Risks of Managed Care 884
Conclusion 884

**CHAPTER 46—COMMON OPERATIONAL PROBLEMS IN MANAGED
HEALTH CARE PLANS** **886**

Peter R. Kongstvedt

Introduction and Background 886
Common versus Unique Problems or Events 887
Common Problems in Managed Care Organizations 888
Conclusion 903

PART V—FINANCE AND UNDERWRITING **905**

CHAPTER 47—OPERATIONAL FINANCE AND BUDGETING **907**

Dale F. Harding

Background 907
Financial Statement Components 908
Balance Sheeet 915
Regulatory Reporting Considerations 917
Budgeting and Financial Forecasting 919
Conclusion 921

CHAPTER 48—TAX ISSUES RELATING TO HEALTH RISK-BEARING ENTITIES **922**

Phillip G. Royalty and Terry A. Jacobs

Taxable Health Risk-Bearing Entities 922
Tax Exempt Health Risk-Bearing Entities 927
Appendix 48–A—*Internal Revenue Service Manual Exempt ORganizations Handbook—*
    Chapter 27: Health Maintenance Organizations 935

**CHAPTER 49—UNDERWRITING AND RATING FUNCTIONS
COMMON TO MOST MARKETS** **945**

Stephen M. Cigich and Michael G. Sturm

Underwriting 945
Rating 947
Conclusion 951

CHAPTER 50—UNDERWRITING AND RATING FUNCTIONS BY MARKET **952**

Michael G. Sturm

Individual Nongovernment Market 952
Commercial Group Market 954
Medicare Supplement 967
Medicare Risk 968

Medicaid Risk 969
Conclusion 970

CHAPTER 51—ACTUARIAL SERVICES IN AN INTEGRATED DELIVERY SYSTEM 971

Stephen M. Cigich

Summary of Actuarial Services 971
Identifying and Realizing Opportunities 972
Creating Incentive Structures 974
Measuring Results 975
Conclusion 975

CHAPTER 52—OPERATIONAL UNDERWRITING IN MANAGED CARE ORGANIZATIONS 977

Gregory J. Lippe

Historical Overview 977
Sales and Underwriting Collaboration 979
Management Information System 979
Regulation 980
Major Risk Factors 981
Underwriting As an Internal Control 982
Employer Group Underwriting 983
Key Employer Group Data 984
Market Factors and Trends 985
Community Rating Methodologies 986
Underwriting Principles 994
Administrative Service Only Underwriting 997
Effective Underwriting: Lessons Learned 997
Conclusion 999

CHAPTER 53—PROVIDER EXCESS LOSS COVERAGE 1000

Scott A. Walker

Introduction 1000
Capitation—The Need for Protection 1001
PEL under Provider Risk Contracting 1003
Types of PEL Coverage 1004
Specific Excess Rate Development 1004
Experience-Specific PEL Rating 1016
Aggregate Excess Rate Development 1023
PEL Policy Coverage Form 1025
Coverage Availability 1032
Conclusion 1032
Appendix 53–A—Sample PEL Policy Language 1034

PART VI—SPECIAL MARKET SEGMENTS 1041

CHAPTER 54—THE FEDERAL EMPLOYEES HEALTH BENEFITS PROGRAM AND MANAGED CARE 1043

Christine C. Rinn

The Application Process 1044
Premium Contribution and Benefit Design 1044

Patients' Bill of Rights and Responsibilities 1045
Premium Rating under the FEHBP 1045
OPM Audits and Appeals 1051
FEHBP and False Claims Liability 1054
OPM's Policy on Error Reporting 1055
Miscellaneous Contracting Issues 1055
Quality Assurance 1057
Conclusion 1057

CHAPTER 55—MEDICARE AND MANAGED CARE 1060

Carlos Zarabozo and Jean D. LeMasurier

Introduction 1060
Organization of the Chapter 1061
Who Is Eligible for a Medicare Risk Contract? 1061
The Exception in State Licensure: Provider-Sponsored Organizations 1062
Other New Options 1063
Muddying the Waters: Plans versus Organizations 1065
Federal Preemption 1072
What the Contract Requires (Finally!) 1073
Limitations on Physician Incentive Plans 1075
Consumer Protections 1076
Provider Protections and Rights: Conscience Protection 1077
Information Dissemination 1078
Enrollment 1078
Marketing Rules 1081
Interactions with Your Government 1081
The Contracting Process 1082
Web Resources and Other Contacts 1083
Future Direction of the Program 1083

CHAPTER 56—MEDICARE + CHOICE: THE HEALTH PLAN'S VIEW 1086

Craig S. Schub and Nick Franklin

Introduction 1086
Today's Elderly 1086
The Demographic Imperative: Aging Population and Unpredictable Health Care Costs 1088
Public Policy Initiatives: From 1965 to the Balanced Budget Act 1088
Evolving Challenges and Opportunities of Medicare + Choice (Risk) Contractors 1092
Changing Dynamics of the Delivery System 1096
Future Trends 1103

CHAPTER 57—MEDICAID MANAGED CARE 1105

Robert E. Hurley and Stephen A. Somers

Introduction 1105
Medicaid—Origins and Evolution 1106
Medicaid Managed Care—Background and Models 1107
Operational Features 1108
Successes of Medicaid Managed Care 1113
Shortfalls of Medicaid Managed Care 1116
The Challenging Contemporary Context 1119
Longer Term Questions and Concerns 1120
Conclusion 1122

CHAPTER 58—CHAMPUS AND THE DEPARTMENT OF DEFENSE MANAGED CARE PROGRAMS 1124

Steve Lillie and Larry Sobel

Legal Authority and Responsibilities 1125
The Military Medical Benefits Program 1125
Eligibility for TRICARE 1126
TRICARE Options 1126
TRICARE Benefits 1126
TRICARE Cost Sharing 1127
TRICARE Beneficiary Assistance 1127
Origins of TRICARE—Managed Care Demonstrations 1127
The TRICARE Program 1130
Managed Care Support Contracts 1131
Comparing TRICARE and Medicare Managed Care 1131
Conclusion: Next Steps for the TRICARE Program 1132

CHAPTER 59—MANAGED CARE ORGANIZATIONS IN RURAL AREAS 1133

Keith J. Mueller

Status of Managed Care in Rural Areas 1134
Appreciating the Rural Context for Managed Care 1135
Reasons To Expect Managed Care Development in Rural Areas 1137
Building Successful Managed Care in Rural Areas 1137
The Future 1142
Conclusion 1144

CHAPTER 60—MANAGED CARE DENTAL BENEFITS 1146

Fred L. Horowitz, Bruce H. Safran, Wayne A. Paul, and Evelyn F. Ireland

Dental HMOs 1146
Dental PPOs 1147
Referral Plans 1149
The Dental Delivery System 1149
Recruiting 1150
Credentialing 1150
Compensation 1150
Utilization Review 1151
Quality Improvement 1151
Specialty Care 1152
Accreditation 1152
Conclusion 1152

CHAPTER 61—WORKERS' COMPENSATION MANAGED CARE: THE SEARCH FOR INTEGRATION 1154

Alex L. Swedlow and Gregory L. Johnson

Introduction 1154
Workers' Compensation: The Origin of the Social Contract 1154
Early Controls on Medical Costs 1155
Key Success Factors 1157
Twenty-Four Hour Coverage: A Solution in Search of Customers 1157

Addressing Worker Expectations 1158
Developing Protocols for Case Management 1159
The Employer Perspective: Changing the Corporate Culture 1159
The Next Step: Comprehensive Medical Events Management 1159
Conclusion 1160

PART VII—REGULATORY AND LEGAL ISSUES **1163**

CHAPTER 62—LEGAL ISSUES IN PROVIDER CONTRACTING **1165**

Mark S. Joffe

General Issues in Contracting 1166
Contract Structure 1167
Common Clauses, Provisions, and Key Factors 1168
Conclusion 1181
Appendix 62–A—Sample Physician Agreement 1182
Appendix 62–B—Sample Hospital Agreement 1194

**CHAPTER 63—ANTITRUST REMEDIES FOR MANAGED CARE: ATTACKING
BARRIERS TO FREE MARKETS** **1203**

William G. Kopit and Robert Hudock

Introduction 1203
Enforcement of the Antitrust and Unfair Competition Laws 1203
The Antitrust Laws 1204
Provider Networks 1207
Physician Unions 1211
Virtual Mergers 1213
Exclusive Dealing Arrangements by Competitors 1214
Most Favored Nation Clauses 1214
Section 2 of the Sherman Act 1215
Conclusion 1219

**CHAPTER 64—LEGAL LIABILITY RELATED TO MEDICAL
MANAGEMENT ACTIVITIES** **1221**

James L. Touse

Obligations To Conduct Medical Management Activities 1222
Common Law Medical Management Liability Actions 1223
Contract Actions Related to Medical Management Activities 1224
Negligence Actions Related to Medical Management Activities 1229
Recommendations 1235
Conclusion 1239

CHAPTER 65—LEGAL ISSUES IN INTEGRATED DELIVERY SYSTEMS **1241**

Jerry R. Peters

Definitions 1241
IDS Models 1242
Provider-Sponsored Organizations 1243
Governance 1244
Committees 1244

Delegated Board Authority 1245
Advisory Committees 1245
Conflict of Interest Policy 1246
Tax Exemption and Charitable Benefit 1247
Physician Compensation 1248
Practice Acquisitions/Valuation 1249
Medicare/Medicaid Provider Numbers 1250
Antitrust Law 1250
Independent Contractor Status 1251
Covenants Not To Compete 1255
Conclusion 1255

CHAPTER 66—ERISA AND MANAGED CARE **1257**

Jacqueline M. Saue and Gregg H. Dooge

Documentation, Reporting, and Disclosure Requirements 1257
Plan Design Considerations 1259
Amendment of Plans 1262
Fiduciary Duties 1263
Challenges to Benefit Denials 1264
ERISA's Civil Enforcement Scheme and Remedies 1267
ERISA Preemption 1267
Conclusion 1280

**CHAPTER 67—THE HEALTH INSURANCE PORTABILITY AND
ACCOUNTABILITY ACT OF 1996** **1285**

Charles N. Kahn III, Dean A. Rosen, Marianne Miller, and Kathleen H. Fyffe

Introduction 1285
Overview 1286
Provisions: Portability and Access 1287
New Access Initiatives 1293
Amendments to HIPAA Portability and Access Provisions 1294
Provisions: Administrative Simplification 1295
HIPAA Administration and Enforcement 1299
An Early Report on the Effects of HIPAA Portability and Access Provisions 1300
Conclusion 1304

CHAPTER 68—HEALTH PLAN CORPORATE COMPLIANCE PROGRAMS **1306**

Mike Treash

Corporate Compliance on Paper 1306
Corporate Compliance in Operation 1307
Structure 1308
Leadership 1309
Education and Development 1311
Measures and Incentives 1311
Staffing 1312
Communication 1313
Conclusion 1320

CHAPTER 69—STATE REGULATION OF MANAGED CARE 1322

Richard I. Smith and Kristin Stewart

Introduction 1322
State Oversight: The Regulatory Process.. 1323
State Regulation of Other Products 1330
Managed Care Legislation 1334
Regulation by Market Segment... 1341
The State Experience—Conclusion 1343

EPILOGUE—MANAGED HEALTH CARE AT THE MILLENNIUM 1346

Peter R. Kongstvedt

Introduction—The Rollercoaster That Never Stops 1346
Using the Magic Eight Ball: The Answer Is Hazy—Try Again Later....................... 1347
They Were Right All Along—Managed Health Care *Is* in Chaos 1347
Reversing Entropy with a Little Help from Professor Heisenberg—Predicting,
    Leading, and Acting in a Chaotic Managed Health Care Environment 1349
Handicapping the Field—The Stratification of Predictability 1350
Driving the Nitroglycerine Truck on a Foggy Night—Leadership, Strategy, and
    Action in the Chaotic World 1353
Door Number One, Two, or Three—Choosing Strategic Options 1355
Conclusion—Shake the Magic Eight Ball and Try Again 1356

GLOSSARY OF TERMS AND ACRONYMS 1357

INDEX 1378

About the Editor

Peter R. Kongstvedt, M.D., F.A.C.P.
Partner
Health Consulting Services
Managed Care

Dr. Peter Kongstvedt is a partner in the international accounting and consulting firm of Ernst & Young, LLP. Ernst & Young has one of the largest health care consulting practices in the United States. Based in the firm's Washington, D.C. office, Dr. Kongstvedt serves as one of the key leaders of the managed care practice. His client work includes such activities as development of strategic direction and tactical planning, assessment of overall operational capabilities, creation of portfolios for operational improvements, restructuring of management, evaluation of product design, reimbursement strategies, HIPAA compliance, and setting of future strategies for e-commerce in managed health care. Dr. Kongstvedt is also heading up the development of the firm's HIPAA-related services and products.

In addition to working with the firm's larger clients, Dr. Kongstvedt serves as a thought leader on managed care for the firm, and is a frequent speaker, as well as the author of numerous articles for health care and consumer publications. Dr. Kongstvedt is the primary author and thought leader behind several innovative monographs for the firm, including a new method for describing health care market places, new methods for strategic planning in chaotic health care environments, leadership in complexly adapting environments, strategies for dealing with the top issues facing managed care executives today, managed care benchmark measures, and the annual payor web-site survey.

Dr. Kongstvedt has 20 years of operational leadership and experience at the senior most levels in progressively larger managed care organizations, including the past six years as a partner at Ernst & Young. In these leadership roles, he has specialized in turning around troubled organizations, defining and achieving strategic goals, conceiving and executing new products, creating and installing new reimbursement methodologies, and developing innovative approaches to care management and health plan operations. He has also focused on HIPAA-related issues and opportunities and the movement of managed health care into the connected economy.

Contributors

Frederick B. Abbey, MPA
Partner
Ernst & Young LLP
Washington, DC

Donald F. Anderson, PhD
Principal
William M. Mercer, Incorporated
San Francisco, California

G. David Baker, MSW
Regional Director
Home Care Services
St. John Health System
Detroit, Michigan

Jeffrey L. Berlant, MD, PhD
Senior Consultant
Mental Health and Substance
    Abuse Services
William M. Mercer, Incorporated
Assistant Clinical Professor
Department of Psychiatry
University of Washington
Seattle, Washington

Pamela J. Byrnes, PhD
Principal
Wellspring Associates
Niantic, Connecticut
Assistant Clinical Professor
Department of Community
    Medicine and Health Care
University of Connecticut Health
    Center
Farmington, Connecticut

Stephen M. Cigich, FSA,
    MAAA
Principal and Consulting Actuary
Milliman & Robertson, Inc.
Brookfield, Wisconsin

Richard J. Coffey, PhD
Director
Program and Operations Analysis
and
Director
Research and Planning
University of Michigan Health
    System
Adjunct Associate Professor
Industrial and Operations
    Engineering
University of Michigan
Ann Arbor, Michigan

Gregg H. Dooge, JD
Partner
Foley & Lardner
Milwaukee, Wisconsin

Anne C. Dye, MHSA
Manager
Health Care Consulting
Ernst & Young LLP
Tampa, Florida

Robert S. Eichler
Vice President
Scheur Management Group, Inc.
Peterborough, New Hampshire

Peter D. Fox, PhD
President
PDF Incorporated
Chevy Chase, Maryland

Nick Franklin, JD
Senior Vice President
Public Affairs
PacifiCare Health Systems, Inc.
Santa Ana, California

Kathleen H. Fyffe, MHA
Federal Regulatory Director
Health Insurance Association of
    America
Washington, DC

Terri Goens
Consultant
Mental Health and Substance
    Abuse Prevention and
    Treatment Services
William M. Mercer, Incorporated
Phoenix, Arizona

Norbert I. Goldfield, MD
Medical Director
3M Health Information Systems
Wallingford, Connecticut

Kathleen M. Griffin, PhD
President and CEO
Valley Consultants, Inc.
Scottsdale, Arizona

Dale F. Harding, CPA
Project Manager
Core Integration Team
Aetna US HealthCare
Blue Bell, Pennsylvania

Geri Hempel, RN, BA
Senior Manager
Ernst & Young LLP
Tampa, Florida

Fred L. Horowitz, DMD
President and Managing Member
Affiliated Network Services
Chicago, Illinois

Robert Hudock
Law Student
Cornell University School of Law
Ithaca, New York

Robert E. Hurley, PhD
Associate Professor
Department of Health
    Administration
Medical College of Virginia
Virginia Commonwealth
    University
Richmond, Virginia

Ann Huston, MHS
Partner
Health Care Consulting
Ernst & Young LLP
Cleveland, Ohio

Evelyn F. Ireland, CAE
Executive Director
National Association of Dental
    Plans
Dallas, Texas

Terry A. Jacobs, JD, CPA
National Director
Insurance Tax Services
Ernst & Young LLP
Washington, DC

Richard J. Jacobsen, PhD
Principal
Birch & Davis Health
    Management Corporation
Niantic, Connecticut

Casey Jason, MD, FACEP
Assistant Clinical Professor
Internal Medicine
Georgetown University Medical
    Center
Medical Advisor
STAR Health Systems/Base
    Technologies, Inc.
McLean, Virginia

Mark S. Joffe, JD
Law Offices of Mark S. Joffe
Washington, DC

Gregory L. Johnson, PhD
Partner
Strategic Change Practice
Pricewaterhouse Coopers
San Francisco, California

Charles N. Kahn III, MPH
President
Health Insurance Association of
    America
Washington, DC

**Meera Kanhouwa, MD,
MHA**
Chairman
Department of Emergency
    Medicine
Prince George's Hospital Center
Associate Clinical Professor
Department of Emergency
    Medicine
George Washington University
    Medical Center
Washington, DC

Sean D. Kenny
National Director
Managed Care Consulting
Ernst & Young LLP
St. Louis, Missouri

**Peter R. Kongstvedt, MD,
FACP**
Partner
Ernst & Young LLP
Washington, DC

William G. Kopit, Esq., JD
Chair
Antitrust Group
Epstein, Becker & Green
Washington, DC

Jean D. LeMasurier
Deputy Director
Health Plan Purchasing
    Administration
Center for Health Plans &
    Providers
US Department of Health &
    Human Services
Baltimore, Maryland

Sarah S. LeRoy, RN, MSN
Clinical Nurse Specialist
C.S. Mott Children's Hospital
University of Michigan Health
    System
Ann Arbor, Michigan

Steve Lillie
Associate Director
Program Design and Innovation
TRICARE Management Activity
US Department of Defense
Falls Church, Virginia

Gregory J. Lippe, MBA
Principal
Ernst & Young, LLP
Milwaukee, Wisconsin

Jennifer H. Lofland, PharmD
Project Director
Thomas Jefferson University
Philadelphia, Pennsylvania

Jacqueline A. Lutz, MBA
Associate Director
Health Care Strategy and Strategic
    Planning
Ernst & Young LLP
Chicago, Illinois

Rick Majzun, MHA
Regional Practice Director
BJC Medical Group
St. Louis, Missouri

William R. Maloney, MA
Principal
Information Planning Group
William M. Mercer, Incorporated
Phoenix, Arizona

Gail Marcus, MBA
Senior Vice President,
    Project Management
CIGNA Healthcare
Hartford, Connecticut

Danna Mauch, PhD
President
Magellan Public Solutions
Magellan Health
Burlington, Massachusetts

Robin L. McElfatrick
Vice President
Scheur Management Group, Inc.
Timonium, Maryland

Marianne Miller, MA
Director
Federal Regulatory Affairs and
   Policy Development
Policy and Information
   Department
Health Insurance Association of
   America
Washington, DC

Keith J. Mueller, PhD
Professor
Preventive and Societal Medicine
University of Nebraska Medical
   Center
Director
Nebraska Center for Rural Health
   Research
University of Nebraska
Omaha, Nebraska

**Catherine M. Mullahy, RN,
   CRRN, CCM**
President
Options Unlimited
Huntington, New York
Director
National Board of Directors
Chair, Ethics Committee
Case Management Society of
   America
Chair, Commission for Case
   Manager Certification

David B. Nash, MD, MBA
Associate Dean and Director
Office of Health Policy and
   Clinical Outcomes
Jefferson Medical College
Philadelphia, Pennsylvania

Robert P. Navarro, PharmD
Principal
NavarroPharma, LLC
Morrisville, North Carolina

Margaret E. O'Kane, MHS
President
National Committee for Quality
   Assurance
Washington, DC

Wayne A. Paul, MA
Executive Vice President
United Concordia Companies, Inc.
Towson, Maryland

Jerry R. Peters, JD
Partner and National Chair
Health Care Practice Group
Latham & Watkins
San Francisco, California

Britton L. Pim
Manager
Health Consulting Practice
Ernst & Young LLP
St. Louis, Missouri

Michael Pine, MD, MBA
President
Michael Pine & Associates, Inc.
Research Associate, Cardiology
University of Chicago
Chicago, Illinois

David W. Plocher, MD
Partner
Ernst & Young LLP
Minneapolis, Minnesota

Robert G. Reese
Partner
East/Great Lakes Consulting
   Practice
Ernst & Young LLP
Detroit, Michigan

Christine C. Rinn, JD
Principal
Michaels & Bonner, PC
Washington, DC

**Peggy H. Rodebush, BS, RN,
   MSN**
Partner
Consulting Services
Ernst & Young LLP
Tampa, Florida

James A. Rodeghero, PhD
President
Rodeghero Consulting Group, Inc.
Los Angeles, California

Dean A. Rosen, JD
Senior Vice President
Policy and General Counsel
Health Insurance Association of
   America
Washington, DC

Phillip G. Royalty, JD, CPA
Partner and Director
National Tax Department
Health Industry Group
Ernst & Young LLP
Washington, DC

**Bruce H. Safran, DDS, MBA,
   MHP**
Executive Vice President
National Marketing
Healthplex
Uniondale, New York

Jacqueline M. Saue, JD
Partner
Foley & Lardner
Washington, DC

Barry S. Scheur, JD
President
Scheur Management Group, Inc.
Newton, Massachusetts

Craig S. Schub
President
Secure Horizons USA
Santa Ana, California

Hindy J. Shaman, MBA
Associate Director
Health Consulting Practice
Ernst & Young LLP
Washington, DC

Judith Shea, MMHS
Principal
Wellspring Associates
Branford, Connecticut

Pamela B. Siren, RN, MPH
Vice President
Quality Services
Neighborhood Health Plan
Affiliate of Harvard Pilgrim
   Health Care
Boston, Massachusetts

James S. Slubowski
Vice President
Information Services
Priority Health
Grand Rapids, Michigan

Richard I. Smith, JD
Vice President
Public Policy and Research
American Association of Health
    Plans
Washington, DC

Larry Sobel, JD
Director
Special Programs and
    Demonstrations
TRICARE Management Activity
US Department of Defense
Falls Church, Virginia

Leif I. Solberg, MD
Associate Medical Director for
    Care Improvement Research
HealthPartners Research
    Foundation
Associate Medical Director
HealthPartners Medical Group
Minneapolis, Minnesota

Terry Sollom
Publications Manager
Public Policy and Research
American Association of Health
    Plans
Washington, DC

Stephen A. Somers, PhD
President
Center for Health Care Strategies,
    Inc.
Visiting Senior Research Scholar
    and Lecturer
Woodrow Wilson School of
    Public and International Affairs
Princeton University
Princeton, New Jersey

Nancy W. Spangler
President
Spangler Associates, Inc.
Prairie Village, Kansas

Jean C. Stanford
Assistant Director
Health Care Consulting
Ernst & Young LLP
Washington, DC

**Katherine O. Sternbach,
    MED, MBA**
Principal
William M. Mercer, Incorporated
San Francisco, California

Kristin Stewart, MHA
Director
Private Market Issues
Public Policy and Research
American Association of Health
    Plans
Washington, DC

**Michael G. Sturm, FSA,
    MAAA**
Actuary
Milliman & Robertson, Inc.
Brookfield, Wisconsin

Alex L. Swedlow, MHSA
Principal
Applied Outcomes Research
Sacramento, California

Michael J. Taylor, MA, MS
Principal and National Managed
    Care Consultant
Towers Perrin
Boston, Massachusetts

John C. Thomson
Senior Vice President
Head of Disability Products
Aetna US Healthcare
Hartford, Connecticut

Daniel Thornton
Senior Policy Analyst
Public Policy and Research
American Association of Health
    Plans
Washington, DC

James L. Touse, JD
Vice President and General
    Counsel
BlueCross BlueShield of
    Tennessee
Chattanooga, Tennessee

Mike Treash
Senior Manager
Health Care Advisory Services
Ernst & Young LLP
Washington, DC

Eric R. Wagner, MBA
Vice President
Managed Care
MedStar Health
Columbia, Maryland

Scott A. Walker
Senior Manager
Managed Care Services
Health Care Management Division
AIG Consultants, Inc.
Atlanta, Georgia

Laura L. Waltrip, RN, BSN
Manager
Consulting Services
Ernst & Young, LLP
Tampa, Florida

John Weeks
Editor
*The Integrator for the Business of
    Alternative Medicine*
Principal
Integration Strategies for Natural
    Healthcare
Seattle, Washington

H.G. Whittington, MD
National Medical Director
MenningerCare Systems of Texas
Plano, Texas

Wendy L. Wilson, MD, MSE
Senior Manager
Health Care Consulting Practice
Ernst & Young LLP
Cleveland, Ohio

**Barbara J. Youngberg, BSN,
    MSW, JD, FASHRM**
Vice President
Insurance, Risk, Quality and Legal
    Services
University HealthSystem
    Consortium
Oak Brook, Illinois

Carlos Zarabozo
Social Science Research Analyst
Office of Strategic Planning
Health Care Financing
    Administration
US Department of Health and
    Human Services
Washington, DC

Preface

With each new edition of *The Managed Health Care Handbook*, the size of the book roughly doubles. This *Fourth Edition* is no exception to that trend. The doubling in size is not the result of a perverse desire to produce a book requiring wheels and a handle to carry it around. Successive doubling in size is due to the continual expansion of knowledge and complexity in this industry; the need to address new topics as well as significant expansions and revisions of topics addressed in previous editions. Of equal importance, other sectors of the health care industry continually change as well, often as a response to managed health care. Physicians do not exhibit the same types of practice behaviors prevalent a decade ago, hospital usage rates have declined across the nation (though not to uniform levels), new diagnostic and therapeutic interventions have appeared, and more. The influence of all sectors of the health care industry, including managed health care, cause change in the other health sectors, and those changed sectors in turn cause change to managed health care. Turbulence remains a prominent dynamic.

Change is a requirement of life, and an integral part of all complex endeavors of society, including the financing, provision, and organization of health care services. The path chosen by the United States, that of combining a single payer system (i.e., Medicare, Medicaid, and other federal health programs) with private health insurance is unique in the industrialized world. The result includes high health care costs as a percentage of the gross domestic product or GDP,[1] seen by many as a severe failing, but it has also resulted in advanced medical interventions and high access to care (i.e., little queuing and early treatment) that leads much of the rest of the world. The current system has also resulted in the greatest percentage of uninsured or underinsured citizens of any industrialized nation, and access to health care by the poor remains a problem. No simple solution exists to maintain the good while eliminating the bad.

The reality is that the health care delivery and financing system existing in the United States is incredibly complex, and that complexity is accelerating, not slowing, nor even increasing at a steady pace. As a result, it is neither possible to describe a steady state nor even a reliably predictable state. In a word, the health care system is chaotic—not using the dictionary definition of chaos as meaning total disorder, but using the word chaos in terms of the new science of chaos theory. More accurately stated, the delivery, organization, and financing of health care is a complexly adapting system. The concept of complexity is useful to bear in mind throughout the book. By doing so, the reader will maintain a sense of the true vibrancy of managed health care, and will not fall into the trap of thinking that managed health care is monolithic, simplistic, or that there is only one way to do something. This concept and its implications are ex-

_____

[1] It should also be noted that the GDP is the manifestation of a hugely robust economy as of 2000.

plored further in the Epilogue as we consider what the future might hold for managed health care in the new millennium.

Everything you read here is a reflection of managed health care in 2000. An immediate and practical effect of the complex health care environment is that changes will continue to occur in this industry, and some of those changes will not have been anticipated in this book. Therefore, it is incumbent on the reader to ascertain for herself or himself the applicability and accuracy of the information presented in the *Handbook*, particularly in regard to federal and state laws. The fundamental concepts and attributes of managed health care nonetheless remain, regardless of such changes. The environmental forces that led to the creation and continued evolution of managed health care still exist and are in many ways even greater than in the past.

Despite continual change and increasing complexity in this industry, the primary mission of *The Managed Health Care Handbook, Fourth Edition* remains unchanged: to provide a strategic and operational resource for managers in the field. It is based as much as possible on actual operations of managed care plans, rather than on purely theoretical models. In a field this complex, many topics may be discussed, but not always to the degree one would like nor with the emphasis that all would agree with. Information in this book is not intended to be the total, final, or best answer to any issue in managed health care. Rather, what is presented are descriptions of the various aspects of managed health care from operational points of view, possible solutions and multiple approaches to issues, and other information that managers need to understand. While practically oriented, the *Handbook* is also intended to be of value to a wider audience as well. Attention has been focused on the needs of academicians and students in advanced programs, regulators, law professionals, practicing physicians, and managers of most types of provider organizations. Finally, material is presented in as accessible a style as possible for each subject area, so as to facilitate its use by any reader.

While the best approach for understanding the information contained in the *Handbook* is to proceed in the order it is presented in, this is not a requirement. In addition to its primary role as a resource to managers and its secondary role as an educational text, this is also a reference text. That means that material is included which will likely be of lesser importance to some readers. As such, it is clearly not necessary that all chapters be read by all readers in order to gain a practical level of understanding. To aid the reader, chapters cross-reference each other when necessary. There is also a glossary found in the back of the book for those times when the acronyms run heavy, the terms are obtuse, or fresh neologisms are blithely used.

In the end, if there is one overall way to characterize *The Managed Health Care Handbook, Fourth Edition*, it is the intent to provide practical knowledge and advice based on the experiences, both first-hand and observed, of managers and experienced consultants in the industry as it exists today. The intent to provide practical knowledge necessitates that some of what is presented is also biased: my biases as well as those of contributing authors. There is no shortage of impassioned opinions in this industry, and many of those opinions are held with near-religious zeal. That means that there will be some who have differing opinions or experiences than what is found here. Specific efforts, therefore, have been made to present varying opinions when appropriate, along with the occasional editorial comment when such is warranted. Still, the information in this book has been created with an overriding single and consistent focus: to enable the reader, regardless of his or her place in the health care system, to better succeed in the world of managed health care.

Peter Reid Kongstvedt
McLean, Virginia

Acknowledgments

I wish to acknowledge and thank the following individuals for their help during the creation of this new edition of *The Managed Health Care Handbook*. First, I want to thank Sandy Cannon and Kalen Conerly at Aspen Publishers for providing support and clearing obstructions from the path, allowing me to concentrate on the writing and editing. I also thank Loretta Haught for her help in collecting research information, and for tracking and assisting the progress of the book throughout its many stages of creation. Ruth Bloom carried out the difficult task of copy editing the text and finding the errors and vagaries that I missed in compiling the manuscript; her efforts are much appreciated.

Although I cannot name them all since to do so would double again the size of this book, I thank my many colleagues and friends in the managed care and consulting industries with whom I have had the pleasure to both work beside and compete with over the years. Words are insufficient to express the appreciation and gratitude I feel to my neglected wife and son for putting up with me during the many months I was locked away every night and weekend in the writer's dungeon during the creation of this text. Lastly, I want to give sincere thanks to the many readers of previous editions of this book for their support, kind words, observations, and suggestions that have fueled my ability to do it once again.

PART I

Introduction to Managed Care

"You know more than you think you do."

Benjamin Spock, M.D.
(1903–1998)
Baby and Child Care, [1945]

CHAPTER 1

An Overview of Managed Care

Peter D. Fox

INTRODUCTION

Managed care is rapidly dominating the health care financing and delivery system in the United States. To illustrate, health maintenance organization (HMO) enrollment reached 81.3 million by January 1, 1999. Although estimates are less reliable, by all accounts the number of persons enrolled in preferred provider organizations (PPOs) and their variants rivals the number enrolled in HMOs.[1] Even traditional plans are adopting principles of managed care; for example, hospital precertification and large case management, daring innovations as recently as a decade ago, have become the norm in indemnity insurance. Public sector, notably Medicare and Medicaid, reliance on managed care is growing rapidly, as discussed in Chapters 55–57.

Managed care has also become a big business. As of 1998 some 61.5 million HMO enrollees were in multistate firms, including nonprofits such as Kaiser and the HMOs owned by the various Blue Cross and Blue Shield plans (which operate largely autonomously).[2] Many of the large managed care companies are traded on the New York Stock Exchange and other stock exchanges, and the general business press regu-

larly reports their profits along with the compensation of the chief executive officers, which can amount to millions of dollars annually.

When one thinks of managed care, one should distinguish between the *techniques* of managed care and the *organizations* that perform the various functions. Managed care can embody a wide variety of techniques, which are discussed throughout this book. These include various forms of financial incentives for providers, promotion of wellness, early identification of disease, patient education, self-care, and all aspects of utilization management.

A wide variety of organizations can implement managed care techniques, of which the HMO has the potential to align financing and delivery most closely by virtue of enrollees' being required (with some exceptions) to use network providers. Managed care techniques can also be employed directly by employers, insurers, union management (Taft-Hartley) trust funds, and the Medicare and Medicaid programs. They can also be implemented by PPOs, organizations that allow enrollees to be reimbursed for care delivered by nonnetwork providers, although the enrollees face higher out-of-pocket payments (that is, cost sharing) if they do. Finally, a variety of hybrid arrangements has evolved. One example is the point-of-service (POS) program, which operates as a PPO except that, to receive the highest level of benefits, the enrollee must obtain a referral from a primary care physician who is part of the contracted network. Increasingly, the arrangements are diffi-

Peter D. Fox, PhD, is an independent consultant, located in Chevy Chase, Maryland, specializing in managed care. His clients include HMOs, PPOs, provider groups, employers, Taft-Hartley trust funds, government agencies, and foundations. He is the author of numerous articles and books.

cult to characterize, let alone profile statistically, in a meaningful manner.

MANAGED CARE: THE EARLY YEARS (PRE–1970)

Whatever its role today, managed care had humble origins and struggled to survive in its early years. To some extent it still struggles today, as evidenced by the controversies, mostly at the state level, surrounding "any willing provider" legislation and other legislative proposals that constrain the development of managed care (see Chapter 69). Rather than focusing on techniques, this section addresses the development of HMOs and other managed care organizations.

The Western Clinic in Tacoma, Washington, is sometimes cited as the first example of an HMO, or prepaid group practice as it was known until the early 1970s.[3] Starting in 1910, the Western Clinic offered, exclusively through its own providers, a broad range of medical services in return for a premium payment of $0.50 per member per month. The program was available to lumber mill owners and their employees and served to assure the clinic a flow of patients and revenues. A similar program was developed by Dr. Bridge, who started a clinic in Tacoma that later expanded to 20 sites in Oregon and Washington.

In 1929 Michael Shadid, MD, established a rural farmers' cooperative health plan in Elk City, Oklahoma, by forming a lay organization of leading farmers in the community. Participating farmers purchased shares for $50 each to raise capital for a new hospital in return for receiving medical care at a discount.[4] For his trouble, Shadid lost his membership in the county medical society and was threatened with having his license to practice suspended. Some 20 years later, however, he was vindicated through an out-of-court settlement in his favor of an antitrust suit against the county and state medical societies.[5] In 1934 the Farmers Union assumed control of both the hospital and the health plan.

Health insurance itself is of relatively recent origin. In 1929 Baylor Hospital in Houston, Texas, agreed to provide some 1,500 teachers prepaid care at its hospital, an arrangement that represented the origins of Blue Cross. The program was subsequently expanded to include the participation of other employers and hospitals, initially as single hospital plans. Starting in 1939 state medical societies in California and elsewhere created, generally statewide, Blue Shield plans, which reimbursed for physician services. At the time, commercial health insurance was not a factor.[6]

The formation of the various Blue Cross and Blue Shield plans in the midst of the Great Depression, as well as that of many HMOs, reflected not consumers demanding coverage or nonphysician entrepreneurs seeking to establish a business but rather providers wanting to protect and enhance patient revenues. Many of these developments were threatening to organized medicine. In 1932 the American Medical Association (AMA) adopted a strong stance against prepaid group practices, favoring, instead, indemnity-type insurance. The AMA's position was in response to both the small number of prepaid group practices in existence at the time and the findings in 1932 of the Committee on the Cost of Medical Care—a highly visible private group of leaders from medicine, dentistry, public health, consumers, and so forth— that recommended the expansion of group practice as an efficient delivery system. The AMA's stance at the national level set the tone for continued state and local medical society opposition to prepaid group practice.

The period immediately surrounding World War II saw the formation of several HMOs that remain prominent even today. They encountered varying degrees of opposition from local medical societies. They represent a diversity of origins with the initial impetus coming, variously, from employers, providers seeking patient revenues, consumers seeking access to improved and affordable health care, and even a housing lending agency seeking to reduce the number of foreclosures. The following are examples of other early HMOs:

- The Kaiser Foundation Health Plans were started in 1937 by Dr. Sidney Garfield at the behest of the Kaiser construction company, which sought to finance medical care, initially, for workers and families who were building an aqueduct in the southern California desert to transport water from the Colorado River to Los Angeles and, subsequently, for workers who were constructing the Grand Coulee Dam in Washington state. A similar program was established in 1942 at Kaiser shipbuilding plants in the San Francisco Bay area. Kaiser Foundation Health Plans now serve 12 states and the District of Columbia and, as of July 1, 1998, had 8.4 million members.

- In 1937 the Group Health Association (GHA) was started in Washington, DC, at the behest of the Home Owner's Loan Corporation to reduce the number of mortgage defaults that resulted from large medical expenses. It was created as a nonprofit consumer cooperative, with the board being elected periodically by the enrollees. The District of Columbia Medical Society opposed the formation of GHA. It sought to restrict hospital admitting privileges for GHA physicians and threatened their expulsion from the medical society. A bitter antitrust battle ensued that culminated in the U.S. Supreme Court's ruling in favor of GHA. In 1994, faced with insolvency despite an enrollment of some 128,000, GHA was acquired by Humana Health Plans, a for-profit, publicly traded corporation.[7] Since that time, it has been divested by Humana and the membership incorporated into Kaiser Foundation Health Plan of the Mid-Atlantic.

- In 1944, at the behest of New York City, which was seeking coverage for its employees, the Health Insurance Plan (HIP) of Greater New York was formed. HIP is licensed in New York, New Jersey, and Florida and, as of January 1, 1999, had 1.1 million members.

- In 1947 consumers in Seattle organized 400 families, who contributed $100 each, to form the Group Health Cooperative of Puget Sound. Predictably, opposition was

encountered from the Kings County Medical Society. Group Health Cooperative remains a consumer cooperative as of the time of publication.

Only in later years did nonprovider entrepreneurs form for-profit HMOs in significant numbers. The early independent practice association (IPA) type of HMOs, which contract with physicians in independent fee-for-service practice, was a competitive reaction to group practice-based HMOs. The basic structure was created in 1954, when the San Joaquin County Medical Society in California formed the San Joaquin Medical Foundation in response to competition from Kaiser. The foundation established a relative-value fee schedule for paying physicians, heard grievances against physicians, and monitored quality of care. It became licensed by the state to accept capitation payment, making it the first IPA model HMO.

THE ADOLESCENT YEARS: 1970–1985

Through the 1960s and into the early 1970s HMOs played only a modest role in the financing and delivery of health care, although they were a significant presence in a few communities, such as the Seattle area and parts of California. In 1970 the total number of HMOs was between 30 and 40, the exact number depending on one's definition.[8] The years since the early 1970s represent a period of vastly accelerated developments that are still unfolding.

The major boost to the HMO movement during this period was the enactment in 1973 of the federal HMO Act. That act, as described below, both authorized start-up funding and, more important, ensured access to the employer-based insurance market. It evolved from discussions that Paul Ellwood, MD, had in 1970 with the political leadership of the U.S. Department of Health, Education, and Welfare (which later became the Department of Health and Human Services).[9] Ellwood had been personally close to Philip Lee, MD, assistant secretary for health during the presidency of Lyndon Johnson (and again in the Clinton administration), and participated in designing the Health Planning Act of 1966.

Sometimes referred to as the father of the modern HMO movement, Ellwood was asked in the early years of the Nixon administration to devise ways of constraining the rise in the Medicare budget. Out of those discussions evolved both a proposal to capitate HMOs for Medicare beneficiaries (which was not enacted until 1982) and the laying of the groundwork for what became the HMO Act of 1973. The desire to foster HMOs reflected the perspective that the fee-for-service system, by rewarding paying physicians based on their volume of services, incorporated the wrong incentives. Also, the term *health maintenance organization* was coined as a substitute for prepaid group practice, principally because it had greater public appeal.

The main features of the HMO Act were the following:

- Grants and loans were available for the planning and start-up phases of new HMOs, as well as for service area expansions for existing HMOs.
- State laws that restricted the development of HMOs were overridden for HMOs that were federally qualified, as described below.
- Most important of all were the "dual-choice" provisions, which required that employers with 25 or more employees that offered indemnity coverage also offer two federally qualified HMOs, one of each type—that is, the closed panel or group or staff model, or the open panel or IPA/network model—if the plans made a formal request* (the different model types are discussed in Chapter 3). Most HMOs were reluctant to exercise the mandate, fearing that doing so would antagonize employers, who would in turn discourage employees from enrolling.

The statute also established a process under which HMOs could elect to be federally qualified. To do so, the plans had to satisfy a series of requirements, such as meeting minimum benefit

package standards set forth in the act, demonstrating that their provider networks were adequate, having a quality assurance system, meeting standards of financial stability, and having an enrollee grievance system. Some states emulated these requirements and adopted them for all HMOs that were licensed in the state regardless of federal qualification status.

Obtaining federal qualification has always been at the discretion of the individual HMO, unlike state licensure, which is mandatory. Plans that requested federal qualification did so for four principal reasons. First, it represented a "Good Housekeeping seal of approval" that was helpful in marketing. Second, the dual choice requirements ensured access to the employer market. Third, the override of state laws—important in some states but not others—applied only to federally qualified HMOs. Fourth, federal qualification was required for the receipt of federal grants and loans that were available during the early years of the act. In 1998 37.3 percent of HMOs nationally, accounting for 59.8 percent of all enrollment, were federally qualified.[10] Federal qualification is less important today than it was when managed care was in its infancy and HMOs were struggling for inclusion in employment-based health benefit programs, which account for most private insurance in the United States.

Ironically, in its early years the 1973 legislation may have retarded HMO development, earning it the nickname of the "Anti-HMO Act." This occurred for two reasons. The first stems from a compromise in Congress between members having differing objectives. One camp was principally interested in fostering competition in the health care marketplace by promoting plans that incorporated incentives for providers to constrain costs. The second camp, while perhaps sharing the first objective, principally saw the HMO Act as a precursor to health reform and sought a vehicle to expand access to coverage for individuals who were without insurance or who had limited benefits. Imposing requirements on HMOs but not on indemnity carriers, however, reduced the ability of HMOs to compete.

Of particular note were requirements with regard to the comprehensiveness of the benefit

---

*For workers under collective bargaining agreements, the union had to agree to the offering.

package, as well as open enrollment and community rating. The open enrollment provision required that plans accept individuals and groups without regard to their health status. The community rating requirement limited the ability of plans to relate premium levels to the health status of the individual enrollee or employer group. Both provisions represented laudable public policy goals; the problem was that they had the potential for making federally qualified HMOs noncompetitive because the same requirements did not apply to the traditional insurance plans against which they competed. This situation was largely corrected in the late 1970s with the enactment of amendments to the HMO Act that reduced some of the more onerous requirements. The federal dual-choice provisions were "sunsetted" in 1995 and are no longer in effect.

The second reason that HMO development was retarded was the slowness of the federal government in issuing the regulations implementing the act. Employers knew they would have to contract with federally qualified plans. Even those who were supportive of the mandate, however, delayed until the government determined which plans would be qualified and established the processes for implementing the dual-choice provisions.

The Carter administration, which assumed office in 1977, was supportive of HMOs. In particular, Hale Champion, as undersecretary of the U.S. Department of Health and Human Services, made issuance of the regulations a priority. As can be seen from Figure 1–1, rapid growth ensued, with enrollment rising from 6.3 million in 1977 to 29.3 million in 1987.

Politically, several aspects of this history are interesting. First, although differences arose on specifics, congressional support for legislation promoting HMO development came from both political parties, and there was no widespread state opposition to the override of restrictive state laws. In addition, most employers did not actively oppose the dual-choice requirements,

Figure 1–1 Number of people receiving their care in HMOs, 1976–1997. 1995 estimate based on Group Health Association of America's 1994 HMO performance report. *Source:* American Association of Health Plans (formerly GHAA/AMCRA). *Patterns in HMO Enrollment,* p. 3 (Washington, DC, 1995), and AAMP Annual HMO Industry Survey (not published).

although many disliked the federal government in effect telling them to contract with HMOs. Perhaps most interesting of all has been the generally positive interaction between the public sector and the private sector, with government fostering HMO development both through its regulatory processes and also as a purchaser under its employee benefits programs.

Other managed care developments also occurred during the 1970s and early 1980s. Of note was the evolution of PPOs. PPOs are generally regarded as originating in Denver, where in the early 1970s Samuel Jenkins, a vice president of the benefits consulting firm of the Martin E. Segal Co., negotiated discounts with hospitals on behalf of the company's Taft-Hartley trust fund clients. Starting in 1978, Jenkins negotiated discounts with physicians.[11] PPO enrollment is difficult to estimate accurately but now rivals that of HMOs.

Although there is no widely accepted legal definition, PPOs are generally regarded as differing from HMOs in two respects. First, they do not accept capitation risk; rather, risk remains with the insurance company or self-insured employment-based entity (employer or Taft-Hartley employer-union trust fund). Second, enrollees may access providers that are not in the contracted network, but they face disincentives for doing so in the form of higher out-of-pocket liabilities (although POS plans provide out-of-network benefits as well). A third, though not exclusive, definitional difference is that PPOs do not require the enrollee to use a primary care physician "gatekeeper" to access specialty services (though so-called open-access HMOs do not require that either). Intermediate between the HMO and the PPO is the POS plan. It is sometimes categorized as a gatekeeper PPO. To avoid financial penalties under POS, the enrollee must designate a primary care physician, who in turn authorizes any referral services. Self-referral to a specialist, including one who participates in the network, generates higher out-of-pocket liabilities.

As noted in Chapter 3 and in many other chapters in this book, there are no clear distinctions between health care plan types anymore, although various attributes are discussed further throughout this text.

Utilization review evolved outside the HMO setting between 1970 and 1985, although it has earlier origins:

- In 1959 Blue Cross of Western Pennsylvania, the Allegheny County Medical Society Foundation, and the Hospital Council of Western Pennsylvania performed retrospective analyses of hospital claims to identify utilization that was significantly above the average.[12]
- Around 1970 California's Medicaid program initiated hospital precertification and concurrent review in conjunction with medical care foundations in that state, starting with the Sacramento Foundation for Medical Care.[13]
- The 1972 Social Security Amendments authorized the federal Professional Standards Review Organization (PSRO) program to review the appropriateness of care provided to Medicare and Medicaid beneficiaries. Although its effectiveness has been debated, the PSRO program established an organizational infrastructure and data capacity upon which both the public and private sectors could rely.
- In the 1970s a handful of large corporations initiated precertification and concurrent review for inpatient care, much to the dismay of the provider community.

Developments in indemnity insurance, mostly during the 1980s, included encouraging persons with conventional insurance to obtain second opinions before undergoing elective surgery and the widespread adoption of large case management—that is, the coordination of services for persons with expensive conditions, such as selected accident patients, cancer cases, and very low-birthweight infants.

Also during the 1980s worksite wellness programs became more prevalent as employers, in varying degrees and varying ways, instituted such programs as:

- screening (for example, for hypertension and diabetes)
- health risk appraisal

- promotion of exercise (whether through supplying gyms, conveniently located showers, or running paths, or simply by providing information)
- stress reduction
- classes (for example, smoking cessation, lifting heavy weights, and the benefits of exercise)
- nutritional efforts, including serving healthy food in the cafeteria
- weight-loss programs
- mental health counseling

For both employers and managed care organizations, wellness and prevention have become integral components of managed care (see Chapter 17).

MANAGED CARE COMES OF AGE: 1985 TO THE PRESENT

Fifteen years has seen a combination of innovation, maturation, and restructuring. These are briefly discussed below.

Innovation

Three areas of innovation are discussed. First, in many communities hospitals and physicians have collaborated to form physician-hospital organizations (PHOs), principally as vehicles for contracting with managed care organizations. PHOs are typically separately incorporated, with the hospital and the physicians each having the right to designate half the members of the board. Most PHOs seek to enter into fee-for-service arrangements with HMOs and PPOs, although an increasing number accept full capitation risk. Other variants on integrated delivery systems are described in Chapter 4.

Whether PHOs are an important development or little more than a transitional vehicle is hotly debated. Some have been successful as provider units of health care plans, particularly those that have accepted capitation risk from HMOs. The skeptics argue, however, that most PHOs are hospital and specialty dominated, whereas one of the success factors in managed care is a strong

primary care orientation. Other reasons for skepticism are that most PHOs allow all physicians with admitting privileges at the hospital in question to participate rather than selecting the more efficient ones, and that the physicians are commonly required to use the hospital for outpatient services (for example, laboratory tests) that might be obtained at lower cost elsewhere, hence hurting the ability of the PHO to be price competitive. Finally, some PHOs suffer from organizational fragmentation, inadequate information systems, inexperienced management, and a lack of capital.

A second innovation has been the development of carve-outs, which are organizations that have specialized provider networks and are paid on a capitation or other basis for a specific service, such as mental health (see Chapter 25), chiropractic, and dental (see Chapter 60). The carve-out companies market their services principally to HMOs and large self-insured employers. Similar in concept are groups of specialists, such as ophthalmologists and radiologists, that accept capitation risk for their services (sometimes referred to as subcapitation) through contracts with health plans and employer groups. One controversy surrounding carve-out arrangements is whether they result in fragmented care for the patient. Such specialty-based networks are also discussed in Chapter 11.

A third set of innovations is those that have been made possible by advances in computer technology. Vastly improved computer programs, marketed by private firms or developed by managed care plans for internal use, have become available that generate statistical profiles of the use of services rendered by physicians. These profiles serve to assess efficiency and quality and may also serve to adjust payment levels to providers who are paid under capitation or risk-sharing arrangements to reflect patient severity. These topics are discussed in greater detail in Chapter 32.

Another example of the impact of computer technology is a virtual revolution in the processing of medical and drug claims, which is increasingly being performed electronically rather than by paper submission and manual entry. The result has been dramatically lower administrative costs and far superior information; an example of the latter is allowing the pharmacist at the time a prescription is dispensed to receive information about potential adverse effects. Management information systems can be expected to improve in the next few years as providers, almost universally, submit claims electronically. In addition, providers are likely to be assigned unique identification numbers, enabling profiling systems to combine data across multiple payers. Electronic data interchange and management information systems are discussed further in Chapters 35 and 36.

Maturation

Maturation can be seen from several vantage points. The first is the extent of HMO and PPO growth. Between 1992 and 1997 HMO enrollment rose 96 percent, reaching 81.3 million.[14] As mentioned earlier, PPO enrollment is difficult to estimate but approximates that of HMOs. Employers have come to rely on managed care at the expense of traditional indemnity insurance, as seen in Figure 1–2, with many no longer offering traditional insurance at all.

Medicare and Medicaid (see Chapters 55–57) have also increasingly relied on managed care. Many HMOs regard Medicare risk contracting

(that is, capitation arrangements that HMOs enter into with the Medicare program) as an essential part of their business strategy, although the penetration is considerably below that of the working-age population. In April 1999 more than 6.1 million Medicare beneficiaries were enrolled in HMOs having "Medicare + Choice" contracts, that is, capitation contracts from the Health Care Financing Administration, the federal agency that administers Medicare and Medicaid. This represents more than a tripling in enrollment since 1994 (see Figure 1–3). In addition, the number of plans with Medicare + Choice contracts increased from 118 in 1994 to 336 in 1998 but declined to 300 in 1999 (see Figure 1–4).

The reasons for health plan interest in contracting with Medicare include the realization that doing so can be profitable; the desire by employers to provide HMO options for retirees; a reluctance to ignore a major market at a time when HMOs are consolidating and, in some cases, fighting for survival; and the belief that the plans that account for a high proportion of a provider's revenue will acquire a competitive advantage because they have leverage in negotiating reimbursement arrangements. The reasons for the decline in 1999 are related to changes in the Balanced Budget Act (BBA) of 1997, which reduced payment levels in most of the country below the rate of increase in medical costs and

Figure 1–2 Market share by health plan type, 1988 and 1999. *Source:* Courtesy of KPMG Peat Marwick, LLP, Health Benefits in 1998, Washington, DC.

Figure 1–3 Medicare risk enrollees (month of April). *Source:* Data from *Managed Care Contract Reports,* Health Care Financing Administration, Baltimore, Maryland.

imposed new administrative burdens. The BBA also calls for "risk adjustors," which adjust payment levels to reflect the relative health status of enrollees, to be phased in starting in 2000; they are expected to further constrain payment and, also, for at least several years make revenues less predictable than before. The reimbursement constraints are causing a pattern whereby plans are increasing premiums and reducing benefits, which can be expected to slow, if not reverse, the rate of enrollment growth.

State Medicaid programs, too, have turned to managed care, and, like employers, many are removing the fee-for-service option. As of June 1997 19.5 million beneficiaries were in managed care, representing more than half the total Medicaid population, an increase from 11 percent just five years before.[15] Some 8.4 million of the 19.5 million beneficiaries were in HMOs, with the balance being under less restrictive arrangements, mostly so-called primary care case management (PCCM) programs, which entail ben-

Figure 1–4 Medicare risk contractors (month of April). *Source:* Data from *Managed Care Contract Reports,* Health Care Financing Administration, Baltimore, Maryland.

eficiaries' electing a primary care physician, who must authorize any referrals to specialists and other services. Under the PCCM programs, providers are generally paid fee-for-service, except that the primary physician may receive a small (for example, $2.00) monthly case management fee. It should be noted that only a small percent of beneficiaries who are dually eligible for both Medicare and Medicaid are in managed care because of various barriers in the Medicare program. Some 17 percent of Medicare and 19 percent of Medicaid beneficiaries are dually eligible.

Another phenomenon is the maturation of external quality oversight activities. Starting in 1991 the National Committee for Quality Assurance (NCQA; see Chapter 44) began to accredit HMOs. The NCQA was launched by the HMO industry in 1979. It became independent in 1991, with the majority of board seats being held by employer, union, and consumer representatives. Many employers are demanding or strongly encouraging NCQA accreditation of the HMOs with which they contract, and accreditation has come to replace federal qualification as the "seal of approval." In 1999 roughly 55 percent of HMOs, accounting for 75 percent of enrollees, were accredited.

In addition, performance measurement systems (report cards) are evolving, although they are at an early stage. The most prominent is the Health Plan Employer Data and Information Set (HEDIS; see Chapters 35 and 44), which was developed by the NCQA at the behest of several large employers and health plans. The indices of quality that are part of the performance measurement system are incomplete but will be improved over time. Shortcomings include a focus on what is easily measurable and the lack of health outcome measures.

In a related development, several consumer-oriented magazines regularly carry articles rating HMOs in their respective communities. As more and more of the insured lose access to traditional indemnity plans, the issue of HMO performance will become more salient.

Another form of maturation is the focus of cost management efforts, which used to be almost exclusively inpatient hospital utilization. Practice patterns have changed dramatically in the last 20 years, however, and inpatient utilization has declined significantly. Although hospital utilization still receives considerable scrutiny, greater attention is being paid to ambulatory services, such as the use of prescription drugs, diagnostics, and specialists.

Restructuring

Perhaps the most dramatic development is the restructuring that is occurring and that reflects the interplay between managed care and the health care delivery system. The definitional distinctions are blurring as managed care organizations undergo a process of hybridization. Staff and group model HMOs, declining in number and faced with limited capital and a need to expand into new territories, are forming IPA components. Meanwhile, some IPAs have created staff model primary care centers while continuing to contract with physicians in independent practice for specialty services. HMOs are offering PPO and POS products, and some PPOs are obtaining HMO licenses. HMOs are also contracting with employers on a self-funded rather than a capitated basis, whereby the risk for medical costs remains with the employer. There are also a variety of hybrid arrangements. In short, the managed care environment is becoming more complicated.

Another change, and a natural evolution of managed care, is the increased role, if not the dominance, of the primary care physician, who assumes responsibility for overseeing the allocation of resources. Most managed care organizations regard gaining the loyalty of primary care physicians as critical to their success. The "food chain" analogy has become a popular one, with primary care physicians rising above specialists and hospitals in the "food chain" hierarchy. Contributing to this role reversal is the excess supply in many specialties, with primary care physicians being in tight supply, a phenomenon that varies geographically. The role reversal has been a mixed blessing for primary care physicians, who may feel caught between pressure to reduce costs on the one hand and, on the other hand, the need to satisfy the desires of consumers, who may question whether the physician has their best interests at heart in light of the financial incentives to limit resource consumption.

Finally, consolidation is notable among both health care plans and providers. The multistate managed care firms, including the Kaiser plans but excluding the Blue Cross and Blue Shield plans that operate largely autonomously, accounted for 75.6 percent of all enrollment nationally in 1999.[16] Mergers are continuing to occur, as exemplified in the late 1990s by Aetna's acquisition of US HealthCare, NYLCare, and Prudential; CIGNA's purchase of HealthSource; and several of the mergers among Blue Cross and Blue Shield plans.

FUTURE ISSUES FACING MANAGED CARE

This chapter concludes with observations regarding managed care and how it has, and will, evolve with regard to the interplay between the public and private sectors; the role of quality in the new competitive, and managed care-dominated, environment; the locus of decision making on coverage of expensive and marginally effective technologies; and how the nation will address problems that managed care and competitive delivery mechanisms cannot solve and may exacerbate, notably access to coverage for the uninsured and the financing of graduate medical education.

Interplay between the Public and Private Sectors

One of the themes of this chapter is the generally positive interplay between the public and private sectors, although this has been less true in recent years. HMOs, which are private entities, have proven themselves to be viable mechanisms for delivering care to Medicare and Medicaid beneficiaries. At the same time, government at all levels has contributed much to managed care growth. One of the earliest examples of a large employer contracting with HMOs on a dual-choice basis was the agreement between the U.S. Office of Personnel Management and Kaiser Foundation Health Plans setting forth the terms under which Kaiser would be offered to federal employees. Today, federal, state, and local (including school district) government employees constitute the largest accounts of many HMOs. In addition, the HMO Act of 1973 provided a major impetus for HMO development. Even before then, the California Medicaid program represented one of the first examples of inpatient precertification and concurrent review. Also, many private plans have adopted diagnosis-related groups for hospital reimbursement and the resource-based relative value scale for physician reimbursement, both developed by Medicare for its fee-for-service program.

The relationship between the public and the private sector worsened in the late 1990s. The stresses that have evolved may reflect the success of managed care, to the point that many employees do not have access to a traditional indemnity program or, if they do, they resent having to pay the cost sharing and high premium costs, preferring HMO paid-in-full benefits and relatively lower premium costs. The stresses also reflect a concern with managed care practices, the frequency of which is a matter of dispute, of denying claims inappropriately, such as when a patient uses the emergency room, based on symptoms that warrant access, later to be denied coverage on the grounds that it was not ultimately a true emergency (addressed by "prudent layperson" laws in many states, as discussed in Chapter 69). Issues have also arisen around whether managed care organizations interpret the medical necessity guidelines in an overly restrictive manner, whether the composition of the drug formulary is overly limited, and whether the hurdles to access a specialist are set too high.

Providers concerned with the perceived interference into their practice, administrative burden, and impact on their incomes have pressed for protections. Ironically, many in the provider community, which is hardly unified, now look to the government for protection, such as by lobbying for laws that limit the ability of managed care plans to select the providers that are in their networks. A significant segment of the provider community appears to prefer government regulation to marketplace competition

The result has been a spate of proposals before state legislatures and in Congress, some of which have been enacted, designed to protect consumers. Whether these in fact do so, or simply serve to increase health care costs, is hotly debated.

Role of Quality

The role of quality in employer contracting decisions as well as in consumer choice among plans is unclear. HMOs pay considerable attention to enrollee satisfaction and regularly conduct surveys of both enrollees and disenrollees. Satisfaction may not equate to technical quality, however. Managed care should have maximizing value as its objective, not minimizing cost. The degree and manner in which quality in the future will enter into employer contracting decisions and consumer choice, thereby affecting financial performance and market share, are unclear. Quality is discussed further in Chapter 30, while issues affecting employer purchasing decisions (including the effect of quality measures) are discussed further in Chapter 41.

Of particular concern to some is how the chronically ill, especially those with rare conditions requiring specialized care, will fare under capitated arrangements. By one estimate, chronic illness accounts for 80 percent of all medical costs.[17] HMOs pay considerable attention to the more prevalent conditions, such as diabetes and asthma, in their disease management programs (see Chapter 23), and these same conditions are also the focus of HEDIS measures. Beyond defined chronic diseases, how good is their performance in caring for persons with complex or rare chronic conditions? Unfortunately, the research literature has little to say on this question, which should be a matter of empirical study, not anecdotes or preconceived views.

Also debated is the role of the specialist versus the primary care physician in caring for persons with certain chronic conditions, such as congestive heart failure and chronic obstructive pulmonary disease, both prevalent among the elderly in particular. Should the cardiologist or pulmonologist be allowed to serve as primary care physician for patients with these respective conditions? This issue is discussed further in Chapters 18 and 23.

Technology Assessment and the Coverage Determination Process

Another issue is the technology assessment or coverage determination process, that is, the process for making decisions about when new procedures or services are no longer experimental, as well as when procedures in general, some in use for many years, are not effective. For example, when is a particular form of transplantation no longer experimental? Subscriber and employer contracts, whether indemnity or HMO, routinely exclude coverage of procedures that are investigational or experimental, yet there is no uniform set of guidelines or a review process for determining when a procedure is no longer investigational or experimental. As a result, coverage denials are often litigated. Whether the courts are the best locus of decision making about what should be accepted medical practice is doubtful. This issue is not new with the advent of managed care, occurring in all forms of health insurance, but has increased dramatically with the rapid increase in medical treatment advances.

Increasingly, states have legislated that there be external reviews, and in those states that have not done so, a significant number of health plans have voluntarily adopted an external review process. They find that although only a small percent of enrollees actually take advantage of the review process, it reduces the fear generally that a health plan might deny the service for financial rather than medical reasons. Also, it may reduce the likelihood that the enrollee will subsequently bring a lawsuit.

Financing Access for the Uninsured and for Graduate Medical Education

Finally, the growth of competitive delivery systems affects the nature of public policy debate for a broad gamut of issues. Even matters such as priorities for biomedical research are not immune. Managed care, however, places into particularly sharp relief the question of financing of access for the uninsured and graduate medical education. With regard to access, on the one hand managed care provides a vehicle for covering all populations efficiently; on the other hand, it reduces the financial capacity of providers, operating in a more price competitive environment, to care for the uninsured. The Health Insurance Portability and Accountability Act of 1996 (HIPAA; see Chapter 67) has provided modest relief as regards access to health insurance, but significant barriers remain.

Much of the cost of graduate medical education has traditionally been financed through higher fee-for-service billings. These costs are principally stipends to residents and interns, along with the costs of supervision and those associated with services and procedures that are principally didactic in nature. Medicare reimburses hospitals for their share of these costs. Until 1997 these costs were incorporated into the county-specific rates at which Medicare pays HMOs.[18] The topic of academic health centers and managed care is also discussed in detail in Chapter 13.

CONCLUSION

Whatever the criticisms of managed care in some circles, a return to an open-ended and unmanaged fee-for-service system that characterized health care financing until a few years ago will not be tolerated by either public or private purchasers. Furthermore, supporting the suspicions of widespread waste are the large unexplained variations in practice patterns across delivery systems that do not correlate with health status differentials. Also, the excesses in provider supply, such as in the number of specialists and hospital beds, will continue to generate competition among providers that purchasers of care and managed care companies will seek to exploit.

Because medical care is such a personal matter, managed care will continue to generate anxiety among some consumers and raise issues of societal values and public policy. Although the major impetus for managed care is competition between health plans, managed care has always existed within a regulatory framework. Critical to the future of managed care is whether the government and the health plans can reach a better understanding of each other's legitimate roles and objectives. This, in turn, may pave the way for managed care to enjoy a high level of public confidence.

REFERENCES AND NOTES

1. American Association of Health Plans, unpublished data. These figures include PPO and point-of-service products of HMOs as well as pure HMO products. The principal sources of data on HMO enrollment are the American Association of Health Plans and InterStudy. They differ slightly in the data collected and the numbers reported. Both are regarded as generally reliable.

2. InterStudy, Competitive Edge 9.2 (Part II: HMO Industry Report), October 1999.

3. T.R. Mayer and G.G. Mayer, HMOs: Origins and Development, *New England Journal of Medicine* 312 (1985): 590–94.

4. G.K. MacLeod, "An Overview of Managed Care," in *The Managed Care Handbook*, 2d ed., ed. P.R. Kongstvedt (Gaithersburg, Md.: Aspen Publishers, 1993), 3–11.

5. Mayer and Mayer, HMOs: Origins and Development.

6. P. Starr, *The Social Transformation of American Medicine* (New York: Basic Books, 1982), 295–310.

7. InterStudy, Competitive Edge.

8. Mayer and Mayer, HMOs: Origins and Development.

9. G.B. Strumpf, "Historical Evolution and Political Process," in *Group and IPA HMOs,* ed. D.L. Mackie and D.K. Decker (Gaithersburg, Md.: Aspen Publishers, 1981), 17–36.

10. InterStudy, Competitive Edge (Part II: Industry Report), 9, 1 (July 1998).

11. J.J. Spies et al., "Alternative Health Care Delivery Systems: HMOs and PPOs," in *Health Care Cost Management: Private Sector Initiatives,* ed. P.D. Fox et al. (Ann Arbor, Mich.: Health Administration Press, 1984), 43–68.

12. J.E. Fielding, *Corporate Cost Management* (Reading, Mass.: Addison-Wesley, 1984).

13. Ibid.

14. American Association of Health Plans, unpublished data.

15. Health Care Financing Administration (HCFA), *National Summary of Medicaid Managed Care Programs and Enrollment* (Washington, D.C.: HCFA, 1994).

16. InterStudy, Competitive Edge (Part II: Industry Report), 4, 1 (1999).

17. K.N. Lohr et al., Chronic Disease in a General Adult Population: Findings from the Rand Health Insurance Experiment, *Western Journal of Medicine* 145 (1986): 537–545.

18. For a discussion of the managed care issues facing academic health centers, see P.D. Fox and J. Wasserman, Academic Medical Centers and Managed Care: Uneasy Partners, *Health Affairs* 12 (1993): 85–93.

SUGGESTED READING

Clark, W.D., and Hulbert, M.M. 1998. Research Issues: Dually Eligible Medicare and Medicaid Beneficiaries, Challenges and Opportunities. *Health Care Financing Review* 20, 2 (Winter): 1–10.

Davis, K., Collins, K.S., and Morris, C. 1991. Managed Care: Promise and Concerns. *Health Affairs* 13 (4): 3–46.

Iglehart, J.K. 1993. The American Health Care System. *New England Journal of Medicine* 328 (12): 896–900.

CHAPTER 2

Managed Care's Regulatory Evolution: Driving Change in the New Century

Frederick B. Abbey

Legislative and regulatory policy decisions and the debates leading up to them continually shape the evolution of managed care. Their far-reaching impact affects the decisions managed care executives make. They also help drive the responsibilities of payers and providers and determine the services health care consumers receive. In recent years, as the nation looks to managed care to provide affordable and effective health care, these debates have become increasingly public. At the dawn of the twenty-first century, congressional debate and action center around three primary issues:

- financing the cost of health care for the growing number of aging Americans as policy makers deal with the projected bankruptcy in 2015 of the Medicare Hospital Insurance (HI) Trust Fund (Medicare Part A)
- assessing the intended and unintended consequences of the Balanced Budget Act of 1997 (BBA)
- keeping Medicare solvent, particularly with projected budget surpluses, and decid-

ing whether to expand benefits or ensure the program's long-term solvency

In addition to these issues, the nation's dynamic economic scenario at the end of the 1990s allowed legislators' focus to shift to other issues including:

- expanding consumer choice
- enacting patient protection measures
- ensuring the privacy and confidentiality of health care information
- covering outpatient prescription drugs for the first time under Medicare

How should managed care organizations view these issues? This chapter presents the forces driving federal health care policy, specifically those most relevant to managed care. It also illustrates incremental policy steps Congress has taken and may take in the future to move more Americans toward a managed care system that balances the consumer's, provider's, and payer's frequently competing needs.

FORCES DRIVING FEDERAL HEALTH POLICY

Trust Fund Solvency—Medicare and Social Security

In recent health care policy debates, one issue has generated the most interest and concern: how to deal with the impending bankruptcy of the Medicare HI Trust Fund. In 1997, Congress passed the BBA (see also Chapter 55), which,

Frederick B. Abbey is a partner in the Washington, DC office of Ernst & Young LLP. He is the Director of Ernst & Young's Center for Health Policy and Strategy. For eight years he served as a federal official in policy development at the U.S. Department of Health and Human Services and the Health Care Financing Administration.

Ernst & Young staff members Marcella Wolfe, Pamela Pepe, Mike Treash, Sherry Hayes, and Kimberly Medland contributed to this chapter.

through changes to the Medicare program, reduced the rate of growth in HI expenditures and extended the solvency of the Trust Fund through 2015. In the early years of the new century, federal policy will continue to focus on the vast number of baby boomers entering the Medicare and Social Security programs, a trend with the potential to overwhelm the nation's health care and social systems. Between 2010 and 2030, Medicare enrollment is projected to grow by 2.4 percent a year—up from the 1.4 percent average annual growth projected through 2007. In 1999, Medicare had 39 million enrollees, nearly 7 million of whom were enrolled in Medicare managed care plans. By 2030, Medicare enrollment will have doubled to 75 million people.[1]

The BBA made more changes to federal health care programs than at any time since Medicare was enacted in 1965. In addition to significant changes in payment methodologies for home health agencies, skilled nursing facilities, and hospital outpatient services, the BBA continued Medicare down the path in which managed care organizations assume a greater role in the financial risk of the program. Congress' long-term assumption is that the fee-for-service (FFS) system will slowly erode in favor of the Medicare + Choice program, which currently enrolls about 16 percent of Medicare beneficiaries.[2]

Through its combination of measures, between 1998 and 2002, the BBA was projected to reduce Medicare program outlays by a total of $115 billion. However, the savings, for a variety of unforeseen factors have been significantly greater. When the BBA was debated, Medicare was growing at an annual rate of 7.9 percent and insolvency of its Trust Fund was seemingly imminent. Since then, however, the economic boom of the late 1990s dramatically eased the pressure on both the Social Security and Medicare trust funds. As a result of those and other factors, the growth rate of Medicare program outlays has dropped dramatically from 1.5 percent in 1998, and a precedent-setting negative 1.2 percent in 1999.[3]

Since the BBA was enacted, much has changed. In July 1999, the Congressional Budget Office released further revisions to its budget outlook, depicting even larger-than-expected surpluses from those it released 6 months earlier (Table 2–1).

Compared with the gloomy economic forecasts predicted during the BBA debate when only deficits appeared on the horizon, Congress now has the task of allocating projected surplus dollars. The options include:

- shoring up the long-term solvency of Medicare—for some period of time beyond its projected insolvency date of 2015—by dedicating some percentage of the projected surplus
- expanding the current benefits package available to Medicare beneficiaries through the addition of outpatient prescription drugs
- returning the surplus dollars to the American public through a series of tax cuts

---

Table 2–1 Federal Budget Surplus (In billions of dollars)

Fiscal Year	2000	2001	2002	2003	2004	2005	2006	2007	2008	2009
Baseline Total surplus	161	193	246	247	266	286	334	364	385	413
On-budget*	14	38	82	75	85	92	129	146	157	178
Off-budget†	147	155	164	172	181	195	205	217	228	235

*On-budget surpluses exclude the Postal Service and Social Security Trust Fund revenues.
†Off-budget surpluses include the Postal Service surplus and the Social Security Trust Fund.
Source: Reprinted from The Economic and Budget Outlook: An Update, Congressional Budget Office, July 1, 1999.

- buying down some of the nation's debt using surplus funds
- using some combination of these options

As a result of recent annual budget surpluses, discussions over the long-term financial stability of federal health care programs are now cast as much or more in political terms rather than in economic terms. The Democrats will want to extend solvency by dedicating a significant portion of the budget surplus while also adding options such as prescription drug coverage if financially possible. The Republicans would prefer to refund the budget surplus to Americans through a series of tax cuts, while continuing to shift risk for the Medicare and Medicaid programs from the federal government to the private sector through managed care organizations.

Predicting Federal Health Program Outlays

Knowing exactly how much money is needed to pay for federally funded health care and accurately predicting this amount from year to year has been a major challenge facing Congress. With the current system, the government cannot support the type and cost of services beneficiaries will consume in a given year. Premium support is increasingly embraced as a means to manage federal outlays. Under a premium support proposal, Medicare beneficiaries receive a government payment to purchase a health insurance policy. The federal government would then pay managed care plans a defined monthly contribution for each beneficiary they enroll. The plans would then assume the risk for providing care to members within that amount.

A premium support model would convert Medicare from a "service reimbursement" system as it is run today. Today, Medicare is an *entitlement*, with most beneficiaries participating in the FFS program. Any health care charge incurred by a Medicare beneficiary is paid by the federal government, subject to annual deductibles and copays by the beneficiary, as long as the services provided are (1) medically necessary and (2) in Medicare's "defined benefit package." With Medicare managed care plans,

per-beneficiary payment rates are set annually and then multiplied by the number of beneficiaries enrolled in the program that year. Nearly 18 percent of beneficiaries are now enrolled in Medicare managed care programs that more closely model the premium support concept.

Premium support is fundamentally a Republican concept, although it has the support of some Democrats. It would dramatically alter Medicare's current funding methods. In theory, some defined benefits package could be retained under premium support, but health plans would have the flexibility to design packages for markets as they saw a need, and seniors would have the freedom to enter the marketplace and select the plan that best meets their needs. For instance, Medicare managed care plans have sometimes distinguished themselves from the FFS program by offering low-cost prescription drug benefits, which Medicare otherwise does not cover. Under premium support, it is argued that benefit packages would be designed to offer even greater flexibility if health plans had the opportunity to develop packages suited to the diverse range of beneficiaries.

Increasing the Number of Consumer Choices

Congress has also begun to debate how and whether to make federal health care programs, particularly Medicare, more like the health plans offered to private sector workers. For instance, most workers covered by employer-sponsored health plans today have access to preventive services such as physicals, well-baby care, and cancer screenings—none of which Medicare has ever covered. Workers also routinely have access to vision care and outpatient prescription drug benefits, whereas Medicare beneficiaries do not unless they are enrolled in a managed care plan that offers such a benefit or qualify for Medicaid prescription drug coverage because of limited income.

There is a growing recognition that the one-size-fits-all nature of a defined benefit package is increasingly outdated for the Medicare population. Healthy 65-year-olds need different services than do frail 90-year-olds with complex, chronic health conditions. Therefore, increasing the number of options available to those covered by federal health plans has support in Congress, provided it can be done without significant increases in beneficiary premiums or annual federal budget outlays.

The most frequently mentioned expansion option during 2000–2001 is the coverage of outpatient prescription drugs (Medicare currently covers only those drugs administered by a physician in a hospital). This option is desired because of the ever-increasing use of pharmaceuticals as treatment therapy, along with growing evidence that many seniors have inadequate resources to purchase the drugs that have been prescribed for them.

However, Congress is hesitant to create an environment in which those seniors who already have drug coverage (for example, through such means as employer-sponsored retirement plans, Medicaid, and Medigap) instead become dependent on Medicare funding for their medication. The Congressional Budget Office projects the administration's prescription drug proposal will cost Medicare $260 billion and Medicaid $19 billion between 2003–2010.[4] This represents a 5 percent to 25 percent increase in the annual cost of the program, depending on the number of beneficiaries with access to the benefit, the copays per prescription, and the annual limit on coverage. To proceed with such a significant benefit expansion, legislators must determine how big the budget surpluses really are, assuming they are to be tapped to help pay for the expansion, as well as how much beneficiary premiums would have to be increased.

Managed Medicare Competition—Medicare + Choice Information Campaign

Driven by the need to balance the federal budget and protect Medicare from insolvency, policy makers built into the BBA incentives to increase the number of Medicare beneficiaries enrolled in managed care—now referred to as the Medicare + Choice program. To help establish this new program, Congress created a model

that promotes consumer empowerment through Medicare + Choice information campaigns. To understand the impact of these campaigns, it is important to relate them to other changes designed to create a competitive Medicare managed care market.

For example, Medicare + Choice strives to adopt private-sector health plan options, such as health maintenance organizations (HMOs), provider-sponsored organizations, preferred provider organizations, private indemnity plans (PIs), and medical savings accounts (MSAs). The goal of policy makers in this action is to improve beneficiaries' choices, thus expanding the number enrolling in managed care. If successful, the influx of new plans into an already competitive Medicare market will stimulate the demand for information to help them compare plans.

To meet this demand for 2001, the administration has requested $150 million from user fees for Medicare to distribute Medicare + Choice health information, recognizing that Medicare beneficiaries require better information to be responsible health care consumers. The BBA requires the Health Care Financing Administration (HCFA) to develop and provide a range of consumer information, including:

- product comparison charts
- Medicare + Choice membership rules
- quality outcome measurements
- member satisfaction data
- quality-of-life indicators
- disenrollment rates

Not only did the BBA include incentives to increase the use of managed care in Medicare, but it also changed the Medicare + Choice payment system with the goal of:

- stimulating growth in smaller markets with little or no managed care penetration
- ensuring that Medicare is saving money in private health plan contracting
- rewarding health plans for marketing and retaining higher risk individuals

Revisions to the *average adjusted per capita cost* (AAPCC) payment formula constrained future rate increases in urban markets that have the highest managed care penetration (although those areas have potential for even greater penetration given the percentage of Medicare beneficiaries still enrolled in FFS rather than managed care). While doing this, it increased the rates for smaller and rural markets. The questions now are how successful the AAPCC payment revisions will be in increasing managed care presence in nonurban areas and to what degree will managed care continue to grow in urban markets as more beneficiaries leave the FFS market.

In addition to issues concerning Medicare, a broad range of managed care legislative and regulatory issues apply to all health care consumers enrolled in managed care plans, not just those who receive their care through Medicare. Consumer protection, ensuring the privacy and confidentiality of health care information, and preventing fraud and abuse in health care are three of these and are discussed in the following section.

MAJOR AREAS OF POLICY DEVELOPMENT

In this environment managed care efforts in Congress are likely to focus on a few key areas:

- making technical changes to the BBA to address any unintended consequences stemming from the legislation
- deciding to what extent the projected federal budget surpluses are real and whether or how best to use them to either expand Medicare benefits or shore up the program's long-term solvency
- protecting consumers from perceived managed care abuses through patient protection legislation
- determining whether to enact federal privacy standards through legislation or regulation to protect the confidentiality of an individual's personally identifiable health information
- continuing a systematic approach to eliminating fraud and abuse in the health care system

Balanced Budget Act

Although Congress made modest adjustments through the Balanced Budget Refinement Act (BBRA) of 1999, Congress will continue to revisit the BBA in areas in which payment changes are believed to have had unintended consequences. For instance, academic medical centers and rural hospitals report being unduly hard hit by the BBA. Further, hospitals complain that in the upcoming years, the profits from their inpatient hospital services will be woefully inadequate, threatening the viability of numerous institutions. In addition, many home health agencies have closed as a result of the financial impact of the interim payment system and skilled nursing facilities are suffering through implementation of the new prospective payment system (PPS).

The development of adjusters is underway for managed care plans, and HCFA continues to look at so-called demonstration projects as a way to include patients with chronic diseases in managed care. One project is currently underway to assess the viability of incorporating patients with end-stage renal disease (ESRD) in Medicare + Choice plans. Sorting out the long-term implications of the BBA could easily take several years, since the data collection in most federal health care programs lags so far behind the fiscal year in which Congress is working.

Consumer Protection Measures

With the growth of managed care, both in the private sector and in federal health programs, Congress increasingly hears from constituents about the limitations of managed care in providing health care. As a result, managed care consumer protection laws continue to be hotly debated in Washington and in state legislatures. Policy makers recognize that helping to contain health care costs and improving the quality of care depends on addressing many of the concerns managed care has raised. These include impeded access to care, a lack of information to help consumers compare among health plans, and the problem of "risk selection," or health plans attracting and retaining only healthy populations.

Exhibit 2–1 Provisions of the Patients' Bill of Rights

- Information disclosure
- Choice of providers and plans
- Access to emergency services
- Participation in treatment decisions
- Respect and nondiscrimination
- Confidentiality of health care information
- Complaints and appeals
- Consumer responsibilities

Source: Reprinted from President's Advisory Commission on Consumer Protection and Quality in the Health Care Industry.

Provisions such as those in the Patients' Bill of Rights (Exhibit 2–1), developed by President Clinton's Advisory Commission on Consumer Protection and Quality in the Health Care Industry, are the direct result of public support for increased consumer protection.

To address many of these concerns, Congress has debated a series of "patient protection" bills, which include provisions for:

- ensuring the patient's right to an external appeal for denied care or coverage
- allowing small businesses to pool together to offer health coverage through association health plans
- allowing parents to select a pediatrician as their child's primary caregiver
- creating a Commission to recommend model health insurance guidelines and whether new health benefit mandates are needed
- banning gag clauses in managed care contracts
- requiring health plans to cover emergency care if patients have to go "out of network" because of circumstances beyond their control
- requiring health plans to disclose clearly worded, easy-to-read information on covered benefits and other policies, as well as patient satisfaction and clinical outcome measurements

Although there is near-universal agreement on a number of these provisions, patient protection legislation frequently is held up by disagreement between Republicans and Democrats over other issues, such as increasing health plan liability. In general, Democrats believe plans should be held liable for both economic and punitive damages resulting from their actions, whereas Republicans generally oppose creating plan liability for punitive damages. Without a doubt, this issue will consume significant time and debate as Congress considers how best to structure managed care in the twenty-first century.

Protecting the Privacy and Confidentiality of Health Care Information

Although the Internet and information technology bring health care organizations, and the consumers of their services, unprecedented access to knowledge and communication, they also raise many questions about how to protect the privacy of personal health care information. An increase in both the quantity and quality of electronic health care transactions, particularly for managed care organizations that possess significant amounts of health data, can potentially create greater administrative and clinical efficiencies, reduce costs, and improve consumer relations. However, ensuring privacy and confidentiality is one of the largest impediments to this increased use.[5] It is also ironic that while technology is driving such changes health care lags significantly behind other industries such as banking and commerce in the degree to which payers, providers, suppliers, and consumers are connected electronically.

To address the ever-increasing need to protect individual health information Congress enacted the Health Insurance Portability and Accountability Act of 1996 (HIPAA; see also Chapter 67). HIPAA mandates two fundamental changes in the collection, use, and dissemination of *individually identifiable health information*. First, through a process known as administrative simplification, any entity capturing health information must do so in a way that complies with HCFA regulations. Second, HIPAA mandates that either Congress, through legislation, or the Secretary of Health and Human Services, through regulation, develops federal privacy standards, laying out required protections for maintaining the privacy of personal health information and penalties when those standards are violated. Creating those privacy protections and implementing administrative simplification will consume significant legislative and regulatory resources well into the twenty-first century.

Preventing Fraud and Abuse in Health Care

In the mid 1990s Congress became increasingly concerned about the reported increases in fraud and abuse, such as *upcoding* of Medicare charges (billing for a higher level of service than was actually provided). In 1998, the Department of Health and Human Services' Office of Inspector General (OIG) concluded that the Medicare program overpaid health care providers more than $12 billion, or 7.1 percent of Medicare payments, because of a variety of reasons, ranging from inadvertent mistakes to fraudulent and abusive activities.[6] The OIG could not quantify what portion of the error rate was attributable to fraud.[7]

As a result, Congress provided additional funding to the OIG to hire new investigative staff, tasked with identifying and eliminating fraud and abuse. Detecting and punishing health care fraud and abuse activities is the number two law enforcement priority for the federal government, second only in importance to the prosecution of violent crime. Increased funding will be provided to the federal government to continue and expand its investigations and activities in this area. Providers found to be noncompliant could face hefty fines, temporary and permanent exclusions from the Medicare and Medicaid programs, and criminal prosecution and imprisonment.

Providers of all types have been found guilty of fraudulent and abusive activities. Many investigations have been high-profile and have involved significant monetary settlements. In its work plan for 2000, the OIG of the U.S. Department of Health and Human Services named the focus areas for the review of managed care organizations serving Medicare and Medicaid clients. These areas are as follows:

Medicare

- audit of new adjusted community rate proposal process
- general and administrative costs
- cost-based managed care plans
- enhanced managed care payments
- HMO profits
- investment income earned by risk-based HMOs
- physician incentive plans
- usefulness of Medicare+Choice performance measures
- managed care additional benefits
- enrollment incentives and disincentives
- enrollee access to emergency services
- chiropractic services
- Medicare managed care prescription drug benefit
- managed care organizational closings

Medicaid

- Medicaid dually eligible FFS payments
- Emergency services to enrollees of Medicaid managed care

Increased government efforts to prevent health care fraud and abuse and recoup fraudulently billed funds will continue to help protect Medicare solvency and prevent jeopardizing the quality of care patients receive. These efforts have strong public backing because many consumers believe that fraud and abuse are still a large problem—despite government efforts to address rising health care costs through antifraud and anti-abuse efforts. Nearly 70 percent of consumers surveyed in a poll by the American Association of Retired Persons said they believe that the Medicare program would not go broke if fraud and abuse were eliminated.[8] Americans' support of antifraud and anti-abuse efforts is also evidenced in their approval of federal legislation addressing fraud issues—HIPAA and the BBA—and will continue.

Public Opinion Shapes Policy

Public opinion will continue to play an important role in congressional action addressing each topic covered in this chapter and shaping managed care's future evolution. Although research shows that most Americans are satisfied with the care they receive from their health plan,[9] the Patients' Bill of Rights and related congressional debates are driven by concern with managed care organizations expressed by constituents and in the media. This concern is being driven by two "publics": the relatively small group reporting direct problems with their plans and the broader public without direct experience that perceives dramatic and threatening events taking place in managed care plans. People in the latter group fear that no matter how well their health plan performs today, it may not make available—or pay for—the care they need in the future should they become very ill. The patient protection provisions that Congress legislates in response to these concerns depend on the state of the economy and the measures plans have already self-imposed to ensure the provision of quality care.

As these provisions are debated, Congress uses public polling data as one of many tools for gauging Americans' views on health care. In a major study conducted by the League of Women Voters (LWV) and the Kaiser Family Foundation, a total of 6,500 participants gave their views on how best to reform Medicare. Participants said they recognized that the number of beneficiaries accessing Medicare will grow substantially over the next several years and that people in general are living longer and thus consuming more services. However, they were reluctant to consider *any* reforms until the federal government better controls the "perceived rampant fraud, abuse and waste in Medicare."[10]

Specifically for managed care, some study participants cited the potential for beneficiaries to have greater access to services through HMOs, particularly for "preventive care and possibly prescription drugs." Others, however, had "serious concerns about losing their doctor, about the referral and authorization process, and about being denied care when they are sick." Overall, study participants expressed a neutral position on the benefit of enrolling more Medicare beneficiaries in HMOs.[11]

Because of the prevalence of opinions such as these on managed care, Congress is beginning to explore other alternatives to meet the public's health care needs, including premium support. A poll by the American Academy of Actuaries (AAA), released the same month as the LWV study, shows that 64 percent of respondents favor changing the Medicare program to a premium support model, including 71 percent aged 50 and over and 70 percent of the respondents less than the age of 35.[12] Participants expressed concern, however, that premium support could cause Medicare beneficiaries' out-of-pocket expenses to increase significantly. As a result, it may take time and effort to gain the support needed to make premium support part of Medicare.

Poll results such as these by the LWV and the AAA are important to managed care organizations for two main reasons. First, they express patient and enrollee experiences in the health care system that provide insight managed care organizations can use in shaping their organizations' future. They are also an important gauge as to what is important to American voters. The longer these issues remain in the forefront and the more they lead to requests for action, the greater the likelihood that they will become public policy issues. This is how the Patients' Bill of Rights became one of the leading topics of debate in Congress at the end of the 1990s.

Beyond the Bill of Rights, Congress will legislate other issues that public opinion interjects into the public policy debate. These opinions also drive Medicare reforms, which will in turn have an impact on managed care organizations. ***These potential reforms include:***

- raising the minimum age requirement from 65 to 67
- means-testing (requiring affluent seniors to pay a greater share of their health care costs)
- continuing to reduce the rate of growth in provider and practitioner rates of reimbursement
- moving to a premium support-style payment method

- deciding whether to increase the current HI payroll tax to preserve and strengthen the Medicare program

Convincing a frequently skeptical public of the need for any of these reforms will require serious leadership, particularly in light of the huge budget surplus projections. Clearly, Congress has much work to do to mold public opinion in support of any reform plan. Nevertheless, the American public has demonstrated considerable commitment to preserving Medicare because of its importance to older Americans and their quality of life. Americans, whether covered by Medicare or private payers, have made it clear that they intend to be vocal and active in making known how managed care is meeting their health care needs—and should be changed to better do so.

OUTLOOK

The health care environment is volatile and dynamic, creating issues that will remain in the forefront of the public policy arena. Congress always will try to respond to voters' needs and reactions to managed care. Furthermore, as managed care organizations respond to meet marketplace demands, there will also be public reactions to those changes. More outcry to Congress will result. This evolutionary spiral can best be characterized as one in which change management is essential.

It is vitally important that managed care organizations develop their capacity to manage the changes driven by congressional response to public response to managed care. The changes that must be addressed consist of tactical initiatives that respond to congressional action and governmental regulation coupled with long-term strategic initiatives that shape their organization's long-term evolution. The matrix in Exhibit 2–2 summarizes a variety of public policy issues managed care organizations face today and will face heading into the future. These issues are divided into four quadrants: short-term tactical, long-term tactical, short-term strategic, and long-term strategic. Exhibit 2–2 details each quadrant's issues.

Exhibit 2–2 Managing Major Legislative and Regulatory Change

	Pace of Change	
	Short Term **6–12 months**	**Long Term** **12–24 months**
Tactical	• Corporate compliance program • Medicare + Choice regulation & data collection • HIPAA AS, portability, & privacy/security • Delegation oversight • Financial stability of provider contractors • State consumer protection enforcement • Provider fraud and abuse	• Medicare + Choice payment policy • Compliance effectiveness • Privacy, confidentiality, & security • Internet security • Medicare intermediate sanctions • Medicare compare
Strategic	• Medicare + Choice competitive pricing demonstration • Medicare + Choice growth • Risk-based capital • Legal liability • Anti-managed care backlash • Consumer protection regulation trend	• Consumer empowerment • Regulation of ERISA plans • E-commerce role • Long-Term Care/Programs of All-Inclusive Care for the Elderly (LTC/PACE) • Medicaid growth • New competitors/new entrants

continues

Exhibit 2–2 continued

Short Term/Tactical

- *Corporate compliance programs*. Implementing a corporate compliance program in accordance with the Office of Inspector General's guidance (see Chapter 68).
- *Medicare + Choice regulation and data collection*. Implementing and developing compliance monitoring tools supporting the new Medicare + Choice regulatory requirements with special attention to the new data reporting requirements that could subject the health plan to the federal False Claims Act.
- *HIPAA administrative simplification, portability, and privacy/security requirements*. Implementing the regulation standards and ongoing compliance monitoring. The administrative simplification standards include electronic transmission standards, standard data sets, and unique identifiers. The portability requirements, already in place, are subject to increased scrutiny by state regulators. The privacy and security standards are being incorporated into the pending federal health care privacy legislation (see Chapter 67).
- *Delegation oversight*. Managing the increased regulators on health plan accountability for processes delegated to providers and vendors (see Chapter 4).
- *Financial stability of risk-assuming providers*. Increasing essential risk management protection to avoid situations such as occurred with the insolvency of HIP of New Jersey (see Chapters 4 and 46).
- *State consumer protection regulation*. Complying with emerging state consumer protection requirements and enforcement. States such as New York and California are aggressively enforcing consumer protections requirements (see Chapter 69).
- *Provider fraud and abuse*. Detecting and investigating provider inappropriate billing and other illegal activities (see Chapter 38).

Short Term/Strategic

- *Medicare + Choice competitive pricing demonstration*. Participating in the demonstration of applicable, long-term implications for Medicare + Choice contracting.

- *Medicare + Choice enrollment and profitability growth*. Balancing enrollment growth targets with Medicare + Choice profitability realities given the increased regulatory requirements and the changed payment policy.
- *Risk-based capital*. Assessing the impact of movement to the new fiscal solvency requirement and compliance to its data capture standards (see also Chapter 49).
- *Legal liability*. Reducing liability to legal cases, especially those involving medical necessity and other coverage decisions, Federal False Claims Act, and federal racketeering laws (see Chapters 63 to 65).
- *Anti-managed care backlash*. Avoiding high-publicity legal and regulatory issues that may feed the public's negative perception of the managed care industry (see Chapter 6).
- *Consumer protection regulation*. Assessing the impact of state and federal consumer protection standards on the business model, compliance activity, and internal audit planning.

Long Term/Tactical

- *Medicare + Choice payment policy*. Assessing the impact of Medicare + Choice payment policy, financial risk adjusters, and competitive pricing on profitability in the market.
- *Compliance effectiveness*. Developing performance measures to demonstrate the effectiveness of the corporate compliance program.
- *Privacy, confidentiality, and security*. Implementing the federal health care privacy principles in policy, operations, and compliance oversight. Includes consumer disclosure and consent forms, disclosure accounting, technical security standards and compliance activities.
- *Medicare intermediate sanctions*. Assessing the federal government's increasing ability to impose penalties for noncompliance and the imperative to reduce culpability through the development of an effective corporate compliance program.
- *Medicare Compare*. Optimizing opportunities created by Medicare's Internet-based tool for consumers to compare health plan benefit and performance measures. The tool is representative of the federal government's efforts to instill greater competition into the health care market.

continues

Exhibit 2–2 continued

Long Term/Strategic

- **Consumer empowerment.** Anticipating efforts by state and federal government to increase and improve consumer decision making in health care (see also Chapter 43).
- **Regulating ERISA plans.** Assessing federal policies that could impact the size and profitability of the ERISA self-funded employer market (see Chapter 66).
- **E-commerce.** Understanding and harnessing the Internet and information technologies to improve customer relationships (see Chapter 37).

Courtesy of Ernst & Young, LLP, 2000, Washington, DC.

- **Long-term care.** Planning for the growth of the long-term-care market and the integration of health insurance, especially coverage of chronic conditions in programs such as the Program of All-inclusive Care for the Elderly (PACE).
- **Medicaid growth.** Assessing market and profitability growth in Medicaid given the continued gradual expansion of the program to deal with the problem of the uninsured (see also Chapter 57).
- **New competitors/new entrants.** Assessing new competitors in Medicare such as association plans, unions, and MSAs and legislation allowing competition from the financial services industry.

It is easy for organizations to be distracted by government initiatives that fall into the short-term tactical quadrant of this matrix and essentially be left devoting their time to complying in a reactionary mode to government regulations imposed on them. The leaders of managed care organizations can better serve their customers by distributing time among the issues of all four quadrants of this matrix with an eye on the organization's *long-term strategic goals.*

In implementing the decisions made in each sector of this matrix, organizations' success in the marketplace depends on balancing efforts among all the quadrants—not just having a focus on the immediate tactical issues. Meeting and anticipating government requirements is the mere minimum for success. Successful managed care organizations will display the ability to allocate time and resources in each of these quadrants in a balanced way. By doing so, they will have demonstrated their ability to learn and adapt to a changing environment, collaborate with health care providers and practitioners for mutual benefit, and successfully manage their own growth and evolution in the changing and dynamic managed care marketplace.

REFERENCES AND NOTES

1. IICFA, *A Profile of Medicare,* 1998 Chart Book.
2. S.M. Lieberman, Executive Associate Director, Congressional Budget Office, testimony on Medicare + Choice before the U.S. Senate Finance Committee, June 9, 1999.
3. U.S. Department of Treasury, 1999.
4. Congressional Budget Office, An Analysis of the President's Budget Proposal for Fiscal Year 2001, March 2000.
5. A. Westin, *The Era of Consensual Marketing Is Coming,* Louis Harris and Associates, December 1998.
6. U.S. Department of Health and Human Services, Press Release, Office of the Inspector General, February 9, 1999.
7. U.S. Department of Health and Human Services, Press Release, Office of the Inspector General, February 9, 1999.
8. American Association of Retired Persons, *Health Care Fraud Survey,* March and September 1997.
9. Is There a Managed Care Backlash? Kaiser Family Foundation and Harvard University National Survey of Americans' Views on Managed Care, Nov. 5, 1997.
10. *How Americans Talk about Medicare Reform: The Public Voice,* Publication #1092, League of Women Voters, 1999.
11. *How Americans Talk about Medicare Reform,* 1999.
12. Premium Support Solution Is Favorite Medicare Fix, a Yankelovich Partners omnibus survey sponsored by the American Academy of Actuaries (AAA), May 26, 1999, http://www.actuary.org.

CHAPTER 3

Types of Managed Care Organizations

Eric R. Wagner

Attempting to describe the types of organizations in a field as dynamic as managed care is not easy. The U.S. health care industry is in a period of significant change. By the time these words are committed to print, the industry is certain to have evolved further. Nevertheless, distinctions remain between different managed care organizations (MCOs), and many are rooted in the historic differences between different forms of managed care. As a result, it is useful to understand the different types of organizations, even though some types may no longer exist in the pure form.

Eric R. Wagner is Vice President for Managed Care at MedStar Health, President and Executive Director for the WHC Physician-Hospital Organization, and President of Helix Family Choice.

His responsibilities include development of managed care strategy, negotiation of participation agreements, oversight of managed care products, and maintenance of relationships with managed care plans for all MedStar Health entities. In addition, he has operations responsibility for the WHC Physician-Hospital Organization and Helix Family Choice, and he chairs the Finance and Operations Committee for Capital Community Health Plan.

Previously, Mr. Wagner was with the health care strategy and managed care practice of an international professional services firm. He has more than 20 years of experience in the health care industry specializing in managed care strategy, development, operations, and finance and has published several books, chapters, and articles on managed care evaluation, development, negotiations, and provider compensation.

It also is worth noting that recent research suggests that though most Americans are enrolled in an MCO, they do not believe that they receive their health care coverage through managed care. According to the 1999 Health Confidence Survey conducted by the Employee Benefit Research Institute, almost two-thirds of the 87 percent of workers who are covered by managed care think they have never been in a managed care plan.[1] This finding suggests that the industry has done a poor job of conveying information about the different organizational types.

About a decade ago, the various types of MCOs and traditional forms of health insurance were reasonably distinct. Since then, the differences between them have narrowed to the point where it is very difficult to tell whether an entity is an insurance company or an MCO. Ten years ago, MCOs were often referred to as "alternative delivery systems," but managed care is now the dominant form of health insurance coverage in the United States, and relatively few people receive their health insurance through a more traditional form of coverage. Figure 3–1 shows how much enrollment in managed care plans grew between 1993 and 1998.

Originally, health maintenance organizations (HMOs), preferred provider organizations (PPOs), and traditional forms of indemnity health insurance were distinct, mutually exclusive products and mechanisms for providing health care coverage. Today, an observer may be hard pressed to uncover the differences between products that bill themselves as HMOs, PPOs, or

Figure 3–1 U.S. Employee Health Plan Enrollment in Managed Care, 1993–1998. Courtesy of William M. Mercer, Inc., San Francisco, California.

managed care overlays to health insurance. For example, most HMOs, which traditionally limited their members to a designated set of participating providers, now allow their members to use nonparticipating providers at a reduced coverage level. Such point-of-service (POS) plans combine HMO-like systems with indemnity systems, allowing individual members to choose which systems they wish to access at the time they need the medical service. Similarly, some PPOs, which historically provided unrestricted access to physicians and other health care providers (albeit at different coverage levels), have implemented primary care case management or gatekeeper systems and have added elements of financial risk to their reimbursement systems. Finally, almost all indemnity insurance (or self-insurance) plans now include utilization management features and provider networks that were once found only in HMOs or PPOs.

As a result of these recent changes, the descriptions of the different types of managed care systems that follow provide only a guideline for determining an MCO's form. In many cases, the MCO will be a hybrid form.

Further confusing this is the emergence of integrated delivery systems (IDSs) or organized delivery systems that accept substantial risk for medical costs (e.g., provider-sponsored organizations [PSOs]). In the never-ending movement to render taxonomy of MCOs as difficult to understand as hieroglyphics, some of these types of IDSs require licensure from the state (e.g., a "limited Knox-Keene" license in California) or from the federal government (e.g., a PSO that does not already have state licensure). For more on IDSs, see Chapters 4 and 65.

Some controversy exists about whether the term "managed care" accurately describes the new generation of health care delivery and financing mechanisms. Those commentators who object to the term raise questions about what it is that is managed by an MCO. Is it the patient's medical care, or the composition and reimbursement of the provider delivery system that is being managed? Observers who favor the term "managed care" believe that managing the provider delivery system can be equivalent in its outcomes to managing the medical care delivered to the patient. In contrast to historical methods of financing health care delivery in the United States, the current generation of financing mechanisms includes far more active management of both the care delivery system and the medical care itself. Although the term "managed care" may not perfectly describe this current generation of financing vehicles, it provides a convenient shorthand description for the range of alternatives to traditional indemnity health insurance. The term also has gained widespread use in popular discourse and in the general media, even though a majority of Americans clearly do not understand what it means.

A simplistic but useful concept regarding managed care is the continuum, illustrated in Figure 3–2. On one end of the continuum is managed indemnity, with simple precertification of elective admissions and large case management of catastrophic cases, superimposed on a traditional indemnity insurance plan. Similar to indemnity is the service plan, which has contractual relationships with providers addressing maximum fee allowances, prohibiting balance billing, and using the same utilization management techniques as managed indemnity (the nearly universal examples of service plans are Blue Cross and Blue Shield plans). Further along the continuum are PPOs, POSs, open-panel HMOs (independent practice associations [IPAs]), and finally closed-panel (group and staff model) HMOs. Moving from left to right on the continuum, there are new and greater elements of control and accountability, greater complexity and overhead required to operate the plan, and greater potential control of cost and quality.

This chapter describes the different types of MCOs. In addition, the chapter discusses the basic forms of HMOs—the original MCOs—and their relationships with physicians.

TYPES OF MCOs

With the firm understanding that there are really no firm distinctions or boundaries between them, what follows is a discussion of the main types of MCOs. Throughout this book, these types of MCOs may be referred to in such a way as to conform to what follows in this chapter; in other cases a chapter author will simply throw in the towel and use "MCO" to cover the whole array of plan types. But distinctions between types of MCOs are not mere historic relics; there are differences that matter, and the terms themselves still enjoy wide usage (or misusage in some cases).

Managed Care and Indemnity Insurance

The perceived success of HMOs and other types of MCOs in controlling the utilization and cost of health services has prompted entrepreneurs to develop managed care overlays that can be combined with traditional indemnity insurance, service plan insurance, or self-insurance ("indemnity insurance" is used to refer to all three forms of coverage in this context). These managed care overlays are intended to provide cost control for insured plans while retaining the individual's freedom of choice of provider and coverage for out-of-plan services.

The following types of managed care overlays currently exist:

Figure 3–2 Continuum of Managed Care. Courtesy of William M. Mercer, Inc., San Francisco, California.

- *General utilization management.* These companies offer a complete menu of utilization management activities that can be selected by individual employers or insurers. Some offer or can develop panels of participating providers within individual markets and bear strong resemblances to PPOs (see below).
- *Specialty utilization management.* Firms that focus on utilization review for specialty services have become common. Mental health (see Chapter 25) and dental care (see Chapter 60) are two common types of specialty utilization management overlays.
- *Catastrophic or large case management.* Some firms have developed to assist employers and insurers with managing catastrophic cases involving all specialties. This service includes screening to identify cases that will become catastrophic, negotiation of services and reimbursement with providers who can treat the patient's condition, development of a treatment protocol for the patient, and ongoing monitoring of the treatment. See Chapter 22 for a detailed discussion of case management.
- *Workers' compensation utilization management.* In response to the rapid increases in the cost of workers' compensation insurance, firms have developed managed care overlays to address what they claim are the unique needs of patients covered under workers' compensation benefits. Managed care and workers' compensation programs are discussed in detail in Chapter 61.

Many indemnity insurance companies have carried these concepts several steps farther along the continuum by transforming themselves through acquisitions into MCOs. In fact, all of the major indemnity insurance companies that existed at the beginning of the decade have either sold their health insurance business lines to other companies or acquired major managed care companies. In the process, these companies have become the largest MCOs in the country, surpassing the original managed care companies

or free-standing HMOs in size and geographic coverage.

PPOs

PPOs are entities through which employer health benefit plans and health insurance carriers contract to purchase health care services for covered beneficiaries from a selected network of participating providers. Typically, participating providers in PPOs agree to abide by utilization management and other procedures implemented by the PPO and agree to accept the PPO's reimbursement structure and payment levels. In return, PPOs often limit the size of their participating provider panels and provide incentives for their covered individuals to use participating providers instead of other providers. In contrast to traditional HMO coverage, PPO coverage allows individuals to use non-PPO providers, although higher levels of coinsurance or deductibles routinely apply to services provided by these nonparticipating providers.

PPOs occasionally are described as preferred provider arrangements (PPAs). The definition of a PPA is usually the same as the definition of a PPO. Some observers, however, use the term "PPA" to describe a less formal relationship than would be described by a PPO. The term "PPO" implies that an organization exists, whereas a PPA may achieve the same goals as a PPO through an informal arrangement between providers and payers. "PPA" is now largely archaic.

The key common characteristics of PPOs include the following:

- *Provider network.* PPOs typically establish a network by contracting with selected providers in a community to provide health services for covered individuals. Most PPOs contract directly with hospitals, physicians, and other diagnostic facilities. Providers can be selected to participate on the basis of their cost efficiency, community reputation, and scope of services. Some PPOs assemble massive databases of information about potential providers, including costs by diagnostic category, before they make their contracting decisions.

Negotiated payment rates. Most PPO participation agreements require participating providers to accept the PPO's payments as payment in full for covered services (except for applicable coinsurance or deductibles). PPOs attempt to negotiate payment rates that provide them with a competitive cost advantage relative to charge-based payment systems. These negotiated payment rates usually take the form of discounts from charges, fixed fee schedules, all-inclusive per diem rates, or payments based on diagnosis-related groups. Some PPOs have established bundled pricing arrangements for certain services, including obstetrical services, open-heart surgery, and some types of oncology.

Rapid payment terms. Some PPOs are willing to include prompt payment features in their contracts with participating providers in return for favorable payment rates. For example, a PPO may commit to pay all clean claims submitted by its providers within 15 days of submittal in return for a larger discount from charges.

Utilization management. Many PPOs implement utilization management programs to control the utilization and cost of health services provided to their covered beneficiaries. In the more sophisticated PPOs, these utilization management programs resemble the programs operated by HMOs.

Consumer choice. Unlike traditional HMOs, PPOs generally allow covered beneficiaries to use non-PPO providers instead of PPO providers when they need health services. Higher levels of beneficiary cost sharing, often in the form of higher copayments, typically are imposed when PPO beneficiaries use non-PPO providers.

Exclusive Provider Organizations

Exclusive provider organizations (EPOs) are similar to PPOs in their organization and purpose. Unlike PPOs, however, EPOs limit their beneficiaries to participating providers for any health care services. In other words, beneficiaries covered by an EPO are required to receive all their covered health care services from providers that participate in the EPO. The EPO generally does not cover services received from other providers, although there may be exceptions.

Some EPOs parallel HMOs in that they not only require exclusive use of the EPO provider network but also use a gatekeeper approach to authorizing non–primary care services. In these cases, the primary difference between an HMO and an EPO is that the former is regulated under HMO laws and regulations, whereas the latter is regulated under insurance laws and regulations or the Employee Retirement Income Security Act (ERISA; see Chapter 66) in the case of self-funded plans. Most state insurance departments have now eliminated the distinction between an HMO and an EPO, though the term may still be used in the marketplace, and in the case of an ERISA plan, the MCO can use any type of designation it wants since it is not subject to state insurance regulation.

EPOs usually are implemented by employers whose primary motivation is cost saving. These employers are less concerned about the reaction of their employees to severe restrictions on the choice of health care provider and offer the EPO as a replacement for traditional indemnity health insurance coverage. Because of the severe restrictions on provider choice, only a few large employers have been willing to convert their entire health benefits program to an EPO format. When EPOs originally surfaced as a form of health coverage, some observers predicted that they were the wave of the future and would be adopted by many large employers. In reality, some of those who established EPOs have abandoned them in favor of insurance vehicles that offer more choice to beneficiaries.

POS Plans

Primary Care PPOs

Primary care PPOs are hybrids of more traditional HMO and PPO models, though they are licensed as PPOs. The following are characteristics of these types of plans:

- Primary care physicians (PCPs) may be reimbursed through capitation payments (i.e., a fixed payment per member per month) or other performance-based reimbursement methods (see Chapters 8 and 10). In some states, capitating the PCP would require the plan to be licensed as an HMO (see below); in those cases, the PCP is paid under a fee-for-service system.
- There may be an amount withheld from physician compensation that is paid contingent upon achievement of utilization or cost targets. Some states restrict the ability of MCOs to establish withholds, and they have become less common over time.
- The PCP acts as a gatekeeper for referrals and institutional medical services.
- The member retains some coverage for services rendered that either are not authorized by the PCP or are delivered by nonparticipating providers. Such coverage is typically significantly lower than coverage for authorized services delivered by participating providers (e.g., 100 percent compared to 60 percent).

Traditional HMOs may offer similar benefit options through an out-of-plan benefits rider or POS option.

POS HMOs

Many HMOs have recognized that the major impediment to enrolling additional members and expanding market share has been the reluctance of individuals to forfeit completely their ability to receive reimbursement for using nonparticipating providers. These individuals consider the possibility that they would need the services of a renowned specialist for a rare (and expensive to treat) disorder and believe that the HMO would not refer them for care or reimburse their expenses. This possibility, no matter how unlikely, overshadows all the other benefits of HMO coverage in the minds of many individuals. It also has precluded most employers from limiting health benefit choice to a single HMO.

An expanding number of HMOs (and insurance carriers with both HMOs and indemnity operations) have adopted a solution to this problem: They provide some level of indemnity-type coverage for their members. HMO members covered under these types of benefit plans may decide whether to use HMO benefits or indemnity-style benefits for each instance of care. In other words, the member is allowed to make a coverage choice at the *point of service* when medical care is needed.

The indemnity coverage available under POS options from HMOs typically incorporates high deductibles and coinsurance to encourage members to use HMO services within network instead of out-of-plan services. Members who use the non-HMO benefit portion of the benefit plan may also be subject to utilization review (e.g., preadmission certification and continued stay review). Despite the availability of out-of-network benefits, studies have found that most POS plans experience between 65 percent and 85 percent in-network usage, thus retaining considerable cost control compared to indemnity-type plans.

As discussed in Chapter 42, this hybrid form of health benefit coverage represents an attractive managed care option for many employers and their covered employees, particularly when the employer is looking toward POS as a consolidation of existing indemnity coverage and multiple HMOs in the group (i.e., total replacement coverage). HMO POS plans had been the fastest-growing segment of health insurance until recently as a result of their attractive features. More recently, PPOs have regained popularity and have overtaken HMO-based products in enrollment growth.

HMO MODELS

HMOs are organized health care systems that are responsible for both the financing and the delivery of a broad range of comprehensive health services to an enrolled population. The original definition of an HMO also included the aspect of financing health care for a prepaid fixed fee (hence the term "prepaid health plan"), but prepaid fixed fees, though still common, are no longer used by all HMOs.

In many ways, an HMO can be viewed as a combination of a health insurer and a health care delivery management system. Whereas traditional health care insurance companies are responsible for reimbursing covered individuals for the cost of their health care, HMOs are responsible for providing or coordinating health care services for their covered members through affiliated providers who are reimbursed under various methods (see Chapters 8 through 12).

As a result of their responsibility for providing covered health services to their members, HMOs must ensure that their members have access to covered health care services. In addition, HMOs generally are responsible for ensuring the quality and appropriateness of the health services they provide to their members.

The commonly recognized models of HMOs are staff, group, network, IPA, and direct contract. An additional model is the open access plan, which has characteristics of an HMO and a PPO. The major differences between these models pertain to the relationship between the HMO and its participating physicians. At one time, individual HMOs could be neatly categorized into a single model type for descriptive purposes. Currently, many (if not most) HMOs have different relationships with different groups of physicians. As a result, many HMOs cannot easily be classified as a single model type, although such plans are occasionally referred to as mixed models. The HMO model type descriptions now may be more appropriately used to describe an HMO's relationship with certain segments of its physicians.

The following paragraphs provide brief descriptions of the five traditional HMO model types, followed by a brief description of the mixed model, the open access model, self-insured and experience-rated HMOs, and specialty HMOs.

Staff Model

In a staff model HMO, the physicians who serve the HMO's covered beneficiaries are employed by the HMO. These physicians typically are paid on a salary basis and may also receive bonus or incentive payments that are based on their performance and productivity. Staff model HMOs must employ physicians in all the most common specialties to provide for the health care needs of their members. These HMOs often contract with selected subspecialists in the community for infrequently needed health services.

Staff model HMOs are also known as closed-panel HMOs because most participating physicians are employees of the HMO and community physicians are unable to participate. There have been many well-known examples of staff model HMOs (e.g., Harvard-Pilgrim Health Plan, Group Health Association of Washington, D.C. [no longer in existence], FHP [no longer in existence]). In most cases, these plans "spun off" the physician component as a private medical group, though the group was initially subsidized by the HMO parent. The track record of these suddenly free-standing groups has not been good, and some of them are now gone. Those staff model HMOs that still exist are incorporating other types of physician relationships into their delivery system. And while insurance companies that dabbled in the creation of staff model systems (e.g., Aetna's Healthways) have abandoned them, there are still some IDSs that use a staff model approach (e.g., organizations in the Twin Cities).

Physicians in staff model HMOs usually practice in one or more centralized ambulatory care facilities. These facilities, which often resemble outpatient clinics, contain physician offices and ancillary support facilities (e.g., laboratory, radiology) to support the health care needs of the HMO's beneficiaries. Staff model HMOs usually contract with hospitals and other inpatient facilities in the community to provide nonphysician services for their members.

Staff model HMOs can have an advantage over other HMO models in managing health care delivery because they have a greater degree of control over the practice patterns of their physicians. As a result, it can be easier for staff model HMOs to manage and control the utilization of health services. They also offer the convenience of one-stop shopping for their members because the HMO's facilities tend to be full service (i.e., laboratory, radiology, and other departments are in the facilities).

Offsetting this advantage are several disadvantages of staff model HMOs. First, staff model HMOs are usually more costly to develop and implement because of the small membership and the large fixed salary expenses the HMO must incur for staff physicians and support staff. Second, staff model HMOs provide a limited choice of participating physicians from which potential HMO members may select. Many potential members are reluctant to change from their current physician and find the idea of a clinic setting uncomfortable. Third, many staff model HMOs have experienced productivity problems with their staff physicians, which has raised their costs for providing care. The former Group Health Association of Washington, D.C., was forced to sell itself to Humana and convert to a group model plan partially because of physician productivity concerns; eventually, Humana in turn sold its entire D.C. plan to Kaiser. Finally, it is expensive for staff model HMOs to expand their services into new areas because of the need to construct new ambulatory care facilities. These disadvantages have led to steadily eroding presence in the market, as depicted in Figure 3–3.

Group Model

In pure group model HMOs, the HMO contracts with a multispecialty physician group practice to provide all physician services to the HMO's members. The physicians in the group practice are employed by the group practice and not by the HMO. In some cases, these physicians may be allowed to see both HMO patients and other patients, although their primary function may be to treat HMO members.

Physicians in a group practice share facilities, equipment, medical records, and support staff. The group may contract with the HMO on an all-inclusive capitation basis to provide physician services to HMO members. Alternatively, the group may contract on a cost basis to provide its services, in which case it shares attributes of a staff model described above.

There are two broad categories of group model HMOs, the captive group and the independent group.

Captive Group

In the captive group model, the physician group practice exists solely to provide services

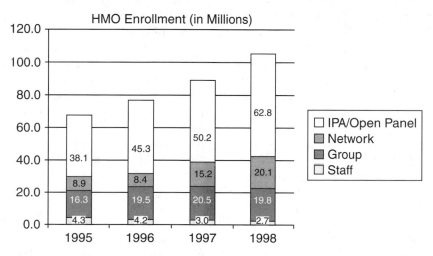

Figure 3–3 HMO Enrollment (in Millions). *Source:* Reprinted with permission from Hoechst Marion Roussel Managed Care Digest Series, *HMO-PPO Digest 1999,* © 1999 Hoechst Marion Roussel, SMG Marketing Group Inc.

to the HMO's beneficiaries. In most cases, the HMO formed the group practice to serve its members and recruited physicians and now provides administrative services to the group. The most prominent example of this type of HMO is the Kaiser Foundation Health Plan, where the Permanente Medical Groups provide all physician services for Kaiser's members. The Kaiser Foundation Health Plan, as the licensed HMO, is responsible for marketing the benefit plans, enrolling members, collecting premium payments, and performing other HMO functions. The Permanente Medical Groups are responsible for rendering physician services to Kaiser's members under an exclusive contractual relationship with Kaiser. Kaiser is sometimes mistakenly thought to be a staff model HMO because of the close relationship between itself and the Permanente Medical Groups.

Independent Group

In the independent group model HMO, the HMO contracts with an existing, independent multispecialty physician group to provide physician services to its members. In some cases, the independent physician group is the sponsor or owner of the HMO. An example of the independent group model HMO is Geisinger Health Plan of Danville, Pennsylvania. The Geisinger Clinic, which is a large, multispecialty physician group practice, is the independent group associated with the Geisinger Health Plan.

Typically, the physician group in an independent group model HMO continues to provide services to non-HMO patients while it participates in the HMO. Although the group may have an exclusive relationship with the HMO, this relationship usually does not prevent the group from engaging in non-HMO business. These types of group models may or may not also contract with other, independent physicians in the community in order to broaden the network for marketing reasons.

Common Features of Group Models

Both types of group model HMOs are also often referred to as "closed-panel HMOs" because physicians must be members of the group practice to participate in the HMO; as a result, the HMO is considered closed to physicians who are not part of the group. Both types of group model HMOs are like staff model HMOs in that it is somewhat easier to conduct utilization management because of the integration of physician practices and in that broad services are provided at the HMOs' facilities. In addition, group practice HMOs may have lower capital needs than staff model HMOs because the HMO itself does not have to support the large fixed salary costs associated with staff physicians.

Group model HMOs and staff model HMOs have many disadvantages in common. Like staff model HMOs, group model HMOs provide a limited choice of participating physicians from which potential HMO members can select. The limited physician panel can be a disadvantage in marketing the HMO. The limited number of office locations for the participating medical groups may also restrict the geographic accessibility of physicians for the HMO's members. The lack of accessibility can make it difficult for the HMO to market its coverage to a wide geographic area. Finally, certain group practices may be perceived by some potential HMO members as offering an undesirable clinic setting. Offsetting this disadvantage may be the perception of high quality associated with many of the physician group practices that are affiliated with HMOs.

As illustrated in Figure 3–3, group model HMOs have also suffered an erosion of market share during the last decade, but not to the same degree as have staff model plans. Kaiser Permanente has helped keep group model percentages up, but other group models (as of the time of publication) such as those operated by the Geisinger Clinic, the Marshfield Clinic, and the Carle Clinic also contribute.

Network Model

In network model HMOs, the HMO contracts with more than one group practice to provide physician services to the HMO's members. These group practices may be broad-based, multispecialty groups, in which case the HMO resembles the group practice model described above. An example of this type of HMO is Health Insurance Plan of Greater New York, which contracts with many multispecialty physician group practices in the New York area.

Alternatively, the HMO may contract with several small groups of PCPs, in which case the HMO can be classified as a primary care network model. In the primary care network model, the HMO contracts with several groups consisting of 7 to 15 PCPs representing the specialties of family practice and/or internal medicine, pediatrics, and obstetrics/gynecology to provide physician services to the HMO's members. Typically, the HMO compensates these groups on an all-inclusive physician capitation basis. The group is responsible for providing all physician services to the HMO's members assigned to the group and may refer to other physicians as necessary. The group is financially responsible for reimbursing other physicians for any referrals it makes. In some cases, the HMO may negotiate participation arrangements with specialist physicians to make it easier for its primary care groups to manage their referrals.

In contrast to the staff and group model HMOs described previously, network models may be either closed or open panel. If the network model HMO is a closed-panel plan, it will contract with only a limited number of existing group practices. If it is an open panel plan, participation in the group practices will be open to any physician who meets the HMO's and group's credentials criteria. In some cases, network model HMOs will assist independent PCPs with the formation of primary care groups for the sole purpose of participating in the HMO's network.

Network model HMOs address many of the disadvantages associated with staff and group model HMOs. In particular, the broader physician participation that is usually identified with network model HMOs helps overcome the marketing disadvantage associated with the closed-panel staff and group model plans. Nevertheless, network model HMOs usually have more limited physician participation than either IPA model or direct contract model plans.

IPA Model

IPA model HMOs contract with an association of physicians—the IPA—to provide physician services to their members. The physicians are members of the IPA, which is a separate legal entity, but they remain individual practitioners and retain their separate offices and identities (see also Chapter 4). IPA physicians continue to see their non-HMO patients and maintain their own offices, medical records, and support staff. IPA model HMOs are open-panel plans because participation is open to all community physicians who meet the HMO's and IPA's selection criteria.

Generally, IPAs attempt to recruit physicians from all specialties to participate in their plans. Broad participation of physicians allows the IPA to provide all necessary physician services through participating physicians and minimizes the need for IPA physicians to refer HMO members to nonparticipating physicians to obtain services. In addition, broad physician participation can help make the IPA model HMO more attractive to potential HMO members.

IPA model HMOs usually follow one of two different methods of establishing relationships with their IPAs. In the first method, the HMO contracts with an IPA that has been independently established by community physicians. These types of IPAs often have contracts with more than one HMO on a nonexclusive basis. In the second method, the HMO works with community physicians to create an IPA and to recruit physicians to participate in it. The HMO's contract with these types of IPAs is usually on an exclusive basis because of the HMO's leading role in forming the IPA.

IPAs may be formed as large communitywide entities where physicians can participate without regard to the hospital with which they are affiliated. Alternatively, IPAs may be hospital based and formed so that only physicians from one or two hospitals are eligible to participate in the IPA.

Hospital-based IPAs are sometimes preferred by HMOs over larger community-based IPAs for at least two reasons. First, hospital-based IPAs can restrict the panel of the IPA to physicians who are familiar with each other's practice patterns. This familiarity can make the utilization management process easier. Second, by using several hospital-based IPAs, an HMO can limit the impact of a termination of one of its IPA agreements to a smaller group of physicians.

Most HMOs compensate their IPAs on an all-inclusive physician capitation basis to provide services to the HMO's members. The IPA then compensates its participating physicians on either a fee-for-service basis or a combination of fee-for-service and primary care capitation. In the fee-for-service variation, IPAs pay all their participating physicians on the basis of a fee schedule or a usual, customary, or reasonable charge approach and withhold a portion of each payment for incentive and risk-sharing purposes.

Under the primary care capitation approach, IPAs pay their participating PCPs on a capitation basis and pay their specialist physicians on the basis of a fee schedule. The primary care capitation payments are based on fixed amounts per member per month and usually vary depending on the HMO member's age and sex. The IPA may withhold a portion of both the capitation and fee-for-service payments for risk-sharing and incentive purposes. Compensation for primary care is discussed in Chapter 8.

IPA model HMOs overcome the disadvantages associated with staff, group, and network model HMOs. They require less capital to establish and operate. In addition, they can provide a broad choice of participating physicians who practice in their private offices. As a result, IPA model HMOs offer marketing advantages that staff and group model plans do not.

There are two major disadvantages of IPA model HMOs from the HMO's perspective. First, the development of an IPA creates an organized forum for physicians to negotiate as a group with the HMO. The organized forum of an IPA can help its physician members achieve some of the negotiating benefits of belonging to a group practice. Unlike the situation with a group practice, however, individual members of an IPA retain their ability to negotiate and contract directly with managed care plans. Because of their acceptance of combined risk through capitation payments, IPAs are generally immune from antitrust restrictions on group activities by physicians as long as they do not prevent or prohibit their member physicians from participating directly with an HMO (see also Chapter 63).

Second, the process of utilization management can be more difficult in an IPA model HMO than it is in staff and group model plans because physicians remain individual practitioners with little sense of being a part of the HMO. As a result, IPA model HMOs may devote more administrative resources to managing inpatient and outpatient utilization than their staff and group model counterparts. Notwithstanding this historical disadvantage, recent analyses suggest that some IPA model HMOs have overcome the challenge and succeeded in managing utilization at least as well as their closed-panel counterparts.

Direct Contract Model

As the name implies, direct contract model HMOs contract directly with individual physicians to provide physician services to their members. With the exception of their direct contractual relationship with participating physicians, direct contract model HMOs are similar to IPA model plans and are included within the IPA classification for reporting purposes. At least at the time of publication, direct contract is the most common type of HMO model.

It is also common for this type of model to be referred to as an IPA, even though it is not legally an IPA. It is not the intent of this chapter, or this book, to proselytize purity of terminology. If individuals wish to refer to a direct contract model HMO as an IPA, that is their business. But the reader should be aware of the differences, since the presence or absence of an actual IPA has an effect on the HMO and its management needs.

Direct contract model HMOs attempt to recruit broad panels of community physicians to provide physician services as participating providers. These HMOs usually recruit both PCPs and specialist physicians and typically use a primary care case management approach (also known as a gatekeeper system).

Like IPA model plans, direct contract model HMOs compensate their physicians on either a fee-for-service basis or a primary care capitation basis. Primary care capitation is somewhat more commonly used by direct contract model HMOs because it helps limit the financial risk assumed by the HMO. Unlike IPA model HMOs, direct contract model HMOs retain most of the financial risk for providing physician services; IPA model plans transfer this risk to their IPAs.

Direct contract model HMOs have most of the same advantages as IPA model HMOs. In addition, direct model HMOs eliminate the potential of a physician bargaining unit by contracting directly with individual physicians. This contracting model reduces the possibility of mass termination of physician participation agreements.

Direct contract model HMOs have several disadvantages. First, the HMO may assume additional financial risk for physician services—more than in an IPA model HMO, as noted above. This additional risk exposure can be expensive if PCPs generate excessive referrals to specialist physicians.

Second, it can be more difficult and time-consuming for a direct contract model HMO to recruit physicians because it lacks the physician leadership inherent in an IPA model plan. It is more difficult for nonphysicians to recruit physicians, as several direct contract model HMOs discovered in their attempts to expand into new markets.

Finally, utilization management may be more difficult in direct contract model HMOs because all contact with physicians is on an individual basis and there may be little incentive for physicians to participate in the utilization management programs.

Mixed Model

Many HMOs or MCOs are actually mixes of different model types. It is far more common for closed-panel types of MCOs to add open-panel components to their health plan than the reverse, but there are examples of large open-panel HMOs adding a staff model component via a contract with an IDS, for example.

Over the years, the marketplace has caused a shift in the popularity of different types of HMOs. As illustrated in Figure 3–4, the movement has clearly been toward open-panel MCOs.

Open Access HMOs

An "open access HMO" does not use a PCP or gatekeeper approach to managing access and

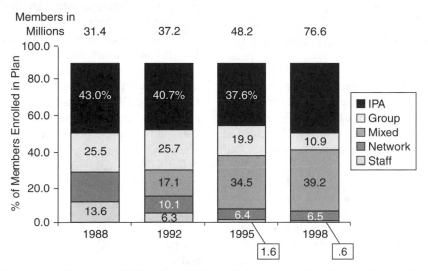

Figure 3–4 Preference Changes in HMOs. *Note:* POS enrollment is excluded. *Source:* Reprinted with permission from Interstudy 1991, 1993, 1997, 1998. © InterStudy Publications, Excelsior, Minnesota.

utilization. As discussed in Chapters 18, 19, and 23, there are clearly instances in any MCO where having a specialty physician manage a case is better than requiring a PCP to do so. But in an open access HMO, there is no requirement at all to go through a PCP to access a specialist. It is common for the copayment to be different (i.e., lower to see a PCP, higher to see a specialist), and there may be other mild economic incentives to use PCPs preferentially, but there is no requirement. In other words, there is a somewhat higher element of cost sharing with the member than exists in the typical HMO.

In this regard, open access HMOs bear some resemblance to PPOs, except that a PPO usually does not have different copayments or coinsurance for different specialty types. Open access plans also frequently put the physicians at some level of financial risk for medical costs, as discussed in Chapter 8. Lastly, these types of plans reportedly depend heavily on their ability to create meaningful physician practice profiles to allow medical managers to focus on problem areas (see Chapter 32).

Open access HMOs are not common as of the time of publication, and many have failed in the 1970s and 1980s. However, new ones appeared in the late 1990s, and it is not possible to tell at this time how successful they will be in managing cost and utilization.

Self-Insured and Experience-Rated HMOs

Historically, HMOs offered community-rated premiums to all employers and individuals who enrolled for HMO coverage. The federal HMO Act (no longer in force) originally mandated community rating for all HMOs that decided to pursue federal qualification. Many states had similar requirements.

Community rating was eventually expanded to include rating by class, where premium rates for an individual employer group could be adjusted prospectively on the basis of demographic characteristics that were associated with utilization differences. Such characteristics often included the age and sex distributions of the

employer's work force and the standard industrial classification of the employer.

Although community rating by class provided HMOs with some flexibility to offer more attractive rates to selected employer groups, many employers continued to believe that their group-specific experience would be better than the rates offered by HMOs. Some HMOs developed self-insured or experience-rated options in response to the needs expressed by these employers.

Under a typical self-insured benefit option, an HMO receives a fixed monthly payment to cover administrative services (and profit) and variable payments that are based on the actual or incurred expenses made by the HMO for health services. There is usually a settlement process at the end of a specified period, during which a final payment is calculated (either to the HMO by the group or to the group by the HMO). Variations in the payment arrangement exist and are similar in structure to the different forms of self-funded insurance programs.

Under experience-rated benefit options, an HMO receives monthly premium payments much as it would under traditional premium-based plans. There typically is a settlement process where the employer is credited with some portion (or all) of the actual utilization and cost of its group to arrive at a final premium rate. Refunds or additional payments are then calculated and made to the appropriate party.

The HMO regulations of some states preclude HMOs from offering self-insured or experience-rated benefit plans. HMOs avoid these prohibitions by incorporating related corporate entities that use the HMO's negotiated provider agreements, management systems, utilization protocols, and personnel to service the self-insured line of business.

Rating methodologies are discussed in detail in Chapters 49 through 52.

Specialty HMOs

Specialty HMOs have developed in some states to provide the benefits of the HMO model to limited components of health care coverage.

Dental (see Chapter 60) and vision care HMOs have become common as an option to provide coverage within these limited specialty areas. Specialty HMOs serving other health care needs (e.g., mental health; see Chapter 25) have also developed in certain states where they are permitted under the insurance or HMO laws and regulations. One challenge to the formation of such HMOs is that state laws usually specify a broad range of health services that are required to be offered by licensed HMOs.

CONCLUSION

Managed care is on a continuum, with a number of plan types offering an array of features that vary in their abilities to balance access to care, cost, quality control, benefit design, and flexibility. During the last 10 years, managed care has gone from being a relatively small part of the health care system synonymous with "alternative delivery system" to being the manner in which most employer-insured individuals obtain their care.

MCOs will continue to evolve, with features from one type of plan appearing in others and new features continually being developed. The march toward "bigger is better" in health insurance is likely to continue, which will blur the lines further. There is no one single definition of the term "managed care" that has endured in the past or will survive into the future.

REFERENCE

1. Americans Confused about Managed Care, Survey Finds. Employee Benefit Research Institute, press release #497, September 21, 1999.

CHAPTER 4

Integrated Health Care Delivery Systems

Peter R. Kongstvedt, David W. Plocher, and Jean C. Stanford

INTRODUCTION

The first hurdle one faces when discussing integrated delivery systems (IDSs) is how to define them. At the very least, an IDS involves more than one type of provider coming together in some type of legal structure to manage health care and, in most cases, to contract with payer organizations such as health maintenance organizations (HMOs), preferred provider organizations (PPOs), and health insurance companies. Beyond that, there is little agreement over what

---

David W. Plocher, MD, is a Partner in Ernst & Young's Health Care Consulting Practice and has 20 years of experience in the managed care field. His early areas of expertise include national point-of-service program administration and the development of the centers of excellence product known as "Institutes of Quality." More recently, he has designed and implemented integrated delivery systems and advanced care management programs including demand and disease management. In addition, he has worked on quality audits and accreditation with both the Joint Commission for Accreditation of Healthcare Organizations and the National Committee for Quality Assurance.

Jean C. Stanford is the associate director of health care consulting at Ernst & Young in Washington, DC. She is a specialist in health care delivery markets and how they are evolving across the United States. She was the technical lead for the development of the spider model for the analysis of health care markets, for internal IDS analysis, for governance, and for physician integration. Previously, Ms. Stanford worked for IBM and a number of health care organizations, including the George Washington University Medical Center.

constitutes an IDS. This chapter will discuss the most common types of IDSs.

The concept of integrated health care delivery is neither new nor novel. Kaiser Permanente Health Plans, Group Health of Puget Sound, the Henry Ford Health System, and other organizations have operated as IDSs (albeit as HMOs rather than as providers) for many years, in some cases for more than half a century. Even before managed care came to play as dominant a role as it does today, an increase in vertical integration was predicted by Paul Starr in 1982 in *The Social Transformation of American Medicine*, though he predicted a form of care somewhat different from what is currently prevalent.[1]

The health care marketplace is continuing to evolve, but it is not clear at all that there is any consensus on the "right" way to configure health care services in the current market environment. Some IDSs have succeeded, but many others have either languished or failed altogether. In particular, many observers believe that many IDSs have not succeeded in meeting their original goal: improved efficiency in managing health care delivery. This leaves some health care executives at a loss; there is no bandwagon to jump onto, no "safe" way to organize. After the frenzied merger and acquisition activities of the last few years, IDS boards in particular are not sure which road to take.

There are many types of organizations that may be called IDSs, and the differences between them are neither clear nor stable: There are physician-hospital organizations (PHOs), indepen-

42

dent practice associations (IPAs), management services organizations (MSOs), provider-sponsored organizations (PSOs), physician practice management companies (PPMCs), and others. The managed care industry involves so many types of organizations, with so many different acronyms, and many with vague or overlapping definitions (see also the Glossary for a mind-numbing excursion through acronym land).

Unlike managed care organizations (MCOs) such as health insurance companies, HMOs, or PPOs where size does matter, IDSs have not always found that bigger is better. Large IDSs may have more leverage in negotiations but have not proven more efficient or easier to manage. And despite much pontificating by pundits about the virtues of various forms of IDSs, it is not clear that there is any superior form of IDS.

According to a survey published by Jantzen and Loubeau, "Managed care's presence was the only significant factor moving hospitals from a standalone status to network membership. The decision to share financial risk was influenced not only by managed care pressures, but also by the level of local hospital competition and the severity of the inpatient case mix."[2(p.83)] Hospitals have continued to combine, but it is not clear that these combinations are working as well as expected. The volume of mergers and acquisitions among hospitals is also falling as of the time of publication. This may be because the most desirable entities have merged or been acquired already; there may be slim pickings for the rest. In fact, there are a number of instances where health system mergers have been called off or even undone.

As to the general low level of success of IDSs, Burns et al. state:

> There are several reasons why the benefits of IDSs may not be readily or soon observed. First, only 25 percent to 50 percent of U.S. hospitals have any type of organizational vehicle to promote integration with their physicians. Second, most of these vehicles are small scale (e.g., few managed care contracts), recently established,

or both. Third, the most prevalent IDS vehicle (the PHO) is designed primarily for managed care contracting but lacks any developed managerial infrastructure. Fourth, in the health care systems that have aggressively pursued integration, most of the gains to date have been on the administrative side, with fewer achievements in the integration of physicians or clinical activities.[3(p.70)]

And a particular form of IDS, the PSO, enabled by federal legislation in the Balanced Budget Act of 1997 (BBA) has not proven to be popular or particularly successful.

Yet all IDSs have not been abject failures. Clearly, many IDSs have met their market objectives. Certain attributes that increase the likelihood of success are discussed in this chapter.

The arena of regulation and oversight is highly complex. The following chapters offer further discussions on regulation, financial and solvency issues, and legal issues: 48, 55, 62–65, 68, and 69. In addition, Chapters 36, 45, 46, 49, 51, and 53 discuss operational issues specific to IDSs.

HIGHLY INTEGRATED DELIVERY SYSTEMS

In a largely successful attempt to define what constitutes a highly integrated IDS,* the SMG Marketing Group and Hoechst Marion Roussel have stated that in order to be considered highly integrated:

> These systems must either own or contract with three or more components of health care delivery, including at least one acute care hospital, at least one physician component (e.g., PHO, IPA, PPMC, or physician practice) and at least one other component (e.g., HMO, nursing home, home health agency, or surgery center). They must also have at

---

*Please excuse the apparent redundancy in this sentence; you know what we mean.

least one systemwide contract with a payer.[4]

Based on this definition, Hoechst Marion Roussel and SMG Marketing Group determined that there were 266 highly integrated IDSs as of 1998 and that the number of such systems has been steadily increasing (see Tables 4–1 and 4–2). If one takes a less structured view of what constitutes an IDS (e.g., physician-only systems as described later in this chapter, or PHOs without any other component), then the number increases, but to what extent it increases is unknown.

MARKET CHARACTERISTICS

Heavily Penetrated Markets

Heavily penetrated markets (i.e., markets in which HMO or point-of-service [POS] plan enrollment is 25 percent or more of the total population) are often dominated by a few health plans. Entry by new plans is difficult, although possible. Likewise, the IDSs in a heavily penetrated market have usually undergone major consolidations. It is remarkable to look across the heavily penetrated markets and watch the back-and-forth balancing of power between the IDSs and MCOs. When one gains greater negotiating strength, the other takes whatever actions necessary to regain the balance of power. Sifferman et al. of Moody's Investors Service say that "To counteract the increasing influence of managed care payers, many health care deliv-

Table 4–1 Components of 266 Highly Integrated IDSs

Component	Number of IDSs with Component
Acute care hospital	All
Physician component (e.g., PHO, IPA, MSO, PPMC, staff physicians)	All
Home health agency	220
Nursing home	144
HMO/PPO	128
Outpatient surgery center	115

Note: To be considered a highly integrated IDS, the IDS must have the first two components and at least one of the others.

Source: Reprinted with permission from Hoechst Marion Roussel Managed Care Digest Series, *Integrated Health Systems Digest,* 1999; © 1999 Hoechst Marion Roussel, and SMG Marketing Group Inc.

ery systems will continue to merge and grow rather rapidly."[5(p.2)]

Underpenetrated Markets

Underpenetrated markets (i.e., markets with less than 20 percent HMO and POS enrollment) have relatively limited experience with advanced managed care activities. In such markets, there is a much greater impetus to consider creative options by both MCOs and IDSs. Partnering with providers may fast-track an

Table 4–2 Number of Components in Highly Integrated IDSs

Number of Components	Year			
	1995	1996	1997	1998
3	35	44	42	57
4	60	66	87	106
5	47	57	70	71
More than 6	17	22	29	32
Total	159	189	228	266

Source: Reprinted with permission from Hoechst Marion Roussel Managed Care Digest Series, *Integrated Health Systems Digest,* 1999; © 1999 Hoechst Marion Roussel, and SMG Marketing Group Inc.

MCO's market entry ahead of its competitors. However, in today's environment, it is not safe to assume that markets will inevitably convert to traditional managed care. They might instead convert to PPOs or another, as yet undefined, hybrid system. So it would not be wise to bet the farm on one payer model.

TYPES OF IDSs

As noted earlier, it is quite difficult to define and categorize types of IDSs. That is the task at hand, however, and it will be the focus of this section. The taxonomy presented below is that in general use at the time of publication. It is expected that, because this is an area in continual evolution (as is managed care in general), these terms and definitions will not remain constant. Even if the nomenclature changes, however, many of the concepts discussed here will remain valid.

IDSs may be described as falling into three broad categories: systems in which only the physicians are integrated, systems in which the physicians are integrated with facilities (hospitals and ancillary sites), and systems that include the insurance functions. Within the context of the first two categories, IDSs fall along a rough continuum of increasing degree of integration and potential ability of the organization to operate effectively in a managed care environment. Also, the complexity of formation and operation, required capital investment, and political difficulties increase from one end of the continuum to the other. The primary political difficulty encountered in the development of these systems, or at least the systems that are tightly managed, is that not all providers can participate. This can present a significant challenge for both hospital and physician leadership that, if not addressed deftly, can result in a career-limiting move by the responsible executive.

For most IDSs, the motivation for forming various physician integration organizations in the last decade has been the recognition that some mechanism was needed to align the economic incentives of providers with that of the hospitals if they were to succeed in joint contracting with MCOs. The various physician or-ganizations developed many ways to compensate physicians, from discounted fee-for-service systems, to capitation, to withholds, to case rates. According to Alexander et al., the evolving physician-hospital organizational structures differ from the faculty practice model or employed physician model in the following ways:

- formal, contract-based structure
- corporate character
- include physicians who are outside of the hospital's paid medical staff[6]

Note that some IDSs offer a variety of integration vehicles (e.g., IPA, PHO, MSO) to physicians in their communities. This allows the physician to gradually become more integrated with the IDS without feeling roped into a too-restrictive relationship too quickly.[7]

IPAs

IPAs, a form of IDS, have existed for several decades and were codified to some degree by the original HMO Act of 1973. The IPA is a legal entity whose members are independent physicians who contract with the IPA for the primary purpose of having the IPA contract with one or more HMOs. IPAs are usually not for profit, although that is not an absolute requirement. The term "IPA" is often used synonymously (and inaccurately) with terms for any type of open-panel HMO (see Chapter 3); although this use of "IPA" is now widespread, it is not technically accurate. The true IPA is discussed here.

According to a study by the Managed Care Information Center, some 130,000 physicians were members of IPAs in 1998. California has the highest physician-owned IPA penetration, with 61 IPAs, followed by Texas with 25, Illinois with 24, New Jersey at 18, and Massachusetts with 17.[8]

In its common incarnation, the IPA negotiates with the HMO for a capitation rate inclusive of all physician services (for detailed discussions of such forms of reimbursement systems, see Chapters 8 through 12). The IPA in turn reimburses the member physicians, although not necessarily using capitation. The IPA and its member physicians are at risk for at least some portion of medical costs in that if the capitation payment is lower than the required reimbursement to the physicians, the member physicians must accept lower income. It is the presence of this risk sharing that stands the IPA apart from a negotiating vehicle that does not bear risk. It is also the reason that true IPAs generally are not subject to antitrust problems (unless the IPA was formed solely or primarily to keep out competition; see also Chapter 63). Usually, an IPA is an umbrella organization for physicians in all specialties to participate in managed care. Recently, however, IPAs that represent only a single specialty have emerged; specialty IPAs and PPMCs are also discussed in Chapter 11.

The IPA may operate simply as a negotiating organization, with the HMO providing all administrative support, or it may take on some of the HMO's duties, such as utilization management (UM), network development, and so forth. Large, mature IPAs and some others may also adjudicate claims. The IPA generally has stop-loss reinsurance, or the HMO provides such stop-loss coverage, to prevent the IPA from going bankrupt (see Chapters 8 and 53).

The history of IPAs in the early years of HMOs was variable, and a number of IPAs did indeed go out of business. The hospital usually has no role in a traditional IPA, although some hospitals have begun sponsoring IPA development as an alternative to a PHO structure (discussed below).

Advantages of an IPA

The first advantage of an IPA is in the marketplace: IPAs generally offer a broad choice of physicians to enrolled members. There is also a current, although undocumented, resurgence of interest in IPAs as a vehicle for private physicians to contract with managed care plans. IPAs stop well short of full integration but have more ability to share risk and obtain HMO contracts than many PHOs. IPAs are more easily understood and accepted by many managed care executives than less traditional models. The newly dominating IPAs are those that allow more convenient geographic access, have succeeded in bearing risk, and have limited specialist membership. They may be the only model available

in nonurban areas, where one- to two-physician offices are the norm. Finally, in contrast to other models, IPAs require much less capital to start up and operate, and some managers feel that IPAs motivate their physicians more successfully than models that depend on salary.

Other factors that may lead to expansions of IPAs are the trend to have open referrals within a network (ending the gatekeeper model). Some plans are willing to allow patients to self-refer within an IPA. They see the gatekeeper as a transitional device. Now that specialists are accustomed to managed care, they can control costs effectively in an IPA environment with aligned incentives. "Specialists have become more and more diversified in the kinds of patients they see," says Henry Loubet. "Practice patterns have changed. Specialists don't require the oversight they once did. In fact, the difference between our HMO and our PPO in bed days per thousand has gone from 40 or 50 percent five years ago to 10 to 20 percent today."[9(p.17)]

As discussed below, since PPMCs are deconstructing and hospital systems are shedding physician practices, IPAs may become refuges for physicians who need a contracting vehicle for negotiating with MCOs.

Disadvantages of an IPA

The IPA is inherently unwieldy because it is usually made up of a large number of independent physicians who have only the contracting vehicle of the IPA in common. While IPAs help to preserve private practice, they are unable to leverage resources, achieve economies of scale, or change behavior to the greatest degree possible. Many IPAs contain a surplus of specialists, resulting in upward pressure on characteristic resource consumption.

An IPA that accepts a high degree of risk for medical costs will likely be subject to risk-based capital requirements (see Chapters 49, 51, and 69) or may be found by the state insurance commissioner to be an HMO and be required to become licensed, with all the issues that go along with being a licensed health plan (see Chapter 69). In many states, IPAs that bear considerable financial risk for medical costs are required to obtain a limited form of license that allows them to accept that risk but also creates more of a regulatory and oversight framework.

Finally, as one article put it:

> Physicians in IPA/network HMOs face maddening complexity. In California, they typically contract with fifteen different managed care plans, each of which may establish its own referral requirements and employ formularies not developed by the treating physicians. This makes it impossible to master all of the rules and procedures that apply. Physicians in IPA/network HMOs typically face more interference in medical decision making from utilization managers than do physicians in group models such as Kaiser Permanente, who monitor their own utilization. Physicians deal with IPA/network insurers at arm's length, if not as adversaries.[10(p.95)]

PPMCs

PPMCs arrived on the integration scene in the mid-1990s. PPMCs may in some ways be viewed as variants of MSOs, but unlike MSOs, PPMCs are physicians only. In other words, there is no involvement by the hospital. Some managed care taxonomists refer to these organizations as physician-only MSOs, but that convention is not the predominant one as this chapter is being written. The operations of a full MSO are described later in this chapter.

Most major PPMCs have failed, either going through bankruptcy or exiting the business altogether. Tom Ducro, vice president of administration for the Cincinnati multispecialty practice Group Health Associates, says that "independence may be the route that more physician groups take, as national firms and hospitals discover that consolidation won't necessarily turn them into big-money generators. Within a practice, most of the profits go into compensation. After you take out compensation, staff and overhead, there's really not a lot left—the margins aren't there."[11 (p.1)]

For-Profit, Comprehensive PPMCs

Private or proprietary PPMCs were also acquiring physician practices throughout the mid-to-late 1990s. Usually organized on a for-profit basis, these PPMCs planned to achieve more efficient management and economies of scale, thereby producing a profit while maintaining physician income. These PPMCs, like hospitals, saw practice acquisitions as giving them a stronger negotiating position with MCOs, at least when the company represented a substantial part of the physician marketplace in an area. Many PPMCs were also seeking capitation contracts, but in general they desired to cut out the hospital from any profit and control.

In a melding of Wall Street and the physician's office, entrepreneurs have capitalized for-profit PPMCs operating independent of hospitals. These have most often purchased physician practices, beginning with primary care groups but including certain large specialty groups as well, and have signed multiyear contracts with those physicians. The physicians are given varying degrees of equity participation in the PPMC (the equity model PPMC) and a voice in governance. In some cases, the PPMC may not necessarily offer equity to all physicians. The PPMC may offer equity only to those physicians who are early participants, or it may offer equity in exchange for the value of the acquired practice but not offer equity if it pays cash for the practice.

In general, the PPMC provides management for all support functions (e.g., billing and collections, purchasing, negotiating contracts) but remains relatively uninvolved with the clinical aspects of the practice. In many cases, the physician remains an independent practitioner, although the PPMC owns all the tangible assets of the practice. The PPMC usually takes a percentage of the practice revenue, often at a rate equal to or slightly below the physician's previous overhead. The physician agrees to a long-term commitment as well as noncompete covenants.

These entities attracted some practitioners who, exasperated by the business pressures of practice, preferred selling to an entity specializing in managing physician practices rather than a hospital because he or she did not trust the hospital or did not feel it was capable of managing a practice. Unfortunately, in most cases, these physicians have been disappointed with the PPMC's lack of management expertise and with being treated like an employee, with all the motivational concerns that can go along with it.

PPMCs have fallen to ruin in large numbers. The most prominent failure was FPA, which flew high in the stock market but then had to file for bankruptcy in 1998. Many other prominent PPMCs (e.g., MedPartners, Coastal) followed suit, either going into bankruptcy or simply exiting the business after massive losses. These failures meant trouble for investors. In addition, most of the MCOs that had global risk contracts with PPMCs were forced to make good on payments to providers that the PPMC failed to make, despite having received capitation payments. Physicians were left without practice support or even offices and staff in many cases. Hospitals and MCOs rushed to provide that support and prevent the PPMC failures from affecting members, but the situation was chaotic and discouraging.

Despite the terrible track record of PPMCs, it is not easy to articulate clear advantages and disadvantages of PPMCs. Compared with hospitals and insurers acquiring practices, the PPMC is theoretically able to be more nimble and is better able to give physicians an investment return. There are also examples of PPMCs that are doing well, so it is not appropriate to dismiss the concept out of hand. But there is no escaping the vision of PPMCs rocketing up into the financial stratosphere, only to come hurtling back to earth, leaving deep, smoking craters.

Physicians themselves are showing little interest in getting back into the physician practice management business: "Physician practice management companies and hospitals are putting practice assets on the selling block, and the price for physician groups is dropping precipitously—more than 90% over two years, in one case. Still, doctors appear reluctant to open their wallets . . . negotiators say it's easier to get physicians to agree to be sold to an outside party than to invest their own money in buying practice assets."[12(p.62)] It can be done, though. Twenty-one physicians

at Axminister Medical Group in Los Angeles, California, were acquired by FPA Medical Management for $16.2 million in stock in 1997.* They reacquired their practice in December 1998 for $1.35 million—a 92 percent discount off the 1997 price.[13]

Specialty PPMCs

A variation on the comprehensive PPMC theme, the specialty PPMC has taken most of the comprehensive PPMC features into consideration for a single specialty's market share preservation or expansion. The most common specialties involved are oncology, cardiology, nephrology, and endocrinology (focused almost exclusively on diabetes as a function of disease management—see Chapter 23); multistate networks are now in place. Other specialties frequently involved include ophthalmology, radiology, anesthesiology, and occupational medicine. The specialty PPMC is a variant of a specialty network, which is also discussed in Chapter 11.

The early experience with this PPMC variant is somewhat better than the experience with the comprehensive PPMCs. Success will be sustained, however, only if two conditions exist: the PPMCs are able to bear financial risk, and the PPMCs' customers are willing to deal with another carve-out vendor. Although the first condition is a managed care fundamental, the second may need clarification. The emergence of disease management vendors is a valuable model. The vendors that are concentrating narrowly on rare, expensive diseases, such as hemophilia, have made some inroads. The typical HMO medical director may be willing to carve that out and devote internal case manager skill to more common specialties (e.g., oncology, orthopaedics). (Note that disease management vendors—those specializing in hemophilia, for instance—usually do not employ their own hemophilia experts but rather contract with them and provide more customized care manage-

*Of course, it did not take long for the $16.2 million in FPA stock to become wallpaper, but it is likely that the group received other financial benefits along the way.

ment.) The potential ability of a specialty PPMC that is not highly focused on a single disease to survive is enhanced by the presence of a less aggressive buyer, such as a PPO. Alternatively, if the specialty PPMC happens to have its network in place in a given city before the HMO provider relations manager begins recruiting specialists, this specialty PPMC could become the dedicated specialist network for the HMO. Finally, an HMO may choose to use such a specialty PPMC because it allows the HMO to improve quality and lower cost compared with using a less organized network of private specialists.

Advantages of a PPMC

The primary advantage of a PPMC is that its sole purpose in business is to manage physicians' practices. This means that it will either have or obtain expertise that is not usually resident in either a hospital or a payer (other than a group or staff model HMO). Also, the PPMC has the ability to bring substantial purchasing power to bear though combining the purchasing needs of several hundred (or potentially more) physicians. The PPMC can also provide a greater sense of ownership to the participating physicians in an equity model, thus helping align incentives and goals. A specialty PPMC has more potential advantages since it is able to be more focused and more able to concentrate management on specific diseases or clinical care.

As noted earlier, the advantages of PPMCs have proven less than compelling.

Disadvantages of a PPMC

PPMCs have been crippled by their track record of failure. The impressive loss of wealth associated with PPMC failures has created an atmosphere of distrust, and that makes it harder for a PPMC to grow and to obtain contracts with MCOs.

Another disadvantage is that the PPMC may not achieve sufficient mass in the market to influence events substantially or to negotiate favorable terms. Also, the physicians may chafe under the long terms usually required and may not change their practice habits sufficiently to be truly effec-

tive in managed care; this last issue becomes especially critical if the PPMC is seen more as a vehicle to negotiate fees than as a system to lower costs and improve quality. These PPMCs often lack strong physician leadership; business leadership comes from nonphysicians who may be more talented at attracting investor financing than running physician practices. Finally, investor-owned PPMCs are businesses that are expected to return a substantial profit; they are not philanthropic institutions. Investors seeking profit demand action, some of which may not be palatable to the participating physicians.

These disadvantages and others have resulted in the failures described above.

Group Practices without Walls

The group practice without walls (GPWW), also known as the clinic without walls, is a step toward greater integration of physician services. The GPWW does not require the participation of a hospital and, indeed, is often formed as a vehicle for physicians to organize without being dependent on a hospital for services or support. In some cases, GPWW formation has occurred to leverage negotiating strength not only with MCOs but with hospitals as well.

The GPWW is composed of private practice physicians who agree to aggregate their practices into a single legal entity, but the physicians continue to practice medicine in their independent locations. In other words, the physicians appear to patients to be independent, but to a contracting entity (usually an MCO) they are a single group. This is differentiated from the for-profit, physician-only MSOs described later by two salient features: first, the GPWW is owned solely by the member physicians and not by any outside investors, and second, the GPWW is a legal merging of all assets of the physicians' practices rather than the acquisition of only the tangible assets (as is often the case in an MSO).

To be considered a medical group, the physicians must have their personal income affected by the performance of the group as a whole. An IPA will place a defined portion of a physician's income at risk (that portion related to the managed care contract held by the IPA), and the group's income from any source has an effect on the physician's income and on profit sharing in the group. But in IPAs, an individual physician's income is likely to be affected most by individual productivity.

The GPWW is owned by the member physicians, and governance is by the physicians. The GPWW may contract with an outside organization to provide business support services. Office support services are generally provided through the group, although as a practical matter the practicing physicians may notice little difference in what they are used to receiving.

Advantages of a GPWW

The GPWW enjoys an advantage over some other models in that it has the legal ability to negotiate and commit on behalf of all the members of the group. Unlike a PHO, where the physicians remain independent private practitioners, the GPWW is a legal group and can legitimately bargain with MCOs or other organizations. The GPWW also has the ability to achieve some modest economies of scale, similar to those found in MSOs. The most common subset of these services includes centralized billing, centralized scheduling, group purchasing, and data sharing. Less often, the GPWW centralizes recruiting and can help with employee leasing. The GPWW is free of hospital influence (at least theoretically) and therefore has greater flexibility.

Perhaps the key advantage of the GPWW is that income is affected by the performance of the group as a whole. Therefore, the GPWW has some ability to influence practice behavior. If a member physician's practice patterns adversely affect the group, considerable peer pressure can be brought to bear. The group can even expel a physician member if the problems are serious and are not rectified.

Disadvantages of a GPWW

The primary disadvantage of the GPWW is that the physicians essentially remain in independent practice. The physicians generally continue to practice in the manner to which they have become accustomed. The ability of the

group to manage practice behavior is thus seriously limited to only those elements that are gross outliers (e.g., exceptionally long lengths of stay). Thus, optimal efficiencies are not achieved. Although there is some alignment of incentives, disparate goals still exist.

The ability of a GPWW to accept risk-based reimbursement (e.g., capitation) is enhanced but is not optimal. The GPWW is potentially capable of negotiating with MCOs for such contracts, but distribution of income and risk usually defaults to those methods used by IPAs (see also Chapters 8 and 9). If this issue is not addressed properly, regulatory authorities (including Medicare) may determine that the GPWW is simply a front and does not represent a true medical group. Penalties usually follow such a determination.

The very feature that attracts many physicians, independence from a distrusted hospital, is also a source of GPWW weakness. That is, new sources of capital, information systems, and management expertise must be explored (e.g., an insurance partner, an MSO).

Finally, the GPWW structure generally does not have as strong a leadership as is seen in a true medical group. This, along with the other disadvantages noted, may lead to a relative instability in the structure. Some managers in the industry believe that the GPWW concept is part of a transition to a more traditional medical group. Furthermore, although sharing of certain administrative services represents an improvement in overhead, there are many more economies of scale to be found in a true, or consolidated, medical group practice.

The GPWW is a model that has not become common, much less dominant.

CONSOLIDATED MEDICAL GROUPS

A consolidated medical group, or medical group practice, is a traditional structure in which physicians have combined their resources to be a true medical group practice. Unlike the GPWW, in which the physicians combine certain assets and risks but remain in their own offices, practicing medicine as they always have, the true medical group is located in a few sites and functions in a group setting; in other words, the physicians occupy the same facility or facilities. This means that there is a great deal of interaction among members of the group and common goals and objectives for group success.

Traditional medical groups are totally independent of hospitals. Even so, it is common for groups to identify strongly with one or more hospitals. Although this is good for the hospital as long as relations are good, it can be devastating to a hospital if relations sour or if the group changes hospitals for any reason. Some hospitals sponsor medical groups, but those operate more like other models discussed later in this chapter.

The group is usually a partnership or professional corporation, although other forms (e.g., a limited liability partnership) are possible. Usually the more senior members of the group enjoy more fruits of the group's success (e.g., higher income, better on-call schedules, and so forth), although one hopes not to an abusive degree. New members of an existing group who pass a probationary period often are required to pay a substantial contribution to the group's capital to join, which can create an entry barrier to growth. Other groups employ new physicians for a lengthy period to control the finances of the group as well as to give all parties the opportunity to see whether the new physicians fit in. In any event, it is common for the group to require physicians to agree to a noncompete clause in their contract to protect the group from having a physician defect and take patients away from the group. A discussion of the general management of medical groups is beyond the scope of this chapter. Physician compensation in such groups is discussed in Chapter 9.

Advantages of a Medical Group

Medical groups are able to achieve substantial economics of scale, to influence physician behavior, and to have good leverage in negotiations. Groups are usually attractive to MCOs because they not only deliver a large block of physicians with one contract but also have the ability to manage their own resources. The group can also decide to make a change (e.g., change hospitals) that can have a rapid and substantial positive effect on managed care.

Although the capital investment required of partners or group shareholders can be an entry barrier, it is also an exit barrier. An additional exit barrier is the noncompete clause required of member physicians. Both of these exit barriers promote stability, which appeals to MCOs. Medical groups are often able to recruit new physicians relatively easily because they offer immediate cash income (critical for a new physician faced with heavy educational debt) and a better lifestyle than solo practice offers at first. On the whole, when working with managed care, physicians in medical groups are better off than physicians in other arrangements and independent private practices.

Disadvantages of a Medical Group

Medical groups can certainly have serious problems, such as uncontrolled overhead or poor utilization patterns. If these problems are not rectified, the impact of failure is much bigger than it is when an independent physician or small group fails. If the group has markedly disproportionate compensation or lifestyle differences between the senior members and the new physicians, the turnover of new members can be unacceptably high. Medical groups can also inflate their own opinions of their worth, impeding effective contracting.

Medical groups can become calcified in their ways and be less able to change than individual physicians. This is a serious problem if compounded by the group being top heavy with subspecialists and, in turn, treating primary care physicians (PCPs) as second-class members. If the group is unwilling to consider redistributing the rewards to the PCPs, it may suffer defections of those physicians, which will make the group less desirable from a managed care standpoint.

Another potential disadvantage of group practices is that they may not have the time, inclination, or capital resources to really understand their costs of delivering care. As they sign contracts with MCOs, they may be negotiating themselves into a fiscal hole without even being aware of it. This seems to be what happened in California and it can certainly happen elsewhere.

Physician practices were purchasing and merging with other practices in order to gain market share, provide for increased coverage of clinical conditions and backup (e.g., on-call responsibilities). More important from a managed care standpoint, large groups, especially primary care groups or multispecialty groups with strong primary care, are expected to have an increased negotiating strength and a greater ability to accept risk. A prominent example of a large group of this kind, Brown and Toland of California, recently gave up its Knox-Keene license, which allowed it to take full risk for hospitalization as well as physician fees. Management decided that it simply was not practical to manage full risk themselves.[14]

California leads the way in the movement to capitate physician groups for medical services (20 million covered lives) and in managing physician group bankruptcies (115 bankruptcies since 1996). A 1999 report from the California Medical Association states that "even as the cost of living and health-care costs rose steadily throughout the 1990s, the amount of money paid by health plans to physician groups to take care of patients dropped, from a high of $45 per patient each month in the period from 1990 to 1993 to a low of $29 from 1997 to 1999."[15(p.A-1)] If these numbers are accurate, then it is not surprising that many California medical groups are now in financial difficulty.

PHOs

The PHO is an entity that, at a minimum, allows a hospital and its physicians to negotiate with third-party payers. PHOs may do little more than provide for such a negotiating vehicle, although this could raise the risk of antitrust. PHOs may actively manage the relationship between the providers and MCOs, or they may provide more services, to the point where they may more aptly be considered MSOs (see below).

PHOs often form as a reaction to market forces from managed care. PHOs are considered the easiest type of vertically integrated system to develop (although they are not actually that easy, at least if done well). They also are a vehicle to provide some integration while preserving the independence and autonomy of the physicians.

PHOs had been considered necessary vehicles for hospitals and physicians to band together to extract the best possible contracting terms from MCOs. However, research by Kaufman "showed no correlation between a hospital's physician integration strategy and its payments under managed care. There is, however, a high correlation between a hospital's payments under managed care and its institutional market position. Dominant hospital systems got paid better than marginal hospitals regardless of whether they had a PHO."[16(p.78)]

It is important to consider the market's phase of managed care development when putting together a PHO. For example, a group of physicians in one location put together a PHO on the premise that local HMOs would capitate them in return for administrative efficiencies and better care management. But they found that most HMOs in their area felt that they had the necessary administrative and quality systems in place already and thus did not need help from the PHO.[17]

By definition, a PHO requires the participation of a hospital and at least some portion of the admitting physicians. Often, the formation of the PHO is initiated by the hospital, but unless the leadership of the medical staff is also on board it is unlikely to get far. It is not uncommon for a PHO to be formed primarily as a defensive mechanism to deal with an increase in managed care contracting activity. It is also not uncommon for the same physicians who join the PHO already to be under contract with one or more managed care plans.

In its weakest form, the PHO is considered a messenger model. This means that the PHO analyzes the terms and conditions offered by an MCO and transmits its analysis and the contract to each physician, who then decides on an individual basis whether to participate.

In the simplest and more common version of a PHO, the participating physicians and the hospital develop model contract terms and reimbursement levels and use those terms to negotiate with MCOs. The PHO usually has a limited amount of time (e.g., 90 days) to negotiate the contract successfully. If that time limit passes, then the participating physicians are free to contract directly with the MCO; if the PHO successfully reaches an agreement with the MCO, then the physicians agree to be bound by those terms. The contract is still between the physician and the MCO and between the hospital and the MCO. In some cases, the contract between the physicians and the MCO is relatively brief and may reference a contract between the PHO and the MCO.

The PHO is usually a separate business entity, such as a for-profit corporation. This requires thorough legal analysis for the participating not-for-profit, tax-exempt (Internal Revenue Code 501c [3]) hospital because the hospital could lose its tax-exempt status if access to tax-exempt financing confers an advantage to the PHO's balance sheet (see Chapters 48 and 65).

Initial capitalization and ownership arrangements vary, but most strive to give the physicians and the hospital equal ownership. The hospital may put up the majority of the cash, however. Physician equity is thought to increase practitioner motivation. A large physician equity position also has a dangerous side, however. In the event of a capital call (not an uncommon event) for purposes of covering losses or investing in infrastructure, the physicians are rarely able to step up to their portion of the call. This leads to high tensions between the hospital and physician owners and suboptimal solutions if the hospital partner is a not-for-profit corporation.

The simplest form of PHO may not concern itself with ongoing revenue because the entity could serve only as a cost center for the hospital. As the PHO takes on various MSO functions, however, participating providers pay a fee for those services. Third-party payers also may pay an access fee.

Governance can evolve similarly. That is, in its simplest form hospital administrators may run the entity. Most PHOs are establishing formal governing boards, however. Board composition is usually equally divided between hospital administrators and physicians, with attention being given to primary care representation within the physician component. Board composition does not have to reflect equity position. Indeed, failure to attend to the needs of the medi-

cal staff may be a serious career-limiting move on the part of the hospital chief executive officer (CEO). In light of this, some PHOs have permitted more than half the board seats to be occupied by physicians, although some are hospital-based physicians. In the case of not-for-profit PHOs, however, physicians may not represent more than 20 percent of the governance, regardless of the hospital's desire (see Chapter 65 for a discussion of this issue).

One last note regarding PHOs: The "PO" portion of a PHO may be a different model entirely. For example, a GPWW or an IPA could represent the physician portion of the PHO. Although the most common model at the time of publication is one in which the physicians remain independent and contract individually with the PHO, use of IPAs has been increasing, and there are other methods of organization as well.

PHOs fall into two broad categories: open and closed. These are described separately because MCOs often view them distinctly differently.

Open PHOs

The open PHO is one that virtually any member of the hospital medical staff may join. There will sometimes be minimum credentialing requirements (see Chapter 7). Open PHOs are almost universally specialty dominated; in other words, there are disproportionately more specialists in the PHO than there are PCPs. The creators of the open PHO are often the specialists themselves, who become concerned that MCOs are selectively contracting, thereby reducing the amount of business that the specialists (as a group) are doing. The medical staff members then approach the hospital administration to form the PHO primarily to allow all the members of the medical staff to participate with MCOs. In this situation, PCPs are usually courted but may still be relegated to secondary citizenship, even if unconsciously.

Some open PHOs claim that, although they began in an open format, the ultimate goal will be to manage the membership and remove those physicians who are unable to practice cost-effectively. MCOs view such claims with skepticism, although the claims are not unrealistic. The political reality of an open PHO is that it is quite difficult to bring sufficient discipline to bear on medical staff members who wield a high level of influence. This is currently complicated by the continued dichotomy of payment mechanisms, in which a certain portion of reimbursement to the hospital rewards cost-effectiveness (e.g., prospective payment, capitation, package or bundled pricing), whereas other forms of reimbursement reward the opposite (e.g., fee-for-service payments, simple discounts on charges).

Closed PHOs

The primary difference between a closed PHO and an open one is the proactive decision to limit physician membership in the PHO. This is clearly more difficult politically than an open model, but it carries greater potential for success. The two general approaches to limiting membership are by specialty type and by practice profiling.

The more common limitation is the number of specialists, to address the imbalance of PCPs and specialists found in an open PHO. In fact, it is not uncommon to find closed PHOs having a disproportionate number of PCPs on the governance board as well as in the membership. Although an extreme demonstration of this concept is the primary care–only PHO that simply subcontracts with certain specialists, the PHO usually places limits on the number of specialists of any specialty for equity sharing and/or membership status. This limitation on the number of specialists is most often accomplished by projecting the number of lives that the PHO is expected to cover over the next several years and then recruiting specialists according to predetermined ratios of specialists to covered lives.

The second type of limitation involves practice profiling and is more difficult to carry out for technical reasons. This type of limitation requires the PHO to examine some objective form of practice analysis (it could be a subjective analysis, but that would probably raise a restraint of trade issue). If the PHO has access to adequate data during the formation stage, which is most uncommon, then based on that analysis, certain physicians are invited to join the PHO. The closed PHO may be impeded in its quest to demonstrate selectivity by those states enacting any willing provider legislation and needs to be aware of any possible antitrust issues (see Chapters 63 and 65 for further discussion of both issues).

As part of ongoing recredentialing, the PHO also regularly reevaluates the number of physicians required in each specialty. If the PHO has the ability to capture and analyze data regarding practice behavior and clinical quality (see Chapters 30 through 32), the data may be used in managing the physician membership and, ultimately, in ending the participation agreement with any physicians who repeatedly depart from the PHO's practice guidelines. Such analyses are difficult to perform properly. It is important for the PHO (or for any type of IDS, for that matter) that accepts full risk to negotiate the right to receive claims data on all members for whom the PHO has the full capitated risk; without the claims data, the PHO will not have sufficient information to analyze all medical costs.

Advantages of a PHO

The primary advantage of a PHO is its ability to negotiate on behalf of a large group of physicians allied with a hospital. This advantage can be ephemeral if no MCO wishes to negotiate (see below), but it may be very real if the hospital and key members of the medical staff are attractive to MCOs and are not already under contract. Closed PHOs are more attractive to MCOs than open ones. Of course, if the providers have already contracted with the MCO and threaten to pull out (i.e., boycott the MCO) unless the MCO uses the PHO, a serious antitrust problem may arise. If the MCO has not already contracted with the providers, the PHO may be an expeditious route to developing a delivery system capability. Even when a contract already exists, contracting through the PHO may be more appealing than direct contracting (e.g., the PHO may be willing to provide performance guarantees). Finally, physicians may view the PHO as a facilitator in landing direct contracts with self-insured employers, with the Health Care Financing Administration for Medicare risk contracts, and with the state for managed Medicaid contracts.

A second advantage of a PHO is its theoretical ability to track and use data and to manage the delivery system, at least from the standpoints of UM and quality management. Once again, this advantage is more likely to be found in a closed PHO than in an open one, primarily because a closed PHO has a greater concentration of events over fewer physicians.

The third advantage of a PHO is that it is the first step to greater integration between a hospital and its medical staff. Although a PHO by itself may result in improved relations, those relations can quickly sour if the PHO consumes time, energy, and money but fails to yield results. If the PHO does result in a better ability to contract or yields economic rewards, then its mission is successful, at least for the near term. If the PHO does not succeed, or if success appears to be short-lived, then the PHO may be the base from which a more integrated model may be built.

A fourth potential advantage (that is seldom realized) is the possibility that, by combining forces, hospitals and physicians may avoid competing against each other for the lion's share of the premium dollar. In theory, they can bid together and then come up with an equitable distribution internally. In practice, the premium dollars are seldom distributed in such a fashion that both the hospital and the physicians feel fairly rewarded. The competition moves from the MCO contract negotiating table to the hospital boardroom.

Disadvantages of a PHO

According to Nathan Kaufman, publishing in *Healthcare Financial Management*, "Many PHOs are either unprofitable, unsuccessful at developing new business, or stalemated by politics. Acquired physician practices are depleting hospital resources as their productivity decreases and overhead increases."[18(p.79)]

The chief disadvantage of a typical PHO is that it often fails to result in any meaningful improvement in contracting ability. In many cases, MCOs already have provider contracts in place and see little value in going through the PHO.

Even worse, an MCO may see the PHO as little more than a vehicle for providers to keep their reimbursement high.

Open PHOs are at a significant disadvantage if the MCO (or employer, in the event that the PHO chooses to contract directly with employers) does not want all the physicians in the PHO to be participating with the health plan. MCOs often want the right to select the providers and are unlikely to give up that ability. Even closed PHOs may suffer from this problem if the MCOs specifically wish to avoid contracting with certain physicians who are members of the PHO.

MCOs may view the PHO as a barrier to effective communication with the physicians and a hindrance to fully effective UM. Unless the PHO has a compelling story to tell regarding its ability to manage utilization, the MCO may believe that it can do a better job without the PHO's interference. Alternatively, if the health plan has relatively unsophisticated UM capabilities, or if the plan is too small to be able to devote adequate resources to UM, the PHO may represent an attractive alternative.

Because PHOs are relatively loose in their structure, and because the physicians may still be completely independent, the PHO's ability to affect provider behavior is rather limited. This can have an impact not only on UM but also on getting the entire organization to make necessary changes.

Many PHOs have not invested in infrastructure in any meaningful way. They may depend on the MCO to perform most or all of the administrative functions, which is a perfectly acceptable way to handle that aspect of operations. But it is not acceptable for the PHO to take on responsibility for functions that it is not able to perform. For example, some PHOs have insisted on doing their own claims processing, using an outside third-party administrator (TPA) or a small, internal (or custom-programmed) system; in many of these cases, the PHO is unable to keep up with demand, unable to generate proper data, and, finally, unable to discharge its obligations. This causes a slow spiral into financial disaster that requires management to undertake significant and costly performance improvement, or it leads to failure.

Regrettably, there have been a few cases where a hospital and medical staff with existing managed care contracts formed a PHO with the intent of using the PHO to improve their negotiating strength, only to lose the existing managed care contract and be unable to replace it with anything better. In other words, the PHO actually harmed them because it was considered undesirable by the MCO. Because most PHOs do allow the participating physicians to contract directly with the MCO in the event that the MCO does not offer terms agreeable to the PHO, this risk is usually minimal.

Specialist PHOs

A recent variant of the PHO has emerged over the past few years: The specialist PHO is a closed PHO with only one type of specialist. Common specialties involved are cardiology and pediatrics; psychiatric PHOs also have existed for many years. Their track record is too brief in most cases for definitive observations about their performance, but since they do not carry the baggage of maintaining a purchased physician practice and investor financial returns, their ability to succeed may be better than that of PPMCs.

MSOs

An MSO represents the evolution of the PHO into an entity that provides more services to the physician. The MSO offers not only a vehicle for negotiating with MCOs but also additional services to support the physician's practice. The physician, however, usually remains an independent private practitioner. The MSO is based around one or more hospitals. The reasons for the MSO's formation are generally the same as for the PHO's formation, and ownership and governance issues are similar to those discussed earlier.

In its simplest form, the MSO operates as a service bureau, providing basic practice support services to member physicians. These services include such activities as billing and collection, administrative support in certain areas, and electronic data interchange (e.g., electronic billing).

The physician can remain an independent practitioner under no legal obligation to use the services of the hospital on an exclusive basis. The MSO must receive compensation from the physician at fair market value, or the hospital and physician could incur legal problems (discussed in Chapter 65 as well as elsewhere in this chapter). The MSO should, through economies of scale as well as good management, be able to provide those services at a reasonable rate.

The MSO may also be considerably broader in scope. In addition to providing all the services described above, the MSO may actually purchase many of the assets of the physician's practice; for example, the MSO may purchase the physician's office space or office equipment (at fair market value). The MSO can employ the office support staff of the physician as well. Furthermore, MSOs can incorporate functions such as quality management, UM, provider relations, member services, and even claims processing. This form of MSO is usually constructed as a unique business entity, separate from the PHO. Because the MSOs are their own corporations, legal advisors are finding advantages in characterizing these as limited liability corporations, but alternatives exist.

The MSO does not always have direct contracts with MCOs for two reasons: Many MCOs insist on having the provider be the contracting agent, and many states will not allow MCOs (especially HMOs) to have contracts with any entity that does not have the power to bind the provider. The physician may remain an independent private practitioner under no contractual obligation to use the hospital on an exclusive basis. It should be noted here that there are IDSs that operate under the label of MSO that actually do purchase the physician's entire practice (possibly including intangible values such as goodwill) and function much like a more fully integrated system, as discussed later in this chapter.

Advantages of an MSO

The primary advantage of an MSO over a PHO is the ability of the MSO to bind the physician closer to the hospital, although not as a contractual obligation to use the hospital on an exclusive basis. The MSO certainly has the ability to bring economies of scale and professional management to the physician's office services, thus potentially reducing overhead costs. The MSO may have the potential ability to capture data regarding practice behavior, which may be used to help the physicians practice more cost-effectively. This situation develops when the MSO involves more advanced functions, such as UM and claims processing.

While MSOs that have purchased physicians' practices face many of the same problems described earlier (in the discussion of PPMCs), an MSO is also usually far closer to the local market than the typical PPMC. This allows the MSO to observe market conditions and to evaluate and respond to opportunities on a local basis.

Disadvantages of an MSO

The disadvantages of an MSO are similar to those of a PHO in that the physician may remain an independent practitioner with the ability to change allegiances with relative ease. Also, when the MSO does not employ the physician, it has somewhat limited ability to effect change or to redeploy resources in response to changing market needs.

Special problems arise with MSOs, problems that can be compounded when MSOs purchase assets from a physician's practice. These are the problems of the transaction being perceived as inuring to the benefit of the physician illegally and of fraud and abuse for federally funded patients. (These issues are briefly discussed later in this chapter and in detail in Chapter 65.) Other disadvantages arise when the hospital management mindset is applied to physician practices: "Since many hospital-affiliated practices are viewed as just 'another hospital department,' hospitals may allocate institutional overhead to acquired physician practices, negatively affecting the practices' final performance."[19(p.84)]

FOUNDATIONS

A foundation model IDS is one in which a hospital creates a not-for-profit foundation and actually purchases physicians' practices (both tangible and intangible assets) and puts those practices into the foundation. This model usually occurs when, for some legal reason (e.g., the hospital is a not-for-profit entity that cannot own a for-profit subsidiary, or there is a state law against the corporate practice of medicine), the hospital cannot employ the physicians directly or use hospital funds to purchase the practices directly. It must be noted that to qualify for and maintain its not-for-profit status, the foundation must prove that it provides substantial community benefit.

A second form of foundation model does not involve a hospital. In that model, the foundation is an entity that exists on its own and contracts for services with a medical group and a hospital. On a historical note, in the early days of HMOs, many open-panel plans were formed as foundations, not IPAs; the foundation held the HMO license and contracted with one or more IPAs and hospitals for services.

The foundation itself is governed by a board that is not dominated by either the hospital or the physicians (in fact, physicians may represent no more than 20 percent of the board) and includes lay members. The foundation owns and manages the practices, but the physicians become members of a medical group that, in turn, has an exclusive contract for services with the foundation; in other words, the foundation is the only source of revenue to the medical group. The physicians have contracts with the medical group that are long term and contain noncompete clauses.

Although the physicians are in an independent group and the foundation is separate from the hospital, the relationship among members of the triad is close. The medical group, however, retains a significant measure of autonomy regarding its own business affairs, and the foundation has no control over certain aspects, such as individual physician compensation (see Chapter 9).

Advantages of a Foundation

The primary advantages of this model pertain to legal constraints that require the foundation to be created. Because the construction of this entity is rather unwieldy, it is best suited to those states in which it is required due to state law so that a not-for-profit hospital can proceed with a fully integrated model. That said, the foundation model provides for a greater level of structural integration than any other model discussed to this point. A not-for-profit foundation may also be better able to access the bond market for capital in an advantageous manner.

Because the foundation clearly controls the revenue that the medical group will get, it has considerable influence over that group. The foundation also has the ability to rationalize the clinical and administrative resources required to meet obligations under managed care contracts (and fee for service, of course) and can achieve greater economies of scale. If the foundation consolidates medical office locations, these economies are improved, as is the foundation's ability to provide more comprehensive services to enrolled members. A foundation also has the ability to invest required capital to expand services, recruit PCPs, and so forth. For these reasons, a foundation model may be viewed quite favorably by a contracting MCO.

Disadvantages of a Foundation

The primary disadvantage of the foundation model is that the physicians in the medical group are linked only indirectly to the foundation and the business goals of that foundation. Although that indirect link is quite strong, the medical group remains an intermediate organization (vaguely analogous to an IPA) that can operate in ways that are potentially inconsistent with the overall goals of managed care. One medical group might be seriously overloaded with specialists and treat PCPs like second-class members. Another group might compensate member physicians based on fee for service or other measures that are easily gamed, leading to less than optimal control of utilization and quality.

Related to this issue is a built-in potential for conflicts between the governance boards of the hospital and the medical group. If the goals and priorities of those two organizations are not completely aligned (and they rarely are), then it is possible for serious disputes to arise, impeding success.

The last main disadvantage is the not-for-profit status of the hospital and foundation. To maintain its status, the foundation must continually prove that it provides a community benefit. The risk of private inurement (discussed below) is also heightened. As this book is going to publication, several not-for-profit hospitals, to compete against foundation models, have formed PHOs and MSOs (both for-profit and not-for-profit entities) allowing well over 20 percent board representation by physicians. These developments have been permitted by a favorable interpretation of regulatory requirements, although their ultimate corporate stability is still undetermined (see Chapter 65).

STAFF MODEL

Not to be confused with the staff model HMO (see Chapter 3), the staff model discussed in this chapter is an IDS owned by a health system rather than by an HMO. The difference is whether the primary business organization is a licensed entity (e.g., an HMO) or primarily a provider. This distinction is not always clear, and in some cases the only way to make any distinction is to look at the genesis of the parent organization: Was it founded to be a health plan or founded to be a provider? If the distinction rests on history only, then it is meaningless.

The staff model is a health system that employs the physicians directly. Physicians are integrated into the system either through the purchase of their practices or by being hired directly. The system is often more than a hospital; it is a larger, more comprehensive organization for the delivery of health care. Because the physicians are employees, the legal issues that attach to IDSs using private physicians are attenuated.

Advantages of a Staff Model

Staff model IDSs are theoretically in a good position to be able to rationalize resources and to align goals of all the components of the delivery system. Physicians are almost always paid based on a salary, and incentive programs can be designed to reward the physicians in parallel with the goals and objectives of the system (see Chapters 8 through 10). Far greater economies of scale are achievable, and capital resources can be applied in a businesslike manner. Staff models also have a greater ability to recruit new physicians because there is no cost to the new physician and the income stream to the new physician begins immediately. The ability to manage the physicians in the system is also at least theoretically enhanced. The problems of taxable status, private inurement, and fraud and abuse are greatly diminished. MCOs generally consider staff model IDSs as desirable business partners, assuming that cost, quality, and access are acceptable; the exception would be if the staff model IDS chooses to pursue obtaining its own HMO license, thus becoming a direct competitor and threat to a contracting MCO.

Disadvantages of a Staff Model

One key problem with staff models occurs when management assumes that because physicians are employees, they can be managed in a manner similar to that of other employees of the system; that is a false and unproductive assumption. Physicians are highly intelligent and highly trained professionals who must operate clinically with considerable autonomy. Any health system that does not recognize this is bound to have difficulties with its medical staff.

Staff models do run into problems with physician productivity, however. Some salaried physicians may not feel motivated to see high volumes of patients, as they were in the fee-for-service system. Staff models may be most attractive to physicians who do not wish to practice full-time or who wish to limit their hours. Productivity problems at some staff model HMOs have at least partially eroded the economies of scale that are possible in tightly integrated systems. Staff models, although having a somewhat easier time recruiting than medical groups, suffer from the doppelgänger of easy entry, easy exit. Physicians in staff models often feel little loyalty and are more easily recruited away than physicians who have an investment in a group.

The last disadvantage is the high capital requirement to build and operate the system. Once there is adequate patient volume, staff models can have excellent financial performance. Until then, however, they are heavily leveraged. Expansion of an existing system likewise requires a great deal of capital investment.

PHYSICIAN OWNERSHIP MODEL

The physician ownership model refers to a vertically integrated system in which the physicians hold a significant portion of ownership (i.e., equity) interest. In some cases, the physicians own the entire system; in other cases, the physicians own less than 100 percent but more than 51 percent. The physicians' equity interest is through their medical group(s). Physicians holding equity as simple shareholders could raise problems with Medicare fraud and abuse (see below and Chapter 65). It is theoretically possible for physicians to own equity through a limited partnership, although that format would require serious legal review. It is also possible to craft a model in which physicians own less than 50 percent as a group, but it is not clear whether that model would survive legal scrutiny (see below) or whether it would confer the same advantages as the model described here.

The physician ownership model has features of both the staff model and the MSO. Unlike the situation with the staff model, the medical groups have a strong role in the overall management of the system, and the physicians (at least those physicians who are partners in the group) have a clear vested interest in the system's success.

Advantages of a Physician Ownership Model

The advantages of the physician ownership model are similar to those of the staff model. But the physician ownership model has one powerful advantage that the staff model lacks: total alignment of goals of the medical group and the health system. Because the physician owners' success is tied directly to the overall success of the entire organization, there is far less of a problem with conflicting goals and objectives (within the boundaries of human nature). Because of this alignment, strong physician leadership is present, which is more effective in managing the medical groups. Finally, organizations following this model can choose either to contract with or to own the hospital rather than being dominated by the hospital.

Disadvantages of a Physician Ownership Model

The primary disadvantage of the physician ownership model is the high level of resources required to build and operate it. Large capital resources are required to acquire the personnel, facilities, and practices necessary to provide comprehensive medical services, an adequate level of managerial support, and the required infrastructure. The source of this capital is primarily the physicians' practices, although outside access to capital is certainly possible. Related to that issue is the generally high buy-in cost to new physician partners, which may keep some physicians from joining the group as anything other than employees.

At this time, it is unknown whether models in which physicians are significant equity holders will face problems with the fraud and abuse provisions discussed below and in Chapter 65, but it is possible that the models will. This is because the physicians receive an economic reward for patient services that is unrelated to their own services. Readers are urged to review recent regulatory and legal rulings on this issue as appropriate.

In physician ownership models that involve joint equity arrangements with hospitals, the physicians contribute equity into for-profit entities that may take the form of a procedure lab (e.g., an ambulatory heart cath lab) or a specialty "hospital within a hospital." For-profit, single specialty hospitals using this equity sharing option have attracted great interest recently.

However, leaders of these equity models must pay particular attention to the Office of the Inspector General's July 8, 1999, Special Advisory Bulletin, which outlaws gain sharing using revenues from fee-for-service Medicare or Medicaid patients. These equity joint ventures must be constructed with due diligence and advice from legal counsel. For example, here are a few caveats to consider.

- No documents, contracts, or bylaws can include wording that suggests there is an inducement for referrals or that physician income will be directly proportional to cost savings.
- The proceeds to a physician owner must be directly proportional to that physician's equity.
- If the physician secures a loan to fulfill the equity contribution, that loan must be fully collateralized, such as with the corresponding medical practice.

PSOs

A PSO is generally a cooperative venture of a group of providers who control the venture's health service delivery and financial arrangements. In effect, a PSO is an integrated provider system engaged in *both* delivery and financing of health care services. PSO activity is focused on the Medicare population but could theoretically expand to include commercial and Medicaid populations. As PSOs were created by federal legislation on Medicare, they are discussed in greater detail in Chapter 55. To better understand this unique form of IDS, readers should look at that chapter.

The BBA that created Medicare + Choice contains the following definition of a PSO:

"A PSO is a public or private entity that is a provider or group of affiliated providers that provides a substantial portion of health care* under the contract directly through the provider or affiliated group of providers, and with respect to those affiliated providers that share, directly or

---

*A substantial portion of health care services in an urban area is 70 percent or more of health care services (as measured by expenditures) that must be provided directly or through affiliated providers (but only 60 percent in a rural area).

indirectly, substantial financial risk, have at least a majority interest in the entity."[20]

Structure

A PSO is an eligible Medicare-contracting organization provided it is organized and licensed to offer prepaid Medicare health services or benefits coverage on a capitated basis. Physician services must be provided by the organization's own physicians or contracting physicians who are assuming full financial risk on a prospective basis for the health care services. A PSO must provide a substantial proportion of the health care items and services under the contract directly to beneficiaries through its own providers or through an affiliated group of providers.

A provider is considered "affiliated" with another if—through contract, ownership, or other arrangement—one provider, indirectly or directly, controls, is controlled by, or is under control of the other; each provider is a participant in a lawful combination under which each provider shares, directly or indirectly, substantial financial risk in connection with the operations.

Unlike Medicare risk HMOs, for organizations meeting the BBA definition of a PSO, the minimum precontract enrollment requirement is reduced to 1,000 members (500 in a rural area), a requirement that may also be waived.

Licensure

PSOs were licensed initially by the Department of Health and Human Services, allowing them to bypass state licensure requirements (state licensure is a requirement of traditional Medicare risk HMOs). Beginning on January 1, 2002, states may regulate PSOs if the financial solvency and capital adequacy standards (see below) for licensure of the organization under the state laws are identical or "substantially equivalent" to federal standards.

Solvency

A PSO may be determined to be "fiscally sound" by the Secretary of Health and Human Services if the organization has a net worth that is not less than the required net worth and has established adequate claims reserves.

A "required net worth"—for an organization with a full risk contract—will not be less than the greatest of the following three items:

1. $1.5 million at the time of application and $1 million thereafter
2. the sum of 8 percent of the costs of health services not provided directly by the organization or affiliated providers to enrollees *and* 4 percent of the estimated costs of the annual costs of health services provided by the organization or affiliated providers
3. three months of uncovered expenditures (organizations with partial risk-sharing arrangements will have lower percentages to reflect a lower level of risk).

The PSO must have "adequate claims reserves," which means reserves for claims that are incurred but not reported, or reported but unpaid.

In determining net worth, the Secretary will treat as "admitted assets" land, buildings, and equipment of the organization used for the direct provision of health care services; any "receivables" from government programs due for more than 90 days; and any other assets designated by the Secretary. PSOs are allowed to include assets in their net worth that MCOs are not (see Chapters 47 and 69). This has been a contentious issue in the industry, but given the poor track record of early PSOs, these more lenient net worth requirements have not conferred a significant advantage.

Advantages of a PSO

The advantages of a PSO were a large part of the debate that led to their creation. During the debate that led to the BBA, arguments were put forward that provider systems were far more capable of running their own medical risk business with a defined population of Medicare beneficiaries than was a "middleman" organization. The providers would be closer to the treatment decisions, would be able to better coordinate care, and would have aligned economic incentives. It was also argued vigorously that a provider system did not need the same level of financial reserves or minimum net worth as a conventional MCO since the risk it took on was for the services that it delivered itself, not for payments to others.

These advantages have been insufficient to overcome the disadvantages of PSOs, however.

Disadvantages of a PSO

PSOs have several disadvantages. Like many other IDSs, PSOs often did not have the managerial or systems capability to administer the plan.

The need for reserves has proven to be grossly underestimated, as medical costs in a PSO are very real. This problem has two components. First, there is payment for services from noncontracting providers. Not all providers in a medical community necessarily contract with a PSO, and not even all physicians (particularly scarce subspecialists) who could potentially contract with the PSO choose to do so, leading to care being rendered by noncontracted physicians. A variant on this issue is care rendered out of area (e.g., for "snowbirds") or emergency care. Second, the internal payment structure of the PSO itself can create problems. Many PSOs set up internal reimbursement systems based on fee for service and quickly depleted the fixed revenue paid to the PSO by Medicare.

Another highly significant problem for PSOs, a problem shared by many other forms of IDSs that directly market to enrollees, is adverse selection. Often the first members to sign up for the PSO are the sickest and most in need of the benefits that a PSO, like a Medicare risk HMO (see Chapters 55 and 56), offers. In other words, patients of the physicians of the PSO enroll sooner and in higher proportion than do members who have no connection or experience with the health system sponsoring the PSO. Said one more way, the proportion of members to patients is heavily skewed toward patients, not members who use few medical resources.

In the end, many PSOs that started up as demonstration projects ended up closing down, and there have been few new ones applying for licensure. Whether this form of IDS will be resurrected in the future is unclear. But it still exists as a possible form of IDS focused on Medicare.

VIRTUAL INTEGRATION

Goldsmith argues that it is possible, and even likely, that many of the structurally rigid vertical integration models are not going to succeed.[21] He concludes that success will be more probable with models of virtual integration, in which more or less independent parties come together for the purpose of behaving like an IDS under managed care but retain their own identities and mission. This virtual integration requires an alignment of financial incentives and business purpose for all parties.

In a virtual integration, each of the major segments of the health care system—the physicians, the institutional providers, the payers/MCOs, and the ancillary providers (e.g., pharmacy)—act in concert for a common cause, but none is an employee or subdivision of another. This allows each party to manage its own affairs and meet its own financial goals without being managed by another segment of the industry. In this model, there is greater horizontal integration (e.g., among hospitals, among physicians), with each of those horizontally integrated systems then forming relationships with other parts of the health care system.

GLOBAL CAPITATION

Global capitation applies to IDSs that are capable of accepting full or nearly full risk for medical expenses, including all professional and institutional services and many ancillary services as well. This differs from the full capitation (described in Chapter 8) in which primary care groups accept full risk for all professional services but not for institutional or ancillary services. Global capitation includes institutional as well as professional services, and the party accepting the capitation payment is a large, vertically integrated organization with presumably greater resources. But this is not necessarily an easy exercise for an IDS. For example one PHO in Florida took on several capitated contracts that it could not actually fulfill at the price quoted. It lost $5.6 million in 1998 and had to cancel or renegotiate its contracts.[22]

Even though the IDS has accepted global capitation, it often purchases reinsurance to protect it against catastrophic cases; that reinsurance is either provided by the HMO or purchased by the IDS from a reinsurer, as discussed in detail in Chapter 53.

Many IDSs accept a percentage of premium revenue from an HMO rather than a fixed capitation. Although these forms of revenue are similar, they are not the same. A percentage of premium may be affected by underwriting and marketing issues, primarily in commercial enrollment; in Medicare and Medicaid, percentage of revenue and capitation are nearly the same, though not identical (and unlike in PSOs, which receive revenue directly from Medicare). As discussed in Chapters 49 through 51, if underwriting is poor and there is a revenue shortfall from the standpoint of covered lives, the percentage of that shortfall passed on to the IDS will mirror the percentage of revenue it is receiving from the MCO.

Although the HMO may have capitated the IDS, the IDS still faces the issue of how to divide up the revenue and risk among the parties. In a sense, global capitation simply transfers the burden of payment and management from the HMO to the IDS, but the fundamental issues remain. If the IDS employs physicians, then it is relatively easier to distribute income.

Many IDSs, however, are combinations of private and employed physicians. Even hospitals that employ physicians usually still rely on private physicians for at least some services, and often the genesis of the IDS was to allow the hospital and private physicians to remain competitive in a managed care environment. Therefore, the IDS that accepts global capitation must still figure out how to allocate risk and reward. The managers of the IDS must be realistic and recognize that individual physicians will be unable and unwilling to bear a high level of financial risk (e.g., how many individual physicians could afford to pay $200,000 as their share of overutilization?) but will usually demand a disproportionate share of financial reward. Although risk

and reward are always related, the IDS management must be careful to give the physicians proper incentives as well as to avoid the legal problems of private inurement and fraud and abuse regulations. Reimbursement of physicians is discussed in Chapters 8 through 11.

The last major issue in global capitation is who is actually the licensed health plan. If an IDS accepts global capitation, then a state's insurance department may require the IDS to become licensed as an HMO. This issue is discussed below and in detail in Chapter 69. Regulation of IDSs accepting full-risk capitation is undergoing considerable change, and the reader will need to keep aware of applicable regulations and laws.

Providing the Insurance Function

Until this point, this chapter has concentrated on vertical integration of practitioners and facilities. The MSO and PHO models are examples of delivery systems that can expand horizontally (by finding other PHO partners and forming a regional network—the super PHO—with convenient geographic access) and then become independently capable of direct contracting with self-insured purchasers. This capability requires incorporating most of the typical insurance functions. These usually begin with claims processing but may extend to ownership of the insurance license itself.

Options for an IDS to converge with insurance functions include the following: The insurer buys the hospital and physician groups, an integrated provider network buys or builds the insurance function, or the insurer and the integrated provider network form a joint venture with shared ownership (or perhaps a looser relationship). An integrated provider network may also rent an insurance function; for example, it may pay several dollars per subscriber per month for TPA functions and possible insurance licensure fronting services.

Clearly, when dealing with purchasers that are not self-insured, the IDS or MSO needs to incorporate all the classic insurance functions, including underwriting and actuarial rate development, as it takes on risk. The IDS also needs to have an insurance license. Many small insurance companies and TPAs are willing to price their role in this scheme competitively and are capable of avoiding the double-digit overhead associated with the largest insurance companies. One must be cognizant, however, that many of these TPAs are not capable of carrying out sophisticated managed care functions. It is also possible for an IDS to contract with an insurer to front the license, that is, to use the insurer's license to back up the IDS's activities.

Advantages

A joint venture between an IDS and an insurer or MCO has several advantages. Both parties bring assets to the venture (at least theoretically). The IDS brings a network, some medical management, the ability to accept some level of risk for medical expenses, and a framework for contracting. The insurer or MCO brings a license and its ability to meet the attendant capital and regulatory needs, possibly an enrolled subscriber base, and expertise in functions such as claims processing, member services, and the like.

Disadvantages

The main disadvantage of an IDS assuming the insurance functions is that it may fail to carry them out competently, and failure would have far-reaching effects. The activities of an insurance company or MCO go well beyond medical management, and it would be naive for the management of an IDS to believe that those functions do not require expertise or that they are not fraught with complexities.

In fact, the fundamental flaw in any provider-owned (hospital-owned) HMO is that hospital and HMO leaders have different goals. This has resulted in an impasse in multiple sites across the country over recent years, resulting in unchecked HMO financial losses. Ultimately, many hospital CEOs have reflected on their central mission and core competency, resulting in HMO divestitures.

The pursuit of the insurance partner requires great caution. Too many insurance entities are configured as indemnity claims processors, incapable of understanding the subtleties associated with managing care. Significant capital may be required to structure the new entity. A large organization perceived to have deep pockets that has gotten closer to the provision of care will also need to evidence due diligence in credentialing providers to minimize the risk associated with negligent credentialing.

Governance of a joint venture may be a sensitive area. Although joint representation on the board is likely to be required, controlling representation may become a contentious issue. Control is generally subject to the Golden Rule (whoever has the gold makes the rules), but supermajority rights may help address control concerns by the minority partner.

Finally, these relationships often begin as nonexclusive. When the stakeholders have multiple alliances, true allegiance and true alignment of motivation are difficult to achieve. Gradually, consolidation will require a deliberate "choosing up sides."

ACQUISITION OF PHYSICIAN PRACTICES

One common approach to integrating providers and payers in the recent past has been the outright acquisition of provider practices or provider facilities by MCOs such as HMOs and Blue Cross/Blue Shield plans or by IDSs. Primary care practices were purchased at an astonishingly fast pace. This enthusiasm for PCP practice acquisition was based on the recognition of the central role of these physicians in an HMO and as the gateway at the POS. This was reinforced by the requirement for PCP selection during open enrollment.

Acquisition of Physician Practices by IDSs or Hospitals

The organizations that purchased perhaps the most physician practices were hospitals. The chief reasons for acquiring practices were to control the primary care referral base, intended to enhance the hospital's ability to negotiate with MCOs, and to prevent a competing hospital from acquiring the practices. Hospitals also hoped that, by controlling primary care practices, they would be in a better position to obtain and successfully manage capitation.

These purchases generally turned out to be (to put it mildly) a disappointment for hospitals. "You have to stay focused on what you do best. Clearly that doesn't mean owning and controlling physicians," Columbia HCA senior vice president Victor Campbell told the *Nashville Tennessean*. "We realize that, for us, that's a horrible strategy."[23 (p.A1)] At its peak, Columbia employed 1,500 physicians. Now, at least 900 of these physicians are working for some other entity. Industry analysts quoted by the Dow Jones News Service believe that Columbia was losing $100 million a year on its physician practices.[24] This level of loss is not uncommon among hospital-owned practices.

The premises that drove the physician acquisitions have not been borne out by experience: There is little empirical evidence that hospital-physician integration alone provides health care organizations with the market leverage or cost structure needed to operate successfully. PHOs and other partially integrated provider organizations give hospitals minimal protection from revenue loss. According to Kaufman, there is "no correlation between a hospital's physician integration strategy and its payments under managed care. There is, however, a high correlation between a hospital's payments under managed care and its institutional market position. Dominant hospital systems got paid better than marginal hospitals regardless of whether they had a PHO."[25(p.78)]

Typically, when hospitals or IDSs tried to manage physician practices, the following things happened:

- *Hospital executives underestimated the difficulty of running physician practices.* This type of retail medicine requires different management skills, spread over a dispersed geography, than does running a hospital campus. A common first move by hospital managers was to fire highly paid physician office staff. Usually this resulted in confusion in the offices, uncollected copayments, and general chaos. The physi-

cians, in turn, were definitely not happy and felt powerless to correct the administrative chaos developing around them.

- *Physician billing and administrative systems were all different.* Much effort went into standardizing them, with little positive effect. More chaos (and unhappy physicians) ensued. Some hospitals centralized billing and administration for all physician offices but could not integrate the various systems fast enough to keep from losing money and also did not work out effective means of remotely collecting claims data from physicians and copayments from patients.

- *The hospital rapidly stripped out any ancillary services from the physicians' offices (e.g., diagnostic testing, laboratory, radiology, certain clinical procedural capabilities) in order to direct those services to the hospital's services.* While this has the theoretical advantage of bringing economies of scale, it generally eliminated the profitability of the physicians' practices.

- *Physicians were perceived as "coasting" once they were on salary and no longer financially motivated based on productivity.* Some physicians hotly contest this perception and claim that if hospital executives paid physicians with bonuses and incentives the way they pay themselves, the problem would be solved. That argument cannot be easily answered, but the reader is referred to Chapter 9 for a detailed discussion of this issue.

- *Physicians did not necessarily steer their patients to the sponsoring hospitals, as expected.* This was a major disappointment to some systems.

MCO Ownership of Physician Practices

As described in Chapter 3, HMOs have historically relied on contracting with private physicians (in open panels), contracting with large medical groups (in group and network models), or employing physicians directly through recruiting efforts (in staff models). HMOs were also acquiring practices in the early to mid-1990s, as open-panel plans became mixed models through practice acquisition, or group and staff model plans absorbed practices into existing structures. HMOs acquired practices for several reasons. The HMO may have perceived a need to expand its delivery system to meet access needs, to rapidly increase membership by acquiring a group, or (not insignificant) to prevent other parties from increasing their negotiating leverage at the HMO's expense. HMOs have not proved to be any more proficient than hospitals or PPMCs at running physician practices, however. Most are divesting.

So, the bottom line is that there is now an opportunity to reorganize physicians into viable contracting units for the purpose of actually managing care—as well as cost. But no obvious consolidators have stepped up to the plate. Wall Street has lost interest, so it is unlikely that new PPMCs will get venture funding. Yet the need remains to consolidate physicians to obtain and manage network contracts. While there has been a slow but steady increase in the number and size of physician group practices, this has not attained broad acceptance. It is therefore not clear how physician reorganization will evolve, though group practice appears to have the greatest likelihood of long-term success.

Whether owned by a hospital or an MCO, these acquired practices are now going through various levels of divestiture.

LEGAL PITFALLS FOR IDSs

There are many legal pitfalls in the development and operation of IDSs, and this chapter cannot possibly address them all. A few particular legal problems are especially worthy of note. Two related issues are the problems of private inurement and fraud and abuse; the other two especially noteworthy issues are problems of antitrust and licensure requirements. Readers are urged to review these and other legal issues in Chapters 63 through 65 and 69 and in the numerous other sources of material available in the literature. More important, competent legal counsel should be obtained before and during any operational activities involving these types of IDSs or any other integration activity not discussed here.

Private Inurement

This issue is raised primarily by the Internal Revenue Service (IRS), which has set rules against the inurement of private benefits from activities of a tax-exempt organization. The tax-exempt organization pertinent to these discussions is usually a hospital but could be any tax-exempt vehicle. The issue at hand is that a tax-exempt organization cannot do any business that provides more than incidental monetary benefit to private individuals. Specifically, if a hospital provides services to a physician at less than fair market value, provides a below-market (or forgiven) loan to a physician, or purchases a practice at greater than fair market value, then the physician has benefited in a manner not allowed by the IRS. The composition of board representation by physicians in a PHO could also be considered an organization created for the private inurement of the physicians. This topic is discussed in Chapter 65.

Fraud and Abuse

The federal government, through Medicare and Medicaid, has developed regulations regarding what it considers fraud and abuse* in the provision of services to federally funded patients. These regulations are extensive, and this chapter will not be able to review them. One pertinent portion of these regulations is similar to the issue discussed above, that of hospitals providing a financial benefit to physicians over what would be considered fair market value. In this case, the federal government views such an offense as fraudulent payments in return for referrals of federally funded patients to the hospital—in other words, kickbacks. This problem would apply to any hospital or provider that serves Medicare or Medicaid patients, regardless of the taxable status of the provider.

A key to avoiding this problem (including the problem of private inurement), in addition to hir-

---

*The terms "fraud" and "abuse" are rarely used separately by governmental agencies, leading to the functional neologism: fraudandabuse.

ing competent legal counsel, is paying or charging only fair market value. If a hospital purchases a physician's practice, it must have that practice valued by an independent firm that is competent to conduct valuation studies. If a hospital provides services to a physician (e.g., facilities, billing and collection), it must charge fair market value and manage those services in a businesslike fashion. The exact same caveat applies to a hospital system infusing capital into physicians' practices or into an IDS: The capital infusion must be based on reasonable business terms and must be recovered over time, just like any investment. It must be stressed that even strict adherence to these guidelines may not guarantee that there will be no problem with charges of fraud and abuse; the federal government is likely to examine each situation on its merits.

A special problem under the fraud and abuse regulations of the federal government relates to prohibitions against self-referral by physicians, the so-called Stark I amendments.* Although self-referral is easily avoided in some situations (e.g., a private physician cannot refer a Medicare or Medicaid patient to a radiology facility that the physician owns), the application of these regulations is not necessarily as clear as it might be to a physician-owned IDS. There are Safe Harbor provisions for some licensed HMOs and for certain clinical activities that are an integral part of a physician's practice, but whether these provisions would apply to certain forms of IDSs that are owned or controlled (even partially) by physicians is unclear. The other Stark amendments, Stark II, also place restrictions on physician payment incentives for MCOs or IDSs serving Medicare or Medicaid recipients. These are evolving areas of law that have not been fully clarified; competent legal counsel is critical here because the penalties for noncompliance with these federal regulations can be severe.

---

*These amendments are named after California Representative Fortney "Pete" Stark; the actual provisions are included as amendments to the Omnibus Budget Reconciliation Act of 1993.

Antitrust

It is well beyond the scope of this chapter to discuss antitrust law in any depth, but a general point may be made. If an IDS is perceived to have been formed primarily to stifle competition, then it may be found in violation of antitrust provisions. Examples of so-called per se violations of antitrust law would include competitors agreeing to fix prices (either minimums or maximums), sharing pricing information, and agreeing to divide the market among themselves. Although per se violations refer to actions that are clearly wrong, other activities may be subject to the rule of reason, in which there are good procompetitive reasons for the activity even though there may be some elements that could be perceived as antitrust. For example, an IDS may encompass greater than 20 percent to 30 percent of the total number of providers in a community but be able to demonstrate clearly that resources are rationalized and competition has increased. Again, competent counsel is required to review this issue. Antitrust issues are also discussed in Chapter 63.

Licensure Provisions

Except in situations where the IDS is part of a joint venture with a licensed insurer or MCO or is a qualified PSO, if an IDS takes on too much risk for medical expenses, the state insurance department may conclude that the delivery system should be the licensed entity, not the HMO or insurance company that contracted with the delivery system. This problem has occurred in some states in which well-organized IPAs or PHOs took full capitated risk, and the insurance department forced the IPA or PHO to cede back a portion of that risk to the HMO or else obtain an HMO license of its own. In a number of states, the IDS may obtain a limited license that allows it to accept and manage risk (including subcontracting capitation contracts with other providers) but not to carry out other functions such as marketing. How much risk is too much in the eyes of a state insurance department? That issue is still not totally clear. The reader is referred to Chapters 65 and 69 for greater discussion of this issue.

The costs associated with becoming a licensed entity are not trivial and can easily exceed several million dollars, including capital necessary to meet statutory reserve requirements. Furthermore, compliance with licensure regulations is a resource- and capital-consuming task that many provider organizations will not willingly accept.

CRITICAL SUCCESS FACTORS FOR IDSs*

By this point in the chapter, some readers may be feeling rather pessimistic about the ability of IDSs to succeed. Certainly there are plenty of examples of IDSs that never achieved their goals or simply failed. But as Tables 4–1 and 4–2 show, there are also IDSs that have succeeded.

Some successful IDSs have been studied and opinions have been expressed about the determining factors in their success; many others have simply been noted in the trade press or known primarily only to those that have business interests in common with them or are in the same communities. Many reported reasons for success are in fact quite localized (e.g., the IDS has a formidable share of the provider market, or the local MCOs are generally weak). But beyond this, there are certain critical success factors for IDSs. For purposes of clarity, these have been categorized into 10 specific questions, illustrated in Exhibit 4–1. Exhibit 4–2 expands on Exhibit 4–1.

It must be stressed that there is no single right answer to any of these questions (with the exception of some of the financial treatment and methodology questions; see Chapter 47 for discussion of these). What is important is that the IDS be able honestly to assess each question and have an effective approach or answer to each one. The ability of the IDS to address each question in a realistic and

---

*This section is adapted and updated from an earlier publication: *Ten Critical Success Factors for Integrated Delivery Systems*, Kongstvedt & Gates, Copyright Ernst & Young LLP, used with permission; Aspen Publishers, 1996. That monograph remains largely relevant, and the reader is referred to it for a more detailed discussion of the issues discussed in this section.

Exhibit 4–1 Ten Critical Success Factors for IDSs

1. What are the core values and goals of the IDS and its sponsoring organizations?
2. What does the internal and external environment look like?
3. What will the IDS organizational model look like?
4. How will the IDS access the marketplace and access revenue, and why is such an approach preferable? How will this approach differ from the ways that participants currently access the marketplace and revenue?
5. How will the IDS perform medical management?
6. How will the IDS perform nonmedical management?
7. How will the IDS measure and manage performance?
8. How will the IDS manage the money and distribute positive and negative financial results?
9. How will the IDS provide sufficient financial and nonfinancial incentives for physicians and nonphysicians?
10. How will the IDS manage change and the future?

Source: Copyright © Ernst & Young LLP, used with permission. Aspen Publishers, 1996.

---

unbiased way is what changes the question into a critical success factor. If the question is glossed over or answered in such a way as to be emotionally satisfying but essentially useless (e.g., an agreement that the physicians do not need to do serious medical management because their real goal is to avoid it), then the question becomes a critical failure factor.

IDSs that avoid addressing these issues in a meaningful way are almost sure to fall short of success unless they enjoy such market power that they need not do more than negotiate for higher payments.

For discussion of these issues beyond the outline format presented in Exhibit 4–2, see *Ten Critical Success Factors for Integrated Delivery Systems* by Kongstvedt and Gates, listed in Suggested Reading.

Exhibit 4–2 More on the Ten Critical Success Factors for IDSs

What are the core values and goals of the IDS and its sponsoring organizations? What role will each sponsoring organization play in the IDS? Examples include the following:
- Preservation or growth of patient base
- Maintenance of control
- Maintenance of income
- Maintenance of clinical availability in a geographic area
- Ability to sustain a special program or mission
- Improvement of quality of care
- Preservation of jobs

What do the internal and external environment look like?
- External environment
  1. HMO and/or MCO penetration
  2. Insurer demographics
  3. Forward integration of insurers into provision of health care services
  4. Competitive delivery system formation and initiatives
- Internal environment
  1. Provider development of risk-bearing entities
  2. Domain expertise
  3. Historical foundation
  4. Market segment focus
- Need to assess environment objectively
  1. Use of a third-party organization
  2. Need to recognize and neutralize internal biases and beliefs

What will the IDS organizational model look like?
- Corporate structure
  1. Not-for-profit corporation
  2. Not-for-profit taxable corporation
  3. For-profit corporation
  4. Limited liability corporation
  5. Limited liability partnership
  6. General partnership
  7. Limited partnership
- Ownership in equity or for-profit model
- Relationship of investment to equity
- Ability to separate equity from meeting needs and goals of participants (e.g., physicians may not actually need to hold equity to meet their needs)

- Board structure and governance
- IDS corporate focus:
  1. geographic area
  2. market
  3. service focus
- Role of participants
  1. Role in direct patient care provision
  2. Role in distribution of patient care dollars and resources
  3. Role in asset allocation
  4. Role in management of system participants
- Contingencies
  1. Need to define contingencies
  2. Need to recognize contingencies early
  3. Need to plan to manage contingencies

How will the IDS access the marketplace and access revenue, and why is such an approach preferable? How will this approach differ from the ways that participants currently access the marketplace and revenue?
- By form of revenue
  1. Percentage of premium
  2. Capitation
  3. Fee for service
  4. Bundled pricing
- Through what channels
  1. Self-insured employers
  2. Joint venture with MCOs
  3. Contracts with existing payers
- For what market segments
  1. Commercial
  2. Specific health plans
  3. Employers, via direct contracts
  4. Medicare
  5. Medicaid
- For what clinical services
  1. All services
  2. Defined services
- How will the IDS distribute revenue in accordance with the goals and needs of the IDS?

How will the IDS perform medical management?
- Need for realistic assessment of how much medical management is really required
- Need to neutralize political pressures on effective medical management
- Utilization management

continues

Exhibit 4–2 continued

- Quality management
- Access to primary and tertiary care, including care from physicians who are not members of the IDS
- Access to care outside of the IDS system
- Credentialing and participant selection
- Leveraging of participants' capabilities
- Building internal resources versus contracting for external resources

How will the IDS perform nonmedical management?
- Financial
  1. Revenues
  2. Treatment of prepaid (i.e., capitated) revenues as liabilities
  3. Accounting techniques for revenue in the risk business
  4. Treatment of medical benefits costs
  5. Management of reinsurance
  6. Administrative expenses
  7. Accurate capture and reporting of administrative expenses
  8. Allocation issues of overhead between the parties
  9. Financial reporting
  10. Statutory reporting—SAAP
  11. Standard reporting—GAAP
  12. Operational reporting
  13. Budget development
  14. Forecasting and projecting financial results
  15. Need for accurate projections
  16. Problems of incurred but not reported claims
  17. Problems of inaccurate cost estimates during periods of high growth or shrinkage in enrolled membership
- Management information systems
  1. Need for specialized information systems
  2. Buy versus lease versus outsource
- Support operations

How will the IDS measure and manage performance? What will the IDS consider as requiring measurement and management? How will the IDS avoid measuring and managing performance that is actually irrelevant to overall organizational success? Examples of potential areas for measurement and management include the following:

- Preventive care activities
- Access to PCPs
- Patient satisfaction
- Utilization rates and resource consumption (inpatient, outpatient, total)
- Health status and quality outcomes
- Cost efficiencies (ability to achieve economies of scale in practice management and nonmedical management)
- Market growth
- Percent of revenue to medical costs, administrative costs, and financial return
- Financial return to partners

How will the IDS manage the money and distribute positive and negative financial results?
- Accessing capital
  1. Internal versus external capital
  2. Treatment of capital contributions or capital loans
  3. Need for extra caution by not-for-profit entities such as hospitals
- Basis for distribution of profits and losses
  1. Profit-sharing considerations
  2. Use as a source of motivation and incentive for IDS participants
  3. Widespread participant desire to share in profits
  4. Need for retention of some earnings for reinvestment or as protection against potential future losses
  5. Potential for downward restatement of profits from prior periods and its effect on distributed profit sharing
  6. Taxation issues
- Loss-sharing considerations
  1. Recognition that not every profit-sharing participant has the same ability to absorb losses
  2. Realization that physicians have a strong desire to share in profits but limited ability to absorb significant losses
  3. Role of retaining earnings to provide a cushion for losses, carrying losses forward, or offering interest-bearing notes payable
- Absolute need to spell out the mechanism for funding losses in early stages, before losses are incurred.

continues

Exhibit 4–2 continued

How will the IDS provide sufficient financial and nonfinancial incentives for physicians and nonphysicians?
- Physicians
    1. Need for alignment with overall financial goals of the IDS
    2. Need to accommodate multiple physician and IDS reimbursement methods
    3. Capitation
    4. Fee for service
    5. Bundled or package pricing
    6. Salary and bonus plans
    7. Need to conform to federal and state regulations regarding incentive programs, including the OIG Special Advisory Bulletin on Gainsharing, July 1999
    8. Stark II laws
    9. Private inurement issues
    10. Fraud and abuse regulations

- Nonphysicians
    1. IDS executive incentive programs
    2. Potential for conflict between incentive programs for hospital executives based on high occupancy and high revenues versus IDS incentives to lower hospital utilization and medical costs

How will the IDS manage change and the future? No matter how an IDS is created today, it will face an ever-shifting health care environment. This requires the IDS to incorporate the following:
- flexibility in the organizational structure
- fair and impartial processes for reevaluation of IDS positioning
- an "opt-out" plan that defines terms for leaving the IDS
- organizational change management principles to support the IDS's need to evolve with the market

Source: Copyright © Ernst & Young LLP, used with permission. Aspen Publishers, 1996.

CONCLUSION

IDSs have existed for quite some time, but under current pressures they are evolving rapidly. The more a system is truly integrated, and the more the goals and objectives of all stakeholders can be aligned, the greater the likelihood of success. IDSs may provide a viable vehicle for managed care plans to deliver services to their members, but no one should assume that the presence of an IDS does not also bring a large set of challenges, both managerial and legal. If those challenges cannot be overcome or managed, the downside of failure in an IDS is potentially more severe than if smaller, unintegrated medical groups fail. When designed and implemented well, however, the IDS can have advantages over many conventional managed care models.

REFERENCES

1. P. Starr, *The Social Transformation of American Medicine* (New York: Basic Books, 1982).

2. R. Jantzen and P.R. Loubeau, Risk Sharing Integration Efforts in the Hospital Sector, *Health Care Management Review,* April 1, 1999: 83.

3. L.R. Burns et al., Managed Care and Processes To Integrate Physicians/Hospitals, *Health Care Management Review,* October 1, 1998: 70.

4. Hoechst Marion Roussel Managed Care Digest Series, *Integrated Health Systems Digest* (Kansas City, MO, Hoechst Marion Roussel and SMG Marketing Group, 1999).

5. K. Sifferman et al., *Volatility Ahead for Health Care Industry* (Moody's Investors Service, 1998).

6. J.A. Alexander et al., An Exploratory Analysis of Market-Based, Physician-Organization Arrangements, *Hospital & Health Services Administration,* Fall 1996: 43.

7. Burns et al., Managed Care, 70.

8. Managed Care Information Center, Some 130,000 Physicians Now IPA Members, press release, February 10, 1998.

9. J. Lawrence, Are We Unmanaging Care? *Managed Care,* December 1997: 9.

10. A.C. Enthoven and S.J. Singer, The Managed Care Backlash and the Task Force in California, *Health Affairs,* July 1, 1998: 95.

11. G. Verna, Entrepreneurial Docs Are Back, *Cincinnati Business Courier,* August 31, 1998: A-3.

12. B. Cook, Thinking First: Many Doctors Are Avoiding the Risks of Repurchasing Their Assets, *Modern Physician,* April 1, 1999: 62.

13. Cook, Thinking First, 62.

14. K. Bole, Doctors Toss License, Gain Fiscal Health, *San Francisco Business Times,* July 5, 1999: 2.

15. S. Bernstein, California Faces "Epidemic" of Bankruptcies, Medical Association Official Says, *Los Angeles Times,* September 2, 1999: A-1.

16. N.S. Kaufman, Market Dominance of PHO Entities Is Key to Achieving PHO Success, *Healthcare Financial Management,* August 1, 1998: 78.

17. A. Moorse, Spark Hasn't Caught for Provider Alliances, *Capital District Business Review,* April 26, 1999: 2.

18. Kaufman, Market Dominance of PHO Entities, 78.

19. Kaufman, Market Dominance of PHO Entities, 78.

20. Public Law 105–33, *The Balanced Budget Act of 1997.*

21. J.C. Goldsmith, The Illusive Logic of Integration, *Healthcare Forum Journal,* September/October 1994: 26–31.

22. K. Hundley, Doctor's Group, Patients Suffering, *St. Petersburg Times,* April 28, 1999: A-4.

23. Dow Jones News Service, Columbia/HCA Removing Hundreds of Doctors from Payroll, August 27, 1999.

24. Dow Jones News Service, Columbia/HCA.

25. Kaufman, Market Dominance of PHO Entities, 78.

SUGGESTED READING

Beckham, J.D. 1995. Redefining Work in the Integrated Delivery System. *Healthcare Forum Journal,* May/June: 76–82.

Boland, P. 1994. Organized Delivery Systems. *Managed Care Quarterly*: 2(4).

Burns, L.R., and Thorpe, D.P. 1993. Trends and Models in Physician–Hospital Organizations. *Health Care Management Review* 18: 7–20.

Coddington, D.C., Moore, K.D., and Fisher, E.A. 1994. *Integrated Health Care: Reorganizing the Physician, Hospital, and Health Plan Relationship.* Englewood, CO: Center for Research in Ambulatory Health Care Administration/MGMA.

Coile, R.C. 1994. Year 2000 Scenario for Physician–Hospital Organizations. *Topics in Health Care Financing* 20, no. 4: 75–83.

Conrad, D., and Hoare, G., eds. 1994. *Strategic Alignment: Managing Integrated Health Systems.* Ann Arbor, MI: Health Administration Press/AUPHA.

Dasco, S.T., and Dasco, C.C. 1996. *Managed Care Answer Book.* New York: Panel Publishers.

DeMuro, P.R. 1994. Integrated Delivery Systems. *Topics in Health Care Financing:* 20(3).

Ernst & Young LLP. 1995. Physician–Hospital Organizations: Profile 1995. Washington, DC.

Fine, A. 1993. *The Integrated Health Care Delivery Systems Manual.* New York: Thompson Publishing Group.

Fine, A., ed. 1995. *Integrated Health Care Delivery Systems: A Guide to Successful Strategies for Hospital and Physician Collaboration.* New York: Thompson Publishing Group.

Kongstvedt, P.R., and R. Gates. 1996. *Ten Critical Success Factors for Integrated Delivery Systems.* Gaithersburg, MD: Aspen Publishers.

Korenchuk, K.M. 1994. *Transforming the Delivery of Health Care: The Integration Process,* 2nd ed. Englewood, CO: Center for Research in Ambulatory Health Care Administration/MGMA.

Traska, M.R. 1996. *Managed Care Strategies 1996.* New York: Faulkner & Gray.

CHAPTER 5

Elements of the Management Control and Governance Structure

Peter R. Kongstvedt

It is not really possible to address comprehensively the topic of governance and management control structure in one chapter of a book. There are myriad courses, texts, and other learning resources that deal with the basic elements of management in depth. This chapter assumes that readers have a working knowledge of business and management, so it does not explain certain fundamental aspects of management (e.g., how to read a balance sheet, write a job description, or construct an organizational chart). Ironically, there is no standardization of management governance or control structure in managed care; for example, the function, or even the very presence, of a board of directors will vary from plan to plan. The function of key officers or managers, as well as of committees, will likewise vary depending on the type of organization, the ownership, and the motivations and skills of the individuals involved. Because each plan will construct its own management control structure to suit its needs, only a few of the most common elements are described in this chapter. Further, there are many legal and regulatory requirements (state and federal) that vary depending on many other aspects of a health plan (e.g., whether it is a for-profit or not-for-profit plan; the state in which the plan is located; whether the plan is provider owned; and whether the plan offers commercial, self-funded, Medicare, or Medicaid products).

The legal and regulatory aspects are discussed in the appropriate chapters elsewhere in this book, not here. Detailed discussions of operational activities are likewise covered elsewhere in this book. What follows in this chapter is a brief overview of certain management control elements as they pertain specifically to managed health care.

BOARD OF DIRECTORS

Many, although not all, types of managed care plans will have a board of directors. The makeup and function of the board will be influenced by many factors (discussed below), but the board has the final responsibility for governance of the operation.

Examples of plans or managed care operations that would not necessarily have their own boards would include the following:

- preadmission certification and medical case management operations of insurance companies
- preferred provider organizations (PPOs) developed by large insurance companies
- PPOs developed for single employers by an insurance company
- health maintenance organizations (HMOs) set up by a single company for purposes of serving only the employees of that company
- employer-sponsored and -developed plans (PPOs, precertification operations)
- HMOs or exclusive provider organizations set up as a line of business of an insurance company

Most of these operations or plans are subsidiaries of larger companies; those companies do have boards of directors, but their boards are involved with oversight of the entire company and not the subsidiary operation. PPOs or HMOs that are divisions of insurance companies may be required to list a board on their licensure forms, but that board may have little real operational role. The one exception noted above is an HMO set up by a single company for purposes of serving only the employees of that company; that is considered a form of self-funding and is regulated by labor laws, not insurance laws.

Board Composition

All HMOs (except the one type noted above, and that type will not be discussed further) have boards, although not all those boards are particularly functional. This is especially true for HMOs that are part of large national companies. Each local HMO is incorporated and required to have a board, but it is not uncommon for the chains to use the same two corporate officers (perhaps with one local representative—see below) as the board for every HMO. Again, the board fulfills its legal function and obligation, but the operation of the HMO is controlled through the management structure of the company rather than through a direct relationship between the plan director and the board.

The legal requirements for boards, particularly for HMOs, are spelled out in each state's laws and regulations. In the past, it was common for states to require an HMO to have at least one-third of the board be consumer representatives, but this is no longer the case. The same requirement used to exist for federal qualification, but that requirement no longer exists either.

Board composition will also vary depending on whether the plan is for-profit, in which case the owners' or shareholders' representatives may hold the majority of seats versus not-for-profit, in which case there will be broader community representation. Some not-for-profit health plans are organized as cooperatives, in which case the board members are all members of the plan. Not-for-profit plans that are not co-

operatives are generally best served by board members that are truly independent and have no potential conflicts of interest. The use of outsiders rather than plan officers as directors in any case will be dictated by local events, company bylaws, and laws and regulations (including the tax code for not-for-profit health plans). Provider-sponsored not-for-profit plans are not allowed to have more than 20 percent of their board seats held by providers. Provider-sponsored for-profit plans may have majority representation by providers and so must take special precautions to avoid antitrust problems.

Function of the Board

As stated earlier, the function of the board is governance: overseeing and maintaining final responsibility for the plan. In a real sense, the buck stops with the board. Final approval authority of corporate bylaws rests with the board. It is the bylaws that govern the basic structure of power and control not only of the plan officers but of the board itself.

The fiduciary responsibility of the board in an operating plan is clear. General oversight of the profitability or reserve status rests with the board, as does oversight and approval of significant fiscal events such as a major acquisition or a significant expenditure. In a for-profit plan, the board also has fiduciary responsibility to protect the interests of the stockholders.

Legal responsibilities of the board also may include review of reports and document signing. For example, a board officer may be required to sign the quarterly financial report to the state regulatory agency, the board chairperson may be required to sign any acquisition documents, and the board is ultimately responsible for the veracity of financial statements to stockholders.

Setting and approving policy is another common function of an active board. This may be as broad as determining the overall policy of using a gatekeeper system, or it may be as detailed as approving organizational charts and reporting structures. Although most policies and procedures will be the responsibility of the plan's officers, an active board may set requirements regarding what operational policies must be brought to the board for approval or change.

In HMOs and many other types of managed care plans, the board has a special responsibility for oversight of the quality management (QM) program, and therefore bears ultimate responsibility for the quality of care delivered to members. Usually, this responsibility is discharged through board (or board subcommittee) review of the QM documentation, including the overall QM plan and regular reports on findings and activities, and through feedback to the medical director and plan QM committee.

In free-standing plans, the board also has responsibility for hiring the chief executive officer (CEO) of the plan and for reviewing that officer's performance. The board in such plans often sets the CEO's compensation package, and the CEO reports to the board.

Active boards have committees to take up certain functions. Common board committees may include an executive committee (for rapid access to decision making and confidential discussions), a compensation committee (to set general compensation guidelines for the plan, set the CEO's compensation, and approve and issue stock options in for-profit plans), a finance committee or audit committee (to review financial results, approve budgets, set and approve spending authorities, review the annual audit, review and approve outside funding sources, and so forth), and a QM committee (as noted above).

Board Liability Issues

Any board faces the issue of liability for its actions. This is especially so in a board made up of outside directors and in a board of a not-for-profit organization. This is not to say that a board must always make correct decisions (it may make an incorrect decision in good faith), although being right is often considered superior to being wrong. Rather, it is to say that a board should act in ways to reduce its own liability, and such actions will also be consistent with good governance. It is beyond the scope of this chapter to fully discuss board liability and prevention, but a few general concepts are impor-

tant to bring out. Examples given in this section do not constitute legal opinions but are simply provided to help illustrate possible issues. Readers are urged to consult competent legal counsel as needed to fully understand board liability.

It is of utterly paramount importance that board members exercise their duties to the benefit of the plan and not in their own self-interest. Conflict of interest is a very difficult problem, and it can surface more readily than one might suppose. Examples of such conflicts would include actions that preferentially profit the board member, actions that are more in the interest of the board member than the plan (e.g., influencing how services are purchased by the plan), taking advantage of proprietary information in order to profit, and so forth. It is certainly possible for an action to benefit both the plan and the board member, but extra care must be taken to ensure that the action is first in the interest of the plan. Board members with an obvious conflict of interest should abstain from voting on an issue, or even absent themselves from discussing the issue at all.

The board must also take care that it operates within the confines of the plan bylaws. In other words, the board cannot take any action that is not allowed in the bylaws of the organization. Examples of such actions might include payment to an individual beyond the normal reimbursement policies, entering into an unrelated line of business, and so forth.

Board members must also perform their duties with some measure of diligence. For example, if plan management provides board members with information needed to properly decide on a course of action or a policy, it is incumbent on the board members to read and understand what is being provided and to ask however many questions are necessary to gain an adequate understanding to make an informed decision. Related to this is a duty to attend board meetings; while this would seem obvious, some board members may be so lax in their attendance as to provide virtually no governance or oversight. In all events, thorough documentation of the decision-making process is valuable, and this documentation should be maintained for an appropriate length of time.

As mentioned earlier, the board's primary responsibility is to the plan or organization (and to the shareholders if the plan is for-profit). The board may also have some measure of responsibility to other individuals or organizations if the plan acts in such a way as to illegally harm another party. For example, if a health plan knowingly sets a policy to not credential physicians and a panel physician commits malpractice, it is possible that the board (which either agreed to the policy or failed to change it) may have some liability.

Regardless of how the board is made up, it is important for there to be adequate director and officer liability insurance as well as insurance for errors and omissions. The need for such insurance may be attenuated by certain provisions in the company's or plan's bylaws holding the board members and officers harmless from liability. This issue requires review by legal counsel, preferably external legal counsel.

KEY MANAGEMENT POSITIONS

The roles and titles of the key managers in any plan will vary depending on the type of plan, its legal organization, its line of business, its complexity, whether it is free-standing or a satellite of another operation, and the local needs and talent. There is little consistency in this area from plan to plan. How each key role is defined (or even whether it will be present at all) is strictly up to the management of each plan. What follows, then, is a general overview of certain key roles.

Executive Director/CEO

Most plans have at least one key manager. Whether that individual is called a CEO, an executive director, a general manager, or a plan manager is a function of the items mentioned earlier in this chapter (e.g., scope of authority, reporting structure of the company). For purposes of discussion, the key manager will be referred to as an executive director in this section.

The executive director is usually responsible for all the operational aspects of the plan, although even that is not always the case. For example,

some large companies (e.g., insurance companies or national HMO chains) have marketing reporting vertically to a regional marketing director rather than through the plan manager. A few companies take that to the extreme of having each functional area reporting vertically to regional managers rather than having all operations coordinated at the local level by a single manager; thus, reporting is a function of the overall environment, and there is little standardization in the industry.

In free-standing plans and traditional HMOs, the executive director is responsible for all areas. The other officers and key managers report to the executive director, who in turn reports to the board (or to a regional manager in the case of national companies). The executive director also has responsibility for general administrative operations and public affairs.

Medical Director

Almost by definition, managed care plans will have a medical director. Whether that person is a full-time manager or a community physician who comes in a few hours per week is determined by the needs of the plan. The medical director usually has responsibility for provider relations, provider recruiting, QM, utilization management, and medical policy.

Some plans (e.g., simple PPOs) may use the medical director, or a medical consultant, only to review claims or perhaps to approve physician applications and to review patterns of utilization. The spectrum of medical director involvement parallels the spectrum of medical management activities. Usually the medical director reports to the executive director.

As a plan grows in size, particularly if it is a complex plan such as an HMO, the need for the medical director to leverage time becomes crucial. If the medical director gets bogged down in day-to-day minutia, the ability to provide leadership in the critical areas of utilization, quality, network management, and medical policy is dramatically reduced.

There are two approaches commonly employed to deal with this problem. The most common is the addition of an associate medical director. An associate medical director position usually starts as part-time, but as the plan grows in size and complexity, the position evolves into a full-time function, and in fact there may be many associate medical directors in large plans. The duties of the associate medical director are often a subset of the overall duties of the medical director; for example, an associate medical director may focus primarily on utilization management or QM. This concept of adding qualified staff is not different from basic management practices for any specialized activity, but health plan managers are occasionally slow to realize the value of adding physician managers when they may be quick to realize the value of adding multiple layers of management in other operational areas.

The second approach to the issue of leveraging medical management in a large plan is to decentralize certain functions. For example, in a closed-panel plan (e.g., a staff model HMO, or a multisite group practice), it is common to assign management responsibilities to a physician at each geographic site. This on-site physician manager may have responsibility for utilization and staffing at the site or other duties as necessary. In an open-panel setting (e.g., an open panel HMO), the network may be divided up into regions, and associate medical directors may be assigned responsibilities for designated regions. In either case, management must be realistic about the time and resources required for these associate medical directors to do their jobs. The skills, motivations, and compensation for decentralized or delegated medical management must be carefully thought through, and of course the medical director retains ultimate accountability.

The third approach to leveraging medical management in a large plan is precisely the opposite: centralize functions to a very high degree. This approach is often found in national insurance companies. For example, all precertification of hospital cases, all referral authorizations, and all report generation may occur at a single, national level. Also frequently found in large national companies is a parsing of responsibilities from the medical director to a nonmedical executive. For example, all provider contracting and network management may report to a nonclinical company officer, and the medical director would have no responsibilities for those functions.

Finance Director

In free-standing plans or large operations, it is common to have a finance director or chief financial officer. That individual is generally responsible for oversight of all financial and accounting operations. In some plans, that may include functions such as billing, management information system (MIS), enrollment, and underwriting as well as accounting, fiscal reporting, and budget preparation. The finance director usually reports to the executive director, although once again some national companies use vertical reporting.

Marketing Director

The marketing director is responsible for marketing the plan. Responsibility generally includes oversight of marketing representatives, advertising, client relations, and enrollment forecasting. A few plans have marketing generating initial premium rates, which are then sent to finance or underwriting for review, but that is uncommon. The marketing director reports to the executive director or vertically, depending on the company.

Operations Director

In larger plans, it is common to have an operations director, or COO. This position usually oversees claims, MIS, enrollment, underwriting (unless finance is doing so), member services, office management, and any other traditional backroom functions. The operations director usually reports to the executive director.

Director of Information Systems

The director of information systems, or chief information officer (CIO) has responsibility for the computer hardware and software used by the plan, as well as the telephone systems and electronic communications. Responsibility for the technical aspects of the plan's electronic commerce capabilities also usually rests with the CIO. This position may report to the chief executive officer (CEO), chief operating officer (COO), or vertically, depending on the company,

Corporate Compliance Officer

As discussed in detail in Chapter 68, health plans with a Medicare + Choice risk contract (see Chapter 55) need a corporate compliance officer. This officer's responsibility is to ensure that the plan operates in compliance with applicable regulatory requirements. There are a variety of duties that are specifically assigned to this officer, as discussed in Chapter 68.

Although the corporate compliance officer is a requirement for those plans that have a Medicare + Choice risk contract, there is a similar function required under the Health Insurance Portability and Accountability Act of 1996 (HIPAA; see Chapter 67): an official responsible for privacy policies and procedures. Specifically, HIPAA requires the following:

- designation of a privacy official who will be responsible for the development and implementation of the privacy policies and procedures
- training for all members of the work force who obtain protected health information (PHI), including an attestation every three years that the employee will honor the covered entity's privacy policies
- administrative, technical, and physical safeguards to protect the privacy of PHI, including procedures for verifying the identity and authority of requesters of information
- detailed specifications of what must be documented to ensure compliance with the regulation

As of early 2000, these requirements had not been finalized. But it is a reasonable assumption that the requirements noted here will be put into place over the next several years.

COMMITTEES

Again, there is little consistency from plan to plan regarding committees. Nonmedical committees are often ad hoc, convened to meet a specific need and then dissolved. Most plans tend to have standing committees to address management issues in defined areas, but that varies from plan to plan. An example of a common type of nonmedical committee is a consumer or member advisory committee; though having no voting rights or governance powers, this committee provides consumer or member input to plan managers.

In the medical management area, committees serve to diffuse some elements of responsibility (which can be beneficial for medical-legal reasons) and allow important input from the field into procedure and policy or even into case-specific interpretation of existing policy. These aspects are discussed in greater detail in Chapter 64.

Some examples of common medical management committees are given below. The formation, role, responsibility, and activity of any committee vary from plan to plan. More information about each of these areas may be found in the pertinent chapters of this book.

QM Committee

QM, discussed extensively in Chapter 30, is one area where a committee is essential. The QM committee will oversee setting of standards, review of data, feedback to providers, follow-up, and approval of sanctions. A peer review committee may be a subset of the QM committee, or it may be separate.

Credentialing Committee

The committee on credentialing—a topic discussed in Chapters 7, 63, and 65—may also be a subset of the QM committee, or it may be separate. In new plans with heavy credentialing needs, it is probably best for the committee to be separate. In states that require "due process" for provider termination (see Chapter 69), this is the committee most likely to take on that responsibility.

Medical Advisory Committee

Many plans have a medical advisory committee whose purpose is to review general medical management issues brought to it by the medical director. Such issues may include changes in the contract with providers, compensation, and changes in authorization procedures. This committee serves as a sounding board for the medical director. Occasionally it has voting authority, but that is rare because such authority is really vested with the board. In national companies, this committee may have input to local medical management issues, but medical issues that cross all plans (e.g., medical policy for new technology) are generally provided from a corporate-level medical policy committee.

Utilization Review Committee

The utilization review committee examines utilization issues brought to it by the medical director. Often this committee approves or reviews policy regarding coverage. This committee is also the one that reviews utilization patterns of providers and approves or reviews the process of sanctioning providers because of their utilization.

Sometimes this committee gets involved in resolving disputes between the plan and a provider regarding utilization approval and may be involved in reviewing cases for medical necessity. In large plans, this function may be further subdivided into various specialty panels for review of consultant utilization. This committee may be a subset of the medical advisory committee, or it may be free-standing.

Pharmacy and Therapeutics Committee

Plans with significant pharmacy benefits often have a pharmacy and therapeutics committee. This committee is usually charged with developing a formulary, reviewing changes to that formulary, and reviewing abnormal prescription utilization patterns by providers. This committee is usually free-standing. In national plans, the formulary may or may not be subject to local input, depending on the type of plan benefit (e.g., tiered copayments). (Pharmacy is discussed in Chapter 24.)

Medical Grievance Review Committee

In most states (and possibly the nation—Congress is considering the issue at the time of publication), a separate committee panel must be established to review member grievances regarding medical management or coverage determinations. This committee must be made up of health professionals of a specialty appropriate to the medical condition under review. This means that most health professional members of this committee will attend meetings only if their specialty is related to the type of grievance being reviewed. The medical professionals should not have been involved in the member's medical care, and if the grievance is significant, they may also be required to not be participating physicians in the plan.

Related to this is the process for external review of appeals. In those states that do not require this appeal process, this activity may be handled by a contracted group of independent physicians. In those states that require such an appeal process, an independent review organization is usually defined by the state and is not part of the plan's committee structure. It is not known at the time of publication whether the federal government will require this process as well, but it is under active debate by Congress as of early 2000, and has a high likelihood of enactment.

Discussion of both of these processes may be found in Chapter 69.

Corporate Compliance Committee

The corporate compliance committee is a function of the plan's corporate compliance program, as noted earlier in the description of the corporate compliance officer. Detailed discussion of this committee is found in Chapter 68.

MANAGEMENT CONTROL STRUCTURE

Control structure refers to issues such as reporting responsibility, spending (and other commitment) authority, hiring and firing, the conduct of performance evaluations of employees, and so forth. Each plan will set these up to fit its situation and needs. Although these issues are too diverse to be addressed in this chapter, a wealth of material on all these functions can be found in the general management literature.

One item that is of special significance is the monthly operating report (MOR). Most tightly run managed care plans develop an MOR to use as the basic management tool. The typical MOR reports the month- and year-to-date financial status of the plan. Those data are backed up with details regarding membership, premium revenue, other revenue, medical costs (usually total and broken out into categories such as hospital, primary care, referral care, ancillary services, and so forth), marketing costs, administrative costs, other expenses, taxes (if appropriate), and the bottom line. Results are generally reported in terms of whole dollars and per member per month. If the plan is not producing an MOR, it is probably not managing optimally. This is discussed in detail in Chapter 47.

How much detail is reported routinely or on an ad hoc basis is a local call. The point here is that managed care, especially in tightly run plans, is so dynamic that managers cannot wait for quarterly results. Managers must have current and reliable data from which to manage. Sutton's Law dictates that you must "go where the money is," and that can only be done if the MOR tells you where to look. In the case of hospital utilization, one cannot even wait for the MOR but must have daily reporting (see Chapter 18).

As discussed in Chapters 32, 35, and 36, many plans are now using a data warehouse. The data warehouse provides an accessible repository of data (both raw data and information that has been created from those data) to managers so as to allow them to understand the metrics of the plan without having to continually order special reports to be run at the expense of other necessary systems activities.

Related to this is a type of reporting system often referred to as an executive information system, or EIS. The EIS allows executives to obtain reports from a large selection of available information. Again, this does not require special reports to be run on the main system, nor does it require the executive to design a report or choose the data to populate the report. Various other types of reports are described throughout this book. What reports and routine reviews a manager needs to run the business is a decision each plan must make.

To paraphrase J. Edwards Deming, you can't manage what you can't measure.

CONCLUSION

The basic functions of governance and control in HMOs are similar to those in any business, although the specifics regarding the board of directors, plan officers, responsibilities of key managers, and committees vary tremendously from plan to plan.

CHAPTER 6

Examining Common Assertions about Managed Care

Richard I. Smith, Daniel Thornton, and Terry Sollom

INTRODUCTION

American health care has experienced dramatic changes in the past two decades, with managed health care principles and organizations leading the way toward a system based on new concepts in care management and service delivery. Some observers view managed health care as a direct response to a health care cost crisis whose persistence threatened the viability of the American economy. Others view managed care as a response to serious, well-documented health care quality problems—specifically, prevalent patterns of underuse, overuse, misuse, and geographical variation in medical services—that characterized much of American health care.

Both statements accurately portray the factors that brought about the widespread adoption of managed health care in this country; however, they do not capture the countless institutional and personal adjustments that have been required to accommodate such a transformation. Although change is a necessary response to a faltering system, it is rarely easy. As a leading agent of change in the American health care system, managed care

has made health coverage more affordable and created a new emphasis on quality, but not without attendant controversy.

The long process of fostering needed change in the health care system has been accompanied by extensive debates. These discussions have been fueled by statements that do not reflect how managed care actually works.

When consumers are asked directly about the quality of their personal health care, they express positive attitudes. For instance, national surveys have reported high levels of consumer satisfaction with managed care health plans. In a 1998 analysis of public attitudes, the president of the Roper Center for Public Opinion Research at the University of Connecticut stated that "huge majorities say they are satisfied with their health care, including their ability to get a doctor's appointment and the most sophisticated medical treatment."[1] A 1998 comprehensive review of surveys on public attitudes toward managed care concluded that "there is little evidence of widespread or serious dissatisfaction with health care arrangements among those who have coverage."[2] The same review also found that most people enrolled in managed care would recommend their plan to others.

Much of the political debate about managed care has been conducted around claims concerning how particular individuals' cases were handled. Recently, some media organizations have started to more closely examine these claims. For instance, in August 1998, *The Washington Post* ran a front-page story by Howard

Richard I. Smith, JD, is Vice President, Public Policy and Research, Daniel Thornton is Senior Policy Analyst, and Terry Sollom is Publications Manager at the American Association of Health Plans (AAHP). The authors gratefully acknowledge contributions from AAHP colleagues Mark Stanton and Kristin Stewart.

Kurtz, the Post's media critic, headlined "Some Managed-Care Sagas Need Second Exam."[3] Kurtz recounts several of the stories that were being covered by multiple national news organizations, including *The Washington Post*, and reported that upon further examination "such stories are often more complicated than they seem at first."

Kurtz's story cited the news media's inclination to simplify stories because "tales of woe are more compelling than abstract debates about cost and liability." In addition, confidentiality laws, Kurtz pointed out, prevent health plans from telling their side of the story: "Much of the coverage of HMOs and their alleged shortcomings is driven by personal anecdotes—or 'horror stories,' as they are known in the trade—that dramatize the supposed heartlessness of cost-cutting HMOs. Journalists and politicians rarely get the other side because health plans are barred by confidentiality laws from discussing individual cases. The patients who have publicly complained to the Clinton Administration or news organizations can waive the confidentiality of their medical records, but often refuse to do so." Kurtz verified that in at least one case, the Clinton Administration stopped talking about a breast cancer patient whose story was challenged by her health maintenance organization (HMO).

As the debate over the direction of the nation's health care system continues, it is essential that claims about how the system is working be subjected to critical analysis. If our understanding of health care in America is allowed to be based on unsubstantiated assertions and incomplete information, both the problems we define and the solutions we devise will be wrong. In this chapter, the authors seek to advance the discussion about managed care by examining just a few of the claims commonly heard in debates.

MANAGED CARE MYTHS

Health Insurance Choices

Critics of managed care claim that the growth of managed care health systems in the United States

has restricted choice. In fact, managed care has expanded health insurance coverage options available to consumers. Before the advent of HMOs, preferred provider organizations (PPOs), and other managed care plans, individuals were limited to traditional indemnity coverage. Health plans developed as a new choice for consumers, providing them access to coverage with features such as preventive care, low cost sharing (deductibles and copayments), credentialed practitioners, and quality assurance programs.

Along the same lines, a common belief prevails that health plans impose unprecedented financial penalties for use of non-network providers in point-of-service (POS) and PPO plans. In reality, high cost sharing is one of the defining characteristics of indemnity plans, whereas POS and PPO enrollees have the option to use in-network providers at lower cost sharing or non-network providers at higher cost sharing. The option of cost sharing arrangements available to POS and PPO enrollees allows greater flexibility in determining the level of financial payment—an option that individuals with indemnity coverage do not have. Fee-for-service (FFS) enrollees face higher cost sharing burdens no matter where they seek care and are not given the opportunity available to POS and PPO members to have lower cost sharing if they seek care from participating providers.

In a report commissioned by the American Association of Health Plans (AAHP), data gathered by the Barents Group LLC in 1996 show that almost two-thirds of employees offered health coverage had a choice of more than one health plan.[4] Furthermore, 92 percent of U.S. workers who received coverage through their employer were offered at least one plan (POS, PPO, or indemnity) that covered care provided by out-of-network physicians and hospitals.[5]

A misconception also exists that even when offered a choice, employers make indemnity premiums unaffordable to steer employees into choosing health plans. But analyses of employer health care subsidies show otherwise. For instance, on average, in dollar and percentage terms, employers with 200 or more employees required their employees in 1996 to pay *more* in premiums for managed care plans than for FFS.[6] And, even though employers charged employees higher premiums when they chose health plans, the percentage of employees choosing an HMO far exceeded the percentage whose employers offered HMOs but no other types of plans. Slightly less than 2 percent of all employees in firms with 5,000 or more employees were offered only one or more HMOs in 1996, but 38 percent of all employees in firms with more than 5,000 employees enrolled in HMOs.[7]

In the public sector, employees make similar choices. In 1996, public employees in 45 states were offered a choice between an HMO or a POS product and an FFS plan: 43 percent of these states' active employees chose an HMO or POS plan; and, in 11 states, the proportion of state government employees enrolled in either HMO or POS health plans surpassed 70 percent (in the previous year, only four states had more than 70 percent of their active employees in HMOs).[8]

Health Care Quality

In the public debate, managed care plan members often are portrayed as receiving lower quality care than is available through traditional indemnity coverage. Notwithstanding this portrayal, a pattern of largely positive findings about quality of care in HMOs has been documented in comprehensive literature reviews published in 1994 and 1997 and has continued to hold true in studies published since early 1997.[9] A review of 15 studies on the quality of care published between late 1993 and early 1997 found that for 18 of 24 indicators of quality of care, HMO care was better than or as good as care provided in other settings.[10] Another, earlier review of 16 studies on quality of care issued between 1980 and 1993 found that for 14 of 17 indicators of quality of care, HMO care was better than or equal to care provided in other settings.[11]

Among the numerous studies (in addition to the literature reviews mentioned earlier) documenting that consumers with health plan coverage receive superior or comparable quality care than those with FFS coverage are the following:

- A review of 17 studies published between 1987 and 1995 examining the quality of cardiovascular care found that the process and outcomes of care in HMOs were better than or equal to care in non-HMO settings.[12] For example, researchers included process measures in the areas of preventive care, hypertension, acute chest pain, congestive heart failure, stroke, and hypercholesterolemia. Of the 107 measures studies, 35 measures (33 percent) showed better performance by HMOs, 67 (63 percent) showed no difference between HMO and non-HMO settings, and only 5 (5 percent) yielded better performance by non-HMO settings.

- A study of more than 88,000 intensive care unit admissions in 1992 showed that both elderly and nonelderly HMO patients had a statistically significant lower level of mortality than patients enrolled in FFS plans.[13]

- A study examining outcomes of home care after hospitalization for HMO and traditional Medicare patients with any of 6 different conditions discharged during 1988 and 1989 showed that both groups had similar functional status and rehospitalization rates at six weeks and six months.[14]

- A study comparing treatment and mortality risk of almost 1,000 prostate cancer patients receiving care in FFS and HMO settings in Washington state from 1981 to 1989 found the mortality risk was lower for the HMO patients over a six-year period; the difference was greatest for patients in the lowest income category.[15]

Utilization Review and Medical Necessity

Critics of managed care claim that utilization review personnel routinely overrule doctors' decisions on necessary treatment. In fact, coverage denial rates for physician recommendations are very low. Refuting these oft-repeated claims is a national survey of more than 2,000 physicians caring for patients in plans that use managed care techniques that revealed the final coverage denial rate for physician recommendations within eight categories of care was at most 3 percent and much less for most categories of care.[16] Initial denial rates were somewhat higher, but between one-half and two-thirds of initial denials were reversed by the health plan, resulting in the lower rates. Coverage for hospitalization was denied only 1 percent of the time; surgical procedures 1.2 percent; and specialist referrals 2.6 percent.[17]

Utilization review programs are developed with extensive input from physicians and other clinical experts.[18] Recognizing the quality problems that managed care strategies are designed to address, private-sector accreditation bodies have established requirements for monitoring underutilization and overutilization of health services.[19] In addition, these accreditation organizations and many states require that all denials based on medical necessity be made or reviewed by physicians.[20]

Utilization review frequently is said to rely on rigid protocols that fail to take individual patient needs into account. AAHP has examined this claim as it pertains to inpatient hospital lengths of stay. A 1997 AAHP analysis of MEDSTAT Group data from 1995 compared a set of Milliman & Robertson (M&R) guidelines (that represent utilization targets reflective of an ideal delivery system for patients without complications) to actual length of stay in HMO and FFS plans for specific procedures. The M&R guidelines for these procedures were identified in a survey by the American College of Surgeons (ACS) as examples of "coverage limits" used by health plans.[21] The analysis showed that the proportion of HMO admissions that met or exceeded the range recommended by surgeons was nearly identical to the proportion of FFS admissions. AAHP's analysis found that 91.9 percent of HMO admissions and 92.3 percent of FFS admissions had lengths of stays that were equal to or greater than M&R guidelines.[22]

As expected, within each diagnosis-related group (DRG), length of stay for HMO members varied. For example, within DRG 105 (cardiac valve procedures without cardiac catheterization), two-thirds of the 52 admissions had a length of stay ranging from 3 to 10 days (the range reported as appropriate in the ACS survey), and 29 percent had a length of stay exceeding 10 days. Four percent had a length of stay ranging from one to two days, and 29 percent had a length of stay ranging from 11 to 26 days. These findings are a clear indication that "rigid" guidelines are not dictating length of stay.

Managed Care and Physician Liability

Health plans are sometimes said to expose physicians to increased medical malpractice claims by limiting the services that are covered. First, plans do not "limit" services; rather, they provide coverage that purchasers choose to include in their contracts with health insurers. Second, as more physicians have contracted with managed care plans and as health plan enrollment has grown, physician liability claims and malpractice insurance premiums have decreased.

Between 1985 and 1996, HMO enrollment increased from 18.9 to 67.5 million individuals. Over the same period, the American Medical Association reports that liability claims per 100 physicians dropped from 10.2 to 9.0.[23] Furthermore, the percentage of physicians incurring professional liability claims decreased from 8.5 percent in 1985 to 7.7 percent in 1996.[24] This was occurring during a time when the percentage of physicians with any managed care contracts grew from 61 percent (in 1990, earlier years not available) to 88 percent (in 1996).[25]

Hospital Length of Stay and Site of Care

Federal and state regulation and legislative proposals pertaining to hospital length of stay for specific conditions have been prompted by concerns that managed care plans are not providing coverage for the full medically necessary length of hospital stay. The facts are dramatically at odds with this portrayal.

As discussed earlier, an analysis of length-of-stay patterns among commercially insured patients in 1995 shows there is a gap between rhetoric and reality. Using MEDSTAT Group data, AAHP determined that 95 percent of both HMO and indemnity hospital admissions had a length of stay that fell within the length-of-stay range, or exceeded the high end of the range, recommended by surgeons surveyed by the ACS.[26] The other 5 percent of admissions fell below the recommended length-of-stay range for both HMO and indemnity enrollees. The analysis looked at only those admissions with DRGs that included at least one of the procedures used in the ACS survey.

Another prevalent misconception is that health plans require mastectomies to be performed on an outpatient basis and disallow any inpatient care. Data from two states prove otherwise. The New York Department of Health reported that of the 124 outpatient mastectomies in the state in 1995, 72 procedures (58 percent) were performed for women in FFS Medicare; 2 (1.6 percent) for women in Medicare HMOs; and 15 (13 percent) in HMOs serving commercial, non-Medicare enrollees.[27] Similarly, data from the Maryland Health Services Cost Review Commission show that the largest number of outpatient mastectomies was performed for women in Medicare FFS. Of the approximately 540 outpatient mastectomies in the state in 1996, 201 were performed for women in traditional Medicare, none for women in Medicare HMOs, 189 for private FFS subscribers, and 107 in private non-Medicare HMOs.[28] An analysis of commercial market data by The MEDSTAT Group prepared for AAHP found that, overall, there was not a statistically significant difference in outpatient mastectomy rates among women in indemnity, HMO, PPO, and POS plans in 1993 and 1994.[29]

The history of the outpatient mastectomy procedure is instructive in looking at how widespread assertions about managed care have prevailed despite evidence to the contrary. Although outpatient mastectomy is attributed to managed care in the public debate, in fact the procedure was originated by physicians outside of a managed care context. For instance, in the early 1990s, physicians and clinical researchers at the Johns Hopkins University Breast Center were part of a pioneering group that developed a protocol for outpatient mastectomies, for certain types of breast cancer, after determining that women released early from the hospital experienced lower infection rates and high levels of satisfaction with care.[30] Other researchers have

found similar results: Henry Ford Hospital in Michigan reported that recuperation at home led to accelerated physical recovery, earlier return to occupational activities, and numerous psychological advantages,[31] and the New Jersey College of Medicine found lower rates of postoperative infection and high levels of satisfaction.[32] Of the 600 women who went to the Hopkins Breast Center in 1996 for mastectomies and lumpectomies, 83 percent left the same day.[33] It was during this time period that managed care plans began to offer this Johns Hopkins–style of care for limited types of breast cancer.

Health Status of Managed Care Enrollees

Critics of managed care contend that health plans achieve the quality and positive outcomes they do because they enroll a healthier population. Although critics claim that health plans avoid enrolling sick patients, research shows that HMOs and indemnity plans enroll similar proportions of members who are in poor health.

The Congressional Research Service reported that physician visits differed only slightly in 1994 between people of all age groups enrolled in HMOs and those with FFS because the two groups' "average health status"—as measured by the percentage of people who have chronic health problems—differed very little.[34] Furthermore, according to the U.S. National Center for Health Statistics, 37 percent of people enrolled in indemnity insurance plans and 37 percent of those in HMOs reported that they had a medical condition of any kind in 1994.[35] Among those covered by indemnity plans, 30.7 percent reported one or more chronic medical conditions versus 29.9 percent of those in HMOs.[36]

Furthermore, while individuals in low-income families have been found to generally be in poorer health than higher income individuals,[37] HMOs enroll a higher proportion of individuals in low-income households than indemnity plans. For example, a survey of 165,000 households in 1997 found that 40 percent of insured individuals younger than 65 in families with annual incomes less than $25,000 were enrolled in HMOs, whereas only 18.6 percent of individuals in such families were enrolled in FFS.[38]

Access to Specialty Care

A widely repeated charge against managed care plans is that enrollees have a difficult time accessing specialty care. However, research studies published in the last five years show that health plan members have good access to specialists.

- According to researchers from Johns Hopkins University, who analyzed National Ambulatory Medical Care Surveys from 1989 to 1994, primary care visits in HMOs were 66 percent more likely than such visits by indemnity patients to lead to a referral: 6.3 percent of all HMO member office visits to primary care physicians resulted in a referral being made during the visit compared with just 3.8 percent of indemnity plan members receiving a referral.[39] This demonstrates the accessibility of specialty care within HMOs, which often require referrals for such care.

    The researchers also reported that from 1989 to 1994 the percent of primary care physician visits that resulted in a referral increased by 58 percent for HMOs, compared to just 27 percent for indemnity plans. In addition, referrals from specialist to specialist occurred with about the same frequency in HMOs and indemnity plans: Among HMO members, 2.8 percent of specialist visits led to a cross-referral to another specialist, compared to 2.5 percent in indemnity plans.[40]
- A 1999 physician survey conducted by the journal *Medical Economics* showed that in eight of nine non-primary care specialty areas, HMO patients had as many or more office visits per patient than non-HMO patients. For example, 87 percent of gastroenterologists surveyed said they participated in HMOs in 1998: HMO enrollees accounted for 26 percent of their patients and 28 percent of their office visits.[41]
- A study of the Medicaid program in Wisconsin found that 25.9 percent of HMO beneficiaries in 1993 saw a specialist physician at least once within the year, compared to only 8.8 percent of FFS beneficiaries.[42]

- A national survey of more than 11,000 individuals in households with annual incomes less than $15,000 found that low-income individuals enrolled in HMOs and PPOs were as likely to have seen a specialist (64.1 percent and 63.1 percent) within the last year as those enrolled in FFS plans (63.3 percent).[43]
- An Arthritis Foundation–sponsored study of HMO patients with rheumatoid arthritis found no significant difference in number of office visits with rheumatologists, number of outpatient surgeries, or number of hospital admissions when compared with FFS patients.[44]

Likewise, the quality studies cited earlier in this chapter cover numerous areas, such as cardiovascular care and intensive care, in which specialty care predominates.

Women's Health Care

Although some policymakers have proposed to legislate the details of specialty care for women's services on the basis of notions that women do not have effective access to obstetrical and gynecological care, data show that women in HMOs are more likely to obtain the benefits of obstetrics/gynecology (OB/GYN) examinations than their counterparts in indemnity plans. In many categories of care, health plans lead the market in covering and providing preventive, as well as diagnostic and therapeutic, services for women.

Cancer Screening and Treatment

Women in Medicare HMOs from 1988 to 1993 were more likely to have had their breast cancer diagnosed at an earlier and therefore more treatable stage than women in Medicare FFS, according to research published in 1999 and sponsored by the federal Health Care Financing Administration and the National Cancer Institute.[45] Women in HMOs were more likely to obtain mammograms, Pap tests, and clinical breast examinations than were women in indemnity plans (62 percent versus 50 percent, 65 percent versus 53 percent, 71 percent versus 61 percent), according to a 1994 report by the federal Centers for Disease Control and Prevention on cancer screening among women.[46] A 1997 study of 10-year survival and treatment rates among women aged 65 and older with breast cancer revealed that women enrolled in two large Medicare HMOs had survival outcomes at least equal to and possibly better than women in Medicare FFS.[47] In addition, use of breast-conserving surgery, the recommended treatment for early-stage breast cancer, was found to be more frequent for the HMO enrollees.[48]

Prenatal Care

A study of more than 24,000 births in the early 1990s in six HMOs showed that HMO prenatal care surpassed the national average in several key areas: For example, 87 percent of HMO women had their initial prenatal care visits during the first trimester compared with a national average of 76 percent; and 93 percent of HMO women had their blood pressure checked at each visit compared with a national average of 67 percent.[49]

Well-Woman Care

In the early 1990s, studies began documenting health plans' predominance in offering preventive services for women. As of 1993, 99 percent of HMOs covered annual gynecological examinations, compared with 49 percent of large-group indemnity plans.[50] In addition, 100 percent of HMOs covered annual Pap tests compared with 67 percent of indemnity insurers; and 98 percent of HMOs covered chlamydia (the most common sexually transmitted disease among women) cultures, compared with 70 percent of large-group indemnity insurers.[51] A 1998 Commonwealth Fund survey found that women in managed care plans are more likely than women in FFS plans to identify a particular doctor as their regular source of care (87 percent versus 78 percent), to have seen an OB/GYN as their primary care physician (66 percent versus 61 percent), and to have received a Pap smear in the last three years (74 percent versus 67 percent).[52]

Reproductive Health Services

As of 1993, 93 percent of HMOs provided contraceptive coverage compared with 51 percent of typical policies offered by large-group indemnity plans.[53] Furthermore, 90 percent of HMOs routinely cover infertility diagnostic procedures compared with 61 percent of indemnity plans.[54]

Involvement in Clinical Trials

A report released by the U.S. General Accounting Office (GAO) in September 1999 highlighted the current state of affairs affecting patient participation in National Institutes of Health–sponsored clinical trials.[55] Findings in this report are contrary to claims that health plans cause poor enrollment in clinical trials. In general, research shows that health plans often cover the routine patient care costs of clinical trials and that enrollment in these trials is more than adequate to conduct studies.

The GAO report found that almost all of the insurers surveyed examine the appropriateness of coverage for trials on a case-by-case basis. When insurers determine that coverage is in a patient's best interest, they typically cover the cost of the routine care associated with the trial and care that would have been otherwise provided. Moreover, the Congressional Budget Office estimates that health plans currently pay at least 90 percent of clinical trial-related patient care costs.[56]

In concluding that it found no evidence to support claims that managed care has impeded participation in clinical trials, the GAO noted that there are a number of impediments to the enrollment process that are independent of how care is financed. Despite the significant increase over time in the number of trials being conducted, the GAO reported that enrollment in these trials often meets or exceeds expectations. Given that managed care enrollment has grown over time, current clinical trial enrollment trends demonstrate that patient access to such trials has not been reduced by the growth in managed care.

Physician-Patient Interaction

Critics of managed care organizations assert that physicians are forced to see too many patients and spend too little time with each patient.

In fact, physicians are spending more time with patients. According to calculations based on data reported by the American Medical Association, physicians spent more time on patient care activities per patient visit in 1998 (29.5 minutes) than in 1985 (26.3 minutes).[57] This encompasses patient visits in all settings, including hospitals, clinics, and other visits.

Physician-Health Plan Contract Provisions

In the mid-1990s, the issue of "gag rules" came to the forefront of the managed care debate. Some policymakers asserted that health plans used such rules to restrict physician-patient communication about available treatment options. Contrary to these claims, a GAO survey conducted in 1997 found that among 1,150 physician contracts with 529 HMOs none used contract clauses that specifically restricted physicians from discussing all appropriate medical options with their patients. Moreover, 67 percent of the contracts that had business clauses (such as nondisparagement, nonsolicitation, or confidentiality clauses) included specific "anti-gag" provisions, which encourage discussion of all appropriate medical options between physician and patient.[58]

Physician Income and Industry Profits

The public debate often includes claims that managed care plans sacrifice quality of care to generate large profits. But a comparison of profit margins both within the health care industry and across multiple industries does not substantiate the notion of managed care as a high-profit type of business. A Standard & Poor's (S&P) analysis of profit margins from 1993 to 1997 in different industries determined that managed care ranked "29" out of 39 industries, with "1" having the highest margin.[59] Within the health care industry, managed care's profit margin ranked "9" out of 12.

A related misconception is that the increased presence of health plans has caused hospitals to lose money. In fact, from 1993 to 1997, profit margins for hospitals in "high" and "low" managed care markets were similar and increased each year except in 1996. For example, in 1993, hospital profit margins were 3.1 percent and 3.7 percent for high and low markets; in 1995 they were 4.6 percent and 4.2 percent; and in 1997, 5.1 percent and 5.2 percent.[60]

Recent federal and state legislative activity concerning attempts to allow physicians to collectively bargain for reimbursement rates and working conditions has focused renewed attention on physician income. The perception is that physician income has decreased because of managed care; however, as HMO enrollment has grown, income has increased. Between 1987 and 1997, HMO enrollment grew 177 percent, from 29.3 to 81.3 million enrollees; during this same period, mean physician net income rose 50.9 percent.[61]

CONCLUSION

The claims made by opponents of managed care are often simply wrong, whereas other claims are provided without any of the context needed to evaluate them properly. By examining some of the more common assertions about managed care, it becomes clear that an informed debate cannot take place without a reasoned discussion of all the facts and a thorough evaluation of not only managed care but of the other components of the American health care system.

REFERENCES AND NOTES

1. E. Ladd, Health Care Hysteria, Part II, op ed., *New York Times*, July 23, 1998.

2. K. Bowman, *Health Care Attitudes Today*, American Enterprise Institute, 1998.

3. H. Kurtz, Some Managed-Care Sagas Need Second Exam, *The Washington Post*, August 10, 1998.

4. Barents Group LLC, *Characteristics of Health Plan Choices Available to Employees Through Employer-Based Health Benefits 1996*, June 1997.

5. Barents Group, *Characteristics of Health Plan Choices*.

6. KPMG Peat Marwick, *KPMG Survey of Employee Health Benefits*, 1997.

7. Barents Group, *Characteristics of Health Plan Choices.*

8. The data do not include enrollment in PPOs. American Association of Health Plans calculation based on Segal Company data from *1996 Survey of State Employee Health Benefit Plans*, 1997.

9. R. Miller and H. Luft, Managed Care Plan Performance Since 1980, *Journal of the American Medical Association*, May 1994; R. Miller and H. Luft, Does Managed Care Lead to Better or Worse Quality of Care, *Health Affairs*, September/October 1997.

10. R. Miller and H. Luft, *Health Affairs*, September/October 1997.

11. R. Miller and H. Luft, *Journal of the American Medical Association*, May 1994.

12. J. Seidman et al., Review of Studies That Compare the Quality of Cardiovascular Care in HMO versus Non-HMO Settings, *Medical Care*, December 1998.

13. D. Angus et al., The Effect of Managed Care on ICU Length of Stay, *Journal of the American Medical Association*, October 1996.

14. J. Holtzman et al., The Effect of HMO Status on the Outcomes of Home-Care After Hospitalization in a Medicare Setting, *Journal of the American Geriatrics Society*, May-June 1998.

15. H. Greenwald and S. Henke, HMO Membership, Treatment and Mortality Risk among Prostatic Cancer Patients, *American Journal of Public Health,* August 1992.

16. D. Remler et al., What Do Managed Care Plans Do To Affect Care, *Inquiry*, Fall 1997. A recent survey conducted by the Kaiser Family Foundation (KFF) found that 87 percent of doctors reported that they have experienced "some type of denial" of coverage for health services by a health plan over the last two years (KFF and Harvard University School of Public Health, *Survey of Physicians and Nurses*, July 1999). However, these results are not comparable to the results of the Remler study because they are not expressed as a statistical "rate" of denial. Instead, the KFF survey indicates the number of physicians who experienced "some type of denial," without reporting the total number of physician recommendations and thus gives no indication as to the actual percentage of services recommended that are denied. Consequently, in the KFF survey, if one physician experienced one coverage denial out of approximately 10,000 patient visits during the two-year period, then that one denial was included in the 87 percent finding. (Number of patient visits is based on calculations from the American Medical Association's *Physician Socioeconomic Statistics 1999-2000* publication, which states that physicians have an average of 105 patient visits per week, translating into more than 5,000 visits per year, assuming a 48-week work year.)

17. D. Remler et al., What Do Managed Care Plans Do?

18. M. Schlesinger et al., Medical Professionalism under Managed Care: The Pros and Cons of Utilization Review, *Health Affairs*, Jan./Feb. 1997.

19. National Committee for Quality Assurance, *2000 Surveyor Guidelines for the Accreditation of Managed Care Organizations*, 1999, 183.

20. National Committee for Quality Assurance, *2000 Surveyor Guidelines*, 142; National Association of Insurance Commissioners, *Utilization Review Model Act*, 1996.

21. American Association of Health Plans, *An Analysis of Inpatient Hospital Lengths of Stay for Selected Diagnosis Related Groups*, Oct. 1997.

22. American Association of Health Plans, *An Analysis of Inpatient Hospital Lengths of Stay.*

23. American Medical Association, *Socioeconomic Characteristics of Medical Practice 1996–1997*, 1997.

24. American Medical Association, *Socioeconomic Characteristics 1996-1997.*

25. American Medical Association, *Socioeconomic Characteristics 1996-1997*; American Medical Association, *Socioeconomic Characteristics of Medical Practice 1994-1995*, 1995.

26. American Association of Health Plans, *An Analysis of Inpatient Hospital Lengths of Stay.*

27. Of the remaining procedures, 3 were performed on women in traditional Medicaid, 2 were for women in Medicaid HMOs, 15 for Blue Cross indemnity subscribers, 10 for other commercial indemnity subscribers, 3 for people who self-paid, and 2 were "other." Data from the New York State Department of Health, Bureau of Quality Management and Outcome Research.

28. Of the remaining procedures, 12 were performed on women in traditional Medicaid, 6 or fewer for women in Medicaid HMOs, and 25 were "other." Data from the Maryland Health Services Cost Review Commission.

29. MEDSTAT Group, *An Analysis of Outpatient Mastectomy Procedures 1993–1994.*

30. L. Shockney, Testimony before the U.S. Senate Finance Subcommittee on Health Care on Senate Bill 249, "Women's Health and Cancer Rights Act," Nov. 5, 1997.

31. A. Kambouris, Physical, Psychological, and Economic Advantages of Accelerated Treatment for Breast Cancer, *The American Surgeon,* February 1996.

32. M.H. Seltzer, Partial Mastectomy and Limited Axillary Dissection Performed as a Same Day Surgical Procedure in the Treatment of Breast Cancer. *International Surgery*, *80* (1) (1995): 79–81.

33. A. Goldstein, Rise in Outpatient Mastectomies Drives Legislation but Little Basic Research, *The Washington Post*, Nov. 19, 1997; Johannes, More HMOs Order Outpatient Mastectomies, *Wall Street Journal*, Nov. 6, 1996.

34. Congressional Research Service (CRS), Health Insurance and Medical Care: Physician Services under Managed Care, *CRS Report for Congress*, March 1998.

35. U.S. National Center for Health Statistics, *1994 National Health Interview Survey*, 1996.

36. U.S. National Center for Health Statistics, *1994 National Health Interview Survey*.

37. U.S. National Center for Health Statistics, *Health—United States—1998*, 1998.

38. U.S. National Center for Health Statistics, *1994 National Health Interview Survey*.

39. C.B. Forrest and R.J. Reid, Passing the Baton: HMOs' Influence on Referrals to Specialty Care. *Health Affairs* (1997, November/December): 157–62.

40. C.B. Forrest and R.J. Reid, Passing the Baton.

41. K. Terry, *Medical Economics*, Dec. 6, 1999.

42. K. Piper and P. Bartels, Medicaid Primary Care: HMOs or Fee-for-Service? *Public Welfare*, Spring 1995.

43. National Research Corporation, *Healthcare Market Guide*, Sept. 1997.

44. E. Yelin et al., Health Care Utilization and Outcomes among Persons with Rheumatoid Arthritis in Fee for Service and Prepaid Group Practice Settings, *Journal of the American Medical Association*, October 2, 1996.

45. G. Riley et al., Stage at Diagnosis and Treatment Patterns among Older Women with Breast Cancer, *Journal of the American Medical Association 285* (1999).

46. U.S. Center for Disease Control and Prevention/National Center for Health Statistics, *Advance Data No. 254*, August 1994.

47. A. Potosky et al., Breast Cancer Survival and Treatment in HMO and Fee for Service Settings, *Journal of the National Cancer Institute*, November 1997.

48. Potosky, Breast Cancer Survival and Treatment.

49. Y. Murata et al., *Archives of Family Medicine*, January 1994.

50. Alan Guttmacher Institute, *Uneven and Unequal: Insurance Coverage and Reproductive Health Services,* 1994.

51. Alan Guttmacher Institute, *Uneven and Unequal*.

52. The Commonwealth Fund, *Health Concerns Across a Woman's Lifespan: 1998 Survey of Women's Health,* May 1999.

53. Alan Guttmacher Institute, *Uneven and Unequal*.

54. Alan Guttmacher Institute, *Uneven and Unequal*.

55. U.S. General Accounting Office, *NIH Clinical Trials: Various Factors Affect Patient Participation*, September 1999.

56. Congressional Budget Office, *Cost Estimate for H.R.3605/S.1890, the Patients' Bill of Rights Act of 1998*, July 16, 1998.

57. American Medical Association, *Socioeconomic Characteristics of Medical Practice 1997–1998*, 1998; AMA, *Physician Socioeconomic Statistics 1999-2000*, 1999. The time spent per patient was calculated by dividing the mean number of hours spent in patient care activities per week by the mean number of total patient visits per week (1985: 51.3 and 117.1, respectively; 1998: 51.7 and 105.0, respectively).

58. U.S. General Accounting Office, *Explicit Gag Clauses Not Found in HMO Contracts, But Physician Concerns Remain*, August 1997.

59. U.S. General Accounting Office, *Explicit Gag Clauses Not Found in HMO Contracts*.

60. American Association of Health Plans, *Standard & Poor's DRI Analysis of Managed Care Industry Profit Margins*, February 1999.

61. American Medical Association, Socioeconomic Characteristics of Medical Practice 1997–1998 (1998).

PART II

The Health Care Delivery System

"When one's all right, he's prone to spite
The doctor's peaceful mission.
But when he's sick, it's loud and quick
He bawls for a physician."

Eugene Field
(1850–1895)
Doctors, st. 2, [1890]

CHAPTER 7

Primary Care in Managed Health Care Plans

Peter R. Kongstvedt

INTRODUCTION AND DEFINITIONS

In all types of health care delivery and health plans, the role of the primary care physician (PCP) is important. Even in the absence of a health plan design that requires enrollees to access their PCP in order to obtain either direct care or referral authorization for specialty care (so-called gatekeeper or coordinating physician types of health plans), a great deal of the regular health care of Americans is provided by PCPs. So the place to begin is with definitions of what specialties are considered primary care. In virtually all systems, care rendered by physicians in the specialties of family practice, internal medicine, and pediatrics is considered primary care. General practitioners (i.e., physicians who have not obtained full residency training beyond their internships) may also be considered PCPs, but their use by managed care organizations (MCOs) is quite low except in rural or underserved areas where there may not be sufficient residency-trained PCPs.

Many specialists in obstetrics and gynecology (OB/GYN) feel that they deliver primary care to their patients. They argue that they are often the only physician a young woman sees for many years. This is true in the case of generally healthy young women, but it is not always so when medical problems not involving the female reproductive tract occur. In at least one program designed to retrain OB/GYN physicians to provide a broader range of primary care, the results were disappointing, with a very high drop-out rate and a high level of dissatisfaction with broad primary care expressed by the OB/GYNs.[1]

Most plans allow direct access to OB/GYNs for female members;* this includes plans that capitate primary care or otherwise use PCPs as case managers (i.e., use a gatekeeper system). In that case, the PCP and the OB/GYN split the care (and often the capitation, if that is the reimbursement system in use). Plans that capitate must define what services are to be delivered by each. For example, the OB/GYN may be seen without referral for Pap smears and pelvic examinations, pregnancy, sterilization procedures, and so forth. For clinical care that is out of the scope of normal OB/GYN practice, the member must see the PCP for either treatment or referral to specialist.

While it is common for PCPs to be trained in primary care, there are certain clinical circumstances when it is better for a specialist to act as the PCP; this is discussed below and in Chapters 18 and 23. There are also a few plans that use what they refer to as a *flexible gatekeeper,* a term applied to those MCOs that require a member to choose a PCP to coordinate and authorize services but allow that PCP to be a specialty physician. For example, a member may choose a cardiologist as a PCP, since the cardiologist is also an internist. This allows for members to choose PCPs according to their primary medical needs,

---

*It should be noted that in addition to simple marketplace demands, many states have passed laws requiring health plans to allow direct access to OB/GYNs.

although it increases the likelihood of adverse selection to the panels of those specialty physicians in the event that the PCP is capitated; this may therefore require some adjustments (see Chapter 8).

Unlike previous editions of *The Managed Health Care Handbook*, this edition does not include a separate chapter dealing with recruiting and staffing issues in group and staff model health maintenance organizations (HMOs). This is due to the dramatic decline in the number of them still operating as such (Kaiser Permanente and a few others not withstanding, many HMOs that were once group or staff model plans no longer have the physician component). The focus is on open-panel MCOs, although some staffing issues in closed-panel MCOs or manged care medical groups are also included later in this chapter. Many of the other topics discussed are equally germane to any HMO model type.

RECRUITING

Young or newly forming plans will concentrate primarily on initial network development. Mature plans will concentrate more on network maintenance (discussed later in this chapter), although recruiting to fill in areas with suboptimal access will always be an ongoing process, particularly during periods of high growth or expansion into a new service area.

The ease of recruiting is influenced by many factors. Markets that are heavily saturated with managed care plans may have difficulty recruiting PCPs (or specialists) if those providers see no need to sign up with yet another plan. Conversely, competition may be so fierce, or there may be so many (underutilized) providers, that recruiting will be easier. In any event, recruiting and credentialing PCPs is best done by means of an orderly approach in order to avoid unnecessary delays or failure to recruit in the areas of highest need.

Access Needs

Consider geographic requirements first. This generally breaks down into three main needs: to

target potential new members, to provide good access to areas with high concentrations of members (discussed below), and to use contracted hospitals.

In the first case, primary target markets should already have been identified (e.g., a large and growing suburban-industrial community). In the second case, the plan should be analyzing access needs on a regular basis, as noted below. In the third case, recruiting physicians from the medical staff of a contracting hospital is required, rather than physicians who practice only at a noncontracting hospital, even if it is in the targeted area. Priorities will also be affected by the availability, acceptability (to plan managers, potential members, and the rest of the medical panel), scope of practice, and practice capacities of physicians in target areas.

In addition to the broad geographic and hospital-related needs, it is important to consider accessibility in general. There are a number of ways to do this. One method is to look at the number of physicians per 1,000 members. The composition of a health plan's provider network is determined by marketing considerations and by need for coverage. With respect to marketing needs, it is generally accepted that the broader the network, the more desirable it will be in the marketplace. Provider network need may also be calculated using specialty-specific ratios of physicians per 1,000 enrollees. A 1991 source suggests plan networks typically had a physician-to-enrollee ratio of 0.8 primary care physician per 1,000 enrollees and 1.3 total physicians per 1,000 enrollees.[2] A more recent source cites two mature staff model HMOs with 1.8 total physicians per 1,000 enrollees; this is a significantly more generous level of staffing than the typically "lean" staffing of HMOs and is close to the national average physician-to-population ratios.[3]

In a large-scale report using 1997 data,[4] HMOs nationally on average reported 10.4 PCPs per 1,000 members (or 220 members per PCP), with a range of 155 members per PCP in open-panel or independent practice association (IPA) HMOs, to 779 members per PCP in staff model plans; the average number of PCPs per 1,000 represented a 30 percent increase in one year. The ratio of specialists to primary care physicians was 2.2, with 23.9 specialists per 1,000 members. The average HMO had 3,044 physicians, up 13.7 percent from 2,768 in 1996. However, ratios vary widely by plan model type, scope of physician practice, and plan size.

It is more useful to look at the number of members each physician must accept (on the basis of contractual terms, see Chapter 62). The ratios of physicians to members in open panels can vary tremendously depending on age of the plan, geographic access needs, the product lines being sold (e.g., a Medicare risk product may require a higher number of physicians than will a commercial), maturity of the marketplace in general, number of open practices, and marketing needs.

Another useful measure is geographic accessibility. This is generally calculated through one of two methods: drive time or the number of PCPs by geographic availability. Drive time refers to how long members in the plan's service area have to drive to reach a PCP (or a PCP with an open practice, that is, one still accepting new patients). In general, drive time should be no more than 15 minutes, although 30 minutes may be appropriate for certain rural areas. A drive time of 20 minutes may be acceptable for access from a purely medical viewpoint, but it may not be as acceptable in a heavily urbanized market.

Analyzing the number of PCPs by geographic availability is also useful. Generally, there should be at least two PCPs within 2 or 3 miles of each ZIP code from which the plan will be drawing members (the density is usually greater in urban areas and less in rural areas). Another measure of geographic availability is the radius from where the members live (e.g., two PCPs within an 8-mile radius for urban areas and two PCPs within a 20-mile radius for rural areas). Again, these ratios may represent a minimum configuration and will not necessarily be acceptable in a specific marketplace.

Closed Panel Access Needs

While the focus of this chapter is on open-panel MCOs, it is still worthwhile noting some data from closed-panel plans. These data help il-lustrate the types of access needs found in the most saturated type of managed care setting (i.e., the physicians only see members of the HMO).

Based on research published in 1995, there appears to be some differences in staffing ratios between "large" and "small" closed-panel HMOs, with the difference occurring when the HMO has approximately 80,000 members. In plans with less than 80,000 members, the weighted mean PCP staffing ratio (rounded) was 0.89:1,000, with a standard deviation of 0.68; for plans with more than 80,000 members, the weighted mean PCP staffing ratio (rounded) was 0.66:1,000, with a standard deviation of 0.51. The weighted mean staffing ratio for all physicians (not just PCPs) was 2.8:1,000 for small plans and 1.2:1,000 for large plans. The majority of closed-panel HMOs increased their staffing ratios for Medicare members to a mean of 1.6:1,000 Medicare enrollees.[5]

These data compare with data published in 1992 that were obtained at an earlier point in time from essentially the same sources, in which large, closed-panel plans serving a primarily commercial population had an average PCP staffing ratio of 0.8:1,000 and an average physician staffing ratio of 1.3:1,000. Smaller plans had more than twice those ratios. In the 1992 data the ratios per 1,000 members, by specialty type, were 0.3 for full-time general/family practice, 0.3 for internal medicine, 0.2 for pediatrics, and 0.1 for OB/GYN.[6] When looking solely at general pediatricians for *pediatric* enrollees (as opposed to all enrollees, which is what the other ratios look at), recent data report 0.54:1,000 for large plans and 0.79:1,000 for small plans.[7]

NONPHYSICIAN OR MIDLEVEL PRACTITIONERS

Nonphysician or midlevel practitioners (MLPs) in primary care include physician assistants (PAs) and nurse practitioners (NPs). There are several different types of NP designations, each having a different focus and training; those include advanced practice nurses (APNs), nurse midwives (NMs), nurse anesthetists (NAs), and clinical nurse specialists (CNSs).

More than 60,000 NPs practice in 48 states and the District of Columbia as of 1999. NPs practice independent of physicians in 25 states and prescribe independently in 17. More than 35,000 PAs prescribe in 44 states and the District of Columbia. In a survey of more than 2,000 physicians by Scott-Levin Associates, 26 percent use NPs and 17 percent use PAs. NPs are more likely to work in OB/GYN practices; PAs are more prevalent in general and family practices, general surgery/surgical subspecialties, and emergency medicine.[8] Table 7–1 provides a view of the association of MLPs with physicians; note, however, that the definition of MLPs

used in Table 7–1 is broader than that used in this section. Note, too, the relationship between medical group size, the use of capitation, and the association of MLPs with physicians' practices.

Although the data are old, closed-panel (group and staff model) health plans are more likely to use nonphysician providers to deliver some medical care to their members. In a previously cited study, 65 percent of closed-panel plans reported the use of nonphysician providers, with a mean ratio of 0.08:1,000.[9] In a 1992 report, 86 percent of closed-panel plans reported using nonphysician providers (compared with 48 percent of open-panel plans), 52 percent of plans used PAs, 52 percent of plans used NPs, and 28 percent of plans used certified nurse-midwives.[10]

Well-qualified nonphysician practitioners are a great asset in managed care in that they are able to deliver excellent primary care, provide more health maintenance and health promotion services, spend more time with patients, and receive generally good acceptance from most members. Nonphysician providers may also play an important role in the management of chronically ill patients. They may provide the primary locus of coordination of care or case management for patients with diseases such as chronic asthma, diabetes, and the like. In a similar vein, nonphysician providers may take a key role in managing high-risk patients, using practice protocols for prevention and health maintenance in this population. Certified nurse-midwives may not only provide services for routine deliveries but may in fact provide primary gynecological care using practice guidelines and protocols.

The availability of nonphysician providers varies widely from state to state and is strongly correlated with a "favorable state practice environment."[11] The practice environment includes such variables as the ability to write prescriptions, to practice in a (relatively) autonomous manner for certain situations, and to receive direct reimbursement. In some locations MCOs are contracting directly with NPs for primary care services, although that remains infrequent as of 2000.

Table 7–1 Staffing, Midlevel Providers

Size	Median MLP Staffing per FTE Physician	Percentage of Groups with MLPs
10 or fewer	0.28	66.7
11–25	0.14	73.2
26–50	0.15	83.0
51–75	0.20	93.9
76–150	0.20	94.9
151 or more	0.26	100.0

Percentage of Capitation Revenue

No capitation revenue	0.17	77.0
1–10%	0.16	77.2
11–50%	0.21	85.4
51–100%	0.18	94.1
All Groups	**0.18**	**80.5**

Note: Midlevel providers are specially trained and licensed nonphysician providers who can provide medical care and billable services. Examples of midlevel providers include audiologists, certified registered nurse anesthetists, dietitians/nutritionists, midwives, nurse practitioners, occupational therapists, optometrists, physical therapists, physician assistants, podiatrists, psychologists, social workers, speech therapists, and surgical technicians. Size is the number of full-time equivalent physicians.

Source: Reprinted with permission from Medical Group Management Association Cost Survey: 1997 Report Based on 1996 Data © 1997 and 1996 Report Based on 1995 Data © 1996; *Hoechst Marion Roussel Managed Care Digest Series* 1998, Medical Group Practice Digest.

TYPES OF CONTRACTING SITUATIONS

In developing a network, an open-panel MCO may have to deal with a number of possible types of contracting situations. The subject of the contract itself is addressed in Chapter 62, and reimbursement is discussed in Chapter 8. This discussion focuses on the types of physician organizational situations that may present themselves, regardless of specific contracting and reimbursement issues.

Individual Physicians

Individual physicians comprise the most common category of contracting in open panels. This is not surprising given the large number of solo practitioners in many parts of the country. In this model the physician contracts directly with the health plan and not through any third party or intermediary. The advantage to the plan is that there is a direct relationship with the physician, which makes it cleaner and simpler to interact. The disadvantage is that it is only one physician, and therefore the effort to obtain and maintain that relationship is disproportionately great.

Medical Groups

While not substantially different from the individual physician category, small groups (i.e., 2–10 physicians) usually operate relatively cohesively. The advantage to the plan is that the amount of effort to obtain and maintain a small group is approximately the same as for individual practitioners but yields a higher number of physicians. Plans generally prefer to contract with small groups for that reason. The disadvantage is that if the relationship with the group needs to be terminated (for whatever reason, theirs or yours), there is significant disruption in patient care.

Multispecialty groups represent a special category. Relatively uncommon in certain parts of the country, they are occasionally the dominant practices in certain areas. The advantage of contracting with multispecialty groups is that both PCPs and specialty physicians are obtained. This provides for broader access (including specialists to whom other PCPs may refer) and allows for existing referral patterns to continue.

One disadvantage is that multispecialty groups sometimes are dominated by the specialty or referral physicians in the group, which may lead to inappropriate overutilization of referral services. Another potential disadvantage is the case where, by accepting the group, you are forced to accept a specialist whose cost or quality is not what you desire (although not so bad as to prevent contracting with the group). Again, as a general rule, if relations with large groups founder, there is a increased likelihood that there will be disruptions in patient care.

The most significant effect on physicians of network selection activity may actually be the organization of physicians into medical groups. Between 1988 and 1998 the percentage of non-institutional physicians practicing in groups increased from 50.7 percent to 63.7 percent.[12] Another significant effect is the increase in the number of physicians who have become employed by medical groups, health systems, or practice management companies. Between 1985 and 1998 the percentage of physicians who were employed increased from 24.0 percent to 36.1 percent.[13] These trends toward group practice and employment have been associated with physicians seeking to gain an advantage in contract negotiations with managed care companies, reducing individual administrative burden, and/or gaining market share.[14]

Independent Practice Associations

The IPA is the original form of an open-panel plan. In the early 1970s it was envisioned that open-panel plans would all be IPA model plans. In this situation, there is actually a legal entity of an IPA, which contracts with physicians; in turn, the IPA contracts with the health plan. The advantage to the plan is that a large number of providers come along with the contract. Furthermore, if relations between the IPA and the health plan are close, there may be a confluence of goals, which benefits all parties.

There are two primary disadvantages to contracting with IPAs. The first is that an IPA functions somewhat like a union. If relations between the IPA and the health plan become problematic, the IPA can hold a considerable portion (or perhaps all) of the delivery system hostage to negotiations. This fact has not been lost on the U.S. Justice Department. IPAs that function as anticompetitive forces may encounter difficulties with the law (see Chapter 63).

The second disadvantage is that the plan's ability to select and deselect individual physicians is much more limited when contracting through an IPA than when contracting directly with the providers. If the IPA is at risk for medical expenses, there may be a confluence of objectives between the plan and the IPA to bring in cost-effective and high-quality providers and to remove those providers whose cost or quality is unacceptable. However, the IPA has its own internal political structure, so that defining who is cost effective or high quality, as well as dealing with outliers, may not match exactly between the plan and the IPA. If the plan has the contractual right to refuse to accept or to departicipate individual providers in the IPA, that obstacle may be avoided, although the purely political obstacles remain.

Integrated Delivery Systems

Many hospitals have been exploring methods of developing organizations that will legally and structurally bond the physicians to the hospital. Sometimes these are referred to as physician-hospital organizations (PHOs) or management service organizations (MSOs). In addition to hospital-based integrated delivery systems (IDSs), there are physician-only MSOs. These and other forms of IDSs are discussed in further detail in Chapter 4. The positive and negative ramifications that apply to IPAs are similar to those for IDSs (including their antitrust risk) and have been discussed above. In addition to those issues, there are two other broad issues that relate specifically to hospital-based organizations.

First is the link between a hospital's own willingness to do business with a plan and the plan's willingness to do business with the PHO or MSO. In other words, the hospital may refuse to contract with the plan or may not provide favorable terms unless the plan brings in the PHO, perhaps even on an exclusive basis. That removes control of that entire portion of the delivery system (physicians and hospital), leaving the plan at the mercy (or abilities) of the PHO or MSO to achieve the plan's goals. If the PHO or MSO is at significant risk for medical expenses, there may be confluence of goals.

The second issue relates to the reasons that the PHO formed in the first place. If the hospital has the goals of keeping beds filled and keeping the medical staff happy and busy, then the selection process for choosing which providers are in the PHO may be weighted toward those physicians who admit a lot of patients to the hospital. This criterion is not ideal from the plan's perspective. In addition, if the PHO formed specifically to resist aggressive managed care, then there may be a mismatch between how the plan wants to perform medical management and how the PHO will allow it to occur. Issues of control of utilization management, quality management, and provider selection then become difficult to resolve.

Nonetheless, hospital-centered organizations can function effectively. If the organization is formed with a genuine understanding of the goals of managed care; a genuine willingness to deal with difficult issues of utilization, quality, and provider selection; and a willingness to share control with the health plan, it is possible to work together.

Physician practice management companies (PPMCs), also discussed in Chapter 4, were for a brief period a viable contracting entity. The PPMC often accepted global risk from the MCO, with the intent of managing utilization and keeping the savings rather than sharing with a hospital system. By 1999, however, most general PPMCs had failed, many in a spectacular display of self-immolation. Many entered bankruptcy, and physicians either were not paid or left on their own. Specialty PPMCs, discussed briefly in Chapter 11, still remain to some extent, and there are still a few general or primary care PPMCs as well. But PPMCs have become largely irrelevant to contracting except for instances of specific specialty services.

The primary advantage to a health plan in contracting with an IDS is the ability to have a network in rapid order. This may be a primary driver in the case of a plan entering into a new market, or one that is already competitive, and may in fact be the only way an MCO can get a network. This last issue will be especially true if a large number of physicians have sold their practices to hospitals or proprietary MSOs. A plan that needs to quickly expand its medical service area, or is expanding into entirely new geographic areas, may find that contracting through IDSs allows it to achieve its expansion goals and be first to market.

An additional advantage may occur if the IDS is willing to provide a substantial savings to the plan, better than that which would be available on a direct contract basis. If the plan is entering into a new product line (e.g., Medicare risk or Medicaid), then the plan may desire to share the risk for medical costs through aggressive capitation with the IDS.

It should be noted that in certain states HMOs are not allowed to contract solely with the IDS; they must have contracts directly with the physicians. The individual physician contract may be brief and encompass no more than standard "hold harmless" language (see Chapter 62) and then reference the contract between the IDS and the physician, and the contract between the IDS and the plan. This requirement is meant to ensure that each individual physician understands and agrees to certain provisions required under state law, such as the prohibition on balance billing. See Chapter 65 for more discussion on legal issues in IDSs.

Faculty Practice Plans

Faculty practice plans (FPPs) are medical groups that are organized around teaching programs, primarily at university hospitals. An FPP may be a single entity or may encompass multiple entities defined along specialty lines (e.g., cardiology or anesthesiology). Plans generally contract with the legal group representing the FPP rather than with individual physicians within the FPP, although that varies from plan to plan.

FPPs represent special challenges for various reasons. First, many teaching institutions and FPPs tend to be less cost effective in their practice styles than private physicians. This probably relates to the primary missions of the teaching program: to teach and perform research. Cost-effectiveness is a secondary goal only (if a goal at all).

A second challenge is that a FPP, like a medical group, comes all together or not at all. This again means that the plan has little ability to select or deselect the individual physicians within the FPP. Related to that is the lack of detail regarding claims and encounter data. Many FPPs simply bill the plan, accept capitation, or collect encounter data in the name of the FPP rather than in the name of the individual provider who performed the service. The plan then has little ability to analyze data to the same level of detail that is afforded in the rest of the network.

A third major challenge is the use of house officers (interns and residents in training) and medical students to deliver care. In teaching hospitals, the day-to-day care is delivered by house officers rather than by the attending faculty physician, who functions as a teacher and supervisor. House officers and medical students, because they are learning how to practice medicine, tend to be profligate in their use of medical resources; they are there to learn medicine, not simply to perform direct service to patients. Furthermore, experience allows physicians to learn what is cost effective, and house officers and medical students have yet to gain such experience. Nevertheless, there is some evidence that intensive attention to utilization management by faculty can have a highly beneficial effect on house staff.[15]

The last major issue with teaching programs and FPPs is the nature of how they deliver services. Most teaching programs are not set up for case management. It is far more common to have multiple specialty clinics (e.g., pulmonary, cardiology, or vascular surgery) to which patients are referred for each specific problem. Such a system takes on characteristics of a medical pinball machine, where the members ricochet from clinic to clinic, having each organ system attended to with little regard for the totality of care. This leads to enormous run-ups in cost as well as continuity problems and a clear lack of control or accountability.

Despite these difficulties, there are good reasons for health plans to contract with teaching programs and FPPs other than the societal good derived from the training of medical practitioners. Teaching programs and FPPs provide not only routine care, but also tertiary and highly specialized care, which the plan will have to find means to provide in any event. Teaching programs also add prestige to the plan by virtue of their reputation for providing high-quality care, although that can be a two-edged sword in that the participation of a teaching program may draw adverse selection in membership.*

Most teaching programs and FPPs recognize the problems cited above and are willing to work with plans to ameliorate them. For example, they may be willing to extend a deep discount to a managed care plan in the recognition that the plan's ability to control utilization is limited and therefore must be made up on price. Teaching programs may occasionally be willing to accept a high level of risk for medical expenses, but that can be a problem for them because of the risk of adverse selection mentioned above. Risk for defined services (e.g., laboratory or radiology) may be more acceptable.

See Chapter 13 for a detailed discussion of academic medical centers and managed care.

CREDENTIALING

It is not enough to get physicians to sign contracts. Without performing proper credentialing,

---

*In other words, if there is more than one health plan competing in a single group account (i.e., an employer group) for membership, members with serious illnesses may choose the health plan affiliated with a teaching program to ensure access to high-quality tertiary care. That means that sicker members join that health plan and less sick members join the health plan that does not have such an affiliation. This issue does not come up if the plan is the sole carrier in an account or if all the competing plans use the teaching program, but it is a clear problem if there are multiple plans competing freely for members in a single account.

the MCO will have no knowledge of the quality or acceptability of physicians, nor whether a physician will actually be an asset to the plan. Furthermore, in the event of a legal action against a physician, the plan may expose itself to some liability by having failed to carry out proper credentialing. In one well-known study, up to 5 percent of physicians applying for positions in ambulatory care clinics misrepresented their credentials in their applications;[16] how that might translate into an HMO or other MCO where physicians are likely to be more stable in their community is unknown. In most plans, the medical director bears ultimate responsibility for credentialing along with a credentialing committee, although the activities of credentialing are usually carried out by the provider relations department.

The credentialing process is a critical one and should be carried out during the recruiting process and, if necessary, after the contract or letter of intent is signed. Periodic recredentialing (usually every 2 years) should also take place. Recredentialing may be less extensive than primary credentialing, but more sophisticated plans are adding new elements to the recredentialing process, including looking at measures of quality of care, member satisfaction, compliance with plan policies and procedures, and utilization management.

A third-party credentialing verification organization (CVO) may also be used. The CVO performs primary credentialing on a physician, and then the HMO or PPO relies on the CVO for that credentialing verification. The purpose of this is to reduce the need for an individual physician to be required to provide identical credentialing data to numerous MCOs; in addition, the MCO can obtain the data in a more timely fashion, and it will be complete on the first pass. The chief problem with this approach is the requirement by many regulators and outside accreditation agencies that the HMO conduct primary source verification (i.e., obtain the information directly rather than relying on another party to obtain it). The National Committee for Quality Assurance (NCQA; see Chapter 44) has created a CVO certification program to allow third-party CVOs to meet NCQA standards in credentialing in order to perform credentialing for MCOs.[17]

The elements illustrated in Exhibits 7–1 and 7–2 are examples of data that should be captured in the credentialing process.

Verification of Credentialing Data

Primary verification of the elements in Exhibit 7–1 should also be performed as appropriate. Verification of data may be obtained from a number of sources, including the National Practitioner Data Bank (NPDB) (see below), as well as sources noted in Exhibit 7–3.

Federal Databases

Special types of credentialing checks have been created by the federal government. One, the NPDB, has been in existence since 1989, while the other, the Healthcare Integrity and Protection Data Bank (HIPDB) was created in 1999. Both data banks have an impact on how health plans credential providers, although the NPDB is currently the most important, since the HIPDB has little data as of 2000.

THE NATIONAL PRACTITIONER DATA BANK

The NPDB was created by the Health Care Quality Improvement Act of 1986 (HCQIA),[18] with final regulations published in 1989.[19] The HCQIA provides for qualified immunity from antitrust lawsuits for credentialing activities as well as professional medical staff sanctions when the terms of the act are followed. Information reported to the NPDB is considered confidential and may not be disclosed except as specified in the final regulations. The NPDB requires reporting of, and serves as a central repository of, information for:

- malpractice payments made for the benefit of physicians, dentists, and other health care practitioners
- licensure actions taken by state medical boards and state boards of dentistry against

Exhibit 7–1 Basic Elements of Credentialing

- Training (copy of certificates)
  —Location of training
  —Type of training
- Specialty board eligibility or certification (copy of certificate)
- Current state medical license (copy of certificate)
  —Restrictions
  —History of loss of license in any state
- Drug Enforcement Agency number (copy of certificate)
- Hospital privileges
  —Name of hospitals
  —Scope of practice privileges
- Malpractice insurance
  —Carrier name
  —Currency of coverage (copy of face sheet)
  —Scope of coverage (financial limits and procedures covered)
- Malpractice history
  —Pending claims
  —Successful claims against the physician, either judged or settled
- National Practitioner Data Bank status
- Medicare, Medicaid, and federal tax identification numbers
- Social Security number
- Location and telephone numbers of all offices
- Yes/no questions regarding:
  —Limitations or suspensions of privileges
  —Suspension from government programs
  —Suspension or restriction of DEA license
  —Malpractice cancellation
  —Felony conviction
  —Drug or alcohol abuse
  —Chronic or debilitating illnesses

physicians and dentists and other health care practitioners who are licensed or otherwise authorized by a state to provide health care services

- professional review actions primarily taken against physicians and dentists by hospitals and other health care entities, including HMOs, group practices, and professional societies

Exhibit 7–2 Additional Elements of Credentialing

- Hours of operation
- Provisions for emergency care and backup
- Use of midlevel practitioners (e.g., physician's assistants or clinical nurse practitioners)
- In-office surgery capabilities
- In-office testing capabilities
- Languages spoken
- Work history—past five years
- Areas of special medical interest
- Record of continuing medical education

- actions taken by the Drug Enforcement Agency
- Medicare/Medicaid exclusions

Hospitals are required to query the NPDB every two years. Health care entities such as HMOs, preferred provider organizations, and group practices may query under the following circumstances:

- when entering an employment or affiliation arrangement with a physician, dentist, or other health care practitioner
- when considering an applicant for medical staff appointment or clinical privileges
- when conducting peer review activity

To be eligible, such entities must both provide health care services and have a formal peer review process for the purpose of furthering the quality of health care.

By December 31, 1998, the end of its one hundredth month of operations, the NPDB contained reports on 202,033 reportable actions, malpractice payments, and Medicare/Medicaid exclusions involving 131,679 individual practitioners. Of the 131,679 practitioners reported to the NPDB, 72.1 percent were physicians (including MD and DO residents and interns), 14.9 percent were dentists (including dental residents), and 13.0 percent were other health care practitioners. During 1998 approximately 69.5 percent of all reports concerned malpractice payments, although cumulatively, malpractice payments comprised 76.4 percent of all reports.[20]

Exhibit 7–3 Credentialing Data Verification Sources

Graduation from medical school (any one of the following):
- Confirmation from the medical school
- American Medical Association Master File of Physicians in the United States
- Confirmation from the Association of American Medical Colleges
- Confirmation from the Educational Commission for Foreign Medical Graduates, for international medical graduates licensed after 1986
- Confirmation from state licensure agency, if the agency performs primary verification of medical school graduation

Valid license to practice medicine (any one of the following):
- State licensure agency
- Federation of State Medical Boards
- Primary admitting facility, if the facility performs primary verification of licensure

Completion of residency training (any one of the following):
- Confirmation from the residency training program
- American Medical Association Master File of Physicians in the United States
- Confirmation from the Association of American Medical Colleges
- Confirmation from state licensure agency, if the agency performs primary verification of residency training

Board certification (any one of the following):
- American Board of Medical Specialties Compendium of Certified Medical Specialists
- American Osteopathic Association Directory of Osteopathic Physicians
- Confirmation from the appropriate specialty board
- American Medical Association Master File of Physicians in the United States
- Confirmation from state licensure agency, if the agency performs primary verification of board status

While hospitals, which are required to query the NPDB every two years, make up the majority of queriers, HMOs are the most active of the voluntary queriers. HMOs represent 7.3 percent of all "active" entities registered with the NPDB as of December 31, 1998, but they made 33.7 percent of all queries cumulatively, and 36.4 percent of all queries during 1998. During 1998 a total of 374,002 matches were made on entity queries, representing almost 11.9 percent of all entity queries resulting in a match.[21]

The HCQIA also states that any hospital, HMO, preferred provider organization, or group practice may contact the NPDB to obtain information about a physician and that, if the hospital or health plan fails to do so, it will be assumed that it did so anyway. In other words, there is a potential for liability on the part of the plan if it fails to check with the NPDB and contracts with a physician who has a poor record as reported in the NPDB, and there is a malpractice problem later.

HEALTHCARE INTEGRITY AND PROTECTION DATA BANK

The secretary of the U.S. Department of Health and Human Services (DHHS), acting through the Office of Inspector General (OIG), was directed by the Health Insurance Portability and Accountability Act of 1996 (HIPAA; see also Chapter 67) to create the HIPDB to combat fraud and abuse in health insurance and health care delivery. At the time of publication, it had just started functioning.

The HIPDB is a national health care fraud and abuse data collection program for the reporting and disclosure of certain final adverse actions (excluding settlements in which no findings of liability have been made) taken against health care providers, suppliers, or practitioners. It is to contain the following types of information:

- Civil judgments against health care providers, suppliers, or practitioners in federal or state courts related to the delivery of health care items or services
- Federal or state criminal convictions against health care providers, suppliers, or practitioners related to the delivery of health care items or services

- Actions by federal or state agencies responsible for the licensing and certification of health care providers, suppliers, or practitioners
- Exclusion of health care providers, suppliers, or practitioners from participation in federal or state health care programs
- Any other adjudicated actions or decisions that the secretary establishes by regulations[22]

The HIPDB is a tracking system that serves as an alert function to users, indicating that a comprehensive review of the practitioners, providers, or suppliers past actions may be prudent. HIPDB information should be used in combination with information from other sources to make determinations on acceptance or rejection of a provider into the network. In addition to federal and state agencies that purchase health care services (e.g., Medicare, Medicaid, the Department of Defense, and so forth), health plans are also eligible to query the HIPDB. For purposes of this database, a health plan is defined as:

- A policy of health insurance
- A contract of a service benefit organization
- A membership agreement with an HMO or other prepaid health plan
- A plan, program, agreement, or other mechanism established, maintained, or made available by a self-insured employer or group of self-insured employers, a practitioner, provider or supplier group, third-party administrator, integrated health care delivery system, employee welfare association, public service group or organization, or professional association
- An insurance company, insurance service, or insurance organization licensed to engage in the business of selling health care insurance in a state and that is subject to state law that regulates health insurance[23]

At the time of publication, the operational functions of both the NPDB and the HIPDB are conducted for the Division of Quality Assurance of the DHHS by Systems Research and Applications, Inc. Further information is available via their website at: *www.npdb-hipdb.com*.

Information about the NPDB may be obtained via the Internet site noted above, or by writing to:

National Practitioner Data Bank
P.O. Box 10832
Chantilly, VA 20151
1–800–767–6732

Office Evaluation

If the plan is contracting directly with physicians, it will likely desire to perform a direct evaluation of the physician's office. If the plan has contracted through an IDS, it is more likely to forgo such a review if the IDS has already performed the review to the satisfaction of the plan. In some cases, the plan may choose not to perform an office review due to the associated cost, the need to get the network up quickly, or fear of offending physicians; these are inadequate reasons.

There are two main items to evaluate in a physician's office: capacity to accept new members and office ambiance. In addition, the plan or IDS may review the office from the standpoint of a quality management process, compliance with Occupational Safety and Health Administration (OSHA) guidelines, presence of certain types of equipment (e.g., a defibrillator), and so forth. If capacity and ambiance are the only review areas, the evaluation is best accomplished by having the recruiter visit the office and may be performed in one fairly short visit. A more detailed review will require a trained health professional, usually a nurse, and may take an hour or two.

In addition to asking physicians directly how many new members they will accept (and usually including that in the contract), the recruiter should ask to examine the appointment book. In this way, the recruiter can get a reasonably good idea of how much appointment availability the physician has. For example, if there are no available appointment slots for a physical examination for six weeks or more, the physician may be overestimating his or her ability to accept more work.

The recruiter can also get an idea of how easy it is for a patient with an acute problem to be put on the schedule. This may be examined by looking at the number of acute slots left open each day and by looking at the number of double-booked appointments that were put in at the end of each day.

In addition, the recruiter can assess less tangible items such as cleanliness of the office, friendliness of the staff toward patients, and general atmosphere. Hours of operation can be verified, as can provisions for emergency care and in-office equipment capabilities.

Medical Record Review

Many plans require a review of sample medical records by the medical director. This is to assure the medical director that physicians do, indeed, practice high-quality medicine and that their practice is already cost effective. Some physicians object to submitting to this review, but if it is required for participation, and if the physician is assured that it is strictly confidential and not a witch hunt, there should be few problems. Since the physician presumably has no plan members whose charts may be reviewed, care will need to be taken to protect the identity of the patients and to maintain privacy, as the plan has no legal right to access confidential medical records.

If the plan already has a quality assurance program that involves chart review, a physician should agree to the initial review as a matter of course. Sometimes objections by the physicians are not the impediment to this review but rather the embarrassment of the medical director in having to perform it.

Electronic Connectivity

Many MCOs are beginning to consider electronic connectivity as a crucial aspect of recredentialing and renewal of provider contracts. While not common as of 2000, as pressures to lower administrative costs continue and the need for more accurate and efficient business transactions becomes acute, some MCOs are considering requiring electronic communication of basic transactions (e.g., claims billing, authorizations, encounter data) as a condition of contract renewal.[24] This is not dissimilar to the requirements that the Health Care Financing Administration (HCFA) currently has for participating providers to submit electronic claims for Medicare (requirements that are largely met via the use of third-party billing services). There are currently ANSII standards in existence for these types of electronic transactions, as described in Chapter 35. These standards are mandated under HIPAA, thereby eliminating confusion and enabling greater electronic commerce.

COMPENSATION

The compensation of PCPs is discussed in detail in Chapters 8 and 9.

ORIENTATION

In all enterprises, time invested in the beginning to ensure real understanding is time well spent. Therefore, a planned approach to orientation of a newly added PCP will yield improved compliance with the plan's procedures and policies, increased professional satisfaction on the part of the PCP, and increased member satisfaction. Orientation is aimed at two audiences: the PCP and the PCP's office staff. Exhibit 7–4 lists some topics to consider in orienting physicians; Exhibit 7–5 lists some topics for orienting their office staff.

NETWORK MAINTENANCE

Maintenance of the professional relationship with physicians in the network has assumed a far greater role in managed care than at any previous time in the industry's history. The saturation of managed care plans in some communities, coupled with increasing interventions by third-party payers (commercial insurers, Medicare, and Medicaid) limiting providers' ability to shift costs to other fee-for-service payers, has placed increasing strain on physicians and has clearly colored how they view participation with managed care plans. Failure to service the network

Exhibit 7–4 Suggested Topics for Physician Orientation

- Plan subscription agreement and schedule of benefits
- Authorization policies and procedures
- Forms and paperwork
- Utilization and financial data supplied by plan
- Committees and meetings
- Quality management program and peer review
- Recredentialing requirements
- Member transfer in or out of practice
  —Member initiated
  —Physician initiated
- Plan member grievance procedure
- Schedule of compensation from plan
- Contact persons in plan
- Affiliated providers
  —Primary care
  —Consultants
  —Institutions
  —Ancillary services

properly can lead to defections or closure of practices to the plan, difficulty with new recruiting, and a slow downward spiral. Even for those plans that have not properly maintained their networks, however, it is never too late to put in the effort because it is certainly possible to recover from a poor history.

If the plan contracts with an IDS for its network, that does not mean that obligations to maintain the network cease. Many of the issues discussed here remain under the control of the plan and will continue to exert a strong influence over the physicians in the contracted network. The IDS will have the burden of responsibility for network maintenance and must therefore also pay attention to these issues. Both the plan and the IDS must pay close attention to network maintenance and not rely solely on one party for this vital function. If both parties are not actively involved, there is the strong possibility of network problems degenerating into finger pointing, in which case both parties lose.

Many of the key elements in network maintenance are discussed in Chapter 33, which fo-

Exhibit 7–5 Suggested Topics for Orientation of Office Staff

- Plan subscription agreement and schedule of benefits
- Authorization policies and procedures
- Forms and paperwork
- Member transfer in or out of practice
  —Member initiated
  —Physician initiated
- Plan member grievance procedure
- Member eligibility verification
- Member identification card
- Current member list and eligibility verification
- Affiliated providers
  —Primary care
  —Consultants
  —Institutions
  —Ancillary services
- Contact persons in plan
  —Names
  —Telephone numbers
- Hours of operation

---

cuses on changing provider behavior, because that involves many issues important to network maintenance. The issues of data and feedback, the use of positive feedback, translation of goals and objectives, autonomy needs, quality of care, role conflict, understanding the insurance functions of the plan, plan differentiation in the marketplace, and discipline and sanctioning will not be repeated here.

In most plans, there are individuals who are solely responsible for maintaining communications with the physician panel, both PCPs and consultants, and both the physicians and their office staff. The roles of these provider relations representatives are to elicit feedback from the physicians and office staff, update them on changes, troubleshoot, and generally keep things running smoothly.

The function of provider relations is similar to customer relations, but it is closer to that of business partner. In customer relations, the customer is always right; in a health plan, neither the plan nor the physician is always right. It is perhaps more useful to strive to be seen as a reliable and desirable business partner to the providers with whom the plan does business under contracts and agreements. Provider relations must therefore be proactive rather than simply reactive.

In addition to the items discussed in Chapter 33, the plan should have a well-developed early warning system for troubleshooting. Such a system could include regular on-site visits by provider relations staff (and occasionally by the medical director) and regular two-way communications vehicles. Changes in patterns, particularly patterns in utilization and compliance with plan policy and procedure, will often be a sign that the relationship is going awry. Last, close monitoring of the member services complaints report can yield crucial information; physicians will often tell their patients what they think and what they intend to do long before they tell the plan.

INTERNET-BASED ACTIVITIES

Electronic commerce (e-commerce), discussed in greater depth in Chapters 35 and 37, can also be considered an important part of maintaining and managing the network. The more the Internet can be used for activities that currently either require a lot of time-consuming effort or that do not exist at all, the more the MCO has to offer to the physicians. Two of the most common categories of MCO-physician e-commerce are discussed below.

Physician Directories

It has become common for MCOs to provide access to provider directories to members via the Internet, using the World Wide Web. In the simplest case, this means a static look-up function whereby a member can search the directory to find a physician that meets specialty and geographic needs. In more advanced settings, this may include more detailed information, such as a photo, a brief curriculum vitae, cultural information (e.g., languages spoken or a special focus on certain cultural needs), the ability to create and print out a map to the office, and other useful information. Such advanced systems also allow members to choose or change their PCP. All these functions, while member oriented, also provide greater opportunities for the physicians to gain membership from the health plan.

While still uncommon, some MCOs are also providing consumers with a rating of a medical group via the web, based on several criteria. In the case of one California MCO, an index of clinical quality measures included cervical cancer screening, eye exams for diabetics, and drug treatment for congestive heart failure. Service measures included satisfaction with physician group and PCP, primary care access complaints, and transfers out of medical groups. Groups received a "best practices" designation for each of 12 categories in which they scored in the ninetieth percentile or above.[25]

Not only MCOs have such websites. There are any number of private sites that provide directories of physicians to consumers. Many of these sites include information similar to that noted above, as well as a listing of the health plans that the physician participates in. Some sites even provide a "rating" of the physician, based on publicly available data and input from other consumers (who are encouraged to rate the physician based on their personal experience).

Physician Interaction with the Plan

The Internet is also being used in network maintenance and management by allowing physicians and the health plan to communicate via the Internet. This does not refer to simple electronic mail (e-mail), but to greater interactions. The most common types of interactions include claims submissions, referral authorization submissions, electronic payments, and so forth. But more advanced capabilities are appearing. For example, in 1999 some MCOs provided web-based capabilities to allow providers to look up the status of individual claims, check member/patient eligibility, access drug formularies, and more.

While such capabilities remain new at the time of publication, it is anticipated that in just a few years after the publication date, Internet interactions between physicians and MCOs will be routine and will encompass significant functionality.

REMOVING PHYSICIANS FROM THE NETWORK

Beyond the elements referred to above, another function of network maintenance is the determination of who not to keep in the plan. In any managed care plan, there will be physicians who simply cannot or will not work within the system and whose practice style is clearly cost ineffective or of poor quality. Quality is discussed in Chapter 30, and sanctions for reasons of poor quality are discussed in Chapter 64; quality-related actions will not be repeated here, except to note that removal of a physician from the network for quality reasons must follow the process described in the HCQIA, and such removal must be reported to the NPDB as well as the medical licensure boards in many states.

A plan may also choose to terminate physicians because the physician panel is too large, though this is rarely an issue with PCPs since most plans can always use wider access to primary care for both medical delivery and marketing reasons. The exception in primary care is likely to occur when a plan makes a wholesale commitment to an IDS, and as part of that commitment agrees to terminate any PCPs that are not part of the IDS. In this situation, plans will usually resist terminating existing PCP relationships, but they may agree to no longer recruit new PCPs that are not part of the IDS (unless the IDS cannot provide sufficient PCPs in a geographic region).

Regarding the issue of unacceptably costly practice style, the plan must develop a mechanism for identification of such practitioners that uses a combination of severity-adjusted claims and utilization data (see Chapter 32) and some type of formal performance evaluation system. If identified providers are reluctant to change even after the medical director has worked closely with them, then serious consideration should be given to terminating them from the panel.

There are any number of objections to removing a physician from the panel. Asking the members to change physicians is not easy or pleasant, benefits managers get upset, and invariably the physician in question is in a strategic location. The decision often comes down to whether the plan wants to continue to subsidize that physician's poor practice behavior from the earnings of the other physicians (in capitated or risk/bonus types of reimbursement systems) and from the plan's earnings, or drive the rates up to uncompetitive levels. If those are unacceptable alternatives, then the separation must occur.

Various states have enacted legislation that requires "due process" or "fair procedure" protection for instances when a provider is terminated from participating in a health plan. This type of legislation also requires health plans to show cause, provide reasons in writing, and/or allow for appeal or review of criteria for practice profiling or utilization/cost performance when providers are terminated from participation in a health plan's network. For example, a California ruling in the case of *Potvin v. Metropolitan Life Insurance* goes as far as barring health plans from invoking no-cause termination clauses in cases where doctors have a significant number of patients in a given plan.[26]

The scope of the due process laws varies by state. In New Jersey, for example, a law put into effect in March 1998 requires HMOs to provide in writing an explanation of the reason for termination if the physician requests it. Also, as part of that law, the doctor may appeal the deselection to a three-member panel, and health plans must reveal practice profiling or utilization/cost performance criteria to physicians when they initially contract with the HMO. By comparison, a much weaker law passed in Maryland requires plans to provide utilization criteria, but explanations or appeals are not required.[27] Of course, these state laws are current as of 2000, and can change with any state legislative session.

Some HMOs contractually require a physician to participate until the physician's entire panel of members has had a chance to change plans (which may take a year unless the physician's member panel is small), but that op-

tion can be quite costly because the physician will have no incentive to control cost once he or she has been notified of termination.

There is little good data about how often a plan either denies a contract to, or terminates a PCP. In one 1998 survey of 947 physicians in California, approximately 22 percent of the physicians in 13 urban counties had been denied a contract or terminated from an IPA or HMO, with somewhat more than twice as many denials as terminations. However, this did not prevent their participation in managed care totally, as only 10 percent had no managed care contracts. Between 30 percent to 40 percent of the respondents did not report being given any reason for denial of a contract or termination; the majority of the remainder reported the reason being excess supply of the physician's specialty, policy conflict with the IPA or HMO, training requirements not met, and (for IPAs) exclusive contract required. The study found physician characteristics such as age, sex, or race did not have high predictive value in terms of the rate of contract denial or termination. Larger practices were less likely to experience denial or termination than were solo or small practices. However, where physicians had high uninsured populations, there was a higher rate of denial or deselection.[28]

CONCLUSION

Network development requires an orderly project management approach, whether such development is undertaken by a health plan or by an IDS. It is equally important to invest in proper orientation of new physicians and their office staff. Maintenance of the relationship between the physicians and the plan is a key element of success that is gaining increasing importance as plans become ever more competitive in the marketplace. The plan or IDS must be willing to departicipate a provider in certain circumstances to deliver the proper combination of quality and cost-effectiveness that is a requirement of managed care.

REFERENCES AND NOTES

1. T. Defina, Educating Physicians in Managed Care, *Health System Leader* (May 1995).

2. Group Health Association of America (GHAA), *HMO Industry Profile,* Vol. 2: *Physician Staffing and Utilization Patterns* (Washington, DC, GHAA, 1991).

3. L.G. Hart and Eric Wagner, Physician Staffing Ratios in Staff-Model HMOs: A Cautionary Tale, *Health Affairs* (January–February 1997): 55–70.

4. Hoechst Marion Roussel, *Managed Care Digest Series HMO-PPO/Medicare/Medicaid Digest* (Kansas City, MO: Hoechst Marion Roussel, 1998).

5. T.H. Dial, S.E. Palsbo, C. Bergsten, et al., Clinical Staffing in Staff- and Group-Model HMOs, *Health Affairs* 14 (Summer 1995): 168–180.

6. GHAA, *HMO Industry Profile,* Vol. 2.

7. Dial et al., Clinical Staffing in Staff- and Group-Model HMOs.

8. Scott-Levin Associates (*www.scottlevin.com*), reported in Nurse Practitioners, Physician Assistants: Rising Forces in Pharmaceutical Marketplace, *Business Wire* (October 11, 1999).

9. Dial et al., Clinical Staffing in Staff- and Group-Model HMOs.

10. J. Packer-Thursman, The Role of Midlevel Practitioners, *HMO Magazine* (March/April 1992): 28–34.

11. E.S. Sekscenski, S. Sansom, C. Bazell, et al., State Practice Environments and the Supply of Physician Assistants, Nurse Practitioners, and Certified Nurse-Midwives, *New England Journal of Medicine* 331, no. 19 (1994): 1266–1271.

12. American Medical Association (AMA), Socioeconomic Characteristics of Medical Practice, 1997/98, 21. *Physician Socioeconomic Statistics, 1999–2000 ed.* (Chicago: American Medical Association, Center for Health Policy Research, 1999), 131.

13. AMA, Socioeconomic Characteristics of Medical Practice, 17.

14. D. Colby, Doctors and Their Discontents, *Health Affairs* (November–December 1997): 112.

15. J.R. Woodside, R. Bodne, et al., Intensive, Focused Utilization Management in a Teaching Hospital: An Exploratory Study, *Quality Assurance Utilization Review* 6 (1991): 47–50.

16. W.A. Schaffer et al., Falsification of Clinical Credentials by Physicians Applying for Ambulatory Staff Privileges, *New England Journal of Medicine* 318 (1988): 356–357.

17. NCQA, CVO Certification Program 1995–1996, National Committee for Quality Assurance, Washington, DC.

18. Health Care Quality Improvement Act of 1986, Public Law 99–660, November 14, 1986.

19. *Federal Register* 45 CFR, Part 60.

20. Department of Health and Human Services, Division of Quality Assurance, 1999.

21. Ibid.

22. *Federal Register* 45 CFR, Part 61.

23. Section 1128E of the *Social Security Act* (Public Law 104–191), the Health Insurance Portability and Accountability Act of 1996.

24. Ernst & Young, personal communication.

25. H. Larkin, Doctors Starting To Feel Report Cards' Impact, *American Medical News* (July 26, 1999).

26. K. Terry, No-cause Terminations: Will They Go Up in Flames? *Medical Economics* (January 12, 1998): 131.

27. Terry, No-cause Terminations.

28. A. Bindman, K. Grumbach, M.A. Vranizan, et al., Selection and Exclusion of Primary Care Physicians by Managed Care Organizations, *JAMA* (March 4, 1998): 675–679.

CHAPTER 8

Compensation of Primary Care Physicians in Managed Health Care

Peter R. Kongstvedt

INTRODUCTION

This chapter provides an overview of the most common methods managed care organizations (MCOs) use to reimburse primary care physicians (PCPs).* MCOs, primarily health maintenance organizations (HMOs), frequently use some form of performance or risk-based reimbursement to pay physicians, especially PCPs. Specialty care physicians (SCPs) may also be paid under some form of risk-based reimbursement, although with less frequency than occurs with PCPs; reimbursement of SCPs is discussed in Chapter 11.

The primary focus here is on direct contract model health plans (that is, the contract between the health plan and the physician is direct, rather than through an intermediary; see Chapter 3). This is distinct from the compensation of individual physicians in organized groups, staff models, or integrated delivery systems (IDSs). It is possible and even common to use these meth-

ods of reimbursement on an individual physician basis in such groups, but not necessarily. Many medical groups and independent practice associations (IPAs) blend forms of capitation, fee for service (FFS), and salary for the compensation of individual physicians even though the IPA* accepts capitation from the HMO (i.e., the IPA is a distinct intermediary between the MCO and the individual physicians).[1,2] In the case of such organized groups, this chapter discusses only the reimbursement of the group by the MCO, rather than any one physician in that group. Compensation of individual physicians under such circumstances is discussed in detail in Chapter 9.

A reimbursement system is simply one of the many tools available in managed care and has limited ability to achieve desired goals in the absence of other tools, such as competent management of utilization and quality. Those whose knowledge about managed health care is superficial often make the erroneous assumption that managed care equals capitation, with little else involved. As will be shown, reimbursement of PCPs (as well as other physicians and hospitals) in managed health care is anything but homogeneous. The objective of any of these reimbursement systems is to better align the compensation of physicians with the overall goals of managed

---

*Primary care physicians are assumed to be in the specialties of family practice, internal medicine, and pediatrics; general practice (that is, nonboard certified general practitioners) are also considered primary care in those plans that contract with general practitioners. Obstetrics and gynecology, while sharing some attributes of primary care, are generally treated as specialty physicians by HMOs, even when members have direct access to OB/GYN. Physician extenders such as physicians assistants and clinical nurse practitioners are generally treated as being associated with primary care physicians, and so are not discussed separately.

---

*The term *IPA* is often used to describe any HMO that uses private physicians practicing in their own offices (as opposed to a group or staff model HMO), but, in fact, the term *IPA* technically refers to an actual legal entity. See Chapter 4.

health care. By itself, it is unlikely that any compensation system will have much of an impact.[3]

Managed care is marked by a high degree of continual change and variation, and never more than is occurring at the time of publication. Change occurs through market forces, changes in managed health care practices, new laws or regulations (especially in Medicare and Medicaid as is discussed later in this chapter, but also at the state level such as is seen in Texas), and uncountable other forces. As a result, the divisions by provider type and the reimbursement mechanisms described here are rarely found in a pure state.

BASIC MODELS OF REIMBURSEMENT

At a simplistic level, there are two basic ways to compensate open-panel PCPs for services: capitation and FFS. There are many varieties of these two ways, as will be discussed. There are also other methods of reimbursement that are discussed in Chapters 9, 10, 11, and 12, and there are surely ways of paying physicians that defy any easy explanation. This chapter focuses

on the types of reimbursement methods used by the vast majority of MCOs.

Surveys over the past decade have reported that between 60 percent and 75 percent of MCOs use capitation to pay PCPs, as is illustrated in Figures 8–1 and 8–2. This distribution of reimbursement methods has been relatively stable for the past decade, although the most recent data available at the time this chapter was written demonstrated a modest increase in the use of capitation.[4–7] It is not clear if this represents a trend or not, since the year prior demonstrated a modest decrease in the amount of capitation. The data also show a marked increase in the use of FFS by MCOs, which further illustrates the heterogeneity of reimbursement models.

In past years, an MCO tended to use one form of reimbursement or the other. Now, the opposite is more frequently the case. There are many reasons for this, including:

- consolidation of health plans has led to broader geographic coverage, requiring different reimbursement methods in differing locales based on local norms

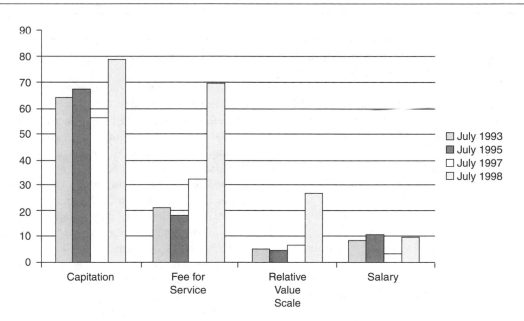

Figure 8–1 Percentage of HMOs Using Primary Care Physician Reimbursement Methods. *Source:* Reprinted with permission from *The Interstudy Competitive Edge: HMO Industry Report* 9.1, © 1999, InterStudy publications.

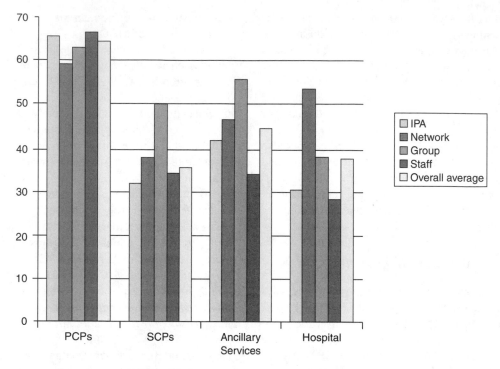

Figure 8–2 Average Percentage of Contracts Reimbursed through Capitation. Multiple reimbursement types exist for most HMOs, therefore total exceeds 100 percent. *Source:* Reprinted with permission from Hoechst Marion Roussel Managed Care Digest Series, *HMO-PPO Digest 1999,* © 1999 Hoechst Marion Roussel, SMG Marketing Group Inc.

- consolidation has also led to the combination of different reimbursement methods used by formerly separate, but now merged MCOs
- different products offered by the same MCO, using the same PCPs, but requiring different reimbursement methods (for example, capitation for an HMO or Medicare risk product, FFS for a preferred provider organization product, and performance-based FFS for a point-of-service [POS] product)
- self-funded employer health plans (see Chapter 66) that prefer FFS so as to better capture utilization data and pay only for what they need
- a mixture of capitation for some services and FFS for other services within the same plan
- PCPs desiring one form of reimbursement over another, such as a large medical group

desiring capitation, while independent PCPs prefer FFS

It is also worth noting some other changes that occurred as the decade closed that had an effect on reimbursement methods. Changes in the regulatory and legal climate have had, and are having, an impact, and this is discussed later in this chapter. There is also geographic variation in the amount of capitation, as illustrated in Table 8–1. The decline of the group and staff model HMOs has also meant that MCOs are now predominantly made up of large, often loose networks of independent physicians; this is discussed in Chapter 3, and figures for enrollment in the different model types are illustrated in Figure 3–3 in that chapter.

One of the most significant changes occurred in the late 1990s, when many physician practice management companies (PPMCs) and IDSs

Table 8–1 Percentage of PCP Capitation in Selected Metropolitan Statistical Areas (MSAs)

MSA Name	Managed Care Penetration	Percent Primary Capitation
Atlanta	27.0	39.6
Boston	49.3	22.3
Chicago	25.9	69.0
Dayton	56.1	27.0
Denver	43.2	48.3
Los Angeles	45.7	92.7
New York City	32.5	35.9
Phoenix	33.7	48.9
Philadelphia	46.5	32.0
Toledo	46.7	100.0
Tulsa	26.2	88.1

Courtesy of HCIA-Sachs, 1998, Evanston, Illinois.

sought out global risk (that is, capitation for all medical costs) with the belief that substantial and easy profits were to be had.* Many of these PPMCs have failed (discussed in Chapter 4), and many of the IDSs no longer accept global risk. This has affected managed care reimbursement in several ways. First and most obvious, there arc fewer provider organizations that seek or accept global risk. Second, when these PPMCs failed, the MCOs had to pay the physicians and cover the loss in order to keep the network intact, and that has resulted in a higher degree of hesitation by MCOs in even considering delegation of global risk. Third, individual physicians had to recontract with the MCOs once the PPMC went out of business or the IDS stopped accepting capitation, and this new and direct contract may have been through capitation or FFS (and may ac-

---

*When these PPMCs and IDSs did accept global risk, the MCO would report that medical costs were capitated, which was true. However, the PPMCs and IDSs often paid their physicians using FFS or salary, and so reported that they did not use capitation, which was equally true. Thus the same MCO, physicians, and product would produce two different but accurate views of the amount of capitation in place.

count for some of the increase in levels of capitation reported by physicians who were formerly paid via FFS or salary by the PPMC or IDS).

CAPITATION

Capitation is prepayment for services on a per member per month (PMPM) basis. In other words, a PCP is paid the same amount of money every month for a member regardless of whether that member receives services or not and regardless of how expensive those services are. There are many different forms and variants of capitation, the most common of which are discussed in the sections that follow.

Scope of Covered Services

To determine an appropriate capitation, it must first be defined what will be covered in the scope of primary care services and what will not. Defining the scope of covered services forms the basis for estimating the total costs of primary care.

Include all services that the PCP will be expected to deliver, including preventive services, outpatient care, and hospital visits. Certain areas require special attention in defining, for example, diagnostic testing, prescriptions, and surgical procedures. Selected diagnostic testing (for example, office urinalysis or electrocardiograms) may be included in the capitation, but other lab testing is sent out to an outside reference lab (see Chapter 20) and the capitation covers only the blood drawing.

The cost of prescription drugs is also an area that has seen great pressure recently, with differing opinions about whether or not to include that cost in the capitation amount. Since prescription drugs are not a service delivered directly by the PCP, those costs are considered financial risk and are discussed separately from service risk later in this section.

As for surgical procedures, what if the same procedure is performed by the PCP and by a referral physician? Under capitation, the PCP may be incented to refer the patient out rather than incur the expense; however, paying a capitated PCP FFS for that procedure (referred to as a carve-out, discussed below) also carries the risk of overutilization.

Other services such as immunizations are easy to define but still may or may not be covered by the capitation payment if the cost of the service is volatile. In the case of immunizations, the schedule of immunizations is frequently changed as new vaccines are released, and the cost of the vaccine may fluctuate as well.

Many performance-based compensation systems also hold the PCP accountable for nonprimary care services, either through risk programs or positive incentive programs, both of which are discussed later in this chapter. For such programs, the same exercise of categorizing what and how services are defined should be carried out for specialty or referral services, institutional care, and ancillary services. Essentially, costs need to be estimated for each of the categories that will be capitated or tracked for at-risk PCPs.

If a plan is unable to define primary care services easily, a good reference is published by Milliman and Robertson, a national actuarial services firm.[8]

Calculation of Capitation Payments

The issue of expected costs in defined categories is beyond the scope of this chapter; so detailed discussion may be found in Chapters 49 and 50. Most plans use an actuary to set these cost categories initially on the basis of the plan's geographic area, the benefits plans in place, and the medical management and cost controls in place. If the plan has been in operation for some time and has a data system capable of tracking the detail, estimating costs in categories is simply a matter of collating the existing data. Even then, most MCOs use an actuary to calculate the amounts.

A plan wishing to convert from a FFS system to capitation will have to calculate the capitation equivalent of average FFS revenues for the physicians. In other words, calculate what physicians would receive from FFS for that membership base, assuming appropriate utilization.* For purposes of this calculation, the actuaries must

also choose what fee allowance system they will use. Fee allowance systems are discussed later in this chapter.

As a rough example, if a physician receives approximately $45.00 per visit (collected, not just billed) and a reasonable estimated visitation rate is 3 primary care visits per member per year (PMPY), then multiplying 3 x $45.00 and dividing the result by 12 (to get the revenue per month) yields $11.25 PMPM. That could approximate the capitation rate. This example is crude and does not take into account any particular definition of scope of covered services, actual visitation rates for an area, visit rate differences by age and sex, average collections by a physician, effect of copayments, or differences in mean fees among different specialties, so this figure should not be used in capitating primary care services.

If the plan uses a risk/bonus arrangement, it is useful to be able to demonstrate to physicians that if utilization is managed they will receive more than they would have under FFS. For example, if the plan uses a blended capitation rate of $11.25 PMPM and there are in fact 3 visits PMPY, and if good utilization management yields a bonus of $2.00 PMPM from the risk pools, then the physician receives a year-end reconciliation that blends out to $13.25 PMPM, or $53.00 per visit. Also, pure luck (good or bad) will have an effect on the ultimate per visit payment, as discussed later.

Variations by Age and Gender

Capitation systems vary payments by the age and gender of the enrolled member to take into account the differences in average utilization of medical services in those categories. For example, the capitation rate for a member younger than 18 months of age might be $31.00 PMPM

---

*In other words, if high utilization is one of the primary reasons to convert from FFS, it would not be appropriate simply to memorialize the high utilization rates when calculating a capitation equivalent; it is more appropriate to calculate the capitation on the basis of what utilization should be.

to reflect the high utilization of services by newborns.* The capitation rate may then fall to $10.00 PMPM for members 1 to 2 years of age, $8.00 PMPM for members 2 to 18 years of age, $7.00 PMPM for male members 18 to 45 years of age, and $12.00 PMPM for female members 18 to 45 years of age (reflecting the higher costs for women in their childbearing years), and so forth. As an end result of this, the actual PMPM payment to a physician may fluctuate each month depending on the demographics of their enrolled panel of members.

Variations by Other Factors

It is possible, although not yet common, to vary capitation by factors other than age and sex. The most prominent issue here is adjustment based on current health status. As discussed in Chapter 32, it is possible to profile patient panels in such a way as to adjust for health status (generally referred to as risk adjustment). As Medicare moves to a risk-adjusted methodology of paying risk-bearing MCOs, this becomes more important to deal with when capitating PCPs. In the commercial population, it is a much smaller subset of the enrolled membership that would be categorized as high risk and high cost. Many MCOs in fact do identify those patients, and either make special provisions for payment of the PCP or do not even include those patients in the PCP's panel, since the care of complex patients is often best done by a specialist (this issue is further discussed in Chapters 18, 22, and 23). However, in that case there is still no adjustment to the capitation, but rather removal of the highly complex patient from the panel of patients covered by capitation. In all cases, including risk adjustors in the calculation of capitation is highly complex compared to simple age and sex adjustments and, while not the norm for most MCOs, will likely increase in the future.[9]

Another relatively easily analyzed factor is geography. Even in the same statistical metropolitan area, there may be considerable differences in utilization. For example, in the Baltimore-Washington, D.C. metropolitan statistical area, there are highly significant differences in utilization among some counties in Maryland, Northern Virginia, and the District of Columbia.[10] In such situations, it may be appropriate to factor in geographic location when capitation payments are calculated.

Practice type may occasionally be a legitimate capitation factor. As an example, internists argue that the case mix they get is different from the case mix family practitioners get. This has not generally been borne out in studies, but there is some evidence that even in the same strata of age and sex, specialty internists (for example, cardiologists) have sicker patients than general internists.[11] The actual mix of services delivered in the office may also differ by specialty type.[12] University teaching programs tend to attract adverse selection from the membership base and may have a legitimate claim in that regard (see Chapter 13).

A theoretical, but rare example would be to vary capitation on the basis of actual cost experience of each commercial account group. In other words, if an account had an unusually healthy population of enrollees (for example, all healthy, young, vegetarian, nonsmoking aerobics instructors who use seat belts and advocate nonviolence), the capitation would be factored downward. The reverse would be true for a group with an unusually unhealthy population of enrollees (for example, all hypertensive, overweight asbestos workers who smoke, and drink heavily before racing on their motorcycles, sans helmets, to buy illegal drugs).

There may be straightforward business adjustments to capitation as well. One example that occurs in certain plans is an adjustment for exclusivity. In this case, the plan pays a higher capitation rate to those providers who do not sign up with any other managed care plans (there are usually no restrictions against participating with government programs or indemnity carriers). Such arrangements may raise the potential for antitrust actions, but that is dependent on the particular situation.

---

*This may include immunizations, unless the plan carves immunization costs out of the capitation rate; this is discussed later in the chapter.

In any event, if factors other than age and sex are to be used to adjust capitation, the calculations become highly complex, and communicating these factors to the participating providers becomes far more difficult. The plan must also guard against an imbalance in factors that lead to a higher than expected (or rated for) capitation payout over the entire network. In other words, adjustments must lead not only to increases in capitation but to decreases as well in order to remain budget neutral.

Carve-Outs

Capitation systems usually allow for certain services delivered by the PCP to be carved out of the capitation payment. The most common example as noted earlier is the cost of immunizations, which is not paid under capitation but is reimbursed on a fee schedule. As a general rule, carve-outs should only be used for those services that are not subject to discretionary utilization. In the case of immunizations, the medical guidelines for administering them are clear-cut but subject to change (for example, there may be an increase in the number of immunizations that are to be given in the first years of life), and there is little question about their use. That would not be the case, for example, for office-based laboratory testing in which there is a high degree of discretion about how much testing is necessary, and which may be considered a profit center by the practice.

Risk

There are two broad categories of risk for capitated PCPs: service risk and financial risk. Service risk refers to the PCP receiving a fixed payment for his or her own professional services, but not being at risk in the sense of having potentially to pay money out or not receive money due to him or her. Service risk is essentially the fact that if service volume is high, then the PCP receives relatively lower income per encounter, and vice versa. While the PCP may not be at obvious financial risk, the PCP loses

the ability to sell services to someone else for additional income in the event that his or her schedule fills up with capitated patients at a rate that is higher than that used to calculate the capitation. This issue is irrelevant if PCPs have slack time in their appointment book, but can be an issue if the PCPs are extremely busy. It is common for PCPs to feel that their capitation patients are "abusing" the service by coming in too frequently, but the perception often is more grievous than the reality.

Financial risk refers to actual income placed at risk, regardless of whether or not the PCP has a service risk as well (that is, the risk/incentive models discussed here may also apply to performance-based FFS as discussed later in this chapter). There are two common forms of financial risk: withholds and capitated pools for nonprimary care services. Figure 8–3 illustrates relative percentages of MCOs that, as of 1994, used withholds and incentives as part of their capitation of PCPs. A more recent study, although confined to California, found that of all PCPs contracting with HMOs, 29 percent had financial incentives of some type (collectively referred to as "bonuses," but inclusive of withholds and risk pool distributions).[13] However, on a broad scale, it appears that risk/bonus arrangements had increased in 1997 (regardless of whether capitation or FFS is used to pay PCPs) but experienced a striking decrease in 1998, as illustrated in Figure 8–4. Confusing this picture, however, is the fact that some of the 1997 data were collected during the period when many PPMCs and IDSs were contracting for full or global risk, which would by definition include risk/bonus amounts. Since most large PPMCs are no longer operating or accepting global capitation, and many IDSs no longer accept it either, it is possible that this dynamic had an effect that appeared in 1998; however, there are no data to definitively explain why the percentage of physician financial risk programs declined, nor is it yet possible to determine a trend.

Of special note, an MCO with a Medicare or Medicaid Risk Contract (see Chapters 55 and 56) should be aware of regulations that limit the

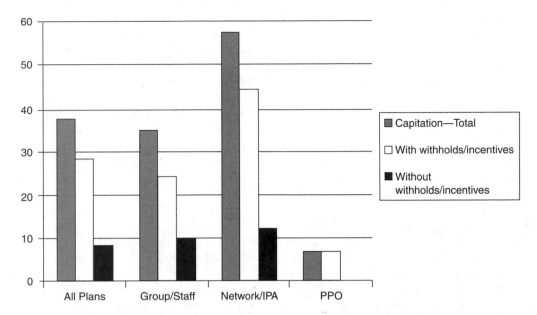

Figure 8–3 Primary Care Capitation and Risk. *Source:* Reprinted from Mathematica Policy Research, Inc. and The Medical College of Virginia for the Physician Payment Review Commission, 1994, MedPac, Government Services Administration.

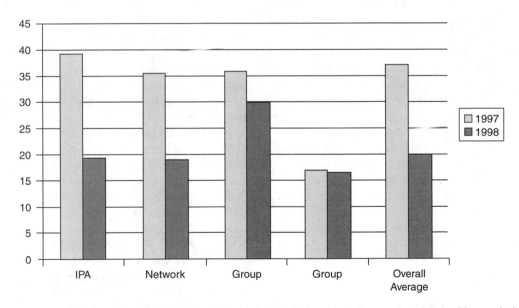

Figure 8–4 Percentage of HMOs Using Withholds/Risk Pools 1997–98. *Source:* Reprinted with permission from Hoechst Marion Roussel Managed Care Digest Series, *HMO-PPO Digest 1999,* © 1999 Hoechst Marion Roussel, SMG Marketing Group Inc.

amount of risk a physician may be at for a Medicare or Medicaid member. These regulations are discussed later in this chapter.

WITHHOLDS AND RISK/BONUS ARRANGEMENTS

One common risk arrangement is the withhold. A withhold is simply a percentage, for example, 20 percent, of the primary care capitation that is withheld every month and used to pay for cost overruns in referral or institutional services. In the earlier example of $11.25 PMPM, a 20 percent withhold would be $2.25. The PCP would actually receive a check each month for the difference between the capitation rate and the withhold, in this case $9.00; the withhold is held by the plan and used at year end (or whenever) for reconciliation of cost overruns, with the remainder returned to the PCP, as discussed below. The amount of payment withheld varied from 5 percent to 20 percent in one older survey, with few plans reporting routine withholds greater than 20 percent.[14]

Some plans also have a clause in their physician's contract that states that the plan may increase the amount of withhold in the event of cost excesses beyond what is already being withheld. For example, the withhold can be increased from 20 percent to 30 percent if referral costs are out of control. This is now quite uncommon, however, for a variety of reasons. The foremost reason is that there is a growing belief that this type of move has little positive effect on utilization and serves only to reallocate a small amount of money from payment of a PCP to payment of specialists. While generating a great deal of ill will, the total dollars saved by the plan in such cases are best described as "decimal dust." MCOs have become more sophisticated in medical management and practice profiling, and are far less reliant on financial incentives to control utilization.

CAPITATION POOLS FOR REFERRAL AND INSTITUTIONAL SERVICES

When capitation exists for primary care services and the PCP is also on a risk/bonus program for other medical costs, payment for referral services and institutional services is often made from capitation funds or pools as well. The services themselves may be paid for under a number of mechanisms (FFS, per diem, capitation, and the like), but for accounting purposes the expense is drawn against a capitated fund or pool. There are a variety of ways that HMOs handle these types of risk pools, and some common methods will be described. It must be stressed that the illustration that follows generally no longer exists in the real world exactly as it appears here. In HMOs that do use this approach, there is considerable variation; the illustration also reflects models that were more prevalent roughly a decade ago, while mature HMOs have undergone considerable changes since then.[15] Nevertheless, the illustration provides a common basis for understanding this type of model.

Figure 8–5 illustrates schematically how some of these risk pools operate. Based on at least one recent study, financial risk for the one-third of HMO PCPs who had financial risk or bonus is roughly evenly spread between specialty costs and institutional costs, as well as other measures such as quality, member satisfaction, and pharmacy costs.[16]

There are three broad classes of nonprimary care risk pools: referral (or specialty care), hospital (or institutional care, regardless of whether or not it is inpatient, outpatient, or emergency department), and ancillary services (for example, laboratory, radiology, pharmacy, and so forth, although it is also common for pharmacy to be considered a separate risk pool). Many HMOs also have a fourth pool, usually called "other," in which they accrue liabilities for such things as stop-loss or malpractice, and in which the physicians have no stake (see below). Some HMOs combine the ancillary services into the "other" pool, which is the model illustrated in Figure 8–5. It is not uncommon for these risk pools to be handled in different ways regarding the flow of funds and levels of risk and reward for the physicians and the plan.

As an example, the PCP receives an $11.25 PMPM blended capitation rate for primary care services (in other words, the blend of all the age

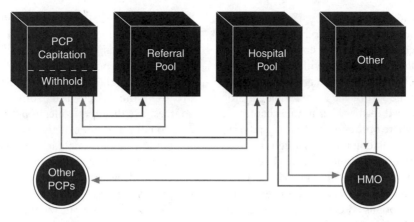

Figure 8–5 Capitation Risk Pools.

and sex capitation rates for that physician's membership base comes out to $11.25 PMPM). For each member, $29.00 PMPM is added to a capitated pool for all specialty referral services, and $50.00 PMPM is added to a capitated pool for hospital or institutional inpatient and outpatient services. The PCP does not actually receive the money in those pools; the plan holds on to it. Any medical expenses incurred by members in that PCP's panel will be counted against the appropriate pool of funds. At the end of the year, a reconciliation of the various pools is made (see below).

As with primary care, the scope of covered services must first be defined. For example, will home health be covered under institutional or referral (probably institutional because it reduces institutional costs), and will hospital-based professionals (radiology, pathology, and anesthesia) be covered under institutional or referral? The same exercise is carried out with any category for which capitated funds will be accrued. Specific carve-out services, such as behavioral health, must also be accounted for.

What if not all the withhold is used or there is a surplus in either the referral pool or the institutional services pool? First, any surplus in a pool is generally first used to pay for any excess expenses in the other pool. For example, if there is money left in the referral pool but the institutional pool has cost overruns, the extra funds in the referral pool are first applied against the excessive expenses in the hospital pool, and vice versa.

After both funds are covered, any excess money is shared with or paid to the physicians. In general, only those physicians with positive balances in their own risk pools receive any money. For example, a PCP has referral services funds tracked for his or her own patients. If the cost of services for those members leaves a positive year-end balance in the referral pool, and if there is also money left in the institutional services pool on a planwide basis, the PCP receives a pro rata share of the money. In other words, risk is shared with all physicians in the plan, but reward may be tracked individually. In another example, some plans disburse positive balances in referral and institutional funds on the basis of both utilization and measures of quality and member satisfaction; a discussion of such incentive programs is found in Chapter 10.

The degree to which an individual PCP's pools will have an impact on year-end bonus disbursements may vary. If the decision is to minimize risk to individual PCPs but not eliminate the risk pools entirely, then a low stop-loss protection level must be set to minimize or even stop tracking expenses against an individual PCP's pools while those expenses are still low.

For example, if a PCP has a member with an expensive chronic disease, the referral expenses will be paid either out of the planwide referral capitation pool, out of a separate fund for disease management costs, or out of a separate stop-loss fund and will not count against the individual

PCP's referral a set amount (e.g., risk fund after referral expenses have reached $2,500). In this way, high-cost cases, which could wipe out an individual PCP's risk pool, will have less effect than that PCP's ability to manage overall referral expenses in the rest of the member panel. Stop-loss is discussed further later in this chapter.

In plans where both a referral and hospital risk pool is used, it is common, although not absolute, for a plan to pay out all extra funds in the referral pool but only half the funds in the hospital pool. In some cases, there is an upper limit on the amount of bonus a PCP can receive from the hospital pool. The justification for this is that the plan stands a considerably greater degree of risk for hospital services and therefore deserves a greater degree of reward. Furthermore, it is often a combination of utilization management and effective negotiating that yields a positive result, and the plan does the negotiating.

Pharmacy Costs

A specific category of expense has become an area of high disagreement in recent years: the risk for the cost of pharmaceuticals. With 1997–98 drug costs varying between $10.50 and $15.00 PMPM[17,18] and drug cost inflation being reported at 14–18 percent in 1999,[19] MCOs have employed a variety of means to manage it. Examples include changing the benefit to a three-tier copayment, increased use of drug utilization review, precertification of selected drugs, the use of formularies, contracting for favorable terms, and other techniques. The reader is referred to Chapter 24 for a detailed discussion on the variety of approaches taken by MCOs and medical managers in addressing this issue, and those will not be further addressed here.

There is one specific approach that does require discussion in this chapter, and that is the increase in the use of financial risk/incentives based on drug costs. As noted earlier, many MCOs do not include drug costs in any financial risk/incentive programs, although most MCOs provide data and feedback to network physicians on drug utilization and cost (see Chapters 24 and 33). But the use of risk/incentives specific to drug cost, or inclusion of drug costs in the

physician's overall capitation rate, has escalated, as illustrated in Table 8–2. The reader should note that the percentages illustrated in Table 8–2 do not match the percentages for overall financial risk programs illustrated in Figure 8–4; these data are from two different sources, use different collection methodologies, and do not represent exactly the same physician population. While one can speculate why risk for pharmacy expenses has increased (difficulty with controlling drug benefits costs) and broader risk has decreased (multiple reasons noted earlier), there is no obvious reconciliation between these two data sets. If nothing else, this helps to illustrate that compensation of physicians is anything but monolithic.

There is no evidence at all that the presence or absence of financial incentives has a negative effect on quality or has led to inappropriate prescribing. One can debate whether or not the use of financial risk/incentives has any real effect on drug costs, but two recent studies have failed to show such an association.[20,21] With the high levels of variation in prescribing patterns and habits, it is theoretically sound to place drug costs into a risk/incentive program along with the other aspects of managing this benefit cost.

Table 8–2 HMO Physician Incentives Specific to Drug Cost and Utilization, 1996–99

Separate Drug Withhold Risk/Pool	
1996	24
1997	28
1998 (est.)	40
1999 (est.)	40
Drug Reimbursement Included in Capitation	
1996	22
1997	28
1998 (est.)	46
1999 (est.)	44

Note: Although pharmacy directors indicated physician report cards and peer review as the more prevalent methods, they forecasted the greatest growth through 1999 in more financial incentives, including establishing separate drug withholds/risk pools and drug reimbursement inclusion in capitation contracts.

Source: Data from 1998 and 1999 Novartis Pharmacy Report, Novartis Pharmaceuticals, Inc., East Hanover, New Jersey.

However, as new and superior pharmaceuticals are released into the market, the number of medications taken by Americans increases, the cost of those new drugs increases, the risk of litigation increases (see the example cited in the section on Civil Liability in Physician Compensation Programs, below), and pressure from patients increases, physicians argue that the level of cost volatility is simply too high. Without being able to substantiate this opinion via research, this author believes that only large medical groups or IDSs, not individual physicians or small medical groups, are in a position to manage the cost of drugs effectively and therefore capable of managing the financial risk. The reader should understand, though, that there are many experienced managers in the managed health care industry who take the opposite stance. Further research may shed light on this contentious conundrum.

Medical Expenses for Which the Primary Care Physician Is Not at Risk

Even in plans that use withholds and risk-and-reward arrangements, there are sometimes certain medical expenses for which PCPs will not be at risk. For example, a plan may negotiate a capitated laboratory contract; laboratory capitation is then backed out of the referral and primary care capitation amounts and accounted for separately. If the PCP orders laboratory services from another vendor, that cost is deducted from his or her referral pool; otherwise, lab cost and use have no effect on the PCP's compensation.

Other examples of such nonrisk services might include any type of rider benefit (for example, vision or dental) or services over which PCPs have no control, such as obstetrics. Another example would be defined catastrophic conditions (for example, persistent vegetative state or certain chronic diseases, as discussed in Chapter 23), where the PCP is taken out of the case management function by the plan and the plan's disease or case management system takes over the coordination of care. It is important to use clear and consistent definitions of what types of cases will be treated this way. Otherwise there will be pressure from PCPs to include too much

in this category, thereby eroding the entire concept of capitation. Once a service has been taken out of the at-risk category, it is exceedingly difficult to put it back in.

Reinsurance and Stop-Loss Protection

The degree of risk to which any physician is exposed needs to be defined. As mentioned earlier, it is common for a plan to stop deducting expenses against an individual PCP's pool after a certain threshold is reached for purposes of the year-end reconciliation. There are two forms of stop-loss protection: costs for individual members and aggregate cost protection.

As an example of individual case cost protection, if a PCP has a member with leukemia, after the referral expenses reach $2,000 they will no longer be counted against the PCP's referral pool, or perhaps only 20 percent of expenses in excess of $2,000 will be counted against the referral pool; the uncounted expenses will be paid either from an aggregate pool or from a specially allocated stop-loss fund.

It is possible to vary the amount of stop-loss protection by the size of a PCP's member base to reduce the element of chance. For example, if a PCP has fewer than 300 members, the stop-loss is $2,000; if the PCP has more than 800 members, the stop-loss is $4,000. It is equally common for a stop-loss to exist for hospital services, although the level is much higher (for example, $30,000). As alluded to earlier, the lower the stop-loss, the less the impact of high-cost cases on individual capitation funds; also the greater the effect of overall medical management on cost. On the other hand, if it is too low, theoretically there may be a perverse incentive to run up expenses to get them past the stop loss. Multitiered stop-loss, a useful way to deal with differing panel sizes, creates an artificial barrier to the PCPs' acceptance of new members. For example, if the stop-loss for 300 members or fewer is less than that for 301 members or more, PCPs may resist adding members above the 300 limit so as to protect the lower stop-loss level. Tiered stop-loss can be time limited to prevent this problem.

As an example of aggregate protection, the plan may reduce deductions to 20 percent or even stop deducting referral expenses entirely after total expenses for an individual PCP reach 150 percent of the capitation risk pool amount. Providing aggregate stop-loss protection on the basis of a percentage of total capitation allows such protection to be tied to the membership base of the PCP. Since most MCOs limit the total risk that a PCP is placed at (for example, 20 percent of the PCP's capitation amount, as noted above), as well as regulatory limits in Medicare and Medicaid MCOs (as noted below), aggregate stop-loss is useful primarily in large groups or IDSs.

The combination of stop-loss protection and risk sharing across the physician panel (discussed below) serves to reduce any individual PCP's exposure to events outside his or her control. It is frustrating to manage properly all your cases but receive no incentive because one seriously ill patient had high expenses.

In any case, providing stop-loss protection to an individual physician who is at financial risk for medical costs beyond their own services, is a necessity, and the plan must budget for its cost. Although such stop-loss protection can theoretically be paid from the aggregate of all the physician's referral funds, that ensures that there will always be a draw on the withhold. Therefore, it is preferable to budget a line item for stop-loss expense, and to adjust the referral allocations by that amount if the cost of the stop-loss has not already been budgeted in the capitation build-up.

It is likewise important for there to exist a mechanism for peer review of excess expenses to determine whether they were due to bad luck or poor case management. In the latter situation, the plan may have contractual recourse to recovering part (up to the contractually agreed upon maximum individual physician risk) of the excess costs from a physician who failed to provide proper case management.

Lastly, as is mentioned briefly later in this chapter and discussed extensively in Chapter 53, only the largest MCOs can afford to carry the total financial risk of stop-loss protection, and provider groups are rarely able to do so. Provider groups at risk, as well as small to mid-sized MCOs, therefore purchase commercially available stop-loss insurance.

Individual versus Pooled Risk

All forms of financial risk are affected by how the HMO handles the issue of individual risk versus pooled risk. In other words, to what degree is an individual physician at risk for his or her own patient panel's medical costs, versus the degree that the risk is shared with some or all other PCPs? It is human nature to wish to share the downside risk (and pain) with others, but keep the upside (profit) for oneself.

In one large survey, 25 percent of plans reported using individual risk pools, 12 percent reported using risk pools of 2 to 50 physicians, and 63 percent used risk pools of more than 50 physicians.[22] In those plans that track risk pools individually, it is more common for only one pool (usually referral) to be tracked on an individual basis while the withhold, if any, and hospital pool are aggregate. In fact, it is exceedingly rare for the hospital risk pool to be at the individual physician level.

While many HMOs contract directly with PCPs, there are many that contract through the vehicle of an IPA, physician-hospital organization (PHO), management services organization (MSO), or another form of IDS (see Chapter 4 for discussions of these organizations). The HMO capitates the IPA or IDS, but that organization may or may not capitate the PCPs. As noted earlier, many of these organizations pay the PCPs on a FFS basis, using one or more of the performance-based FFS reimbursement methods described below.

Even when there is no intervening organization, the issue of determining actually who is being capitated, and for what, still remains. Is it the individual PCP? Is it a subset of the total network of PCPs (that is, pools of doctors, [PODs])? The entire network of PCPs? The answers may not be the same for each category or risk. For example, a plan may wish to capitate PCPs individually for their own services, combine them into PODs for purposes of referral services, and use the performance of the entire network for purposes of hospital services.

A plan can also choose to use different categories for risk and for reward. For example, a plan may spread risk across the entire network, but only reward a subset of PCPs. An example was given earlier in which positive balances in withholds or referral pools were used to offset deficits in the hospital pool; any remaining surplus balance would be paid only to those PCPs with a positive balance.

Issues with Individual Risk

There are common and predictable issues with individual risk. The majority of those relate to the issue of small numbers. As noted earlier, luck can have as much or more of an impact on utilization as does good management, at least in small member panels. As a PCP's panel grows to more than 500 members, this problem starts to lessen but still persists. This is one of the most important reasons that an HMO will contractually require a PCP to not close their practice to the HMO until that PCP has at least 250 or more members (see Chapter 62); it is also the identical reason that a PCP should desire to have a large panel enrolled. When a PCP has good utilization results, they generally desire to keep the reward for their hard labors; when results are poor, they frequently feel that they have been dealt an abnormally sick population of members and should not be held accountable for the high medical costs. This is a common and usually unfounded complaint, but a sophisticated practice profiling system (see Chapter 32) is able to quantify this.

The larger the dollars at stake, the more danger the problem of small numbers becomes to an individual PCP. While stop-loss and reinsurance somewhat ameliorate the problem, the problem remains. This is the reason that plans may be willing to use individual pools for referral services but will not do so for hospital services, where the dollars are substantially higher.

The other major issue with individual risk is the ability of some PCPs to game the system. In other words, in order to enhance income, the PCP manages to get his or her sickest patients to transfer out of the practice, with a resulting improvement in that individual PCP's medical costs. While all plans prohibit a PCP from kicking a member out of his or her practice due to medical condition, the rare unethical PCP can find a way to do so and remain undetected.

Related to that last issue is the concern that individual risk incents a PCP to withhold neces-

sary medical care. While this charge has been leveled at the HMO industry for many years, it has never been demonstrated. This topic is discussed below.

Finally, there have been cases of HMOs requiring an individual PCP (or small group) to actually write a check to the plan to cover cost overruns in medical expenses (as opposed to simple reconciliation of accounts held by the MCO). This has usually occurred when the plan agreed to not actually keep the withhold (in response to the PCP's plea to improve cash flow) but to track it nonetheless. Whenever a PCP is required to pay money back to the plan due to medical costs, a severe problem in provider relations is likely to occur, and it is a poor idea that is bound to lead to trouble.

Issues with Pooled Risk

If the plan chooses to pool risk across the entire network, then the flip side of individual risk occurs: the impact of any individual PCP's actions are diluted so much as to be undetectable. If a PCP is having good results, then he or she may resent having to cover for the problems of colleagues with poor results (of course, no one objects to being helped out when one's own results are poor). If the plan does not track individual results, then it will have little capability of providing meaningful data to individual physicians to help them better manage medical resources.

Because of these two extremes, many plans have chosen to use PODs for at least some financial risk management. PODs are a subset of the entire network, although there is no standard size. PODs may be a large medical group, an aggregation of 10 to 15 physicians, or may be made up of all participating PCPs in an entire geographic area. A POD could also be made up of the physicians in a PHO or MSO that accepts risk. The common denominator is that there are sufficient members enrolled in practices in the POD to allow for statistical integrity, but small enough to still allow the POD to make changes that will be seen in utilization results. The chief risk is that PODs require support from the plan in the form of timely data and utilization management. PODs cannot run in the dark and be expected to get anywhere.

It should not be assumed that PODs are a panacea; they are not. If a POD fails, the repercussions are greater than if an individual physician fails, since far more members are affected, and the dollars are higher. There are times when individual risk and reward is best, times when the entire network should be treated as a single entity, and times when PODs will make sense. Medical managers should be aware that there is some evidence from older studies (but no useful current studies) that individual risk/bonus arrangement elicits behavior changes, while aggregated risk/bonus arrangements do not.[23]

FULL PROFESSIONAL RISK CAPITATION

Full professional risk capitation* refers to the PCP or primary medical group receiving money for all professional services: primary and specialty, but not hospital services (although the group may still be on an incentive program regarding hospital utilization management). This should be distinguished from global capitation, which is discussed in Chapter 4 regarding IDSs and refers to capitation for all medical costs, not just professional.

In some cases, the PCP not only authorizes the referral but also has to write checks to SCPs for specialty services. This was once marginally popular but is currently rare, since there were problems in the past when the PCPs were unable to pay for specialty costs and members were exposed to balance billing. This was because the capitation funds arrived on a prepaid basis, but costs were not incurred until sometime later (that is, the cash arrives on Day 1, but the expenses do not occur until Day X). As cash built up, PCPs sometimes failed to understand that the bulk of that cash was actually a liability (for specialty services to be incurred sometime in the future) and needed to be treated as such. So they used the cash and had insufficient funds when they

needed to write the checks to the SCPs. Also, if they had not purchased adequate stop-loss insurance (Chapter 53), they were exposed to the cost of catastrophic cases.

There has been a recent resurgence of interest in this form of capitation, as PCPs band together into large groups or other forms of collective activity, such as IPAs, PHOs, and MSOs. Full professional risk capitation is generally not supportable by other than a large group or organized system of PCPs. If the organized group is large and well capitalized, has good information systems, and is able to manage the funds and risk-based accounting (Chapter 47) via their business office, this may be acceptable. At an individual or small group level, it is unacceptable. To the degree that the primary care group can capitate SCPs for services, the less the danger of having insufficient funds. However, many state insurance departments will not allow a provider to subcapitate without a special license; that is, the insurance department believes that only a licensed HMO or specialty HMO, not another provider, may capitate a provider (see Chapter 69). As an example, in California this would take the form of a "Limited Knox-Keene License," which is a form of MCO license that limits the provider organization to contracting with other providers, but prohibits it from marketing or other activities that a fully-licensed MCO does.

Any group accepting full professional risk capitation needs strong financial management skills and good computer systems support. Of considerable interest, one substantial study looked at how physicians at such a form of financial risk managed their own utilization: the physicians employed techniques identical to traditional HMO utilization management, including the use of a PCP gatekeeper, an authorization system, practice profiling, clinical guidelines, and managed care education (see Chapters 18, 19, and 20 for discussions of these techniques).[24] It should be noted that many HMOs are reluctant to enter into full risk arrangements unless they are convinced that the physicians will be able to manage utilization, since they do not wish to be exposed to the risk of failure such as occurred with the PPMCs.

---

*The term *full professional risk* **capitation** is one of convenience in this chapter. There is no consistent term for this in the real world.

REASONS TO CAPITATE

The first and most powerful reason for an HMO to capitate providers is that capitation puts the provider at some level of risk or incentive for medical expenses and utilization. Capitation eliminates the FFS incentive to overutilize and brings the financial incentives of the capitated provider in line with the financial incentives of the HMO. Under capitation, costs are more easily predicted by the health plan (although not absolutely predictable because of problems of out-of-network care and catastrophe cases). Capitation is also easier and less costly to administer than FFS (for example, fewer claims to adjudicate), thus resulting in lower administrative costs in the HMO and potentially lower premium rates to the member.

The most powerful reasons for a provider to accept capitation from an HMO are financial. Capitation ensures good cash flow: the capitation money comes in at a predictable rate, regardless of services rendered, and comes in as prepayment, thus providing positive cash flow.

Also, for physicians who are effective medical case managers as well as cost-effective providers of direct patient care, the profit margins under capitation can exceed those found in FFS, especially as FFS fees come under continued pressure.

In 1998 and 1999 profitability of capitation fell, however, as illustrated in Figure 8–6. The results shown in Figure 8–6 do not differentiate the causes for this fall in profitability, but the financial losses of the HMO and health insurance industry are parallel and probably due to the same forces (for example, downward market pressure on premiums in the face of rising medical costs, especially in pharmacy). The levels and effects of various risk/incentive arrangements are not differentiated and may account for much of the erosion in margin. The reader should not conclude, based on this figure, that capitation is a losing proposition; historically it has not been, and the events of 1998 and 1999 do not necessarily predict a trend. At the same point in time, downward pressure has been exerted on

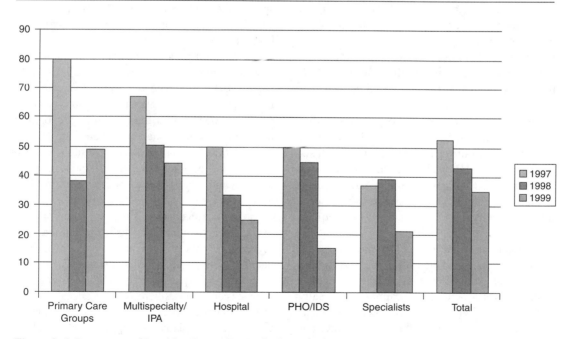

Figure 8–6 Percentage of Providers Reporting Capitation as Profitable. *Source:* 1999 Capitation Survey, Copyright © 1999 by National Health Information, LLC, Atlanta, GA. For further information on this and other NHI publications, call 800-597-6300 or visit www. nhionline.net.

all forms of physician reimbursement, including fees from Medicare and Medicaid as well as fee allowances from commercial health insurers.

PROBLEMS WITH CAPITATION SYSTEMS

The most common problem with capitation involves chance. As mentioned earlier, a significant element of chance is involved when there are too few members in an enrolled base to make up for bad luck (or good luck, but nobody ever complains about that). Physicians with fewer than 100 members may find that the dice simply roll against them, and they will have members who need bypass surgery, have cancer, have acquired immune deficiency syndrome (AIDS), or a host of other expensive medical problems. The only way to assuage that is to spread the risk for expensive cases through common risk-sharing pools for referral and institutional expenses and to provide stop-loss protection for expensive cases.

The problem of small numbers is especially acute in the early period of a PCP's participation with the MCO (unless the MCO is failing to grow, in which case both physician and MCO have a problem). In order to deal with this, as well as a way to entice PCPs to participate, some HMOs have offered to pay the PCP on an FFS basis for the first six months or until the PCP has more than 50 enrollees, whichever comes first. A few HMOs have offered to pay capitation but have guaranteed that the PCP would receive the higher of capitation or FFS in that first six months. A few HMOs have even agreed to pay FFS until the PCP has more than 50 members, without any time limit, but that is unwise since it may disincent the PCP to enroll an adequate number of members.

Another frequent problem is in the perception of the physicians and their office staff. Although many practices have now acclimated to capitation, there is a feeling that capitation is really funny money. When PCPs are receiving a capitation payment of $11.25, this is sometimes unconsciously (or consciously) confused with the office charge. In their minds, it appears as though everyone is coming in for service and demanding the most expensive care possible, all for an office charge of $11.25. It is easy to forget that many of the members who have signed up with that physician are not even coming in at all. It takes only 10 percent of the members to come in once per month to make it seem as if there is a never-ending stream of entitled demanders in the waiting room. The best approach to this is to make sure that the plan collects data on encounters so that the actual reimbursement per visit can be calculated.

The last major perceived problem is inappropriate underutilization. An argument made against capitation in general and risk-and-reward arrangements in particular, is that the MCO is paying physicians to not do something, and that is dangerous.[25-35] Despite these concerns, a very large body of literature shows that managed care systems have provided equal or better care to members than uncontrolled FFS systems, even while lowering costs.[36-59]

In an unmanaged FFS system, there is a direct and immediate relationship between doing something and getting paid for it; under capitation, the reward is temporally remote from the action. In other words, the capitation check does not change each month depending on services. Furthermore, by carefully constructing a stop-loss protection program, the effect of high-cost cases on capitation funds is attenuated. Spreading the risk over more than one physician can lower the effect of single cases on a physician's reimbursement, but at the cost of not recognizing individual performance. In addition, it must be kept in mind that HMOs, with their lack of deductibles and high levels of coinsurance, lower economic barriers to care, thus improving access to care.

In the final analysis, it is the obligation of plan management to monitor the quality of services and to ensure that there is no inappropriate underutilization of services. One can argue that in a well-managed plan, identification of poor quality is easier because there is more access to data and a tighter quality assurance system, and that is exactly how the plan must approach this issue.

One last issue should be raised, although it is not a problem per se but something to be aware of: in a capitated system, savings from decreased utilization may not always result in direct savings to the plan. In other words, if primary care services undergo a reduction in utilization, the capitation payments will not go down, just as they will not go up when there is increased utilization.

EFFECT OF BENEFITS DESIGN ON REIMBURSEMENT

Benefits design may have a great effect on reimbursement to PCPs in capitated programs, although the effect is felt in any reimbursement system that relies on performance. The three major categories of benefits design that have such an impact are reductions in benefits, copayment levels, and POS plans.

Benefits Reductions

Because many managed care plans have adopted greater flexibility in benefits design in response to marketplace demands, the underpinnings of actuarial assumptions that are used to build capitation rates have become more variable and complex. The impact of benefits reductions on primary care services is usually not so great as to warrant changing previously acceptable capitation rates, but that is not an absolute.

Benefits changes have a greater impact on risk pools. For example, if mental health and chemical dependency coverage are carved out of the PCP managing system and turned over to a dedicated management function (a common occurrence in managed care; see Chapter 25), then concomitant reductions in the referral and hospital risk pools are warranted. The same is true if an account wanted to carve out pharmacy services to another vendor (for example, a national company that administers a card and mail order program).

Copayment Levels

Copayment levels can have an immediate impact on capitation rates, both for PCP capitation and for risk pool allocations. The amount of capitation due a PCP will be different with a $5.00 copayment compared to a $10.00 copayment. For example, if a capitation rate were calculated to be $11.25 on the basis of three visits PMPY at $50.00 per visit and a $5.00 copayment ($50.00 − $5.00 =

$45.00; 3 visits × $45.00 = $135.00; $135.00 ÷ 12 = $11.25 PMPM), then application of a $10.00 copayment would reduce the capitation amount to $10.00 ($50.00 − $10.00 = $40.00; 3 visits × $40.00 = $120.00; $120.00 ÷ 12 months = $10.00 PMPM).

The same issue applies for calculating contributions to referral risk pools and hospital risk pools. For example, if consultant care has a $15.00 copayment, then estimated consultant visit costs would have to take the copayment into account. The same is true for hospital care if copayments of $100.00 or $200.00 are applied.

The effect of copayments and cost sharing on utilization is real, although it differs with respect to the health status of an individual as well as the amount of out-of-pocket expense to which the member is exposed.[60–62] It should be noted, however, that cost sharing does not necessarily selectively reduce inappropriate hospitalization (in other words, although total utilization may be reduced with cost sharing, the change in utilization may not reflect a change in whether the utilization was appropriate in the first place).[63] Deciding whether to adjust capitation rates on the basis of expected utilization differences from copayments is difficult. Explaining such adjustments to PCPs is no easy or enjoyable task either because changes in utilization are population based, and any individual member may or may not change his or her behavior.

Adjusting capitation rates for copayments is not easily done if there are widespread differences in copayment amounts among different accounts. For example, if 50 percent of the members have a $5.00 copayment, 35 percent have a $10.00 copayment, and 15 percent have a $15.00 copayment for primary care services (not to mention different copayments for referral services), calculating the appropriate capitation is complex. Even so, it is necessary to do unless the variations are exceedingly minor or infrequent.

Point-of-Service Plans

For the purposes of this discussion, POS plans are those that allow members to obtain a high level of benefits by using the HMO or gatekeeper system while still having insurance-

type benefits available if they choose to use providers without going through the managed care
system. For further discussion of POS, see
Chapters 3 and 41.

Because members with POS benefits are not
totally locked in to the managed care plan, utilization occurs both in and out of network. Although the plan can actuarially determine the
level of in- and out-of-network use for the entire
enrolled group, that cannot be said for an individual physician's member panel. This has an
obvious impact on capitation rates.

When POS plans were first introduced in the
1980s, some plans attempted to adjust capitation
rates on the basis of prospective in-network utilization. The capitation rate was thus reduced, further exacerbating the problem of luck (good or
bad). Because of the problem of small numbers
noted earlier. When one adds the probability of
out-of-network usage, chance becomes an even
greater force. One PCP might find that all of his
or her members access services exclusively via
the PCP (resulting in severe underpayment by
the reduced capitation amount), while another
PCP may find that the majority of his or her
members go out of network (resulting in capitation overpayment due to the low visit rate). In
those MCOs that place the PCP at some level of
financial risk for specialty services, the same
problem existed, although in reverse (members
staying in network resulted in better financial results in the risk pool than occurred when members went out of network).

Other plans at that time attempted to make
adjustments on a retrospective basis, actually
asking a PCP to refund a percentage of the capitation payment they had received all year (corresponding to the percentage of out-of-network
costs above that predicted actuarially) or increasing the withhold to high levels to recover
the money. The ability of the PCP to write that
check was usually poor due to the chronic cash
flow problems that most physicians face (they
need to pay their staff, the rent, supplies, insurance, and so forth); even if they did pay the
MCO back, it often meant financial hardship.
These two approaches created terribly difficult
exercises in provider relations, were generally

perceived as unfair (a perception shared by this
author), and are now uncommon.

An alternative approach was not to reduce the
capitation rate. That meant that the MCO paid
twice for some out-of-network costs (specifically
those services that the PCP was capitated for but
were delivered by out-of-network physicians). It
also created windfall profits for the PCP whose
POS members never came in for services (or, on a
more pernicious note, for the PCP who did not
provide adequate access for POS members,
thereby driving them out of network for services).
As noted earlier, if the PCP also was at some level
of risk/incentive for nonprimary services, the reverse dynamic occurred.

The problem of using capitation with POS has
become so difficult that many plans capitate PCPs
for pure HMO (that is, not POS) members and pay
FFS (without using any risk pool) for POS members. This creates problems due to the schizophrenic reimbursement systems and results in
what psychologists refer to as cognitive disso-
nance. But it is viable and is used. Many MCOs
with high levels of POS membership simply do
not capitate at all and use FFS exclusively.

Figure 8–7 illustrates relative percentages of
MCOs that, in 1994, used different reimbursement systems for different product types, illustrating the high heterogeneity of payment systems. One may safely assume, based on data
presented earlier regarding levels of capitation
and incentive programs in place in 1998–99, that
this heterogeneity is even more pronounced than
was the case in 1994.

As stated above, POS makes it difficult to
measure performance of PCPs. For example, if
performance is based only on in-network utilization, one good way to look like a stellar performer is subtly to encourage POS members to
seek services out of network. If PCPs are held
accountable for all services, both in and out of
network, then they may argue that it is not fair
that they are held accountable for cost and utilization that is completely out of their control.

Although this issue is not easily resolved,
some plans have chosen to fold out-of-network
utilization into the performance-based reimbursement system, whether capitation or FFS.

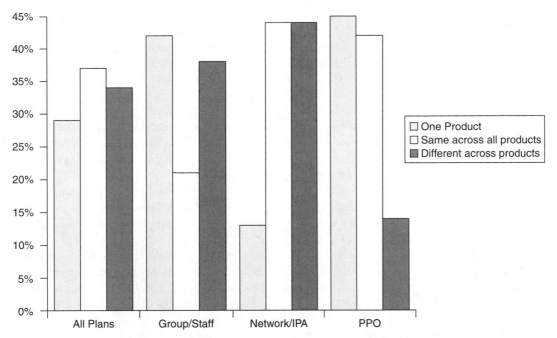

Figure 8–7 Variation in Reimbursement Model by Product. *Source:* Reprinted from Mathematica Policy Research, Inc. and The Medical College of Virginia for the Physician Payment Review Commission, 1994, MedPac, Government Services Administration.

To attenuate the problem of lack of control by an individual PCP, the risk or reward system is spread out among groups of PCPs or the entire network, thereby maintaining actuarial integrity. In other MCOs that choose to maintain a performance-based reimbursement system that includes POS, the incentive may be based primarily on nonutilization factors (for example, quality measures, member satisfaction, efficient use of electronic commerce, and other measures) and only secondarily on cost or utilization measures. In these programs though, the funding for nonutilization incentives may be derived from medical cost savings, in which case incentives are paid only if surpluses are generated. Nonutilization-based incentive programs are the focus of Chapter 10.

While capitating individual PCPs is a challenge with POS, it is certainly possible to capitate a large group or an IDS. In most cases, a prospective adjustment is made to the capitation rate based on the actuary's best estimate of in- versus out-of-network utilization. Out-of-net-

work claims are paid by the plan from the funds that had been backed out of the capitation rate. Surpluses (or a percent of surpluses) in that pool of funds may be returned to the group or IDS in order to encourage them to find ways of getting their enrolled members to seek care in network, thus reducing out-of-network utilization.

FEE FOR SERVICE

There are some veterans of managed health care who hold that the FFS system of American medicine is the root of all the problems we have historically faced with high costs. Although that is simplistic, there is some truth to it, particularly when there were no controls in place. In a system where economic reward is predicated on how much one does, particularly if procedural services pay more than cognitive ones, it is only human nature to do more since it pays more. The reward is immediate and tangible: A large bill is made out, and it usually gets paid. Doing less results in getting paid less.

On the other side of the argument, FFS results in distribution of payment on the basis of expenditure of resources. In other words, a physician who is caring for sicker patients will be paid more, reflecting that physician's greater investment of time, energy, and skills.

In a managed health care plan, FFS may be used to compensate physicians and may be the method of choice in certain situations. For example, in a simple preferred provider organization (PPO; see Chapter 3), FFS will be virtually the only option available, except in the oxymoronic "capitated PPO". The reasons for an HMO to use FFS reimbursement are varied and have not been systematically studied. One dynamic is that FFS is frequently more acceptable to physicians, so many HMOs use FFS in order to get more physicians to sign up, at least in an HMO's initial period of development. This is especially true in markets where managed care penetration is low; where managed care penetration is high, PCPs often prefer capitation. As noted earlier, HMOs may also capitate IPAs or PHOs, but those organizations actually pay FFS to the physicians. Also as noted earlier, certain products such as POS also are difficult to capitate and lead many MCOs with a large POS enrollment to use FFS. Some HMOs simply believe that FFS is the best way to reimburse PCPs and have operated that way for more than 20 years.

It is worth noting in passing that for years the concept of paying FFS to PCPs but capitation to SCPs has been bandied about. The theoretical advantage of this approach is that it encourages PCPs to see their managed care patients rather than refer them out, since they otherwise do not get paid. Capitating SCPs, on the other hand, reduces the FFS pressure to do more and charge more. It is an excellent concept but has proven difficult to put into place. There are no studies that illuminate the reasons why this idea has not successfully taken root. Conjecture would include:

- the large number of SCPs in any market coupled with the market's demands for access to a large specialty network makes capitating SCPs difficult due to the requirement for larger panels of members assigned to the SCP to achieve actuarial integrity

(i.e., patients visit surgeons far less frequently than they do PCPs, so the base number of members must be much higher just to get an adequate number of total visits to the surgeon)
- resistance by SCPs or even PCPs
- problems with the plan's information system in administering the program
- problems installing this reimbursement system in the face of highly variable benefits designs
- all the problems associated with POS and other non-HMO products
- corporate inertia at the MCO level.

In order to still try to apply this idea despite the above noted problems, some plans and IDSs have used contact capitation. This uncommon reimbursement methodology is discussed further in Chapter 11.

Fee-for-Service Categories

There are two broad FFS categories: straight FFS and performance-based FFS. Performance-based incentive programs unrelated to cost or utilization are discussed separately in Chapter 10.

The first category, straight FFS is less common in HMOs, although nearly universal in PPOs, Blue Cross Blue Shield (BCBS) service plans, and indemnity insurance. In some cases, an HMO may not even be allowed to use straight FFS, since the PCPs are required to be at some level of financial risk in order for the HMO to qualify for licensure.

Performance-based FFS simply refers to the fact that the fees that the PCPs (and perhaps the SCPs) ultimately receive will be influenced to some degree by performance. Whether performance refers to overall plan performance, performance of only one segment of medical costs (professional costs, for example), or performance of the individual PCP is quite variable. How performance affects the fees is likewise variable. The no-balance-billing clause (Chapter 62) is critically important to a managed FFS plan. This clause states that the physician will look only to the plan for payment of services and will accept payment by the plan as payment in full. In other words, if the plan has to reduce or otherwise alter the amount of payment, the physician will not look to the member for any additional fees. The use of FFS by MCOs has increased dramatically in recent years, as illustrated earlier in Figure 8–1.

Determination of Fees

Usual, Customary, or Reasonable

The historical method of fee determination is the usual, customary, or reasonable (UCR) fee. The exact definition of the term *UCR* has undergone a subtle change in the past 10–15 years. It used to be defined as "usual, customary, *and* reasonable." It is now defined as "usual, customary, *or* reasonable." The definition of reasonable is one made by the payer, not the provider, and may actually be quite a bit lower than any of the prevailing charges for certain procedures that payers determine to be grossly overpriced. For example, when the charges for a procedure like cataract removal and lens implantation were first set, it was new, complex, took a long time to do, and required skills in rare supply. Now, that procedure is considered routine, is a high-volume procedure, takes little time, and is performed by a great number of ophthalmologists; the historical basis for the charge is no longer valid. Therefore, many payers (MCOs, health insurance companies, and governmental agencies) pay far less than the prevailing charges.

There is little uniformity to UCR across the country because UCR represents what physicians usually bill for defined services, and there can be tremendous discrepancies among physician's fees for the same service. One common methodology for determining UCR is to collect data for charges by current procedural terminology (CPT) code, calculate the charges that represent the 25th, 50th, 90th, and 95th percentiles, and then choose which percentile represents the UCR maximum. The MCO's customer (that is, an employer contracting with the MCO), sometimes determines the percentile used and may even choose different percentiles for different types of services (for example, basic medical-surgical, behavioral health, preventive care, and so forth). It is by far most common, however, for the MCO to make the determination.

It is uncommon for plans to generate all the UCR data themselves unless they are very large in a geographic area. If they have a very large database, they can achieve statistically meaningful numbers. Most plans do not have that amount of concentrated data, however. Large, national managed care companies may have a large amount of data, but they are spread across wide geographic areas. In that case, they may have sufficient data to set the maximum UCR for certain CPT codes, but not others. MCOs usually purchase a commercially available database. The two most common are the MDR™ database, owned by Ingenix, Inc., of Salt Lake City, Utah; and what was popularly known (and is often still called) the HIAA* database, renamed the Prevailing Healthcare Charges System™ (also owned by Ingenix after their 1998 acquisition of it). Both databases provide information based on geographic region. As of 1999 the MDR™ database incorporates some statistical analysis, while the Prevailing Healthcare Charges System™ database is primarily based on prevailing charges.

In the simplest form of indemnity insurance, when a claim is submitted it is paid in full if it is lower than the UCR maximum. If the claim is higher, it is paid at the UCR maximum. All claim payments are subject to coinsurance, deductibles, and overall benefits determination.

A SPECIAL REQUIREMENT FOR REIMBURSEMENT WHEN COINSURANCE IS IN PLACE

For any benefits plan in which the member must pay coinsurance (i.e., a *percentage* of the total) to a contracted FFS provider, an important policy must be put in place. This policy is the result of numerous lawsuits by state's attorneys general and concerns the base that the coinsurance is calculated on. It applies to any charges from any type of provider, but not to capitation systems or benefits plans that use copayments rather than coinsurance.

---

*The acronym of the Health Insurance Association of America, the original developer of the database.

In past years, some insurance companies (for example, some BCBS plans or other predominantly non-HMO plans) that contracted with providers for reduced fees or charges, calculated the member's coinsurance requirement on the charged amount, not on the negotiated amount. For example, if a member was subject to a 20 percent coinsurance requirement and a physician charged $100 but the plan's negotiated fee was $75, the member had to pay 20 percent of $100 (or $20), not 20 percent of $75 (or $15).

This was determined to be fraudulent by the courts, since the member was required to pay a percentage of the total actual cost, not of charges that exceeded the total. As illustrated above, the member was in fact paying more than the designated percentage of the total payment to the contracted provider. Since then, any plan using FFS or charge-based reimbursement (including many of the forms of reimbursement of hospitals and institutions discussed in Chapter 12) must apply the coinsurance percentage to the actual reimbursement amount to contracted providers, not the charge. The net effect of this was to reduce the total amount of money received by the providers, but it provided better protection and greater value for the members.

This issue only applies to payments to contracted providers whose charges are higher than the total payment they agree to accept as payment in full. It does not apply to any charges by noncontracted providers, even when the plan's payment is less than the charges, as discussed next.

OUT-OF-NETWORK FEES

The way a health plan determines fees to be paid to noncontracting physicians, while not the direct focus of this chapter, is a topic that deserves brief mention. In any service plan, PPO, POS, or even HMO, members will incur charges out of network. In the case of HMOs, that will generally only occur in emergencies or when the member is travelling far from the service area and needs care. For other types of plans, out-of-network care is expected and is part of the benefits package. In the case of HMOs that do not have out-of-network benefits, costs for true emergencies or out-of-network care authorized by the HMO are usually paid in full.

Other than for pure HMO products, what an MCO will actually pay for out-of-network charges is not as simple as it appears on its face. For example, a POS plan may provide for a 30 percent coinsurance for out-of-network care, but that does not mean that the plan will actually pay 70 percent of the charge. Unless the benefits state specifically that the plan will pay at those levels, the most common approach is to pay at 70 percent of what the POS plan considers *reasonable* (see note above). In some cases, reasonable may be defined using a UCR schedule as described earlier. In other cases, reasonable is defined using the fee schedule that the plan uses to reimburse in-network providers. In the latter case, depending on the level of discount the plan has with contracting providers, the difference between the "allowed" charge and what the patient was charged can be considerably less than 70 percent. For example, the charge from the non-contracting provider is $100.00, but the health plan's fee allowance for contracting providers is $60.00. Coverage is therefore 70% of $60.00, or only $42.00 (.07 × $42.00), *not* $70.00 (0.7 × $100.00). Since the out-of-network provider is not subject to no-balance billing, the patient is liable for the difference between what the plan pays and what the provider charged.

Marketing literature and benefits contracts must explain this policy. However, not all members read such literature, nor understand it if they do read it. But as a simple matter of actuarial fact, the more generously a plan pays for out-of-network care, the more cost it will incur and the more out-of-network care will be rendered—and the more costly the premium of the product.

Since the focus of this chapter is not on benefits design, further discussion of coverage issues is not warranted.

DISCOUNTS, NEGOTIATED FEE SCHEDULES, FEE MAXIMUMS, OR FEE ALLOWANCES

In some plans (i.e., service plans or PPOs that are fast fading from the scene), the negotiated payment rate to contracted providers is simply a percentage discount off the UCR or the submitted claim, whichever is lower. The advantage to using this approach is that it is extremely easy to obtain. Most physicians will gladly accept a discount on fees if it ensures rapid and guaranteed payment. The problem is that there is nothing to prevent a physician whose fees are below the UCR maximum from increasing his or her fees up to the UCR maximum, which they will promptly do unless they are totally asleep at the wheel. Some plans require the physician to notify the plan of a fee hike, but in truth there is little that the plan can or will do if it has no real clout.

Related to the use of UCR, many plans that pay FFS have a maximum fee allowance schedule. This schedule is created using a combination of UCR data and internal plan data, and is subject to policy decisions by the medical department. In other words, some of the fee maximums are set by policy, not by historical charge data. For example, both UCR and local prevailing fees for a certain procedure may be high, but plan medical managers set a much lower fee maximum based on decreases in the cost, complexity, and volume of the procedure that reflect current reality, not past experience.

In provider-sponsored MCOs or IDSs, it is important that the physicians who participate in the plan not be the ones to set the fee schedules or relative value scale (RVS—discussed next). To do so courts an antitrust violation. In such organizations, it is necessary to employ an outside firm to create the fee schedules and RVS.

RELATIVE VALUE SCALES

The use of an RVS has gained widespread popularity in FFS plans. In this system, each procedure, as defined in CPT, has a relative value associated with it. The plan pays the physician on the basis of a monetary multiplier for the RVS value. For example, if a procedure has a value of 4 and the multiplier is $12, the payment is $48. In the past, RVSs merely reflected prevailing fee schedules or UCRs, but had the advantage of allowing for easy modifications to the fees overall by simply changing the multiplier. This could be done uniformly for all types of procedures or differently for classes of procedures (for example, the multiplier for office visits could be raised more than the multiplier for cataract removal and lens implantation).

A classic problem in using an RVS and negotiating the value of the multiplier has been the imbalance between procedural and cognitive services. As in FFS in general, procedures have higher charges than cognitive services. In other words, there is less payment to a physician for performing a careful history and physical examination and thinking about the patient's problem than for doing a procedure involving needles, scalpels, or machines. This is why the use of simple RVSs has been giving way to the resource-based relative value scale (RBRVS).

Resource-Based Relative Value Scale

The RBRVS was developed on behalf of the Health Care Financing Administration (HCFA) for Medicare. By looking at the amount of resources actually required to provide each service (including not only tangible resources such as materials, clinical settings, and time, but also the resources invested by the physician in training), a relative value was assigned to each CPT code in use by Medicare. That meant that many CPT codes not commonly used by Medicare (for example, pediatric procedures) were not originally affected by RBRVS, but it has since broadened to cover more codes.

RBRVS has addressed to some extent the imbalance between cognitive and procedural services, lowering the value of invasive procedures (for example, cardiac surgery) and raising the value of cognitive ones (for example, office visits). HCFA has imposed this on all physicians for Medicare recipients, and uses it to limit the amount that even nonparticipating physicians may charge Medicare beneficiaries, using a complicated formula not germane to this discussion.

Many large insurers and MCOs have followed suit in setting their determination of reasonable fees. They usually do not pay the same amount as Medicare but use the same RBRVS schedules. The percent above or below a Medicare payment is partly determined by geography and partly by competition. For example, in 1999 the average percentage of Medicare fees that commercial plans considered as the maximum fee allowance was 119 percent of the Medicare fee. In different parts of the country, that percentage was higher or lower, and in some locales with steep competition and a surplus of physicians, the percentage of the Medicare fee allowance was under 90 percent.

GLOBAL FEES

A variation on FFS is the global fee. A global fee is a single fee that encompasses all services delivered in an episode. Common examples of global fees include obstetrics, in which a single fee is supposed to cover all prenatal visits, the delivery itself, and at least one postnatal visit; and certain surgical procedures, in which a single surgical fee pays for preoperative care, the surgery itself, and postoperative care. Although the subject of this chapter is compensation of PCPs, it is worthwhile discussing the application of global fees in both the SCP and PCP settings in order to provide an adequate picture.

Global fees may encompass more than one provider if the providers themselves are organized to manage it. The most common example of this is the management of a patient with coronary artery disease. The MCO and providers negotiate a global fee that covers multiple services for this disease. For example, cardiac testing, coronary angiography, and the coronary surgical procedure are all part of the single global fee. In some cases, the diagnostic workup will be uncomplicated and the patient will have a transluminal coronary angioplasty; in other cases, the patient will have complex disease and require multivessel coronary artery bypass surgery. Unless the volume of such cases referred to the contracted providers is high and therefore evens out (actuarially speaking), it is common to also negotiate an outlier "trim point" where the costs so exceed the global fee that the MCO pays an additional amount, usually a fixed amount per day or some form of fee schedule.

The concept is applicable to chronic, nonsurgical care as well, though not as often as for surgical care. The most common examples are in diseases such as insulin-dependent diabetes, AIDS, end-stage renal disease, and others that are similar in their chronicity. In these types of situations, the SCP or the organized provider system (for example, a nephrologist, a dialysis center, and other physicians, such as ophthalmologists and podiatrists) are paid a fixed fee on a regular basis. This can be monthly or quarterly, but it is not advisable to lengthen the time period beyond that, since these patients are not necessarily stable. For this type of global fee to work, the services must be well defined, similar to what is done under capitation. Services beyond what are included in the global fee (for example, acute hospitalizations) are paid separately by the MCO. This approach is well suited to disease management programs (see Chapter 23), especially in MCOs that remove such chronically ill patients from a PCP's member panel so that care is managed by an SCP of the appropriate specialty.

Global fees are useful in any type of reimbursement system used for PCPs. They may be used to pay for nonprimary care services regardless of the use of capitation, FFS, or any other system to compensate PCPs. Having said that, some plans use a form of global fees to cover primary care as well. In this case, the plan must statistically analyze what goes into the average primary care visit in order to calculate the global fee. That analysis must include the range of visit codes as well as all covered services that occur during primary care visits (for example, electrocardiography, simple laboratory tests, spirometry, and so forth). The analysis will vary by specialty type (that is, internal medicine, family practice, or pediatrics).

The analysis then builds by specialty a composite type of visit. The average type of visit for internal medicine, for example, may be an intermediate visit, and 20 percent of the time an electrocardiogram is performed, 30 percent of the time a urinalysis is performed, and so forth (these figures are fictitious and should not be used for actual fee calculations). The plan then builds up the global fee by putting together the pieces, for example, $42 for the office visit, $7.00 for the electrocardiogram ($35.00 × 0.2), and so forth.

Plans that use global fees for primary care may also tie the fees to performance. For example, utilization targets may be set for some or all medical services. How a PCP or group of PCPs performs against these targets may be used to set the global fees. For example, PMPM targets are set for primary care, referral care, institutional care, and ancillary services. Performance of a group or POD of PCPs is measured against those targets on a rolling 12-month basis, and performance against those targets is used to adjust prospectively the next quarter's global fee up or down. Targets are of course modified by age, sex, product type (for example, pure HMO versus POS), or any other variables that are appropriate. Targets are also modified for the effect of stop-loss against catastrophic cases. In other words, measurement of performance is similar to that used in capitated systems but does not involve actual capitated risk pools or withholds. What the PCP gets as the global fee is what they get, period.

The chief value of a global fee is that it protects against problems of unbundling and upcoding. With unbundling, the physician now bills separate charges for services once included in a single fee; for example, the office visit is $45.00, the bandage is $10.00, starch in the nurse's uniform is $3.00, and so forth. Upcoding refers to billing for a procedure that yields greater revenue than that actually performed; an example is coding for an office visit that was longer than the time actually spent with the patient. In the primary care setting, global fees offer no protection against churning, which is the practice of generating more bills by seeing patients more often than is medically necessary. In fact, global fees, if not managed correctly, may exacerbate a problem with churning, and that is a form of utilization that requires monitoring by the MCO.

A global fee system is really a hybrid of capitation and FFS. Like capitation, PMPM targets in all categories of medical expense are monitored, and there is a statistical buildup to determine the global fee. Also like capitation, it transfers some level of risk to the provider and provides for some stability in costs to the MCO.

Unlike capitation, there are generally no payouts from capitated risk pools (for example, referral pools), so there is no dollar-for-dollar relationship between utilization and reimbursement. Like FFS, payment is made only if services are rendered, and no payments are made if there are no services. Thus, even though some level of risk has been transferred to the provider, it is based on known medical conditions that are more clearly within the purview of the contracted provider(s).

This last feature makes such systems attractive to employer groups that have much lower than normal utilization (that is, those that have healthy employees and dependents who require fewer services than a typical capitation calculation assumes). It is also attractive to POS plans where the plan desires to reward performance but needs to address both in- and out-of-network utilization. As discussed earlier, under capitation the MCO runs the risk of paying twice for services under POS: once through capitation and again through out-of-network claims. It is attractive to providers since it has some of the advantages of capitation (cash flow, known reimbursement, and less paperwork) as well as some of the advantages of FFS (it is based on services rendered and defined medical conditions that the provider has expertise in managing).

Withholds

As with capitation, many plans that use FFS withhold a certain percentage of the fee to cover medical cost overruns. For example, the plan may be using a negotiated fee schedule that amounts to a 20 percent discount for most physician fees. The plan then withholds an additional 20 percent in a risk pool until the end of the year. In effect, physicians receive what amounts to 60 percent of their usual fee but may receive an additional 20 percent at the end of the year if there were no excess medical costs.

It is possible to create profiles of physicians' utilization patterns to distribute more equitably the withhold funds in the event that some, but not all, of the withhold is used to cover extra medical costs. This is difficult in an FFS system using a withhold if there is no gatekeeper model in place. In that case, most plans simply return remaining withhold funds on a straight pro rata basis, although some plans return withhold on a preferential basis to PCPs as opposed to SCPs.

Mandatory Reductions in All Fees

In an HMO where risk for medical cost is shared with all the physicians and where straight CPT codes are used to reimburse on an FFS basis, there must exist a mechanism whereby fees may be reduced unilaterally by the HMO in the event of cost overruns. This concept may be employed in a strongly managed PPO as well.

For example, the plan may be using a fee schedule that is equivalent to a 20 percent discount on the most common fees in the area. In the event that medical expenses are over budget and there is not enough money in the withhold fund (if present) to cover them, all physicians' fees are reduced by a further percentage, say an additional 10 percent, to cover the expenses. At this point, the effective discount is 30 percent, although this would really be 50 percent in the event that a withhold system was in place, all of the withhold funds had been used, and there were still excess medical liabilities. The major policy decision to be made when things go awry is setting how low fee reductions will go before they will not be further reduced. For example, the plan may set the lowest possible fees at 60 percent of Medicare, though if the plan reaches that point, there will not be too many physicians left in the network to pay.

Budgeted FFS

Related to mandatory fee reductions, budgeted FFS is used in a few plans. In this variation, which is somewhat like contact capitation (discussed in Chapter 11 as it applies to SCPs), the plan budgets a maximum amount of money that may be spent in each specialty category. This maximum may be expressed either as a PMPM amount (for example, $7.50 PMPM) or as a percentage of revenue (for example, 5.6 percent of premium revenue). As costs in that specialty category approach or exceed the budgeted

amount, the withhold in that specialty—but not across all specialties—is increased. In addition, the fees for that specialty—but not all specialties—may be reduced.

This approach has the advantage of focusing the reimbursement changes on those specialties in which excess costs occur rather than on all specialties in the network. The disadvantage is that this is not individual provider specific; in other words, all specialists are treated the same, and there is no specific focus on individual outliers. Plans that do not use gatekeepers to manage care may find this type of approach useful. This type of system usually only works when there are regular reports and practice profiles provided to the physicians (see Chapters 32 and 33). Budgeted FFS also requires an excellent computer system and reliable data—both of which may not be readily available.

Sliding Scale Individual Fee Allowances

Related to budgeted FFS is the sliding scale individual fee allowance. In this model, PCP performance is again measured against benchmark targets in all categories of medical expense, with appropriate protection for expensive outlier cases. On the basis of performance, the PCP's reimbursement, for example, may vary from 70 percent of allowable charges up to 110 percent if performance exceeds targets.[64] Although this system still allows for upcoding and unbundling, it does vary by individual on the basis of performance and could be applied to groups of physicians as well as to individuals. The effects of chance and small numbers apply to this concept even more than they do to capitation, since reimbursement may be lowered more than would occur under a fixed capitation system. This method also requires a lot of computer as well as timely and reliable data.

Point of Service and Performance-Based FFS

As discussed earlier, a central issue facing plan management in applying performance-based reimbursement under POS is determining whether to include out-of-network costs in the performance evaluation of PCPs. The issues are identical no matter if capitation or performance-based FFS is used.

PROBLEMS WITH FFS IN MANAGED HEALTH CARE PLANS

There are two significant problems with using FFS in managed health care plans. These problems can become markedly exacerbated if the plan starts to get into financial trouble. The best approach to both of these problems requires the MCO to have excellent data management and profiling capabilities (see Chapter 32). Without good profiling and data management capabilities to identify and manage issues early, as well as provide feedback to the PCPs, managers are more likely than not to experience these problems.

The first problem is churning. This simply means that physicians perform more procedures than are really necessary and schedule patient revisits at frequent intervals. Because most patients depend on the physician to recommend when they should come back and what tests should be done, it is easy to have a patient come back for a blood pressure check in two weeks instead of a month and to have serum electrolytes measured (unless laboratory services are capitated) in the physician's office at the same time. Few patients will argue, and the physician collects for the work.

Few physicians consciously churn, but it does happen, even if unconsciously. The serious problem comes when the plan reduces the fees because of medical expense overruns. When this happens, a re-visit frenzy can occur. In effect, physicians start to feel that they have to get theirs first. If the fees are lowered 10 percent this month, what might happen next month? Better to get in as many visits as possible this month because next month may bring a 20 percent fee reduction. This creates a self-fulfilling prophecy, and the inevitable downward spiral begins.

The only effective approach to churning is tight management (or switching to capitation). Some plans develop physician peer review committees to review utilization. These committees have the authority to sanction physicians who abuse the system. This has some slowing effect

if there are enough reviewers and not too many physicians to review. The actions of such committees should follow a process that includes warnings and a probationary period in which expectations for improvement are clearly outlined. Other plans apply differential withholds selectively on those providers whose utilization is clearly out of line, although defining that takes some care.

Better still is to manage the plan such that few sanctions are necessary. This means managing referrals, managing hospital and institutional utilization, and negotiating effective discounts with providers and hospitals. It also means closely monitoring utilization and billing patterns by PCPs and acting when necessary. Performance-based programs such as those described earlier can also be applied to lessen the impact of churning, but this problem still remains in any FFS plan.

On the other hand, if cost overruns bring fees down to grossly unacceptable low levels, utilization may decrease simply because the plan does not pay enough to get providers to do the work. That is a serious situation that can lead to inappropriate underutilization.

The second major problem set is upcoding (sometimes referred to as CPT creep) and unbundling. As mentioned earlier, upcoding refers to a slow creeping upward of CPT codes that pay more; for example, a routine office visit becomes an extended one, a Pap smear and pelvic examination become a full physical examination, or a cholecystectomy becomes a laparotomy. Unbundling refers to charging for services that were previously included in a single fee without lowering (or lowering sufficiently) the original fee.

These problems are best monitored by the claims department in coordination with whichever department is responsible for data analysis. There are two useful approaches. The first is to look for trends by providers. Individuals who are trying to game the system will usually stand out. If there is one physician who has 40 percent extended visits compared to 20 percent for all the other physicians in the panel, it may be worth further review. The second approach is to automate the claims system to rebundle unbundled claims and to separate for review any claims that appear to have a gross mismatch between services rendered and the clinical reason for the visit (this topic is addressed in Chapter 38).

There are also software programs in existence that automatically recode claims based on statistical norms. Using the above example, a PCP with 40 percent extended visits may have 20 percent of them lowered to routine visits by the system, using some type of criteria to choose which visits get lowered. The use of these programs is not widespread as of 2000 and there has been considerable objection to the use of these types of programs. As of the time of publication, lawsuits had been filed against the MCOs that used these programs, but the outcome is not known.

The problems of upcoding and unbundling may also be addressed through the use of global fees, as discussed earlier in this chapter.

LEGISLATION AND REGULATION APPLICABLE TO PHYSICIAN INCENTIVE PROGRAMS

In recent years, many states and the federal government have passed laws and created regulations that affect physician incentive programs (referred to here as PIPs in keeping with federal acronyms). These apply primarily to capitation programs and to incentive programs under which a physician's income may be affected by performance, particularly utilization and medical cost performance. Of course, there are no such regulations placed upon FFS under which a physician is rewarded for doing more, not less, with the unsubstantiated thought being that there is less danger from providing more care rather than less care. The issue of whether or not capitation or incentive programs have an effect on quality is addressed elsewhere in this chapter.

Other measures of performance may also fall under these laws and regulations, such as quality and member satisfaction (see Chapter 10), but usually not, and specifically not under federal regulations for Medicare or Medicaid MCOs. But even these types of programs may benefit from legal review by the plan's attorneys in the event that state laws might apply.

It is difficult to discuss state laws and regulations that apply to physician compensation and incentives under managed health care. Not all states have passed such laws or promulgated such regulations, and those that have show little consistency from one state to another. In general, when states have such laws, they focus on disclosure of financial incentives. For example, as of 1999 the following states had some form of disclosure law (although this is not consistent among the states): Arizona, California, Connecticut, Georgia, Kentucky, Maine, Minnesota, New Jersey, New York, Oregon, Pennsylvania, Rhode Island, Virginia, Vermont, Washington, and Wyoming.[65] Some states also have laws restricting the types or the scope of financial incentives that an MCO may use, generally focusing on financial incentives tied to utilization or medical cost (Texas is one such state).

For a discussion of state regulation in general, the reader is referred to Chapter 69, although that chapter does not specifically address physician incentives. With the rapidly changing environment, it is necessary to investigate each state's laws and regulations on as current a basis as possible. Because of this lack of consistency and stability at the state level, little discussion of state issues is included in this section.

The remainder of this section focuses on the federal regulations, since those are consistent and also serve to illustrate the approaches taken by some states. Also, in the event that federal legislation occurs on a broader level (for example, the "Patient's Bill of Rights" debated in the 1999 Congress), it is likely that HCFA's regulations would form the basis for a broader application.

HCFA has implemented regulations that place limits on PIPs in Medicare and Medicaid MCOs. First enacted in 1987, they have been modified several times, and as of the time of publication, the "final" regulations had been in effect since 1998. The final regulations may be found in the *Federal Register*.[66]

The reader is also referred to Chapters 55 and 56 for further discussion of Medicare and managed health care and to Chapter 57 for a discussion of Medicaid and managed health care.

Significant Financial Risk

HCFA first determines whether or not a physician or medical group is at "significant* financial risk" (SFR) for medical costs. For purposes of this regulation, medical costs are only those costs applicable to Medicare or Medicaid beneficiaries. The determination of SFR is as follows:

> The amount at risk for referral services is the difference between the maximum potential referral payments and the minimum potential referral payments. Bonuses unrelated to utilization (for example, quality bonuses such as those related to member satisfaction or open physician panels) should not be counted towards referral payments. Maximum potential payments is defined as the maximum *anticipated* total payments that the physician/group could receive. If there is no specific dollar or percentage amount noted in the incentive arrangement, then the PIP should be considered as potentially putting 100 percent of the potential payments at risk for referral services. The SFR threshold is set at 25 percent of "potential payments" for covered services, regardless of the frequency of assessment (that is, collection) or distribution of payments. SFR is present when the 25 percent threshold is exceeded.

The following Incentive arrangements should be considered as SFR:

- Withholds greater than 25 percent of potential payments.
- Withholds less than 25 percent of potential payments if the physician or physician group is potentially liable for amounts exceeding 25 percent of potential payments.

- Bonuses that are greater than 33 percent of potential payments minus the bonus.
- Withholds plus bonuses if the withholds plus bonuses equal more than 25 percent of potential payments. The threshold bonus percentage for a particular withhold percentage may be calculated using the formula: Withhold percent = -0.75 (Bonus percent) + 25 percent.
- Capitation arrangements, if the difference between the maximum potential payments and the minimum potential payments is more than 25 percent of the maximum potential payments; or the maximum and minimum potential payments are not clearly explained in the physician's or physician group's contract.
- Any other incentive arrangements that have the potential to hold a physician or physician group liable for more than 25 percent of potential payments.[67]

Any service that a physician does not provide him or herself, or that is not provided by another member of the physician's group, should be considered a referral service. If the physician group refers patients to other providers (including independent contractors to the group) to perform the ancillary services, then those services are considered referral services. If the physician group performs ancillary services, then those services are not considered referral services. Whether or not such referrals contribute to the financial risk borne by the physician will depend on whether his or her compensation arrangements are such that referrals for those services or supplies could impact upon the physician's income.

Stop-Loss Protection

Stop-loss protection must be in place to protect physicians and physician groups to whom SFR has been transferred by an MCO. Either aggregate or per patient stop-loss may be acquired.

*The definition of "significant" is a legislative one, not one based on any particular research.

The rule specifies that if aggregate stop-loss is provided, it must cover 90 percent of the cost of referral services that exceed 25 percent of potential payments; physicians and groups can be held liable for only 10 percent. If per patient stop-loss is acquired, it must be determined based on the physician or physician group's patient panel size and cover 90 percent of the referral costs that exceed the per patient limits noted in Table 8–3.

HCFA has also set criteria for when an MCO, physician, or physician group may pool patients for purposes of determining stop-loss levels. To determine the patient panel size in Table 8–3, specific criteria are stated in the regulations. Any entity that meets all five criteria required for the pooling of risk will be allowed to pool that risk in order to determine the amount of stop-loss required by the regulation. Those five criteria are:

- Pooling of patients is otherwise consistent with the relevant contracts governing the compensation arrangements for the physician or group (that is, no contracts can require risk be segmented by MCO or patient category).
- The physician or group is at risk for referral services with respect to each of the categories of patients being pooled.
- The terms of the compensation arrangements permit the physician or group to spread the risk across the categories of pa-

tients being pooled (that is, payments must be held in a common risk pool).
- The distribution of payments to physicians from the risk pool is not calculated separately by patient category (either by MCO or by Medicaid, Medicare, or commercial).
- The terms of the risk borne by the physician or group are comparable for all categories of patients being pooled.[68]

Pooling and stop-loss requirements applicable to a group cannot be extended to a subcontracting level. In other words, if a group meets pooling requirements for a high stop-loss, but subcontracts with physicians who are at SFR with smaller patient panels, then the stop-loss requirements for the smaller panels apply to those subcontracted physicians. If an MCO uses PODs as described earlier in this chapter, then the pooling criteria may still be met by the POD if the incentive program for the POD physicians meets the criteria noted above, even though the POD is not an actual legal entity. In other words, the concept of sharing risk and reward via a POD system may be considered pooling for this purpose.

An MCO, medical group, or physician may combine commercial membership with Medicare and Medicaid membership for purposes of pooling if the financial risk is applicable to all members, but may not do so if the risk arrangements are different between those types of pa-

Table 8–3 Limits on Referral Costs Based on Patient Panel Size in Medicare or Medicaid MCOs

Patient Panel Size	Single Combined Limit	Separate Institutional Limit	Separate Professional Limit
1–1,000	$6,000*	$10,000*	$3,000*
1,001–5,000	$30,000	$40,000	$10,000
5,001–8,000	$40,000	$60,000	$15,000
8,001–10,000	$75,000	$100,000	$20,000
10,001–25,000	$150,000	$200,000	$25,000
> 25,000	none	none	none

*"In these situations, stop-loss insurance would be impractical. Not only would the premiums be prohibitively expensive, but the protections for patients would likely not be adequate for panels of fewer than 500 patients. MCOs and physician groups clearly should not be putting physicians at financial risk for panel sizes this small. It is our understanding that doing so is not common. For completeness, however, we do show what the limits would be in these circumstances."
Source: Reprinted from PIP Regulations 1998, Health Care Financing Administration.

tients. If such pooling is appropriate but stop-loss is still required, then the stop-loss arrangement need only cover Medicare and Medicaid members, not commercial members.

Interestingly, HCFA has stated in a listing of frequently asked questions (which, as of early 2000, may be found at *www.hcfa.gov/medicare/physincp.htm*) that arrangements between MCOs and PHOs (see Chapter 4) are not subject to the stop-loss arrangements because the PHO is not a physician group. The physicians in the PHO would be subject to stop-loss arrangements, however, and unless all the physicians in the PHO pool the risk, then the PHO patient panel would not meet the criteria for pooling of risk. For example, if a PHO accepts a percentage of premium from an MCO and in turn passes that on to several medical groups, then pooling and the determination of SFR would take place at the level of the medical groups, not the PHO.

As is made clear in the footnote to Table 8–3, HCFA takes a dim view of putting physicians at SFR when their panel size is less than 500–1,000 members. As discussed earlier in this chapter, the degree of financial risk for medical costs that a physician with a small panel would face is usually limited by the MCO in any event. Many MCOs that use capitation for PCPs will use FFS for physicians with small panels, at least during the initial period when the physician is new to the plan. In cases where a physician with a small panel might be placed at SFR, the MCO can provide stop-loss protection by adjusting the capitation payment or fee schedule so as to budget for the cost of the stop-loss (in other words, treat it as an insurance premium).

Finally, for those medical groups with large panels of enrollees, or for IDSs that pool risk, either the MCO may provide stop-loss coverage at a competitive premium rate or commercial stop-loss insurance is available from third parties. Commercial provider excess stop-loss insurance is discussed in great detail in Chapter 53.

Disclosure Requirements

HCFA requires disclosure to both itself and to members or beneficiaries of the Medicare or Medicaid MCO. This disclosure applies to all providers in the network if they are at any financial risk. For example, if an MCO capitates an IPA, and the IPA in turn capitates a medical group, then both financial arrangements are subject to disclosure. If that medical group in turn subcapitates other medical groups, that too is subject to disclosure. IPAs that contract only with individual physicians and not with physician groups are considered physician groups under this rule.

The following pieces of information are required by the regulation to be provided to HCFA:

- whether referral services are covered by the PIP (if only services furnished directly by the physician or group are addressed by the PIP, then there is no need for disclosure of other aspects of the PIP)
- type of incentive arrangement (for example, withhold, bonus, capitation)
- percent of total income at risk for referrals
- amount and type of stop-loss protection
- panel size and whether enrollees were pooled in order to achieve the panel size
- if the MCO is required by this regulation to conduct a customer satisfaction survey, a summary of the survey results.[69]

The survey and stop-loss protection requirements are discussed below.

At Medicare or Medicaid beneficiaries' request, MCOs must provide information indicating whether the MCO or any of its contractors or subcontractors use a PIP that may affect the use of referral services, the type of incentive arrangement(s) used, and whether stop-loss protection is provided. If the MCO is required to conduct a survey, it must also provide beneficiary requesters with a summary of survey results.

The MCO is only required to provide to a beneficiary a summary statement or letter outlining all the incentive arrangements in place throughout the MCO. A beneficiary will not necessarily be able to tell from the required MCO disclosure whether or not a specific physician has a PIP, or the amount or type of risk that individual physician might experience. However, there is nothing in federal statute or regulation to prevent an MCO or individual physician from providing physician-specific information to a beneficiary who requests it.

HCFA has a document entitled *Guidance on Disclosure of Physician Incentive Regulation* that may be used by the MCO or IPA to develop its beneficiary disclosure document. As of 1999 further information, including suggested language, may be found at *www.hcfa.gov/medicare/physincp/beneinfo.htm.*

The issue of disclosure appears deceptively simple. It is not, as even HCFA admits in its many documents on the subject. While there now appears to be some general agreement among the managed health care industry, regulators and governments, and consumer groups endorsing some form of disclosure of reimbursement methods as worthwhile, the details of how to provide that disclosure engender much debate and uncertainty. HCFA has dealt with this problem by issuing guidelines about what to say in enrollee literature. These guidelines may be useful in some situations, but will require interpretation or judgment in others; but in all cases, the MCO must follow the guidelines. Similar, if far messier, approaches are taken in many states, and recent court cases add to the pressure.

Disclosure of reimbursement methods is not as simple as many lawmakers, regulators, or consumer advocates would like to believe. The form of reimbursement can mutate rapidly as money passes from one organization to another. For example, an MCO may capitate an IPA, which in turn subcapitates some medical groups while paying FFS to others; the medical group may pay salary with a bonus potential to the individual physicians; the IPA may use different levels of withholds for different medical groups or individual physician members based on panel size or past performance; the MCO may have direct contracts with individual physicians not associated with the IPA and pay some of them using capitation and others using FFS (with or without a withhold). Other reimbursement systems, such as the use of POPs or bundled case rates, further complicate explanations.

By requiring disclosure only of managed care related financial incentives, it leaves the erroneous impression that only incentives to manage the amount of health care services lead to problems in care.* Disclosure policies also have substantial unresolved issues, such as the scope of disclosure, the effect of disclosure on the physician-patient relationship, how to make disclosure understandable in relatively simple terms, and the need to provide such disclosure without being required to use language that makes any reimbursement system other than FFS appear to be evil (evil being considered a distinct competitive disadvantage).[70] But debates over policy and philosophy have only limited room in this already crowded chapter and are thus left to the readers to ponder and discuss among themselves.

Customer Satisfaction Survey

HCFA requires that MCOs conduct a customer satisfaction survey of both enrollees and disenrollees (that is, Medicare or Medicaid members who have disenrolled within the past 12 months of the compliance date) if any physicians or physician groups in the MCO's network are at SFR for referral services, as defined above. If a survey is required, it must be conducted within one year of the MCO's compliance date for disclosure. The compliance date is when the MCO contract either renews or a new contract is made effective. As long as physicians or physician groups are placed at SFR for referral services, surveys must be conducted annually thereafter. The survey must address enrollees' and disenrollees' satisfaction with the quality of services provided and their degree of access to the services.

---

*Before the ubiquitous presence of managed health care, the literature focused almost exclusively on how unfettered FFS led to high levels of inappropriate procedures and care, with attendant health risks.

As of early 2000, there is no single survey that HCFA has designated as the "official" survey instrument. The final rule did not specify that MCOs must conduct a specific survey for this regulation because most plans already administer surveys that meet the requirements of this regulation. MCOs may also satisfy their requirement for enrollee surveys by participating in HCFA's national administration of the Consumer Assessment of Health Plan Study survey.[71]

At present, most consumer satisfaction surveys use a random sample of enrollees within an MCO, so that at best, MCO to MCO comparisons can be made. MCO participation in the administration of customer satisfaction surveys at the MCO level appears to meet the letter of the regulation's requirement for MCOs to perform satisfaction surveys when physicians or physician groups are placed at SFR for referrals. But it is possible or even likely that in the future HCFA will require these surveys to take place at the level of the physician or physician group at SFR.

MCOs will be expected to compile, analyze, and summarize survey data within a reasonable period of time after conducting the survey. Generally, this would mean summary survey results should be available to beneficiaries and provided to regulators within four months of conducting the survey. Frequently, satisfaction information has been presented to consumers in a "report card" format and sent by direct mail to the enrollees, displayed in newspapers or magazines, and appearing on Web sites. It must also be provided to prospective enrollees upon request.

CIVIL LIABILITY IN PHYSICIAN COMPENSATION PROGRAMS

In cases where an MCO, IDS, or medical group does not have Medicare or Medicaid risk business, and there are no state laws or regulations governing physician compensation or incentives, managers should note that potential liability still remains in civil court. Physician incentives in managed health care have largely withstood legal challenges in the past, but beginning in the late 1990s, there have been a few court cases where MCOs have been successfully sued based on their physician compensation system. Regardless of the facts or merits of incentive systems, some judges and juries have expressed their opinion in judgment that financial incentives to management utilization or cost are injurious to patients. This is a different issue than utilization management (see Chapters 45 and 64) and does not even require that a member be injured in order for a plaintiff's attorney to file a suit; the very existence of an incentive program is postulated as reason enough. In early 2000, this issue was taken to the Supreme Court of the United States; though a final ruling had not been issued at the time of publication, the initial questions and comments from the justices clearly revealed an attitude that physician incentives are the domain of the Congress, not the courts.

At the end of 1999, two states, Texas and Georgia, had passed legislation to make it easier for members to sue MCOs. In October 1999 Harris Methodist Health Plan in Texas reached a $4.7 million settlement with plaintiff's attorneys, who had filed two class-action lawsuits against the HMO because it did not disclose that capitation payments included prescription costs, thus, they argued, incenting physicians to limit prescribing. No actual evidence of harm to a patient was provided; and the settlement is believed to be the first in the nation in which uninjured patients recovered cash (approximately $50 per member after legal fees) because the HMO failed to disclose such incentives.[72] Several similar lawsuits have been filed by plaintiff's attorneys who specialize in large, class-action lawsuits, but the outcome is unknown at the time of publication.

Exposure to lawsuits regarding financial incentives is not necessarily confined solely to individual plaintiffs. In 1998 the former attorney general of Texas, citing a 1997 state law prohibiting financial incentives "that act directly or indirectly as an inducement to limit medically necessary services," filed a suit in a state district court, asking the court to fine six HMOs and prevent them from offering financial incentives to physicians. Harris Methodist Health Plan of Texas, the same HMO cited above, was fined $3.5 million in that action; and in April 2000, other MCOs agreed to eliminate all financial incentive programs (except FFS) despite no evidence that harm was caused.*

CONCLUSION

To be effective, an MCO (HMO, IDS, or any type of risk-assuming managed care system) must align the financial incentives and goals of all the parties: the health plan and the providers who deliver the care. Capitation and, to a somewhat lesser extent, performance-based FFS do that in ways that traditional FFS plans do not.

In a closely managed plan such as an HMO, capitation is often considered to be more consistent with the overall goal of managing costs. Although capitation is initially harder to calculate, and is sometimes harder to gain acceptance for it

_____

*At least as of early 2000, Texas is not a nurturing environment for managed health care.

from physicians, this system has less likelihood of leading to overutilization than FFS. Problems of inappropriate underutilization must be guarded against with effective monitoring and an effective quality management system.

FFS can be used as well but requires a different set of management skills as well as good data and profiling systems. It is easier to install and is often more acceptable to physicians, but it can quickly get out of control unless managed carefully. New products such as POS are better suited to FFS than is capitation. Global fees offer a middle ground, at least in some circumstances. New products also require new approaches to reimbursement because classic approaches are not ideally suited. As managed care evolves, reimbursement may be expected to evolve further.

The reimbursement system is a tool, and like any tool it has limitations. Just as a hammer is the correct tool for pounding and removing nails, it is a poor tool for cutting wood and drilling holes. A reimbursement system is an effective tool, but it can only be effective in conjunction with other managed care functions: utilization management, quality management, network contracting, provider relations, and the many other activities of a well-run managed care organization.

REFERENCES AND NOTES

1. J.C. Robinson, Blended Payment Methods in Physician Organizations under Managed Care, *JAMA* 282, 13 (October 6, 1999): 1258–1263.

2. A.L. Hillman, W.P. Welch, and M.V. Pauly, Contractual Arrangements between HMOs and Primary Care Physicians: Three-tiered HMOs and Risk Pools, *Medical Care* 30, 2 (February 1992): 136–148.

3. D.A. Conrad, C. Maynard, A. Cheadle, et al., Primary Care Physician Compensation Method in Medical Groups, *JAMA* 279, 11 (March 18, 1998): 853–858.

4. Group Health Association of America, *HMO Industry Profile, Vol. 2: Physician Staffing and Utilization Patterns* (Washington, DC: GHHA, 1991).

5. M. Gold, R. Hurley, T. Lake, et al., Arrangements between Managed Care Plans and Physicians: Results from a 1994 Survey of Managed Care Plans, Washington, DC: Mathematica Policy Research, Inc., 1996.

6. *HMO Industry Reports 9.1,* InterStudy Publications, St. Paul, MN.

7. SMG Marketing Group Inc., Hoechst Marion Roussel Managed Care Digest Series, *HMO-PPO Digest 1998.*

8. R.L. Doyle and A.P. Feren, *Healthcare Management Guidelines: Ambulatory Care Guidelines,* Milliman & Robertson, published periodically.

9. J.B. Fowles, J.P. Weiner, D. Knutson, E. Fowler, A.M. Tucker, and M. Ireland, Taking Health Status into Account when Setting Capitation Rates: A Comparison of Risk-Adjustment Methods, *JAMA* 276, 16 (October 23, 1996): 1316–1321.

10. Blue Cross Blue Shield of the National Capital Area, unpublished data, 1989–1992.

11. R.L. Kravitz, S. Greenfield, W. Rogers, et al., Differences in the Mix of Patients among Medical Specialties and Systems of Care: Results from the Medical Outcomes Study, *JAMA* 267, 12 (March 25, 1992): 1617–1623.

12. Blue Cross Blue Shield of the National Capital Area, unpublished data, 1989–1992.

13. K. Grumbach, D. Osmond, K. Vranizan, et al., Primary Care Physicians' Experience of Financial Incentives in Managed Care Systems, *New England Journal of Medicine* 339, 21 (1998): 1516–1521.

14. A.L. Hillman, M.V. Pauly, K. Kerman, and C.R. Martinek, HMO Managers' Views on Financial Incentives and Quality, *Health Affairs (Millwood)* 10, 4 (Winter 1991): 207–219.

15. N. Schlackman, Evolution of a Quality-Based Compensation Model: The Third Generation, *American Journal of Medical Quality* 8, 2 (1993): 103–110.

16. K. Grumbach, D. Osmond, K. Vranizan, et al., Primary Care Physicians' Experience of Financial Incentives in Managed Care Systems, *New England Journal of Medicine* 339, 21 (1998): 1516–1521.

17. SMG Marketing Group, Inc., in Hoechst Marion Roussel, Managed Care Digest Series, *Integrated Health Systems Digest* (1999).

18. A.L. Hillman, M.V. Pauly, J.J. Escarce, K. Ripley, et al., Financial Incentives and Drug Spending in Managed Care, *Health Affairs (Millwood)* 18, 2 (March–April 1999): 189–200.

19. L.W. Hann, Best's Review—Life-Health Insurance Edition (February 1998).

20. R. Popovian, K. Johnson, M. Nichol, and G. Liu, The Impact of Pharmaceutical Capitation to Primary Medical Groups on the Health-Care Expenditures of Medicare HMO Enrollees, *Journal of Managed Care Pharmacy* (September–October 1999).

21. A.L. Hillman, M.V. Pauly, J.J. Escarce, K. Ripley, et al., Financial Incentives and Drug Spending in Managed Care, *Health Affairs* 18, 2 (March–April 1999): 189–200.

22. A.L. Hillman, M.V. Pauly, K. Kerman, and C.R. Martinek, HMO Managers' March/April 1999 Views on Financial Incentives and Quality, *Health Affairs* 10, 4 (Winter 1991): 207–219.

23. L. Debrock and R.J. Arnould, Utilization Control in HMOs, *Quarterly Review of Economics and Finance* 32, 3 (Autumn 1992): 31–53.

24. E.A. Kerr, B.S. Mittman, R.D. Hays, et al., Managed Care and Capitation in California: How Do Physicians at Financial Risk Control Their Own Utilization? *Annals of Internal Medicine* 123, 7 (October 1, 1995): 500–504.

25. A.L. Hillman, Health Maintenance Organizations, Financial Incentives, and Physician's Judgments, *Annals of Internal Medicine* 112, 12 (June 15, 1990): 891–893.

26. A.L. Hillman, Financial Incentives for Physicians in HMOs—Is There a Conflict of Interest? *New England Journal of Medicine* 317, 27 (December 31, 1987): 1743–1748.

27. A.L. Hillman, M.V. Pauly, and J.J. Kerstein, How Do Financial Incentives Affect Physicians' Clinical Decisions and the Financial Performance of Health Maintenance Organizations? *New England Journal of Medicine* 321 (1989): 86–92.

28. D.F. Levinson, Toward Full Disclosure of Referral Restrictions and Financial Incentives by Prepaid Health Plans, *New England Journal of Medicine* 317, 27 (December 31, 1987): 1729–1734.

29. Medicare: Physician Incentive Payments by Prepaid Health Plans Could Lower Quality of Care. General Accounting Office publication GAO/HRD-89–29, Washington, DC, 1988.

30. S.D. Pearson, J.E. Sabin, and E.J. Emanuel, Ethical Guidelines for Physician Compensation Based on Capitation, *New England Journal of Medicine* 339, 10 (September 3, 1998): 689–693.

31. Helen Schauffler and Sara McMenamin, Reforms Are Needed To Increase Quality of Care and Health Plan Accountability in California. University of California Berkley School of Public Health, *California Managed Health Care Improvement Task Force Survey,* 1997; reported on Managed Care On-Line.

32. K. Grumbach, D. Osmond, K. Vranizan, et al., Primary Care Physicians' Experience of Financial Incentives in Managed Care Systems, *New England Journal of Medicine* 339, 21 (1998): 1516–1521.

33. J.J. Escarce, J.A. Shea, and W. Chen, Segmentation of Hospital Markets: Where Do HMO Enrollees Get Care? *Health Affairs (Millwood)* 16, 6 (November–December 1997): 186–187.

34. T.E. Miller and W.S. Sage, Disclosing Physician Financial Incentives, *JAMA* 281, 15 (April 21, 1999): 1424–1430.

35. C.J. Simon and D.W. Emmons, Physicians' Earnings at Risk: What Physicians Don't Know about Managed Care Capitated Contracts Could Place Them—and Their Patients—at Risk, *Health Affairs (Millwood)* 16, 3 (May–June 1997): 120–126.

36. J.E. Ware, R.H. Brook, W.H. Rogers, et al., Comparison of Health Outcomes at a Health Maintenance Organization with those of FFS Care, *Lancet* 1, 8488 (May 3, 1986): 1017–1022.

37. I.S. Udvarhelyi, K. Jennison, and R.S. Phillips, Comparison of the Quality of Ambulatory Care for Fee-For-Service and Prepaid Patients, *Annals of Internal Medicine* 115, 5 (September 1, 1991): 394–400.

38. E.M. Sloss, E.B. Keeler, R.H. Brook, et al., Effect of a Health Maintenance Organization on Physiologic Health, *Annals of Internal Medicine* 106, 1 (January 1987): 130–138.

39. C.M. Clancy and B.E. Hillner, Physicians as Gatekeepers—The Impact of Financial Incentives, *Archives of Internal Medicine* 149, 4 (April 1989): 917–920.

40. N. Lurie, J. Christianson, M. Finch, and I. Moscovice, The Effects of Capitation on Health and Functional Status of the Medicaid Elderly: A Randomized Trial, *Annals of Internal Medicine* 120, 6 (March 15, 1994): 506–511.

41. P. Braveman, M. Schaaf, S. Egerter, et al., Insurance-Related Differences in the Risk of Ruptured Appendix, *New England Journal of Medicine* 331, 7 (1994): 444–449.

42. A. Relman, Medical Insurance and Health: What about Managed Care? *New England Journal of Medicine* 331, 7 (1994): 471–472.

43. J.P. Murray, S. Greenfield, S.H. Kaplan, and E.M. Yano, Ambulatory Testing for Capitation and FFS Patients in the Same Practice Setting: Relationship to Outcomes, *Medical Care* 30, 3 (March 1992): 252–261.

44. R.A. Dudley, R.H. Miller, T.Y. Korenbror, et al., The Impact of Financial Incentives on Quality of Health Care, *Milbank Quarterly* 76, 4 (1998): 649–686.

45. Robert H. Brook, Managed Care Is Not the Problem, Quality Is, *Journal of the American Medical Association* 278, 19 (1997): 1612–1614.

46. L.C. Baker and J.C. Cantor, Physician Satisfaction Under Managed Care, *Health Affairs Supplement* (1993): 258–270.

47. Michael D. Weiss, Capitation Can Be Beneficial to Providers and Patients, *Maryland Medical Journal* 46, 4 (1997): 170–171.

48. R.H. Miller and H.S. Luft, Does Managed Care Lead to Better or Worse Quality of Care? *Health Affairs* (Millwood), 16, 5 (September–October 1997): 7–25.

49. J.J. Seidman, E.P. Bass, and H.R. Rubin, Review of Studies That Compare the Quality of Cardiovascular Care in HMO Verses Non-HMO Settings, *Medical Care* 36, 12 (December 1998): 1607.

50. Richard Bruno and Bradley Gilbert, In California, Medi-Cal Managed Care Is Superior to Medi-Cal Fee-for-Service, *Managed Care Quarterly* 6, 4 (1998): 7–14.

51. Heidi Whitmore, Comparing Outcomes in Managed Care, *HMO Magazine* (January–February 1996): 75.

52. F.J. Hellinger, The Effect of Managed Care on Quality, *Archives of Internal Medicine* 158, 8 (April 27, 1998): 833–841.

53. D.M. Berwick, Quality of Health Care, V: Payment by Capitation and the Quality of Care, *New England Journal of Medicine* 335, 16 (October 17, 1996): 1227–1231.

54. G.F. Riley, A.L. Potosky, J.D. Lubitz, and M.L. Brown, Stage of Cancer at Diagnosis for Medicare HMO and Fee-for-Service Enrollees, *American Journal of Public Health* 84, 10 (October 1994): 1598–1604.

55. D.M. Carlisle, A.L. Siu, E.B. Keeler, et al., HMO vs. Fee-for-Service Care of Older Persons with Acute Myocardial Infarction, *American Journal of Public Health* 82, 12 (December 1992): 1626–1630.

56. P. Braveman, V.M. Schaaf, S. Egerter, et al., Insurance Related Differences in the Risk of Ruptured Appendix, *New England Journal of Medicine* 331, 7 (August 18, 1994): 444–449.

57. T.S. Carey, J. Garrett, A. Jackman, et al., The Outcomes and Costs of Care for Acute Low Back Pain among Patients Seen by Primary Care Practitioners, Chiropractics, and Orthopedic Surgeons, *New England Journal of Medicine* 333, 14 (October 5, 1995): 914–916.

58. E.H. Yelin, L.A. Criswell, and P.G. Feigenbaum, Health Care Utilization and Outcomes among Persons with Rheumatoid Arthritis in Fee-for-Service and Prepaid Group Practice Settings, *JAMA* 276, 13 (October 2, 1996): 1048–1053.

59. Collaborating with Managed Care Organizations for Mammogram Screening and Rescreening, Center for Disease Control, Atlanta, GA, 1997.

60. M.F. Shapiro, R.A. Hayward, H.E. Freeman, S. Sudman, and C.R. Corey, Out-of-Pocket Payments and Use of Care for Serious and Minor Symptoms, *Archives of Internal Medicine* 149, 7 (July 1989): 1645–1648.

61. J.P. Newhouse, W.G. Manning, C.N. Morris, et al., Some Interim Results from a Controlled Trial of Cost Sharing in Health Insurance, *New England Journal of Medicine* 305, 25 (December 17, 1981): 1501–1507.

62. K.F. O'Grady, W.G. Manning, J.P. Newhouse, and R.H. Brook, The Impact of Cost Sharing on Emergency Department Use, *New England Journal of Medicine* 313, 8 (1985): 484–490.

63. A.L. Siu, F.A. Sonnenberg, and W.G. Manning, Inappropriate Use of Hospitals in a Randomized Trial of Health Insurance Plans, *New England Journal of Medicine* 315, 20 (1986): 1259–1266.

64. D.E. Church, A. Bokor, and D.D. McCain, An Alternative to Primary Care Capitation in an IPA-Model HMO, *Med Interface* (November 1989): 37–42.

65. F.J. Hellinger, Regulating the Financial Incentives Facing Physicians in Managed Care Plans, *American Journal of Managed Care* 4 (1998): 663–674.

66. Legislative action to regulate physician incentive plans (PIP) was first enacted in the Omnibus Budget Reconciliation Acts (OBRA) of 1986 and 1987. In 1990 these laws were superseded by a new OBRA. Statutory authority for this regulation can be found in sections 1876(I)(8), 1903(m)(2)(A)(x), and 1903(m)(5)(A)(v) of the Social Security Act (the Act) and Part C of the Balanced Budget Act of 1997. A final rule on PIP for Medicare and Medicaid Managed Care Organizations was published in the *Federal Register* on March 27, 1996. Corrected final rules were published in the *Federal Register* on September 3 and December 31, 1996. PIP regulations are at 42 CFR 422.208/210 of the June 26, 1998, regulations that implement Part C.

67. *Federal Register* 42 CFR 422.208/210, June 26, 1998.

68. Ibid.

69. Ibid.

70. T.E. Miller and W.M. Sage, Disclosing Physician Financial Incentives, *JAMA* 281 (1999): 1424–30.

71. For additional information on the survey and data requirements, see HCFA Operation Policy Letter 99.078, available via the HCFA website at *www.hcfa.gov*.

72. *Ingram vs. Harris Health Plan*, No. 98-CV-179 (USDC E.D. Texas, settlement filed Oct. 12, 1999).

CHAPTER 9

Physician Compensation in Medical Groups and Health Systems

James A. Rodeghero

BACKGROUND

Many of the factors affecting, and affected by, physicians' reward programs under managed care continue to evolve in response to market, economic, professional, and cultural changes. This fourth edition of the *Managed Health Care Handbook* reflects many of those changes. Interestingly, although the techniques, formulas, and overall economics of physicians' rewards under managed care continue to evolve, the underlying fundamentals have changed little in the recent past.

Three fundamental issues continue as anchors for this discussion of physician compensation. First, there is an unstoppable trend for physicians to practice medicine as employees or in structured contexts where reimbursement and compensation are externally managed rather than based on their own efforts. Further reinforcing this phenomenon is the recent push for col-

lective organization (i.e., unionization) of these employed physicians. Second, as society addresses increasing health care costs, physicians' incomes continue to be scrutinized by employers, payers, and patients challenging the value of medical services. Third, the very nature of compensation theory and practice presumes that compensation itself (i.e., monetary rewards) is a primary determinant of and/or a reward for the practice of medicine and should be a central factor in the management and reward of physicians.

The day-to-day challenges in managing physician compensation are grounded in the changing health care system context and each organization's situation. In response to this context, large numbers of physicians have become employees or contracted with payers, hospitals, and other provider organizations in recent years. The trend to consolidate and integrate the industry is continuing despite the absence of a clearly superior operating or financial model. But other trends indicate that large-scale integration of physician practices will not succeed. For example, the FPA bankruptcy and MedPartners' exit from the medical management arena suggest that the national practice model is in trouble. In this context one would expect physicians to move into roles with more impact outside their traditional clinician responsibilities. Many integrated delivery and financing systems have found the value of bringing physicians into central nonclinical roles where they assume more responsibility for structuring and managing care. But the continuing pressures to contain

James A. Rodeghero, PhD, is President of the Rodeghero Consulting Group, Inc., which specializes in the design of reward, governance, and human resources programs in health care organizations. Rodeghero is a recognized expert and author in the areas of physician and executive compensation in health care and has served as a Partner with Ernst & Young and a Senior Principal with the Hay Group. He has worked in all areas of the health care industry, including acute care hospitals, HMOs and managed care organizations, and freestanding group practices. He is experienced in the design and implementation of management and reward systems for all levels of health care industry providers, executives, and employees.

health care costs find clinical physicians, as high earners, continuing as a focal point of cost-cutters, regulators, and payers.

Despite the mixed successes for integrating physicians into delivery systems as employed clinicians, the trend continues. The broad movement of physicians into the employed/contracted context reinforces an important shift in physicians' roles in health care delivery. Having moved beyond being owner-operators of cottage enterprises—and having lost the primary entrepreneurial motives for efficiency and profitability—physicians no longer exercise broad independence in either the medical or the business aspect of their practices. Furthermore, although physicians are surrendering much of their prior independence, they are assuming new risks under managed reimbursement. As physicians assume economic risk, they essentially underwrite the medical risks of increasingly large populations of managed care plan members.

In this context, the overall economics of medical care should be shifting from volume to effective risk management. In many practices the metrics driving rewards are shifting from individual effort/volume to the selective delivery of care, from effective management of a small business (medical practice) to satisfaction of employment standards in large organizations, and from independent judgment to compliance with protocols. Factors such as patient (i.e., customer) satisfaction, resource management, and organizational compliance are new to physicians and the source of confusion and frustration as they seek success in their practices.

This chapter explores the background, mechanics, and outcomes of various approaches to rewarding medical practice. The impact of the changing health care industry on physician earnings and the reciprocal impact that employed and contracted physicians are creating are discussed. The "best" physician reward plan continues to elude employers, payers, attorneys, and consultants, but a number of traditional and evolving approaches to physician rewards are surveyed and the pros and cons that may shed light on efforts to restructure and align physician compensation are discussed.

It is important to note that this discussion differentiates between compensation and reimbursement, the latter referring to organizational level payments or direct premium payments. Although reimbursement may often constitute the physicians' compensation plan (as with direct distribution of per member per month [PMPM] payments) or define an aggregate contractual agreement between entities (as in independent practice associations [IPAs], foundations, or other structural relationships), the current discussion focuses on compensation, defined as the individual physician level pay plan. The reader is also encouraged to review physician compensation issues from a managed care plan's perspective as discussed in detail in Chapters 8, 10, and 11.

TRADITIONAL CONCEPTS IN PAY PLAN DESIGN

Before proceeding with a discussion of specific issues in rewarding physicians, let us review the basic concepts and assumptions in compensation plan design and the implications for physicians. One lesson in recent years from structuring and restructuring physician reward plans is that the basic fundamentals apply in almost all cases. Admittedly, many traditional industrial compensation models will not apply with physicians, but we can learn some useful techniques, and avoid making some mistakes, from the traditional rationales.

At its simplest, three basic factors drive the design of rewards in any context: need, desire, and ability. These factors apply to both the employer/contractor physician and provide a simple and reliable reference point when designing compensation programs. First and foremost, there will always be a clear need for the employer or contractor to provide a market wage for any labor services. Calibration of physician incomes to market norms to establish the need-to-pay level will require a common denominator for the services being priced, and although it may be straightforward to define a common standard for many labor classifications, the practice of medicine has historically represented an exceptionally robust range of behaviors, resource requirements, and outcomes. As a simple example, primary care physicians' market values are reported across a range of more than 200 percent. This range is a reflection of the wide variation among physicians' activities, effort levels, market demands, and practice contexts.

Second, we can discuss the rationale and design of reward systems in terms of the employer's desire to provide a certain level of rewards. These goals are often described in terms of market norms, and less frequently in terms of ensuring a motivating pay level. Market targets, such as the median or third quartile, help to reinforce the market linkages discussed above. But organizations espousing a relatively high competitive pay level are often challenged to ensure sufficient funding. For example, those organizations targeting physician salaries at above-average market levels may find it impossible to fund incomes under discounted or capitated reimbursement. And the cost structures in many integrated delivery systems (IDSs) are higher than in free-standing medical groups,

so delivering a competitive percentage of collections as pay to physicians in IDSs is often impossible (unless the parent corporation subsidizes or otherwise supports the physician entity).

Analysis of market data should underlie any effort to ensure that physicians' salary and total compensation levels reflect actual market practices. Figure 9–1 highlights the variability in market pay comparisons based on different subgroup breakdowns. It also highlights how a hybrid market norm may be drawn from the comparative data to support the broadest level of competitiveness.

The organization's ability to fund physician labor costs may be the most critical factor in pay plan design. Under fee-for-service and discounted procedure-based reimbursement, the ability to fund physician labor is directly measurable. The final physicians' pay pool equals net collections minus costs. Capitated reimbursement blurs the direct linkage between volume and individual physicians' contributions. This leads some managed care organizations to

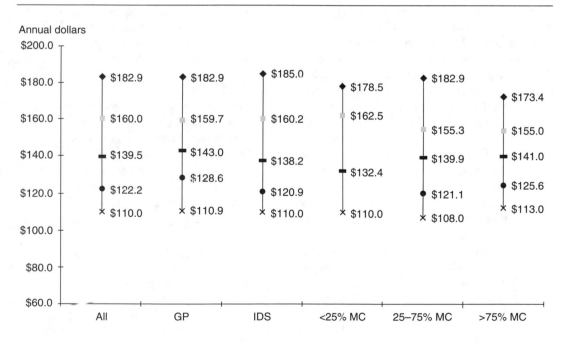

Figure 9–1 A Market Chart of Total Cash Compensation, Internal Medicine. *Source:* Data from *1999 Ernst & Young Physician Benchmarking Survey*; data presented for total sample (all), Group Practices (GP), Integrated Delivery Systems (IDS), and by percentage of managed care (MC) reimbursement.

define pay plan goals not in terms of competitive rates but rather in relation to internal economics. These economic ratios most often are structured around the organization's realities and not market benchmarks since the normative amount of operating revenue/income delivered as physician cash compensation is so often inclusive of subsidies and other revenue sources not found in all practices.

Funding issues in physician compensation hold an importance not seen in traditional employment situations. Under traditional (indemnity) reimbursement and in independent practices, physicians' incomes are funded directly from collected professional (and technical) fees. The resulting range of individual earnings is largely within physicians' control, so that the range of their earnings is considered an accurate reflection of productivity. But under managed reimbursement and when the physicians are practicing as employees or contractors, the economics of the practice is largely driven by external forces. Under many forms of managed care reimbursement, increased physician clinical volume increases costs, thus eroding profitability. Whereas budgeting for physician labor costs may be straightforward under fee for service, accounting for the value of physicians' labor under capitated reimbursement raises the paradox of establishing the remunerative value of a commodity that, by its very exercise, raises costs.

Finally, the context of medical practice may challenge some of our most fundamental assumptions about the role of monetary rewards in linking behaviors, results, and economics. Many of the pay models discussed herein implicitly assume that rewards will shape behavior. While there is broad evidence that compensation for sales representatives, piece-rate workers, and other classifications will effectively change behavior, there is little empirical evidence that pay drives behavior among professionals.

While the debate over the role of monetary rewards in behavior change will not be resolved easily, the various approaches to rewarding physicians can be considered. But it should be recognized that monetary rewards may be best considered for their role in recognizing behavior changes and accomplishments, not for their potential impact in changing behavior. Conventional wisdom says that incentives will work—but it is often found that they work too well (e.g., increasing productivity under capitation becomes overutilization) and many physician practices are returning to a focus on professional standards to manage behavior with less emphasis on cash compensation.

PAY PLAN DESIGN ISSUES

In actual practice, there will be relatively few basic pay plan designs from which to choose. Any physicians' pay plan development effort seeking the best model for a specific context will depend on a few primary considerations:

- *Practice context.* The physicians' practice setting and relationship to the payers or contracting organization may define the amount and type of compensation. Free-standing contracted groups, with or without management service organizations (MSOs), physician-hospital organizations (PHOs), IPAs, or preferred provider organizations (PPOs), and hospital-based practices all require different reward schemes. These types of organizations are discussed in Chapter 3.
- *Available remunerative elements or pay vehicles.* Options for delivering rewards to physicians may be chosen from fixed or variable cash compensation (salaries and bonuses/incentives), equity-based, profit sharing, or dividend income (in some settings), benefits, and perquisites. The use of nonmonetary rewards (recognition, research opportunities, and the like) is often an overlooked reward component and is becoming more important in structuring total remuneration packages.
- *Regulatory and payer considerations.* Special restrictions in tax exempt settings may limit the ability to use some income deferral vehicles or share profits and may create special reporting issues. The Health Care Financing Administration's (HCFA's)

so-called Stark fraud and abuse regulations and recent rulings from the Office of the Inspector General (OIG) further restrict IDSs' and hospitals' ability to reward physicians for cost containment, risk management, and other important contributions.

- *Risk and economics.* Although the trend to pay physicians with direct capitation split seems to be slowing, physicians' roles in managing risk continue to grow. This shifts the focus from the traditional volume/productivity metrics to the more complex arena of risk management. Establishing a prudent and appropriate funding model becomes difficult in this context, as is the design of an equitable and motivating distribution formula.

In a mature industry with predictable revenue and cost structures, these issues can be addressed in an integrated fashion to develop a balanced (even optimal) solution. But the continuing changes in the health care industry mean that the design of physician pay plans occurs more often under a transitional state with imperfect information, limited strategic clarity, and immediate operational or financial needs. An example (current at the time this chapter was written) is the pending expiration of employment or professional services agreements that were based on acquisition agreements many years ago. The market and economic contexts have changed, but physicians expect to receive income continuity as their contracts change. Balancing the external and internal realities with physicians' expectations in these contexts is almost impossible under traditional approaches to pay plan design.

First, the impact of practice context on physician pay plan design will be explored. Many contextual factors, such as the type and size of the business unit, will directly affect physicians' rewards. For example, large clinical settings lend themselves to operational and scheduling economies that make it easier to structure workloads around common standards.

An increased ability to manage the level and amount of physician work allows a more structured approach to pay, such as the use of salaries

rather than variable pay. Conversely, in multiple sites contracting with many different payers and with mixed (capitated, discounted, private, federal, state) reimbursement, the organization may want to use higher levels of variable (at-risk) pay. This approach reflects the variability among physician practices and allows the employer/contractor to build variability into compensation commensurate with reimbursement mix. But the variability in revenues may lead physicians to desire more stability instead of the opportunities offered under higher incentive levels.

Other factors will affect the level and type of variable or risk-based pay in a physician plan, and the risk and economics that define the reimbursement profile should be tightly integrated with the physicians' reward plan. Risks associated with the effect of resource management on compensation are the most typical in managed care practices, and most plans have one or more mechanisms to pass risk through to the physicians.

For example, many salary-based care pay plans under primarily risk-based reimbursement put some of the physicians' base rate at risk through withhold amounts. This compensation plan mirrors many group level PMPM reimbursement plans. A physician's annual pay rate may be set at $140,000, but a flat amount or percentage (e.g., 20 percent, reducing the effective salary to $112,000) may be held back until year end to cushion cash flow and hedge against utilization overruns. The amount of at-risk pay is generally calibrated to the total contracted amount of revenue risk, and other measures of physician contribution may affect payouts.

The structure of this at-risk compensation should be balanced to reflect both the physicians' risk profile and the employer's/contractor's expectation that variable pay will affect behavior. Also the reality of differential specialty overall pay rates will affect the design of any variable pay component: Cash flow and lifestyle factors may preclude large relative amounts (e.g., 40 percent or more) of at-risk pay for primary care providers, but many high earners can bear, and perhaps will be better motivated by, relatively large incentives.

The level of risk in the pay plan should also reflect the extent to which physicians' efforts and outcomes reflect true manageable variability. Behaviors and outcomes that are expected from all individuals are best managed and rewarded through fixed compensation (i.e., salary). For example, if physicians' schedules can be managed to result in similar visit volumes, then that component of pay is best compensated within the salary component. Similarly, call coverage (always a source of pay plan distress) is most easily rewarded by requiring all clinicians to assume equal call schedules and assuming the rewards are included in salaries.

Payers and provider organizations continue to try to standardize the practice of medicine, and some recent trends suggest a new openness to protocols and pathways. But the nature of professional medical practice probably precludes full standardization. The extent to which physicians' practices can be standardized will be determined both by organizational systems and controls and by physicians themselves. Most organizations would, if given the opportunity, opt to standardize as many behaviors as possible to support their cost containment and quality assurance strategies. But many physicians would prefer the income security of a steady practice volume and salary. Physicians will also balk at what they see as the practice of "cookbook medicine" under such managed situations. Most important, the nature of the practice of medicine will always include activities and responsibilities that cannot be standardized across clinical settings, practitioners, patients, and illnesses despite payers' and others' desire to standardize behavior, outcomes, and reimbursement.

The primary regulatory and payer considerations in structuring physician pay plans are centered in restrictions on tax exempt organizations in distributing profits, and federal restrictions on referrals and incentive structures. Restrictions in tax exemptions include the need to justify the reasonableness (or fair market value) of compensation levels and plan design, the expected use of caps (maximums) in administering physician earnings, and sanctions against inurement or private benefit. Restrictions on pension and

deferred rewards in tax exempts may limit the organization's ability to deliver long-term rewards, security, and tax advantages. Taxation issues, particularly at the organizational level, are further discussed in Chapter 48.

The primary restrictions created by HCFA and the OIG focus on proscriptions against self-referrals within physicians' practices, the ability of physicians to derive direct income from ancillary or technical services, and the use of incentives that may be construed as rewards for limiting care. Both Internal Revenue Service (IRS) and HCFA guidelines prescribe substantial fines for violations, and recent investigations and indictments underscore the importance of compliance. The government's guidelines also define a number of safe harbors within which physicians and groups may operate.

Restrictions on distribution of ancillary revenues are a major issue for physicians who historically derived a large amount of income from laboratory or imaging operations. While these practices, now integrated into an IDS, may still generate a large amount of fee-for-service professional and technical revenue, the ancillary revenue is not a liability under managed care. Pharmacy risk has become a significant new factor under many managed care contracts and many physician groups find that their projected pharmaceutical risk exceeds their full monthly capitation payment. Practices with large ancillary components either have been forced to accept reduced incomes from divesting ancillary operations or have redistributed these earnings in compliance with the regulations.

The effect of the Stark regulations has been to reduce distributable income in a practice with significant ancillary income if the practice is forced to divest any ancillary business interests. Even though these revenues may remain elsewhere in the IDS, direct distribution to physicians is illegal. Even in primarily fee-for-service practices, these factors are creating a more "managed care-friendly" reward context as the relative importance (i.e., amount) of ancillary income is diluted.

Fraud and abuse regulations have another indirect impact on managed care physician compensation. As might be expected, as practices have lost or been forced to redistribute ancillary revenues, their willingness to enter into integrated service agreements via contracts, acquisitions, or mergers increases. IDSs may be able to retain the ancillary revenue sources in other business units and may have the financial ability to compensate physicians at historical levels based on compensable outcomes other than volume of technical or referral fees. As long as indemnity reimbursement motivates increased technical charges, however, retaining ancillary services in mixed reimbursement practices may be dysfunctional.

GENERAL DESIGN ALTERNATIVES

Although the above discussion of the general issues facing physician pay plan design may seem to present impossible challenges, most approaches to physician compensation reflect relatively few different designs. Each of these is reviewed separately.

Productivity Plans

Traditional productivity-based pay plans, including income distribution schemes in group practices, have direct implications for structuring physicians' rewards under managed care. These fully variable plans' greatest, and most problematic, impact comes from the historical psychological impact of decades of piece-rate pay. Few occupations or professions have enjoyed such high relative earnings coupled with immediate linkages between productivity and rewards. Coupled with physicians' innate achievement orientation, this reinforcement scheme gets much of the credit (or blame) for the high levels of productivity, technology advancement, and tertiary outcomes reflected in the U.S. health care industry. The emphasis on production and volumes under traditional pay plans becomes dysfunctional under managed care and may confuse physicians' motives in IDSs. Certainly, increased resource utilization and patient visits are problematic under capitation and are increasingly being negatively rewarded under discounted reimbursement.

Results from the Ernst & Young 1999 Benchmarking Survey show that 97 percent of medical practices measure and reward productivity, and that most of these groups focus on traditional volume metrics.[1] In fact, most groups continue to measure gross charges (or equivalents) even though the actual relationship between gross charges and actual practice income is increasingly distorted by reimbursement contracts, collection rates, and managed care agreements.

Many physician practices are using productivity surrogates to provide the feel of a production-based system under mixed reimbursement, and some find such plans effective under full capitation. The most typical of this genre use relative value units (RVUs) to calibrate each physician's productivity. The total RVUs, or the physician's relative contribution to total group RVUs, are then used to distribute available labor funds or to establish incentive payouts. Differential conversion factors (pay dollars per RVU) are often used to reward fee-for-service versus capitated volume. This approach is attractive when the practice wants to send a clear signal about the relative "value" of fee-for-service and capitated clinical work, but it may be problematic due to the complexity of the required information systems and calculations.

The apparent return to productivity pay plans in medical groups may seem anachronistic in a world racing to managed care, but most groups are finding that their physicians understand clinical volume and respond well to this approach. Even though productivity-based pay plans are enjoying great popularity, they risk significant problems when not coupled with strong resource management programs under managed care reimbursement. More than one group has experienced the negative impact of diluted or nonexistent risk pools due to overutilization. When physicians feel motivated to increase their earnings by increasing their RVUs under managed care, they may take two steps forward and one step back (or, worse yet, one step forward and two steps back) by increasing their individual percentage of a diluted income pool.

The use of productivity-based pay plans may even affect a group's ability to contract for capitated members when a payer organization feels that production pay plans may lead to overutilization or quality problems. It is always in a payer's best interest for physicians to be satisfied with their pay plan and pay levels simply because motivated physicians can provide better and more personable patient care. Enlightened payers therefore seek those medical groups where the physicians are not demotivated by the inverse impact of productivity-based pay under fixed reimbursement.

Direct Distribution Plans

The managed care era equivalent of the productivity-based pay plan model is demonstrated in full capitation models where net premium income is distributed directly to physicians. As in productivity plans, the total net income attributable to individual physicians is computed and allocated. Income sources typically include all PMPM revenue plus net risk-pool distributions. In this plan, reimbursement is paid directly to the physicians, thus providing the linkage between the plan's goals and the physicians' reinforcement.

Computing each physician's PMPM income is usually based on paneled members, member months, or a visit/encounter measure. Risk-pool distributions may be similarly based, or they may be computed based on tabulation of each physician's resource, inpatient, and specialty utilization. These latter computations may become complex under multiple plans. A blended rate is the most frequent approach under multiple contracts. The available revenue may also be recalibrated based on productivity if there are wide variations in clinical activity across similar numbers of contracted members within a specialty. In this context, risk pools are often distributed on the physician's volume (members and visits), which is adjusted based on a moderator variable, such as a rating of resource management outcomes.

The direct distribution approach provides a direct link between net pay and each individual physician's total volume and managed care effectiveness. It assumes an individual (rather than group) level of service delivery, however, and in

its purest form puts the individual physician fully at risk for underwriting health care costs for the covered members, or at least those costs for which the physician is receiving capitation.

As discussed in Chapters 8, 11, and 32, for the small number of members (whether active patients or not) that are associated with a single physician, chance is likely to play as strong a role in resource use as is medical management; in other words, it is difficult to adjust for illness burden of a panel of patients at the individual physician level. See Chapter 32 for a detailed discussion of the challenges of risk adjustment in provider profiling.

Salary-Only Plans

In some contexts, physicians are best rewarded with fixed compensation only. For example, physicians entering practice from residency are best paid a straight salary if they cannot yet produce sufficient volumes to participate in incentive-based pay. Physicians moving to new sites with underdeveloped patient populations, or when physicians are involved in a "turnaround" practice, are other examples that may be best rewarded with fixed pay. Some managed care organizations have used salary-only plans under structured practice contexts, and government facilities have historically paid physicians via salary alone. Hospital-based practitioners are another group that is often paid only in fixed pay. But overall, the prevalence of salary-only rewards is declining, with 79 percent of groups in the Ernst & Young Benchmarking Survey sample using a combination of salary and incentives.

Salary-only plans are most attractive for their administrative simplicity and for those practitioners who are not able or willing to accept compensation risk. Although it may seem unlikely that physicians would prefer fixed compensation, many find that, as patient populations shift among payers and volumes become unpredictable, their best option is the security of a salary-only pay package.

The primary drawbacks to salary-only plans are the high fixed-cost basis created by physician salaries and the absence of linkages between physicians' behaviors and overall practice outcomes. In salary-only models, productivity, resource utilization, and quality assurance must be managed through other (nonmonetary reward) mechanisms.

Salary Plus Variable Pay Plans

Most organizations recognize that a pure productivity model creates too much pay risk for physicians, and salary-only models remove all linkages to variable outcomes. Therefore, most organizations embrace a combination of both fixed and variable pay. The design of the salary/fixed component in these pay plans must reflect a concern not only for salary levels, which may be defined in relation to market norms or funding ability, but also for the relative level of incentive or variable pay. Salary setting (both for policies ranges and actual individual rates) can be structured as a forward or reverse engineering exercise.

In all cases, salary and incentive levels (i.e., target amounts) should be set within an a priori structure based on market norms, the organization's funding ability, and historical physician earnings (or a combination thereof). For example, the employer may, based on historical earning trends, specify a targeted salary level at the market median for most practitioners. Market-sensitive hiring rates will be set, with caps or maximums being set high enough to reward those who exceed basic expectations.

These pay targets are generally structured as a range (i.e., a minimum—target/midpoint—maximum), often with steps that provide rapid early career growth slowing in later years. This approach provides a good link to market norms, and midpoints are often the employer's "philosophical" pay goal—typically the market median. But this approach presupposes adequate funding for the aggregate fixed labor cost of all employed physicians. Also, when setting salaries based on market norms, one must isolate salaries and total cash compensation (salaries plus bonuses and incentives) in survey data to ensure accurate analysis. Assuming that the targeted salary level is economically prudent, incentive opportunities are then designed as incremental earnings.

The level (amount) of potential incentive earnings should have administrative caps in tax-exempt delivery systems and will ultimately be limited in all organizations to available funding. When a physician's practice has operating losses (the norm in IDSs), the available funding often includes subsidies from the parent organization. This reality is being challenged as a business model and may create compliance issues in tax-exempt IDSs.

In organizations with high relative salaries, the ability to structure and fund incentives is limited. As noted earlier, the relative impact is quite different at the primary care level compared with the subspecialist pay level. It is often necessary to provide high fixed compensation in competitive markets, but these high salaries may limit the organization's ability to fund incremental (incentive) earnings. In practices where some physicians may be able to generate high volumes under fee-for-service or discounted procedure-based reimbursement, however, this approach can provide significant upside motivation.

Conversely, salaries and incentives can be reverse engineered by starting with available labor funds and backing into the relative amount of pay in fixed and variable components. Alternatively, the design can be anchored in market norms for total cash compensation, with the respective elements being computed as percentages of the total. For example, available income (from all sources) for a clinic, department, or single specialty may provide an average of $160,000 cash compensation for each of 10 physicians. If 20 percent of the available cash is allocated to incentives, then physicians' salaries will average $128,000. Conversely, salaries and incentives could be anchored using absolute dollar amounts across all specialties. For example, all physicians may have a $20,000 incentive opportunity regardless of specialty. Base rates would be adjusted to reflect this withhold amount.

Another design option for setting salaries and incentive opportunities is afforded in practices where high volumes, favorable reimbursement, and low relative costs allow competitive salaries plus significant incentive opportunities. One might expect this set of conditions to occur only under fee-for-service reimbursement, but many predominantly managed care practices find that they can fund such programs where their physicians generate high patient volumes with effective specialty and ancillary utilization.

MEASUREMENT ISSUES

The adage, "We measure what we can, and we get what we measure," applies as much to designing pay plans as to other aspects of business. Under fee-for-service reimbursement, measuring a physician's productivity or value is easy and direct. In transitioning from fee-for-service to managed care reimbursement, the measurement of physicians' contributions and productivity must change. The shift in measures simply reflects the changing (appropriate) practice behaviors, but the direct link between pay and the measures creates special pressures.

The most typical first-generation productivity measures (as managed care reimbursement becomes significant to the practice) use a form of fee-for-service equivalent, RVUs, visits/encounters, or paneled members. Any or all of these measures may be effective in calibrating total volume/productivity for the purposes of allocating performance-based rewards.

As noted earlier, most performance measures continue to focus on productivity or utilization. But new measures are being designed to capture better the full value that physicians provide to managed care plans and delivery systems. But the linkages between pay, behaviors, outcomes, and performance measures may not be as obvious as assumed. Ernst & Young's 1999 Benchmarking Survey finds that physician practices that measure specific productivity metrics for purposes of setting pay do not consistently demonstrate higher levels of those measured factors. This suggests that compensation may not actually "drive" behavior, although this may be a good way to recognize appropriate behavior.

Under predominantly managed care reimbursement, measuring physicians' performance must move beyond traditional volume-based measurement. In practices where fixed (capitated) reimbursement is reallocated based on RVUs or fee-for-service equivalent charges, there is the risk of overdistribution. That is, available funding may be depleted as a result of poor resource management, thereby limiting upside incentive opportunities.

This impact may justly be felt by the highest producers if they achieved that status by churning or other dysfunctional activity. Even appropriate practice behaviors can be negatively reinforced, however, when managed care reimbursement is distributed based solely on individual productivity. Again, only when effective resource management and quality assurance programs are in place can productivity-based pay plans ensure the appropriate rewards for the right practice behaviors under managed reimbursement.

Measurement issues affect the design and administration of both fixed compensation and incentives. Most fixed-pay plans assume a nominal or threshold level of activity as justification for receiving the base salary of the fixed-pay component. This assumption may be operationalized as predefined production/volume levels as preconditions for receipt of the full-time equivalent (FTE) salary.

The transition away from traditional productivity-based measurement under managed care presents the greatest current challenge in ensuring prudent and motivating physician pay plans. As noted above, historical approaches to productivity assessment (professional collections) and transitional approaches (RVUs) carry the risk that physicians will maximize their incomes via inappropriate activity and resource utilization. But many groups have shifted their focus from a search for the ultimate transitional measures to a return to traditional considerations. Many of the most successful practices with substantial capitated reimbursement simply pay physicians for productivity but manage utilization, minimal standards (hours, members, and so on) through the medical management process without direct linkages to cash compensation (other than the implicit impact of these factors on total compensation funding).

THE ROLE OF BENEFITS IN TOTAL COMPENSATION

As physicians find themselves increasingly in employed status, the value and structure of benefits packages become more important. Most employed physicians enjoy competitive benefits, traditionally structured to include the following:

- *Health and welfare benefits*, including medical, dental, and prescription benefits
- *Disability and survivor benefits*, including short- and long-term disability and life insurance
- *Retirement and savings plans*, including qualified or nonqualified retirement plans, 401(k) or 403(b) (in tax exempt organizations) savings plans, annuities, and other programs (see below)
- *Employment benefits*, including paid time off (vacations, holidays, etc.), business expense reimbursement, and so forth (many groups are finding that time off benefits are more important than many others, especially in two wage-earning households)
- *Medical malpractice coverage*, often including tail coverage for physicians entering employment from existing practices
- *Professional expense accounts*, including reimbursement for continuing medical education, professional development, memberships, certifications, licensure, subscriptions, and other qualified expenses

Basic benefits programs vary widely in actual costs as a result of coverage, structure, and population differences, but the basic provisions in these plans are relatively similar. In many contexts, physicians are necessarily covered by existing employee benefits packages. For example, hospitals acquiring medical practices generally extend their current benefits plans to cover the physicians and their staffs. Benefits programs may add from 15 to 30 percent to direct (cash compensation) labor costs, depending on the provisions and cost structure. Benefits plans in large organizations, especially those with union employees, may be significantly more costly than those in free-standing medical practices. These employers are often challenged to demonstrate the value of any increase in costs to physicians who would not incur such expenses in their own businesses. Many medical practices in IDSs also find that these newer higher benefits costs contribute significantly to the negative overall practice net income.

Retirement and deferred income benefits warrant special discussion. This class of benefits continues to be a critical component in structuring competitive pay plans for employed physicians. Physicians in private and group practice have generally enjoyed the benefits of business ownership as reflected in their ability to defer income and structure retirement plans to meet individual tax, security, and income needs.

The use of individual retirement accounts, Keogh accounts, trusts, and annuities in medical groups generally allows a higher level of retirement plan funding than in typical employer plans. Considerations in tax exempt organizations further restrict the ability to structure such plans for highly paid individuals (i.e., executives and physicians). Finally, qualified retirement plans are limited to contributions based on a current maximum of $160,000 in cash income (salaries and incentives/bonuses). Whereas employers can provide supplemental benefits to offset this regulatory cap, the potential costs for large numbers of employed physicians may limit employers' ability to fund such plans broadly.

The net effect of the regulatory and economic context in employment settings is to limit the level of income deferral and retirement funding options. Legal, administrative, risk management, and financial issues keep many organizations from providing special supplemental benefits for physicians, although such programs are gaining wider appeal. Employers may directly supplement retirement or deferred benefits for physicians in for-profit entities or through the use of intermediary financial devices, such as insurance or trusts, in tax exempts. Supplemental benefits in tax exempt organizations must be subject to a risk of forfeiture and other constraints, making these plans generally unattractive to physicians.

COMPENSATING MEDICAL DIRECTORS AND ADMINISTRATIVE PHYSICIANS

The expanding numbers of practicing physicians in employed contexts and IDSs with substantial managed care reimbursement are creating parallel growth in the numbers and types of nonclinical physician roles. These roles, while highly variable, can be categorized across the range of organizational structures as follows:

- *system level, systemwide,* responsibility for all physician management (typically the "chief medical officer")
- *system level, single function/service area,* such as quality assurance, professional relations, or regional operations (often a "vice president of medical affairs")
- *entity level, entity wide,* usually within a hospital or clinic (typically the "medical director")
- *entity level, single function/service area,* such as the head of contracting within a facility
- *entity level, single department/unit area,* typically structured as the traditional chair, chief, or unit manager role

These roles may be in any type of organization, including hospitals, IPAs, PPOs, MSOs, HMOs, and medical groups. Administrative physician roles are compensated with a variety of approaches, generally reflecting the organization's relative level of sophistication and maturity in the utilization of physicians in such roles. Many organizations with less than full-time administrative roles simply provide hourly reimbursement for meetings and functional activity. This approach is simple but may not provide rewards for the actual value of the services rendered. More than one employer has found that time spent in meetings increases when it is compensated but that outcomes may not improve.

Many organizations are moving to the use of formal compensation arrangements for nonclinical physicians in which the amount, type, and value of services are calibrated to pay levels. Such plans may also use multiple pay elements, such as salaries plus incentives, to link activities to rewards. This approach can be adapted to a wide variety of physician roles and for full- or part-time responsibilities.

The structure of medical director compensation packages is often anchored in the physician's historical practitioner earnings. Although most organizations would agree that administrative roles should be rewarded based on actual responsibilities and not the incumbent physician's prior practice income, attracting qualified practitioners into administrative roles often demands compensation levels above those available for clinical practice.

When administrative physicians maintain an active clinical practice, administrative compensation should be structured to represent accurately the relative amount of effort and time committed to the nonpractitioner role. Many organizations put limits on the medical director's practitioner earnings, especially if this income is based on productivity, to ensure that energies are not diverted from critical administrative duties.

Structuring medical director pay packages around the relative value of the job should begin with a definition of all core ongoing responsibilities, including documentation of activities, time commitments, authorities and controls, and expected outcomes. This core job can then be priced in relation to external and internal benchmarks to set a fixed salary that covers all ongoing duties. Incentives may be appropriate for motivating extra effort, rewarding special projects or initiatives, or producing incremental operational/financial results.

Under this approach, compensation packages for medical directors may take on the nature of typical executive pay plans (except for any clinical compensation component). This approach will afford the opportunity to align medical directors' incentives with organizational priorities. As in any executive pay plan, however, defining performance standards and expectations and measuring results may present new challenges.

Performance indicators for administrative physicians may be based on process goals, such as chairing meetings or developing and administering policies. As physician roles become more directly linked to the organization's management and clinical activities, pay can be linked to measurable outcomes. For example, incentives for medical directors with quality assurance or utilization management responsibilities can be linked to the total practice's performance on the same quality assurance and utilization management measures used in individual physicians' incentives. It should be noted, however, that regulatory guidelines and specific court cases make it clear that a medical director cannot be financially rewarded to deny payment for specific cases or for moving referrals or patients to the employer's facility.

COMPENSATING HOSPITAL-BASED PRACTITIONERS

Hospitals have traditionally provided some level of reimbursement/compensation for some specialties operating within hospital units. Such arrangements may be structured as direct compensation agreements when the physicians are employed or as contracts between the institution and a hospital-based medical group. Pathology, radiology, anesthesiology, and emergency medicine are the units most often providing compensation to hospital-based practitioners.

Compensation to hospital-based specialists is most often linked to administrative, quality assurance, and other nonpractitioner duties. Under typical relationships, the physicians bill and collect separately for the professional fee revenue from their practice. The level and structure of compensation from the hospital may range from token payments to recognize the physicians' administrative presence to significant amounts tied to broad management responsibilities. Unfortunately, the general level of documentation of these roles and the sophistication of the economic linkages suggest that many such relationships are not truly structured as reward plans.

Many hospitals are shifting these payments from fixed payments to more complex group level pay plans similar to those described above for medical directors. By structuring some or all of the hospital-based specialist group's income

as incentives linked to predefined goals, the hospital can begin to shift physicians' focus as both administrators and as practitioners.

This shift is largely in reaction to the recognition that hospital-based specialists can have a significant impact on resource management efforts but that incentives to these physicians to comply with cost containment initiatives may negatively affect their own professional incomes. Physicians whose professional reimbursement is calibrated in fee-for-service or other volume measures present special problems for hospitals and MSOs being paid under capitation or other fixed reimbursement arrangements.

Examples of incentive programs for hospital-based medical groups may include specified bonus opportunities linked to achievement of predefined utilization or quality goals. Arrangements where physicians share directly in cost reductions have been popular in recent years, and many were designed as "gain-sharing" programs that split cost savings with the physicians who helped the hospital achieve the financial goals. But these plans have been deemed illegal in a recent OIG ruling (see box, "Beyond Gainsharing") and must be unwound.

COMPENSATION IN FACULTY PRACTICE PLANS UNDER MANAGED CARE

Special considerations apply when one is compensating practitioners in faculty practices under managed reimbursement. Because faculty practices often represent the higher levels of care (tertiary or quaternary) and the highest cost basis in a community, they may not always be perceived as the best locus for managed health care, but faculty plans find themselves increasingly seeking participation in managed care plans to ensure their patient base.

Physicians in many faculty practices are paid with salaries plus bonuses tied to patient care volumes, academic achievement (teaching and research), and other professional contributions. Funding may be from mixed sources, including academic stipends (i.e., tuition), research grants, and professional fees. The relative mix of fund-

---

Beyond Gainsharing

One of 1999's most significant events in relation to physicians compensation programs was the OIG's advisory ruling related to gainsharing programs. These programs, which share a portion of cost savings from joint medical management programs, have become popular as a way to involve physicians in hospitals' quality improvement and cost containment efforts. The OIG ruling makes it clear that, from their perspective (which is not shared by the IRS, the other major federal regulator of physicians' compensation plans), these gainsharing plans are illegal and should be discontinued as soon as possible.

While the attorneys sort through the details and prepare opinions on the viability of gainsharing variants, providers must deal with unwinding current plans and with many physicians' expectations to be included in (and paid for) joint programs. Without pushing the legal envelope, there are clear alternatives for a hospital to work with physicians on these strategic programs. Moving beyond the simple gainsharing model, these hospitals can:

- Reward physicians for program design and implementation, and provide incentives for continuing achievement of non-financial outcomes. It may be illegal to link incentives to cost savings, but lump-sum payments for successful implementation of programs, or for continuing improvements in clinical outcomes or patient satisfaction are possible.

- Contract with physicians for quality improvement and implementation of clinical protocols. While it may be illegal to contract with physicians for economic benefits (i.e., cost savings), physicians can be paid to design, implement, and administer programs that support improvements in clinical quality.
- Pay fair market value for any nonclinical services rendered. Again, any payments for outcomes must be linked to nonfinancial results. But payment for services (for example, program design or consulting) is legitimate as long as the amounts reflect the fair market value of services rendered.

Many gainsharing plans were flawed from the outset since their intent was to capture physicians' energies (and loyalties and patients) through sharing cost savings. Since physicians (and patients, and the OIG) may be legitimately concerned that these cost cutting efforts may compromise care, the typical gainsharing plan runs the risk of moving physicians' focus from quality to cost management. The new guidelines provide a clear, and many believe superior, roadmap for contracting with physicians to improve clinical outcomes through consistent adherence to normative protocols. These incentives are well aligned with physicians' primary professional motives. And most hospital executives recognize that a consistently administered quality improvement program will inevitably lead to better patient care and lower ongoing costs.

---

ing sources may not be well defined for individual practitioners, and total physician labor costs may not be fully self-funded from internally generated revenues. These pay plans are not well suited for the distribution of managed care reimbursement. The lack of incentives for effective resource utilization or high-volume patient loads limits the typical faculty practice pay plan under managed reimbursement.

Operational changes and a shift in practice behaviors are often required to align faculty practices with the new protocols in managed care. Considerations such as scheduling and staffing models may have more impact on the ability to design appropriate physician pay plans than other issues. As operating practices change in response to shifting reimbursement, faculty practices will increasingly adopt pay plans similar to those in managed care medical groups. Many faculty groups have explicitly isolated the clinical component in their pay plans and restructured all clinical rewards around the same principles used in other managed care practices.

EXAMPLES

Implementing an RVU Plan

The simplest path to an RVU-based pay plan measures existing RVUs as reflected in the Medicare resource-based relative value scale tables. All patient encounters and procedures are coded for RVU credit, and the resulting totals supplant fee-for-service collections as the measure of physician productivity. Compensation may be paid fully on numbers of RVUs (i.e., 100 percent incentives) or may also include a salary component.

As an example, in a mostly primary care organization (with only a few selected specialists), an RVU plan will usually set thresholds for full-time salaries and minimal clinical productivity. Funding for the RVU-based incentives will blend market norms with the practice's economic resources. RVUs are tracked for all patient care activity, and special RVUs are often added to recognize the value of nonclinical duties such as board or committee assignments. No distinctions are typically made for different types or levels of reimbursement, but it is possible to design different conversion factors for different revenue streams.

Most such plans include a basic or salary component, with rates set against market norms by specialty. Caps are set relatively low (below market medians) to focus physicians on achieving minimal productivity levels and become eligible for incentives. Salaries are standardized for all "journeyman" practitioners operating as FTE providers. FTE is most often defined through a combination of schedule, members, and other factors.

When the practice group produces excess net income after all expenses, including physician salaries and benefits costs, the excess is distributed to all physicians as an extra conversion factor payment for RVUs produced. This approach may demand significant investments in information systems and medical management systems, but these investments are needed in today's delivery context regardless of pay plan design. This approach allows the practice to reward physicians based on their bottom-line results, including (or excluding) any subsidies or investments from a parent organization. Integration of the reward plan with ongoing medical management, peer review, quality assurance, and other professional activities adds the ability to link a variety of factors—often changing annually—to the payment formula.

Multispecialty Group Rewards under Managed Care

Many large multispecialty groups have embraced (or been forced to participate in) managed care plans. Some have developed, acquired, or merged with health plans. Managing the reward plan across specialties ranging from pediatrics to neurosurgery under mixed reimbursement presents special problems. Although the short-term reimbursement context may include substantial fee-for-service opportunities for some subspecialties, most physicians are experiencing pricing and volume decreases. Staffing models may require substantial revision under managed care as fewer specialists and more primary care practitioners are required to service the patient population.

For example, a large multispecialty group (more than 150 physicians) has integrated with a community hospital, has created a proprietary health plan with 35,000 lives, and contracts for 55,000 more (most are for full risk). A majority (more than 75 percent) of professional fees come from capitation. The parent system is tax exempt, creating limits on pay levels and plan designs as well as new reporting requirements.

Many specialists continue to receive substantial fee-for-service referrals, whereas most primary care physicians' practices are now mostly capitated. All physicians' productivity is tracked as fee-for-service equivalent collections by imputing the average reimbursement amount per procedure or visit for capitated patients.

Salaries are set based on an annual analysis of group trends (productivity and costs), group and system budgets, and market norms (collected in a proprietary survey of similar practices). Salary targets for each specialty are linked to the norms, within internal budgetary funding limits, commensurate with relative productivity. That is, if fee-for-service obstetrics/gynecology equivalent productivity is at the third quartile of the benchmark, the target salary for these physicians is set at the competitive cash compensation third quartile.

Total budgeted salaries are set below projected net income both to ensure a cash flow cushion and to increase the group's ability to fund the incentive pool. This is analogous to the group's prior partnership plan that provided a "draw" against projected annual productivity income. Adjustments are made to the target rate to reflect individual physician performance, citizenship, and other metrics from the health plans. When net income exceeds budgeted levels, an incentive pool is funded and distributed based on relative productivity and on professional criteria. The Compensation Committee makes these distribution decisions within general policy guidelines but is empowered to exercise judgment as appropriate.

This approach generally suffers from initial problems related to high utilization among specialists, but most problems can be resolved by staffing adjustments, professional review and feedback, or (in drastic cases) through salary reductions. Internal committees reviewing quality and resource utilization must be linked with those in health plans and integrated hospitals, creating multiple review points to recognize problems early.

DESIGNING PERFORMANCE MEASURES

Any non–productivity-based pay-for-performance plan will require formal measurement of physician performance and, ideally, outcomes. Although job performance measurement is a relatively mature exercise in traditional employment contexts, the technology for reliably measuring a physician's performance is still evolving.

As noted earlier, the most significant trend in performance metrics is the return to classic productivity measures. Other measures are used in a number of groups as well (see Figure 9–2). Other measures relying on industry standards (e.g., HEDIS) or payer feedback (e.g., patient satisfaction) are used variously, but physicians generally balk at external metrics that do not capture the "special" nature of their practices.

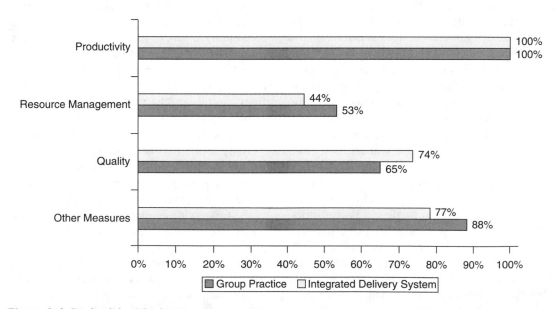

Figure 9–2 Productivity Metrics: Prevalence of Performance Measures Used in Physicians' Compensation Programs. Courtesy of Ernst & Young, 1999, Physician Benchmarking Survey.

A physician profile is often used to measure an individual physician's performance and to benchmark against a predefined set of standards. These profile ratings can be linked to incentive calculations. Because profiling standards generally include professional qualifications and behaviors as well as comparisons with similar practitioners within the group, physicians may be more receptive to this approach than to purely subjective evaluations or financial measurement only. Physician profiling is discussed in greater detail in Chapter 32.

Steps for building a profiling tool for compensation purposes may include the following:

- *Develop performance categories.* Performance categories should be developed based on the most important input and output factors directly affected by physician behavior. Examples might include productivity or volume, resource utilization, quality of care and service, financial performance, and professionalism.
- *Define measures.* Specific measures must be defined for each performance category, ideally emphasizing objective measurement or behaviorally anchored ratings. Using the above examples, typical measures could include those listed in Figure 9–3.
- *Define data collection method.* Ratings scales, data reporting and recording formats, and administrative protocols should be carefully defined to maximize the accuracy and reliability of the profiling information. When possible, data should be taken directly from available sources, such as system reports on patient volumes, costs, and referral tracking. Any data elements collected via subjective ratings should be anchored with behavioral indicators. For example, peer ratings of work habits should be grounded in specific indicators, such as attendance and communication, not wholly subjective ratings.
- *Develop standards for comparison.* Profiles should be compared among physicians and with normative data when possible. Most organizations track internal historical trends as one key benchmark.

- *Build a reporting protocol.* The success of any profile plan will depend largely on the timeliness, accuracy, and user-friendliness of the reports used to track and manage results. Implementing a good profiling plan may require a significant investment in computer and accounting systems as well as implementation and ongoing communication with physicians. Because these measurements will affect the physicians' incomes and be instrumental in guiding their behaviors, the organization should recognize the need for both competent technical design and effective communications.
- *Link to rewards.* The final step includes building linkages to physicians' earnings. Minimal standards for profile scores are typically used to determine continued employment and eligibility for salary increases. Profile scores are also typically used to define incentive payouts.

The link between profile scores and incentive earnings will depend on the structure of the incentive plan itself. If incentives are either targeted at a percentage of salary or based upon the retrospective distribution of withheld earnings, profile scores above a predefined threshold may trigger a full incentive distribution. Similarly, scores above or below the expected standard may increase or decrease payouts. The ratings and linkages to the incentive payouts can be varied to reflect different ratings schemes, and different measures on the profile can be weighted to reflect relative importance. It is also possible for a managed care plan to engage in this type of performance-based compensation system, as is discussed in greater detail in Chapter 10.

CONCLUSION

An effective physician compensation model will reflect a thoughtful application of general compensation plan concepts, benchmarks for successful plans in similar contexts, and organization-specific business strategies to the individual practice context. The variety of situa-

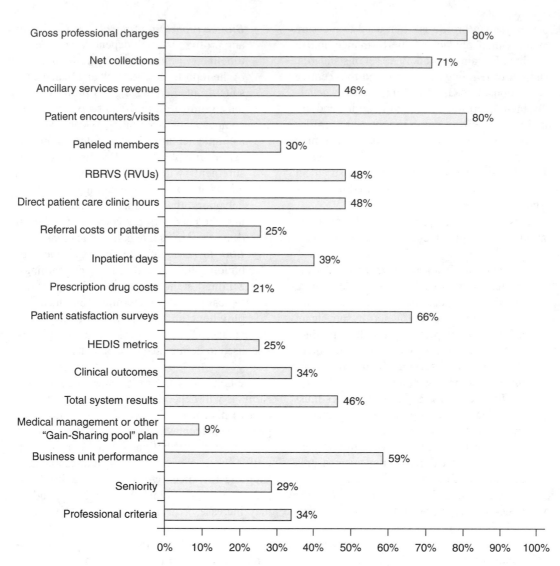

Figure 9–3 Productivity Performance Measures for Use in Profiling. Courtesy of Ernst & Young, 1999, Physician Benchmarking Survey.

tions encountered as IDSs move further to managed care limits the ability to adopt a "one size fits all" model, and any new pay plan must include significant flexibility to deal with individual physicians and cope with changes in the marketplace.

The most prevalent current trend in pay plans is the use of salary plus incentives and the reliance on traditional productivity-focused performance metrics. Linkages to funding models are

slowly becoming more typical, but since most practices have negative net income, the subsidies and investments included in funding physician pay pools make accurate financial determinations problematic.

Integration of the physicians' pay plan with other organizational strategies, such as developing stronger physician leadership in nonclinical roles, appears to be an evolving best practice. The importance of information systems technology in providing performance feedback, tracking results, and improving practice efficiencies is growing exponentially.

The trend toward simpler approaches to physician compensation models may be the best near-term response to the industry's unpredictable state. Many organizations have experimented with complex formulas that combined productivity, risk management, and outcomes measures. But these approaches usually failed due to complexity and a lack of fundamental economic linkages among the metrics. In the absence of these relationships between funding and individual physician income, simpler models that reward clinical productivity may be the best compromise until market factors stabilize and provider organizations find ways to optimize physician practice operations.

REFERENCE

1. Ernst & Young LLP, Physicians' Benchmarking Survey (Los Angeles: Ernst & Young LLP, 1999).

CHAPTER 10

Nonutilization–Based Incentive Compensation for Physicians

Peter R. Kongstvedt

INTRODUCTION

Physician compensation is an area with a great deal of variation. Basic methods of compensation of primary care physicians (PCPs) are addressed in Chapter 8, specialty care physicians (SCPs) in Chapter 11, and compensation of physicians in medical groups and integrated delivery systems (IDSs) is addressed in Chapter 9. Although those chapters do give the reader a sense of the complexity of reimbursement issues, it is often believed by many that physician compensation in managed care focuses solely on issues of utilization and cost. It is accurate to state that the alignment of financial incentives between the managed care organization (MCO) and the physicians is important in managed care, but it is inaccurate to state that there is no interest in aligning physician incentives with goals that are based on performance other than utilization. Therefore, although many MCOs combine utilization and nonutilization financial incentives, this chapter focuses on incentive compensation programs that rely on standards of performance outside of utilization management.

The use of financial incentives applied to measures such as patient satisfaction and quality is found in many MCOs. A large study published in 1995 reported that 36 percent of MCOs used member satisfaction surveys for purposes of adjusting physician payments, and 56 percent of MCOs used quality measures.[1] Looking at the same issue from the perspective of physicians who receive income from MCOs, another study,

using 1996 and 1997 data, reported 23 percent of physicians having financial incentives based on patient satisfaction, and 18 percent having incentives based on quality of care such as preventive care measures; PCPs were more likely to have such financial incentives than were specialists.[2] Further detail from the physician study is illustrated in Table 10–1.

Obviously, there are significant differences between closed-panel health plans (i.e., group and staff model HMOs) or medical groups, and open-panel plans. In closed panels and medical groups, it is easier to observe behavior, a greater reliance on subjective evaluations is possible, and the financial incentives usually include both PCPs and SCPs who are members of the group. Indeed, formal performance evaluations in closed-panel managed care plans, similar to what is discussed in this chapter, have been in use for many years.[3]

In open panels, there is no real opportunity to directly observe practice behavior, and so measures must rely on broad approaches to data gathering. Measuring quality and satisfaction in open panels is also more difficult when a physician has a small number of members because the measures will be based on a small base. In open panels, the focus is usually on PCPs, but it is certainly possible to construct an open panel performance evaluation program for SCPs and PCPs, and the principles will be the same.

It is not clear from published studies that financial performance incentives have a long-term effect, although many health care organiza-

Table 10–1 Factors Considered in Physician Compensation* (Physicians for whom the following factors are considered in determining their compensation in managed care systems)

	Patient Satisfaction Surveys	Measures of Quality of Care	Practice Profiles
Boston, Mass.	22%	17%	12%
Cleveland, Ohio	34†	28†	23†
Greenville, S.C.	25	18	16
Indianapolis, Ind.	21	13†	13
Lansing, Mich.	21	14†	20
Little Rock, Ark.	13†	11†	13
Miami, Fla.	26	27†	19
Newark, N.J.	29	21	15
Orange County, Calif.	44†	37†	33†
Phoenix, Ariz.	31	23	23†
Seattle, Wash.	23	10†	12
Syracuse, N.Y.	21†	17	13
Metropolitan areas >200,000 population	24	19	17
United States	23	18	16

*Physicians in the survey sample totaled 9,264, of whom 5,160 are primary care physicians. Physicians who were full owners of a solo practice (30 percent of the sample) were not asked about these compensation factors and are excluded from this table.
†Site value is significantly different from mean for metropolitan areas >200,000 population.
Source: Factors Considered in Physician Compensation, 1996 and 1997 Physician Survey, from *The Community Tracking Study,* Center for Studying Health System Change, Data Bulletin Number 8, Fall, 1997. Reprinted with permission of the Center for Studying Health System Change, Washington, D.C.

tions use them.[4] Even when such incentive programs are used, they usually undergo continual retooling in a quest to improve effectiveness.[5] If for no other reason, financial incentives based on quality and member satisfaction help to make it clear that the health plan is serious about rewarding those physicians that demonstrate high performance in those two areas. This chapter focuses on PCPs, looks at both closed and open panel programs, and provides examples that may work in one or the other. Although most performance evaluation systems have been applied to PCP managing plans (i.e., gatekeeper plans such as an HMO or a point of service plan), it is also possible to apply them to preferred provider organizations.[6]

PROBLEMS WITH EVALUATION SYSTEMS

Evaluating physician performance is unique in managed health care. As mentioned earlier, traditional fee-for-service has a straightforward reward system: The more you do, the more you are rewarded. Although rewarding productivity is useful and often necessary, traditional fee-for-service incentives often work in opposition to the goals of managed care, so different criteria are required.

At first, it would appear that simply reversing the economic reward would work. In other words, the less physicians use services, the more money they get. Unfortunately, that method not only fails to take into account certain behaviors that have no direct impact on utilization (such as member satisfaction, participation with the quality management [QM] program, or compliance with administrative procedures) but may also be subject to inappropriate manipulation or, worse yet, inappropriate underutilization.

Objective Criteria

The use of strictly objective criteria has recognized drawbacks. Examples of strictly objective criteria include utilization rates (e.g., hospital rates, referral rates, and ancillary testing), overall medical cost (e.g., per member per month [PMPM] cost), productivity (e.g., visits per day), and so forth. The major problem with strictly objective criteria is that they can be "gamed." The two major games played with objective criteria are (1) churning and (2) turfing.

Churning is the major complaint against fee-for-service medicine but can be equally prevalent in some managed care environments that rely heavily on productivity measures. Churning is simply increasing the revisit rate of existing patients more than is medically necessary. For example, it is just as easy to schedule a hypertension recheck in 4 weeks as 8 weeks. Furthermore, a revisit is a lot easier than a new patient, so the temptation can occur to see many revisits rather than allow the time for lengthy visits from new patients. Of course, if productivity is *not* tracked and rewarded in a staff model plan or medical group, overhead and costs will rise, and productivity will decline, as will member access. Therefore, nothing in this section should be interpreted as advocating not using productivity as a fundamental performance measure for medical groups and staff model plans.

Turfing refers to a physician's culling sick patients out of the practice to make the utilization profiles look better—in other words, transferring the sickest patients to other physicians for care to look like a low-utilizing provider. Turfing can occur in any plan with an undue emphasis on low utilization and when the compensation and reward structure for physicians is heavily weighted toward individual physicians having low utilization profiles.

This problem is not to be confused with the common excuse for failing to control utilization, the excuse of "But I've got all the sick patients!" A good risk-adjusted practice profiling tool (Chapter 32) can address that problem, and it is up to the medical director to determine whether the complaint has validity. Turfing refers specifically to physicians trying to "dump" their high-cost patients on to other physicians.

Subjective Criteria

Strictly subjective criteria are just as problematic as strictly objective criteria. Examples of strictly subjective criteria can include judgments about attitude, professionalism, demeanor, and the like. The principal problems with subjective criteria are the variability of interpretation and charges of favoritism and bias.

The very nature of subjective criteria demands variability in interpretation. Although a subjective category may be defined, performance in that category will be judged on the basis of the evaluator's opinion rather than on a set of numbers. This is certainly legitimate because presumably the manager making the judgment has a reasonably good idea of what he or she wants to see. It is still true, however, that different managers may judge the same behavior in different ways.

Charges of favoritism and bias are much more serious. If strictly subjective criteria are used, and if a negative evaluation is given to a physician, the manager may find that the physician does not accept the results, and charges of favoritism or bias may ensue. This can be of great concern if disciplinary actions are necessary and could theoretically lead to legal action unless good documentation has been kept for some time.

CATEGORIES FOR EVALUATION OF PHYSICIAN PERFORMANCE

If the use of strictly objective or subjective criteria can cause problems, then using both types of evaluation criteria in assessing physician performance provides balance. There are clearly objective items that can be measured and evaluated, items that a medical manager will consider important, such as utilization or productivity. The same is true for subjective measures such as participation, attitude, and so forth. The real issue is to combine objective with subjective in such a way as to avoid as much as possible the disincentive aspects of concentrating too heavily on any one category. Examples of evaluation categories are discussed, but it must be emphasized that not all of these categories should be used at the same time. Any incentive program that involves a high number of measures will dilute the effect of all of them and create confusion or diffidence to the program. Plan managers should use those few that are important to the plan's particular situation.

Categories for Evaluation in Closed Panels

This section briefly discusses potential categories for evaluation of physician performance in closed panels. These categories are listed in Exhibit 10–1 and are discussed in the following paragraphs.

It is important that the physicians in the group buy in to the process and not feel that it is being forced on them. It is up to management to decide what behaviors to motivate and then to present the concept to the practicing physicians. Allowing the physicians to have input into developing the criteria against which their performance will be judged is valuable toward gaining acceptance and cooperation with the program.

What follows are areas that one may wish to consider for evaluation of closed-panel physician performance. General ideas of how the categories are defined are also given, although before using these categories one would want to

---

Exhibit 10–1 Possible Categories for Evaluation in Closed Panels

- Productivity
- Medical charting
- Dependability and efficiency
- After-hours call duty
- Medical knowledge
- Management of patient care
- Management of outside resources
- Patient relations
- Staff relations
- Attitude and leadership
- Participation

---

define more specifically just what aspects of behavior would be evaluated.

Productivity

Productivity looks at volume of work and efficiency. Whatever standard a plan sets, such as number of visits per week, hours worked, and so forth, would be used as judgment criteria. One could add an element of time management as well. This very important measure is discussed further in Chapter 9.

Medical Charting

Medical charting would evaluate a physician's outpatient charts for legibility, timeliness, thoroughness, and compliance with whatever system is being used (e.g., chart format, face sheets, medication sheets).

Dependability and Efficiency

Dependability and efficiency would include arriving on time for work, sticking to the schedule, and complying with administrative aspects of the plan, such as properly using the forms.

After-Hours Call Duty

After-hours call duty looks at responsiveness, appropriate use of emergency medical resources, proper documentation, ensuring continuity of care through follow-ups or transfer of care to the appropriate primary physician, and any other aspects of care delivered through the after-hours on-call mechanism.

Medical Knowledge

Medical knowledge evaluates the level of medical knowledge, amount of technical skills, evidence of proper medical judgment, awareness of limitations in skills and knowledge, and appropriate use of continuing medical education opportunities.

Management of Patient Care

Closely related to the category of medical knowledge, the category of management of patient care looks at how the basic medical skills are translated into action and how that relates to cost-effectiveness. This category would include both outpatient and inpatient care. Examples would include logical and efficient plans for diagnosis and treatment, proper discharge planning, appropriate follow-up intervals, and so forth. The common thread is how patient care is handled by the physician being evaluated rather than by a consultant.

Management of Outside Resources

Management of outside resources looks at a physician's use of outside resources, including consultants and ancillary services, both diagnostic and therapeutic. Evaluations of appropriateness, cost-effective use, and maintenance of continuity would be made.

Patient Relations

Patient relations looks at a physician's ability to communicate effectively with patients, the quality of patient relations, and any concerns regarding member satisfaction. Member surveys may be conducted to obtain the opinions of members after their encounter; telephonic surveys generally yield more data than do mail-based surveys.

Staff Relations

Staff relations looks at a physician's ability to communicate and cooperate with other members of the medical staff, including a physician's working relationship with support staff.

Attitude and Leadership

Attitude looks at a physician's enthusiasm, interest, commitment, flexibility, responsiveness, and so forth. Although essentially this is a measure of positive attitude, one may wish to add those specifics about what is considered most important in judging attitude. Leadership refers to a physician's ability to train others and to motivate and lead and to his or her decision and communication skills in nonmedical matters.

Participation

Closely related to attitude, participation refers specifically to participation in plan committees and meetings. This looks at attendance, contribution, and initiative in taking responsibility.

Categories for Evaluation in Open Panels

This section discusses possible categories for formal performance evaluation in open panels. Again, this list is not exhaustive, and a plan should not use all the categories. These categories are much more objective than subjective, in keeping with the management structure of open panels. They are listed in Exhibit 10–2 and are discussed in the following paragraphs.

Utilization

Utilization is included in this section, but not in any detail. It is included only because many open-panel plans that have incentive programs include utilization data as part of the total program and do not necessarily separate them from the final incentive result. Issues such as adjustments for case mix and severity are important, and data use in medical management and practice profiling is discussed in greater detail in Chapters 32 and 33. More commonly, non–utilization-based incentives are funded solely via savings in medical costs. Thus, utilization management provides the funds, while distribution of that money is at least partly a function of non–utilization performance measures.

Exhibit 10–2 Possible Categories for Evaluation in Open Panels

- Utilization
- Access
  - Access
  - Panel size and status
- Compliance with administrative procedures
  - Cooperation with precertification and authorization requirements
  - Compliance with use of the plan network
  - Cooperation with other plan policies and procedures
- Electronic transactions and e-commerce
- Quality management
- Patient relations and member satisfaction

Access

Access. Accessibility may be measured in several ways. One easy measure is the total number of office hours available, and the plan may wish to reward the availability of increased office hours, especially nights and weekend hours. The plan may also perform on-site office reviews and examine the appointment book of the physician to determine how long it takes to get an appointment.

Panel Size and Status. Some plans want to provide incentives to large panels and will therefore provide incrementally higher incentives to larger panels (up to a limit; the plan does not want to provide incentives to panels so large that access is hampered). The plan may also want to encourage the physician to keep the panel open to new members of the plan and will provide incentives for the PCP to keep the panel in an open status. Because most plans require a PCP to keep the panel open up to a set number of members (e.g., 250 members), this incentive may be used only for panels with greater than the minimum required number of members.

Compliance with Administrative Policies and Procedures

In addition to clinical behavior, the plan benefits from high compliance with administrative policies and procedures. Examples of these are as follows.

Cooperation with Precertification and Authorization Requirements. This measures the physician's compliance with the plan's requirements for precertification and authorization of services and is measured as a percentage. For example, 88 percent of admissions for a physician are precertified, and 95 percent of referrals are prospectively authorized. There is no value that can be too low.

Compliance with Use of the Plan Network. This measures a physician's use of the plan network, both consultant and hospital. The more a physician uses nonparticipating providers, the worse the compliance. A certain amount of background noise (e.g., from out-of-area emer-

gencies) is to be expected, especially with point-of-service plans.

Cooperation with Other Plan Policies and Procedures. Beyond the policies and procedures for precertification and authorization, this measures compliance with encounter tracking, participation in meetings and committees, fee structures, and so forth. This measure may be somewhat subjective.

Electronic Transactions and E-commerce

Electronic communications between the plan and the physicians improves efficiency and timeliness. Therefore, it is appropriate to provide an incentive to practices that communicate electronically for defined activities such as encounters, authorizations, claims, and reimbursement. This may be accomplished through the use of an intermediary company or directly by means of the Internet. As the transaction standards mandated by the Health Insurance Portability and Accountability Act (HIPAA; see Chapters 35 and 67) become the norm, the ability of physicians to conduct e-commerce with the plan is significantly enhanced, and the plan has a great deal to gain by increasing its use.

Quality Management

Quality management looks at a physician's cooperation with the QM program and the results of actual audits and focused chart reviews. Failure to cooperate would result in either no points or a negative score or evaluation. Standards of care for such things as health maintenance or common problems (e.g., hypertension) would be evaluated, and a cumulative score would be developed. For example, 85 percent compliance with standards for a particular audit would yield a result equal to 85 percent of the maximum possible score.

Patient Relations and Member Satisfaction

Patient relations and member satisfaction data are obtained from member services reports (see Chapter 40). Evaluations could include the rate at which members transfer out of the practice, the rate at which the physician asks to remove members from the practice, and complaints or grievances about the physician. Another source for member satisfaction data is member surveys. Periodic mail or telephone surveys with a well-designed survey instrument can yield valuable information about patient satisfaction and perceived quality of service.

MEASURING THE CATEGORIES AND PRODUCING A RESULT

To use a financial incentive system that is predicated on nonutilization measures, it is still necessary to use numeric results to calculate how much to pay out. To facilitate this, it is sometimes helpful, although not required, to assign relative weights to each category. These weights would reflect the importance of that category in the overall scheme of things. Regardless of whether a weighting factor is used, it is necessary to translate the evaluation of performance in each category into a numeric value or score; for example, a scale of 1 to 5 or 1 to 10. If weighting factors are being used, the score is multiplied by the weight to achieve a numeric result. For example, if a score of 5 is given and the weight is also 5, the score would be 25.

The last step is to tabulate the results. For example, in an evaluation system with five categories, a scale of 1 to 5, and no weighting factor, the highest possible result or score would be 25. The numeric result is then used to calculate the amount of payout as illustrated in the examples provided in the following.

Closed Panel Example

The following example will illustrate the use of a formal evaluation system for allocation of bonuses in a group or closed-panel plan. Assume that there are 50 physicians eligible to participate in a year-end incentive equal to $500,000. Assume also that the medical leadership has chosen to focus on the following areas of concern, and with the following weights: Productivity (weight = 5), utilization management and re-source use (weight = 3), member satisfaction (weight = 3), and attitude and participation (weight = 2). Each category is evaluated on a scale of 1 to 5, so the highest possible score would be 65 for any single physician ($[5 \times 5]$ + $[5 \times 3]$ + $[5 \times 3]$ + $[5 \times 2]$ = 65). After all the physicians are evaluated, the total number of points for each physician are added together to yield a maximum number of points. In this case, assume that grand total equals 1,250 (an average score of 25 for the 50 eligible physicians). Therefore, each point is worth $400 ($500,000 ÷ 1,250). Multiplying each physician's score times $400 results in the incentive payment; for example, a score of 50 would result in an incentive payment of $20,000. The medical leadership may also choose to pay no incentive to any physician with a score less than a certain amount (e.g., lower than 15), thus slightly increasing the amount available to those who remain eligible.

Open Panel Example

How complex one makes an incentive program will depend on the plan's goals for the program, the level of sophistication in the physician panel, the size of the panel to be covered under the program, and the amount of money available for incentive compensation. Some plans pay incentive compensation from utilization-based risk pools (such as referral or institutional risk pools); other plans budget incentive compensation as a separate line item independent of utilization. In open panels, it is also useful to look at both behavior and the size of the membership base a physician is responsible for, with greater potential rewards going to those physicians who demonstrate desired behavior and whose panel size is large.

In a small, stable, and sophisticated independent practice association, one may use many of the above-mentioned categories for evaluation. In a large and heterogeneous direct contract model open panel, the focus may be more narrow. The following examples illustrate some different ways to approach an open panel.

In one example, payment of performance-based incentive compensation is not influenced by utilization results or the status of any utilization-based risk/bonus pool. The incentive compensation is funded on a PMPM basis as a distinct line item in the budget. Points are assigned for each category, and a minimum score (for example, 50 percent of the total possible points) must be achieved for the physician to participate in the incentive compensation program.

In this example, assume that there are 180 PCPs in a direct contract, open-panel HMO. Because of problems with member satisfaction, it is decided to pay out incentive compensation based 40 percent on member satisfaction and 30 percent each on compliance with administrative procedures and QM. For simplicity's sake, assume that that translates to 40 possible points for member satisfaction and 30 possible points each for compliance and QM. Funding is at $0.30 PMPM, and there are 60,000 members in the HMO, so there is $216,000 potentially available (60,000 × 12 × $0.30) at year end.

Member satisfaction is measured by telephone surveys of members who have seen the PCP in the past 6 months, transfer rates out of the practice, and member complaints and concerns.

Compliance with administrative procedures is measured by looking at compliance with precertification requirements (measured as a percentage of hospital admissions and outpatient surgeries that are precertified), encounter form submission (measured against a statistical average, 3.2 visits per member per year, for example), and compliance with the referral authorization system (measured by timeliness and completion of the referral authorization form and use of participating providers).

QM is measured by compliance with standards of care set by the QM committee for both routine health maintenance and disease-specific process audits. For example, a set number of charts is audited for a fixed set of criteria; if the PCP meets the criteria 90 percent of the time, the score would be 90 percent of the maximum number of possible points. If a PCP refuses to participate in the QM program, or if the PCP has been sanctioned by the QM committee, no participation in the incentive program is allowed.

The plan may choose to pay out only on the basis of the PMPM allocation to any individual PCP,

or it may choose to pay out the entire incentive pool but only to those PCPs who are eligible to participate. In other words, if half the network qualifies, the plan must choose whether to pay out only half the incentive pool (on the basis of the assumption that PCPs who fail to qualify increase the overhead cost to the plan because of their poor habits) or to pay out the entire incentive pool but only to half the network.

In the case of only paying out an individual PCP's allocation, the plan simply pays out the individual PCP's PMPM allocation times the total member months for a qualifying physician, times the percentage of the maximum score received. For example, assume that a single PCP has 700 members and has achieved a rating of 85 percent on member satisfaction, 75 percent on compliance, and 80 percent on QM. The calculation would then be ($0.30 × 700 × 12) × ((0.4 × 0.85) + (0.3 × 0.75) + (0.3 × 0.8)) = $2,028.60.

In a situation in which the entire fund is to be paid out to qualifying PCPs, the following calculations illustrate disbursement of incentive compensation. First, membership must be factored into the score. One simple method is to multiply the score by the membership base the PCP covers; for example, if a PCP has achieved results as noted previously, the total score would be (700 × 12) × [(0.4 × 0.85) + (0.3 × 0.75) + (0.3 × 0.8)] = 6,762. Next, the entire incentive fund must be divided by the total number of available points to assign a value to each point; for example, if 70 PCPs qualified to participate and the aggregate point value of those 70 PCPs is 444,500, then each point is worth ($216,000 ÷ 444,500) = $0.486. Last, each PCP has his or her individual total points multiplied by the point value; in our example that would be (6,762 × $0.486) = $3,286.33.

Some managers believe that if a PCP has already received a substantial bonus from the utilization risk/bonus pools (in a capitated system), then incentive compensation should be reduced, and they therefore include a negative factor for bonus already received. In that way, the incentive program preferentially rewards PCPs who were good case managers but who experienced more than their share of bad luck in terms of adverse selection. This method of adjustment is not common.

CONCLUSION

Most managed care products have similar benefit designs. As efficiencies standardize across plans, price competition intensifies and creates a marketplace where plans can only distinguish themselves on service, and the plans that thrive will be those that motivate health care providers to provide cost-effective and high-quality service to members. Professional behavior may be evaluated with a combination of objective and subjective criteria. Formal evaluations of physician performance can and should be made in a managed care plan and appropriate financial incentives provided.

REFERENCES AND NOTES

1. M.R. Gold, R. Hurley, T. Lake, T. Ensor, and R. Berenson, A National Survey of the Arrangements Managed-Care Plans Make with Physicians, *New England Journal of Medicine* 333, 25 (1995): 1678–83.

2. T.K. Lake, and R.F. St. Peter, Payment Arrangements and Financial Incentives for Physicians. Community Tracking Study, Center for Studying Health System Change, Data Bulletin No. 8, Fall, 1997.

3. R.M. Cooper, Formal Physician Performance Evaluations, *Journal of Ambulatory Care Management* 3 (1980): 19–33.

4. R.A. Dudley, R.H. Miller, T.Y. Korenbrot, and H.S. Luft, The Impact of Financial Incentives on Quality of Health Care, *Millbank Quarterly* 76, 4 (1998): 649–85.

5. E.S. Ogrod, Compensation and Quality: A Physician's View, *Health Affairs* 16, 3 (1997): 82–86.

6. M. McGuirk-Porell, G.A. Goldberg, D. Goldin, et al., A Performance-Based Quality Evaluation System for Preferred Provider Organizations, *Quality Review Bulletin* November (1991): 365–73.

CHAPTER 11

Contracting and Reimbursement of Specialty Physicians

Peter R. Kongstvedt

INTRODUCTION

This chapter discusses the reimbursement of specialty care physicians (SCPs)* and common issues involved in SCP network contracting, reimbursement, and development and contracting. In prior years, some health maintenance organizations (HMOs) had difficulties contracting with SCPs. More recently, the oversupply of SCPs in some markets, along with the increasing penetration of managed care organizations (MCOs), has led SCPs in those markets to actively pursue contracts with MCOs. Concomitant with that shift in attitude, many HMOs and other forms of MCOs, such as preferred provider organizations (PPOs) and even some integrated delivery systems (IDSs; see Chapter 4), have closed their panels to new SCPs and have even de-participated some SCPs with existing contracts but a low level of usage by plan members. In other markets, SCPs remain in strong financial positions, may not be overrepresented (at least not as regards desirable candidates), or managed care may not yet be in a strong market position.

HOW MANY SPECIALTY CARE PHYSICIANS?

How many SCPs of each type are necessary to contract with is not an easy question to answer. Many plans have between two and three times as many SCPs as primary care physicians (PCPs), while some aggressive systems in the western United States have equal numbers of SCPs and PCPs. Certain specialties, such as general surgery, orthopaedics, and obstetrics and gynecology (OB/GYN), and some of the medical subspecialties, such as cardiology and gastroenterology, need to be adequately represented at each major hospital with which a plan contracts. Other specialties, such as neurosurgery or cardiothoracic surgery, need only be represented at those hospitals to which the plan refers members for appropriate treatment.

In one widely cited article, the number of SCPs required is estimated at between 80 and 110 SCPs per 100,000 population depending on the type of MCO, as illustrated in Table 11–1 (adjustments for Medicare and Medicaid are noted in the source).[1] There was, however, considerable variation in staffing ratios for all types of plans and all specialties. When the figures in Table 11–1 are translated into metrics more common in the managed care industry, they are 0.68 to 0.8 per 1,000. Another study has used group model HMOs to project the number of covered lives needed for each of a variety of specialists in nonrural areas (see Exhibit 11–1).[2] More recently, highly complex formulas have

---

*For purposes of this discussion, SCPs refer not only to physician SCPs but to nonphysicians as well, such as psychologists, physical therapists, and the like. The chapter is most germane, however, to physician specialists.

Table 11–1 Physician Requirements per 100,000 Population

Sector	Overall	Primary Care	Specialty Care
Staff/Group HMO	146.4	65.9	80.5
IDS and IPA	124.4	55.9	68.5
"Managed" FFS	171.0	61.6	109.4
Open FFS	180.1	64.8	115.3

Notes: HMO, health maintenance organization; IDS, integrated delivery systems; IPA, independent practice association; FFS, fee-for-service.

Source: Reprinted with permission from JP Weiner, Forecasting the Effects of Health Reform on US Physician Workforce Requirements: Evidence From HMO Staffing Patterns, Journal of the American Medical Association, 272 (3): 222–230, © 1994, American Medical Association.

been developed to determine optimal physician staffing needs in HMOs, taking into account several different scenarios; in this model, SCPs per 1,000 population (excluding PCPs but including OB/GYN) range from 0.13 to 0.24 per 1,000.[3] In all these cases, the projections are based on maximally efficient use of SCPs, not on other considerations as discussed below. These very low ratios of SCPs to members there-

Exhibit 11–1 Group Model HMO-Covered Lives per Physician

Family practice and general internal medicine	2,250
Pediatrics	6,000
Obstetrics/gynecology	7,000
General Surgery	15,000
Anesthesiology	17,000
Radiology	20,000
Orthopaedics	20,000
Mental health	20,000
Ophthalmology	25,000
Ear, Nose, and Throat	35,000
Cardiology	35,000
Dermatology	35,000
Cardiovascular surgery	35,000
Gastroenterology	50,000
Neurosurgery	150,000

Source: Data from New England Journal of Medicine 328 (January 14, 1993): 148–52.

fore represent a grossly unrealistic reduction in the need for SCPs than actually exists or is likely to exist in the United States, even in nonurban markets.

An MCO or IDS must balance between a low number of SCPs preferred for purposes of medical management, and a higher number of SCPs required for purposes of access and marketing. In most all cases, an MCO or IDS will have a higher number of SCPs than would be required to provide specialty services in the most efficient manner, in order to provide good access to SCPs, thus improving satisfaction and retention of both members and PCPs. Unlike the tight ratios found in group and staff model HMOs, the number of SCPs per 1,000 members in a study of 19 large MCOs (covering 27 million people) averaged between 11 to 18 per 1,000 for general commercial HMOs and point-of-service (POS) plans (for in-network SCPs), and 113 to 131 per 1,000 for Medicare risk plans.[4] In fact, the average total number of SCPs used by HMOs has been steadily increasing, with 1998 levels illustrated in Table 11–2. For PPOs the ratio of SCPs per 1,000 *employees* has been reported as 200.5, which equates to approximately 83 per 1,000 to 91 per 1,000 members, using imputed family sizes of 2.4 and 2.2 respectively.[5]

PRIMARY VERSUS SPECIALTY CARE DESIGNATION

It is not uncommon, especially in open panel HMOs and in IDSs, for the same physician to

Table 11–2 Average Number of Specialists Used by an HMO by Model Type

IPA	Network	Group	Staff	Overall Average
2,964	3,016	2,061	1,241	2,825

Source: Reprinted with permission from Hoechst Marion Roussel Managed Care Digest Series, *HMO-PPO Digest 1999,* © 1999 Hoechst Marion Roussel, SMG Marketing Group Inc.

desire to be designated as both a PCP and an SCP. The usual argument is that the SCP, almost always a medical subspecialist, performs a significant amount of primary care, perhaps as much as half of his or her practice time. In some cases, the same physician also wishes to be able to see a member for primary care, then refer that member back to himself or herself at a later time for specialty services (that is, get paid first to see the member as a PCP, then get paid a second time to see the same member as an SCP). It is uncommon and foolhardy to allow physicians to be able to authorize referrals back to themselves and get paid twice to provide care for the same member.

In some cases, a plan will make the decision based on criteria, such as an objective review of a physician's practice, and thereby designate the physician as a PCP or an SCP. In other cases, the plan may allow a medical subspecialist to self-designate but will prohibit that physician from being both a PCP and an SCP. It is also possible for a physician to be a PCP for his or her own panel of members, but take referrals as an SCP from other PCPs who are not associated with that physician in some way, such as in the same multispecialty group.

This has commonly been done through the use of different provider ID numbers for the same provider depending on the type of service. However, under the requirements of Health Portability and Accountability (HIPAA, see Chapter 67), all provider IDs will be replaced by a National Provider ID (NPI). Each provider will be issued only one NPI number, which will complicate the ability of the MCO to have a provider designated as both a SCP and a PCP. New logic will be required in the MCO's computer system to deal with this change.

SCPs as Primary Physicians

There is conflicting evidence on how costly SCPs are versus PCPs in overall use of medical resources to deliver similar episodes of care. Several studies support the notion that SCPs are more costly than PCPs in managing routine care and common chronic conditions, without any difference in outcomes.[6]

It is certainly possible that at least some of the variation even in routine care is caused by a different mix of cases and severity, since SCPs get sicker patients on average than do PCPs.[7] Added to this, there is at least one recent study reporting that approximately 25 percent of PCPs felt that the scope of care they were expected to provide was greater than it should be, with a slight rise in the percentage reporting this feeling among PCPs functioning as "gatekeepers" in HMOs.[8] There is also evidence that medical specialists may be more efficient in their use of resources than are PCPs for certain serious chronic conditions as well as many acute episodes of inpatient care.[9] It should be noted, however, that these studies (and several others not cited here) focused on the care of defined clinical conditions, not the overall health care needs of the individual.

It is not at all unreasonable for a specialty-trained internist to function as a PCP, especially in an open panel type of MCO or in an IDS. As managed care increases its penetration in the health care market, this issue takes on even greater importance.

The point of this discussion is not to assert that either SCPs or PCPs are superior in their performance of primary medical care. In most instances, it is appropriate for a PCP to serve as the primary caregiver and coordinator of health care. However, in certain cases of serious, chronic conditions, it will be preferable for an SCP to play that role.

CREDENTIALING

Credentialing of SCPs is performed the same way as it is for PCPs and will not be repeated here. It should be noted that many MCOs require SCPs to be fully board certified or board eligible, without exception. Credentialing is examined in detail in Chapter 8.

TYPES OF REIMBURSEMENT ARRANGEMENTS

This section discusses reimbursement of SCPs on the basis of the direct financial relationship between the plan and the SCPs. It is possible that a contracting entity, such as a group or a management service organization (MSO), may accept reimbursement from the plan but compensate individual physicians in a separate manner. The compensation of physicians in medical groups and IDSs is discussed in Chapter 9.

Exhibit 11–2 lists the methods for reimbursing SCPs in managed health care plans. The most appropriate method for use in any given situation will be predicated on the goals of the plan, the SCP, and each party's ability to actually manage within the terms of the agreement. As illustrated in Figures 11–1 and 11–2, most MCOs use combinations of capitation and fee-for-service (FFS) systems to reimburse SCPs, with a clear predominance of FFS. Table 11–3 illustrates the relative fluidity of these reimbursement methods over the past several years.

Exhibit 11–2 Models for Reimbursing SCPs in Managed Health Care Plans

- Charges
- Discounts (straight sliding scale)
- Fee allowances
- Global fees
- Performance-based FFS
- Capitation (with and without carve-outs)
- Contact Capitation
- Retainer
- Hourly and salary
- Outpatient and professional diagnosis-related groups, or ambulatory patient groups
- Withholds
- Penalties
- Periodic interim payments or cash advances

Charges and Discounts

The simplest arrangement to understand, though highly unsatisfactory, is straight FFS. The SCP sends a claim and the plan pays it. Then why bother to contract at all? The answer is to get the SCP to agree to the National Association of Insurance Commissioners' sole source of payment clause (see Chapter 62). While certainly not a preferred arrangement, occasionally it is all an MCO can get, particularly in high-cost specialties (such as neurosurgery) when there may not be good alternatives, or in small start-up plans without a significant enrollment. Paying straight charges is uncommon.

Another simple arrangement is discounted FFS. There are two variations here: first, a straight discount on charges, such as 20 percent; and second, a discount based on volume or a sliding scale. In the latter type, the degree of discount is based on an agreed-upon set of figures. For example, for an obstetrician who performs up to five deliveries per month there is a 10 percent discount, for six to ten per month there is a 15 percent discount, and so forth. Many plans combine a discount arrangement with a fee maximum. The fee maximum is a fee allowance schedule (see below); the plan pays the lesser of the SCP's discounted charges or the maximum allowance.

Relative Value Scale or Fee Allowance Schedule

The most common form of FFS is the relative value scale (RVS), such as the resource-based relative value scale (RBRVS) or a fee allowance schedule. The RBRVS is discussed in Chapter 8. The difference between the RVS and fee allowance schedule is that when RVS is used, each procedure is assigned a relative value, usually on the basis of listings in *Current Procedural Terminology,* fourth edition (CPT-4); that value is then multiplied by another figure (the conversion factor) to arrive at a payment. Rather than negotiate separate fees, one negotiates the conversion factor. In a fee allowance schedule the fees for procedures (again, usually on the basis of CPT-4) are explicitly laid out, and the SCP

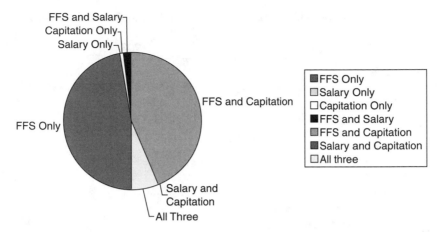

Figure 11–1 Percentage of Plans Using SCP Reimbursement Model. Courtesy of AAHP Annual Industry Survey, 1998, American Association of Health Plans, Washington, DC.

agrees to accept those fees as full payment unless the discounted charges are less than the fee schedule, in which case the plan pays the lesser of the two. The majority of MCOs that use FFS use the RBRVS, and the majority of those set the conversion factor somewhat higher than that used by Medicare.[10]

The real utility with RBRVS or a fee allowance schedule is the avoidance of unanticipated fee hikes. If the plan has simply negotiated a discount on charges, the discount can easily be made up by raising fees. This may be partially offset by contractually requiring notice for any fee increases, assuming that the stray fee hike

Figure 11–2 Percentage of SCPs Compensated by Various Methods. Courtesy of AAHP Annual Industry Survey, 1998, American Association of Health Plans, Washington, DC.

Table 11–3 Percentage of HMOs Using Specialty Physician Reimbursement Methods

	July 1993	July 1998
Primary Care Physicians		
Capitation	69.3%	78.7%
Fee for Service	59.8%	69.7%
Relative Value Scale	11.1%	27.2%
Salary	13.7%	9.8%
Specialty Care Physicians		
Capitation	30.2%	56.4%
Fee for Service	61.7%	75.5%
Relative Value Scale	12.6%	32.2%
Salary	6.1%	3.3%
Hospitals		
Fee for Service	68.1%	71.7%
Per Diem Rates	90.8%	86.2%
Diagnosis Related Groups (DRGs)	39.4%	49.5%
Capitation	18.0%	32.5%

Source: Reprinted with permission from *The Interstudy Competitive Edge: HMO Industry Report* 9.1, © 1999, InterStudy publications.

can and will actually be spotted, but that still leaves the problem of administering a jumble of different agreements. It is far preferable to have one uniform method of handling claims.

Performance-Based FFS

Performance-based FFS for SCPs is similar to that discussed for PCPs in Chapter 8. The most common examples are withholds and fee adjustments in an independent practice association (IPA), in which all physicians are treated the same, regardless of whether or not they are PCPs or SCPs. A few IPAs and IDSs have attempted to adjust fees based on each specialty, so called budgeted FFS. In this approach each specialty has a per member per month (PMPM) budget (for example, $3.25 PMPM for cardiology), and actual costs for that specialty service in the IPA are measured against that budget. If costs exceed budget, then fees are lowered, but only for that specialty, and vice versa if costs are better than budget. While this is an interesting variation, it takes a highly sophisticated tracking system, sound actuarial analysis, and a very large mem-

bership base to ensure statistical integrity and that utilization patterns are based on provider behavior rather than on random chance. Contact capitation, which is discussed later in this chapter, is similar to budgeted FFS. Other variations on FFS are global fees, flat rates, and case rates, all of which are discussed later.

Capitation

SCP capitation is in general simpler than PCP capitation as discussed in Chapter 8. Capitation refers to a fixed payment PMPM for services (unlike contact capitation, discussed later). The capitation payment may be adjusted for age, sex, and product type, but not as universally as is found in PCP capitation. The capitation amount must calculate the expected volume of referrals, the average cost, the ability to manage utilization, and the relative negotiating strengths of each party. A large plan may have past data to guide it, but more commonly needs to depend on an actuary to derive the correct capitation amount. Calculations of capitation and utilization rates are discussed more fully in Chapters 49–51. Table 11–4 illus-

Table 11–4 Percentages of 1998 SCP Income Source, by Specialty

Specialty	HMOs	PPOs	Capitation
Anesthesiologists	38	28	24
Cardiologists	19	19	14
Cardiothoracic surgeons	24	14	14
Gastroenterologists	22	23	12
General surgeons	24	19	20
Obstetricians/gynecologists	36	32	15
Opthalmologists	22	20	15
Orthopaedic surgeons	21	24	14
Plastic surgeons	18	19	21
Psychiatrists	24	20	27

Note: Figures exclude physicians with no HMO, PPO, or capitation contracts.
Source: Copyright © 1999 by Medical Economics Company. Reprinted by permission from *Medical Economics* Magazine.

---

trates an example from a survey of the relative percent of capitation in various specialties.

In some cases, particularly in plans with Medicare + Choice risk contracts (though not confined to Medicare), the capitation amount may be based on a percent of premium revenue, rather than a hard PMPM dollar amount. This is not unreasonable in Medicare and Medicaid MCOs, since the premium revenue is set by the government and presumably has the appropriate mix of specialty services already in the total; this will potentially become more visible (and problematic) under the risk-adjuster rating methodologies currently planned by Medicare (see Chapters 55 and 56). For commercial plans, however, the case of percent of premium is not as clear. Premiums are set as much by market pressures as they are by actuarial build up, and a plan forced to market low premiums will end up passing along that reduced income in exact proportion to the percentage of premium payment the SCP group has negotiated. In addition, if the MCO has poor underwriting procedures (Chapter 52), a PMPM premium shortfall may occur, which will also be passed on to SCPs under a percentage of premium arrangement. In other words, true capitation is a fixed amount, while percentage of premium varies based on the amount of premium the MCO actually collects.

While theoretically the same utilization issues apply to specialty care as they do to primary care, the numbers involved in SCP capitation are often significantly smaller for any given specialty, even though specialty PMPM costs as a whole are usually one and a half to two times higher than total costs for primary care. For example, PCP capitation may average $14 PMPM, while the capitation for neurology may be $0.55. Thus adjustments based on demographic variables become very small indeed and may not be worth the effort. Because the capitation amounts are smaller, an SCP requires a much higher number of members in their panel for capitation to have meaning. Where a PCP may achieve relative stability in capitation at a membership level of 400 to 600, an SCP may require triple that number or more in order to avoid the problem of random chance having more effect than medical management on utilization.

Capitation clearly has the advantages of allowing the plan to budget for expected medical costs and to place a degree of risk and reward on the SCP; the financial incentives encourage the SCP to be a more active participant in controlling utilization. Capitation also "locks in" a membership base and revenue source for the SCP, as well as providing positive cash flow. If done properly, capitation can be valuable both to the SCP and to the plan. If done poorly, it can be a chronic headache.

An issue that usually requires clear definition is that of carve-outs. This topic is discussed later in this chapter, but the point here is that for all except the largest and best organized SCP medical groups, there will always be a set of procedures that are highly expensive and/or not performed by all SCPs of the same specialty type. This usually means adding a second form of reimbursement on top of the capitation program, for example, FFS, case rates, or global fees.

Capitating SCPs While Paying PCPs via FFS

As a side note, the concept of paying PCPs FFS and capitating SCPs has been around for a long time. In theory this rewards PCPs for actually seeing their patients rather than automatically referring them to SCPs, while at the same time using capitation to limit the variability in specialty care costs. While a great theoretical concept, it has met with limited success in those few MCOs that have attempted it. For one thing, if the MCO capitates specialty care to any great degree, it may find that it has obligated more money than intended to SCP capitation, to the detriment of primary care and hospital funds. In addition, the problems noted above of needing a larger membership base for SCPs than for PCPs still exist, and since most MCOs have such large SCP panels, achieving that level of actuarial integrity is nearly impossible for all but a few specialties.

In nongatekeeper types of HMOs as well as POS plans, this problem is acute. As discussed in Chapter 8, it is difficult to capitate PCPs in any type of MCO other than a gatekeeper-style HMO. Proponents of contact capitation, discussed below, believe that this method provides one way of accomplishing this goal. Those same proponents also believe that it allows an MCO to achieve the goal of capitating SCPs while paying PCPs on an FFS basis. These are good theoretical arguments, but there are several difficulties with implementing contact capitation, as discussed in the next section.

Contact Capitation

Contact capitation bears some resemblance to the budgeted FFS method noted earlier. As of 2000, this form of SCP reimbursement is undergoing a small upswing in popularity, and warrants additional discussion. As with any other form of reimbursement, contact capitation does not have a single definition of how it works and is subject to a variety of local variations.

Like budgeted FFS, contact capitation begins with a capitated (that is, budgeted, based on PMPM calculations) pool of money for each major specialty. And like other forms of capitation, provisions in the calculations are made for product design, the effect of copays and coinsurance, the effect of stop-loss insurance for catastrophic cases, and the effect of other party liability offsets. These basic reasons for adjustment are discussed in Chapters 8, 39, and 51.

The plan then tracks each member contact with each specialist; that is, regardless of whether that member/patient sees the SCP once or 100 times, it is counted as a single contact. This is tracked over a set period of time, such as a year, a quarter, or semiannually. Once the period is over, the counters are reset to zero and it begins again. The plan pays out the total capitated pool of money to the SCPs based on the distribution of the contacts. For example, if one cardiologist has 8 percent of the total number of cardiology contacts (that is, unique, nonduplicated patients), that cardiologist receives 8 percent of the total capitation pool. It is usually assumed that once a patient makes contact with that SCP, the patient will remain with the SCP. Of course, this is not something that can be guaranteed, and so provision should (but may not) be made for patients that change SCPs during the course of the tracking period.

It is common for certain procedures to be carved out of the capitation consideration. The reason for this is that those SCPs that perform high-cost procedures will be relatively disadvantaged compared to SCPs that perform only less expensive office-based care. Of course, this is a dynamic that many proponents of contact capitation desire to achieve: the removal of FFS incentives to do more (and more expensive) procedures. Nevertheless, like most other forms of capitation, certain defined procedures will end up being paid via FFS, outside of the contact capitation mechanism.

Some contact capitation programs have an additional layer of complexity when calculating the distribution of the capitation payouts. While not going so far as to be budgeted FFS, some systems take into account levels of complexity and acuity of illness and give those factors weighting in calculating the ultimate payout of the capitation pool. For example, a cardiologist who only cared for patients with stable angina would have a different morbidity and complexity profile than would a cardiologist who cares primarily for patients with acute cardiac conduction disorders or congenital heart disease. In that case, even if each cardiologist saw 8 percent of total contacts, the cardiologist with the sicker patients would receive some type of additional consideration in calculating the payout. If the plan is highly sophisticated, it may be able to take advantage of some of the new risk-adjuster methods as discussed in Chapter 32; if not, it may be forced to use a peer review format to make such decisions.

The timing of payouts under contact capitation is highly variable, unlike more common forms of capitation. Since the payout is a factor of the total percentage of contacts in a period of time, it cannot occur until adequate encounters have occurred to allow for a calculation; in other words, it is not actually prepayment, so the time value of money is therefore not present. Most systems that use contact capitation use an entire 12-month period to make the adjustments, while others do so on a quarterly or semiannual basis. Some form of interim payment mechanism must therefore be in place (as no one would expect physicians to receive no reimbursement for a year). This interim payment may be a form of discounted FFS, it may be a monthly "capitation" payment based on the distribution of contacts each month or to-date, or it may be by some other means. In all cases, this adds a layer of complexity to the ultimate calculation.

Contact capitation may work for large, organized groups that use it to distribute income within the group. Likewise, highly organized IPAs, specialty-specific or broad, in which the SCPs are able to work together well and have active peer review, may be better suited to this methodology. Contact capitation systems require a strong internal management structure by the SCPs themselves. This is generally through a peer review type of mechanism that will look at individual patterns of care, note any extraneous circumstances, and take remedial action when required.

In all cases, a highly sophisticated information system is required, as are excellent reporting and practice profiling capabilities (Chapter 32). Financial management to support contact capitation is of a higher level of complexity as well. The ability to produce highly accurate statements, handle incurred but not reported costs, manage the effect of copayments or reinsurance, and manage provider excess stop-loss coverage (see Chapter 53) must also be present.

There are no good data regarding how many SCPs are under contact capitation arrangements, nor is there any way to predict the long-term viability of this form of capitation. Due to its complexity, its requirement of sophisticated information systems, and the need for a high level of understanding by the physicians, it is the opinion of this author that contact capitation will serve a few markets that are able to support it but will not soon become a major methodology.

Subcapitation of SCPs by Other SCPs

There are occasions when a specialty group or IDS will accept capitation for defined specialty services, and in turn contract with other SCPs on a subcapitation basis to deliver at least some of those services. This is sometimes referred to as "downstreaming." This issue has drawn the attention of state and federal regulators as well as MCO executives. By making the risk-sharing aspect one step removed from the relationship between the MCO and the capitated medical group or organization, the ability of the MCO to monitor the quality of care and the ability of the subcapitated group to manage the financial risk become less well known. In some states, a provider group undertaking subcapitation must itself have a limited form of a license in order to do so. In Medicare + Choice risk plans, subcapitated providers are the responsibility of the primary organization, and all of the same requirements apply to the subcapitated providers as well. It takes a higher level of management expertise and information systems by the capitated group to be able to manage a subcapitated arrangement.

ORGANIZATIONAL MODELS FOR CAPITATING SPECIALTY SERVICES

How a plan capitates for specialty services has some complexities when compared to PCP capitation. When capitating PCPs, a member must choose a PCP and it becomes a straightforward issue of tracking that membership. Specialty capitation is different, in that any given SCP will provide care to patients of multiple PCPs, and there is no requirement on the part of a member to choose an SCP.* Because of these issues, HMOs must use alternate methods to determine how to capitate SCPs. Some of these methods are described as follows.

Organized Groups

The easiest form of SCP capitation is through organized medical groups. In some cases, the group is a multispecialty group, inclusive of primary and specialty care. In that case, it is assumed that any member assigned to a PCP in that group will likewise be assigned to the SCPs in the group.

---

*The common exception to this last point is OB/GYN. Nearly all HMOs as well as all non-HMO MCOs allow members to self-refer to OB/GYNs, although in HMOs those OB/GYNs generally do not have the authority to refer the member to another specialist. HMOs that capitate OB/GYNs generally require all female members over the age of 12 to choose an OB/GYN, and the plan in turn capitates that OB/GYN based on that enrolled panel.

Organized single specialty groups are also good candidates for capitation. If the group is large enough, then the group may even be capitated for the entire network. If it is not large enough to cover the entire medical service area, then the group may be capitated for that portion of the geographic medical service area that it can cover.

Geographic Distribution

Geographic distribution is closely related to the way an organized medical group is capitated. The reason to discuss it separately is that it involves the same principle applied to a smaller group. In essence, a small (for example, two or three) physician specialty group accepts capitation for all relevant specialty services in a defined portion of the medical service area but not the entire service area. For example, a group of general surgeons might be capitated to cover all services rendered at a single hospital. In an urban area, a capitated SCP might cover all PCP practices located in a particular set of ZIP codes. Since it is not uncommon for PCP (or SCP for that matter) practices to have multiple locations, assignment is based on whatever office is considered the physician's principal office.

Specialty IPAs

Specialty-specific IPAs have become somewhat more common than in the past, and the recent increase in IDSs has led to an increase in interest in this form of specialty capitation. The specialty IPA operates similar to a standard IPA as described in Chapter 8. The specialty IPA accepts capitation from the HMO but usually pays FFS to the participating specialists. Capitation of individual SCPs within the specialty IPA is certainly possible but not usually seen because specialty IPAs are often created in order to preserve the opportunity for multiple, unrelated SCPs to participate with aggressive HMOs. In specialty IPAs that are highly organized, contact capitation may be a viable approach. Whether or not specialty IPAs become more prevalent is unknown.

Disease Management Organizations

A new variation on single group capitation is capitation for single specialty services to a specialty organization (for example, a vendor that specializes in cancer services or cardiac care). This is most commonly a company or corporation that employs physicians and support staff and provides facilities and ancillary services, i.e., a form of physician practice management company (PPMC; see Chapter 4). It can also be an organization created by a large, comprehensive provider system as an internal unit. In this model, the organization is then responsible for providing all specialty services within the MCO's medical service area. This approach is best suited to specialty care that is not usually associated with emergencies, unless the vendor's employed physicians are on staff at all of the HMO's participating hospitals.

Discussed in more detail in Chapter 23, disease management organizations focus on those chronic conditions in which a broad, integrated approach can make a difference in outcomes and/or cost of care. Because it is more comprehensive, the capitation calculation must take into account a somewhat larger set of factors, such as:

- inpatient costs and utilization
- outpatient costs and utilization
  - by service type
  - by location
- physician costs and utilization
- nonacute care costs
  - inpatient facilities, such as skilled nursing facilities
  - outpatient or alternative settings, such as hospice
- pharmaceutical costs and utilization
  - those agents included as a routine part of medical surgical benefits, such as injectibles
  - the cost of outpatient or chronic drugs if the disease management organization is to be at risk for their use
- frequency of the disease state
  - new occurrences expected by age and sex categories
  - existing cases[11]

Single Specialty Management or Specialty Network Manager

An uncommon method, this involves the HMO contracting with one single entity to provide all services within a single specialty, but that entity does not actually provide all the services. There are two basic approaches within this method.

In one approach, an HMO capitates a single specialist (that is, an individual physician) to manage all services in that specialty for all HMO members, even though the SCP cannot personally provide the services. This contracted SCP, the specialty network manager, must then subcontract with other specialists to provide services throughout the medical service area. The specialty network manager either makes or loses money depending on how efficiently specialty services are managed. The specialty network manager may subcapitate with other SCPs, if that is allowed by the state insurance department (many states will not allow a provider to capitate another provider; see Chapter 54), or may pay FFS. In all events, the primary SCP acts like a second "gatekeeper" in that PCPs need to work through the primary SCP in order to access specialty care for members. Sometimes the primary SCP receives the full capitation payment and must pay the other SCPs directly, or the HMO may administer the claims payments and provide the accounting and reporting for the primary contract holder. In fact, the HMO may wish to do so in order to track performance on a real-time basis, as well as protect members from possible nonpayment of claims by the primary contract holder.

In the other approach, an HMO contracts with a single institution for single specialty services (for example, the HMO contracts with a local university faculty practice plan for all cardiology services). The contracted institution is then responsible to arrange for specialty services that it cannot provide itself. The primary specialty contract holder receives the capitation payment and must then administer payment to subcontractors. In some cases, the administrative cost to the primary contractor may be greater than the total capitation payment, since it is often a manual process.

By PCP Choice

A theoretically interesting though seldom used method of capitating SCPs is through the mechanism of PCP choice. This model requires each PCP to choose which SCP from the applicable specialties will be used on an exclusive basis. The presence of choice means that multiple SCPs have agreed to a capitation rate, but no single SCP has exclusive rights. The plan is then required to track the members assigned to those SCPs by virtue of being on the PCP's panels, and pay the SCP capitation based on that. While this is interesting and has good logic, most HMO management information systems are not capable of handling it, and the administrative headache would be great.

COMMON PROBLEMS WITH SPECIALTY CAPITATION

The pressure to capitate frequently comes as a result of uncontrolled utilization. Referrals are high, expenses are out of control, and there is high negative variance to budget. The pressure to capitate is to prevent costs from going even higher and to bring some predictability to medical expenses. This is often the wrong time to capitate. Be assured that the SCP knows exactly how much the HMO has been paying and will not eagerly agree to a capitation rate that amounts to a substantial discount, unless the plan and the PCPs are willing to change SCPs. It is far preferable to manage utilization before negotiating a capitation rate. If not, the plan will be locked in to the higher rate for at least a year.

Management of Referral Volume

Another common problem is being able to control the flow of referrals. It is easy to assume that once a deal has been made with an SCP, all that is needed is to notify the PCPs and/or members, and all problems are solved. This is not so. Disrupting old referral patterns is tough, and many physicians do not have the system capabilities to respond proactively to referrals outside the capitated system. Furthermore, the capitated SCP may not be able to provide adequate geographic or emergency coverage. When referrals go outside the capitated system, the plan is essentially paying for them twice; once in the capitation payment; and again in fees to SCPs outside the capitated system. This problem virtually defines a POS plan, which is why capitating SCPs in a POS plan is problematic.

One possible approach to the geographic coverage problem is to capitate only for an appropriate geographic primary care base. Unless the capitating specialty group has wide coverage, this balkanization of the specialty base frequently is more acceptable.

Potential To Increase Utilization

Capitation may actually serve to increase utilization. If the PCPs who are managing the referrals, and perhaps even the medical director of the plan, see capitation as putting a lid on expenses, there is far less pressure to control utilization because it appears that the service costs the same regardless of use; it could almost be said that it is free! If utilization of capitated services is not controlled, there will be a most unpleasant surprise when the contract comes up for renegotiation. Most SCPs will keep track of what they would have made in FFS equivalents. If utilization was not controlled, the capitation rate may be equivalent to an unacceptable discount on charges, leading the SCP to demand a large increase in the capitation rate. The plan members either have to give in, find a new SCP, or hang tough. In each of those cases, someone loses.

The other problem with high levels of SCP utilization is the increase in other forms of utilization as well. As noted in earlier references, there is evidence that for many routine types of conditions, SCPs use more resources than do PCPs. Increases in institutional and ancillary services may follow increases in SCP referrals.

Capitation in Point of Service and Other Non-HMO Plans

Capitation in POS plans (Chapter 3) is difficult to accomplish. Since the POS plan is designed to include benefits for in-network and out-of-network care, it becomes difficult to determine the proper amount of capitation for any SCP. Proponents of contact capitation believe that form of reimbursement is useful in POS plans, but this author disagrees, since the difference in coinsurance between in- and out-of-network benefits has such a great impact on the capitation rate. The degree of information systems sophistication is generally beyond the capabilities of most MCOs, even now.

Carve-Outs from Capitation

The last major problem encountered in capitation is the issue of carve-outs. A carve-out is a particular service that the SCP does not include in the capitation rate. For example, ophthalmologists may capitate for all services except cataract extractions, for which they will give a 25 percent discount on charges; the plan may then find itself with an unexplainably high rate of cataract extractions. If the service is one that only the SCP can reasonably judge the need for, and that service is a carve-out, the plan has this potential problem. In all fairness, it is unlikely that the plan will be a victim of outright fraud, but it still makes for a significant problem.

A variation of the carve-out problem arises when the SCP cannot or will not handle all the services. If a plan capitates for all services, but the SCP refers out for the delivery of some of those services, it is best to consider deducting those costs from the capitation payment. There are no consistent guidelines here. If the service is one that the SCP truly cannot perform (for example, an ophthalmologist who does not do retinal surgery), then the plan can probably budget properly and not roll that expense into the capitation rate, thereby avoiding having to adjust the rate frequently. On the other hand, if the SCP can perform the service but simply does not (for example, an ophthalmologist who is never available on Wednesday afternoons), then it is appropriate to deduct those expenses from the capitation payment. If the plan intends to do so, it must be clear about those intentions from the start, and place appropriate language in the contract.

Inability of the Capitated Organization To Manage or Withstand Financial Risk

The inability to manage and withstand financial risk is primarily a problem when capitating an organization for a broad level of financial risk. It is particularly problematic for organizations capitated for services that are delivered by providers other than the organization accepting the capitation (for example, a specialty management company that contracts with hundreds of independent SCPs). In the late 1990s there were many failures of large IDSs and PPMCs due to inability to deliver services within the capitation amount or to manage the financial risk aspect. This is discussed further in Chapter 4, and the reader is urged to understand those dynamics.

OTHER FORMS OF SPECIALTY PHYSICIAN REIMBURSEMENT

Retainer

The retainer is a rare form of reimbursement outside of closed-panel HMOs and organized medical groups or IDSs. It is identical to what is commonly used with law firms. The MCO simply pays a set amount to an SCP every month and reconciles at periodic intervals on the basis of actual utilization, either as a prenegotiated fee schedule or on some other objective measure. This ensures availability of the SCP to members and provides for the steady income desired by the SCP, while still allowing payment on the basis of actual utilization. One issue to address early is whether the reconciliation goes both ways or whether it only goes up. That issue surfaces more often than would be expected.

Hourly and Salary

With hourly and salary arrangements the plan pays an SCP an hourly rate or salary for performing services. In essence the MCO is buying block time, most commonly for direct care but potentially for emergency care or on-call coverage. In addition to closed-panel HMOs and organized medical groups or IDSs, this type of arrangement is common in emergency departments or other settings when a physician needs to be available for a defined time period. Likewise, it is common in those plans using a hospitalist model for inpatient coverage (see Chapter 18).

Case Rate, Global Fee, or Flat Rate for Procedures

As discussed in Chapter 8, case rates, global fees, or flat rates are single fees that are paid for a procedure, and the fee is the same regardless of how much or how little time and effort are spent. In obstetrics, for example, many plans use the same flat rate for either a vaginal delivery or a Caesarean section, thereby eliminating any financial incentive to perform one or the other; this has been associated with a decrease in the Caesarean section rate,[12] although there may be other factors affecting the section rate as well.

Related to the flat rate is the global fee. A global fee is a flat rate that encompasses more than a single type of service. For example, a global fee for surgery may include all preoperative and postoperative care as well as one or two follow-up office visits. A global fee for obstetrics may include all prenatal and postnatal care.

Global fees must be carefully defined as to what they include and what may be billed outside them. For example, if ultrasound is billed by OB/GYN outside the global fee for a delivery, the plan will need to monitor its use to determine whether any providers are routinely using (and billing for) an abnormally high number of ultrasounds per case.

Bundled Case Rates or Package Pricing

Bundled case rates refer to a reimbursement that combines both the institutional and the professional charges into a single payment. For example, a plan may negotiate a bundled case rate of $20,000 for cardiac bypass surgery. That fee covers the charges from the hospital, the surgeon, the pump technician, and the anesthesiolo-

gist as well as all preoperative and postoperative care. Bundled case rates sometimes have outlier provisions for cases that become catastrophic and grossly exceed expected utilization.

Diagnosis-Related Groups and Ambulatory Patient Groups

Diagnosis-related groups and ambulatory patient groups (APGs) are important topics for hospital reimbursement but currently have limited utility in SCP reimbursement other than through bundled case rates, as discussed above. Some MCOs, however, are using APGs more commonly than in the past for most procedures regardless of the location of service. Further discussion on these methods is found in Chapter 12.

Periodic Interim Payments and Cash Advances

Occasionally a plan may use periodic interim payments (PIPs) or cash advances with SCPs. In the case of PIPs, the plan advances the provider a set amount of cash equivalent to a defined time period's expected reimbursable charges. As claims come in from that SCP, the claims are taken against the PIP, but the PIP is routinely replenished. In this way, the SCP gets a positive cash flow as well as the use of the plan's money interest free. Cash advances are simply that: The plan advances the provider a set amount of cash and then carries it as a receivable on the books. In the event that the relationship between the SCP and the plan terminates, the final claims are taken against the cash advance.

Neither of these techniques can be recommended for routine use. In either case, the advanced cash may not be treated as a liability by the SCP but rather simply as a payment, which makes it difficult to recover the funds. Capitation will accomplish much of what a PIP is intended to accomplish and is a preferred method. It is possible that in a plan using contact capitation, this method may be employed, but even then it is something that must be approached with caution due to the potential for reconciliation difficulties.

RISK AND REWARD

In addition to whatever reimbursement arrangement is made with an SCP, there are times when it is mutually advantageous to add an element of risk and reward. This is frequently done in the context of utilization but can be tied to other objectives, such as quality and access as well (see Chapter 10). These types of arrangements are best suited to those specialties in which the SCPs themselves control a major aspect of utilization and in which there is a sufficient volume of referrals to rule out random chance playing too large a role in the results. Risk and reward arrangements are far easier to do in a pure HMO environment than in a PPO (where they generally are not allowed by state regulations) or a POS plan.

In setting risk and reward levels, keep in mind that the risk or reward must not be so great as to have the potential of serious negative impact on clinical decision making. It is better policy to devise a reimbursement mechanism that fairly compensates an SCP up front for appropriate and judicious use of clinical resources and then sets a risk or bonus level that, while still being of value, is not potentially seriously injurious to the fiscal health of the SCP.

As discussed in Chapter 8 regarding PCP risk and bonus arrangements, a plan with a Medicare + Choice risk contract must be aware of the limitations on the total amount of risk a physician may be at without requiring the plan to undertake detailed member surveys. In addition, stop-loss provisions are equally germane to the reimbursement of SCPs as they are to PCPs. The reader is urged to review the relevant sections of Chapter 8 for further discussion of this issue.

CONCLUSION

Medical care delivered by SCPs is a crucial element in the cost and quality of health care. This is due not only to the costs associated with specialty care, but more importantly to the costs and medical utilization generated by the SCP during the course of care. The roles of the SCP are continuing to evolve in managed care, as are the organizational structures that SCPs are using to contract for services. Reimbursement arrangements and contracts are tools that codify and clarify the responsibilities of each party to the other. A reimbursement system will not solve any problems by itself and cannot take the place of good management. Remember: A discount will not make up for poor utilization management, and nothing will make up for poor quality of care.

REFERENCES AND NOTES

1. J.P. Weiner, Forecasting the Effects of Health Reform on U.S. Physician Workforce Requirements: Evidence from HMO Staffing Patterns, *JAMA* 272, 3 (1994): 222–30.

2. R. Kronick, D.C. Goodman, J. Wennberg, and E. Wagner, The Marketplace in Health Care Reform: The Demographic Limitations of Managed Competition, *New England Journal of Medicine* 328 (1993): 148–52.

3. J.R. Vitiello and R.R. Levary, Determining the Optimal Physician Mix in Health Maintenance Organizations, *Journal of Medical Systems* 21, 4 (1997): 249–66.

4. Ernst & Young proprietary data from the Managed Care Benchmarking Studies, 1998 and 1999.

5. SMG Marketing Group Inc., Hoechst Marion Roussel Managed Care Digest Series, *HMO-PPO Digest* (1999).

6. S. Schroeder and L. Sandy, Specialty Distribution of U.S. Physicians: The Invisible Driver of Health Care Costs, *New England Journal of Medicine* 328, 13 (1993): 928–33; S. Greenfield, E.C. Nelson, M. Zubkoff, et al., Variations in Resource Utilization among Medical Specialties and Systems of Care: Results from the Medical Outcomes Study, *JAMA* 267, 12 (1992): 1624–30; A.W. Murphy, G. Bury, P.K. Plunkett, et al., Randomized Controlled Trial of General Practitioner versus Usual Medical Care in an Urban Accident and Emergency Department, *British Medical Journal* 312 (1996): 1135–42; S. Greenfield, W.

Rogers, M. Mangotich, et al., Outcomes of Patients with Hypertension and Non-insulin Dependent Diabetes Mellitus Treated by Different Systems and Specialties, *JAMA* 274 (1995): 1436–44; T.S. Carey, J. Garrett, A. Jackman, et al., The Outcomes and Costs of Care for Acute Lower Back Pain among Patients Seen by Primary Care Practitioners, Chiropractors and Orthopedic Surgeons, *New England Journal of Medicine* 333 (1995): 913–17.

7. R. Kravitz, Differences in the Mix of Patients among Medical Specialties and Systems of Care: Results from the Medical Outcomes Study, *JAMA* 267, 12 (1992): 1617–23.

8. R.F. St. Peter, M.C. Reed, P. Kemper, and D. Blumenthal, Changes in the Scope of Care Provided by Primary Care Physicians, *New England Journal of Medicine* 341 (1999): 1980–85.

9. M. May, Resource Utilization in Treatment of Diabetic Ketoacidosis in Adults. *American Journal of Medical Sciences* 306, 5 (1993): 287–94; E.J. Zarling, F. Piontek, L. Klemka-Walden, and D. Inczauskis, The Effect of Gastroenterology Training on the Efficiency and Cost of Care Provided to Patients with Diverticulitis, *Gastroenterology* 112 (1997): 1859–62; J.B. Mitchell, D.J. Ballard, J.P. Whisnant, et al., What Role Do Neurologists Play in Determining the Costs and Outcomes of Stroke Patients? *Stroke* 27 (1996): 1937–43.

10. M. Gold, R. Hurley, T. Lake, et al., Arrangements between Managed Care Plans and Physicians: Results from a 1994 Survey of Managed Care Plans; Washington, D.C., 1995. Mathematica Politica.

11. K.T. LaPensee, Pricing Specialty Carve-Outs and Disease Management Programs under Managed Care, *Managed Care Quarterly* 5, 2 (1997): 10–19.

12. E.B. Keeler and M. Brodie, Economic Incentives in the Choice between Vaginal Delivery and Cesarean Section, *Milbank Quarterly* 71, 3(1973): 365–404.

Negotiating and Contracting with Hospitals and Institutions

Peter R. Kongstvedt

INTRODUCTION

Hospital contracting is one of the most important tasks that an executive director and other appropriate health plan managers face. Hospital executives likewise need a thorough understanding of the issues involved in contracting with managed care organizations (MCOs). Although there are a few states (e.g., Maryland) that are so heavily regulated that there is little or no latitude allowed in reimbursing hospitals, in general this represents an area of great potential for creativity.

HOSPITAL NETWORK DEVELOPMENT

The development of a hospital network can be viewed from two primary perspectives: new network development and renegotiation with existing network participants. In the past, new network development was a common occurrence as new MCOs entered the marketplace. However, despite the continued growth in managed health care, there are relatively few MCOs starting up as new organizations because of the already high number of existing plans as well as the consolidation that is occurring. New startups still do take place (e.g., in a market with low managed care penetration and few existing plans), just not as often.

The basic concepts of network development still apply to existing plans. If an MCO is expanding its geographical service area, that will be much like a new network development

project. Likewise, the addition of a new hospital or system to a network will require the same fundamental approach.

Renegotiating existing contracts is the most common event that any MCO will face. This occurs through the regular contracting cycle but may also be instigated by one party or the other because of a change in circumstances. Consolidation provides a common cause for renegotiation. If two MCOs merge, their legacy networks may not be compatible, there may be contractual clauses in existing contracts that automatically terminate the hospital contract in the event of a change of control, or negotiating leverage may have changed. The same principle applies to the creation of a large hospital system through mergers or affiliations. The new system may have more negotiating leverage, may rationalize clinical services, and so forth. In almost all cases of consolidation, the reimbursement terms are not exact matches (i.e., the terms between the premerged MCOs are not the same for the same hospital, and the terms between premerged hospitals are not the same for the same MCO).

Whether renegotiation is a routine matter or caused by a significant event, approaching it using the same concepts as applied in new network development will generally yield positive results. The effect on existing business of any change in terms, including possible severance of the relationship, is the greatest difference and therefore weighs heavily in the decision-making process during renegotiation.

Because of these similarities in approach, this chapter will use the process of network development as the primary vehicle for discussion.

Selecting Hospitals

Selecting which hospitals for an MCO to approach is done by balancing a number of variables. In a small or rural market there may be limited or even no choices (see Chapter 59). In most cases, though, there will be some latitude. Before beginning the selection process, plan management must first decide how much they are willing to limit the choices in the plan.

Generally, the more the MCO is willing to limit the number of participating hospitals, the greater the leverage in negotiating. Limiting the number has significant disadvantages as well. If the MCO strictly limits itself to just a few hospitals, it will have a competitive disadvantage in the marketplace because prospective members and accounts often use hospitals as a means of judging whether to join an MCO; therefore, if the plan fails to include a sufficient selection of hospitals, it may see disappointing marketing results. On the other hand, if the MCO refuses to limit the number of hospitals, it will have considerable difficulty in extracting favorable agreements and in managing utilization.

A certain number of hospitals will be required to cover a medical service area effectively. In some small communities, a single hospital may be able to serve the entire population, but that is rare. It is important to map out the hospital locations relative to the defined service area and to look for overlap among competing hospitals.

Selecting which hospitals to approach first in a service area is a combination of hard data—such as occupancy, cost, and services offered—as well as judgment about the hospital's willingness to negotiate and the perception of the public and physician community about the hospital's quality. It does little good for an MCO to make an agreement with a hospital that is perceived as inferior. Likewise, it is less than optimal to contract with a hospital that does not do high-volume obstetrics if there is a regional competitor

that does, because the MCO will then be less attractive to young families.

In some instances, the presence of a well-run integrated delivery system (IDS; see Chapter 4) will make a particular hospital attractive. This is most likely to be the case if a plan is a new entrant to the market, is introducing a new service line, or has been unable to create an attractive network from a marketing standpoint. The IDS may be in a position to accept considerable financial risk, such as total capitation, which may be desirable to an HMO that wishes to limit financial risk.

If the hospital is a sponsor or joint venture partner in an MCO, the choice factors become rather clear. If a hospital is an enthusiastic supporter of the MCO or if there is a long history of a good working relationship, that should also be taken into consideration. Of course, the reverse is equally true: if a hospital or IDS owns a health plan that competes, an MCO may choose not to subsidize that competitor by channeling business to the parent hospital or IDS.

Last, consolidation in the hospital industry has been occurring at a rapid pace. In many cases, this leads to the creation of a system with multiple hospitals. The MCO is then in a position of negotiating a broader contract with the system for services at multiple sites. The system may also demand a higher level of preference or even exclusivity in exchange for favorable terms. Although consolidation does not always bring value, the potential of cost reduction and rationalization of clinical services may allow the new system to provide care far more efficiently than individual hospitals, thus allowing for a considerable price advantage.

General Negotiating Strategy

An MCO's ability to negotiate successfully with hospitals will depend on a number of things. Chief among them are the personal abilities of the negotiator, the size of the plan, the MCO's ability actually to shift patient care, and the past track record of the MCO in being able to deliver what was promised. A new startup operation has considerably less clout than an existing large plan. If the new startup can demonstrate genuine potential for significant growth, that may help offset the weakness of having little to offer but promises.

Setting an overall strategy is important to the ultimate success of an MCO's hospital network. It is certainly possible to approach hospital negotiations by using the managerial equivalent of Brownian motion, but the end results will be tepid.

The strategy should address both regional and planwide issues. There may be one set of criteria for primary care services in a service area and a different set for tertiary services. After plan management has selected the hospital they wish to approach first, they must then select the hospitals to approach next if the initial hospital either is unwilling to come to agreement or offers too little to make the agreement worth the risk. The plan may also find that it will want to approach some hospitals for tertiary services on a much wider regional basis than for primary care. If the MCO does not intend significantly to restrict its hospital panel, then those hospitals with the most marketing value should be selected first.

Data Development

After selecting individual hospitals to approach, a worksheet should be made for each, and one for the entire service area as well. The hospital's occupancy rate (these data may be available from the local or state health department or the American Hospital Association[1]) and operating margin (this too may be available at the health department or may be published in the hospital's annual report) should be estimated.

The total number of bed days the plan currently has in the hospital should be estimated. If the plan is a new startup, the total number of bed days the medical director believes can be controlled and over what time span should be estimated (be honest here). The number of bed days the plan can realistically shift into the hospital or if necessary, away from the hospital should be estimated as well. This estimate will be affected by geographical accessibility and acceptability of such case shifting by members and physi-

cians. It is helpful to both parties if the bed days are categorized at least into broad categories such as medical/surgical, obstetrics, intensive care, mental health, and so forth.

Last, the whole dollars associated with all the preceding estimations or facts should be calculated. Plan management will want to know what whole dollar amount the plan represents to the hospital now and in the future. What happens if utilization shifts into and out of the hospital and what percentage of the hospital's gross income that would represent should be calculated.

Goal Setting

Markets with Low Managed Care Penetration

In markets that do not have high levels of managed care penetration (e.g., where managed care, primarily HMOs and point-of-service (POS) plans account for less than 30 percent of *total* health coverage), it is axiomatic that medical services are bought at the margin. As with purchasing an automobile or furniture, it is unusual to pay the sticker price. This goes for primary care, consultant care, and, most important, hospital services. If a hospital ward is fully staffed but running at less than full occupancy, the marginal cost of filling another bed on that ward is minor compared with the revenue. It is unlikely that the hospital will call in extra nurses, hire extra support staff, buy new equipment, or take out more insurance to care for a 10 percent increase in bed days; those costs are relatively fixed. The marginal costs (such as laundry, food, drugs and supplies, and the like) are a fraction of the fixed overhead.

Because of this, a hospital has room to maneuver in negotiating. This does not mean that a hospital will reduce its charges by half (unless its charges are grossly inflated to begin with), but an MCO can reasonably expect effective discounts of 20 percent to 30 percent if it is able to deliver sufficient volume. Certain for-profit hospitals are actually managed to show a profit at less than 50 percent occupancy. In those cases, even greater discounts may sometimes be obtained because much of the added revenue to the hospital goes right to the bottom line. Conversely, such high-margin hospitals may feel little pressure to increase their occupancy if they have a good market share, and may be difficult to deal with because they hope to freeze the MCO out.

After developing the worksheet referred to earlier, take the assumptions regarding how much can be shifted into the hospital and apply the desired discount. If a hospital has a low occupancy rate or if it has less than a full occupancy rate but is enjoying healthy profit margins (or reserves if it is not-for-profit) and the MCO can deliver or remove a significant volume of patients, it may be able to achieve a good reimbursement rate. If the hospital is running more than 90 percent occupancy, the prospects of substantial savings are not so good.

Outpatient procedures should be included in the calculations. It is common to find that outpatient procedures, if paid on a discounted charges basis, are actually substantially more expensive than identical procedures done in an inpatient setting. Hospital managers have not been idly watching utilization shift to the outpatient department; they have adjusted charges to manage revenues.

Markets with High Managed Care Penetration

In markets with high levels of managed care penetration, the dynamics may look considerably different. In those markets, the margin has been reduced and few payers are paying full charges. Public sector fee-for-service reimbursement (i.e., Medicare and Medicaid) certainly does not pay full charges, and if managed care accounts for most of the rest, as well as a considerable portion of the public sector, then charges become relatively meaningless, and a hospital's ability to absorb payment differentials is diminished. In such markets, MCOs, especially HMOs, are most likely to use a reimbursement system that is unrelated to charges (discussed later). The MCO and the hospital must then balance the actual cost to provide the service (if the hospital has a cost-accounting system, which is not always the case), the ability to

provide volume to offset fixed costs, the market presence and desirability of the parties, and the cost of not doing business together.

Markets with high managed care penetration also tend to have high levels of hospital consolidation. This changes the dynamic as noted earlier. In addition, the levels of sophistication increase on all sides. More creativity comes into play, and the MCOs and hospitals find themselves operating more as business partners (or at least close acquaintances) and less as arm's length contracting entities. Although price and clinical services are still the most important factors, the ability of the parties to operate together becomes of greater importance. The ability to interface administratively, the ability to resolve operating problems, and so forth play heavily in the negotiating strategy.

In high penetration markets, there is sometimes a desire on the part of the hospitals, usually through their IDSs, to accept greater amounts of risk for medical expenses because there is the perception that there is greater margin in that form of reimbursement. As discussed in Chapter 4 though, the acceptance of global risk for medical expenses has not been totally successful in all markets, and many IDSs have failed because of an inability to manage the risk. This has led to a decrease in the desire to accept such risk and even the undoing of existing global capitation contracts to revert to an earlier form of reimbursement. These financial failures of IDSs have also resulted in a decreased desire by some MCOs to delegate such risk. But there is often a cyclic nature to reimbursement methods, and so the reader should not assume that global capitation is disappearing in managed care markets.

Responsibilities and Roles of Plan Management

The key players in hospital negotiations from the health plan side are the executive director, the medical director, and the finance director. In large national companies, these functions may be the responsibility of a network manager, but the concepts are the same.

It is the responsibility of the executive director or network management to initiate the contact, set the stage or tone, and be sure that the executive director of the hospital feels comfortable with the plan's commitment to proceed fairly, openly, and honestly. It is not always necessarily the role of the executive director actually to negotiate the details of the agreement because it is unlikely that the executive director of the hospital will be doing so. However, a relationship between the chief executive of the MCO and the chief executive of the hospital is important to establish. Large MCOs may have an officer who is specifically responsible for managing relations with hospitals, and that individual may also be the senior-most person in the plan who will manage the process. In small plans or sometimes for political reasons, the executive director may end up carrying the ball all the way through.

The role of the finance director is to work closely with the plan's executive director (or the officer responsible for hospital contracting) and the hospital's finance director or controller. In many cases, the actual negotiation takes place at this level. The finance director should not have the authority actually to sign off on the agreement because the controller of the hospital will surely not have this authority, and it further serves a useful purpose to be able to break the negotiations to confer with the executive director back at the plan. Because the hospital may not believe the numbers produced by the plan, it falls to the finance director of the plan to present those numbers in a credible and understandable way (not only the numbers now but also the numbers the plan expects).

In addition to evaluating the quality of the institution and helping understand the political climate, the medical director needs to be able to convince the hospital administrator that the plan will genuinely shift the patient caseload as necessary. If the medical director cannot persuade the hospital that the plan is able to move patients in or out, the plan will have lost a key advantage in the negotiations. This need not be done in a heavy-handed way or as a naked threat. It suffices for this issue to be brought out in a businesslike and unemotional way.

It is important to set a realistic time schedule. The degree to which plan management achieves success in their hospital negotiations will be reflected in the amount of effort put into the negotiating process. It is not realistic to think that one can obtain favorable pricing and contracts with a number of hospitals in less than two or three months (and perhaps considerably longer). It will take time to do the preplanning work for the hospital to digest what is being proposed, for the hospital to make a counter offer, and for the plan to counter that, and so on. After that, each side's lawyers will want to review the contract language.

Conversely, try not to let too much dust collect on the proposal before either following up or approaching another hospital as an alternative. If the plan has proposed a reduction in what it is currently paying, the hospital will obviously prefer to keep collecting revenue under the existing terms as long as possible unless the plan is promising a sizable increase in volume that it is not now getting. There is no reason for the hospital to hurry the process unless it believes that to delay will mean losing the contract.

Responsibilities and Roles of Hospital Management

The chief executive officer (CEO) or executive director of the hospital must set the overall strategy for managed care contracting. In most major markets, managed care is far too important to delegate to a lower level individual in the organization. Many hospital CEOs may not be comfortable with this role because their training and experience are in the operations of the clinical facility, and they may choose to delegate the development of managed care strategy to another officer or director. This is perfectly acceptable and may even be necessary, but the CEO should be fully knowledgeable about the terms and strategies and accept ultimate responsibility for them. In many cases, it is important for the hospital CEO to establish a good working relationship with the CEO of the MCO to indicate the level of importance that the hospital holds for the MCO and to work through any obstacles in the negotiating process. It also allows the

CEO to better understand the goals and strategies of the MCO.

As noted previously, it is common for a hospital to appoint a high-level individual to be the primary source of managed care relations. This individual may have primary responsibility for all aspects of the negotiation, including financial analysis, operational issues, and reimbursement terms. It is a serious mistake for the hospital to use an individual who is not sufficiently senior in the system or one who cannot make any decisions. The MCO will become frustrated in dealing with a lower level functionary, and this will impede success.

The hospital's finance director must be closely involved in the process as well. Unless the MCO is of trivial size, managed care revenues need to be carefully analyzed as described in the preceding section (and if the MCO is of trivial size, there better be a pretty compelling reason for the hospital to provide it with favorable terms). Of special concern is the ability of the hospital to meet its direct costs for providing care; if the MCO's reimbursement terms do not even cover direct cost, then the hospital is in trouble. How much the MCO's terms contribute to the hospital's indirect costs and margin is at the core of the negotiation, along with the usual issues of market strength, services offered, and ability to shift volume.

The hospital should have a medical director involved as well. In the past, hospital medical directors were primarily involved with issues of credentialing and privileges, clinical services, recruiting, and so forth. In a market with high levels of managed care penetration, the medical director needs to be heavily involved in clinical aspects of the relationship with the MCO, including clinical efficiency, utilization management, quality management, and member satisfaction. The hospital must be able to provide quality services efficiently and to manage its costs to prosper under managed care reimbursement terms.

As noted above, it is common for hospitals to have some form of IDS, and the MCO may or may not be willing to contract with it. In the event that the IDS does indeed accept a significant level of risk for medical expenses, then the IDS and hospital will need to apply managed care utilization management (UM) techniques or face a negative financial result.

TYPES OF REIMBURSEMENT ARRANGEMENTS

There are a number of reimbursement methods available in contracting with hospitals, except in those rare states where regulations diminish or prohibit creativity. Exhibit 12–1 lists a number of methods that have been used by plans, but it is not exhaustive. Table 12–1 and Figure 12–1 provide data on relative distribution of the more common types of reimbursement methods. It is common to find more than one reimbursement method present in a single relationship as illustrated in Figures 12–2 and 12–3.

Management on either side of the equation must have the internal ability to manage these financial terms in their information systems. The more one is dependent on manual intervention and adjustment, the higher the error rate, the higher the cost

---

Exhibit 12–1 Models for Reimbursing Hospitals

- Charges
- Discounts
- Per diems
- Sliding scales for discounts and per diems
- Differential by day in hospital
- Diagnosis-related groups (DRGs)
- Differential by service type
- Case rates
  - Institutional only
  - Package pricing or bundled rates
- Capitation
- Percent of premium revenue
- Contact capitation
- Bed leasing
- Periodic interim payments or cash advances
- Performance-based incentives
  - Quality and service incentives
  - Penalties and withholds
- Ambulatory patient groups (APGs) and ambulatory payment classifications (APCs) for outpatient care

Table 12–1 Percentage of HMOs Using Specialty Physician Reimbursement Methods

	July 1993	*July 1998*
Primary Care Physicians		
Capitation	69.3%	78.7%
Fee for Service	59.8%	69.7%
Relative Value Scale	11.1%	27.2%
Salary	13.7%	9.8%
Specialty Care Physicians		
Capitation	30.2%	56.4%
Fee for Service	61.7%	75.5%
Relative Value Scale	12.6%	32.2%
Salary	6.1%	3.3%
Hospitals		
Fee for Service	68.1%	71.7%
Per Diem Rates	90.8%	86.2%
Diagnosis Related Groups (DRGs)	39.4%	49.5%
Capitation	18.0%	32.5%

Source: Reprinted with permission from *The Interstudy Competitive Edge: HMO Industry Report* 9.1, © 1999, InterStudy publications.

of administration of the contract, and the greater the need for reconciliation.

Straight Charges

The simplest (albeit least desirable) payment mechanism in health care is straight charges. It is also obviously the most expensive, after the option of no contract at all. This is a fallback position to be agreed to only in the event that one is unable to obtain any form of discount at all, but it is still desirable to have a contract with a no balance billing clause in it (see Chapter 62) for purposes of reserve requirements and licensure.

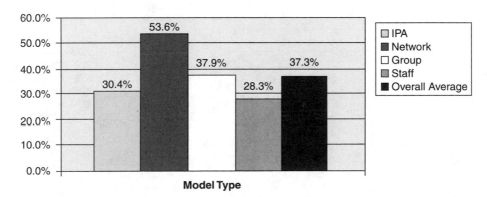

Figure 12–1 Average Percentage of Hospitals under Capitation. *Source:* Reprinted with permission from Hoechst Marion Roussel Managed Care Digest Series, *HMO-PPO Digest 1999,* © 1999 Hoechst Marion Roussel, SMG Marketing Group, Inc.

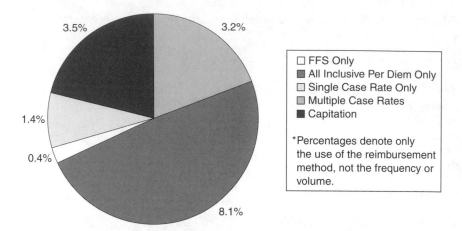

Figure 12–2 Percentages of HMOs Using Hospital Reimbursement Type*—1997. Courtesy of AAHP Annual Industry Survey, 1998, American Association of Health Plans, Washington, DC.

Straight Discount on Charges

Another possible arrangement with hospitals is a straight percentage discount on charges. In this case, the hospital submits its claim in full and the plan discounts it by the agreed-to percentage, and then pays it. The hospital accepts this payment as payment in full. The amount of discount that can be obtained will depend on the factors discussed

earlier. This type of arrangement is more common in markets with low levels of managed care penetration but is uncommon in markets with high levels of managed care.

Sliding Scale Discount on Charges

Sliding scale discounts are an option, particularly in markets with low managed care penetra-

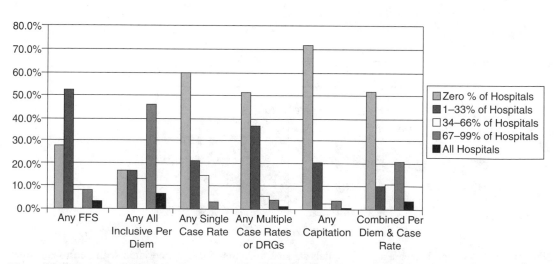

Figure 12–3 Percent of Hospitals Compensated by Various Methods for HMO's Largest Commercial Product. Courtesy of AAHP Annual Industry Survey, 1998, American Association of Health Plans, Washington, DC.

tion but some level of competitiveness between hospitals. With a sliding scale, the percentage discount is reflective of total volume of admissions and outpatient procedures. Whether to lump the two categories together or deal with them separately is not as important as making sure that the parties deal with them both. With the rapidly climbing cost of outpatient charges, savings from reduction of inpatient utilization could be negated by an unanticipated overrun in outpatient charges.

An example of a sliding scale is a 20 percent reduction in charges for 0 to 200 total bed days per year, with incremental increases in the discount up to a maximum percentage. An interim percentage discount is usually negotiated, and the parties reconcile at the end of the year on the basis of the final total volume. The time periods for measurement are also negotiable. For example, the discount could vary on a month-to-month basis rather than yearly. The sliding scale could track total bed days, number of admissions, or whole dollars spent. The most important thing is to be sure that it is a clearly defined and easily measurable objective.

The last issue to look at in a sliding scale is timeliness of payment. It is likely that the hospital will demand a clause in the contract spelling out the plan's requirement to process claims in a timely manner, usually 30 days or sooner. In some cases, the plan may negotiate a sliding scale, or a modifier to the main sliding scale, that applies a further reduction on the basis of the plan's ability to turn a clean claim around quickly. For example, an additional 4 percent discount may be negotiated for paying a clean claim within 14 days of receipt. Conversely, the hospital may demand a penalty for clean claims that are not processed within 30 days. Many states have laws and regulations that require timely payment before the imposition of penalties and interest payments (see Chapter 69), and so the additional discount based on rapid payment must be negotiated using that as the base level.

Straight Per Diem Charges

Unlike straight charges, a negotiated per diem is a single charge for a day in the hospital regardless of any actual charges or costs incurred. In this most common type of arrangement, the plan negotiates a per diem rate with the hospital and pays that rate without adjustments. For example, the plan will pay $900 for each day regardless of the actual cost of the service.

Hospital administrators are often reluctant to include days in the intensive care unit or obstetrics to the base per diem unless there is a sufficient volume of regular medical-surgical cases to make the ultimate cost predictable. In a small plan, or in one that is not limiting the number of participating hospitals, the hospital administrator is concerned that the hospital will be used for expensive cases at a low per diem and competitors will be used for less costly cases. In such cases, a good option is to negotiate multiple sets of per diem charges on the basis of service type (e.g., medical-surgical, obstetrics, intensive care, neonatal intensive care, rehabilitation, and so forth) or a combination of per diems and a flat case rate (see later) for obstetrics.

The key to making a per diem work is predictability. If the plan and hospital can accurately predict the number and mix of cases, they can accurately calculate a per diem. The per diem is simply an estimate of the charges or costs for an average day in that hospital minus the level of discount. For example, if the plan has a per diem arrangement that pays $900 per day for medical admissions and the total allowable charges (billed charges less charges for noncovered items provided during the admission) for a five-day admission are $6,200, the hospital is reimbursed $4,500 for the admission ($900 per day × 5 days).

A theoretical disadvantage of the per diem approach, however, is that the per diem must be paid even if the billed charges are less than the per diem rate. It has been anecdotally reported that some large, self-insured accounts have demanded the lesser of the charges or the per diems for each case (i.e., laying off the upper end of the risk but harvesting the reward). Such demands are to be avoided because they corrupt the integrity of the per diem calculation.

A plan may also negotiate to reimburse the hospital for expensive surgical implants provided at the hospital's actual cost of the implant.

Such reimbursement would be limited to a defined list of implants (e.g., multichannel cochlear implants) where the cost to the hospital for the implant is far greater than is recoverable under the per diem or outpatient arrangement.

Sliding Scale Per Diem

Like the sliding scale discount on charges discussed previously, the sliding scale per diem is also based on total volume. In this case, the plan negotiates an interim per diem that it will pay for each day in the hospital. Depending on the total number of bed days or admissions in the year, the plan will either pay a lump sum settlement at the end of the year or withhold an amount from the final payment for the year to adjust for an additional reduction in the per diem from an increase in total bed days or admissions. It may be preferable to make an arrangement whereby on a quarterly or semiannual basis the plan will adjust the interim per diem so as to reduce any disparities caused by unexpected changes in utilization patterns.

Differential by Day in Hospital

This simply refers to the fact that most hospitalizations are more expensive on the first day. For example, the first day for surgical cases includes operating suite costs, the operating surgical team costs (nurses and recovery), and so forth. This type of reimbursement method is generally combined with a per diem approach, but the first day is paid at a higher rate. For example, the first day may be $1,100 and each subsequent day is $650.

Diagnosis-Related Groups

As with Medicare, a common reimbursement method is by diagnosis-related groups (DRGs). There are publications of DRG categories, criteria, outliers, and trim points (i.e., the cost or length of stay that causes the DRG payment to be supplemented or supplanted by another payment mechanism) to enable the plan to negotiate a payment mechanism for DRGs on the basis of Medicare rates or, in some cases, state-regulated

rates. DRGs as used by the Health Care Financing Administration (HCFA) are not severity adjusted at the time of publication. As discussed in Chapter 32, there are some systems that recategorize DRGs on the basis of severity, but their use in reimbursement is uncommon.

If high utilization rates are prevalent, a reduction in unnecessary utilization will not necessarily provide concomitant savings when using straight DRGs. If the payment is fixed on the basis of diagnosis, any reduction in days will go to the hospital and not to the plan. Furthermore, unless the plan is prepared to perform careful audits of the hospital's DRG coding, it may experience code creep. On the other hand, DRGs do serve to share risk with the hospital, thus making the hospital an active partner in managing utilization. DRGs are perhaps better suited to plans with loose controls than plans that tightly manage utilization.

Service-Related Case Rates

Similar to DRGs, service-related case rates are a cruder cut. In this reimbursement mechanism, various service types are defined (e.g., medicine, surgery, intensive care, neonatal intensive care, psychiatry, obstetrics, and the like), and the hospital receives a flat per-admission reimbursement for whatever type of service the patient is admitted to (e.g., all surgical admissions cost $6,100). If services are mixed, a prorated payment may be made (e.g., 50 percent of surgical and 50 percent of intensive care).

Case Rates and Package Pricing

Whatever mechanism a plan uses for hospital reimbursement, it may still need to address certain categories of procedures and negotiate special rates. The most common of these is obstetrics. It is common to negotiate a flat rate or case rate for a normal vaginal delivery and a flat rate or case rate for a Caesarean section or a blended rate for both. In the case of blended case rates (which are much preferred over separate rates for the two types of deliveries), the expected reimbursement for each type of delivery is multiplied by the expected (or desired) percentage of utilization. For example, a case rate for vaginal delivery is $2,500 and for Caesarean section it is $3,500. Utilization is expected to be 80 percent vaginal and 20 percent Caesarean section; therefore the case rate is $2,700 ($2,500 × 0.8 = $2,000; $3,500 × 0.2 = $700; $2,000 + $700 = $2,700).

Other common areas for case rates are specialty procedures at tertiary hospitals, for example, coronary artery bypass surgery, heart transplants, or certain types of cancer treatment. These procedures, although relatively infrequent, are tremendously costly.

A broader variation is package pricing or bundled case rates. The package price or bundled case rate refers to an all-inclusive rate paid for both institutional and professional services. The plan negotiates a flat rate for a procedure (e.g., coronary artery bypass surgery or cataract surgery), and that rate is used to pay all parties who provide services connected with that procedure, including preadmission and postdischarge care. Bundled case rates are not uncommon in teaching facilities where there is a faculty practice plan that works closely with the hospital.

Capitation or Percentage of Revenue

Capitation refers to reimbursing the hospital on a per member per month basis to cover all institutional costs for a defined population of members. The payment may be varied by age and gender but does not fluctuate with premium revenue. Percentage of revenue refers to a fixed percentage of premium revenue (i.e., a percentage of the collected premium rate) being paid to the hospital, again to cover all institutional services. The difference between percentage of revenue and capitation is that percentage of revenue may vary with the premium rate charged and the actual revenue yield.

Although capitation and percent of premium revenue are essentially the same for public sector programs (i.e., risk contracts for Medicare and Medicaid), that is not the case for the commercial sector. For commercial products, percentages will vary most commonly based on benefit plan design (e.g., the level of copayments the member must make), but there are other reasons as well. In the event the plan fails

to properly develop rates or perform underwriting (or gets caught up in a price war), a proportionate percentage of that shortfall will be passed directly to the hospital.

In all cases, the hospital stands the entire risk for institutional services for the defined membership base; if the hospital cannot provide the services itself, the cost for such care is deducted from the capitation payment. For this type of arrangement to work, a hospital must know that it will serve a clearly defined segment of a plan's enrollment and that it can provide most of the necessary services to those members. This also means that the primary care physician is clearly associated with just one hospital. If the plan is dealing with a multihospital system with multiple facilities in the plan's service area, it may be reasonable to expect that the hospitals in the system can care for the plan's members on an exclusive basis.

Closely related to hospital capitation is the idea of global capitation, in which an IDS accepts capitation or percent of premium revenue in exchange for total risk for medical services. This is discussed in Chapter 4.

There must be a clear definition of what is covered under the capitation payment and what is not. For example, the capitation may include outpatient procedures, but the plan and hospital need to account for outpatient procedures that are being performed outside the hospital's domain. Will home health be part of the capitation, and if so, what agency? It is preferable not to place the hospital at risk for services it cannot control, as long as there is a clear definition of what those services are.

The hospital must also perform aggressive UM to see any margin from capitation; if UM is carried out so as to ruffle the least number of feathers of attending staff, the hospital will pay a stiff price. More advanced methods of managing utilization will also clearly be in the hospital's financial benefit. For example, advanced disease management results in a general reduction of inpatient hospital stays. It is therefore in the interests of the hospital to ensure that such programs exist and are optimally managed. The various forms of medical management are discussed in detail in Part III.

The hospital also needs to have stop-loss insurance to protect it against catastrophic cases. This stop-loss coverage may be provided by the MCO; for example, the plan may reimburse the hospital at a low per diem for all days of a case after it has been in the hospital for a number of days (e.g., beyond 30 days in a year). Alternatively, the plan may pay a percent of charges after a certain charge level has been reached, and the plan's own reinsurance comes into play. For capitated hospitals, if the MCO does not provide the stop-loss, then it should be purchased from an outside company specializing in such products, as discussed in Chapter 53.

POS plans with an out-of-network benefit make capitation methods difficult to use. As discussed in Chapter 8, capitation in POS may mean having to pay twice for a service, once under capitation and again if the member seeks service outside the network. In areas where there are no real alternatives to a certain hospital (e.g., a rural area or an area where a hospital enjoys a monopoly), this problem may not be material, but that is the exception. Contact capitation, as noted later, may also attenuate this problem. The alternative is to deduct out-of-area costs from the capitation payment.

The advantage of capitation to an MCO is that it is not only budgetable but also results in laying off much of the risk for institutional expenses. The hospital becomes a full partner in managing utilization, and the plan has less need to intervene. A disadvantage is that the plan will see none of the savings for improved utilization control. Another problem can arise if the hospital refuses to share any of the savings (calculated as though there were a per diem or discounted charges model) with the physicians who are controlling the cases.

The most important problem to note is that some hospitals are simply not able to manage the financial risk associated with capitation. The financial management tools and expertise, UM, and data and information management capabilities in a hospital may not be adequate to manage the risk associated with a broad population of members. In situations where there is a small base of capitated lives, then chance becomes equally or even more important than clinical management. In the event that capitation results

in severe financial results, nothing but harm and poor future relations will result. It should therefore be a requirement that when an MCO capitates a hospital or IDS, the MCO is able to ascertain whether the provider system has the capabilities, and a mechanism for regular monitoring of results must be in place.

Contact Capitation

Contact capitation of hospitals is similar to contact capitation for specialty physicians, as discussed in Chapter 11. Like contact capitation for specialty physicians, this method of reimbursement is not common. In short, the capitation is tied to the percentage of admissions to a hospital, with adjustments for the type of service. As an example (not adjusting for service type), the overall capitation rate is $40 per member per month. The plan has 100,000 members, and 50 percent of admissions go to a particular hospital system that month. The payment to that system therefore is $40 \times (100,000 \times 0.5) = $2,000,000.

Adjusting for service type is usually required as well, unless it is clear to all parties that there is no relevant reason for such adjustments (e.g., the population covered by capitation is large, the number of hospitals participating is low, and the services offered are equal between the different hospitals). Type of service adjustment simply means more categories in which the percentages must be calculated or an adjustment takes place in the payment by some factor that accounts for the acuity. As an example, using the same base capitation and population size noted previously, if hospital A has 10 percent more intensive care days in its mix than does hospital B, and intensive care days are considered twice as costly as other days, then the percentage of the capitation payment is adjusted by that amount; in this case, hospital A receives $2,400,000, and hospital B receives $1,600,000. [Adjusted percentage = actual percentage plus or minus the percentage adjustment. Hospital A is $40 \times (100,000 \times (0.5 + (0.5 \times 0.1)) = $40 \times (100,000 \times 0.6) = $2,400,000. Hospital B is $40 \times (100,000 \times (0.5 - (0.5 \times 0.1)) = $40 \times (100,000 \times 0.4) = $1,600,000.]

Such adjustments can quickly become complicated, particularly when there are more than two types of service type adjustments to be made. Like contact capitation for specialty physicians, this approach requires sophisticated information systems and is often not an easily automated function, thus requiring manual administration. Unlike specialty physician contact capitation though, the number of participants is lower and is therefore at least theoretically more manageable.

As noted earlier, this form of reimbursement can also be combined with case rates or other capitation rates. Obstetrics is the most common reason for having an additional reimbursement system, with the cost of obstetrics being carved out of the basic capitation rate, and payment for obstetrical services occurring either by means of case rates or a separate capitation.

Bed Leasing

A rare reimbursement mechanism is bed leasing. This refers to a plan actually leasing beds from an institution, for example, paying the hospital $350 per bed for 10 beds regardless of whether those beds are used or not. This ensures revenue flow to the hospital, ensures access to beds (at least some beds) for the plan, and is budgetable. It is perhaps best used in those situations in which a plan is assured of a steady number of bed days with little or no seasonality. The problem with bed leasing is that there is no real savings from reducing utilization unless contract terms allow the plan to lease back the beds to the hospital if they are not being used. Bed leasing, which was never common, has declined along with the decline of the group and staff model HMO, although it may be used by a large, globally capitated medical group (see Chapter 4).

Periodic Interim Payments and Cash Advances

Once common but now rare, periodic interim payments (PIPs) and cash advances are methods whereby the plan advances cash to cover expected claims to a hospital. This cash advance is periodically replenished if it gets below a certain amount. Claims may be applied directly against the cash advance or may be paid outside of it, in which case the cash advance serves as an advance deposit. The value of this to a hospital is obvious: positive cash flow. PIPs and cash advances are quite valuable to a hospital and will generate a discount in and of themselves.

This is also a mechanism that has great application in those cases where an MCO's claims systems are overwhelmed or the MCO is otherwise unable to process payments in a timely manner. The cash advance allows the MCO to meet timely payment provisions and keeps the hospital financially sound, while allowing additional time for the MCO to clean up its payment systems.

Performance-Based Reimbursement

The largest portion of reimbursement to hospitals is likely to be done under one or more of the methods described previously. Capitation is clearly an example of performance-based reimbursement, in that the hospital only profits if it can provide services at a low cost and a high level of quality. Beyond that, there are other forms of performance-based reimbursement, although they are not common.

Penalties and Withholds

As with physician services (see Chapters 8 and 11), penalties or withholds occasionally are used in hospital reimbursement methods. As an example, a plan may negotiate with a hospital to allow the hospital's own UM department to perform all the UM functions (see Chapter 18). As part of that negotiation, goals are set for average length of stay and average admission rate. Part of the payment to the hospital may be withheld, or conversely the plan may set aside a bonus pool. In any event, if the goals are met or exceeded, the hospital receives its withhold or bonus, and vice versa. One complication with this is the possibility that a hospital can make its statistics look good by simply sending patients to other hospitals; this is similar to problems encountered with physician capitation. If a service area is clearly defined or if the hospital is capitated, it may be easier to apply a risk or reward program. The reader should be aware, however, that there is evidence that financial penalty models applied to hospitals have little or no effect on utilization or physician performance.[2] Furthermore, utilization-based performance payments may be considered to be a liability from the standpoint of risk management, as discussed in Chapter 45.

Service and Quality Incentives

An alternative, and in the opinion of this author, superior approach to financial risk/bonus payments associated with utilization is to provide the hospital incentives for improving its quality and service, as well as its business operations. In one model, hospitals receive an incentive payment that is affected by three broad variables: satisfaction of services (measured by surveys of patients and physicians), clinical care (measured by looking at complication rates, average length of stay, and other measures), and business structural support for managed care (e.g., electronic data interchange, case management support, and other aspects).[3] In another case, hospitals receive modest incentives based on outcomes for certain clinical procedures.[4]

OUTPATIENT PROCEDURES

As mentioned earlier, the shift from inpatient to outpatient care has not gone unnoticed by hospital administrators. As care has shifted, so have charges. It is not uncommon to see outpatient charges exceeding the cost of an inpatient day unless steps are taken to address that imbalance.

Discounts on Charges

Either straight discounts or sliding scale discounts may be applied to outpatient charges. Some hospitals argue that the cost to deliver highly technical outpatient procedures actually is greater than an average per diem, primarily because the per diem assumes more than a single day in the hospital, thereby spreading the costs over a greater number of reimbursable days. Some plans have responded by simply admitting patients for their outpatient surgery, paying the per diem, and sending the patient home. Many plans negotiate the cost of outpatient surgery to never exceed the cost of an inpatient day, whereas other plans concede the problem of front-loading surgical services and agree to cap outpatient charges at a fixed percentage of the per diem (e.g., 125 percent of the average per diem).

Package Pricing or Bundled Charges

Plans may negotiate package pricing or bundled charges for outpatient procedures. In this method of reimbursement, all the various charges are bundled into one single charge, thereby reducing the problem of unbundling and exploding (i.e., charging for multiple codes or brand-new codes where previously only one code was used). Plans may use their own data to develop the bundled charges, or they may use outside data (one such source is published by Milliman and Robertson,[5] a national actuarial firm). Bundled charges are generally tied to the principal procedure code used by the facility. Bundled charges may also be added together in the event that more than one procedure is performed, although the second procedure is discounted because the patient was already in the facility and using services.

Related to this approach are tiered rates. In this case, the outpatient department categorizes all procedures into several different categories. The plan then pays a different rate for each category, but that rate covers all services performed in the outpatient department, and only one category is used at a time (i.e., the hospital cannot add several categories together for a single patient encounter).

Ambulatory Visits

There are two main classification systems developed and used in the reimbursement of ambulatory visits or encounters: ambulatory patient groups (APGs) and ambulatory payment classification (APCs). APGs were developed as a forerunner and are quite similar to APCs. Both are in the public domain. The APCs are being (as of the time of publication) implemented by HCFA for outpatient prospective payment in hospital outpatient departments and ambulatory surgery centers for Medicare patients.[6] APGs are already used by a variety of payers (for example, Medicaid and several Blue Cross Blue Shield plans).[7] More than one may be billed if more than one procedure is performed, but there is significant discounting for the additional charges.

APGs are already used by a variety of payers (for example, Medicaid and several Blue Cross Blue Shield plans).[7] More than one may be billed if more than one procedure is performed, but there is significant discounting for the additional charges.

APGs and APCs are to outpatient services what DRGs are to inpatient ones, although APGs and APCs are based on procedures rather than simply on diagnoses, contain a greater degree of adjustment for severity, and are considerably more complex. A few processing systems

support these, and a number of companies produce mainframe and/or desktop versions of add-on software for these classification systems. With the use of APCs by HCFA, plans will need to be able to support APGs and APCs, since cost-shifting is bound to occur otherwise.

CONCLUSION

As with all provider payment systems, reimbursement mechanisms and contracts with hospitals are tools. The importance of these tools cannot be overestimated, and an MCO must craft these tools with all the skills they have available. It is possible and desirable to develop mutually advantageous contracts between MCOs and hospitals, and that can be a pivotal issue in the ultimate success of a plan.

REFERENCES AND NOTES

1. American Hospital Association. *American Hospital Association Guide to the Health Care Field.* (Chicago: American Hospital Association), 1999.

2. L. Debrock and R.J. Arnould, Utilization Control in HMOs. *Quarterly Review of Economics and Finance* Autumn 32 (1992): 3, 31–53.

3. C. Sennett, A.P. Legorreta, and S.L. Zata, Performance-based Hospital Contracting for Quality Improvement. *Journal on Quality Improvement* 19 (1993): 9, 374–383.

4. Presentation by Blue Cross Blue Shield of Minnesota, 1993.

5. R.L. Doyle and A.P. Feren, *Healthcare Management Guidelines: Ambulatory Care Guidelines.* Milliman & Robertson. Published and updated periodically.

6. R.F. Averill et al. *Design and Evaluation of a Prospective Payment System for Ambulatory Care, Final Report.* Health Care Financing Administration Cooperative Agreement No. 17-C-99369/1-02.

7. S. Larose, Preparing for Ambulatory Patient Groups. *Capitation & Medical Practice* March 1 (1995), 9.

CHAPTER 13

Academic Health Centers
and Managed Care

Jennifer H. Lofland and David B. Nash

Academic health centers (AHCs) have long symbolized the great technological advancements and specialization in patient care that have occurred in this century. They have been successful in their classic mission to train health professionals, foster basic and clinical research, and provide the highest quality of patient care.

However, these traditional ways are facing an uncertain future in today's rapidly changing health care environment. Public generosity toward research and education is tempered by a strong deficit-lowering sentiment in the nation. Furthermore, with the failure of comprehensive health reform, medical educators have lost confidence in the certainty of future public support for education, research, and patient care in the academic setting. This would not be an insurmountable problem as long as the historical subsidization of education and research by profitable clinical activities continued indefinitely. It is clear, however, that this cannot continue as the purchasers of health care seek continued cost

Jennifer H. Lofland, PharmD, is a Project Director in the Office of Health Policy and Clinical Outcomes at Thomas Jefferson University, Philadelphia, Pennsylvania.

David B. Nash, MBA, MD, is Associate Dean and the Director of the Office of Health Policy and Clinical Outcomes at Thomas Jefferson University, Philadelphia, Pennsylvania.

containment through managed care. Therefore, the AHCs are forced to compete in the marketplace on cost and quality. This may leave little support for less profitable activities and require the transformation of the current AHC structure.

An understanding of the complex interaction among patients, physicians, hospitals, insurers, employers, and government agencies is necessary before a strategy for the managed care market can be developed. The traditional role played by each party is constantly changing. Providers, including hospitals and physicians, deliver care to patients. Insurers provide various financing arrangements as defined by a specified benefits plan for purchasers and beneficiaries (or patients). The purchasers of health care include patients, employers, and government agencies, such as Medicare and Medicaid, which pay premiums to insurers or pay providers directly for services. Managed care is the integration of financing with the delivery of health care services. Therefore, managed care organizations (MCOs) provide plans or products that integrate the health care financing activities of insurers with the delivery of care by providers for purchasers. Some insurers are becoming MCOs since they go beyond simply paying for services rendered in a fee-for-service (FFS) system to managing provider activity and arranging the delivery of care. In addition, providers are becoming MCOs by providing financing and delivery of health care services when contracting directly with purchasers. Some MCOs, such as the staff model* health maintenance organizations (HMOs), provide financing and delivery within one system and assume both the provider and insurer role. With the rapid changes in the health care industry, this terminology is rather artificial. Further discussions of the evolving taxonomy of MCOs and integrated provider systems are found in Chapters 3 and 4.

This chapter defines the challenges to academic medicine regarding changing market mechanisms and financial support for AHCs, and demonstrates how the unique AHC organizational and cultural environment contributes to problems of the AHC and therefore obstructs potential solutions. Potential strategies must integrate primary and specialty care with network formation to secure a solid patient base. Furthermore, the AHC must create and cultivate stakeholders in its mission to support necessary but nonprofitable activities. Internal changes to meet these new demands require innovation and leadership in realigning incentives, managing information and outcomes, and reinventing education and research. Finally, anticipating change to improve market position and profitability will prove valuable as rapid change continues.

DIMENSIONS OF THE PROBLEM

With the rapid growth of managed care, AHCs face multiple financial challenges that threaten their ability to perform their traditional academic mission. The potential loss of public funds that directly and indirectly support medical education, research, charity, and care take on new implications in the context of the challenges presented by managed care. It is important to

*The number of staff and even group model HMOs has been steadily diminishing over the past decade. However, there remain certain similarities between staff model HMOs and other forms of organized medical delivery systems that accept global risk for health care expenses. These issues are discussed further in Chapters 3 and 4.

recognize that managed care is a reflection of the change in societal values and attitudes. Managed care is a response to two decades of runaway medical inflation caused by a cost-plus system that encouraged unlimited use of medical services. Although the AHCs benefited immensely in this environment, continued reliance on the structure and culture of the past is the real threat to the viability of AHCs. The answer lies in recognizing that "they can no longer operate as specialty-driven institutions largely divorced from the trends that favor lower costs, less hospitalization, and more primary care."[1] The dimensions of the problem will be examined here in terms of the interaction between the barriers to organizational change and the changes in market mechanisms and financial support for academic medicine. (For a discussion of the broad forces at play in managed care see Chapters 1, 2, and the Epilogue.)

Change in Market Mechanisms

Many feel that the multiple roles of AHCs make them noncompetitive in this changing environment. Excluding the direct cost of teaching, the average cost of care per AHC admission is $6,000 compared with $4,400 for nonteaching hospitals.[2] Because clinical activities under capitation become cost centers, managed care plans avoid contracting with teaching hospitals. The University HealthSystem Consortium (UHC), an alliance of 70 AHCs, studied the impact of managed care penetration and concentration on AHC hospitals. A UHC analysis showed that hospitals moving from a Stage 3 (provider consolidation) health care market to a Stage 4 (managed competition) health care market experienced a 7.2 percent decline in net hospital revenue per discharge.[3] Given that an average of 40 percent of medical school revenues are derived from professional and hospital services, academic funding is suffering considerably under these conditions.[4]

Many MCOs have used telephone calls and medical chart abstraction as a means to micromanage the delivery of care by providers. Recently these techniques have been replaced by a system of risk shifting that forces clinicians and hospitals to assume the responsibility for the costs of the care provided.[5] This risk pool-based system may change the activities of AHCs in two ways. First, referring clinicians that are at risk for the cost of patient care may not send patients to specialists of the AHC because they may be more costly. Second, AHCs are reviewing their financial, operational, and clinical processes to understand their costs and determine if they can continue to provide indirect support for clinical research from the limited reimbursements.

Another change in the market affecting AHCs is the shift in the types of institutions conducting industry-sponsored clinical research. In 1988 the pharmaceutical industry spent more on research and development than the entire National Institutes of Health budget, and these expenditures were 40 percent higher in 1994.[6] Before 1980 most industry-sponsored research was conducted at AHCs. Recently for-profit contract research organizations have played a major role in industry-sponsored research by conducting Phase I–III trials outside AHCs. Therefore, the use of AHCs in industry-sponsored research trials fell to 68 percent in 1993 from 82 percent in 1989. The loss of such valuable support for research has had a tremendous impact on the revenue and academic mission of many AHCs.

To respond to the threat of declining revenues and potential closure of academic medical centers, academic leaders must focus on the market mechanisms that create the environment in which they will operate. The paradigm shift in health care toward cost containment occurred in 1982, when prospective payment was introduced for Medicare. Although this did not control the growth of medical expenditures, a clear message was sent that the 20-year era of cost-plus medicine was over. However, real changes in cost containment occurred only with an increasing role of the purchasers of health care and the subsequent shift in financial risk allocation from these purchasers to insurers, providers, and patients.

Increasing Role of Purchasers

The importance of the purchasers, who bear the burden of health insurance premiums, cannot be overstated. The separation of the consumer (patient) from the provider by third-party payers (insurers) has removed the normal economic mechanism that controls utilization, namely cost to the consumer. The vast majority of Americans are sheltered from the direct cost of rising premiums because health care is a benefit funded either by their employer through pretax payroll deductions or by the taxpayer through Medicare and Medicaid.[7] Rampant medical inflation increased this responsibility immensely and forced these purchasers to be the most significant catalyst for the movement toward managed care.

Because the consumer is sheltered from the rising cost of health care premiums and the direct medical care costs, there is no market mechanism to control demand for health services and, in turn, total costs. Total medical expenditures depend on the product of the volume of services and the price for these services. Although discounted FFS and price controls in the form of diagnosis-related groups (DRGs) for hospitals slowed the rate of medical inflation for Medicare, true cost reduction in the absence of demand control requires a reduction in the volume of services provided. For years after DRGs were introduced, AHC revenues were not drastically threatened because physicians still controlled the flow of patients into the system and could therefore continue to generate volume in an atmosphere of price control. Intense use of services continued along with a shift toward FFS outpatient services.

Private industry, Medicare, and Medicaid are increasingly attracted to managed care.[8] Since 1990, HMO enrollment has increased by 85 percent. In 1996 the total number of HMO members grew by an estimated 8.4 million people, to 67.5 million—approximately one in four Americans.[9] In 1997 approximately 81 percent of employees of large firms were enrolled in managed care plans.[10] This was an increase from 65 percent in 1994.[11] In contrast, 18 percent of employees remain in FFS plans.[12] Even though this is an employer decision rather than a beneficiary preference, reports indicate a high level of patient satisfaction.[13] A study of consumers enrolled in HMOs nationwide found an increase in satisfaction with managed care rising from 56 percent in 1995 to 59 percent in 1997.[14] Many states have followed the example set by employers and now encourage managed care for Medicaid beneficiaries. From 1993 to 1998 the number of Medicaid recipients enrolled in Medicaid managed care plans more than tripled from 4.8 million to 16.5 million, while 14.3 million beneficiaries were enrolled in FFS.[15] (See Chapter 57 for a discussion of Medicaid and managed care.) Since the early 1980s, the Health Care Financing Administration (HCFA) has also encouraged HMO enrollment for Medicare beneficiaries. Although enrollment in HMO Medicare is growing at an annual rate of 12 percent, the projected growth, by 1994, was only 6 percent of the estimated 36 million beneficiaries.[16] (See Chapters 55 and 56 for a discussion of Medicare and managed care.)

Utilization control is the result of increasing purchaser involvement in cost containment. Purchasers have long noted regional variation in practice patterns as well as lower levels of spending per capita in other industrialized countries. As the level of medical inflation has continued to rise, purchasers have turned to managed care as a mechanism for removing "fat" from the current system. The government considered regulatory mechanisms and forms of universal health care used in other nations to control total expenditures. Instead, the private market concentrated on changing incentives from FFS that produced independent profit centers to managed care with annually capitated cost centers.[17] The result was minimal premium increases and some reductions by 1995.[18]

This distinct change from the previous culture of overutilization is the fundamental threat to the AHC. The decline in the utilization of high technology and other AHC services directly reduces revenues that have traditionally subsidized "unprofitable" or indirect activities, such as education, research, and unreimbursed patient care. Academic leaders must also recognize that eco-

nomics is not the only factor promoting managed care. Although health spending decreased by 1 percent for American industry in 1994, employers are not yet satisfied.[19] They want further information about quality and experience to improve their purchasing decisions. Purchasers and their beneficiaries are concerned with determining quality and appropriateness of care based on definable outcomes and physician accountability. MCOs are responsive to these needs, and the managed care culture supports deliberate evaluation of outcomes, accountability, utilization control, primary care, disease management, and integration of care for defined populations.[20] If viewed broadly as the integration of financing with the delivery of services, whether through capitation or a combination of financial mechanisms, managed care is seen by purchasers as essential for transforming medicine into an efficient, high-quality industry for the twenty-first century (see Chapter 42 for additional discussion of the topic of what employers want from managed care).

Shift in Financial Risk Allocation

The most important factor in the proper allocation of resources is the allocation of financial risk among patients, purchasers, insurers, and providers. When patients assume risk, they gain in the form of savings through demand control. When insurers and providers assume risk, profit is achieved by more efficient delivery of fewer services. Insurers are in the best position to assume risk for catastrophic conditions, whereas providers are in the best position to control utilization on a case-by-case basis.

Purchaser involvement led to utilization control by shifting financial risk to insurers and providers. The ideal strategy is to allocate financial risk to the party that is most able to manage utilization and outcomes effectively. Even though purchasers are the least able party to manage processes and outcomes, they assumed the greatest risk under a cost-plus FFS system in the form of ever-increasing insurance premiums or direct costs for self-insured businesses. Additionally, AHCs, like all providers, could profit from overutilization while passing along all costs resulting from inefficiencies. Under managed care, capitation allows for a fixed budget and transfers financial risk to insurers and providers. Future attempts to distribute more risk to employees through increased deductibles and copayments are likely.[21]

Change in Financial Support

Three interrelated factors directly threaten the support for the academic mission. First, employers are selecting health plans largely on the basis of cost because there is little information available about differences in quality.[22,23] The perceived superiority of care in AHCs no longer guarantees continued utilization or funding of their services. In effect, the focus on price by purchasers has transformed medicine into a commodity market. Second, with the failure of legislative health care reform in late 1993 (see Chapters 1 and 2), AHCs are facing the threat of diminishing revenues under managed care. Third, the loss of federal support, in the context of the purchaser shift toward a commodity view of health care, has led to the loss of financial support obtained from the clinical revenues of academic providers.

Medicine As a Commodity

Most types of insurance have traditionally acted as commodities in the market. Because commodities are usually indistinguishable, commodity businesses compete solely on price and cannot keep market share at prices above others in the marketplace. Conversely, health insurers, and especially Blue Cross/Blue Shield and indemnity plans (see Chapters 1 and 3), as well as providers such as AHCs, have enjoyed a noncommodity identity. In the past they could increase prices without losing market share. Profitable organizations were high-cost producers. The shift toward competition based solely on price suggests that medical care has transformed into a commodity in which the products offered are virtually indistinguishable. Reports indicate that patients are willing to change plans for a price differential as low as $5.00.[24] Unless services can be distinguished through measures of quality, AHCs must become

low-cost producers in order to survive in the current health care environment.

Studies have shown that the quality of care provided by MCOs is equal to or exceeds that provided by FFS plans.[25] Investigations have demonstrated that MCOs perform better in preventive care with a greater proportion of mammography,[26] prenatal care, and immunizations.[27] Even more important, these results are disseminated in the financial papers and general media, exposing purchasers to data suggesting that care provided to managed care enrollees is indistinguishable from that provided through traditional indemnity insurance.[28] Therefore, academic pursuits are not immune to economic forces, and the feeling of superior quality of care at AHCs cannot be taken for granted. Private insurers, Medicare, and Medicaid will not pay higher prices to support increased costs incurred by AHCs for teaching, research, and indigent care because such payments cannot be justified.[29]

Graduate Medical Education

The academic mission has been subsidized by an illogical process and through the improper allocation of society's resources. Public support for education, indigent care, and research has traditionally been hidden in Medicare payments as adjustments for graduate medical education (GME). To promote the training of physicians, Medicare assumed partial responsibility for the financing of GME. Initially, Medicare paid for these programs on a cost-reimbursement basis. However, with the enactment of the Consolidated Omnibus Budget Reconciliation Act of 1985, Medicare changed its medical education funding scheme into two types of payments: direct medical education (DME) and indirect medical education (IME) adjustments.[30]

Direct medical education payments cover the added direct costs of physician training, including salaries and fringe benefits for trainees, as well as faculty, classroom space, clerical staff, and a segment of the institution overhead.[31] The Medicare program has also made payments for the increased operating costs of AHC hospitals through the IME adjustment. The IME adjustment, covering the additional costs associated with the infrastructure of the academic setting and treating indigent patient populations, was factored into DRG payments to hospitals with resident training. However, there were two unanticipated results from these hidden indirect payments.

First, there was a dramatic rise in accredited programs for GME, increasing by 21 percent from 1983 to 1991.[32] Second, these hidden payments supported managed care profits. When HCFA targeted payments to MCOs at 95 percent of projected FFS levels as defined by geographic area, it included direct and indirect support for GME in these capitated payments. There was no obligation for MCOs to pass along these funds for educational activities.

In the past, private health plans indirectly contributed to GME by using AHC hospitals and paying them an increased rate for patient care. However, over time, as MCOs use more community hospitals and negotiate lower reimbursement rates with AHCs, this indirect GME funding has decreased.[33] The federal government has never supported undergraduate medical education, and the failure of health care reform eliminated assurances of continued support for GME. In conjunction with diminishing federal support, an avoidance of AHC services by purchasers and insurers resulting from the shift in belief that health care is a commodity leads to a divergence of the medical center and medical school goals.

Historically, medical schools and their associated teaching hospitals have prospered by supporting each other. The linkage of GME support to Medicare payments resulted in a mutual financial dependence between the medical school and academic providers. The academic hospital and its physicians gained surplus revenues for the teaching they provided in two ways. First, they benefited directly from inflated Medicare payments. Second, higher prices and volume were achieved from the perception that the "professor" is the expert and delivers the highest-quality care. In return, physicians and hospitals provided the medical school with financial support and a large, comprehensive patient base for students and residents.

In hopes to create more equitable GME funding streams, the 1997 Budget Reconciliation Act Agreement enacted significant changes to Medicare's assistance of GME funding. The agreement states:

1. DME and IME payments will be based on a rolling average of full-time equivalent residents on duty.
2. IME payments will be reduced by approximately 25 percent over five years.
3. Funding will be provided for training in nonhospital settings.
4. IME payments will be made directly to AHCs.
5. DME and IME payments to AHCs will be based on utilization by Medicare MCO enrollees.
6. Access to care for low-income persons will be provided.[34]

This new legislation represents substantial change for GME and sends a number of clear, striking messages to AHCs. The agreement caps the total number of positions in each AHC eligible for Medicare DME and IME, thus discouraging the expansion of residency programs.[35] There are incentives to encourage the downsizing of the number of trainees while maintaining primary care capacity. Training in ambulatory settings is encouraged, and MCOs will no longer receive GME payments unless they provide GME training.

With the introduction of managed care, divergent needs exist between academic providers and medical schools. Association with the medical school may no longer provide the hospital and faculty the benefit of increased payments through Medicare and increased referrals through reputation. As described earlier, lack of outcome measures showing better quality converts medicine to a commodity market based on price. Therefore, academic providers can no longer maintain higher prices. Conversely, the medical school benefits less from association with the hospital. The health care system of the future will not revolve around the hospital. The inpatient environment does not provide the education needed for the ambulatory, managed care setting. Instead of handling all aspects of care, hospitals will care only for those patients who cannot be cared for in other settings. With the changes in GME payments along with declining revenues, medical schools cannot rely on hospitals for continued financial support. In addition, the association of the medical school with the hospital will present a conflict of interest when attempting to increase the teaching patient base or find new sources of support by aligning with MCOs.

As hospitals and medical schools realign their goals for survival, common areas for continued collaboration will emerge. The paradigm shift suggests that the two need not remain linked.[36] Acting independently, they will be free to pursue alliances with other competing organizations. Unless the teaching hospital and academic faculty pursue a strategy that addresses proper training for managed care, the medical school needs to look at other venues for an appropriate teaching environment. Even with successful adaptation to managed care, hospitals alone cannot support the academic mission. The survival of AHCs to continue the pursuit of graduate education and research is dependent on academic leaders to be creative and find new means for funding and new partners.

Barriers to Organizational Change

The unique organizational and cultural structure of the traditional AHC is an impediment to adaptation to a competitive environment. Although the AHC has been tremendously successful under the FFS system, its present structure does not allow it to adapt to the rapid changes affecting the industry. The changes in market mechanisms and financial support provide an incredible challenge for the AHC. How can the AHC create a cultural and organizational structure that improves competitiveness, fosters education and research, contributes to efficient use of resources, and maintains a high level of technical quality? The traditional culture, based in physician autonomy, presents the strongest barrier to collaboration. A market in transition further prevents changes by providing conflicting incentives to providers. Finally, the current information structure, based in a billing function, does not allow for accurate determination of cost bases, processes, and outcomes for services and education.

Traditional Culture

The structure of the AHC is the product of a culture that fostered great clinical and technical advances over the last half century. This structure is based in a culture or system in which the physician is the focus. The hospital is the physician's workshop; the medical school is the physician's classroom. Autonomy of the individual physician results from revenue generation. In FFS the individual physician controls access, and therefore generates revenue for the AHC. Within the inpatient setting, specialists generating a large volume of services through procedures and hospital admissions have developed a great deal of power. This system defines the physician as the knowledgeable decision maker. However, individual autonomy is so important that bias and habits often replace true evidence-based decision making (see Chapter 33).

Because the culture of the AHC is centered on the individual physician, it revolves around the needs of the departments of various specialties. From the frustration that many feel in dealing with the divergent needs of different departments, these departments have often been described in a derogatory manner as "fiefdoms." This political entrenchment prevents beneficial change, and individual power struggles destroy the ability of the AHC to act in a rational, cohesive manner. Given that purchasers increasingly insist on cost-effectiveness, a culture that obstructs fundamental change may be the ultimate demise of the AHC. The present structure forms a bias against primary care, population focus, evidence-based decision making, and sound business principles. Most AHCs use a model of educating medical students and resident physicians that is oriented to the subspecialty dominated, university affiliated, and inpatient environments. Therefore, this educational setting is largely responsible for a physician work force in which less than 30 percent of physicians are primary care clinicians, such as family practitioners, general internists, or general pediatricians.[37]

The Transition Market

The profits of today are a barrier and threat to the profits of tomorrow. Continued revenue for individuals and autonomous departments, because of incomplete capitation and utilization control, obstruct attempts at changing the traditional culture of the AHC. With this dichotomy in place, the AHC remains a revenue center, while increasing capitation and its resulting shift in financial risk transform it to a cost center. The AHC still needs the individual physicians, in particular the specialists, to generate revenues in the current hybrid environment. Therefore, the needs for future viability of the AHC do not coincide with the needs for today's profitability. A transition market dictates that the timing of strategic actions takes on great importance. Additionally, change that precedes the arrival of fierce competition requires leadership that will alter the traditional culture by creating a common vision for those with a stake in the AHC.

Information Structure

The absence of information regarding clinical processes and cost structures is a significant barrier to effective competition. For the majority of physicians, current information systems perform a billing function and do not provide information about clinical processes and underlying cost structures. A few hospitals have internal cost accounting systems that can be used to evaluate physician practice patterns and overall institutional averages by diagnosis. However, these hospitals do not usually have this information available in a timely manner for immediate clinical use and feedback.

As AHCs assume increased financial risk and the economics begin to resemble a commodity market, internal cost and process accounting becomes necessary for success. Profit under capitation can occur only at the margin between revenues and costs of services provided, and only

the low-cost provider in a commodity market can profit because there is little price flexibility. This involves creating higher margins that result from cost controls and aggressive cost analysis. Information systems of the future must combine clinical resources such as guidelines and protocols with accurate cost data to manage process and outcome effectively.[38]

With improved information management, medical centers can withstand poor economic environments and strengthen their market positions by driving weaker competitors from the market. Problems in operations can be identified more easily as well. In addition, improved profit margin allows growth without debt and accumulation of funds for the academic mission. Management information systems and the use of data for medical management are discussed in Chapter 32.

STRATEGIES FOR SUCCESS

Attempts at uniformity and standardization aimed at reducing variability in treatment are a first step toward lowering costs within AHCs. As purchasers shift their focus from cost to value, the health care industry requires a new system or culture that promotes decentralized decision making and accountability to purchasers. Impediments to cooperation are especially strong from the physician perspective. Hospital administration has always depended on physicians to provide care for patients. Physicians, however, have not relied on outside parties for strategy, marketing, capital allocation, and cost structure. Success with cultural change in the AHC will depend more on effective leadership than traditional corporate management to create a clear mission and vision, foster cooperation and collaboration, and promote appropriate physician education.

Since managed care will ultimately limit the number and types of specialists and reduce hospital overcapacity, AHCs must alter their training and culture. Success will depend largely on leadership and its ability to find innovative ways to maintain a patient base, transform the traditional culture, and create new stakeholders in the academic mission. In addition, the AHC must reinvent education and research in the context of these strategies. Because the literature on this subject is largely anecdotal, a framework for potential solutions must be based on common trends in the industry. As a result of rapid changes in the industry, current information often comes from non–peer-reviewed journals and news sources.

Innovation and Leadership

Given the speed with which the market is evolving, successful strategies will not be known until they are tried and tested. Projects attempting to delineate strategies for dealing with educational funding have begun. The Council on Graduate Medical Education released its sixth report specifically dealing with the effect of managed care on the physician work force and medical education in 1995. The report recommended that with the rapid changes in the health care environment, AHCs and MCOs are encouraged to collaborate to produce physicians within the requisite numbers, specialty mix, and competencies to the current societal needs.[39] In addition, the council recommended that MCOs and all other third-party payers need to share in the cost of paying for medical education, through an all-payer fund, and by developing mechanisms to support and encourage training and evaluation of medical students and residents in their practice sites.

The University HealthSystem Consortium commissioned two task forces that conducted research in an attempt to identify effective organizational structures and models for the delivery of care in the evolving managed care environment. They determined that a quick and radical response to the eventual dominance of managed care and integrated delivery systems (IDSs; see Chapters 4 and 65) is needed to maintain the clinical income required to support the academic mission.[40] Although a complete review and analysis of this work are beyond the scope of this chapter, it is apparent that survival for the AHC will ultimately depend on innovation and a re-

sponsiveness to change within the marketplace.

Managed care is rooted in the notion that health care can be managed. Who makes up the management ranks in an AHC, and how do you manage highly skilled people in an information-oriented industry? Traditional management evolved from the industrialization of manufacturing. Before industrialization, craftsmen produced goods while educating apprentices, a process similar to medical education today. By simplifying production processes into small, definable tasks, less skilled workers could produce similar goods more efficiently. Labor became more interchangeable, simplification of the processes meant skilled labor was no longer required, and apprentices disappeared. Unfortunately, innovation and creativity were effectively removed from the labor force. In the end, thinking resided with management and anything but obedience by workers led to chaos in production.

The industrialization of medicine parallels that of manufacturing. In medicine there is a drive toward standardization with guidelines, protocols, and benchmarking. Standardization implies simplification and the need for less skilled labor. In addition, the lure of standardization is that the generalist will be able to replace the specialist without needing the same knowledge or experience. Medicine, however, is a complex, knowledge-dependent process. Although improved information capabilities foster the industrialization of medicine, they also require a different form of management.

Systems play an important role in defining management and producing outcomes. Traditional corporate culture has defined the manager as the knowledgeable decision maker while traditional medical culture has given this role to the physician. In the past, without experience or training in financial and managerial skills, physicians could "manage" medicine successfully, although inefficiently, because price and ultimately cost were unimportant. Today, in a commodity business, where aggressive cost control and differentiation are essential, management takes on greater importance. Similarly, managed care executives who have successfully capitalized on overcapacity, negotiating substantial price discounts, believe that they can "deskill," simplify, and control processes they cannot fully understand.

As with any imperative, the outcome is inevitable regardless of individual or group opposition. The market imperative for change created by the health care purchasers leads to the industrialization of medicine. Network formation is clearly necessary in the evolution of medical organizations. Network formation does not automatically lead to system improvement, however, and a primary care strategy for negotiating capitated contracts does not intrinsically lead to greater physician productivity and competitiveness (see Chapters 8 and 9). The ultimate challenge for the AHC will be what to do with networks once they are formed. Furthermore, what role will the primary care physician hold within a newly created system?

Innovative ways of maintaining the AHC patient base, and in turn clinical revenue, are a top priority. Strategies for integrating hospital, generalist, and specialist services into functional networks are essential for successful positioning in the marketplace. Concurrently, the creation and cultivation of stakeholders in the academic mission are of paramount importance to supplement revenues that cannot be maintained as a result of the changes in support for GME. Collaboration with new stakeholders can reinvent education and research in the academic environment. Although innovation is necessary for survival in the short run, anticipating change is essential for prosperity in the end.

Maintaining a Patient Base

Maintaining a patient base is fundamental for the financial survival of academic physicians and hospitals. For the university, it is mandatory for maintaining quality educational and training programs. As a result of the market forces discussed earlier, total inpatient and specialty service volume is declining as care shifts away from AHCs and toward less expensive settings. To remain profitable, AHCs must focus on gaining covered lives through risk sharing and capitated contracts as well as on sustaining their share of the remaining FFS market. In addition, in an environment of capitation, providers want and need more members than patients because most of the money in a capitated system comes from members of health plans who use few or inexpensive medical services. This issue is especially important for AHCs, which stand a greater than normal risk of adverse selection in an enrolled population (see Chapters 50 through 52 for detailed discussions of risk selection).

Consolidation between academic and nonacademic hospitals has occurred and the remaining institutions are in a stronger financial position. Furthermore, declining support for AHCs may lead to a reduction in the number of medical schools and residency programs, leaving the remaining institutions with potentially more funding. Current strategies for maintaining a patient base by an AHC rest upon network formation in combination with primary and specialty care strategies.

Network Formation

Maintaining clinical revenues requires satisfying the demands of health care purchasers for access, low cost, appropriate care, ease of contracting, and patient satisfaction. The marketplace response has been the formation of networks that can eventually serve as the backbone for IDSs. Positioning by insurers, hospitals, and AHCs to create service networks of primary care physicians and specialists has reached a rapid pace.[41] Blumenthal and Meyer describe the network formation strategy as involving "the development of integrated healthcare systems that are capable of providing a full range of health care services, hopefully at competitive prices."[42] This may involve the addition of physician practices, other hospitals, and ambulatory sites, and depends on the market demands, managed care pressure, leadership of the AHC, and the culture within the AHC. Shortell et al. demonstrated that there are similar expansion strategies for AHCs.[43] Although AHCs are building networks through diversification into home health care, nursing homes, and ambulatory units, the majority of AHCs placed their greatest emphasis on enlarging their primary care physician practice base.[44]

Networks provide access to geographic areas, reduce the cost of capital, and foster information systems development. Therefore, network formation is expected to increase market share and reduce operating costs. Networks are useful to AHCs in preserving the academic mission by educating primary care physicians and retraining specialists in a managed care environment.[45] Additionally, an IDS allows the creation of insurance products that can be marketed directly to purchasers. By integrating the financing and the delivery of care with networks, AHCs may become MCOs in their own right and may profit from greater risk sharing.

Large networks do not always equate with purchaser satisfaction, however. After encouraging market consolidation into three large HMOs, employers in Minnesota decided to negotiate contracts directly with smaller groups of physicians and hospitals. This move occurred for two simple reasons. First, the health plans were engaging in price wars instead of focusing on medical care. Second, employers and health plans wanted to get "out of the middle" between patients and their physicians.[46] This example gives providers such as AHCs an opportunity to develop networks that eliminate the "middleman." Yet, within any delivery system, care will continue to be influenced, if not managed, by parties other than individual physicians. Therefore, elimination of MCOs that have provided value through innovative management of care in combination with the creation of delivery systems may be shortsighted. This example reinforces that networks must satisfy purchasers by providing measurable quality care to patients.

AHCs can form primary care networks, hospital networks, or a combination. Primary care networks often require significant capital compared with hospital networks. Positioning in the marketplace can range from forming networks providing a full range of services for a capitated population to providing secondary and tertiary specialized services to other networks, employers, and insurers. These strategies are not mutually exclusive and will probably coexist in the future. A network can be created by acquisition of hospitals or physician practices, partnering with established MCOs, and undertaking joint ventures with local physician groups and community hospitals.[47] (See Chapter 4 for more discussion of these options.)

Primary Care Strategy

Current thinking stresses the importance of a primary care strategy for success in a market dominated by managed care. Whether loosely associated or acquired, physicians who will accept capitated payments for defined populations are the prerequisite for negotiating broader arrangements. The adoption of a primary care strategy by the AHC has other important benefits. Besides revenue generation through capitated payments, an environment is created within the academic setting for education and research in managed care.

Some options for gaining covered lives through primary care include purchasing existing practices, affiliating with existing practices or MCOs, or forming a teaching staff model HMO. Each option has different risks and rewards. For those AHCs with sufficient resources, acquisition of primary care practices is one possible strategy. The University of Pennsylvania Health System (UPHS) and Duke University have acquired practices in the areas of and surrounding Philadelphia and Duke respectively.[48] Using operating income from its profitable teaching hospital, the University of Pennsylvania has already acquired 150 of the planned 300 community-based, physician practices.[49] This capital-intensive strategy is anticipated to cost $100 million.[50] The university is not competing directly with insurers but is providing a full range of services to MCOs in the area. In addition to the University of Pennsylvania, the Allegheny Health System, in Philadelphia and Western Pennsylvania, employed the strategy of primary care practice acquisition.

However, it appears that the primary care acquisition strategy is not a financially successful means to increase and maintain covered patient lives. The Allegheny Health System is now nearly defunct. The system's Philadelphia-area hospitals are bankrupt and were sold in November 1998 to a for-profit hospital firm, Tenet

Healthcare Corporation. It appears that the University of Pennsylvania is not immune to the financial woes of primary care acquisition. In a sign of the deepening pressures on AHCs, the UPHS announced in May 1999 that it was decreasing its total health care workforce by 9 percent. Then, in July of that same year, UPHS hired a consulting firm known for slashing jobs and reshaping hospitals. This marked another ominous sign of financial difficulty for one of the largest health care institutions in the Philadelphia area.

Another option for obtaining covered lives is forming an alliance with a partner that has resources available for physician acquisition. Tulane lacked the necessary funds to build its own physician network; therefore it sold 80 percent interest in its hospitals to Columbia/HCA.[51] However, few AHCs may desire giving up their autonomy in such a situation.

Unlike the University of Pennsylvania's strategy of acquisition, Thomas Jefferson University Hospital and Mainline Health System, of the Philadelphia metropolitan area, created the Jefferson Health System using a collaborative strategy.[52] This is a less expensive strategy for affiliating with generalists who can eventually assume risk for defined populations. However, there is no evidence to date that using this collaborative strategy of an IDS is a more successful approach for obtaining covered lives. Another approach might consist of collaboration with a strong MCO and taking a role as its sole provider. By reducing the fixed cost per covered life and avoiding the complexity of managing primary care, the risk created by building the infrastructure needed for primary care is avoided.

There are a few caveats when forming a primary care strategy. First, primary care providers cannot be used as a mechanism to provide patients for continued specialty and tertiary care. This will continue to encourage overutilization, raising premiums for insurers and purchasers and resulting in poor competitiveness.

Second, the AHC must attract healthy members to profit on capitated contracts. Converting the present patient population to a risk contract will be financially dangerous if the patients are an older or sicker group. Excellence in well baby care, sports injuries, and general obstetrics and gynecology may attract younger and healthier enrollees.[53] A focus on the ability to treat complex cases may be a disadvantage, leading to adverse risk selection by patients requiring access to costly tertiary care.

Third, the AHC must recognize that the immediate importance of primary care physicians in network formation is gaining covered lives. Competitiveness based on expected reductions in specialist use or improved population health through preventive care will depend on primary care physicians of the future.[54] Although health care expenditures for American industry decreased in 1994, it is unclear whether managed care as it exists today lowers overall costs or just allows a selection bias, reducing the proportion of sick and elderly in these plans.[55] There is no doubt that fierce competition leads to lower prices. Continued price reductions based on real changes in the delivery of health services, however, will depend on increased physician productivity created with a combination of system improvements and innovative physician training.

Specialty Strategy

The role of the specialist in managed care and network formation is a more challenging issue. FFS, global packaging, and capitation arrangements will probably remain in varying combinations. Further growth of managed care is expected to lead to continued decreases in the use of specialty and tertiary services. To maintain current levels of specialist revenue, AHCs need to serve larger populations. The number of managed care enrollees needed to support current levels within any particular AHC would differ depending on whether the AHC provides all the specialty services needed by a defined HMO population or only a portion of referral services for the members of various managed care plans. Furthermore, the number of enrollees needed to support revenues varies widely among specialties.[56] Examples of such numbers can be found in Chapter 11.

Options for specialist providers include broader than normal geographical linkages with community providers and insurers as well as increased referrals within their primary service areas. A reliance on referrals from community physicians to teaching hospitals is not viable as the market moves increasingly toward managed care.[57] Primary care cannot be viewed as a means to support specialist and tertiary services, and a specialty strategy should be structured to support market needs for such services. AHCs must recognize that, although the current goal of MCOs is to reduce specialty use, elimination is impossible. The goal is the elimination of inappropriate utilization. Although fewer high-priced specialists will be needed, this area can continue to provide a large portion of revenue for the AHC. It is possible that AHCs will have a long-run competitive advantage in situations requiring complex care or the use of new technology for chronic, difficult-to-manage conditions. Real differences would allow lower per member per month premiums for covered lives within AHC integrated networks. In addition, consolidation among AHCs may parallel consolidation of specialty services. The remaining providers will be a combination of low-cost providers and providers of excellence who can demonstrate superior results at a reasonable premium. This may allow the expansion of local and broader referral bases. Arbitrary designations as "centers of excellence" in the absence of superior results, however, will require aggressive marketing in an attempt to differentiate services from the competition.

The battle between producing services within the organization or network versus subcontracting to providers that are more efficient is a fundamental challenge to all organizations within managed care. Therefore, centers of excellence and integrated networks are not mutually exclusive. Outsourcing often allows more efficiency and less risk for organizations. If the AHC can package specialty and tertiary care for a price below the marginal cost for other networks and MCOs, it can create revenues outside of its own capitated contracts. This requires aggressive tertiary marketing that segments and satisfies different customer needs. Unfortunately, adverse risk selection to plans offering these services may eliminate AHC competitive advantage and

make these services unappealing to other organizations. Therefore, centers of excellence may exist only for a minority of complex cases or procedures such as transplantation.[58]

Transforming the Traditional Culture

AHCs must compete with service-oriented community providers to survive. Clearly, the clinical faculty must offer price-competitive and user-friendly services. Clinical training needs to focus on more relevant and emerging practice situations. Finally, the AHC must delineate funding streams and identify cross-subsidies taking place among teaching, research, and patient care enterprises. This can strengthen clinical training and the financial positions of the AHC and faculty.[59] Leadership is essential for overcoming the barriers to such organizational changes. By stressing the inevitability of managed care, academic leaders can use market imperatives to begin the process toward transforming the traditional culture. The system must encourage centralized capital allocation and information management in the context of flexible, decentralized delivery of care. Focusing attention on accountability to purchasers for the cost and quality of care is an important first mechanism for fostering cooperation within the AHC. Next, managing outcomes through information and aligning incentives can promote a common vision within the AHC. New organizational structures will depend on functional production rather than departmental orientation, and the traditional risk-averse culture must evolve to take financial risk. Ultimately, though, the challenge for academic leaders is to prepare for the inevitable external jolt of fierce competition that can unite powerful internal interest groups and successfully guide their institutions to a competitive position.[60]

Accountability

Although the traditional academic culture based on physician autonomy presents a barrier to collaboration, the threat of extinction will be the ultimate catalyst forcing cooperation. The need for provider accountability to purchasers is one market imperative for change within the AHC. As Millenson states, "A company can set performance standards for a health plan and demand that it hold doctors and hospitals accountable for those standards. A number of leading employers are starting to demand quality report cards from health plans...."[61] Normal market mechanisms always make the seller accountable to the buyer, but the presence of third-party payers and purchasers has altered these normal market forces and eliminated provider accountability. By altering the physician's ability to control the stream of revenues, managed care has taken the once autonomous physician and made him or her accountable to the market. Interference in autonomy through imposed practice guidelines and utilization review is a function of providers' past unwillingness to be accountable for the resources they use. Physician accountability assumes that individual physicians determine outcomes, and the question of whether provider accountability and autonomy are mutually exclusive is left to be determined.

Providers assume that, by engaging in risk contracts, they may retain their autonomy while becoming accountable to the consumer. Problems defined in terms of individual physicians, however, often lead to inappropriate solutions. Therefore, defining the challenges faced by AHCs as a function of systems as opposed to individuals implicitly alters the culture. Essentially, good people can have bad results depending on the system in which they operate. This was clearly demonstrated in the 1994 cardiac surgery report cards released in New York state.[62] As a result of a poor report card, a system flaw was found and corrected at one hospital in the study. Yet ranking this particular surgeon last implied that the problem was with the individual physician.

As the New York report card indicates, defining the problem in terms of individuals is too simplistic. The assumption of financial risk under capitation by individuals creates accountability for outcomes that may depend on institutional structures or societal issues, such as violence, pollution, lifestyle, diet, alcohol, tobacco, and illicit drug use. By emphasizing the need for group accountability, a common goal is created, and a cultural shift that embraces managed care can begin.

Information Sharing and Outcomes

Response to external pressure for proof of value by purchasers is another market imperative for cooperation within the AHC. Employers want information about value based on measures of cost and quality. AHCs have always claimed superior results. Now they must be able to document these results to justify higher fees for their services. Current information systems perform a billing function and do not provide information about clinical processes and their underlying cost structures. As AHCs assume increased financial risk and the economics of the health care system more resemble those of a commodity market, information about internal cost and process becomes necessary for success. Information systems of the future must combine clinical and financial data to manage process and outcome effectively.[63]

The 1994 report cards released for cardiac surgery in New York again provide insight into the motivation for cooperation. Because the results suggested problems with individual physicians, purchasers may view report cards as a mechanism to improve care by eliminating poorly performing physicians. The usual argument against the use of such information is that it is not statistically significant for the individual physician and low-volume providers. This fact will not end requests for better outcomes measurements. Although providers will continue to block the release of outcomes data because they fear that the results may be misleading to the public, the marketplace will prevail. Successful integration provides statistically significant samples from which outcomes can be measured. Good results will promote increased market share for providers who are willing to cooperate.

Besides creating valid report cards, linking process to outcomes improves quality and controls costs. There is tremendous variation in the clinical and economic performance of individual providers.[64] Continuous internal evaluation involves separating practice bias and habits from truly effective clinical principles. Ideally, there is a method to promote the best health possible for each individual patient. Medicine, once impervious to standardization because of its complexity, can benefit from application of newer information techniques. The process of identifying best practices is a result of normal industrialization. Although clinical intuition cannot be ignored, a database that knows how 100,000 patients responded to a particular treatment compares favorably with a physician who has seen 100 patients. The initial step toward coordinating efforts at creating clinical pathways and practice protocols depends on elucidation of unexplained clinical variability that increases costs without improving outcomes. Information management using clinical pathways can determine the best of a multitude of alternatives. Using these breakthroughs in information technology and statistics, "complex calculations incorporating the clinical variability that physicians have struggled with for centuries" may provide the ability to determine best practices.[65] In the ideal, one clinical approach will be better, more cost effective, and less risky than another. When raw data are transformed into comparative clinical information, the decision process, management structure, and processes of the institution transform as well.

Many MCOs are using information with traditional management techniques that control, instead of improve, processes. Although the technology to examine complex variables in care exists, the information gained is only as good as the data used and the people who interpret them. Real gains in productivity will result from greater provider use of information in managing processes and outcomes rather than standardization and managerial control.[66] Protocols should be viewed as a way of gaining feedback to improve quality. By evaluating the current processes and adjusting practice patterns to align with cost containment and quality goals, overall value can be optimized. Information transforms opinion and clinical bias into the rational weighing of alternatives. Information also shifts control of process to the point of service.

AHCs cannot rely on MCOs for information. Controlling data is strategically important and operationally essential. Fundamentally, it is an important core competence regardless of strategy. There is evidence to show that, as MCOs become more sophisticated with information management, they are less likely to share financial risks and rewards with providers. Since they profit from retaining financial risk and controlling utilization, decapitation occurs because MCOs often choose discounted FFS options over global packaging and capitation.[67] Aggressive utilization management with a per diem fee schedule in lieu of capitation allows an MCO to retain the financial benefits of lowered utilization. MCOs may also fear that shifting financial risk to providers eliminates their major function as insurers. Once at risk, providers can obtain their own licenses, bypass MCOs, and contract directly with purchasers. With or without capitation, information management using efficient systems and meticulous records is vital for continuous internal evaluation within the AHC. Academic leaders must stress that technological and information demands have become too complex and require a collaborative framework between the medical staff and hospital administration.

Reinventing Education and Research with New Stakeholders

Since hospitals and medical schools do not know the true costs of their activities, there is disagreement as to whether residents are a burden providing inefficient care or an inexpensive source of highly trained labor. One health care plan has estimated that residents' training requires 20–25 percent more space, 20–25 percent more personnel than would be needed otherwise, and residents reduce productivity by 25–33 percent.[68] However, the expense of teaching is viewed as proportional to residents' experience, with the health plan losing money on a first-year resident, breaking even the second year, and generating a surplus in the third. Clearly, residents enhance productivity after an initial learning period. Residents are less effective as substitutes for ambulatory care, and there is pressure to keep them in the hospital, where low cost and high skill allow a competitive advantage.[69] But is it ethical to train people for jobs that will not exist?

Education must parallel, and prepare students for, the work force as it is, not as it has been. Because the current trend is toward ambulatory and primary care, physicians must be trained with these skills and in these settings. Effective management should lead to improved education. Controlling the desire to use all available technology requires more oversight and teaching on the part of faculty. Although current educational efforts are based on advancement of medical knowledge, future education will include a focus on efficient and effective delivery of quality care.

The introduction of managed care has created divergent needs between academic providers and medical schools. Although alterations in the culture of the AHC may lead to improved financial strength and an improved patient base, the real cost of education and research may place an insurmountable burden on clinical support for these activities. Tulane University sold 80 percent of its hospital to Columbia/HCA Hospital Corporation while continuing to channel its 20 percent share of the profits to support the academic mission.[70] Meeting the challenges created by managed care involves reconciling the academic mission with the demands of the marketplace. In addition, communication of the importance of the academic mission by academic leaders can foster the creation and cultivation of new stakeholders with an interest in the educational and research value provided by the AHC.

The traditional sources for support of GME—clinical activities of the medical center and the federal government—will remain important. With the creation of Medicare, the federal government has supported GME, and it is likely that this support will continue in some form. As seen in the 1997 Budget Reconciliation Act Agreement, there is heavy political negotiation of the proper allocation of resources for medical education funding. AHCs can gain public support for endeavors that promote the public good, but not as a proxy to continue inefficiencies. In light of the recent changes in GME support, AHCs need to formulate a GME strategy that is responsive to the organization's mission and recognizes future GME financing challenges.

In a recent experience, one AHC recognized that the development of an effective, institution-wide GME strategy would involve:

- analysis of the current status of the institution's GME programs
- assessment of the financial impact of the 1997 Balanced Budget Act on the AHC
- development of criteria by which the GME programs could be assessed
- formulation of a GME strategy specific to the institution's needs[71]

However, the authors caution that each AHC's GME strategy will be different, but it is important for institutes to develop such strategies so they may better face the challenges of the future.

State-based experiments to develop new strategies for GME funding are increasing. In February 1997, HCFA announced a Medicare GME demonstration project in New York state. Under this demonstration project, New York state teaching hospitals that agreed to downsize their residency programs over the next five years would have their GME payments reduced more slowly than the actual cuts in residency positions.[72] To participate in the project, teaching hospitals had to agree to decrease residency positions by 25 percent or by 20 percent if they agree to increase the number of general clinician positions. It is anticipated that this project will save $300 million in Medicare GME payments over five years.[73]

This project complements changes made in the 1996 New York State GME policies. The total payments for GME were decreased from $1.8 to $1.4 billion. In addition, a $54 million pool was created to provide financial inducements for decreasing the number of trainees and increasing training in primary care disciplines, ambulatory sites, and underserved areas.[74] However, as of the writing of this chapter, no AHCs in New York state have agreed to downsize their residency programs as outlined in the demonstration project. This lack of action reflects the AHCs' naïveté of the seriousness of the GME funding issues. Academic health centers need to demonstrate their willingness and ability to respond to change in order to successfully help lead the reformation of GME funding.

With these recent changes, AHCs need to promote discussions of public policy issues, such as undergraduate and GME, research funding, and care for the indigent.[75] In addition, federal action will be extremely important to help ensure that hospitals and physicians in the academic setting are properly reimbursed for cases that are more complex. However, AHCs must be able to prove that their patient population has greater needs that require additional support.

Support from clinical operations will also continue. Systems that remain fully integrated with the university can profit from and support the academic mission only if education is also fully integrated and adds value to the system. This may be the crux of reinventing education. Academic providers may find that association with the medical school helps recruit and retain top physicians.[76] Therefore, the institution will have an opportunity to select and recruit the best and brightest before its competition.

In an effort to bring the AHC and managed care cultures together, in July 1996 the Pew Charitable Trusts awarded a three-year, $8.3 million grant to Harvard Pilgrim Health Care (HPHC) to oversee the Partnerships for Quality Education (PQE) project.[77] This initiative was part of a decade-long commitment and was designed to encourage joint ventures between AHCs and MCOs in the development and implementation of innovative models for training physicians to provide quality, cost-effective, managed care. It is hoped that the partnerships created through this initiative will produce new models for jointly developed curricula, new methods for training community-based physicians as preceptors and faculty, and innovative models for shared governance and allocation of resources between partners.

At the center of the initiative were eight medical school-managed care collaborations.[78] The six selected partnerships included HPHC with Harvard Medical School; Henry Ford Health System with Case Western Reserve University School of Medicine; Tufts Managed Care Institute; Cornell University Medical College and New York Hospital with Empire BlueCross BlueShield (BCBS); Georgetown University

Medical Center with Kaiser Permanente; and the Legacy Health System with Regence BCBS of Oregon and the Northwest Group. Each of the six partnerships received between $450,000 and $1.2 million to create initiatives aimed at improving training in managed care and encouraging education and research relationships. In addition, two additional partnerships, the University of Pennsylvania with Independence Blue Cross and the Lovelace Health System with the University of New Mexico School of Medicine, were selected to be associate partners. In addition to funding eight partnerships, the PQE project supported a number of collaborative projects as well.

This timely initiative between AHCs and MCOs offered medical education at least three benefits:

1. encourage a broader educational focus than that offered by traditional FFS sites
2. permit medical students and residents to gain real-world experience in settings similar to those they will encounter in the future
3. enhance the medical students' and residents' awareness of the need to measure quality and outcomes of care[79]

Realizing these potential benefits, Harvard Medical School and HPHC collaboratively founded the medical school's new Department of Ambulatory Care and Prevention, based at HPHC.[80] This was the first medical school department to be based in a free-standing HMO, turning the teaching hospital structure into a "teaching HMO" that created a practice setting for education and research in a managed care environment.[81] This teaching HMO laid the groundwork for Harvard's medical students to perform clerkships within an ambulatory care, managed care, setting. The three-year PQE project is complete; however, a PQE II initiative has been established to continue the mission and vision of the original program.

With the changes in health care, besides developing new strategies for training physicians for the ambulatory, managed care environment, AHCs need to engage in the revision of their organizational structures and operational practices.[82] Within many AHCs there are health policy centers that have the knowledge and expertise to assist with this effort. Many health policy centers are involved to some degree in areas such as medical school curriculum development, clinical practice guidelines, and the use of physician report cards—areas that are drivers of the changes in today's health care environment.[83]

Aside from government and clinical subsidies, the most likely stakeholders in the academic mission are MCOs, pharmaceutical manufacturers, and medical device companies. By providing new avenues for income and investment, new stakeholders reduce university reliance on clinical and federal funds. With joint ventures, universities are already forming relationships with other stakeholders in the academic mission. Collaboration with these new organizations gives industry access to academic experience and resources. For example, Duke University has formed a business unit called the Duke Clinical Research Center. It competes directly with private companies that perform clinical trials for drug and medical device companies. Other ventures will promote the development of information tools that improve the quality and cost-effectiveness of care.[84]

A NEW ROLE FOR MCOs

Few MCOs have formal relationships with AHCs other than through contracts for tertiary services. First, MCOs find that it is difficult to provide the cost-effective care needed to survive under the influence of the needs and culture of teaching hospitals.[85] This is especially true because MCOs seek to limit specialist use, while the traditional academic culture encourages its use. Second, university medical centers in urban areas offer few services that are not available in community hospitals and from specialists in private practice.[86] A change in the AHC culture is important to overcome barriers to collaboration with outside MCOs. It is also clear, however, that MCOs will need to embrace the advantages of supporting academic endeavors. As the chief executive officer of a major insurer commented,

"We recognize that AHCs have educational costs. We just aren't going to pay for them."[87]

Nevertheless, there are powerful reasons for MCOs to collaborate with AHCs. Simply put, education and research will become more critical in transforming managed care and medicine in the future. The major benefits from managed care have come through macro-management, which has reinvented the financing of health services. The resulting change in financial incentives has promoted a population-based, cost-effective perspective that rests with defining appropriate care. In response, provider organizations are adopting management techniques that were previously used only by insurers.[88] Innovation in the future, however, will increasingly depend on micro-management of the delivery of care. Reports of increasing physician management of care at the clinical level represent a fundamental transformation in the practice of medicine.

Undoubtedly, MCOs and providers will struggle in defining their respective roles in decision making. This is a fundamental conflict between management and labor in highly technical, specialized service industries. Given the importance of knowledge in today's information society, however, the power of implementation ultimately lies with the service provider.[89] The role of capital assets in the delivery of services will continue to diminish. At the same time, labor's transformation from an expense to an asset requires a dedicated investment.[90]

Consequently, provider education and training are important in creating value for managed care. The quality of primary care graduates is already a concern to MCOs that employ them, and shortages of primary care physicians have been reported as a limiting factor in the growth rates of staff and group model HMOs in particular.[91] An unwillingness to support education could have deleterious long-term effects for MCOs. Without new financial supporters, current educators could dramatically decrease the training of their competition, ultimately raising expenses for MCOs. Partnerships with medical centers will allow greater input into the training needs of an MCO and ensure an adequate supply of well-trained physicians. This is not an abstract concept; as private practices affiliate or merge, the ability of an MCO to purchase practices or to contract with existing groups becomes more difficult. If an MCO has an established and good relationship with an AHC that is training the types of physicians most attractive to the MCO, then recruiting becomes easier.

Next, the growth of managed care has highlighted the need for outcomes research while simultaneously diminishing the funds available. The philosophy of managed care emphasizes appropriate care based on outcomes analysis. Yet (with some exceptions) MCOs do not support research in this area.[92] In an effort to promote research within MCOs, the Agency for Health Care Research and Quality (AHRQ) has cosponsored the HMO Research Network. The AHRQ is the lead federal agency charged with supporting and performing health services research. The HMO network is comprised of researchers working in HMO research centers at 11 sites. One of the principal aims of the HMO network is to create opportunities for HMO researchers to collaborate on multisite research projects.

The fight for survival may provide the impetus for innovative management techniques within successful AHCs. Through association with medical centers, MCOs can benefit from continued improvements that result from systematic research on best practices and outcomes measurements. Furthermore, as MCOs have increasing responsibility for older and sicker populations, they will require further advances in basic and clinical resources.[93] Many AHCs have extensive experience with complex cases, Medicare populations, and indigent populations, which are becoming a greater source of revenue for MCOs. The AHC provides a legitimate source for research into health service delivery, with dissemination of literature that influences the definition of medically acceptable and appropriate care.

Examples of support for the academic mission by MCOs appear regularly. A collaborative investigation evaluating the outcomes of migraineurs among an MCO, GlaxoWellcome, Inc., and Office of Health Policy and Clinical Outcomes at Thomas Jefferson University proved to be a successful relationship that supported the academic mission of the AHC.[94] This collaboration allowed an AHC to perform research using real-world population-based data while the MCO was able to determine ways to improve care for its patients with migraine. A joint research venture between the Fallon Healthcare System and the University of Massachusetts Medical Center showed that research between MCOs and AHCs can prove mutually beneficial.[95]

Despite long-term benefits for the support of AHCs by MCOs, fierce price competition may leave little excess revenue for such direct support. The collaboration between Sanus Health Systems, a subsidiary of New York Life Insurance, and Duke University Medical Center goes beyond direct support for the academic mission and transforms the relationship between MCOs and AHCs from contractor and contracted to equal partners. The new health management and benefits company, WellPath Community Health Plans Holdings, splits ownership and decision making between the two organizations. Sanus sees this partnership as an opportunity to take advantage of the excellent relationships already established between the AHC and hospitals and physicians in the community. However, the success of the venture focuses on effective community-based care and is not a mechanism for steering patients to Duke for specialized care. Contracts will be created with other hospitals, including other tertiary care centers.[96] MCOs interested in creative approaches to contracting with AHCs must recognize the importance of shared ownership and decision making with academic centers and providers.

In addition to the above, many MCOs have developed attractive primary care networks and affiliations with community hospitals. An MCO, newly entering the market or entering a new line of business, such as Medicare or Medicaid, may find contracting with the AHC and its network an efficient means of getting into the market. In addition, negotiating a global capitation (with stop-loss protection) is an equally efficient way to attenuate the risk for health care costs. As AHCs learn more about health care resource management, they are more willing to accept that level of risk, especially in partnership with an MCO that can provide the data and support necessary for the AHC to succeed.

CONCLUSION

The threat to the traditional financing of the academic mission by the spread of managed care presents many serious challenges for AHCs. This is an incredibly turbulent time within health care for the AHC. Change is rippling through the health care system, and no individual or institution is immune to its effects. Within the last three years the academic medical community has seen the bankruptcy of an AHC in Philadelphia, an initiative to encourage the development of innovative models for physician training, and significant federal legislation restructuring the allocation of GME funding. However, opportunities exist for improved patient care amid all the physician doom and gloom. Individuals with a stake in this mission need to respond to the challenges outlined in this chapter. Academic health centers must accept and face these challenges now if they are to remain the centerpiece of American medicine.

REFERENCES AND NOTES

1. J.K. Iglehart, Rapid Changes for Academic Medical Centers: Second of Two Parts, *New England Journal of Medicine* 332 (1995): 407.

2. J.K. Iglehart, Rapid Changes for Academic Medical Centers: First of Two Parts, *New England Journal of Medicine* 331 (1994): 1391–95.

3. D.A. Burnett, Evolving Market Will Change Clinical Research, *Health Affairs* 15 (1996): 90–92.

4. University Hospital Consortium, Responding to a Dynamic Health Care Marketplace: Implementation Strategies for Academic Health Centers. Paper presented at the University Hospital Consortium 1995 Research Conference, St. Petersburg, FL, February 2–3, 1995.

5. Burnett, Evolving Market Will Change Clinical Research.

6. Ibid.

7. Office of National Cost Estimates, Health Care Financing Administration, *1991–1992 Hospital Fact Book* (Sacramento, CA: California Association of Hospitals and Health Systems, 1992).

8. R.S. Brown et al., *Does Managed Care Work for Medicare? An Evaluation of the Medicare Risk Program for HMOs* (Princeton, NJ: Mathematica Policy Research, Inc., 1993); D.G. Clement et al., Access and Outcomes of Elderly Patients Enrolled in Managed Care, *JAMA* 271 (1994): 1487–92; and Managing Medicaid, *American Medical News* (December 19, 1994): 11.

9. Managed Care Facts: American Association of Health Plans, January 1998.

10. Ibid.

11. University Hospital Consortium, Responding to a Dynamic Health Care Marketplace.

12. Managed Care Facts: American Association of Health Plans.

13. J.P. Kassirer, Academic Medical Centers under Siege, *New England Journal of Medicine* 331 (1995): 1370–71.

14. CareData of New York, Health Market Survey, September 29, 1997.

15. National Summary of Medicaid Managed Care Programs and Enrollment, Health Care Financing Administration, 1998, *www.hcfa.gov/medicaid/trends98.htm*.

16. HMOs Are Changing the Face of Medicine, *New York Times* (January 11, 1995): A1.

17. U.E. Reinhardt, The Bounty Hunters, *Imaging Economics* (July/August 1995): 9–10.

18. A.J. Slomski, Employers to Doctors: It's Time for REAL Savings, *Medical Economics* (August 1995): 34–48.

19. Reinhardt, The Bounty Hunters.

20. University Hospital Consortium, Responding to a Dynamic Health Care Marketplace.

21. A.J. Slomski, Employers to Doctors—Demand Management: A "New" Strategy To Solve Our Health Care Ills, *Managed Care Update* (July 1995): 3–10.

22. Reinhardt, The Bounty Hunters.

23. Managed Care Maelstrom, *American Medical News* (July 25, 1994): 1.

24. University Hospital Consortium, Responding to a Dynamic Health Care Marketplace.

25. R. Miller and H. Luft, Does Managed Care Lead to Better or Worse Quality of Care? *Health Affairs* 16 (1997): 7–25; R. Miller and H. Luft, Managed Care Plan Performance since 1980: A Literature Analysis, *JAMA* 271 (1994): 1512–19.

26. L. Nelson, *Health Affairs* (March–April 1997).

27. The State of Managed Care Quality, National Committee on Quality Assurance 1999, *www.ncqa.org/docs/*reports/somcq2.*doc*

28. Large Study Finds Certain Patients Fare as Well in HMOs as in Insurance Plans, *Wall Street Journal* (November 8, 1995): B13.

29. R.A. Culbertson, How Successfully Can Academic Faculty Practices Compete in Developing Managed Care Markets? *Academic Medicine* 71 (1996): 858–70; M.R. Gold, Effects of the Growth of Managed Care on Academic Medical Centers and Graduate Medical Education, *Academic Medicine* 71 (1996): 828–38.

30. J.Q. Young, Overview of Graduate Medical Education: Funding Streams, Policy Problems, and Options for Reform, *Western Journal of Medicine* 168 (1998): 428–36.

31. J.R. Boex, Factors Contributing to the Variability of Direct Costs for Graduate Medical Education in Teaching Hospitals, *Academic Medicine* 67, no. 2 (1992): 80–84.

32. University Hospital Consortium, Responding to a Dynamic Health Care Marketplace.

33. Young, Overview of Graduate Medical Education.

34. Ibid.

35. Ibid.; J.L. Wray and S.M. Sadowski, Defining Hospitals' GME Strategy in Response to New Financial and Market Challenges, *Academic Medicine* 73, no. 4 (1998): 370–79.

36. K. Pallarito, New York's Academic Medicine Goes Ape, *Modern Healthcare* (August 28, 1995): 34–41.

37. M.R. Weitekamp and J.T. Ziegenfuss, Academic Health Centers and HMOs: A Systems Perspective on Collaboration in Training Generalist Physicians and Advancing Mutual Interests, *Academic Medicine* 70 (1995): S47–53.

38. S.R. Craig, Practicing Medicine under Capitation: One Group's Experience, *Internist* (May 1995): 8–9.

39. Council on Graduate Medical Education, sixth report, September 1995.

40. University Hospital Consortium, Responding to a Dynamic Health Care Marketplace.

41. Iglehart, Rapid Changes for Academic Medical Centers: Second of Two Parts; J.K. Iglehart, Academic Medical Centers Enter the Market: The Case of Philadelphia, *New England Journal of Medicine* 333 (1995): 1019–1023.

42. D. Blumenthal and G.S. Meyer, Academic Health Centers in a Changing Environment, *Health Affairs* 15 (1996): 200–15.

43. S.M. Shortell, R.R. Giles, D.A. Anderson, K.M. Erickson, and J.B. Mitchell, *Remaking Health Care in America: Building Organized Delivery Systems* (San Francisco: Jossey-Bass, 1996).

44. Blumenthal and Meyer, Academic Health Centers in a Changing Environment.

45. University Hospital Consortium, Responding to a Dynamic Health Care Marketplace.

46. Employer Groups Rethink Commitment to Big HMOs, *Wall Street Journal* (July 21, 1995): B1.

47. University Hospital Consortium, Responding to a Dynamic Health Care Marketplace.

48. Iglehart, Academic Medical Centers Enter the Market: The Case of Philadelphia.

49. Iglehart, Rapid Changes for Academic Medical Centers: Second of Two Parts.

50. Iglehart, Academic Medical Centers Enter the Market: The Case of Philadelphia.

51. Academic Centers—and GME—Face Growing Market Pressure, *American Medical News* (September 18, 1995): 1.

52. Iglehart, Academic Medical Centers Enter the Market: The Case of Philadelphia.

53. Craig, Practicing Medicine under Capitation.

54. B. Starfield, Is Primary Care Essential? *Lancet* 344 (1994): 1129–33.

55. Brown et al., *Does Managed Care Work for Medicare?*

56. J.E. Billi et al., Potential Effects of Managed Care on Specialty Practice at a University Medical Center, *New England Journal of Medicine* 333 (1995): 979–83.

57. Iglehart, Academic Medical Centers Enter the Market: The Case of Philadelphia.

58. University Hospital Consortium, Responding to a Dynamic Health Care Marketplace.

59. J.E. Kralewski et al., Can Academic Medical Centers Compete in a Managed Care System? *Academic Medicine* 70 (1995): 867–72.

60. Ibid.

61. M.L. Millenson, *Demanding Medical Excellence: Doctors & Accountability in the Information Age* (Chicago: University of Chicago Press, 1997).

62. Death-Rate Rankings Shake New York Cardiac Surgeons, *New York Times* (September 6, 1995): A1.

63. M. Clare et al., Reducing Health Care Delivery Costs Using Clinical Paths: A Case Study on Improving Hospital Profitability, *Journal of Health Care Financing* 21 (1995): 48–58.

64. HMOs Are Changing the Face of Medicine, *New York Times* (January 11, 1995): A1.

65. Medicine's Industrial Revolution, *Wall Street Journal* (August 21, 1995): A8.

66. E.J. Proenca, Why Outcomes Management Doesn't (Always) Work: An Organizational Perspective, *Quality Management in Health Care* 3 (1995): 1–9.

67. M. Gold et al., Behind the Curve: A Critical Assessment of How Little Is Known about Arrangements between Managed Care Plans and Physicians, *Managed Care Research and Review* 52 (1995): 307–41; University Hospital Consortium, Responding to a Dynamic Health Care Marketplace.

68. M.R. Gold, Effects of the Growth of Managed Care on Academic Medicine Centers and Graduate Medical Education, *Academic Medicine* 71 (1996): 828–38.

69. P. Fox and J. Wasserman, Academic Medical Centers and Managed Care: Uneasy Partners, *Health Affairs* 272 (1993): 85–93.

70. Academic Centers—and GME—Face Growing Market Pressure, 1.

71. Wray and Sadowski, Defining Hospitals' GME Strategy.

72. Young, Overview of Graduate Medical Education.

73. Ibid.

74. Ibid.

75. Reinhardt, The Bounty Hunters.

76. Market Changes Hasten Oversupply of Physicians, *American Medical News* (August 8, 1994): 1.

77. J.J. Cohen, Pew Catalyzes Education Partnerships with Managed Care Organizations. *Academic Medicine* 72 (1997): 372; E.L. March and G.T. Moore, Allied for Good: Academic Medicine and Managed Care Form Educational Partnerships, *New Medicine* 1 (1997): 179–82.

78. S. Karp et al., The Need for Comprehensive Data on Educational Affiliation between AHC and MCO, *Academic Medicine* 72 (1997): 341–46; March and Moore, Allied for Good.

79. Cohen, Pew Catalyzes Education Partnerships.

80. Karp, The Need for Comprehensive Data.

81. G.T. Moore et al., The "Teaching HMO": A New Academic Partner, *Academic Medicine* 69 (1994): 595–600; Managed Care and Academia Join To Build "Teaching HMOs," *ACP Observer* (April 1995): 1.

82. *Mission Management: A New Synthesis,* executive summary (Washington, DC: Association of Academic Health Centers, 1998).

83. D.B. Nash, P. Chodoff, and S. C. Sauereisen, *The Role of Health Policy Centers in Academic Health Centers: Meeting the New Challenge, 1998* (Washington, DC: Association of Academic Health Centers).

84. Getting Down to Business at Duke's Medical School, *Wall Street Journal* (August 29, 1995): B1.

85. Fox and Wasserman, Academic Medical Centers and Managed Care.

86. Kralewski et al., Can Academic Medical Centers Compete in a Managed Care System?

87. University Hospital Consortium, Responding to a Dynamic Health Care Marketplace.

88. E.A. Kerr et al., Managed Care and Capitation in California: How Do Physicians at Financial Risk Control Their Own Utilization? *Annals of Internal Medicine* 123 (1995): 500–04.

89. P.F. Drucker, The Coming of the New Organization, *Harvard Business Review* (January/February 1988): 45–53.

90. B.J. Reilly et al., Traditional Decision-Making Questioned: It's Time for New Thinking for a New Age, *Business Forum* (Winter/Spring 1993): 25–30.

91. Moore et al., The "Teaching HMO."

92. HMOs Value Research—If Others Pay for It, *American Medical News* (November 20, 1995): 1.

93. Academic Centers—and GME—Face Growing Market Pressure; Managed Care and Academia Join To Build "Teaching HMOs."

94. J.H. Lofland et al., Changes in Resource Use and Outcomes for Migraine Patients Treated with Sumatriptan: A Managed Care Perspective, *Archives of Internal Medicine* 159 (1999): 857–63.

95. D.C. Donahue, B.E. Lewis, I.S Ockene, and G. Saperia, Research Collaboration between an HMO and an Academic Medical Center: Lessons Learned, *Academic Medicine* 71 (1996): 126–32.

96. Sanus Offers Multiple-Option Plan with N.C. Academic Medical Center, *Managed Care Outlook* (November 17, 1995): 1–3.

SUGGESTED READING

Kleinke, J.D. 1998. *Bleeding Edge.* Gaithersburg, MD: Aspen Publishers, Inc..

Millenson, M.L. 1997. *Demanding Medical Excellence: Doctors and Accountability in the Information Age.* Chicago: University of Chicago Press.

Nash, D.B. 1994. *The Physician's Guide to Managed Care.* Gaithersburg, MD: Aspen Publishers, Inc.

Weitekamp, M.R., and Ziegenfuss, J.T. 1995. Academic Health Centers and HMOs: A Systems Perspective on Collaboration in Training Generalist Physicians and Advancing Mutual Interests. *Academic Medicine* 70, no. 1: S47–S53.

CHAPTER 14

Community Health Centers and Managed Health Care

Pamela J. Byrnes, Judith Shea, and Richard J. Jacobsen

INTRODUCTION

During the 1990s, the health care system in the United States underwent a profound restruc-turing of corporate and financial relationships at a rapid pace. Questions of control over many aspects of the health care system are unsettled and shifting daily, with mergers, acquisitions, and

Pamela J. Byrnes, PhD, specializes in the organizational development, operations, program design, implementation, and evaluation of community health centers as well as community- and population-based health care access and health status research. She has worked with public and private nonprofit community-based providers to expand their ability to care for the underserved. Her recent work centers on managed care systems and developing innovative affiliations between community-based primary care and institutional providers.

Dr. Byrnes was appointed to the Connecticut Health Care Access Commission and the Advisory Committee of the Office of Health Care Access. She serves as health policy advisor to consumer and provider groups at the state and national levels and is a funded consumer advisor to the National Association of Insurance Commissioners.

She is an Assistant Clinical Professor in the Department of Community Medicine and Health Care at the University of Connecticut School of Medicine, where she teaches epidemiology and health systems theory; and a principal of Wellspring Associates, a firm that specializes in health and human services consulting for nonprofit corporations.

Judith Shea, MMHS, has an extensive history of work with Community Health Centers at the national, state, and local levels. Her professional expertise includes policy development, needs assessment, delivery systems analysis, program design, implementation, and organization operations. She was the Director of Primary Care Association Relations and Director of the National Immunization Campaign for the National Association of Community Health Centers. Ms. Shea served on the "Every Child By Two" Immunization Advisory Committee, headed by Mrs. Roslyn Carter and Mrs. Betty Bumpers. Ms. Shea was the Executive Director of the Connecticut Primary Care Association as the CHCs entered the Medicaid managed care marketplace and was instrumental in Connecticut CHC operations transitions. Ms. Shea is a principal of Wellspring Associates, a firm that specializes in health and human services consulting for nonprofit corporations.

Richard J. Jacobsen, PhD, is a Principal with Birch & Davis Health Management Corporation. He presently serves as Deputy Project Manager on a multiyear contract overseeing Rhode Island's Medicaid managed care program, RIte Care. He previously played a central role in the startup of, and served for four years as Chief Executive Officer of, Community Health Network of Connecticut, a 38,000-member community health center–sponsored health maintenance organization. Dr. Jacobsen also served for eight years as Executive Director of the Connecticut Primary Care Association. He has over 15 years' experience in the design, development, and operation of community-based systems of care for low-income and uninsured populations and participated extensively in statewide health policy task forces, particularly those dealing with strategies for coverage of the uninsured. Dr. Jacobsen is an Assistant Clinical Professor in the Department of Community Medicine at the University of Connecticut School of Medicine.

significant movements in private and public sector arrangements. Controlling primary care, the entry point into the health care system, becomes ever more important for those seeking successful positioning in this system. Community Health Centers (CHCs) are relatively new to this game of competition and control.*

The health care system, particularly after the passage of Medicaid, has run in two parallel streams. One side is the private sector commercial marketplace. In this stream, fee-for-service medicine combined with the fastest-growing sector of the U.S. post–World War II economy: pharmaceuticals and medical technology. Over time, with the entry of large-scale finance capital through insurance companies and managed care organizations (MCOs), the entrepreneurial aspect of the health care industry has increased. On the other side is the publicly financed provision of health care to uninsured, publicly insured, and medically disenfranchised populations. People who are homeless, people who are uninsured and uninsurable, people who have acquired immune deficiency syndrome and tuberculosis, and others who lack access to the private sector are treated by CHCs and other safety net providers who are funded primarily through public insurance reimbursements and public and private grants. CHCs, in effect, participate in a system of care for vulnerable and disenfranchised people through the provision of comprehensive, family-oriented primary care and linkages to public and charity hospitals.

There have always been fundamental tensions within this parallel system. On the one hand, our

---

*"CHC" will be used in this chapter to include all federally qualified health centers (FQHCs) and FQHC look-alikes. While the discussion is directed toward these providers, it is important to note that similar effects have been experienced by other safety net providers such as maternal and child health programs, homeless health programs, school-based health services, and primary care services run by public health departments. These other provider groups, however, have not necessarily been able to benefit from the types of strategies the CHCs have been able to undertake and find themselves in a relatively disadvantageous position.

nation has professed the belief that health care is a right for all citizens. On the other hand, there is the belief that providing health care for people who are disadvantaged should not cost much and should not affect significantly the way "most" Americans experience health care. As the health care system has grown and changed in response to new technologies and increasing costs, CHCs have adapted, always staying with their mission to serve all regardless of ability to pay.

Managed care, in the form of health maintenance organizations (HMOs), arose initially as a health care delivery model based on the premise that primary care providers tending to the whole patient could best coordinate an individual's care and provide an entryway into specialty care, thereby containing the need for specialists. The financing aspects of managed care—the sharing of risk and controlling of costs through risk-based contracting, utilization review, and provider oversight—have moved to the forefront in the present climate of cost control, often subordinating the original concerns for patient health management. Risk-based MCOs, until recently, were mainly in the realm of the private sector commercial marketplace. CHCs, and the poor and uninsured people they serve, were by and large unaffected by these new arrangements. Stress on state and federal health care budgets increased rapidly in the 1980s, creating pressure to find new approaches to predict and control costs. Over the past several years, through the use of federal waivers, most states have moved their Medicaid programs to a managed care structure and have mandated that recipients enroll in managed care plans to access health care.

These shifts have altered the playing field for CHCs and their patients. CHCs are now separated from patients, who are actually members of a plan first, and then CHC patients. The relationship between the CHC and its patients and the ultimate payer (the state) is mediated through a third party who controls to a large extent both the conditions and financing of the CHC's services. While their funding and access to the patients have been privatized, CHCs still live under federal statutory requirements about how CHCs are managed, who governs them, what services are offered, and which populations are to be served.

Increasing Tensions in a Shifting Landscape

The social conditions that helped spawn CHCs and the development of the social safety net continue to push the health care system into new arrangements. During the past five years, welfare reforms have been widely enacted throughout the nation, with most legislation affecting not only the conditions of cash payments and housing subsidies, but access to Medicaid as well. In many states, the initial cutoff period is approaching at the time this is being written, and it is anticipated that significant numbers of people will lose their cash benefits. While most states allow for continuation of medical benefits for a period of time after the cutoff, most safety net providers are anticipating increases in uninsured patients. Unfortunately, it is not necessary to wait for welfare reform–related uninsurance problems: CHCs are already experiencing a shift toward uninsured patients. After a declining trend in the early 1990s, the number of people without health insurance has increased annually in the United States. According to the Agency for Health Care Policy and Research, 17 percent of the U.S. population, or 44.8 million people, had no health insurance in 1996.[1] This phenomenon has occurred in spite of an improving economy and low unemployment rates. Much of the increase is related to a sharp decline in employer-based health insurance, particularly for dependents. Corporate streamlining and downsizing have led to increased employee contributions to health coverage, often pricing low-wage workers out of insurance for themselves as well as for their children and spouses. From 1995 to 1996, the percent of people uninsured in the country rose from approximately 14.5 percent to 17 percent, while the percent of CHC patients that were uninsured rose from 35 percent to 46 percent.[2]

The increase in uninsured people and decrease in persons eligible for Medicaid and other public welfare programs has a significant impact on CHCs and other safety net providers. At the same time that pressures from the state to reduce costs and competition in the marketplace are intensify-ing, CHCs are finding themselves confronted with a shift in payer mix toward the uninsured. These contradictory pressures place CHCs in the untenable position of having to support more uncompensated care with leaner revenues.

COMMUNITY HEALTH CENTERS

History

In the mid-1960s, with a rising tide of sentiment against the Vietnam military action, the fight against segregation, the public outcry against poverty, and the push for civil rights, a mood that favored the social good was also rising. The Great Society and the War on Poverty initiated by President Johnson heralded new resources for addressing the unmet needs of the nation's poor. The Economic Opportunity Act, the cornerstone of the War on Poverty, was passed by Congress in 1964 along with funding for the Community Action Programs. These federal initiatives established the cornerstone of the future CHC movement.[3]

Concurrently, Congress passed legislation for two public insurance plans: Medicare, comprehensive health care for those over age 65 (see Chapter 55); and Medicaid, the medical care program for people on welfare, including Aid to Families with Dependent Children (AFDC; see also Chapter 57). The Medicaid legislation authorized and institutionalized annual federal and state expenditures and a specified set of health care services for women and children eligible for AFDC. This created a demand for primary care services for women of childbearing age, pregnant women, infants, and children in today's terms, a new market entrant, where the door remained outside the entrenched private practice, fee-for-service health care system.

The passage of Medicaid in 1965, while addressing the payment issues related to health care for the poor, did not resolve the problem of who would actually provide health care to these people. Private providers remained largely out of reach for welfare recipients because neither they nor their patients were prepared to deal with a population that was so different and needy. In rural and urban ghetto areas, there simply were no physicians at all. In response to the continued lack of access to care for the poor, the Office of Economic Opportunities (OEO) provided funds for a pilot program to establish two CHCs, a rural one in Mississippi and an urban one in Massachusetts, to address the need for community-based health care for people without insurance. The OEO wanted to ensure that health care was available to people who, for whatever reason, could not access traditional office medical practices. In the South, segregation and denial of medical care exacerbated this condition. Rural areas had no means to attract or support a physician practice. Urban areas had marginalized vulnerable populations, for whom access to mainstream medical services was restricted.

CHC Model

CHCs, which are required by statute to be 501(c)(3)-approved nonprofit entities, use a comprehensive primary health care model based on an understanding of social medicine and the social causes and correlates of illness. This includes emphasis on prevention, outreach, and community responsiveness. The service model is guided by epidemiological analysis of the health needs of a whole community and by a conscious effort to attain an integrated program of services. The model is carried forward by a commitment to serve all people—particularly the most vulnerable—and accountable to bona fide community governance. Further, CHCs are required to serve all persons, regardless of ability to pay or insurance status.

Service Model

The CHC service delivery model is based on community-oriented primary care, which is different from the medical model more characteristic of private practice medicine. Assessments are conducted in targeted communities and populations to determine community need. Data on health status indicators, race and ethnic composition, health professional shortages in primary care, mental health and dentistry, clinical needs and gaps in available services, emergency room usage, continuity of care, and other pertinent measures are used to develop services to meet the needs of the specific population. Quality

health services are then delivered to the targeted community and/or population in accessible settings (e.g., homeless shelters, school-based clinics, picking fields where migrant workers labor, urban office facilities).

The breadth of the CHC bundle of services has helped make one-stop health care a reality for many patients. The family-oriented practice model is built on continuity of care from birth to old age through a lifecycle care plan. Care is provided by family practice physicians, internists, pediatricians, obstetrics and gynecology board-certified or -eligible physicians, nurse practitioners, and physician assistants. Specialty services may be obtained on site by appointment or off site by referral; social, mental health, and nutrition services are provided on site. Dental services are available at larger sites and by referral at sites without facilities. Laboratory, X-ray, and pharmacy services are also frequently available at larger sites.

Governance

Unique within the U.S. health care system is the CHC's governance structure. This structure is designed by statute to ensure that the needs of the community remain paramount in policy and operations. Boards of directors are required to include at least a 51 percent majority of persons who are ongoing patients of the health center. The remaining 49 percent (or less) of members are drawn from the larger community and bring additional expertise to the boards. No more than half of the nonuser board members can derive more than 10 percent of their incomes from health care–related activities. Each member is a volunteer committed to fiduciary and policy responsibility and oversight for the CHC. Boards are expected to be representative of the ethnic and racial composition of the local community. Having consumer-based boards helps CHCs meet the requirement that they remain accountable to their local community.

PUBLIC POLICY AND SUPPORT

Federal Funding

Since 1965, CHCs have enjoyed bipartisan support in Congress. Both Republican- and

Democrat-initiated congressional appropriations for health care for uninsured and poor populations have continued a sporadic growth since that time. Original funding came from War on Poverty legislation in 1964. In 1975, CHCs became a separate categorical grant program in the Department of Health, Education, and Welfare, gaining their own "line item" in the congressional budget. To date, the primary source of operating funding for CHCs, other than reimbursements, comes from federal funding under section 330 of the Public Health Service Act. Federal funding for support of CHCs has increased from $758.1 million in fiscal year 1996 to $825.0 million in fiscal year 1998.[4] Revenues from Medicaid, Medicare, and other third-party payers as well as state-level appropriations and public and private grants also support CHCs. In 1998, health care was provided to 9.3 million individuals, including over 3.8 million uninsured persons, at over 800 CHCs with nearly 3,600 service delivery sites.[5]

State Funding

States have initiated a myriad of approaches to assist CHCs. Prior to managed care, some states had developed their own budget "line items" for subsidizing health care for the uninsured and other special populations receiving care at CHCs. Several states have uncompensated care pools that are funded through sources such as hospital surcharges, general revenues, or other assessments. Usually, funds from these pools are distributed according to a formula based on amount of care to uninsured people. Brick and mortar funding through bond initiatives and special health center capital expansion allotments may be available along with special appropriations for statewide development of CHCs and safety net infrastructures. Specific to managed care participation, several states have developed transitional payment systems to ease the financial impact on CHCs. These payments may be in the form of add-ons to the per member per month capitation payments or enhanced payments according to patient case mix.[6]

Policy Initiatives

The delivery costs of primary care required by the 330 Public Health Services CHC authorization was far in excess of Medicaid reimbursement rates as set by the states. The Omnibus Budget Reconciliation Act (OBRA) of 1989 and 1990 rectified this problem with the authorization of FQHCs and concomitantly guaranteed reimbursement for reasonable costs for a defined set of services. At this time, FQHC "look-alikes" were also authorized. These are facilities such as free-standing clinics and hospital-based clinics that do not receive 330 funding but do meet the core set of statutory requirements set for CHCs (e.g., consumer governance, serving all regardless of ability to pay). OBRA recognized that the required FQHC bundle of services was extraordinarily comprehensive in that it included access barrier reduction requirements such as transportation, outreach, translation services, case management, and other broadly defined health services. The cost-based reimbursement (CBR) mandate implicitly recognized that in most instances the level of reimbursement paid by Medicaid agencies was well below the actual cost of services. For other providers, cost shifting to other payers might be possible. For CHCs, given the commitment to the uninsured, there was no other payer that could offset losses. The FQHC rates further recognized that the comprehensive bundle of services provided by CHCs would now be compensated on the basis of the calculation of reasonable costs. Associated rate increases enabled CHCs to expand their services. Rates paid by Medicaid under FQHC reasonable costs are now higher than those typically paid, even in the commercial market. This has been a major issue as managed care has entered the CHC environment. CBR is scheduled to be phased out over the next three years. Recent federal budget negotiations have reestablished the wraparound payment through 2003, albeit with reduced proportional payments relative to actual costs each year.

Legislation that established the National Health Services Corps (NHSC) assists FQHCs through designation of health professional shortage areas and medically underserved areas that qualify for Public Health Service clinical recruitment and retention assistance. The ability to access physicians through the NHSC significantly improved recruitment for CHCs. In response to federal cutbacks, some states have enacted their own loan repayment programs, which allow physicians and other licensed providers to have some loans forgiven for service in CHCs and other safety net provider sites. Passage of the Federal Torts Claims Act reduced CHC operating costs by moving clinical malpractice liability from the costly realm of market-driven insurance to the auspices of the U.S. Justice Department.

With the advent of managed care, federal and state policy has focused most broadly on shaping the relationship between CHCs and MCOs and trying to sustain CHCs and other safety net providers in the new environment. Federal Medicaid waivers (1915b and 1115), which enable states to waive selected Medicaid program requirements, contain specific safeguards to protect the position of CHCs. For example, states with 1915b waivers are required to pay CHCs cost-based reimbursement, whereas 1115 waivers allow for waiving this requirement. Several state waivers require MCOs participating in Medicaid to contract with CHCs and other safety net providers. However, this requirement and many others can be waived if the MCOs can prove they are providing adequate access and appropriate services to the population. Federal funding initiatives have helped groups of CHCs and/or their state associations to form their own MCOs and integrated delivery systems (see Chapter 4).

Some states have also adopted rules to support CHCs under managed care. Required contracting with CHCs and other community providers has been legislated in several states, and most at least require MCOs to show openness to contracting with safety net providers. A similar approach, without actually mandating contracting, is to increase MCOs' bid scores if they establish formal linkages with safety net providers in their provider networks. The assignment methodology for people who do not select a plan voluntarily may also encourage contracting with CHCs:

"Default" assignments can be directed solely to plans that meet certain contracting and linkage requirements.

Though alone not enough to make comprehensive, affordable health care available to all, federal and state resources are the bedrock upon which health care for the poor and uninsured exists. These public sector resources are the major contributors to the care of the 46 percent of CHC patients who are uninsured.

Technical Assistance

As part of the strategy to ensure the successful transition to managed care of these essential parts of the safety net, the federal government provides a broad range of technical assistance and training to support CHCs in adapting to managed care through the Bureau of Primary Health Care (BPHC) and the Center for Managed Care in the Health Resources and Services Administration (HRSA). Direct assistance programs focus primarily on helping CHCs upgrade their operations, information management systems, and practice management to be able to function efficiently and productively in the managed care environment. A collaborative effort among the health-related agencies within the Department of Health and Human Services is being developed around their shared priority of assisting community providers in adapting to managed care.

Many of these programs are implemented in conjunction with the National Association of Community Health Centers (NACHC), the national advocacy, education, and support organization for CHCs. The BPHC and HRSA conduct ongoing research on the impact of managed care on CHCs. Analysis is also conducted by numerous academic and private research organizations and foundations, data from which are used to develop further technical assistance programs and to highlight areas for policy modification.

ENTRY INTO MANAGED CARE

Throughout the 1990s, states moved Medicaid beneficiaries from fee-for-service to managed care arrangements. In 1991, Medicaid managed care enrollment stood at 2.7 million persons. By June 30, 1998, enrollment of Medicaid recipients in managed care had increased more than sixfold, to include 16.6 million persons, representing 53.6 percent of total Medicaid enrollment.[7] The large majority of these people were eligible for Medicaid through programs targeted to families and children rather than older people and people with disabilities. By June 1998, 21 states and Medicaid jurisdictions (including Puerto Rico and the District of Columbia) had enrolled more than two-thirds of their beneficiaries in managed care. Only 11 states and jurisdictions had enrolled fewer than one-third of their beneficiaries. The large majority of these beneficiaries were enrolled in risk-based managed care programs; approximately 4 million were in primary care case management programs.

In many states and counties, once begun, the movement of the Medicaid population from fee for service into managed care was very rapid, often largely accomplished within 12 months. These changes dramatically transformed the environment in which CHCs had traditionally functioned in a very short period of time. In part, this was because of the substantial involvement of CHCs in providing care to Medicaid beneficiaries. Nationally, in 1998 Medicaid represented the largest single source of revenue for CHCs. Medicaid-eligible patients represent fully one-third of the total CHC patient population and one-third of total revenues (grant revenues accounted for 26 percent of revenue).[8] Fewer than 20 percent of CHC patients have commercial insurance or Medicare. In some states and markets, the portion of revenue attributable to Medicaid is substantially higher.

Additionally, however, the move to managed care also transformed the environment through the entry of commercial HMOs and direct competition into the marketplace at levels previously not present. By June 1998, 585 health plans were participating in Medicaid managed care. Though it was clear that important changes were coming, most CHCs had little experience upon which to gauge the ways in which they would be affected. CHCs across the country examined their own options for participation in Medicaid managed care programs.

CHCs faced many critical decisions as state-mandated Medicaid managed care and scarce organizational resources collided. These decisions have resulted in both independent and collaborative strategies to meet open market competition for Medicaid managed care–eligible patients and to retain the historic CHC niche and mission.

OPERATIONAL AND STRATEGIC RESPONSES TO MANAGED CARE

Like any organization facing paradigm shifts in the marketplace and social will, CHCs were faced with the need to rapidly restructure their operating systems. Financial systems, clinical systems, and management information systems (MIS) needed altering. New strategic plans that encompassed administrative operations, staffing, non–managed care patient services, and the integration of managed care plan requirements had to be implemented.

Health center analysis, tracking and monitoring of finances, and clinical operations were often archaic and carried out by MIS designed specifically for CHCs. These systems contained modules that captured and sorted data elements required by the BPHC to monitor usage and application of federal funds to provide health care to the uninsured (e.g., unduplicated users per year).* The recently implemented Uniform Data Set (UDS) moved CHCs into using common procedural coding systems such as the International Codification of Diseases and current procedural terminology codes, which have been the

---

*Until recently, basic demographic and reimbursement source information was provided under the BPHC's Bureau of Common Reporting Requirements and included numbers of unduplicated users, numbers and types of visits, numbers and types of clinicians, payer mix, and other stipulated data. In recognition of the more complex environment CHCs were moving into as well as the stepped-up competition and cost consciousness of the marketplace, a new reporting system was implemented in 1997. The Uniform Data Set is more extensive in its reporting requirements and incorporates information related to costs, provider productivity, and operating efficiency.

industry standard for patient utilization tracking and billing. However, even the UDS does not require the level of information and detail necessary for CHCs to monitor and assess the practice management details essential for on-site care, referrals, hospitalizations, and continuity of care. Information management systems in CHCs have had to become far more sophisticated in their ability to monitor patient and provider experiences. Clinical performance data need to give detailed information about clinic visits, specialty care and hospital utilization, and clinical and provider efficiency. This information will then be used to determine patient utilization costs and health center efficiency and productivity.

The advent of CHC managed care capitated payments at negotiated per member per month rates was in stark contrast to fee-for-service cost-based reimbursement. With managed care, billing and collections functions for Medicaid enrollees, which averaged 35 percent of the patient population, became relatively obsolete. Moreover, the previous financial systems, adequate under the less complex conditions of fee for service, were not sufficient to monitor costs and revenues for multiple capitated contracts, grants, uncompensated care, sliding fee schedules, and other financial indicators. Health centers lacked the capacity to assess and monitor patient utilization in environments outside the CHC.

CHC-Level Responses

The slim financial margins within which CHCs operate set significant constraints on their capacity to upgrade to state-of-the-art financial and clinical data management systems. In 1998, Medicaid managed care patients were 34 percent of the over 9 million users, while the uninsured were 41 percent, yet the need for accurate data and complex information systems was driven by the smaller proportion of the patient base. Furthermore, CHCs in many cases lost Medicaid market share as more traditional providers accepted Medicaid patients through MCO contracts and as welfare-to-work programs further reduced the number of Medicaid recipients.

CHC responses to the pressures of financial, clinical, and MIS retooling and restructuring have been varied. Many educational and technical assistance opportunities were made available, initially through the BPHC. Senior CHC staff participated in BPHC and NACHC training modules for MIS and clinical practice. Centers used self-assessment tools to determine managed care readiness, clinical capacity, quality assurance, and compliance with National Conference on Quality Indicators (NCQI) standards. Administrative staff composition was changed to incorporate the new managed care expertise required by centers, often by recruiting chief financial officers, establishing managed care departments, and adding claims expertise. A redistribution of the Medicaid population into traditional service streams caused an erosion of the historic patient base and therefore required the CHCs to realign staff through position changes and staff reductions.

Delivery of ancillary services was addressed by many CHCs. In some cases, on-site laboratory, X-ray, and/or pharmaceutical services were closed down; yet some CHCs added selected ancillary services. Again, each CHC chose what it perceived as the most advantageous strategy for its community and organization.

CHCs realized that administrative changes were needed to operate in a competitive environment. These changes generally included operations streamlining, directed customer service activities such as patient satisfaction surveys, reengineering activities, appointment management systems, patient recall systems, and a centralized patient referral system. It was widely accepted that facility upgrades were necessary to attract new patients to CHCs and to penetrate to the mainstream health care market of commercially insured people.

Concomitant with the systems changes was the need to educate and train CHC senior staff and boards of directors, who, under articles of incorporation and bylaws, are liable for the fiduciary operations of a CHC and answerable to the community for the services the CHC provides. Most critical to the organization was the capacity to analyze and understand costs, revenues, and degrees of risk for each patient plan. This capacity would position CHCs to determine effective contracting strategies and to conduct negotiations with plans.

Many CHCs used the delivery system shifts to make their relationships with hospitals and other managed care providers mutually beneficial. CHCs began to form strategic alliances with hospitals to expand or develop facilities, develop collaborative services, expand their patient base into other underserved areas, and carry out other health initiatives. A potential win-win situation was then established for CHCs and hospitals as new patients, i.e., plan members, entered the system through primary care centers and could be referred on to allied hospitals.

Network-Level Strategies of CHCs

In the early 1990s, the BPHC recognized the need for CHCs to prepare to enter the managed care arena as the safety net provider for Medicaid recipients. The BPHC initiated several avenues for CHC market entry. Educational modules were developed by acknowledged mainstream managed care experts and made available through NACHC, state primary care associations, and other appropriate vendors. Early modules included training in MIS, managed care readiness assessment, clinical practice analysis, and managed care operations and procedures. On-site technical assistance and network development assistance were part of the early package.

The opportunity for CHCs to develop networks came when the BPHC announced Integrated Service Network (ISN) grants in 1994 as the first phase of its Integrated Services Delivery Initiative (ISDI). The funds were for the planning, development, and operation of the ISNs. Each ISN is organized and structured to meet local needs, leading to a broad variety as opposed to a universal ISN blueprint.[9] One state, for example, chose to develop a management services organization (MSO) that would serve as contract negotiator for member CHCs with all licensed HMOs, MCOs, and vendors. Another statewide network chose to develop a certified, licensed MCO when mandated Medicaid managed care was implemented. All members of the MCO network board of directors were CHCs, so the CHCs controlled the strategies and fiscal and policy decisions that would directly impact the centers.

In 1997, the emphasis of the ISDI shifted toward the integrated delivery systems designed to increase the efficiency and effectiveness of CHCs by having them share specific functions. Many of these MSOs provide a portfolio of services that may include joint purchasing, administration services, human resources and clinician recruitment, facilities management, and billing and collections. This collaboration would make the CHCs stronger in contract negotiations and reduce their cost of operations, ultimately making them more competitive in the marketplace.

The CHCs' loss of patient base to other providers through patient self-selection or default enrollment was a signal to the BPHC that CHCs' niche for comprehensive primary care service delivery to those living below 200 percent of the federal poverty level was in jeopardy. The ISDI then supported the development of managed care networks (MCNs) and practice management networks (PMNs) in 1998. In its Policy Information Notice 99–05, BPHC states that it "anticipates BPHC funded managed care networks will play a vital role in the ability of health centers to maintain and enhance their base of patients with public insurance."[10(p.2)] The BPHC expects that all MCNs funded in 1999 will be involved in arrangements in which financial risk is assumed.

The PMN projects are intended to catalyze the development and operation of truly integrated and efficient health care delivery systems that maximize the quality of services and access to care. BPHC expectations for each PMN include one or more of the following: cost efficiencies, economies of scale, use of interdisciplinary provider teams, joint development of standards and protocols, shared expertise, and common or relational systems (e.g., billing and collections, claims management, utilization management, credentialing). Grants were awarded to 32 CHCs for network development in 1998. Table 14–1 shows the distribution and type of networks funded.

Network formation and CHC affiliations with health care entities such as teaching hospitals, universities, and tertiary care hospitals are strictly governed by HRSA regulations. CHC affiliation regulations that permit vertical network

Table 14–1 CHC Networks

Type*	MCN	PMN
Horizontal 1	4	11
Horizontal 2	3	10
Vertical	1	6

*Horizontal 1 = horizontal with other BPHC-funded centers; Horizontal 2 = horizontal with other primary care providers (non-BPHC funded); Vertical = vertical with other types of health care providers and/or entities (e.g., hospitals).

Source: Reprinted from Bureau of Primary Health Care, Health Resources and Services Administration, Department of Health and Human Services.

formation were most recently defined. The regulations were crafted with significant recognition of the threat to the viability of CHCs in the competitive marketplace and the knowledge of the current and future necessity for the community-based CHC system of care as safety net providers. The capacity to participate in vertical network affiliations as well as horizontal networks among 330-funded CHCs and/or 330-funded CHCs and 330 look-alike organizations has created vital opportunities for CHCs. These newly formed networks, combined with the existing 25 CHC-sponsored MCOs, help make CHCs more competitive.

FORMATION OF CHC-SPONSORED HEALTH PLANS

Rationale

For many CHCs, formation of a CHC-sponsored health plan represented both the most desirable and the most far-reaching strategic option. Many CHCs felt that formation of a full-risk MCO would provide the greatest opportunity to determine their own future and improve their opportunity for long-term success. As is noted below, this strategy has often worked. Some potential perceived benefits for CHCs include the following:

- Participation as a managed care plan could enhance the CHC's ability to participate in key policy arenas on issues affecting Medicaid, uninsured people, and CHCs.

- CHCs see themselves as providing high-quality, cost-effective care and seek to retain the benefits of that effectiveness within the CHC system rather than have those benefits inure to an outside party.
- Having a health plan could help CHCs retain the CHC Medicaid patient base. Increased competition—from health plans and from private and institutional providers—threatens the Medicaid patient base and the financial viability of the CHCs.
- Having a health plan would ensure that CHCs received higher reimbursement rates for services than would be obtained from other MCOs.
- CHCs would be able to exercise substantial control over the policies of the health plan.
- To the degree that the health plan generated an operating surplus, there would be an opportunity for additional distributions to CHCs.
- Full participation in the health plan provides opportunities to give shape to the system in ways that are consistent with the core mission of CHCs.

Plan Formation

It is one thing to want to establish a CHC-sponsored health plan but still another to succeed. Many groups of CHCs actively pursued the option. For a variety of reasons (e.g., shortage of capital, lack of CHC readiness where state implementation of Medicaid managed care moved at a rapid pace, regulatory obstacles, divisions among health centers), not all of these CHCs have been successful. Nonetheless, as of June 1999, CHCs had played a key role in establishing 25 MCOs. In some cases, the founders were groups of CHCs that collaborated in the establishment of the health plan. In other cases, a single CHC was the primary actor. In still other cases, CHCs joined with other providers with a strong commitment to provision of services to Medicaid beneficiaries. In all of these situations, the CHC presence was significant, most typically with a majority position on the governing board.

Plan Characteristics, Strengths, and Challenges

For-Profit versus Not-for-Profit

One of the core decisions for most plans was whether to be for-profit or not-for-profit. Both approaches have been utilized. The for-profit option depends heavily upon the ability to secure capital. Some CHCs have felt that not-for-profit status is more consistent with the CHC mission.

HMO vs. Alternate Type of Risk-Bearing MCO

Licensing and certification regulations vary from state to state. CHC-sponsored health plans may be fully licensed HMOs, they may serve commercial and/or Medicaid markets, or they may exist under alternative arrangements. CHC MCOs vary in structure. In New York State, for instance, several CHC-sponsored plans have operated as Provider Sponsored Health Plans (see Chapter 4).

Enrollment

Of the 25 plans, 23 were operational in 18 states. Combined enrollment in June 1999 was just below 1 million members, according to information provided by the BPHC in June 1999. Enrollment in these plans tends to be fairly small, with a median enrollment of 36,800. Three plans have over 100,000 members, with the highest enrollment shown at 143,000. Table 14–2 shows the distribution of plans by enrollment.

Financial Strength

Although no systematic information is available, a key issue for many CHC-sponsored plans is the level of available capital reserves that can be used to (1) meet statutory requirements, (2) ride out periods of financial losses, (3) support investments in new product development or strengthen position in the current market, and (4) invest in infrastructure needs (e.g., information systems).

Table 14–2 CHC-Sponsored Health Plans by Enrollment Level

Members	Plans
<20,000	5
20,000–40,000	10
40,001–60,000	3
60,001–80,000	2
80,001 and above	3

Source: Reprinted from Bureau of Primary Health Care, Health Resources and Services Administration, Department of Health and Human Services.

Potential Tensions within Provider-Sponsored Plans

Virtually all provider-sponsored plans will encounter some tension between the business and financial pressures faced by the provider sponsors and the business and financial pressures faced by the organization they have created, the MCO. The immediate and long term business and strategic interests of the MCO may not correspond with those originally envisioned by the sponsors. The sponsors, as members of the governing boards, need to confront the dual roles that they play as contracted providers and the MCO stewardship role they play as a governing board. The MCO has to determine the degree to which its business objectives and strategic niche are shaped by the worlds of the CHCs and Medicaid. There is a need to balance the expectations of the different participants in the MCO's strategic objectives. **Areas where potentially divergent needs of CHCs and the MCO can arise include:**

1. The proportion of the premium dollar which is allocated to primary care payments to CHCs versus retained for other purposes, including targeted end-of-year surplus
2. Circumstances where shorter term financial needs of sponsoring CHCs create pressures for dollar distributions instead of longer term investment in growth or in building financial reserves
3. The degree to which the primary care network of the MCO is built around the CHC

to the exclusion of other local primary care providers

4. The degree to which the marketing and support services investments of the MCO are focused more narrowly on the CHCs versus more broadly in the marketplace
5. The degree and conditions under which the MCO is the favored managed care business partner of the CHCs
6. Whether the MCO pursues growth strategies and markets that are not tied to the CHCs.

These types of concerns over MCO focus, in fact, reflect the core reasons why the CHCs considered it important to form their own plans. At the same time, if the MCO does not address its business needs, it may face risk of failure in a very competitive and unforgiving environment.

Mission versus Margin

Over the last several years, it has been common for Medicaid agencies to both lower capitation payments and increase contractual requirements. For these and other reasons that affect investment return, many stockholder-held health plans have opted to exit the Medicaid market. CHC-sponsored plans are more fundamentally rooted in the Medicaid market, both by business base and by core commitment. The CHC-sponsored plan does not typically require the same level of return as a publicly traded company to meet its business objectives. However, the CHC cannot sustain a negative margin (in the aggregate—that is, inclusive of all sources of revenue and costs) for a significant period of time and still be able to deliver necessary services.

Need To Achieve Strong Brand-Name Image

An obstacle for many plans to overcome is the lack of an established positive brand-name image in the market. Name and product recognition has to be achieved. Other plans tend to connote middle-class status and good quality. Medicaid and CHC-based plans can have difficulty achieving a comparable level of product acceptance.

Just as member recruitment can be a challenge, provider recruitment is not always easy. Plans may lack the ability to bring other, better reimbursed business to providers.

Concentration of the Medicaid Market and Membership Base

Enrollment in the CHC-sponsored plans is heavily weighted toward Medicaid managed care and other public sector programs (e.g., Children's Health Insurance Plans(CHIP)). More than 80 percent of members of most plans are eligible for Medicaid. It is common for 60 percent or more of the enrollment to be based at CHCs.

The combined concentration in the Medicaid marketplace and in the CHCs reflects the success of the plans in achieving their initial objectives and highlights some of the difficulties they may face in growing their membership. Many plans have struggled with the issue of identity and focus. Does the plan aspire to be a larger MCO with aggressive business strategies to grow beyond its initial base in Medicaid and CHCs? Or does the organization maintain a primary focus in its established market niche? On the one hand, the issue is a pragmatic one. Small size limits a plan's negotiating ability in a variety of contexts and provides less economy of scale for administrative costs. To the degree that the targeted Medicaid population is fully enrolled in managed care, growth opportunities can be few. Entry into commercial markets may offer an avenue for growth, but success can be both expensive and difficult to achieve.

Beyond the pragmatic issue may be that of the organizational mission and marketplace and political niche. Focus on the Medicaid market is consistent with CHC origins. Success in the Medicaid market is largely built on the partnership with the CHCs. Movement into other markets can shift the focus away from the core business and core providers and create tension. Further, many CHC plans are favorably situated in their state's political and regulatory landscape. As one health plan chief executive officer (CEO) commented, "We are short on financial capital but long on political capital."

Whether to focus on Medicaid or diversify is a core decision for many plans and will be largely affected by conditions in the local marketplace. The Medicaid managed care marketplace continues to evolve. In several cases, CHC plans have been able to achieve membership growth within Medicaid as other plans have left the market.

Similarly, the concentration of membership at the CHCs is an issue. To the degree that the primary care provider network is dominated by CHCs, growth opportunities may be limited. Startup enrollment for plans may have been driven by an exclusive contracting relationship with CHCs. Efforts to move significantly beyond that base can alter the ways in which the business operates. The CEO of one of the larger and older plans has observed that the plan has had to examine why it is in business. CHCs are aware that if their needs are not met through the plans, they have other contractual options. The plan's strategy is to ensure that the CHCs continue to see the plan as their preferred managed care business partner.

Medicaid Marketplace Changes

The Medicaid managed care marketplace continues to evolve. Though states need to be able to offer Medicaid recipients a choice of plans, the number of participating health plans has declined in many states. Between 1996 and 1998, the number of commercial plans participating in Medicaid declined by 20 percent.[11] CHC-sponsored plans can serve as committed partners to state programs. At the same time, those plans are particularly vulnerable to financial reverses and to adverse changes in capitation rates.

Further Collaboration among CHC-Sponsored Plans

In their individual settings, the CHC-sponsored health plans have largely succeeded in achieving their initial objectives. As participants in Medicaid managed care, they present an important option for beneficiaries. They continue to play an important role in supporting the CHC safety net. At the same time, with small size, limited financial resources, and concentration in a single product line, the plans can be highly vulnerable to subtle shifts in regulatory, fiscal, and contracting arrangements.

Located in different states and markets and joined by common origins and missions, many of these plans have begun to explore the opportunities for product enhancement and long-term success that could be achieved through joint efforts. Combined, the plans' membership was just below 1 million in June 1999. In late 1999, several of the health plans were actively preparing to establish an association of CHC-sponsored plans. This decision followed long discussions about the core commitments and purposes of the plans and their roots in the founding CHCs. It was not expected that all plans would join, reflecting differences within the group.

In moving forward, three preliminary objectives were identified.

First, plans would address the federal policy arena. As individual state-based plans, there is limited visibility at the national level. As one CEO remarked, "With a stroke of the pen Congress could put us out of business without even noticing." Plans agree that the role being played by CHC-sponsored plans in sustaining the safety net and strengthening state managed care programs must be recognized. There is an interest in having federal regulatory and financial policy informed by a greater understanding of this system.

Second, plans seek to leverage their combined experiences to enrich quality of care by developing and sharing best practices for Medicaid safety net plans. Third, plans want to pursue opportunities for greater cost and service effectiveness through joint purchasing (e.g., pharmacy services, reinsurance).

THE IMPACT OF MANAGED CARE AND CHALLENGES FOR THE FUTURE

The entrance of managed care into the Medicaid arena has had a significant impact on CHCs, their patients, and the overall health care sector. This impact is evident throughout CHCs.

Financial Impact and Operations

On the financial side, the movement to managed care is, in effect, the privatization of the financing of health care for the poor. Under the fee-for-service reimbursement system, the dollars flowed from the state directly to the nonprofit providers and generally reflected the costs to the providers for each service. The move to managed care shifted the dollar flow from a direct line from payer to payee, to an indirect line from payer to fiscal intermediary to payee. The managed care companies became recipients of the money and, just as important, managers of the delivery system. The shift away from fee for service has meant that reimbursements to CHCs are not based on the costs of delivering services but on the negotiated amount that MCOs are willing to pay and CHCs are able to extract. As the cost-based reimbursement "wraparound" (discussed above) indicates, reimbursements to health centers under most managed care agreements have not covered the cost of care.

A second financial impact is the shifting payer mix being experienced by CHCs. Prior to managed care, Medicaid visits represented the dominant portion of CHCs' reimbursements. Most CHCs could anticipate that at least 60 percent of their visits would be with Medicaid recipients. Managed care has had a number of influences on this payer mix. First, as Medicaid has assigned people into MCOs, people's choice of provider is dictated by the MCO provider panels. The impact of this has been varied in different states depending on the organization of CHCs and the approach to assigning enrollees. In states where CHCs have been very organized about either becoming MCOs or contracting with MCOs, the centers have been able to retain a greater portion of Medicaid patients. In states where CHCs have been less organized or less successful in contracting, greater losses have been experienced. Similarly, in states where default assignments

are made on a rotating or equal basis, CHCs have tended to fare better in retaining their Medicaid patients than in states where default assignment is limited to one or two MCOs.

The impact of the loss of Medicaid patients is significant, considering that the other major payer in most CHCs is the self-paying patient. These people are overwhelmingly uninsured and ineligible for medical assistance. As managed care has moved more of the insured poor people out of CHCs, their payer mix has shifted significantly toward visits from those who can pay little if anything at all. In many CHCs, visits by uninsured people have grown to represent nearly half of all visits, with Medicaid visits dropping to one-third. As noted above, the number of uninsured is growing and will continue to do so as welfare reform cutoffs begin to be implemented in the coming years. At the same time, in many settings capitation rates are being ratcheted down and MCOs are negotiating more aggressively.

Operational Analysis and Efficiency

A counterpoint to the financial losses experienced by CHCs is the need to examine operating systems and become more efficient organizations. Since their beginning, CHCs have tended to view financial troubles as problems to be solved in the political realm by garnering greater appropriations and higher public reimbursement rates. This dynamic may have led to a laxness on the part of some centers in the area of organizational efficiency. The concept of health center as business enterprise, with the concomitant exigencies of "lean and mean" operations, was frequently looked at with disdain. The mission of providing for the poor and disenfranchised, with the extreme pressures of serving populations with very stressful lives and complex health problems with minimal resources, did not lend itself to making operational efficiency a priority. The small size of many centers made it particularly difficult to achieve operating efficiency. The near-bankrupting of state governments by Medicaid in the 1980s, which gave rise to the managed care era, was an important wake-up call to CHCs and other safety net providers to become more savvy in managing their businesses and develop their financial and operating systems. A positive outcome, then, has been increasingly sophisticated information management and practice management systems, more provider productivity analysis, more attention to costs, and the development of professional administrative and financial systems. CHCs have also paid renewed attention to their physical plants, striving to be more attractive to MCOs and patients alike.

Quality of Care and Credentialing

The need to compete with private sector providers and to engage MCOs in meaningful dialogue has meant that CHCs must measure their own performance on the same scales as private sector institutions, and credentialing and accreditation have improved. While CHCs have always provided high-quality care, many are requesting accreditation reviews from the Joint Commission on Accreditation of Healthcare Organizations (Joint Commission) and other organizations. An initiative involving the NACHC, the Joint Commission, and the BPHC is accelerating the number of BPHC-funded provider sites undergoing a new combined Joint Commission/Primary Care Effectiveness Review accreditation survey. This process, which requires in-depth systems analysis, will enable CHCs to better recognize infrastructure development needs, to increase integration of long-term strategic planning goals with daily operations, and to set quantifiable, time-bound goals and objectives against which progress and performance can be measured. Health centers and their patients will benefit from these efforts to upgrade and streamline operational and clinical systems and performance improvement programs.

Delivery System Integration

Managed care has forced CHCs and other safety net providers to develop systems of care that are better integrated. Given their broad man-

date of services, CHCs have always sought referral and contractual partners in social services and medical specialties. Managed care has encouraged health centers to work more closely with mainstream providers to assess population needs and find ways to fill gaps through coordinated and creative program development. Many more affiliations are being formed with hospitals and other institutional providers that enable joint ventures, with each provider offering several services. For example, where previously a hospital outpatient clinic may have been in direct competition with a CHC, now it is likely that the two will partner and open a multispecialty clinic, with the CHC offering the primary care and dental services and the hospital providing behavioral and mental health care services. These affiliations have to be carefully structured to protect the governance and other statutory requirements of CHCs and to maintain the delicate balance of power between the two institutions. However, with these safeguards, integration of services can lead to more efficient and coordinated care delivery.

Structural Change

The shift to managed care critically changed the structure in which CHCs and other safety net providers exist. Dollars no longer flow from the state directly to the providers; now they flow along a system of pass-through private financing and management. The state maintains oversight of and accountability for publicly financed health care for the poor but loses its direct connection with providers and their function as maintainers of the safety net. The managed care companies have, in effect, replaced CHCs as the apparent safety net providers through their pivotal intermediary role.

The same confusion that exists in private sector health care (i.e., Who is making health care decisions? Who is liable? Who is the actual health care provider?) exists in the public sector. Under the present system, the MCO basically becomes the Medicaid provider, with actual delivery of care being provided through agents (e.g., private physicians, hospitals, CHCs). As manager of this system, the state will take the position that contracted MCOs are accountable for seeing that beneficiaries are receiving care. At the same time, CHCs and other community providers are also held accountable for providing care to the underserved and are expected to continue to fulfill the safety net function. This dynamic leads to confusion over who is actually responsible for health care to the underserved, specifically Medicaid recipients: the MCO as the Medicaid contractor or the CHC as the actual health care provider? Further complicating the issue is that many Medicaid recipients continue to visit CHCs, regardless of their plan enrollment.

CHCs are caught in a paradoxical situation as, on the one hand, they are expected to direct people to the appropriate contractual provider while, on the other hand, they are expected to serve all people that present themselves for care. CHCs do not have the mindset to turn people away, so they increasingly find themselves providing uncompensated care to publicly insured people.

Although some states have required some level of contracting with safety net providers, it is overwhelmingly apparent that CHCs are having problems being cut into the pie. At the most basic level, CHCs find that some commercial MCOs will refuse to enter into contracting discussions. Many of these MCOs, while carrying on apparent negotiations, submit numerous credentialing and accreditation requests that are insurmountable for the CHCs. The sense on the part of many safety net providers is that an endless series of barriers is thrown up, impeding the contracting progress. The situation is eased in places where CHCs have successfully implemented collaborative contracting strategies and CHC-owned MCOs.

When contracting does succeed, there remain many issues related to costs. Despite the efficiency and operations concerns discussed above, the calculation of appropriate rate and the need for cost-based reimbursement may have less to do with inefficiency or other provider delivery and organizational issues as it does with the breadth of services that health centers provide and the nature

of the populations they serve. It costs more to provide transportation, ensure translation services, and case manage people whose lives are extraordinarily complex and whose resources are minimal. By federal statute, CHCs are required to develop a comprehensive bundle of primary care services that address the specific needs of a delineated population. CHCs must continuously assess the needs of the people through community health assessments in which health is broadly defined to include housing, food, employment, literacy, and other subsistence needs.

CHCs have to identify and develop leadership in the community through their governing board requirements. They must prove that they are responsive to the input of their patients and communities. CHCs must develop lengthy and complex justifications for receiving funding, requiring significant use of resources. And they must do this all without creating any financial barriers to care. The recognized special needs of people disenfranchised from the private health care system—needs that led to the creation of CHCs—are what is creating the most severe tension for the CHCs.

CONCLUSION

CHCs and other safety net providers are competing in two different worlds. They provide health care to millions of people, many of whom have no health insurance, under the most difficult conditions while maintaining their mission to be community governed and accountable, and at the same time they are confronted with an environment that demands that they be increasingly competitive with providers who have only the strain of dealing with the private health care system (a daunting task in its own right!). Safety net providers in general, and CHCs specifically, find themselves caught in the tension between mission and margin in an increasingly competitive and commercial health care industry.[12]

The system continues to move in the direction of private financing and delivery, and the pressures to decrease health care costs are increasing. In the private sector, recently announced premium increases by several major insurers hark back to the double-digit increases of the early 1990s. Medicaid managed care plans and providers will have to face starker state financing and still serve more people. According to a recent analysis, changes already under way in many states will increase pressure on providers of health care to the poor: decreases in capitation rates, more competitive contracting, expanded enrollment of more medically complex recipients (e.g., persons dually eligible under Medicare and Medicaid), and reduced financial protections for CHCs.[13] The study further concluded that future pressures could very likely lead to a lessening of the number of providers

and plans participating in Medicaid, cutbacks in support for enabling services, and a reduction in service to the uninsured.

However, there still are poor and uninsured people with special needs that no one else wants to help and who require extra attention and health care (broadly defined). As long as we, as a nation, profess to believe in the right to health care, and as long as private sector institutions are reluctant to respond to the needs of this population, CHCs and other safety net providers will be needed. As the health care environment continues to change, CHCs and other traditional providers to the underserved will have to develop new strategies for survival.

REFERENCES

1. Agency for Health Care Policy and Research, *The Uninsured in America—1996* (Rockville, MD, 1997).
2. Lewin Group, *Evaluation of the Impact of the Medicaid Waivers on Consumers and Services of Federally Qualified Health Centers* (Fairfax, VA, 1997).
3. H.H. Schauffler and J. Wolin, Community Health Clinics under Managed Competition: Navigating Uncharted Waters, *Journal of Health Politics, Policy and Law* 21, no. 3 (1996): 461–488.
4. Bureau of Primary Health Care, Health Resources and Services Administration, *Community Health Center Program* (Bethesda, MD, 1999).
5. J. Meyer et al., *Current Policy Issues Affecting Safety Net Providers* (Washington, DC: Economic and Social Research Institute, 1999).
6. D. Lipsen, "Medicaid Managed Care and Community Providers: New Partnerships," *Health Affairs,* July/August 1997, 91–107.
7. Health Care Financing Administration, HCFA Medicaid Managed Care 1996 Enrollment Report and Medicaid

Managed Care 1998 Enrollment Report, http://www.hcfa.gov/medicaid.
8. K. Davis et al., *Policy Brief: Community Health Centers in a Changing U.S. Health Care System* (New York, NY: Commonwealth Fund, 1999).
9. M. Harrington et al., *Medicaid Managed Care and FQHCs: Experiences of Plans, Networks, and Individual Health Centers* (Washington, DC: Mathematica Policy Research, 1998).
10. Bureau of Primary Health Care, Health Resources and Service Administration, U.S. Department of Health and Human Services, Policy Information Notice 99–05 (Bethesda, MD, 1999).
11. *State Health Watch* 6, no. 10 (Atlanta, GA: American Health Consultants, 1999): 6.
12. Meyer et al., *Current Policy Issues.*
13. S. Felt-Lisk et al., Medicaid Managed Care: Does It Increase Primary Care Services in Under-Served Areas? *Mathematica* (Washington, DC, November 1997).

SUGGESTED READING

Dievler, A., and Giovannini, T. 1998. Community Health Centers: Promise and Performance. *Medical Care Research and Review* 55: 405–431.

Hawkins, D.R., Jr., and Rosenbaum, S. 1998. The Challenges Facing Health Centers in a Changing Health Care System. In *The Future U.S. Healthcare System: Who Will Care for the Poor and Uninsured?* eds. S. Altman et al. Chicago: Health Administration Press.

Complementary and Alternative Medicine Integration: Trends, Structures, and Challenges

John Weeks

INTRODUCTION

In November 1997 George Lundberg, MD, then editor of the *Journal of the American Medical Association (JAMA)*, stated that the "bamboo curtain" that has separated conventional medicine from what has become known as complementary and alternative medicine (CAM) in the United States "is beginning to splinter."[1]

Lundberg's use of a cold war metaphor suggests a pent-up demand for greater discourse and exploration. The value of the metaphor is underscored by the intensity of activity as mainstream health care organizations work to find a place in their offerings for a movement that was scorned only recently as quackery. The bomb that began the splintering process was the publication in the *New England Journal of Medicine (NEJM)* in early 1993 of results of a survey of consumer use of what the researchers called "unconventional medicine."[2] The findings, reported below, placed the popular movement on the doorstep of conventional medicine. A concurrent trend in health

---

John Weeks is publisher and editor of *The Integrator for the Business of Alternative Medicine* (www.onemedicine.com), a monthly newsletter devoted to offering practical reports, trends, and insight to those integrating complementary and alternative medicine into the payment and delivery system. He is a principal with Integration Strategies for Natural Healthcare, Seattle, Washington, and he writes, consults, and presents workshops on coverage and integration issues.

care's mainstream, toward market competition and patient-centered care, opened the door.

Since publication of the survey, leaders of many health systems, health maintenance organizations (HMOs), and public agencies have been pioneering strategies for incorporating CAM. Structures for integration are emerging, together with clarity on challenges identified by these initial forays. This chapter is an evidence-based exploration of the emerging models for integration. The perspectives rely heavily on the documented case reports, business developments, and surveys reported by the author in *The Integrator for the Business of Alternative Medicine*, a monthly newsletter that started in July 1996.[3] The first section provides data regarding use and integration by leading stakeholders. Focus then shifts to an evaluation of the dominant strategies for inclusion. The context of CAM integration is dynamic. Most observers agree that CAM integration will unfold in U.S. health care over decades, not years. This chapter ends with a look at emerging approaches that reach beyond the present, consumer-oriented models toward CAM integration into core decisions regarding the effectiveness and cost-effectiveness of care.

ORIENTATION: STAKEHOLDER ACTIVITY

Institutions undertaking CAM integration are moved by diverse interests. Top among these are the *consumer* (see also Chapter 43), and the consumer in wolves clothing, otherwise known to health plans and integrated delivery systems as legislative *mandates* (see also Chapter 69). A corollary motivation is *market competition*: creating CAM products and services in response to offerings by other payers and providers who are themselves responding to perceived consumer demand (see also Chapter 41).

None of these leading motivations for CAM product development requires close connection with the core challenge of medicine: offering services that are optimally clinically effective and cost effective. CAM providers, however, argue that their services can have a positive impact on the bottom line. In fact, significant subsets of mainstream decisionmakers, particularly those with personal experience of CAM, agree with this assertion. This section provides an overview of the present interest among leading stakeholders, together with available evidence on the consumer, cost, and effectiveness motivators for their CAM-related activities.

Consumers

Defining the level of consumer use of CAM is to shoot at a moving target. The *NEJM* survey referenced above was followed by a similar examination by the same team of Harvard researchers in 1997.[4] As illustrated in Table 15–1, during the 1990–1997 interval the percent of

CAM users jumped from 34 percent to 42 percent. Roughly two-thirds of use represented self-care applications. Estimates of total dollars spent rose even more significantly, nearly doubling from $13.7 billion to $27 billion, and remaining largely out-of-pocket by the users. Total office visits to CAM providers, such as chiropractors, relaxation therapists, and massage practitioners jumped from 427 million to 629 million.

That these data are controversial is clear from other studies. A team of researchers at Yale in 1997 found use of CAM providers lower (8.8 percent) than the Harvard team's 1990 data.[5] At the other end of the spectrum, researchers at Stanford presented data from 1998 that suggested that 69 percent were using some CAM, through self-care or CAM providers.[6]

Variation is partly explained by study methodology. The Stanford data, like that by the Harvard group, include self-care. The most significant increases were found in use of herbal medicines and vitamin therapies. Yet the Stanford group found that roughly 15 percent had used chiropractic and a similar percent had used massage. While a clear understanding of differences in outcomes is not available, health systems and HMOs that have undertaken their own proprietary studies tend to find between 40–60 percent of their members have used CAM in a given year.[7] Notably, two analyses of use by se-

---

Table 15–1 Comparative Consumer Use of Complementary and Alternative Medicine, 1990 and 1997

Finding/Therapy	1990	1997
Total expenditures	$13.7 billion	$27 billion
Total visits	427 million	629 million
Total use: All therapies	34%	42%
Relaxation techniques	13.1%	15.3%
Chiropractic	10.0%	11.1%
Acupuncture	0.4%	1.0%
Massage	6.9%	11.1%
Homeopathy	0.7%	3.4%
Herbs	2.4%	12.1%
Vitamin therapy	2.4%	5.5%

Source: Eisenberg et al., 1993; Eisenberg et al., 1998.

niors, undertaken as exploration of possible Medicare + Choice benefits, similarly found use in the 40–50 percent range.[8,9]

Self-care treatment, led by relaxation treatments, vitamin therapy, and herbs, represents a significant percentage of consumer use. Chiropractic and massage lead provider-delivered services. With acupuncture, chiropractic and massage are the provider-delivered services most often favored by seniors.

Employers and HMOs

One sign of the appreciation for a growing role of CAM in mainstream payment and delivery is the mere fact that, beginning in 1998, questions seeking baseline data on CAM offerings were included in major, ongoing surveys of employers, hospitals, and managed care organizations.[10,11] Table 15–2 reports CAM-related findings in an annual survey of employers by William M. Mercer/Foster-Higgins. Table 15–3 includes CAM-related findings from an ongoing survey of HMOs by InterStudy.

Most observers of the CAM integration process agree that the findings in Tables 15–2 and 15–3 are, in the words of the Mercer consultant assigned to the study, "skewed upward."[12] That an employer or HMO is "offering" a CAM service may not mean that the service is a covered benefit. Even an affirmative response on coverage may be misleading. For instance, "coverage" of acupuncture by one HMO may mean that the payer has approved coverage of services provided by a certain physician who sometimes uses acupuncture for a limited percentage of his pain patients. From a consumer's perspective, the likelihood that an acupuncture treatment by a chosen provider for a specific health concern is covered may remain slim to nonexistent. Similarly, coverage of chiropractic may be limited to acute low back pain following referral from a gatekeeper. While some plans have elected to take a more expansive approach toward CAM services, for a CAM consumer a "yes" by an HMO or employer is still likely to mean "no."

Motivations

Available evidence regarding motivation for CAM coverage points squarely to the consumer. At 38 percent each, consumer or employer inter-

---

Table 15–2 Employers Saying They Offer CAM

Plan Type	Percentage of Employers Offering				
	Acup	*Bio*	*DC*	*Hom*	*MT*
PPO					
500+ workers	19%	8%	65%	8%	9%
10–499	10%	4%	56%	8%	10%
Point of Service					
500+	15%	8%	59%	7%	9%
10–499	14%	9%	44%	11%	8%
HMO					
500+	9%	5%	45%	4%	6%
10–499	11%	6%	41%	10%	9%
Traditional Indemnity					
500+	17%	10%	65%	5%	8%
10–499	14%	8%	53%	7%	10%

Note: Acup (acupuncture/acupressure), Bio (biofeedback), DC (Chiropractic), Hom (Homeopathy), MT (Massage Therapy), PPO (preferred provider organization).

Courtesy of William M. Mercer, Incorporated/Foster-Higgins, National Survey of Employer-Sponsored Health Plans, 1998, San Francisco, California.

Table 15–3 Percentage of CAM Offerings in Two HMO Surveys

Therapy	1998	1999
Chiropractic	58%	65%
Acupuncture	33%	31%
Massage	14%	11%
Naturopathy	8%	2%
Homeopathy	6%	4%
Herbs	5%	4%
Hypnotherapy	7%	2%
Biofeedback	24%	2%
Guided Imagery	3%	4%

Source: Data from Landmark Healthcare, Sacramento, California and InterStudy, Minneapolis, Minnesota.

est and state mandates figured in one study as the most important factors in HMO coverage decisions.[13] Mandates of some sort for chiropractic currently exist in 42 states, for acupuncturists in eight states, for naturopathic physicians in four, and for massage therapy in one. Creating more effective care led decisionmaking for just 8 percent of those surveyed. No plan listed "cost-effectiveness" as a chief motivation.

While clarity on the percent of consumers using CAM may currently be difficult to pin down, significant majorities of those surveyed in all three studies believed that coverage and inclusion would grow in years ahead. Two demographic trends are often referenced that support anticipated growth. One is the aging of the "baby boomers." The boomers are expected to look to CAM approaches to maintain quality of life while living with chronic conditions during their anticipated longer lifespans. The second trend is the shrinking of the labor force, behind the boomers, which will put pressure on employers to do all they can to attract and maintain work forces. CAM is expected to be useful to employers as an enticement to employees.[14]

Physicians and Medical Schools

Dynamism in physician interest in CAM is underlined by data that prompted the statement by former *JAMA* editor Lundberg cited above. A 1996 *JAMA* survey of priorities of medical journal editors for articles in the organization's family of publications placed alternative medicine sixty-eighth among 73 topics. Just 12 months later, the editors ranked CAM second among 86 topics.[15]

Published surveys on physician use of CAM in their own practices as well as proprietary reports by health systems uniformly find significant and growing physician interest in CAM. A Kaiser Northern California survey discovered that 89 percent had "used or recommended" CAM in their practice.[16] Relaxation techniques (67.6 percent), acupuncture (57 percent), support groups (58 percent), meditation (48.9 percent), massage (42.5 percent), chiropractic (33.6 percent), biofeedback (31.9 percent), and acupressure (30.9 percent) were all noted by more than 30 percent. Seventy-five percent said they were "interested" in CAM, and 35 percent said they were "very interested." Physician interest is not only a function of acknowledging patients' interest. A survey of primary care physicians (PCPs) in the Seattle area found that 38 percent believed that appropriate CAM integration could lead to "more effective care," while 30 percent believed such an undertaking would create more "cost-effective" care.[17] A significant percentage thought dollars could be saved under capitated contracts with appropriate integration. In studies, proximity generally makes the heart grow fonder; those who have had personal experience of CAM are more likely to believe more highly in the value of CAM.

Individual physician behavior is both stimulating and creating an expanding place for CAM in conventional medical schools and continuing medical education courses. Seventy-five of the nation's medical schools (64 percent) had at least one course in CAM in 1997, up from just a handful at the time Eisenberg's survey was taken in 1990.[18] These data, while useful as a sign of movement, may also be best viewed, like that on HMO and employer offerings above, as soft. Most of the courses are surveys, often taught by community providers. Little evidence is presently available that any medical school is ensuring that the literature on the potential value of CAM modalities or providers is routinely integrated throughout the medical school curriculum. However, physicians interested in reeducation in CAM can now find intensive, medical school-endorsed continuing medical education in diverse CAM areas. Included here are medical acupuncture, botanical medicine, body-mind approaches, therapeutic nutrition, and homeopathy.[19] Leading medical schools are claiming turf as the recognized purveyors of 2- to 5-day conferences on CAM applications for diverse specialties, such as pediatrics, rehabilitation, and oncology.

Hospitals and Health Systems

The annual *Health Statistics Survey* published by the American Hospital Association (AHA) added a CAM question for the first time in 1998. The core finding: 9 percent of the respondents said they offered some CAM services. The finding stimulated the industry organization to announce, in August 1999, a memorandum of understanding with a CAM program at the State University of New York, Stony Brook, to provide AHA members with information which would "help hospitals and other institutions learn about and develop complementary and alternative medicine programs."[20] Models for integration are discussed in a later section of this chapter.

Federal Research and Agency Activity

One major outcome of the splintering of the bamboo curtain between CAM and the medical mainstream is that the polarizing assertion by skeptical mainstream stakeholders that CAM is without a scientific basis is increasingly accepted as more prejudice than evidence-based conclusion. A useful published literature on some CAM modalities, such as mind-body approaches, clinical nutrition, acupuncture, massage, and some botanicals, is becoming widely accessible. Numerous private venture initiatives are cropping up to make the evidence on CAM that currently exists readily available to physicians and consumers through newsletters, books, CD-ROM, Internet, and Intranet technologies. Concomitant awareness of shortfalls in research support for many conventional interventions brings balance to the discussion.

Knowledgeable lambasting of CAM's scientific basis is increasingly a precision sport. Major information gaps continue to exist, especially regarding critical implementation questions on costs and cost-offsets.

The turning point in CAM's relationship to the mainstream research and scientific infrastructure was the decision by the U.S. Congress in 1991 to fund CAM research inside the National Institutes of Health (NIH). The combination of public interest and available funds converted CAM into a legitimate research arena. This federal initiative has steadily grown and is now the independent National Center for Complementary and Alternative Medicine (NIH NCCAM) with a budget for fiscal year 2000 of $69 million—roughly 35 times the original funding. A separate NIH Office of Dietary Supplements began contracting $8 million center grants in late 1999. CAM research affiliations of $2 million or more have been established at more than 15 distinct academic centers. Foci range from pediatrics to geriatrics, and from HIV/AIDS to natural therapies used by ethnic minorities.

The importance of federal funding of research in natural health care is underscored by the nonpatentable nature of most natural health care modalities—from counseling and dietary adjustment, to acupuncture and massage, to vitamins and botanicals. Without ownership, CAM lacks a significant, interested, private funding source for research. A case has been made by this author that in order to ensure that natural health approaches achieve their appropriate place in U.S. medicine, they must be viewed not as owned by no one, but by all of us.[21] Viewed as a part of a broader public health responsibility, CAM may be positioned for increased governmental research support.

NIH funds also underwrite numerous educational programs and conferences, from clinical applications to ethical and operational concerns. In October 1996 the NIH linked with the U.S. Agency for Health Care Policy and Research to explore coverage issues associated with CAM.[22] An August 1999 program explored CAM in liver disease, cosponsored with the American Association of Naturopathic Physicians. The most influential of these gatherings was a November

1999 Consensus Conference on Acupuncture.[23] The panel concluded that definitive research supports the use of acupuncture for four conditions (postoperative nausea, chemotherapy-induced nausea and vomiting, nausea of pregnancy, and postoperative dental pain) and suggested value in a half-dozen others (addictions, stroke rehabilitation, headache, menstrual cramps, tennis elbow, fibromyalgia/general muscle pain, low back pain, carpal tunnel syndrome, and asthma).

While NIH NCCAM actions dominate federal CAM activity, explorations are also underway in diverse agencies. The Health Care Financing Administration (HCFA) is looking into acupuncture. A demonstration project on a mind-body program for cardiac rehabilitation was contracted in 1999. CAM expertise is also being developed inside the Substance Abuse and Mental Health Services Administration, Centers for Disease Control and Health Promotion, Health Resources Services Administration/Bureau of Primary Health Care, Veterans Health Administration (VHA), and the Department of Defense. Outcomes of these explorations may have significant downstream effects on coverage. A late 1999 consultant report to the VHA, for instance, recommended partnerships between the VHA and local health systems.[24]

CAM Professions and Organizations

Another critical stakeholder in the CAM integration movement is the licensed CAM professional. When consumer use awakened conventional interest, many mainstream decision-makers were surprised to discover the extent to which the distinctly licensed CAM professionals had been busy creating internal standards during the previous two decades. Table 15–4 shows the progress of CAM professions in this intensive period of standard setting. In short, mainstream investigators discovered that, in states where these providers are licensed, core credentialing requirements (such as educational standards, recognized accreditation, standardized licensing exam, and availability of malpractice insurance) were more or less in order. However, this nominal clarity is confounded by significant differences that still exist in state-to-state scope of practice, as well as individual practice styles.[25]

One estimate of the growth of these professions concludes that by 2010 distinctly licensed acupuncturists, chiropractors, and naturopathic physicians will represent 17 percent of "direct

Table 15–4 Development of Standards by the Complementary Professions

Profession	Accrediting Agency Established	U.S. DOE Approves	Recognized Schools	Standardized National Exam	State Regulation*	Malpractice Insurance Available	Total Estimated Practitioners
Acupuncture	1982	1990	30	1982	37	1980s	10,000
Chiropractic	1971	1974	16	1963	50	1950s	50,000
Massage	1982	In application	**	1994***	29	1993	60,000
Midwifery****	1990s	—	1st school 1995	1994	18	spotty	—
Naturopathy	1978	1987	4	1986	11	1988	1,750

*For chiropractors and naturopathic physicians, this category uniformly represents licensing statutes; for acupuncture, massage, and midwifery, a mixture of licensing, certification, and registration.

**Roughly 120 massage schools meet the 500-hour requirement recommended for accreditation by the leading massage school accrediting body.

***The exam is recognized by the quasi-governmental National Organization for Competency Assurance, the leading third-party reviewer of certification organizations.

****This is European-style, direct entry midwifery.

Courtesy of Integration Strategies for Natural Healthcare, Seattle, Washington.

care providers," up from 11 percent in 1994.[26] One indicator of this growth was that, in 1999, the number of naturopathic medical students in the three U.S. residential, four-year, federally recognized programs (e.g., Bastyr University, National College of Naturopathic Medicine, Southwest College of Naturopathic Medicine) was roughly equivalent to the total number of licensed naturopathic physicians.[27]

MODELS AND CHALLENGES: NETWORK DELIVERED SERVICES

Managed Care Strategies

The nonmandated movement to integrate CAM into managed care plans began in earnest with the late 1996 announcement by then-thriving, Connecticut-based Oxford Health Plans. The core elements of the Oxford strategy provide the broad outlines of typical integration approaches by other health plans into the payment system in the subsequent three years.

- *Rider.* A CAM rider is offered through a credentialed network of licensed providers (typically chiropractors, acupuncturists, and naturopathic physicians, where licensed, and, in some instances, massage practitioners); generally only offered to groups (21 or more, 51 or more, etc.) in order to limit adverse selection; usually allow direct access without referral from a physician; benefit limits against which the price of the rider is pegged (either a total dollar figure, typically $500 to $2,000, or annual number of visits, typically 12–30); and a higher than usual copayment, perhaps up to 50 percent.
- *Discount product.* A noncovered, "affinity" product, through which all members have access to a network that includes the abovementioned categories, plus a variety of other providers and services (in Oxford's case, massage and yoga practitioners), all of whom provide their services at a discount, or based on a contracted fee schedule, to members who must still pay cash.
- *Natural products.* Natural products, such as herbs and vitamins, together with educa-

tional materials, are available through a catalog, 1–800 number, or online.

Most plans mix and match these components, refining and altering them, based on local market factors, regulatory requirements, and health plan mission. Table 15–5 describes one such hybrid product, offered beginning in 1999 by an Oxford competitor in the Northeast, Physicians Health Services (PHS). Some notable characteristics of this product include:

- subcontracting with a CAM network firm—"buying" rather than "building"— for access to credentialed providers
- online availability of natural products, via a limited product line through which the network seeks to have more control over product quality
- mixed access to CAM providers (direct for acupuncture and naturopathy, where offered; both direct and via referral for chiropractic)
- an unusual, nonmandated, core, covered benefit for acupuncture, which, however, features a high copayment, to decrease the plan's financial exposure.

The PHS covered benefit distinguishes itself from most recent managed care CAM activity by the plan's east coast location and the decision to offer acupuncture as a part of the HMO's core benefit. United Health Care plans in Colorado and Georgia, Aetna-US Health nationally, Kaiser Health Plans in Hawaii and Oregon, and Blue Cross Blue Shield plans in Georgia, North Carolina, Maryland, Pennsylvania, Illinois, Texas, California, and Massachusetts are among the major providers that have entered the nonchiropractic CAM arena through affinity products as of 1999. Nonmandated covered CAM benefits, when offered, are more often than not on the West Coast. When offered, they are usually only available, unless otherwise mandated, as riders, and usually involve only chiropractic, or chiropractic and acupuncture. In the 11 states where licensing for naturopathic physicians exists, this category is usually also included.

Table 15–5 Physicians Health Services CAM Services

Covered Services	Chiropractic, Acupuncture
Acupuncture	Needles, electro-acupuncture, cupping, moxibustion
Chiropractic	Examinations, manipulation, X-rays, hot packs, electrical stimulation
Discount only services	Massage, nutritional supplements
Massage	Network in directory
Supplements	Via Landmark's arrangement with Leiner Health Products, available online
Eligibility	All new groups and renewing groups as of January 1, 1999
Benefit limits	For acupuncture: $20 co-pay, 20 visits; varies based on plan and state mandates
Geographic area	New York, New Jersey, Connecticut
Network size	Plan 20% of eligible providers, by county
Access	Most acupuncture is direct
	DC varies by state (90% direct in New York, 80% in Connecticut; most via referral in New Jersey)
PMPM rate	Not disclosed
Naturopathic services	As "direct access specialist," via internal PHS network developed in 1995

Source: Reprinted with permission from J. Weeks, THE INTEGRATOR *for the Business of Alternative Medicine,* Vol. 3, #11, May 1999.

Growing Role of CAM Network Businesses

Recent managed care activity has been stimulated in part by aggressive development and national expansion of CAM network businesses that carve out CAM services. Managed CAM can be offered without the plan developing significant internal expertise in how to either credential CAM providers or manage CAM services. The network firms offer to take over all provider credentialing, manage benefits, and take risk on products. They often promote benefit models that offer the plan's members direct access to CAM providers.

Table 15–6 includes some results from a late 1998 CAM network chief executive officer (CEO) executive survey. Most of the 16 network executives in the survey represent chiropractic networks that subsequently added other CAM services. Others are venture businesses founded to seize a perceived business opportunity.

Credentialing

The first section of this chapter and Table 15–4, on the development of standards by the distinct CAM professions, outline the internal standard setting by chiropractors, acupuncturists, naturopathic physicians, and massage practitioners that provides the foundation for provider credentialing. Beneath these standards, considerable challenges remain.

- *Scope of practice variations.* Multistate plans must be aware that the scope of practice for these provider categories may differ. Chiropractors may be general practitioners of natural medicine in one state and be limited to adjustment of the spine in others. In some states, naturopathic doctors may have broad prescriptive rights or be allowed to perform acupuncture under their naturopathic license. The title "physician" is accepted in certain jurisdictions but not in others. The CAM professions face the challenge of standardizing their scope of practice across jurisdictions. Such efforts may be charged with significant philosophic differences among providers.
- *Individual practice variations.* In addition, CAM practitioners may show substantial

Table 15–6 The Developing CAM Network Industry: Findings of a CEO Survey

Measured	Result
Began as chiropractic network with business still principally chiropractic	9/16
Began offering nonchiropractic CAM before 1997	6/16
Over 10 contracts[1]	8/16
Over 5 contracts that include CAM in addition to chiropractic	3/16
Networks in over five states by December 1999	8/16
Offer affinity/discount products	13/16
Go at-risk on covered benefits[2]	9/16
Over 100,000 covered at-risk lives	6/16
Credential 4 or more types of CAM providers	10/16
Credentialing requires primary source verification, site visits[3]	12/15
Have MD/DO CAM providers in network[4]	8/16
Offer natural products[5]	5/8
Have greater than $5 million in revenues in 1998[6]	8/11
Have greater than 30 employees[7]	6/9
Have institutional investors	5/15
Anticipate significant growth in 1999[8]	8/11

Note: Sixteen firms were included in this survey. Some firms did not respond to certain questions for proprietary reasons. Total respondents to the question are listed in the denominator. Findings in this chart have been altered in minor ways to reflect more recent knowledge. Responses are self-reported and were not independently verified. The original survey took place in the fall of 1998.

[1] Tops were two with 60–80 health plan contracts.

[2] Virtually all are chiropractic only.

[3] Information from other sources suggests this figure probably overstates actual site visiting.

[4] Most are MD/DO acupuncturists, one area where a reasonable credentialing criterion exists.

[5] Most non-respondents have no natural products offerings.

[6] Two firms that didn't respond are probably in this category.

[7] All but one non-respondent probably had less than 30 employees.

[8] Among non-respondents, many expected 1999 to be a year of dynamic growth.

Surveyed networks included: Alignis, ACN/ACCN, American Specialty Health Plans, American WholeHealth Network, ChiroServices, Complementary Healthcare Plans, Landmark, Sierra Chiropractic, Triad, AcuCare, Alternare, Commonwell, Consensus, FCQA, Holisticos, Optimum.

Source: Reprinted with permission from J. Weeks, THE INTEGRATOR *for the Business of Alternative Medicine,* Vol. 3, #5-6, December 1998, January 1999.

variation in the nature of the services they offer. One acupuncturist may use only needles in a practice that focuses on treatment of pain, while another will engage the general practice of traditional Chinese medicine, operating in many respects as a general practitioner. Some CAM providers specialize in one modality or certain conditions, while others define their practices more broadly.

In states where these providers are not licensed, the status of some of these professionals, from a credentialing perspective, appears to be equivocal. Plans must first be aware that, without formal standards, some individuals may practice without having achieved the professional standards represented in Table 15–4. Some delivery systems are comfortable working with CAM providers who are unlicensed when they are directly supervised by licensed physicians. In such a situation, one strategy for guaranteeing a level of competency is to require that the practitioner has passed the profession's national exam. Alternatively, the practitioner may be required to have secured and maintain a license in a state that licenses their provider type. However, state laws in some jurisdictions expressly forbid such practices. The National Committee for Quality Assurance (see Chapter 44) has not established standards in this arena, except for chiropractic care.

Restrictive Strategies of Some Plans

The blend of CAM services is, depending on perspective, either *richer* with diversity or more *fraught* with diversity, than even the individual practice styles listed here. Some health plans that credential complementary providers have established additional, restrictive standards to cull a subset from the group of available providers. Often these additional credentialing criteria are directed at ensuring that the CAM providers are comfortable working in a collaborative fashion with the conventional medical community. Examples include:

- continuing education beyond that which may be required for licensing

- evidence that the complementary provider has working relationships with conventional medical professionals
- a minimum number of years of practice, especially in lieu of a residency
- evidence that one or more conventional medical professionals will agree to consult when patient needs are beyond the scope of the CAM provider's practice or the provider's legal ability, such as hospital admissions

One interesting example of special criteria is the Regence Blue Shield of Washington strategy relative to naturopathic physicians. Regence allows naturopathic physicians to act either as PCP gatekeepers or as specialists. Those who wish to be in the Regence network as PCPs are required to show, in their application, that they are: (1) willing to perform immunizations, (2) have plans for 24-hour coverage, and (3) have a relationship with a conventional physician (M.D. or D.O.) who will handle hospital admissions for them. (No Washington state hospitals allow naturopaths to admit.) Naturopathic physicians who do not meet these criteria, but meet the other Regence credentialing requirements, can be listed as specialists who are available only on referral.

Finding Good CAM Providers Who Are Prepared for Participation

Processes for including CAM providers in health system or managed care offerings may also encounter informal barriers. CAM providers are often not prepared for participation in managed care from the perspective of capital (malpractice, office staff, computers, etc.) or experience. Unless their practices are geared around workers compensation claims in states in which their services are mandated, most have limited experience with insurance practices, and even less with managed care. CAM providers typically desire more education about referral procedures, utilization management, how insurance works, capitation, medical recordkeeping, medical necessity and technology assessment process, and the role of the gatekeeper.

Plans optimally will provide educational programs to these providers upon bringing them into networks.

Another useful strategy is an elaborate provider preselection process. The plan or network may request information on typical billing rates, most frequently seen conditions or codes utilized, number of patients, number of support staff, use of computers for office management, and their comfort with the integration processes. Plans may also begin by finding a few trusted providers, or consultants familiar with the CAM profession, then build a network based on their recommendations (with care taken to avoid potential antitrust problems as discussed in Chapter 63).

Credentialing Conventional Providers Who Use CAM Therapies

Credentialing processes are paradoxical for medical doctors and other conventionally trained and licensed medical professionals who use complementary methods. On the surface—with licensing in all 50 states, and very similar scopes of practice—core standards are easily met by these providers. But if the intent of credentialing is to ensure that providers meet standards *for the delivery of CAM*, the picture shifts.

- *Medical education.* Most conventional medical, nursing, physician assistant, and dietetics educational programs do not include complementary therapeutics in their core curriculum or as electives. Clinical training is rare.
- *Licensing examination.* Conventional providers are not tested in these skill areas as part of their examination process prior to attaining licenses.
- *Malpractice insurance.* Malpractice insurance carriers typically offer policies with the expectation that conventional providers will practice within the community standard of care. Most complementary approaches are outside this standard and therefore may not be covered by the

provider's policy. Some policies are available, however, that specifically cover alternative methods.

At the present time, most alternative medical doctors gain their education in CAM through a nonstandardized composite of lectures, books, tapes, conferences, collegial relationships, and clinical experimentation. A medical doctor may be exceptionally well skilled in one or more complementary therapies. Yet objective, verifiable standards for medical education, licensing and examination, the backbone of managed care credentialing, are limited. Thus the conventionally trained categories of providers with which the health plan is familiar, and with which it may be most comfortable, may be the least qualified, from a credentialing standpoint, to provide complementary services.

The recent growth in education programs in complementary medicine inside conventional medical schools and nursing schools may eventually lead to development of traditional credentialing standards. Courses on specific areas of CAM that offer continuing education credits through, or in partnership with, academic medical centers, are beginning to fill the gap. The standout example is acupuncture training offered through an extension program at the University of California at Los Angeles. However, neither standardization of these programs nor inclusion of a routine testing in complementary medicine in licensing examinations is expected soon.

No accrediting agencies for managed care have put standards for the delivery of complementary therapeutics by conventional providers to a credentialing test. Therefore, no clarity on the leniency these agencies might show has been established. Until the conventional medical professions establish verifiable standards, intermediate steps may fill the void:

- Requesting full documentation of all complementary education, including the background of the teaching faculty.
- Investigating the extent to which the education offered includes a clinical component.

- Requesting information on any education that has led to a certificate of completion, or which led to an examination.
- Requesting information on the status, if any, the certificate program has achieved with an independent review organization.
- Requesting evidence that the provider's malpractice carrier is aware of the provider's complementary practices and will cover these services.

Credentialing Unregulated Providers

A subset of CAM services is often provided by individuals who have no accredited health care training but who have undertaken to educate themselves, sometimes extensively, in one or more complementary medicine modalities. Included in this category are lay homeopaths, herbalists, and some types of nutritionists, bodyworkers, yoga, Qigong and Tai Chi instructors, and nutritional counselors.

Health plan accreditation standards would not appear to allow such individuals to provide services for an accredited health plan. Again, quite a bit of flexibility seems to be allowed here—perhaps again because the potential for harm is believed to be low. Some integrated clinics may offer such services under the aegis of a medical doctor. In addition, some plans will offer some of these services as part of health education or wellness, and not as nominally clinical services.

Per Member Per Month Pricing of Network Delivered Services

The dynamism in the marketplace has created uneven and dramatically shifting pricing. While little published information is available, industry sources reveal the following picture:

- A significant CAM preferred provider contract in which the network managed all payments on covered products to an HMO with more than 250,000 lives, but was not at risk, went for $0.08 per member per month (PMPM). Pricing on direct-to-employer contracts (100–1,000 employees), providing similar services, will run substantially higher, at $0.50 to $1.50 PMPM.

- An early affinity product for a large HMO was priced as high as $0.30 PMPM. The firm originally had no competition. Later, competitive contracting drove rates down.
- Network contracts in 1999 for large affinity contracts with more than 100,000 lives were generally awarded for bids as low as $0.00–$0.03 PMPM. The networks provide their credentialed CAM networks to managed care organizations with little cost, or for free, on discount products to position themselves in a marketplace for covered benefits that may develop in the future. In addition, such networks increasingly focus their efforts on sales of natural products through online and catalog channels as their core revenue source when accepting affinity contracts. In effect, the CAM network becomes a loss-leader to access the HMO's membership base to sell product. Estimates of one consultant, while deemed high by some, place PMPM revenue at $0.30 and up from natural product sales.[28]
- PMPM rates in large HMOs contracting with a network that goes at-risk on a standard chiropractic benefit ($10 copayment, 20 visit limit) are generally at $0.75–$2.50 PMPM, depending on the marketplace. A significant factor in utilization is requiring referral from gatekeepers who have little training or experience in the CAM approaches. A Milliman and Robertson report states that use of chiropractors could go down as much as 75 percent based on this factor.[29]
- In West Coast markets that most often offer nonmandated riders, health plans frequently add a premium of 50 percent to 250 percent for "retailing" the network's "wholesale" product, a significant inflation that means the price to the employer may have little relationship to the price of actually delivering the CAM services.
- Competition stirred by national ambitions of regional networks has created an environment full of cross-accusation that others are "buying business"—taking business at a loss in order to establish marketplace presence.

For managed care organizations, the growth of the CAM network industry has two significant outcomes: First, the health plan can develop a method for responding to consumer interest without developing significant internal competence in CAM. Second, with regional dominance by individual networks eroding as venture capital drives national network expansions, the purchase of network CAM services has become a buyer's market.

The emergence of noncovered affinity products, together with the growing competitiveness in the network industry, creates challenges for the CAM network firms. Most business plans assumed more substantial growth in the covered benefits that are the bread-and-butter of a network's revenue stream.[30] Development of a business infrastructure that can support such critically needed functions as research and data collection are almost impossible on the PMPMs in affinity contracts. Provider participation in data gathering is also limited when no direct financial relationship exists between the network and the credentialed provider. Finally, the economic imperative of networks that bid contracts at very low prices, unless they can stand to take losses for a long period of time, is to cut fees to providers or limit access to care. The former hastens cynicism of already skeptical CAM providers, while the latter may be especially inappropriate given the consensus view that member interest in CAM services is growing.

As noted above, most leading networks are seeking to insulate themselves from financial shortfalls through promoting sales of natural products through catalogs, 1–800 numbers, and significant website and internet investment.

Experience Data on Utilization, Cost, and Cost-Offsets

An executive of a plan that pioneered a CAM product in 1995 spoke of the plan's actuary taking a "leap of faith" in pricing the CAM product.[31] A limited amount of experience data is beginning to emerge that at least shortens the jump across the chasm of uncertainty in developing network-based CAM benefits.

One source of early data is Washington state, where an unusually broad 1995 mandate required all health plans to include every category of providers as part of a plan's core benefits. An unpublished study, reported at a Health Forum conference, compared utilization rates and costs in two benefit models for combined acupuncture, massage, and naturopathic physician services, in the second year of the benefit.[32] One plan was a relatively unmanaged, direct access preferred provider organization (PPO) benefit with a $1,000 maximum, shared equally by the plan and member, with medical necessity as the only requirement. Providers were paid on a fee schedule. While outside actuaries estimated that the price of covering CAM could run as high as 11 percent of total premiums, actual costs were at less than 1 percent. Only 1.2 percent of members used services that were reimbursed by the plan. Average cost to the health plan per user on this PPO model was less than $200.

The second model was in a heavily managed, staff-model HMO. Coverage was limited to just six to eight conditions for each of the three provider types. Services could only be accessed following referral from a PCP. Providers were paid on the same fee schedule as the PPO plan. In the gatekeeper environment, just over 0.5 percent of eligible members utilized services of the three provider types that were covered in the study period. The average cost to the plan was less than $350 per member using the covered services.

A third example is from a Colorado HMO that proactively entered the CAM market with a CAM rider, delivered through a broad, internal network of credentialed CAM providers, with a cap of $250 during the benefit year.[33] First year utilization was low. Early analysis suggested that total costs of covering the CAM users was roughly the same as members who did not use CAM services. The HMO, which distinguishes itself by a desire to explore whether, and in what contexts, CAM may provide more effective or cost-effective care, responded by converting the CAM benefit into part of its core offering. The HMO also created new strategies to increase utilization in order to add a more robust charter to the firm's internal research.

Many CAM providers argue that use of CAM services will prove cost effective through reducing the use of conventional medical services and procedures. Little definitive information is yet available on this core question. Researchers from Yale concluded that those using CAM services tended to have as many emergency department visits, conventional physician visits, and hospitalizations. The researchers speculated that the CAM user profile may reflect the profile of high-utilizers of conventional medical services.

A significantly different picture is created by a series of surveys of CAM users reported in 1998.[34] When asked for their perceptions as to whether CAM use had diminished use of conventional services, between 30 percent and 65 percent answered in the affirmative. The perception appears to increase with the level of intervention. For instance, one study found that just 20 percent of users of "vitamin therapy" believed that this frequently self-administered CAM treatment had a limiting effect on use of conventional care, while 55 percent to 64 percent of those who saw highly trained CAM providers—acupuncturists and chiropractors—perceived a lowering of use of conventional care. The only survey that was limited to users of covered CAM services—a segment of the Washington state members in the study referenced above—found a parallel perception. Users of massage perceived lower offsets than users of acupuncturists and naturopathic physicians. Of the latter group, 55 percent believed that their use of CAM diminished use of their conventional providers, and nearly 65 percent believed CAM use lowered their use of prescription drugs.

Clearly, more elaborate studies, comparing these perceptions against actual utilization, and over a significant period of time, must be completed before conclusive evidence for or against offsets is produced. While some network executives claim that such research is underway in partnership with their significant HMO clients, no outcomes have yet been publicly available. The

Washington experience, while not definitive on cost-offsets, suggests that the otherwise low cost of initially covering CAM services may be lowered even further if even 50 percent of perceived reduction is proven. Explorers of CAM benefits may have a slightly more financially comfortable playing field in which to work.

Limits of Network-Delivered Services As an Integrative Model

From a health plan's perspective, network-delivered CAM discount products and riders have many attractions.

- Initial investment is minimal. Other than a product development specialist who oversees research and contracting, little internal competence needs to be built or acquired.
- The PMPM price of a discounted product is minimal; a rider is covered through additional fees. In fact, as noted above, serving as a middle-entity between a purchasing employer and a CAM network may even return a nice margin to the contracting HMO.
- With a direct-access product, the HMO need neither engage the cross-professional challenges of working with conventional providers who may express reluctance toward integration, nor sort out the relationship building that might lead to optimal integration.
- Meantime, the plan can market its CAM product to members as evidence of the plan's commitment to promoting healthy behavior and being responsive to the expressed wishes of its members.

In this scenario, the basic economic interest of the network is aligned with this status quo. The more an HMO develops internal competence in CAM, the less the services of the network may be required. In short, network delivered CAM offerings, while nominally representing an integration of CAM into the mainstream payment and delivery system, may be viewed as disintegrative administratively, financially, and clinically. Unless organizations develop policies to mediate against these nonintegrative tendencies, the following can be viewed as expected side-effects of outsourcing as a mechanism for offering CAM services.

- Neither the conventional nor CAM providers, because they may be in separate organizations, have substantial organizational incentives to learn to work closely together and understand when CAM is most appropriate.
- If the outside contractor does a good job, CAM will not receive much internal attention.
- The leadership of the health plan will have little reason to assess whether CAM actually *replaces* or limits conventional services—and thus might be best considered as a core benefit—or is merely an add-on benefit and thus reasonably paid for by additional fees.

Interestingly, CAM providers and many CAM consumers believe that better integration of CAM will lead to more cost-effective treatment. They believe that CAM methods can help the health care system toward a more fundamental health-oriented focus that they believe is true reform. However, these characteristics suggest that outsourcing CAM services, as typically managed today, may limit the extent to which the health care payment and delivery system discovers and optimizes CAM in delivery of effective and cost-effective care.

CHALLENGES AND MODELS: HOSPITALS AND HEALTH SYSTEMS

The response of hospitals and health systems to CAM integration has centered around four areas:

- ***Expansion of wellness and fitness offerings.*** Stores and pharmacies stock herbs and botanical medicines, additional vitamins, minerals, enzymes, and natural health-oriented self-care educational materials favored by CAM users. Tai chi and

Qigong classes may be added to more traditional fitness offerings. Public education classes include speakers on CAM topics. Health systems may sponsor or cosponsor community-based CAM-oriented conferences or events.

- *Cross-training of conventional physicians in CAM services.* Some systems support the cross-training of respected medical doctors in CAM modalities. Medical acupuncture tops the list.

The last two areas, integration of body-mind therapies into inpatient and outpatient services and development of integrative clinics, represent the most significant exploration and warrant a more detailed examination.

- *Integration of body-mind approaches into inpatient and outpatient services.* Leaders of many health systems view CAM as an extension of a corporate mission that may already acknowledge the importance of treating the whole person, and of the role of spirituality in health care. CAM is also viewed by some as aligned with the so-called healing health care and patient-centered care movements that began in the mid-1980s and expanded in the early 1990s. The champions are typically individuals responsible for mission, and nursing executives. One or more medical doctors may be advisers or necessary advocates with the medical staff, yet nurses tend to drive these programs.

The leading therapies under exploration in inpatient settings are massage, therapeutic touch, music therapy, reflexology, aromatherapy, hypnosis, relaxation techniques, meditation, acupressure, support groups, educational materials, and guided imagery. Services are usually provided by nurses. Medical conditions for which these services may be offered as complements to conventional treatment vary widely and include cancer and cardiac rehabilitation. Therapies are used for preparation of preoperative patients and pain reduction in postoperative care. Initial data from a New York hospital with a combined inpatient-outpatient program using these services found an average pain reduction of 57 percent and stress reduction of 69 percent among users of a combination of mind-body services. Potential financial outcomes include more rapid wound healing time and diminished length of stay.

A leading outpatient mind-body approach is multiweek, interactive programs in which participants are trained in a rich mixture of approaches. Programs typically link education about the condition and scientific literature on mind-body interventions with experiential self-care training in nutrition, meditation, stress reduction, cognitive restructuring, and exercise. Some programs are condition-specific, ranging from fibromyalgia and premenstrual syndrome to various cancers and heart disease. Another approach is not condition-specific, but focuses on medical symptom reduction. Targeted clinical outcomes are typically pain reduction, increased functionality, enhanced self-care abilities, and other quality of life betterment. Financial outcomes center around diminished use of other hospital or physician services.

- *Development of integrative clinics.* The most visible of health system forays into CAM integration is the so-called integrative clinic in which conventional and CAM providers are linked in a single setting or adjacent settings. No data are currently available on the number of hospitals and health systems that have established, or are establishing, these facilities, but activity and interest are exploding. Many models are emerging, based on local factors, varying levels of system commitment, and physician leadership. At one end of the spectrum are integrative practices that feature cross-trained medical acupuncturists, who may work with a whole-foods oriented dietitian and a nurse or psychologist trained in body-mind approaches. The clinic may use not more than 1,000 square feet. At the other end of the spectrum are clinics in which systems have invested substantial funds in 10,000-square-foot-plus facilities that link a diverse set of a dozen or more providers.

Experience data are not available on which models bring the highest likelihood of financial and clinical success. Table 15–7 provides an overview of diverse models discovered in an ongoing benchmarking survey. The key finding to date from the project is that most health system clinics, despite their sponsorship, continue to operate in a referral and payment structure that reflects alternative medicine practices in the preintegration era. Physicians account for more than 20 percent of referrals in just 4 of 12 health system clinics, while the self-family-friend combination of referral sources was greater than 70 percent in 6. Most payment remains on a cash basis. Managed care contracting accounts for greater that 20 percent of revenues in few clinics. While health system clinics may have substantially more overhead than a usual alternative medicine practice, new sources of referrals and revenues that may make up the difference are generally not yet well tapped.

CONCLUSION: EXPLORATORY INTEGRATION FOR MOVING CAM OUT OF QUARANTINE

The first phase of CAM integration into the mainstream payment and delivery system may

Table 15–7 Sample Data Sets: Integrative Clinic Benchmarking Survey

Question	Total	By Type	By Size
Total clinics involved	20	12 HS, 8 PV	10 SM, 10 LG
Less than 2,500 sq. ft. (SM)	10	8 HS, 2 PV	—
Greater than 2,500 sq. ft. (LG)	10	4 HS, 6 PV	—
Opened before January 1, 1997	5	3 HS, 2 PV	2 SM, 3 LG
Include chiropractors	6	3 HS, 3 PV	3 SM, 3 LG
Include licensed acupuncturists/OMD	12	4 HS, 8 PV	5 SM, 7 LG
Include naturopathic physicians	8	2 HS, 6 PV	1 SM, 7 LG
Include massage practitioners	18	10 HS, 8 PV	9 SM, 9 LG
Services principally by MD providers	6	6 HS, 0 PV	4 SM, 1 LG
Have MDs on site	12	8 HS, 4 PV	5 SM, 5 LG
Group, multiweek condition special programs	14	8 HS, 6 PV	6 SM, 8 LG
Routinely see patients as a team	9	6 HS, 3 PV	5 SM, 4 LG
Have regular case review	11	6 HS, 5 PV	5 SM, 6 LG
Formal list of community CAM providers	11	6 HS, 5 PV	6 SM, 5 LG
Have relationships with CAM labs	11	4 HS, 7 PV	2 SM, 9 LG
Have a natural product dispensary	15	7 HS, 8 PV	6 SM, 9 LG
Have an outcomes component	12	8 HS, 4 PV	7 SM, 5 LG
Exploring add-on vs. replacement	10	7 HS, 3 PV	7 SM, 3 LG
Referral from self-family-friend > 70%	10	6 HS, 4 PV	4 SM, 6 LG
Referral from MD < 20%	4	4 HS, 0 PV	4 SM, 0 LG
Managed care revenue > 20%	4	2 HS, 2 PV	3 SM, 1 LG
Anticipated to be revenue source	12	5 HS, 7 PV	5 SM, 7 LG
Broke even within 12 months	5	2 HS, 3 PV	3 SM, 2 LG

Sponsoring organizations: Community Hospital of Indiana, Presbyterian Healthcare (N.C.), Catholic Healthcare West/Arizona Centers for Health and Medicine (Ariz.), Harvard Vanguard Medical Associates (Mass.), Hennepin Medical Center (Minn.), California Pacific Medical Center, UCSF-Stanford, University of Arizona, Mercy Health Partners (Ohio), Kaiser Permanente Mid-Atlantic (Md.), Advocate Healthcare (Ill.), and Columbia Hospital for Women Medical Center (D.C.). The other eight clinics are all venture or private capital-backed.

Data are self-reported. Some respondents viewed information as proprietary, or too early or unknown, and left spaces blank.

Note: HS, Health System; PV, Private Venture; <2,500 sq. ft., SM; >2,500 sq. ft., LG.

Source: Reprinted with permission from J. Weeks, THE INTEGRATOR *for the Business of Alternative Medicine,* Vol. 4, #7-8, 1999, Vol. 3, #3, October 1998.

be summarized as inclusion, but in a kind of quarantine.

- Medical schools are beginning to offer CAM education, but the courses are most often electives and the focus is less on the role CAM may have in serious conditions than on education about consumer use. Instructors are typically brought in from outside. The CAM literature and approaches are not usually integrated into general coursework.
- Managed care models focus on carving out services to external networks, with the greatest activity, outside mandated, usually chiropractic benefits, in noncovered affinity products in which consumers must continue to pay cash out-of-pocket. Most management models feature direct consumer access.
- The concept of a carve-out also characterizes the integrative clinic movement in health systems: integration activity centers on single or multiple site delivery, rather than the diverse applications that may exist to complement or replace conventional treatment across the health care spectrum. Referrals by physicians and managed care payment for services remain low.

In summary, initial CAM integration strategies have taken significant steps to begin to meet consumer interest. Yet most do not directly engage more substantial challenges in changing conventional practice patterns than would be implied if CAM integration were viewed as a helpful approach to creating more effective and cost-effective care.

A brief in favor of more aggressive strategies to integrate CAM more deeply into the mainstream payment and delivery system has a strong, impressionistic case. The argument begins with perception: surveys of consumers, physicians, employee benefits managers, and HMO executives find that significant percentages of these stakeholders who are users of CAM services believe that CAM can be both effective and create cost-offsets. The argument ends with the generally accepted knowledge that conventional medicine excels in reacting to crisis but has proved less successful in creating health in the populations served, particularly in the area of chronic conditions. CAM professionals, meantime, state that the latter is the forte of the health care paradigm they represent. Naturopathic physicians, the most thoroughly educated of general practitioners of natural medicine, state this case succinctly: their core mission is "treating disease by restoring health."

What is missing in the middle of this brief are definitive data proving that by intensifying integration of CAM into the mainstream payment and delivery system, the perceptions of the CAM users and beliefs of CAM providers will be confirmed. Undaunted CAM advocates will argue that a definitive basis for clinical and cost decisions is more the exception than the rule in most all of medicine, alternative or conventional. Experts on the scientific basis of conventional medicine conclude that as little as 15 percent of what is offered in conventional medicine is based on controlled, scientific research.[35]

A remarkable smorgasbord of integration experiments is percolating among managed care organizations and health systems that are exploring extension of CAM's role beyond the mere response to consumer interest. Some examples of these initiatives as of 1999 follow:

- ***Primary Care.*** Are natural therapies not just secondary resources but might they instead represent first-line tools of general practice? CAM providers argue that such is the correct "therapeutic order" that, while time intensive, leads to enhanced self-care, fewer conventional drug prescriptions (and their adverse effects), and diminished high-end referrals and hospitalizations. Experiments by Richard Sarnat, MD, with Alternative Medicine, Inc. and Blue Cross/HMO Illinois, and by Washington's Regence Blue Shield, with CAM-oriented PCPs (broad scope chiropractors and licensed naturopathic physicians, respectively) and the services of integrative-MDs in primary care-oriented clinics will test these claims. If the postulate is proven, reverberations may be felt through HMOs, clinical practice, and medical school curricula.

- *Group-focused services.* At HealthEast, Chris Foley, MD, and a local PPO are teaming to offer covered, integrative clinical services, physician-delivered to groups of clients rather than one-to-one. This concept of group-focused CAM services draws on mainstream experiments at Kaiser Permanente facilities, plus the work of CAM and body-mind professionals like Michael Smith, MD, at Lincoln Hospital in the Bronx, N.Y. The approach may be perfectly matched with CAM's core principles: integrative care groups alleviate provider time pressures, underscore the collective etiology (diet, stress, exercise, and lifestyle) of many chronic conditions, and place patients firmly in the center of the intervention. Says Smith: "If you want to empower patients, put more patients than physicians in the room."[36] Groups may prove to be the optimal locus of most integrative clinical care, with one-to-one short visits largely introductory and adjunctive.

- *Cost offsets.* Some CAM networks are partnering with HMO clients to analyze claims data on whether CAM has cost-offsets. A few academic centers, like the Center for Alternative Medicine Research, led by David Eisenberg, MD, at Harvard University, are showing willingness to move out of the ivory tower and engage in the more messier research on which many real-world coverage decisions are made. One potential treasure: insurance records in states where broad mandates have left decades of unexamined data.

- *Communication: Internet and information.* The transformation of conventional practice may be hastened through readily accessible information platforms. Organizations like Micromedex, Integrative Medicine Communications (publisher of *The Integrator*), and HealthNotes are creating licensable databases on CAM research that are available through Internet and Intranet technologies.

- *Natural product/drug substitution.* Portland, Oregon-based Tyler Encapsulations argues a savings to HMOs of $47 per converted user per month on a well-researched fish-oil option to typical cholesterol lowering drugs. Significant savings may be gained even if these and other scientifically supported natural alternatives were made available only to consumers who would prefer to explore a CAM option. Experts in research outcomes on natural products hold that similar savings might be found with at least a dozen other, consumer-directed substitution interventions.

- *Clinical pathways.* At Group Health Cooperative of Puget Sound, a CAM provider was invited into the HMO's development of an outcomes-based sinusitis guideline. Providers from both sides of the aisle—each attuned to the other's research shortcomings and relatively blind to their own—found the effort humbling. Three natural agents—zinc, Echinacea, and Vitamin C—made the grade. Bringing CAM providers into such processes will enhance cross-education on appropriately integrative care.

- *Creating relationships.* In organizations like HealthPartners, Kaiser Northern California, Hennepin Faculty Associates, and Harvard Vanguard, CAM providers work side-by-side or in near proximity, with medical staff. Trust and clinical creativity are stimulated by exchanges in hallways, lunchrooms, and face-to-face joint case review.

- *CAM coding.* A New Mexico business, Alternative Link, has developed an extensive CAM procedure coding system, similar to CPT codes, linked to relative value units and compatible with HCFA and health system software. This patented coding system may provide an information infrastructure for comparing experience across systems and geographic areas.

- *Tertiary care.* New York Presbyterian Hospital offers diverse CAM therapies as complements to inpatient care. Cancer Treatment Centers of America goes a step further: Naturopathic physicians, whose medical training fills voids in MD education—therapeutic nutrition, botanical medicine, homeopathy, and mind-body approaches—directly co-manage patients with oncologists. Insights into co-management and complementary use of natural approaches for high-end treatment may be gained.

- *Public health.* Region X of the U.S. Public Health Service, led by regional administrator Richard Lyons, MD, has engaged a long-term relationship with Bastyr University, a leading research and education center for natural medicine, through which

CAM organizations are invited into public health campaigns: cosponsored education on integrative diabetes care, population-based programs, and even immunization education strategies. Participants are discovering significant common ground.

Initiatives such as these will, with publication of outcomes, help us clarify optimal models for CAM integration, not just as a service to consumers, but also as components of the payment and delivery system's challenging work of creating optimally effective and cost-effective treatment.

REFERENCES AND NOTES

1. G. Lundberg, cited in *USA Today*, November 25, 1997.

2. D.M. Eisenberg, R.C. Kessler, C. Foster, et al., Unconventional Medicine in the United States: Prevalence, Costs and Patterns of Use, *New England Journal of Medicine* 328 (1993): 246–52.

3. Published continuously since July 1997, originally by St. Anthony Publishing, Reston, Va., and presently by Integrative Medicine Communications (onemedicine.com), John Weeks, publisher-editor, Newton, Mass.

4. D.M. Eisenberg, R.B. Davis, S.L. Ettner, et al., Trends in Alternative Medicine Use in the United States, 1990–1997: Results of a Follow-Up National Survey, *JAMA* 280 (1998): 1569–75.

5. B. Druss and R. Rosenheck, Association between Use of Unconventional Therapies and Conventional Medical Services, *JAMA* 282 (1999): 651–56.

6. Stanford University/American Specialty Health Plans, Understanding Consumer Trends in Complementary and Alternative Medicine: A National Survey. Paper presented at a conference at Stanford University, September 18, 1998.

7. J. Weeks, Structure for CAM Integration, in *Best Practices in Medical Management*, edited by P.R. Kongstvedt and D.W. Plocher (Gaithersburg, MD: Aspen Publishers, Inc., 1998).

8. W. Alles, What Is Complementary and Alternative Medicine? Paper presented at the National Managed Health Care Congress East, Atlanta, GA, March 28, 1999.

9. J. Weeks, Open Enrollment: Two Sample New Products, *The Integrator for the Business of Alternative Medicine* 3, 5 (December 1998): 8, 12.

10. National survey of employer sponsored health plans, William Mercer/Foster Higgins, 1998.

11. The Competitive Edge 8.2, Part II: HMO Industry Report, InterStudy, St. Paul, MN, 1998.

12. J. Weeks, CAM in Employer and HMO Benefits, Mercer/Foster Higgins and InterStudy, *The Integrator for the Business of Alternative Medicine* (May 1999): 4–5.

13. The Landmark Report II: HMOs and Alternative Care, Landmark Healthcare, Sacramento, CA, 1999.

14. Health Benefits for Alternative Medicine: Is There a Fit? International Society of Certified Employee Benefit Specialists, 1999.

15. P. Fontanerosa and G. Lundberg. Alternative Medicine Meets Science, *Journal of the American Medical Association* 280(18) (1998): 1618–1619.

16. N.P. Gordon, D.S. Sobel, and E.Z. Trazona, Use of and Interest in Alternative Therapies among Adult Primary Care Clinicians and Adult Members in a Large Health Maintenance Organization, *Western Journal of Medicine* 169 (1998): 153–61.

17. J. Weeks and R. Layton, Integration as Community Organizing: Toward a Model for Optimizing Relationships between Networks of Conventional and Alternative Providers, *Internal Medicine* 1 (1998): 15–25.

18. Eisenberg et al., Unconventional Medicine in the United States.

19. J. Weeks, Education Opportunities Expand and Diversify, *The Integrator for the Business of Alternative Medicine* (August–September 1999): 1–5.

20. American Hospital Association release, August 1999.

21. J. Weeks, Moving CAM out of Quarantine, *Health Forum Journal* (September–October 1999): 29–30, 32.

22. Complementary and Alternative Medicine: Issues Impacting Coverage Decisions. Invitational Workshop cosponsored by the NIH Office of Alternative Medicine,

U.S. Agency for Health Care Policy and Research, and the Arizona Prevention Center at the University of Arizona Health Sciences Center, October 9, 1996.

23. National Institutes of Health, Consensus Conference on Acupuncture, November 3–5, 1997.

24. Veteran Health Administration, Report on Complementary and Alternative Medicine Therapy: Assessment of Current VHA Practice and Future Opportunities, prepared by Klemm Associates, 1999.

25. J. Weeks, Operational Issues in Incorporating Complementary and Alternative Therapies and Providers in Benefit Plans and Managed Care Organizations. Unpublished paper developed for the Complementary and Alternative Medicine workshop, October 9, 1996.

26. R.A. Cooper and S.J. Stoflet, Trends in the Education and Practice of Alternative Medicine Clinicians, *Health Affairs* (Fall 1996): 226–38.

27. American Association of Naturopathic Physicians, 1999.

28. J. Weeks, Special Report: The Evolving Economics in CAM Network Delivered Services, *The Integrator for the Business of Alternative Medicine* (November 1999): 1–6.

29. T.D. Snook, Considerations in the Design and Pricing of an Alternative Medicine Benefit, Milliman & Robertson, Inc., 1999.

30. J. Weeks, 1998 CAM network executive survey, Part 1, *The Integrator for the Business of Alternative Medicine* (December 1998): 1–7.

31. Sandy Mathee, vice president, American Medical Security, personal communication, 1997.

32. P. West and J. Weeks, A Word from the Epicenter: Complementary and Alternative Medicine Integration in Washington State. Presentation at Healthier Communities Best Practices Forum, conference sponsored by Health Forum, Honolulu, Hawaii, 1999.

33. J. Weeks, Sloans Lake: Spiritual Care and CAM in Core Benefits, *The Integrator for the Business of Alternative Medicine* (May 1999): 1–3.

34. J. Weeks, Is CAM an Add-on or Replacement? A Call for Significant Claims-Based Research, *The Integrator for the Business of Alternative Medicine* (December 1998): 1–2.

35. Healthcare Management Guidelines: Questions and Answers, Milliman & Robertson, Inc., 1998, pp. 3–4.

36. M.O. Smith, Using Complementary Medicine in the Inner City. Presentation at Healthier Communities Best Practices Forum, conference sponsored by Health Forum, Honolulu, Hawaii, 1999.

Part III

Medical Management

"You can't always get what you want.
But if you try sometimes
You just might find
You get what you need."

Mick Jagger [1969]

CHAPTER 16

Care Management and Clinical Integration Components

David W. Plocher, Wendy L. Wilson, Jacqueline A. Lutz, and Ann Huston

THE CONTEXT FOR ADVANCED CARE MANAGEMENT

Managed care dynamics motivate many organizations to assemble historically fragmented components of the health care system—hospitals, physicians, managed care organizations (MCOs) and health maintenance organizations, postacute services, and so forth—into integrated delivery systems (IDSs). Integration can be defined as the optimization of interactions among components of a system to provide health services of high value to those served.[1] It is predicated on economic theory that suggests that an organization achieves a competitive advantage by controlling or managing, through ownership or contract, as large a span of the health care value chain as possible.

As markets evolve toward more aggressive forms of managed care, clinical delivery systems

David W. Plocher, MD, is a Partner in Ernst & Young's Health Care Consulting Practice and has 20 years of experience in the managed care field. His early areas of expertise include national point-of-service program administration and the development of the centers of excellence product known as "Institutes of Quality". More recently, he has designed and implemented integrated delivery systems and advanced care management programs including demand and disease management. In addition, he has worked on quality audits and accreditation with both the Joint Commission for Accreditation of Healthcare Organizations and the National Committee for Quality Assurance.

Wendy L. Wilson, MD, MSE, is a senior manager in Ernst & Young's Health Care Consulting Practice. Prior to joining Ernst & Young in October 1996, Wendy worked in a variety of academic medical settings. She was a member of a group practice in Physical Medicine and Rehabilitation at MetroHealth Medical Center (then a 750-bed hospital system, affiliated with the Cleveland Clinic in a network including nine regional hospitals). Her past experience includes: Chair, System-wide Outcomes Measurement Team; Appointee, Greater Cleveland Health Quality Choice, Functional Status Outcomes System Advisory Panel. She recently completed a fellowship in Outcomes Measurement and Disease Management at Thomas Jefferson University.

Jacqueline A. Lutz, MBA, is an Associate Director in the Chicago office for Ernst & Young's Health Care Strategy and Strategic Partnering practice. She has more than 10 years' experience in the health care industry, and specializes in partnering strategies and the development of integrated delivery systems. She is currently responsible for the development of the practice's strategic partnering methodology and related tools and processes.

Ann Huston, MHS, is a Partner in the Health Care Consulting practice. She has over 10 years' experience, including a variety of senior-level, corporate and operational roles within health care systems, community and large teaching hospitals. Ann's health care experience lies in the areas of strategy formation, integrated delivery and financing design and development, physician integration, and strategic partnering. During her consulting career, Ann has assisted a wide variety of clients ranging from academic health centers, urban and rural community hospitals, health plans, and large, multispecialty physician groups.

come under greater pressure to reduce and manage costs. Future success in this environment, however, cannot be achieved by simply cutting costs; rather, a cost-competitive position must be reached through effective clinical integration and resource management. A number of common initiatives—advanced care management, process and system redesign, change management—are complex efforts aimed at reducing costs and increasing quality and value by transforming organizational processes, resource utilization, and service delivery.

A recent *Hospital and Health Services Administration* article[2] on clinical integration notes that "simply forming an IDS, even one with all the needed components, while necessary for ... integration, is not sufficient to actually achieve it." However, progress toward integration can be assessed according to four criteria:[3]

1. coordination of clinical activities and services among operating units
2. avoidance of unnecessary duplication of clinical facilities and services
3. appropriate sharing of clinical services among operating units
4. integration of clinical services and facilities to achieve cost-effective patient care

Considerable effort has gone into trying to define the functional requirements and competencies for successfully meeting these criteria. Since the ability to accept and manage capitated or fixed risk for medical costs is a common goal for MCOs and IDSs, advanced care management* invariably appears as one of the critical success factors for MCOs and IDSs.

Advanced care management refers to a comprehensive, integrated program that allows an

organization to effectively assess and manage (1) the clinical performance of its providers and (2) the health status of the insured population. In this context care management refers to the program components, competencies, processes, and infrastructure necessary to manage and deploy the clinical resources within the system.

The rationale for adoption of an advanced care management system extends far beyond the pure economic advantages. Excellence in clinical quality and consumer satisfaction are anticipated to become significant market drivers in the near future and have become significant forces in the shaping of health care in advanced markets. The establishment of an advanced care management system allows for optimization of outcomes on several axes, all of which are key denominators in future success of large systems.[4] Key outcomes important to future system success are well described in the clinical value compass as developed by Batalden et al. Those outcomes include:

- business/financial outcomes, depicted here as "total costs"
- classical medical outcomes, typically morbidity and mortality, depicted here as "clinical outcomes"
- recently developed outcomes systems, including a broad variety of functional, health status, quality of life, and patient-referenced outcomes, depicted here as "functional health status"
- patient/member satisfaction, driving member retention, employer purchasing, and those market trends that are impacted by member choice and consumerism, depicted here as "satisfaction against need" (this axis can also encompass poly-customer and provider satisfaction as well)

DEFINING ADVANCED CARE MANAGEMENT

The primary objective of advanced care management is to ensure each enrollee receives the appropriate level of care (including preventive services), at the lowest cost, with optimal outcomes.

Advanced care management is a term used to differentiate from more basic forms of utilization management, quality management, and medical management. As demonstrated in this book, advanced care management is clearly focused on issues of utilization and quality (as distinct from other administrative or clinical activities involved in the provision of health care), but in a far more comprehensive manner than has occurred in past years.

Advanced care management goes beyond traditional utilization or stand-alone case management programs by evaluating care in all settings against a more comprehensive set of criteria (e.g., quality, cost, patient satisfaction, and health promotion) and within more aggressive time frames (e.g., prospective as opposed to retrospective review). Figures 16–1 and 16–2 outline a single model for advanced care management, but seen from two different perspectives. The model provides a framework for developing and structuring comprehensive care management systems.

As illustrated in Figures 16–1 and 16–2, advanced care management is comprised of a number of specific program elements that are designed to move patients to the most appropriate setting for their health care services. In this way care management programs reflect the full continuum of care, in terms of settings and scope of services. Two program elements—disease management and case management—seek to coordinate activities across various elements of the broader program. Conventional case management typically addresses inpatient cases and attempts to streamline activities associated with a particular inpatient admission. Disease management encompasses a broader spectrum of health care settings and focuses on integrating services for a particular disease state, such as asthma, congestive heart failure, or diabetes.

Other components of care management that help transform the program from a series of independent elements to a truly integrated system capable of managing care and resources include information technology and systems, network management, and the integration model for the delivery system.

INTEGRATING THE COMPONENTS OF CARE MANAGEMENT

In many health care systems, current care management activities are predominantly insur-

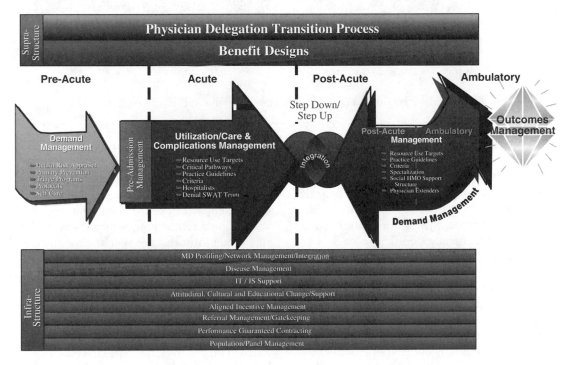

Figure 16–1 Care Management Components, Payer-System Perspective. Courtesy of Ernst & Young LLP, 2000, Washington, DC.

W = well, C = chronic, T = terminal, A = acute

Figure 16–2 Care Management Components, Patient/Member-Population Perspective.

---

ance focused. The various components are designed to respond to external demands for utilization controls and retrospective review. As a result, the system and processes do not encourage sharing information among providers, caregivers, utilization management staff, social workers, discharge planners, and so on. In addition, the focus of the activities is typically the inpatient arena. Care management, under this scenario, is a support function for patient care.

Care management models typically evolve from insurance-focused programs, to care delivery models, and eventually to continuum of care models. This evolution is outlined in Exhibit 16–1. What truly differentiates the continuum of care model from the other models is that care manage-

ment *drives* patient care. It is no longer a support function but a core business of the health system. This is a subtle but significant difference.

The evolution of care management systems is neither simple nor linear. Organizations must invest in the core program elements, develop the supporting infrastructure (i.e., disease management, information systems), and determine the appropriate integration model to convert the program elements into an integrated care management system. The development of the program requires consistent and continuous effort over a significant period of time. However, as illustrated in Figure 16–3, the more advanced models have significantly more impact on the ability of the health system to manage resources and

Exhibit 16–1 The Evolution of Care Management Models

Insurance Model	Care Delivery Model	Continuum of Care Model
• Utilization review and quality assurance functions • Inpatient focus • Compliance and access orientation • Driven by insurance benefit parameters and national practices • No integration among components or patient care providers and settings	• Development and use of standard tools, such as critical pathways, care plans • Inpatient focus with some attention given to preadmission and postadmission service requirements • Exception-based review • Driven by medical staff buy-in and system integration efforts (e.g., PHO) • One-dimensional (linear)	• Community health care requirements drive program • Focus on appropriate provider and optimal care site • Continuous quality improvement (CQI) • Driven by promotion of wellness and community health status • Balances cost, access, and quality by managing across the entire continuum • Multidimensional

Courtesy of Ernst & Young LLP, 2000, Washington, DC.

health status, thereby providing an appropriate "return on investment."[5]

In order to truly appreciate Figure 16–3, one simply has to consider the theory and practice of the IDS (see also Chapter 4). The theory driving organizational integration is that controlling all the inputs to the health care process can achieve improved quality and service, lower cost structure, and achieve the critical mass necessary to survive as a dominant player in the market. Yet, in practice, results to date appear less than stellar. For most IDSs, clinical integration has yet to be achieved. Systems have not yet realized anticipated cost reductions. The market does not yet recognize significant improvements in quality and health status.

Yet systems are still investing time and resources into integration. Perhaps the answer lies in another conceptual "arrow." Figure 16–4 defines the evolution of integrated systems. Most IDSs are in the early stage of collecting assets. These systems are trying to build a continuum of care in a market region through vertical and horizontal integration. The transition stage requires systems to define and develop new competencies—many of which were not required in traditional fee-for-service markets. These competencies—which include care management—are complex, multidisciplinary processes. During the transition stage, an organization begins to develop an understanding and definition of "systemness."

The four criteria for assessing progress toward integration (discussed earlier) can be incorporated into a number of key characteristics for integrated care management. In this way we can differentiate between the components or program elements, and an advanced care management system.

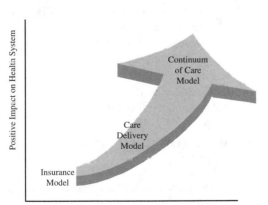

Figure 16–3 The Impact of Care Management Models on Integrated Systems. Courtesy of Ernst & Young LLP, 2000, Washington, DC.

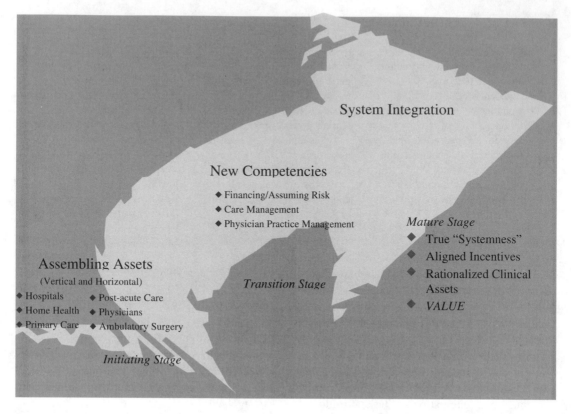

Figure 16–4 The Evolution of Integrated Delivery Systems

Key Characteristics of Advanced Care Management

- Multidisciplinary teams (e.g., physicians, nurse managers, hospital administration) drive the development and ongoing operation of the care management system. Physicians are well integrated into these teams.
- Communication and documentation are enhanced throughout the system.
- Patient care and service across the different settings and departments are well coordinated.
- Processes are streamlined and resources are effectively managed to improve service and reduce costs.
- There is a marked reduction in the duplication of clinical and administrative efforts.

- Services are redesigned to allow departments and operating units to share resources, as appropriate.
- Internal and external customer satisfaction improves throughout the health system.
- Within the health care organization, care management is functionally and structurally situated as a core business.

THE ROLE OF PHYSICIANS IN CARE MANAGEMENT

The successful development and management of a care management system is highly dependent on a "partnership" between the health system and its affiliated physicians. Currently, physicians remain the primary providers of patient care services and, as such, manage the overall health of their patients; are a critical element in providing patients with information related to wellness programs; and determine diagnoses, care settings, treatment plans, and follow-up. As providers, therefore, physicians largely drive the use of clinical resources within the health system.

Although care management requires a multidisciplinary team composed of physicians, other clinical practitioners, administrative personnel, and external (e.g., payer) representatives, physicians perform a number of critical roles in care management.

- As providers, physicians must collaborate with the patient care team regarding the overall care plan.
- Physicians retain the technical knowledge needed to develop a number of the tools used in care management (e.g., pathways and guidelines).
- Physicians are primary users of care management systems.
- Physicians document care, thereby generating a considerable amount of data that should be retained within the care management system. Ongoing management and improvement of the care management system depends, in part, on information access and management.
- Physicians act as advisors within the care management system by resolving clinical practice issues and serving as technical resources for case managers and other care management providers.
- Physicians are primary intermediaries with payers, providing clinical information critical to resolving care and benefit issues.
- Finally, physicians have clinical leadership and administrative roles within the health system. In these roles, physicians help define the direction and priorities of the health system.

The following section of this chapter broadly outlines a typical process for developing a care management system. Because of the many roles physicians play within this system, it is critical that they provide leadership and input throughout the development process.

BUILDING AN ADVANCED CARE MANAGEMENT SYSTEM: A TYPICAL PROCESS

Building an advanced care management system is typically a four-phase process:

1. elaboration of mission and vision, current state assessment
2. future state design, including the benchmarking of leading practices
3. construction of the model and long-term plan
4. staged implementation

Classically, such a system is built sequentially. With the rapid evolution of corporate change processes, nonlinear design/implementation processes are becoming popular, leading to a variety of accelerated process methods. A classical design/implementation process is described below, contrasted with examples of accelerated methods.

Phase 1: Mission and Vision, Current State Assessment

Early in the building process, it is important to relate the emerging care management model to overall mission and vision of the integrated system. Different priorities and structures would be built, for example, if the primary current developmental aim of the integrated system were to achieve access and care for vulnerable and disadvantaged populations rather than to build components of the system to serve an affluent population that demands alternative/complementary medicine and wellness programs from its care providers.

It is also important to define the current state of the system with regard to overall system maturity, financial health, market pressures, population served, and position in the evolution of care management systems. Examples are:

- A very mature system may have little need for length of stay reductions and remodeling of inpatient case management, and much more need to refine its delivery of care to capitated populations across the continuum at multiple sites of care.

- An integrated system that is new or economically fragile may choose to focus on care management initiatives that improve quality while concurrently reducing cost with a rapid rate of return on investment (such as a congestive heart failure disease management program, which can yield up to a 10 percent net cost reduction in 90 days). By contrast, a solvent and mature system may choose to implement care management initiatives that are "the right things to do," that attract and retain key populations but require an investment that may or may not yield a pure financial return, especially in the short term (such as extended health risk assessment and outreach among well populations).

- A large system that has been recently integrated may have profound needs to achieve clinical integration across its multiple sites, ramifying best practices within the overall system and facilitating the formation of a learning organization across multiple sites of care.

Depending on what aspects of care management are being redesigned and implemented, it may be important to complete a detailed current state assessment, including the following:

Assessment of hospital-based processes

- discharge planning
- infection control
- social service
- quality management
- risk management
- guest relations
- points of access
- scheduling
- ancillary services
- regulatory requirements

Assessment of ambulatory practice and extended continuum processes (Figures 16–5 and 16–6)

- processes that are general across the system and affect all patient populations (access, scheduling, documentation, etc.)

- care of specific populations along the continuum (well care, chronic care, terminal care)
- care of patients/members with specific diseases (disease management)
- current state of attempts to reduce demand in the system (demand management, including nurselines and health risk assessment and outreach)

Assessment of current infrastructure design and current organizational change processes

- information systems and technology
- outcomes measurement and feedback
- care management infrastructure, roles, responsibilities, and organization of providers
- facilities: physical configuration and geographic proximity
- approach to organizational change: organizational structure and alignment of incentives

This phase is typically completed through a series of interviews, facilitated sessions, and data analysis. It may be abbreviated and consolidated considerably in accelerated delivery by combining aspects of it with later phases in accelerated sessions. For example, there are methodologies for facilitating this in small (i.e., fewer than 20) and large (i.e., up to 200) numbers of participants. Very large group facilitation (up to 1,000 to 2,500 organizational participants) is useful for "whole scale change" in large organizations and is applicable to a variety of needs (strategic planning, business planning, process redesign/transformation).

Phase 2: Benchmarking and Future State Design

Taking into account key aspects of organizational mission and vision and opportunities as defined in the current state assessment, this phase further defines the initiatives to be undertaken based on where the strongest opportunities lie. Both internal and external systems and information should be used to develop an analysis of leading practices. The elements typically targeted include:

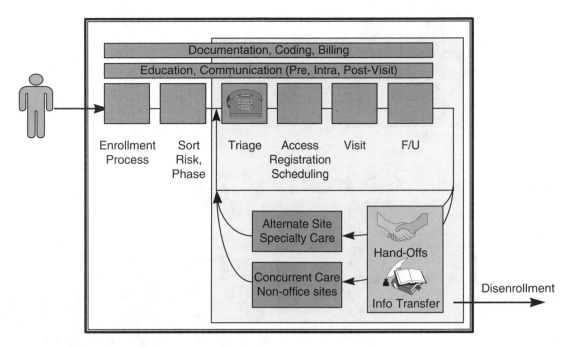

Figure 16–5 Processes Affecting All Patients

- cost: length-of-stay data, resource utilization, per member per month (PMPM) and procedure costs (defined across key populations and diseases)
- classical medical outcomes: morbidity and mortality data (complications, deaths, and so on)
- functional and health status outcomes
- poly-customer satisfaction and retention rates

The possible opportunities are contrasted against the organizational "gaps," such as where significant deviations from best practice lie, and where they correspond to areas where improvement is relatively easy to achieve and is possible to achieve. Again, the mature and financially healthy organization that lives on the leading edge of change may well decide to undertake initiatives that do not have a defined return on investment and are relatively experimental but are either "the right thing to do" or the next logical, although unproven, step in the organization's evolution.

This phase is typically completed in facilitated sessions and workgroups in classical design/implementation methods and can readily be combined with aspects of other phases in accelerated change design.

Phase 3: Construction of the Model and Long-Term Plan

Design of the care management model will include both a high-level design to achieve clinical integration across multiple sites and key "ground level" care management initiatives, with key infrastructure development and organizational change management support.

The infrastructure design, again tailored to market, organization maturity, and approach, includes designing where support personnel (such as case managers and physician extenders) will "live" and how they will be paid. Examples include:

- Will such disease-specific case managers live at the "corporate level" and be funded

Note: L = low, M = medium, H = high

Figure 16–6 Detail Risk Stratification Process Population/Disease Management

by "corporate moneys" or will they live in the individual physician practices and be paid by those practices?

- Will the system have, for a given geographic area, a "practice without walls" of leading providers for caring for its diabetic population, for example, or will it have a common protocol to be implemented through numerous primary care providers who then refer to key specialists per protocol?

Infrastructure development also includes definition of key areas such as information support, how outcomes will be measured and disseminated, and incentives alignment design.

In addition to infrastructure, design and implementation must include components targeted toward physician/clinical team behavior change. A definitive answer to the question "Why do you want to do this?" must be provided. The answer must be compelling enough to overcome resistance to the change. Depending on the position of the organization and individual providers relative to market pressures, a motivational platform can be constructed using a variety of "push-and-pull" approaches: the burning platform versus the manifestation of a compelling vision. Once the message is defined, a systemwide communication program must be put in place, with key data and outcomes delivered at critical moments as the model is implemented. Development and/or dissemination of an approach to change behavior and process that is relatively easy to implement must follow closely.

Finally, ground-level design and implementation must be planned. The key preventive, disease management, and demand management programs to be implemented are prioritized and defined. Key population and panel management programs likewise are prioritized and defined. The organization answers the questions, relative to key care management initiatives:

- What do we want/need to achieve in one year?
- What do we want/need to achieve in five years?
- What will we achieve this quarter?

The system will need to incorporate tools for some process standardization, outcomes measurement, reporting, and variance documentation, such as:

- interdisciplinary clinical guidelines
- outcomes measurements
- variance tracking documentation tools
- methods for variance analysis and reporting
- methods for data feedback and communication of progress relative to need

Measurements will need to be developed to provide feedback on the integrated care management program. Examples of these include patient functional status, patient clinical indicators, patient satisfaction survey results, physician satisfaction survey results, return on investment, and resource consumption or utilization.

The new care management system will create new skill and resource requirements within the health system. Clearly, a key element of the future transition is that we will develop a variety of new positions and responsibilities. Staffing, operations support, and roles and responsibilities are key elements of ground-level redesign.

The formulation of a long-term plan becomes essential at this stage. The probable initiatives to be undertaken in the next 3–6 months are defined, in the overall context of the long-term plan. This plan will need to be revisited and changed on an ongoing basis as it is referenced to a rapidly and fundamentally changing target.

This phase is typically conducted through the formation of a variety of work teams under the purview of a "steering committee." Again, it can be effectively consolidated with the previous phases through any variety of accelerated methods. Such methods typically combine the individuals involved at the steering committee level with ground-level workers for effective and rapid design sessions, typically spanning 3–5 days for a defined initiative followed by the implementation phase (which can be conducted in classical or accelerated form).

Phase 4: Staged Implementation

Implementation is a key component of the care management system and deals largely with the development and training of the staff who will take on new roles within the organization as well as guiding existing personnel through changes in their processes and existing roles. Transition to these changed roles and processes is often challenging, and the training and communication provided can ease the progression to meet the new expectations.

The training and communication program for physicians, case managers, and new physician extenders, as well as those whose current roles will be directly affected by the new model, should be developed during the design phase of the process.

Typically, a number of initiatives are selected for design and implementation in a given quarter. For example, an organization might choose to develop the following program in a given quarter:

1. *system coordination*
   - key aspects of care management infrastructure: development of specialty case manager "pods"
   - key aspects of information systems development
   - key aspects of incentives alignment/design
2. *organizational change and communication*
   - physician/clinical team motivational platform construction and communication
   - definition of key organizational and clinical team outcomes and ongoing reporting/communication
3. *care process redesign/implementation*
   - development of coordinated system-wide disease management pilot
   - development of selected Medicare health risk assessment pilot

With the appropriate allocation of resources, this program could be accomplished, in part, with classical methods, and probably in full with accelerated methods.

DEFINING THE FUTURE STATE OF CARE MANAGEMENT

It is anticipated that the future state of care management will reclaim some of the personal touches and advantages that were present under the previous fee-for-service, non–risk-bearing environment. One of the difficulties for physicians and caregivers in moving into an advanced care management model is that it feels "impersonal" to treat an individual patient as a "member of a population" with "defined population-based outcomes." The n:1 model lacks the 1:1 touch (Figure 16–7).

In migrating to an advanced care management system, there will be significant shifts in provider roles and the nature of care delivery as we have known it. Inevitably, there will be a radical increase in the numbers of nonphysician providers. There will also be increased intrageneralist specialization of physicians along new lines, creating the role of the hospitalist, among others. Postacute services will move to expanded coverage with many patients directly admitted, seven days a week, to the subacute environment for what was previously acute care (stroke, heart failure, diabetes). Observation units will stabilize another group of patients who were previously admitted to the acute environment (encompassing such diagnoses as diabetic ketoacidosis, congestive heart failure, pyelonephritis, and so forth). These patients will be rapidly stabilized and their exacerbations treated in as little as 10–12 hours.

It is also anticipated that the future state of care management will garner greater control and extension across the continuum of care. It will extend beyond the continuum as it exists in most

Figure 16–7 Models of Care Delivery and Targeted Aims

environments today to encompass the health and well-being of the community. Systems will begin to rationalize programs and services relative to the need of the community. The services in the continuum will also expand beyond what has been considered conventional and strictly medical to encompass the world of holistic and alternative medicine and nonmedical interventions in the community as an extension of the system itself. And perhaps most pivotally, the nature of relationships within the system will be substantially altered as provider/patient relationships deepen, perhaps to the point of opening the window of risk from the payer to the provider and ultimately to the patient/customer.

In order to move across these radically extended boundaries, philosophically and physically, care management design will demand new tools and new implementation depths. System-

wide care management design has often been "high level" or "lofty," existing high above the care environment itself. To meet the future, care management will need to be designed at the level of the smallest replicable unit of care,[6] efficiently and effectively leveraging advantage across the system. A corresponding infrastructure will be necessitated at the system or multi-system level. Bilevel design (at the level where the work occurs and at the level where system integration occurs) will allow for true clinical integration and system transformation, with design and change at the 1,000-foot level inextricably linked to the vision at the 200,000-foot level, delivering personalized care community-wide.

Relationships, in their character, will be altered substantially, moving as leadership has moved in the last decade to being principle-centered, for the purpose of incorporating patients/

Table 16–1 Value Proposition for Care Management

Investments	*Benefits*

• **People**
  1. project manager
  2. staff support for design/implementation
  3. medical and other clinical leadership
    —Role
    —Technology
• **Technology**
  1. laptop computers for care coordinators
    —Information systems interface—financial data
  2. on-line clinical documentation
  3. on-line interface with payers/providers
  4. on-line interface to claims payment system
  5. Internet interface with patients (variety of e-commerce applications)
  6. software support
    —clinical practice guidelines
    —case finding
    —case tracking and monitoring
    —best practice measurement
	• **Capital**
	  software/hardware to support operations
	• significant decrease in clinical resource use
	  1. decreased length of stay/ equivalent dollars
	  2. decreased cost per member per month
	• full-time equivalent reductions realized through elimination of duplication of effort within facilities and among facilities
	• savings related to process improvement
	  1. dollar reduction through skill mix changes
	  2. savings through capacity management
	  3. increased provider/patient satisfaction
	• ability to deliver and manage care under a fixed payment system

Courtesy of Ernst & Young LLP, 2000, Washington, DC.

members as partners. In disease management, something is done *to* the patient, and the patient stands as host to the disease. In prevention programs and in demand management, we do something *for* the patient, generally delivering educational materials. To shift a portion of responsibility to the patient level, something must be done *with* the patients, and enter into true partnerships at a systemwide level: patient self-management or comanagement.

Similarly, in conventional managed care relationships, physicians are managed from above, doing things *to* them and *for* them based on data they do not hold or originate and holding them to requirements and protocols typically dictated externally. Future care management systems will likely provide infrastructure, relationships, and processes to allow physicians and teams to self-manage in alignment with multiple priorities (individual, system, regulatory and man-

aged care)—the system operating in partnership, *with* them.

CONCLUSION

In summary, the development of a comprehensive, integrated care management system requires a significant and essential investment. The requirements of the managed care marketplace are clear, unambiguous, and unavoidable: the ability to efficiently and effectively manage health care resources will determine the success—and the viability—of today's health care organizations. Despite the necessity of this investment, however, it is important to understand the potential benefits resulting from the investment. Many of the benefits can be quantified, once current and target levels of resource utilization are determined. An example of such investments and benefits is provided on Table 16–1.

REFERENCES AND NOTES

1. D. Berwick, Continuous Improvement as an Ideal in Health Care. *New England Journal of Medicine* 320, 1 (1989): 53–56.

2. D. Young and D. Barrett, Managing Clinical Integration in Integrated Delivery Systems: A Framework for Action. *Hospital and Health Services Administration*, 1997.

3. R. Gillies, S. Shortell, D. Anderson, L. Mitchell, and K. Morgan, Conceptualizing and Measuring Integration: Findings from the Health Systems Integration Study, *Hospital and Health Services Administration* 38, no. 4 (1993): 467–89.

4. E.C. Nelson, J.M. Mohr, P.B. Batalden, and S.K. Plume, Improving Health Care: Part 1. The Clinical Value Compass, *Joint Commission Journal on Quality Improvement* (April 1996); E.C. Nelson, P.B. Batalden, S.K. Plume,

and J.M Mohr, "Improving Health Care: Part 2. Clinical Improvement Worksheet and Users Manual," *Joint Commission Journal on Quality Improvement* (August 1996).

5. Care management initiatives result in significant reductions in *utilization*. The net revenue impact depends on (1) current utilization levels, (2) scope of care management programs, (3) level of centralized administration, (4) scope of clinical services and settings, (5) method of reimbursement, and (6) portion of premium dollar controlled.

6. P. Batalden, J. Mohr, E.C. Nelson, et al., Continually Improving the Health and Value of Health Care for a Population of Patients: The Panel Management Process, *Quality Management in Health Care* 5, no. 3 (1997): 31–41; J.B. Quinn, *The Intelligent Enterprise* (New York: Free Press, 1992).

Description of the Components of the Advanced Care Management System

Following are brief descriptions of the various components of the advanced care management system. Far more detailed discussions and examples of these components (as well as additional components that some organizations will want to consider) are provided elsewhere in this book. For now, consider the following components as basic to any advanced care management program.

PROGRAM ELEMENTS OF MEDICAL MANAGEMENT

Health risk assessment is designed to identify individuals who could benefit from targeted health promotion programs or appropriate interventions, thus helping them become aware of the risks of their unhealthy habits and motivating them to change. The health risk assessment can also be used to track the progress of members who have taken steps to change their behavior.

Primary prevention refers to wellness programs and other interventions/screenings (e.g., yearly exams, well-baby care, immunizations, regular screenings, and so on) typically provided, in a managed care setting, by the primary care physician. Within a care management program, primary prevention involves the development of appropriate recommendations for the type and frequency of these primary care services.

Demand management is designed to encourage the appropriate utilization of health services by offering triage programs and providing patients with information about their disease, disease process, and desired outcomes, thereby en-

abling them to participate in self-care and the selection and utilization of health services. Demand management programs, in addition to increasing member and physician satisfaction, typically reduce the nonurgent cases at emergency rooms, urgent care settings, and primary care facilities.

Triage refers to the process for sorting out member requests for services into those that need to be seen right away, those who can wait a little while, and those whose problems can be handled with advice over the phone. Because of the military origins of the term *triage,* many MCOs and IDSs use alternate terms for the same activity.

Basic utilization management is the coordination of the various tools capable of managing resource utilization (e.g., length of stay for inpatients) within specific care settings. Tools that support utilization management include:

- *Protocols*—specify the care that is to be provided to a patient undergoing a particular treatment. Protocols are often used in clinical research. They are strict management directives and more binding than clinical guidelines.
- *Resource use targets*—designed to facilitate optimum resource use and outcomes by outlining "leading practice" methodologies and protocols for the treatment of inpatients and outpatients.
- *Referral guidelines*—indicate the appropriateness of referral to or consultation with

a specialty physician from a primary care physician or other specialty physician managing the patient.

- *Practice guidelines*—systematically developed statements to assist practitioner and patient decisions about appropriate health care for specific clinical conditions.
- *Pathways*—an optimal sequencing and timing of interventions by physicians, nurses, and other staff for a particular diagnosis or procedure. Pathways are designed to minimize delays, resource utilization, and unit costs and to maximize the quality of care.

Outcomes reporting is designed to improve the effectiveness of health care services by examining measures of health care quality, utilization, and cost, including underutilization, readmission, and recidivism rates; levels of improvement in clinical status; functional performance; morbidity; mortality; and satisfaction.

Provider profiling using a denominator-based population to develop measurements that monitor the impact of the care management system on provider practice patterns.

SUPPORTING INFRASTRUCTURE

Conventional case management is a collaborative multidisciplinary process designed to manage an individual's care for a specific illness or episode. Case management streamlines all the services provided and focuses on the achievement of quality outcomes within a defined time frame using appropriate resources in a cost-effective manner.

Disease management is designed to produce optimal clinical outcomes in a cost-effective manner through a system-based, proactive, disease-specific approach to delivering health care services. This process spans the entire continuum of care and focuses on the natural course of chronic diseases and at-risk populations (e.g., asthma, AIDS, cancer, chronic renal failure, congestive heart failure).

Conventional case management and disease management can be differentiated as described in Table 16A–1.

ADDITIONAL PROGRAM ELEMENTS BEYOND MEDICAL MANAGEMENT

Table 16A–2 describes the further differentiation between medical management and premium management and between medical management and practice management.

Premium management refers to the development of specific financial services relating to contracting and risk adjustment across the system, between internal and external entities.

Practice management refers to the development of support structures and practices that optimize physician coordination and effectiveness across the system, provide for aligned incentives, and support the practice effort of the physician enterprise.

Table 16A–1 Conventional Case Management versus Disease Management

	Case Management	*Disease Management*
Goal	streamline components	integrating components
Emphasis	treatment of sickness	prevention and education
Setting	inpatient	all settings
Timing	concurrent	prospective
Guidelines	generic	customized to diagnosis

Courtesy of Ernst & Young LLP, 2000, Washington, DC.

Table 16A–2 Comparison of Premium, Medical, and Practice Management

Premium Management	Medical Management	Practice Management
• payer contracting • provider contracting • risk adjustment • re-insurance • actuarial services • premium allocation/risk sharing • legal services • financial services	• disease management • demand management and self-care • utilization and referral management • outcomes management • case management • health risk appraisal • practice profiling and credentialing • population-based management • panel management • critical pathways • clinical/practice guidelines	• organization/governance • practice management • faculty practice • MD leadership and training • physician network transformation • physician productivity • physician compensation • incentive alignment • documentation redesign • billing, accounts receivable

Network management refers to the development and management of the overall clinical delivery system. The intent is not only to acquire the clinical services necessary to provide a full continuum of care but also to build the administrative and organizational infrastructure to manage the strategic and operational activities ongoing within the system.

Information system and technology (IS/IT) refers to a comprehensive system capable of accessing, integrating, and processing data, real-time, throughout the delivery system. IS/IT is a critical success factor for advanced care management. Typical technology enablers include: automated clinical information systems, automated medical records, clinical decision support systems, health maintenance surveillance systems, comparative databases, technology-based education tools, and e-commerce applications.

Integration model refers to provider organizational structure and processes that help trans-form the individual program elements into a truly integrated care management system. A simple example is a physician-hospital organization (PHO).* The PHO attempts to integrate providers for the purpose of accepting risk-based managed care contracts. If under capitated contracts the hospital and physicians share financial risk, the PHO frequently encourages development of more sophisticated medical management programs. The structural link of the PHO provides the health system an opportunity to share information critical to managing contracts negotiated by the PHO.

---

*The authors recognize that many PHOs have not been successful and do not intend by the example in this chapter to necessarily endorse one structure over another.

CHAPTER 17

Primary Prevention in Managed Health Care

Leif I. Solberg

INTRODUCTION

Mary Jones was already favorably inclined toward health maintenance organization (HMO) X because she had heard about its goal of reducing heart attacks by 25 percent and its success in reducing preterm births. She had seen its clever television counter-advertising discouraging teenage smoking. Therefore, when her employer offered HMO X as one of the alternatives for her health care, she chose that plan. She was pleasantly surprised when she was given the opportunity to complete the plan's health risk assessment survey at work. She was even more pleased when a health education counselor called from HMO X to discuss how HMO X could help Mary with the weight and exercise concerns she had identified in the survey. The counselor told her about the relevant health promotion pro-

grams they had developed at her workplace and about other community resources. The counselor also explained that the HMO provided various counselors who could assist her over the telephone. And when the staff at the primary clinic she had chosen took advantage of her visit to identify her disease prevention needs and to recommend specific services for Mary and her family, she knew she would never willingly go anywhere else for care.

Corny? Impossible? Such a scenario is occurring daily at HealthPartners, and various elements of it are a growing part of other leading managed care organization (MCO) programs around the country. HealthPartners is an 800,000-member MCO with one-third of the members served by a staff model medical group and two-thirds served through contracts and partnerships with 47 primary care medical groups and about 2,500 consultants. It is concentrated in the Minneapolis-St. Paul metropolitan region of Minnesota, where about 80 percent of the population is covered by managed care. This chapter is designed to encourage the spread of health promotion and disease prevention (HP/DP) activities by explaining why they are important and increasingly prevalent in MCOs, to provide conceptual frameworks for these activities, and to describe examples of them. Although most examples are drawn from the experience of HealthPartners, other MCOs are doing similar things.

Leif I. Solberg, MD, is the Director for Care Improvement Research at HealthPartners Research Foundation and an Associate Medical Director and practicing family physician in the HealthPartners Medical Group. His research interests include disease prevention (especially tobacco cessation), chronic disease management, and quality improvement. He has published more than 75 peer-reviewed journal articles and 17 book chapters and is particularly interested in conducting research that addresses care delivery concerns and in translating research lessons back into patient care.

WHY SHOULD AN MCO DO PREVENTION?

Because It Is Possible

When HMOs were first conceived, Ellwood et al. called them health maintenance organizations because they thought that the prepaid economics and the integrated care system would make it both attractive and feasible to shift health care from an illness-based approach to one that emphasizes preventing disease and maintaining health.[1] Although they did not foresee the high turnover of members, which makes it less obvious that prevention services will pay off financially, MCOs still have the advantages of a large, defined population and an integrated comprehensive care system. They also have data about the health and health care of that population. These elements make it possible to address prevention in a way that was nearly impossible in a fragmented fee-for-service (FFS) marketplace.

Unfortunately, it has become common to ridicule the term *health maintenance organization* as if these plans provide no more prevention actions than the typical FFS plan. Studies comparing members of HMOs with those in indemnity insurance plans have mostly confirmed that HMO members receive more clinical preventive services, even when (as in the classic RAND study) those services are free for FFS members.[2] However, there have been no good studies comparing other types of HP/DP services. Nevertheless, there is reason to doubt that this potential has been widely exploited, and some of the HMO advantage may have been due to selection bias.

Because It Is Becoming Necessary

Although there is a growing proportion of the population that, like Mary Jones above, values prevention, we have still not reached the point where prevention activities determine the choices of most potential MCO members. However, the purchasing decisions are still being made largely by employers, employer groups, and governments, and they are increasingly wanting evidence of effective prevention programs. This is demonstrated by purchaser data comparisons like the Health Plan Employer Data and Information Set (HEDIS) measures, many of which are prevention indicators.

Rundall and Schauffler have suggested that the ability, necessity, and extent of managed care prevention activities will depend upon the evolutionary stage of the local health care marketplace.[3] Table 17–1 illustrates their ideas about this association between market stage and prevention for MCOs. The Twin Cities are well into Stage 4, expecting that the next stage will only increase the need to devote attention and resources to prevention. Where is your marketplace in this picture?

TYPOLOGY OF HP/DP ACTIVITIES

Regardless of the stage of your marketplace, it is useful to have a conceptual typology when establishing the plan's prevention activities. A modification of Rundall and Schauffler's typology seems as good as any, building on the same evolutionary sequence shown in Table 17–1.

Clinical Preventive Services

Clinical preventive services are provided primarily in the clinical care setting, essentially all the screening, counseling, and immunization activities considered by the U.S. Preventive Services Task Force.[4] They include efforts to reduce risks for both asymptomatic individuals and those with existing diseases. Because the opportunity to build prevention around clinical care is so important and because it is a key distinction between MCOs and insurance plans, this will be expanded upon later in this chapter.

Health Data Systems

This involves taking advantage of existing administrative, financial, and utilization data sys-

Table 17–1 Market Stage and Prevention

Stage	Description	Prevention
1	Largely fee-for-service and provider groups that are not allied.	Prevention gets little attention and is limited to clinical preventive services.
2	Prepaid care and mergers develop.	There is more concern about appropriateness of preventive services and with development of health data systems and some health promotion activities.
3	Prepaid care covers 30 percent to 50 percent of the population; purchaser alliances may develop.	MCOs are being held accountable for quality, services, and access, including prevention. This requires plans to improve, to collect data about health status and risks, and to address community health and collaborative actions.
4	Most of the population is covered by prepaid care, and purchaser alliances demand both cost reduction and quality.	Population-based and public policy aspects of HP/DP become increasingly important along with much more active attention and accountability for all aspects of prevention.

Source: Data from T.G. Rundall and H.H. Schauffler, Health Promotion and Disease Prevention in Integrated Delivery Systems: The Role of Market Forces, *American Journal of Preventive Medicine,* Vol. 13, pp. 244–250, © 1997, American College of Preventive Medicine, Association of Teachers of Preventive Medicine.

tems as well as creating and integrating systems that capture population-based health-related information, such as outcomes, risks, use of preventive services, and various epidemiologic data.

Population-Based (Member) Programs

Here, HP/DP services are provided to individuals and groups in schools, workplaces, and other venues. These services include health education classes, group behavior change programs, and direct MCO outreach to members through mail or phone systems. They often involve relationships with various community organizations.

Community Programs

These programs are aimed at the entire community and are intended to influence health or health behaviors of large numbers of people, regardless of whether they are members of the MCO. Most involve media campaigns or public information and may require partnerships or collaborations, sometimes with competitors.

Public Policy

This covers the advocacy for public policies aimed at protecting or improving the health of the entire population. It requires policy analysis and participation in the political process, usually in collaboration with other organizations.

A FRAMEWORK FOR ACTION

Being able to categorize prevention activities is a necessary but insufficient foundation for carrying them out. The other and more important precondition is a strong commitment to prevention from senior leadership. In the absence of such leadership desire, active support, and commitment of major resources, it may not be possible to achieve much.

Once MCO leaders decide to make prevention an organizational priority, they should establish specific public objectives and designate authority, responsibility, and resources to achieve those objectives. Ideally, those objectives should be information-based and measurable, and they should require such a large effort that many will doubt they can be accomplished. The eight goals established at HealthPartners to be accomplished within 4 years are listed in Table 17–2. When these goals were established, HealthPartners announced them in a very public way, making it hard to avoid trying its best to reach them.

In order to accomplish these goals and to increase the ability to promote health, many separate programs and initiatives have been developed. Most of these efforts have relied on quality improvement concepts and techniques, using a variation of the well-established plan-do-study-act (PDSA) approach to developing new processes and improving existing ones. The original approach at HealthPartners involved following an organized process improvement approach with the seven steps illustrated in Figure 17–1. However, that process required building a complete new system before testing or implementing it, leading to long development periods and some frustration.

We have evolved toward an approach closer to that described in articles by Nolan and by Berwick and illustrated in the Institute for Healthcare Improvement Breakthrough Series.[5] Although strong leadership, systems thinking, and measurement are important to both approaches, the new one emphasizes moving much more quickly toward repeated small tests of change that are combined and expanded to produce an overall improved system. However, the biggest challenge is not in proving that changes can work in small tests, but disseminating successful models of new systems widely throughout one's organization. This is the real test of an organization's leadership and its ability to implement the changes needed to deal with challenging times.

TAKING ADVANTAGE OF THE CLINICAL SETTING

It is both logical and important to start planning managed care prevention interventions in

Table 17–2 HealthPartners Prevention Goals for a Four-Year Period

Goal	Topic	Specifics
1	Heart disease	Reduce by 25% the number of heart disease events (e.g., heart attacks).
2	Breast cancer	Reduce by 50% the number of cases that reach an advanced stage before detection and increase to 85% the number of women ages 50–74 who are screened at least biennially.
3	Diabetes	Reduce by 25% the progression from high-risk to active disease and reduce by 30% the onset and progression of eye, kidney, and nerve damage resulting from diabetes.
4	Childhood injuries	Reduce by 25% the number of childhood (ages 0–14) injuries severe enough to require medical attention and by 10% the number of those requiring hospitalization.
5	Childhood immunization	Increase from 75% to 95% the number of children fully immunized by the age of two.
6	Pregnancy	Reduce by 30% the infant and maternal complications of pregnancy.
7	Dental caries	Reduce by 50% the number of new dental caries in all age groups among dental members.
8	Abuse	Increase by 50% the screening for domestic violence among women seen for preventive services or relevant presenting symptoms.

Courtesy of HealthPartners, Minneapolis, Minnesota.

Figure 17–1 Continuous Quality Improvement Model. *Source:* Reprinted from L. Solberg, Prevention in Managed Care, in *Best Practices in Medical Management,* Peter R. Kongstvedt, David W. Plocher, eds., pp 37–44, © 1998, Aspen Publishers, Inc.

the clinical care setting. Members are already present for face-to-face interventions, often at times when they are particularly ready to make changes in their health risks. Moreover, members are more likely to pay attention to recommendations for preventive services or behavior changes if the recommendations come from their personal clinician. For example, the most common reason given by women for not having had a mammogram is that their physician has not encouraged them to do so.

On the other hand, there are also factors that make it difficult to use these prevention opportunities. The most important barriers are clearly time constraints and the need to focus on the presenting problem.[6] In addition, both physicians and patients have traditionally regarded the routine "physical," not other types of visits, as the time for prevention, even though many patients do not schedule routine physicals and physicals center on an examination that has been found to be of little preventive value. Thus, patients who need important clinical preventive services usually do not receive recommendations for them during acute care visits and are only somewhat more likely to receive them during physicals.[7] This is especially true for identifying behavioral

risk factors and for providing counseling to modify those behaviors.

Much research has been done on this problem over the last 10 years, resulting in a gradually developing consensus that the main way to improve the above problems is to institute the systematic, organized prevention approaches that are typically absent from clinical settings. Most existing clinic systems are designed to support only acute care, in part because most physicians have not considered care for populations to be their responsibility. A recent report by members of the American Cancer Society Advisory Group on Preventive Health Care Reminder Systems came to the conclusion that office systems and extensive delegation to office staff are needed to improve clinical preventive services.[8] The supporting literature has summarized and described the major features of such an office prevention system.[9] In addition, we have documented that those system features are currently absent in most primary care practices.[10]

It is helpful to think of an overall prevention system as a single system composed of separate processes. Each of these processes is a series of step-by-step actions designed to accomplish a particular overall task (e.g., summarizing information about the current status of many preventive services for each patient). However, as with any system, those individual processes must be well integrated; if they are not designed to serve the needs of all preventive services, they will not result in patients receiving needed services consistently. Exhibit 17–1 describes 10 of the main processes in the prevention system.

These processes describe only the supports needed for providing preventive services, not who needs to actually recommend and perform those services. It is increasingly clear that the more that nonclinician staff can be involved in recommending and performing preventive services (through standing orders), as well as in handling all other processes, the more likely it is that the system will work consistently. The trick

is to increase delegation wherever possible without losing the valuable agenda-setting and reinforcing role of the clinician-patient relationship.

The real challenge for a managed care plan that wishes to improve the delivery of clinical preventive services in its care delivery settings is how to facilitate the development, implementation, and maintenance of such prevention systems. This is no small challenge. Nevertheless, the task is so important that it requires substantial attention. For example, routine physicals fill 20 percent of the appointment schedule in our staff model medical group, and nationally physicals are the most common medical visits, despite the fact that routine physicals do not address preventive needs very well.

Exhibit 17–1 Processes in a Prevention System

---

1. Guidelines: The process by which a clinical organization develops, obtains broad buy-in, and updates a specific uniform set of preventive services for defined age/gender/risk groups. Without organizational agreement on the recommended services, effective and efficient prevention systems cannot be developed.

2. Screen: The process of obtaining health risk and previous preventive service information in a standard way about all patients of a clinic in order to identify their specific prevention needs.

3. Summarize: The process of organizing and updating the information obtained in the screening process so that it is all in one place and can easily be reviewed by those needing to know the current prevention status of a particular patient. Without a continuously updated summary of each patient's preventive service status, it is not possible to keep members up to date on the recommended services.

4. Cue/Remind: The process of reminding clinic staff and clinicians about their need to undertake necessary prevention system tasks.

5. Follow-Up: The process of communicating to patients the results of preventive services along with appropriate explanations and recommendations.

6. Resources: The process of selecting, gathering, organizing, and maintaining patient education and referral information needed by both patients and clinic personnel.

7. Counsel: The process of assisting patients and their families to make needed changes in their behavior.

8. Track and Recall: The process of reminding patients, especially those patients without acute care visits, about their needs for specific preventive services.

9. Patient Activation: The process of encouraging patients to take greater responsibility for their own preventive services and behavior changes.

10. Prevention Visits: The process of providing all of the preventive services needed by a patient during a single visit designed and organized for that purpose. This special visit may not be necessary in the future for many patients who have their preventive service needs met during other visits.

Source: Reprinted with permission from L.I. Solberg et al., Delivering Clinical Preventive Services Is a Systems Problem: The Paradigm Shift of Improvement, *Annals of Behavioral Medicine,* Vol. 19, No. 3, pp. 271–278, © 1998, Society of Behavioral Medicine.

Primary versus Secondary Prevention

Traditionally, textbooks of disease prevention have distinguished between primary and secondary prevention activities.

- primary = efforts to prevent the occurrence of conditions in individuals without them (e.g., smoking cessation to prevent cancer)
- secondary = efforts to detect a condition early enough or to manage it so well as to improve the likelihood of a good outcome (e.g., Pap smears to detect early cervical cancer or lipid reduction treatment in patients with known heart disease)

There is little practical reason for an MCO or care system to separate these activities, either conceptually or programmatically. Both will occur predominantly in the primary care setting, although secondary prevention activities will often involve some coordination with specialty consultants. Those patients who have conditions that are complicated enough to require ongoing supervision exclusively in specialty clinics will need to have their overall prevention needs addressed there as well. This means that those clinics will also need to have supportive office systems, since subspecialists are traditionally even less likely to address preventive needs that lie outside their area. The same is true for disease management programs.

Helping Clinics Create Prevention Systems

Creating such systematic ways to support the provision of preventive services appears to require that certain conditions be present in care systems and care delivery sites. The conditions are listed in Exhibit 17–2. Some might add another condition to this list—minimal distracting turmoil or financial pressure. However, turmoil can also force a medical group to change, and waiting for tranquil times may be as futile as waiting for Godot.

If these conditions are present in an individual medical group or clinical site, they will be able to greatly improve preventive services delivery. However, if an MCO wants consistent preventive services delivery to be implemented in all its delivery settings and for all its members, then

Exhibit 17–2 Environmental Preconditions for Prevention Success

1. Prevention is identified as a high priority for the organization.
2. Effective, strong leadership is present and supports that priority.
3. There is an ability to facilitate organizational change.
4. Leadership has a clear systems-oriented vision.
5. Measurement and data are recognized as crucial to the identification of needs and the improvement of the process.
6. Creativity and innovation are valued and rewarded.

Source: Reprinted from L. Solberg, Prevention in Managed Care, in *Best Practices in Medical Management,* Peter R. Kongstvedt, David W. Plocher, eds., pp. 37–44, © 1998, Aspen Publishers, Inc.

the MCO itself will need to have these conditions as well. It will also need to work hard at facilitating the development of these conditions in its care delivery sites.

Once both settings are in the right stage of readiness, an MCO can do many things to facilitate change in the medical groups and sites that provide care to its members, regardless of whether the relationship is through ownership or contract:

- facilitate the development of explicit evidence-based guidelines for preventive services that have substantial clinician involvement and buy-in
- provide accurate accountability comparison data for care groups and sites
- provide financial incentives for those that achieve desired prevention targets
- provide opportunities for training and collaboration in the improvement process

HealthPartners has sponsored a medical group collaborative for the development and implementation of clinical guidelines called the Institute for Clinical Systems Improvement (ICSI). This organization is governed by the participating groups, so they have sufficient ownership to invest their time and energy in it. An outcomes recognition program (ORP) has also been created to provide financial bonuses to medical groups that achieve specific performance targets.

However, even when there is an environment in which the health plan and most of its contracting medical groups want to improve prevention and are working at doing so, there are still challenges. The following are some lessons learned from attempting to facilitate change:

- It is not easy!
- It will take time and considerable effort to get past the initial suspicion that many clinicians and medical groups have about the motives and capabilities of the MCO with which they contract.
- It is not necessarily easier to make change in a large group than in a small one. Although the larger group may have more resources, it may have more inertia, and making changes may be more complicated.
- It is not any easier to make change in an "owned" staff clinic than in a contracted one.
- Clinician leaders with the skills and vision identified in Exhibit 17–2 are rare—treasure and support them.
- Data knowledge and skills are as rare as they are important—work to provide training and support for their development.
- Training, consulting, and networking with peers in other medical groups are each valuable—provide or facilitate them.
- The medical groups that seem to be making the most progress are those that have at least one skilled staff person dedicated to the task.

HEALTH DATA SYSTEMS

It is a common misperception that managed care plans have an enormous amount of data about their members that are easy to use for planning, programs, and research. Unfortunately for prevention, that is not true. The data have been collected for administrative reasons and are not easy to use for other purposes, either because the data desired have not been collected, are not sufficiently accurate or up-to-date, or are not easy to link the various databases. For example, HealthPartners has been creating and sending to clinics "at-risk" lists of members who are believed to need various preventive services. Most clinics have not found these lists useful directly, because the members are either inappropriate for the service or they have received it and that information is not in the MCO records. Similarly, in order to operate the ORP described above for comparison of service rates between medical groups, HealthPartners has had to do its own primary data collection through chart audits.

Another problem with taking advantage of MCO data systems is not clear until one understands the differences between data that are used for improvement from data that are for accountability or research.[11] When an outside party uses data for accountability, it is likely to create a defensive and critical reaction from the accountable sites that makes it virtually impossible for them to use the same data for improvement. In fact, it tends to poison the well of cooperation with the source of that data for any mutual improvement actions.

POPULATION-BASED (MEMBER) PROGRAMS

MCOs, especially those with staff model care systems, have long provided health promotion programs directly or by contract with community groups at a discounted fee. Recently, MCOs in Stage 4 markets have found it necessary to become much more creative and assertive in order to identify risk factors and facilitate needed behavior changes by members. Pronk has described these programs at HealthPartners, including collaborative efforts with worksites and phone line consulting services.[12]

COMMUNITY OUTREACH PROGRAMS

HealthPartners has taken very seriously the fact that tobacco use is by far the most important preventable cause of death and disease. In order to reach beyond their membership to try to influence the entire community's attitude about tobacco, they have undertaken some major counter-advertising initiatives.

- A dragon-themed smoking cessation calendar with encouragement and quit tips for each day after quitting was distributed throughout the state as a supplement in newspapers.
- A version of this popular calendar is being developed for similar distribution to teenagers.
- Television and radio ads were developed with extensive teen input. These ads, called "Garbage-face," feature a smoking teen girl's face being morphed into a variety of garbage collages as she talks about the approach of a boy she idolizes, only to be spurned by him as he tells her to get breath mints. These ads have garnered a lot of favorable attention.

PUBLIC POLICY INITIATIVES

HealthPartners has long been an active sponsor of the Minnesota Coalition for a Smoke-Free 2000. In the past few years, however, HealthPartners made antitobacco legislation one of their lobbyists' highest priorities. In addition, a phone tree of employee volunteers has been used at several critical points in the legislative process to generate large numbers of legislator contacts on short notice. These efforts have been fairly successful and have generated both favorable attention for the company and important health promotion changes for the community. Finally, HealthPartners has joined with another MCO in its community to sue the tobacco companies.

CONCLUSION

The goal of this chapter was to heighten the interest of MCOs in addressing disease prevention and health promotion issues, as well as to provide a framework for doing so and some concrete examples of how one plan is going about it. These issues are an important part of the future, and although some regions might still be in earlier market stages (see Table 17–1), farsighted plans will start to work now on what will increasingly become a necessity.

REFERENCES AND NOTES

1. P.M. Ellwood, N.N. Anderson, J.E. Billings, R.J. Carlson, E.J. Hoagberg, and W. McClure, Health Maintenance Strategy, *Medical Care* 9 (1971): 291–98.

2. T.G. Rundall and H.H. Schauffler, Health Promotion and Disease Prevention in Integrated Delivery Systems: The Role of Market Forces, *American Journal of Preventive Medicine* 13 (1997): 244–50; R.H. Miller and H.S. Luft, Managed Care Plan Performance Since 1980—A Literature Analysis, *Journal of the American Medical Association* 271 (1997): 1512–19; W.G. Manning, A. Leibowitz, G.A. Goldberg, W.H. Rogers, and J.P. Newhouse, A Controlled Trial of the Effect of a Prepaid Group Practice on Use of Services, *New England Journal of Medicine* 310 (1984): 1505–10.

3. Rundall and Schauffler, Health Promotion and Disease Prevention.

4. U.S. Preventive Services Task Force, *Guide to Clinical Preventive Services*, 2nd ed. (Baltimore: Williams & Wilkins, 1996); U.S. Department of Health & Human Services, *Clinician's Handbook of Preventive Services* (Washington, DC: author, 1994).

5. T. Nolan, Accelerating the Pace of Improvement: An Interview with Thomas Nolan, *Joint Commission Journal of Quality Improvement* 23 (1997): 217–22; D.M. Berwick, From Measuring to Managing the Improvement of Prevention, *American Journal of Preventive Medicine* 11 (1995): 385–87; C.M. Kilo, A Framework for Collaborative Improvement: Lessons from the Institute for Healthcare Improvement's Breakthrough Series, *Quality Management in Health Care* 6 (1998): 1–13.

6. T.E. Kottke, M.L. Brekke, and L.I. Solberg, Making "Time" for Preventive Services, *Mayo Clinic Proceedings* 68 (1993): 785–91.

7. T.E. Kottke, L.I. Solberg, M.L. Brekke, A. Cabrera, and M. Marquez, Preventive Services Rates in 44 Midwestern Primary Care Clinics: Room for Improvement, *Mayo Clinic Proceedings* 72 (1997): 515–23.

8. L.S. Leininger, L. Finn, L. Dickey, et al., An Office System for Organizing Preventive Services, *Archives of Family Medicine* 5 (1996): 108–15.

9. L.I. Solberg, T.E. Kottke, M.L. Brekke, S.A. Conn, C.A. Calomeni, and K.S. Conboy, Delivering Clinical Pre-

ventive Services Is a Systems Problem, *Annals of Behavioral Medicine* 19, no. 3 (1998): 271–78.

10. L.I. Solberg, T.E. Kottke, and M.L. Brekke, The Case of the Missing Clinical Preventive Services Delivery Systems, *Effective Clinical Practice* 1, no. 1 (1998): 33–38.

11. L.I. Solberg, G. Mosser, and S. McDonald, The Three Faces of Performance Measurement: Improvement, Accountability, and Research, *Joint Commission Journal of Quality Improvement* 23, no. 3 (1997): 135–47.

12. N.P. Pronk, Outreach from the Managed Care Organization to the Population, in *Best Practices in Medical Management*, ed. P.R. Kongstvedt and D.W. Plocher (Gaithersburg, MD: Aspen Publishers, Inc., 1998).

SUGGESTED READING

Batalden, P.B., Mohr, J.J., Nelson, E.C., and Plume, S.K. 1996. Improving Health Care, Part 4: Concepts for Improving any Clinical Process. *Joint Commission Journal of Quality Improvement* 22: 651–59.

Centers for Disease Control and Prevention. 1996. Prevention and Managed Care: Organizations, Purchasers of Health Care, and Public Health Agencies. *JAMA* 275, no. 1: 26–29.

Langley, G.J., Nolan, K.M., and Nolan, T.W. *Improvement Guide: A Practical Approach to Enhancing Organizational Performance.* San Francisco: Jossey-Bass.

Schauffler, H.H., and Rodriguez, T. 1993. Managed Care for Preventive Services: A Review of Policy Options. *Medical Care Review* 50: 153–98.

Schoenbaum, S.C. 1990. Implementation of Preventive Services in an HMO Practice. *Journal of General Internal Medicine* 5 (suppl.): S123–S127.

Thompson R.S., Taplin S.H., McAfee, T.A., Mandelson, M.T., and Smith, A.E. 1995. Primary and Secondary Prevention Services in Clinical Practice: Twenty Years' Experience in Development, Implementation, and Evaluation. *JAMA* 273: 1130–35.

CHAPTER 18

Managing Basic Medical-Surgical Utilization

Peter R. Kongstvedt

INTRODUCTION

The tremendous amount of variation observed in many areas of medical practice suggests some degree of inappropriate use of health care resources: patients may be overtreated, undertreated, or treated with the wrong interventions. A principal objective of the management of utilization is the reduction of practice variation by establishing parameters for cost-effective use of health care resources. The techniques used in utilization management (UM) programs serve to manage resource utilization within those parameters to contain cost while ensuring appropriate care is provided.[1] When utilization guidelines and disease management programs are incorporated into health delivery, the degree of practice variation and the amount of inappropriate care are reduced. This affects even the nonmanaged care patients of physicians who have significant managed care practices; for example, inpatient utilization in nonmanaged care patients is observed when managed care presence is high.[2]

The management of utilization has many facets. As managed care has become prevalent, the divisions between the management of specialty physician care, inpatient care, outpatient care, case and disease management, preventive care, and indeed all aspects of health care delivery have become progressively blurred. Many aspects of UM are discussed in this book in separate chapters; however, there is a core set of activities that may be considered fundamental to managing utilization of medical and surgical services. This chapter's purpose is to provide an overview of that core set. The topics addressed in this chapter overlap information presented in greater detail in other chapters; if anything, this attribute helps to underscore the fact that management of medical services is not made up of discrete activities unrelated to each other. Interested readers should understand that although other chapters of this book go into depth on some of the other activities of care management, many more cannot be addressed in this text because of practical limitations on space. For more detailed information on both the topics discussed in this book and the myriad others not addressed here, the reader is referred to a companion book of this series, *Best Practices in Medical Management*.[3]

RETURN ON INVESTMENT IN MANAGEMENT OF MEDICAL COSTS

Experienced health maintenance organization (HMO) managers know well that investment in UM is well leveraged in the classic sense of the word. That is, there is a high rate of return for money spent in this activity in the form of lower health care costs. The degree of leverage in the past has been severalfold. It is more difficult to measure that economic return now because few models of *un*managed care are left. How one di-

The author thanks Karen Davis and Alyssa Williamson for their help in compiling some of the research referenced in this chapter. In addition, David Plocher provided information used in the prevention and health appraisal sections of this chapter.

vides the management activities (and associates an economic value to those activities) makes it difficult to know which particular medical management activities provide the greatest return on a plan-to-plan basis. Of course, because all medical management activities are interrelated, the synergy obtained by performing multiple aspects of medical management well also plays into the discussion.

In two comprehensive studies of 1,000 benchmark data and associated statistical correlations in large managed care organizations (MCOs) covering a total of 26 million lives, Ernst & Young LLP found a strong linear relationship between higher investments in medical management and lower medical costs, with a consistently positive return on the investment (although there was variability in the amount of that economic return).[4,5] What was striking about this finding was that although that linear correlation was strong, there was low consistency in *what* the medical managers in the studied MCOs actually did. The methods and techniques used for effective medical management varied between geographical regions, reflecting differences in local and regional medical practice environments. In other words, a particular activity that is effective in Southern California is not necessarily effective in the Eastern United States. Table 18–1 provides additional examples of savings for selected aspects of medical management.

DEMAND MANAGEMENT

Demand management refers to activities of a health plan designed to reduce the overall requirement for health care services by members. In addition to helping to lower health care costs, these services also may provide a competitive advantage to a plan by enhancing its reputation for service and giving members additional value for their premium dollar. Demand management services fall into five broad categories that are briefly discussed to place them in context to the basic medical-surgical UM functions. For an in-depth discussion of self-help and nurse advice line services, the reader is referred to *Best Practices in Medical Management*.[6]

Nurse Advice Lines

Nurse advice lines provide members with access to advice regarding medical conditions, the need for medical care, health promotion and preventive care, and numerous other advice-related activities. Such advice lines have been in use in closed-panel HMOs for many years, where they are occasionally referred to as "triage"* nurse lines. Plans may staff these lines with their own nurses, or they may purchase the service from any one of a number of commercial services. Hours of operation are almost always extended, and it is now common for coverage to be 24 hours per day, 7 days per week (especially if a plan uses a commercial service). A geographically large plan or a commercial service will use a toll-free line to make it easier for members to access the service.

Special market segments such as Medicare and Medicaid may benefit from dedicated programs. Attention to the special problems and concerns of seniors will go a long way toward improving health status and can be a major contributor to the overall management of care in this population. Easy access to medical advice in the Medicaid population may allow these members to avoid a trip to the emergency department.

As noted in Table 18–1, a study completed by Ernst & Young, LLP, demonstrated savings of $2.69 to $3.81 per dollar spent for a nurse advice line program.[7] In another study, the combination of a 24-hour nurse advice service combined with a self-care program (see following) resulted in a savings of $4.75 per dollar invested, whereas the self-care program alone resulted in a savings of $2.40 per dollar invested.[8] Other studies have documented similar results.

---

*The use of the term "triage nurse" is not recommended if for no other reason than its military history. Triage is a term used in battlefield medicine that refers to the separation of casualties into three categories: immediate attention required, attention can be delayed, and casualty is beyond hope and only will be given palliative care.

Table 18–1 Return on Investment (ROI) for Medical Management Programs

Component	ROI
Inpatient management	Early studies indicated savings on inpatient total costs of 6% because of UR of admissions. In relatively unmanaged markets, reductions in days/1,000 of approximately 10% the first year can be achieved through inpatient management. Less dramatic reductions will be achieved in subsequent years. ROI is improved through targeting by diagnostic category and/or provider/facility to decrease the administrative costs of the program.[1,2]
Ambulatory review including referral management	One study for specific types of DME documented a 2.6:1 ROI. Procedural reviews have been measured more commonly in reduction in rates of procedures with rates reductions from 1%–15%, depending on the procedure and variation at onset of review program. Studies of preauthorized reviews are limited, but sentinel effect combined with a review process has decreased rates for these services by as much as 5%–10%.[3,4]
Case management	Studies have documented savings of 4–7.8:1 in periodicals and studies in specific settings. A 4:1 savings ratio should be attainable.[5,6]
Demand management	A recent study completed by Ernst & Young LLP demonstrated savings of $2.69–$3.81:1 with the Access Health demand management program. Other studies have documented similar results.[7]
Disease management	Savings vary by program and by disease. Example: Diabetes Treatment Centers of America (DTCA) reports a return of 3.75:1 for its diabetic program. Many programs are measured as before and after costs per member rather than on a ROI basis[8]; example: DCTA (the same firm as noted above) reports in press interviews, between $50 and $75 PMPM savings for diabetic patients.[9] Savings for a large variety of conditions are discussed in more depth in Chapter 20 and in *Best Practices in Medical Management*.

[1]L. Citrome, Practice Protocols, Parameters, Pathways, and Guidelines: A Review, *Administration and Policy in Mental Health* 25(3), 257–269.

[2]T.M. Wickizer, The Effects of Utilization Review on Hospital Use and Expenditures: A Covariance Analysis, *Health Services Research,* April 27 (1992) (1), 103–121.

[3]T.M. Wickizer, Controlling Outpatient Medical Equipment Costs Through Utilization Management, *Medical Care,* 33(4), 383–391.

[4]E.A. Kerr et al., Managed Care and Capitation in California: How Do Physicians at Financial Risk Control Their Own Utilization? *Annals of Internal Medicine* 123 (7), (1995): 500–504.

[5]D. Huggins and K. Lehman, Reducing Costs Through Case Management, *Nursing Management* (December 1997): 34–36.

[6]B.H. Warren et al., Cost Effectiveness of Case Management Experiences of a University Managed Health Care Organization. *American Journal of Medical Quality* (Winter 1996): 173–178.

[7]Ernst & Young, LLP, Study: Return on Investment of a Nurseline Telephone Triage System, Press Release, 1998.

[8]D.W. Plocher and R.S. Brody, Disease Management and Return on Investment. In: P.R. Kongstvedt and D.W. Plocher, Eds., *Best Practices in Medical Management* (Gaithersburg, MD: Aspen Publishers, 1998).

[9]High Start-Up Costs of Disease Management Programs Offset by Improved Outcomes, Lower Utilization, Reduced Costs, *Managed Care Week* (June 21, 1999): 6–7.

Courtesy of Ernst & Young, LLP, 2000, Washington, DC.

Self-Care and Medical Consumerism Programs

This activity refers to the provision of information to members to allow them to provide care for themselves or to better evaluate when they need to seek care from a professional. Member newsletters with medical advice are used extensively by HMOs. The most common example of a more proactive approach is a self-care guide provided by the plan and available via ths plan's web site. These books are generally written in an easy-to-understand manner, and they provide step-by-step advice for common medical conditions and preventive care. Information about the wise use of medical services or how to be an informed consumer would fall into this category as well.

Self-care programs have been evaluated since the early 1980s. Typical results have shown $2.50 to $3.50 saved for every dollar invested.[9] In one structured study in a staff model HMO, the targeted use of self-care manuals resulted in decreased outpatient visits and a 2:1 return on the cost of the program.[10] A fever health education program at Kaiser decreased pediatric clinic utilization by 35% for fever visits and 25% for all acute visits.[11] Other studies have reported savings of $2.40 to $2.77 per dollar invested.[12]

Shared Decision-Making Programs

This activity refers to making the member an active participant in choosing a course of care. Although this general philosophy may be prevalent in the routine interactions between patients and physicians, shared decision programs are more focused. They provide patients with in-depth information on specific procedures. By providing this information, patients gain a deeper understanding of not only the disease process but also the treatment alternatives. Some HMOs that use this type of program will not finalize authorization for certain elective procedures (e.g., transurethral resection of the prostate) until the member has completed the shared decision-making program.

A number of commercial services have appeared in the past few years to produce these programs. Many use interactive CD-ROMs, videotapes, computer programs, and even Internet websites to provide information. Supplemental access to a nurse advice line, as well as the ability to discuss the alternatives with the physician after the patient has reviewed the material, is also routine.

Medical Informatics

Medical informatics is a broad term that applies to the use of information technology in the management of health care delivery. The broader topics on the use of data in medical management are discussed in Chapter 32. For purposes of this chapter, medical informatics refers to the use of information technology in helping to manage demand for services. It must be emphasized here that the use of data and informatics in medical management is now subject to considerably heightened standards for security and privacy. The most important and comprehensive force behind this is the Health Insurance Portability and Accountability Act of 1996 (HIPAA), which is discussed in Chapter 67. These new standards become mandatory for all MCOs, providers, and business partners most likely in 2002 or 2003. HIPAA also mandates conformance with certain data definitions, as described in Chapter 35. Although HIPAA is beyond the scope of this chapter, the reader is encouraged to refer to those chapters.

An MCO may use information systems to anticipate demand for services or to analyze how demand for services can be better managed. For example, an analysis of the use of urgent care or emergency services may be related to hours of operation, location of primary care, work patterns at a large employer, and so forth. By looking for patterns, the plan may be able to develop strategies for lowering demand for one type of service by substituting another type of service.

Most MCOs now provide services to members such as health, wellness, and self-care information, in addition to some administrative capabilities (e.g., obtaining a new identification card) through their websites on the Internet. MCOs and health care delivery systems are also using the Internet to support medical education and management of utilization and quality.

The Internet itself also has become a source of health-related information that is totally unregulated or monitored for quality. It is very common now for patients to bring print-outs from web sites when they see their physicians. The constitutional right to free speech is necessarily silent about the issue of publishing drivel, even potentially dangerous drivel. Therefore, medical managers will want to stay abreast of at least the most popular health information websites and make the locations of high-quality sites known to the plan's membership (along with a note that advice can vary from one source to another and still be of good quality).

All these activities that are Internet related fall under the general category of electronic commerce (e-commerce), which is discussed in Chapter 37. E-commerce is accelerating rapidly, and medical managers must expect that the Internet will play an increasingly important role in managing utilization in the future.

Preventive Services and Health Risk Appraisals

Preventive services, which are a hallmark of the HMO industry, are discussed in detail in Chapter 17. In addition, further discussion of prevention activities is found in *Best Practices in Medical Management*.[13] Only a brief mention of some of these activities is provided here.

Common preventive services include immunizations, mammograms, routine physical examinations and health assessments, and counseling regarding behaviors that members can undertake to lower their risk of ill health (e.g., smoking cessation and stress reduction). Counseling and education also may be directed toward specific clinical conditions. For example, one managed indemnity plan studied an employer's on-site prenatal education program. The study found that participants had an average cost per delivery that was $3,200 less than that of nonparticipants.[14] Another study of modifiable health risks (e.g., tobacco use and physical activity) and short-term health care costs found an increase in charges over an 18-month period, ranging from $1,500 to $2,500 per patient, when comparing low-risk behavior with high-risk behavior.[15]

The health risk appraisal (HRA) is a tool designed to elicit information from a member regarding certain activities and behaviors that can influence health status. HRAs are commonly used by HMOs, and are also widely available on the Internet. Self-reported information about obvious behaviors (e.g., smoking and alcohol use) and less obvious behaviors (e.g., seatbelt use and gun ownership) is obtained. That information then is used to produce a profile of an individual's health risks and what modifications of behavior may improve that individual's life expectancy. Typically, this information is provided to the member's primary care physician (PCP), who is in a better position to counsel the member.

HRAs may be broadly classified into three categories:[16]

- **Risk-based HRA:** It is the earliest type of HRA. It focuses on patient behavior and its effect on health risk.
- **Habit-based HRA:** It is similar to the risk-based HRA. It not only looks at habits that create increased health risk but also incorporates elements of health education and behavioral change.
- **Utilization-based HRA:** A form of HRA that focuses on predictors of utilization. It has not been as predictive as expected.

In plans that have a large Medicare enrollment, the plan may take extra steps in performing an initial assessment. The most common extra activity is an in-home assessment of the new Medicare member. A trained nurse or medical social worker may determine, for example, that if the plan gives the new Medicare enrollee a bath mat or shower chair that it will significantly reduce the risk of a hip fracture from falling in the bathtub. An inventory of the member's diet also may yield valuable information that will enable the new member's provider to improve health status by lowering sodium intake or saturated fats in the diet. This activity not only improves the quality of care for these members but also yields considerable savings. In one case, Kaiser Permanente in Denver reported a $70 per member per month (PMPM) drop in cost within 6 months of implementing a Medicare health status and risk screening program.[17] HealthPartners of Southern Arizona reported savings of $65,000 per 1,000 Medicare enrollees per year from its screening and early intervention program.[18]

MEASUREMENTS OF UTILIZATION

It is not possible to manage utilization well unless there is a means to measure it. Though the topic of using data and information for medical management is discussed in depth in Chapter 32, some basic measurements need to be noted here to bring perspective to basic medical-surgical UM. This brief discussion will focus on the broadest types of utilization measurements only, but these measures are the ones commonly reported by MCOs and reviewed by both medical managers and other senior executives.

Tables 18–2 and 18–3 present common, high-level measures of HMO utilization, but sort the data in somewhat different ways. Table 18–2 provides 1997 data, whereas Table 18–3 presents 1998 data. Note that utilization levels (using essentially the same cohort of plans) decreased between 1997 and 1998 in all basic measures. Table 18–4 provides comparative data on preferred provider organizations (PPOs) for 1997 only. It is important to bear in mind that utilization data reported by PPOs is likely to have far less precision than those reported by HMOs. Thus, the data in Table 18–4 must be viewed with caution.

Physician Utilization Data

A basic tenet of managed health care, primarily in HMOs, is to provide low-cost and unlimited access to primary care, but require referral for specialty services. Recent legislation in several states has required open access to a variety of specialty providers, but there is little uniformity between states about what types of providers are given such privileges. Obstetrics/gynecology (OB/GYN) is the only specialty that is commonly granted open access under managed care.

Measurement of physician visits, or encounters, is shown in Tables 18–2 and 18–3, but these numbers are not separated by primary or specialty care. With the steady blurring of managed care models, the increase in specialty-specific open access requirements under state laws, and the fact that many physicians perform both roles, it is difficult to make these distinctions.

In those plans that use a PCP referral authorization system (as discussed in the following), measurement of referral rates may be useful. There is no set standard for reporting data on referral utilization as there is for hospital utilization. Nevertheless, managers use certain measures frequently and find them useful. In HMOs that do not pay benefits for services provided without an authorization from a PCP, a useful measure is referrals per 100 encounters per PCP.

Table 18–2 1997 Annual Utilization Rates of HMOs*

HMO Utilization Measure	Average for HMOs in Systems	Average for HMOs Not in Systems	Average for All HMOs
Number of HMO enrollees per plan	190,326	99,372	110,546
Hospital days per 1,000 non-Medicare members	236	230	231
Hospital days per 1,000 Medicare members	1,465	1,508	1,501
Hospital admissions per 1,000 non-Medicare members	63	61	61
Hospital admissions per 1,000 Medicare members	239	257	254
Physician encounters per non-Medicare member	3.52	3.17	3.21
Physician encounters per Medicare member	7.50	7.04	7.11
Ambulatory visits per non-Medicare member	1.66	1.27	1.32
Ambulatory visits per Medicare member	2.68	2.56	2.58
ALOS per non-Medicare hospital admission	3.79	3.73	3.74
ALOS per Medicare hospital admission	6.08	5.79	5.84

*HMOs are considered to be integrated health systems if they are part of a system by virtue of ownership or contractual arrangements. HMOs are not considered to be in integrated health systems if they hold only provider network contracts with systems. Utilization data exclude psychiatric care.

Source: Reprinted with permission from Hoechst Marion Roussel, *Managed Care Digest Series* 1999, *Integrated Health Systems Digest,* 1999 © 1999 Hoechst Marion Roussel, SMG Marketing Group Inc., 1999.

Table 18–3 1998 HMO Utilization Data* for Commercial HMO Members

	Hospital Days/ 1,000 Members	Hospital/ Admissions/ 1,000 Members	Average Length of Stay	Physician Encounters Per Member
HMO model type				
IPA	210.5	57.6	3.7	4.3
Network	207.0	60.5	3.6	3.8
Group	200.6	56.6	3.8	3.4
Staff	215.3	66.8	3.9	4.1
HMO ownership				
Corporate owned	206.7	57.3	3.6	4.2
Corporate managed	238.1	70.5	4.0	6.1
Corporate affiliated	202.2	55.3	3.7	4.2
Hospital owned	236.5	66.7	3.8	4.2
Independent	217.5	65.2	3.6	3.6
HMO membership				
Under 15,000	210.0	59.9	3.6	4.5
15,000–24,999	202.6	58.1	3.6	3.7
25,000–49,999	206.0	58.9	3.6	4.5
50,000–99,999	208.3	57.1	3.6	3.6
100,000–249,999	213.7	58.8	3.6	4.1
250,000 and over	207.5	57.0	3.7	4.1
Overall average	209.0	57.3	3.6	4.5

*HMOs are considered to be integrated health systems if they are part of a system by virtue of ownership or contractual arrangements. HMOs are not considered to be integrated health systems if they hold only provider network contracts with systems. Utilization data exclude psychiatric care.
Courtesty of SMG Marketing Group, Inc., 1999, Chicago, Illinois.

This figure correlates to a referral percentage. For example, 11 referrals per 100 encounters per PCP equates to a referral rate of 11 percent.

The referral rate per 1,000 members per year is used more commonly. Like the measurement of hospitalization rate, this figure looks at an annualized referral rate for every 1,000 members. Although it is less directly related to a PCP encounter than are referrals per 100 primary care encounters, the nomenclature is standard across many types of plans.

It is important to know what is being counted: initial referrals or total visits to a referral specialist. In other words, counting only the initial referral or authorization may result in missing a large portion of the actual utilization. It is common, especially in loosely managed systems, for a single referral to generate multiple visits to a specialist. For example, if a PCP refers a member with the request to evaluate and treat, it is

carte blanche for the specialist to take over the care of the patient. Succeeding visits will be to the specialist, not to the PCP.

Hospital Utilization Data

Definition of the Numbers

It is important to choose what is to be measured and to define that measurement precisely. Most plans measure bed days per 1,000 plan members per year (the formula is given later). Deciding what to count as a bed day is not always straightforward, however.

In some plans, outpatient surgery is counted as a single day in the hospital. It is done on the assumption that an outpatient procedure will cost the plan nearly the same as or sometimes more than a single inpatient day. Some plans count skilled nursing home days in the total, whereas others add commercial, Medicare,

Table 18–4 1997 PPO Utilization Data* for Commercial PPO Members

PPO Size	Hospital Days/ 1,000 Members	Average Length of Stay	Physician Encounters Per Member
Under 19,000	253.0	4.1	4.2
20,000–99,999	243.0	4.1	3.0
100,000–499,999	271.8	4.2	3.2
500,000–999,999	365.0	4.9	4.7
1,000,000+	294.3	3.8	3.4
Overall average	252.0	4.1	3.2

*Excluding psychiatric/substance abuse.

Source: Reprinted with permission from Hoechst Marion Roussel, *Managed Care Digest Series,* 1998, © 1998, Hoechst Marion Roussel, SMG Marketing Group Inc., 1998.

Medicaid, and fee for service into the total calculation. In some plans, the day of discharge is counted; in most it is not (unless the hospital charges for it). A decision must be reached on whether to count nursery days in the total when the mother is still in the hospital or only if the newborn is boarding over or in intensive care.

As a general rule of thumb, most plans count commercial days separately from any other days, especially Medicare days. If there is a significant Medicaid population, that should be tracked both separate from and together with commercial days. Most plans do not count outpatient surgery as an inpatient day but break out that number separately. Likewise, most plans report skilled nursing days separately.

How to count nursery days is not straightforward. Under the assumption that skilled nursing days are not counted as hospital days because the cost is so much less, the same assumption may be made for nursery days while the mother is in the hospital. In most hospitals, the nursery charges for a normal newborn are relatively low. If the newborn requires a stay beyond the mother's discharge, the charges usually are higher. If the neonate is in the intensive care unit, charges will be quite high. If the MCO has negotiated an all-inclusive per diem rate or a case rate that takes normal nursery days into account while the mother is in the hospital, there may be no need to count them separately. If the MCO must pay a high rate for nursery days, then they should be counted in the total.

Further discussion about utilization reports may be found in Chapter 32.

Formulas To Calculate Institutional Utilization

The standard formula to calculate bed days per 1,000 members per year is straightforward. It may be used to calculate the annualized bed days per 1,000 members for any chosen time period (e.g., for the day, the month to date, the year to date).

When calculating bed days per 1,000, the assumption of a 365-day year as opposed to a 12-month year should be used to prevent variations that are due solely to the length of the month. The formula is as follows:

$$[A \div (B \div 365)] \div (C \div 1,000)$$

where A is gross bed days per time unit, B is days per time unit, and C is plan membership.

This calculation may be broken into steps. Exhibit 18–1 illustrates the calculation for bed days per 1,000 on a single day, whereas Exhibit 18–2 presents the calculation for bed days per 1,000 for the month to date.

VARIATIONS IN UTILIZATION

There is a substantial body of evidence that hospital utilization and procedure rates vary significantly from one geographical area of the country to another in the absence of explanations

Exhibit 18–1 Example of Bed Days for a Single Day

Assume: Current hospital census = 10
          Plan membership = 12,000

Step 1: Gross days = 10 ÷ (1 ÷ 365)
                   = 10 ÷ 0.00274
                   = 3,649.635

Step 2: Days per 1,000 = 3,649.635 ÷ (12,000
                         ÷ 1,000)
                       = 3,649.635 ÷ 12
                       = 304 (rounded)

Therefore, the days per 1,000 for that single day equal 304.

caused by sociodemographic or morbidity factors. Table 18–5 presents examples of geographic variations in hospital utilization.

As far back as 1982, Wennberg and Gittelsohn coined the term "surgical signature" to describe a regional practice pattern of surgical rates within an area that cannot be explained by differences in population morbidity or other market phenomena.[19] According to Wennberg

Exhibit 18–2 Example of Bed Days for the Month to Date (MTD)

Assume: Total gross hospital bed
           days in MTD = 300
         Plan membership = 12,000
         Days in MTD = 21

Step 1: Gross days MTD = 300 ÷ (21 ÷ 365)
                       = 300 ÷ 0.0575
                       = 5,217.4

Step 2: Days per 1,000
        in MTD = 5,217.4 ÷ (12,000 ÷ 1,000)
               = 5,217.4 ÷ 12
               = 435

Therefore, the days per 1,000 for the MTD equal 435.

and Caper, the rate of some treatments does not vary much from one market to the next; however, the variations in rates across markets can be fourfold to fivefold for other treatments with no population-based explanation for the differences.[20] In a follow-up to a landmark study of the differences in utilization between Boston and New Haven,[21] Fisher and associates found that significant variations continue to exist.[22] Findings of geographical variation and avoidable hospitalizations have been supported by other, more recent studies.[23–26] Such variations are not limited to private health care; substantial geographical variations in inpatient and ambulatory utilization in the Veterans Affairs hospitals and clinics also have been reported, with a clear knowledge that physician income is unaffected by utilization.[27]

Research by the RAND Corporation also has revealed that geographical variations exist in the type and use of different treatments by physicians across the country.[28] This phenomenon can be explained in various ways, including the hypothesis that variations in health care and treatment are "caused by variability in prevalence of physicians who are enthusiasts about the use of the services whose use varies."[29] In addition, other evidence supports the theory that those health care markets with a higher than average number of hospital beds and physicians tend to have correspondingly higher utilization rates.[30,31]

The National Center for Health Statistics, Centers for Disease Control and Prevention, performed a study of variance in hospitalizations and reported that 12 percent of all hospitalizations in the United States were avoidable. Unlike other studies, these hospitalizations did not vary greatly by region (i.e., range of 11 percent to 13 percent); differences were primarily tied to sociodemographic factors. Low-income to middle-income and minority segments of the study population had higher hospitalization rates, and admissions of people age 65 and older accounted for almost half of the avoidable hospitalizations. The authors suggested that this variation was linked to disparities in access to primary care that might have prevented acute disease and subsequent hospitalization.[32]

Table 18–5 Managed Care Characteristics of Selected Metropolitan Statistical Areas

MSA Name	Percent Managed Care Penetration	Percent HMOs Using Primary Capitation	Utilization in Days/1,000
Atlanta	27.0	39.6	452.0
Boston	49.3	22.3	598.0
Chicago	25.9	69.0	601.0
Dayton	56.1	27.0	544.0
Denver	43.2	48.3	390.0
Los Angeles	45.7	92.7	411.0
New York City	32.5	35.9	1,039.0
Phoenix	33.7	48.9	420.0
Philadelphia	46.5	32.0	740.0
Toledo	46.7	100.0	658.0
Tulsa	26.2	88.1	446.0

Courtesy of HCIA-Sachs, 1998, Evanston, Illinois.

Practice variation also is evident in the management of various diseases. Several research findings that are not focused on managed care present evidence that although medically accepted approaches for the management of particular diseases exist, the implementation of these approaches varies widely. Three illustrative examples are:

- In 1993, one researcher found rates of inappropriate treatment ranged from about 15 percent to 30 percent, reaching as high as 40 percent for particular procedures at individual institutions.[33]
- Treatment of pneumonia in the elderly indicates administration of antibiotics within 8 hours of admission, and blood cultures within 24 hours of admission are related to higher patient survival rates. Actual practice differs significantly across geographical areas, with a variance of 49 percent to 90 percent for antibiotics given within the 8-hour guideline and a variance of 46 percent to 83 percent for the blood culture guideline.[34]
- Rates of prescribing beta-blockers after acute myocardial infarction (AMI) remain low despite widespread education efforts.

One study comparing regional variation in the management of cardiovascular patients showed that patients receiving prescriptions for beta-blockers after AMI ranged from 55 percent to 81 percent.[35]

Variations reflect inappropriate overtreatment or undertreatment that may be attributable to multiple factors, including the practice of "defensive medicine," training biases, and lack of access to the most current medical practice information. Variations also may occur as a result of fee-for-service incentives that reimburse providers for more care or financial incentives under capitation that reward providers for less care. In addition, variations may result when there is an oversupply of providers trying to do more for fewer patients. Sex, race, insurance status of patients, and access to technology also contribute to variation.[36,37]

Despite generally low utilization in HMOs and other forms of managed care plans, some researchers believe that a significant amount of unnecessary utilization remains even now. The most aggressive of these is found in a report by Milliman and Robertson.[38] Table 18–6, adapted from that report, lists "optimally managed" admits per thousand and days per thousand for commercial and Medicare enrollees.

Table 18–6 Optimal Utilization Levels (July 1,1997)

Category of Service	Optimally Managed			
	Commercial (Under Age 65)		Medicare	
	Admits per 1,000	Days per 1,000	Admits per 1,000	Days per 1,000
Inpatient hospital				
Nonmaternity				
Medical	19.4	57.4	118.7	402.3
Surgical	9.7	35.2	57.8	289.0
Psychiatric	1.6	6.2	0.9	4.2
Alcohol/drug	0.8	2.9	0.8	3.4
SNF/ECF*	2.4	12.0	65.5	765.8
Maternity				
Mother	13.2	19.1	0.0	0.0
Well newborn	11.1	13.6	0.0	0.0
Nondelivery	0.8	1.2	0.0	0.0
Total (excluding SNF/ECF)	45.5	122.0	178.2	698.9
Total (including SNF/ECF)	47.9	134.0	243.7	1464.7

*SNF, Skilled Nursing Facility; ECF, Extended Care Facility.
Courtesy of Milliman & Robertson, 2000, Brookfield, Wisconsin.

Examining medical appropriateness does not clarify the issue substantially. Medical appropriateness has been studied by a number of investigators, and most found that there is a considerable amount of care that is delivered inappropriately because of overuse, underuse, or misuse (the wrong procedure or therapeutic intervention). Studies of actual medical practice compared with the judgments of medical experts find a high percentage (i.e., 10 percent to 50 percent) of care is inappropriate.[39] This finding emphasizes that the judgment of any individual physician does not in all cases represent the most appropriate care. Other studies have been more difficult to interpret.[40]

Examples of appropriateness investigations also include a study by researchers from the RAND Corporation, the University of California, and Fink & Kosekoff, Inc. The investigators reviewed medical record data on rates of inpatient and outpatient upper gastrointestinal endoscopy procedures and found that 65 percent were appropriate, 24 percent were inappropriate, and

the appropriateness of 11 percent could not be determined on the basis of clinical findings (i.e., the highest rated indicator of appropriateness was indeterminate).[41]

In a nationally representative sample of Medicare patients, a study by Brook and others found 17 percent of coronary angiographies, 17 percent of endoscopies, and 32 percent of carotid endarterectomies were inappropriate (i.e., represented overuse); 9 percent, 11 percent, and 32 percent of the procedures were classified as of equivocal benefit, respectively. The authors were unable to explain appropriateness on the basis of information related to patient symptoms (e.g., rates of stenosis, surgical high risk, history of transient ischemic attacks), patient demographics, physician characteristics (e.g., board certification, training), or hospital characteristics (e.g., teaching status, bed size).[42] The authors did conclude, however, that how well a procedure is performed is not a proxy for whether it needs to be performed.

Numerous studies have been done to support the preceding conclusions,[43-45] but the point is made. To a large degree, UM seeks to reduce this high level of variation to promote good outcomes (outcomes are discussed in detail in Chapter 31) while also managing costs.

THE ROLE OF ELECTRONIC COMMERCE

Electronic commerce, or e-commerce, is an area that has not been exploited to any substantial degree for purposes of UM. Other than basic transactions such as authorizations and claims, e-commerce for UM as of 2000 has been restricted to the provision of clinical protocols, directories of providers, formularies, and other such static "look-up" functions. It is expected that e-commerce will be successfully applied over the next several years, however. The ability to apply expert decision-making algorithms and rapid response by means of electronic communications is feasible.

Most physicians are not taking advantage of e-commerce at the time of publication. Even the most simple of functions such as electronic claims submission has not been widely adopted by physicians. Because most e-commerce in this industry has taken place by means of proprietary systems, it is not surprising that physicians have been reluctant to take on multiple systems. That will change by 2002 or 2003 because of HIPAA. All the basic data standards that are involved in an e-commerce application of UM are defined in HIPAA, and their use is mandated for any electronic interchange. E-commerce is discussed in greater depth in Chapter 37. However, currency of information about e-commerce is nearly impossible to maintain in a book because of the nature of this rapidly evolving field, so the reader will continually need to seek out fresh sources of information.

AUTHORIZATION OR DENIAL OF PAYMENT FOR SERVICES

Many of the approaches to UM have imbedded within them the concept of an authorization system. This topic is sufficiently important to warrant its own chapter (Chapter 19), and so is dealt with here only in the context of the overall approach to UM. Certain elements of authorization systems are focused on later when discussing the management of referral services, but not the entire array of elements. When discussing management of institutional utilization, it is assumed that an authorization system is in place and is therefore not specifically addressed at all.

It would be misleading, though, to fail to underscore the importance of an authorization system in supporting management of utilization. It is through the mechanism of approving or denying payment for services that many UM activities are effective. The other primary approaches to managing utilization include the uses of data and information (Chapter 32) and direct interactions between network physicians and medical managers (Chapter 33). Beyond managing utilization, the other main approach is to manage price, which refers to contracting issues that are discussed in Chapters 8 through 12.

An important adjunct to the topic of authorization systems is how disputes over authorization between providers and the plan or between members and the plan are managed. In other words, if MCO medical managers deny an authorization, which means denying payment for the service, and the network physician or member disagrees with that decision, there must be in place a means of resolving that disagreement. This is referred to as an appeal, and an MCO must have the policies and procedures in place to deal with appeals expeditiously.

In many states, and under debate at the federal level at the time of publication, the right to an external review of an upheld appeal is mandatory. Fixed timelines are established for review and determination of appeals for Medicare members, as well as in many states, whereas an expedited appeal process must be in place for times when the authorization dispute is over services currently being provided. Internal dispute resolution and external appeals are highly important for medical managers to fully understand and to comply with. The reader is referred to Chapter 40, where appeals policies, including external appeal rights, are addressed in the context of member services. No one involved with medical management can afford not to be thoroughly familiar with this topic, even though it is not addressed in this chapter.

MANAGING UTILIZATION OF SPECIALTY SERVICES

Management of medical services requiring authorization is discussed in greater detail in Chapter 19, but a subset of that discussion is presented here. The reader will want to review both chapters to gain a reasonably broad understanding of this category of care management.

Managing the utilization of referral and specialty services (both physician and nonphysician) is important in medical management. In most managed health care plans, the costs associated with non–primary care professional services will be substantially greater than the cost of primary care services, often between 1.5 and 2.0 times as high. This difference arises from the increased fees associated with specialty services and from the hospital-intensive and procedure-intensive nature of those services. The associated utilization costs generated by specialists are often overlooked. It is not only the fees of the specialists themselves that add to the cost of care but also the cost of services ordered by specialists, such as diagnostic studies and facility charges for procedures.

These costs are not routinely added to the cost of specialist services when data are compiled, but management of specialist services will often lead to management of these outside services as well. In one study, the savings generated by managing specialty physician services was actually twice the amount generated from hospital UM (adjusted for severity and case mix).[46]

Definition of Specialist Services

Referral or specialist services are those professional services not considered primary care; in other words, all physician services that are not from general internists, family physicians, and general pediatricians. If OB/GYN is considered primary care, it must be defined which OB/GYN services (e.g., surgery, routine Pap smears, pelvic examinations, colposcopy) are included as primary care and which are specialty care.

Most managed care plans count specialist physicians and nonphysician professionals (e.g., psychologists) in the specialist cost category, and ancillary services (e.g., laboratory, radiology, pharmacy) are dealt with separately. In keeping with that philosophy, management of ancillary and pharmaceutical utilization are addressed separately in Chapters 20 and 24, respectively.

Selection of Referral and Consulting Providers

The ability to select providers on the basis of a demonstrated pattern of practice can have a considerable impact on referral expenses. There are large differences in the efficiency of practice between providers within each specialty. If patients are preferentially sent to those specialists who demonstrate cost-effective practice, the plan can achieve considerable savings.

It is especially important in plans that allow self-referral to specialists by members, such as PPOs, point-of-service (POS) plans, and "open-access" HMOs. If a plan allows open access to any specialist at any time other than through selection of providers, there will be little control of utilization or cost except perhaps by making fee adjustments after enough documentation of overutilization has been accumulated. The problem with using fee adjustments to control utilization (i.e., adjusting a specialist's, or the entire provider panel's, fees downward as utilization goes up) is that it can lead to an "I'd better get mine first" mentality. In that situation, providers may begin churning visits and increasing utilization to increase revenues, worried that next month the fees may be adjusted even lower.

Evaluating and managing specialty practice behavior are not easy tasks and must be done over a long period of time on a significant number of events. Those plans that have the size and capability to collect data and create useful information are better positioned to manage specialty utilization than are plans lacking those two requirements. Chapters 32 and 33 discuss this topic further.

Authorization System

An authorization system in the context of this section is mentioned here because without one, there is a diminished opportunity to effectively manage referral utilization. Educational and data feedback techniques may be used, and an MCO may be able to select specialists through practice pattern analysis. These actions will result in some improvement in referral expenses, but not to the same degree that a PCP authorization system will create. A PCP referral authorization system accomplishes two primary tasks: to ensure that the need for referral to a specialist is determined by a physician and to provide the structure for creating data and information to better manage utilization overall.

The corollary to this is the possibility that a PCP is able to deliver many of the same services as a specialist, but at considerable savings and in a more appropriate setting. Even in non–managed care systems, PCPs manage a substantial proportion of their patients' care.[47] In recent years, though, some PCPs have been feeling uncomfortable about providing some services, with one large survey reporting that nearly one in four PCPs believed that the scope of care they were expected to provide was greater than it should be.[48] It is in no one's interest for patient care to be rendered by a physician who is not comfortable doing so. If a sizable segment of the PCP network feels such discomfort, it is advisable for medical managers to re-evaluate policies and procedures around what is normally expected to be in the scope of primary care and what is more appropriately provided by a specialty physician.

The remainder of this section assumes that there is some type of authorization system in place, regardless of whether it is rigid or loose.

Methods To Manage Specialty Services

A medical director or medical group may apply many methods to manage the cost and volume of specialty physician services. Some of those methods, such as the use of a PCP acting as a care manager or gatekeeper, single visit authorization, and a prohibition on secondary referrals

(discussed later), are designed to achieve the most management over specialty costs. Those methods may or may not be appropriate, however, depending on plan design, market forces, and other internal or external factors. As managed health care has grown and evolved and physicians' practice behaviors have incorporated many of the overall goals of managed health care, some of the methods described in this section have become archaic and now provide lowered value. There will be some environments in which these earlier techniques are still appropriate for medical managers to use, but the return in improved performance versus the cost to carry out the function and the extra burden placed on the physicians is a determination that must be made periodically by each MCO.

In addition to these methods, there is the general issue of modifying the practice behavior of physicians. The goal for medical managers is to bring about appropriate practice behavior change so that physicians provide high-quality care at lower costs. Chapter 33 focuses on this important topic; therefore it is not dwelt on here.

Occasionally, a genuine clinical disagreement will exist between the medical director and either the PCP or the specialty physician regarding authorization for services. These disagreements, which may or may not be acute in nature, must be dealt with promptly and fairly. The resolution of such disputes is discussed later in this chapter because the topic can apply equally to specialty referrals, procedures, and hospitalizations.

THE ROLE OF THE PRIMARY CARE PHYSICIAN IN SPECIALTY SERVICES MANAGEMENT

The general role of the PCP is discussed in Chapter 7. It is necessary, however, to discuss some aspects of the PCP's role in managing utilization here because the PCP plays a significant role in managing specialty services in most HMO and POS plans. It is done primarily through the use of an authorization system in which a member may go to a PCP without any barriers to access; but to see a specialist, an authorization from the member's PCP must be obtained. Failure to obtain such an authorization may result in no payment for unauthorized services (in an HMO) or payment at a lower level (in a POS plan). This chapter provides an overview of how an authorization is generated and how a plan manages the authorization system, and Chapter 19 provides an in-depth discussion of these topics.

Female members commonly do not need to obtain an authorization to see an OB/GYN, although the OB/GYN may or may not have the ability to authorize additional services. As noted in Chapter 7, some plans allow (or are mandated by the state) for OB/GYNs to act as PCPs, although that is less common than providing members direct access to OB/GYNs not acting as PCPs. For direct member access to OB/GYN care, the scope of services provided by the OB/GYN that are considered primary care (e.g., routine Pap smears, pelvic examinations, colposcopy) versus those that are considered consultant care (e.g., surgery) must be defined.

A few plans use "flexible gatekeepers," a term applied to those MCOs that require a member to choose a PCP to coordinate and authorize services but allow that PCP to be a specialty physician. For example, a member may choose a cardiologist as his or her PCP because a cardiologist is also an internist. Thus, members can choose PCPs according to their primary medical needs. It does increase the likelihood of adverse selection (i.e., a higher share of members who are sicker than average) to the panels of those specialty physicians, but this is only relevant if the PCP "flexible gatekeeper" is capitated.

Studies examining the ability of PCP-model HMOs to lower costs and maintain quality were most often done in the late 1980s or early 1990s.[49-52] Although the overall medical environment has changed considerably since then, recent literature continues to show value for this model. One recent study found that ambulatory charges were $21 lower per person per year in the PCP model as a result of 0.3 fewer visits per year to specialists.[53] A more comprehensive study recently confirmed lower rates of specialist use in a PCP model and suggested that referrals from PCPs to specialists may reflect different patterns of referral compared with indemnity models, rather than simply lower rates of referral. The study, a National Ambulatory Medical Care Survey (NAMCS) study of 1989 to 1994 data, examined referrals for managed and indemnity patients (Medicare and Medicaid excluded) by community-based physicians.[54] Referral patterns, including PCP-referred, self-referred, and specialist-to-specialist-referred, suggested the following:

- Lower use of specialists by HMO patients may be a consequence of less patient self-referral and fewer patient visits once a referral is made (more one-time visits/consultations).
- PCP-referred patients had a higher level of severity than self-referred (as evidenced by a higher hospitalization rate).
- Some increases in the rate of PCP referrals have been observed over time, suggesting restrictions in referrals to specialists may be decelerating.
- Self-referral in HMOs occurred for 31.3 percent of newly referred patients compared with 49.5 percent of newly referred indemnity patients.
- Self-referral occurred with variable frequency across most specialties with the exception of dermatology, OB/GYN, ophthalmology, and psychiatry. These four specialties have the highest rate of indemnity self-referral as well.

Assuming hospitalization rate as a proxy for severity, the data suggest PCPs referred patients who were more acute; therefore, the PCP role is seen as appropriately managing less sick patients and referring higher acuity patients to specialists.

A study of 3,000 Medicaid enrollees managed within a primary care gatekeeper model revealed similar findings: (1) PCPs tended to provide more of the care than specialists, and (2) enrollees tended to see fewer providers over the course of a year, potentially resulting in greater continuity of care.[55] Medicaid managed care is specifically discussed in Chapter 57.

Although specialty referral rates are somewhat lower in PCP-model HMOs, a review of

data for referrals to specialists suggests that denial rates have also been relatively low. A study
of 2,000 physicians revealed a denial rate of 3
percent for eight categories of referrals; these
rates are measured after appeals, however, with
initial denial rates slightly higher. Other denial
rates in this study were 1 percent for hospitalization, 2.6 percent for specialist referrals, 1.25 percent for surgical procedures, 0.7 percent for cardiac catheterizations, and 3.0 percent for mental
health referrals.[56]

There has been some level of controversy
about the value of the PCP gatekeeper role in
managed care and how the interaction between
the PCP model and the reimbursement or financial incentive systems has affected utilization.
Physician attitudes also have been variable over
recent years, and one study serves as an illustration. In that study, physicians reported that a
PCP gatekeeper model was effective in controlling costs and other aspects of care, but those
physicians had complaints about the imposition
of administrative requirements and issues of access to specialists, testing, and other measures.
Although decidedly a mixed group of opinions,
overall 72 percent of physicians thought that the
gatekeeper model was better than or comparable
to traditional care arrangements.[57]

Some HMOs have chosen to do away with the
gatekeeper authorization model and simply use
different levels of copayment for specialty physician visits compared with visits to PCPs.
Those plans anecdotally report that overall costs
are roughly the same, but it must be noted that
there are some markets where this open-access
model is not considered suitable, even by those
plans that use the model frequently. MCOs that
choose this route must have good data and profiling systems (see Chapter 32) that allow them
to manage specialty utilization through other
means. One major national managed care company has adopted this strategy for many, but not
all, of its markets, citing market immaturity in
some metropolitan areas. It is still too soon to
know whether this model will ultimately be as
cost-effective as the PCP model. In light of this
model, it is interesting to note that even in situations that do not involve managed care, there is

evidence that PCPs still function as the primary
case managers for a large number of patients.[58]

SINGLE VISIT AUTHORIZATIONS ONLY

An authorization system that allows only one
visit per authorization is one that provides the
highest degree of management, even if it is not
ultimately the type of system a plan chooses to
use for reasons addressed later (as well as in
Chapters 3 and 41). In essence, every time a
member is referred to a specialist, the PCP
gatekeeper must issue a unique authorization.
That authorization is good for one visit and will
be used to pay only one claim. Claims submitted
by a specialist that list multiple charges will be
compared with what was authorized, and only
the authorized services will be reimbursed.
Common exceptions to single visit authorization
requirements exist even in MCOs that use this
system and will be addressed shortly.

The single visit authorization approach
sounds strong in theory, and it is. It is also sometimes difficult to enforce, and it may not always
be desirable from a member relations standpoint.
A mechanism for review of claims that do not
exactly match the authorization must be put in
place so as not to penalize members and specialists if the PCP fails to document the authorization correctly. It also is sometimes difficult in
practice to separate out overcharges or add-ons
to a claim, particularly when the claims adjudi-
cators get overworked. Finally, recent legislation in some states and at the federal level provides for direct access to certain specialists for
patients with particular diseases, and this requirement must be accommodated in the UM
system. Nonetheless, a single authorization system is both workable and required for optimal
results if cost is the paramount factor.

It is necessary to inform members through full
and fair disclosure of such a system before they
enroll in a plan and continuing thereafter. The
usual methods of informing members include
enrollment literature, new member kits, the
identification card issued by the plan, the evidence of coverage certificate issued to members,

the referral form itself, the plan newsletter, and even signs in specialists' offices. Specialists will usually agree to allow signs in their offices when they understand that improving compliance with authorization procedures will enhance their revenue both by speeding up claims processing and by decreasing bad debt load.

As mentioned earlier, there are very common exceptions to the rule of one authorization per visit. These exceptions include chemotherapy and radiation therapy for cancer, obstetrics, mental health and chemical dependency therapy, physical therapy, and rehabilitation therapy. Other exceptions also commonly exist, such as automatically allowing one or two home health visits after short-stay obstetrics when a member and her physician choose the short-stay option.

Even for these exceptions, however, it is not wise to have open-ended authorizations. There should be an absolute limit on the number of visits that can be authorized at once. For example, a referral for physical therapy should be limited to an initial number of visits, after which the therapist must discuss the case with the physician before any further authorizations are issued. For chemotherapy cases, the oncologist should discuss the case with the PCP or case manager (see Chapters 22 and 23) and outline the course of treatment, which could then be authorized all at once. The overriding principle is that open-ended authorizations are simply blank checks.

SPECIALTY PHYSICIANS AS PRIMARY PHYSICIANS

In certain clinical circumstances it is better for a specialist to act as the PCP (i.e., in the role of primary provider and coordinator of care as well as the "gatekeeper" function). This occurs in those instances in which a member has a complex and chronic disease, and routine care is beyond the typical scope of primary care medicine. For such patients, it is good case management (CM) to have a specialist act as the PCP because the specialist is not only more experienced at managing that condition but is also better able to provide cost-effective care. As noted earlier, in some states there is legislation that actually requires this for defined diseases.

Clinical conditions that fall into this category are typically those managed using a disease management approach (Chapter 23) or a large CM approach (Chapter 22). For example, a patient with active and symptomatic acquired immune deficiency syndrome (AIDS) is likely to be better managed by a physician who specializes in that disease. The same may be said for a variety of other chronic and complex diseases such as severe diabetes,[59] chronic rheumatic and musculoskeletal diseases,[60] or debilitating congestive heart failure.[61] In these cases, the appropriate specialist has the same level of authorization authority as a PCP (i.e., is not subject to limitations on being able to authorize services other than those that apply to all PCPs).

It may be clear in some cases that a specialist is better able to manage a patient with a chronic and complex illness, but it is sometimes difficult to know when that is the preferred approach. Patients that benefit from this approach are clearly those with a high severity of illness, but in many cases that represents the final stages of a long-term condition. For example, a PCP may easily manage a patient with cardiovascular disease, with referrals to a cardiologist as appropriate. That same patient may have congestive heart failure develop over the course of years, until it becomes debilitating and beyond the scope of most PCPs. At what point is it appropriate for the specialist to assume the role of that patient's PCP? Because there is no clear-cut way to define that point, each potential case will need to be evaluated individually. The need for such an assessment may be prompted by the patient's PCP, the specialist, the plan's disease management personnel, or the member and their family.

Advocates can be found who will argue for early transition to a specialist (or elimination of the PCP role altogether), whereas others will argue for the effectiveness of PCPs in all but the most serious cases. There are many studies that conclude that a specialist is better at treating a specific condition than is a generalist, and these are well summarized by Cram and Ettinger.[62] The problem that many of these studies illustrate is that a specific condition will more likely be treated effectively by specialists using the most recent therapeutic approach than it will be by PCPs.

That is quite different from providing or coordinating the entire spectrum of medical needs, though. The primary argument that can be made from at least some of these studies is that PCPs need to be more current in their knowledge of common diseases and to know when referral is appropriate, not that a specialist who treats a particular clinical condition well is in any better position to manage overall medical needs than is a PCP.

PROHIBITION OF SECONDARY REFERRALS AND AUTHORIZATIONS

A related facet of managing referral utilization is the prohibition of secondary referrals by specialists. This means that a specialist cannot authorize other referrals for a member. In other words, if a specialist feels that a patient needs to see another specialist, then that judgment must be communicated back to the PCP, who is the only one able to issue an authorization for services.

This requirement may extend to revisits to the specialist and tests and procedures. For example, if a specialist has an expensive piece of diagnostic equipment in the office, there may be a subtle pressure to use it to make it pay for itself. One widely cited study looking at physician ownership of radiology equipment documented a fourfold increase in imaging examinations and significant increases in charges among physicians who used their own equipment compared with physicians who referred such studies to radiologists.[63] Similar results have been reported for laboratory services[64] and a wide variety of ancillary services.[65]

The issue of physician-owned diagnostic and therapeutic equipment or services is a difficult one to address and one that is coming under increasing pressure from government regulation, at least for Medicare.[66] Perhaps the best method for dealing with this issue is simply to prohibit or markedly restrict the use of such services. Most managed care plans contract with a limited number of vendors for such ancillary services and may limit referral to only those vendors. The topic of ancillary services is discussed in Chapter 20.

Even in the absence of those types of pressures, secondary referrals may simply be unnecessary. For example, an endocrinologist may be concerned about a referred patient's chest pain and may refer the patient to a cardiologist when in fact the patient's PCP had worked up the problem and was tracking it carefully. This situation happens more often than one might think because patients do not always communicate or even understand what previous care they have received, and the PCP may not have considered it necessary to put that information into the referral letter or form.

It is important to emphasize here that such restrictions cannot be applied to those diagnostic and therapeutic services that are routine for the specialist. It would be absurd to prohibit a cardiologist from performing an electrocardiogram or an orthopaedist from performing radiographic studies. These and similar examples of medical policy, as applied to payment provisions of the plan, are necessary to define and must ensure that there is no barrier to the ability of the specialist to use appropriate technology. Having said that, there also are also examples in which a specialist should not automatically be paid for doing a procedure; rather, the specialist should be required to obtain additional authorization. Of course, this issue is moot if the original authorization was for the specialist to perform the procedure as part of his or her overall evaluation, but the authorization system should note that in the referral. The plan's data information and profiling systems (Chapter 32) can be used to look for aberrant or inappropriate practice patterns.

REVIEW OF REASONS FOR REFERRAL

It is the responsibility of the medical director to review the reasons for referrals by PCPs. In the tightest of all systems, this review takes place before the actual referral is made. In other words, the medical director or associate medical director must approve any authorization prospectively. This system is grossly cumbersome, prohibitively expensive, and is seen as demeaning to PCPs, but it is definitely tight. Plans using this type of review and approval system are now relatively rare, and its routine use is not advocated. It is perhaps most suitable for a tightly managed closed panel or a training program where interns and residents are involved. It also is appropriate for selected types of referrals where the plan may wish to ensure that sufficient reason exists before it authorizes the service (e.g., some plans categorize referrals to sleep laboratories as needing this type of review).

Retrospective review of referrals is more acceptable. Here, the medical director or associate medical director reviews referral information after the fact, although preferably not long after. Reviews may encompass all referrals, which achieves tight control but is unrealistic, or just randomly selected referrals, which is less tight but still useful. Most useful and cost effective from the plan's standpoint is to evaluate PCP referral rates and patterns, as well as utilization patterns of referral physicians to determine where retrospective review will have the greatest potential. As noted several times throughout this chapter, the topic of information and profiling systems is discussed in Chapter 32.

Several potential sources of information exist for retrospective review of referrals. How technologically advanced an MCO is in e-commerce, as well as how much the physicians use e-commerce in their interactions with the plan, will determine the sources of information. MCOs that depend on paper-based authorizations will have reams of forms that a medical director can churn through, but that exercise will produce more paper cuts than valuable information.

In an earlier era of managed care, when closed panel HMOs were more prevalent, referral authorization forms would contain clinical information useful both to the specialist and to a reviewing medical director. This is still often the case in organized medical groups with a high level of peer review. In today's large open panels though, it is considered successful if the form can even be read and nearly miraculous if the form can be scanned in by optical character recognition. In large open panels, unless targeted specifically to a single physician and looking for a specific problem (e.g., self-referral), review of paper-based forms yields little value.

Telephonic-based systems provide for more current capture of data and possibly more uniform data entry but are unable to capture much clinical information that will be of any use in retrospective review. The usefulness of telephonic

authorization systems is in the timely entry of data to support more accurate processing of claims, and it provides no appreciable added value for retrospective review other than better data capture.

MCOs with advanced e-commerce capabilities, combined with physicians willing and able to take advantage of those capabilities, do have potential to provide some improvement in information value. If e-commerce is used solely to capture the same data that a paper-based or telephonic authorization system does, there is no particular added value other than timeliness of the data and ease of performing automated analyses. If the e-commerce capabilities extend to some application of expert systems, pattern detection may occur much sooner than if it depends on accumulating large amounts of historical data. The ability to use different levels of monitoring is also of value, allowing the medical director to focus attention where it will have greater return. E-commerce too has its limitations. HIPAA mandates (Chapters 35 and 67) regarding data definitions including referral authorizations, the new provider identification number system, and other items will provide for greater uniformity and simplicity of data and transactions but also will restrict what information may be required.

The other significant impact of HIPAA in this area of discussion is a result of the privacy requirements. This refers not only to data security issues but also to policies and procedures about who is allowed access to patient-identifiable data, for what purpose, when it is allowed, when a specific signed release from the patient is required before medical information may be accessed by another party, and what safeguards are in place. The overall intent is to protect the privacy of medical information of citizens, not to prevent medical management. At the time of publication, the proposed privacy regulations for HIPAA provided specific allowances for the management of utilization and quality, as well as other clinically valuable activities. However, those proposed regulations cannot be considered final, so the reader must ascertain the impact of the final regulations on medical management activities. Medical managers also will need to put in place a compliance program consistent with the overall privacy compliance program required under HIPAA.

Periodic chart review, similar to a quality assurance audit (see Chapter 30), is also of value. This is a time-consuming and labor-intensive activity but provides a higher level of information about how clinical decision making occurs in an individual practice. Chart reviews are required for some external accreditation programs (Chapter 44) and are routine in most HMOs, even large open panels. If the goal is overall network behavior change, random sampling of individual physicians will suffice. The other use of chart review is when practice pattern analysis of referrals raises the possibility of inappropriate referral management by an individual PCP, either by overreferring or by underreferring.

Medical managers need to bear in mind the limitations on chart review. The chart may contain insufficient information to form an opinion about reasons for referral, or it may contain documentation that is ambiguous for purposes of review. Therefore, chart review should be considered as one additional method of gathering information, not as a sure means of finding definitive answers.

When the medical director finds problems in the use of referrals by a PCP, it is not necessary to reprimand or embarrass the physician. It is more appropriate to discuss the case clinically and suggest options that the PCP might use to be more appropriate in the use of referrals. The ultimate goal of these discussions is to foster an internal questioning behavior in the PCP so that the medical director will not have to do it. The goals are for the PCP to consider the options before making a referral, to make referrals count, and to refer when appropriate. It often means breaking old habits, but then that is what medical management is about.

Self-Referrals by Members

In managed care plans with authorization systems, members referring themselves to specialists for care is a common occurrence. In open-access HMOs and POS plans that have benefits for self-referral, plan design allows this to occur. In either a traditional HMO or a POS plan, new members who are not used to the system and who signed up because of the benefits offered may not recall or note the requirements for authorization. These individuals are more apt to self-refer and later be surprised that there is reduced or no coverage for the service. This problem is particularly evident in new Medicare enrollees.

In these situations, it is useful to have a policy regarding the first time it occurs with a new member. Many HMOs will pay for the first self-referral by a new member and document that the member was educated about the referral authorization system, so that benefits for self-referral may be denied on subsequent occurrences. Most POS plans do not cover any self-referrals at the higher level of benefits even on first occurrence, but most will remind the member by way of the explanation of benefits statement that the benefits would have been higher if the member had obtained authorization.

There is a particular problem that appears to fall into this category but is actually a problem of synchronizing the claims (Chapter 38) and authorization systems (Chapter 19). This is the situation in which a PCP refers a member to a specialist, and the specialist sees the patient and submits a claim promptly, often electronically. The authorization, however, is not electronic or even telephonic, but rather paper based, and it does not arrive at the plan until *after* the claim has been received and processed. This results in either a denial of payment (for a traditional HMO) or a lower level of benefits (for a POS plan), although it is clearly an incorrect payment that requires rectification (at considerable hassle to the member and the physician and great aggregate expense to the plan). Therefore, if a plan uses a referral authorization system, it is important to bear this potential complication in mind and take it into account in operations.

INSTITUTIONAL UTILIZATION MANAGEMENT

Utilization of hospital (or more accurately institutional) services may account for 40 percent or more of the total expenses in a managed health care plan. That amount can be even greater when utilization is excessive. Management of these expenses is therefore prominent among most managers' priorities.

The expense of any medical service is a product of the price of that service times the volume of services delivered. Simple reduction of bed days may be of value but can lull the inexperienced manager into a sense of complacency. Management of institutional utilization is therefore to be understood in context with management of other areas of utilization as well. It is possible to reduce inpatient utilization and actually experience a rise in cost, as is discussed later in this chapter. Pricing for institutional services is discussed in Chapter 12.

COMMON METHODS FOR MANAGING UTILIZATION

Management of institutional utilization may be best presented by discussing the key categories for managing the process: prospective, concurrent, and retrospective review, and large (i.e., catastrophic) case management (LCM, as discussed in greater detail in Chapter 22). *Prospective review* means review of a case before it even happens, *concurrent review* means review occurs while the case is active, and *retrospective review* occurs after the case is finished. *LCM* refers to managing cases that are expected to result in very large costs, so as to provide coordination of care that results in both proper care and cost savings.

Prospective Review

Precertification

Precertification refers to a requirement on the part of the admitting physician (and often the hospital) to notify the plan before a member is admitted for inpatient care or an outpatient procedure. There is a widespread and rather erroneous belief that the primary role of precertification is to prevent unnecessary cases from occurring. Although that may occasionally happen (particularly in workers' compensation cases, see Chapter 61), it is not the chief reason for precertification and has not been so for a long time.

There are three primary reasons for precertification. The first is to notify the medical management system that a case will be occurring. In most plans, this refers to the software decision support systems that specialize in medical management, creating substantial leverage for the case managers, UM nurses, and the medical director. Also, UM will be able to prepare discharge planning ahead of time and look for the case during concurrent review rounds. In some instances, the LCM function may be notified if the admission diagnosis raises the probability that the case will be expensive (e.g., a bone marrow transplant).

The second major reason for precertification is to ensure that care takes place in the most appropriate setting. Perhaps an inpatient case is diverted to the outpatient department, or a case is diverted from a nonparticipating hospital to a participating one or to a facility that has been designated as a center of excellence for a selected procedure.

The third reason is to capture data for financial accruals. Although it is unlikely that a plan can capture every case before or while it is taking place, a mature plan that is running well can capture most cases, perhaps 90 percent to 95 percent. By knowing the number and nature of hospital cases and potential or existing catastrophic cases, the plan may more accurately accrue for expenses rather than have to wait for claims to come in. It allows financial managers to take action early so as to avoid nasty financial surprises, as well as properly manage reinsurance. Accrual method is discussed in Chapter 47.

In any case, for inpatient cases the plan usually assigns a length of stay (LOS) guideline at the time the admission is certified, as will be discussed shortly. The plan will also use the precertification process to verify the member's eligibility for coverage and to communicate that to the provider, although most plans have a disclaimer stating that ultimate eligibility for coverage will be determined at the time the claim is processed. Eligibility determination is another example of a standardized and defined electronic data definition under HIPAA.

In the case of an emergency or urgent admission, it is obviously not possible to obtain precertification. In that event, there is usually a contractual requirement in the provider contracts to notify the plan by the next business day or within 24 hours if the plan has UM staffing 24 hours per day. Most plans have contractual language with both physicians and hospitals whereby financial penalties are imposed (e.g., a percentage of their fee or a flat penalty) for failure to obtain certification. In plans that allow members to seek care from noncontracted providers (e.g., in POS plans), the responsibility to contact the plan rests with members if they choose not to access care through the in-network system. In such cases, most plans impose benefits penalties (e.g., a higher coinsurance or a flat penalty rate) on members who fail to obtain proper precertification.

Preadmission Testing and Same-Day Surgery

One of the easiest and ubiquitous methods for cost control is preadmission testing and same-day surgery. A member who is going to be hospitalized on an elective basis has routine preoperative tests done as an outpatient and then is admitted the same day as the surgery is to be performed. Both these policies are confirmed at the time of precertification.

For example, if a member has elective gallbladder surgery scheduled for 10:00 AM on Thursday, then on Tuesday the member goes to the hospital for preoperative tests. The results are made available to the admitting physician, who performs the admission history and physical as an outpatient and either delivers the results to the hospital or calls them in to the hospital's transcription department. The member arrives at the hospital at 6:00 AM on Thursday, is admitted, and has the surgery as scheduled.

In many health plans, the plan arranges for laboratory work to be done with a contracted laboratory at reduced rates or has in-house capabilities to perform the laboratory work. Occasionally, a hospital will refuse to accept the results of these laboratories. If the laboratory is accredited and licensed, the hospital has little grounds to require use of its laboratory, electrocardiography, and radiology services for preoperative admission testing. In these cases it falls to the plan's management team to discuss this issue with the hospital administrator and negotiate an agreement for the hospital to accept laboratory work or to agree to perform the work at equivalent costs. If the hospital refuses to cooperate, the medical director needs to decide whether to direct the elective cases to another, more cooperative hospital.

Mandatory Outpatient Surgery

It has become standard for health plans to produce mandatory outpatient surgery lists. These are lists of procedures that may only be performed on an outpatient basis unless prior approval is obtained from the plan's medical management function. These lists are used by so many third-party payers that one does not need to make it from scratch; simply look at what a similar plan or even Medicare is using or purchase it from an outside source. One byproduct of the popularity of these lists is that no two are identical, which causes at least occasional confusion with physicians and hospitals. Although consensus exists on most common procedures (e.g., a carpal tunnel release), there are always procedures that are migrating from inpatient to outpatient (e.g., outpatient cardiac catheterization has become popular in the past several years). That confusion probably tends to encourage the use of outpatient surgery when physicians are in doubt.

As mentioned earlier in this chapter and elsewhere, it is important to ensure that the desired savings are achievable before instituting mandatory outpatient surgery requirements. In some cases, hospitals or freestanding outpatient surgery facilities have charges that are equal to or greater than those for an inpatient day. In other cases, the facility charge may be lower, but the unbundled charges for anesthesia, recovery, supplies, and so on can drive the costs higher than anticipated. These issues are discussed in Chapters 11 and 12.

Concurrent Review

Concurrent review means managing utilization during the course of a hospitalization (as opposed to an outpatient procedure). Concurrent review results in more effective management of inpatient utilization than does retrospective review.[67] Common techniques for concurrent review involve assignment and tracking of LOS, review and rounding by UM nurses, and discharge planning. The roles of the medical director, the PCP, and the attending or consulting physicians are briefly discussed as well, as is the relationship between concurrent review and CM.

Maximum Length of Stay

A common approach to hospital utilization management is the assignment of a maximum allowable LOS (referred to as MaxLOS here for convenience) that sometimes appears in the guise of an estimated LOS. With the MaxLOS, the plan assigns a LOS on the basis of the admission diagnosis and that stay is all the plan will authorize for payment. For example, an admission for a particular surgical procedure may be assigned 3 days, and it is assumed that the patient will be admitted on the day of surgery and go home on the third day. Any costs beyond that day are not covered unless clinical circumstances support the additional stay. In those plans that cannot or will not restrict payment, the MaxLOS is used only to trigger greater involvement by the medical director. It is worth noting that reduced inpatient utilization is now due more to reductions in LOS than it is to reductions in admission rates.

The MaxLOS is determined by International Classification of Diseases, Ninth Revision, Clinical Modification (ICD-9-CM) code, or diagnostic code, although diagnosis-related groups (DRGs) are similar in concept. Selecting a norm for the MaxLOS is not always easy given the regional variations. Looking at the local fee-for-service experience is usually not helpful, and indeed will not accurately represent prevalent utilization standards, particularly in markets with high levels of managed health care. It has become common now for plans to purchase LOS guidelines from third parties and modify them as required for local variations.

The advantages of using MaxLOS designations are threefold. First, it allows the plan to cover a relatively large geographical area with few per-

sonnel. Second, such a list has the power of legitimacy and does not require continual negotiation. Third, it is a relatively mechanical technique and requires less training of plan personnel. This last advantage may be true for the person issuing the MaxLOS designation, but it is still important to verify, usually through the UM nurse, that the diagnosis is accurate and that there are no serious mitigating factors that will affect the LOS.

The problems with using MaxLOS designations also are threefold. First, it is easy to get complacent. By choosing certain values for MaxLOS designations, medical managers may fail to evaluate continually whether those are in fact the correct values, and there is less incentive to evaluate critically every day in the hospital for appropriateness and alternatives if plan personnel and the physician believe that there is still time on the meter. Second, the use of such a mechanical system often achieves less than optimal results. Management of inpatient utilization by the UM nurses and the medical director should produce a reduction in LOS. Third, if each case is not monitored, a MaxLOS may create undue consternation when the patient has a high illness burden or is highly complex.

An assigned MaxLOS may not adequately take into account concurrent or comorbid conditions. There is no one MaxLOS that will be applicable to all patients for any given reason for admission. This is not to say that the presence of comorbidity should automatically result in longer inpatient stays, but rather that this must be taken into account as part of inpatient UM.

The consequences of exceeding the MaxLOS must be defined. In many plans, exceeding the MaxLOS results in either a denial of payment for services rendered after the MaxLOS has been reached or a reduction in payment, usually by a percentage amount. If the MCO has failed to inform its membership of a MaxLOS program and the plan does not have sole source of payment clauses with its providers and hospitals (see Chapter 62), it may not be able to enforce a MaxLOS designation easily.

Role of the Utilization Management Nurse

The one individual who is crucial to the success of a managed care program is the UM nurse. It is the UM nurse who is the eyes and ears of the medical management department, who is able to apply clinical knowledge to cases, who will coordinate the discharge planning, and who will facilitate all the activities of UM.

Staffing levels for UM nurses will vary depending on the size of the geographical area, the number of hospitals, the size of the plan, and the intensity with which UM will be performed (e.g., by on-site hospital rounding). A common rule of thumb is for plans to staff one UM nurse for every 6,000 to 8,000 members, assuming that the UM nurses will be making rounds on all hospitalized patients and that utilization is tightly managed, but not on a 24-hour-per-day basis. Staffing ratios have considerable variation, however, with one study reporting the average number of full-time nurse reviewers at 0.16 per 1,000 enrollees, with a range of 0.01 to 0.8 per 1,000.[68] In a comprehensive 1999 study of large MCOs covering an aggregate of 26 million lives, staffing ratios for UM were further subdivided as illustrated in Table 18–7.[69] Plans that perform telephone review only may staff at ratios that are half the average. It also is necessary to provide clerical support to do intake, to follow up on discharge planning needs, to take care of filing, and so forth.

The scope of responsibilities of the UM nurse will vary depending on the plan and the personalities and skills of the other members of the medical management team. In some plans, the role simply involves telephone information gathering. In other plans, there will be a more proactive role, including frequent communication with attending physicians, the medical director, the hospitals, and the hospitalized members and their families; discharge planning and facilitation; and a host of other activities, including active hospital rounding.

Information Gathering. The one fundamental function of the UM nurse is information gathering. Information about hospital cases must be obtained in an accurate and timely fashion. It falls to the UM nurse to be the focal point of this information collection effort and to ensure that it is obtained and communicated to the necessary individuals in medical management and the claims department. Necessary information includes admission date and diagnosis, the type of hospital service to which the patient was admitted (e.g., medical, surgical, maternity), the admitting physician, specialists, planned procedures (type and timing), expected discharge date, needed discharge planning, and any other pertinent information the plan managers may need.

Telephone Rounding. In some plans, information gathering is done strictly by telephone; in other plans, hospital rounding is done in person by the UM nurse. When the telephone is used, it is used first to check with the admitting office to determine whether any plan members were admitted and then to check with the hospital's own UM department to obtain any further information.

Table 18–7 Staffing Ratios in Large MCOs in 1999

Staffing Ratio for UM Personnel as FTEs per 1,000 Members	25th Percentile	Mean	75th Percentile
FTEs dedicated to all UM functions	0.19	0.26	0.31
FTEs dedicated to hospital precertification and concurrent UM	0.13	0.18	0.24
FTEs dedicated to case management	0.04	0.04	0.05
FTEs dedicated to referral authorization	0.02	0.03	0.04
FTEs dedicated to ambulatory diagnostic testing and procedure authorization	0.001	0.002	0.003

Courtesy of Ernst & Young LLP, 2000, Washington, DC.

Telephone rounding is usually done in locations where there is too much geographical area to cover and the plan cannot yet justify adding more UM nurses (e.g., in a start-up individual provider association or PPO covering five counties). It also may be done in those rare instances in which a hospital refuses to give the UM nurse rounding privileges on hospitalized plan members. There are certainly instances in which a plan may delegate rounding and review to the hospital's UM department, but they are not common; examples include arrangements in which the hospital is at significant financial risk (e.g., through capitation or diagnosis-related groups). Telephone rounding also is used when tight controls on utilization do not exist and the UM function looks for clear outliers rather than tries to achieve optimal utilization management.

Hospital Rounding. Rounding in person is far superior to telephone rounding. When rounds are conducted daily by a UM nurse on every hospitalized member, the medical director will obtain the most accurate and timely information and will have information that might not otherwise be obtainable. For example, in a good quality management program (Chapter 30), the rounding UM nurse can watch for quality problems or significant events that would trigger a quality assurance audit. A rounding nurse also can pick up information about a patient's condition that may affect discharge planning—information that the attending physician may have failed to communicate (e.g., home durable medical equipment that must be ordered).

The UM nurse also can detect practice behavior that increases utilization simply for the convenience of the physician or the hospital. For example, a patient may be ready for discharge but the physician may have missed making rounds that morning and will not be back until the next day, or the hospital may have rescheduled surgery for its own reasons and the patient will have to stay an extra, unnecessary day. In situations such as these, the UM nurse must not be put into an adversarial position but rather should refer such matters to the medical director.

Personal rounding by the UM nurse has the added advantage of increasing member satisfaction. Many people feel uncomfortable talking to physicians and welcome the chance to express their fears or feelings to the UM nurse. In other cases, inquiring about how members are feeling can let them know that the plan cares about them as people and is not only interested in getting them out as fast as possible.

Occasionally, hospitals will refuse to grant rounding privileges to a UM nurse, the typical excuse being that the hospital already has a UM department. The hospital UM department is usually inadequate for the needs of an MCO that truly manages care and also does not address the specific member satisfaction and quality assurance needs of the plan. Another frequent excuse is the need to protect the confidentiality of patients. That excuse does not hold if the plan's UM nurse is only rounding on plan members and is properly performing utilization and QM; even the privacy requirements under HIPAA recognize the need for these functions and allow access to protected medical information to qualified personnel. If a hospital refuses to cooperate on allowing the plan's UM nurse to round, then the plan must seriously question its willingness to do business with that hospital. Fortunately, most hospitals and MCOs are able to accommodate this activity without difficulty.

Review against Criteria. An important feature of concurrent review is the evaluation of each hospital case against established criteria. Many plans, especially open-panel plans and PPOs, use published or commercially available criteria for such reviews[70–73] to facilitate evaluation by UM nurses. Experienced nurses use such criteria as an aid in managing utilization, but they do not blindly depend on them. It is possible to keep a patient in the hospital for less than adequate reasons but still meet criteria; the seasoned UM nurse is able to evaluate each case on its own merits.

Most plans have automated this function to improve the efficiency of the UM nurse. Software allows the MaxLOS to be generated automatically from the admission diagnosis or procedure. Member and benefit eligibility are checked, diagnostic and procedure codes are generated from entered text, review criteria are automatically displayed for both admission and concurrent review, unlimited text may be entered to allow tracking, census reports are produced, statistics are generated, and so forth. It is commonly done not only at the MCO but also at remote locations by means of dial-up connection or laptop computers that exchange information with the main system. UM software also links to the claims and enrollment systems so that claims can be properly processed and also take into consideration any special instructions from the nurses.

Discharge Planning and Follow-Up. Good discharge planning starts as soon as a patient is admitted to the hospital or even before. The physician and the UM nurse should be considering discharge planning as part of the overall treatment plan from the outset. This planning includes an estimate of how long the patient will be in the hospital, what the expected outcome will be, whether there will be any special requirements on discharge, and what needs to be facilitated early on.

For example, consider the example of a patient admitted with a fractured hip. If it is known from the outset that many weeks of rehabilitation will be necessary, it is helpful to contact the rehabilitation facility to ensure that a bed will be available at the time of transfer. If it is known that a patient will need durable medical equipment, the equipment should be ordered early so that the patient does not spend extra days in the hospital waiting for it to arrive.

An aspect of discharge planning that is often overlooked is informing the patient and family. If the patient and family do not know what to expect, they may be surprised when the physician tells them that the patient is being discharged. This is especially true if the patient has received hospital care in the past and has certain expectations. Informing the patient and family from the start about when they can expect discharge, how the patient will be feeling, what they might need to prepare for at home, and how follow-up will occur will help to smooth things considerably.

In the case of short-stay obstetrics, the government has mandated that the minimum length of stay is 2 days. However, a 1-day LOS for obstetrics is still acceptable if the patient, the physician, and the plan all agree. In the case of short-stay obstetrics, the patient and family must be prepared for the homecoming. Active discharge planning for short-stay obstetrics patients is crucial. Plans must offer home health visits to mothers who are discharged after a short-stay delivery.

Discharge planning is an ongoing effort beginning with admission or preadmission screening. The UM nurse is in the ideal position to coordinate discharge planning. In addition to making sure that all goes smoothly to effect a smooth and proper discharge from the hospital, the UM nurse can follow up with the member by telephone after discharge to ensure that all is well.

Primary Care Physician's Responsibilities

There are three basic models for managing hospital cases: a model in which the PCP remains active in the care of the patient; a model in which inpatient care is entirely managed by a specialist, with little or no involvement by the PCP; and a model requiring the use of a designated rounding physician or "hospitalist." In the PCP model, PCPs are expected to manage the hospital care of their patients even when patients are hospitalized for care delivered primarily by specialists. Examples include patients hospitalized for surgery, for severe medical conditions (e.g., a myocardial infarction), or for prolonged courses of treatment (e.g., recovery from a stroke). In the PCP model, the most important functions of the member's PCP are also the most obvious: to make rounds every day and to coordinate the patient's care.

In the example of care from a specialist, it is important for the PCP to round daily for a number of reasons. First, it helps ensure continuity of care while the patient is in the hospital (i.e., the PCP may be able to add pertinent clinical information as needed). Second, it provides a comforting presence for the patient, a presence that results not only in better bonding between physician and patient but also in providing emotional support. Third, it allows for continuity after discharge because the PCP is aware of the clinical course and discharge planning.

UM by the PCP is effective in the setting of a member receiving hospital care from a specialist. The PCP is able to discuss the case with the specialist and suggest ways to decrease LOS (e.g., home nursing care) that the specialist might not usually consider. Presumably the PCP will know the patient well enough to determine the patient's capability to do well in alternative situations.

The PCP also will be able to communicate effectively with the specialist in the event that the specialist failed to see the patient on rounds. For example, if a busy surgeon misses a patient on rounds because the patient was in the bathroom, the surgeon, because of a heavy operating room schedule, may not make it back to see that patient until late at night. If the patient is actually ready for discharge, the PCP can communicate with the surgeon that morning and arrange for discharge.

There will be situations in which the PCP is unable to make rounds in person. This happens most frequently when a member is admitted to a tertiary hospital where the PCP does not have privileges. For example, cardiac bypass surgery may be done at a teaching hospital with a closed medical staff. In these situations, it is important for the PCP to be in frequent telephone contact with the attending physician to keep up with developments and to aid in the discharge planning process. In that example, the PCP may be comfortable in accepting the patient back in transfer during the recovery period or may be able to suggest home nursing care. In addition to managing utilization, this helps ensure continuity of care, and the attending physician will almost always remark to the patient how attentive the PCP has been.

Equally important to good medical management is for the PCP to avoid the trap of "That's the way it's always been done, and I see no reason to change." The PCP and the specialist must be open to evaluating new methods of treatment and considering high-quality but cost-effective ways of caring for people.

As a corollary, PCPs must be confident and assertive about their own abilities. It is an unfortunate byproduct of the highly specialized nature of medicine that there are times when a PCP is looked down on by a specialist. Certainly a specialist who depends on the PCP for referrals will not knowingly exhibit behavior that the PCP will find offensive, but there remains an unspoken agreement that the specialist will call the shots once the patient is admitted.

There are a number of objections that a PCP may raise concerning getting involved with patients admitted to a specialist's service. First, the PCP may feel intimidated by the specialist's knowledge about the medical problem. When this happens, the PCP can certainly research the subject, at least in a major medical text, and ask questions. Also, it is the PCP's patient, and the specialist is a consultant. It is the role and responsibility of the PCP to follow the care of the patient and to be aware of the medical issues involved. The simple act of asking the specialist questions about care is appropriate and necessary. It will frequently result in improved understanding by all parties and improved UM.

The possibility exists that the PCP will view such questioning as confrontational and will be unwilling to question the specialist. It is important to point out that the PCP is not questioning the specialist's competence (assuming that the specialist is indeed competent) but rather is discussing the case and asking the specialist his or her opinion about alternatives. The fear of such confrontations is far greater than the reality. The PCP has nothing to be shy about. PCPs are trained physicians specializing in primary care, and the specialist is helping care for the PCP's patient, not vice versa.

Specialist Physician Model

Even in a PCP model, there will be many cases that are managed totally by a specialist, with no real involvement by the PCP. Unlike the hospitalist model described next, in this model the managing specialist may be any specialist in the network that the PCP has referred the admission to.

In this model, the interaction between specialist and PCP remains highly important to good medical management and should be expected in all cases. Beyond that, the UM personnel and the medical director work directly with the managing specialist. This applies to most types of managed care by specialists. For example, it has been shown that even in intensive care units—where little discretion would be expected in treatment decisions—HMOs have 30 percent to 40 percent lower utilization (measured by LOS, charges, and use of ventilators) compared with fee for service even when adjusted for case mix.[74] This finding points out that specialists, particularly specialists in a managed care environment, have considerable effect on resource use.

Clear expectations should be communicated from the plan to the specialists. First, all specialists should be expected to be aware of and to cooperate with the plan's policy on testing, procedures, and primary care CM. Second, plans that use PCPs as gatekeepers or managing physicians should expect specialists to be in communication with PCPs about their patients and to provide written reports on consultations (some plans go as far as to refuse payment to a specialist until the PCP receives a written report). Third, care should be directed back to the PCP as soon as it is appropriate to do so (except in those uncommon cases in which the specialist is acting as the PCP), and the specialist will reinforce the plan's philosophy of primary care. Last, the specialist will not subauthorize nonurgent followup care for the member without first discussing the case with the PCP involved. The PCP may already have worked up a problem that the specialist is seeing for the first time, or the PCP may be able to perform the medical duties that the specialist is requesting.

In a loosely managed plan there will be fewer expectations of the specialist than in a tightly managed one. As has been mentioned numerous times, the better the management of utilization, the more one must deal with practice patterns and physician behavior. Specialists are able to add significantly to the cost of care not only from their own fees but also from additional fees generated by extra days in the hospital and through tests, procedures, and secondary referrals to other specialists.

Hospitalist Model

In the hospitalist model, sometimes called the *designated admitting physician* or *rounding physician* model, one physician is designated to care for all admissions of a group or health plan to a given hospital or hospital service (e.g., to a medical service). This model is found in some group-model and staff-model HMOs, large organized private medical groups, and has also appeared in some open-panel HMOs. The primary feature of this model is that the PCP or specialist who was providing care in the outpatient setting relinquishes responsibility for the admission, and the hospitalist assumes it.

The term *Hospitalist* is relatively new, and was coined by Wachter and Goldman in an article in the *New England Journal of Medicine*.[75] They describe a "new breed of physicians we call 'hospitalists'—specialists in inpatient medicine—who will be responsible for managing the care of hospitalized patients in the same way that primary care physicians are responsible for managing the care of outpatients."

Shy of a fully implemented hospitalist model, a rounding or designated physician model may be in place. In this case, the rounding physician may be on site on a full-time basis or may simply carry a lighter outpatient load and can devote more time to rounding on hospitalized patients. In the large closed panels and medical groups, as well as the open-panel plans that have adopted this system, it is more common for the designated physician to be on site at the hospital full time. In this setting, the responsibility is rotated among members of the medical group, but the group may also use a hospitalist who only practices in the hospital. On a secondary note, large groups find that the use of a hospitalist increases the group's overall efficiency because this model avoids many physicians going into the hospital for just one or two visits.

Some large organized medical groups have gone so far as to create entire hospital care groups that include not only a hospitalist physician but also a physician's assistant or clinical nurse practitioner, a dedicated rounding nurse, and other clinical team members (e.g., a clinical pharmacist or a social worker). This may best be described as a hospitalist team and is most suited for medical groups or hospitals that provide care for a large number of patients with serious and complex conditions.

Some open-panel MCOs have adopted a model in which the plan or the hospital employs the full-time hospitalist, and all admissions are managed by him or her. Although very uncommon, some MCOs have made this a mandatory requirement even when the PCP or specialist who determined that admission was necessary does not wish to relinquish responsibility for the inpatient care. In most cases, it is voluntary, and the PCP may manage the case or choose to have the hospitalist do so. The imposition of mandatory hospitalist use has met with resistance, even if it did result in improved efficiency of inpatient care. For that reason, some MCOs that once mandated that all inpatient care be managed by a hospitalist now make that a voluntary option.[76] The hospitalist managing the case will coordinate with the PCP or specialist as necessary, but the PCP will not be reimbursed for making rounds.

The reasoning behind the hospitalist model is that a dedicated, on-site physician will be closer to the care that the patient is receiving, in a better position to coordinate needed services, and able to monitor care for quality and appropriateness. A dedicated hospitalist is better able to obtain diagnostic study reports, consultations, and so forth in a timely manner. The hospitalist also is available any time of day, rather than once or twice per day, which is the norm when private practice physicians care for inpatients. Of course, there will be many clinical conditions in which the hospitalist is not at all in a primary caregiver situation (e.g., in the early stages of an AMI, during chemotherapy, for obstetrics, for surgical procedures). Even in these cases, however, the hospitalist will follow the case in a fashion similar to that described earlier for the PCP.

The hospitalist model may work best in a capitated environment in which the medical group and the hospitalist all share in the same capitation payment. Alternatively, if a hospital system is receiving global capitation for services, it may wish to employ the hospitalist to manage and monitor cases, even when the outside medical group has no direct financial stake in the cost of institutional services.

Medical Director's Responsibilities

In addition to monitoring all the elements discussed in this chapter, there are a few specific functions that the medical director should perform.

Communications. The medical director is involved in the most difficult cases from a management standpoint. The difficulty is not necessarily medical but rather may be a problem with a PCP, a specialist, a hospital, a member, or a member's family. There are times when the medical director must deal with uncooperative individuals, and this responsibility certainly can be difficult. The medical director must take a compassionate, caring, but firm stance when dealing with difficult people. Often it is easiest simply to give in, but that can only be done so many times before it becomes a habit that damages the plan's effectiveness. The ability to empathize and sympathize with someone's point of view and to recognize what the real issues are in a dispute is not always the same as acquiescing. Although there are indeed times when the medical director will want to loosen the reins, it is important for the medical director to remain firm when the situation is clear and to back up his or her subordinates and the PCPs when they are right.

If the medical director is heard from only when there is a problem, his or her effectiveness will be diminished. It is important for the medical director to be in frequent contact with PCPs and important specialists even when all is well. This practice can be especially useful when discussing cases. If the medical director discusses cases and suggests alternatives even when there is no pressing need to make a change, the participating plan physicians will be much more accepting of the medical director's opinions when change is needed (assuming that the medical director has useful opinions in the first place, of course).

The usefulness of frequent contact cannot be underestimated. By asking thoughtful questions in a nonthreatening manner and by constantly stimulating thought regarding cost-effective clinical management, the medical director may slowly reinforce appropriate patterns of care. The most successful outcome of such contacts occurs when physicians begin asking themselves the questions the medical director would ask and begin improving their practice patterns on that basis.

Daily Review of Utilization. For optimal management of utilization, the medical director or associate medical director should review the hospital log daily. This task may seem onerous—and it can be—but it is the only way the medical director can consistently spot problems in time to do something about them. If possible, it is even better for the medical director to review the hospital log with the UM nurse early in the day. Such a review enables meaningful action to be taken before noon, the time when many hospitals automatically charge for another day. Large plans with highly competent UM nurses and UM departments may get to a point where the medical director or associate medical directors do not need to review every case every day, focusing instead on problem cases or outliers. Even in these situations, the medical director should periodically review every case to be certain that the UM department is performing as well as expected.

Retrospective Review

Retrospective review occurs after the case is finished and the patient is discharged. Retrospective review takes two primary forms: claims review and pattern review.

Claims Review

Claims review refers to examining claims for improprieties or mistakes. Most MCOs use soft-ware to screen for and identify claims that are incorrect, misleading, or falsified. The most common problems are the result of coding errors by providers, such as diagnosis-procedure mismatch. Other common problems might include upcoding (i.e., submitting a claim using the code for a procedure or diagnosis that is more complex than what was actually the case, but will result in higher reimbursement) and unbundling (i.e., submitting multiple claims by separating out various components and charging for each). Some plans take this process one step further and use the software to automatically change claims that are determined to be problematic. For example, the software will rebundle unbundled claims and pay only the appropriate reimbursement. A more forceful step is to use the software to automatically down-code claims on the basis of statistical norms; in other words, reduce the payment by reducing the type of code on the basis of how often those types of codes appear under normal circumstances. This last activity has resulted in legal action by the providers in some cases and should be used judiciously.

It is routine for plans to review large claims to verify whether services were actually delivered or whether mistakes were made in collating the claims data. In such large cases, the plan may actually send a representative on site to the hospital to review the medical record against the claims record. In most cases, this results in some level of payment reduction when information supporting the charges cannot be found.

Pattern Review

Pattern review refers to examining patterns of utilization to determine where action must be taken. This is different from the software-based reviews described previously, in that pattern review in this context refers to patterns on the basis of actual services and utilization, not on claims errors or falsifications. For example, if three hospitals in the area perform coronary artery bypass surgery, the plan may look to see which one has the best clinical outcomes, the shortest LOSs, and the lowest charges. The plan may then preferentially send all such cases to that hospital. Pattern review also allows the plan to focus UM efforts primarily on those areas needing greater attention.

One other use of pattern review is to provide feedback to providers. Although not as powerful as active UM by the plan's own department, feedback sometimes can have an effect in and of itself.[77] When combined with other management functions and financial incentives, feedback is a useful management tool (see Chapters 32 and 33 for in-depth discussion of the use of feedback in modification of physician behavior).

ALTERNATIVES TO ACUTE CARE HOSPITALIZATION

There are many instances in which patients are ill or disabled but not to the extent that they need to be in an acute care hospital. Yet, an acute care hospital is where they often stay for a variety of reasons. In some cases, the patient initially needed the services of an acute care hospital (e.g., the patient had surgery but the recovery phase requires far fewer resources than the hospital offers). In other cases, there is simply no place for the patient to go (e.g., a patient who lives alone is recovering from a broken femur). In a few cases, the patient is kept in the hospital for the convenience of a physician who does not want to make house calls or rounds at another institution. Last, there are times when the patient is kept in the hospital simply because "That's the way I want to do it."

Subacute Care: Skilled or Intermediate Nursing Facilities

One alternative to consider is the skilled or intermediate nursing facility or subacute facility. This is most suited for prolonged convalescence or recovery cases. For example, if a patient with a broken femur requires more traction than can be provided safely at home and requires many months to recover, the cost for a bed day in a subacute facility will be much less than in an acute care hospital. The same goes for rehabilitation cases such as stroke or trauma to the brain when the damage is too extensive for the patient to go home immediately.

Over the past several years, the subacute care industry has focused on making their facilities a practical alternative to an acute care hospital for a larger variety of medical cases. For example, some subacute care facilities provide a cost-effective location for the administration of chemotherapy that requires close supervision. The treatment of many medical conditions such as acute pneumonia or osteomyelitis when the patient is too sick to be cared for at home may be done in a subacute facility. In some cases, the patient may be able to be cared for at home, but it is still more cost-effective to deliver the therapy in the subacute facility because of more favorable pricing achievable through economies of scale. For a subacute facility to vie effectively for this type of business, it must transform itself into something other than a nursing home.

The main problem with the use of subacute facilities or nursing homes is objection from the patient or the family, particularly in the case of young patients. There is a stigma attached to nursing homes, even if they are renamed subacute facilities, that makes some people associate them with warehouses for the elderly. To overcome this stigma, a proactive approach is required.

First, contract only with those subacute facilities that meet the plan's (and implicitly the plan's members') needs for pleasant surroundings. There may be a better price elsewhere, but try to imagine one's loved ones staying at the facility for a month and see if it would be acceptable. A good subacute facility will be interested in working with the plan to make this option acceptable. For example, the facility might ensure that the plan's members are given a private room (a private room in a nursing facility is still less costly than a semiprivate bed in an acute care hospital) or are placed in a room with a patient with a similar functional status.

Second, discuss the alternative with the patient and the family well in advance of the actual move. Nothing is as distressing as suddenly finding out that you will be shipped out in the morning to a nursing home. If possible, have the family visit the subacute facility to meet the staff and see the environment before the patient is transferred.

Last, do not abandon the patient. In other words, have someone, preferably the physician and the UM nurse, visit the patient on a regular basis. It is easy to rationalize that because the patient is in the subacute facility for long-term care, there is no need to visit often. Although that may be true from a medical standpoint, it is not true from a human relations standpoint.

How the use of subacute facilities is handled will have an impact on sales and marketing. If it is perceived that people are coldly shunted into a subacute facility simply to save money, the plan will rapidly get a reputation for placing its financial needs over those of the members. Members will complain to their benefits managers or to other potential members, and growth will be affected. If, however, this option is handled with compassion, taking the time to alleviate the emotional distress that may be caused, most people will be quite understanding and accepting of this alternative.

The other issue to consider in the use of subacute facilities is monitoring the case in regard to the plan's benefit structure. It is easy for a case to go from prolonged recovery to permanent placement or custodial care. Facing the end of coverage benefits can be an emotionally wrenching experience both for the member's family and for the medical managers involved. The problem of who will pay for long-term custodial care is a national dilemma, and it becomes personal when a family is faced with high costs because the benefits the plan provides do not continue indefinitely. If it is possible or likely that benefits will end, it is wise to make the benefits structure clear to the family early on. This notification does not have to be done in a cold and calculating manner but rather in a way that lays out all the possibilities so that the family can begin early planning.

Step-Down Units

As an alternative to free-standing nursing facilities, many hospitals with excess capacity have developed step-down units. Even if they have not, many hospital administrators are willing to consider this option in negotiations.

In essence, a step-down unit is a ward or section of a ward that is used in much the same way as a skilled nursing facility. A patient who requires less care and monitoring, such as someone recovering from a hip replacement (after all the drains have been removed), may need only bed rest, traction, and minimal nursing care. In recognition of the lesser resource needs, the charge per day is less.

The step-down unit has the advantage of being convenient for the physician and UM nurse and is more acceptable to the patient and family. It also does not require transfer outside the facility. Although the cost per day is sometimes slightly more than that of a subacute facility, the difference may be worth it in terms of member acceptability.

Outpatient Procedure Units

In many instances, performing a procedure in an outpatient unit is less expensive than admitting a patient for a 1-day stay. This is not always true because some hospitals have raised their outpatient unit charges to make up the revenue lost because of the increased popularity of outpatient surgery and the increased complexity of outpatient procedures. As discussed in detail in Chapter 12, careful attention must be paid to outpatient charges when negotiating with hospitals.

Free-standing outpatient facilities also are an alternative. They may be affiliated with a hospital or they may be independent. As with hospitals, the charge structure must be negotiated so that cost savings in outpatient surgery are realized.

Hospice Care

Hospice care is that care given to terminally ill patients. It tends to be care that is supportive to the patient and the family. Much hospice care is outpatient or home-care based, but inpatient forms of hospice are also available and is used most often when such care cannot be given in the home. It is not always covered by the schedule of benefits, but it may take the place of acute care hospitalization and should be considered for exceptional coverage when appropriate. Care of the terminally ill patient has not been a focus of most medical management programs, even though it can be considered a form of disease management or CM (Chapters 22 and 23). The reader is referred to Chapter 28 for focused discussion of end-of-life and hospice care.

Home Health Care

Home health care, discussed in depth in Chapter 26, is a frequent alternative to inpatient care and has become common in MCOs. Services that are particularly amenable to home health care include nursing care for routine reasons (e.g., checking weights and changing dressings), home intravenous treatment (e.g., for osteomyelitis, certain forms of chemotherapy, or home intravenous nutrition), home physical therapy, respiratory therapy, and rehabilitation care.

There should be little trouble negotiating and contracting with home health agencies for services. It is becoming popular for hospitals to have home health care services to aid in caring for patients discharged from their facilities, and those services may be negotiated with the overall contract. Furthermore, as Medicare continues to tighten down on payments for home care, many agencies are looking for alternative sources of revenue. As with hospitals or any other providers of care, home health and high-technology home care agencies need to be evaluated for more than simple pricing breaks. An active quality management program, the presence of a medical director, and evidence of attention to the changes that are constantly occurring in the field are all requisites for contracting.

A caution about home health services is in order. Because the physician and UM nurse seldom visit the patient receiving home health care, it often defaults to the home health nurse to determine how often and how long the patient should receive services, and this practice can lead to some surprising costs. It is advisable to have a firm policy regarding the number of home health visits covered under a single authorization and a requirement for physician review for continued authorization.

CASE MANAGEMENT

CM (also referred to as large or catastrophic CM) refers to specialized techniques for identifying and managing cases that are disproportionately high in cost. This subject is covered in detail in Chapter 22 and so is only discussed briefly here within the context of overall management of basic medical-surgical utilization.

Identification of large cases may be straightforward because patients are hospitalized the first time they are identified, as in the case of trauma. Other cases may be identified before the patient is hospitalized. For example, examining the claims system for use of dialysis services may identify a patient with end-stage renal disease. Proactively contacting patients with potentially catastrophic illnesses not only can save the plan considerable expense by managing the care cost-effectively but also can result in better medical care because the services are coordinated.

Prenatal care is a specialized form of CM because active coordination occurs before the newborn is delivered. Prenatal CM involves identification of high-risk pregnancies early enough to intervene to improve the chances of a good outcome. With the staggering costs of neonatal intensive care, it takes only a few improved outcomes to yield dramatic savings. Methods for identifying cases include sending out information about pregnancy to all members, reviewing the claims system for pregnancy-related claims, asking (or requiring) PCPs and obstetricians to notify the plan when a delivery is expected, and so forth. After the UM department is informed of the case, the member may be proactively contacted, and a questionnaire may be given to assess for risk factors (e.g., very young maternal age, diabetes, medical problems). If risk factors are noted, the plan can coordinate prenatal care in a proactive manner. Although it is impossible to force a member to seek care and to follow up on problems, it is possible to increase the amount and quality of prenatal care that is delivered. A special problem exists when the pregnant patient is also abusing drugs; close coordination with the substance abuse program must then occur.

The degree to which the plan can become involved in CM is in part a function of the benefits structure. In a tightly run managed health care plan, it is common for the UM department to be proactive in CM; in simple PPOs, CM is often voluntary on the part of the member (in other words, if the member chooses not to cooperate, there is little impact on benefits). Even in situations requiring strictly voluntary cooperation by the members and physicians, it is common for CM to be highly effective.

In addition to the standard methods of managing utilization, CM often involves two other techniques. First is the use of community resources. Some catastrophic cases require support structures to help the member function or even return home. Examples of such support include family members, social service agencies, churches, and special foundations.

The other common technique is to go beyond the contractual benefits to manage the case. For example, if the benefits structure of the group has only limited coverage for durable medical equipment, it may still be in the plan's interest to cover such expenses to get the patient home and out of the hospital. In self-funded groups, the group administrator may actually be willing to fund extracontractual benefits simply as a benefit for an employee or dependent who is experiencing a terrible medical problem.

In all events, the hallmark of CM is longitudinal management of the case by a single UM nurse or department. Management spans hospital care, rehabilitation, outpatient care, professional services, home care, ancillary services, and so forth. It is in the active coordination of care that both quality and cost-effectiveness are maintained.

CONCLUSION

The provision of basic medical-surgical services involves a broad continuum of care. Managing utilization of these services must focus on managing basic demand, referral and specialty services, and institutional services.

The management of referral and specialty services affects not only professional expenses but also costs associated with tests and procedures, including hospitalization, that may be generated by the specialist. The ability to select only those consultants and referral specialists who practice cost-effectively can yield cost savings, but optimal management depends on an authorization system. The lack of such a system will hamper the plan's abilities to decrease utilization in a meaningful way over the long term.

The management of hospital or institutional utilization is one of the most important aspects of managing overall health care costs. The methods used to manage hospital utilization vary from relatively weak and mechanical to tightly managed, longitudinally integrated, and highly labor intensive. The management of hospital utilization is a function that must be attended to every day to achieve optimal results, and special attention must be paid to CM to produce the greatest savings.

REFERENCES AND NOTES

1. L. Citrome, Practice Protocols, Parameters, Pathways, and Guidelines: A Review, *Administration and Policy in Mental Health* 25, 3 (1998): 257–269.

2. R.L. Van Horn, L.R. Burns, and D.R. Wholey, The Impact of Physician Involvement in Managed Care on Efficient Use of Hospital Resources, *Medical Care* 35 (1997): 873–889.

3. P.R. Kongstvedt and D.W. Plocher, Eds., *Best Practices in Medical Management* (Gaithersburg, MD: Aspen Publishers, 1998).

4. *Managed Care Measures: Results of the 1999 Benchmarking Study* (Washington, DC and Walnut Creek, CA: Ernst & Young LLP, 2000). The full results from this study are proprietary to Ernst & Young, and only summary findings and correlations are reported in this publication.

5. *Critical Calibration: Metrics and Benchmarking in Managed Care* (Washington, DC: Ernst & Young LLP, 1999). The full results from this study are proprietary to Ernst & Young, and only summary findings and correlations are reported in this publication.

6. Kongstvedt and Plocher, *Best Practices in Medical Management*.

7. Ernst & Young, LLP Study: *Return on Investment of a Nurseline Telephone Triage System* [press release], 1998.

8. Ernst & Young, LLP, Study on Investment.

9. D.M. Vickery, H. Kalmer, and D. Lowry, Effect of a Self-Care Education Program on Medical Visits, *JAMA* 250 (1983): 2952–2956.

10. V.D. Elsenhans, C. Marquardt, and T. Bledsoe, Use of Self-Care Manual Shifts Utilization Pattern, *HMO Practice*, 2 (June 9, 1995): 88–90.

11. J.S. Robinson, M.L. Schwartz, K.S. Magwene, et al., The Impact of Fever Health Education on Clinic Utilization, *American Journal of Diseases of Children* 143, 6 (June 1989): 698–704.

12. Robinson et al., *The Impact of Fever*.

13. Kongstvedt and Plocher, *Best Practices in Medical Management*.

14. W.N. Burton and D.A. Hoy, First Chicago's Integrated Health Data Management Computer System. *Managed Care Quarterly* 1, 3 (1993): 18–23.

15. N.P. Pronk, M.J. Goodman, P.J. O'Connor, and B.C. Martinson, Relationship Between Modifiable Health Risks and Short-term Health Care Charges, *JAMA* 282 (1999): 2235–2239.

16. W.S. Elias, Introduction to health risk appraisals. In P.K. Kongstvedt and D.W. Plocher, Eds., *Best Practices in Medical Management* (Gaithersburg, MD: Aspen Publishers, 1998).

17. M. Ringle, Implementing Health Status Measurements, *Health Care Leadership Review* (February 1998): 12.

18. Study proves $6,500 saved per patient thanks to risk assessment program. In: Editorial Staff of National Health Information LLC, *Medical Management under Medicare Risk* (Marietta, GA: National Health Information, LLC, 1998: 22–23.

19. J.E. Wennberg and A. Gittelsohn, Variations in medical care among small areas, *Scientific American* 246, 4 (1982): 120–134.

20. J. Wennberg and P. Caper, Medical Practice: Why Does It Vary So Much? *Hospitals* 59, 5 (1985): 89.

21. J.E. Wennberg, J.L. Freeman, and W.J. Culp, Are Hospital Services Rationed In New Haven or Overutilized In Boston? *Lancet* 1 (1987): 1185–1189.

22. E.S. Fisher, J.E. Wennberg, T.A. Stukel, and S.M. Sharp, Hospital Readmission Rates for Cohorts of Medicare Beneficiaries in Boston and New Haven, *New England Journal of Medicine* 331 (1994): 989–995.

23. J. Restuccia, M. Shwartz, A. Ash, and S. Payne, High Hospital Rates And Inappropriate Care, *Health Affairs (Millwood)* 15, 4 (1996): 156–163.

24. E.J. Graves, National Hospital Discharge Survey: Annual Summary, 1993. Vital and Health Statistics, Series

13, No. 121 (Washington, DC: Government Printing Office; 1995). U.S. Department of Health and Human Services Publication PHS 95-1782.

25. A.B. Bindman, K. Grumbach, D. Osmond, et al., Preventable Hospitalizations and Access to Health Care, *JAMA* 274 (1995): 305–311.

26. J.S. Weissman, C. Gatsonis, and A.M. Epstein, Rates of Avoidable Hospitalization by Insurance Status in Massachusetts and Maryland, *JAMA* 268 (1992): 2388–2394.

27. C.M. Asthon, N.J. Petersen, J. Souchek, et al., Geographic variations in utilization rates at Veterans Affairs hospitals and clinics, *New England Journal of Medicine* 340, 1 (1999): 32–39.

28. J.P. Kahan, S.J. Bernstein, and L.L. Leape, Measuring the Necessity of Medical Procedures, *Medical Care* 32, 4 (1994): 357–365.

29. M.R. Chassin, Explaining geographic variations: the enthusiasm hypothesis, *Medical Care* 31, 5 (1993): Suppl., YS37–YS44.

30. J. Wennber, M. Cooper, J. Birkmeyer, et al., *The Dartmouth Atlas of Health Care* (Chicago: American Hospital Publishing, 1998).

31. J.D. Moore, Market Pressures Say What? *Modern Healthcare* 28 (1998): 26, 150, 156, 168.

32. G. Pappas, W.C. Hadden, L.J. Kozak, et al., Potentially Avoidable Hospitalizations: Inequalities in Rates Between US Socioeconomic Groups. *American Journal of Public Health* 87, 5 (1997): 811–816.

33. C. Phelps, The Methodologic Foundations of Studies of the Appropriateness of Medical Care, *New England Journal of Medicine* 329, 17 (1993): 1241–1245.

34. T.P. Meehan, M.J. Fine, H.M. Krumholz, et al., Quality of Care, Process, and Outcomes in Elderly Patients with Pneumonia, *JAMA* 278, 23 (1997): 2080–2084.

35. L. Pilote, R.M. Califf, S. Sapp, et al., Regional Variation across the United States in the Management of Acute Myocardial Infarction, *New England Journal of Medicine* 333, 9 (1995): 567–572.

36. C.R. Gaus and C.M. Clancy, Research at the Interface of Primary and Specialty Care, Adapted from the Agency for Health Care Policy and Research, *JAMA* 274, 18 (1995): 1419.

37. C.L. Bryce and K.E. Cline, The Supply and Use of Selected Medical Technologies, *Health Affairs (Millwood)* 17, 1 (1998): 213–224.

38. Milliman & Robertson Health Cost Guidelines, 1997.

39. D.M. Eddy, Balancing Cost and Quality in Fee-For-Service Versus Managed Care, *Health Affairs (Millwood)* 16, 3 (1997): 162–173.

40. M.R. Chassin, J. Kosecoff, R.E. Park, et al., Does Inappropriate Use Explain Geographic Variations in the Use of Health Care Services? A Study of Three Procedures, *JAMA* 258 (1987): 2533–2537.

41. K. Kahn, M.R. Chassin, M.T. Flynn, et al., Measuring the Clinical Appropriateness of the Use of a Procedure. Can We Do It? *Medical Care* 26, 4 (1998): 415–422.

42. R.H. Brook, R.E. Park, M.R. Chassin, et al., Predicting the Appropriate Use of Carotid Endarterectomy, Upper Gastrointestinal Endoscopy and Coronary Angiography, *New England Journal of Medicine* 323, 17 (1990): 1173–1177.

43. L. Leape, R.E. Park, D.H. Soloman, et al., Relation Between Surgeons' Practice Volumes and Geographic Variation in the Rate of Carotid Endarterectomy, *New England Journal of Medicine* 321, 10 (1989): 653–657.

44. E. Guadagnoli, P.J. Hauptman, J.Z. Ayanian, et al., Variation in the Use of Cardiac Procedures after Acute Myocardial Infarction, *New England Journal of Medicine* 333, 9 (1995): 573–578.

45. G.T. O'Connor, H.B. Quinton, and N.D. Traven, Geographic Variation in the Treatment of Acute Myocardial Infarction, *JAMA* 281, 7 (1999): 627–633.

46. A.B. Flood, A.M. Fremont, K.B. Jin, et al., How Do HMOs Achieve Savings? The Effectiveness of One Organization's Strategies, *Health Services Research* 33, 1 (1998): 79–99.

47. A.J. Dietrich, E.C. Nelson, J.W. Kirk, et al., Do Primary Physicians Actually Manage Their Patients' Fee-for-Service Care? *JAMA* 259 (1988): 3145–3149.

48. R.F. St. Peter, M.C. Reed, P. Kemper, and D. Blumenthal, Changes in the Scope of Care Provided by Primary Care Physicians, *New England Journal of Medicine* 341 (1999): 1980–1985.

49. J.E. Ware, R.H. Brook, W.H. Rogers, et al., Comparison of Health Outcomes at a Health Maintenance Organization with Those of Fee-for-Service Care. *Lancet* 10 (1986): 1017–1022.

50. I.S. Udvarhelyi, K. Jennison, and R.S. Phillips, Comparison of the Quality of Ambulatory Care for Fee-for-Service and Prepaid Patients, *Annals of Internal Medicine* 115 (1991): 394–400.

51. E.M. Sloss, E.B. Keeler, R.H. Brook, et al. Effect of a Health Maintenance Organization on Physiologic Health, *Annals of Internal Medicine* 106 (1987): 130–138.

52. C.M. Clancy and B.E. Hillner, Physicians as Gatekeepers—The Impact of Financial Incentives, *Archives of Internal Medicine* 149 (1989): 917–920.

53. D.P. Martin, P. Diehr, K.F. Price, and W.C. Richardson, Effect of a Gatekeeper Plan on Health Services Use and Charges: A Randomized Trial, *American Journal of Public Health* 79, 12 (1989): 1628–1663.

54. C.B. Forrest and R.J. Reid, Passing the Baton: HMOs' Influence on Referrals to Specialty Care, *Health Affairs (Millwood)* 16, 6 (1997): 157–162.

55. R.E. Hurley, D.A. Freund, B.J. Gage, et al., Gatekeeper Effects of Patterns of Physician Use, *Journal of Family Practice* 32, 2 (1991): 167–174.

56. D.K. Remler, K. Donelan, R.J. Blendon, et al., What Do Managed Care Plans Do To Affect Care? *Inquiry* 34, 3 (1997): 196–204.

57. E.A. Halm, N. Causine, and D. Blumenthal, Is Gatekeeping Better Than Traditional Care? *JAMA* 278 (1997): 1677–1681.

58. A.J. Dietrich, E.C. Nelson, J.W. Kirk, et al., Do Primary Physicians Actually Manage Their Patient's Fee-for-Service Care? *JAMA* 259 (1988): 3145–3149.

59. K.E. Quickel, Managed Care and Diabetes, With Special Attention to the Issue of Who Should Provide Care. *Transactions of the American Clinical and Climatological Association* 108 (1997): 184–199.

60. Committee of the American College of Rheumatology Council on Health Care Research, Role of Specialty Care for Chronic Diseases: A Report from an Ad Hoc Committee of the American College of Rheumatology, *Mayo Clinic Proceedings* 71 (1996): 1179–1181.

61. D. Bello, N.G. Shah, M.E. Edep, et al., Self-reported Differences Between Cardiologists and Heart Failure Specialists in the Management of Chronic Heart Failure, *American Heart Journal* 138 (1999): 100–107.

62. P. Cram and W.H. Ettinger, Generalists or Specialists—Who Does It Better? *The Physician Executive* January–February (1998): 40–45.

63. B.J. Hillman, C.A. Joseph, M.R. Mabry, et al., Frequency and Costs of Diagnostic Imaging in Office Practice—A Comparison of Self-Referring and Radiologist-Referring Physicians, *New England Journal of Medicine* 323 (1990): 1604–1608.

64. Office of the Inspector General. *Financial Arrangements between Physicians and Health Care Businesses: Report to Congress* (Washington, DC: U.S. Department of Health and Human Services; 1989). U.S. Department of Health and Human Services Publication OAI-12-88-01410.

65. State of Florida Health Care Cost Containment Board. *Joint Ventures among Health Care Providers in Florida* (Tallahassee, FL: State of Florida; 1991) 2.

66. The Ethics in Patient Referrals Act—Omnibus Budget Reconciliation Act of 1989.

67. B. Santos-Eggimann, M. Sidler, D. Schopfer, and T. Blanc, Comparing Results of Concurrent and Retrospective Designs in a Hospital Utilization Review, *International Journal for Quality in Health Care* 2 (April 9, 1997): 115–120.

68. S.K. Kelley and J.J. Trutlein, A Survey of Human Resources in Managed Care Organizations. *Physician Executive* 18, 6 (1992): 49–51.

69. *Managed Care Measures: Results of the 1999 Benchmarking Study* (Washington, DC and Walnut Creek, CA: Ernst & Young LLP, 2000). The full results from this study are proprietary to Ernst & Young, and only summary findings and correlations are reported in this publication.

70. R.L. Doyle, *Healthcare Management Guidelines, Vol. 1: Inpatient and Surgical Care*, Milliman & Robertson.

71. *The ISD-A Review System with Adult Criteria* (Chicago: InterQual, 1991).

72. *Surgical Indications Monitoring SIM III* (Chicago: InterQual, 1991).

73. *Managed Care Appropriateness Protocol (MCAP),* (Wellesley, MA: Utilization Management Associates, 1991).

74. J. Rapoport, S. Gehlbach, S. Lemeshow, and D. Teres, Resource Utilization among Intensive Care Patients: Managed Care Vs. Traditional Insurance, *Archives of Internal Medicine* 152 (1992): 2207–2212.

75. R.M. Wachter and L. Goldman, The Emerging Role of "Hospitalists" in the American Health Care System, *New England Journal of Medicine* 335, 7 (1996): 514–517.

76. Aetna To End Prudential Doctor Plan. John Murawski in The Palm Beach Post pg. 8D, 02/11/2000.

77. J.E. Billi, G.F. Hejna, F.M. Wolf, et al., The Effects of a Cost-Education Program on Hospital Charges, *Journal of General Internal Medicine* 2 (1987): 306–311.

CHAPTER 19

Clinical Services Requiring Authorization

Peter R. Kongstvedt

One of the (relatively) definitive elements in managed health care is the presence of an authorization system. This may be as simple as precertification of elective hospitalizations in an indemnity plan or preferred provider organization (PPO) or as complex as mandatory authorization for all nonprimary care services in a health maintenance organization (HMO; except for the so-called "open-access" HMO discussed later). It is the authorization system that provides a key element of management in the delivery of medical services.

There are multiple reasons for an authorization system. One is to allow the medical management function of the plan to review a case for medical necessity. A second reason is to channel care to the most appropriate location (e.g., the outpatient setting or to a participating specialist rather than a nonparticipating one). Third, the authorization system may be used to provide timely information to the concurrent utilization review system and to large case management. Fourth, the system may help finance to estimate the accruals for medical expenditures each month.

It is important to note here that important information on this subject is also found in Chapter 18, which addresses basic medical-surgical utilization. The reason for this is the interdigitated nature of how medical services are actually delivered. Chapter 18 focuses on specialty physician services, and information from that chapter will only be briefly referenced in this chapter. This chapter focuses on the methods for managing authorization systems; therefore, the reader will want to read Chapter 18 to obtain an aggregate understanding of this topic.

DEFINITION OF SERVICES REQUIRING AUTHORIZATION

The first requirement in an authorization system is to define what will require authorization and what will not. This is obviously tied to the benefits design and is subject to the full and fair disclosure marketing requirements; i.e., if services require authorization, the plan must make that clear in its marketing literature.

There are no managed care systems that require authorization for primary care services. PPOs and HMOs require members to use providers on their panels, and most HMOs require members to choose a single primary care physician (PCP) to coordinate care, but this does not require an authorization. Defining what constitutes primary care services is another issue and is addressed in Chapter 7.

The real issue is determining what nonprimary care services will require authorization. In most HMOs (other than open access HMOs, discussed later), most services not rendered by the PCP require authorization. In other words, any service from a referral specialist, any hospitalization, any procedure, and so forth requires specific authorization. There are certain conventional exceptions such as an optometry visit or a routine gynecology visit. In less tightly managed systems, such as many PPOs and most indem-

331

nity plans, the requirements are less stringent. In those cases, it is common for authorization to be required only for elective hospitalizations and procedures, both inpatient and outpatient.

The tighter the authorization system, the greater the plan's ability to manage utilization. An authorization system per se will not automatically manage utilization, although one could expect some sentinel effect. It is the management behind the system that will determine its ultimate effectiveness. If the medical director is unable or unwilling to deal with poor utilization behavior, an authorization system will have only a marginal effect. If the claims department is unable to back up the authorization system, it will quickly be subverted as members and providers learn that it is little more than a burdensome sham.

In any plan there will be times when a member is unable to obtain prior authorization. This is usually due to an emergency or to an urgent problem that occurs out of the area. In those cases, the plan must make provision for the retrospective review of the case to determine whether authorization may be granted after the fact. Certain rules may also be defined regarding the member's obligation in those circumstances (e.g., notification within 24 hours of the emergency). Be careful that such requirements do not allow for automatic authorization if the plan is notified within 24 hours but only for automatic review of the case to determine medical necessity, even though the plan uses a "reasonable layperson's standard."

Many states have passed laws placing some limits on the need to obtain authorization for services. In some states, certain types of providers have successfully achieved the ability for a member to access them directly. For example, chiropractors are allowed direct access in a few states. More commonly, direct access to obstetrics/gynecology is allowed, which is common for most HMOs in any event. Other examples of state (and federal) laws that have an impact on authorizations include payment for emergency services, applying a "prudent layperson" standard. These issues are discussed in Chapter 69.

The last issue to note here is that there are clinical situations in which a non-PCP will act as a patient's primary provider. This occurs in patients with significantly serious, chronic illnesses that are far better managed by a specialist than a generalist. For example, a patient with severe congestive heart failure will often be better managed by a cardiologist than a general internist or family physician. This approach is discussed more in Chapters 18, 22, and 23. For the remainder of this chapter, no additional distinction will be made between PCPs and specialty physicians acting as PCPs.

DEFINITION OF WHO CAN AUTHORIZE SERVICES

The next requirement of an authorization system is to define who has the ability to authorize services and to what extent. This will vary considerably depending on the type of plan and the degree to which it will be medically managed.

In addition to most HMOs, PPOs that are tightly managed may have a requirement for PCP authorization; these are often referred to as "gatekeeper" PPOs. In loosely managed PPOs and in managed indemnity plans, there is usually only a requirement for authorization for elective hospitalizations and procedures, but that authorization comes from plan personnel and not from the PCP or any other physician.

For example, if a participating surgeon in a non-PCP type of plan wishes to admit a patient for surgery, the surgeon (or more likely the surgeon's assistant) first calls a central telephone number and speaks with a plan representative, usually a nurse. That representative then asks a number of questions about the patient's condition, and if predetermined criteria are met, and after the member's eligibility is confirmed, an authorization is issued. In most cases, the surgery must take place on the day of admission, and certain procedures may be done only on an outpatient basis.

It is common practice in HMOs to require that most or all medical services be authorized by the member's PCP. Even then, however, there can be some dispute. For example, if a PCP authorizes a member to see a referral specialist, does that specialist have the ability to authorize tests, surgery, or another referral to himself or herself or to another specialist? Does a PCP require authorization to hospitalize one of his or her own patients?

A relatively common exception to this practice is in the area of mental health and substance abuse (MH/SA). As discussed in detail in Chapter 25, MH/SA services are unique and often lend themselves better to other methods of authorization. Plans, or even the accounts themselves, may carve out MH/SA from the basic health plan and treat it as a stand-alone function.

Another exception to the PCP-only concept occurs in HMOs that allow specialists to contact the plan directly about hospitalizations. In these cases, the referral to the specialist must have been made by the PCP in the first place, but the specialist may determine that hospitalization is required and obtain authorization directly from the plan's medical management department. Plans that operate this way generally do so because the PCPs have no real involvement in hospital cases anyway and because there is no usefulness in involving them in that decision.

There is a fundamental split in MCOs that require PCP authorization for nonprimary care services: whether or not the PCP's authorization needs secondary review by a utilization management committee (UMC). From the mid-1980s until the mid-1990s, it was common for many MCOs to require that the PCP's authorization first go to a UMC for additional review. If the UMC approved the authorization request, then it was valid and the member and the PCP were so notified (or just the PCP was notified) and the referral went forward; if the UMC decided that the referral was medically unnecessary, investigational, or not a covered benefit, then the authorization would be denied and the PCP so notified. Then the PCP had the much coveted task of explaining that decision to the member.

Although this type of secondary review system still exists in some MCOs, it has been abandoned in favor of a model in which the PCP's authorization is valid immediately. Why the change of procedure? In earlier times (defined as a decade or more ago*), MCOs did not have the data systems to perform practice profiling properly (see Chapter

32); in addition, PCPs were generally not used to their role as care coordinators and were more likely to refer cases. As managed care has become more prevalent, information systems have improved and PCPs have become much more experienced with managed care.

Unless secondary review by a UMC is required because utilization is grossly and inappropriately high, the benefits of not requiring the use of a UMC are obvious: administrative costs are much lower, physician satisfaction is higher, member satisfaction is higher, and it is likely that member retention in the MCO will be higher (although that is conjecture). However, this does require the use of a reasonably sophisticated profiling system that is able to detect patterns, adjust for severity of illness, and provide usable feedback to the plan's medical management and to the PCPs.

In any type of managed care plan, there may be services that will require specific authorization from the plan's medical director. This is usually the case for expensive procedures such as transplants and for controversial procedures that may be considered experimental or of limited value except in particular circumstances. This is even more necessary when the plan has negotiated a special arrangement for high-cost services. The authorization system not only serves to review the medical necessity of the service but ensures that the care will be delivered at an institution that has contracted with the plan.

The last area that commonly requires authorization from the plan is the use of certain pharmaceutical agents. As discussed in Chapter 24, it is common for an MCO that provides drug benefits, which almost all do, to have a short list of a dozen or so drugs that require prereview by the medical director or the plan's pharmacy and therapeutics committee. These are usually drugs that have use for treating both actual disease states and use for cosmetic or lifestyle reasons. For example, growth hormone replacement therapy is clearly indicated for children with deficiency of growth hormone; what is less easy to

---

*Managed care time apparently exists in dog years.

determine is growth hormone's use in children with normal levels of the hormone but who are small in stature.

CLAIMS PAYMENT

A managed care health plan does not exist as a dictator, preventing a member from accessing services. The only recourse a plan has is to deny full payment for services that have not been authorized. This pertains equally to services obtained from nonparticipating providers (professionals or institutions) and to services obtained without required prior authorization. The counter argument to this concept is that refusal to pay equates to a member's inability to access that service at all. Although this argument has little merit for routine types of services that are affordable even in the absence of insurance, it carries more weight when the services are very expensive.

In an HMO, payment can be completely denied for services that were not authorized. Point of service (POS) is unique and is discussed later. In most PPOs and in indemnity plans, if a service is not authorized but is considered a covered benefit, payment may not be denied, but the amount paid may be reduced. For example, a plan pays 80 percent of charges for authorized services but only 50 percent of charges for nonauthorized services or perhaps imposes a flat dollar amount penalty for failure to obtain authorization.

In certain cases, a plan may deny any payment for a portion of the bill but will pay the rest. For example, if a patient is admitted the day before surgery even though same-day admission was required, the plan may not pay the charges (both hospital and physician) related to that first day but will pay charges for the remaining days.

In a PPO in which a contractual relationship exists between the provider and the plan, the financial penalty may fall solely on the provider, who may not balance bill the member for the amount of the penalty. In the case of an indemnity plan (or a PPO in which the member received services from a nonparticipating provider), the financial penalty falls on the member, who must then pay more out of pocket.

Point of Service

POS is a special challenge for authorization systems and claims management (a thorough discussion of claims management is found in Chapter 38). It is necessary to define what is covered as an authorized service and what is not, because services that are not authorized will still be paid, albeit at the lower out-of-network level of benefits. Because POS is sold with the express intent that members will use out-of-network services, it is not always clear how a service was or was not authorized. Common examples of this issue are illustrated as follows.

If a PCP makes a referral to a specialist for one visit and the member returns for a follow-up, was that authorized? If a PCP authorizes three visits but the member goes four times, does the fourth visit cascade out to an out-of-network level of benefits? If a PCP refers to a specialist and the specialist determines that admission is necessary but the member is admitted to a nonparticipating hospital, is that authorized? What if the member is admitted to a participating hospital but is cared for by a mix of participating and nonparticipating physicians? What if a member is referred to a participating specialist who performs laboratory and radiology testing (even though the plan has capitated for such services); is the visit authorized but not the testing? What if the member claims that he or she had no choice in the matter?

Many other examples of these types of policy questions can be found, and the list of "what ifs" is a long one. Most plans strive to identify an episode of care (e.g., a hospitalization or a referral) and to remain consistent within that episode. For example, the testing by the specialist referenced earlier may be denied payment and the specialist prohibited from balance billing, or an entire hospitalization would be considered either in network or out of network. In any case, the plan must develop policies and procedures for defining when a service is to be considered authorized (and when it is considered in-network in the case of hospital services that require precertification in any event) and when it is not.

A special problem bedevils POS plans: sometimes the claim arrives before the authorization.

This can easily occur in any plan that has a high rate of electronic claims submission, but that depends on a paper-based authorization system. In a typical HMO in which only authorized, in-network benefits are available, this situation usually results in the HMO's claims system "pending" (i.e., holding) the claim to wait and see if the authorization comes in. But POS is specifically designed to allow for out-of-network, so a claim that does not have an associated authorization immediately cascades down to be processed as a nonauthorized service with lesser benefits; and in some cases, *then* the authorization arrives. The member and/or provider complains, the plan has to rework the claim, and the overall cost of rework, to say nothing of the high level of irritation by the member and provider, is a negative event. As electronic commerce becomes more ubiquitous (see Chapters 35 and 37), particularly with the adoption of the ANSI X 12N standards for claims and authorizations (see Chapter 35), both the claim and the authorization will arrive in the same time frame, along with verification of eligibility for the providers, and this problem will be lessened. But at this point, it will remain a steady irritant for several years to come.

CATEGORIES OF AUTHORIZATION

Authorizations may be classified into six categories:

- prospective
- concurrent
- retrospective
- pended (for review)
- denial (no authorization)
- subauthorization

There is value in categorizing authorization types. By examining how authorizations are actually generated in the plan, management will be able to identify areas of weakness in the system. For example, if all elective admissions are thought to be receiving prospective authorization but it turns out that in fact most are being authorized either concurrently or worse yet, retrospectively, then medical management will be unable to intervene effectively in managing hospital cases because they do not know about them in a timely manner.

A brief description of the authorization categories follows.

Prospective

Sometimes referred to as precertification, this type of authorization is issued before any service is rendered. This is commonly used in plans that require prior authorization for elective services. The more prospective the authorization, the more time the medical director has to intervene if necessary, the greater the ability to direct care to the most appropriate setting or provider, and the more current your knowledge regarding utilization trends.

Inexperienced plan managers tend to believe that all authorizations are prospective. That naive belief can lead to a real shock when the manager of a troubled plan learns that most claims are actually being paid on the basis of other types of authorizations that were not correctly categorized. This is discussed further later.

Concurrent

A concurrent authorization is generated at the time the service is rendered. For example, the utilization review nurse discovers that a patient is being admitted to the hospital that day. An authorization is generated, though by the nurse and not by the PCP. Another example is an urgent service, such as setting a broken leg. In that case, the PCP may contact the plan, and the referral or authorization is made at the same time.

Concurrent authorizations allow for timely data gathering and the potential for affecting the outcome, but they do not allow the plan medical managers to intervene in the initial decision to render services. This may result in care being inappropriately delivered or delivered in a setting that is not cost-effective, but it also may result in the plan's being able to alter the course of care in a more cost-effective direction even though care has already begun. This is especially true when large case management is appropriate (see Chapter 22).

Retrospective

As the term indicates, retrospective authorizations take place after the fact. For example, a patient is admitted, has surgery, and is discharged, and only then does the plan find out. On the surface, it appears that any service rendered without authorization would have payment denied or reduced, but there will be circumstances when the plan will genuinely agree to authorize services after the fact. For example, if a member is involved in a serious automobile accident or has a heart attack while traveling in another state, there is a clear need for care and the plan could not deny that need.

Inexperienced managers often believe not only that most authorizations are prospective but that, except for emergency cases, there are few retrospective authorizations. Unfortunately, there are circumstances when there may be a high volume of retrospective authorizations. This commonly occurs when the PCPs or participating providers fail to cooperate with the authorization system. A claim for a referral service comes in cold (i.e., without an authorization), and the plan must create one after the fact if it finds out that the service was really meant to be authorized. The plan cannot financially penalize the member because it was really the fault of the PCP, so that claim gets paid.

Most plans have a *no balance billing* clause in their provider contracts (see Chapter 62) and may elect not to pay claims from contracted providers that have not been prospectively authorized, forcing the noncompliance providers to write off the expense. That will certainly get their attention, but it comes at some cost in provider relations. Even so, sometimes it becomes necessary if discussions and education attempts fail.

If the plan's systems allow an authorization to be classified as prospective or concurrent regardless of when it is created relative to the delivery of the service, it is a sure thing that retrospective authorizations will occur but not be labeled retrospective; for example, the PCP or specialist will say "I really meant to authorize that" or "It's in the mail" and call the authorization concurrent. Another possibility is that claims clerks may be creating retrospective authorizations on the basis of the belief that the claim was linked to another authorized claim (discussed later).

In a tightly managed plan, the ability to create a retrospective authorization is strictly limited to the medical director or utilization management department, the ability to create prospective authorizations does not exist once the service has actually been rendered, and concurrent authorizations cannot be created after 24 hours have passed since the service was rendered.

Pended (For Review)

Pended is a claims term that refers to a state of authorization purgatory. In this situation, it is not known whether an authorization will be issued, for there is a question as to coverage for a service, and the case has been pended for review. This refers to medical review (for medical necessity such as an emergency department claim or for medical policy review to determine whether the service is covered under the schedule of benefits) or to administrative review. As noted previously, if a plan is having problems getting the PCPs or participating providers to cooperate with the authorization system, there will be a significant number of pended claims that ultimately lead to retrospective authorizations.

Denial

Denial refers to the certainty that there will be no payment forthcoming. As has been discussed, one cannot assume that every claim coming into the plan without an associated authorization will be denied because there are multiple reasons that an unauthorized claim may be paid.

Subauthorization

This is a special category that allows one authorization to hitchhike on another. This is most common for hospital-based professional services. For example, a single authorization may be issued for a hospitalization, and that authorization is used to cover anesthesia, pathology, radiology, or even a surgeon's or consultant's fees.

In some plans, an authorization to a referral specialist may be used to authorize diagnostic and therapeutic services ordered by that specialist. For example, a referral to an orthopedist automatically allows for authorized payment for radiological services, a referral to a cardiologist allows for electrocardiograms, and so forth. Some care must be taken to manage this, however. If not, the phenomenon of linking will occur.

Linking refers to claims clerks linking unauthorized services to authorized ones and creating subauthorizations to do so. For example, a referral to a specialist is authorized, and a claim is received not only for the specialist's fees but for some expensive procedure or test as well, or a bill is received for 10 visits even though the PCP intended to authorize only one. The claims clerk (who is probably being judged on how many claims he or she can process per hour) may then inappropriately link all the bills to the originally authorized service through the creation of subauthorizations, thereby increasing the costs to the plan. Fully automated claims systems will have algorithms in place to determine payment for real or imputed subauthorizations, and exceptions will be pended and require manual review.

STAFFING

Plan personnel required to implement properly an authorization system are the medical director, an authorization system coordinator (whatever that person's actual title), and the utilization review nurses. Various clerks and telephone operators will also be required; the number of these depends on the size of the plan and the scope of the system. In plans that are able to use electronic communications for these functions, staffing needs will be relatively low in terms of clerks and telephone operators, but the need for clinically trained personnel to review exceptions will remain.

The medical director has three primary roles. The first is to interact with the plan's PCPs and specialty physicians to ensure compliance with the authorization system. Second, the medical director is responsible for medical review of pended claims. That does not mean that the medical director will have to review every claim personally, but that it is ultimately the medical director's responsibility. In some instances the case will be reviewed by the member's PCP; in others, it will be more appropriate for a nurse reviewer or even the medical director (or designate) to perform the primary review. Third, the medical director will sometimes have interactions with members when payment of a claim is denied. Although the claims department usually sends the denial letters and responds to inquiries, it is common for members to demand a review of the denied claim on the basis of medical necessity or a belief that the PCP really authorized the service. It has become common in most MCOs (required in many states and under active consideration by the Congress as of 2000) to have an outside review of disputed authorization requests (see Chapter 18), and in those cases, the medical director will be involved.

The authorization system needs a coordinator to make sure that all the pieces fit together. Whether that responsibility falls to the claims department, the utilization department, the medical director's office, or general management is a local choice. In a small plan, the role of coordinator usually falls to a manager with other duties as well, but as the plan grows, it is necessary to dedicate that function.

The coordinator's primary purpose is to track the authorization system at all its points. Any system can break down, and the coordinator must keep track of where the system is performing suboptimally and take steps to correct it. In some cases, that will require the intervention of others because an authorization system has ramifications in the PCP's office, the hospitals, the utilization review department, the claims department, member services, and finance. If no one is in charge of maintaining the authorization system, people will tend to deny their responsibilities in making it work.

Some thought must be given to the relationship of the authorization system to the utilization review coordinators. Specifically, how much can the utilization review coordinator authorize? It makes sense to allow some ability to create authorizations, especially subauthorizations for hospital services, but the medical director must decide whether the utilization review coordinators will be allowed to create primary authorizations, particularly for hospital cases. It is common in large HMOs for nurse case managers involved in large case management and disease management programs to have the ability to authorize services without the need to go through a PCP (see Chapters 22 and 23 for discussion of this activity).

COMMON DATA ELEMENTS

New Electronic Standards

With the passage of the Health Insurance Portability and Accountability Act of 1996 (HIPAA, see Chapters 35 and 67), standards have been set for the electronic transmission of authorization data. These standards are part of the overall ANSI X 12N standards mandated by HIPAA; specific to this chapter is the 278 set for referral and authorization standards.

These standards are far more complex than older, manual standards, and at the time of publication were about to be finalized. In addition to the ANSI X 12N 278 standards, there are additional standards, referred to as HL7, that apply to clinical information systems that communicate directly with each other. The HL7 standards are not mandated at this time but may end up being commonly used for these transactions. Additional ANSI X 12N standards are referenced in Chapters 35 and 67.

Because these standards are both highly complex, no exhibit is provided here. However, the reader can readily obtain information by means of the Internet.* Good places to start are:

- http://aspe.os.dhhs.gov/admnsimp/
- http://www.ansi.org/
- http://www.wedi.org/

---

*Website addresses can change faster than any book can keep up with, so these addresses are not guaranteed. Fortunately, official government sites have a bit more stability, so the reader has a better than average chance of finding these sites still active.

The website that has the actual standards available for purchase or free download as of the time of publication is: http://www.wpc-edi.com/HIPAA_40.asp

These electronic standards are mandated for use by any provider, payer, or third party that uses electronic transmission (e.g., an electronic claims clearinghouse, an Internet company that serves as an intermediary for physicians), or practice management software designed to transmit electronically to managed care organizations (MCOs). The date that the mandate becomes effective is 24 months after finalization of the regulations (which are likely to be finalized in the late spring of 2000, but that is not exactly known at the time of publication) for large organizations and 36 months for small (i.e., less than 5,000 members) MCOs. Providers that rely on paper-based communications are not affected by these standards, however, so it is possible and even likely that there will remain a large cohort of physicians that will continue to rely on paper or telephonic authorizations systems as described later.

Manual or Nonelectronic Data Elements

HIPAA, though not finalized at the time of publication, will mandate the ANSI X 12N standards including those for referral authorization, for electronic transmissions as of some time in 2002 or 2003. However, HIPAA does not address non-electronic data capture such as paper-based, telephone-based, or fax-based. Since it is most unlikely that all physicians will be using electronic transmission for all activities by 2002, the other means of capturing authorization data are briefly described below, and common data elements captured in non-electronic authorization systems are illustrated in Exhibit 19–1.

In systems where there are clinical requirements for authorization, the system then must determine what the requirements are on the basis of the diagnosis. For example, if a plan has pre-set criteria for authorization for cataract surgery, those requirements may be reviewed with the physician at the time of authorization. The same issue applies to mandatory outpatient surgery: if admission is being requested, the procedure may

Exhibit 19–1 Data Elements Commonly Captured in a Non-Electronic Authorization System

- Member's name
- Member's birth date
- Member's plan identification (ID) number
- Eligibility status
- Commercial group number or public sector (i.e., Medicare and Medicaid) group identifier
- Primary care physician (PCP) ID number
- Referral provider
  - Name
  - Specialty
  - ID number
- Outpatient data elements
  - Referral or service date
  - Diagnosis (*International Classification of Disease*—9th Edition, Clinical Modification [ICD-9-CM], free text)
  - Number of visits authorized
  - Specific procedures authorized (*Current Procedural Terminology*—4th Edition [CPT-4], free text)
- Inpatient data elements
  - Name of institution
  - Admitting physician
  - Admission or service date
  - Diagnosis (ICD-9-CM, diagnosis-related group, free text)
  - Expected length of stay or discharge date
- Subauthorizations (if allowed or required)
  - Hospital-based professionals
  - Other specialists
  - Other procedures or studies
- Free text to be transmitted to the claims processing department

be compared with an outpatient surgery list to determine whether the physician needs to justify an exception. Such reviews should be done only by medically trained personnel, usually nurses. In the case of disagreements with the requesting physician, the medical director must be able to contact the physician at that time or as soon as possible. External review in the case of an unresolvable disagreement may also be required, as noted earlier. It becomes less common for a plan to deny authorization on the basis of medical necessity as the plan matures and the participating physicians become more conversant in definitions of medical necessity; however, the other values of the authorization system remain important.

When an authorization is made, the system also must be able to generate and link an authorization number or identifier to the data, so that every authorization will be unique. In tightly managed plans, any claim must be accompanied by that unique authorization number to be processed.

METHODS OF DATA CAPTURE AND AUTHORIZATION ISSUANCE

There are three main methods of interacting with an authorization system: paper based, telephone based, and electronic.

Paper-Based Authorization Systems

Paper-based systems generally work in plans that allow the PCP to authorize the service without prospective review by the plan. If plan preapproval is necessary before an authorization is issued (except for infrequent services such as transplants), a paper-based system will not be responsive enough. If, however, the PCP has the authority to authorize services, a paper-based system will be adequate, although far from state-of-the-art.

This type of system depends on the PCP (or other authorizing provider), or more commonly the PCP's office staff, to fill out an authorization form, which may be used as a referral or admission form as well. A copy of the form is sent to the plan, which enters the authorization data into its system. Claims submitted to the plan may or may not require a copy of the authorization form, depending on plan policy.

The advantages of paper-based systems are as follows. They are less labor intensive than telephone-based systems and therefore require less overhead for the plan. Although electronic systems are even more labor efficient, electronic systems require a higher level of sophistication and support than paper-based systems and must now also be HIPAA compliant. Manual data entry can be done in batch mode because there is little need for real-time interaction. Paper-based systems also tend to be acceptable to physicians because they are less intrusive regarding clinical decision making, run less risk of violating patient confidentiality, and do not have the problem of busy signals or a physician's being placed on hold during a busy day in the office.

The disadvantages of paper-based systems are as follows. There is less opportunity to intervene at the time the authorization is made. Once an authorization is issued, it is nearly impossible to reverse it. Medical managers may be able to alter future behavior, but neither physician nor member will easily accept an after-the-fact reversal of an authorization. Another disadvantage is that it increases the administrative burden on the physician, particularly if he or she is participating in multiple plans, each with its own complicated set of forms. Paper authorizations can also get lost in the mail (or mail room) and lend themselves to data entry errors (e.g., digit transpositions). Last, paper-based authorizations may arrive at the plan well after an electronic claim has been received, resulting in a processing error and a required re-issuance of a payment.

Telephone-Based Authorization Systems

Telephone-based systems rely on the PCP or office staff to call a central number and give the information over the phone. If clinical review is required, it is done at that time. Telephone-based systems have the built-in potential of clogging up and leading to poor service. If the system is unresponsive or if PCPs get frequent busy signals or are put on hold, they will stop calling. The investment in a responsive telephone-based system will be paid back in a reduction of pended claims and retrospective authorizations.

Collecting the data and issuing an authorization number may be done either manually or by an automated system (referred to as interactive voice response, or IVR; see Chapter 35). Because authorization is linked to claims payment, there must be an interface between the telephonic authorization and the claims payment systems.

One approach is simply to print out all the telephonically collected data on manual logs and then enter them into the claims system through batch processing. Another more common and more reasonable approach is to automate the entire process. If the MCO has the systems capabilities to do so, it is best to have the authorization clerks or nurses enter the data directly into the computer. Be aware, though, that computer systems can cause delays with slow screens, complicated menus and entry screens, down time, training problems, and a host of other problems. Some computer systems are made for batch entry, making real-time entry too inefficient. In those situations, the plan may wish to use a manual log for data capture and authorization issuance until the automated system is well tested. One should also be able to use a manual system as a backup on a moment's notice.

It has also become common for the software or systems support for utilization management to be a separate system from the main system, but electronic linkages usually are created.

The advantages of telephone-based systems are that they can be more responsive and timely, have greater potential for directing care to the appropriate location and provider, and have the potential of reducing the administrative burden on the PCP's office staff. The disadvantages are that they increase the administrative burden on the plan and, if not run efficiently and responsively, can generate great ill will with the PCPs.

Electronic Authorization Systems

Electronic authorization systems are still not as common as paper- or telephone-based systems, but their popularity is rapidly growing. Electronic-based systems require participating physicians and hospitals to interface electronically with the plan, usually through a personal computer, a dumb terminal in the office, or an intermediary (e.g., an electronic claims company or a physician support Internet company). Electronic commerce between MCOs and providers has traditionally focused on claims submission and payment, but authorizations have become more common, as well as other high volume e-commerce transactions such as eligibility verification.

Electronic authorization standards are defined by the ANSI X 12N 278 standards noted earlier and scheduled for mandatory implementation (only for those entities that use electronic interchange) by 2002 at the earliest. An electronic authorization system may be more useful than the simple transmission of data, however. For example, the system should be able to check fields to ensure that the referral or admission is to a participating provider, provide automatic information transfer (e.g., member status and demographics), automatically notify all affected parties, and so forth. It is also possible for an electronic system to gather clinical information and to compare that with protocols before processing the authorization, but currently that is not a common feature of such systems. However, as noted in Chapter 18, the use of algorithms and expert systems will become more common in the future.

AUTHORIZATION SYSTEM REPORTS

The reports needed from an authorization system will depend on the complexity of the system and the needs of medical management. Obviously, the one absolutely necessary report function is linking incoming claims to authorized services.

Hospital logs and reports are discussed in greater detail in Chapters 18 and 32. The authorization system should be able to provide a report indicating prospective admissions and procedures, current admissions and procedures, and retrospectively authorized cases. Cases pended for review should also be reported, with data indicating when the claim was received, when it was reviewed, and its current status.

Outpatient reports from the authorization system could include summaries of authorizations by type for each PCP expressed as ratios; for example, total authorizations per 100 encounters per PCP or per 1,000 members per year (annualized), with a breakdown of prospective compared with concurrent compared with retrospective, and so forth. Authorization categories may also be expressed as a percentage of the total number of authorizations for that PCP. For example, the total authorization rate may be eight per 100 encounters per PCP with 50 percent prospective, 40 percent concurrent, 6 percent retrospective, and 4 percent pended (if it is denied, it is not an authorization, although it is still useful to report denial statistics by provider as well).

A valuable report is a comparison of authorization categories to paid claims. This is basically looking at the percentage of claims that have been authorized prospectively, concurrently, and so forth. This is valuable in determining the plan's ability to capture the data in a timely fashion. It will be inversely proportional to the plan's rate of incurred but not reported claims (IBNRs).

These reports will allow managers to identify noncompliant providers or providers who comply but not in a timely fashion. The medical director will be able to focus on those providers who either do not obtain authorizations or who do so in a way that does not allow for active medical management by the medical director (if that is needed). These reports, along with a report on the number and nature of open authorizations (i.e., authorizations for services for which a claim has not yet been received), will also allow the finance department to calculate more accurately the accruals and IBNR factor for the plan, reducing the chances of nasty surprises later.

OPEN ACCESS HMOs

As noted early in this chapter, there are some HMOs that do not require a member to go through a PCP to access a specialist (thus the term "open access"—access to specialists is open to members). These types of plans were quite popular in the late 1970s and early 1980s, but a string of failures led to their near extinction. However, a few did survive, and as of the time of publication, they have regained a degree of presence in the health care market. This is most prominent with certain managed care companies that have chosen the open access model as their preferred model, at least in markets that have relatively high levels of managed care penetration (and thus have physicians and hospitals that are more experienced with managed care principles).

The phoenix-like resurrection of open access HMOs is usually predicated on one or both of the following reasons. First, market research indicates that members prefer to access specialists directly without having to go through a PCP. Second, many plans find that they rarely deny a request for a referral to a specialist from a PCP, and that the PCP-based authorization system therefore may be creating unnecessary visits for no good reason.

There are potential flaws in these two lines of reasoning. First, it did not require too much research to know that members would prefer direct access to specialists since that does not prevent them from visiting a PCP, but does not require it either. This type of model is embodied in indemnity insurance, PPOs, and POS; and the costs of such systems have usually been higher than that found in HMOs. The second issue, that of not denying authorization requests, is also not quite on point because the denial rates of HMOs are quite low (see Chapter 6). The real issue is that the request comes from a physician, not from a member who has no medical training.

Even in open access plans, certain services will probably still require authorization. For example, highly expensive diagnostic studies, inpatient care, surgical procedures, and so forth may still be required, even though it would be the specialist who now requests them. Also, certain services may be carved out even in open access plans, such as behavioral health and chemical dependency treatment.

Some open access HMOs limit the number of self-referrals that a member may make per year (e.g., a member may self-refer up to three times per year). This option is rather difficult to track from an information systems standpoint, and issues such as follow-up visits must be clarified (i.e., does a follow-up visit count as part of the original self-referral, or is it a second self-referral?), as well as the ability of the specialist to initiate diagnostic or institutional based services. More commonly, these plans use economic barriers (i.e., high copayment requirements for specialty access) in lieu of a PCP referral system but still require authorization notification for services such as hospitalization.

SPECIALTY-PHYSICIAN BASED AUTHORIZATION SYSTEMS

As noted earlier and in several other chapters in this book, there are a number of advanced MCOs that use specialist physicians in the primary physician role as regarding care coordination and authorization for services. When one encounters this type of care management authorization system, it is usually in a plan that is relatively experienced in overall care management and that has a reasonably good management information system.

Not all members of the plan would be under this type of system; in fact, most would still use PCPs as their main coordinators of care. However, it is clear that in many cases, specialists are both more efficient and provide higher quality of care for certain clinical decisions. Common examples of this would include patients diagnosed with human immunodeficiency virus, certain forms of cancer, certain neurological diseases, certain cardiovascular diseases, brittle diabetes mellitus, and so forth. In these instances, the plan determines that the member falls into the category of one of these disease states and then removes that member from the usual PCP care management system and assigns the member to the appropriate specialist for care coordination.* For an in-depth discussion of disease management, see Chapter 23.

NON-PHYSICIAN-BASED AUTHORIZATION SYSTEMS

A few plans have been using a system in which requests for authorization for services come directly from members to the plan; in almost all cases these requests are directed to a

---

*Of course, the member chooses the specialist he or she wants from the plan's participating specialist list. In some cases, however, the plan may have selected a specialty provider to care for all of the members with that diagnosis, in which case the member's choice is limited to physicians in that group.

registered nurse (RN) who is specially trained in evaluating such requests. In these types of plans, the member calls a central telephone number to request an authorization and speaks with an RN. The member tells the RN on the telephone the reasons for the request for authorization for nonprimary care services, the RN then accesses computerized algorithms to verify the appropriateness of the request for a referral for specialty services and either authorizes the referral or refers the member back to the PCP. In this type of plan, the PCP may have no influence or input into whether the plan authorizes the referral and may find out only after the event has occurred.

Although this type of system looks attractive on its surface, there are some issues that are worthwhile considering before adopting it. First, are the clinical algorithms appropriate and adequate? Such algorithms can be purchased, but the plan may find it difficult to put them into place if the PCPs have had little or no input into them. More importantly, this type of authorization system is always done by telephone, with no information available based on a history or physical examination; therefore, the RN making the evaluation can rely only on information reported by the member. Although this is often adequate, that is not always the case. Therefore, it is likely that authorization for specialty services will occur more often than if PCPs are making that decision. Counterbalancing that is the improved member satisfaction that the plan enjoys from this more relaxed type of authorization system.

CONCLUSION

An effective authorization system is a requirement of any managed care plan. Whether that system is all encompassing or pertains only to certain types of services depends on the type of plan. Key elements to address are what services require authorization, who has the ability to authorize, whether secondary plan approval is required, what data will be captured, how they will be captured, and how they will be used.

CHAPTER 20

Ancillary Diagnostic and Therapeutic Services

Peter R. Kongstvedt

INTRODUCTION

This chapter addresses those medical services that are generally considered ancillary services by most managed care organizations (MCOs). These are a collection of services that are provided as an adjunct to basic primary or specialty services and include almost everything other than institutional services (although institutions can provide ancillary services).

ANCILLARY SERVICES

Ancillary services are divided into diagnostic and therapeutic services. Examples of ancillary diagnostic services include laboratory, radiology, nuclear testing, computed tomography, magnetic resonance imaging, electroencephalography, electrocardiography, and cardiac testing (including plain and nuclear stress testing, other cardiac nuclear imaging, invasive imaging, echocardiography, and Holter monitoring). Examples of ancillary therapeutic services include cardiac rehabilitation, noncardiac rehabilitation, physical therapy (PT), occupational therapy, and speech therapy.

Pharmacy services are a special form of ancillary services that account for a significant measure of cost and have been subject to recent price and use inflation; this topic is discussed in detail in Chapter 24. Mental health and substance abuse services may also be considered ancillary from a health plan's standpoint but are really core services, albeit discreetly defined; those services are discussed in Chapter 25.

Ancillary services are unique in that they are rarely sought by a patient without a referral by a physician. For example, it is certainly possible that an individual could self-refer to a rehabilitation center, but it is likely that the center would require a referral from a physician before accepting the individual into the program. Diagnostic studies almost universally require physician referral. One exception is the freestanding diagnostic center that has medical staff whose sole purpose is to guide a patient through the diagnostic workup that the patient seeks (e.g., a freestanding cardiac testing center whose advertisements appeal to people who want those tests done). Because those types of centers are out of a plan's control, as are freestanding urgent/convenience care centers, the only real way to control them is economic. If those centers do not have a contract with the plan or if the plan requires authorization from a contracted physician to pay in full, then the plan does not have to pay such freestanding centers. In the case of a health maintenance organization (HMO), the plan does not have to pay at all. For a preferred provider organization (PPO), a point-of-service (POS) plan, or a managed indemnity plan, the plan may or may not have a partial payment liability, depending on the service agreement and schedule of benefits.

Because most ancillary services require an order from a physician, it is logical that managing the cost of such services depends on changing

344

the utilization patterns of physicians. As discussed later, the other primary method of controlling costs of ancillary services is to contract for such services in such a way as to make costs predictable. In fact, many MCOs rely far more heavily on favorable contracting terms to manage the cost of these services than they do on managing utilization. Even with favorable contracts, however, managing utilization of ancillary services by physicians remains an important ingredient to long-term cost control.

PHYSICIAN-OWNED ANCILLARY SERVICES

Compelling evidence exists that physician ownership of diagnostic or therapeutic equipment or services, whether owned individually or through joint ventures or partnerships, can lead to significant increases in utilization of those services. Several studies documented this phenomenon in diagnostic imaging,[1] laboratory,[2] and a remarkably wide range of other services.[3] Physician self-referral has been restricted by the Health Care Financing Administration (HCFA) for Medicare services.[4] MCOs that enroll Medicare or Medicaid members must adhere to HCFA requirements as well. Most MCOs have followed suit and restrict physician self-referral as a routine requirement of plan participation by physicians, clearly prohibiting physician self-referral in their provider contracts (unless expressly allowed by the plan). The MCO contract also requires the physician to disclose any fiduciary relationship with such ancillary service providers.

Actually tracing ownership or fiduciary relationships is not always easy to do, however. The ancillary services may have a completely separate provider name and tax identification number, may have a separate billing address (perhaps not even in the same geographical area), and may otherwise appear to be an independent vendor. Tracking unusually high rates of referral to a given provider of ancillary services (see Chapter 32) may be the only clue to such potential abuse.

In coming years, another source of information will be the national Healthcare Integrity and Protection Data Bank (HIPDB). The Secretary of the U.S. Department of Health and Human Services, acting through the Office of Inspector General, was directed by the Health Insurance Portability and Accountability Act of 1996 (see Chapter 67) to create the HIPDB to combat fraud and abuse in health insurance and health care delivery. The HIPDB is a national health care fraud and abuse data collection program for the reporting and disclosure of certain final adverse actions (excluding settlements in which no findings of liability have been made) taken against health care providers, suppliers, or practitioners. Although focused primarily on actions such as fraud convictions and exclusion from state or federal programs, actions taken by HCFA around physician self-referral would be included. At the time of publication, the HIPDB had just started functioning.[5]

It is neither practical nor desirable to place too heavy a restriction on a physician's ability to use appropriate services or equipment that they own to deliver routine care within their specialty. For example, orthopaedists cannot properly care for their patients if they cannot take radiographs. In some cases, a physician may be the only available provider of a given service (e.g., in a rural area). In other cases, it may actually be more cost-effective to allow physicians to use their own facility.

Managed care plans deal with this issue in a number of ways. One method is to have an outright contractual ban on self-referral other than for specifically designated services. For example, a cardiologist may be reimbursed for performing in-office exercise tolerance testing but be prohibited from referring to a freestanding cardiac diagnostic center in which he or she has a fiduciary relationship. Another method is to reimburse for such physician self-referred services at a low margin (not so low as to cause the physician to lose money but low enough to prevent any profit) or to include it in the capitation payment. The last common method is to contract for all ancillary services through a very limited network of providers and require the physicians and members to use only those contracted providers for ancillary services; this is discussed later in this chapter.

The advent of integrated delivery systems (IDSs; see Chapter 4) has complicated this issue somewhat. It is not always clear if the ancillary services are owned by the physician or the IDS, and those services may be included in an all-encompassing global capitation rate in any event. However, the regulatory environment is changing in this arena, which is particularly important for those MCOs that are contracting for public sector business (Medicare and Medicaid). Chapter 65 further addresses legal issues in IDSs.

DATA CAPTURE

The ability to manage utilization of ancillary services will be directly related to the ability to capture accurate and timely data. An MCO with a tight authorization system (see Chapter 19) may get prospective data. If the claims management system is capable, the MCO should be able to get retrospective data. If there is no way to capture data regarding ancillary services, there will be difficulty controlling utilization. Lack of data will also make contracting problematic because no vendor will be willing to contract aggressively without having some idea of projected utilization (at least not on terms that will be beneficial to the plan or medical group responsible for the cost).

Data elements that need to be captured include who ordered the service. This is sometimes different than the physician of record; for example, a member may have signed up with a primary care physician (PCP), but the referral physician ordered the tests. Additional data to capture include what was ordered, what is being paid for (in other words, is the plan paying for more than was ordered?), and how much it is costing.

The ability to look at patterns of use in ancillary services is quite valuable. For example, it would be useful to know that of 10 family practitioners there is one who routinely orders double the number of radiographs compared with the other nine. There may be a perfectly good reason for this, but medical managers will never know unless they can identify that pattern and look for the reasons.

FINANCIAL INCENTIVES

Ancillary services utilization is commonly incorporated into primary care reimbursement systems that are performance based (e.g., capitation or performance-based fee-for-service). For example, in one study, capitation with risk-sharing, combined with education and feedback (see later) led to a clear reduction in the use of ambulatory testing, while having no adverse impact on outcomes.[6] The topic of financial incentives is discussed in Chapter 8.

FEEDBACK

The issue of monetary gain leading to excessive use of ancillary services has been discussed earlier in this chapter, but there are a number of nonmonetary causes of excessive testing. Such causes include the quest for diagnostic certainty, peer pressure, convenience, patient demands, and fear of malpractice claims.[7]

There is evidence that physicians will modify their use of ancillary services when given feedback on their performance. Simple feedback regarding test-ordering behavior has led to modest reductions in use.[8] This response has been confirmed for simple feedback, and somewhat greater decreases have been seen when feedback was combined with other written guidelines or peer review.[9,10]

Feedback to physicians regarding their use of ancillary services is therefore a worthwhile endeavor. Feedback should include comparisons to their peers and should be properly adjusted for factors that affect utilization (e.g., age and sex of patients, specialty type, adjustments for acuity or severity). Feedback should also contain adequate data to allow a physician to know where performance may be improved. See Chapters 32 and 33 for further discussion about using reports and practice profiling.

CONTROL POINTS

Irrespective of physician self-regulation of the use of ancillary services, many plans apply additional controls over ancillary utilization.

The most common of these are briefly discussed as follows.

Indications for Use

One control point is indications for use of services. This is not an easy means of controlling ancillary services, but it has the potential of producing the most control and fostering high quality. In essence, this means using standards of care. Like protocols and clinical pathways (see Chapter 29), standards of care outline the events and thought processes that should occur before physicians refer for ancillary or consultant services.

Indications for use or standards of care are useful in certain types of services. Theoretically, one could develop standards of care for virtually any service, but because review of such standards is time consuming, it is utterly impractical for routine diagnostic testing. For example, unless a plan is experiencing a tremendous cost overrun connected with urinalyses, there will be no marginal benefits to developing a protocol for when a urinalysis is required and when a urine dip test will do.

Cardiac testing is another matter. Cardiac testing, particularly stress testing and imaging, is generally both expensive and common. Indications for cardiac testing have been published in medical journals, and texts and algorithms are available, but the ordering of cardiac testing sometimes defies rationality. As mentioned earlier in this chapter, a scattershot approach may be used by some physicians that results in test ordering simply as an effort to turn something up. Concentration on this service by means of chart reviews for appropriateness as an aspect of the quality management program (see Chapter 30) may yield interesting results and provide direction in developing standards for ordering.

There are now multiple sources for clinical protocols, including the federal government at www.guideline.gov. In the example of cardiac testing, a reasonable approach is to enlist several highly respected cardiologists to use published protocols as a beginning and then tailor the algorithms, protocols, or standards rather than simply impose the protocol without input from plan physicians. A well-reasoned, referenced, and well-presented approach to diagnostic cardiac services will benefit the patient and result in lower costs.

Limits on Services Authorized

Another standard feature of managed care is limiting the number of visits for therapy without prior approval. This refers not only to having a limitation on the total number of visits that are covered in the schedule of benefits but to having a limitation on the number of visits that a member may receive without reauthorization.

For example, up to three or four visits to PT may be routinely allowed, but for any more the PCP must receive a case report or the therapist must discuss the case with the physician or the plan's case manager. At that point a treatment plan is developed and the appropriate number of visits is authorized.

There will be exceptions to the concept of requiring regular reauthorizations. In cases in which the absolute treatment need is known, authorization for the entire course of treatment may be made. Examples include radiation therapy or home intravenous treatments. In such cases, the treatment plan is worked out in detail before therapy is initiated. The number of treatments required and their duration is known and may be authorized at the beginning.

Failure to control prospectively the use of ancillary therapy may result in the number of treatments or visits required in a particular type of therapy exactly equaling the level of benefits the plan offers. Much preferred is a rational approach to treatment with review of the case by the member's physician or the plan's case management function (as appropriate) and a definite treatment plan with periodic reassessments required.

CONTRACTING AND REIMBURSEMENT FOR ANCILLARY SERVICES

Contracting and ancillary services network development is one of the first and most important approaches an MCO takes in dealing with costs in this area. Many ancillary services are among the first to be "carved out" of the main medical delivery system, with the risk transferred to another organization that is able to achieve economies of scale and manage the overall cost and quality.

Closed panel plans, large medical groups, and IDSs have the option of providing certain ancillary services in house. It is up to management to do the cost/benefit analysis to determine whether that is the best course of action. One thing to keep in mind, though, is that managing utilization is no less difficult when the service is in house because referral for that service is often seen as free and certainly as convenient.

For open panel plans or closed panels that do not have the services in house, the services must be contracted for. A plan usually has its choice of hospital-based (sometimes that is the only choice), freestanding or independent, or office-based service. The choice will be made on the basis of a combination of quality, cost, access, service (e.g., turnaround time for testing), and convenience for members. Unlike physician services, ancillary services usually may be limited to a small subset of providers. This allows for greater leverage in negotiating and greater control of quality and service.

In HMOs or plans that have absolute limitations on benefits for ancillary services, such ancillary services often lend themselves to capitation. When capitating for ancillary services, one needs to calculate the expected frequency of need for the service and the expected or desired cost and then spread this over the membership base on a monthly basis. Plans that allow significant benefits for out-of-network use (e.g., a POS plan) may still capitate but only for the in-network portion; out-of-network costs will have to be paid through the regular fee allowances. If the capitated provider strictly limits access or cannot meet demand, the plan will end up paying twice—once through capitation and a second time through fee-for-service. If the MCO has a large membership base, the ability to forecast cost and use even under POS may be possible, but if the MCO has a small enrollment base, capitation for benefits plans other than a pure HMO plan may not be feasible.

Although relatively uncommon, a POS plan may have no out-of-network benefits for some ancillary services, thus more easily allowing for capitation. For insured products though not for self-funded programs, this may be difficult from a regulatory standpoint if the ancillary services are clearly part of the basic medical benefit. Simple PPOs generally are unable to capitate and must therefore depend on fee allowances or other forms of episode-related reimbursement.

Capitating for ancillary services clearly makes the provider of the service a partner in controlling costs and helps the MCO budget and forecast more accurately. The benefit to the provider of the service is a guaranteed source of business and a steady income. In diagnostic services, great economies of scale will often be present (this is especially true for diagnostic laboratory services). In those services where the provider delivering the service may be determining the need for continued services (e.g., PT), capitation will remove the fee-for-service incentives that may lead to inappropriately increased utilization. As with all capitation contracts, medical managers must be sure that they can direct all (or at least a defined portion) of the care to the capitated provider and not allow referrals to noncontracted providers.

Certain types of ancillary services require greater skill in capitating than others. If an ancillary service is highly self-contained, it is easier to capitate; for example, PT usually is limited to therapy given by the physical therapists and does not involve other types of ancillary providers. Home health, on the other hand, is often a combination of home health nurses and clinical aids, durable medical equipment, home infusion and medication delivery (which includes the cost of the drug or intravenous substance and the cost to deliver it), home physical therapy, and so forth. A number of plans have successfully capitated for home health services, although those have tended to be larger plans with sufficient volume to be able to accurately predict costs in all of these different areas. Other plans have been able to capitate only parts of home health (e.g., home respiratory therapy) but have had less success in other forms. In those cases, a combination of capitation and fixed case rates (e.g., for a course of chemotherapy) may yield positive results.

A recent variant on capitation is similar to the single-specialty management organization or specialty network manager. In this case, a single entity accepts capitation from the plan for all of a particular ancillary service (e.g., PT). That organization then serves as a network manager or even an independent practice association. The participating ancillary providers may be subcontractors to the network manager and be paid either through subcapitation or through a form of fee-for-service, but in all events, the network manager is at risk for the total costs of the capitated service (the participating ancillary providers are usually at risk as well through capitation, fee adjustments, withholds, and so forth).

Some plans that capitate for ancillary services are using risk and reward systems to ensure high levels of quality and satisfaction. For example, a plan may withhold 10% of the capitation or set up an incentive pool to ensure compliance with service standards such as accessibility, member satisfaction, turnaround time for results, responsiveness to referring physicians, and documentation.

Plans that do not have the option of capitating may still achieve considerable savings from discounts. Many diagnostic ancillary services are high-volume services, so it is usually not difficult to obtain reasonable discounts or to have a negotiated fee schedule. Related to that for therapeutic ancillary providers are case rates or tiered case rates. In this form of reimbursement, the ancillary provider is paid a fixed case rate regardless of the number of visits or resources used in providing services. For home health that is inclusive of high-intensity services such as chemotherapy or other high-technology ser-

vices, the plan may pay different levels of case rates depending on which category of complexity the case falls into. These types of reimbursement systems are appealing but are often quite hard to administer, requiring manual administration by both the plan and the provider.

The exception to being able to obtain substantial discounts and savings is when there are a limited number of providers offering the service. Outside of exotic testing and therapy, this is usually not the case unless the plan is located in a rural area. In general, high savings can be achieved through good contracting.

CONCLUSION

The management of ancillary diagnostic and therapeutic services requires a multifaceted approach. The first approach is through the behavior of the physicians ordering the ancillary services. Through the use of profiling and feedback, direct discussions between the medical director and physicians who appear to be highly excessive in their use of ancillary services, and the use of capitation, reasonably effective results may be obtained. The second, and far more important, approach is by contracting for these services on a favorable basis. Capitation is well suited to ancillary services in HMOs and sometimes POS plans, but in all cases, substantial savings are to be had from favorable contracting. This is predicated on the MCO using a restricted network and on the ability to steer services to the contracted entity. Requirements for quality and service on the part of the ancillary services provider are also important to address in the contract, and this performance should be tied to financial incentives.

REFERENCES AND NOTES

1. B.J. Hillman, C.A. Joseph, et al., Frequency and Costs of Diagnostic Imaging in Office Practice—A Comparison of Self-referring and Radiologist-referring Physicians, *New England Journal of Medicine* 323 (1990): 1604–08.
2. Office of the Inspector General, *Financial Arrangements between Physicians and Health Care Businesses: Report to Congress*. Department of Health and Human Services Publication No. OAI-12-88-01410 (Washington, DC: Department of Health and Human Services, 1989).
3. State of Florida Health Care Cost Containment Board, *Joint Ventures among Health Care Providers in Florida* (Tallahassee, FL: State of Florida, 1991), 2.

4. The Ethics in Patient Referrals Act—Omnibus Budget Reconciliation Act of 1989.

5. The operational functions of the HIPDB are conducted for the Division of Quality Assurance of the DHHS by Systems Research and Applications (SRA), Inc. Further information is available via their website at http://www.npclb-hipdb.com/.

6. J.P. Murray, S. Greenfield, S.H. Kaplan, and E.M. Yano, Ambulatory Testing for Capitation and Fee-For-Service Patients in the Same Practice Setting: Relationship to Outcomes, *Medical Care* 30 (1992): 3, 252–61.

7. J.P. Kassirer, Our Stubborn Quest for Diagnostic Certainty: A Cause of Excessive Testing, *New England Journal of Medicine* 320 (1989): 1489–91.

8. D.M. Berwick and K.L. Coltin, Feedback Reduces Test Use in a Health Maintenance Organization, *JAMA* 255 (1986): 1450–54.

9. K.I. Marton, V. Tul, and H.C. Sox, Modifying Test-ordering Behavior in the Outpatient Medical Clinic. *Archives of Internal Medicine* 145 (1985): 816–21.

10. A.R. Martin, M.A. Wolf, L.A. Thibodeau, et al., A trial of Two Strategies To Modify the Test-ordering Behavior of Medical Residents, *New England Journal of Medicine* 303 (1980): 1330–36.

CHAPTER 21

The Emergency Department and Managed Care

Casey Jason and Meera Kanhouwa

OVERVIEW

At present, health care expenditures make up more than 14 percent of the domestic gross national product. Managed care has moderated the rate of rise in health care inflation over the past 15 years, but the ability to achieve the dramatic savings that were seen in the past is no longer as easily achieved. Managed care organizations (MCOs) have approached controlling costs by using the approaches discussed in the other chapters in this section, with special emphasis on the use of preventive services, reducing hospital admissions and length of stay (LOS), the application of case and disease management for chronic conditions, and favorable contracting. To keep premiums low and remain competitive in today's marketplace, additional solutions to keep quality high and expenditures under control are continually being sought. MCOs have always placed focus on the use of emergency services, but that focus has increased in recent years because of this increased pressure.

The established use of the emergency department (ED) has been one of unrestricted access to patients for unscheduled medical care. In the effort to reduce ED costs, managed care has increasingly experienced conflicts with the emergency health care system. Methods of preauthorization for treatment, retrospective denial, and/or limitations on treatment already given have reduced consumer trust in the health care system.[1] Areas of conflict include the following:

- The definition of an emergency medical condition used to determine appropriate use of the ED
- The requirement of preauthorization calls by ED staff and the effects of these calls on ED operations
- Safety and outcome of patients for whom preauthorization is denied
- Disagreements with regard to the need for ancillary services such as diagnostic laboratory tests, radiological imaging, specialty consultation, and transfer to other facilities
- What constitutes fair reimbursement and how to define it for various levels of ED service
- Cost shifting by the hospital and emergency physicians to cover the costs of uncompensated care[2]

The lack of consistency in managed care guidelines has made all aspects of caring for a patient in the ED more difficult. This chapter will deal with methods to achieve a more uniform approach to managed care in the ED.

Casey Jason, MD, FACEP, is Assistant Clinical Professor of Internal Medicine at Georgetown University Medical Center and Medical Advisor at STAR Health Systems/Base Technologies.

Meera Kanhouwa, MD, MHA, is Chairman of the Department of Emergency Medicine at Prince George's Hospital Center and Associate Clinical Professor of Emergency Medicine at George Washington University Medical Center.

CHALLENGES SHARED BY MANAGED CARE AND EMERGENCY MEDICINE

The Definition of an Emergency

What constitutes an "emergency medical condition?" The answer to this seemingly innocuous question has perplexed emergency medicine, patients, and managed care. EDs are in the unique position of trying to assess whether the "prudent layperson's assessment" of his or her emergency condition is truly prudent.[3] One author has suggested that this evaluation depends on whether prospective versus retrospective classification methods are used in the analysis.[4] Currently available prospective classification methods reveal that only 15 to 30 percent of the ED visits are nonurgent,[5,6] whereas retrospective studies show that 40 to 55 percent of patients evaluated in EDs have nonurgent medical conditions.[7,8] Currently available triage methods lack the sensitivity to prospectively determine acuity in a reproducibly defensible fashion representing the current standard of care for the area.

What Is the Federal Law?

The Consolidated Omnibus Budget Reconciliation Act/Emergency Medical Treatment and Active Labor Act (COBRA/EMTALA) was passed by the federal government in 1985 to prevent transfer or "dumping" of uninsured patients by private hospitals to public hospitals. This antidumping legislation dictates that all patients presenting to any hospital ED must have a medical screening examination performed by qualified personnel, usually the emergency physician (EP). The medical screening examination cannot be delayed for insurance reasons: either to obtain insurance information or to obtain preauthorization for examination.

Specific language in EMTALA states, "An emergency medical condition means a medical condition manifested by acute symptoms of sufficient severity (including severe pain) that the absence of immediate medical attention could reasonably be expected to result in: a) placing the patient's health in serious jeopardy; b) serious impairment to bodily functions; or c) serious dysfunction of any bodily organ or part."[9] In

other words, EMTALA is an unfunded mandate to EDs regarding *all* patients who come to the ED requiring the ED to medically screen and medically stabilize life- and limb-threatening medical conditions.

Although EMTALA was originally developed to protect the unborn, its domain has become the largest unfunded federal health care program. It is so confusing that an EMTALA working group[10] was formed by the Health Care Financing Administration and convened from 1996 to 1998 to refine the definition of an emergency medical condition. After 2 years of work, there were still significant problems defining the following:

- Medical screening examination—How much and by whom is enough?
- Stabilization—How stable is stable enough for transport? Should it rest with the ED physician?
- Transfer—Lateral transfers, although allowed with COBRA, become difficult or prohibited with EMTALA.

Rather than supplying funds to support any health care delivery program, EMTALA is the punitive arm requiring hospitals and physicians to obey confusing legislative guidelines. An alleged violation of EMTALA carries a potential death blow to both the hospital and physician. It includes:

- Suspension of hospital Medicare provider status
- $25,000 to $50,000 hospital fine per violation
- Exclusion of physician from Medicare/Medicaid participation
- Physician fine of $5,000 per violation

Preauthorization

Any preauthorization for emergency medical system (EMS) transport or emergency care presents a risk both to patient and MCO. Preauthorization calls are often made by ED staff who are not clinicians and received, in some cases, by MCO staff who may or may not be clinicians.[11,12] Calls made for authorization to call 911 or to access emergency care can cause delays in obtaining medical treatment with potential detrimental outcomes.

However, even if the MCO denies authorization for emergency care, EMTALA mandates that all patients coming to the ED undergo a medical screening examination to rule out an emergency medical condition. An MCO denial simply means that ED services will not be reimbursed but does not obviate the need for a medical screening examination to be performed by the ED staff.

At the time of publication, 26 states and the District of Columbia are considering or have passed "prudent layperson" legislation that more closely resembles the balanced budget amendment legislation for Medicare and Medicaid (see Table 21–1). Prudent layperson legislation allows patients to determine for themselves if a medical condition exists that requires emergency medical evaluation. The Access to Emergency Medical Services Act (HR 815/S356) allows for a prudent layperson determination of an

Table 21–1 1999 List of States Having Prudent Layperson Legislation

Alabama		April 1999
Arkansas	SB 671	April 19, 1995
Colorado	Ins. Reg. 4.2.17	July 1, 1997
Connecticut	HB 6883	May 21, 1997
Delaware	HB 366	April 1998
District of Columbia		May 1998
Georgia	HB 1575	April 8, 1996
Hawaii	SB 2037	July 21, 1998
Idaho	SB 1150	July 1, 1997
Indiana	SB 364	March 24, 1998
Kentucky	HB 315	May 1, 1998
Louisiana	HB 2206	June 19, 1997
Maine	Ins. Rules, Chapter 850	April 28, 1997
Maryland	SB 701	May 27, 1993
Minnesota	SB 346	December 1995
Missouri	HB 335	June 25, 1997
New York	SB 7553	June 1996
North Carolina	SB 455	January 1, 1998
Ohio	SB 361	December 18, 1997
Oregon	SB 21	October 1997
South Carolina	HB 3889	June 8, 1998
Tennessee	SB 3244	May 20, 1998
Texas	SB 385/386	May 22, 1997
Virginia	HB 2583	March 16, 1995
Washington	HB 2018	October 1997
West Virginia	HR 4043	June 14, 1998
Wisconsin	AB 652	March 1998

American College of Emergency Physicians' (ACEP's) "Definition of Emergency Medicine" Policy Statement–January 1, 1994
National Association of Insurance Commissioners Model Legislation–February, 1995
AMA Council on Legislation–Adopted April, 1995
Date of ACEP/Kaiser Agreement–August 19, 1996
American College of Emergency Physicians®
External sites are not endorsed by ACEP
Source: Reprinted with permission from *Definition of Emergency Medicine Policy Statement,* January 1, 1994, the American College of Emergency Physicians.

emergency without gatekeeper authorization. The inevitable problem of MCO determination of actual acuity by the ED for reimbursement purposes then becomes important.

In one study of triage decision making, the ability for nurses and physicians to correctly predict the need for admission was only fair, and with a tested computer system, little better than chance.[13] From this study, one might conclude that managed care gatekeepers would have difficulty predicting the need for emergency treatment and admission. Some MCOs use gatekeepers to reduce ED use, but studies in which the accuracy of gatekeeper ED diversion has been examined are absent in the ED literature. As one EP describes this situation, "This may be the first time in history that physicians have been required by law to deliver care but prohibited …from receiving payment for their services.[14]

According to a study by the Kaiser Family Foundation,[15] one of the top five concerns by consumers is access to emergency care. In this study, 79 percent of Americans surveyed favored an ED access law, whereas 62 percent favored an ED access law even if it meant increased insurance premiums. In another study,[16] a representative 1,018 adult sample of the general public was asked to choose among the four categories of emergency as to what constituted an "emergency."

- 50 percent of this representative population believed that the ED was a 24-hour convenience clinic.
- Forty-eight percent chose the EMTALA definition.
- Seventeen percent chose the EMTALA definition plus after-hours care.
- Thirty-two percent chose being seen for any condition at any time.
- Three percent chose the EMTALA definition plus any conditions preventing work.

The lay person's ability to separate the serious from the nonserious medical condition is even worse in the areas of headache, chest pain, difficulty breathing, uncontrolled bleeding, and the inability to walk. An average person can learn to differentiate the serious from the nonserious medical condition with a great deal of education. This type of education is lacking and difficult to administer because of the variety of possible clinical situations. Patient sorting and severity screening most appropriately occurs at triage within the ED.

Payment for Emergency Services

Many policymakers in health care believe that most ED visits are inappropriate for the level of care needed. This raises two issues: Does it make financial sense to see these people in the ED? Is it logical to treat nonemergency cases in the emergency setting?

Estimates of marginal ED costs[17,18] and the assumption that the cost shifting from the uninsured does not materially affect the cost for insured patients is questionable. Marginal costs—which include the facility, the staff, and care for low-income people—materially affect the cost of seeing the ambulatory, nonemergent insured patient, estimated at more than $5 billion in "excess" per year.[19] Given the overcrowding at many EDs and the adverse medical and financial effects that the crowding has on having truly emergent patients treated efficiently,[20] the ambulatory patients qualifying for care would be better served in a lower acuity setting.

The efficient use of the ED can occur only if several important steps occur. First, uniform, scientifically defensible triage capable of comparison among institutions must precede the patient's physician evaluation and treatment. Second, prompt evaluation and continuing care in the proper setting must take place. Third, the appropriate personnel, including physician staff, must be present to care for the patient.

EMTALA mandates that EPs must examine patients and provide a medical screening examination; it does not provide for any reimbursement of ED care, nor does it establish what a reasonable reimbursement would be for such services. Denying reimbursement on a retrospective basis for the extent of triage and its resulting expense reflects the inability of the present systems to prospectively predict the acuity of illness and probability of requiring specific interventions. To address this, some states are creating legislation to prevent downcoding or denial of care on the basis of final diagnosis, but better efforts are needed to objectively characterize presenting symptoms and expected care.

CREATING EFFICIENCIES AND IMPROVING PRODUCTIVITY

The Current State of Emergency Medicine

The prediction for ED visits as managed care matured was that the total number of ED visits would decrease as MCO primary care networks became more facile in managing the continuum of care and keeping their patients from accessing the "expensive" ED. In 1994, ED utilization did decrease by 12.2 percent in California, whereas, nationally, ED visits decreased by only 2.2 percent. The reality, however, has been divergent from predictions in the early 1990s.

ED visits have increased across the nation. For example:

- Fairfax Hospital in Fairfax County, VA, increased its ED volume 14 percent from 1992 to 1997.
- Harris Methodist Hospital in Ft. Worth, TX, increased its ED volume 45 percent between 1992 and 1997.
- Torrence Memorial ED increased its ED volume from 2,400 per month to 4,000 per month since 1995.
- Medica Health Plan's (Minneapolis, MN) ED visits were up 20 percent in 6 years despite rigorous cost-cutting efforts.
- Sinai Health System in Baltimore, MD, had an increase of 21 percent in 1998 alone.[21]

In 1988, there were 81 million ED visits per year. By the end of 2000, there will be more than 100 million ED visits per year. With decreased revenue across the health care industry, smaller and financially insolvent hospitals will close, increasing the burden on surrounding EDs. As the number of uninsured also continues to rise, the ED will continue to remain as the only safety net

for medical care for the indigent, uninsured, and underinsured: a safety net subsidized through other federal programs such as Medicare, Medicaid, and by managed care.[22] Although losing Medicare payments can close a hospital, the subsidy generated for indigent care from Medicare needs to be critically evaluated. Realistically, surplus Medicare dollars are probably only a small portion of the greater than $30 billion of uncompensated care estimated by the Congressional Budget Office.

By definition the uninsured population receives little or no preventive health care. Given that there is no EMTALA equivalent for doctors' offices, this means that the ED becomes the default center for health care delivery.

Independent of any other considerations, the American College of Emergency Physicians estimates the current EDs to be approximately 4,700 and the average number of patients per ED to be 20,000. If the number of indigent patients were spread evenly over those numbers, the problem would be troublesome but not overwhelming, but this is not the case. Rather, urban, particularly inner-city community hospitals, inner-city teaching hospitals, and rural hospitals with fewer than 50 beds bear the brunt of this patient load. For these, Medicare, a shrinking Medicaid-eligible population, and managed care assume the lead role for offsetting indigent health care costs; and these sources of revenue are increasingly unable or unwilling to accept this cost-shifting.

Where should the dollars of uncompensated health care come from? No groups at the federal, local, or private level address the issue of payments from the working uninsured. Current measures to offset indigent health care costs include:

- Taxes on health care providers
- Surcharges on health plan payments
- Vice taxes (tobacco, alcohol)

How does a hospital or physician group shift costs to subsidize indigent care without upcoding or raising facility rates above the usual and customary rates for these services? Physician groups must look to supplemental revenue streams to offset losses because uncompensated care is marginally advantageous to the facility but not to the professional sector.

Current possible avenues have included the following:

- Using federal subsidies through
  — Resource-based relative value systems
  — Tax incentives
- Increasing the patient population enrolled under existing Medicaid programs

Although these areas for revenue need to be developed, managed care is under pressure not only to deliver high-quality and efficient care but also to help subsidize indigent care. This occurs through health plan surcharges and hospital cost shifting on services and medications, supplies, and so forth. As negotiated MCO contracts use strict guidelines, the number of appeals and even litigation for denied LOS and hospital services could be expected to rise. With more Medicare/Medicaid patients joining managed care, the pressure for uncompensated cost shifting will shift further from the federal to the private sector. In 1999 with reimbursements for Medicare patients falling and nearly 100 MCOs opting out of the Medicare risk program, it has become obvious that a serious cost reimbursement mismatch is occurring.

Given the current climate at the state and federal levels, what are the means available to managed care to offset regulatory actions? Possibilities include:

- Methods to ensure that high-quality care appropriate to the clinical situation is delivered
- Tools to ensure that triage is reflective of the current standard of care and will be reflected in the subsequent care
- Means to compare ED triage and performance with established standards of care
- Better cooperative efforts with EDs for systems development
- Methods to maximize the efficiency of ED operations

The challenge for emergency medicine in the next decade will be to maintain high-quality pa-

tient care while continuing to treat an ever-increasing volume of patients within greater financial constraints.

The Service Edge

Improving ED service to key customers such as patients, medical staff, ED staff, and managed care will not only improve patient outcomes but also improve the quality of health care delivered at lower cost. Increasingly across MCOs, hospitals, and EDs alike, patient satisfaction is becoming the venue for measuring service excellence, a topic also discussed in Chapters 40 and 43. Patients expect qualified, trained personnel to deliver the care they receive in the ED. Technical expertise is a given because most patients do not feel qualified to judge the technical merits of their health care. Patients do judge their care by other dimensions that they can "see, feel, understand, and personally value."[23]

How important is patient satisfaction in the ED? The national admission rate is 15 to 20 percent of those seen, which means that nearly 80 percent of all patients are treated and discharged. Whether that patient returns to the department for his or her future unscheduled care or future inpatient care will depend largely on the first impression in the ED. The factors that have the most direct impact on patient satisfaction in the ED are relatively well understood. The foremost determinant of patient satisfaction in the ED is wait time[24] (or from a patient perspective, "neglect" time; i.e., the patient feels neglected during this time period). In one study, it was found that the primary reason for patients leaving without being seen was prolonged waiting time.[25] Patients come to the ED for immediate attention for their medical problem and naturally get tired of waiting when they have to:

- Wait for the triage nurse, then
- Wait for registration, then
- Wait to go back to an examination room, then
- Wait for the treatment nurse, then
- Wait for the doctor, then
- Wait for the doctor to finish the physical examination and history, then

- Wait for the doctor to decide what diagnostics to order, then
- Wait for the nurse to draw the blood, then
- Wait for the blood test result, then
- Wait for the x-ray film to be taken, then
- Wait for the x-ray result, then
- Wait for the doctor to analyze the blood and x-ray results, then
- Wait for the primary care doctor to call back, then
- Wait for the EP to make a diagnosis and a disposition, and finally
- Wait for the nurse or an aide to deliver the discharge paperwork

Average LOSs in an ED are 200 minutes, which breaks down to 150 minutes on average for a discharged patient and 280 minutes for an admitted patient. It is axiomatic that patients do not care how much you know until they know how much you care. When a patient has to wait for extended periods of time, the perception is that the caregivers do not care; therefore, the patient feels neglected and ignored, which leads to increased patient dissatisfaction.

Patient turnaround times are receiving intensifying attention from payers and governmental regulatory bodies. In the state of Maryland, for example, the Maryland Quality Indicators Project tracks and reports on the rate of ED stays greater than 6 hours for all EDs in the state. Currently though, there are no national standards to guide hospitals as to what constitutes acceptable turnaround times in the ED.[26]

Counter to the preceding, in one study (reported in two parts) the investigators found that neither the physician wait time nor the total wait time were predictive of patient satisfaction.[27,28] Their study demonstrated that patient satisfaction was greater when health care providers were more expressive and provided continued information throughout the emergency encounter. Expressive qualities assessed included an impression of competence, professionalism, and caring; and information provided was both verbal and written. Another author concluded that "Patients desire 'high touch' over 'high tech.'"[29] Patients seem to respond more from the caring aspects of treatment (high touch) rather than the curing (high tech) aspects of treatment. These studies have implications for practitioners in emergency medicine. Although the physicians and nurses may not be able to control increased patient volume on a busy day, by effectively managing patients' waiting time expectations, providing information, and showing caring, patient satisfaction may still be an achievable outcome.

What Is Being Done To Increase Efficiency and Productivity?

Serial processing of patients creates queuing in the ED. As long as the processes in the ED function in the traditional manner, efficiency and increased productivity will never become a reality. At present, most EDs around the country are engaged in changing the process of patient throughput from a serial process to a parallel process. A parallel process allows for stacking of times for the various actions that must be completed before the patient has obtained emergency care. This approach leads to an overall decrease in total waiting time. Parallel processing of patients in the ED requires changes in every aspect of emergency care delivery, from changing the manner in which a patient is registered to the ordering of tests and x-ray films.

Often in the ED, the same information is collected multiple times by different people and recorded in different areas of the patient chart. A good example of this is the triage process. Initially, the triage nurse performs a history and physical assessment on the patient coming to the ED, but the treatment nurse later repeats this once the patient is in the examination room. Efforts to reduce redundancy of work and data collection will increase efficiencies in the patient throughput process.

Time studies are an important and standard method of identifying bottlenecks in ED patient care delays and inefficiencies. In one ED, time study analysis done over a 5-year period showed continued and incremental improvements in patient care efficiency as bottlenecks were identified, analyzed, and solutions implemented.[30] The main processes examined included triage presentation to completion of registration, completion of registration to ED treatment area entry, ED treatment area entry to initial medical assessment, triage presentation to initial medical assessment, initial medical assessment to disposition order, and disposition order to patient discharge from the ED.

Other industries have been using industrial quality management techniques to improve service delivery for many years. Health care as an industry has not adopted a rigorous quality management ethic as of yet, but is beginning to do so.[31,32]

Triage

Triage is derived from the French trier, "to sort," and was adopted into English after the Napoleonic wars. The purpose of triage is to rapidly sort patients to prioritize the timing and location of service in the ED.[33] The function of triage is to ascertain that the sickest patients are seen first, with queuing occurring on the basis of severity of illness. Traditional triage systems are largely poorly standardized and institution specific. By convention, current triage categories are emergent, urgent, or nonurgent. It is important to remember that a triage examination does not qualify for the purposes of a medical screening examination as mandated by EMTALA.

Since the advent of EMTALA, the triage process occurs before the registration process during which insurance information is taken, and any co-pays required by third-party payers are collected. Before EMTALA, in many EDs the registration process occurred as the first step in the patient care process. However, EMTALA specifically stipulates that insurance cannot be a determinant in a patient's access to emergency care; thus EDs have had to change their practice over the years to comply with federal legislation.

At present, little is known about the accuracy and reliability of prevalent triage methods.[34] One author attempted to compare triage categorization by a physician, nurse, and computer program. The results indicated that great variability existed between physicians, nurses, and the computer program with regard to triage decisions. In fact, none of the three groups performed well in predicting

which patients required admission. This study underscored the need for triage methods to be standardized and validated and that in the existing state triage decisions should not be used to determine the timeliness of access to emergency care. Ideally, criteria-based triage systems should be developed, standardized, and validated. This information should be readily available to hospitals, payers, regulators, and providers of emergency medical care.

Although no validated computer triage programs are currently commercially available for use in the ED, work is progressing. Work at STAR Health Systems has demonstrated that linear regression/neural network modeling to assess acuity and probability for selected clinical procedures and outcomes on the basis of a given clinical presentation is a powerful tool. These probabilities for specific outcomes would be based dynamically on the current standard of care. Although not commercially available at this time, work such as this represents a much-needed approach to standardizing the expectations for subsequent ED care. Given the fact that triage is presently inexact and is not yet a scientifically validated patient care process, many EDs have found immediate efficiencies by greatly reducing the extent of the triage nursing evaluation or eliminating it altogether.

In addition to "quick" or limited triage, EDs are using protocols to enable triage nurse ordering of tests before the physician sees the patient. Studies that have examined the role of the triage nurse in extremity radiograph ordering have shown excellent agreement with physicians.[35–38] One study of triage nurse test ordering found substantial correlation with physician ordering of x-ray films, electrocardiograms, and urinalysis.[39] Results such as these can be further improved with the use of test-ordering guidelines.

Registration

Historically, the registration process has been a major cause of delay in delivering patient care. The purpose of the registration process is to collect insurance and financial information, and the process generally results in the generation of an account number or a visit number correlated with a unique medical record number for each patient. In most EDs, registration is a laborious process, requiring the completion of multiple screens of data. Registration clerks usually sit at a registration terminal, requiring the patient go to that discrete location away from the patient care area. Most importantly, however, no portion of the clinical evaluation can begin until an account number is generated. Laboratory tests and x-ray films cannot be ordered without an account number. Electrocardiograms need an account number to be entered into monitors, old medical records cannot be ordered without a medical record number, and in most EDs generation of the paper chart depends on the completion of the registration process.

An immediate efficiency booster is the implementation of bedside registration with a "mini-registration" screen. Instead of collecting all demographic information before the patient visit, a mini-registration allows the registration clerk to enter just 4 or 5 data elements such as name, date of birth, chief complaint, and primary care physician (PCP). This brief information can be used to quickly generate an account number, thus preempting delays in ordering critical diagnostic interventions.

The registration clerk can return to the patient's bedside with a rolling laptop computer or a hand-held computer to collect the rest of the information sometime during the patient's stay in the ED. These rolling laptops or hand-held computers communicate with the base computer or server by either radiofrequency technology or docking stations conveniently located throughout the ED. By shifting the timing of registration until after the patient is in the examination room, the first available provider that is free to see the patient does so. This could be the registration clerk, the nurse, or the EP, all processes occurring in parallel.

Some EDs have ambulatory patients stop at a discharge area after ED evaluation to complete the registration process. This also has its advantages. When the remainder of the registration process is shifted to the end of the patient care process, there is an additional opportunity to increase patient satisfaction, answer questions, and intervene in a positive manner.

The only problem with solving front-end delays in the ED is the issue of bed/examination room availability. Bed availability largely depends on the number of patients waiting for diagnostic studies to be completed or patients waiting for admission to an inpatient bed. Front-end reforms will not be effectual unless the entire clinical process is optimized.

Expediting Diagnosis and Treatment

The surest method for expediting diagnosis and treatment is to gain an in-depth understanding of subprocesses that affect rapid diagnosis, and to streamline and simplify them whenever possible. Redundant activities should be obliterated from the process, and duplicate information gathering should be weaned from the system as well. Process change in these areas generally requires a multidisciplinary approach involving either the laboratory or radiology, the ED medical director, the ED nursing director, the administrator responsible for the ancillary functions, and a dedicated team of ED staff that will spearhead the process change.

The EP spends most of his or her time in tedious, nonclinical tasks.[40,41] On a per hour basis, 39 percent is related to direct patient care, and 61 percent is related to indirect patient care. Of the nonclinical time, nearly all of it is spent looking for information (e.g., the current ED chart, the old medical record, laboratory results, and x-ray results), making phone calls to MCOs and PCPs, charting the paper chart, analyzing test results, and a full 15 percent of this time is spent just walking around the department looking for various critical pieces of information. Obviously, this traditional "hunter-gatherer" approach to emergency diagnosis and treatment is inefficient, outmoded, and outdated. To have the time to focus on "high touch" the EP's time must be freed up from these more mundane tasks.

A charting scribe has been used by some health systems in the ED as a means for the EP to decrease the amount of time spent charting.[42] A charting scribe is essentially a personal note taker, trained for 6 to 8 weeks in the basics of physical assessment and patient history. Other systems include dictation systems, voice recognition systems, and chief complaint–based template-charting systems, all of which variably reduce the physician's charting time.

Busy EDs may also use a dedicated communications nurse to manage all incoming telephone calls from PCPs, family members, and MCOs. This reduces total telephone time for the EP.

Because most nonclinical time is spent looking for clinical information, it only makes sense to develop strategies to accelerate providing completed laboratory and x-ray results to the EP. As an example, an easy process change is for x-ray films to be placed in a central location within the ED, giving the EP the ability to take a "quick look" at all x-ray films before the radiograph is viewed by the radiologist. This saves time spent searching for misplaced x-ray studies and waiting for a radiologist reading of the film. Patient care will not be compromised by this approach because studies have shown that there is relatively little disagreement between EPs and radiologists' reading of plain films.[43–46] Examples of other methods used by EDs to expedite information transfer include maintaining a charge nurse without clinical duties who monitors ancillary status and notifies the EP as diagnostic tests are completed. Often, EDs will free up beds by having ambulatory and less ill patients wait for results in a diagnostic waiting area, which frees beds of ancillary wait times.

Increasingly, physician groups are using physician profiling as a method to affect physician test-ordering behavior (Chapter 32).[47] Physician profiling consists of documenting and tracking physician ancillary use and giving this information back to the practitioner. Most physicians do not know how their practice patterns relate to their peers. An opportunity not yet optimized exists within emergency medicine physician management groups to develop databases of clinical ancillary test ordering by physician, chief complaint, level of service, ICD-9 code, and geographical region. Such a database could also track outcomes and become the basis for the development of evidence-based data-centric practice guidelines in emergency medicine.

In addition to the "traditional" practice of emergency medicine, advances in technology are enabling EPs to increase their scope of practice considerably. In the past, EPs were not allowed to administer thrombolytics to patients with acute myocardial infarction. As the benefit of rapid thrombolytic therapy has become paramount in the cardiology and emergency literature, EPs now administer this drug primarily. In fact, the decreased mortality of acute myocardial infarct patients is now largely due to interventions by EPs.

Just as an EP could not perform rapid sequence intubation as recently as 1990 in some hospitals, EPs now do this as a routine part of their practice along with conscious sedation, fiberoptic laryngoscopy, and other procedures previously limited to anesthesiologists.

Another new development in the diagnostic armamentarium for EPs is the ultrasonogram. It is currently believed that within the next few years, ED ultrasonography will become the standard of care.[48,49] Ultrasonography is a powerful tool to enable rapid diagnosis and facilitate procedures. The American College of Emergency Physicians has adopted a position statement supporting the immediate availability of ED ultrasonography on a 24-hour basis for physicians trained and credentialed in its use. Bedside ultrasonography enhances patient diagnosis, decreases the need to obtain emergency scans, decreases the need to send patients to other areas of the hospital that are not equipped to manage hemodynamically unstable patients, and may result in a shorter decision time for patient transfer to a trauma center when indicated.

Admissions Process

A successful admissions process will directly increase ED capacity, decrease patient turnaround times, increase patient satisfaction, and decrease staff stress. Long ED LOSs for admitted patients increases the LOS for all patients in the ED.[50] Unfortunately, the admissions process is often the most laborious and emotionally exhausting process in evaluation of the emergency patient. The basic steps needed to admit a patient include the following:

- EP decides to admit patient
- EP calls PCP or MCO
- EP waits for PCP or MCO to call back
- EP and PCP or MCO discuss case
- EP orders additional diagnostic tests per PCP or MCO request
- EP calls back PCP or MCO after additional diagnostics are completed
- PCP gives orders to the nurse, MCO makes arrangements for transfer to MCO participating facility, or MCO sends admissions gatekeeper to ED to evaluate patient
- ED nurse submits bed request to bed control
- Bed control contacts floor/unit with bed request
- Floor/unit charge nurse contacts bed control with bed assignment
- Bed control contacts ED with bed assignment
- ED nurse attempts to call floor/unit to give report
- Inevitably, floor/unit refuses to take report for some reason, usually "nurse busy"
- ED nurse attempts to call floor/unit to give report
- ED nurse takes patient to floor

This process can take more than 2 hours, with some institutions reporting maximal waits of several *days* before an inpatient bed is assigned.[51] Methods to decrease delays in the admissions process involve giving the EP admit authority (granted in medical staff bylaws: i.e., the EP makes the decision to admit where and to whom, but does not write admission orders), requesting beds immediately after the decision to admit has been made (while concurrently placing a call to the PCP or MCO), engendering nurse to nurse bed requests and bypassing bed control, and decentralizing bed availability (secret) information.

The most successful EDs have access to inpatient bed status availability by means of a computerized bed-tracking system. This prevents much of the delay that occurs as a result of individual inpatient floors delaying admissions. Other EDs may adopt a no-delay nurse report, with a faxed nurse report copy being sent to the floor/unit,[52] only one phone call attempt, and the patient is immediately delivered.

Another strategy is to eliminate discharge holding of patient beds. Discharge holding occurs when discharged patients continue to occupy bed space while awaiting a family member or transportation. In addition, housekeeping services must be readily available to clean beds at a moment's notice. In one ED, a housekeeping team remains in the ED for the sole purpose of going to the floor/unit to rapidly clean a vacated bed soon after it is available.

Many hospitals also choose to create an admissions holding unit for patients waiting for inpatient beds. This is a powerful strategy because it facilitates rapid ED bed turnover. Rapid ED bed turnover will in turn decrease ED diversion or reroute status and increase ED patient throughput. Administrators and chief executive officers (CEOs) of hospitals must realize that whenever the ED is forced to go on diversion because of overcapacity (often because of admissions being held indefinitely in the ED), ambulance traffic no longer comes to the ED. Diversion of ambulances has an effect not only on the admission rate or volume to the hospital (a primary concern to a hospital CEO) but may also result in patients being diverted to a hospital that does not participate with the MCO (a primary concern to the MCO medical managers).

Flexible Staffing Options

At some point every day of the week in any ED in the country, patient volume becomes overwhelming, patient wait times increase, patient LOS increase, and staff become overwhelmed. To address this problem, the ED must adopt some flexibility in staffing. For example, one ED actually planned for a staffing solution to the seasonal increase in ED patient census related with influenza outbreak.[53] It developed a protocol for an additional team of personnel who were called to work if the hourly ED census was 25 percent or more of the past year's hourly patient volume. Extra examination rooms were made available, and the left-without-being-seen rate decreased in this study by 37 percent. This example of a flexible staffing option represented a statistically significant improvement in ED efficiency and quality of care.

Others use volume triggers to activate the "backup" system of calling in an extra nurse or physician. The accepted volume trigger is 5 percent of the daily volume.[54] In other words, if this number of patients is reached, the charge nurse may call in the next scheduled physician early or ask the current physician(s) to stay from 2 to 4 hours past their shift until the backlog of patients has been cleared. The charge nurse may also call in any additional nurses required to care for the increased volume.

Clinical Pathways

The three most validated clinical pathways currently in routine use in emergency medicine are for ankle and knee radiographs,[55–65] chest pain,[66–76] and asthma.[77–79] Many individual EDs develop conjointly with nursing individualized clinical protocols and pathways for use in their particular ED to expedite and standardize care. Continuing research in this area will produce greater standardization of care delivery and increase appropriate resource utilization to optimize patient care delivered in the ED. The reader is referred to Chapter 29 for an in-depth discussion of this approach to care.

Nonurgent (Fast Track) Care

With the appropriate triage system, responsible choice of alternative treatment sites will be possible. These will include urgent care centers within EDs, urgent care centers at a location away from the hospital, or even committed physician offices. Alternative treatment locations become important as overflow because unavail-

able office appointment times during the day and after-hours illness remain an ongoing problem. Urgicenters represent a well-recognized and appreciated source of low overhead care,[80] although cost is better contained by a physician's office that offers extended hours.[81] *With regard to urgicenter or office alternatives, a number of important issues must be considered:*

- Location
  - They must be convenient and easily accessible from the patient's home.
  - Reasonable access to a higher level of care must be available.
- Personnel/equipment
  - Proper personnel and equipment should be present, with particular attention being given for those who might deteriorate during their stay.
  - A pleasant, well-lit environment should greet the patient.
  - Proper computer/electronic systems should be available to transmit clinical and billing information.
  - Minimum standards of care should be established for physicians and staff.
- Quality management
  - Documentation should be equal to the standard of emergency medicine.
  - Adverse outcomes should be reported to the health care plan and the PCP.
  - Clinical summaries including 24- and 72-hour return rates should be reported.
  - PCP notification of clinical condition and disposition should occur.
  - Regular quality assurance reports for both health care plan patients and summary total should be reported to the plan on a regular basis.
  - Standard operating procedures should be established.

In summary, the same high standard of care should be present whether the location is an ED, an urgent care center, or a physician's office. Board certification in the appropriate primary care field, such as internal medicine or family practice, should be required, although emergency medicine would be an appropriate alternative. The best use of the ED for these nonurgent cases would be avoiding it altogether if the appropriate acuity were present and a facility available. Alternative treatment facilities fitting the preceding standards must be made available onsite or offsite from the ED.

MCO executives need to bear in mind, however, that urgent care centers have the potential to be used for convenience care rather than truly urgent care. In other words, it is more convenient for members to access care through the urgent care center than from their primary physician during normal office hours. This is a positive attribute from the standpoint of member satisfaction (especially for families with two working spouses) but a potentially negative attribute from the standpoint of efficiency and continuity of care. This dilemma may be partially addressed through the uses of differential copayments for routine care, urgent care, and care received through an actual ED. In any event, it is important for clinical information from the urgent care center to be provided efficiently to the member's primary physician.

TECHNOLOGY IMPACT

The current state of ED management systems lags far behind that of other industries. Emergency medicine processes are still largely manual, paper-based, human-input dependent, and replete with all the inadequacies and errors characteristic of such a system. In addition, many of the software systems that exist today do no more than automate the poor manual processes currently in use.[82] EPs are essentially knowledge workers, and their practice revolves fundamentally on the rapid interpretation of large amounts of data. Patient care in the ED depends on the EP having information immediately available to make rapid clinical decisions.

Most emergency medicine information technology experts agree that rapid information retrieval is the key to improved EDs and quality of care in the next decade.[82–88] Ubiquitous computing will characterize the ED of the near future (5 years). Given the rapid pace and acute nature of

emergency care, the focus of technology implementation in the next several years should be on how to acquire, save, transfer, manage, and present clinical information in the required amount at the exact time needed to make a clinical decision. Information retrieval will be characterized by the right amount of information at the right time for the right person whenever and wherever it is needed.

Although there are hospital systems currently in place that automatically store and collect patient data from the hospital information database, this information is rarely available to the EP at the time needed to aid in clinical decision making. In fact, most hospitals have multiple disparate software systems that do not communicate with each other.

The problem is, of course, that the true clinical patient record does not reside within any one given system. The patient's clinical information resides partially in the laboratory database; in the radiology database; in the pharmacy database; in the admissions, discharge, transfer database; in the hospital financial database; in the outpatient clinic database; and so on. Health care costs are high, in part, because no one system at the time of this writing can provide physicians with useful, complete, up-to-date information regarding patient care at the point of service. Thus, medical evaluations are repeated, health care personnel enter information multiple times, medical errors are made because of lack of complete information; ultimately, costs increase and patient care suffers.

The amount of rework and redundancy exhibited in today's management of patient information is staggering. Vital signs must be documented not only by the triage nurse, but by the physician, by the treatment nurse, and multiple times by every health care worker that has contact with a patient. Even if it takes only 3 minutes to gain vital signs information manually, by the time six people have documented the same information, 18 minutes of patient care time have been lost. However, systems currently exist that enable automatic physiological information to be documented into a patient's medical record as often as needed without human intervention or human documentation. For an ED that sees 200 patients per day, 18 minutes × 200 patients amounts to a significant increase in the amount of time available for direct patient care.

At present, many ED systems are configured such that direct data entry by the clinician or nurse provider is required. Such systems function adequately when the ED is not busy. However, because most EDs today are over capacity and extremely busy, in many cases manually entered data will not get entered at all by providers. Thus the quality of data in such a system is suspect. Purchasers of software systems must realize that any system that requires clinical providers to become data entry personnel is bound for failure. Manually entered data will continue to exhibit similar inadequacies to paper-based systems, replete with errors, inadequate documentation, lack of consistency, and so forth. Multiple technologies exist today that enable automatic data collection, and the use of these technologies is currently not optimized in the ED or health care setting.

Federal Express has become a multibillion dollar enterprise because of only one trait: its ability to track its processes. Federal Express has revolutionized the use of inexpensive bar code technology in its processing of packages by using a proven technology that is inexpensive and reliable and that makes information readily available to anyone that might need it. In 2000, any consumer with a computer can track his or her package within seconds; however, the ED physician has trouble locating a patient chart that might be within 20 feet.

Moving patients through an ED or through a health care system has at least some attributes in common with moving boxes from one location to another. A patient could be easily tracked through the process of ED care with a simple bar code system. This process would be automatically time-stamped and personnel-stamped as well. One ED studied the use of bar code technology in patient triage and found that accuracy was maintained under all conditions for longer than when written by hand.[89] A few other examples would include the automation of order entry, nursing documentation, process of man-

aging laboratory specimen flow, and delivery of medications. Bar code technology can be used to efficiently track any process in the ED with minimal capital investment.

Actual patient and personnel tracking can be accomplished with inexpensive off-the-shelf technologies available and widely used by other industries. An inexpensive infrared or radio frequency badge worn by staff and patients could be used to track physician-patient and nurse-patient interaction times automatically. Patient tracking in the ED would become automatic as sensors captured patient movement through the department, to and from x-ray, etc. No longer would the nurse have to hand write "Patient left for x-ray," "Patient back from x-ray," and so forth.

Technology use in the ED should be geared toward enabling processes to occur at any location within the ED. Often, specific areas become bottlenecks in patient flow. If the patient must wait at the registration desk for initial registration, then that physical area becomes a bottleneck. Use of portable 8 1/2 × 11 hand-held computers with radiofrequency capability allows the patient to be registered in any location within the ED and enables bedside registration. Biometric devices such as iris scanning, fingerprint, or hand morphology can also be used in a portable fashion for instant registration and identification of patients. Similarly, point of care testing or bedside testing for laboratory blood tests can be achieved with the use of a simple hand-held I-Stat device. In fact, bedside testing is now available for previously complicated laboratory tests such as cardiac enzymes to enable rapid evaluation of patients with chest pain. Thus, the physical location of the laboratory no longer has to create a bottleneck for patient flow through the ED.

Technology use in the ED should also be geared toward automating routine communications required to deliver patient care. Physicians and nurses should not need to waste time "hunting and gathering" patient-relevant information given the technologies that exist today. One commercially available ED tracking system automatically pages the physician (or nurse) when laboratory results have been completed,[90] and those results are immediately available on computer. Another system functions as a complete clinical information database, with patient information from multiple sources available with just a single mouse click.[91] Most ED tracking systems also have the ability to automatically electronically transfer information regarding the ED visit to the patient's PCP.

Technology implementation must result in higher quality patient care. Improvements in patient care and patient outcomes should be the natural reason for any process improvement undertaken in a hospital or ED setting. ED systems will have to be well integrated with all possible sources of patient information to avoid errors that could otherwise cause detrimental patient care. Pharmacy systems must be "smart" such that the system can automatically alert clinicians for any potential drug interactions or allergies. These systems should also be able to automatically suggest more efficacious medications given the information that already exists regarding a particular patient. Tracking systems should automatically alert the physician or charge nurse when time limits have been exceeded for diagnostic evaluations to avoid delays in patient care. Advanced computer-assisted triage systems should help initiate diagnostic tests and indicate the need for necessary treatment on the basis of clinical guidelines. Authorization and payment for emergency care from third-party payers should occur automatically (and electronically) in real time on the basis of the medical evaluation and available data while the patient is in the ED.

No discussion of technology is complete without reference to the Internet. The single biggest problem with the current process of patient care in the ED is lack of current and correct clinical information at the time of patient presentation for care. Appropriate information in the appropriate manner at the time of patient evaluation is the key to improving care delivery in the ED setting. This requires not only that disparate systems within one hospital communicate and interchange data but that hospitals and EDs across the country communicate and interchange patient relevant data in real time as well. Add to this the ability to access MCO eligibility information and pro-

vide the MCO with data regarding the encounter, and the Internet serves as the means to facilitate communication between the multiple potential parties to an ED encounter.

A revolution in information sharing will take place out of necessity within the upcoming decade. Patient information will be shared by clinicians in a manner that is Web-based such that it is immediately accessible at any time to any provider with Internet access.

Even now, patients are accessing the Internet before visiting the ED for a particular illness. It is not uncommon for patients to come to the ED with articles downloaded from their favorite healthcare portal regarding the symptoms they have been experiencing. To quote the futurist Alan Kay, "The best way to predict the future is to invent it." Those who understand how information is best managed to optimize timely patient care need to create the future of information technology in emergency medicine. The technologies necessary to complete this task are currently available, although not well organized.

The use of the Internet, along with any use of electronic communications between different parties involved in either clinical care or the business of health care, will need to conform to the mandates under the Health Insurance Portability and Accountability Act (HIPAA) (Chapters 35, 36, and 67). These mandates require policies and procedures for maintaining high levels of data security and privacy, with special focus on protected health information about individual patients or members of an MCO. Standards for most of the business transactions (e.g., eligibility checking, claims, authorizations) are also mandated under HIPAA, as are new standards for identifier coding for providers and health plans. These mandates will not come into effect until 2002 at the earliest, at which time conformance will be required by all providers using electronic data interchange (including the ED) and the MCO. The presence of these mandated transactions and identifier codes should go a long way toward simplifying electronic communications between parties through the Internet and facilitating appropriate care and business relationships.

OPPORTUNITIES WITH MANAGED CARE

As managed care penetration grows nationwide, EPs have an opportunity to partner with MCOs in providing improved patient care delivery. Under capitated contracting arrangements, EDs can strategically position themselves to be proactive. Demand management programs (Chapter 18) are becoming more commonplace and include limited use of telephone triage programs, ED nurse screening programs, and EMS stratified response programs.[92] It is logical for emergency medicine to take the lead in providing demand management services. Physicians are already present 24 hours per day, and the nursing staff are already trained to perform initial assessments. By championing demand management, EPs could be viewed as partners with managed care rather than adversaries.[93] Additional discussion around 24-hour medical advice lines may be found in Chapter 11, "Nurse Advice Services," by Barry Wolcott in *Best Practices in Medical Management* (Aspen, 1998, Kongstvedt and Plocher, Editors).

Other areas currently being evaluated by emergency medicine experts include observation medicine. Recent studies in the medical literature have shown that patients with many clinical conditions that routinely used to be admitted may now safely be discharged home after a period of observation in the ED. The best current example is the chest pain observation protocol that many EDs use for low-risk patients with normal electrocardiograms. Patients are evaluated with three sets of serial enzymes drawn 4 hours apart followed by a stress test. If all are negative, the patient can safely be discharged home. A successful observation unit can be used to increase diagnostic accuracy as in the case of chest pain, and it can reduce the need for an inpatient admission without exposing the patient to medical risk.[94] Additional discussion around "fast track" EDs and chest pain observation units

may be found in Chapter 13, "The Fast Track Emergency Department," by Angela Zotos, and Chapter 14, "Chest Pain Centers" by Suzanne White, in *Best Practices in Medical Management* (Aspen, 1998, Kongstvedt and Plocher, Editors).

A substantial opportunity exists for managed care to partner with emergency medicine. Despite managed care growth over the last 5 years, nationwide the total number of ED visits has continued to escalate. MCOs understand that a significant consumer demand exists for provision of unscheduled medical care. In many cases, patients come to the ED for convenience (i.e., consumers want convenience in accessing the health care system, just as they do other services in their lives). Managed care should continue to partner with emergency medicine in providing unscheduled medical care by rewarding higher performing EDs with contracts to deliver nonurgent care at a favorable rate, while reimbursing appropriately for bona fide emergencies. In areas such as development of statistical methods for triage where both the ED and managed care benefit, managed care should take the lead in development and implementation.

MCOs have a significant opportunity when it comes to optimizing use of technology in delivering online real-time insurance verification and/or authorization for admissions. MCOs can also aid in the delivery of health care by making clinical information available at the point of service. If a database of clinical information exists, MCOs should attempt to make this information available to providers of emergency or unscheduled medical care. EDs in turn should provide the MCO and the patient's physician with real-time (or nearly real-time) information about the ED encounter. The advent of mandated standards under HIPAA should serve to significantly enhance the ability to provide this electronic, two-way communication by means of the Internet, as well as ensure that proper security and privacy are maintained.

REFERENCES AND NOTES

1. G.L. Larkin, Ethical Issues in Emergency Medicine: Ethical Issues of Managed Care, *Emergency Medicine Clinics of North America* 17, 2 (1999): 397–415.

2. R.W. Derlet and G.P. Young, Managed Care and Emergency Medicine: Conflicts, Federal Law, and California Legislation, *Annals of Emergency Medicine* 30, 3 (1997): 292–300.

3. R.W. Derlet and A. Ledesma, How Do Prudent Laypeople Define an Emergency Medical Condition? *Journal of Emergency Medicine* 17 (1999): 413–418.

4. R.W. Derlet and L. Ray, Emergency Department Acuity: Who Is Really Non-urgent? *Academic Emergency Medicine* 3 (1996): 499.

5. M. Afilalo, A. Guttman, A. Colacone, et al., ED Use and Misuse, *Journal of Emergency Medicine* 13 (1995): 259–264.

6. R.W. Derlet, D.J. Kinser, L. Ray, et al., Prospective Identification and Triage of Nonemergent Patients out of an ED, *Annals of Emergency Medicine* 25 (1995): 215–223.

7. U.S. General Accounting Office: *Hospital EDs: Unevenly Affected by Growth and Change in Patient Use* (Washington, DC: U.S. Government Printing Office, 1993).

8. U.S. Department of Health and Human Services, Office of Inspector General: *Controlling Emergency Room Use: State Medical Reports* (Washington, DC: Office of Evaluations and Inspections, 06-90-00181, 1993).

9. *The Emergency Medical Treatment and Active Labor Act.* 42, USC 1395 dd (1986) Pub. L. No. 99-272, 9121, 1986.

10. American College of Emergency Physicians, American Hospital Association, Public Citizen, American Association of Retired Persons, EMTALA Working Group, 1996–1998.

11. G.P. Young and D. Sklar, Health Care Reform and Emergency Medicine, *Annals of Emergency Medicine* 25 (1995): 666–674.

12. R.W. Derlet and B. Hamilton, The Impact of HMO Care Authorization Policy on an ED before California's New Managed Care Law, *Academic Emergency Medicine* 3 (1996): 338–344.

13. J.C. Brillman, D. Doezema, D. Tandberg, et al., Triage: Limitations in Predicting Need for Emergent Care and Hospital Admission, *Annals of Emergency Medicine* 21, 4 (1996): 493–500.

14. H.H. Osborn, Health Maintenance Organizations: Managed Care or Mismanaged Care? *Annals of Emergency Medicine* 27, 2 (1996): 225–228.

15. Kaiser Family Foundation/Harvard University National Survey of Americans' Views on Consumer Protection in Managed Care, January 1998.

16. R.W. Derlet and A. Ledesma, How Do Prudent Laypeople Define an Emergency Medical Condition? *Journal of Emergency Medicine* 17 (1999): 413–418.

17. R.M. Williams, The Cost of Visits to Emergency Departments, *New England Journal of Medicine* 334 (1996): 642–646.

18. R. Steinbrook, ed., The Role of the Emergency Department, *New England Journal of Medicine* 334 (1996): 657–658.

19. L.C. Baker and L.S. Baker, Excess Cost of Emergency Department Visits for Nonurgent Care, *Health Affairs* 13 (1994): 162–171.

20. P. Krochmal and R. Tamrah, Increased Health Care Costs Associated with ED Overcrowding, *American Journal of Emergency Medicine* 12 (1994): 265–266.

21. Emergency Care: The State of the Union. The Advisory Board Company, 1998.

22. W. Fields, ed., Defending America's Safety Net, American College of Emergency Physicians 1998–1999 Safety Net Task Force Report (Dallas, TX: ACEP, 1999).

23. J.W. Kenagy, D.M. Berwick, and M.F. Shore, Service Quality in Health Care. *JAMA* 281, 7 (1999): 661–665.

24. A.J. Booth, C.J. Harrison, G.J. Gardener, et al., Waiting Times and Patient Satisfaction in the Accident and Emergency Department, *Archives of Emergency Medicine* 9 (1992): 162–168.

25. K.J. McNamara, Patients Leaving the ED without Being Seen by a Physician: Is Same Day Follow Up Indicated? *American Journal of Emergency Medicine* 13 (1995): 136–140.

26. A.C. Southall, and V.V. Harris, Patient ED Turnaround Times: A Comparative Review. *American Journal of Emergency Medicine* 17, 2 (1999): 151–153.

27. D.A. Thompson, P.R. Yarnold, D.R. Williams, and S.L. Adams, Effects of Actual Waiting, Perceived Waiting Time, Information Delivery and Expressive Quality on Patient Satisfaction in the Emergency Department, *Annals of Emergency Medicine* 28, 6 (1996): 657–665.

28. D.A. Thompson, P.R. Yarnold, S.L. Adams, and A.B. Spacone, How Accurate Are Waiting Time Perceptions of Patients in the Emergency Department? *Annals of Emergency Medicine* 28, 6 (1996): 652–656.

29. K.D. Bopp, How Patients Evaluate the Quality of Ambulatory Medical Encounters: A Marketing Perspective, *Journal of Health Care Marketing* 10 (1990): 6–15.

30. D.N. Kyriacou, V. Ricketts, P.L. Dyne, et al. A 5-Year Time Study Analysis of Emergency Department Patient Care Efficiency, *Annals of Emergency Medicine* 34, 3 (1999): 326–335.

31. P.E. Pisek, Section 1: Evidence Based Quality Improvement, Principles, and Perspectives—Quality Improvement Methods in Clinical Medicine, *Pediatrics* 103, 1 (1999): 203–214.

32. R.H. Brook, E.A. McGlynn, and P.D. Cleary, Quality of Health Care. Part 2: Measuring Quality of Care, *New England Journal of Medicine* 335 (1996): 966–970.

33. L.A. Johnson, Triage: Limitations and Opportunities, *Annals of Emergency Medicine* 28, 3 (1996): 372–374.

34. D.A. Wachter, J.C. Brillman, J. Lewis, and R.E. Sapien, Pediatric Telephone Triage Protocols: Standardized Decisionmaking or a False Sense of Security? *Annals of Emergency Medicine* 33, 4 (1999): 388–394.

35. D.C. Seaberg and B.A. MacLeod, Correlation between Triage Nurse and Physician Ordering of ED Tests, *American Journal of Emergency Medicine* 16, 1 (1998): 8–11.

36. L. Ropp, R. Blouin, C. Dulberg, et al., Radiograph Ordering: Agreement between the Triage Nurse and the Physician in a Pediatric Emergency Department, *Journal of Emergency Medicine* 8 (1990): 697–700.

37. T.P. Klassen, L.J. Rott, T. Sutcliffe, et al., A Randomized, Controlled Trial of Radiograph Ordering for Extremity Trauma in a Pediatric Emergency Department, *Annals of Emergency Medicine* 22 (1993): 1524–1529.

38. I.G. Stiell, G. Greenberg, R.D. McKnight, et al., Triage Nurse Use of Decision Rules for Radiography in Ankle Injuries, *Annals of Emergency Medicine* 22 (1993): 948 (abstract).

39. C.L. McArthur and M. Thomas, Comparison of Triage Nurses Versus Emergency Physician Ordering of Extremity Radiographs, *American Journal of Emergency Medicine* 13 (1995): 248–250.

40. J. Hollingsworth et al. How Do Physicians and Nurses Spend Their Time in the Emergency Department? *Annals of Emergency Medicine* (January 1998): 87–91.

41. L. Graff et al. Emergency Physician Workload: A Time Study, *Annals of Emergency Medicine* (July 1993): 1156–1163.

42. D. Witt, Transcription Services in the ED, *American Journal of Emergency Medicine* 13, 1 (1995): 34–36.

43. K.C. Lufkin et al., Radiologists' Review of Radiographs Interpreted Confidently by Emergency Physicians Infrequently Leads to Changes in Patient Management, *Annals of Emergency Medicine* 31, 2 (1998): 202–207.

44. L.A. Nitowski et al., The Rate of Clinically Significant Plain Radiograph Misinterpretation by Faculty in an Emergency Medicine Residency Program, *Academic Emergency Medicine* 3, 8 (1996): 782–789.

45. J.E. Brunswick et al., Radiographic Interpretation in the Emergency Department, *American Journal of Emergency Medicine* 14, 4 (1996): 346–348.

46. M.C. Gratton et al., Clinically Significant Radiograph Misinterpretations at an Emergency Medicine Residency Program, *Annals of Emergency Medicine* 19, 5 (1990): 497–502.

47. E.A. Ramoska, Information Sharing Can Reduce Laboratory Use by Emergency Physicians, *American Journal of Emergency Medicine* 16, 1 (1998): 34–36.

48. T.K. Tandy and S. Hoffenberg, Emergency Department Ultrasound Services by Emergency Physicians: Model for Gaining Hospital Approval, *Annals of Emergency Medicine* 29, 3 (1997): 367–374.

49. W. Durston, M.L. Carl, and W. Guerra, Patient Satisfaction and Diagnostic Accuracy with Ultrasound by Emergency Physicians, *American Journal of Emergency Medicine* 17, 7 (1999): 642–646.

50. J. Bazarian et al., Do Admitted Patients Held in the Emergency Department Impact the Throughput of Treat-and-Release Patients? *Academic Emergency Medicine* December (1996): 1113–1118.

51. Personal experience at current facility, 1999–2000.

52. L.M. Vescio, S.P. Donahoe, and C. Gentile, An Organization-Wide Approach to Improving ED Patient Satisfaction: One Community Teaching Hospital's Experience, *Journal of Emergency Nursing* 25, 3 (1999): 192–196.

53. K.N. Shaw and J.M. Lavelle, VESAS: A Solution to Seasonal Fluctuations in Emergency Department Census, *Annals of Emergency Medicine* 32, 6 (1998): 698–702.

54. Personal communication with Dr. James Espinosa, Chairman, Overlook Hospital, New Jersey, July 1999.

55. I.G. Steill, G.H. Greenberg, and R.D. McKnight, A Study To Develop Clinical Decision Rules for the Use of Radiography in Acute Ankle Injuries, *Annals of Emergency Medicine* 21 (1992): 384–390.

56. I.G. Steill, G.H. Greenberg, and R.D. McKnight, Decision Rules for the Use of Radiography in Acute Ankle Injuries: Refinement and Prospective Validation, *JAMA* 269 (1993): 1127–1132.

57. E.C. Pigman, R.K. Klug, and S. Sanford, Evaluation of the Ottawa Clinical Decision Rules for the Use of Radiography in Acute Ankle and Midfoot Injuries in the Emergency Department: An Independent Site Assessment, *Annals of Emergency Medicine* 24 (1994): 41–45.

58. I.G. Steill, G.H. Greenberg, and R.D. McKnight, The "Real" Ottawa Ankle Rules, *Annals of Emergency Medicine* 27 (1996): 103–104.

59. G.R. Auleley, L. Keroull, P. Durieux, et al., Validation of the Ottawa Ankle Rules in France: A Study in the Surgical Emergency Department of a Teaching Hospital, *Annals of Emergency Medicine* 32, 1 (1998): 14–18.

60. R.J. Markert, M.E. Walley, T.G. Guttman, et al., A Pooled Analysis of the Ottawa Ankle Rules on Adults in the ED, *American Journal of Emergency Medicine* 16, 6 (1998): 564–567.

61. G. Nichol, I.G. Steill, G.A. Wells, et al., An Economic Analysis of the Ottawa Knee Rule, *Annals of Emergency Medicine* 34, 4 (1999): 438–447.

62. I.G. Steill, G.A. Wells, I. McDowell, et al., Use of Radiography in Acute Knee Injuries: Need for Clinical Decision Rules, *Academic Emergency Medicine* 2 (1995): 966–973.

63. I.G. Steill, G.H. Greenberg, G.A. Wells, et al., Derivation of a Decision Rule for the Use of Radiography in Acute Knee Injuries, *Annals of Emergency Medicine* 26 (1995): 405–413.

64. I.G. Steill, G.H. Greenberg, G.A. Wells, et al., Prospective Validation of a Decision Rule for the Use of Radiography in Acute Knee Injuries, *JAMA* 275 (1996): 611–615.

65. I.G. Steill, G.A. Wells, R.H. Hoag, et al., Implementation of the Ottawa Knee Rule for the Use of Radiography in Acute Knee Injuries, *JAMA* 278 (1997): 2075–2079.

66. R.J. Rydman, R.J. Zalenski, R.R. Roberts, et al., Patient Satisfaction with an Emergency Department Chest Pain Observation Unit, *Annals of Emergency Medicine* 29, 1 (1997): 109–115.

67. R.J. Zalenski, R.J. Rydman, M. McCarren, et al., Evaluation of a Short-Stay Diagnostic Protocol for an Emergency Department Chest Pain Observation Unit, *Annals of Emergency Medicine* 29 (1997): 99–108.

68. R.J. Zalenski, R.J. Rydman, R.R. Roberts, et al., Ruling Out AMI in a Chest Pain Center without Hospital Admission: Potential Utility of a Protocol Requiring Exercise Testing (abstract), *Academic Emergency Medicine* 2 (1995): 365.

69. L.G. Graff, J. Dallara, M.A. Ross, et al., Impact on the Care of the Emergency Department Chest Pain Patient from the Chest Pain Evaluation Registry (CHEPER) Study, *The American Journal of Cardiology* 80, 5 (1997): 563–568.

70. H.P. Selker, R.J. Zalenski, E.M. Antman, et al., An Evaluation of Technologies for Identifying Acute Cardiac Ischemia in the Emergency Department: A Report from a National Heart Attack Alert Program Working Group, *Annals of Emergency Medicine* 29, 1 (1997): 13–87.

71. H.P. Selker, R.J. Zalenski, E.M. Antman, et al., An Evaluation of Technologies for Identifying Acute Cardiac Ischemia in the Emergency Department: Executive Summary of a National Heart Attack Alert Program Working Group, *Annals of Emergency Medicine* 29, 1 (1997): 1–12.

72. L. Goldman, E.F. Cook, D.A. Brand, et al., A Computer Protocol To Predict Myocardial Infarction in Emergency Department Patients with Chest Pain, *New England Journal of Medicine* 318 (1988): 797–803.

73. L. Goldman, M. Weinberg, M. Weisberg, et al., A Computer-Derived Protocol To Aid in the Diagnosis of Emergency Room Patients with Chest Pain, *New England Journal of Medicine* 307 (1982): 588–596.

74. L. Goldman, E.F. Cook, P.A. Johnson, et al., Prediction of the Need for Intensive Care in Patients Who Come to Emergency Departments with Acute Chest Pain, *New England Journal of Medicine* 334 (1996): 1498–1504.

75. W.B. Gibler, G.P. Young, J.R. Hedges, et al., Acute Myocardial Infarction in Chest Pain Patients with Nondiagnostic EKGs: Serial CK-MB Sampling in the Emergency Department, *Annals of Emergency Medicine* 21 (1992): 504–512.

76. A. Qamar, C. McPerson, J. Babb, et al., The Goldman Algorithm Revisited: Prospective Evaluation of a Computer-Derived Algorithm Versus Unaided Physician Judgment in Suspected Acute Myocardial Infarction, *American Heart Journal* 138, 4 (1999): 705–709.

77. R. Goldberg, L. Chan, P. Haley, et al., Critical Pathway for the Emergency Department of Acute Asthma: Effect on Resource Utilization, *Annals of Emergency Medicine* 31, 5 (1998): 562–567.

78. S.E. Emond, P.G. Woodruff, E.Y. Lee, et al., Effect of an Emergency Department Program on Acute Asthma Care, *Annals of Emergency Medicine* 34, 3 (1999): 321–325.

79. S.E. Emond, C.A. Camargo, and R.M. Nowak, Advances, Opportunities, and the New Asthma Guidelines, *Annals of Emergency Medicine* 31 (1998): 590–594.

80. J.C. Wong, Efficiency and Effectiveness in the Urgent Care Clinic, *Postgraduate Medicine* 99 (1996): 161–166.

81. C.B. Forrest and B.S. Starfield, The Effect of First Contact Care with Primary Care Clinician on Ambulatory Health Care Expenses, *Journal of Family Practice* 43 (1996): 40–47.

82. T.B. Taylor, Emergency Department Automation and Informatics, 1995, www.acep.org

83. R. SoRelle, ED of the Future: The Next Generation, *Emergency Medicine News* XXII (2000): 1, 1, 32.

84. M.S. Smith, and C.F. Feied, The Next Generation Emergency Department, *Annals of Emergency Medicine* 32, 1 (1998): 65–74.

85. J.M. Teich, The Benefits of Sharing Clinical Information, *Annals of Emergency Medicine* 31, 2 (1998): 274–276.

86. J.M. Teich, Emergency Medical Informatics, *Annals of Emergency Medicine* 30, 5 (1997): 667–669.

87. T.B. Taylor, The Emergency Department of the Future, 1998, www.acep.org

88. D.A. Pollock, D.L. Adams, L.M. Bernardo, et al., Data Elements for Emergency Department Systems, Release 1.0 (DEEDS): A Summary Report, *Annals of Emergency Medicine* 31, 2 (1998): 264–273.

89. G.J. Noordergraaf, J.H. Bouman, E.J. Van Den Brink, et al., Development of Computer-Assisted Patient Control for Use in the Hospital Setting during Mass Casualty Incidents, *American Journal of Emergency Medicine* 14, 3 (1996): 257–261.

90. Medhost, Inc.

91. Personal communication with Craig Feied, MD, Director National Center for Emergency Medicine Informatics, 1999.

92. L.A. Johnson and R.W. Derlet, Conflicts between Managed Care Organizations and Emergency Departments in California, *Western Journal of Medicine* 164 (1996): 137–142.

93. S.J. Dresnick, The Future of the Private Practice of Emergency Medicine, *Annals of Emergency Medicine* 30, 6 (1997): 754–756.

94. H.S. Luft, How Do Health Maintenance Organizations Achieve Their Savings? *New England Journal of Medicine* 298 (1978): 1336–1343.

CHAPTER 22

Case Management and Managed Care

Catherine M. Mullahy

THE CASE MANAGER'S ROLE

Managed care and *case management* are not interchangeable concepts. Managed care is a system of cost containment programs; case management is a process. It is one component in the managed care strategy.

The following definition of case management has been adopted by the developers of the leading credentialing process for case managers, the Commission for Case Manager Certification (CCMC), previously the Certification of Insurance Rehabilitation Specialists Commission (CIRSC): "Case management is a collaborative process which assesses, plans, implements, co-

ordinates, monitors, and evaluates the options and services required to meet an individual's health needs, using communication and available resources to promote quality, cost-effective outcomes." The credentialing group went on to clarify the role by stating that case management is not episodic but "occurs across a continuum of care, addressing ongoing individual needs" rather than being restricted to a single practice setting.[1]

Case managers work in the provider sector in hospitals, rehabilitation facilities, managed care organizations (MCOs), home health agencies, infusion care companies, and other practice settings, as well as in the payer sector, representing employers through third-party administrators (TPAs) or self-administered programs, employed within health maintenance programs or by major insurance carriers. Independent case managers, professionals working outside the medical care provider and claims payer systems, can be found in any of the practice settings mentioned and may also be working directly for a patient or other family member.

Case managers are not the claims police. Though they work to ensure cost-effective treatment, case managers are not overrated number crunchers who review treatment simply to find the cheapest scenario. Case managers are coordinators of care, catalysts, problem solvers, facilitators, impartial advocates, and educators.[2] They are professional collaborators with physicians and negotiators with durable medical equipment providers, home health care agen-

Catherine M. Mullahy, RN, CRRN, CCM, is a consultant and spokesperson for the case management industry. She is founder and president of Options Unlimited, a medical case management and benefits consulting firm in Huntington, New York. Mullahy is chair for the Commission for Case Manager Certification (CCMC) and its executive committee, and has served on ongoing expert panels in connection with the development of the CCM credential since its inception. On the national board of the Case Management Society of America, she chairs its ethics committee and is editor of *The Case Manager* magazine. The second edition of her book, *The Case Manager's Handbook*, published in 1998, was named a 1998 "Book of the Year" by the *American Journal of Nursing*.

This chapter is adapted from C.M. Mullahy, Case Management and Managed Care, in *Best Practices in Medical Management*, ed. P.R. Kongstvedt and D.W. Plocher, pp. 187–217, © 1998, Aspen Publishers, Inc.

cies, therapists, and many other providers. They make certain that the patient is following the treatment plan prescribed by the physician and that the equipment delivered to the home is the equipment that was ordered—not the same bed's super-deluxe version, which costs $400 more per week. As a liaison with insurance claims staff, case managers clarify claims information. With benefits personnel, and in the best interests of the patient and the payer, they sometimes pursue alternatives to the plan package.

PATIENT PROFILE: NOT EVERY CASE NEEDS A CASE MANAGER

For years, it has been known that most health care costs are generated by the 3 percent to 5 percent of patients that are at high risk, critically injured, or suffering from a chronic disease. As an example, in one 10-month period, one firm spent more than $1.8 million in health care benefits for its employees and their dependents (2,520 covered lives). Half of that cost was distributed to 30 individuals (4 percent of the employees). This means that half of the benefit dollars spent—more than $900,000—was focused on 1.1 percent of the total covered population. Twenty-two employees spent $588,702; expressed differently, 3 percent of the employees accounted for 33 percent of the group's total in paid claims, or 0.9 percent—*less* than 1 percent of those covered—spent 33 percent of the dollars.[3]

In an insurer's review of its plan year covering 11,000 employees, a report showed health benefits expenditures of $36 million. A program designed to flag each case totaling more than $50,000 produced 35 cases responsible for $5 million in benefits. Those 35 cases represented 0.3 percent of the employees; less than one-half of 1 percent of the group spent 14 percent of the group's dollars.[4] This is the central message of this chapter: you do not have to manage all of the patients all of the time. You do have to track those complex cases, those patients who are most likely to fall through the cracks in our health care delivery system because of the layers of care they require.

By developing systems to identify and manage the high-risk, high-cost cases (cancer, acquired immune deficiency syndrome [AIDS], stroke, transplant, head injury, severe burns, high-risk pregnancy, neonates, spinal cord injuries, neuromuscular diseases, and so on) from day one, case management promotes quality care and contains costs. By wrapping the case management approach around all lines of medical coverage, case managers can be appropriately attentive to potentially problematic cases, more creative in problem solving, and better able to address spiraling expenses before they take off. The cost-to-savings ratio will vary depending on the case. (If a case manager is not saving any money, he or she is doing something wrong.) At the low end, savings might be 1:3; at the high end, for a well-managed traumatic brain injury or premature baby case, savings of 1:30 to 1:50 can be expected. As a bonus, case management also tackles other problem areas that push up health care costs and concerns: patient compliance, prevention of complications, patient satisfaction with medical services, and timely return to work. According to the National Pharmaceutical Council's Task Force on Noncompliance, the annual cost of noncompliance alone exceeds $100 billion every year.[5] A case manager's professional intervention and guidance improves patient outcomes and morale by providing direct communication and personal attention, helps make the best use of limited benefit dollars, and helps eliminate repeated occurrences of the same afflictions.

Throughout the course of care, the case manager will work in four major areas of activity: medical, financial, behavioral/motivational, and vocational.

Medical Activities

This area encompasses all those activities a case manager performs to ensure that the patient receives the most effective medical and nursing care, including the following:

- contacting the patient in the hospital, in the rehabilitation unit, or at home to assess the patient's condition, understanding of his or her injury and its ramifications, and ability or predisposition to follow the treatment plan

- contacting the members of the medical treatment team (the physician, nursing staff, clinical practitioners, rehabilitation therapists, etc.) to discuss the patient's course of progress and needs, utilizing the information in discharge planning and the initial needs assessment
- arranging for all services required for discharge or relocation (equipment, home nursing care, therapy, transportation, transfer to another facility, home utilities, and so on); coordinating efforts with the primary registered nurse (RN), discharge planner, or social services administrator to eliminate duplication of service and conserve benefit dollars
- visiting with the family to ascertain its understanding of the patient's diagnosis and prognosis, and its ability to provide caregiver support
- checking the home for safety factors and architectural barriers and arranging for any needed safety aids and modifications
- on follow-up, reevaluating equipment, ensuring supplies are replenished, monitoring home nursing services, and arranging for equipment repair; evaluating activities of daily living, home programs, and modifications to treatment
- identifying problems, anticipating complications and acting to avoid them, providing health instruction to the patient and family, and referring the patient back to the physician or other health team member when appropriate
- identifying plateaus, improvements, regressions, and depressions; counseling accordingly or recommending help
- making personal visits or contacting the physician or other appropriate practitioner to clarify the diagnosis, prognosis, therapy, activities of daily living, expected permanent disability, and so on
- assisting in obtaining payer authorizations for any modalities of treatment recommended; investigating and suggesting alternative treatments when appropriate

- assisting in obtaining information and forms regarding a living will, health care proxy, do-not-resuscitate order, and so on
- acting as a liaison between the physician and the insurance company when necessary
- sharing pertinent information about the patient with the physician and working with the physician to achieve the best outcome

Financial Activities

Some of the specific financial services a case manager might contribute on behalf of a patient include:

- assessing the patient's benefit plan (indemnity, group medical, managed care, workers' compensation, disability, auto, dental, disease-specific) for coverage and limitations; negotiating with the plan for out-of-plan coverage as appropriate to make best use of the plan's financial resources
- negotiating for more cost-effective rates for provider services
- suggesting medically appropriate alternatives (a timely move from an acute care facility to a skilled nursing facility or home care, for example) to accomplish treatment plan goals more cost effectively
- counseling the patient or family on budgeting and notifying creditors
- identifying financial distress and referring the patient or family to appropriate community resources
- helping the patient or family sort and prioritize unpaid bills
- acting as a liaison among the insurance company, stop-loss carrier, referral source, employer, patient, and family to alleviate financial and other problems or misunderstandings
- educating the payer regarding the risk (financial exposure) of noncompliant, untreated, or unmanaged cases, and the documented success rates medical case management achieves; protecting payer funds

Behavioral/Motivational Activities

A case manager might aid a patient and family in dealing with such behavioral activities as:

- exploring the patient's feelings about him- or herself and his or her injury or illness and helping the patient with the associated trauma and frustration
- monitoring the family's feelings regarding the patient's illness and observing the family's ability or inability to manage new emotional stress
- offering reassurance and information about the patient's condition
- if qualified, counseling in the areas of marital discord, role reversal, dependency, and sexual problems arising from the injury or illness

Vocational Activities

A case manager may work with a patient on such vocational issues as:

- obtaining a history of past education, employment, hobbies, and job skills and uncovering vocational interests and future goals
- if appropriate, overseeing psychovocational testing, work evaluations, schooling, on-the-job situations, transportation, and anything else needed to assist the patient in becoming or remaining gainfully employed
- assisting the patient in using the recuperative period in a constructive fashion (studying, upgrading skills, preparing for job interviews, and so on)
- visiting the patient's place of employment and talking with the personnel director or immediate supervisor about the employer's expectations and the patient's needs
- completing a job analysis and discussing the possibility of the patient's return to work in the same job, perhaps after job modification or lightening of duties
- sharing the above information with physician at appropriate times[6]

ON-SITE VERSUS TELEPHONE-BASED CASE MANAGEMENT

Case management is not a hands-on role. Case managers are not actively practicing nurses, clinicians, or caregivers. They do not diagnose an ailment, prescribe a medication, or set the course of treatment. They do offer their expertise and observations to suggest alternative care options. Using on-site visits and information-gathering conversations, a case manager can make sure a noncompliant patient is following the treatment plan outlined by the physician or note the possible complications from the medications recommended by one of the patient's specialists but never mentioned to his or her other physicians.

Although case managers do not offer hands-on care, they cannot be truly effective if every case is addressed in a totally hands-off manner. Telephone work is necessary for maintaining lines of communication without driving up costs. Case management over the telephone is particularly effective for preventive and case screening measures and for tracking low-intensity patients or patients who have improved to the point where in-person case management is no longer needed. However, when all communication among the case manager, patient, family, physician, and payer occurs over the telephone, oversights in care can result, especially in cases where the patient is noncompliant, undereducated, or poor. The vulnerability of the patient coupled with the legal and monetary exposure of the provider and payer may call for, at the least, a minimum of on-site interactions.[7]

Case management by telephone is almost always less expensive than on-site case management, and its use has grown in our current managed care environment. The increasing practice of telephone-based case management is not in itself alarming; however, the increasing prevalence of poor-quality telephone-based case management is a problem. Much information can be lost over the telephone unless the individual is skilled and devoted to the particulars of the job. Callers are encouraged to get beyond the "no" by asking questions that demand more than a "yes" or "no" answer and to explore answers by asking leading questions. The question is not, "Are you taking your medication?" but rather, "What medications are you taking and when?"

Many case managers are hard pressed to convince payers that on-site assessment is necessary. But if it can be established that care decisions were based only on lowering costs, then employers, providers, payer groups, and case managers could be held liable in a wrongful action suit. To protect their interests and liabilities, it behooves each party to be fully aware of how care decisions are made. It is the case manager's responsibility to say, "No, I must be on site to review this case," or "No, I'm unable to put that plan into action," if she or he feels the level of care being provided is substandard or places the patient at too great a risk. Further, providers need to maintain accurate outcomes data and can use case managers as their eyes and ears.

CASE MANAGERS IN MANAGED CARE

An integral part of the managed care process, case managers are introduced to patients and cases in a variety of ways. They may be a member of the discharge planning team employed on site at a hospital; part of a major insurer's in-house case management team; an independent case manager working on contract for an employer or TPA; a community-based social worker/case manager; or on staff at a rehabilitation facility, infusion therapy company, home health agency, or other provider location. The referral source might be an insurance company with clients covered under workers' compensation, auto, or group medical plans; a TPA that is paying claims for a client company; or a corporate human resources manager. It might be a state Medicaid office with case management services within a line of insurance or a population segment, such as high-risk newborns or children who are dependent on technological medical assistance. Case managers are also contacted directly by families seeking to monitor the care of an out-of-state relative or friend, for example. There are individuals and firms providing a broad range of case management services, and those specializing in specific diseases or patient groups, such as premature babies, individuals with diabetes, or those suffering from Alzheimer's disease, AIDS, or breast cancer.

For optimum outcomes, a case manager will be called in on the case as early as possible. If case management services are strategically coordinated with preadmission review and concurrent review services, early intervention and its benefits often occur. However, there are times when a case manager is not notified until a case has reached a threshold of $30,000—a little late in the game, but not past the point of no return.

Although many MCOs employ case managers as part of their utilization management departments, in other situations case management services are outsourced to an independent case management service. Services are customarily billed on an hourly or a flat-fee basis, where a set fee is established for each review conducted. More frequently, with the increased use of managed care strategies, case management services are being purchased at a capitated rate, similar to preadmission and concurrent review services. In a capitated rate structure, a per case, per month fee is established, and it is up to managers of a case management department to accurately predict the caseload and needs of the covered lives.

Case management services may be covered by language in the benefit plan or requested as an alternative to policy benefits. Sometimes part of a comprehensive managed care program, case management services are offered in conjunction with preadmission review and concurrent review. In these cases, all three services might be offered at a capitated rate or on a stand-alone (per service, per case) basis.

CASE MANAGEMENT WORK FORMAT AND PROCESS

Money is pouring into our health care system. But improved treatment and services are not flowing out at the same rate. Case management is a catalyst that pushes performance to more cost-effective levels, promoting better outcomes and the maintenance of quality care. (See the case management flowchart presented in Figure 22–1.)

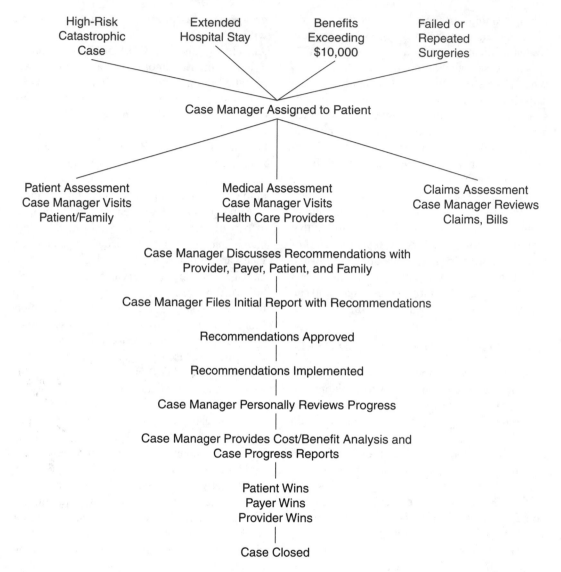

Figure 22–1 Case Management Work Format Flowchart. Courtesy of Options Unlimited, Case Management Services Division, Huntington, New York.

Gathering and Assessing Information

A case manager's approach to a new case is influenced by the referral source (generally the payer) and the line of insurance; her or his latitude in creatively and effectively managing a case will vary with the amount the payer has at risk. Generally, the self-insured employer, paying dollar-for-dollar for benefits, is more interested in and involved in the case management process and more readily approves out-of-plan benefits to make the most of benefit dollars. On the other hand, a large employer paying a capitated, one-rate-fits-all fee to a major insurer for its employees' health benefit coverage is often less inclined to work with a case manager on an individual case.

Appropriate and effective case management is possible only when the information gathered is accurate and thoughtfully analyzed. This gathering process will include conversations with the major players—the referral source or payer, patient, family, physicians, and other key members of the medical treatment team. The case manager will introduce him- or herself and explain the role of case management, making certain that each person understands what the case manager will focus on. Medical records must be consulted; employers and attorneys must be contacted as needed. The right questions must be asked: Does the wheelchair fit through the doorjambs in the patient's home? Does the cardiac patient think hypertension occurs only when he has a headache, and does he take his medication accordingly? Is the wife of the man who had a massive cardiovascular accident (CVA) expecting him to be up and back in the office in a month?

Furthermore, all data must be carefully considered. Too often case managers fall into the habit of transferring information from their notes to a report without asking themselves the same direct questions they should be asking their patients, payers, and providers: What is hindering better progress here? What can be done to encourage the patient's family to help with the care? Should I aggressively pursue this seemingly necessary service on an out-of-plan basis?

Initial Assessment

The words *initial needs assessment* carry a variety of meanings, depending on the listener. An initial needs assessment is the case manager's first activity, undertaken to prepare a report to the referral source (payer) that will include a description of the patient; the patient's condition, diagnosis, and prognosis; and the case manager's recommendations. Some organizations think of an initial needs assessment as a four-page document prepared by the case manager following on-site visits with the claimant, family, physician, and employer. Others feel a thorough telephone conversation will cover their needs (and their liability) or request that the case manager visit with the patient but not with other participants in the care plan when conducting an initial needs assessment.

Talking with the Referral Source

Before beginning an initial needs assessment, the case manager should know if the patient is covered under the specific line of insurance paying for case management. To determine the client's responsibility on this case, for this individual, under this policy, it is not too rudimentary to start with the basics: What is the line of insurance? Is this patient covered under this policy? Suppose the case manager works in the preadmission and concurrent review department of a health care provider group and receives a call that James Jones has just been admitted to the hospital with which the provider group is affiliated. Upon checking, the case manager determines that James' father, John, is covered by a plan in which the group's practitioners are participating physicians (or member physicians) and that James is listed as a dependent on his father's plan. However, the case manager discovers that James' injury occurred at work, making it a workers' compensation case. James is not eligible for benefits under his father's group medical plan but may be covered under workers' compensation. (This topic is discussed in detail in Chapter 61.)

To assess the case for possible high-risk or long-term cost factors, the case manager will ask how long the patient has been ill. Even with minimum description—"The car accident occurred two years ago"; "It's a spinal cord injury"; "This is his third hospitalization in eighteen months"—the case manager begins to get a clear picture of short- and long-term needs and can begin considering any required adjustment to the treatment plan, the potential requirement for long-term case management, or a closer case review. The person in a coma rarely jumps up during week two to return to his or her normal lifestyle; hence, a long-term case management plan would be in order. If an individual citing lower back pain has been in physical therapy for three years, a wake-up call to the treating physician might be in order.

Other questions for a case manager to put to a payer include:

- What dollars are available for how long?
- Are there any limits or restrictions on the type of care provided?
- Type of care facility?
- Length of stay?
- Is there coverage for a skilled nursing facility versus an acute care center?
- Does the provision for home nursing services include 24-hour care or is it limited to one four-hour shift each day?

The line of insurance itself indicates certain questions to a case manager. In workers' compensation cases, one such question is: How did the injury happen? This might be one in a series of injuries at the same workstation, causing the case manager to urge the employer's risk manager to investigate that job procedure and workstation before another employee is disabled and before the employer is facing a wrongful injury lawsuit.

More details about the case manager's conversation with the referral source are presented in Exhibit 22–1.

Talking with the Patient

When interviewing the patient, the case manager is trying to obtain an overview of the patient's current medical history, the particular individual, and the situation, as well as to encourage the patient to be participatory in his or her own care program. Initial questions will center on the patient's understanding of his or her medical diagnosis and prognosis. How does the patient view the situation? The individual might answer, "My doctor told me I have lupus." The case manager must then ask, "What do you think that means? Will it affect your lifestyle?" By listening carefully to patient responses, a case manager will be able to determine the individual's level of understanding and acceptance (or denial) of the problem.

Exhibit 22–1 Communicating with Referral Sources

1. A referral is made to the case manager by the payer, employer, hospital discharge planner, attending nurse, or the MCO's precertification department.
2. The case manager gets the appropriate details and confirms the needs of the referral source (e.g., expectations, fees, format and time frame for reports, etc).
3. The case manager requests case background (e.g., the status of the patient, the diagnosis and the prognosis, the type of insurance coverage, the patient's eligibility under the policy, the policy benefit limits, the plan's flexibility, the restrictions on care, etc.).
4. The case manager confirms the initial needs assessment and report parameters in writing to the referral source and/or payer.
5. The case manager makes a follow-up call to review the confirmation letter.
6. The case manager documents all conversations.

Source: Reprinted from C.M. Mullahy, *The Case Manager's Handbook,* 2nd ed., p. 160, © 1998, Aspen Publishers, Inc.

The case manager should never assume that a patient has the ability to understand the diagnosis; the ability to accept the diagnosis; or enough information and understanding of that information to be a cooperative, compliant participant in the health care plan. Perhaps the family is withholding information from the patient in a misguided effort to protect the patient. Perhaps the referral source, the physicians, and the case manager all have a clear understanding of the patient's condition—a malignant tumor that has already metastasized to other organs—but the patient and family have no concept of how this will affect their future. They might have heard the information but chosen to edit it to a version more easy or convenient to accept—"I had a growth, but it was removed and I'm fine now"; "Dad can go back to his job in two weeks, and my college tuition will be no problem."

A case manager also needs to be able to spot those who want to be lifelong members of the health care delivery process. Turning a chronic headache pattern into an undetectable brain tumor allows one some respite from life's greater responsibilities.

A crucial line of questioning, often overlooked by all members of the medical system, including case managers, centers on medications. There is a gap—the distance between life and death—between what a patient perceives as a problem and what the medical profession knows is a problem. Whether the patient takes an interest in his or her medications or not, the case manager should ask to see all pills and medications being taken, including over-the-counter capsules and herbal supplements. The case manager should also ask related questions: Which of these are you taking? How often are you taking them? What do you think they are for? Sometimes patients halve their doses, stop taking medications midway through the course of treatment, or take medications only on the days when the presenting problem is noticeable. In some cases, this medical manipulation has no significant consequences. In other cases, the ill effects are harrowing.

Also important are questions regarding the patient's vocation and avocations. Is this person actively involved in a church? If yes, perhaps other church members might provide the family with care respite. Is he or she an avid golfer, fisher, or skeet shooter? Does he or she enjoy working? An optimistic person, fully experiencing life, is more likely to be a cooperative patient than the individual who is not participatory by nature. Someone seeking to get back to all of life's business will follow a treatment plan; someone who was recently laid off may choose a "disability mentality," where the illness becomes his or her job and social life.

At the end of the interview, the case manager should obtain a signed consent form (Exhibit 22–2) from the patient or the patient's guardian. This will enable the case manager to review the patient's medical records and to share information regarding the patient with his or her physician(s) and attorney, if the case is in litigation.

Talking with the Family

Families affected by an injury or illness often will experience role changes, dependency shifts, anxiety, anger, and an inability to make decisions, particularly in long-term cases. Because of this, it is helpful for a case manager to interview the family early on to determine family dy-

---

Exhibit 22–2 Patient Consent Form

CONSENT

Date:_____

To ensure appropriate medical case management services, I, _____, authorize any physician, hospital, or other professional involved in my treatment to disclose medical, hospital, vocational, or related information. I authorize that the information may be shared with other professionals, agencies, or insurance companies that may be involved in the provision or payment of necessary services.

A copy of this authorization may be accepted, if necessary.

Signed _____

Guardian _____

Witness _____

Source: Reprinted from C.M. Mullahy, *The Case Manager's Handbook,* 2nd ed., p. 160, © 1998, Aspen Publishers, Inc.

namics. Is the family taking an overprotective stance with the patient? Is the family spokesperson speaking for the patient unnecessarily? "He needs to eat more." "She isn't sleeping well." Is there so much fear associated with this illness that other members of the family are developing symptoms, having emotional outbursts, or relying on alcohol in an effort to regain a feeling of balance or control in their lives?

In many ways, the patient's health will be supported by the emotional and physical health of the family. The case manager will want to not only gauge the strength of the family structure but also compile a medical family tree. Do certain illnesses run in the family? Does the 42-year-old man recuperating after a heart attack have a family with a history of cardiac disease and middle-age deaths?

The case manager needs answers to the following questions:

- What was the prime caretaker's role in the family prior to this illness?
- Did he or she run the household?
- Did he or she hold down a job?
- Does the caretaker still have those responsibilities in addition to caring for the patient?
- How is the caretaker reacting to the illness?
- Is the caretaker physically and emotionally capable of supporting and caring for the patient?[8]

All these elements will influence the case management plan and sometimes even dictate what the case manager can hope to accomplish. For example, the family with three active, inquisitive, dial-turning children under age seven, plus an infant who requires oxygen, is going to need part-time home nursing assistance following discharge; also helpful will be an oxygen system with outdoor tanks, removing the siblings' temptation to tamper.

Talking with the Treating Physician

When a case manager works as a collaborative partner with a physician, as well as all other members of the medical team, there is greater opportunity to track a patient's progress, ensure that the patient is and remains participatory and compliant, and check that each element of the treatment plan is carried out appropriately. To build such partnerships, a case manager should schedule a personal meeting with the physician at his or her convenience when the case is complex. In less medically complex or physically distant cases, a telephone conversation with the treating physician is effective.

The case manager will ask questions such as:

- What is the diagnosis?
- What is the treatment plan and prognosis?
- What do you think will be the outcome for this person, both short term and long term?
- Do you anticipate any complications?
- What have you told the patient?
- What do you think he or she understands?[9]

This last question is important because the patient, the physician, and the case manager all need to be speaking the same language. Patients often choose to forget the components of conditions that they have difficulty accepting. This impacts the treatment plan. It is the case manager's job to make certain the patient has all the information necessary to cooperate and follow the treatment plan.

If the case manager knows up front that there is a limit on care dollars, he or she has the responsibility to make the physician aware of the limit and share in the goal of using the money in the best way possible. Although some care options may be ideal, the expenses connected with them make them poor first choices. A good alternative may not be perfect, but it will not pose any risk to the patient and may cover care and services over a longer period of time.[10]

Independent Medical and Second Opinion Exams

In some cases, an independent medical exam or a second opinion exam will be requested. A case manager's involvement depends on the type of exam performed. An independent medical exam is generally used by insurance carriers to determine the diagnosis, the need for continued treatment, the degree of disability (partial or total), the duration of a disability (temporary, long-term, or permanent), and the patient's ability to return to work. Independent medical exams are requested when treatment appears excessive, when the recovery time appears overly extended, or when there is a delay in the patient's return-to-work schedule. They are also employed upon request to authorize surgery, expensive equipment, or unusual diagnostic testing, or when there is an increase in the number of treating professionals. The physician conducting the exam most often remains in a nontreating role. A case manager may assist in setting up the exam and may accompany the patient but in most instances will not be present at the exam.

Also used to determine a diagnosis, a second opinion exam is often performed to help clarify a complex medical outlook or to prepare alternatives to the current or proposed treatment. In group medical plans, a second opinion exam is sometimes required prior to certain surgical procedures that the carrier or the latest utilization review statistics show to have a high usage rate (such as hysterectomies, hip replacements, cardiac bypass, magnetic resonance imaging scans, disc surgery, etc.). Such exams are also called for when there is a conflict between potential treatment plans, when a questionable treatment is in place, or when the existing treatment plan is not achieving the expected outcome. The case manager who arranged for the second opinion exam is usually in attendance, and the physician conducting the exam often will become a treating physician.

To get greater benefit from independent medical exams and second opinion exams, a case manager should thoroughly understand the purpose of any exam ordered and be specific about what the physician's report should address. The examining physician should be given as much information as possible (operative reports, diagnostic test reports, X-rays, computed tomography [CT] scans, etc.) and be given enough time to review all the data prior to the actual exam. After reviewing the physician's report to confirm that it is responsive to the initial request for information, the case manager should speak to the physician to discuss findings and clarify any unanswered issues.[11]

Talking with Service and Equipment Providers

Many case managers find it helpful to work with one representative at a durable medical equipment, home medical equipment, or home health care agency. In this way equipment, services, contracts, and billing can all be reviewed in one phone call. In addition, it helps case managers get answers when they need them, and very often answers are needed immediately (especially on Friday afternoons, when it seems every patient in the country is simultaneously declared ready for discharge).

Prior to selecting providers or arranging for services, a case manager should review the benefit plan contract to make certain that its language supports the use of home nursing visits, durable medical equipment, and so on. It is the case manager's responsibility to verify that the contract she or he arranges agrees with plan language and will be approved when the bill for the services/equipment finally arrives in a claims department.

There are many questions case managers should ask:

- What are the options included with this piece of equipment?
- What specifically is it designed to do?
- What are the terms—lease, rent, rent with option to buy, outright purchase?
- This patient will be using this equipment for at least six months; what discount will you offer for a long-term rental?
- Is repair service available 24 hours a day?
- What are the costs for various levels of service?
- What services do your homemakers provide, and how do they differ in price and services from the home health aides?

Talking with Community Resources

The case manager need not spend benefit plan money just because it exists. There are numerous local, state, and national agencies—as well as disease-specific organizations, foundations, and philanthropic groups—that may provide services, guidance, and equipment free of charge. The United Way, Meals on Wheels, and "I Can Cope" programs and loaner wheelchairs from the American Cancer Society are examples of available assistance. Easter Seals offers support on a sliding scale for children and adults with crippling diseases. Some local volunteer fire departments provide ambulance services at no charge.[12]

Planning

Case management is a process of identifying and solving problems. The first and key issue is whether the treatment is appropriate and being provided in the best possible setting. If the patient is not being well served, the case manager can help create a better system of care. The case manager's evaluation of the patient's current status will be the foundation for the case management plan. The case manager must look at what the patient's needs are and how they can best be met in terms of quality and cost. One factor should never drive the others; there must be equilibrium among needs, quality, and cost. Given the patient's diagnosis, current medical status, and prior medical history, is the treatment plan attaining the most desirable results? Does it appear that it will lead to an eventual recovery or have there already been too many complications? Is the treatment plan sound? Is it appropriate, reasonable, and really necessary for this patient? Is it forcing the patient into any undue hardship or discomfort?

Is the patient in the most appropriate and most cost-effective setting for his or her problem? Imagine that John is in the hospital, his surgery has been completed, and now he is being observed and given medication, physical therapy, or pain or infusion care services. Does he have to remain in the hospital? Once patients can be effectively managed without all the expensive support services of an acute care facility, they should be moved to a more appropriate and less costly arena for care— the home or another setting.

During assessment and planning, the case manager will also be evaluating the money available and the exposure faced. Whose pocket is it, and how large is the pocket? If unlimited dollars are available, should they be spent whatever way the providers want, regardless of necessity? Sometimes this attitude prevails. Case managers need to look for the "value-locked dollar" for a demonstration that the treatment is necessary, reasonable, and will achieve good results and that the treatment plan is the most cost-effective way to provide the requisite care.[13]

Reporting

A case manager's report back to the referral source, payer, or internal department head should reflect those issues that most concern the payer or facility. If the case manager is on staff at a health maintenance organization (HMO) and the lines of insurance are predominantly group medical, reports will address medical issues for the most part. In a disability case where the client is the employer, the case manager needs to focus on return-to-work issues. A case manager in a rehabilitation facility will detail patient progress and outcomes information, and relate it to cost. In a workers' compensation case, carriers are responsible for both medical costs and lost earnings. This payer will want to know the extent of medical involvement, the severity of injury, and the likelihood of some permanent incapacitation. When reporting to a claims supervisor, the case manager will want to include specific medical information and parenthetical explanations to help the reader interpret the medical terms (and to help educate him or her about information likely to appear in other reports regarding the diagnosis or prognosis). The desired frequency and length of case management reports should be confirmed with the referral source.

Reports should be written at least once a month. All pertinent case activity should be recorded in a specific, regular format. Readers should not be punished with a stack of casework, and payers should not be put off with the attached large invoice. By reporting in manageable increments of 3 to 4 weeks, case managers gain better control of client files, outcomes tracking, and invoicing and keep the payer up to date on the case. Significant activities or events requiring clarification should be reported in a timely fashion, first by phone and subsequently through written documentation (within a few days).

How extensive should reports be? Some payer organizations have specific guidelines, limiting initial report writing time to 2 hours or even a half an hour. Others request a verbal report, asking that the case manager not even take the time to send a document, even a fax. In this type of situation, the case manager needs to educate the referral source. Case management reports have practical and legal value as documents chronicling case management activity.

Suppose the case manager, during a phone conversation, reports to the payer a previously undocumented call to the patient or the physician. Will either of them remember this exchange of information? What if the case moves into litigation? What if the patient takes a turn for the worse? Especially when planning services, negotiating services, or putting alternative plans in place, case managers need to document—in writing—decisions and their implementation. This is just good case management administration.

Case management reports should follow a certain format and contain the name of the referral source, the mailing address and phone number for reporting, the line of insurance, the date of occurrence of the accident or injury, a code for the name of the insured, and a code for the name of the claimant or patient. In addition, the report should include any pertinent information obtained from the payer, patient, family, employer, medical records, physician(s), and other medical professionals; a review of the policy coverage and limits; any suggested alternative treatment program; and a discussion of relevant community resources.[14] In their own best interests, case managers should also use these reports to educate readers on the positive impact of case management on outcomes and costs.

Obtaining Approval from the Payer

Once the case management plan has been devised and the report has been sent to the client, the case manager must then obtain approval to proceed with the recommendations in the report. There are always going to be times when case managers have to use their own judgment and consider whom they are representing. An employer or referral source might say directly, "I want John out of that facility; it's too expensive." If case managers feel that patients are in the most appropriate center and that there is no less costly setting, they cannot allow the client to override their professional judgment. The case manager cannot service the client first and the patient last; the interests of the patient must always predominate. Case managers are not in the business of slashing away at the federal or corporate health budget while sacrificing patients' well-being and safety.[15]

Coordinating and Monitoring: Putting the Plan into Action

Plans are sometimes put in motion as early as the initial evaluation stage. Case managers may not have completed gathering all the information or submitted a report when they get the go-ahead to put services in place. When an involved case has been referred from a company the case manager has worked with before, the company might request a verbal report from on-site. During that phone conversation, the case manager might obtain approval to begin the recommended intervention.

The case manager not only has the responsibility to put appropriate services in place but also should make certain that the services and treatments put in place remain cost effective, of good quality, and necessary; the case manager should monitor the case. Sometimes a client company will want a case manager to make a one-time visit, arrange for services, and be done with the case. Then who is watching for changes in the patient's needs or tracking and assisting with increases or decreases in services—the home infusion company or home care agency that obviously has a stake in the case's progression? Who is tracking the continued adherence to the physician's treatment plan?

The monitoring process varies from case to case. It may include semimonthly home visits by the case manager or periodic phone calls made by the patient to the case manager. In active cases where multiple services are in place, the case manager must make monthly on-site visits. If there are no services in place, but the patient has been discharged and asked to take specific medications or dress a wound a certain way, the case manager will make check-in calls to see how the patient is coping. When a patient sounds poorly or acknowledges problems, the case manager should call the treating physicians and assess the situation. Perhaps the treatment plan needs to be reevaluated.[16]

Evaluating the Plan

Along with monitoring the medical treatment plan and its effectiveness, the case manager will evaluate and reevaluate the case management plan over the course of intervention. Is the treatment working? Have any complications developed? How is the family coping? Does the caregiver need a respite? Each case will go through modification and redevelopment. Changes in patient status will require new measures of care.

The case manager should review the treatment plan and the patient's progress at least once every 30 days. Short-term referrals, which generally run less than 3 months and are characterized by intense activity at the outset that tapers off as the patient improves, are always reassessed prior to the patient's discharge from a facility or program. Long-term programs, such as geriatric care, are evaluated at intervals of 3, 6, or 9 months. In a brain or spinal cord injury case, care may be evaluated at 1-year intervals. Long-term care evaluations can become challenging because the goal of case management is stability; in some cases, things can go smoothly for long periods of time and there will seemingly be nothing to report.

Further, quality of life is less easily measured than the quantity of money spent on care. Is a continuation of the program warranted? Are the dollars spent on John's care every day worth it? Treatment might be necessary for a 6- to 9-month period, but the patient may not require facility services for that entire time. Although making great strides in the first 2 months, the patient may show no further improvement after 3 months. Perhaps the patient has hit a plateau and needs a break from the rigorous therapies. The next step might be to place the patient in a less expensive day program, then perhaps return him or her to the inpatient facility for another round of intensive therapy if improvement again becomes noticeable.

Over the course of care, as a treatment facilitator, the case manager maintains communication with the treating physicians to share concerns and observations regarding developing conditions, and with physical therapists, social workers, community center personnel, employers, and anyone else who may contribute to the patient's care and welfare. The case manager may need to reestablish ties to a specialist to request assistance.[17]

UTILIZATION REVIEW: PREADMISSION AND CONCURRENT REVIEW AND CASE MANAGEMENT

Generally speaking, utilization review (now also known as utilization management) falls into three categories: prospective (before the event, called preadmission or precertification), concurrent (during the event), or retrospective (after the event). Each type of review uses certain criteria to determine whether there is a need for further action, decision, or intervention, and to evaluate the necessity and efficiency of the medical services. In addition to tracking the appropriateness of medical care and expenses, the review process itself can also be used to identify cases for case management if the organization or reviewer is aware of the red flags that indicate a need for case management intervention, such as multiple hospital admissions, certain International Classification of Diseases, Ninth Edition, Clinical Modification (ICD-9-CM) diagnostic codes, claims for apnea alarms, electric hospital beds, infusion care services, and so on. These indicators are discussed further below. From a case management perspective, the opportunity to explore alternatives, assist the patient, and preserve benefit dollars is already missed when the case manager is confronted with a claim for $42,000 resulting from a hospital stay of 28 days. Could the patient have gone to a skilled facility for 2 of those weeks? Were nursing and other services in the home a possibility? With alternatives, would there have been opportunities for fee negotiations? Would fee negotiations have been possible with the hospital itself? The lack of early intervention in this case carried a $42,000 price tag.

It is amazing that carriers, TPAs, employer groups, and even some MCOs often set up preadmission review without linking it to some kind of case management program. Reviews are performed in a management vacuum; it is assumed that there are no savings to be gained. And, except for those savings possibly realized through the denial of a few days in the hospital or avoidance of an inpatient stay, there will not be any savings to record. Without a connection to case management, preadmission review accomplishes nothing more than maintaining a census of inpatient admissions. Preadmission review alone, without concurrent review, is incapable of reducing lengths of stay or allowing alternative care plans to be considered. (Just as problematic—and ineffective, in terms of care and cost management—are those individuals in managed care who are called case managers, or care managers, but in reality provide utilization review services only. Again, a case manager coordinates patient care across the care continuum, through the various care settings, and works in conjunction with the patient, care and service providers, payers, employers, and others to improve outcomes and make the best use of health care dollars.)

The maximum opportunity for success exists when one organization provides preadmission and concurrent review along with case management services. Too often, particularly in large organizations, one company does the reviewing and another provides the case management. The delays that inevitably occur between identifying a high-cost case, referring it for case management, assigning the case, and actually managing the case make the system ineffective instead of the ongoing process of evaluation, identification, assessment, planning, and implementation that would be ideal. The key in case management is how the case manager gets involved and how soon. For example, one has missed an opportunity if a case manager starts working with a patient with an injured spinal cord 20 or 30 days after the initial hospitalization. Earlier involvement could have resulted in a transfer of this patient to a spinal cord injury treatment center and the prevention of some complications that would, after 20 or 30 days, have already occurred, that will be more costly to treat, and that prolong the period of rehabilitation.[18]

Case managers are facilitators who have the expertise to understand complex cases and the ability to effect change. They assist patients by getting information and expediting the delivery of services. To perform effectively, case managers need to work within a system that allows involvement to occur at an optimum time. Because a seemingly simple procedure can unexpectedly become complex and expensive, each admission needs to be reviewed as it occurs. This does not mean that each case will require case management intervention. Most will not. But the strategy of reviewing each will promote better outcomes for patients and payers.

The sample case presented in Exhibit 22–3 was created to illustrate what would probably occur with and without an integrated system in place. Exhibit 22–4 is a letter designed to be sent to plan participants to explain the advocacy role of the case manager and the nature of the case management process.

For example, the author once received a referral from a claims department after it was notified by a provider who had conducted a preadmission review 7 weeks prior and noted a diagnosis of cancer of the stomach. A claims examiner now had the end-of-month printout and had also just received a claim for 1 week of total parenteral nutrition (TPN) and other services totaling $10,000. The examiner thought a case management referral was in order. It was, but it came a little too late. The services continued a second week as arranged; the provider refused to negotiate retrospectively to lower costs because he knew his services were

Exhibit 22–3 Case Samples Without and with Preadmission Review, Concurrent Review, and Case Management

Case A

Scenario—Mr. Jones sustains an injury to his right knee following a fall from a ladder and reports the injury. He is out of work for 1 week, and his supervisor hasn't heard from him or when he's coming back. The worker's family physician is treating the injury conservatively with rest and minimal activity. It's three weeks later and the supervisor now hears from the worker's coworkers that there is now an infection in the knee and the worker is scheduled for a surgical procedure. No date for return to work is known. Another week passes. The worker is out of the hospital but still having problems. The supervisor doesn't know what the problems are but the worker's prolonged absence is increasing the workload on the department, and the supervisor also is behind on his work. It's now six weeks since this "little fall" (in the words of the supervisor) and it has gone on "too long." The treating physician has told the worker that he can go back to "light duty" and maybe his old job in another month. The supervisor tells the claims examiner there is no "light duty" and the worker continues to remain home. Someone sees the worker mowing his lawn, word reaches the employer, who notifies the claims examiner and requests surveillance. It is clear where this is going, isn't it?

Case B

Scenario—Mr. Jones sustains an injury to his right knee following a fall from a ladder. As is required, he reports the injury to his supervisor. The supervisor advises him that a case manager will be contacting him to help him get appropriate care, answer questions he may have, and assist him in returning to work. The case manager contacts the injured worker and learns that he has sustained a four-inch laceration to the knee, which required several stitches in the emergency department. She also learned during her phone assessment with the employee that he is unsure about how to care for the wound, or what dressing is needed and how often it should be changed. He also does not know the signs of infection to check for and has not yet scheduled a follow-up visit with his family physician. Because the case manager asked about prior medical history, she discovered that the worker had a "little bit of diabetes" (in the words of the worker) and was lacking knowledge about this disease and, in fact, was told he had cataracts and that his vision is a little "blurry."

The case manager assessed the following as problems:

- a large laceration requiring daily dressing changes and inspection of the wound
- cataracts, which resulted in blurred vision and the inability to detect subtle changes in the wound
- unmanaged diabetes, which prolongs and complicates the wound healing process

The case manager implemented the following:

- skilled nursing visits daily to inspect the wound, change the dressing, and assess diabetic care needs
- referral to physician the following day (after explaining risk factors for infection to office nurse)
- call to supervisor apprising him of status of employee (during this call, obtained description of employee's job [physical demands, etc], discussed some possible modifications to be considered, and suggested a call to the worker by the supervisor to "touch base"— express concern and good wishes).

Within a week, healing was progressing well and following calls to employee and the treating physician, it was determined that the worker could

continues

Exhibit 22–3 continued

Case A continued

Case B continued
return to work as long as he did not have to use a ladder or work in a crouched position.

The supervisor was able to modify the worker's position (climbing the ladder was needed only occasionally and another worker could do this; crouching position was done rarely and this, too, could be done by another). Employee could also be checked daily by the company nurse, who would also monitor his diabetes.

Eleven days after the injury, the employee returned to a modified form of his job. The case manager maintained contact with all parties, ensured that the wound was completely healed in three weeks and that the worker could then return to all of his duties.

Costs:

Medical: Hospital admission for wound infection and intravenous (IV) antibiotics, wound incisions, and drainage

Hospital @ $1,500 × 7 days = $10,500

Surgery: $2,500

Physical therapy, 3 times a week × 4 weeks (and continuing) = $900

IV antibiotics at home following hospital stay @ $550/day plus nursing visit @ $140/visit × 7 = $4,830

Physician fees: $2,000

Replacement of earnings @ $450/week × 6 = $2,700

Total medical: $20,730 (and continuing)

Total lost earnings: $2,700 (and continuing)

Total costs: $23,430

Indirect costs: decreased productivity, litigation, employee morale

AND IT'S NOT OVER!

Costs:

Medical: Nursing visits for wound care/dressing changes @ negotiated rate of $75 × 10 days = $750

Physician fees: 2 visits for wound care/diabetic management = $200

Replacement of earnings @ $450/week × 2 = $900

Total costs: $1,650*

Results from Case A:

Increased costs

An employee with continuing medical complications

Adversarial relationship between employer and employee

Pending litigation

Decreased productivity

Decreased morale

Results from Case B:

Savings (net): $20,780. Actual costs and case management fees were deducted from costs of case that would have occurred as in Case A.

A productive employee with a better outcome and the recipient of a true advocacy program

A business that can return to its own business needs and goals

*Case management is another cost consideration. In this kind of case, case management started early would cost less than $1,000.

Courtesy of Options Unlimited, Case Management Services Division, Huntington, New York.

Exhibit 22–4 Letter Explaining Case Management to Plan Participants

---

January 15, _____

Dear _____:

Please allow this letter to serve as an introduction and explanation of services that have been requested on your behalf by _____ of Third-Party Administrator (TPA), which is the company administering the health care benefits on behalf of your employer, _____.

_____ is a private consulting firm utilized by TPA on behalf of its insured to assist TPA with the problems resulting from a variety of medical conditions. This service is at no cost to you and is a benefit provided by the company.

Our nurse consultants work with you, your family, and treating physicians in coordinating whatever care and services are necessary in order that you may receive the best results possible. This intervention is not intended to interrupt or interfere with any care you are currently receiving, nor is this a "hands-on" service.

In order to determine just how we may be of assistance, one of our consultants, _____, would like to meet with you at your home. Because our consultants are frequently out of the office, would you please call us COLLECT at (999) 999-9999 in order that we can put _____ in touch with you.

Enclosed please find a brochure that further describes our services. Should you have any questions or concerns, please feel free to contact me directly. Please accept my personal assurance that every effort will be extended on your behalf.

Very truly yours,

Case Manager

cc: Claims Department

Courtesy of Options Unlimited, Case Management Services Division, Huntington, New York.

---

payable at 100 percent. (He knew that the patient's benefit plan would pay full price for his services because he called the claims department and learned this from a customer service representative.) The patient died after a second admission to the hospital. Perhaps the TPN services could have been negotiated more cost effectively. Perhaps a hospice program could have been arranged, allowing the patient to die at home with his family around him. Perhaps money could have been saved. In this instance, there were preadmission and concurrent review and case management and a benefit plan that would have permitted alternatives, yet because each system functioned independently of the others, realizing an alternative was impossible.

When preadmission and concurrent review and case management functions are integrated, the coordination can avoid duplication of involvement, help a claims department manage its workload, assist in the development of prevention and wellness programs, support the evaluation of benefit use, and expose the need to redesign plans.[19]

PREADMISSION AND CONCURRENT REVIEW CASE MANAGEMENT REPORTS

Preadmission and concurrent review summary reports (Exhibit 22–5) and other documentation of case events constitute an ongoing pro-

Table 22–5 Preadmission and Concurrent Review Summary Report

Group #001	Third-Party Administrator	1/1/99–1/31/99				
Date Reported	Employee SSN	Patient Name	Diagnosis	Type	Date of Admission	Date of Discharge
1/2/99	000-00-0000	J Smith	Fracture	Emergency	1/1/99	1/2/99
1/3/99	000-00-0000	C Jones	Normal Delivery	Emergency	1/25/99	
1/5/99	000-00-0000	K Williams	Lump in Breast	Scheduled	1/8/99	
1/7/99	000-00-0000	S Allen	Myocardial Infarction	Emergency	1/11/99	1/18/99
1/12/99	000-00-0000	T Hans	Herniated Disc	Scheduled	1/21/99	1/25/99
1/14/99	000-00-0000	L Mooney	Miscarriage	Emergency	1/13/99	1/14/99
1/16/99	000-00-0000	J Bono	Appendicitis	Emergency	1/15/99	1/18/99
1/18/99	000-00-0000	N Strong	Derangement Knee	Scheduled	1/25/99	
1/25/99	000-00-0000	P Duffy	Depression	Scheduled	1/28/99	
1/28/99	000-00-0000	I Grello	Pregnancy	Scheduled	3/25/99	

Total Admissions for Period = 9   **Total Discharged = 5**   **Total Referred for Case Management = 1**

TOTAL CASES FOR PERIOD = 10

Courtesy of Options Unlimited, Case Management Services Division, Huntington, New York.

file of a case. Case-specific reports (Exhibit 22–6) help establish a case history and can be used to track the details of a case, which can be extremely helpful if the patient moves from low- to high-risk status. Produced for all hospital ad-missions, all scheduled pregnancies, and all emergency cases, case-specific reports incorporate notes made by nurse reviewers. They are valuable for internal use in a preadmission and concurrent review department, provide the ratio-

Exhibit 22–6 Preadmission and Concurrent Review Case-Specific Report

CareWatch ID #: 00676
Date Reported: 08/31/99
Reported by: RENY

Group/Carrier:
Employee Information:
    Name: G. Jones   SSN: 123-45-6789
    Address: 12 Amhurst Street, Mid-Island, NY
    Hire Date: 03/01/91   Effective Date of Coverage: 06/01/91
    Telephone:
Patient Information:
    Name: G. Jones   DOB: 01/25/69   Age: 30
    Relation: Employee   Sex: Male
    Confinement Type: Emergency
    Admission Date: 08/28/99   Length of Stay: 2 days
    Discharge Date: 08/30/99
    Procedure: initial hosp. care/eval. and management
    Hospital: COMM. HOSPITAL
    Address: ROUTE 111
              SMITHTOWN, NY 11787
    Telephone: (516) 555-1234   Fax:
Admitting Physician Information:
    Doctor: Dr. J. Kahn
    Telephone: 555-1212   Fax:
    Diagnosis: hemorrhage—cerebral

CASE REMARKS

9/3/99: t/c to hospital, claimant was discharged on 8/30/99 but could not give me any other info. CTR t/c to MD, spoke Evelyn Spencer, who said that the claimant has an app't. with the MD today and she will call me back after he has been seen by the MD. CTR

t/c to claimant, who said he felt dizzy and went to the ER, he was admitted to ICU and had a CAT scan, was told he had an elevated BP and is on medication. He continues to feel dizzy sometimes and gets tingling in his tongue. Has an appt. today at 12:30 PM, will f/u on 9/8. CTR

9/8/99: t/c to claimant—per family member he is having some type of outpt. test today. f/u with claimant 9/9. IK

9/9/99: t/c to MD—told me that claimant was readmitted to hosp. for one day 9/8 to have arteriogram done. Diagnosis is seizure disorder and AV malformation and he was started on Dilantin. Will be referring him to neurologist. Will f/u with claimant. MF

9/10/99: t/c to claimant—still feels dizzy, has appt. with his MD today. Will f/u with claimant 9/14 for outcome and neuro. appt. IK

9/14/99: T/C to claimant—per his father, he has an appt. with neurologist Dr. Kahn (didn't have no.) tomorrow at 1 PM; he still has dizziness and numbness of tongue. f/u with claimant/MD 9/16. IK

continues

Exhibit 22–6 continued

9/16/99: t/c to claimant—told me that he had appt. with neurologist yesterday and that he referred him to another MD (neurosurgeon?) and that appt. is for next week 9/22 (claimant did not know name of MD offhand). Continues to take Dilantin and continues to feel dizzy, even though he stopped smoking. Claimant mentioned that MD might have to operate on his brain because "there is something wrong with blood vessel in his brain." Obtained Dr. Kahn's phone number 516-555-1212. Will f/u with MD. MF

9/16/99: t/c to MD—not in because of holidays. Will be back in office on 9/21 after 1 PM. MF

9/21/99: t/c to Dr. Kahn—per Sue pt. has AVM, will not be seen again in MD's office until sometime around 10/12, not aware of ref. to another MD, not aware of potential for surg. at this time. f/u with claimant to obtain name and no. of referral MD. IK

9/21/99: t/c to claimant—no answer × 2. IK

9/24/99: t/c to claimant—left message on answering machine. MF

9/30/99: t/c to claimant—no answer. Will try one more time tomorrow if no answer or return call, then will close case. MF

10/01/99: t/c to claimant—no answer × 2. IK. MULTIPLE attempts made to contact claimant; per MD office no further therapy scheduled at this time. Case closed. IK

MONITOR FILES FOR FUTURE CLAIMS*****************

CareWatch ID #: 00954
Date Reported: 11/08/99
Reported by: BARBARA

Group/Carrier:
Employee Information:

Name:	G. Jones	SSN: 123-45-6789
Address:	12 Amhurst Street, Mid-Island, NY	
Hire Date:	03/01/91 Effective Date of Coverage: 06/01/91	
Telephone:		

Patient Information:

Name:	G. Jones DOB: 01/25/69 Age: 30	
Relation:	Employee Sex: Male	
Confinement Type:	Emergency	
Admission Date:	10/30/99 Length of Stay: 4 Days	
Discharge Date:	11/03/99	
Procedure:	initial hosp. care/eval. and management	
Hospital:	COLUMBIA PRESBYTERIAN MED CTR.	
Address:	207 ST & BROADWAY	
	NEW YORK, NY 10032	
Telephone:	(212) 555-1234 Fax:	

Admitting Physician Information:

Doctor:	Dr. Z. Binder
Telephone:	(212) 555-1212 Fax:
Diagnosis:	hemorrhage—cerebral

CASE REMARKS
CASE KNOWN TO OPTIONS FROM PREVIOUS ADMISSION—VERY DIFFICULT TO FOLLOW—CLAIMANT DID NOT RETURN PHONE CALLS.

11/8/99: t/c Dr. Binder office. MD not available. will have secretary (Aline) call me back. vc

11/8/99: t/c to hospital pt info. patient discharged 11/3/99. vc

11/8/99: t/c claimant. no answer. vc

11/8/99: t/c hospital medical records. dept closed (hrs. 9–12, 2–3:45) direct #212-555-1246

continues

Exhibit 22–6 continued

11/9/99: t/c to MD—MD is away, per Aline, residents are following claimant. She will get info. from them and return call. MF

11/9/99: t/c from Aline at Dr. Binder's office—told me that claimant is being followed by Dr. Sachs and that I should speak to Pat his secretary for further info. Number is 212-555-1212. Transferred me to that number—according to Pat, MD is away and she could not tell me about hosp. stay. Claimant does not have a follow-up appt. yet, she has to call him this week and set something up. Told me that claimant did not have surgery and during hosp. stay claimant was under the care of Dr. Frank 212-555-2212. MF

11/9/99: t/c to Dr. Frank—not in yet, left message with secretary, Lisa. MF

11/10/99: t/c to Dr. Frank—not in yet; left message with secretary, Lisa, for MD to call back. BR

11/11/99: t/c to claimant—spoke to man who rents a room from claimant's father. Told me that claimant does not live here anymore. Claimant's father is out right now, he will give him my phone number for him to call me back with number where claimant can be reached. MF

11/11/99: t/c to claims. Renee will pull most recent claims and check on address and call me back. MF

11/11/99: t/c to MD office—spoke to Lisa who told me that she gave the MD the messages. She will speak to him again and try to get info and call me back. Asked if she had claimant's address and phone number and she transferred me to billing to speak to Terry. Per Terry, claimant does not appear to be in computer system at office or with hosp. Check system several times. Told me to call back after 1 PM and speak to Carmen and perhaps she could help. MF

11/12/99: t/c to Dr. Frank. Claimant had a minor cerebral hemorrhage. Dx. is arterial malformation of the brain; Dr. Sachs is performing surgery at a later date; (212)555-1212; individual not in any danger; need to contact Dr. Sachs for more detailed info. JG/br

11/15/99: t/c to Dr. Sachs office/Pat: they have been unable to contact claimant; he needs to see Dr. Sachs & then surgery can be scheduled. BR

11/15/99: t/c to claims. Renee says claimant admitted to Community Hosp. of W. Suffolk on 11/13.

11/15/99: t/c to C.H.O.W.S./UR Dept./Mrs. King—claimant adm. 11/13 via ER with seizures; was in ICU—now on telemetry; under the care of Dr. Zeller, (516)555-1212 has no additional info @ this time. BR

11/15/99: t/c to Dr. Sachs/Pat—given above info; she will inform MD to f/u with Dr. Z; BR

11/15/99: t/c to Dr. Zeller's office—informed of pending consult with Dr. S # given; Dr. Zeller in with patient; will call with claimant when finished. BR

11/15/99: t/c from Dr. Zeller, claimant c/o numbness of tongue which MD feels is seizure activity; Dilantin increased—c/o of dizziness; CAT scan WNL; EEG pending; will be disch. tonight or tomorrow; f/u with Dr. S. BR

11/15/99: t/c to claimant; spoke with father; corrected birthdate obtained (12-06-34): will f/u with claimant tomorrow to schedule CM assessment; in rm 254, father & son work for the same company. BR
CASE REFERRED FOR CASE MANAGEMENT.

Courtesy of Options Unlimited, Case Management Services Division, Huntington, New York.

nale for case management referral, contain important background information for the case manager assigned to the case, and are forwarded to the claims examiner.

The review summary report shows that only 1 patient out of 10 was referred for case management. One review summary prepared by the au-thor showed a surprisingly high incidence of admission for pregnancy complications for one employer group, and it led to the formation of a maternity screening and management program and the prevention of two premature births. The savings to the group far outweighed the costs of the managed care program.[20]

RED FLAGS: INDICATORS FOR CASE MANAGEMENT

Cases that benefit most from case management commonly involve the most expensive services. Use of these services is thus a red flag. Other indicators include a high frequency of admissions in a short period and an unusually lengthy hospital stay. A stay of 10 days or longer for a surgical hospitalization indicates multiple problems or complications now and points to problems down the road as well. This is where a case manager needs clinical knowledge—a feel for what constitutes a big case. Exhibit 22–7 is a sample tip sheet that includes red flags for case management intervention as well as indicators for claims review.

Different red flags should be used for different lines of insurance. Looking for case management indicators, a case manager will not apply the same dollar limit per claim in a workers' compensation case as he or she applies in a group medical case. In workers' compensation, for each lost-time injury there is an established guideline, and if the injured person is still out of work a month beyond the date calculated using the guidelines, then that fact becomes a red flag. Many physicians use *The Medical Disability Advisor: Workplace Guidelines for Disability Duration*, written by Presley Reed and published by Reed Group, as a reference. A six-volume set of care guidelines for hospital admissions and stays, physician's office treatments, home health care, dentistry, recovery times before returning to work, and medicines has been developed by Milliman & Robertson Inc. These guidelines are followed by the health plans of more than 50 million Americans.

Other indicators of a problem: extension of treatment, treatment recommended by a physician at his or her physician-owned facility, a patient receiving physical therapy and chiropractic manipulation at the same time, a variety of practitioners consulting on a seemingly straightforward case, a case that continually bypasses its return-to-work date, and a patient taking large numbers of pain medications or antidepressant medications.

In group medical coverage the concerns will be different. Group plans cover employees and their dependents, and a case manager might target catastrophic illnesses, premature deliveries, cancer cases, plus other chronic and devastating long-term diseases, such as AIDS or multiple sclerosis. Other things to watch for include multiple hospitalizations, multiple physicians, expenses beyond a certain threshold (e.g., $10,000), and particular kinds of services, such as chemotherapy, radiation therapy, and infusion care.[21]

TIMING CASE MANAGEMENT INTERVENTION

At what point in the review process should a referral be made for case management intervention? As discussed earlier, there are some basic indicators or red flags to look for and there are other, more individualized considerations. Some indicators may actually be evident during the very first call from a hospital admissions department, treating physician, or patient's family to a preadmission review department or company. A preterm delivery, a high-risk pregnancy, a CVA suffered by a teenager, a spinal cord injury, or a traumatic brain injury with coma are all conditions for which there is a high probability of a lengthy hospital stay, a need for additional care and services upon discharge, high costs, and benefits to be gained through case management.

Other conditions would also merit an early referral, not because of a particular diagnosis but because of surrounding circumstances. For instance, diabetes is not by itself a condition that would necessarily promote a case management referral, but the fourth hospital admission in 2 months of a patient with diabetes might. Why are these readmissions occurring? Is the patient noncompliant or noneducated? Is the treating physician a retiring family practitioner? Perhaps an endocrinologist is needed?

Consider a patient with an admitting diagnosis of cellulitis. At first glance, this is not a situation appropriate for case management. However, perhaps as the patient's stay in the hospital continues, more is revealed about this 46-year-

Exhibit 22–7 CareSolutions and AccuClaim Red Flags

CareSolutions Red Flags

Diagnosis:	Cancer	Neuromuscular diseases	Head injury	Psychiatric
	AIDS	Spinal cord injuries	Severe burns	Multiple trauma
	Stroke	Alcohol and substance abuse	High-risk pregnancy	High-risk infant
	Transplant	Cardiovascular	Chronic respiratory illness	
Potential treatment:	Ventilator dependent	TPN/enteral	Home care	
	IV antibiotics	Extended ICU	Chemo	

Frequent hospitalizations: 3 admits same year/same or related problem

Cost of claim: Same illness over $10,000 so far this year

Location of claim: Complex care delivered in rural setting, small hospital, or facility with poor outcome history/diagnosis

Patterns of care: Failed or repeated surgeries, hospital-acquired infections, malpractice concerns

Diagnostic codes: ICD-9-CM Case Management Referral Indicators

Code	Description	Code	Description	Code	Description
042–044	HIV infection	358	Myasthenia gravis (repeat hosps.)	800	Fx vault of skull
140–239	Neoplasms (cancer)	359	Muscular dystrophy (repeat hosps.)	806	Fx of vertebral column w/SCI
250	Diabetes with complications	430–438	Cerebral vascular disease, car. hemorrhage	850–854	Intracranial injury excluding those w/ skull Fx
252	(Possible mult. hosps., coma, renal, eye, neuro)	496	COPD	860–869	Internal injury of chest, abdomen, and pelvis
277	Cystic fibrosis, porphyria, metabolic disorders (mult. hosps.)	501–503	Asbestosis and Silicosis	870–879	Open wound of head, neck, and trunk
279	Immunity deficiency disorders (repeat hosps.)	584–586	Renal failure	925–929	Crushing injury (may involve extensive trauma)
286–287	Coagulation defects (repeat hosps.)	644	Early or threatened labor	948	Burns over 25% of body
290–299	Psychoses	655–656	Fetal abnormality	952	SCI without spinal bone injury
300–316	Neurotic, personality and other nonpsychotic mental disorders	710	All collagen (SLE1)	994	Effects of external causes—lightning, drowning, strangulation
330–337	Hereditary and degenerative diseases of CNS (Alzheimer's, Huntington's chorea)	714	Rheumatoid arthritis w/inflammatory polyarthropathies	996–999	Complications of surgical and medical care
340–349	CNS disorders, MS, CP, quadriplegic, paraplegic, anoxic brain damage	740–759	Congenital anomalies, spina bifida, cardiac septal defect		
		760–763	Maternal causes of perinatal morbidity and mortality		
		765.1	Premature birth		

continues

Exhibit 22–7 continued

AccuClaim Red Flags

Surgical and anesthesia claims: All surgery claims over $1,000 and all cases with more than two line items should be referred for a medical review. Alert for GYN, orthopaedic, plastic surgery. If the surgical claim is referred, corresponding anesthesia claims should be referred also to verify complexity of claimed procedure.
Information to obtain: 1) operative report; 2) anesthesia time; 3) R&C charges for EACH CPT code.

Podiatrists: All claims that exceed $800 should be referred.
Information to obtain: 2) operative report if a surgical procedure is being billed; 2) R&C charges for EACH CPT code.

Physical therapy and occupational therapy: Claims that exceed 6 weeks of treatment should be referred.
Information to obtain: 1) PT evaluation; 2) therapy progress notes that include long- and short-term goals and the range of motion results; 3) letter of medical need from treating MD with diagnosis, frequency of treatment, and estimated duration.

Chiropractic care: Claims that exceed $300 should be referred.
Information to obtain: 1) complete copy of the medical records—NO summaries. Include diagnosis, treatment plan, frequency of treatment, estimated duration.

Durable medical equipment: This is an area of extreme abuse and overutilization of services and fees. The following claims should be referred: oxygen concentrators and related equipment, hospital beds, wheelchairs, ANY monitors, respirators/ventilators, requests for home modifications (ramps, etc).

Home health services: All claims for nursing, aides, or related services should be referred.
Information to obtain: 1) itemized bills; 2) nursing notes.

Infusion care services: All claims for the following infusion services should be referred: IV antibiotics and other medications, TPN (total parenteral nutrition), chemotherapy, analgesia (pain medications).
Information to obtain: 1) MD's prescription; 2) itemized billing for medications, nursing, and related services and supplies.

Any of the following should be referred: 1) appeals; 2) difficult providers; 3) ambulatory surgical centers; 4) large hospital bills: over 7 days LOS—to review for LOS, medical needs *vs.* custodial needs.

continues

Exhibit 22–7 continued

Procedure Codes: CPT AccuClaim Referral Indicators

Integumentary system
11000–11044 For cosmetic vs. medical
15780–15791 For cosmetic vs. medical
15810–15840 For cosmetic vs. medical
17304–17310 For cosmetic vs. medical
19318–19500 For cosmetic vs. medical

Musculoskeletal
27290–27295 Amputation
27590–27598 Amputation

Pulmonary system
30400–30630 For cosmetic
31300–31660 Laryngectomy—tracheotomy, etc
32310–32545 Lung surgery

Cardiovascular
33200–33220 Pacemaker surgery
35450–35458 Vascular vs. cosmetic
37799 Unlisted procedure
38999 Unlisted procedure
39599 Unlisted procedure

Digestive
41100–41155 Mouth, tongue (for cancer)
43600–43640 Stomach (biopsy, etc)
44100–44340 Intestinal
47100–47135 Liver

Urinary system
50200–50380 Kidney, incl. transplant
51550–51597 Bladder (especially for cancer)

Maternity
59000–59100 High-risk procedures
59120–59140 High-risk procedures

Nervous system
61304–61576 Craniectomy
62180–62258 Spine
64999 Unlisted procedure

Eye and ear
65771 Radial keretotomy
68899 Unlisted procedure
69300 Cosmetic
69399 Unlisted procedure

Courtesy of Options Unlimited, Case Management Services Division, Huntington, New York.

old woman: she is also hypertensive, had a coronary bypass 2 years earlier, is diabetic, and weighs 250 pounds—clearly morbidly obese for her height of 5 feet, 4 inches. This woman might eventually require a below-knee amputation secondary to her multiple conditions. The potential for this occurrence warrants an assessment by a case management professional. Patients like this woman would likely be overlooked by a system for case management referral that was driven solely by one ICD-9-CM code or one set dollar limit. Each similar case presents such substantial opportunities for improved outcomes, prevention of complications, and reduction of expenses that not referring becomes a costly risk.[22]

BEYOND THE CASE MANAGEMENT BASICS

Case Management's Contribution to Claims Management

By helping identify the small percentage of claimants responsible for generating the majority of claims and the bulk of benefit payouts (those in need of case management intervention) and educating claims administrators regarding medical issues, case managers serve a vital function in claims departments. They help providers, MCOs, insurers, and TPAs look good to employers and payers by better managing benefit dollars; help patients get care approval in a timely fashion; and help speed the claims administration process without losing patients through the cracks in the system.

Nothing speaks more loudly to a client than a report taken from its own group experience. With a claims run, the case manager can show that out of a group of 500, with total claims paid of $200,000, fewer than 20 individuals (4 percent) filed claims totaling 80 percent ($160,000) of that sum. With this information in hand, a case manager can work with the claims administrator and the employer/payer to improve that claims experience. When the few cases are properly managed, the whole group benefits from lower claims costs.[23] (It must be emphasized that a case manager's work is accomplished without compromising the patient/employee's right to privacy. A case manager can save a company big bucks; the chief executive officer has no need to know and will never know the name of the individual in each case.)

Using a computer program, a case manager can conduct a group run, a profile that may include all hospital admissions, all workers' compensation cases, all short-term disability cases, all cases lasting over a year, and so on. The purpose is to begin examining the claims experience of the group to answer the question: Where have the dollars gone?

For one client, the author prepared a group claims run to find those patients in need of case management intervention. For the first check, a wide net was cast—all hospital admissions. (This field could be narrowed later by setting specific length-of-stay parameters.) The first month's claims run showed that 1 percent of the group generated 34 percent of the claims; the next month, 2 percent generated 67 percent of the total. In the third month, 2 percent of the group was responsible for 73 percent of the benefit dollars paid, and 0.3 percent (three employees) accounted for 44 percent of the total. This 3-month run also revealed those cases requiring costly care from month to month—a clear indicator for case management intervention.[24]

Case managers also work with individual reports. The specific limit for this hypothetical report is $15,000. The first patient that the computer identifies has claims for one hospitalization and one major surgical procedure, a colostomy. The surgery was successful, the postoperative problems minor; there was no real opportunity here for case management to have a major impact. The next individual who has reached the $15,000 limit has a series of claims for an unresolved ulcer of the foot, diabetes, hypertension, and vascular disease. This patient is a health care time bomb. What is the real problem here? Why is the ulcer not healing? Is this person receiving appropriate care? When reports break out claims history by ICD-9-CM or current procedural terminology codes, the case manager can ascertain the presenting problems and procedures taken to alleviate problems;

actual claims files will indicate potential difficulties such as complications from the interaction of various medications. Case managers can
use the tools of the claims department to help resolve health issues, while claims departments
can use the skills of case managers to better their
service.[25]

Cost Benefit Analysis Reports

Cost benefit analysis reports are one form of
case management documentation; they illustrate
in financial terms that the costs spent on case
management services (and the services that are
put in place as part of an alternate care plan)
translate into dollar savings, or dollars spent versus dollars saved. The report format can be customized or modified to meet departmental or client company needs, and report citations may
change as a case management program develops. Generally, a cost benefit analysis report
should include an overview of the case management intervention (a brief narrative), a summary
of the intervention, case management fees, savings (avoided charges, potential charges, discounted and negotiated reductions, and reductions in services, products, and equipment),
actual charges, gross savings (potential charges
minus actual charges), net savings (gross savings minus case management fees), and the status of the case (open or closed).

There are many opportunities for case managers to improve treatment quality, outcome, and
lifestyle for patients. Arranging for home care can
increase patient morale and save money; additional savings are realized when a case manager
asks providers for prompt-pay discounts or reduces the level of care or hours of care through
continual assessment of the patient's progress. Reductions, discounts, negotiated rates, all-inclusive
per diem rates, and "freebies" (the free ambulance
service provided by some community fire departments, for instance) are examples of savings reported in a cost benefit analysis report.

Savings achieved by avoiding potential
charges are more difficult to quantify but should
be reported as well. Consider this scenario: A

case manager is referred to a patient who, in
prior months, had an admission every 1 to 2
months for diabetic complications and an emergency hospital stay of 5 to 7 days. The case manager discovers that Julie does not understand her
diagnosis, is minimally compliant, and frequently ignores dietary restrictions and blood
and urine testing. During the case management
intervention of 3 months, the case manager
spoke to Julie's physician regarding these problems, referred Julie for formal education and a
diet counseling program, and involved Julie in
daily monitoring of her own progress. The pattern of admissions and complications was
halted. Over 6 months of case management intervention, there were no further hospital admissions. The dollars in acute care that could have
been spent, but were not, are savings achieved
via avoided or potential charges.[26]

Combined with outcomes data (and including
outcomes data as part of the summary of case
management intervention), cost benefit analysis
reports chart the success of alternative treatment
plans and serve as strong arguments for the effectiveness of case management and managed care.

Wellness Programs

A good case management program should
come full circle, with outcomes data providing
the rationale for wellness programs designed to
address the problems before they arise so employers and payers spend even less money treating them, and patients are relieved of having to
live through the treatments. If a preadmission
and concurrent review program or a claims report sequence is pointing out patients whose illnesses are protracted and all of them are smokers, perhaps a "smoke out" wellness program is
needed. If every third worker in the warehouse
has been out on disability for lower back pain, a
case manager might design a wellness program
incorporating exercise, review of and instruction
on improved lifting patterns, and a facility review to make site modifications as needed to reduce the lifting injuries. As mentioned earlier in
the chapter, effective pregnancy counseling and

case management intervention can prevent premature labor and the problems arising from low-birthweight babies.

Once a company puts a case management program in place, the next step is to begin using the case management outcomes data wisely to reduce the company's exposure and liabilities by addressing those areas where it is most vulnerable.

Twenty-Four Hour Coverage Programs

Like wellness programs, 24-hour coverage programs take the best facets of case management and managed care programs and put them to broader use. Combining total health care and disability management, 24-hour coverage is a program that coordinates all aspects of health care management. This eliminates the oversight, duplication of services, and paper chase that results when care and management of care are split into categories based on whether or not the slip on the ice occurred on the job (workers' compensation) or at home (group medical coverage), includes a jaw injury (dental coverage), or removes the patient from the work force for 3 months (short-term disability). Rather than pass this individual from management system to management system, 24-hour programs coordinate the entire care program as it moves from site to site, and coverage plan to coverage plan. This puts the focus back on the patient and the care, better managing his or her needs and therefore better managing the costs.

Disease Management

As it was defined in early 1995, disease management bore a striking similarity to case management. An article in the *Journal of Subacute Care* called disease management a coordinated care strategy, citing a Blue's National Coordinated Care Management program as an example and calling it "a new strategic direction for managing customer healthcare experience. The program presents an opportunity to enhance patient care and decrease benefit costs by identifying and selecting chronically ill individuals who represent high-cost users of medical care and linking those individuals with appropriate providers and outpatient interventions. The program involves three separate but integrative components: (1) Identification; (2) Intervention; and (3) Monitoring and Evaluation, which are designed to provide a comprehensive approach to the management of an individual patient's care."[27]

Sound familiar? Look again at the description of case management at the beginning of this chapter and the section on the case management work format and process to see just how familiar. The reader is also referred to Chapter 23 for further discussion of disease state management.

In *Medical Marketing & Media* there was less consensus about what disease management covered. However, it was summarized as "a system of viewing health care disease by disease and examining the interrelated elements in the treatment process with outcomes research to improve quality and lower costs."[28] The article further defined disease management as an "integrated system of customized interventions, measurements, and refinements to current processes of care designed to optimize clinical and economic outcomes within a specific disease state by facilitating proper diagnoses, maximizing clinical effectiveness, eliminating ineffective or unnecessary care, using only cost-effective diagnosis and therapeutics, maximizing the efficiency of care delivery and improving continuously."[29]

While the majority of case management programs have focused on the management of the sickest and costliest individuals in a group, most experts would agree that earlier, more creative, nonepisodic management presents far greater opportunities to prevent these health care disasters. Health care organizations and payers have been striving to improve the quality of care, to control costs, and to actively involve plan members in this process. Whereas case management focuses efforts on an individual patient, disease management targets groups of individuals with diagnostic conditions that have historical and financial evidence of being costly and that will be significantly improved with more integrated and systematic management. Several diseases have already been identified as having the greatest potential for change: asthma, diabetes, high-risk pregnancy, and cardiac disease.[30]

The major thrust of effective disease management programs is in the prevention of acute episodes. The Diabetes Treatment Centers of America in Nashville, Tennessee, successfully reduced hospital admission rates for patients enrolled in its program to 67.3 percent below the national average for persons with diabetes nationwide. Another successful program at the Denver-based National Jewish Center for Immunology and Respiratory Medicine reports outcomes that show asthma hospitalizations decreased 83 percent, emergency department visits decreased 45 percent, and hospital days decreased 82 percent for this high-cost patient group.[31]

A LONG-TERM SOLUTION TO A LONG-TERM PROBLEM

Case management was improving outcomes and preserving benefit dollars long before "health reform" became a catch phrase bandied about in political circles, and case management will continue to help maintain quality care while making the most of the dollars available. As an integral part of effective managed care programs, case management is a long-term solution to a long-term problem—the attempt to find a balance in our health care delivery system—for patients, families, physicians, employers, and payers confronted by diverse health care challenges, new medical technologies, broad ethical questions, and cost concerns. As a managed care tool, case management works. As a health care discipline, it is here to stay.

REFERENCES

1. P. McCollom, Position statement by the Interim Commission for Certification of Case Managers (CCM), presented at the meeting of the CCM Interim Commission Committee, Orlando, FL, January 27, 1995.
2. C. Mullahy, *The Case Manager's Handbook,* 2nd ed. (Gaithersburg, MD: Aspen Publishers, Inc., 1998).
3. Ibid.
4. Ibid.
5. G. Dearing, Improving Patient Compliance in the Best Interests of All, *Managed Healthcare News* 12, no. 12 (1996): 1, 15–16.
6. Mullahy, *The Case Manager's Handbook.*
7. Ibid.
8. Ibid.
9. Ibid.
10. Ibid.
11. Ibid.
12. Ibid.
13. Ibid.
14. Ibid.
15. Ibid.
16. Ibid.
17. Ibid.
18. Ibid.
19. Ibid.
20. Ibid.
21. Ibid.
22. Ibid.
23. Ibid.
24. Ibid.
25. Ibid.
26. Ibid.
27. S.P. Falcon, S.S. Berg, and K.C. Kosel, National Coordinated Care Management: Focused Disease Management Strategies for the 21st Century, *Journal of Subacute Care* 3, no. 2 (1995): 16–19.
28. W.G. Castagnoli, Is Disease Management Good Therapy for an Ailing Industry? *Medical Marketing Media* 30, no. 1 (1995): 46–53.
29. Ibid.
30. Mullahy, *The Case Manager's Handbook.*
31. Ibid.

SUGGESTED READING

Books

Benefits Source Book. Updated annually. Marietta, GA: Employee Benefit News, Enterprise Communications.

Blancett, S., and Flarey, D. 1996. *Handbook of Nursing Care Management.* Gaithersburg, MD: Aspen Publishers, Inc.

Center for Healthcare Information. *Case Management Resource Guide.* Updated annually. Irvine, CA: Center for Healthcare Information.

Cohen, E.L., and Cesta, T. 1997. *Nursing Case Management: From Concept to Evaluation*, 2nd ed. St. Louis, MO: Mosby-Year Book.

Kemether, N.A., ed. 1985. *Crisis Management and Catastrophic Care: A Guide for Rehabilitation Specialists.* Richmond, VA: Vocational Placement Services.

Mullahy, C.M. 1998. *The Case Manager's Handbook*, 2nd ed. Gaithersburg, MD: Aspen Publishers, Inc.

Rossi, J. 1998. *Case Management in Healthcare.* St. Louis, MO: Mosby-Year Book.

Schwartz, G.E.; Watson, S.D.; Galvin, D.E.; and Lipoff, E. 1989. *The Disability Management Sourcebook.* Washington, DC: Washington Business Group on Health and Institute for Rehabilitation and Disability Management.

St. Coeur, M., ed. 1996. *Case Management Practice Guidelines.* St. Louis, MO: Mosby–Year Book.

Thorn, K. 1990. *Applying Medical Case Management: AIDS.* Canoga Park, CA: Thorn Publishing.

Periodicals

Business & Health
5 Paragon Drive
Montvale, NJ 07645
(201) 358-7276

Business Insurance
740 North Rush Street
Chicago, IL 60611-2590
(888) 446-1422

Managed Healthcare
7500 Old Oak Boulevard
Cleveland, OH 44130-3343
(440) 243-8100

Case Management Advisor
3525 Piedmont Road NE
Building 6, Suite 400
Atlanta, GA 30305
(800) 688-2421

The Case Manager
10801 Executive Center Drive, Suite 509
Little Rock, AR 72211
(501) 223-5165

Case Review
4676 Admiralty Way, Suite 202
Marina del Rey, CA 90292
(310) 306-2206

Group Practice Managed Healthcare News
201 Littleton Road, Suite 100
Morris Plains, NJ 07950-2932
(201) 285-0855

Journal of Care Management
1903 Post Road
Fairfield, CT 06430
(203) 259-9333

Managed Healthcare News
26 Main Street
Chatham, NJ 07928-2402
(973) 701-8900

The Remington Report
30100 Town Center Drive, Suite 421
Laguna Niguel, CA 92677-2064
(800) 247-4781

Risk & Insurance
747 Dresher Road, Suite 500
Horsham, PA 19044-0980
(215) 784-0860

Risk Management
205 East 42nd Street
New York, NY 10017
(212) 286-9364

Self-Insurer
17300 Redhill Avenue, Suite 100
Irvine, CA 92714
(714) 261-2553

Fundamentals and Core Competencies of Disease Management

David W. Plocher

DEFINITION AND CLARIFICATION

Disease management is a prospective, disease-specific approach to delivering health care for chronic illnesses managed medically. It spans all encounter sites and augments the physician's visits with interim management through nonphysician practitioners, emphasizing education of members (through self-care) and physicians (through guidelines).

Disease management has been the subject of hundreds of publications and conferences since the publication of a chapter on this topic in *The Managed Health Care Handbook,* 3rd edition. This chapter will not attempt to review or summarize that information. Instead, readers are referred to two excellent meta-analyses: a recent text on disease management, edited by Todd and

Nash,[1] and a peer-reviewed document on chronic illness management by Von Korff et al.[2]

Disease management differs from conventional medical management and conventional hospital-based case management. *Characteristics specific to disease management include the following:*

- Physicians are no longer the center of caregiving; instead, they are members of a caregiving team.
- Nonphysician practitioners deliver most of the care.
- Nearly all care is delivered in the ambulatory care setting.
- Guidelines and outcome measures are more condition specific than body system specific.
- Care is delivered more often over the telephone (including interactive voice response) and the Internet and less often via home and office visits. Medicaid subscribers may be an exception to this type of care if they have limited access to telephones.
- To produce positive changes in members' health status, organizations focus more on education—member and physician behavior change—and less on highly advanced, highly technical, invasive medical procedures.
- Conditions that show modifiable variability in resource use (e.g., prescription drug nonadherence) or morbidity (e.g., emergency department visits for asthmatics) are preferred for disease management.

I thank several colleagues for their role in the survey used to create Figure 23–5: Linda Davis, Walter Elias, Nancy Spangler, and Mary Ann Huseth.

David W. Plocher, MD, is a Partner in Ernst & Young's Health Care Consulting Practice and has 20 years of experience in the managed care field. His early areas of expertise include national point-of-service program administration and the development of the centers of excellence product known as "Institutes of Quality". More recently, he has designed and implemented integrated delivery systems and advanced care management programs including demand and disease management. In addition, he has worked on quality audits and accreditation with both the Joint Commission on Accreditation of Healthcare Organizations and the National Committee for Quality Assurance.

- Data must be collected from all sites of care annually (certain conditions may have shorter episode definitions).
- Fee-for-service physicians and hospitals are not financially rewarded for good disease management in most environments, although satisfied patients are less likely to switch physicians, and the contracting arms of purchasers and payers view these lower-cost providers as a better buy.

This list does not mention all components of disease management, such as the fundamentals of guidelines and outcomes. These components, reviewed in the above references, existed long before the term *disease management* was coined. As this list may suggest, renal dialysis centers and certain managed behavioral health services have displayed most of the features of disease management long before the term was conceived.

Disease management is not primary prevention, population health, or community health. The goal of disease management is more modest: to reduce frequency and severity of exacerbations of a chronic illness so that readmission costs are reduced.

Two historic phenomena may clarify the origin of some of disease management's distinguishing features. First, managed care organizations have struggled to improve their medical loss ratios. Our half-century-old group and staff models believed in the virtue of primary prevention, but added major emphasis on secondary and tertiary prevention over the past 10 years, for economic reasons (Figure 23–1). Secondary and tertiary prevention efforts can yield greater savings than primary prevention efforts.

Second, there has been a long-standing tendency to focus medical management on the acute inpatient stay, leaving ambulatory utilization costs unchecked. Figures 23–2, 23–3, and 23–4 offer three separate perspectives supporting this contention. Costs of noncatastrophic recurring care, diagnostic radiograph and laboratory charges, and other costs outside the acute inpatient stay have risen significantly over the past few decades.

In fact, ambulatory visits result in many more physician–member encounters than inpatient

Figure 23–1 The Origins of Disease Management Medical Loss Ratio Management. *Source:* Reprinted from David W. Plocher, Fundamentals and Core Competencies of Disease Management, in *Best Practices in Medical Management,* Peter R. Kongstvedt, David W. Plocher, eds., pp 339–348, © 1998, Aspen Publishers, Inc.

"Rising health care costs may stem more from the proliferation of laboratory tests than from the often-cited budgetary burdens of technological advances or treatment of the gravely ill."

Minnesota Provider Charges

Figure 23–2 The Origins of Disease Management (Analysis in 1983 by Minnesota Medical Association). *Source:* Reprinted from David W. Plocher, Fundamentals and Core Competencies of Disease Management, in *Best Practices in Medical Management,* Peter R. Kongstvedt, David W. Plocher, eds., pp 339–348, © 1998, Aspen Publishers, Inc.

hospitalizations do. The probability of interacting with a member is shown by a mathematic ratio of encounter sites. The average annual interaction with providers is:

- for hospitalization: 70 admissions/1,000 members/year

- for ambulatory MD office visits: 4,000 encounters/1,000 members/year

In addition to learning to focus on ambulatory as well as inpatient care costs, disease management experts are finally learning from models in general industry that describe supply chain man-

Population: 19 Blue Cross Plans
Time Period: 1986–1988
Hospital visits fell 6% while imaging procedures rose 48%

Figure 23–3 Physician Spending, Private Health Insurance. *Source:* Reprinted from Z. Dyckman, Physician Cost Experience under Private Health Insurance Programs, *Health Care Financing Review*, Vol. 13, No. 3, pp. 85–96, 1992, Health Care Financing Administration.

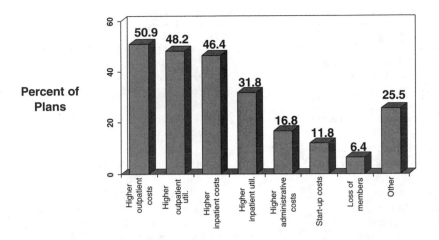

Figure 23–4 Reasons for 1988 Net Loss from Health Maintenance Organization Operations. Courtesy of InterStudy Publications, 1998, Excelsior, Minnesota.

agement with concentration more on annual cost than on unit cost. For example, a heart failure program's prescription drug costs may rise slightly but be more than offset by the larger decrease in total care costs.

BARRIERS AND DRIVERS FOR DISEASE MANAGEMENT

Todd and Nash and Von Korff et al. offer thorough discussions of the barriers to and drivers of disease management programs.[3] Some of the most important barriers include:

- fragmented delivery system
- reimbursement favoring component care delivery
- information system incompatibility

There are many important drivers for disease management programs as well.

- risk-sharing contracting
- information systems that are beginning to collect data across all settings
- a desire for more useful guidelines
- a desire to improve continuous quality improvement techniques

- purchaser and payer interest in and requirements for proof of value
- patients' enthusiasm for self-managing their illnesses

BUSINESS PLAN

A list of key program elements to remember while composing the business plan for the disease management initiative is shown in Exhibit 23–1. From strategic plan/governance to benefit design, marketing and sales issues to education, there is much to consider.

Of these elements, 24-hour access to various services and information must be given higher priority. This forms the basis for patient self-management as well as program-initiated outreach. Telephony and e-commerce represent far less expensive outreach mechanisms than the conventional, nonprioritized home care visit.

The organization must converge reporting lines among personnel conducting utilization review/utilization management discharge planning, social work, and case management. If operating in separate departments, efforts will be duplicated and handoffs will be poorly coordinated.

Exhibit 23–1 Program Elements for Disease Management Business Plan

- Strategic plan/governance
- Provider network development
- Capitalization/ownership
- Benefit design
- Structure/model
  - Emergency department/management observation rooms
  - Inpatient (hospital) management
  - Ambulatory clinic management
  - Pharmacy management
- Marketing and sales
  - Employer groups
  - Local health plans
    1. Fee for service
    2. Capitation
  - Medicaid/Medicare
  - Individuals
- Enrollment, billing, and collection
  - Member verification
  - Claims submission and collection
- Patient access to services
  - 24-hour nurseline/interactive voice response/e-commerce
- Education
  - Telephone-based and mailed information/interactive voice response/e-commerce
  - On-site intervention
- Community intervention and monitoring
  - Community programs
  - Worksite programs
  - School programs
  - Telemonitoring

- Case management and clinical guidelines
  - Inpatient
  - Ambulatory
- Entry/discharge from program
  - Identification/patient profile
  - Education
  - Follow-up
  - Outcome definition
- Information management
  - Ability to identify targeted members through claims, pharmacy data, and risk surveys
  - Disease-specific provider databases
  - Ability to automate reminders
  - Automated tracking of members
- Data collection and outcome evaluation
  - Emergency department visits and hospital days/1,000 members
  - Patient clinical status indicators
  - Patient functional status indicators
  - Patient knowledge and self-management skills
  - Physician/patient compliance with treatment guidelines
  - Patient's perceived value of mailed materials
  - Patient satisfaction
- Reporting
  - Clinical outcomes—ability to generate provider reports
  - Financial outcomes

Courtesy of Ernst & Young LLP, 2000, Washington, DC.

Another high priority is the assembly of data required for program evaluation. The organization's leadership must be provided with an analysis, by the end of the first 12 months at the latest, of the program's return on investment (ROI). In the most ideal circumstances, this ROI analysis should be submitted for independent validation, through external agencies or the peer-reviewed literature.

SURVEY OF DISEASE MANAGEMENT PROGRAMS

A group of researchers and this author recently interviewed the operators of 24 disease management programs. Our questions searched for the characteristics of each site that contributed to its success. Here is a summary of the composite of proficiencies. (Within each proficiency, detailed scoring criteria with numeric thresholds have been developed, but these details are not presented here.)

- *implementation:* speed to market, successful implementation
- *management tools:* automated tracking, ticklers, computer-generated reminders and prompts, guidelines, surveillance for outcomes, provider profiles
- *staff:* adequate staffing ratios for nonphysician practitioners managing a given cohort of patients
- *organizational integration:* roles and processes defined, no duplication of effort, few handoffs, no silos (e.g., case managers, utilization managers, disease managers, and demand managers work together and have systems and tools that connect to each other's activities)
- *marketing and sales:* successfully sold to multiple groups, regionally or nationally
- *targeting tools:* accuracy, predictive validity independently established, automated; optimal use of surveys and pharmacy and claims data

- *stratification tools:* accuracy, predictive validity independently established, designed to prompt customized interventions for optimal outcomes
- *guideline validity:* high quality of evidence
- *member behavior change:* method based on behavior change models including learning style, readiness to change, and efficacy; interventions targeted and tailored; maintenance strategy
- *physician behavior change:* behavior change based on research including aligned incentives, academic detailing, feedback of comparative performance data
- *outcomes collected:* automated collection, both process and endpoints, including utilization, satisfaction, functional status, and clinical indicators
- *reported outcomes:* results frequently reported; sustained or improved outcomes
- *ROI:* costs and benefits measured, positive return within fewer than three years

When studying a new program, a snapshot of strengths and weaknesses can be assembled in the form of a spider diagram, as in Figure 23–5.

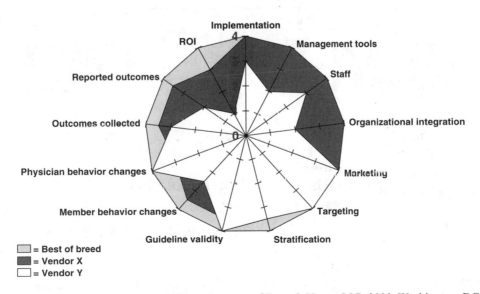

Figure 23–5 Disease Management Capabilities. Courtesy of Ernst & Young LLP, 2000, Washington, DC.

The spider diagram is an easy and clear way to compare health care providers against "best of breed" performance.

We see the next generation of disease management programs evolving with three added characteristics:

1. Care managers will improve coordination of services for a patient with *multiple* chronic diseases.
2. Care managers will become more reluctant to carve out services to a separate, outsourced vendor, believing that the continuity of care for these complex patients is better served with a carved-in model.
3. Care managers and consumers will gain from e-commerce applications, discussed below.

IMPORTANT LINKAGES

In Figure 23–6, the fit for disease management within the spectrum of services following member enrollment is summarized.

The operational detail inside the disease discovery and follow-up processes is exemplified as follows. After the disease is discovered, it should be classified by risk level (mild, moderate, or severe) and appropriate intervention should follow. Risk level is determined by:

- how well the patient understands the disease
- how well the patient learns
- how well the patient cooperates with the provider
- severity of illness measures
- the patient's resource use patterns (incorrect administration of medications, excess emergency department use)
- modifiability of course of disease

Next, in an outbound phone call to the patient, the caller should interview the patient. The number of questions can vary greatly; up to 180 questions (45-minute duration) can occur. The caller should try to determine the patient's level of knowledge and then educate the patient about self-care techniques, symptoms and signs to watch for at home, and whom to call or where to go for help as certain changes occur. Advanced programs retest the patient's fund of knowledge after disease education.

Several types of intervention are possible:

- mild risk—mail education materials
- moderate risk—phone and mail communication to provider

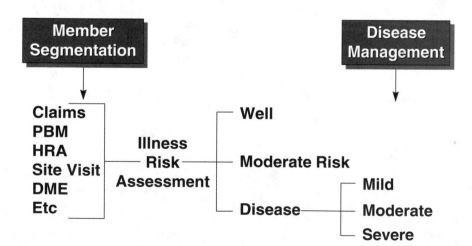

Figure 23–6 Important Linkages. *Note:* DME, durable medical equipment; HRA, health risk appraisal; PBM, pharmacy benefits management. Courtesy of Ernst & Young LLP, 2000, Washington, DC.

- severe risk—dedicated home care team specializing in the disease

SUPPORT FROM ELECTRONIC COMMERCE

Disease management has recently been enhanced by the convergence of health care and the Internet. Electronic commerce is discussed separately in Chapter 36, but it is worthwhile to list some of the applications of e-commerce as they relate to disease management. Increasingly sophisticated applications for health care management via the Internet (e-health) are being developed at a record rate to correct the inefficiencies and deficiencies of the existing model. This relates to the Internet's unique ability to accomplish mass customization, transfer knowledge at trivial cost to users, and take advantage of continuous function that can reduce the time from symptom change to treatment change. The speed advantage is partially due to liberation from "telephone tag." Thus, the patient continues to progress toward being his or her own primary care provider. The following are several examples of typical functionality supported by the convergence of the Internet with health care and disease management:

- *Self-Service Care (Business to Consumer)*
  - medical reference databases
  - health assessment/risk profiles
  - referrals
  - physician directory
  - facility location
  - appointment requests
  - pre-visit patient input
  - discussion groups
  - secure patient/provider messaging
  - prescription refill and prescription refill reminders
  - layman disease protocols
  - diary
  - patient-focused electronic medical record, including progress report/data tracking
  - telemedicine/health
  - advice nurse/pharmacist
  - on-line physician consultations
  - chronic disease management

  - home care televisits and telemonitoring
  - targeted follow-up
  - web-based clinical applications (results viewer)
- *The Virtual e-Health Community (Business to Business)*
  - supply chain consolidation
  - patient, provider, payer linkages (web-based eligibility, authorization, payment, etc.)
  - employer, health plan, insurance, pharmaceutical linkages

The support of disease management using the Internet deserves several notes of caution. Of course, patients will be delighted to have their secure, personalized website, as a repository or hub for communication on their illnesses with their physicians. However, assuming security issues will be adequately addressed, the following concerns continue to need resolution:

- The physician's most precious commodity is time, and responding to a flood of e-mail from patients will extend each workday.
- Responding to e-mail is currently not eligible for reimbursement. However, as some health plans have allowed phone call reimbursement in specific circumstances, it is not out of the question to anticipate a fee schedule for e-mail, as a print of the correspondence is available to document time and effort (more so than a phone call).
- The physician's delivery of e-mail medical advice across state boundaries has fueled an ongoing debate on interstate licensure problems.
- Liability risks are hot discussion topics in e-commerce, including:
  - e-mail advice from physician departing from practice guidelines*

---

*Although nurselines are equipped with well-researched symptom-triage algorithms, with emphasis on ruling out the most catastrophic possibilities first, most physicians do not have such enablements for their e-mail with patients. Furthermore, not all patients are accurate historians, and the physician on e-mail cannot hear the patient's voice inflections, much less interpret body language.

—multiple physicians e-mailing same patient with conflicting advice

—technology failures (applies more to
telemonitoring)

- The primary care physician may have
fewer office visits when e-commerce
works well, impacting fee-for-service revenues

Beyond the e-mail dimensions of e-commerce, disease management stands to gain from
a variety of technologies involving telemonitoring. For example, support for monitoring congestive heart failure (CHF) patients' blood pressure and rhythm,[4] asthma, chronic obstructive
pulmonary disease patients' pulmonary function,[5] and pregnant (high-risk) women's uterine
activity[6] has been encouraging. That is, although
telemedicine is not new and has assisted care in
rural areas, especially for seniors finding travel
difficult, the Internet should enhance the information communicated, from video images to
digitized heart sounds.

More than 100 new companies emerged as of
mid-1999 to create new business models that
serve inadequately met needs of consumers and
health professionals. While their names and revenue streams are rapidly changing and subject to
brisk merger and acquisition activity, three
themes within their operating strategies have
emerged, supported by e-commerce:

- emphasis on knowledge dedicated to self-
care education for consumers and guideline
information to providers
- extension into workflows, helping providers and payers to serve consumers
- facilitation of product acquisition by consumers

A CHF program recently designed by the author with other professionals is summarized in
Exhibit 23–2.*

---

*Detailed perspectives on disease management of
CHF and selected other examples may be found in
Peter R. Kongstvedt and David W. Plocher, *Best
Practices in Medical Management* (Gaithersburg,
MD: Aspen Publishers, Inc., 1997).

CASE STUDY

In this case, a private, 420-bed hospital in the
northeastern United States needed to formulate
its response to new market pressures. The payers were no longer as concerned about length of
hospital stay for CHF as they were about annual care costs. The chief executive officer
chose to fund the start-up of an expanded case
management program with a home care emphasis for CHF.

Multiple site visits for discussions with
physicians, nurses, and ancillary care services,
including training on disease management
fundamentals, were conducted. From these essentials, specifications that were unique for
CHF were developed and agreed upon. A partial list of program elements included:

- structure
- practice guidelines
- data elements
- functional status scale
- behavior change techniques

Initially, the referring physicians were not
supportive. The fee-for-service environment
would result in loss of revenue to them whenever they referred a patient. However, after further educational sessions, some movement began to occur in their attitudes.

The results are encouraging. Over 75 patients have been through the program by late
1998. Preliminary analysis shows that there is
value in directing staff and resources toward
the more severely ill CHF patients. Using the
New York Heart Association classification, it
was found that the 25 Class III patients showed
the largest improvement, reducing by over
50% their hospital admits and total hospital
days. Interestingly, the 25 Class IV patients did
not reduce resource use, perhaps confirming
one of the requirements for disease management offered earlier in the chapter: the circumstances of the patient must be *modifiable* (however, our interventions did not extend into a
program for parenteral inotropes, left ventricu-
lar assist devices, etc.). Similarly, Class I and II
patients (the remaining 25) did not change hospital use, as mildly ill patients are usually managed in the ambulatory setting.

Exhibit 23–2 Design of a CHF Program

THE BEGINNING
- Began in August 1996
- Referral sources:
  - Physicians
  - Discharge planners
  - Home health care
- Multidisciplinary team
  - Pharmacist
  - Dietitian
  - Social worker
  - Chaplain

THE PROCESS
- Initial assessment
  - Registered nurse (RN) collects recent data on patient's use of hospital, emergency department, physician office
  - RN administers the Minnesota *Living with Heart Failure* questionnaire
- Concurrent care
  - RN on call 7 days/week, 12 hours/day
  - Patient calls RN directly
  - RN can do in home
    1. Pulse oximetry
    2. Blood draws
    3. ECG
    4. IV Lasix or Bumex
  - The CHF hotline
  - CHF support group
- Given detailed home diary for events to track and triggers for dialing hotline
- Excerpt of reasons to call RN or physician
  - Gained 2–5 lbs in 2–4 days
  - Swelling ankles or abdomen

- Worsening shortness of breath (SOB)
- Sudden awakening from sleep with SOB
- Needing more pillows to raise head when trying to sleep
- Worsening cough
- Persistent nausea, vomiting, diarrhea
- New or worsening dizziness
- New fatigue with exertion
- Loss of appetite

CASE STUDY
- 86-year-old female with CHF
- Prior to CHF program (6 ER visits in 6 months)
- Following entry into CHF program (no ER visits in 3 months)
- Typical intervention
  - Case manager found 4-lb gain and worsening SOB
  - Home visit did ECG, blood work, oximetry, and IV Lasix

RESULTS
- Patients like it (more comfortable calling in a question to the RN than their physician)
- Physicians liked it—eventually
  - Now referring "difficult" patients
  - Phone call volume to physician reduced
  - Perceived as an extension of physician office rather than a separate home health care or hospital program

HOTLINE TIPS FOR URGENT CARE
(*not* a substitute for 911 for extreme, catastrophic emergencies)

Source: Reprinted from David W. Plocher, Fundamentals and Core Competencies of Disease Management, in *Best Practices in Medical Management,* Peter R. Kongstvedt, David W. Plocher, eds., pp 339–348, © 1998, Aspen Publishers, Inc.

CONCLUSION

I would like to offer a final caution for the attendee of the next disease management conference. Beware the vendor that dusts off its guidelines or outcome database and repackages it in a presentation titled "disease management." Practice guidelines and outcome measurement have been around for decades. Beware the promotion of a single pharmaceutical agent as the only indicated treatment for a condition. Disease managers will allow for continuous innovation, prompt adoption of blockbuster drugs, and continuous reassessment using pharmacoeconomic analyses. The lecture on the pathophysiology of the disease for training physicians to manage the patient in the acute hospital setting is not directly relevant; disease management does not occur in the acute inpatient setting, and patients are not available for teachable moments while they are intubated. Disease management also does not occur during the 8-minute physician office visit, crammed with the technology of laboratory work, imaging, and prescription refills.

Disease management can occur just about everywhere else. Communication technology is the most important kind of technology; multiple media are available for information transfer 24 hours a day, 365 days a year. The most successful caregivers (many of them nonphysicians) are making a difference through their skill in member assessment and behavioral change techniques.

REFERENCES AND NOTES

1. W. Todd and D. Nash, eds., *Disease Management: A Systems Approach to Improving Patient Outcomes* (Chicago: American Hospital Publishing, Inc., 1996).

2. M. Von Korff, J. Gruman, J. Schaefer, S.J. Curry, and E.H. Wagner, Collaborative Management of Chronic Illness, *Annals of Internal Medicine* 127, no. 12 (1997): 1097–02.

3. Todd and Nash, *Disease Management*; Von Korff et al., Collaborative Management of Chronic Illness.

4. D. Shanit, A. Cheng, and R.A. Greenbaum, Tele-cardiology: Supporting the Decision-Making Process in General Practice, *Journal of Telemedicine and Telecare* 2 (1996): 7–13.

5. F. Mair, M. Wilkinson, S.A. Bonnar, et al., The Role of Telecare in the Management of Exacerbations of Chronic Obstructive Pulmonary Disease in the Home, *Journal of Telemedicine and Telecare* 5, suppl. 1 (1999): 66–67.

6. M. Torok, Z. Turi, and F. Kovacs, Ten Years Clinical Experience with Telemedicine in Prenatal Care in Hungary, *Journal of Telemedicine and Telecare* 5, suppl. 1 (1999): 14–17.

CHAPTER 24

Prescription Drug Benefits in Managed Care

Robert P. Navarro

Prescription drugs are a highly coveted and widely used health care benefit and an important cost-effective component of a comprehensive health care benefit program. More than 92 percent of health maintenance organization (HMO) membership has access to a prepaid pharmacy benefit, although historically prescription drugs have been a mandated HMO benefit only in Minnesota.[1] By 1995, third-party payers reimbursed more than 50 percent of all prescriptions dispensed in retail pharmacies in the United States. In the year 2000, IMS Health (web address: http://www.imshealth.com) estimates that third-party reimbursement levels will approach 80 percent of all retail prescriptions in the United States.[2] Clearly, managed pharmacy benefit programs have increased the use of medications by making prescription drugs more affordable and accessible to the members of managed care organizations. However, despite the clinical and economic value of appropriately used pharmaceuticals, managed care and its customers have expressed alarm at the steady double-digit annual increase in pharmacy program costs that is exceeding the cost trend of physician and hospital costs. As a result, managed care and its employer group customers are attempting to minimize the cost and maximize the clinical and economic outcomes of the pharmacy benefit through an evidenced-based approach. The result is an evolution in the benefit design of the pharmacy program that will have a significant impact on future access and use of pharmaceuticals, although the ultimate impact on clinical outcomes and quality of life is yet unknown.

Robert P. Navarro, PharmD, is President of NAVARRO*Pharma*, LLC, a consulting group serving the health care industry on outcomes-oriented, cost-effective pharmacy benefit management programs, and the pharmaceutical industry on training, customer interventions, and strategies to successfully market pharmaceutical products to managed care customers. He has practiced in long-term care, acute care, community pharmacy, as well as 17 years in managed care building and operating prescription drug programs with United HealthCare, Diversified Pharmaceutical Services, Health Net (California), and Express Scripts, Inc.

Navarro was a co-founder and first president of the Academy of Managed Care Pharmacy, now a 4,500 member professional association representing managed care pharmacists. He is a member of the American Society of Health-System Pharmacists and the International Pharmacy Federation. He is chief editor of *Managed Care Pharmacy Practice*, a textbook published in 1999 by Aspen Publishers. He writes and speaks frequently on managed care

FINANCIAL BASIS FOR PHARMACY BENEFIT MANAGEMENT

In the early formative years of managed care, health policy administrators and providers of care recognized that affordable prescription drug benefits were an important health care delivery component that was consistent with the prepaid "health maintenance" concept of HMOs and managed care. In 1970, just before the passage of the HMO Act of 1973, pharmacy costs were just more than 8 percent of total U.S. health care expenses, whereas hospital costs made up 38 percent of total costs, and physician expenses represented 19 percent of expenditures.[3] By the early 1980s, pharmacy costs were typically only 5 percent of an HMO's total health care costs. However, cost containment of all products and services has always been a core responsibility of managed care organizations (MCOs). As a result, after most large HMOs had implemented strategies to contain hospital and physician costs, they began to address pharmacy costs. Figure 24–1 illustrates the percent consumption of hospital, physician, and pharmacy programs of total health care costs from the 1970s through the 1990s. By the mid-1980s, pharmacy costs were showing a steady increase (see Figure 24–2). Although the total pharmacy program costs were relatively small compared with hospital and physician costs, the trend rate became alarming. As a result, managed care be-

gan to aggressively manage pharmacy program benefits.

Pharmacy program cost increases came under relative control from 1990 to 1993 (see Figure 24–3) but have increased steadily since that time. In a 1999 survey of 20 pharmacy benefit managers (PBMs) and HMOs representing more than 161 million lives, pharmacy program costs were increasing at an average annual trend rate of 18 percent (range, 14 to 28 percent).[4] This is in sharp contrast to the cost trend of hospital and physician costs, which have been in the 3 to 5 percent range since 1995. Express Scripts, Inc., a large independent PBM reported that the pharmacy program drug average wholesale price (AWP) on a per-member-per-year (PMPY) basis increased 16.8 percent from 1997 to 1998. The same study found that pharmacy program cost increased 66.6 percent from 1994 to 1998, with half of this growth caused by drugs launched after 1994.[5] The annual pharmacy program increases caused great alarm among payers

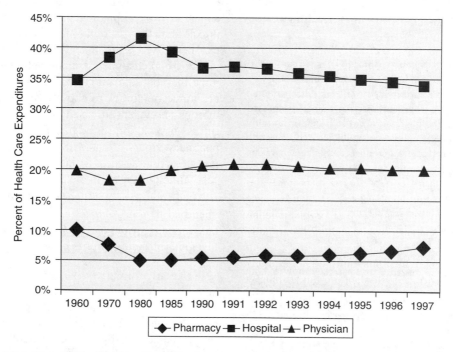

Figure 24–1 Percent Health Care Expenditures of Hospital, Physician, and Pharmacy Services. *Source:* Reprinted from National Health Statistics, 1999, Office of the Actuary, Health Care Financing Administration.

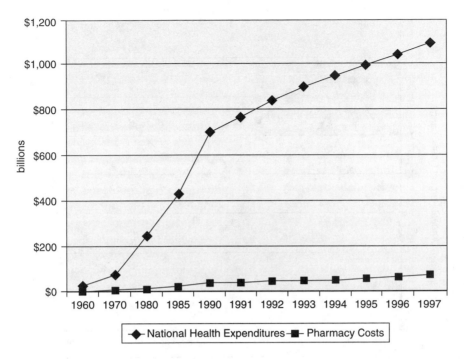

Figure 24–2 Comparison of U.S. National Health Care Expenditures and Pharmacy Costs Trend. *Source:* Reprinted from National Health Statistics, 1999, Office of the Actuary, Health Care Financing Administration.

and pharmacy program managers, especially because the annual cost increases of hospital and physician costs were approximately 3 to 5 percent at the same time (see Figure 24–3).[6]

Unquestionably, an aggressive pharmacy program management can reduce program costs. Figure 24–4 illustrates the difference in long-term program per member per month (PMPM) costs between an HMO that implemented an aggressive pharmacy program management in 1988 and an HMO that did not. There is an approximate $10 PMPM difference between the two plans after 15 years of operation. Note that the cost trend of both programs is positive, but the managed program started at a lower point after implementation of the managed program in 1988 and has a slightly lower slope of the curve.

The growth in the average prescription price provides another metric to measure pharmacy cost increases. The National Association of Chain Drug Stores (NACDS) found that the average retail prescription price increased 7.5 percent from $35.72 in 1997 to $38.43 in 1998.[7] When dissecting the brand versus generic prescription prices, the NACDS found that brand prescription prices increased from $49.55 to $53.51, an 8 percent increase, whereas generic drug prices increased 2 percent, from $16.95 to $17.33 from 1997 to 1998. Clearly, this demonstrates why managed care has mandated the use of generic drugs, when clinically appropriate, as a seminal cost-containment strategy. As will be discussed later, this is also the reason for the tiered copayment structure that provides a financial incentive for the member to accept, or even request, a generic alternative.

PHARMACY PROGRAM COST COMPONENTS

Although the total pharmacy program costs and the annual cost trend are important financial performance measures to follow, these metrics alone do not provide adequate information to

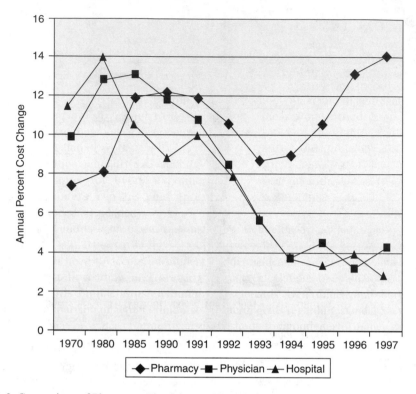

Figure 24–3 Comparison of Pharmacy, Physician, and Hospital Annual Cost Changes. *Source:* Reprinted from National Health Statistics, 1999, Office of the Actuary, Health Care Financing Administration.

develop a comprehensive pharmacy benefit management program. Effective pharmacy benefit managers will dissect their overall cost trend and identify the specific cost drivers so that they may craft a program that addresses the components that contribute to program cost increases. Express Scripts conducted such an evaluation and found that when costs increased 16.8 percent from 1997 to 1998, the primary cost drivers were drug price inflation (5.1 percent), a change in the drug mix (4.4 percent [physicians "trading up" from older, less expensive products to newer, more expensive drugs]), and an overall increase in prescription use (3.8 percent). Other less important drivers were the number of units per prescription and an increase in drug strength (e.g., higher milligrams being dispensed).[8]

Drug price inflation and utilization rate are typically the two components that are most re-

sponsible for pharmacy program cost increases, and most management strategies address these cost drivers. Express Scripts found that the drug price inflation more than doubled between the periods of 1996 to 1997 (2.4 percent increase) and 1997 to 1998 (5.1 percent increase).[9] At the same time, the utilization rate (number of prescriptions obtained PMPY) increased 4.5 percent in the 1996 to 1997 period and actually declined 3.8 percent in the 1997 to 1998 period. However, this 3.8 percent trend represented an increase from 7.4 prescriptions PMPY in 1997 to 7.68 prescriptions PMPY in 1998.

Pharmacy program costs, the utilization rate, and average prescription price are tangible, highly visible, and easily measurable metrics. As a result, payers and health plans naturally focus on costs. However, intellectually we understand that appropriately used pharmaceuticals

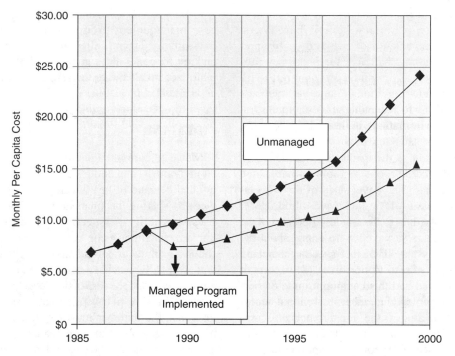

Figure 24–4 Comparison of Managed and Unmanaged Pharmacy Program Costs (Example).

are perhaps one of the most cost-efficient forms of therapy, and we hesitate to control pharmacy benefits excessively. As will be discussed later, it is difficult to judge the clinical or economic impact of drugs due to the challenge of measuring outcomes. From the cost-containment perspective, the pharmacy program manager may be concerned that the increase in prescription use will increase program costs. However, from the perspective of outcomes management, the increase in prescription use may result in better disease prevention or treatment that may ultimately improve the quality of care and total direct medical costs as a result of avoided hospitalizations. The general lack of data to definitively link drug use with medical or economic outcomes is the fundamental reason why pharmacy programs are aggressively managed to contain utilization and costs.

New drugs, often more expensive than older brand and generic drugs, may be restricted or not covered by some MCOs when launched for two primary reasons. First, health plans are reluctant to cover a new drug for several months until the adverse effect profile is well established. Second, new drugs that are more costly may not offer any significant clinical advantages over existing, less expensive products. Health plans will investigate the literature and consult with their specialists to determine whether the new, expensive drug provides greater value than existing formulary products. Express Scripts found that the 50 top drugs by cost that were launched subsequent to 1992 represented 35.6 percent of the total 1998 AWP PMPY costs.[10]

PRINCIPLES OF PHARMACY BENEFIT MANAGEMENT

Health care is a market-driven business, and there is enormous competition among MCOs for employer groups and members. As a result, HMOs, PBMs, and other MCOs providing a pharmacy benefit must do so in a cost-efficient manner. That is, they must provide affordable access to required medications at a cost that is acceptable to pharmacy benefit purchasers. Achieving this balance of cost and quality presents an ongoing challenge for pharmacy program managers as program costs continue to increase (as shown previously) and yet members are less willing to accept higher copayments, restrictions, or limitations in their pharmacy benefit. Member satisfaction is becoming increasingly important as the quality of care delivered by managed care becomes a topic for public and political debate. The cover story of the November 8, 1999, issue of *Newsweek* was titled "HMO Hell."[11] According to the article, 61 percent of the HMO members surveyed were angry about the health care system. The chief specific complaint was high cost of prescription drugs (81 percent of those surveyed had this complaint), and 84 percent of the surveyed members stated that access to affordable drugs is the "most important" component of their health care. This survey verifies the importance affordable prescription drugs are to members of managed care plans.

Recognition of the value of pharmaceuticals (the product of cost and benefit) must not be ignored when making a drug formulary coverage decision. Ideally, we should construct and evaluate the pharmacy program while considering the impact of appropriately used, cost-effective pharmaceuticals on the clinical, economic, and humanistic (quality of life) outcomes.

For example, the least expensive drug may produce a high rate of serious, costly adverse effects that may result in hospitalization (with obvious negative clinical and economic outcomes). However, a newer, more expensive drug may have been much safer, and although the pharmacy budget may increase, the total overall impact on economic and quality of life outcomes would be more positive than with the less expensive drug. Therefore, we must not manage the pharmacy benefits as an isolated component but as an interactive component that has an influence on the outcomes of other components. Unfortunately, until we have complete, integrated clinical or claims data that will allow the overall evaluation of drug use, we will likely continue to manage health care from a compartmentalized,

silo perspective. Pharmacoeconomics and disease management programs, discussed later, have provided some enlightenment in this regard and are focusing more attention on the value of pharmaceuticals rather than simply on their cost.

MANAGING THE SUPPLY AND DEMAND

Managed care attempts to control behavior of all individuals, and entities can influence the supply and demand of health care products and services by sharing the financial risk. From a pharmacy benefit perspective, managed care implements supply side contracts with pharmaceutical manufacturers and dispensing pharmacies that essentially provide a discount on the drug ingredient cost and the dispensing fee. Demand-side controls involve prescription copayment or coinsurance the member must pay to access pharmacy services. Many managed care organizations, especially on the West Coast and in the Northeast, also share the financial risk of the pharmacy benefit with prescribing physicians. The theory behind this strategy is that physicians will prescribe more cost-efficiently if they share in the cost of the drugs they prescribe. Despite the fact that this practice has been criticized for allegedly providing perverse incentives to physicians, pharmacy cost risk sharing with physicians continues and is spreading to other parts of the country. In summary, pharmacy program managers attempt to control the drug ingredient cost and prescription use, obtain discount contracts with all entities that can influence drug cost or the dispensing process, and share the financial cost of the pharmacy program with all individuals that can influence the supply and demand of prescription benefits.

PHARMACY INFORMATION SYSTEMS AND HEALTH INFORMATICS

Similar to any modern business, pharmacy practice and the administration of a pharmacy benefit are critically dependent on data and information systems. The basic information systems involved in pharmacy benefit management include the following:

- Internal MCO systems used for storing member demographic, benefit, and claims adjudication data. Actual claims adjudication may occur within the HMO, a third-party claims processor, or a PBM (if used). See Chapter 38 for additional discussion about claims processing.
- In-pharmacy point-of-service (POS) system dispensing pharmacist uses to determine member and drug coverage information and reimbursement information and adjudicate the claim online and in real time.
- Pharmacy claims analysis system (for drug utilization review, pharmacy program performance analysis, research, patient and physician intervention programs, etc.). This capability often resides within the third-party administrator or the PBM (if used). Larger, sophisticated HMOs may have their own internal analysis system even though they use a PBM. See Chapter 32 for additional discussion about practice profiling.

The presence of an accepted electronic data interchange standard for pharmacy claims transmission and adjudication accelerated the adoption of pharmacy e-commerce. This standard, maintained by the National Council for Prescription Drug Programs (NCPDP), permits the submission of pharmacy claims and the adjudication of those claims in a real-time interactive mode. This universal standard has allowed the pharmacy profession an advanced position in electronic commerce that other segments of the health care industry have not yet achieved. The NCPDP is a nonprofit organization of almost 1,200 members representing almost 600 companies that "establishes, monitors, and maintains standards of information processing for the pharmacy-services sector of the healthcare industry."[12] The NCPDP is recognized by the American National Standards Institute (ANSI) as an American Standards Developer in pharmacy electronic data interchange.

Pharmacy Claims Adjudication Systems[13]

Observation of the NCPDP data standards allows 95 percent of all prescription claims to be processed electronically online and usually in real time. Pharmacists rely on the benefit design and coverage information provided to them through the in-pharmacy POS system. More than 75 percent of patients obtaining pharmacy benefits in many pharmacies are members of MCOs, and because of the highly variable, frequently changing, complex benefit design and coverage rules, pharmacists simply must rely on electronic messaging to process the prescription. When a pharmacist fills a managed care prescription, the required patient, drug, and prescriber data are input into the POS system. Within seconds, the pharmacist is informed if the patient and drug are eligible for coverage, is given the copayment to be collected, is told the level of prescription reimbursement from the MCO or PBM, and is provided any pertinent clinical information (e.g., drug interactions). The pharmacist then "approves" the prescription reimbursement data and within seconds the claim is adjudicated online.

The latest generation of pharmacy management systems provide patient-specific information to the prescriber or dispenser at the point-of-care that will help reduce side effects, drug interactions, dispensing errors, and the improper use of medication. Frequently, systems encourage drug compliance through messaging or other forms of communication directed at the dispensing pharmacist. Although improved compliance may increase drug costs, the goal is to reduce long-term overall medical costs. All these improvements, based on an increase in software complexity, have occurred as a result of better and faster hardware.[14]

Evolving pharmacy management systems are able to select appropriate pharmaceuticals on the basis of submitted diagnosis codes, patient drug histories, or other specific clinical guidelines. Specific evaluations of encounters, not available in the first-generation systems, can enable the pharmacist to influence patient drug use or provide patient-specific counseling strategies.[15] The newest generation of systems often focuses on clinical guidelines on the basis of specific conditions or disease states. Pharmaceutical and medical professionals can design patient management programs that target small, high-risk populations that are driving health care costs. Clearly, the ability to analyze information provided by the online systems is a key to the evolution of prescription benefit management systems.

Other Pharmacy Information Systems[16]

MCO management information systems that store billions of prescription records, member medical history and utilization patterns, provider activities, claims administration, and financial records are generally referred to as online transaction processing systems (OLTPs). These systems and advances in technology have provided the means to collect and store data. Beyond claims adjudication and data storage, there is another challenge to use the data to advance prospective drug utilization review, disease management, incentive-based cost management (rebate programs) to improve cost, and quality outcomes. This requires the development of systems that can transform huge amounts of data and convert them into understandable information for clinical and business decision makers.

This different application requires a different type of information system. Online analytical processing systems (OLAPs) transform the data collected from different sources and delivery systems by the OLTP systems into clinical and business decision support tools. OLAP systems are often called data warehouses, in which data from transaction based systems are collected, integrated, and delivered to end users expressly to support data or clinical analysis activities. The basic requirements of an OLAP system are to assemble and transform raw data into a form that is suitable for analysis, distribute the data, and provide access to the information store in a "datamart" concept accessible to the appropriate user (see also Chapters 35 and 36 for additional discussion about data warehousing and reporting). Protection of patient confidentiality is paramount in successful administration of the data warehouse concept, ever more so with the passage of the Health Insurance Portability and Accountability Act of 1996 (HIPAA; see Chapter 67). Access to integrated pharmacy, medical,

demographic, provider, and financial records supports that ability to manage pharmacy benefits from an integrated perspective and allows the consideration of pharmacy as a source of value rather than only a cost center.

Pharmacy and Medical Claims Integration

Medical and pharmacy data are collected for various financial, administrative, and clinical reasons. However, most delivery system data and information were developed at different times, by different developers, and for independent reasons. As a result, most health plans do not have the ability to easily collect, integrate, and analyze comprehensive patient care records that span all delivery components.

Merging of these medical and pharmacy databases is accomplished through linking the common shared dimensions, such as identifiers for member, physician, and employer group. Because pharmacy coding is very specific and standardized (i.e., a drug's National Drug Code [NDC] number can relate to only one drug entity), drug utilization serves as a surrogate quality of care indicator for many diseases. For example, in asthma treatment, the relative amount of inhaled corticosteroids and beta-agonists used can be an indicator of how successfully the disease is being managed. National Commission for Quality Assurance (NCQA) has established many such "effectiveness of care" indicators through its HEDIS program (Health Plan Employer Data and Information Set), thus forcing MCOs to create merged or linked databases.[17]

Integrated claims databases can be analyzed to observe patterns of medical or drug interventions that produce superior or inferior outcomes. For example, a population of case-mix–adjusted patients with a specific medical condition can be stratified according to severity, age, comorbidity, and so forth, and different antibiotic interventions to compare the clinical and economic outcomes of each cohort. Similarly, physician performance may also be evaluated and compared. A well-constructed, merged database may be used to identify clinical "best practices" that are associated with most cost-effective outcomes.

Electronic Data Interchange and Electronic Commerce

The NCPDP has developed at electronic data interchange (EDI) format called SCRIPT to standardize electronic commerce of prescription data from the physician to the pharmacist. Successful installation of this application will help increase formulary conformance, adherence to drug therapy guidelines, and increase pharmaceutical manufacturer contract performance.[18] Other segments of health care are working under the ANSI Health Informatics Standards Board (HISB) to ensure that the developing standards allow the systems of the various health delivery components will be interactive and share standardized processes, data definitions, and data interchange procedures. Clearly, the incredible pace at which Internet e-commerce is progressing will provide interactive applications for pharmacy benefit administration by exchange of data and pharmacy-related information among the trading partners. See also Chapter 37 for additional discussion about electronic commerce.

Electronic Prescribing[19]

Electronic prescribing is an EDI application that provides physician connectivity with the pharmacy to allow a physician to transmit a prescription order to a pharmacy online. There are several potential financial and patient care advantages to the physician, health plan, pharmacy, and patient. Electronic prescribing (EP) provides the physician the ability to consult an online, point-of-care drug formulary, and/or treatment guideline reference to minimize variation in drug prescribing, as well as providing physicians a complete patient medication history. This point-of-prescribing information supports physician behavior modification by providing instantaneous feedback. Prior authorization or step-care protocols may be recommended or enforced through EP. The EP system can also alert the physician at the point-of-prescribing of any drug interactions, history of adverse events, redundant prescriptions, and incorrect dosages before the patient leaves the physician's office so that they may be corrected before the prescription is transmitted to the pharmacy.[20] Figure 24–5 illustrates one example of the EP process.

Through EP, prescriptions can be transmitted electronically to the pharmacy of choice in a legible format. Alerts and reminders are integrated into such programs to encourage compliance and follow-up and enhance appropriate drug utilization. When the physician makes the diagnosis, the system will provide recommended drug products on the basis of the diagnosis, current patient data, past medical history, known aller-

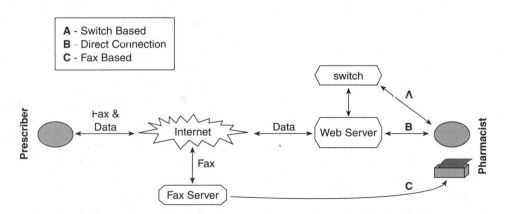

Figure 24–5 Schematic of Electronic Prescribing Transmission. Courtesy of Med Data Healthcare Systems, Inc.

gies, past drug experiences, health plan treatment guidelines, drug use protocols, and comparative drug outcomes research. The system can construct a patient-specific prescription on the basis of these data elements in a real-time basis.

The physician can then transmit the prescription information to the selected pharmacy, alone or with other pertinent patient information, such as diagnosis or drug indication or laboratory or physical findings, that would assist the pharmacist in providing patient counseling or drug monitoring. EP reduces physician office time and costs by transmitting a "clean" prescription to the pharmacy. This eliminates any phone calls from the pharmacy if a nonformulary drug is mistakenly prescribed or if the dosage is unclear or incorrect. EP also reduces the time for the prescription to be filled and may reduce patient time waiting in the pharmacy because the prescription is electronically transmitted to the pharmacy before the patient arrives at the pharmacy. EP can support and enforce prior authorization programs, disease management, drug use guidelines, or step-care protocols that check a patient's drug history to determine whether the required initial drug of choice has been used before a more expensive, second-line drug is prescribed. The EP system can provide immediate prescribing feedback to the physician so that education occurs and behavior is modified and the new learning is reinforced. The physician can send to the pharmacy a message indicating that patient educational material should be customized, printed, and provided to the patient when the prescription is dispensed.

The MCO benefits from EP through increased formulary conformance. One health plan experienced a 12 percent increase in formulary conformance and a 14 percent increase in generic drug use through an EP application.[21] There are a number of pilot projects that use web technology to support EP. Although some state Boards of Pharmacy may have expressed concerns over security and confidentiality of electronically transmitted prescriptions, it appears as if there are enough economic and patient care benefits that EP will become a standard practice in the near future.[22]

Pharmacy Services and Health Telematics[23]

The rapid expansion of information technology presents novel opportunities and challenges for patient communication and intervention related to their pharmacy benefits. The National Association of Boards of Pharmacy defines health telematics as "a composite term for health-related activities, services and systems, carried out over a distance by means of information and communications technologies, for the purposes of global health promotion, disease control and health care, as well as education, management, and research for health."[24] Health telematics, telemedicine, and telepharmacy are all concepts that use information technology and enlightened health care practitioners to advance health care promotion and outcomes. The World Health Organization also endorses these strategies to advance global health development through its Health-for-All Strategy in the twenty-first century.[25]

EDI, physician connectivity and EP, the Internet, and web technology all present a practice platform that is quite different. The success of telemedicine and telepharmacy is based on two fundamental concepts: moving information rather than people, and bringing care to the point of need. Pharmacists in particular will benefit from information technology advancements by having greater access to more patient care data and improved communication to other health care professionals and patients. Pharmacists will have greater access to observing patient behavior so that they may better monitor prescription drug use, provide targeted and specific patient education, implement compliance and persistence interventions, and communicate directly with patients regarding any drug or medical questions they may have. Pharmacists and other health professionals will also be able to input information they learn from or about the patient into the MCO or PBM patient database that can be accessed by the physician when reviewing drug use, prescribing a new drug, or refilling a prescription. Through video conferencing, web technology, and access to the clinical data warehouse, health professionals and caregivers throughout the world can communicate and yet provide personal interaction to individual patients to meet specific patient-care needs.

Internet Patient Marketing

Pharmaceutical manufacturers have used newsprint and television direct-to-consumer (DTC) advertisements quite effectively. Some advertisements are blatantly product based and inspire a patient to request a specific drug product from the physician. Other ads, considered more palatable by managed care, are more educational in nature and provide information about a specific medical condition to urge consumers to seek treatment if they have the condition. However, the rapid expansion of Internet access by a growing number of households has produced another medium for DTC advertisement.

More than 8,000 health-related Internet websites and pharmaceutical manufacturers hoping to influence patient behavior sponsor many of these technological advertisements.[26] The content of the pharmaceutical-related websites provides information on a treatment or medical conditions, and some provide comprehensive consumer-oriented drug information. Some websites are interactive and allow the patient to communicate with the corporate sponsor and request additional information. Many of the websites have established links to other related websites, and some MCO websites recommend health-related websites that are particularly informative and unbiased. It is also possible to provide coupons and discounts to patients through the Internet and even send samples for nonprescription products to patients on request.

PHARMACY BENEFIT MANAGEMENT COMPANIES (PBMs)[27]

Pharmacy benefit management companies, or pharmacy benefit managers, abbreviated as "PBMs," are specialized business entities established to provide a broad spectrum of outsourced pharmacy benefit management services for their private and public payer-customers on a stand-alone or carve-out basis. That is, the management of the pharmacy benefit is "carved-out" from internal management within the health plan and provided by an external PBM. Carve-out services are not unique to pharmacy. It has been very common for HMOs to carve out mental health, dental, and chiropractic services to external management companies. The basic business reasons for an employer group, an MCO, or an insurer to use a PBM are the potential for lower developmental and operational program costs, reduced development time, breadth of flexible data processing services, and other clinical and patient care services provided by the PBM. Certainly an HMO can internally develop the capabilities offered by a PBM. There may be reasons of cost-efficiency to justify using an external PBM rather than building internal pharmacy benefit program capabilities. This is an important concept: If the internally developed pharmacy benefit management program does not offer competitive cost or quality advantages, it may be a wise business decision for the MCO to "buy" PBM services rather than "build" them internally. PBMs exist and thrive because they are highly cost-efficient and flexible in providing customized pharmacy program management because of their specialized pharmacy benefit resources and economies of scale.

Genesis of PBMs

PBMs generally developed as separate, independent companies or from within HMOs. The earliest third-party prescription drug management programs, Prescription Card Services (PCS) and Medco Containment Services, came into existence in the 1970s to provide third-party prescription drug programs primarily for self-insured companies. The second route of PBM development, from within HMOs, occurred as a natural evolution from successfully managed internal HMO pharmacy programs. These HMOs saw an opportunity to commercialize their successful strategies and offer pharmacy management services to external customers without adequate internal resources. In 1987, Diversified Pharmaceutical Services (DPS) was one of the earliest examples of a PBM that grew from within an HMO (United HealthCare [UHC]).

These three early PBMs—PCS, Medco, and DPS—were born from three different heritages and displayed unique benefit management philosophies. PCS developed to offer third-party prescription care benefits primarily to employer groups using a vast network of community chain and independent pharmacies. Medco Containment Services developed for similar reasons but focused on mail service to dispense and distribute prescriptions. DPS developed from the pharmacy department within an HMO and had primarily a clinical focus to its pharmacy benefit management strategies. Therefore, the three early PBMs grew from very diverse origins but eventually evolved to become more similar than dissimilar realizing that they must take advantage of the efficiencies of all types of pharmacy benefit management and distribution strategies to successfully meet the needs of their diverse and evolving customer base. As a result, these three, and other PBMs, became similar in the products and services they offered employer group and HMO customers. However, not all PBMs enjoyed the same performance success.

Soon after the success of United HealthCare's PBM subsidiary DPS, other HMOs with internal pharmacy departments began to offer their programs to noncompeting HMOs, self-insured employers, and government-funded programs, such as the state Medicaid programs. Examples of some of the PBMs that developed as internal HMO pharmacy program management are

found in Table 24–1. By the late 1980s, the term "pharmacy benefit management company" or "pharmacy benefit manager" or "PBM" became popular, although its exact origin is unknown.

PBMs have continued to grow in number and in membership. Table 24–2 displays the larger PBMs and their membership. Although some double-counting may exist (e.g., members obtaining mail order or Internet pharmacy services from one PBM and retain pharmacy services from another), the PBM membership is estimated to be 246 million, or more than 80 percent of the entire U.S. population. The PBM market is dominated by a small number of large companies. According to the reported membership in PBM corporate websites, the combined membership of the six largest PBMs is 219 million or more than 90 percent of all estimated PBM lives.

There has also been much ownership change and consolidation within the PBM industry. For example, PCS Health Systems, Inc. (the PBM's current name), originally an independent company, was purchased by McKesson Drug (a drug wholesaler), then Eli Lilly & Company (a pharmaceutical manufacturer). Rite Aid chain pharmacy company finally purchased it in 1999, and PCS is reportedly again for sale as of the end of 1999. Another example of ownership change occurred with DPS. The PBM developed within the UHC pharmacy department and began offering pharmacy management services to non-UHC health plans in 1987. The drug manufacturer SmithKline Beecham purchased DPS in 1994, and it was subsequently purchased by Ex-

---

Table 24–1 Examples of PBMs Originally Developed from within HMOs

Parent HMO	PBM
United HealthCare	Diversified Pharmaceutical Services
Blue Cross Blue Shield of Minnesota	Pharmacy Gold
Blue Cross of California	WellPoint Pharmacy Management
Blue Cross Blue Shield of Maryland	Advance Paradigm
General American (Sanus; NY Life)	Express Scripts
PacifiCare Health Systems	Prescription Solutions

Table 24–2 Largest PBMs, Ownership Status, and Membership

PBM Company	Membership (millions)
Merck-Merck Managed Care	51
PCS Health Systems	>50
Express Scripts	47
Advance Paradigm	27
MedImpact	26
WellPoint Pharmacy Management	18
Others (est.)	27
Total	246 million lives

Source: Data from PBM websites, January 2000.

press Scripts, Inc., an independent PBM, in 1999. It is interesting to note that PCS and DPS were last sold for approximately one third of their original purchase price.

Rationale for Using a PBM

The decision for an MCO to develop and operate an internal pharmacy program or to contract with an external PBM depends on many factors. Essentially, the MCO must determine whether it can "build" and efficiently operate an internal infrastructure to manage prescription drug benefits or whether it is more efficient to "buy" this service from an external PBM company. In fact, many MCOs will build certain internal management capabilities and buy other operational "commodity" services, such as claims processing, from a PBM

A PBM offers certain advantages in the build versus buy evaluation. The primary advantages of using a PBM to provide pharmacy services are the MCO can save the program development costs, eliminate a significant information system investment, implement the program in a much shorter time frame, and minimize operational expenses. Building and maintaining internal pharmacy management services are expensive and time consuming exercises that require ongo-

ing operational support to maintain system components and provide continuous upgrades.

The services of a PBM can be implemented rapidly. The pharmacy networks, information systems, manufacturer contracts, and other standard program components already exist and can be rapidly implemented flexibly to meet customer-specific requirements. Large MCO customers with multiple products and complex benefit designs may require significant customization, and a PBM may be able to better provide such diverse services because of information system capabilities.

Hybrid Pharmacy Program Management Using PBMs

Even though an MCO has the option of building or buying pharmacy management services, it often decides to take advantage of both options through a hybrid program. Thus, it is quite common for an HMO to build an internal pharmacy *management* program and also use a PBM for specific, basic resource-intensive *operational* services that take advantage of a PBM's economies of scale. The program components that should be built or at least managed internally are those that the MCO or employer group believes it can do in a cost-efficient manner that will provide a long-term, differentiating, competitive advantage. Even though a PBM has the ability to offer a turnkey pharmacy benefit management program and the *à la carte* components, it is important for a PBM customer to be actively involved in design of the benefit and oversight of the program performance to ensure objectives are achieved. Table 24–3 lists the PBM services commonly used by 70 HMOs.[28] These findings demonstrate that HMOs contract with PBMs for core commodity services, especially claims processing, but HMOs often maintain internal control of clinical programs that may provide competitive differentiation.

Reintegrating the Value of PBM Services

PBMs are successful in providing stand-alone pharmacy benefit management because of their singular focus, dedicated resources, experience,

Table 24–3 PBM Services Used by HMOs

PBM Service	Percent of HMOs Obtaining This Service from a PBM
Claims processing	86%
POS edits	76%
DUR programs	54%
Pharmacy network development and management	50%
Formulary management	46%
Physician intervention	34%
Demand management	22%
Disease management programs	16%
Treatment guidelines	15%
Outcomes management	6%

Source: Reprinted with permission from RP Navarro (ed), *Pharmacy Benefit Report Trends & Forecasts,* Issue 21, © 1998, Novartis Pharmaceuticals Corporation.

and economies of scale. However, although carving out the pharmacy benefit for efficient management may achieve pharmacy program cost-containment objectives, this component, or silo management, may cause payers to focus on pharmacy program cost rather than value. As discussed earlier, appropriately used pharmaceuticals provide tremendous clinical and economic value. It is critical that the positive impact the pharmacy benefit can have on other direct medical costs and quality of life are not lost. Therefore, PBMs and their clients are attempting to integrate prescription claims data with medical claims and clinical data so that the interrelationship of the various health care delivery components can be recognized. MCOs, employer groups, and other customers "carve-out" the pharmacy benefit to a PBM for management and "carve-in" the pharmacy outcomes data into their overall health care delivery management process so that the overall value of pharmacy is recognized. This ensures that pharmacy benefit management decisions are consistent with the

overall health care delivery process and not made in isolation. Although component cost will always be important, the reintegration of pharmacy data in overall health care management will help promote drug benefit designs that balance cost and quality of care objectives. This value reintegration philosophy is supported by all stakeholders in the pharmacy benefit management continuum, including pharmaceutical manufacturers, pharmacists, PBMs, and their customers. The primary challenge to achieving this value reintegration goal has been the inadequacies of managed care information systems to capture, merge, and report accurate and complete integrated outcomes data.

In summary, a PBM may offer cost-efficient outsourcing of some or all pharmacy program management components. The HMO or self-insured employer group must consider the advantages of using a PBM and determine what components can be carved out and what should be maintained within the health plan to maximize the efficiencies and resources of each entity.

PHARMACY BENEFIT MANAGEMENT PROGRAM COMPONENTS

Pharmacy benefit management strategies have changed very little in concept over the past 20 years. However, the growth and acceptance of managed care and the expansion of information technology have increased the success with which these concepts can be executed. The success with which they are implemented can also vary greatly among the various MCOs, depending on the aggressiveness of their employer groups and the resources and expertise of the MCO or PBM. Most managed care prescription drug benefits include the following basic components:[29]

- legally enforceable benefit design contract outlining covered benefits
- defined physician provider network under contract with the health plan
- defined pharmacy provider network under contract with the health plan or PBM required to use a POS prescription adjudication system

- enforceable drug formulary
- mandatory generic substitution program
- pharmaceutical manufacturer discounts or rebates
- patient prescription copayment
- retrospective drug utilization review (DUR)

Advanced programs may include additional components, such as drug conversion or switching programs, compliance interventions, and disease management programs.

Pharmacy Benefit Design

The first step in developing a pharmacy benefit is to ensure that a legal contract exists between the parties (i.e., employer group and HMO, HMO and PBM, employer group and PBM). The contract must be filed with the individual state regulatory agency and may be called a Certificate of Coverage, Evidence of Coverage, Certificate of Benefits, or other similar name. It is a legally enforceable contract by which the MCO (i.e., HMO or PBM) agrees to provide explicitly defined prescription drug benefits for a specific price and the purchaser of the benefit (payer) agrees to accept the defined covered benefits according to certain coverage and access rules.

The Certificate of Coverage is a legal document filed with state regulatory agencies that explicitly states the following:[30]

- what persons are eligible for benefits (e.g., employer group employees and their dependents)
- what benefits are covered (e.g., legend drugs requiring a prescription by a physician)
- what benefits are not covered (e.g., nonprescription drugs, injectable drugs, experimental drugs)
- what benefit limitations exist (e.g., prescriptions for up to a 30-day supply through a retail pharmacy and up to a 90-day supply through mail service)

- additional requirements for coverage (e.g., drugs must be included on the health plan's or PBM's formulary)
- how benefits are accessed (e.g., members must obtain a prescription from a plan physician and must have the prescription filled at a plan pharmacy)

A Certificate of Coverage may include other policies and procedures, but the elements listed previously are the most standard types of information included. A member should be able to clearly understand the extent and limits of the benefits by reading the Certificate of Coverage. This document often includes the procedure for resolution of a grievance or for the member to obtain coverage for a nonformulary drug. The Certificate may not be changed without the approval of both signatory parties (e.g., MCO and employer group) and usually changes only at annual contract renewal, although a mid-year contract addendum may be used to change mutually agreeable terms.

Legal Basis of Pharmacy Benefit Management

John Jones of PacifiCare lists the following factors that allow the organization to exercise pharmacy benefit controls:[31]

- Boards of pharmacy in each state regulate pharmacy, individual state agencies regulating controlled substances, the United States Food and Drug Administration, and the United States Drug Enforcement Agency.
- Many states have established regulations governing the operation and administration of HMOs. Most involve enforcement by a regulatory agency such as the state Department of Insurance, Department of Corporations, or Department of Health Services.
- A body of federal law governing the provision of health benefits is the Employee Retirement Income Security Act of 1974 and the rules and regulations passed into law subsequently. They are collectively known

as the ERISA laws. Employer groups, pharmacy benefit management companies, and HMOs are generally protected by federal ERISA laws from liability for their administration of pharmacy benefits designed or selected by the payers for their covered members (although some states are challenging this liability exemption with state legislation).

- PBMs do not prescribe medications or practice medicine; they administer prescription drug benefits according to parameters established by the employer or health plan and according to the physician's prescription.
- Formularies are lists of drugs selected by a pharmacy and therapeutics (P & T) committee through a deliberative process and are administered according to the benefit design by the PBM. Plan members are not prohibited from receiving prescriptions for nonformulary drugs, but the plan is not generally bound to pay for nonformulary drugs unless the plan is bound to cover all medically necessary drugs. Medical necessity is generally determined by the plan according to specific criteria established by the P & T committee or by a pharmacist or physician by means of a prior authorization process or by review during an appeal.
- Beneficiaries are notified that their prescription drug benefits are limited. This notification is generally done through an explanation of benefits (EOB) document that members receive from their health plan or employer. When they file a claim for prescription coverage, the EOB must clearly state which drugs are covered and which are excluded, either naming the drugs individually or by treatment category.
- Some states and occasionally the federal government have established mandatory coverage of certain drug treatment categories that must be included if a pharmacy benefit is offered.
- PBMs contract with pharmacies to provide services to members. The contractual obligations must satisfy state licensure and record keeping requirements.

Some states have strong regulatory agencies that enforce laws created to govern the activities of health plans and protect the consumers. Health plans and the PBMs with which they contract must comply with the laws of those states. Generally, the health plans must provide medically necessary treatment within the guidelines of the health plan benefit policy

PHYSICIAN PROVIDER NETWORK

The health plan may employ physicians, or more likely it will contract with community physicians and medical groups. Community physicians that are under contract with a health plan are often referred to as "participating providers." Health plans employ or contract with physicians to obtain a discounted reimbursement in exchange for allowing the physician to care for the health plan's patients (members). Although a physician provider network is generally not considered part of the pharmacy benefit program, the health plan must include physicians in the pharmacy benefit design because they prescribe the drugs that are to be covered.

Contracts with participating physician providers usually state that they will prescribe drugs in accordance with the plan's drug formulary and other pharmacy benefit policies. If a physician or medical group accepts financial risk for the cost of pharmacy benefits, the physician provider contract will outline this risk-sharing arrangement (see Chapter 8). The contract also details periodic drug prescribing drug utilization review "report cards" that physicians can expect to receive periodically that allow them to compare their prescribing habits and drug costs with other physicians in their specialty peer group. As stated previously, more HMOs are sharing the financial risk of the pharmacy benefit with participating physicians in an attempt to sensitize prescribers to the cost of drugs. This practice is more common on the West Coast and in the Northeast but is increasing in many states. Regrettably, physicians often do not know the details of their pharmacy risk contract, and they frequently lose money on these relationships.

PHARMACY PROVIDER NETWORK

How the member obtains the final prescription product is an important link in the pharmacy benefit process. The MCO or PBM will own or contract with community pharmacy providers, Internet pharmacies, or mail service pharmacies to control both the drug ingredient cost and administrative costs (dispensing fee, packaging, distribution fees, claims adjudication fees, etc.). The MCO will also require the contracted pharmacy distributor to dispense drugs in conformance with the drug formulary to maximize the MCO's discount or rebate contracts with pharmaceutical manufacturers. The health plan must define its prescription distribution channels so that drug costs and dispensing process costs can be controlled effectively. There are three primary channels to distribute pharmaceuticals:

- owned, in-house pharmacies within health plan medical centers (usually staff and group model HMOs)
- independent and chain community retail pharmacies
- mail service pharmacies and Internet pharmacies

Owned, in-house pharmacies and community-based retail pharmacies dispensed more than 85 percent of outpatient prescriptions. Mail order prescription volume has remained relatively constant at about 12 percent of the total retail prescriptions, but its volume is growing by about the same annual percent.

Internet Pharmacies

Internet pharmacies are becoming increasingly popular. In reality, Internet pharmacies may be considered a high-tech mail service pharmacy because they distribute prescriptions by mail or overnight package delivery service. However, they allow access to prescription ordering and refills through the Internet in addition to the telephone or fax (common with all mail service pharmacies). Although the dispensing "back end" of Internet pharmacies may be no different than mail order pharmacies, the "front end" patient health and drug information services and patient access are quite novel. Some traditional mail service and chain pharmacies now offer Internet access for patients to order refills, non-prescription drugs, or health and beauty products similar to Internet pharmacies. Examples of Internet pharmacies as of 2000 include HealthCentralRx.com, PlanetRx.com, YourPharmacy.com, DrugStore.com, and many others. In December 1999, a national concern regarding the lack of adequate regulations governing the operation of Internet pharmacies may result in the FDA licensing or certifying Internet pharmacies. These concerns are largely due to some Internet pharmacies that will mail prescription drugs without a prescription or will offer an "online consultation" with a physician (or someone claiming to be a physician) that will result in a "prescription" being written. Some Internet pharmacies, possibly operating outside of the United States, will distribute unapproved or experimental drugs within the United States.

Internet access to prescription drugs is an extension of the "e-tailing" phenomenon, whereby individuals are becoming increasingly comfortable with Internet shopping. In addition to allowing an interesting and interactive method of communicating, the Internet pharmacies provide a broad array of patient health information, drug education, hot links to other health-related websites, and access to a wide variety of discounted health and beauty products that can be sent by overnight mail. Many pharmacy chains and PBMs have developed their own Internet portals to their pharmacy services, and many have established partnerships with other Internet pharmacies. For example, Express Scripts has announced it has selected PlanetRx as its exclusive Internet pharmacies. The power of the Internet can provide definite patient care advantages, such as access to targeted and comprehensive health and drug information, as well as offering automated refill monitoring to support patient compliance and persistence programs.

Specialized Distribution Networks

A specialized network is developed to accommodate a specific class or type of drug (e.g., interferon, AIDS therapy, injectables) or services available (e.g., anticoagulation clinics or home infusion); such services are frequently associated with disease management programs (see Chapter 23). The services may thus require specialized education in a particular disease state, patient monitoring, or concentrated consultations. It may require the willingness to maintain an inventory of specialized medications or injectables. Credentialing and/or certification may be required to ensure quality and consistency when delivering professional services. Reimbursement can be based on both the product cost and the amount of time necessary to deliver the service.

Prescription distribution channels are not mutually exclusive, and MCOs often use two or more channels. For example, an IPA or network model HMO will contract with community pharmacies to form a pharmacy provider network and may also contract with a mail service pharmacy. A staff or group model health plan may have owned pharmacies within its medical centers in a metropolitan area and augment the owned pharmacies with a community pharmacy network and a mail service pharmacy. Chain pharmacies in the MCOs community network may also provide mail service prescriptions and allow Internet access, as discussed previously.

Physician Dispensing

Some health plans may reimburse physicians for dispensing drugs directly from their office, but this is an uncommon practice and most often occurs only in rural areas without adequate coverage of community pharmacies. In general, health plans will not reimburse physicians for dispensing drugs unless the physician's office agrees to accept the same level of reimbursement as is paid to pharmacies and if the physician's office submits pharmacy claims through a POS terminal. Physician dispensing units often contain a limited amount of acute-care drugs and generally promote the use of generics. Some applications link in-office physician dispensing units for acute care drugs with mail order for chronic care medications.

Retail Community Pharmacy Network

There are currently 50,000 community retail pharmacies (30,000 chain and 20,000 independent). Chain pharmacies dispense 60 percent of all outpatient prescriptions, about 1.6 billion per year, or 400 million per day.[32] The food stores with pharmacies represent the fastest growing retail pharmacy segment, with a 13.8 percent growth in prescription volume from 1997 to 1998. During the same period, chain pharmacy prescription volume increased 8.8 percent, and independent prescription volume increased 1.2 percent.[33]

Health plans and PBMs often contract with a broad network of retail and chain community pharmacies to ensure members have easy access to pharmacy benefits. In an area without significant managed care penetration, MCOs or PBMs may find it necessary to barter members for discounts. That is, pharmacies may be unwilling to accept discounts on prescriptions unless they are members of a relatively exclusive pharmacy provider network and believe they will have access to members because of their participation. Conversely, if they elect not to accept the discounts and not to participate in the provider network, managed care members will likely not patronize their pharmacies because their prescriptions would not be covered at the non-participating pharmacies. Therefore, the MCO or PBM will offer their contracted members to the pharmacies if they agree to accept discounted reimbursement and participate in the network.

When constructing a pharmacy provider network, it is relatively easy to construct a network around chain pharmacies. Generally, they are very willing to accept discounts to lure managed care customers into their stores. In fact, in most metropolitan areas, it is likely that an adequate pharmacy provider network can be constructed of 80 percent chain pharmacies and 20 percent independent pharmacies. However, for competitive purposes, many large MCOs offer a variety of access points for prescriptions through a hybrid distribution network that is focused around community pharmacies but also includes mail service pharmacies or chain pharmacies, both of which may be accessed by way of the Internet. Staff or group model HMOs may also have some in-house pharmacies in owned medical centers.

Pharmacy Provider Contract

All participating pharmacies are bound by a contract (provider agreement) that stipulates that the MCO or PBM will reimburse the pharmacy for approved prescriptions dispensed to their members in accordance with drug benefit and coverage policies. The pharmacy agrees to accept a discounted level of reimbursement and to follow the defined dispensing policies and procedures. These policies are usually detailed in a policy and procedure manual provided to each pharmacy and updated from time to time by the MCO or PBM. A pharmacy provider contract will generally include the following requirements:[34]

- The health plan or PBM agrees to allow their members to obtain prescriptions from the contracted pharmacy only. (Some states with any willing provider laws will allow noncontracted pharmacies to be reimbursed at the contract rate of the dispensed prescriptions to managed care members; see also Chapter 69 for a discussion of state any willing provider laws.)
- The health plan or PBM agrees to pay the pharmacy within a specific period (usually every two weeks or less) for all prescriptions dispensed according to a contracted reimbursement schedule.
- The pharmacy agrees to accept a defined reimbursement for each prescription filled under contract. For example, the contract may stipulate a reimbursement of a 15 percent discount off the AWP for brand-name drugs and 50 percent off the AWP for generic drugs.
- The pharmacy agrees to accept a discounted dispensing fee (e.g., $2.50) for each prescription filled. Typically, up to a 30-day supply is allowed through community pharmacies.
- The pharmacy agrees to accept the patient copayment and health plan or PBM reim-

bursement as payment in full for the prescription. That is, the pharmacy cannot request that the patient pay more than their copayment (called "balance billing"; see Chapter 62 for discussion of this clause).
- The pharmacy agrees to dispense prescriptions according to the drug formulary and the dispensing requirements specified in the policy and procedure manual.
- The pharmacy agrees to use the in-pharmacy POS computer adjudication system to process and bill all health plan or PBM prescriptions. Use of the system benefits both parties. The pharmacy obtains complete coverage and reimbursement information from the system, and, if the prescription data are accepted by the computer, the pharmacy is guaranteed payment within a specific time frame.
- The pharmacy agrees to participate and dispense prescriptions in conformance with the following additional administrative requirements regarding the dispensing process, according to Sterler and Stevens:[35]
  — services and standards such as licensing, certification, and continuing education
  — prior authorization policies that may require the pharmacy to contact the physician in specified circumstances
  — documentation, including the signature log that documents that counseling was performed and the patient or other authorized person accepted the prescription
  — record retention requirements beyond those set by state pharmacy or other laws
  — electronic communication standards requiring transmission and display of all online messages from the claims processor (such as drug formulary compliance, drug interactions, patient eligibility, DUR, DUE) and that appropriate action is taken
  — pharmacy provider insurance standards
  — expectations for online and real-time claim submission in the required format
  — requirements for participation in national pharmacy provider networks
  — taxes that must be collected

— reimbursement policies and accompanying payment reports
— enrollment fees the pharmacy must pay to participate in a network
— audit and inspection rights of the contractor and responsibilities of the pharmacy
— definition of the pharmacy provider records that must be maintained
— advertising and trademarks privileges of the contractor

Participating Pharmacy Policy and Procedure Manual

The provider policy and procedure manual details the specific policies and procedures the participating pharmacies must follow to be in compliance with the provider agreement. According to Sterler and Stephens of PCS Health Systems, the manual must be consistent with the performance criteria outlined in the provider agreement. Typical topics addressed in the manual include the following:[36]

- systems requirements (hardware and software requirements of the POS system [current and future upgrades] and data transmission standards)
- drug formulary dispensing policy
- DUR messages transmitted on the electronic system
- enhancements to electronic messages
- incentive programs associated with dispensing performance requirements
- contract compliance and audits
- operational procedures (e.g., signature log and dispense-as-written [DAW] codes)
- components of performance evaluation

PHARMACY PROVIDER AUDITS

Some degree of fraud and abuse is always present within a large pharmacy provider network but can be minimized with a well-designed and thorough auditing system and an effective provider and member educational program. Fraud and abuse can arise from actions of a member, pharmacy, or prescriber and are usu-

ally unintentional and simply caused by a lack of appropriate education about a certain procedure. The first line of defense is online claims adjudication using automated real-time POS edits to ensure compliance with program coverage and dispensing policies.

The second line of defense is the audit, with two common types.[37] The first is usually the "bench" or desk audit that analyzes reports on the basis of utilization and cost data to identify erroneous billings and confirm that billed drugs were, in fact, dispensed. A more controversial form of desk audit uses pre-established algorithms to indicate the highest boundaries within which a pharmacy's claims may fall. For all claims that fall outside these boundaries, the pharmacy is held responsible for the dollar amount of these claims. This method is referred to as extrapolation. Because the monetary impact is only detected through exception reports, as opposed to an actual review of the claim, this auditing method is more frequently challenged.

The more common audit is the actual field or on-site pharmacy audit. An auditor personally visits the pharmacy and reviews claims, signature logs, and other substantive documentation within the pharmacy. Pharmacies are targeted for a field audit if the claims analysis indicates a potential problem. Possible actions include onsite inspection of pharmacy documentation, a contact with the prescriber-of-record for validation, or a contact with the patient for validation of receipt of the drugs.

Another form of the field audit is an educational audit. Auditors will answer questions about claims processing, inform pharmacists about programs and policies, and relay pharmacists' concerns back to the processor. Educational material is reviewed to help the pharmacy prevent future problems. Following are some common criteria used to screen pharmacies for potential problems:[38]

- usual and customary (U & C) price submission
- claim submission exceeding a specified number of claims per patient per day
- average ingredient cost paid

- average amount paid per prescription filled
- percentage of compounded claims
- percentage of controlled drugs
- percentage of brand name claims for multi-source drugs
- DAW classification
- percentage of refilled prescriptions
- percentage of DAW prescriptions

The pharmacy contract also allows the MCO or PBM to audit the pharmacies in-store records based on possible dispensing or billing irregularities discovered through automated audits of billing records. Pharmacies found to be in violation of the terms of the contract may be terminated from the pharmacy provider network.

DRUG FORMULARY MANAGEMENT[39]

A drug formulary is a preferred list of medications developed by the health plan or PBM to guide physician prescribing and pharmacy dispensing. Formularies are not novel but have been used for decades by hospitals, health plans, and other health care institutions as a method of inventory control and to promote the use of the most cost-effective products.[40] Early formularies in the United States were primarily compilations of formulas and recipes used to prepare medicines. The first hospital formulary, the Lititz Pharmacopoeia (1778), attempted to standardize compounding and dispensing of medicines in military hospitals that were set up during the Revolutionary War.[41] The first civilian hospital formulary, the Pharmacopoeia of the New York Hospital (1816), was the first attempt to incorporate the opinions of the hospital's medical staff in the development of an institutional formulary.[42]

The hospital formulary system, more commonly in place today, had its origins in the 1920s. In 1925, 45 physicians and a pharmacist at Syracuse University Hospital established a scientific basis for drug control and reduction of therapeutic duplications through its drug therapy program. The New York Hospital completed a similar project in 1932.[43]

In the 1960s, the formulary system was established in virtually every hospital in the United States. The publication of the American Hospital Formulary Service (AHFS) in 1959 expanded the use of formularies. The flexibility of the AHFS allowed even the smallest hospital to incorporate a formulary system into its operating policies. Today, the AHFS is a critical component in the formulary system and drug information service of most hospitals and MCO pharmacy departments.

Simply defined, a drug formulary is a list of drugs approved for use within a health care setting. A formulary system is the method and processes used that continually update the formulary's content of prescription medications. The formulary system "...provides for the procuring, prescribing, dispensing, and administering of drugs...."[44] It is a uniquely dynamic system that represents the current body of pharmaceutical knowledge and medical community practice standards resident in the health care setting it serves. Formularies are continuously evaluated by a committee of experts, primarily composed of physicians and pharmacists, working within the health care setting. This committee is most often called the Pharmacy and Therapeutics Committee, or the P & T committee. "The P & T Committee is responsible for developing, managing, updating, and administering the formulary."[45]

The drug formulary is often printed in booklet form and distributed to participating physicians. It is occasionally sent to patients in an abridged form. Drugs that are eligible for coverage and included in the formulary are usually listed by therapeutic category. Additional information included for the prescriber and dispenser include: if the generic and/or brand name form are covered, coverage restrictions, relative cost index (a guide to relative pricing of drugs within the category), and possibly the copayment tier. The copayment tier and especially copayment dollar amount may not be included because of the benefit design differences among the various payer groups that may all seek care from the same provider physicians and pharmacies. Some formularies may include clinical information (e.g., dosing considerations, adverse effects, interactions, age-related dose guidance) and drug use guidelines (e.g., step-care protocols). An example page of a simple drug formulary is found in Exhibit 24–1 (*Note*: copayment dollar amounts are included for illustrative purposes only).

Drug Formulary Selection and Decision-Making Process

The physicians who sit on the P & T committee often represent a wide scope of medical practice by including both primary care physicians and a variety of medical specialties. Other health care professionals, such as nurses, may also be appointed to the committee. Although medicine and pharmacy compose the core of the P & T committee membership, some managed care plans have added additional representatives from a variety of interests, including administration, legal, marketing, or even lay health plan members.

The primary purposes of the P & T committee are to determine drug coverage policy development and enforcement and education to promote safe, effective, and cost-effective pharmaceuti-

Exhibit 24–1 Example of a Drug Formulary Page

5.0 Antidepressant Drugs*				
5.1 *Tricyclic antidepressants*	*Reimbursed* [†]	*Cost Index* [‡]	*Copay Tier/Amount* [§]	
Amitriptline[‖]	Generic	$	Tier I	$5
Imipramine	Generic	$	Tier I	$5
Desipramine	Generic	$$	Tier I	$5
Nortriptyline	Generic	$$	Tier I	$5
5.2 Selective reuptake inhibitors (SRIs)				
Citalopgram (Celexa®)	Brand	$$$	Tier II	$10
Paroxetine (Paxil®)	Brand	$$$$	Tier II	$10
Sertraline (Zoloft®)	Brand	$$$$	Tier II	$10
Note: only the 100-mg strength tablet of Zoloft is eligible for reimbursement.				
Fluoxetine (Prozac®)	Brand	$$$$$	Tier III	$25
5.3 Other antidepressants				
Trazodone	Generic	$$	Tier I	$5
Bupropion (Wellbutrin®)	Brand	$$$	Tier II	$10

Source: Adapted from Michael J. Dillon, Drug Formulary Management, in *Managed Care Pharmacy Practice,* RP Navarro, ed, p 150, © 1999, Aspen Publishers, Inc. Copayment information added by Robert P. Navarro, 2000.

*Drugs listed by therapeutic category.

[†]Generic and brand indicator. This informs the prescriber that if the word "generic" is listed, the drug is subject to a maximum allowable cost (MAC) and only reimbursed at the generic level. If the brand name is included, the brand name drug is included on the formulary and reimbursed.

[‡]Relative cost index. Dollar signs ($) are used to indicate the relative cost of each covered drug within the same therapeutic class. This cannot be used to determine exact dollar cost of a prescription. The greater the number of dollar signs, the more costly the product.

[§]Copay tier and amount. This refers to the copayment tier in which the drug is positioned and the prescription copayment amount to be paid by the patient for each prescription. *Note:* The copayment amount is usually not listed, because it is subject to change and may be different for various payer groups. The copayment amount is included here to illustrate the cost difference among the various drugs on the basis of copayment tier.

[‖]Name of drug. The generic name of all drugs is included. The brand names are also listed for those drugs that are included as brand name drugs on the formulary and are reimbursed as brand drugs.

cals.[46] Policies are established concerning the evaluation and selection of drugs to be included in the formulary and policies regarding drug utilization review and evaluation. These range from policies regarding relationships with the pharmaceutical industry, drug formulary exceptions, and participation in clinical research.

The P & T committee must meet regularly (usually quarterly with interim conference calls as necessary) to continually revise and update to ensure it is a dynamic reference. P & T committees must consider a number of key points when evaluating a new pharmaceutical to determine whether it should be awarded a position in the formulary. In this evaluative process, P & T committees review and consider the following factors, according to Dillon:[47]

- source of supply and reliability of manufacturer and distributor
- pharmacological considerations (e.g., drug class, similarity to existing drugs, adverse effect profile, mechanism of action, therapeutic indications, drug-drug interaction potential, clinical advantages over other products in drug class)
- unlabeled uses and their appropriateness
- bioavailability data
- pharmacokinetic data
- dosage ranges by route and age
- risk versus benefits regarding clinical efficacy and safety of a particular drug relative to other drugs with the same indication
- patient risk factors relative to contraindications, warnings, and precautions
- special monitoring or drug administration requirements
- pharmacoeconomic data
- cost comparisons against other drugs available to treat the same medical condition(s)[48]

P & T committees most commonly consider peer-reviewed clinical literature and information from the pharmaceutical manufacturer when evaluating a new drug. The P & T committee members, given the potential for bias, treat the manufacturer's findings with a slight degree of healthy skepticism. Information provided by the manufacturer is balanced by published research not sponsored by the drug's manufacturer, if possible. An ideal, yet uncommon, occurrence is identifying data from research conducted in a managed care practice in which the patient population matches that of the managed care organization that is reviewing the drug for possible formulary inclusion.

Role of Pharmacoeconomic Data in Evidence-Based Drug Formularies[49]

Pharmacoeconomics is a tool that can mitigate this continuing obsession with cost minimization and broaden the appreciation of payers to the economic and clinical value of pharmaceuticals and pharmacy programs. If this occurs, it would theoretically relieve some of the cost-containment pressure for pharmacy program managers and the pharmaceutical industry. However, payers (and as a result, managed care) will likely never be comfortable with rising costs, and the promise of pharmacoeconomics to allow a relaxation in strident pharmacy benefit controls is a partial delusion. It may likely have a positive impact but less so in the near term.

Pharmacy and medical directors, and P & T committees, have increased their requests for pharmacoeconomic (PE) data from the pharmaceutical industry. There is an intellectual appreciation of the need for such data to demonstrate how the appropriate use of cost-effective pharmaceuticals can contribute value broadly throughout the health care system. Economist Paul Langley suggests a "...systems-based approach...offers an analytic framework that...is likely to contribute significantly to the management of health care systems."[50] However, there is a fundamental challenge that may prevent the widespread dissemination and use of pharmacoeconomic data: many pharmacy and medical directors may not understand the concepts and may be uncertain as to how to implement pharmacoeconomic criteria within their P & T committee drug evaluation process. The Academy of Managed Care Pharmacy is publishing *Pharmacoeconomic Evaluations: Guidelines for Drug Purchasers* in an attempt to advance the understanding and application of pharmacoeconomic evaluation guidelines. Regence Health Plan is taking a proactive approach and requiring all manufacturers to submit a complete drug information dossier, complete with pharmacoeconomic data, before a drug is reviewed by the P & T committee.[51]

In a survey of 51 managed care organizations, Luce and colleagues found that clinical effectiveness remained more important than cost-effectiveness (second most important) or quality of life (third most important) in drug evaluations.[52] In general, there is a lack of understanding of the PE concepts and how to incorporate PE data into the drug formulary evaluation process. Cost minimization is widely accepted and used. Cost-effectiveness analysis (CEA) is generally understood, and if the data are credible and applicable, CEA data may be used. However, cost-benefit analysis, cost-utility metrics, and willingness to pay are concepts somewhat foreign and not widely used in the formulary process, even if the pharmaceutical manufacturer provides these data. There are exceptions, as seen with the comprehensive review and novel formulary treatment of salmeterol at the Dean Clinic.[53] Pharmaceutical manufacturers should continue to invest in PE research for most new drugs (except clearly undifferentiated products), but it must be designed to produce outcomes of interest to managed care.

Data suggest that research conducted in other HMOs or PBMs is used if it is credible and applicable. In early 1998, the Zitter Group conducted a national study of managed care decision makers entitled "Health Economics Leaders Study."[54] Results of the study reported that findings from health economics research conducted outside the managed care organizations were overwhelmingly used to make formulary decisions if it was credible and applicable to managed care.

Acceptance of PE concepts, especially by payers, will help shift the focus from the cost of drugs to the value of drugs. As a result, this evolution will have a positive impact on improving access and use of cost-effective pharmaceuticals. It will be the responsibility of the manufacturer to have credible and applicable PE data to support the launch of novel pharmaceuticals. In the absence of such PE data that clearly demonstrate significant product differentiation, pharmacy and medical directors will assume products are similar (and thus interchangeable) and make formulary coverage decisions on cost rather than outcomes.

A controversy continues between the use of "efficacy" data and "effectiveness" data. Efficacy data are generated from randomized, controlled clinical trials of the genre submitted to the Food and Drug Administration (FDA) for the basis of new drug product approval. Effectiveness data are generated from "uncontrolled" studies often conducted in a managed care environment that reflects the naturalistic use and outcomes associated with the drug. Efficacy is a measure of the ideal performance of a drug product; effectiveness reflects how the drug is likely to perform in an uncontrolled environment. The FDA has required at least two pivotal efficacy studies to support new drug launches or new indications. However, by nature these efficacy studies are controlled and do not reflect how a drug will be used in a "real world" environment.

Therefore, managed care has requested that pharmaceutical manufacturers provide uncontrolled, real-world effectiveness research data and controlled efficacy trial data. Thus far, the FDA has restricted what effectiveness data manufacturers have been able to provide because the FDA seems to only consider controlled efficacy studies as valid. In late 1997, the U.S. Congress passed the FDA Modernization Act of 1997, which will influence the type and amount of PE data provided to P & T committees from pharmaceutical manufacturers.[55] Section 114 of this act (Health Care Economic Information) amends the previous 1992 legislation by adding to Section 502(a) (21 U.S.C. 352(a)) the statement, "Health care economic information provided to a formulary committee, or other similar entity, in the course of the committee carrying out its responsibilities for the selection of drugs—shall not be considered to be false or misleading—if the information directly relates to an indication approved and is based on competent and reliable scientific evidence." The original intent of Section 114 was thought to allow manufacturers greater latitude in providing PE data from uncontrolled research to health plan decision makers and P & T committee members (not any or all participating provider physicians). The interpretation and practice of Section 114 remains controversial and unresolved. Thus far, pharmaceutical manufacturers have infrequently provided information under Section 114, and if it is not used, the right to do so may be rescinded by the FDA.

Paul Langley has the following opinion:[56]

> If our ultimate objective is to ensure that pharmaceutical manufacturers are not discouraged from producing pharmacoeconomic studies that meet the needs of drug purchasers in varied treating environments, then the FTC approach might appear the most appropriate. It still could involve an expert committee to review studies that are considered to be deceptive, but it would not be involved in policing initial proposals for pharmacoeconomic studies or reviewing those undertaken for promotion and marketing by pharmaceutical manufacturers.

> If the FDA takes the view that the phrase "competent and reliable scientific evidence" must be interpreted as evidence based on randomized-controlled experiments, then we are back to square one. If the FDA takes a more eclectic position and refers to accepted standards of professional practice within the appropriate discipline, in this case health care economics, then we can look forward to entering a more information-rich environment—and one that will present some interesting challenges not only to pharmaceutical manufacturers but also to health economists and health care purchasers. Unless a more eclectic regulatory position is taken, it is most unlikely that the discipline of pharmacoeconomics will become anything more than an exercise in generating clinical trial-based cost-outcomes ratios.

Impact of Drug Formularies on Drug Access and Utilization

Overly restrictive formularies may deny patients access to necessary medications. This assertion has prompted criticism of restrictive or closed drug formularies. However, managed care counters that in developing their formularies all necessary drugs are included and, by definition, if a drug is not included in the formulary, it is not necessary and there is an alternate and equally effective product on the formulary. Walser, Ross-Degnan, and Soumerai concluded that the elimination of restrictive Medicaid formularies improved access to 200 of the most prescribed drugs, but most of these popular drugs added no therapeutic benefit.[57] In general, restrictive Medicaid formularies have prevented access to new drug introductions.[58] Very little is known about the ultimate impact on patient outcomes as a result of pharmacy benefit programs.[59,60] Not exclusively a U.S. phenomenon, the European economic community has also found that the rational development of a drug formulary can have positive financial benefits without jeopardizing patient care.[61] Gross found no evidence that the use of formularies adversely affects patients' access to pharmaceutical care.[62]

Drug formularies will continue to be used and will generally grow more restrictive with greater use of NDC blocks, eliminating coverage of certain drug products.[63,64] However, this is not consistent across all health plans, as indicated previously. Many plans will use a combination of NDC blocks and higher and tiered copayments to limit access and influence use of formulary products. Pharmaceutical manufacturers must continue their organization-specific intelligence gathering so that they understand the current and future access and utilization control strategies of their key managed care customers.

Prior authorization (PA) of selected drugs is another formulary control activity that is commonly used to control access and use of expensive products or those drugs that have a high abuse or misuse potential. PA programs are expensive, unfriendly to patients, and administratively cumbersome, and they often cost $5.00 to $15.00 per PA episode. Therefore, we are also seeing PBMs and HMOs use higher and tiered copayments for products normally subject to a PA to eliminate the frustration involved with a physician or pharmacist trying to obtain authorization to prescribe or dispense a drug.

The result of these formulary changes is to shift the financial burden and demand management function to the patient by way of a utilization copayment. This also reduces the objectionable use of noncoverage activities (i.e., NDC blocks or prior authorization). Essentially, patients can have whatever they want, as long as they accept the financial responsibility associated with their decision.

Mandatory Generic Substitution Program

Mandatory dispensing of generic drugs is perhaps the single most effective cost-containment drug formulary component available. Aggressively promoting the use of generic drugs when appropriate can reduce pharmacy program costs by approximately 10 to 15 percent. The National Association of Chain Drug Stores reported that the average price of brand prescriptions was $53.51 in 1998, whereas the average generic prescription price was $17.33, approximately one third the price of branded prescriptions. An MCO with an aggressive generic substitution program can have at least 50 percent of prescriptions dispensed generically without compromising patient care.

To take advantage of the lower acquisition price of generic drugs, the pharmacy program administrator will set the amount of reimbursement for each generic drug product. This may be called the "maximum allowable cost" or MAC. If an MCO or PBM establishes a MAC on a drug product, this means that the pharmacist will only be reimbursed at the MAC, regardless if a generic is dispensed or if the pharmacist dispenses a more expensive brand product. If an MCO or PBM has a "MAC program" and if a pharmacist dispenses a more expensive brand product, the pharmacist will not

receive complete reimbursement. In this situation, the patient will be asked to pay the difference between the brand name drug cost and the generic MAC-level of reimbursement.

Managed care generally supports the use of generic drugs and anxiously awaits the patent expiration of expensive brand medications that are highly used. In 1999, IMS America estimated that approximately $1.2 billion of generic savings could result in the United States from the brand products that will be available as generic drugs for the first time. This number is expected to increase to $5.2 billion in 2000, drop down to $3.7 billion in 2001, and rise to $7.5 billion in 2002.

Role of the Drug Formulary and Treatment Guidelines

Many health plans and PBMs use treatment guidelines or algorithms to minimize treatment variations and to improve outcomes for patients while reducing costs. The purpose of guidelines is to promote the appropriate use of the most cost-effective pharmaceuticals. Guidelines are often derived from medical specialty societies or governmental entities, such as the National Institutes of Health or the Agency for Health Care Policy and Research (AHCPR). Also called clinical pathways or treatment protocols, clinical guidelines are recommendations to practitioners of a course of action concerning diagnosis and treatment of a specific disease or medical condition. Often drug formulary documents include treatment guidelines within appropriate therapeutic category sections. Clinical guidelines are discussed in detail in Chapter 29.

PHARMACEUTICAL MANUFACTURER DISCOUNT AND REBATE CONTRACTS

Health plans and PBMs that can effectively enforce drug formularies and influence physician prescribing and pharmacy dispensing may negotiate discount contracts with pharmaceutical manufacturers. The contracts are often performance based and provide financial rewards to the health plan or PBM if the market share or volume of the products under contract increases. Contracts may provide off-invoice discounts on purchased drugs (for in-house pharmacies that take possession of drugs) or rebates on used drugs (for community-based pharmacy networks). The Omnibus Budget Reconciliation Act of 1990 (OBRA '90) places effective limitations on the level of rebate, usually to approximately 15 percent. Manufacturers must provide equivalent rebates to Medicaid pharmacy programs. Health plans and PBMs may pass on some of the discounts to their payer-customers or to provider physicians or pharmacists as incentives for prescribing and dispensing formulary drugs. Table 24–4 illustrates the potential cost impact of a rebate. As shown, generic drug "A" offers the payer a much lower net cost ($6.50) but offers no rebate income. Brand drug "B" subject to a rebate contract offers a net cost of $15.00 to the payer and a $1.50 rebate income to the PBM (or health plan) that holds the contract with the manufacturer. Brand drug "C" is priced the same as drug "B," but drug "C" does not have a rebate associated with it. As a result, drug "C" is more expensive to the payer ($18.00) and offers the PBM or HMO no rebate income. If drugs "B" and "C" are equivalent, the presence of the rebate would influence the P & T committee to select drug "B" if a brand name drug is preferred. If a generic product is acceptable, drugs "A," "B," and "C" would be subject to a MAC and would all be reimbursed at the same level. As a result, pharmacies would dispense drug "A" only, unless the patient was willing to pay the cost difference between the MAC level of reimbursement and the cost of drugs "B" or "C."

PRESCRIPTION PATIENT COPAYMENTS

Managed care members are usually required by contract to pay a copayment for each prescription they obtain for three reasons. First, the copayment is a method that involves the patient as a financial risk-sharing partner in the quest to control the cost of the prescription drug program. Second, the copayment should influence the patient's behavior to select a lower copayment drug that has a lower cost to the HMO or PBM. Third, a copayment introduces a hesitation factor designed to discourage unnecessary or trivial use of prescription drugs. Traditionally, health plans attempted to set the pre-

Table 24–4 Illustration of the Cost Impact of the Rebate

	Generic A	Brand B	Brand C
Drug AWP*	$10.00	$30.00	$30.00
Drug AWP—15%**	$ 8.50	$25.50	$25.50
Dispensing Fee***	$ 3.00	$ 2.50	$ 2.50
Prescription Subtotal	$11.50	$28.00	$28.00
Tiered Copay	$ 5.00	$10.00	$10.00
Net Subtotal Cost	$ 6.50	$18.00	$18.00
10% Rebate (Drug B)	—	$ 3.00	—
Net Total Cost	$ 6.50	$15.00	$18.00
50% Rebate Share	—	$ 1.50	—
Net Cost to Payer	$ 6.50	$16.50	$18.00
Rebate Income to PBM	—	$ 1.50	—

Source: Robert P. Navarro, 2000.

*AWP = average wholesale price.

**15% is typical discount on published drug ingredient cost (AWP).

***Pharmacist received additional $0.50 fee for dispensing a generic.

scription copayment at approximately 25 percent of the average prescription cost and adjust the copayment annually as the prescription costs increased. Therefore, if the average brand prescription cost is $45.00, the average brand copayment would be $11.25. This general guideline usually holds true, although other competitive factors and rebate contracts may influence in what formulary copayment tiers drug products will be placed. Certain union trusts or state Medicaid programs may choose not to require a copayment or have a very low copayment (e.g., $1.00 per prescription). Copayment must be high enough to achieve the desired financial goals but not too high as to discourage or prevent the appropriate use of cost-effective pharmaceuticals.

Employer groups and managed care have been frustrated by their apparent inability to contain rising pharmacy program costs and now have gone to the ultimate user of health care products and services, the member-patients, in an attempt to control costs and use of pharmaceuticals. Employers and managed care have routinely levied higher and tiered user fees (copayments) on most health care products and services used. Some health benefit programs, such as many Medicare programs or indemnity-style insurance, also have front-end deductibles, benefit maximums, or both as cost-containment features to help limit the financial exposure of the health plan. We will likely see a greater array of benefit designs with different levels of front-end deductibles, copayment tiers, and benefit caps from which members can select on the basis of their health care demands, financial status, and willingness to pay. As this occurs, individual patients will be even more appropriate targets for a direct-to-consumer marketing message.

Economic theory suggests that the demand for prescriptions should fall as the price increases, all else being equal. This assertion is based on Grossman's derived demand model, which contends that the demand for medical care and prescription drugs flows from an underlying demand for health.[65] Other studies have shown a slight or modest reduction in drug use with higher copayments.[66–68] However, there is not universal consistency in the limited number of copayment studies. The demand elasticity is highly variable and depends on a patient's financial abilities, perception of heath needs, perception of the value of the desired resource, the influence of the patient's physician and other external influencers.

Copayment Tiers

Copayments are increasing in dollar amount and becoming increasingly tiered to share costs and influence patient demand. However, despite continuously rising AWP ingredient cost, according to a national survey of 333 employer plan sponsors, retail prescription copays for brand medications rose only 6.6 percent between 1995 and 1997.[69] An unpublished study of 20 MCOs (5 PBMs with an average membership of 20 million lives) and 15 HMOs (average membership of 1.1 million lives) revealed the copayment tier levels shown in Table 24–5.

Not all copayment schemes are effective in shifting costs and influencing patient demand. Consider the example in Table 24–6 in which the copayment results in the member selecting a drug in the next lower copayment (e.g., paying the Tier III nonpreferred brand copayment versus influencing the member to switch to the Tier II preferred brand).

If health plans only shift cost without influencing drug use behavior, they will reduce some costs by shifting some of the drug costs to the patient through copayments but will not experience the full potential of changing patient behavior. As indicated previously, it is preferable to influence the patient to accept a lower tiered product for additional savings. This is particularly important for chronic medications because with each month of use, the plan will save an additional $10 if a Tier II product is used in place of a Tier III product in this example.

Pharmacy directors generally believe that an inter-tier change of at least $10.00 is necessary to influence patient decisions. However, this is highly dependent on patients' socioeconomic levels. There may limited elasticity in the demand of pharmaceuticals from the patients' perspective.

Table 24–5 Copayment Tiers

MCO Type	Average Tier I Generic Copayment (Range)	Average Tier II Formulary or Preferred Brand Copayment (Range)	Average Tier III Nonformulary or Nonpreferred Brand Copayment (Range)
PBM	$5.40 ($5.00–$7.00)	$11.40 ($10.00–$15.00)	$25.00 ($25.00)
HMO	$6.40 ($5.00–$10.00)	$15.40 ($10.00–$25.00)	$32.22 ($15.00–$40.00)
Total	$6.15 ($5.00–$10.00)	$14.40 ($10.00–$25.00)	$26.43 ($15.00–$40.00)

Physician Response to Rising Copayments

Physicians are generally unaware of the copayment level of the products they prescribe because they pay little attention to the multiple printed formularies of the numerous health plans with which they participate. It is generally only if the patient informs the physician on a subsequent visit of his or her concern over the copayment level that a physician would become aware of the copayment (or if a pharmacist contacts the physician on a patient's behalf).

However, by the time the patient has revisited the physician, the drug has likely been used for a

Table 24–6 Financial Impact of Influence on Patient Behavior with Copayments

Formulary/ Copayment Tier	Net Prescription Cost	Copayment Amount	Net Cost to HMO	Net Cost to HMO by Use of Drug One Tier Lower
Tier I (generic)	$15	$5	$10	—
Tier II $50 preferred brand	$50	$15	$35	$10 ($25 savings if Tier I drug is used)
Tier III $70 nonpreferred brand	$70	$25	$45 (if the Tier III product is used) If the Tier III, nonpreferred brand is used, the patient pays $25 copayment, and the HMO has a net exposure of $45 for this $70 product.	$35 ($10 savings if Tier II is used) However, if the patient is influenced because of the high $25 Tier III copayment to accept the Tier II product, the plan "saves" an additional $10 in the net cost of the Tier II product

month or two, and if effective, the patient will likely continue the medication. Medicare members may be an exception. They may be more likely to express concern over high copayment costs if their out-of-pocket expenses introduce a personal hardship or result in personal drug rationing.

Theoretically, in situations in which physicians are at financial risk for pharmacy benefits, there should be alignment of the financial interests of the patient and physician. That is, lower AWP products (preferred by physicians at financial risk) should also be preferred by patients because such products are likely to be in lower copayment tiers.[70]

However, there is a relative inelasticity of demand in this situation because physicians are not often aware of AWP drug prices and generally try to use the most effective product, despite the copayment tier. This is not universal, and some physicians are quite aware of AWP levels and may preferentially use less-expensive products whenever possible.

A confounding element is DTC advertising.[71] Patients may request higher AWP products on the basis of DTC advertising, and the physician may be unable to dissuade the patient without an extensive and time-consuming discussion. It is estimated that when a patient requests a DTC-advertised product, 40 percent of physicians simply prescribe the product without argument, and 40 percent of physicians attempt to convince the patients a less-expensive product is preferable. The introduction of higher copayments for nonpreferred drugs may assist the physician in dissuading the patient from using the DTC-advertised product. However, this is highly variable.

One New York area health plan introduced a higher $50.00 prescription copayment on a nonpreferred, nonsedating antihistamine and experienced almost no change in patient use, presumably because of the impact of effective DTC advertising.

Relationship of Copayments to Formulary Positioning

Increasingly, there is a contractual relationship between the formulary positioning of a drug product and the copayment associated with its use. MCOs and PBMs are using copayments to influence patient drug selection and utilization to increase the market share of contracted products. Contracts may also limit the number of drugs at specific copayment tiers. For example, a rebate contract may allow only two products to be "preferred" in the formulary and available at the second tier copayment. Additional brand products must be positioned in the formulary as "nonpreferred" and available only at the higher, third-tier copayment. Generic products within the category are available at the lowest (first tier) copayment (even though they may be preferred, generics do not violate the rebate contract requirements). This is illustrated in the Table 24–7.

A fourth copayment tier is being introduced for nonformulary products (for plans that do not use NDC blocks) or for noncovered, "lifestyle," or cosmetic drug products (i.e., for alopecia or male impotence). Fourth copayment tiers are frequently percent copayments (coinsurance), such as 50 percent up to a maximum dollar amount. Exhibit 24–1 illustrates how a drug formulary might be constructed to reflect drug copayment.

Table 24–7 Relationship of Contract and Copayment Tier

Drug Product	Formulary Position	Copayment Tier	Copayment Example
Generic	Preferred	First	$6.00
Contracted brand	Preferred	Second	$12.00
Noncontracted brand	Nonpreferred	Third	$25.00

The net result is to allow access to more drugs previously not covered but require the patient who selects them to use these products in the third or fourth tier and to accept the financial responsibility for their decision. Health plans do not consider this an unfair penalty because they consider these third or fourth tier products (especially fourth tier products) to be optional and nonessential drugs for which there are formulary alternatives.

Drug Utilization Review[72]

DUR is a common clinical pharmacy procedure that involves the thorough review of patient drug history records by a pharmacist to determine whether patient's drug use or physician's drug prescribing require intervention. Typically, the patient drug history is reviewed for unnecessary or redundant drug use, drug interactions, adverse effects, noncompliance, and lack of persistence.

DUR is a well-accepted quality assurance and improvement activity and is now mandated by the Joint Commission on Accreditation of Healthcare Organizations (Joint Commission), NCQA, and the federal government (accreditation agencies are discussed in Chapter 44). The purpose of this activity is to ensure appropriate drug therapy. In 1972, Brodie published an important paper that defined the DUR process as the "ongoing study of the frequency of use and cost of drugs, from which patterns of prescribing, dispensing, and patient use can be determined."[73] An effective DUR program must have the authority to review the use of drugs through available information and to compare the observed use to standards identified by knowledgeable professionals.

Stolar furthered the concept of DUR by stating that for a DUR program to ensure the quality of drug use, it must be continuous, authorized, and structured. DUR programs must measure the use of drugs against predetermined criteria and initiate changes in drug use that do not meet these criteria.[74] The added criteria of continuous review and intervention transformed DUR from simply a passive study of drug use patterns to an active evaluation and intervention program with defined outcomes.

DUR programs are qualitative studies with corrective action, prescriber feedback, and re-evaluation. This not only achieves the improved patient care objective but also provides substantial educational benefit to the pharmacist and prescriber. By definition, "retrospective" review is conducted using historical records. However, a retrospective review generally is not timely enough to prevent acute drug use problems. Concurrent review processes are often established to address this problem area and are done by use of online, real-time, POS computer systems. The in-pharmacy POS computer system interacts with patient drug history maintained by the health plan or PBM. The system provides immediate clinical messages that may alert the pharmacist to drug use problems. Regardless of the source of the drug use records, a pharmacist is required to assess information and make contact with the patient's physicians to investigate or correct dangerous drug use patterns.

Application of DUR in Pharmacy Benefit Management

Similar to formularies, DUR is a clinical pharmacy quantitative review process that began in hospitals and migrated to the outpatient, managed care environment because of the need to maximize outcomes and minimize costs. Managed care lends itself quite well to the DUR philosophy because managed care generally is associated with large amounts of data. DUR in managed care is conducted on a population basis, but interventions occur on a patient-specific basis. Hospitals and health care systems will use DUR concepts for accreditation purposes. As noted earlier, the Joint Commission incorporates DUR in its accreditation of hospitals, and the NCQA uses DUR concepts for its health plan accreditation and HEDIS measurements. Effective DUR counseling has been required for all Medicaid patients as of 1993, secondary to the Omnibus Budget Reconciliation Act of 1990. This act provides legislation for federal financial participation (FFP) payment for covered outpatient drugs under the Medicaid program. DUR programs have taken on many different appearances in managed care, but the common theme among all the programs is that they are designed to review physician prescribing, pharmacist dispensing, and patient use of medications in an attempt to minimize treatment variations and optimize patient care outcomes.[75]

ROLE OF PHARMACY PROGRAMS IN DISEASE MANAGEMENT AND QUALITY IMPROVEMENT PROGRAMS

Disease management (DM) programs are integrated patient management activities with the goal of achieving the most cost-effective patient treatment outcomes. The DM programs attempt to improve clinical, economic, and quality-of-life outcomes. Such programs are possible in MCOs that have the ability to collect and merge medical claims and clinical data with pharmacy claims and establish effective management programs to achieve the desired outcomes. DM is discussed in Chapter 23 in greater depth but will be related to the pharmacy program administration here.

DM has been defined in various ways but is often considered to be a patient-focused, comprehensive approach to minimize the treatment variability of a specific disease to improve patient care outcomes and optimize the expenditure of resources.[76] DM programs fit well with pharmacy benefit management because DM concepts will help focus on the value of pharmaceuticals in their role in achieving clinical, economic, and quality-of-life outcomes. DM helps to shift the focus from the cost of drugs to the value of the pharmacy benefit program because DM broadens the focus to direct and indirect economic outcomes rather than only pharmacy component cost management.

This interest in qualitative outcomes was supported by the growth of organizations' quality improvement initiatives in health care, such as the NCQA and other similar quality improvement entities. Payers, health care plans, and vendors saw DM as a tool to implement quality improvement strategies into the delivery of health care services. Because health care is a market-driven business, health plans also saw their ability to document the quality of care provided by their physicians and hospitals as an important marketing tool to grow their membership and reduce enrollee turnover.

DM is a continuous, coordinated evolutionary process that seeks to manage and improve the health status of the affected patient subpopulation over the entire course of the disease.[77] When clinical guidelines deal with the treatment of a disease, DM, or health management, is a comprehensive program that deals with each aspect of health care along the continuum of an identified disease, from detection to treatment to follow-up. Those diseases that are chosen are often chronic diseases in which there is evidence that associated care processes bring about measurable improvements in the patient's health status. Diseases are also targeted that consume a large amount of resources or are associated with a high overall cost. Examples of diseases treated by DM programs include asthma, diabetes, hypercholesterolemia, hypertension, congestive heart failure, diabetes, depression, AIDS, cancer, and osteoporosis. The formulary and clinical guidelines are also involved because the formulary provides the most cost-effective drugs available, and guidelines help ensure they are used appropriately. DM programs can lead to positive economic outcomes that identify those drugs that, when appropriately used, effectively minimize costs and maximize outcomes associated with specific, targeted medical conditions.

QUALITY IMPROVEMENT IN PHARMACY BENEFIT MANAGEMENT[78]

The NCQA established HEDIS as the first organized set of performance measures to evaluate the quality of managed care plans. Specific HEDIS measures are associated with accurate and appropriate delivery of the pharmacy benefit. Often the health plan will "carve out" the pharmacy benefits to a PBM. As an outside vendor of the health plan's services, the PBM is responsible to the health plan for collecting the pharmacy data needed to report these specific

HEDIS measures. These data must then be matched with the health plan's medical claims data because all information for one patient can be scattered across several different databases.

Integrating medical and pharmacy claims data is a challenging process that is necessary to meet HEDIS and NCQA accreditation requirements.[79] Medical conditions and diseases are most often coded by the International Code for Diagnoses (ICD-9 or ICD-10), whereas procedures are coded by the American Medical Association's Physicians' Current Procedural Terminology (CPT). Codes for pharmaceuticals have not been yet standardized into one internationally recognized code. Generic product identifier (GPI) and generic code name (GCN) are just two examples of nationally recognized index codes for pharmaceuticals owned by FirstDataBank, a pharmacy data and information management company. Most of the HEDIS measures do not involve pharmaceuticals, although this is rapidly changing. Some of the current measures that involve pharmacy benefits include those found in Table 24–8. The reader is referred to Chapter 35, and specifically Figures 35–1 and 35–2, for the complete HEDIS measures.

Table 24–8 Examples of HEDIS Measures Requiring Pharmacy Data

Domain	Measure	Description	Pharmacy Data to Report
Effectiveness of care	Beta-blocker treatment after a heart attack	% members ≥35 years who were hospitalized and discharged with a diagnosis of AMI and who received a Rx for β-blockers on discharge	Members who received an outpatient Rx within 30 days before admission for AMI to 7 days after discharge
	Eye examinations for people with diabetes	% members ≥31 years with type I or II diabetes who had a retinal examination within the year	Identification of population: those members dispensed insulin, oral hypoglyce- mics, antihyperglycemics
	Comprehensive diabetes care	% of members 18–75 years with type I or II diabetes who had HbA1c, lipids, eyes, and kidneys monitored during the year	Identification of population: those members dispensed insulin, oral hypoglycemics, antihyperglycemics
	Antidepressant medication management	% members ≥18 years diagnosed with a new episode of depression, treated with medication: acute and continuation phase follow-up	Members diagnosed with a new episode of major depressive disorder treated with antidepres- sant meds
Use of services	Outpatient drug utilization	Summary of drug use: average # and cost of Rx's PMPM, total # and cost of Rx's; stratified by age and payer	"Prescription" is defined as one 30-day (or less) supply of pharmaceuticals *or* one supply requiring a copay

AMI = acute myocardial infarction; Rx = prescription
Source: Adapted from Amelia Goodwin, Quality Improvement Initiatives in Managed Care, in *Managed Care Pharmacy Practice,* R.P. Navarro, ed., p. 300, © 1999, Aspen Publishers, Inc. Copayment information added by Robert P. Navarro, 2000.

MEASURING PHARMACY BENEFIT MANAGEMENT PROGRAM PERFORMANCE

The competitive managed care environment requires that health plan and PBM pharmacy programs are successful from a clinical, patient satisfaction, and economic perspective. The pharmacy program manager will monitor specific performance metrics on a monthly basis (see following) and attempt to modify controllable factors if performance measures suggest costs are rising more than forecast, member satisfaction is declining, drug-related clinical outcomes are being achieved, or other markers of poor pharmacy program performance are indicated.

An MCO tries to accomplish the following objectives to achieve the cost, access, and quality of care goals:

- implement and maintain a comprehensive, cost-effective, and dynamic drug formulary program, including an exception or PA process, to meet all reasonable patient care needs as defined in the certificate of coverage
- develop a responsible pharmacy program member service function to ensure members access pharmacy benefits most effectively
- construct a pharmacy provider network to include a participating pharmacy within a reasonable distance of member homes and offices (usually 1 to 5 miles)
- develop drug utilization review and other quality improvement programs to help optimize drug performance and provide intervention for patients requiring special assistance in achieving pharmacy program outcomes

The pharmacy program must also meet strict budgetary and performance objectives. The basic performance benchmarks monitored usually include the following measurements:

- total prescription program costs (dollars)
- monthly (PMPM) and annual (PMPY) program costs
- prescription utilization (PMPM and PMPY). The PMPY utilization rate for HMOs with managed pharmacy programs is now in the 7 to 9 prescriptions PMPY range for a non-Medicare population.[80]
- administrative and claims processing fees (per prescription and per patient)
- prescription discount or rebate (total amount, per prescription, and per patient)
- generic dispensing rate (overall, by pharmacy, by therapeutic class, and by physician)
- drug formulary conformance rate (overall, by physician, and by pharmacy)
- patient satisfaction and member complaints related to the pharmacy program
- number of drug formulary exception requests and approvals
- trend of all the preceding performance measurements measured monthly, quarterly, and annually

There are many more performance measurements pharmacy directors routinely monitor, especially with more sophisticated programs that may include drug formulary conversion, compliance, and persistence activities. However, with the preceding basic performance measurements, a pharmacy director can evaluate the effectiveness of his or her prescription drug management program.

Budgeting and Planning To Achieve Pharmacy Program Performance Goals

Pharmacy program performance goals can only be achieved with a well-designed and executed pharmacy program plan. By the late summer or early fall, the pharmacy program manager is told the membership, marketing, financial, benefit design, and other plan characteristics that will influence the cost and use of pharmaceuticals in the subsequent year, as well as his or her budget, to achieve specific PMPM and PMPY cost goals. The pharmacy manager must then allocate financial and human resources to appropriate tasks to achieve the forecast budget goals. Because most employer groups renew their contract in January, and the contract is generally in force for 12 months, the pharmacy manager has limitations on what benefit design or copayment changes can be made throughout the year to compensate for higher-than-budget pharmacy cost experience. Therefore, accurate budgeting and planning must occur before the benefit design or premium and copayment levels are established because they often cannot be changed for 12 months.

When a new drug is launched, the pharmacy manager attempts to determine the cost (if not known before launch) and the potential utilization because it is the product of these factors that will determine the total forecast cost impact of the new drug. Hedayati and Kleinstiver propose a novel cost impact model.[81]

FUTURE CHANGES IN PHARMACY BENEFIT MANAGEMENT

The evolution of pharmacy benefit management depends heavily on technological advances, first in the arena of biotechnology, high throughput, combinatorial chemistry that will deliver more effective and efficient but more expensive pharmaceuticals, and the second in the area of information processing and communications.

High throughput and combinatorial chemistry will allow a geometric improvement in the number of chemicals that can be analyzed for potential human value and will allow chemists to develop patient-specific drug therapy that will virtually ensure therapeutic outcomes. The price for these compounds will likely be high, and economic and ethical arguments will occur regarding the patient's, health plan's, and employer group's willingness to pay for such outcomes. The role of health economics will become more important as esoteric concepts such as quality of life and functional status are incorporated into formulary and benefit design coverage decisions.

The information storage and processing advances will allow the ability to identify patient candidates for intervention, monitor outcomes, and conduct population-based outcomes research to refine drug therapy, formulary decisions, and treatment guidelines. Information warehouses will also support economic research regarding the coverage issues of expensive biotechnology products, discussed previously. Advances in communications will provide patient-specific clinical data to the physician at the point of prescribing to maximize outcomes and minimize adverse drug events. The Internet will advance patient access to health and drug information, provide patient-specific monitoring and educational opportunities, allow Internet access to drug distribution channels, and in general increase the health knowledge status of patients. This will likely result in greater individual responsibility for health care outcomes and allow the patient to make better informed decisions on how to spend his or her health care premium and copayment dollars.

CONCLUSION

Prescription drugs are a highly used and aggressively managed health benefit offered by managed care. Purchasers of pharmacy benefits continue to focus on drug costs, especially because of the double-digit pharmacy program annual trend rate of the past few years for many payers. Pharmacy program managers must focus on the value that appropriately used pharmaceuticals can have on total direct economic, clinical, and quality of life outcomes.

REFERENCES AND NOTES

1. R. P. Navarro, ed., *Pharmacy Benefit Report Facts & Figures* (East Hanover, NJ: Novartis Pharmaceuticals, 1998), 3.

2. Anonymous, Ethical Pharmaceuticals: Managed Care Impact. *Medical & Healthcare Marketplace Guide* website, December 10, 1999:2–4.

3. Health Care Financing Administration, Office of the Actuary, National Health Statistics, 29 October 1998.

4. R. P. Navarro, data on file, 1999.

5. F. Teitelbaum, A. Parker, R. Martinez, and C. Roe, *Express Scripts 1998 Drug Trend Report* (St. Louis: Express Scripts, 1999), 3.

6. W. Knight, Too Much or Too Little? The Role of Pharmaceuticals in the Health Care System. *Journal of Managed Care* 5(4) (1999).

7. Anonymous, *National Association of Chain Drug Stores* website (www.nacds.org), December 28, 1999.

8. F. Teitelbaum, A. Parker, R. Martinez, and C. Roe, *Express Scripts 1998 Drug Trend Report*, 6.

9. F. Teitelbaum, A. Parker, R. Martinez, and C. Roe, *Express Scripts 1998 Drug Trend Report*, 7.

10. F. Teitelbaum, A. Parker, R. Martinez, and C. Roe, *Express Scripts 1998 Drug Trend Report*, 23.

11. *Newsweek*, November 8, 1999.

12. D. J. Stanied, D. Goodspeed, L. A. Stember, M. Schlesinger, and K. Schafermeyer, Information Technology: The National Council for Prescription Drug Programs: Setting the Standards for Electronic Transmission of Pharmacy Data. *Drug Benefit Trends* (January 1997): 29–35.

13. J. H. Romza and G. E. Black, "Pharmacy Data and Information Systems. In: R. P. Navarro, ed. *Managed Care Pharmacy Practice* (Gaithersburg, MD: Aspen Publishers, 1999), 141–143.

14. D. Cassak, PBM's Second Generation: From Formularies to Triggers. *IN VIVO*, September 1995.

15. J. H. Romza and G. E. Black, Pharmacy Data and Information Systems, 143.

16. J. H. Romza and G. E. Black, Pharmacy Data and Information Systems, 143–144.

17. HEDIS 3.0 Handbook, Effectiveness of Care.

18. NCPDP web page, January, 1999 (http://www.ncpdp.org).

19. R. P. Navarro, R. Da Silva, and S. Rivkin, Health Informatics Systems. In: R. P. Navarro, ed. *Managed Care Pharmacy Practice* (Gaithersburg, MD: Aspen Publishers, 1999), 313–343.

20. G. D. Schiff and D. Rucker, Computerized Prescribing. *Journal of the American Medical Association* 279 (1998): 13, 1024–1029.

21. S. Rivkin, Opportunities and Challenges of Electronic Physician Prescribing Technology. *Medical Interface* August (1997): 77–83.

22. M. Monane, D. M. Matthias, B. A. Nagle, and M. A. Kelly, Improving Prescribing Patterns for the Elderly Through an Online Drug Utilization Review Intervention. *Journal of the American Medical Association* 280 (1998): 13, 1239–1252.

23. D. Angaran, personal communication, December 19, 1998.

24. National Association of Boards of Pharmacy website, January 1999.

25. World Health Organization website December 23, 1997.

26. D. Goldstein, Marketing Pharmaceutical Products Online to Consumers. *Managed Care Interface* 11 (1998) 2, 50–52.

27. R. P. Navarro and S. S. Blackburn, Pharmacy Benefit Management Companies. In: R. P. Navarro, ed. *Managed Care Pharmacy Practice* (Gaithersburg, MD: Aspen Publishers, 1999), 221–240.

28. R. P. Navarro, ed., Pharmacy Benefit Report Trends & Forecasts, 1998 (East Hanover, NJ: Novartis Pharmaceuticals Corporation, 1998), 21.

29. R. P. Navarro, Pharmacy Benefit Management Principles and Practices. In: R. P. Navarro, ed. *Managed Care Pharmacy Practice* (Gaithersburg, MD: Aspen Publishers), 36–37.

30. R. P. Navarro, Pharmacy Benefit Management Principles and Practices. In: R .P. Navarro, ed. *Managed Care Pharmacy Practice* (Gaithersburg, MD: Aspen Publishers, 1999), 38.

31. J. D. Jones, Pharmacy Benefit Design, Contracting, and Marketing. In: R. P. Navarro, ed. *Managed Care Pharmacy Practice* (Gaithersburg, MD: Aspen Publishers, 1999), 50–51.

32. National Association of Chain Drug Stores website (www.nacds.org), December 28, 1999.

33. National Association of Chain Drug Stores website (www.nacds.org), December 28, 1999.

34. R. P. Navarro, Pharmacy Benefit Management Principles and Practices. In: R. P. Navarro, ed. *Managed Care Pharmacy Practice* (Gaithersburg, MD: Aspen Publishers, 1999), 40.

35. L. T. Sterler and D. Stephens, Pharmacy Distribution Systems and Network Management. In: R. P. Navarro, ed. *Managed Care Pharmacy Practice* (Gaithersburg, MD: Aspen Publishers, 1999), 94–95.

36. L. T. Sterler and D. Stephens, Pharmacy Distribution Systems and Network Management, 95.

37. L. T. Sterler and D. Stephens, Pharmacy Distribution Systems and Network Management, 98.

38. L. T. Sterler and D. Stephens, Pharmacy Distribution Systems and Network Management, 99.

39. M. J. Dillon, Drug Formulary Management. In: R. P. Navarro, ed. *Managed Care Pharmacy Practice* (Gaithersburg, MD: Aspen Publishers, 1999), 145–163.

40. R. B. Goldberg, Managing the pharmacy benefit: the formulary system, *Journal of Managed Care Pharmacy* 3(5) (1997): 565–573.

41. N. M. King, *Pharmacopoeias and Formularies: A Selection of Primary Sources for the History of Pharmacy in the United States* (Madison, WI: American Institute of the History of Pharmacy, 1985), 9–11.

42. J. Iglehart, Health Policy Report: The American Health Care System—Expenditures, *The New England Journal of Medicine* 340 (1999): 1, 75.

43. G. Sonnedecker, *Kremers and Urdang's History of Pharmacy* (Madison, WI: American Institute of the History of Pharmacy, 1976), 259.

44. American Society of Health-System Pharmacists, ASHP Statement on the Formulary System. In: *Practice Standards of ASHP 1997–1998* (Bethesda, MD, 1997).

45. Academy of Managed Care Pharmacy, *Concepts in Managed Care Pharmacy Series—Formulary Management* (Alexandria, VA: 1998).

46. American Society of Health-System Pharmacists, ASHP Statement on the Pharmacy and Therapeutics Committee. In: *Practice Standards of ASHP 1997–1998* (Bethesda, MD: 1997).

47. M. J. Dillon, Drug Formulary Management, 153.

48. T. R .Covington and J. L. Thornton, The Formulary System: A Cornerstone of Drug Benefit Management. In: S. Ito and S. Blackburn, eds. *A Pharmacist's Guide to Principles and Practices of Managed Care Pharmacy* (Alexandria, VA: Foundation for Managed Care Pharmacy, 1995).

49. D. I. Brixner, S. L. Szeinbach, S. Mehta, S. Ryu, and H. Shah, Pharmacoeconomic Research and Applications in Managed Care. In: R. P. Navarro, ed. *Managed Care Pharmacy Practice* (Gaithersburg, MD: Aspen Publishers, 1999), 416–417.

50. P. C. Langley, Meeting the Information Needs of Drug Purchasers: The Evolution of Formulary Submission Guidelines. *Clinical Therapeutics* 21 (1999): 4, 768–787.

51. S. Sullivan, personal communication, July and August, 1999.

52. B. R. Luce, C. A. Lyles, A. M. Rentz, The View from Managed Care Pharmacy. *Health Affairs* 15 (1996): 4, 168–186.

53. D. A. Bukstein, Incorporating Quality of Life Data into Managed Care Formulary Decisions: A Case Study with Salmeterol. *American Journal of Managed Care* 3 (1997): 11, 1701–1706.

54. C. Todd, What Makes Health Economics Research Useful to Decision Makers? *Pharmacoeconomics & Outcomes News Weekly* 170 (1998): 3–4.

55. D. I. Brixner, S. L. Szeinbach, S. Mehta, S. Ryu, and H. Shah, Pharmacoeconomic Research and Applications in Managed Care. In: R. P. Navarro, ed. *Managed Care Pharmacy Practice* (Gaithersburg, MD: Aspen Publishers, 1999), 405.

56. P. C. Langley, Information Requirements of Health Systems as Drug Purchasers: Does the FDA Have a Role in Setting Evidentiary Standards? *Journal of Managed Care Pharmacy* 4 (1998): 6, 593–598.

57. B. L. Walser, D. Ross-Negnan, and S. B. Soumerai, Do Open Formularies Increase Access to Clinically Useful Drugs? *Health Affairs* 15 (1996): 3, 95–109.

58. H. G. Grabowski, S. O. Schweitzer, and S. R. Shiota, The Effect of Medicaid Formularies on the Availability of New Drugs. *Pharmacoeconomics* 1 (1992): Suppl 1, 32–40.

59. H. L. Lipton, D. H. Kreling, T. Collins, and K. C. Hertz, Pharmacy Benefit Management Companies: Dimensions of Performance. *Annual Review of Public Health* 20 (1999): 361–401.

60. K. A. Schulman, L. E. Rubenstein, S. R. Abernethy, D. M. Seils, and D. P. Sulmasy, The Effect of Pharmaceutical Benefits Managers: Is It Being Evaluated? *Annals of Internal Medicine* 15 (1996): 10, 906–913.

61. M. De Smedt, Drug Formularies—Good or Evil? A View from the EEC. *Cardiology* 85 (1994): Suppl 1, 41–45.

62. D. J. Gross, Prescription Drug Formularies in Managed Care: Concerns for the Elderly Population. *Clinical Therapeutics* 20 (1998): 6, 1277–1291.

63. A. Lyles and F. B. Palumbo, The Effect of Managed Care on Prescription Drug Costs and Benefits. *Pharmacoeconomics* 15 (1999): 2, 129–140.

64. H. Grabowski and C. D. Mullins, Pharmacy Benefit Management, Cost-Effectiveness Analysis and Drug Formulary Decisions. *Social Science and Medicine* 45 (1997): 4, 535–544.

65. M. Grossman, *The Demand for Health: A Theoretical and Empirical Investigation.* (New York: Columbia University Press [for the National Bureau for Economic Research], 1972).

66. R. E. Johnson, M. J. Goodman, M. C. Hornbrook, and M. B. Eldredge, The Effect of Increased Prescription Drug Cost-Sharing on Medical Care Utilization and Expenses of Elderly Health Maintenance Organization Members. *Medical Care* 35 (1997): 11, 1119–1131.

67. B. L. Harris, A. Stergachis, and L. D. Ried, The Effect of Drug Co-Payments on Utilization and Cost of Pharmaceuticals in a Health Maintenance Organization. *Medical Care* 28 (1990): 10, 907–917.

68. A. A. Nelson, C. E. Reeder, and W. M. Dickson, The Effect of a Medicaid Drug Copayment on the Utilization and Cost of Prescription Services. *Medical Care* 22 (1984): 8, 724–736.

69. *The Wyeth-Ayerst Prescription Drug Benefit Cost and Plan Design Survey Report: 1998 Edition* (Albuquerque, NM: PMBI Inc., and Wellman Publishing, Inc., 1998).

70. D. Saikami, Financial Risk Management of Pharmacy Benefits. *American Journal of Health-System Pharmacy* 1 (1997): 19, 2207.

71. M. Z. Bloom, Direct-to-Consumer Advertising Provides Challenge to Managed Care. *Journal of Managed Care Pharmacy* 5 (2) (1999): 2.

72. A. M. Peterson and M. D. Wilson, Drug Utilization Review Strategies. In: R. P. Navarro, ed. *Managed Care Pharmacy Practice* (Gaithersburg, MD: Aspen Publishers, 1999), 176–183.

73. D. C. Brodie, Drug Utilization Review/Planning, *Hospitals* 46 (1972): 103–112.

74. M. Stolar, Drug Use Review: Operational Definitions, *American Journal of Hospital Pharmacy* 33 (1978): 225–230.

75. A. M. Peterson and M. D. Wilson, Drug Utilization Review Strategies, 176.

76. R. P. Navarro, D. Christensen, and H. Leider, Disease Management Programs. In: R. P. Navarro, ed. *Managed Care Pharmacy Practice* (Gaithersburg, MD: Aspen Publishers, 1999), 372.

77. Academy of Managed Care Pharmacy, *Concepts in Managed Care Pharmacy Series—Disease State Management* (Alexandria, VA: 1998).

78. A. Goodwin, Quality Improvement Initiatives in Managed Care. In: R. P. Navarro, ed. *Managed Care Pharmacy Practice* (Gaithersburg, MD: Aspen Publishers, 1999), 297.

79. A. Goodwin, Quality Improvement Initiatives in Managed Care, 297.

80. R.P. Navarro, *Pharmacy Benefit Report Facts & Figures*, 5.

81. S. Hedayati and P. W. Kleinstiver, A Predictive Cost Analysis Model for Estimating Formulary Impact of New Products In Managed Care. *Journal of Managed Care Pharmacy* 4 (1998): 6, 585–590.

CHAPTER 25

Managed Behavioral Health Care and Chemical Dependency Services

Donald F. Anderson, Jeffrey L. Berlant, Katherine O. Sternbach, Danna Mauch,
H.G. Whittington, William R. Maloney, and Terri Goens

INTRODUCTION

Management of behavioral health (BH) services has unique characteristics and delivery challenges that stem from the historical development of mental health as a discipline, public perceptions about mental illness, and recent massive changes in ideology, organization, and service delivery. For this chapter, BH is defined as including mental health, substance abuse or chemical dependency, and serious mental illness or brain disorders. ***Special factors influencing managed BH care include the following:***

- advances in medication and psychological therapeutic techniques that have promoted effective treatment of more BH disorders
- greater acceptance of mental illness and chemical dependency as illnesses with biological origins, which has led to a greater willingness on the part of the general public to seek help for these problems
- exclusion of BH benefits from the early HMOs and managed care programs, limit-

Donald F. Anderson, PhD, is a Principal with William M. Mercer, Incorporated, a human resources consulting organization. As the founder of Mercer's Behavioral Health Care Practice, he has extensive experience in the evaluation of managed mental health and substance abuse programs.

Jeffrey L. Berlant, MD, is William M. Mercer, Incorporated's senior consultant for mental health and substance abuse services. He has broad experience in evaluation of both public and private sector managed mental health and substance abuse programs.

Katherine O. Sternbach is a Principal with William M. Mercer, Incorporated's Health & Group Benefit Practice. Her consulting specialty is in the design, delivery, and implementation of managed behavioral health systems of care.

Danna Mauch, PhD, is the President of Magellan Public Solutions, a managed behavioral health care organization. She has extensive experience in strategic planning, operations management, systems evaluation, and the development and implementation of innovative managed care programs.

H.G. Whittington, MD, is the National Medical Director for MenningerCare Systems. Dr. Whittington is a board-certified psychiatrist and a Life Fellow of the American Psychiatric Association. A nationally recognized expert in outcomes research, clinical information management systems, and the cost-effective delivery of clinical services, he has over 30 years' experience in psychiatric practice, outcomes evaluation, clinical information management, administration, and consultation and teaching.

William R. Maloney is a Principal in William M. Mercer, Incorporated's Information Planning Group. His consulting specialty is the evaluation of information management systems for managed behavioral health applications.

Terri Goens is William M. Mercer, Incorporated's consultant for mental health and substance abuse prevention and treatment services. Her consulting specialty is in designing and evaluating managed care substance abuse programs.

ing experience with and access to "managed" BH care

- proliferation of private hospitals during the 1970s and early 1980s as a result of high profit margins, cheap capital investment, elimination of certificate-of-need laws in several large states, and exemption from reimbursement by diagnosis-related groups (DRGs)
- emergence in the 1980s of managed BH care in the employer market and for indemnity insurers for the purpose of cost containment
- significant benefit restrictions for treating serious mental illnesses and addictions, which have prompted a national advocacy strategy to promote parity between mental health and physical health care benefits
- tightening during the 1990s of public sector BH funding at the federal level, which resulted in increasing pressure on local government agencies to contain costs, straining the public mental health service delivery safety net for all individuals, including poor persons with serious mental illness and employed individuals
- increasingly vocal criticism of managed care initiatives for vulnerable populations, which is contributing to intensified regulatory action[1]
- more demands by employers and purchasers to focus on clinical outcomes of services and not solely on cost containment

Underlying these developments is the fact that many BH problems tend to be chronic and recurrent, requiring periodic treatment, sometimes intensive in nature, throughout the lifetime of the affected individual. Finally, BH diagnostic categories do not lend themselves to by-the-book utilization management with standardized lengths of stay and treatment protocols for specified diagnoses. The range of accepted treatment approaches for a given BH diagnosis can be broad, and severity of illness and service requirements cannot be inferred without detailed information about social context and specific symptoms. Thus, the complexity of managing BH care cannot be understated.

HISTORICAL PERSPECTIVE

Managed BH care dates back to the 1960s and the community mental health movement, where the concept of a "single point of accountability" for the organization and delivery of care emerged as a key value in the design and operations of community mental health systems. The community mental health center (CMHC) became a vehicle to deliver a comprehensive array of mental health services to the general population as well as to individuals with serious mental illness.

Over the past four decades, the focus on provision of integrated and comprehensive treatment through CMHCs has been balanced by the need to address specialty treatment issues. Adults with serious mental illness, children with serious emotional disturbance, the child welfare populations, homeless mentally ill individuals, children and adults with addictive disorders, and individuals with developmental disabilities and mental health needs became rallying points around which different constituents organized. Thus, state and federal categorical funding of services increased significantly between 1960 and the early 1980s, and age- and disability-specific organizations began to flourish. State and local governments began to organize their administrative systems categorically in response to funding availability and the desire to address unmet special needs of children and adults with mental health and addictive disorders.

Rising health care costs and the general state of the U.S. economy in the 1980s renewed the focus on managed care. In the public sector, as states began to shift care from institutional to community settings and likewise began to aggressively tap into federal Medicaid mental health resources, there was increasing emphasis on defining (or narrowing) priority populations (individuals with serious mental illness and/or serious emotional disturbance). There was an emphasis on providing care in the least restrictive setting to the most severely ill individuals in most state BH care reform initiatives.[2] Likewise, the emergence of managed BH care in the private sector employer market was an effort to provide cost savings and institute benefit limits. First-generation managed care efforts of the 1980s focused on reducing costs for employers without any real emphasis on managing clinical care.[3]

Substantial efforts at managing BH treatment and costs first emanated from HMOs. Early HMOs, for the most part, were wary of BH coverage. Some plans offered only diagnosis and consultation; others arranged for discounted fee-for-service care for members. The HMO Act of 1973 required only minimal BH benefits, such as crisis intervention and a maximum of 20 visits for outpatient services. No benefits for inpatient care, chronic or recurrent conditions, or chemical dependency were required. Later in the 1970s and 1980s, increasing numbers of HMOs expanded BH benefits as a result of consumer demand and legislation enacted in a number of states that required enriched benefits.[4]

During the late 1970s and 1980s, when insurers and self-insured employers began instituting general utilization management techniques to help control their indemnity plan health benefit costs, it became clear that these approaches were far less effective in controlling BH costs than they were in controlling other medical benefit costs. Thus, the scene was set for development of a niche industry of specialized managed BH organizations to contract directly with HMOs, indemnity insurers, and self-insured employers and to apply specialized techniques in managing these costs. Employers traditionally have been the ultimate payers for most BH treatment managed by specialty BH management entities (whether in-house HMO, insurance carrier–based, or free-standing). Increasingly in recent years, government BH agencies have also become purveyors and/or purchasers of managed BH services as budgets have constricted, federal regulations have been administered more flexibly, and accountability has migrated to local governments.

Since the first flush of the CMHC "revolution," there have been massive changes in ideology, organization, and service delivery. While most early BH reforms were idealistic, based on emerging value systems and improved technology of clinical services, the later phases have been motivated primarily by financial considerations.

Similar changes have buffeted all of medicine.[5] The difference between BH care and general health care lies in the economic systems underlying each: Medicine is technology-intensive, with enormous capital investment in facilities and instrumentation, while BH, with the exception of psychopharmacology, is labor-intensive. *Capital-intensive enterprises tend to prevail in the contest for resources for three reasons:*

1. To the extent that technology reduces labor costs, capital-intensive enterprises have the potential to be more profitable.
2. The capital intensity acts as a barrier to entry of new competitors, allowing a centralization of power and resources.
3. Together, the technology suppliers and the technology users (the medical-industrial complex) can generate enormous political power and dominate decisions about resource allocation.

Professionals must understand the way managed BH care operates within this larger context if they are to help individuals gain fullest access to needed and effective BH services.

This chapter highlights the highest clinical values and provides a map of the BH system. The map is continually changing, however. Nationally and locally, legislative and regulatory bodies are developing models to temper cost containment (and profits) through imposition of quality requirements, using the traditional governmental mechanisms of utility and insurance regulation and the legal remedies of tort and malpractice litigation. In a strong economy with employers competing vigorously for employees, there has also been a rediscovery that it is good business to conserve human resources and nurture human potential through investment in work-based preventive services.

We hope that this chapter helps the reader become knowledgeable about managed BH care as it undergoes transformation and reinvention during an era of ferment and change.

Paradigmatic Shifts in Progress

During the 1990s, the expansion of managed care into public sector BH care systems meant that earlier BH care strategies and methods were being questioned. Government mandates to meet the BH care needs of a more seriously ill population require modification of clinical methods and planning techniques. Brief cognitive interventions requiring high levels of patient motivation and compliance do not meet the needs of individuals with severe mental illness or chemical dependency who, due to the negative symptoms of their disorders, may lack motivation and/or the ability to comply. Rather, managed care systems serving the public sector must encompass a wide range of treatment options, including social support, outreach, and intensive case management. Without appropriate treatment, persons with severe illnesses can have poor clinical outcomes, including higher mortality rates, higher nonelective inpatient utilization rates, and higher medical morbidity and associated costs.

Modifications in medical management approaches to persons with severe mental illness and/or chemical dependency represent more than technical adaptations to special populations. These changes reflect a maturing trend in managed clinical care to refocus systems planning and care management onto the problems of a defined population rather than solely on the care of individual patients. Two initiatives promote the shift toward population-based case management: the growth of capitated and subcapitated reimbursement systems and the increase in population-defined service mandates of public sector systems. The pressure to cap health care expenditures while expanding managed care technologies to (historically underserved) vulnerable populations requires careful consideration of the systemic consequences of managed care technologies.

The most distinctive feature of the shift toward systems planning is the emphasis on examining the consequences, especially the unintended consequences, of changing clinical practices and strategies. For example, studies comparing the unintended consequences of different pharmacy cost-containment strategies find that lower unit costs of apparently similar medication may result in higher system costs. Because there are comparable rates of efficacy for all classes of antidepressants, the least expensive agent would seem to be the rational choice for treatment. Although the direct unit cost of tricyclic antidepressants is considerably lower than for newer agents such as selective serotonin reuptake inhibitors, the overall costs of the use of tricyclics is at least as great and perhaps greater, if additional costs (laboratory, psychiatric and medical office visits, psychiatric and medical hospitalizations) are included.[6–10] Particularly important, negative effects of tricyclic use may include higher costs related to intensive medical care for tricyclic overdoses and falls and accidents due to diminished cognitive clarity.

Another example is the lower overall costs of care for the more expensive, newer atypical neuroleptic agents recently marketed for the treatment of schizophrenia.[11] Due to fewer adverse effects, favorable effects on negative schizophrenic symptoms, and the capacity to treat patients refractory to conventional neuroleptics, these medications result in higher patient acceptance and compliance and better symptomatic improvement. The cost savings result from fewer treatment failures and hospital admissions.

The system effects of using newer psychotropic agents parallel similar findings in primary care medicine in which newer agents, although more expensive on a unit-cost basis, result in cost containment for several common disorders. Even the restricted-formulary use of generic medications in place of newer single-source agents, a commonly used cost-savings method, unexpectedly results in *higher* overall costs due to higher aggregate drug costs and an increase in the number of drugs dispensed. Cost-containment strategies other than drug formulary restriction (e.g., strict gatekeeping, visit copayments) may work better.[12]

The emerging shift to a systems paradigm promotes several other modifications of conventional managed care practice. In the older paradigm, there has been an emphasis on cost containment through minimizing unit costs of individual care, standardizing care methods, and decreasing access to services by controlling the supply of services. In the newer paradigm, there is an emerging emphasis on determining the lowest cost of effective care for a population, promoting and comparing competing clinical care methods, and proactively reducing the need for more costly services. For example, in the older managed care paradigm and prior to legislation curbing the practice, services for alcohol-related disorders such as delirium tremens were often not covered under HMO benefits. In the newer paradigm, trauma-prone persons with alcohol problems are sought out for treatment in order to reduce more costly large-case trauma related to alcohol use, such as automobile or motorcycle accidents, falls, or physical battery.

Previously, the focus was on the service needs of an individual, the selection of efficient techniques for expediting episodes of care, and the avoidance of high-risk patients. In the new paradigm, the emphasis is on determining the service needs of groups within the service population and developing systems for the tightly coordinated management of care on a longitudinal basis, targeting the highest-risk individuals within the population.

Past emphasis was on cost reduction, primarily through reduction of direct point-of-service costs and of service utilization in general. In the newer paradigm, there is an emerging emphasis on enhancing the clinical value of resources invested in services, maximizing cost offsets of services to defray direct costs, and shaping utilization to lower the overall cost of care by enriching care in specific areas.

In the emerging, population-based paradigm for cost containment, several strategic approaches for enhancing clinical value seem prominent:

- Accelerate the onset of response.
- Develop systems to ensure follow-up and continuity of care to avoid waste of high-quality intensive care.

- Eliminate counterproductive, low-quality interventions.
- Prevent illness, especially trauma-related illness, through treatment of predisposing behavioral disorders.
- Enhance medical cost offsets.
- Lower complication rates.
- Lower recidivism rates.
- Improve prognosis for medical disorders and surgical procedures.

Emerging Strategic Approaches

From Carve-out to Carve-in

To reduce costs and produce better outcomes, BH care services are being reincorporated into capitated medical-surgical systems. This newer paradigm counters the historic tendency of general medical-surgical HMOs to distance themselves from BH care and to use specialized "carve-out" utilization review organizations for BH issues. Although pioneering efforts over several decades in using brief behavioral interventions to reduce medical utilization suggested potential savings, little has been done to refine and develop this approach. The advent of automated clinical tracking in more sophisticated systems may facilitate targeting of BH care interventions in a manner previously infeasible.

In Search of Medical Cost Offsets

Recent epidemiological research finds two types of relevant linkages.

1. high prevalence of comorbid depressive and anxiety disorders among several major medical disorders, particularly neurological disorders, certain cancers, diabetes mellitus, and autoimmune disorders
2. depression in particular as an adverse, rapidly modifiable prognostic factor for outcomes of certain medical disorders (e.g., myocardial infarction)

In general, depression is more prevalent in the presence of more severe medical illness. Independently, however, depression as a comorbid factor is associated with lower survival rates, longer and more frequent hospital stays, lower compliance with treatment, diminished ability to care for self, and a lower quality of life.

The potential for modifying service burdens of medical-surgical illness through attending to behavioral disorders is diverse and extensive, so much so that managed care systems need effective mechanisms to identify site-relevant problems and systematically develop intervention programs. Broad-based efforts to detect and treat mood and anxiety disorders in primary practice, however well intentioned, face the difficult challenge of training primary care practitioners to refocus on behavioral disorders and to incorporate diagnostic screenings into already tightly time-limited clinical encounters. Other strategies to supplement broad-based efforts may include targeted surveillance and detection of high resource utilizers and behavioral interventions with high probability for return on resource investment. *Such strategies take the following general form:*

- identifying people with high-cost, high-prevalence medical-surgical care problems as a target group
- identifying behavioral symptoms causing problems or adverse prognosis in the target group
- profiling the distribution of behavioral problems within the target group
- devising therapeutic interventions likely to have low costs and high returns
- identifying specific individuals for targeted intervention
- locating and treating targeted individuals

The reintegration of BH care with medical-surgical care requires an understanding of and special attention to BH treatment methods.

KEY TREATMENT PRINCIPLES

Special Issues and Common Problems

Any managed care organization (MCO) venturing into management of BH care faces the dilemma of how to address potentially large unmet treatment needs that may compete with other medical care specialties for scarce resources. On an operational level, it has been difficult to establish the boundaries of BH service obligations.

The concept of "medical necessity" begins to blur when the causes of the disorder encompass social, personality, and biological factors, and when necessary services often must address stabilization of social supports; these factors are not universally recognized as medical needs.

When an organization is designing a delivery system, this need for social stability as a critical prerequisite for clinical stability requires a broader, more diverse continuum of programs and services than is seen in the general medical-surgical realm.

Due to recent advances in diagnostics, psychopharmacology, and psychotherapeutic techniques, there is a growing demand for powerful new treatment options during a time of shrinking resources. All of these factors enhance the need for incisive management of BH care.

Goals of Treatment

Ideally, the goal of treatment for the health plan should be to improve the BH status of a defined population. A well-managed system should improve the clinical status of a population in terms of symptomatic distress levels and improve life functioning in several areas. A well-managed system should aim to reduce suicide and homicide rates, substance abuse–related impairments, and mortality and morbidity from accidents related to substance abuse or mental disorders.

Another central goal of managed BH care should be conservation and rational allocation of resources to optimize return on expenditures. Finding the correct balance between conservation of resources and provision of the appropriate mixture of effective services is the fundamental task for managed care.

Objectives of Treatment

There are a number of important clinical objectives for a managed care system to pursue:

- rapid symptomatic relief
- protection of the physical safety of the patient and others
- satisfaction of the patient and his or her family
- improved life functioning

To conserve resources, managed care systems need to invest in cost-effective treatments and high-return therapeutic activities and maximize medical-cost offsets (decreased costs for general medical and surgical care).

Strategic Approaches to Treatment

Historically, MCOs have regarded BH care services very cautiously. Coming down strongly on the side of conservation of resources, at least in terms of short-term, direct costs of care, they have pursued two general strategies: controlling demand and controlling supply.

Typical strategies for controlling demand make use of the established fact that demand for mental health services is very price sensitive. Techniques employed that are based on this price sensitivity include setting higher copayments and deductibles, delaying access to treatment, and limiting benefits, including imposing lifetime ceilings on BH benefits. Typical strategies for controlling supply have included benefit restrictions, program limitations, gatekeepers, triage systems, and waiting lists.

Benefit and program restrictions have at times been profound, severely limiting or excluding BH services entirely from the benefit package, excluding certain diagnostic-specific disorders or chronic illnesses, and providing few or no psychiatric inpatient services and little or no long-term outpatient treatment. Some contracts have excluded certain member groups (e.g., people with mental retardation, organic psychoses, alcoholism, or intractable personality disorders) from coverage. Others have limited or refused to provide court-ordered services, thereby reducing liability for uncooperative clients. Some contracts have excluded geriatric patients, violent or assaultive patients, primary substance abusers, heroin-dependent persons, and people with sexual dysfunction, severe learning disabilities, or attention deficit hyperactivity disorder. Virtually all managed care plans use some form of utilization review. Although many use primary care practitioner gatekeeping, large HMOs (over 200,000 enrollees) usually allow self-referral. Large-case or catastrophic management is also used.

Beyond a certain point, however, limitations on services can result in underservice of legitimate needs. To better meet the BH care needs of a population, MCOs are exploring strategies for improving the clinical value received for each BH dollar.

From a clinical perspective, managed care should favor the following strategies:

- using multiple clinical pathways, providing simpler treatment plans for uncomplicated cases and more intensive treatment plans for more intensive cases
- developing a network of effective, efficient providers selected and retained on the basis of demonstrated superior clinical performance
- assessing comprehensively the types and intensity of services needed
- matching the treatment problem with the optimal provider(s)
- selecting treatment innovations and clinical best practices to optimize effective and efficient patient response
- minimizing disruption of patients' everyday social role obligations
- treating at the least restrictive but effective level of care, favoring community-based over facility-based services
- coordinating all the patient's BH services
- measuring and tracking clinical performance, focusing on clinical outcomes, management of resources, and efficiency of response
- using systematic methods for assisting treatment of refractory patients to gain access to highly skilled, specialized services, including the use of centers of excellence for specific problems
- reducing relapse through identifying and planning for ongoing support for therapeutic and social needs

Finally, there is a need for the collective management of aggregate clinical expenditures in comparison to budgeted resources, concurrently identifying reasons for unexpected excessive expenditures and incisively constructing corrective action plans. It is a powerful strategic concept in managed care to tie useful clinical information to financial information so that changes in clinical practices can target high-risk areas.

Methods of Treatment

Specialized managed BH care is rooted in four key principles of clinical treatment: alternatives to psychiatric hospitalization, alternatives to restrictive treatment for substance abuse, goal-directed psychotherapy, and crisis intervention.

Alternatives to Psychiatric Hospitalization

Partial hospitalization (day, evening, and/or weekend nonresidential) programs have proven to be effective alternatives to hospital inpatient treatment in many outcome studies.[13,14] In a plan with adequate coverage for alternatives to inpatient services, and with informed decision making as to which patients can benefit from these alternatives, economical and effective treatment can be provided to acutely ill patients in a partial hospital setting.

Alternatives to Restrictive Treatment for Substance Abuse

Research does not provide evidence that inpatient or residential substance abuse treatment is superior to outpatient or partial hospitalization approaches.[15,16] The central question of which patients truly need inpatient treatment and which can benefit equally well from outpatient or partial hospitalization has yet to be answered definitively. In the absence of support for the superiority of inpatient programs for the general treatment population, specialized managed BH systems tend to emphasize the more economical alternatives.

Goal-Directed Psychotherapy

The research literature supports the effectiveness of brief, goal-directed psychotherapeutic approaches for a number of problems.[17,18] Specialized managed BH care systems generally emphasize an interpersonal rather than an intrapsychic focus of therapy. These systems also place emphasis on therapy that is designed to be brief and time limited and not just a truncated version of long-term therapy.

Crisis Intervention

Successful managed BH systems are designed to make use of crisis intervention as a key service in the overall constellation of services. Research has demonstrated that short-term, intensive support of individuals during life crises or periodic acute episodes of psychiatric illness is an effective way to diminish the incidence of future crises and can substantially reduce the inappropriate use of psychiatric care.[19]

Additional clinical methods, utilized especially when applying managed care principles to the care of severely ill persons, include the following:

- accurate behavioral diagnosis and attention to potential medical and neurological diagnostic issues
- detection and management of substance abuse
- prompt access to services for high-risk clients
- effective management of safety issues
- coordination of services from other agencies and multiple providers
- prevention of relapse through specialized clinical and case management services and adoption of a longitudinal treatment perspective for chronic disorders
- integrated use of multidisciplinary providers for exceptional cases, driven by a coherent, comprehensive treatment plan
- intensive community treatment of high-risk patients
- use of social stabilization measures to reduce relapse

The Ideal Continuum of Care

Despite the separation of substance abuse and mental health treatment programs in the past, effective systems integrate treatment programs that tailor the appropriate mix of services to each individual's treatment needs.

Entry into the system requires an intake function, not necessarily geographically centralized, to triage cases, gather initial data, establish the presence of a BH disorder requiring treatment, determine the clinically appropriate level of care and mix of service types, and refer the patient to appropriate services. Immediate access to emergency evaluation services is also essential.

Mobile emergency services should also be available on a 24-hour basis for on-site evaluations of the need for acute inpatient services and to provide stabilization services as an alternative to hospitalization. Other important emergency services include the capacity to schedule next-day outpatient appointments and to provide psychiatric nursing backup for problems that might arise after hours.

Patients not stabilized despite on-site interventions may require 24-hour observation and assessment by a multidisciplinary team in a short-term behavioral crisis unit providing one to five days of 24-hour voluntary or involuntary observation, containment of assaultive or self-destructive behavior, and treatment of acute psychiatric emergencies.

Because of the high prevalence of dual diagnoses, chemical dependency detection and treatment protocols as well as staff with specialized training in both chemical dependency and mental disorders should be standard components for all basic services, as well as for inpatient and residential programs.

Treatment Services

Substance Abuse Services

Few patients with substance abuse problems require inpatient treatment. Patients with mild to moderate withdrawal symptoms who need more than social support to maintain abstinence can be referred for ambulatory detoxification with daily medical management and monitoring by a physician–nurse practitioner team, including administration of medications as needed. Patients with more severe problems need at least three types of alternative treatment levels:

1. social detoxification centers for those who require removal from their usual living en-

vironment due to an inadequate support system
2. residential rehabilitation for medically supervised detoxification when moderate withdrawal symptoms are present or there is a problem with compliance with instructions
3. inpatient medical detoxification, usually in a general hospital setting, for patients with severe withdrawal symptoms of an imminently life-threatening nature, such as delirium tremens or withdrawal seizures

A full spectrum of nonintensive outpatient chemical dependency treatment services should be available, including brief alcohol and substance abuse treatment, maintenance counseling for individuals who need long-term support, and medication services for those requiring longer-term chemical stabilization.

Most patients unable to control substance use despite outpatient efforts can benefit from a partial hospital or intensive outpatient program, including standardized, systematic group education and therapy, core information about chemical dependency, and development of peer supports. Standard treatment packages may include an initial intensive phase with at least 20 evenings of treatment, followed by progressively less intensive treatment for the remainder of at least a year. Drug counselors in the intensive outpatient program discourage dropout by contacting patients who fail to attend meetings to determine whether relapse is occurring and to encourage return to treatment.

For those patients who relapse despite the best therapeutic efforts and completion of treatment in the intensive phase of an intensive outpatient program, the continuum of care needs to provide several levels of care and therapeutic programs:

- There should be residential chemical dependency rehabilitation with 24-hour supervision during initial rehabilitation treatment in order to identify and correct factors interfering with the ability to receive successful treatment at an outpatient level. Once these factors have been removed, discharge to an intensive outpatient program can proceed.

- There should be relapse prevention programs providing specialized, more individualized techniques to address unmet treatment needs and specialized after-care for those for whom standard methods are ineffective.
- There should be therapeutic halfway houses, linked to participation in a relapse prevention program, for those who repeatedly fail outpatient efforts.

Basic Mental Health Services

The vast majority of patients with mental health problems need only outpatient therapy services, including brief (less than 12 sessions) individual, group, and family psychotherapy; medication management services; and, for those at risk of relapse and deterioration, long-term supportive therapy. Complicated cases need a designated primary therapist who is responsible for formulating and implementing a master treatment plan and for coordinating referrals to other outpatient services. Very complicated cases may require individualized services, such as on-site clinical case management assistance, social service interventions, and wraparound services.

Patients unable to succeed by using only outpatient therapy services need access to intensive outpatient services. These may consist of crisis services such as daily intensive individual, group, or family therapy sessions or outpatient medication visits; home-based or school-based therapeutic services, including in-home family therapy; or modular outpatient programs with an array of psychoeducational modules combined with specialized individual outpatient services and interdisciplinary treatment team involvement.

For more severely ill patients who cannot be adequately served by outpatient or intensive outpatient services, multidisciplinary partial hospital programs (PHPs) provide several hours per day of structured, integrated, modular treatment and psychoeducational services throughout the week and weekend. PHPs have the range and intensity of services previously found in inpatient psychiatric programs, except for 24-hour supervision and security.

Some patients require brief removal from troubled environments for stabilization of potentially life-threatening situations or situations that may cause family disintegration. Crisis/respite house services may avert the need for a more restrictive and intensive facility placement. Such settings provide brief removal from a destructive or dangerous social situation or from an excessively strained family system for periods up to two weeks to allow stabilization of the living environment, placement in a more suitable living arrangement, or investigation by protective service agencies. This level of care would be appropriate for runaway adolescents with oppositional behavior and limited substance abuse problems, battered spouses with highly disruptive adjustment disorders, self-mutilating nonpsychotic patients, and chronically mentally ill patients with families needing respite from excessive care needs or unremitting levels of conflict.

Despite intensive efforts, return home is infeasible in some situations due to excessive long-term danger related to family violence or conflict, risk of violence by the patient, or predatory sexual behavior on the part of the patient. For such patients, community-based residential treatment services, such as a range of residential alternatives for out-of-home placement, need to be available, including therapeutic homes under the care of a family with parenting training and therapeutic group homes for small groups of adolescents and chronically ill adults with frequent disruptive behavior or without the skills to live independently or semi-independently.

Some children or adults may require placement in conventional large residential treatment centers for modification of subacute dangerous behaviors that exceed the skills, capacity, and security of community-based therapeutic services. Such centers provide 24-hour, tightly coordinated behavioral modification and medication treatment services, preferably with programs designed to prepare patients as rapidly as possible for placement in less restrictive therapeutic settings.

Psychiatric acute care facilities remain essential for patients requiring high-security and very highly intensive treatment for imminently life-threatening conditions.

Dual Diagnosis Services

The combination of substance use disorders with major mental disorders, usually referred to as "dual diagnosis," has emerged as a central clinical focus for managed care approaches to public sector BH care. Systems for treating each type of disorder have evolved along separate lines in the past, resulting in limited competencies for treating individuals who have both disorders. Dual diagnosis, often a marker for poor treatment compliance, resistance to medication interventions, and multiple social problems, represents a disproportionate burden on resource utilization. The introduction of managed care into public sector psychiatry has prompted attention to the long-standing system failures for treating these difficult cases, resulting in the creation of specialized integrated dual diagnosis treatment programs and even the reorganization of separate agencies responsible for different types of disorders. In addition to having specialty units for the integrated treatment of individuals with primary mental and substance use disorders, there is growing interest in integrating well-targeted BH services into mainstream managed health care.

To address the treatment needs of the large population of patients with both mental disorders and substance abuse disorders, the continuum of care should include two general types of program elements: (1) routine surveillance and cross-training in both disciplines at all levels of care, and (2) specialized dual diagnosis programs to facilitate simultaneous treatment of both types of disorders. Treatment of individuals with dual diagnosis should be integrated and not sequential; that is, treatment should address the underlying mental disorder and the substance use conjointly.

For more severely ill patients with dual diagnoses, outpatient programs need to address abuse of a wide range of substances since polysubstance abuse is highly prevalent among dual diagnosis patients. Intensive day and evening programs are needed for motivated patients with dual diagnoses, including psychotic mental disorders without severe residual symptoms, personality disorders without severe behavioral disturbance, and moderately severe coexisting anxiety, mood, and post-traumatic stress disorders. In these specialized dual diagnosis treatment programs, abstinence may be a goal rather than a prerequisite for entry. An ideal system will make provision for programs integrating interventions from both psychiatric and substance abuse treatment camps: continuous treatment teams, monitored medication compliance, behavioral skills training to prevent both psychiatric relapse and lapses into substance abuse, close monitoring of drug abuse, modified 12-step groups, behavioral reinforcement programs (such as a token economy) to reward abstinence and healthier behaviors, and assertive case management to reengage noncompliant participants.

Specialized dual diagnosis treatment programs may exist at the level of crisis houses, social detoxification houses, behavioral crisis units, partial hospitals, community therapeutic residential programs, large-scale residential treatment centers, and acute inpatient services.

BENEFIT PLAN DESIGN

Benefits design for services, including BH services, is beyond the scope of this chapter and this book, but it will be discussed briefly here. Until passage of the 1996 Mental Health Parity Act,[20] the design of BH services almost always involved a substantial difference between benefits for basic medical-surgical services and those for BH. The parity legislation, effective January 1998, requires group health plans that have annual or lifetime dollar limits for medical or surgical benefits to also have the same dollar limits on mental health benefits, thereby promoting parity between physical and mental health care. In addition to extending mental health coverage (substance abuse treatment is not covered by the Mental Health Parity Act), the law provides a venue to accurately document the financial impact of mental health treatment and to identify cost savings attributable to medical cost offset by managed mental health programs. Within this context, BH benefit design, like all health benefit design, needs to address two key issues: coverage limits and incentives.

Coverage Limits

Coverage limits are essentially a fail-safe to limit benefit cost by establishing levels beyond which the plan will not pay, even for medically necessary, cost-effective treatment. Coverage limits can include maximum days, visits, or dollar amounts and can be based on levels of care (e.g., inpatient, partial hospitalization, structured outpatient), types of disorders (e.g., acute psychiatric, chronic, custodial, specific diagnoses), types of treatment (e.g., psychosurgery, psychoanalysis, nutritionally based therapies), and/or types of providers (e.g., physician; psychologist; social worker; marriage, family, and child counselor [MFCC]). The optimal benefit design for a managed BH program will provide adequate coverage for inpatient treatment and its alternatives as well as for treatment providers from various professional disciplines. Federal and state parity laws provide for equity between physical and BH care benefits and dollar limits; however, many employers and insurers are reinstituting session or day limits, to minimize liability for coverage. This, in effect, neutralizes the impact of parity legislation, and the national advocacy community is lobbying for legislative modifications.[21]

Levels of Care

Traditional indemnity plans and many HMO plans limit coverage to inpatient hospital care and minimal outpatient care for mental health problems and inpatient detoxification. To support a comprehensive managed BH program, the benefit should cover a number of levels of care (Exhibit 25–1).

Types of Disorders

Another way that some managed BH plans limit plan liability is through limiting covered disorders. Respondents to a survey indicated considerable variation in the types of disorders

Exhibit 25–1 Managed Mental Health Benefits: Covered Levels of Care

Mental Health
- Hospital inpatient services
- Nonhospital residential treatment
- PHP/day treatment
- Individual/group outpatient treatment
- Crisis intervention
- Outreach services

Substance Abuse
- Detoxification (inpatient, noninpatient residential, and outpatient)
- Hospital rehabilitation
- Nonhospital residential rehabilitation
- Intensive outpatient rehabilitation
- Individual/group outpatient rehabilitation

Source: Reprinted from DF Anderson et al., Managed Behavioral Health Care Services, in *Best Practices in Medical Management,* Peter R. Kongstvedt and David W. Plocher, eds. pp. 407–432, © 1998, Aspen Publishers, Inc.

covered by plans featuring BH management (Table 25–1).

Some plans also exclude coverage for specific *Diagnostic and Statistical Manual IV (DSM IV)* diagnostic categories (e.g., learning disorders, autism) as well as medical diagnoses with potential psychiatric treatment regimens (e.g., obesity).

Table 25–1 Typical Coverage of Disorders in Plans with Specialized Mental Health/Substance Abuse Management

Category of Disorder	Percentage of Plans Offering Coverage
DSM diagnoses	100
Chronic mental disorders	71
Sexual addiction	21
DSM V codes	7
Codependency	7
Nicotine addiction	7
Custodial care	0

Courtesy of William M. Mercer, Inc., San Francisco, California.

Types of Treatment

Many plans built around specialized BH management limit specific treatments covered. Table 25–2 indicates variation among respondents as to coverage of selected types of treatment. Many plans also exclude from coverage such treatments as biofeedback and electroconvulsive therapy.

Types of Providers

Many traditional indemnity plans have covered only the services of physicians and PhDs for outpatient BH psychotherapy. HMOs and managed indemnity BH plans have expanded coverage to a broader range of mental health professionals. Table 25–3 indicates patterns of provider coverage for plans with specialized BH management. Some plans also cover pastoral counselors and family practitioners for BH services. For public sector managed care initiatives, an even broader range of providers is necessary. These networks usually include CMHCs, substance abuse treatment agencies, and other specialty organizations that typically receive funding through state and local initiatives.

Incentives

The greater the incentives to access and comply with the managed BH system, the greater the

Table 25–2 Typical Coverage of Treatment Types in Plans with Specialized Mental Health/Substance Abuse Management

Category of Treatment	Percentage of Plans Offering Coverage
Brief problem-focused therapy	93
Long term psychodynamically oriented therapy	64
Psychosurgery	15
Nutritionally based therapies	7

Courtesy of William M. Mercer, Inc., San Francisco, California.

Table 25–3 Typical Coverage of Provider Types in Plans with Specialized Mental Health/Substance Abuse Management

Category of Provider	Percentage of Plans Offering Coverage
MD	100
PhD psychologist	93
MA social worker	87
MA psychiatric nurse	87
MFCC	83
MA psychologist	73
Certified alcoholism counselor	57

Courtesy of William M. Mercer, Inc., San Francisco, California.

impact. Most employers are not comfortable with a plan that offers no BH coverage outside the managed system. For this reason, most managed BH plans tend to offer point-of-service choice where patients can select a network provider or an out-of-network provider. Point-of-service coverage usually has a higher deductible and coinsurance. The typical managed indemnity plan offers a $0 deductible in-network benefit with a coinsurance of 20 percent. Out-of-network coverage typically will feature a deductible of $250 with 50 percent coinsurance.

An optimal coinsurance differential may be 40 percent (e.g., 10 percent in network and 50 percent out of network). Managed BH plans typically do not publish a preferred provider list. For practical purposes, then, coverage differentials actually apply to the plan member accessing a gatekeeper and accepting channeling to a network provider rather than accessing a provider directly without going through the gatekeeper.

UTILIZATION MANAGEMENT

Utilization management in specialized BH programs falls into two general categories: utilization review (UR) and case management. In practice, distinctions between the two functions often become blurred, but it will be instructive to discuss them separately.

UR

In the mid-1980s, when an increasing number of employers had installed UR systems to help contain costs of indemnity plans, it became clear that UR conducted by nonspecialized staff with general medical backgrounds was ineffective when applied to BH cases. As a response, specialized BH UR developed that employed specialized staff applying BH-specific utilization criteria. Specialized UR typically includes preadmission certification of inpatient BH cases and concurrent review of inpatient and residential cases (and sometimes of outpatient cases) to determine the medical necessity of treatment.

Operational characteristics of effective specialized UR programs are as follows:

- Telephone-based treatment review is conducted by credentialed BH professional reviewers, usually MA-level psychiatric nurses, MA-level social workers, and PhD- or MA-level psychologists.
- Reviewers as a group are trained and experienced in inpatient and outpatient treatment for BH adults, adolescents, and children.
- Initial and concurrent review episodes involve direct contact with the primary clinician instead of, or in addition to, the facility UR nurse.
- There is readily available high-level clinical supervisory staff as backup for frontline reviewers. Such backup staff members include, at a minimum, board-certified adult and child/adolescent psychiatrists and a certified addictionologist.
- Medical necessity/level of care criteria employed by reviewers are age and diagnosis specific and behaviorally descriptive and encompass all levels of care, including, for example, nonhospital residential programs and partial hospitalization. Criteria are tested and retested continually and modified as needed.

UR construed narrowly as determination of medical necessity is typically installed as a means of protecting against abuses in a traditional fee-for-service plan. Although specialized

BH UR has proved to be somewhat more effective in containing costs than nonspecialized UR, utilization management has been far more effective in conjunction with a specialized BH network with point-of-service choice.[22] This comprehensive approach to managing BH care generally invokes case management as the utilization management tool of choice.

Case Management

As comprehensive managed BH programs have evolved during the late 1980s and early 1990s, the case management function has crystallized as a focal point for promoting cost-effective, high-quality BH care. BH case management encompasses traditional UR but extends beyond into a broader form of patient advocacy, addressing the longitudinal course of care as well as discrete episodes of intensive treatment.

Comprehensive case management includes four overlapping components:

1. *promoting correct diagnosis and effective treatment:* assisting plan members to access the best level, type, and mix of treatment; keeping alert to opportunities for enhancing the quality and efficacy of care; acting to make provider and patient aware of these opportunities (UR strives to exclude payment for unnecessarily intensive treatment, whereas case management strives to direct patients into effective forms of treatment at appropriate levels of intensity.)
2. *promoting efficient use of resources:* helping the patient and family access the most effective resources with the minimum depletion of family finances and finite available insurance dollars (Directing patients into effective care may be the most potent cost-saving method.)
3. *preventing recidivism:* monitoring progress subsequent to intensive treatment episodes; encouraging and, if necessary, helping arrange for interepisode care to prevent recidivism
4. *monitoring for and containing substandard care:* identifying potential quality of

care defects during treatment; investigating and, when needed, intervening to ensure remediation

Comprehensive case management goes beyond determination of medical necessity and seeks to promote enhancement of the quality, efficacy, and continuity of care. As such, it is a more demanding discipline than simple UR. Optimally, case management services should employ qualified front-line clinicians with a minimum of 5 to 10 years of relevant clinical experience who are thoroughly trained in case management techniques. These clinicians generally have access to readily available doctoral-level advisors with relevant clinical experience (including managed care experience) and have the support of well-articulated systems to assist with the case management task. Examples of such systems include the following:

- *Triage systems.* Every managed BH system must devise a mechanism for directing cases to the proper case manager. This includes, for example, ensuring that cases with medical issues are directed to a psychiatric nurse rather than to a social worker and that substance abuse cases are directed to case managers specifically qualified and experienced in this area.
- *Quality screens.* Diagnosis-based criteria delineating typical best practice patterns of high-quality care for specific problems as well as screens for common quality of care defects should be employed routinely as cases are reviewed. Such screens assist in early identification of mismatches between treatment plans and diagnoses as well as pinpoint more subtle opportunities to enhance quality and efficacy of care (e.g., when providers may be unaware of or unwilling to use superior treatment methods).

CHANNELING MECHANISMS

A key aspect of any managed BH system is a channeling mechanism to assess initially and direct an individual to the appropriate type and intensity of treatment. This gatekeeper function is crucial to the effectiveness of the managed BH program and is fraught with potential implementation problems. Who should conduct the initial assessment to determine whether there is a BH problem for which an evaluation and treatment plan are in order? Who should conduct a thorough clinical evaluation and formulate a treatment plan? Who should carry out the treatment plan? Playing some role in the gatekeeper function may be an employee assistance program (EAP), a primary care physician (PCP) in a general managed medical system, and/or a specialized BH case manager and designated assessor clinician belonging to a contracted BH provider network.

In practice, the gatekeeper role in a managed BH system is often divided among a number of system participants. EAP counselors may be credentialed to make direct treatment referrals for certain types of cases but may be required to review decisions with a case manager before making other types of referrals. PCPs may have full authority to treat mental health problems, may have authority to refer cases directly for BH treatment with notification to the BH managed care system, or may yield all authority over BH treatment to the BH manager. Protocols detailing roles and responsibilities of all concerned must be carefully worked out, understood, and agreed to.

The EAP As Gatekeeper

EAPs play a unique role in corporate America, serving as a wide-open point of access for employees and dependents with various problems and concerns. Before the advent of specialized BH systems, EAPs were often the only reliable source of information and guidance for individuals needing BH services. In this role, the EAP assesses an individual's BH status and if necessary makes a referral for treatment.

The positive aspect of involving EAP counselors as gatekeepers for the managed BH benefit is that they are numerous, are generally knowledgeable, and cast a wide net. They are likely to come in contact with people early, when problems of living have not necessarily grown to become major BH problems. Drawbacks of assigning gatekeeper responsibilities to EAP counselors include the fact that not all are clinically credentialed and qualified, virtually none have the medical background to enable identification of medical and medication problems that may mimic or underlie BH problems, and some may not be philosophically in tune with the goals of the managed BH program.

The PCP As Gatekeeper

Many managed medical care programs (including many HMOs) restrict direct access to mental health practitioners and require the approval of the PCP before mental health specialists may be consulted. In some managed care programs, the PCP is expected to diagnose and treat common, uncomplicated mental disorders.

The advantage of investing gatekeeping responsibility in the PCP is that it encourages continuity of care and concentrates authority over preventing unnecessary use of all specialty services in the hands of one person. A major disadvantage of using PCPs as gatekeepers for BH services is that medical clinicians have been shown to be dramatically less likely to detect or treat mental disorders than mental health specialists.[23] Historically, HMOs have gradually acknowledged the value of allowing direct access to mental health services.

The Mental Health/Substance Abuse Case Manager and Assessor As Gatekeepers

Most specialized managed BH systems are organized to utilize some combination of case managers and designated assessor-clinicians within the contracted provider network as gatekeepers/channelers to appropriate treatment. Some systems rely on case managers to conduct a fairly detailed initial assessment over the telephone and to make referrals for treatment on that basis for all but the most complex cases, which are referred to a field clinician for further evaluation. Other systems routinely channel virtually every case to one of a group of specially designated assessors for detailed face-to-face evaluation and treatment planning.

In either instance, important triaging occurs at the outset. Many systems are able to case match referrals to assessors or treatment clinicians on the basis of the therapist's specialty interests, gender, language, ethnicity, and so forth. Among systems that encompass a broad spectrum of mental health providers (e.g., MD, PhD, MSW, RN), few have developed a practical theory or usable criteria for matching cases to specific provider disciplines.

Provider Networks

Assembling and administering a specialized BH provider network involves a more labor-intensive selection and monitoring process than is usually required for a general medical provider network. Some of the criteria could apply to any network: geographic accessibility, inclusion of a full continuum of care, willingness to negotiate favorable rates in exchange for channeling of patients, willingness to cooperate with utilization management procedures and standards, and structural evidence of quality, such as appropriate credentials, current licensure, and certification. Some other issues related to continuum of services, practice patterns, and practice philosophy are uniquely relevant to specialized BH networks. Therefore, although network formation is not the subject of this book, a brief discussion of pertinent aspects of a BH provider network is warranted. Generally, managed BH organizations adhere to a network development process that is similar to other network development processes but has a few unique aspects.

Size and Scope of the Network

To pinpoint the size and scope of the network, the organization must take into account the benefit design to be administered (i.e., the array of services and the range of provider types covered), the demographic characteristics of the population to be served, area geographic characteristics (e.g., physical or psychological barriers to provider access), and any specific payer requirements related to the size and composition of the network. ***Certain general rules of thumb apply across most specialized BH networks:***

- No plan member has driving time of more than
  1. 1 hour to a full-service hospital
  2. 30 minutes to an emergency room
  3. 30 minutes to an outpatient substance abuse program
  4. 30 minutes to an individual provider or program
  5. 30 minutes to an assessor
- Network coverage ratios should be at least
  1. one individual provider per 1,000 covered members
  2. one assessor per 3,000 covered members
- The distribution of network providers by discipline generally falls within the following ranges:
  1. up to 30 percent psychiatrists
  2. 0 percent to 30 percent PhD psychologists
  3. 40 percent to 60 percent MA-level providers (psychologists, social workers, nurses, MFCCs).

Selection Criteria

Many providers completing the application typically are eliminated as a result of failure to pass the screening process (most BH organizations have a formalized set of screens that are applied to applications to narrow the field of eligible network participants). Virtually all organizations conduct an in-person site visit to facility-based programs before approving them for network membership. With individual providers, there is considerably more variation. Many organizations rely completely on written applications, some include a telephone interview, some conduct face-to-face site visits/interviews for selected providers, and a few require site visits/interviews for all providers admitted to the network. Some common selection criteria for facilities and individual providers are listed in Exhibit 25–2.

For public sector–oriented agencies such as CMHCs, chemical dependency organizations, and other specialty services organizations, network admission criteria are variable. Virtually all MCOs require state licensure of specialty service programs and professional staff, as well as documented qualifications of nonlicensed staff who may provide valuable support services for which a professional license is not required. Beyond that, state and local governments usually promulgate regulations and standards for public sector managed care networks.

PROVIDER STRUCTURES FOR INTEGRATED DELIVERY SYSTEMS TO MEET MANAGED CARE OBJECTIVES

The preceding section focused on aspects of network formation from the perspective of MCOs. Market changes are rapidly moving the BH delivery system toward mergers of providers themselves into vertically or horizontally integrated systems and toward the integration of providers and MCOs. Therefore, this section will focus on aspects of network formation from the point of view of such emerging systems.

Importance of Planned Integrated Delivery Systems

The nature of psychiatric and addiction disorders and the secondary disabilities that manifest as a result of the severity and persistence of these disorders underscore the importance of integrated delivery systems. A range of treatment interventions must be simultaneously available to address numerous and discrete demands for crisis intervention, stabilization and relief of acute symptoms, and continuing treatment and psychoeducational support for recovery and relapse prevention.

Historic Structures: Public and Private

Integrated service delivery systems can offer better access and accountability while safeguarding against clinical risk and cost shifting.

Exhibit 25–2 Common Selection Criteria for Providers

Facilities
- Must provide a continuum of levels of care (not only acute inpatient)
- Average length of stay for acute inpatient cases <10 days

Psychiatrists
- Accustomed to filling medication management role in conjunction with other therapists handling individual therapy
- Usual practice pattern involves referring patients to psychologists and social workers for individual therapy
- Work primarily with serious, complicated conditions

Psychologists
- Usual practice pattern involves referring to physician for medication evaluation when appropriate
- Do not routinely test all patients unless specifically indicated

Social workers
- Demonstrated experience in treating sociofamilial issues
- Experienced with assessment, especially in community mental health center settings

Nurses
- Some general medical nursing experience
- Demonstrated current knowledge of psychopharmacology

All practitioners
- Knowledge, experience, and training in goal-focused, brief therapy techniques
- Experienced in multidisciplinary treatment approaches
- Routinely use peer support system to discuss difficult cases
- Demonstrated familiarity with community resources

Courtesy of William M. Mercer, Inc., San Francisco, California.

In the past, BH delivery structures in the private sector were one dimensional (a hospital) or two dimensional (a hospital and an outpatient clinic). These limited structures were inadequate to address the heterogeneity of the client population and its needs. Interventions more intensive than an outpatient visit were either carried out in expensive hospital settings or not available. Public care systems began to develop a broader range of services in the 1960s under the umbrella of comprehensive CMHCs.

Until the advent of managed care, CMHCs represented the majority of comprehensive and integrated care systems. Managed BH care organizations adopted community mental health approaches and became leaders in creating integrated service delivery networks, initially for the private sector and more recently for Medicaid and Medicare recipients.

Move to Provider Networks

Integrated service delivery systems have a comprehensive array of services organized to meet the needs of a defined population and geographic base. Fully integrated systems in BH care comprise acute and intensive care services, continuing care and relapse prevention, and community support and long-term care. Integrated care systems provide a single point of clinical and fiscal accountability to patients and payers, promoting access, managing utilization, and ensuring quality.

Integration has been achieved through consolidation and/or affiliation of providers into defined delivery networks. The model of a physician-hospital organization, familiar to health practitioners, is less common in BH care. More common are preferred provider organizations designed to link individual and small group practitioners and established by hospitals, insurers, and MCOs. Horizontal networks composed of provider organizations in similar lines of business (e.g., hospitals, CMHCs, *or* residential providers) are most often formed to consolidate a broader geographic and client base, to achieve management efficiencies, and to position the combined organizations to compete for managed care business. Vertical networks incorporate hospitals with ambulatory service providers. In the BH arena, this may include acute care services or a combination of acute, continuing, and long-term care services (e.g., hospitals, CMHCs, *and* residential providers).

"Carve-in" and "Carve-out" Strategies

In order to succeed in the current reimbursement environment, BH networks require the capacity to integrate internally across programs and facilities and externally with primary health care providers. Carve-out approaches, where both reimbursement and management of BH benefits are separate from those of broader health benefits, persist where payers believe that separate administration strengthens accountability, lowers cost, and/or improves access to care. Carve-outs are most common in the private sector in areas where benefits were historically generous, utilization was high, and the provider community was well developed. In the public sector, the strategy has been focused most often on people with disabilities, who represent the greatest clinical and financial risk.

Carve-in approaches are most frequently found in HMOs that provide all health and BH services for a single capitated rate and limit even specialty service utilization to providers within the organization or network. Carve-in strategies are viewed as useful in controlling inappropriate health utilization driven by behavioral disorders and in promoting more integrated care. BH delivery systems must organize to accept payment on a carve-out basis as well as on a carve-in basis if volume is to be maintained and growth achieved. This capacity is particularly important in the short term to preserve continuity with clients whose insurance coverage may shift and to mitigate the financial impact of low HMO expenditures and subcapitated payments for BH. The capacity to play on both terms is considered essential to positioning for the long term, for which the forecast is greater integration between physical health and BH.

QUALITY ASSURANCE

Quality management (QM) refers to activities designed to prevent and/or correct quality problems. (QM in basic medical-surgical care is discussed in Chapter 30.) In managed BH systems, core QM activities are focused on the qualifications and behavior of case managers and providers and (to some extent) on the treatment results achieved by providers. This section discusses common elements of internal QM programs for managed BH organizations.

UR/Case Management

Internal QM programs should include the following elements designed to ensure quality in the UR/case management process:

- *Credentialing/recredentialing.* Typical requirements are that case managers have at least MA-level BH clinical credentials, have a minimum of 3 to 5 years of clinical experience, and maintain current licensure and certification to practice. Many organizations consistently exceed these standards in practice; for example, it is not uncommon for incumbent case managers in a given setting to average 10 to 15 years of clinical experience at various levels of care.
- *Clinical rounds.* Staff must participate in educationally oriented interdisciplinary conferences that include senior clinical staff.
- *Formal supervision.* Provision must be made for regular direct supervision and coaching of case managers by clinically qualified supervisors.
- *Clinical audits.* Routine internal audits of case management notes must be performed with attention to administrative and clinical

performance, routine feedback to case managers, and individualized remedial activities when standards are not met.

- *Analysis of patient complaints/grievances.* An ongoing process to review complaints and grievances must be available and focus on clustering complaint categories, analyzing implications for policy/procedural modifications, and giving feedback to clinical and administrative personnel.
- *Patient/consumer satisfaction surveys.* Written tools for obtaining recommendations and measuring patient satisfaction with both the process and outcomes of care must be distributed to a sample of patients and analyzed at least annually.
- *Data tracking.* Staff- and diagnosis-specific outcome data (e.g., average length of stay) must be tracked with comparison to norms, analysis of implications for case management technique, and feedback to case managers.
- *Inservice training.* Inservice training programs for case managers must be shaped and driven by the findings of the internal QM monitoring system.

Network Providers

Internal QM systems in BH programs should include the following elements to ensure quality in the provider network:

- *Credentialing/recredentialing.* Minimum requirements usually include academic credentialing, licensure, certification, confirmation of criterion-level malpractice insurance, and clearing of malpractice history. Some organizations independently check licensure directly with state licensing boards and perform direct checks on legal actions concerning malpractice. Recredentialing should be done on a continual basis (e.g., every 2 years), including systematic reminders to providers when current licensure or insurance is about to expire.
- *Case manager ratings.* Routine global ratings of providers by case managers per con-

tact episode must be based on cost-effectiveness, quality of care, and degree of cooperation with the managed care system.
- *Provider profiling.* Diagnosis-based provider profiling must be based on measures of cost and utilization with feedback to providers on network norms. This topic is also addressed in Chapter 32.
- *Treatment chart audits.* There must be routine audits of provider treatment charts, often focused on profile outliers, with feedback to providers.
- *Provider communications.* These include bulletins, newsletters, and memoranda to network providers. The materials address administrative and clinical issues; issues are chosen based on findings of the internal QM system.
- *Provider education.* Provision must be made for formal education programs for providers driven by findings of the internal QM system.
- *Provider satisfaction surveys.* The plan must conduct routine monitoring of network provider satisfaction with clinical and administrative requirements of the managed care system and provide the opportunity for constructive suggestions for system changes.
- *Outcome monitoring.* There must be diagnosis- and provider-specific tracking of outcome measures, including patient satisfaction, recidivism/relapse, mental and/or physical health status change, mental and/or physical claims costs, and functional change (through employer-based data such as absenteeism rates and productivity measures).

External Quality Assurance Monitoring

It has been suggested that the incentives and conflicts of interest inherent in a managed BH program are too great to be overcome entirely by internal self-regulation. In recognition of this problem, some state and federal regulatory agencies and employers/payers have instituted routine external quality monitoring of managed BH systems. In addition, the National Committee for

Quality Assurance has incorporated BH measures to some extent in the Health Plan Employer Data and Information Set (see also Chapters 35 and 44).

The results of such external auditing activities reveal considerable variation in performance among managed BH organizations and within organizations over time and at different service delivery locations.

Routine monitoring of the quality of patient care services may be a useful check and balance mechanism. Audits of treatment records and case management records can reveal significant areas for improvement in the service delivery system not otherwise detected by internal quality assurance methods. Determining these areas may help improve the MCO's quality of care and its competitive position. Following are some examples of variation and common weaknesses in systems.

Utilization Criteria

Most organizations have criteria that specify clear behavioral criteria for various levels of care. Some organizations, however, have adopted criteria that do not provide clear guidance to the case manager. In these cases, general, nonbehavioral criteria are difficult to apply with any precision. In some other instances, criteria are clear but inefficient. For example, some organizations use published 50th percentile norms to assign initial lengths of stay, thus missing the opportunity to influence cases for which earlier discharge would be reasonable and achievable.

As specialized BH MCOs have matured, there has been a growing consensus among organizations concerning the essential criteria for inpatient care. There has also been serious attention paid to indications for outpatient care and elaboration of UR criteria for intermediate levels of care in the continuum of care.

While there is increasing emphasis on the use of "evidence-based" practice guidelines and medical necessity criteria in both utilization management and case management functions, definition of practice guidelines and medical necessity throughout the BH field is challenging.[24] Differences among the BH professions, the lack

of science-based evidence of effective treatments, and different schools of thought among practitioners, consumers, and advocates make it especially difficult to institute universally accepted, evidence-based guidelines.[25] Practice or provider guidelines are generally defined as patient care strategies developed to assist clinicians in clinical decision-making and patient management.[26]

Many organizations develop practice guidelines and utilization criteria, but these guidelines often reflect the vested interests of the developers: providers, professionals, pharmaceutical companies, and MCOs. Furthermore, the criteria may be suited to one population served by the plans (e.g., commercial contracts) but not be suited to other recipients (e.g., Medicaid consumers). The Federal Substance Abuse and Mental Health Services Administration's pivotal role in sponsoring the national Planning Summit on Scientifically-Based Behavioral Health Practice Guidelines and the Practice Guidelines Coalition's (PGC's) effort to develop evidence-based treatment guidelines through broad consensus are positive initiatives. PGC's focus is on high-frequency and/or high-impact conditions, including behavioral disorders such as depression and bipolar disorders, clinical problems such as marital or work stress, suicidal crises, and the behavioral aspects of acute and chronic illness, such as smoking cessation and weight reduction.[27]

Development of guidelines for the treatment of schizophrenia has been a priority of the University of Maryland's Center for Mental Health Services Research and the Johns Hopkins University School of Public Health, funded by the Agency for Health Care Policy and Research and the National Institute of Mental Health. However, one consumer/professional critic indicates that this study emphasizes "maintenance approaches and does not include primary consumers or reference consumer-operated recovery-oriented programs in their literature review."[28(p.596)]

The difficulty in agreeing upon and developing performance-based practice guidelines and utilization criteria pales in comparison to the challenge of implementing guidelines. Often the availability or lack of availability of a certain type of service is a better predictor of utilization than adherence to practice guidelines. Also, clinicians with different orientations may interpret clinical evidence differently.[29] Clinicians within the same organization vary in their application of criteria based on their clinical background, personal traits, or differential understanding of the expectations of the purchaser. Because criteria are designed to be guidelines and applied in conjunction with an assessment of the patient, the possibility of significant variance is substantial.

These challenges, when coupled with the requirements of payers to demonstrate medical necessity of service, present multiple complexities for state and local governments as they plan and implement managed mental health and substance abuse programs. The Office of Inspector General's report (1998) on the Health Care Financing Administration's financial statements for fiscal year 1997 cites the lack of documented medical necessity as the second highest cause of Medicare billing errors. Increased scrutiny of Medicaid payments and the tension between offering flexible Medicaid benefits and ensuring cost-efficiency and budget neutrality contribute to the need for clear practice guidelines and service utilization criteria.

Staff Qualifications

Some organizations lack case managers or even supervisory personnel with a relevant BH background and appropriate experience. Some lack doctoral-level advisors who can engage in matched peer review with doctoral-level providers. Some programs have physicians without a psychiatric or substance abuse background functioning as psychiatric medical directors. This is inappropriate, at best.

Inservice Training

Some organizations select inservice training programs on the basis of apparently random or arbitrary topic selection rather than needs identified through an internal QM system. Many have no inservice training, orientation, or QM oversight applied to doctoral-level advisors. Some

have no discernible inservice training program at all.

Quality of Care Problem Identification

The incidence of quality of care problems such as misdiagnosis, subtherapeutic or toxic medication dosages, unexplored medical complications, mismatch of diagnosis and treatment plan, and mismanagement of dangerous behavior has not diminished over time, and specialized MCOs have yet to devise effective methods for improving care at the point of UR. In general, review programs document detection of and action on these problems in only a small minority of cases, although informal activity is believed to occur in some programs. When problems are identified by case managers in these programs, action by doctoral-level advisors can also be too rare. The potential for conserving resources through methodical improvement of the quality of care has hardly been explored.

Provider Credentialing

In the most minimal level of QM for a provider network, the BH system warrants to payers and direct consumers that all network providers meet certain baseline credentialing standards. Some programs fail to thoroughly document and independently confirm credentialing when providers are admitted to the network, and many programs fail consistently to recredential on a continuing basis to ensure that network members continue to meet basic requirements.

Progress in Outcomes Measurement, Tracking, and Assessment

The ultimate gateway to true continuous quality improvement is keyed to the reliable measurement of treatment outcomes and analysis of the relationship among treatment approach, provider type, case management technique, and treatment outcome. Some BH programs have begun to track treatment outcomes in a number of ways, and joint meetings between MCOs and large provider entities have been held to stimulate consensus on proposed tentative conceptual schemes and data measurement tools. There remains, however, great variation among programs and providers in the degree of conceptual development of these approaches, in the sophistication of information systems available to put data to use, and in the extent of agreement about appropriate measures and methods.

BH INFORMATION SYSTEMS

Managed BH care information systems are a subset of general managed care information systems. Consequently, many of the issues surrounding the automation of BH care processes affect health care systems generally. It is helpful to review BH systems from both perspectives: those areas where BH systems are similar or identical to their general health care counterparts as well as those areas where the greatest contrasts exist. Consequently, this section will review the common challenges that all managed health care systems face while also highlighting those features that make BH care systems unique.

Issues Common to All Health Care Informatics

Health care has lagged behind many other industries in the effective adoption of information technologies, and BH organizations tend to lag furthest behind. There are several reasons for this.

- *Historically, health care has been a fragmented "cottage" industry.* The financing of care has traditionally been separated from the delivery of care, and the delivery system is further divided into thousands of individual providers, clinics, and facilities. While there has been significant consolidation in recent years, the system is still highly fragmented, with few of the players able to make significant investment in information systems.
- *There is a lack of information standards in health care.* While there has been much progress in this area through the American National Standards Institute and other standard-setting groups, there is still considerable work to be completed. The implementation of the electronic standards defined in the Health Insurance Portability and Accountability Act legislation represents another important step forward (see also Chapters 35 and 67).[30]

The development of effective standards is extremely important to all industries. When effectively developed and implemented, standards streamline the processes by which trading partners interact. The best recent example of the power of introducing a standard is the Internet. Electronic networks existed long before the Internet, but it was the agreement by many vendors to use the same standard communication protocols, the Internet and web protocols, that fueled the growth of the Net and the World Wide Web. When standards in health care reach the same level of acceptance and completeness, the impact will be of similar magnitude. This will fuel large advances in the portability of health care information, in the electronic medical record, in the efficiency of the health care delivery and payment systems, and in outcomes, practice, and accountability.

- *In the past, information processing systems have not been seen as critical to the delivery of care.* This is especially true in BH. The main purpose of data systems was for billing and payment, not for collecting clinicians' notes. The concept of a clinician typing during therapy has not been accepted, and systems that could provide the therapist with information (care guidelines or pathways) during therapy are not yet well developed. An interesting factor for BH care is that while traditional methods of therapy have been slow to adopt information systems assistance, technology is fueling the growth of alternative methods. There has been considerable growth in BH-related web sites, and it is now possible to seek psychological advice over the Internet.

Each of these factors has contributed to the slower acceptance of information systems by managed BH health care. While there has been improvement in each area, it may still be many years before information systems will reach their peak of implementation in health care.

Features Required of All Managed Health Care Information Systems

Components of the system may be reduced or eliminated in some situations. For example, if an MCO has mandated that its provider network use only electronic claims, then the need for a mail room and document imaging capability may be greatly reduced. Most MCOs—especially those handling BH care–would insist that their provider network is too diverse to allow such a mandate to be implemented across all providers. Therefore, even an organization with a focus on electronic claims will need to keep some mail room functions.

The functions required by a managed care system include the following:

- *group setup and membership-related functions*
  1. eligibility
  2. enrollment
  3. benefit plan
  4. member services support
  5. client registration
- *claim- and encounter-related functions*
  1. imaging
  2. workflow
  3. electronic claims
  4. electronic funds transfer
  5. claims adjudication
  6. claims processor support
  7. capitation
  8. check printing
- *care management–related functions*
  1. precertification and care authorization
  2. referral management
  3. care guidelines
- *provider-related functions*
  1. provider contracts
  2. provider demographics and billing information

3. provider credentialing
4. provider profiles
- *accounting-related functions*
  1. general ledger
  2. accounts receivable
  3. premium billing
- *reporting-related functions*
  1. executive information system
  2. financial reports
  3. utilization reports
  4. quality reports
  5. episode of care reports

Some of these functions have been web enabled in recent years. For example, people can use enrollment applications on their web browsers to enroll in a health plan and make changes to existing enrollment.

In the future, BH care information standards should link managed care functions more directly to the therapy process. Eventually, symptoms, treatment plans, outcomes, and other measures captured electronically during the therapy process will be matched in real time to the treatment pathways and benefits covered in the client's benefit plan. Both therapist and client will understand how much assistance the insurance coverage will provide in financing a course of treatment as it is being planned and delivered. Similarly, outcome information collected using standard measures can be compared to normative information to determine the effectiveness of the intervention and to compare the client's progress to that of others with similar symptoms. In this future scenario, the information technology provides the therapist with direct assistance in the therapeutic process and handles most of the time-consuming administrative tasks inherent in managed care.

The issues and information system structure described above are applicable to all managed health care. In the next section, the characteristics that distinguish BH systems are investigated in greater detail.

Unique Features of BH Information Systems

An information system designed specifically for BH diverges functionally in several ways from similar medical-surgical systems. Good BH systems will include, for example, *DSM IV* diagnosis codes (including all axes). They will allow for residential and partial care settings, nontraditional treatment alternatives, and BH testing. Many of the most important methods for delivering BH services under managed care involve the use of intensive noninpatient alternative care settings. These alternatives are incompatible with the basic inpatient/outpatient structure and coding schemes of typical medical-surgical information systems. Any information standards developed for health care will not be complete if codes for each of the diverse settings utilized in BH care are not included.

The best BH management information systems developers recognize the more chronic and long-term nature of BH problems and have structured system functions accordingly. These systems smoothly handle issues of multiple and extended authorizations for all levels of care, review and approval of treatment plans, and episodes of care that are routinely longer than those in medical-surgical systems. Contracting and provider modules have well-developed BH credentialing and profiling systems and allow for provider searches on the full range of provider experience, treatment preferences, and education. A wide range of contracting options should be accommodated, and utilization against these contracts should be tracked.

Integration of Health Care and BH Systems

While good BH information systems have many features that distinguish them from typical medical-surgical systems, there are many functions that the BH and corresponding medical-surgical systems can share. More important, there are many functions that by definition must be the same.

Eligibility information, for instance, must be shared by both systems because the BH benefit is usually part of a larger medical benefit. Typically, the BH system relies on the corresponding medical-surgical or employer system for eligibility information. The level of integration can be represented as a continuum, with the highest

level being a single system for both medical-surgical and BH and the lowest level being two independent systems with incompatible eligibility file structures.

At the high-integration end of the continuum, BH processing is accomplished using the medical-surgical information system. Historically, this has led to significant functional compromises in the quality and specificity of the BH data, but it does have the positive effect of making access to the eligibility file simple. Since the BH staff members are using the same system as the medical-surgical staff, they have access to the same eligibility functions and access the same eligibility file. No transfer of eligibility information between systems is required.

At the other end of the integration continuum, there are many independent BH systems that have varying degrees of compatibility with the employer systems or medical-surgical systems from which they must obtain their eligibility data. In the worst case, the BH staff must either access the medical-surgical system themselves for the eligibility data or rely on paper printouts or phone calls to the medical-surgical staff.

The center point of the integration continuum involves maintaining duplicate eligibility files on each system. This requires transferring the data from one system to the other. Duplicating the files leads to new issues, including scheduling the replication process, reconciling the files, and accessing the original file between replications when eligibility questions arise.

The best integration options utilize client/server approaches. In these cases, there is only one eligibility file or object, and it is maintained separately from the medical-surgical and BH applications. When a user of either the medical-surgical system or the BH system checks the eligibility of a client, the respective systems contact the independent eligibility function, which returns with the appropriate eligibility and demographic data. This is transparent to the user, who is unaware that the system has accessed an external resource to answer the query.

This last approach allows the BH system the independence required to preserve its unique BH functions without requiring the duplication of files that need to be accessible to all systems. It also makes it easy to develop BH-specific data files that contain information not required by medical systems. These files can be accessed by the BH client application at the same time as the shared eligibility file. The BH system user receives an answer that contains information from both the unique BH file and the systemwide eligibility file.

As noted above, the development of information standards is a major issue in health care. The eligibility example described above further demonstrates the point. If there were a universal eligibility information set that was used by all health care vendors, including BH vendors, many of the integration challenges described above would be simplified.

Key Information Systems Issues

A successful BH information system both incorporates BH-specific system functions and data and integrates other functions and data with the remainder of the benefit plan. Eligibility is an example of a function that must be well integrated. Other examples include accumulators against benefit plan maximums, integrated claims files, member service systems, and contracting.

Many other system functions and data, as indicated above, must be developed independently. The quality of the service provided is compromised when these functions are combined because the medical-surgical information systems do not support the unique needs of BH care. Treatment planning provides a good example. Medical-surgical applications have not been designed to accommodate treatment plans prior to the delivery of the service. There is much less variability in the possible treatments, and they are typically not delivered over the longer time spans that BH care requires. Consequently, medical-surgical systems do not analyze treatment plans and progress against treatment plans in determining the appropriateness of service delivered. However, in BH this is the main method of precertification and concurrent review. It is much more efficient and effective to develop this and other functions as separate

mental health modules or as an entirely independent system.

PUBLIC/PRIVATE SYSTEMS INTEGRATION

BH is unique in the health care world for the dominant role the public sector has played in the financing and delivery of care. Approximately two public dollars are spent for every private dollar in the financing of psychiatric and addiction treatment services. Moreover, publicly financed and publicly operated systems have more often cared for individuals with the most serious forms of behavioral illness; by contrast, in the medical-surgical arena, the sickest people more often accessed care in the best-staffed teaching hospitals.

The BH field moved from a medical to a psychosocial model of care in the last 30 years to support the decongregation of public psychiatric hospitals and the development of community-based care. New approaches were developed in community mental health and addiction services for the management of care in alternative and less costly settings. Adoption of these practices was key to the success of the early managed BH care organizations.

Managed BH care was formally established in response to private sector demand for an alternative to unrestrained and growing use of inpatient and outpatient care. Emergence of managed care in the public sector has, in the main, been driven by a desire to manage the cost of the benefit, combined with aspirations to improve access, quality, and outcomes of the care provided. Despite the fact that first-generation managed BH care developed from public sector approaches, the advent of managed care in the public sector has been accompanied by the notion that the private sector is more consistent and considered in its approach, which can benefit the public sector. This implied notion has created some misunderstanding and disappointment.

Managed care has also been accompanied by a government privatization effort that has (more than managed care techniques) promoted public/private systems integration. Opportunities for a positive fusion of public and private sector technologies and competence are a great benefit accrued to patients at a time when the amount and cost of service benefits are being reduced. Through privatization and managed care initiatives, those with the most serious disorders now have access to the best hospitals at more affordable rates. At the same time, privately insured persons now have access to less restrictive and broader types of care. Together, public sector community treatment technology and private sector quality improvement and information management hold great promise for consumers of care.

The promise of public/private systems integration can be realized through a deliberate and planned approach to implementation of a reformed system. *Steps to be taken include the following:*

- understanding the shifting roles of government players in the local environment as departments of mental health, public health, and medical assistance reframe their policy, regulatory, financing, and provider roles
- analyzing the case mix characteristics and utilization patterns among publicly insured persons to identify client risk groups and project utilization and cost associated with care for people in these groups
- assessing political and regulatory challenges to implementing new provider arrangements, service models, and reimbursement rates
- evaluating the potential for integration of publicly and privately insured persons at the provider level to reduce segregation, maximize resources, and improve access
- establishing a process and standards for quality assurance and improvement of all care programs
- incorporating the voice and interests of consumers in the planning, delivery, and evaluation of accountable services
- developing benchmarks to guide monitoring of client utilization and professional practice patterns as a safeguard against underservice

- framing agreements and a plan for allocation of savings as a return on public investments

EMERGING ISSUES

As with managed health care in general, the BH field remains highly dynamic, with new issues emerging every year. The most important emerging issues in BH care today are discussed below.

The paradigm shift toward population-based care management challenges the limits of earlier generations of BH managed care. Prompted by poor BH care outcomes and vocal patient/family advocacy, government and employer requirements to address the needs of individuals with more severe mental illnesses are increasing. MCOs face the challenge to refocus systems planning and care management onto the problems of defined and often vulnerable populations.

Involvement of a large advocacy community in the past and the more recent involvement of primary consumers in the public sector advisory process require accommodation by the private sector as more public services are privatized. As noted earlier, the Mental Health Parity Act, effective January 1998, requires that group health plans with annual or lifetime dollar limits for medical or surgical benefits have the same dollar limits on mental health benefits. This national effort to promote parity between physical and mental health care is prompting renewed discussion on the health benefits of integrating physical and behavioral care management and the potential for medical cost offset through BH treatment.

The potential for medical cost offset as a result of timely and targeted psychiatric and addiction treatment is recognized but infrequently measured. As data emerge and the number of full-risk capitation arrangements grows, the demand for behavioral treatment in primary and tertiary care settings increases. A substantial proportion of the highest-cost tertiary care patients have psychiatric and substance abuse disorders that increase morbidity and mortality if left untreated. The implications for redistribution of resources to BH depend upon the ability of the BH field to produce data and educate payers and practitioners.

BH providers are challenged to integrate horizontally to achieve comprehensiveness of service and large geographic base, and to cover public and privately insured populations. They are also challenged to integrate vertically to complete continuums with primary health and tertiary care providers. BH providers and networks must be able to operate as, and accept varying payments on, both carve-in and carve-out bases.

Legal, ethical, cultural, and accountability-related challenges that have been commonplace in public care systems are emerging in managed BH care systems.

- **Legal.** Legally mandated civil commitment is producing uncontrolled expenses in length of stay and legal representation, creating financial risk for capitated systems.
- **Ethical.** Under managed and capitated arrangements, fiscal incentives may promote underservice.

- **Cultural.** Demands for treatments, providers, and programs that are accessible to people of all cultures are increasing as managed care penetration increases, particularly among publicly insured clients.
- **Accountability-related.** Patient and family member advocacy groups are organizing and demanding greater accountability from insurers, employers, and governments.

CONCLUSION

This chapter outlines some of the key components of issues and recent developments in specialized managed care programs addressing BH treatment. BH care efforts present unique management problems that are increasingly being addressed through specialized managed care systems with specific and separate operational guidelines, managed care personnel, provider networks, and QM approaches.

REFERENCES

1. National Alliance for the Mentally Ill, *Stand and Deliver: Action Call to a Failing Industry* (Arlington, VA, 1997).

2. K. Sternbach and R. Waters, Anatomy of a Medicaid Behavioral Managed Care Program: Green Spring's AdvoCare of Tennessee, *Behavioral Health Management* 15, no. 4 (1995): 13–18.

3. B. Bengen-Seltzer, *Fourth Generation Managed Behavioral Health: What Does It Look Like?* (Providence, RI: Manissess Communications Group, 1995).

4. M.J. Bennett, The Greening of the HMO: Implications for Prepaid Psychiatry, *American Journal of Psychiatry* 145 (1988): 1544–1549.

5. P. Starr, *Social Transformation of American Medicine* (New York: Basic Books, 1984).

6. D.A. Sclar et al., Antidepressant Pharmacotherapy: Economic Outcomes in a Health Maintenance Organization, *Clinical Therapeutics* 16, no. 4 (1994): 715–730.

7. S.T. Melton et al., Economic Evaluation of Paroxetine and Imipramine in Depressed Outpatients, *Psychopharmacology Bulletin* 33, no. 1 (1997): 93–100.

8. G.E. Simon et al., Initial Antidepressant Choice in Primary Care: Effectiveness and Cost of Fluoxetine vs. Tricyclic Antidepressants, *JAMA* 275, no. 24 (1996): 1897–1902.

9. Y. Lapierre et al., Direct Cost of Depression: Analysis of Treatment Costs of Paroxetine versus Imipramine in Canada, *Canadian Journal of Psychiatry* 40, no. 7 (1995): 370–377.

10. P.E. Keck, Jr., et al., A Pharmacoeconomic Model of Divalproex vs. Lithium in the Acute and Prophylactic Treatment of Bipolar I Disorder, *Journal of Clinical Psychiatry* 57 (1996): 213–222.

11. H.Y. Meltzer and P.A. Cola, The Pharmacoeconomics of Clozapine: A Review, *Journal of Clinical Psychiatry* 55, suppl. B (1994): 161–165.

12. J.C. Barefoot et al., Depression and Long-Term Mortality Risk in Patients with Coronary Artery Disease, *American Journal of Cardiology* 78 (1996): 613–617.

13. J.S. Rosie, Partial Hospitalization: A Review of Recent Literature, *Hospital and Community Psychiatry* 38 (1987): 1291–1299.

14. L.R. Mosher, Alternatives to Psychiatric Hospitalization, *New England Journal of Medicine* 309 (1983): 1579–1580.

15. H.M. Annis, Is Inpatient Rehabilitation of the Alcoholic Cost-Effective? A Composition, *Advances in Alcoholism and Substance Abuse* 5 (1986): 175–190.

16. L. Saxe and L. Goodman, *The Effectiveness of Outpatient vs. Inpatient Treatment: Updating the OTA Report,*

(Hartford, CT: Prudential Insurance Company, 1988).

17. R. Husby et al., Short-Term Dynamic Psychotherapy: Prognostic Value of Characteristics of Patient Studies by a Two-Year Follow-up of 39 Neurotic Patients, *Psychotherapy and Psychosomatics* 43 (1985): 8–16.

18. M.J. Horowitz et al., Comprehensive Analysis of Change after Brief Dynamic Psychotherapy, *American Journal of Psychiatry* 143 (1986): 582–589.

19. H.G. Whittington, Managed Mental Health: Clinical Myths and Imperatives, in *Managed Mental Health Services,* ed. S. Feldman (Springfield, IL: Charles C Thomas, 1992), 223–243.

20. D. Anderson, How Effective Is Managed Mental Health Care? *Business Health,* November 1989, 34–35.

21. National Alliance for the Mentally Ill, *Legislative Agenda* (Arlington, VA, 1999).

22. K.B. Wells et al., Detection of Depressive Disorder for Patients Receiving Prepaid or Fee-for-Service Care, *JAMA* 262 (1989): 3298–3302.

23. M. Shadle and J.B. Christianson, The Organization of Mental Health Care Delivery in HMOs, *Administration of Mental Health* 15 (1988): 201–225.

24. I. Shaffer, Accountability and Variability, in *Faulkner and Gray 1999 Behavioral Outcomes & Guidelines Sourcebook* (New York: Faulkner & Gray, 1999), 597–598.

25. D.J. Abrahamson, Political Issues in Practice Guidelines Implementation, in *Faulkner and Gray 1999 Behavioral Outcomes & Guidelines Sourcebook* (New York: Faulkner & Gray, 1999), 592–593.

26. D.A. Zarin et al., The Role of Psychotherapy in the Treatment of Depression: Review of Two Practice Guidelines, *Archives of Behavioral Psychiatry* 53 (1996): 291–293.

27. D. Strickland, A Decisive Year Ahead for the Practice Guidelines Coalition, in *Faulkner and Gray 1999 Behavioral Outcomes & Guidelines Sourcebook* (New York: Faulkner & Gray, 1999), 582–586.

28. D. Fisher, Recovery: The Behavioral Healthcare Guidelines of Tomorrow, in *Faulkner and Gray 1999 Behavioral Outcomes & Guidelines Sourcebook,* 594–596.

29. Shaffer, Accountability and Variability, 597–598.

30. *Health Insurance Portability and Accountability Act of 1996,* P.L. 104-191, August 21, 1996.

CHAPTER 26

Home Health Care

Peggy H. Rodebush, Laura L. Waltrip, and G. David Baker

INTRODUCTION

How often are patients sent home from a physician's office or clinic, emergency department (ED), or hospital with prescriptions and follow-up instructions, only to return a short time later with no improvement or in worse condition? How many health care providers are puzzled and frustrated by patients who are noncompliant or simply unable to carry out instructions? Without a good understanding of pa-

---

Peggy H. Rodebush, RN, MSN, is a partner in Ernst & Young's consulting service. Specializing in health care business transformation, she works with leading health care providers across the United States. She is a nationally recognized post–acute care and medical management expert and is a frequent speaker at national conventions.

Laura L. Waltrip, RN, BSN, is a manager with Ernst & Young's consulting practice and assists health care providers with business transformation efforts. She specializes in medical management and integration with post–acute care services. She has spent over 20 years in health care, including more than 10 years in post–acute and home care operations. She has medical management experience in managed care and academic environments.

G. David Baker, MSW, Regional Director of Home Care Services for St. John Health System in Detroit, Michigan, has over 25 years' experience in health care, including 20 years in post–acute care and home care. He has been a manager in Ernst & Young's consulting service and is a nationally recognized expert in home care, frequently speaking at national, regional, and state meetings.

tients' home environment, lifestyle, and family support system, providers are lacking the complete picture necessary for successful medical management.

Home health care has matured and evolved to become a critical component of medical management. It is used successfully in pre– and post–acute care settings and is vital in the existing environment of cost-efficiency pressures and quality measurement through the continuum of care. There are many different types of home health care, including medical and nonmedical care, intermittent and continuous care, custodial and skilled care, and formal and informal care. The limits of each of these categories are usually not driven by the medical needs of the patient but by the financing mechanism available for payment of the services provided. For example, Medicare, as the predominant home care payer, has traditionally consisted of multiple medical disciplines within a highly coordinated plan of treatment. The complete team, if medically necessary, comprises a registered nurse (RN), physical therapist (PT), licensed practical nurse (LPN), occupational therapist (OT), speech therapist, social worker, and home health aide (HHA).

The limits of care are frequently set in the federal code that authorizes payment for the care and describes the conditions that must be met by providers to participate in the federal programs. The goal of the Medicare program is to improve the health and functional status of patients. Medicare approves payment for this care only as long as progressive improvement can be shown and in some specific chronic cases that require skilled nursing follow-up on a long-term basis (such as monthly urinary catheter change).

Older persons receive most home care because of the age criteria of Medicare and older persons' higher health care needs. There is an increasing number of non-Medicare, younger patients receiving home care services, however. This growing younger market is an extension of the improving clinical capabilities of home care providers and the increasing number of third-party payers that recognize home care as a viable medical alternative or adjunct to more expensive acute and subacute care.

WHAT IS HOME CARE?

Home care encompasses a broad range of medical, social, and support services. It involves the delivery of health care at home typically to persons who are disabled, chronically ill, terminally ill, or recovering.

Care may be intermittent or continuous. Continuous care is frequently referred to as "private-duty care," since it is seldom reimbursed by Medicare or third-party payers. This type of care is typically offered by organizations other than those providing intermittent care designed for the capitated Medicare program and for third-party payers who stipulate intermittent care. Continuous and intermittent home care differ in the duration of time for care delivery. Private-duty care is usually for service unit increments longer than 1 hour or service units that are billed relative to the number of hours or shifts spent delivering care. A service unit for intermittent home care is described as a patient visit.

Both continuous and intermittent care have complex and support care components. Continuous care may range from RN support for ventilator-dependent patients to companions for older people or confined persons. Intermittent care requires highly skilled professionals who can work independently in the home, under a physician's orders, with typically much stronger problem-solving and technical skills than the same professionals would have in many inpatient medical settings. Likewise, HHAs provide

intermittent support care, such as bathing, assistance in moving about the home, and meal preparation.

HISTORY OF HOME CARE

Care provided to a member of a household by a recognized health care practitioner or member of the household has been in existence for centuries and preceded institutional care. It started as a local phenomenon focused on the neighborhood, village, or town in which the ill person lived. As practitioners' ability to care for the ill improved, the level of the care provided in the home evolved with it.

Health care focused outside the home began to develop as the involvement of religious and academic organizations in health care increased and formal medical education evolved. As these organizations began to serve ill people, larger, more complex health care organizations began to emerge, providing hospitals where higher levels of care were developed and could be provided.

Home care in the modern sense existed as a cottage industry until the early 1980s, when a lawsuit concerning excessive paperwork and unreliable payment policies led to a revision in the Medicare home health payment policies. With the favorable ruling from that lawsuit in 1986, which clarified expanded coverage for beneficiaries, the Medicare annual benefit outlay and the number of agencies grew significantly until 1997 and 1998. The period of growth and expansion was fueled by a growing demand for care at home as well as recognition that complex medical care could be safely provided in the home, with patient satisfaction frequently increasing. With expansion, the share of the health dollar devoted to home care grew (see Figures 26–1, 26–2, and 26–3).This increase in expenditures received great scrutiny from the federal government and resulted in changes to reimbursement practices. The implementation of the Balanced Budget Act (BBA) of 1997 resulted in severe reimbursement restrictions that continue to have a dramatic impact on the home health care industry. As of 1999, the industry was experiencing a sharp decline in the number of agencies serving

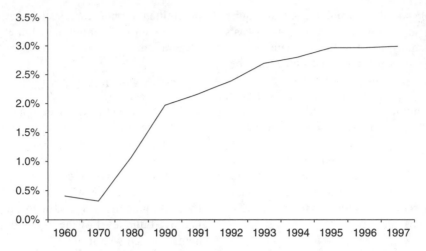

Figure 26–1 Home Care Expenditures as a Percentage of National Health Expenditures. *Source:* Reprinted from OSCAR Report 10, Office of National Health Statistics, Office of the Actuary, Health Care Financing Administration.

patients: in 1997, there were 10,570, but in June 1999, there were only 8,613 (see Figure 26–4). The shrinking numbers of providers has created growing concern that not all those who need home care services will get them, especially in rural areas.

INDICATORS AND PREDICTORS OF HOME CARE DEMAND

There are multiple factors contributing to the evolution and growth of the home care market, including

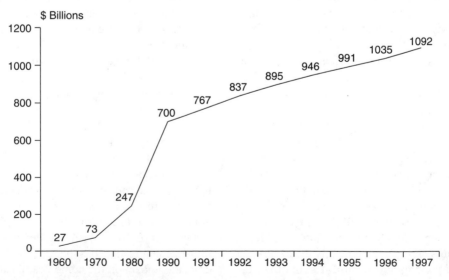

Figure 26–2 National Health Expenditure Trends. *Source:* Reprinted from Office of the Actuary, Health Care Financing Administration.

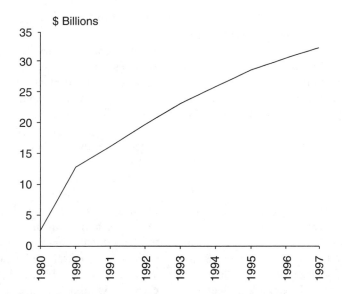

Figure 26–3 Home Health Care Expenditure Trends. *Source:* Reprinted from Office of the Actuary, Health Care Financing Administration.

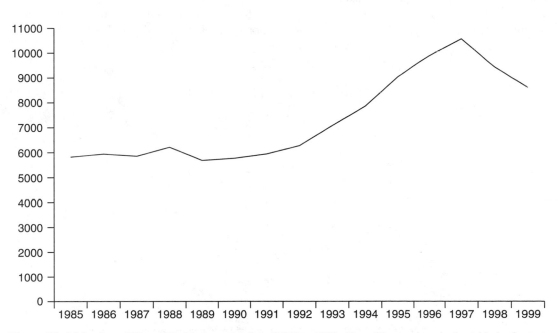

Figure 26–4 Number of Home Health Agencies from 1963 to 1999. *Note:* The numbers in the table in the text cannot be replicated by NAHC. Both the Office of the Actuary and NAHC recognized the numbers above as accurate home health agency totals. Figures for 1999 are through June 4, 1999. *Source:* Reprinted from Office of the Actuary, Health Care Financing Administration.

- demographic shifts (resulting in a greater proportion of older people in the U.S. population)
- the shrinking hospital system (because of cost containment pressures)
- decreased availability of informal caregivers (producing a need for more formal caregivers)
- improved home care technology

Demographic Shifts

The first major factor contributing to the evolution of the home care market is the much-discussed "graying of America." The number of persons reaching retirement age and Medicare eligibility age is increasing and is predicted to grow exponentially in the next few decades. Americans' life expectancy has increased from age 63 in 1940 to age 82 today. By 2100, it is projected that the United States will have 20.1 million residents over 85 years old, 50.6 million over 75 years old, and 89.9 million over 65 years old (Figure 26–5).[1] This growing aged population continues to put tremendous pressure on the health care system.

The Shrinking Hospital System

The hospital industry continues to struggle with an excess of acute care beds in many markets as well as continued pressures to reduce costs and generate positive net income. As a result, hospitals have continued to experience mergers, acquisitions, and consolidations and to downsize. Meanwhile, the number of acute care hospitals and the acute care length of stay continue to decline (see Table 26–1 and Figures 26–6 and 26–7). Many of the patients still need some level of care following hospital discharge. Increasingly, the home care industry has experienced the "sicker and sooner" discharge for acute care, with many being referred to home care agencies. With less costly care available through home care and with sicker patients being discharged sooner, the home care industry has moved forward to fill this void.

Decreased Availability of Informal Caregivers

It is estimated that 9 to 11 million people need home care services. Many of these people will

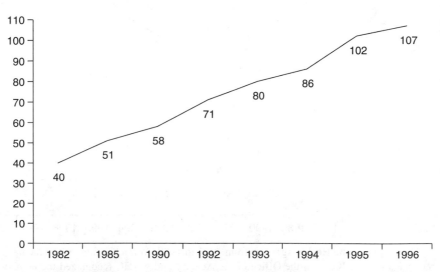

Figure 26–5 Number of Home Health Patients Served per 1,000 Medicare Enrollees. *Source:* Reprinted from 1997 statistics, Health Care Financing Administration.

Table 26–1 Inpatient Beds Trends

Year	Total Hospitals	Average Beds per Hospital	Beds per 100 Enrollees
1975	6,707	1,132	51.5
1980	6,780	1,152	46.9
1995	6,414	1,074	29.4
1996	6,376	1,056	28.4
1997	6,293	1,037	27.0

Source: Reprinted from 1997 statistics. Health Care Financing Administration.

receive care from family members, friends, or others. These "informal caregivers" are not compensated.[2] Due to the breakdown of the nuclear family, the increased mobility and dispersion of extended families, and the fact that many would-be informal caregivers work outside the home and are themselves in need of assistance, there are fewer informal caregivers available. The gap created by the loss of informal caregivers will necessitate a shift to the formal caregiver, and this shift will contribute to the growth in demand for home care services.

Figure 26–6 Persons Aged 65 and Older in the United States. *Source:* Reprinted from 1996 statistics, Health Care Financing Administration.

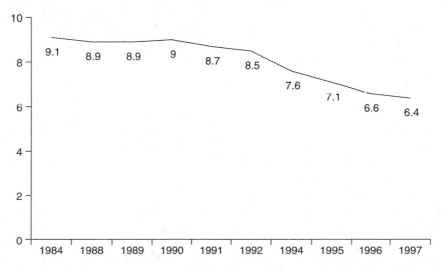

Figure 26–7 Trends in Medicare Average Length of Stay (in Days). *Source:* Reprinted from Office of the Actuary, National Health Statistics Group, Health Care Financing Administration.

Improved Home Care Technology

Telemedicine companies have entered the market in recent years with technology appropriate for the home setting. Their products have evolved from large, robotic machines to smaller, more streamlined monitoring devices. The equipment placed in patients' homes has been extremely expensive in the past. However, recent reductions in the costs of telephone technology and computer hardware and software have made equipment more affordable. For example, adult working children may now have visual contact with aging parents through advances in telephone equipment and resources. This regular contact may be enough to provide peace of mind and prevent placement of a parent in a long-term care facility.

HOME CARE SERVICES AND DISCIPLINES

The home care market is segmented due to the unique nature of the various services as well as differing reimbursement mechanisms for each service type. A single patient can receive care from one or several service areas. *Home care services can generally be divided into the following four groups:*

1. traditional nursing services
2. infusion services
3. medical equipment and supplies
4. respiratory services

Traditional Nursing Services

Traditional nursing services form the largest category of home care services. When most people think of home care, they envision traditional services, which include care provided by RNs, LPNs, HHAs, certified nursing assistants, and medical social workers (MSWs). In-home rehabilitation services, frequently grouped with traditional nursing services, are performed by licensed or registered therapists, including PTs, OTs, dietitians, and speech language pathologists (SLPs).

Infusion Services

Home infusion services are often viewed as a component of traditional care. Infusion services require a higher skill level of nursing, a pharmacy component, and a safe, clean home environment. Types of infusion therapy conducive to home administration include continuous or intermittent chemotherapy, parenteral nutrition support, antibiotics, hydration, and pain control. These services have experienced rapid and sustained growth, and in the last 10 years their fees and quality of service have been scrutinized. In 1996, infusion services in the United States were a $6 billion market.[3]

Medical Equipment and Supplies

Home medical equipment and supplies are generally nonclinical items that consist of durable medical equipment (wheelchairs, walkers, hospital beds, and activities of daily living [ADL] equipment and supplies) and other disposable medical supplies. In 1996, the U.S. medical equipment market was $1.5 billion.[4]

Respiratory Services

Home respiratory services, often viewed as the clinical component of home medical equipment and supplies, consist of home oxygen and respiratory therapy services. This U.S. market was $4.5 billion in 1996.[5]

HOME CARE PROVIDERS

Formal home care services are offered by a multidisciplinary mix of medical and nonmedical professionals.

Nurses

Nurses include RNs and LPNs. These medical professionals provide skilled services—including assessments, injections, intravenous therapy, psychiatric care, wound care, education, disease management, and case management—that certain patients may need. RNs have received 2 or more years of formal education and training and are licensed to practice in individual states. LPNs have 1 year of specialized training. They are also licensed in individual states and must operate under the supervision of an RN.

Physical Therapists

PTs perform treatment to restore loss of mobility and strength caused by physical impairments. They may also be involved in treatment and management of complex wounds. These professionals may use specialized equipment to conduct these therapeutic treatments. An important aspect of therapy is the education of the patient and other health care professionals in proper physical techniques to alleviate pain and prevent initial or future injury. A licensed physical therapy assistant may also provide services under the direction of a PT.

Occupational Therapists

OTs provide treatments similar to physical therapists' but focus on improving the patient's performance of ADLs. ADLs include eating, drinking, dressing, bathing, and performing other routine household duties. An OT often must address the physical, social, and emotional needs of the patient. A certified occupational therapy assistant may also provide services under the direction of an OT.

Speech Language Pathologists

SLPs provide care to diagnose, restore, and improve the speech and swallowing function of patients having dysfunction due to stroke or injury. SLPs work to improve the communication function of these patients by using specialized tools and techniques. These therapists also work with patients suffering from problems with breathing and swallowing.

Respiratory Therapists

Respiratory therapists provide care related to the treatment of patients with pulmonary and res-

piratory dysfunction. This care frequently involves the use of specialized equipment, including ventilators, oxygen concentrators, liquid oxygen dispensing systems, nebulizers, continuous positive air pressure apnea monitors, and other respiratory support equipment and supplies.

MSWs

MSWs assess and help improve patients' psychological and social difficulties. MSWs counsel patients with illnesses or disabilities and their families, helping them understand the resources available to them. These resources include public and private agencies that may temporarily assist the patient and patient's family, providing food, shelter, funds to pay bills, clothing, and so on. Frequently, the MSW will assist in completing the required documentation and coordinating the support needs of more acutely ill patients.

Pharmacists

Pharmacists provide technical and advisory services for home infusion services. Pharmaceutical products must be prepared, and supplies and deliveries must be coordinated with the ordering physician, the nurse, the patient, and often the patient's family. Pharmacy technicians may be utilized under the supervision of a pharmacist. One of the most important roles for the pharmacist is to provide education to patients and other staff members regarding medication administration and compliance and monitoring for adverse side effects. Home care patients, even those not on infusion drugs, are often on a large number of medications. Pharmacists can often assist in evaluating the home medication management process and for that reason are often included in multidisciplinary case conferencing.

Dietitians

Dietitians offer nutritional monitoring and education to those patients needing dietary support services as part of their treatment regimen. Nutritional counseling continues to be critical for management of most chronic conditions, such as diabetes and cardiac disease. It is also required to appropriately manage the medically complex pediatric population.

HHAs

HHAs frequently provide the majority of services in traditional home care agencies. These caregivers may have specialized training and are not licensed by the state, though many states require a certification process. They assist patients with a large variety of support services, including ambulation, bathing, toileting, personal care, and dressing. Under Medicare, these services must be provided under the guidance of an RN.

Nonmedical home caregivers, including HHAs, homemakers, and companions, are an important component of the service mix. HHA services are reimbursed by Medicare as long as a medical plan of treatment is in effect. Some Medicaid programs have waivers that pay some costs of HHA or homemaker services for the very frail or poor ill under certain conditions. However, most types of home care services, although they improve the quality of life and play a major role in raising health status and safety, are not reimbursable by third-party payers.

Homemakers

Homemakers provide support services in the form of general household duties, including meal preparation, laundry, light housekeeping, and shopping. They usually do not participate directly in the care for medical needs.

Companions

Companions are frequently called "sitters." These individuals provide a physical presence and safety net for those patients who should not be left at home alone. These caregivers do not provide medical care and are generally viewed as custodial.

Volunteers

Volunteers provide a vast number of services to the home care patient. Their involvement is determined by their individual capabilities and the needs of the patient. They are used extensively in hospice programs for bereavement care. These professionals operate from a variety of organizations, including home care agencies, hospices, staffing (private-duty) agencies, registries, medical and supply companies, and pharmaceutical and infusion services companies. These organizations may operate independently, vertically through common ownership with hospitals or skilled nursing homes, or horizontally with other home health agencies through partnerships or common ownership.

Physicians

Although they are last in this discussion and receive the smallest share of home care funds, physicians are the gatekeepers for most home care services. In both traditional Medicare and commercial payment scenarios, the physician goes uncompensated for medical supervision of all home care services unless payment is handled indirectly under a full-risk arrangement. The physician is responsible for initiating the plan of treatment and all changes, which can be numerous under Medicare, given the progressive rehabilitation requirement and the generally frail condition of the Medicare population. Additionally, physicians may conduct visits to the patient's home, although this is not common. Physicians do work closely with home care service providers to determine patient needs and which mix and frequency of services best meet those needs. Care plans for Medicare patients under a physician's care must be reviewed every 62 days, or more frequently, as the patient's medical needs change. The home care provider usually reviews these Medicare plans of care as part of a multidisciplinary approach to meeting the patient's needs. In many cases, physician time involvement for home care patients approaches (and sometimes exceeds) that for acute hospitalized patients.

REGULATIONS GUIDING HOME CARE

Home care service providers that participate as Medicare providers are subject to Title 42 of the Code of Federal Regulations. This section of the code describes the Conditions of Participation that home health agencies must comply with to become Medicare-certified agencies and to provide care to Medicare and Medicaid recipients. These regulations establish minimum requirements for management and patient care. These regulations, which have undergone numerous changes, were initially based upon the belief that any reasonable and appropriate caregiver could understand medical instructions and administer progressive rehabilitative care.

Medicare-certified home care services were loosely regulated in the past. HCFA allowed state regulatory agencies to serve as approval authorities for entry and continued participation in the Medicare system. These approvals came in the form of annual state surveys performed by state employees using a combination of local, regional, and national regulations, more often than not subjective and incorrectly interpreted by providers and regulatory agencies alike. The surveys usually lasted 1 to 3 days and consisted of nonstatistical sampling of medical charts for audits, limited visits to patient homes, and reviews of policies, procedures, and other documents. The results of these surveys were discrepancy lists; the agency had a certain amount of time to develop a correction plan and forward it to the regulators. The agency might then be subject to a reinspection.

These regulations were relatively toothless in the past. However, recent legislation has imposed substantial criminal and other penalties for fraud and abuse of the Medicare system. This new breed of regulations includes the Operation Restore Trust initiatives, surety bond regulations, and the BBA of 1997. Additionally, numerous rulings and mandates from HCFA, the Department of Health and Human Services, fiscal intermediaries, and even the President have substantially altered the way home health agencies currently operate and will operate in the near future.

Certification of a Medicare agency is the responsibility of the HCFA. However, most state health departments have attained "deemed status" to conduct on-site surveys and reviews of agencies in their state. Thus, a single review team applies the higher standards or the combined federal and state standards, making Medicare and Medicaid reimbursement possible. In many states, agencies cannot bill commercial carriers without state (and often, therefore, federal) certification and licensure.

If providers do not desire to participate in the Medicare and Medicaid programs, they are subject to existing state requirements. The majority of states do not have specific requirements for nonparticipating providers. Frequently, however, private third-party payers require an agency to be Medicare certified in order to care for their beneficiaries and receive reimbursement.

For patients to qualify for home health coverage under the Medicare system, the following four conditions must be met:

1. The physician must have determined a medical need for home care and developed a plan of care.
2. The care described in the plan of care must be for intermittent skilled nursing, therapy, or speech services.
3. The patient must be homebound.
4. The home health agency delivering care must be certified to participate in the Medicare program.[6]

Once these four conditions are met, Medicare will generally approve the following types of services:

- skilled nursing care on an intermittent or part-time basis, but not full-time
- HHA services on an intermittent or part-time basis, but not full-time
- PT, based on medical necessity
- SLP, based on medical necessity and reasonableness
- OT, based on medical necessity and reasonableness (OT can be provided in the absence of any other skilled care.)
- medical social services
- medical supplies
- medical equipment (Medicare Part B generally pays for 80 percent of the approved amounts, and the patient is responsible for the remaining 20 percent.)[7]

The length of time that care may be delivered is based on the medical reasonableness and necessity of the care to be delivered. Limitations do exist on the number of days and hours of care that may be received.

Part-time care is defined by Medicare as

- 28 hours a week of skilled nursing and HHA care
- services provided 7 days a week if they are provided for fewer than 8 hours per day
- allowable increase to 35 hours if Medicare agrees that the patient's condition merits the change

Intermittent care is defined by Medicare as

- 28 hours per week of skilled nursing care and HHA care, with increase to 35 hours a week if the patient's condition merits the change
- services provided 6 days a week
- in some cases, nursing and HHA services provided for a maximum of 8 hours a day, 7 days a week, for 21 consecutive days, with a defined extension beyond 21 days for extreme cases[8]

These limitations do not apply to therapy services, which may be provided for as long as they are deemed medically responsible and necessary.

The indemnity, health maintenance organization (HMO), and, more recently, large self-insured employer sectors have developed a broader understanding of the value of medically necessary home care. Initially, approvals for reimbursement were on a case-by-case exception basis, led by nurse case managers who arranged for complex long-term care, such as intravenous antibiotic therapy, in the home. The main driver was cost, with the added benefit of customer satisfaction. As these sectors became more creative, programmatic handling of home care began (e.g., supporting earlier discharge of new mothers and babies with one or two home visits and follow-up telephone calls). Hospitals initiated these efforts to differentiate themselves and increase margins under case rate contracts.

Commercial HMOs also followed the path of Medicare HMOs in seeking procedure-specific

(e.g., lumbar laminectomy) or disease-specific carve-outs. Programs focused on specific disease states require highly skilled professionals. Successful implementation of the programs hinges upon close working relationships of the discharge planning teams, which include inpatient and home care program coordinators, payer case managers, and physicians.

FINANCING HOME CARE SERVICES

Health care expenditures have significantly increased in the last 30 years, and the source of payments has undergone a fundamental shift. Private funds were far and away the primary payer source in 1960. In 1997, federal, state, and local funds represented just less than half of total expenditures (see Figure 26–8). Expenditures for home health care services have increased astoundingly since 1980. Home health care has been one of the fastest-growing segments of Medicare system expenditures, until the recent slowdown. It has grown from 2.9 percent of all Medicare payments in 1980 to over 9 percent in 1997. Figure 26–8 shows the growth in home health care expenditures nationally.

Home care services are paid for by a variety of payer sources, from public or private organizations to patients or responsible parties. There has been a shift in home care payer types. In 1980, federal funds accounted for 37 percent of home care payments (Figure 26–9). Private funds, including private health insurance and other private sources, contributed 38 percent. By 1997, federal funds had risen to 48 percent, an 11 percent increase. Medicare represented 83 percent, $12.8 billion, of those federal funds. (The federal fund figures recently declined slightly, from $15.5 billion in 1996 to $15.4 billion in 1997. Medicare's portion declined from $13.2 billion in 1996 to $12.8 billion in 1997.) By 1997, private source funds had declined to 23 percent, a 15 percent decrease from 1980. During the same period, out-of-pocket reimbursement remained the same at 22 percent, and state and local funds contributed 4 percent in 1980 and 7 percent in 1997, a 3 percent increase.

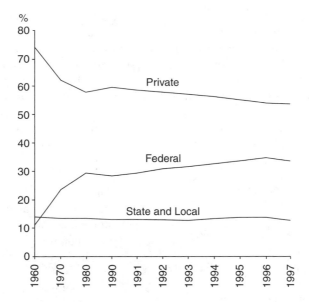

Figure 26–8 National Health Expenditures by Payer Type. *Source:* Reprinted from Office of the Actuary, National Health Statistics Group, Health Care Financing Administration.

Public third-party payers constitute the largest sector of funding sources. These payers include Medicare, Medicaid, the Department of Defense, the Maternal and Child Health Bureau, the Department of Veterans Affairs, Indian Health Services, Social Services Block Grant programs, workers' compensation programs, and other community service organizations.

Though federal programs continue to be the predominant funding source for home health care services, the changes in the reimbursement system made by the BBA of 1997 had a fundamental, lasting impact on home care providers. The BBA contained many provisions designed to reduce the cost of home health services. An interim payment system (IPS) for Medicare was

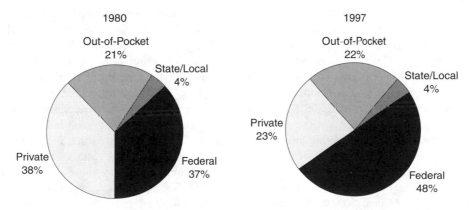

Figure 26–9 Home Health Care Payer Types. *Source:* Reprinted from Office of the Actuary, National Health Statistics Group, Health Care Financing Administration.

created effective October 1, 1997. Medicare reimbursement changed to the lowest of actual allowable costs, per visit cost limits, or agency per beneficiary annual limits (annual unduplicated Medicare admissions multiplied by the agency per beneficiary limit). IPS established the per beneficiary annual limit based on a mix of agency-specific costs and census region costs. The cost was defined from Medicare cost reports filed in 1994.

Additional provisions and clarifications to the BBA were approved by Congress in 1998:

- All agencies below the national median rate would be adjusted based on a formula blending the agency-specific rate and the national median rate.
- Agencies above the national median rate would receive no change.
- New agencies (agencies starting prior to October 1, 1998) would receive 100 percent of the national median rate.
- "New, new" agencies (agencies starting after October 1, 1998) would receive a per beneficiary rate of 75 percent of the national median rate.

Other provisions also illustrate the intent of HCFA to reduce overall expenditures and discourage the growth of new agencies.

- A prospective payment system (PPS) is being developed and becomes fully effective as of October 1, 2000. This will replace the IPS. HCFA is developing the unit of service (reportedly based on episodes of care) and how to apply a case mix adjuster. HCFA had expected to have industry case mix data from Outcomes and Assessment Information Set (OASIS) data. With the OASIS implementation postponed, HCFA reportedly will use limited OASIS demonstration project data.
- Nine census region geographic areas were created.
- A transfer provision from hospitals to skilled nursing facilities and home care agencies was created for 10 diagnosis-related groups and will involved partial reimbursement under certain circumstances.

- Cost limits by discipline were reduced on average 15 percent effective October 1, 1997.
- Cost limits by discipline will be further reduced by 15 percent effective October 1, 2000, regardless of the implementation of PPS.
- Venipuncture, an important qualifying skilled service, was no longer funded by HCFA.
- Provisions were established for proration of annual episodic rate between providers.
- Billing will be based on the site of service, not the location of the billing office or parent corporation, thus preventing agency offices in a higher-reimbursement urban setting from billing for services in a lower-reimbursement rural setting.
- Sequential billing was implemented but then eliminated as of July 1, 1999.
- Visits will be reported in 15-minute increments.
- Periodic interim payments will be eliminated October 1, 2000.

RECENT LEGISLATION AND REGULATORY ISSUES AFFECTING HOME CARE

There has been continuous scrutiny of home health care related to fraud and abuse of the reimbursement system. The focus has been primarily on the Medicare reimbursement system, with its incentives and opportunities for fraud and abuse. Operation Restore Trust (ORT) has been successful in detecting this fraud and abuse. The Secretary of Health and Human Services stated at one point in early 1998, at the height of ORT activities, that 40 percent of all Medicare home health care claims were fraudulent. The statement was reportedly based on results of sample claims audits. This statement and others like it created controversy and mistrust for lawmakers and to some extent the public. The ORT program was expanded from 5 to 12 states and eventually the whole nation. In late 1997, the ORT program introduced wedge audits as another tool in its review of home care.

These quick-hit, limited-focus audits have been particularly injurious to the home care industry. In fiscal year 1997, the Department of Health and Human Services identified $1.2 billion for recovery in collections, fines, settlements, and restitution. This represented a sixfold increase over 1996. Criminal and civil prosecution cases totaled 1,340 in fiscal year 1997, and over 2,700 providers were excluded from participation in federal and state programs. The home care industry has continued to struggle with this sustained level of scrutiny and investigation, with many providers going out of business due to demands for payback of overpayments as a result of ORT-related audits.

The BBA of 1997 contained additional provisions to fight fraud and abuse in home care, including the following:

- new penalties of $50,000 per violation for providers paying kickbacks for referrals
- requirements that providers disclose Social Security numbers and employer identification numbers so that past offenders may be screened out
- requirements for surety bonds from home health agencies
- a clearer definition of what qualifies as skilled services, to prevent unnecessary visits
- authority to deny payment to providers that bill in excess of what other providers bill for similar services

Surety bonds have been put on hold as a requirement for home health agencies, but the requirement is likely to be reinstated in the near future. Other actions by HCFA have included the following:

- Home health agencies are being asked about related business interests before admission as a Medicare provider. This will help determine if there are any previous instances of fraud and abuse and will also help to prevent unauthorized billings through nonexistent or nonapproved companies.
- Home health companies must have provided care to at least 10 patients requiring skilled services before being allowed to provide care to Medicare beneficiaries. At least 7 of those patients must be receiving care at the time of the survey for approval to receive a Medicare provider number.
- Claims review has increased to 25 percent of claims submitted. HCFA has set aside $10 million to perform audits, such as the compliance audits and wedge audits. This is nearly double past expenditures.
- Fiscal intermediaries have hired medical directors to advise claims processors and providers on medical necessity of care.

The provisions outlined herein and the effects of continued fraud and abuse activities have fundamentally changed the home health care industry.

MEASURING QUALITY IN HOME CARE SERVICES

The federal government and the home health care industry are aggressively pursuing initiatives to measure and improve the quality of home care services. Two rulings announced in March 1997 have affected the home health care industry. The first ruling revises Medicare's Conditions of Participation to include

- a requirement that HHAs be subject to criminal background checks
- the expansion of existing HHA qualifications to include only HHAs who have completed nurse aide training or competency evaluations
- active involvement of patients in the planning and conduct of their care through discussions between care providers and patients about expected outcomes of care
- a requirement that home care agencies coordinate all the physician-ordered care for patients

The second regulation requires that home health agencies use the OASIS. This standardized system is designed to monitor patients' condition, levels of function, and satisfaction. This system requires that each new patient receive a standardized assessment within 48 hours of admission. This assessment is designed to determine the patient's care and support needs. It is updated continually to monitor and track changes in the patient's condition. This continuous assessment would end upon discharge of the patient from the home health agency. Home health agencies are required to evaluate the OASIS assessments, track and submit this information, and incorporate changes in their quality improvement programs. These data sets can also be used by inspectors and surveyors to standardize the agency surveys and to identify improvement opportunities related to patient care and satisfaction.

The Joint Commission on Accreditation of Healthcare Organizations (Joint Commission) also monitors home health care organizations through a comprehensive quality survey process utilizing home care–specific standards. The most recent version of standards was published for 1999. The accreditation process is voluntary and conducted in three-year cycles. For home health organizations that are hospital based or affiliated with health systems, the three-year accreditation cycle generally coincides with that of the rest of the health system. The Joint Commission also conducts random, unannounced surveys on approximately 5 percent of accredited agencies.

EXAMPLES OF ADVANCED CLINICAL PRACTICES IN HOME CARE

Leading home care practices are not well documented, yet there are examples of wide variations and innovations. For instance, West Coast agencies have been successful in managing post–total hip replacement care in 6 to 8 visits with outcomes similar to those realized from 8 to 12 visits on the East Coast. Many managed care organizations are utilizing experienced home health clinicians to conduct health risk assessments (HRAs) in the home setting. The accuracy and completeness of the HRAs have been found to be enhanced when done in the home setting, especially when screening for high-risk members.

Recognizing the high incidence of psychosocially driven ED visits, a very large Southern home health agency has become creative in working with a number of hospitals to manage their Medicare risk ED visits. It has developed a triaging program that identifies patients before processing at the hospital and refers them to an adult day care program with after-hours homemaker care to effectively decrease ED visits and their related admissions by 25 percent.

An example of a procedure-specific clinical process that has been developed by another Southern agency for post-lumbar laminectomy using a combination of accelerated postoperative teaching and two home care follow-up visits reduced inpatient hospital stays from 5 or 6 days to 2 days.

The increasing number of frail elderly requiring medical management has led to the establishment of "home hospital" programs in a number of academic settings throughout the country. Typically, these services are overseen by a geriatric service line or a medical center's own home health agency. Patients are maintained at home, even through acute episodes, through a multidisciplinary approach that includes home visits by physicians and other geriatric clinicians, thereby minimizing the complications often seen when the frail elderly enter an institution.

Disease state case management companies have entered the market with a home care model that combines in-home environmental assessments and routine visits with up to daily telephone contact to maximize treatment compliance in chronic diseases such as congestive heart failure. These companies have shown the ability to significantly reduce ED visits, admissions, and overall costs associated with diseases such as congestive heart failure and asthma.

Academic medical centers focusing on medical and/or technological research have been turning to and testing telemedicine approaches. Some managed care organizations, seeking cost-effective alternatives, have begun to invest in telemedicine as a way to closely monitor patients' conditions without costly home visits or office visits. A 1996 study done by a West Coast managed care organization found that "video visits" averaged 18 minutes per patient, while in-person evaluations took an average of 45 minutes plus travel time. A successful telemedicine approach, however, typically involves a combination of actual home visits and telephone contacts.

It is unclear at this time what influence the Internet and Web-based access to information (good and bad) will have on the dynamics of home health care. Some agencies are already utilizing resources available on the Internet for patient education purposes. It will be increasingly important for providers to be aware of the information patients may be accessing in their homes, and to monitor for confusion or conflicting approaches to health care at home.

REFERENCES

1. Health Care Financing Administration, U.S. Department of Health and Human Services, Bureau of Data Management and Strategy, *HCFA Statistics,* publication no. 03394 (Washington, DC: 1996).

2. Health Care Financing Administration, press release, January 13, 1998.

3. K. Schworm and E. Gruenwedel, The Industry's Facts and Figures, *HomeCare,* July 1997, 36.

4. Schworm and Gruenwedel, The Industry's Facts and Figures, 36.

5. Schworm and Gruenwedel, The Industry's Facts and Figures, 36.

6. Health Care Financing Administration—Medicare and Medicaid, U.S. Department of Health and Human Services, *Medicare and Home Health Care,* publication no. 10969 (Washington, DC: 1996).

7. Health Care Financing Administration—Medicare and Medicaid, *Medicare and Home Health Care.*

8. Health Care Financing Administration—Medicare and Medicaid, *Medicare and Home Health Care.*

CHAPTER 27

Subacute Care within the Managed Care System

Kathleen M. Griffin

Subacute care emerged in response to pressures from third-party payers to provide a less costly alternative treatment setting to acute hospital care. Subacute care is provided both in specialty hospitals and in skilled nursing facilities (SNFs) and units. Because of variations in the definition of subacute care and in services furnished by self-named subacute providers, an accurate estimate of the number of subacute beds available in the United States is nonexistent. An industry review from 1995 estimated that, in that year, there were 720 subacute providers supplying 27,050 beds.[1] However, given the rapid growth of the industry between 1995 and 1998, it can be assumed that the number of subacute providers and the number of specialty hospital and SNF beds dedicated to subacute care have increased significantly. Among the 50 national long-term care chains alone, analysts put the current number of subacute beds at between 35,000 and 45,000.[2]

Definitions of subacute care have been prepared by a number of organizations. The definitions developed by two organizations, the National Subacute Care Association (NSCA) and the Joint Commission on Accreditation of Healthcare Organizations (Joint Commission), appear to contain the key components reflected in most other definitions (see Appendix 27–A).

CATEGORIES

In spite of the promulgation of definitions of subacute care by NSCA and the Joint Commission, there remains a great deal of confusion about exactly what subacute care is. This confusion is due to the lack of a federal definition of subacute care and to the fact that subacute care is commonly provided in three different settings: specialty hospitals, hospital-based SNFs, and free-standing SNFs. Each setting tends to focus on one or two of the four categories of subacute care: transitional, general, chronic, and long-term transitional.

Hospital-based subacute skilled nursing units typically focus on the first category, transitional subacute care. Subacute units in free-standing nursing facilities usually can be classified as general subacute or chronic subacute care units. Specialty hospitals (most often long-term care, prospective payment-exempt hospitals) focus on long-term transitional subacute care. Appendix 27–B describes the categories of subacute care, reflecting the key differences in service intensity and length-of-stay parameters.

SUBACUTE PATIENTS

Subacute patients vary in acuity levels and exhibit a variety of problems. *Subacute patients generally include the following:*

Kathleen M. Griffin, PhD, is President and Chief Executive Officer of Valley Consultants, Inc., in Scottsdale, Arizona, and National Director of Post Acute and Senior Services for Health Dimensions Consulting Group, Inc., a member organization of the Benedictine Health System, in St. Paul, Minnesota.

- medically complex patients who are chronically ill or have multiple medical problems or disorders (these patients need medical monitoring and specialized care and can be managed in a subacute setting)
- respiratory care patients who require ventilator weaning or ventilator care programs as a result of a respiratory disease, injury, or impairment or who require medical and nursing care as well as therapies to recover from an acute respiratory episode
- recuperating surgery patients who need rehabilitative therapy but no longer need an acute level of care
- patients who require rehabilitation for a variety of reasons, most frequently after orthopedic surgery or a stroke
- patients with brain injuries as a result of ischemic or hemorrhagic stroke, blunt trauma, or penetrating trauma
- cardiovascular patients who require a cardiac recovery or rehabilitation program, often related to congestive heart failure or cardiovascular surgery
- patients with such medical conditions as septicemia or osteomyelitis who require short-term intravenous therapy
- oncology patients who require radiation oncology services, chemotherapy, pain management, and rehabilitation
- wound management patients with chronic wounds (e.g., pressure ulcers, necrotic wounds, or peripheral vascular disease ulcerations) related to diseases that need management before the wounds will heal

SUBACUTE PROVIDERS

Although managed care organizations are increasingly becoming payers for subacute care, especially with the growth of Medicare risk health maintenance organizations, Medicare continues to be the major payer for subacute services. As a result, provider settings for subacute care, to a great extent, reflect the idiosyncrasies of the health care reimbursement system. Subacute care may be provided in hospital-based SNF units, subacute units in free-standing SNFs,

and in long-term care hospitals. Hospital-based SNF units may be found in acute care hospitals as well as in specialty hospitals.

Hospital-Based Skilled Nursing Facility Units

Hospital-based SNF units allow the hospital to create a continuum of care. Patients who no longer require the intensity of services typically found on the medical–surgical floor of an acute care hospital can be transferred to a subacute unit, where the sophisticated diagnostic, monitoring, and emergency response capabilities are available but the intensity of services is less. Programs in the subacute unit are oriented toward a patient's optimal functional independence at the time of discharge.

To be eligible for favorable reimbursement by Medicare, the hospital-based subacute unit must be licensed as a SNF unit. The result is that the hospital's performance under the Medicare prospective payment system (PPS) is improved. Hospitals reduce their inpatient lengths of stay for Medicare patients by utilizing the subacute SNF unit as a step-down or transitional facility.

For managed care organizations, hospital-based subacute units provide a low-cost alternative setting for patients who are not medically stable enough to be transferred to a subacute unit in a free-standing nursing facility or for patients who simply require a few additional days of inpatient care before being discharged home. The location of the subacute unit in the hospital facilitates patient–physician interaction and enhances the integration of services between the subacute unit and the hospital. For example, although the subacute unit's nursing staff usually will be different from the nurses who cared for the patient on the medical–surgical floor, rehabilitation staff who provided services to the patient while in a hospital bed may continue to provide services to the same patient in the hospital-based subacute unit. The subacute unit also can benefit from the hospital's quality improvement programs, infection control procedures, and management information system.

Although it is clear that there are many system and patient management benefits to hospital-based subacute units, the costs of patient care in these units typically are greater than the costs for care in subacute units in free-standing nursing facilities. In 1996, the latest year for reported data at the time of publication, the average cost per day for Medicare patients in hospital-based SNFs was $443; for Medicare patients in free-standing nursing facilities the cost was $292.[3]

Subacute Units in Free-Standing Skilled Nursing Facilities

The creation of a subacute unit in a free-standing SNF usually involves the establishment of a distinct area within the facility that is separated from the areas of the building dedicated to long-term care services. Subacute units in free-standing SNFs have separate nursing stations, patient rooms, and common areas so that subacute patients and long-term care residents and their families do not mix.

From the provider's perspective, the greatest challenge to the free-standing SNF that has created a subacute unit is to ensure that there is a cultural paradigm shift from a long-term care, custodial focus to a short-term recovery and rehabilitation focus, wherein the patient will be discharged home or to a less costly level of care in one to three weeks. To achieve this conceptual shift, the most successful subacute units in free-standing SNFs have staff who are dedicated to the subacute unit and are separate from the nursing, activities, and social services staff for the long-term care residents. In addition, the successful subacute unit employs a medical director who is different from the administrative medical director for the long-term care facility. Other components of successful subacute units are specific programs of care, outcomes measures, subacute unit-specific admission and discharge criteria, and care protocols that help ensure that patients in the subacute unit receive the services they need in a cost-effective manner.

Long-Term Care Hospitals

Long-term care hospitals are one of the types of hospitals that may be excluded from Medicare PPS reimbursement. Instead of being paid prospectively on the basis of diagnosis-related groups (DRGs), the PPS-exempt long-term care hospitals are paid a specific amount per Medicare discharge. The amount is established based on the individual hospital's costs during its initial year of PPS-exempt operations, subject to certain caps. The Medicare PPS exemption for long-term care hospitals, however, is slated to be discontinued in the future.

Long-term care hospitals provide services to patients who continue to require intensive or other acute inpatient care and have an average length of stay of 25 days or more. Patients in long-term care hospitals usually have complex medical conditions and multisystem failures that require more intensive care, monitoring, and emergency backup resources than are available in subacute units in free-standing nursing facilities. Patients may be admitted to long-term care hospitals either directly or from the intensive care unit (ICU) of an acute care general hospital.

Subacute programs in long-term care hospitals provide more hours of nursing care per patient day (6.5 to 9.0 hours) than are typically provided in subacute programs in hospital-based or free-standing SNFs. Also, average lengths of stay are longer than in SNF subacute care units. Patients in subacute programs in long-term care hospitals have an average length of stay of 32.9 days.[4]

Although the costs of subacute care in long-term care hospitals are higher than in SNF subacute units, long-term care hospitals' costs can be considerably less than those in an ICU in an acute care general hospital.

Specialty Hospital-Based Subacute Skilled Nursing Facility Units

Both long-term care hospitals and PPS-exempt rehabilitation hospitals may create subacute SNF units within the hospital. The subacute unit within a long-term care hospital would focus on medically complex patients who have met certain goals in the long-term care hospital and who no longer need the same intensity of services. Such patients would require continued inpatient care for their medical conditions, however, in order to eventually be discharged home or to a long-term care facility.

Free-standing acute rehabilitation hospitals may create subacute SNF units for patients who either are not medically stable enough to benefit from or unable to tolerate an intensive acute rehabilitation program (e.g., three hours or more of rehabilitation daily). These patients would be able to benefit from a less rigorous, subacute rehabilitation program (e.g., one to two hours daily). Although the average length of stay for patients in the acute rehabilitation hospital is 16 days,[5] the average length of stay for patients in the slower paced, less intensive rehabilitation program in the subacute SNF unit in the rehabilitation hospital may exceed 20 days. Typically, the costs of care in the subacute SNF unit of the specialty hospital would be less than the costs for acute care in the specialty hospital.

SUBACUTE CARE SITES IN THE FUTURE

Medicare payment for subacute care was changed significantly by the Balanced Budget Act of 1997. Prospective payment for SNF subacute providers began on July 1, 1998. The PPS for SNFs involves a case mix-adjusted per diem payment. Although there is a four-year phase-in for the federal per diem payment rates, many hospital-based SNF subacute units are realizing financial losses in their subacute units. The greater costs of hospital-based subacute SNFs are related both to the higher patient acuity level as well as costlier overhead in hospitals. The number of subacute units in hospitals is expected to decline in the future.

Subacute care provided in long-term care hospitals will also be subject to Medicare PPS in the future. Whether or not Medicare PPS will result in a reduction in the number of long-term care hospitals is unknown at this time.

SUBACUTE CARE WITHIN A CONTINUUM OF CARE

Subacute care cannot be viewed as independent from other levels of care within the care con-

tinuum. Appropriate utilization of subacute care requires an effective case management system that ensures that the patient receives the right care, at the right time, in the right setting, and for the right cost. The case management system must focus on the patient's condition and medical needs, level of family and/or other social support systems available, the services available within the continuum, the location of those services, and the health benefits available to the patient. Table 27–1 shows how transitional subacute care and general subacute care fit into a care continuum and contrasts subacute care levels with other components of the care continuum, such as intermediate/custodial care, skilled nursing care, acute rehabilitation, and acute care.

As health care providers in the United States convert from nonaffiliated, independent provider entities into integrated delivery systems, the four categories of subacute care are expected to be components of every system. During the current transition period from multiple independent providers to integrated provider networks, however, utilization of subacute care, as with other postacute health care levels, has tended to be stratified and fragmented. The regulatory requirements for subacute providers within SNFs, whether hospital based or freestanding, have served as barriers to easy transition of patients between the acute and subacute settings. For example, to transfer a patient from an acute hospital bed to a SNF bed in an adjacent unit within the hospital, the patient must be formally discharged from the hospital and formally admitted to the subacute unit. The admission procedures to the subacute SNF unit must comply with federal and state nursing facility regulations. Compliance with these regulations often means the completion of a substantial amount of paperwork related to the admission process.

Nevertheless, active case management within an integrated delivery system, wherein an individual patient's care is managed by the same case manager throughout the continuum, can help ensure that the transfer of a patient to the most appropriate level of care within the continuum occurs as seamlessly as possible.

Table 27–1 Subacute Care within the Care Continuum

	Acute Rehabilitation (from Lowest Acuity to Highest Acuity)					
	Nursing Facilities			Hospital		
Characteristics	Intermediate Care	Skilled Nursing	General Subacute	Acute Rehabilitation	Transitional Subacute	Acute
Patients (residents)	Restorative care	Medically stable/ rehabilitation	Medically stable/ rehabilitation	Medically stable, need acute rehabilitation	Medically sick/ highly complex care	Medically unstable/ invasive procedures/ most complex care
Physician visits	Monthly	Monthly	Weekly to biweekly	Daily	3–7 times/ week	Daily
Nursing (HPPD)	< 2.5, LPN/ CNA	2.5 to 3.5, 1 RN + LPN/ CNA	4.0 to 4.5, RN/LPN/ CNA	5.5 to 7, RNs and nursing assistants	5 to 6, RNs and CNAs	6.5 to 9, RNs and nursing assistants
Rehabilitation	Rarely	3 to 5 times per week	5 times per week	5 to 7 times per week, 3 hours/day	Daily PT, OT, ST	Daily PT, OT, ST
Average length of stay	2 years+	34 days	25 days	16 days	12 days	
Discharge	Death	LTC or home	LTC, home or acute rehabilitation	Home or general subacute	Home or SNF	Home or SNF

Note: CNA, certified nursing assistant; HPPD, hours per patient day; LPN, licensed practical nurse; LTC, long-term care; OT, occupational therapy; PT, physical therapy; RN, registered nurse; ST, speech therapy.

Courtesy of Health Dimensions Consulting Group, Scottsdale, Arizona.

PAYMENT FOR SUBACUTE CARE

Although the majority of subacute patients have Medicare as a primary payer, increasingly managed care organizations are including subacute care in their hospital or health care system agreements. *Managed care organizations and subacute providers negotiate payment under a variety of arrangements (also discussed in Chapter 12):*

- *Discounted fee for service.* The provider typically agrees to furnish subacute care services at a discount from its standard charges. The discount may be a percentage of the standard charge for all services or may be specific to the service or category of service.
- *Per diem.* The managed care organization pays the provider a fixed rate for each day that an enrollee is treated within the provider's subacute facility or unit. The per diem rate may be specified in a contractual arrangement or may be negotiated for each patient admission.
- *Per case.* The managed care organization pays the provider a fixed rate for each case of inpatient treatment. The rate will vary

depending on service category or patient category. This payment methodology is similar to the hospital DRG payment under Medicare.

- *Capitation.* The provider receives from the managed care organization a fixed payment per enrollee per month. For that monthly fee, the provider agrees to furnish specified subacute care to the payer's enrollees. The number of enrollees, as opposed to the utilization of services, controls the provider's revenues.

Today, the most common payment arrangement between managed care organizations and subacute providers is the per diem payment. In the contract between the subacute provider and the managed care organization, certain items and services typically will be included in the per diem rate, and items or services over which the provider has less control often will be excluded. Exhibit 27–1 lists usual inclusions and exclusions from a per diem rate negotiated between a managed care organization and a subacute care provider.

Per diem rates also may vary based on patient acuity as well as resources required by the patient. Subacute care providers often utilize a patient acuity measurement system to define subacute care levels, and each level has a different per diem payment amount. An example of subacute care per diem payment levels is shown in Exhibit 27–2.

Subacute care providers may include a stop-loss provision for patients whose acuity levels increase significantly during their inpatient stay in the subacute care unit or facility. Conversely, the managed care organization may include stipulations in the agreement that the patient will be reviewed weekly to determine whether a less expensive level of subacute care or discharge home or to a long-term care facility is appropriate for the patient.

SELECTING A QUALITY SUBACUTE PROVIDER

In most areas of the United States, managed care organizations have an array of subacute providers from which to select. Certain indicators of quality may be used as benchmarks in the selection process.

Accreditation

The size of the subacute provider marketplace and the number of alternative settings for managed care organizations have spurred the need for an agreed-upon set of national standards against which to judge performance, monitor service delivery, and determine the outcomes of care. While

---

Exhibit 27–1 Items and Service Usually Included in or Excluded from a Per Diem Rate for Subacute Care

INCLUSIONS
- Room and board (semiprivate)
- Nursing and personal services
- Rehabilitation
- Medical social services
- Recreation/activities program
- House toiletries
- Patient/family education
- Surgical dressings
- Dietary consultation
- Case management

EXCLUSIONS
- Special beds
- Ventilators
- Respiratory therapy
- Intravenous antibiotics
- Third generation pharmaceuticals
- Traction equipment
- Prosthetic devices
- Laboratory tests
- Radiology services
- Parenteral formulas, supplies, equipment

Courtesy of Health Dimensions Consulting Group, Scottsdale, Arizona.

Exhibit 27–2 Subacute Care/Per Diem Payment Levels

Level of Care	Level of Payment
Subacute care: special	Special arrangements. Patients with specialized care needs. Averages 6+ nursing hours per patient day and 0–2 hours of rehabilitation per day.
Subacute care: tier III	Patients requiring intense medical or nursing intervention and procedures, and/or rehabilitation. Definition of intense: 4.5–6 nursing hours per patient day and 0–2 hours of rehabilitation per patient day.
Subacute care: tier II	Patients requiring moderate to minimal medical and nursing procedures and moderate rehabilitation. Definition of moderate: 4–4.5 nursing hours per patient day and 0–1.5 hours of rehabilitation per patient day.
Subacute care: tier I	Patients requiring minimal medical and nursing procedures and interventions and minimal rehabilitation. Definition of minimal: 3.5–4 nursing hours per patient day and 0–1 hour of rehabilitation per patient day.
Skilled nursing care:	Patients requiring skilled care, 2.5–3.0 nursing hours per patient day and 0–2 hours of rehabilitation per patient day.

Courtesy of Health Dimensions Consulting Group, Scottsdale, Arizona.

a few states have licensure or Medicaid payment categories specific to subacute care, Medicare does not differentiate subacute care from the skilled nursing benefit for Medicare beneficiaries.

Two accrediting organizations have created standards for subacute providers: the Joint Commission and the Rehabilitation Accreditation Commission (CARF). The Joint Commission's standards related to subacute care are reflected in the standards for accreditation of long-term care facilities.[6] Certain of the approximately 600 standards have a subacute intent and are contained within 11 categories of standards for long-term care facilities:

- resident rights and organizational ethics
- continuum of care
- assessment of residents
- care and treatment of residents
- education of residents
- improving organizational performance
- leadership
- management of environment of care
- management of human resources
- management of information
- surveillance, prevention, and control of infections

CARF is the national accrediting agency that establishes standards for organizations serving persons with disabilities. Subacute providers may be accredited if they demonstrate compliance with the standards for comprehensive integrated inpatient rehabilitation.[7] Comprehensive integrated inpatient rehabilitation programs may be offered in hospitals or SNFs.

In selecting subacute providers, managed care organizations may wish to ascertain whether a provider is accredited by the Joint Commission or CARF.

Programs of Care

The subacute provider should have clearly defined protocols, care paths, or programs for the key categories of patients whom they serve. Admission criteria, continuing stay criteria, and discharge criteria should be delineated for each program. Programs may include one or more of the following:

- *Medically complex/postsurgical.* Patients in this program may require the following types of care:
  1. Active treatment of disease under the direction of a physician (e.g., administering intravenous medications, epidural medications, agents by continuous infusion pump, hypodermatoclysis monitoring/ evaluating signs and symptoms of condition change; teaching care to the patient and/or significant others; providing respiratory therapy and care; performing hemodialysis and peritoneal dialysis; evaluating effective intervention through laboratory values, signs, and symptoms)
  2. Postsurgical care (managing and evaluating drains and tubes, performing complex dressing changes, evaluating and assessing changes in wounds)
  3. Pulmonary care (managing tracheotomized patients)
  4. Nutrition management (enteral and parenteral feedings; monitoring the effect of intervention and therapeutic diets through weight, tissue turgor, wound healing, and laboratory values)
- *Wound management.* Patients in this program may need complex treatment and dressing procedures, whirlpool treatment and debridement, electrical stimulation, specialty beds and pressure-reducing devices, frequent laboratory evaluation, teaching, and ongoing assessment of the effectiveness of treatment by changes in wound status.
- *Rehabilitation.* These patients typically have medical complications or frailties that preclude their ability to tolerate or benefit from acute rehabilitation services. Patients with orthopaedic conditions, strokes, degenerative neurological disorders, and other medical complexities may require the combination of intensive nursing care and a low-intensity rehabilitation program.
- *Cardiopulmonary recovery/rehabilitation.* Patients in this program may have been hospitalized because of congestive heart failure, suspected myocardial infarction, or for cardiovascular surgical procedures. These patients typically are deconditioned as both a cause and an effect of acute treatment, possibly exacerbated by their stay in the ICU or by their course of treatment, resulting in malnourishment, weakness, frailty, and poor physical stamina. Patients also may have complicating co-morbidities that require subacute care following an acute hospitalization.
- *Respiratory.* Patients for subacute care typically have respiratory infections, pneumonias, or chronic obstructive pulmonary disease with medical complications. Some respiratory patients are on ventilators and are admitted to the subacute unit for ventilator weaning, intensive care, and intravenous infusions with antibiotics.

Clinical Staff

Clinical direction of a subacute program should be provided by a physician who is qualified by virtue of training and experience in the area(s) related to the program being offered. In addition to the medical program director, a medical staff of credentialed and privileged physicians should be created so that physicians can serve as either attending or consulting staff in the subacute unit or facility. A dedicated clinical staff for the subacute care unit or facility should report to a program director, who is responsible for the overall management of the subacute program. An interdisciplinary clinical team should include nursing and medical staff, social services staff, rehabilitation therapists, respiratory therapists, dietitians, pharmacists, and, as appropriate, psychologists and pastoral counselors.

Case Management

A case management system should involve appropriate coordination of care, allocation of resources, and an effective communication system with payers, families, physicians, and referral sources. The case management function usually is provided by a registered nurse. The goal of case management is to help the patient attain appropriate goals by the most cost-effective means. Case management is discussed further in Chapter 22.

Outcomes Measurement System

An outcomes measurement system should include an ongoing, organized, systematic method of evaluating the results of interventions and services relative to patient and family goals and expectations. The outcomes to be achieved in a subacute program include the resolution of medical problems and functional improvement. A key outcome for subacute care includes a reduction of rehospitalizations as well as a reduced risk of utilization of health care services after discharge from subacute care. Outcomes measurement and management is discussed further in Chapter 31.

Cost-Effective, Quality Care

The subacute program should incorporate admissions procedures that are as simplified as possible, given the need to comply with regulatory requirements. Throughout the subacute care program, the focus should be achieving optimal results in a reasonable time period so that the patient can be discharged home or to a less costly level of care. Operations should support patient and family dignity, realistic goal setting, and early preparation and planning for discharge.

CONCLUSION

The subacute care industry has rapidly evolved into a recognized niche within health care. Its continued growth will be dependent on a clear demonstration of the cost-saving potential of moving patients out of high-cost acute care hospitals and into low-cost subacute care units and facilities and on patient outcomes that demonstrate that subacute program treatment interventions have positive long-term effects. With the growth of managed care, cost-effective, quality subacute levels of care will continue to be important components of the continuum of health care.

REFERENCES

1. H.M. Ting, *Subacute Care: Analysis of the Market Opportunities and Competition* (Newport Beach, CA: Center for Consumer Health Care Information, 1995).

2. Reprinted from *Consumer Information: Subacute Care* (Washington, DC: American Health Care Association, August 14, 1999).

3. Prospective Payment Assessment Commission, *Medicare and the American Healthcare System, Report to Congress* (Washington, DC: Prospective Payment Assessment Commission, 1997).

4. Medicare Payment Advisory Commission, *Report to Congress: Medicare Payment Policy* (Washington, DC: 1999).

5. Prospective Payment Assessment Commission, *Medicare and the American Healthcare System.*

6. Joint Commission on Accreditation of Healthcare Organizations, *Comprehensive Accreditation Manual for Long Term Care* (Oakbrook Terrace, IL: 1998).

7. Rehabilitation Accreditation Commission, *The 1999 Medical Rehabilitation Standards Manual* (Tucson, AZ: 1999).

SUGGESTED READING

American Association of Critical Care Nurses. 1997. *Subacute Care, An Interdisciplinary Curriculum for the Care of Clinically Compromised Patients.* Aliso Viejo, CA.

Griffin, K.M., ed. 1995. *Handbook of Subacute Health Care.* Gaithersburg, MD: Aspen Publishers, Inc.

Griffin, K.M. 1999. Senior Strategies. *ADVANCE for Providers of Post-Acute Care* 2, no. 4: 38–44.

Griffin, K.M. 1999. Trade Secrets of the Prosperous. *ADVANCE for Providers of Post-Acute Care* 2, no. 2: 71–72.

Levenson, S.A. 1996. *Subacute and Transitional Care Handbook: Defining, Delivering, and Improving Care.* St. Louis, MO: Beverly Cracom Publications.

National Health Information, LLC. *Postacute Payment Report.* 1123 Zonolite Road, Suite 24, Atlanta, GA 30306–2016.

NSCA and Joint Commission Definitions of Subacute Care

The definition of subacute care developed by the National Subacute Care Association (NSCA) is as follows:*

Subacute care is a comprehensive, cost-effective inpatient level of care for patients who:

- have had an acute event resulting from injury, illness, or exacerbation of a disease process and have a determined course of treatment
- though stable, require diagnostics or invasive procedures but not intensive procedures requiring an acute level of care.

The severity of the patient's condition requires:

- active physician direction with frequent, on-site visits
- professional nursing care
- significant ancillary services
- an outcomes-focused interdisciplinary approach utilizing a professional team
- complex medical and/or rehabilitative care

Typically short term, subacute care is designed to return patients to the community or transition them to a lower level of care.

The definition developed by the Joint Commission is as follows:**

Subacute care is comprehensive inpatient care designed for someone who has an acute illness, injury, or exacerbation of a disease process. It is goal-oriented treatment rendered immediately after, or instead of, acute hospitalization to treat one or more specific active complex medical conditions or to administer one or more technically complex treatments in the context of a person's underlying long-term conditions and overall situation. Generally, the individual's condition is such that the care does not depend heavily on high technology monitoring or complex diagnostic procedures. Subacute care requires the coordinated services of an interdisciplinary team including physicians, nurses, and members of other relevant professional disciplines who are trained and knowledgeable in assessing and managing these specific conditions and in performing the necessary procedures. Subacute care is given as part of a specifically defined program, regardless of the site. Subacute care is generally more intensive than traditional nursing facility care and less intensive than acute care. It requires frequent (daily to weekly), recurrent patient assessment and review of the clinical course and treatment plan for a limited (several days to several months) time period, until the condition is stabilized or a predetermined treatment course is completed.

---

*Courtesy of National Subacute Care Association, Bethesda, Maryland.

**Source: © Joint Commission: *Comprehensive Accreditation Manual for Hospitals: The Official Handbook.* Oakbrook Terrace, IL: Joint Commission on Accreditation of Healthcare Organizations, Update 3, August 1999, pp. GL 25–26. Reprinted with permission.

Categories of Subacute Care

TRANSITIONAL SUBACUTE CARE

Transitional subacute care can be described as short-stay (5 to 30 days) hospital step-down care. Nursing care averages 5.0 to 6.5 hours of direct care per patient day. Licensed nurses provide 50 percent to 70 percent of the direct nursing care. Transitional subacute units are utilized for patients who require daily medical care and monitoring; highly skilled nursing care; an integrated program of rehabilitative therapies; and frequent utilization of pharmaceutical and laboratory services. Days in this type of subacute care unit serve as replacement hospital days to effect a significant reduction in acute hospital days. In other words, a transitional subacute unit actually serves as a substitute for continued hospital stays, not as an alternative hospital discharge placement. For example, stroke patients may be transferred to a transitional subacute unit on day four or five of hospitalization in the acute hospital, and coronary bypass patients who are not off the ventilator within four or five days may be transferred for a weaning program. Transitional subacute units typically have a variety of physician program directors or consultants, a dedicated staff of acute or critical care nurses, 24-hour respiratory therapy, and seven-day-per-week rehabilitation therapies.

GENERAL SUBACUTE CARE

General subacute units are most often utilized for patients who require medical care and monitoring at least weekly, short-term nursing care at a level of approximately 4.0 to 4.5 hours per patient day, and rehabilitative therapies that may extend from one to three hours per patient day. Short stay in nature (averaging 20–30 days), general subacute care units focus on patients who require rehabilitation, wound care, or intravenous therapies, often with other medical complications. Although there is some overlap in the clinical programs between transitional subacute units and general subacute care facilities, the key difference is the acuity level of the patients. The goal of both transitional subacute units and general subacute units is to manage the patient's recovery or rehabilitation in a cost-effective manner and to discharge the patient home or, in some cases, to a less expensive level of care, such as long-term care or an assisted-living facility.

CHRONIC SUBACUTE CARE

Chronic subacute units manage patients with little hope of ultimate recovery and functional independence, such as ventilator-dependent patients, long-term comatose patients, and patients with progressive neurological disease. Typically, these patients require nursing care at a level less than that of the general subacute unit (three to five hours per patient day), medical monitoring biweekly to monthly, and restorative therapies, usually provided by nursing staff with guidance from rehabilitation therapists. These patients either will eventually be stabilized so that they can be discharged home or to a long-term care facility or will expire. Their length of subacute stay is in the 60- to 90-day range.

LONG-TERM TRANSITIONAL SUBACUTE CARE

Long-term transitional subacute facilities most often are licensed as long-term care hospi-tals rather than as nursing facilities. Average length of stay is greater than 25 days. These fa-cilities provide care for acute ventilator-depen-dent or medically complex patients. Because they are housed in hospitals, the patients are vis-ited daily by attending physicians. Nursing staff tend to be primarily registered nurses, and nurs-ing hours per patient day may range between 6.5 and 9.0 depending on the types and acuity levels of the patients.

CHAPTER 28

Hospice and End-of-Life Care

Anne C. Dye, Peggy H. Rodebush, and Geri Hempel

MEDICAL MANAGEMENT AND END-OF-LIFE CARE

Introduction

The main focus of health care in the United States during the past 50 years has been the aggressive treatment and eradication of disease and illness to prolong life. Overall, that approach has proven to be very successful. During the past 50 years, experts have created vaccines to eliminate such communicable diseases as polio and smallpox, developed noninvasive surgical inter-

Anne C. Dye, MHSA, is a Manager in Ernst & Young LLP. She holds a master's degree in Health Services Administration from George Washington University and has over 15 years of operational, marketing, and business development experience in health care, including ambulatory, home health, hospice, and long-term care. Ms. Dye has been Director of Business Operations for the nation's largest hospice company, with responsibility for strategic planning, nonclinical operations, fiscal management, budget preparation and maintenance, service line development, and new site development.

Peggy H. Rodebush, RN, MSN, is a Partner in Ernst & Young LLP, where she specializes in health care business transformation. In this role, she works with leading health care providers across the United States. She is a nationally recognized post–acute care and medical management expert and is a frequent speaker at national conventions.

Geri Hempel is a Senior Manager for Ernst & Young in Tampa, Florida.

ventions, and perfected open-heart surgery so it is now routine. Partly because of these medical and public health advances, the population in the United States has increased rapidly. The number of older adults in particular has grown and will be likely to continue to grow at a tremendous rate. In fact, the population aged 65 and over is expected to increase by 35 percent between 1996 and 2015 (Figure 28–1). These demographic changes, an attempt to contain costs, an increasing need for individuals to take control over their own health care, and changing attitudes about death and end-of-life care have influenced medical management decisions over the last 10 years.

Clinicians now face an array of chronic illnesses that progress to terminal phases. These illnesses may be classified by site of care (e.g., acute care facility, nursing home, home, hospice), by disease (e.g., congestive heart failure, cancer), or by intervention (e.g., cardiothoracic surgery, diagnostic radiology). However, dying patients experience illness in a much more fragmented way than dying patients once did. They get care from a number of provider sites, with multiple medical specialists attending to illnesses that cannot be cured. It is a challenge to standardize pain management across providers, and quality of care and outcomes are not adequately measured. According to the Center to Improve Care of the Dying:

> End-of-life care often falls to physician specialists focused on rescue (e.g., oncologists, cardiologists) when

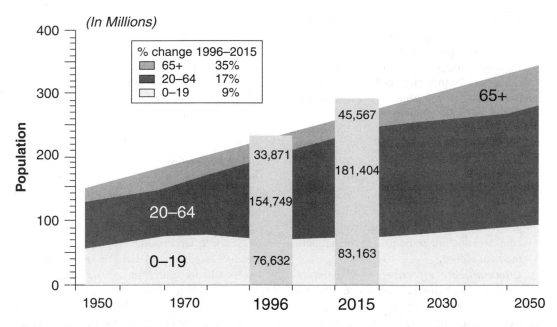

Figure 28-1 Actual and Projected Population Growth, 1950 to 2050. *Source:* Reprinted from U.S. Bureau of the Census, 1996.

multi-disciplinary teams attentive to nursing and social issues could provide more effective and more reliable supportive care. All the evidence suggests that patients and their families have little ability to reshape care to better meet their needs compared with the influence of provider supply and established care patterns.[1]

U.S. health care advances and research are respected throughout the world. However, in the zeal to become the world's greatest healers, U.S. health care providers have failed to sufficiently educate and prepare health care professionals to provide end-of-life care. It is not enough to teach our health care professionals how to identify and refer terminally ill patients to appropriate palliative care providers. Every health professional who deals directly with patients or families needs to know how to deal both compassionately and competently with the seriously ill and dying

patient. Palliative and end-of-life care needs to be incorporated into the traditional care delivery model and into managed medical care.

Most people agree that whenever possible a person should be able to die at home, surrounded by family. However, some health care providers have trouble understanding what the patient and family want and how to assist them during the end-of-life process. It is critical for health care providers to understand that the patient and family members want to be treated with compassion and dignity, to receive support and care, to have adequate pain control, to avoid becoming victims of technological advances, to know when everything that can be done has been done, and to be assured they will not be abandoned by the health care system when the end of life is near.

Given the likelihood that end-of-life care will be given by a variety of health care providers, it is important that there be an interdisciplinary approach to the process. (The concept is quite similar to that discussed in Chapters 22 and 23 regarding case and disease management; medical managers and health care providers should familiarize themselves with those chapters and apply the same principles, which also will be further discussed in this chapter.) *To effectively manage the end-of-life process, the health care team must take the following steps:*

- *Reduce fragmentation of care.* Develop certainty regarding who should care for people with terminal illness, and work from an established plan. Initiate advanced care planning discussions within 24 hours of a patient's admission to a facility or home care, and document the plan in the patient's medical record.
- *Communicate effectively and compassionately with the patient and family.* Assess providers' own feelings, attitudes, and expectations surrounding death, and consider patients' cultural and spiritual diversity. Begin bereavement assistance and support before the patient dies.
- *Assess and treat all dimensions of health.* To improve the quality of life for the terminally ill patient, assess the patient's physical, psychological, emotional, and spiritual well-being.
- *Identify ways to obtain resources.* Assist the patient and family in identifying and accessing all available community resources.
- *Develop and/or adopt standardized tools.* Use standardized tools to assess symptoms experienced by the patient at the end of life. Based on the information obtained from the assessment, develop a plan that provides for intervention and symptom management. Develop pain and symptom management protocols.
- *Collaborate with an interdisciplinary team.* The care provided to the patient should be coordinated and available around the clock, and providers should be sensitive to diversity issues as well as the patient's and family's needs. Each member of the health care team should make a specific contribution, but others should offer assistance. For instance, pain management

is generally in the realm of the physician, but other members of the team should be able to provide insight into pain management as well.
- *Reduce fear and anxiety.* Both pharmacological and nonpharmacological protocols should be developed to manage the patient's symptoms and reduce his or her stress.

It is the health care provider's obligation to help terminally ill patients receive the support and care that they deserve, and it is the obligation of the health plan's medical management function to assist in the process. Americans are not dying well. The Study to Understand Prognoses and Preferences for Outcomes and Risks of Treatment found there is still too much unwarranted aggressive treatment against patients' wishes. Despite advances in pain relief, too many people are still dying without adequate pain control. There is still not enough communication between physicians and patients; many patients (or their families, when appropriate) are never asked about treatment preference. We can and should do better.[2]

Hospice care represents a comprehensive solution that fits many different models of medical care management. It is a mode of care for the terminally ill patient that may or may not encompass facility-based care.

THE BASICS OF HOSPICE CARE

Philosophy

Hospice is a remarkable treatment modality. It often combines state-of-the-art pain management techniques and pharmacology with counseling, personal care, and (when desired) spiritual support to provide comfort to individuals entering the last months of their lives. Because hospice is focused on care for the terminally ill, it encompasses areas not typically considered part of medical management or the health care continuum. Hospice professionals are called upon to aid patients and families in understanding the meaning of their lives, and deaths; to reconcile themselves to death as the natural end to life; and to fulfill last wishes when possible.

As defined by Flexner, hospice is a "medically directed, nurse coordinated program providing a continuum of home and inpatient care for the terminally ill patient and family. It employs an interdisciplinary team acting under the direction of an autonomous hospice administrator."[3] It is also a philosophy of care that accepts death as a natural part of life, seeking neither to hasten nor prolong the dying process, and existing solely to support the terminally ill person and family through the last stages of life. The primary objective of hospice is to provide supportive care and counseling to the dying patient and family. The clinical goals of hospice are oriented toward palliative care, with pain management and symptom control, not curative therapy, as the primary focus of treatment.

Senator James Randolph, in establishing National Hospice Week (SR 170, March 18, 1982), described hospice well: "Hospice is a place, people, and a philosophy. It is a system of care that seeks to restore dignity and a sense of personal fulfillment to the dying. The focus is on the patient and the family, rather than on the disease—and the aim is not to extend life, but to improve the quality of life that remains."

The first hospice in the United States opened its doors in 1974. It began as a grassroots reaction to the depersonalization of care and treatment for the dying patient. Early supporters of hospice recognized a need to isolate the terminally ill patient from the treatment-based philosophy of the acute care setting. Today, hospice has developed into an integral component of the health care continuum.

The majority of hospices in the United States today are designed to provide care in patients' homes. Although services may be provided in a variety of settings and facilities, the home setting is a main component of the hospice philosophy. Providing care in this nontraditional health care setting also helps to contain the costs of care. Care for a terminally ill patient in the hospital setting is expensive, and hospice provides a cost-effective alternative to the high-technology, labor-intensive acute care setting. But more important, the home setting provides the greatest comfort to the dying patient.

Structure and Organization

Hospices in the United States come in all shapes, sizes, and reimbursement models. Programs are located in office buildings, physician offices, and even churches. These programs may have contractual arrangements with other facilities to provide inpatient care. They may be freestanding with their own inpatient unit or may be affiliated with a hospital or an extended care facility. A program may be for-profit or not-for-profit. Currently in the United States, most hospices are not-for-profit. The staffing model may be all paid staff, a combination of paid staff and volunteers, or all volunteer. Volunteers in an all-volunteer model work cooperatively with agencies and other programs to provide the necessary services.

Regardless of the structure of the hospice, standards have been established by both regulatory agencies and the National Hospice Organization (NHO) that serve as the guiding principles for care of patients and families. These standards include requirements that care be available 7 days a week, 24 hours per day, with integrated inpatient and home care services available. Volunteers are used to assist with the patient and family during both the dying process and the bereavement process. An interdisciplinary team guided by a medical director plans and provides the care. The family members and anyone important to the patient participate in hospice care, working closely to support the patient during the final days.

FINANCING AND REIMBURSEMENT

Medical Coverage for Hospice Services

Hospice care is financed through several mechanisms: Medicare, Medicaid, private insurance, private pay, donations, and grants (Figure 28–2). While reimbursement for hospice services increased dramatically in recent years, Medicare remained the primary payer, representing 68 percent of hospice revenues, or $1.2 billion in 1994.[4] Medicaid hospice expenditures

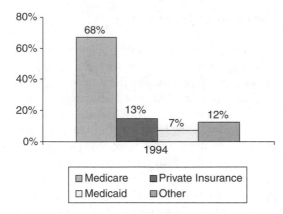

Figure 28–2 1994 Hospice Revenues by Payer. *Note:* "Other" indicates donations, grants, and private pay. *Source:* Data from National Hospice Organization Fact Sheet, 1996.

grew as well, totaling $197.6 million in fiscal year 1994, an increase of 53 percent over the $128.9 million spent in fiscal year 1993.[5]

The Medicare Benefit

The Medicare hospice benefit is available under Part A of Medicare. Medicare reimburses Medicare-certified hospices on a per diem basis by level of care, including routine home care, inpatient care for acute symptom management, continuous care, and respite services for durations of not longer than 5 days per episode. Persons electing hospice must have a terminal diagnosis with a life expectancy of 6 months or less, as certified by a physician. Care is provided in a variety of settings, including inpatient facilities and homes.

Persons electing to use their hospice benefits under Medicare must select this benefit in lieu of traditional Medicare reimbursement for all treatments related to their terminal illness. Services provided include skilled nursing, physician services, home health aides, social workers, home medical equipment, palliative medications, laboratory testing, volunteer services, and bereavement counseling. These services are available 24 hours a day.

Managed Care

The key factors affecting hospice's success within a managed care environment include demonstration of quality, evidence of cost-effectiveness, and willingness to share financial risk.[6] Providers are developing strategies to address these factors, as increasing numbers of hospice programs have begun to compete for managed care contracts. For example, in Baltimore, Maryland, hospice services for patients with acquired immune deficiency syndrome (AIDS) covered by Medicaid are included in an AIDS care capitation program designed by Johns Hopkins AIDS Service, Johns Hopkins HealthCare LLC, the Maryland Department of Health and Mental Hygiene, and health maintenance organizations (HMOs) in Maryland.[7]

Eighty-two percent of managed care plans offered hospice services as part of their benefit package in 1993.[8] Managed care organizations (MCOs) such as Kaiser Permanente, Group Health Cooperative, and AvMed continue to recognize the value of hospice and operate their own hospice programs that serve Medicare, Medicaid, and private clients. However, there is little information published on the managed care dollars spent providing hospice services. Additionally, hospice is still a carve-out for Medicare HMOs, and patients have to disenroll from Medicaid HMOs to receive Medicaid hospice benefits.

SIZE OF THE U.S. HOSPICE INDUSTRY

Agency Characteristics

In 1995, the overall revenues for the hospice market were estimated at $2.8 billion, with Medicare revenues at about 68 percent, or $1.9 billion (unpublished data, A.C. Dye, Ernst & Young, 1997). According to the NHO, there were approximately 3,200 operational or planned hospice programs in all 50 states and Puerto Rico as of April 1998. The Health Care Financing Administration (HCFA) reported that 1,857 Medicare-certified hospice programs provided hospice services to 309,336 Medicare patients in 1995.[9] The average length of stay

(ALOS) for these patients was 59 days. Home health agency–based hospices made up 27 percent of the hospice market, while not-for-profit hospices represented 72 percent of the hospice industry (Figure 28–3).[10]

Patient Information

In 1995, approximately one out of every seven individuals who died in the United States from all causes (not just terminal illness) received care from a hospice program.[11] HCFA statistics show that hospice patients are more likely to be older, married, and living with their spouse.[12] The most prevalent diagnoses at admission were related to cancer (71 percent), diseases of the heart and circulatory system (9 percent), and respiratory conditions (6 percent).[13] The number of hospice patients is expected to more than double between 1990 and 2000 (Figure 28–4).

Still, too few terminally ill persons receive care from hospice services. According to the Hospice Association of America, patients who received care other than hospice often died in the hospital instead of in the comfort of their own homes. Just

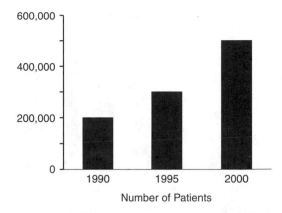

Figure 28–4 Hospice Patient Growth, 1990–2000. *Note:* 2000 figures are projections. *Source:* Data from The Hospice Market, FIND/SVP, 1996.

13 percent of hospice patients were admitted to the hospital two months prior to their death, compared to 41 percent admitted from other care providers during the same period of time.[14]

Growth Projections

The number of Medicare-certified hospices more than doubled between 1990 and 1995, largely as a result of the 1989 congressional mandate to increase reimbursement rates by 20 percent (Figure 28–5). The provider that emerged with clear market dominance was VITAS Healthcare Corporation. Fiscal year 1998 revenues for VITAS were about $220 million; the second largest hospice, VistaCare, reported revenues of only about $75 million for the same period. It is expected that, with the aging of the baby boomer population and the increasing acceptance of hospice, the number of hospice programs will increase rapidly. The House Ways and Means Committee projected an average annual growth rate for hospice at 25 percent through the year 2000.[15]

MAJOR POLICY ISSUES

Ethics

Hospice began as a philosophy of care inspired by volunteer activity. As a philosophy,

Figure 28–3 1995 Ownership Status of Hospice Programs. *Source:* Data from National Hospice Organization Fact Sheet, 1996.

Figure 28–5 Medicare-Certified Hospice Growth by Year. *Source:* Reprinted from Health Care Financing Administration Bureau of Policy Development, 1995.

hospice is straightforward. It accepts death's inevitability and seeks to support the dying person and his or her family and friends through palliative symptom control, counseling, and support. Challenges arise when this philosophy is translated into a program of care that receives third-party reimbursement. The hospice must justify the terminal diagnosis of the population served, provide care and services at a lower cost than most programs oriented toward cure, and be responsible for providing many nontraditional services, such as spiritual support, anticipatory grief counseling, and bereavement care.

Any health care program that limits resources and aims to serve a select group of people must provide justification for the allocation of benefits. Traditionally, the allocation of benefits has been the responsibility of the government, third-party payers, or charities and not the responsibility of the provider. The Medicare regulations established for hospice have set criteria that the hospice must observe for patient selection and restriction of treatment modalities. However, it is the providers' responsibility to define which services a patient receives and which resources are used in caring for him or her.

By its very nature, hospice has the potential to involve ethical and moral dilemmas. The NHO has issued a code of ethics to guide the staff of hospice and palliative care programs through issues such as physician-assisted suicide, confidentiality, removal of artificial nutrition and hydration, and pain control.[16] In order to address these issues, hospices should support the development of internal ethics committees. Ethics committees are a key component in any health care organization and can assist in establishing baseline criteria regarding organizational policy for service provision, patient population, questions regarding suicide and assisted suicide, responsibility for resource conservation and allocation, and responsibility for care for those patients who do not qualify for services. As consumers of health care become more educated regarding the hospice philosophy and hospices develop a major role in the health care continuum, hospice ethics committees will play a vital role in how the medical community provides comfortable, compassionate, and palliative care to the terminally ill.

Legal Issues

In recent years, health care providers have been faced with a growing awareness of and concern regarding the legal and regulatory issues surrounding the industry. Hospice providers may be at a particular disadvantage because of the type of care they provide. Legal issues may arise from a variety of areas, including, but not limited to, malpractice, wrongful death, negligence, and nontreatment. The fact that a hospice is believed to provide a valuable service does not necessarily protect it from potential legal issues. To succeed, a hospice needs to understand the situations that could lead to litigation and have safeguards developed to minimize exposure to liability.

One of the most important safeguards a hospice can have to reduce its exposure to legal issues is a quality improvement program. Properly implemented, a quality improvement program will provide the hospice with tools for continuous improvement throughout the organization, thus reducing potential liability issues. Equally important is a risk management program designed to reduce liability exposure and foster an awareness within the organization regarding legal liabilities. While risk management programs must be tailored to individual organizations, the following basic elements should be included:

- continuing review of insurance to determine adequacy of coverage
- ongoing review of the physical premises and equipment to discover and correct defects
- ongoing personnel performance appraisals and revision of hospice policies so that those policies reflect adequate quality of care measures
- maintenance of systems for investigating adverse incidents to prepare a defense and to develop procedures for avoiding future occurrences
- support of grievance procedures to handle patient and family complaints, solve problems, and prevent litigation[17]

Care Provision

The advent of Medicare certification in 1983 created extensive requirements with which hospice programs must comply to be eligible for federal reimbursement. Currently, Medicare requires hospice programs to be responsible for providing certain core services—including skilled nursing, social work, and counseling—performed by noncontract employees. Noncore services may be provided by contract employees and include physician services, home care aide/homemaker services, physical therapy, speech therapy, occupational therapy, volunteer services, and bereavement counseling. Additionally, the hospice is required to provide all medications, laboratory work, medical equipment, and supplies that relate to the terminal diagnosis. While the Medicare program dictates the scope of services to be provided, the hospice defines how and to what extent services will be provided. Following an in-depth admission process, the hospice admits the patient into the program. Next, during an interdisciplinary team conference, a plan of care is established outlining the services the patient will receive. The care plan is then modified based on the patient's

needs throughout the course of care. Services may be provided in the home or in an inpatient setting.

The hospice recognizes the special needs of the terminally ill patient, and all programs and services are developed to meet those needs. Although hospice programs may provide services in different ways, there are certain fundamental guidelines in developing the care delivery model. These guidelines distinguish hospice from other programs. ***Hospice care is:***

- exclusively for the terminally ill
- focused on the patient and family
- provided to the family through the bereavement period
- provided by an interdisciplinary team
- medically directed
- available 24 hours a day, 7 days a week
- a service that uses volunteers as an integral part of the program

SERVICE MODELS

Hospices may be licensed in several ways, depending on the affiliation of the provider. It is important to model potential cost report and other financial implications before choosing the licensure category for newly licensed programs. Additionally, there are criteria that must be satisfied for each licensure classification.

The Government Accounting Office classifies hospice providers into the types discussed below. There are specific advantages and disadvantages to each model. The community or organization must address all planning issues prior to determining which hospice type is best.

Free-Standing Hospice

The free-standing hospice is a separate facility providing both inpatient and home hospice services. Inpatient services may be provided by the hospice or contracted with a local hospital or nursing home. The considerable start-up costs for a free-standing hospice and the continued operating expenses require aggressive financial planning.

Hospital-Based Hospice

Hospital-based hospice programs are a distinct unit of a hospital that provides inpatient hospice services, also known as a palliative care unit. The program may provide home hospice services through its own hospital-based hospice or through a contracted arrangement with a free-standing program. The hospital unit generally requires remodeling of the physical plant to adapt to the hospice concept. A hospital-based program may have less autonomy than a free-standing program. However, it does have increased access to hospital resources and the medical community. The hospital-based hospice is guided by the governing board of the hospital, and the mission and philosophy of the hospice are generally those of the hospital.

Reimbursement is generally provided through the Medicare hospice benefit and other third-party payers. Due to the hospital affiliation, there may be an enhanced opportunity for inclusion of the hospice in managed care contracts.

Hospice Affiliated with an Extended Care or Skilled Nursing Facility

Some hospice programs are a distinct part of a skilled nursing facility (SNF) or an extended care facility (ECF). Home hospice arrangements are generally provided through a community-based or a facility-based hospice. Many patients in a nursing home have a terminal illness, and the hospice provides the opportunity for the patient and family to take advantage of additional services. The hospice improves the continuity of care offered to the nursing home patient.

The mission and philosophy of the hospice complement those of the ECF or SNF. The hospice is governed by the facility board. Reimbursement is provided through the traditional Medicare hospice benefit and some limited third-party payers. A facility-based hospice may have some opportunities for recruitment of staff and volunteers, depending on the reputation of the facility in the community.

Hospital-Based Hospice Home Care

This type of hospice is a hospital-based home health agency that provides hospice services. Inpatient services are provided either through the hospital's separate part or through a contracted arrangement with an ECF or SNF.

In this arrangement, the mission and philosophy of the hospice complement those of the home health agency and the hospital. The hospice may function as a semiautonomous program of the home health agency. If the inpatient unit is with the hospital, continuity of care is enhanced through the availability of the various programs. This arrangement provides patients with the opportunity to transfer among programs easily. There is the potential, however, for home care and hospice programs to compete for referrals with common hospice diagnoses such as cancer and to question when to refer patients from curative treatments in home care to more palliative hospice programs.

Reimbursement is provided through the Medicare hospice benefit and other third-party payers. The hospital-based hospice has an improved opportunity to obtain other third-party contracts due to the affiliation with the home health agency and the hospital.

Community-Based Home Health Agency Hospice

Part of a community-based home health agency, this type of hospice requires an agreement with a facility to provide inpatient services. The mission and philosophy of the hospice complement those of the home health agency, and the governing board of the agency provides the direction for the hospice. The hospice could function as a semiautonomous program that enhances the services offered through the home health agency. The home health–based hospice can provide services to a patient through a terminal care program of the home health agency prior to admitting the patient to the hospice. Reimbursement of the hospice is generally through the Medicare hospice benefit and other third-party payers.

HOSPICE COST AND STAFFING

The budget structure for hospice is unlike that for many other levels of care, primarily because reimbursement is both per diem and all-inclusive of services provided for the terminal illness. But as with other levels of care, there are direct costs such as employee salaries and fringe benefits, transportation, equipment, and supplies. Indirect costs include public relations, fund-raising activities, volunteer recruitment and training, staff education, and space considerations. *Key statistics to include when developing the budget for a hospice include the following:*

- *Average daily census.* The average daily census is the number of patients that the hospice will care for on a daily basis.
- *Average length of stay (ALOS).* The ALOS is the average number of days a patient will stay on service. The most expensive time during the course of care for a hospice patient is during the admission process and when the patient is actively dying. If patients are admitted to service late in the course of illness, the costs to the hospice will be high. Also, if patients are admitted for a short period of time, the true value of the hospice for the patient and the family is not recognized.
- *Payer mix.* The Medicare hospice option pays a per diem rate. The average daily home rate was approximately $96 as of 1998. Many MCOs may pay a per diem rate or break out the services.
- *Staffing ratio.* Critical to determining the staffing ratio are the ALOS and the level of care needs of the patient. If a hospice's ALOS is less than 30 days, the level of care is greater and therefore the staffing needs will be higher than those for a hospice whose ALOS is greater than 60 days. Patients referred to the hospice who are close to death require more visits and services than patients who stay on the program longer. The NHO indicated that for programs with an ALOS of 60 days, approximately 34.5 visits are made. They were dis-

tributed as shown in Figure 28–6. The NHO recommends the staffing plan shown in Table 28–1.

- *Expenses per patient per day for major costs.* The hospice is required to provide all supplies, equipment, drugs, and treatments directly related to the terminal diagnosis. To accurately determine the cost of operating the hospice, the cost of medical supplies, equipment, drugs, and treatment must be monitored. Typical productivity standards are shown in Table 28–2.

SPECIALTY PROGRAMS

Hospice care continues to be a relatively new field of practice in the U.S. health care system. There are many innovative programs that serve the terminally ill in unique and caring ways. Examples of these programs are described below.

Zen Hospice Project Residence Program

This program operates a four-bed hospice residence. The primary goal of the project is to provide care and support to patients with terminal illnesses in a homelike setting. The residence is a restored Victorian home with high ceilings, fireplaces, and a patio and garden. Services are available to people with AIDS, cancer, and other life-threatening illnesses. Family and friends are encouraged to visit and actively participate in the

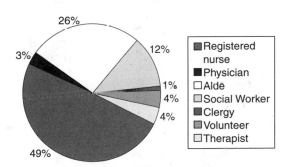

Figure 28–6 Distribution of Staff Providing Visits for Programs with ALOS of 30 Days. *Source:* Data from National Hospice Organization.

Table 28–1 Hospice Staffing Recommendations

Discipline	Daily Census	FTEs*
Registered nurse	8–12	1
Social worker	20–30	1
Chaplain	40–60	1
Home health aide	12–15	1
Volunteer coordinator	60–80	1

*FTE = Full-time equivalent
Source: Data from National Hospice Organization.

patient's care. Medical services are provided 24 hours per day, 7 days per week, through a collaboration with Visiting Nurses and Hospice, a program of the California Pacific Medical Center.

Hospice in Nursing Homes

Florida's Panel for the Study of End-of-life Care reported that in 1997, Florida hospice programs served 46,608 patients, just under 2,000 of which were in nursing homes. While end-of-life care alternatives to the traditional hospice model are being piloted in nursing homes through mechanisms such as Robert Wood Johnson Foundation grants, at least one hospice provider has developed hospice services specifically designed to address the nursing home population. VITAS Healthcare provides long-

Table 28–2 Hospice Provider Productivity Standards

Discipline	Average Visits per Day
Registered nurse	3.7
Licensed practical nurse	4.2
Social worker	2.5
Home care aide	4.5

Source: Data from National Association for Home Care, 1997. Not for further reproduction.

term care (LTC) teams that are dedicated to the care of terminally ill nursing home patients. In addition, it provides assistance to the LTC facility in state surveys, palliative care education for staff, and bereavement support for families and facility staff.

Pediatric Hospice Programs

The death of a parent or a loved one is devastating. However, nothing is more traumatic for a family than the loss of a child. Pediatric hospices are being developed nationwide to provide support and services to this special population. The family of a pediatric patient may be more likely than other families to use the services of a pediatric hospice during both the dying process and the bereavement process. These hospices are designed especially to provide the necessary support and services.

Disease State Management Protocols

Several hospices have begun to provide disease-specific care to terminally ill patients (again, readers are urged to review Chapter 23). VITAS Healthcare has developed an emergency response plan for chronic obstructive pulmonary disease (COPD) hospice patients. The plan is designed to provide immediate intervention in respiratory crises and to decrease emergency department visits and hospitalizations. The Hospice of North Central Florida, in cooperation with 6 other hospices around the country and under direction from Dr. Joanne Lynn of the Center to Improve Care of the Dying, is piloting disease management protocols for COPD and congestive heart failure (CHF). The program focuses on CHF and COPD patients nearing the end of life (the last 2 to 3 years). The goals of MediCaring are to improve care at the end of life by developing appropriate, optimal, cost-effective services that blend the best of palliative care with the best of medical and disease management and to propose sustainable service, financing, and regulatory reform in Medicare through a national demonstration project involving health care provider organizations nationwide (including hospices, large group practices, Medicare MCOs, and the Veterans' Affairs Health Care System).

Florida Palliative Home Care Program

The Florida Palliative Home Care Program is a new Medicare-certified home health agency developed by five hospices serving 16 counties in Florida. It offers care to chronically ill preterminal patients and provides a hospicelike range of care to those not yet eligible for the hospice benefit. It is thought that this model will also increase the length of stay in hospice for this patient population, as patients will be discharged to the participating hospices earlier than from more traditional home health, community, or acute care providers.

Hospice Care of Rhode Island AIDS Case Management Program

Hospice Care of Rhode Island, a partner of the Lifespan Healthcare System, developed an AIDS hospice program using Ryan White Title II funding in the early 1990s, primarily as a response to increasing mortality rates for this population. Recently, it has implemented a case management program in collaboration with the Miriam Hospital Clinic, as treatment advances in recent years have increased the chronicity of the high-risk AIDS population in its service area. It is hoped that this program will avert hospitalizations and improve quality of life for and management of preterminal AIDS patients as they approach hospice-appropriate stages in the disease process.

FUTURE INTEGRATION AND AFFILIATION STRATEGIES

Utilization of hospice care services has increased tremendously in the last 10 years, primarily as a result of the implementation of the acute care prospective payment system in 1982 and the move to increase Medicare hospice reimbursement rates in 1989. Concern about escalating costs and overutilization of services has shaped current reimbursement trends in both the public and the private sectors. Accordingly, the market is beginning to change dramatically as network and provider consolidation continues and strategic integration and affiliation trends accelerate. The next 5 years will see a dramatically changed business and health care environment within the post–acute care industry. The key challenge for hospice care providers will be to develop and implement effective strategies to address these changing factors in an environment increasingly dominated by managed care, including:

- probable shift of Medicare from fee-for-service prospective payment reimbursement structures to Medicare HMO products (a trend that slowed in 1998 and 1999 but is likely to pick up again)
- selective managed care contracting strategies
- vertical integration strategies for post–acute care providers (e.g., nursing homes, rehabilitation centers, home health providers, and hospice providers as integrated service lines)
- increasing need for disease management product line development
- strong information technologies that bridge service lines

It is clear that hospice will continue to provide needed care to the terminally ill and that it will remain an important service to individuals and families, including those in managed care programs. It is equally clear that it will become more integrated with other modalities of care and that the need for hospice will increase for the foreseeable future. Hospice and end-of-life care can no longer be dealt with on a case-by-case basis but must be fully integrated, just as case management and disease management are.

REFERENCES

1. Center to Improve Care of the Dying, http://www.gwu.edu/~cicd/ (accessed 11/2/99).
2. L. Snyder, Die Hard: End-of-Life Care in America, *Pennsylvania Medicine,* July 1996, 10–11.
3. J.R. Flexner, The Hospice Movement in North America—Is It Coming of Age? *Southern Medical Journal* 72 (1979): 248–250.
4. National Hospice Organization, *Fact Sheet* (Arlington, VA: 1996).
5. Hospice Association of America, *Hospice Facts and Statistics* (Washington, DC: 1996).
6. M. Michal, Managed Care: The Characteristics of a Successful Hospice, http://www.rbvdnr.com (accessed October 1997).
7. M. Kusinitz, Johns Hopkins To Announce AIDS Capitated Care Program, http://hopkins.med.jhu.edu/newsmedia/press/1997/january/1997.htm (accessed January 1997).
8. Lewin-VHI, Inc., *Hospice Care: An Introduction and Review of the Evidence* (Arlington, VA: National Hospice Organization, 1994).
9. K. Beebe, *Hospice State Summary* (Washington, DC: Health Care Financing Administration, Bureau of Data Management and Strategy, Office of Health Care Information Systems, 1996).
10. National Hospice Organization, *Fact Sheet*, 1996.
11. National Hospice Organization, *Fact Sheet.*
12. National Center for Health Statistics, *An Overview of Home Health and Hospice Care Patients: Preliminary Data from the 1993 National Home and Hospice Care Survey; Advance Data from the Vital and Health Statistics of the Centers for Disease Control and Prevention,* publication no. 256 (Washington, DC: 1994).
13. National Center for Health Statistics, *An Overview.*
14. P. Lemkin, Hospice: Can It Work within Managed Care? *Caring,* August 1997, 22–28.
15. House Ways and Means Committee, *1996 Green Book* (Washington, DC: 1997).
16. American Health Consultants, Tips for Deciding about a Hospice Ethics Committee, in *The 1996 Hospice Manager's Resource Bank* (New York: 1997).
17. M. Richards, *Medical Risk Management: A Preventive Legal Strategy* (Gaithersburg, MD: Aspen Publishers, 1982).

Clinical Pathways: Linking Outcomes for Patients, Clinicians, Payers, and Employers

Richard J. Coffey and Sarah S. LeRoy

INTRODUCTION

Clinical pathways are important tools that link patients, clinicians, managed care organizations and other payers, and employers and help achieve both high-quality and cost-effective care. Clinical pathways have improved the planning, coordination, and evaluation of care as well as the communication about care. In earlier publications we have referred to clinical pathways as "critical paths."*

This chapter provides an overview of the concepts, approaches, and uses of clinical pathways and offers guidance for developing and implementing clinical pathways based upon the knowledge gained at the University of Michigan Health System (UMHS) and other organiza-

tions. Giffin and Giffin estimate that 60 percent of U.S. hospitals now incorporate some form of clinical pathway into patient care.[1] In a managed care environment, there is greater emphasis on coordination of services and efficient use of resources across multiple settings, such as inpatient settings, outpatient settings, and homes.

Clinical pathways foster collaborative goal setting among multiple care providers for specific case types. Outcomes that have been discussed and agreed upon by a whole team are more likely to be achieved. Changes or variations in outcomes are more likely to be attended to. There is less chance of confusion for the patient, the family, the care providers, and the payer concerning the intent of care, expected activities, and expected outcomes.

When outcomes are related to processes that will lead to achieving those outcomes (the pathway), payers and health care providers are more likely to agree upon resources necessary for care. Pathway development is also based on data from research and benchmarking. Clinical path-

Richard J. Coffey, PhD, is Director of Program and Operations Analysis and Director of Health System Planning at the University of Michigan Health System, an Adjunct Associate Professor in Industrial and Operations Engineering at the University of Michigan, and an Adjunct Professor at the Union Institute in Cincinnati, Ohio. He has authored and coauthored over 45 publications, including three coauthored books and multiple book chapters, for which he has received several book awards. He has given over 120 professional presentations at regional, national, and international conferences.

Sarah S. LeRoy, MSN, RN, is a clinical nurse specialist in pediatric cardiology at C.S. Mott Children's Hospital in the University of Michigan Health System.

*Previous publications include R.J. Coffey et al., An Introduction to Critical Paths, *Quality Management in Health Care* 1, no. 1 (1992): 45–54; R.J. Coffey et al., Extending the Application of Critical Path Methods, *Quality Management in Health Care* 3, no. 2 (1995): 14–29; and R.J. Coffey et al., Critical Paths: Linking Outcomes for Patients, Clinicians, and Payers, in *The Managed Health Care Handbook,* 3rd ed., ed. P.R. Kongstvedt (Gaithersburg, Md.: Aspen Publishers, Inc., 1996), 301–317.

ways help health care providers to have input into the payers' guidelines for "reasonable" care.

BACKGROUND AND TERMINOLOGY

Critical path method (CPM), program evaluation and review technique (PERT), project management, and related approaches have their roots in construction and industrial applications, where there is a need to coordinate multiple contractors and activities to complete a project on time and within limited resources. CPM calculations use estimates of average times, whereas PERT calculations use three time estimates: optimistic, most likely, and pessimistic. Within the health care industry, several different terms are used, including clinical pathways, critical paths, CareMaps® (Center for Case Management, South Natick, Massachusetts), clinical guidelines, clinical protocols, CPM, and algorithms. There are no universally accepted definitions of these terms, although the underlying concepts are very similar. As long as an organization's leaders understand the concepts, they can select whatever terms seem best for their organization. Some operational definitions are offered below.

In 1992, Coffey and colleagues described the basics of critical paths for health care: "A critical path is an optimal sequencing and timing of interventions by physicians, nurses, and other disciplines for a particular diagnosis or procedure, designed to minimize delays and resource utilization and to maximize the quality of care."[2(p.45)] In 1995, they noted that "a critical path is the sequence of activities that takes the most time to complete."[3(p.15)]

When first introduced, the term "critical path" caused some confusion in health care organizations due to multiple interpretations of the word "critical." Clinically, the word "critical" refers to the urgency of a patient's clinical condition. There is the critical care unit, and patients are said to be in critical condition. From the perspective of critical path methodology, however, "critical" refers to the sequence of activities that take the most time. So the term "clinical pathways" has been introduced to represent the application of critical path techniques to health

care. Organizations may choose to use terms such as "time-limiting path," which clarifies that the goal is to coordinate resources and care to minimize the duration of care;[4,5] or CareMaps, which clarifies that the map describes the care provided.[6,7] CareMaps also include outcome information.

Schriefer offers a useful distinction between the terms associated with pathways and those associated with algorithms or guidelines: "The pathway provides an overview of the entire production process from start to finish, not only pieces in the process, and can be used to reduce variation in the production process."[8(p.485)] "Conversely, algorithms often guide clinicians through the 'if, then' decision-making process, such as a variation from a pathway. Algorithms, which were initially developed for handling complex mathematical equations, usually address patient responses to a particular treatment or condition."[9(pp.485–486)]

SCOPES AND USES

Depending upon the nature and requirements of the population whose care is being managed, there are different types of guidelines and clinical pathways.[10] Exhibit 29–1 lists types of guidelines and pathways for populations in different states of health.

Many hospitals, health systems, and managed care organizations have developed guidelines and/or clinical pathways related to one or more of the states of health described in Exhibit 29–1. The distinction between a guideline and a clinical pathway is based upon the type and structure of information. For example, UMHS has developed several evidence-based medical management and disease management guidelines, including guidelines for asthma, diabetes mellitus, essential hypertension, venous thromboembolism, and peptic ulcer disease. These guidelines are available on line to clinicians. UMHS has also developed many clinical pathways. Similarly, the Agency for Health Care Policy and Research has developed and provides over the Internet many types of clinical information and evidence reports (*http://www.ahcpr.gov/clinic*).

Exhibit 29–1 Types of Guidelines or Pathways for Different States of Health

State of Health	Type of Guideline or Pathway
Healthy	Prevention and screening practice guidelines
Stable chronic disease and stable at risk	Stable chronic disease practice guidelines
High-risk or unstable chronic disease	High-intensity management guidelines
Hospitalized	Clinical pathways

Courtesy of Dr. J. Billi, University of Michigan Health System, "Partnership Health: A Partnership between Ford Motor Company and University of Michigan Health System," presented at the 1999 Duke Private Sector Conference on Integrated Health Delivery Systems, March 22-23, 1999, in Winston-Salem, NC.

Most examples used within this chapter are from hospitals because clinical pathways are most often used for episodes of care related to hospital admissions.

Clinical pathways can be applied using different scopes, just as a microscope can be used at different levels of magnification. The use of clinical pathways and guidelines of different scopes is particularly important for managed care organizations. *Sample scopes include the following:*

- *Inpatient care.* Clinical pathways are most commonly used for inpatient care. These pathways are initiated either at the time of admission or at the time of a surgical procedure, and they typically end at the time the patient is discharged. As length of stay is shortened, some clinical pathways now include selected pre- and posthospitalization care as well.
- *Complete episode of care.* These clinical pathways begin at the time the patient presents at the physician's office requiring diagnosis, and they end when the patient has completed all therapeutic care related to that episode of illness. This scope of clinical path addresses care across multiple geographic settings, including inpatient care in a hospital, outpatient care at a clinic or physician's office, and home care.
- *Specialized applications.* Clinical path methods can also be used for specialized

applications such as for ambulatory surgery patients, renal dialysis patients, or patients in an intensive care unit.
- *Life and health management.* For health and medical management, clinical guidelines are more common than clinical pathways. However, clinical pathways can be developed for management of chronic conditions. These might be used to coordinate the care of patients with hypertension, asthma, cancer, and other illnesses and achieve the highest-quality and most cost-effective care practices.

The scope chosen affects the geographic setting of care and the resources involved. The scope for clinical pathways will be addressed again under "Environment" below.

Clinical pathways have many important uses:

- *Clarifying the "big picture" of planned care.* Traditionally within hospitals, physicians write orders each day, but often other members of the care team are unaware of the overall plan for care. The overall plan for care may be even less clear within ambulatory care and other settings, where care providers do not see each other regularly. Lacking knowledge of an overall plan, nurses, pharmacists, therapists, personnel in ancillary departments, and others carry out each day's orders but cannot plan ahead. Hence, breakdowns in communication and delays are common. Clinical pathways direct care toward agreed-upon end-points that are expected outcomes.

- *Planning and coordinating care.* During development of clinical pathways, the teams of physicians, nurses, pharmacists, therapists, and others discuss the coordination of appropriate care based upon data, expert opinion, and consensus. Thus, the different specialties and disciplines are acting in a coordinated, rather than independent, manner.
- *Establishing expectations.* Clinical pathways developed by a multispecialty, multidisciplinary team establish specific expectations about the actions of all personnel, timing, and outcomes of care.
- *Reducing variation of care.* An almost uniform outcome of using clinical pathways is reduction in the variations in clinical care.
- *Educating and orienting.* Clinical pathways provide an excellent tool to educate staff, students, and others regarding treatment plans and expected outcomes. This represents a substantial deviation from the traditional way of educating hospital officers or residents, medical students, nurses, and others. (The traditional approach is for each specialty or profession to educate its own students as actions are taken, with little information about the overall plan or treatments provided by others.)
- *Benchmarking.* Clinical pathways provide an excellent mechanism to study alternative care plans and patient outcomes. Many health care providers and managed care organizations compare clinical pathways and learn which pathways had the best outcomes (see Chapter 31 for further discussion about clinical outcomes).
- *Facilitating communication.* Probably one of the best uses of clinical pathways is to communicate the planned care and expected outcomes among clinicians, patients, families, payers, and others. Managed care organizations, for example, might approve services based upon use of a clinical pathway.
- *Improving the working environment.* The process of developing and using clinical pathways encourages cooperation and mutual understanding of everyone's role in providing high-quality, cost-effective care. This leads to an improved working environment.
- *Clarifying patient responsibilities.* Clinical pathways clarify what is expected of patients on a daily basis. If the patient is expected to ambulate, take medications, do breathing exercises, and do other things, the pathway will clearly state so.
- *Reducing legal exposure.* If a physician is providing care using a clinical pathway or guideline based upon documented clinical evidence and concurrence of several physicians and other clinicians, it is much more difficult for the patient, family, or others to claim negligence on the part of the caregivers (see also Chapter 45).[11]

ENVIRONMENT

Successful development and use of clinical pathways is not just a matter of learning the analytical technique. Clinical and administrative support of this process are crucial to the success of such a program. Time must be dedicated to clinical path development, training, monitoring, and data analysis if pathway outcomes are to be met.

Success is vitally tied to creating the right environment for clinical pathways. *The following conditions will exist in a good environment:*

- *Strong reason to change.* Change occurs only when people perceive that there is a reason to change. Without an understanding that change is necessary, physicians, nurses, other clinicians, payers, and others will continue to practice as they have in the past. Business, government, and payers are seeking to control costs without sacrificing quality of care, and this is driving many of today's changes.
- *Champions.* Involvement of respected clinicians from all disciplines is necessary for broad acceptance of clinical pathways. Look for teams of physicians, nurses, pharmacists, therapists, and others that believe clinical pathways will help them. Working

with the champions to demonstrate success with pilot studies will encourage broader participation.

- *Willingness to challenge current practices and boundaries.* It is very important that the environment encourage clinicians and support staff to challenge current practices, such as current clinical protocols, settings where care is provided (e.g., inpatient, outpatient, home), roles of individuals providing services (e.g., physicians, registered nurses, physician assistants, technicians, family members), and timing of activities. One of the keys to challenging the boundaries is to think about the whole episode of care, not just the inpatient portion. The time in a hospital may be very short, but the total time the patient's care is managed may be substantial.
- *Desire to standardize.* One of the most significant changes facing physicians is the introduction of more standardization of clinical practice and the move away from the independent, autonomous practice of the past. Many physicians consider clinical pathways, algorithms, and other guidelines part of "cookbook medicine." For clinical pathways to succeed, the environment must encourage physicians and other clinicians to standardize care to the extent helpful, then address appropriate exceptions. The idea is to reduce inappropriate and unnecessary variations in care rather than to replace the critical thinking of caregivers. Clearly, caregivers must assess variations in patient condition and progress, known as patient variation, and determine whether deviations from the pathway are appropriate.
- *Same scope of services.* It is important that managed care organizations cover the same scope of services as addressed by the clinical path. For example, a broad-scope clinical path addressing the complete episode of care related to a knee replacement might address prehospitalization care in the physician's office, preadmission testing, inpatient care, outpatient physical therapy, durable medical equipment, and home care.

However, if a managed care company covers only inpatient care and selected outpatient therapy, clinicians will tend to utilize these more expensive services and minimize services that result in direct costs to patients. Thus, managed care organizations should consider extending coverage of services when broad-scope clinical pathways demonstrate cost-effectiveness and quality.

DEVELOPMENT

Clinical pathway development may vary with the organization and the team, but the following steps provide a useful approach to developing a clinical path:

1. *Select the diagnosis, procedure, or condition.* Although this may sound obvious, there are some cautions. As discussed above, there should be a strong reason for change and a champion. In addition, it may be helpful to do an initial sensitivity analysis of where extra costs and problems exist. Comparing length of stay and costs with those of other physicians or organizations will point out areas for improvement. Similarly, look for those services that contribute most to the length of stay and costs. If, for example, 80 percent of the costs for a surgical patient are associated with the surgical procedure, spending large amounts of time on a postsurgical clinical path may address postsurgical length of stay but may miss the major opportunity to reduce costs.
2. *Define the scope.* Will the clinical path address the inpatient stay only, inpatient plus outpatient follow-up care, the whole episode of care, or another scope?
3. *Select a multidisciplinary team.* As with quality improvement projects, the team should include all types of key clinical and nonclinical staff involved with the scope of care included in the clinical path.
4. *Flowchart the process and collect baseline information.* Most clinical path efforts begin by flowcharting the current

processes and noting current practices and outcomes through documentation of clinical practices and review of medical records. This approach helps team members understand the complexities of, precedent relationships (those that define activities that must be completed before other activities can begin) in, and current variations in practice within the process before instituting change. Time estimates for different activities are helpful to clarify understanding. Assembling research and clinical evidence, benchmark information, and clinical pathways from other organizations for the same diagnosis, procedure, or condition is valuable. If another organization is found to achieve similar outcomes with substantially shorter lengths of stay or at substantially lower cost, further information should be gathered about how that organization achieves those results.

5. *Identify outcomes.* When developing a clinical path, it is important to begin by defining the specific desired patient outcomes. Ideally, these outcomes should be defined as final goals relating to the patient's functional status. When defining outcomes, it is helpful to think in terms of what specific outcomes the patient must achieve.

  • Define the outcome criteria to be discharged from the hospital, to return home, and to return to daily activity. The focus here should be on the most important criteria. All clinical activities should be addressed as part of the clinical path, but some are not as important to the overall progress toward the desired outcomes. It is useful to contrast patient outcomes related to physiological progression or functionality with system outcomes, such as patient transfer or discharge. Focusing on the system-generated boundaries may prevent people from finding more creative alternatives to achieving the desired patient outcomes. These same patient out-

comes are used to develop the tool for monitoring variance from the pathway and planned outcomes.

  • Be specific. Use objective, quantitative terms and measures, to the extent practical.

  • Be alert to changes in criteria due to new clinical practices, new technology, changing resources available in different settings, and other changes. For example, UMHS has been able to change the discharge criteria related to stable heart rhythm by using a home care agency with experienced cardiac care nurses to monitor patients at home.[12] In this case, the discharge criteria were achieved earlier in the treatment course and resulted in the emergence of a new clinical path.

6. *Define intermediate patient care objectives.* Although not currently done by most teams at UMHS, the next logical step in defining the clinical path is to define intermediate patient care objectives necessary to achieve the desired outcomes, such as breathing room air or ambulating. Care planning should be based upon the clinical and support activities required to achieve the intermediate patient care objectives leading to the major outcome criteria. To the extent possible, the intermediate objectives should be related to the patient condition rather than system outcomes or constraints.

7. *Determine the activities that are necessary to achieve outcomes.* Next, all the activities required to accomplish the outcomes and intermediate objectives should be identified. There may be some confusion about what are activities and what are events. Activities are actions that require time and resources to complete, whereas events are milestones that have no time factor. Activities are often grouped into categories such as consults, tests, patient activities, treatments, medications, diet, and patient and family education. Including events may be helpful to clarify progress.

8. ***Determine precedent relationships.*** An activity that must be completed before a subsequent activity can begin is called a precedent. Certainly, care providers understand precedent relationships within the scope of their own practice. However, formalizing the sequence of all activities and the precedent relationships is difficult but important, particularly for coordination among professions. In part, this is difficult because care providers have different conceptual frameworks of how care should be organized, different information, and different involvements and priorities for activities. The more formalized definitions of precedent relationships and activity times stimulate important discussions, which often result in more efficient care. To identify the precedents for each outcome, intermediate objective, and activity, providers must ask, "What must be completed before this can begin?" A flowchart/network format showing the steps of the care process helps providers reach consensus and discover opportunities for improvement.

9. ***Question current practices.*** During development and use of pathways, it is very important that all current practices be questioned. Simply replicating current practice in pathways may be an acceptable place to start, but improving practice requires serious questioning of what is done, when it is done, who does it, where it is done, how it is done, and why it is done. What criteria are really necessary for the patient to be discharged? What care can be provided at home or on an outpatient basis? What intermediate patient care objectives or outcomes are really necessary to accomplish the desired outcomes? What activities contribute? What activities are unnecessary or not directly related to the key discharge criteria? Do different practices really result in different outcomes? Asking these questions means analyzing current practices to identify those activities that help attain and improve outcomes and to eliminate or give less attention to those that are less important to outcomes. As a mechanism to create more innovative ideas, it may also be helpful to pose the questions as "Why *can't* we do it another way?" Ask whether hard evidence exists to prove that an approach will not work. Asking the "why not" questions stimulates more creative approaches. If no counterevidence exists, then a new approach can be tested to determine its effectiveness.

10. ***Determine activity times.*** Some health care organizations discuss the time requirements of activities in general but do not determine times for every activity. Discussions of general time requirements may help with understanding of the process. However, the times of all activities must be determined to calculate the time-limiting path. Different approaches can be used to estimate activity times. Initially, most teams develop consensus estimates involving small interdisciplinary efforts. Analyses of medical records can provide frequency data and times of certain events, from which activity times can be estimated. After a pathway is in use, analyses of variations can provide additional data. Formalized time studies are the most accurate but are infrequently done. It should be noted that activity durations can be changed by changing the processes, the productivity, or the amount of resources allocated to an activity. For example, after a coronary artery bypass graft (CABG) procedure, an aggressive monitoring of intake, output, and patient weight can shorten the amount of time needed for the patient to "dry out," or reduce to preoperative weight. One of the distinctions between clinical pathways and medical management and disease management guidelines is that pathways state time expectations rather precisely, whereas guidelines often prescribe care based upon changes in the patient's condition or broad time guidelines.

11. ***Determine the critical path.*** The critical path can be charted by summing the times of the respective activities and intermediate outcomes to calculate the total duration of each path through the network or flowchart. The path with the longest time requirement is the critical path. Because the critical path is intuitive to the clinical team, the formal calculation of the critical path and float/slack times for shorter duration paths may not be done. These calculations are done most easily by computerized project management software such as Microsoft Project, Harvard Project, or InstaPlan.

12. ***Implement and monitor pathways.*** Once consensus is reached on a pathway, it is implemented and monitored. Pathways should be viewed as guidelines for coordinated care that regularly change based upon changes in clinical practice, new technologies, and resources available in different settings. Consequently, it is acceptable to initiate pathways without 100 percent clinician agreement. Clearly, variations in patient condition may require alterations in pathway activities. Outliers are allowed and their outcomes documented. Those data are then used to subsequently review and revise the pathway. By analyzing data comparing variations in practice, costs, and outcomes, clinicians are able to reduce future variations. As with any tool, if the clinical pathways are not regularly used in the care of patients and updated as new evidence is found, the pathways will become obsolete.[13,14]

APPLICATION

In practice, the majority of clinician effort toward clinical pathways involves using them in daily care of patients. Many health care organizations assign a case manager, pathway coordinator, or another member of the health care team to monitor all patients on clinical pathways. Richards and colleagues describe a sample process to initiate and use critical paths, or clinical pathways, for an inpatient care episode.

1. Pathway coordinator is notified of admission.
2. Head nurse/designee assigns appropriate bed on unit.
3. Pathway coordinator initiates patient on pathway by:
   – Documenting in unit log (handwritten or computer database).
   – Entering dates on preprinted orders.
   – Entering dates on pathway.
   – Placing completed pathways in plastic folder on bedside chart and in main chart.
4. Pathway coordinator talks with admitting physician to clarify any questions related to caring for this patient while looking at clinical pathway and preprinted orders.
5. Pathway coordinator talks with the nurse providing care for this patient to clarify any questions.
6. Variance documentation takes place throughout the admission and upon discharge; pathway coordinator completes the variance record and the unit log.
7. Ongoing communication between outpatient and inpatient care providers facilitates smooth transition of patient care through the continuum.[15(p.36)]

The clinical path serves as an important tool for daily communication and coordination about clinical activities, support activities, expected outcomes, and the patient's progress.

The clinical path is only one tool in patient care. Any program that uses a pathway must have a method to evaluate the patients' progress while on the pathway and to evaluate the effectiveness of the pathway. UMHS staff have developed variance tools to assess deviations from the planned pathways.

Variances from expected activity along the clinical path, or inability to meet intermediate objectives, must be monitored. Because these objectives are constantly monitored, action can be taken proactively when a variance is identified. In some cases, knowledge of the pathway allows for corrective action before variances occur. For example, if a physician orders a complete blood count and chemistries to be drawn every day, and the pathway specifies these to be drawn on days 1, 3, and 5 only, timely monitoring can circumvent these labs from ever being drawn by having the orders changed. While retrospective monitoring takes place, it is less than optimal because variances may already have taken place.

It is also necessary to identify clinical events or activities that have a direct impact on pathway outcomes and are schedule dependent. Examples of these are the ordering of needed consults and initiation of discharge planning. While the pathway may describe when to begin these activities, the variance tool describes the last point at which the activities can be initiated before an outcome or resource use will be affected. Another example might be that the pathway states that the patient should begin an ambulation protocol within 6 hours of return from surgery. The outcome is that the patient walks the length of the hallway independently by the time of discharge. The team may decide that an intermediate outcome is that the patient walks at least a certain number of feet by 24 hours after surgery. If the patient cannot meet the intermediate outcome time frame, a consult may be needed, and the consult time must be built in so the patient can still meet the intended discharge on the third day. Still another example of clinical events or activities that affect pathway outcomes is a 5-day course of continuous 24-hour chemotherapy, where completion of 5 days of chemotherapy is one of the pathway outcomes. A critical event or activity that must occur every day is the initiation of each bag of chemotherapy, on time and infused over the appropriate hours, to meet the final outcome of a certain amount of drug given over 5 days, or 120 hours. A variance in this process would be the development of patient toxicities resulting in delay of chemotherapy—a patient variance. On the other hand, if the first day's bag was hung late due to delay in nursing time to initiate, this would be a clinician variance.

Documentation of variances from the clinical path is important both to the care of the patient and to the continued improvement of the care processes and clinical pathways. As Richards and colleagues state:

> When a variance occurs between expected and actual treatment plan of care, documentation should identify the variance, its type (patient, clinician, or system), and its effect on outcomes achievement. This should be followed by a review of aggregate data about multiple patients and the long-term outcomes achieved. Only patient variances should be addressed in the patient record. For legal reasons, clinician and system variances may be tracked and recorded separately as part of a more confidential quality assurance document. Variance data collection routinely has been labor-intensive, especially when the information is collected in narrative form. When variances are collected outside the patient record they should be recorded in a quantitative format that is user-friendly and clear, allowing clinicians to use the data to identify trends requiring timely action plans.[16(pp.35–36)]

ALTERNATIVE FORMATS AND SAMPLE USES

Critical path methods include a number of formats for information displays and associated calculations that can further enhance understanding and provision of health care services. Although some of these formats are not normally used, they offer opportunity for enhancement of clinical pathway applications, particularly as the pathways are computerized. This section briefly summarizes four key formats: the activity/precedent table format, the Gantt chart format, the flowchart/network format, and the resource format as well as an interpretation of float/slack time. A more complete description was provided by Coffey and colleagues.[17] Some computer programs include additional formats or views. All of the formats or views are interrelated. So, if someone changes the number of hours or days required for an activity in one view, the other views change to reflect the longer time period. Also, the same information, such as precedent relationships, can be discussed using different formats. In choosing formats, it is best to use those formats that are easiest to understand and readily allow involvement by members of the team.

Activity/Precedent Format

After defining the desired outcomes, the next step in the methodology discussed above is to define all the necessary activities and their relationships. A sample activity/precedent format appears in Exhibit 29–2. The activity/precedent format is helpful for listing all the activities and their required precedents, durations, and resource requirements. Calculated start times, finish times, and float/slack times may be displayed in this table also. Use of the activity/precedent format forces a formal consideration of the precedent relationships and duration of all activities, which in turn raises questions about availability of ancillary services and other resources to expedite patient recovery. But the relationships among activities are more difficult to understand in this format than in the flowchart/network format, since there is no indication of which activities are on the clinical path. Also, it is difficult to visualize which activities are done on the same day.

Gantt Chart Format

A Gantt chart shows the beginning and ending times for each activity on a bar chart, along a timeline in the units being used. Most health care organizations currently implementing clinical paths use a form of the Gantt chart: listing the activities to be done each day, as illustrated in Exhibit 29–3. This format presents a concise, easy-to-understand picture of the activities, and in some cases expected outcomes, for each day. The activities are typically organized into consults, tests, patient activities, treatments, medications, diet, and patient and family education. The Gantt chart format is particularly helpful in communicating which activities are being done during each time period. It provides an excellent tool for communications among staff, patients, and family members, and it is very useful for teaching, orientation, and education of clinicians related to care requirements. Although it is useful to display activities by day for communication purposes, it may be more useful to use smaller time units, like hours, for planning, coordination, and evaluation.

This format does not work well to illustrate the precedent relationships among activities, nor does it identify which activities are on the critical path. Some computer software programs have partially solved this deficiency by including lines linking the information on the Gantt chart to show precedence.

Flowchart/Network Format

The flowchart/network format graphically illustrates the precedent relationships among activities and shows the time-limiting, or critical, path, as shown in Figure 29–1. This format displays the activities in the care process as a flowchart. A flowchart of the current process may be used as a first step, but it may be refined as precedent relationships and activity durations are revised. It is important to involve direct care providers in creating the flowchart. Using the flowchart may allow creation of the pathway in less time because it is easier to visualize the relationships of activities in a flowchart/network format than in other formats. It is particularly helpful for discussions about existing or changing precedent relationships, clinical practices, and sequences of activities. People can see the clinical path clearly. There may be one or more time-limiting, or critical, pathways of equal duration.

There are some drawbacks to using the flowchart/network format. Flowcharts require more space than tables of activities and can be quite large. This format does not work well to communicate what will be done each day. Manually generated networks seldom have supplemental information such as durations of activities or float times, but some computerized project management programs display this additional information on the flowchart/network format.

Exhibit 29–2 Sample of Activity/Precedent Table for Uncomplicated CABG Patients

ID No.	Activity Name	Duration (Hours)	Precedent Activities
1	Thoracic surgery clinic visit	3	None
2	Anesthesia clinic visit	3	1
3	Physical therapy visit	1	1
4	Preoperative assessment	1	2, 3
5	Preoperative identification of postdischarge caregiver	1	4
6	Pre- and postoperative patient and family teaching	1	5
7	Operative procedure—CABG	6	6
8	Pharmaceutical support	16	7
9	Hemodynamic monitoring	16	7
10	Cardiac monitoring	16	7
11	Ventilator support maintenance	16	7
12	Stabilization of hemodynamics	1	8, 9, 10
13	Discontinuation of hardwire monitoring	1	12
14	Discontinuation of hemodynamic monitoring	1	12
15	Adequate blood gases, with reduced oxygenation	1	11
16	Extubation	2	15
17	Transfer to step-down unit	1	13, 14, 16
18	Cardiac monitoring via telemetry	48	17
19	Discontinuation of telemetry	24	18
20	Normal and preoperative cardiac rhythm	0	19
21	Monitoring of intake and output, vitals, etc. (ongoing)	0	17
22	Diuretic protocol	36	21
23	Weight monitoring	1	22
24	Weight approaching preoperative weight	0	23
25	Increasing activity (and other related activities)	85	17, 27, 28
26	Bowel movement	1	25
27	Weaning to nasal cannula	3	16
28	Discontinuation of nasal cannula	34	27
29	Room air × 24 hours	24	28
30	Tolerance of activity on room air	0	29
31	Discharge	4	20, 24, 26, 30
32	Positive lifestyle activities		31
33	Postoperative appointments kept		31
34	Weight at preoperative level		31
35	Stable cardiac rhythm		31
36	Activity at least at preoperative level		31

Source: Reprinted from R.J. Coffey, J.E. Othman, and J.I. Walters, "Extending the Application of Critical Path Methods," *Quality Management in Health Care,* Vol. 3, No. 2, p. 24, © 1995, Aspen Publishers, Inc.

Resource Format

There are entry and output forms of the resource format. The data entry table, which is sometimes an extension of the activity table, is used to enter the amounts of different resources required for each activity. An output form of the resource format is illustrated in Exhibit 29–4. If the activity duration is significantly altered, it may alter the resource requirements. Like the required activities and precedent relationships, the resource requirements must be carefully chal-

Exhibit 29–3 Sample of Gantt Chart Format for Uncomplicated CABG Patients

Category	Postoperative Period of Operative Day	Postoperative Day 1	Postoperative Day 2
Treatment	Ventilator support until extubation		
	Weaning to nasal cannula	Oxygen by nasal cannula	Room air
			Intake and output monitoring TID
	Hardwire monitoring	Telemetry	Telemetry
	Vital sign monitoring	Vitals every 4 hours	Vitals every 4 hours
	Hemodynamic monitoring		
	Cardiac output every 4 hours		
	Pharmaceutical support	Pharmaceutical support	Pharmaceutical support
	Initiation of diuretic protocol	Continuation of diuretic protocol	Continuation of diuretic protocol
Patient Activity	Bedrest until extubated	Ambulation to tolerance QID	Increase ambulation to tolerance QID
	Being up in chair at bedside		
Diet	NPO	No added salt, low cholesterol	No added salt, low cholesterol
	Advance to clear liquids	Solid diet	Solid diet
Discharge Planning		Assessment of additional home care needs	
		Transfer to step-down unit	
Teaching	Explanation of ICU procedures	Reinforcement of incentive spirometer use	Reinforcement of increasing activity
	Explanation of transfer to step-down unit	Reinforcement of increasing activity	
Medications	Potassium as needed		Potassium as needed
	Magnesium as needed		
	Diltiazem 30 mg TID	Diltiazem CD once a day	Diltiazem CD once a day
	Nitroglycerine 1 mcg/kg		
Tests	Electrolytes (potassium × 3)	Electrolytes	
	CBC		
	Arterial blood gases		
	Chest X-ray		
	Pulse oximetry	Pulse oximetry	

Note: This table is for illustration only and should not be used as a standard of care. TID = three times per day, QID = four times per day, NPO = nothing by mouth, ICU = intensive care unit, CBC = complete blood count.

Source: Reprinted from R.J. Coffey, J.E. Othman, and J.I. Walters, "Extending the Application of Critical Path Methods," *Quality Management in Health Care,* Vol. 3, No. 2, © 1995, Aspen Publishers, Inc.

lenged. For example, activities that may have been previously done by a physician in an intensive care unit might possibly be done by a nurse in an acute care unit, or even by a visiting nurse in a patient's home. The resource requirements by activity differ from the activity times. The activity time is the amount of chronological time required to complete the activity. The resource requirement is the amount of time or resources required during the activity. For example, a CABG patient may need 16 hours of pharmaceutical support, yet the resource requirement during that period may be 1 hour of registered pharmacist time and 1 hour of registered nurse time. As with estimates of activity times, resource requirements may be derived from consensus estimates of the different professionals, from times in patient charts, and from analyses of variances. Although conceptually simple, the calculations related to float time (see below) are detailed and best done by a computer program. Resource requirements by activity are not part of the clinical path work to date in health care. The resource format can be helpful when planning and scheduling resource requirements and evaluating changes in resource use as more patients are put on computerized clinical pathways. Like the Gantt chart, this format does not communicate precedent relationships, nor does it have information about the duration of each activity.

Float/Slack Time

All tasks not on the clinical path have "slack" or "float" time. Float time is the amount of time an activity or task can be delayed without delaying something else. Although this concept is not currently used in health care, knowing the amount of float time is helpful in prioritizing activities, particularly in clinical situations where the path is very constrained. "Free float" is the amount of time an activity can be delayed without delaying any other activity. "Total float" is the amount of time an activity can be delayed without delaying the finish date but possibly cutting into the float time of its successor activity or activities. A path with relatively large float time allows for more tolerance of uncontrollable variation. Clinicians must be extremely vigilant if the float time is zero or small, since delays of these activities will delay the outcomes or discharge.

RESULTS

The results associated with implementing clinical pathways fall into two general catego-

ries. Some results are qualitative. According to the patients, clinicians, and payers involved, clinical pathways and variance tools are useful for focusing and improving planning, coordination, and teamwork. The pathways facilitate communication among clinicians, patients, family members, and payers.

Of particular interest to health care administrators and payers is the second type of results: quantitative results related to length of stay, resource use, costs, and so forth. Based upon the work at UMHS and other health care organizations, clinical pathways do have a positive impact on these quantitative measures. Selected examples are discussed below.

At the C.S. Mott Children's Hospital within UMHS, data were analyzed for a sample of 300 inpatients admitted to the pediatric cardiology service and included on one of the clinical pathways for 19 diagnoses and procedures.[18] Charts were analyzed for 130 patients before the clinical pathways were initiated, and these were compared with results for 170 patients after the clinical pathways were initiated. Cost and readmission data were obtained from patient accounting and admitting, respectively. "After implementation of case management [with critical paths], 76% (130 of 170) of the patients were discharged within the expected length of stay, which increased from 66% (86 of 130) of patients in the pre-case management group (x^2=3.89, p=0.05). . . . Finally, the average length of stay decreased by 0.2 to 1.0 day for 11 of 14 diagnoses/procedures in the case-managed group."[19(p.76)] According to another article, "The incidence of readmissions was not significantly changed after initiation of case management at only 1.2% (2 of 170), as compared with 1.5% (2 of 130) before case management."[20(p.76)] The same article noted that "discharge readiness was not assessed in patients hospitalized less than 72 hours. At the time of assessment before discharge, 97% (67 of 69 [assessed]) of parents reported readiness for their child's discharges within 24 hours. Follow-up assessment approximately two weeks later revealed that parental perception of discharge readiness was highly reliable with 95% agreement (that is, same or bet-

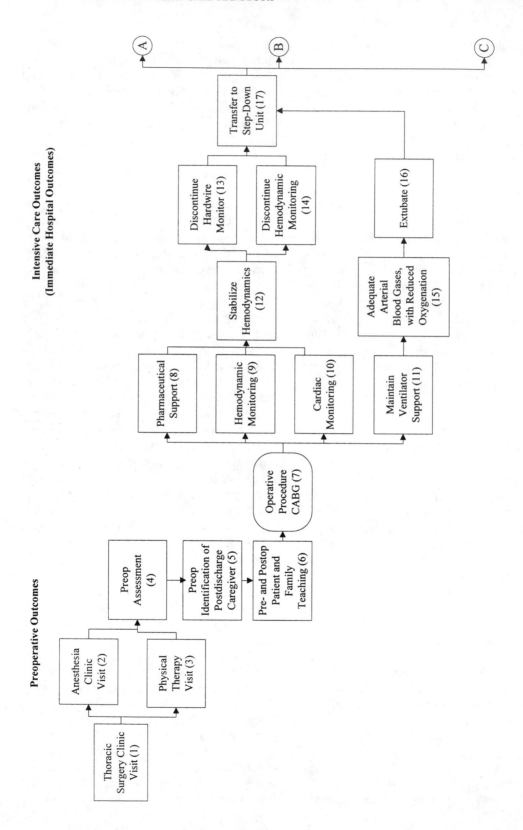

Preoperative Outcomes

Intensive Care Outcomes
(Immediate Hospital Outcomes)

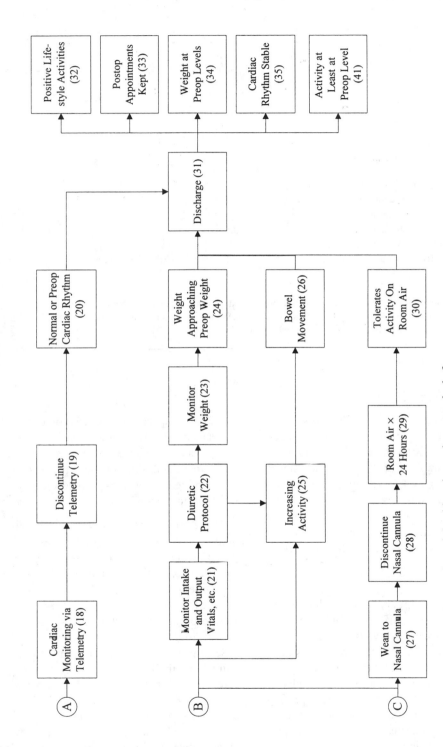

Note: This figure is for illustration only, and should not be used as a standard of care.

Figure 29–1 Excerpt from a Sample Flowchart of Activities and Outcomes for Uncomplicated CABG Patients. *Source:* Reprinted from R.J. Coffey, J.E. Othman, and J.I. Walters, "Extending the Application of Critical Path Methods," *Quality Management in Health Care,* Vol. 3, No. 2, p. 20, 1995.

Exhibit 29–4 Sample Resource Table for Uncomplicated CABG Patients

ID No.	Activity Name	Staff Time Requirements				Equipment	
		Physician Time	Nurse Time	Tech/PA Time	Other Time	Room	Other
1	Thoracic surgery clinic visit	1		0.5	0.75	Exam room	
2	Anesthesia clinic visit	0.5			0.75	Exam room	
3	Physical therapy visit			1		Exam room	Spirometer
4	Preoperative assessment		0.5				
5	Preoperative identification of postdischarge caregiver		0.5				
6	Pre- and postoperative patient and family teaching		0.5				Booklet
7	Operative procedure—CABG	24	12		16	Operating room	

Note: This table is for illustration only and should not be used as a standard of care. PA = physician assistant.

Source: Reprinted from R.J. Coffey, J.E. Othman, and J.I. Walters, "Extending the Application of Critical Path Methods," *Quality Management in Health Care,* 1995, 3(2), p. 24.

ter rating of readiness)."[21(p.77)] With respect to charges for the surgical procedures, however, the "data regarding average billed charges for eight cardiac surgical procedures suggested a mean increase of 13.4%, without adjustment for changes in hospital costs [over a multiyear period]."[22(p.76)]

Multiple clinical services have implemented clinical paths within the adult hospital of UMHS. The following are selected examples of quantitative results.

- For thoracic surgery, average lengths of stay decreased significantly for the four key procedures with pathways, as illustrated in Table 29–1. Some of the procedures have multiple clinical pathways. The changes in other resource use, as measured by relative value units (RVUs) to eliminate pricing changes, varied. For 4 of 7 procedures, resource RVUs decreased, and for 3 of 7, resource RVUs increased.

- For orthopaedic surgery, average lengths of stay decreased significantly for the five key procedures with pathways, as illustrated in Table 29–2. Four of the 5 procedures also experienced decreases in resource use, as measured by RVUs.

A relevant question is whether the clinical pathway is the reason for the decreasing length of stay. Decreases in length of stay have been occurring across the health care industry. Based upon documentation at UMHS, although the length of stay was decreasing before implementing the clinical path, the rate of decrease increased after the pathway was implemented.

Several other authors have documented positive results of implementing clinical pathways. Cardozo and Aherns compared congestive heart failure (CHF) patients over age 65.[23] Ninety five were placed on pathways during 1996 and 1997 and compared to a random sample of 200 CHF patients treated without pathways during 1995.

Table 29–1 Average Length of Stay for Thoracic Surgery Patients

	Length of Stay (Days)	
Unit and Procedure	*Before Critical Path (4/1/90–1/19/91)*	*2 Years after Critical Path (4/1/92–12/31/92)*
Intensive care unit		
Heart transplant	12.10	8.47
CABG (first time)	4.60	2.53
Esophagectomy	3.60	0.80
CABG (revision)	6.29	2.73
Routine unit		
Heart transplant	14.60	10.44
CABG (first time)	8.50	6.90
Esophagectomy	12.70	11.99
CABG (revision)	6.83	6.58

Cardozo and Aherns found that "the patients on the pathway had significant reductions in length of stay and cost of care as well as more effective delivery of processes of care. Mortality rates were unchanged, at 3.5%. However, readmission rates showed a significant increase, from 9.25% to 13.5%, for patients on the pathway."[24(p.12)] They are further investigating the unexpected increase in readmission rate.

Silverstein documented that lost workdays and claims also decreased substantially after pathways were introduced. "One of the most successful areas of the program is the initiation of light duty for employees. This is necessary to save money. If the employee can return to work for light duty this speeds up the process and it costs less for the employer. Physicians also get paid faster when the Care Manager is involved."[25(p.75)] For one local distributor, average cost per claim decreased from $4,332 to $2,915, and lost workdays decreased from 865 to 126, from March 1993 to March 1996.

As stated earlier, clinical pathways can be extended beyond inpatient care. Baker and colleagues documented improvements by using clinical pathways for ambulatory surgery.

The benefits of using the OR [operating room] subpathway were (1) a 78% reduction of incomplete preop-

Table 29–2 Average Length of Stay for Orthopaedic Surgery Patients

	Length of Stay (Days)	
Procedure	*Before Critical Path (1/1/92–12/31/92)*	*After Critical Path (1/1/93–12/31/93)*
Posterior spinal fusion	10.40	8.39
Total knee arthroplasty	6.39	5.65
Total knee arthroplasty (revision)	8.20	6.33
Total hip arthroplasty	7.24	6.52
Total hip arthroplasty (revision)	10.52	9.26

erative charts, (2) a 50% reduction in OR cases that were scheduled for longer times than actually required for the procedure, and (3) a 50% reduction in length of OR delays from 1 hour to less than 30 minutes. The benefits of using the Phase I postanesthesia care unit (PACU) subpathway were (1) elimination of postprocedure chart reviews for completed documentation, (2) provision of a quantifiable method of verbal and nonverbal pain assessment, and (3) improvement of nursing staff and anesthesia staff awareness of pain management.[26(p.3)]

CONCLUSION

Clinical pathways help ensure that care will be both high quality and cost-effective. Effective clinical pathways are focused upon achieving patient care outcomes and intermediate objectives as quickly as possible while avoiding resource waste. Clinical pathways can help people plan and coordinate care; establish expectations about care; reduce variances in care provision; educate and orient staff; ease communication among patients, clinicians, payers, and others; benchmark best practices; and reduce lengths of stay and costs. Successful development and use of clinical pathways depend upon creating the right environment for clinical pathways.

REFERENCES

1. M. Giffin and R.B. Giffin, Critical Pathways Produce Tangible Results, *Health Care Strategic Management* 12 (1994): 17–23.
2. R.J. Coffey et al., An Introduction to Critical Paths, *Quality Management in Health Care* 1, no. 1 (1992): 45–54.
3. R.J. Coffey et al., Extending the Application of Critical Path Methods, *Quality Management in Health Care* 3, no. 2 (1995): 14–29.
4. Coffey et al., Extending the Application, 14–29.
5. S. Wintermeyer-Pingel, Coordinated Care Variance Data Collection: A "Time Limiting Pathway" Approach (Paper presented at the National Leadership Conference Management of Quality: Changing Today for Tomorrow, Ann Arbor, MI, November 1993).
6. K. Zander, Estimating and Tracking the Financial Impact of Critical Paths, *Definition* 5, no. 4 (1990): 1–3.
7. K. Zander, Care Maps: The Core of Cost/Quality Care, *The New Definition* 6, no. 3 (1991): 1–3.
8. J. Schriefer, The Synergy of Pathways and Algorithms: Two Tools Work Better Than One, *The Joint Commission Journal on Quality Improvement* 20, no. 9 (1994): 485–499.
9. Schriefer, *The Synergy of Pathways and Algorithms*, 485–499.
10. Coffey et al., An Introduction to Critical Paths, 45–54.
11. Coffey et al., An Introduction to Critical Paths, 45–54.
12. A. Frantz, Cardiac Recovery in Home: Improving Quality While Reducing Cost, *Remington Report* 7 (1993): 14–15.
13. Coffey et al., An Introduction to Critical Paths, 45–54.

14. Coffey et al., Extending the Application, 14–29.
15. J.S. Richards et al., Clinical Paths and Patient Care Documentation, in *Clinical Paths: Tools for Outcomes Management*, ed. P.L. Spath (Chicago, IL: American Hospital Association, 1994), 33–44.
16. Richards et al., Clinical Paths, 33–44.
17. Coffey et al., Extending the Application, 14–29.
18. K. Uzark et al., The Pediatric Nurse Practitioner as Case Manager in the Delivery of Services to Children with Heart Disease, *Journal of Pediatric Health Care* 8, no. 4 (1994): 74–78.
19. J. Billi, "Partnership Health: A Partnership between Ford Motor Company and University of Michigan Health System," in R. Snyderman and V.Y. Saito, eds., Integrated Health Delivery Systems: 1999 Duke Private Sector Conference (Duke University Health System).
20. Uzark et al., The Pediatric Nurse Practitioner, 74–78.
21. Uzark et al., The Pediatric Nurse Practitioner, 74–78.
22. Uzark et al., The Pediatric Nurse Practitioner, 74–78.
23. L. Cardozo and S. Aherns, Assessing the Efficacy of a Clinical Pathway in the Management of Older Patients Hospitalized with Congestive Heart Failure, *Journal of Healthcare Quality,* May/June 1999: 12–20.
24. Cardozo and Aherns, Assessing the Efficacy.
25. W. Silverstein, Care Management: The Right Balance of Care and Management? *Nursing Administration Quarterly* 22, no. 4 (1998): 66–75.
26. B. Baker et al., Ambulatory Surgical Clinical Pathway, *Journal of PeriAnesthesia Nursing* 14, no. 1 (1999): 2–11.

CHAPTER 30

Quality Management in Managed Care

Pamela B. Siren

INTRODUCTION

Managed care is under tremendous scrutiny. As we embark on a new millennium, a majority of states and the federal government have managed care reform legislation under debate. The central focus of the reform is patients' rights and protection. The legislation advocates for the right of patients to sue managed care organizations (MCOs) for death or injury sustained from poor care or denied treatment. Patient protection clauses include the freedom of choice, the freedom to access urgent care, and the freedom to receive whatever care is necessary in light of a life-threatening illness.

In addition to the rise in consumerism (see also Chapter 43), managed care is experiencing medical cost increases. As of 1999, most parts of the country were experiencing double-digit rate increases. Many managed care plans are dropping entire product lines such as Medicare and Medicaid and are retreating from unprofitable markets. Providing high-quality care and understanding customer needs are more important than ever.

Pamela B. Siren, RN, MPH, is the Vice President of Quality Services with Neighborhood Health Plan in Boston. Her area of expertise is quality management in health care. She has designed approaches to assess organizational performance and developed strategies for improvement in academic medical centers, managed care organizations, group practices, and disease management ventures. She gratefully acknowledges the contributions of Glenn Laffel, MD, PhD, to earlier versions of this manuscript.

The versions of this chapter in prior editions of *The Managed Health Care Handbook* provided a primer for developing a managed care quality management program. This chapter updates that basic primer, providing more discussion of measurement, customer focus, and statistically based decision making.

TRADITIONAL QUALITY ASSURANCE

Advocacy for performance assessment in health care can be traced to E.A. Codman, a surgeon who practiced at Massachusetts General Hospital in the early 1900s. He was among the first advocates of systematic performance assessment in health care. His efforts included evaluation of the care provided to his own patients.

In the 1960s and 1970s, the introduction of computers and large administrative data sets (used initially to support Medicare claims processing) permitted investigators to use powerful epidemiological methods in their analyses of practice variations and related phenomena. In this period, Avedas Donabedian developed three criteria for the assessment of quality that are still used today: structure, process, and outcome.[1] His approach to quality assessment of care has stood the test of time and remains useful in managed care settings.

Structure Criteria

Structural measures of health care performance focus on the context in which care and services are provided. These measures provide inferences about the MCO's ability to provide the services it proposes to offer. Structural measures include board certification of physicians, licensure of facilities, compliance with safety codes, recordkeeping, and physician network appointments. Many such requirements are delineated in federal, state, and local regulations that govern licensing or accreditation and mandate periodic review and reporting mechanisms.

Accreditation and regulatory bodies have traditionally emphasized structural criteria because of their ease of documentation. Purchasers support this tradition by requesting such information in their contract negotiations with MCOs. The role of the MCO's leadership in improving performance is increasing and is evaluated by accrediting agencies through assessment of committee function. The MCO leadership's team needs a complete understanding of the role it plays in performance improvement.

As MCOs form into integrated delivery systems, the structural criterion of performance assessment becomes more complex. The regulations and standards that may govern MCOs, such as those of the National Committee for Quality Assurance (NCQA), may be different from the standards to which member hospitals are held accountable, such as those of the Joint Commission on Accreditation of Healthcare Organizations. Reconciliation of at least the minimal and widely accepted standards within the MCO and across an integrated delivery system is the first step to developing structural measures and evaluating structural performance and its impact on the quality and cost of health care delivery. See also Chapter 44 for a discussion of accreditation agencies.

Structural measures generally do not offer adequate specificity to differentiate the capabilities of providers or organizations beyond minimum standards. In addition, the relationship between structure and other measures of performance, such as outcomes, must be clarified to ensure that enforcing structural standards leads to better results.[2]

In an era of increasing demand by consumers and increasing costs, MCOs must manage their structural resources strategically. For example, some states, in collaboration with MCOs, are streamlining the provider credentialing process through centralization. In Massachusetts, for example, MCOs will be able to purchase provider credentialing information for a subscription fee. The efficiency achieved is twofold: providers have a single application to complete for all of the state's MCOs, and MCOs can reduce resources devoted to credentialing. From a quality perspective, required credentialing criteria can be consistently met with a minimum of variation and error.

Process Criteria

The second traditional criterion for health care quality assessment is process. Langley and Nolan describe a process as a set of causes and conditions that repeatedly come together in a series of steps to transfer inputs into outcomes.[3] Processes of care measures evaluate the way in which care is provided. Examples of care process measures for MCOs include the number of referrals made out of network, health screening rates (e.g., cholesterol), follow-up rates for abnormal diagnostic results, and clinical algorithms for different conditions. Such measures are frequently evaluated against national criteria or benchmarks. Process of service measures are also frequently used. These include appointment waiting times and membership application processing times.

As with structural measures, it is important to link process measures to outcomes. Although the field of outcomes research continues to grow, the link between many health care processes and key outcomes has not always been clearly defined. The relationship between process and outcomes is also addressed in Chapter 31.

Freedom of choice and ease of access to specialty care are common themes in managed care reform legislation. MCOs have been experimenting with open access specialty networks where referrals are not required. MCOs should compare the cost and clinical value of requiring referrals with the cost and clinical value of allowing open access. If referral processing is not embraced as an opportunity for care management, there may be little value and considerable added administrative expense for requiring referrals.

Outcome Criteria

The third traditional category of quality assessment is the outcome of care or service (see also Chapter 31). Traditional outcomes measurements include infection rates, morbidity, and mortality. Relatively poor outcomes performance generally mandates careful review. Exhibits 30–1 and 30–2 illustrate common outcome criteria used to assess quality of inpatient and outpatient care. Unfortunately, although

---

Exhibit 30–1 Examples of Events for Hospitalized Patients That May Indicate Inadequate Quality of Care

Adequacy of discharge planning
- No documented plan for appropriate follow-up care or discharge planning as necessary, with consideration of physical, emotional, and mental status/needs at the time of discharge

Medical stability of the patient at discharge
- Blood pressure on day before or day of discharge: systolic, < 85 mm Hg or > 180 mm Hg; diastolic, < 50 mm Hg or > 110 mm Hg
- Oral temperature on day before or day of discharge > 101°F (rectal > 102°F)
- Pulse < 50 beats/min (or < 45 beats/min if patient is on a beta blocker) or > 120 beats/min within 24 hours of discharge
- Abnormal results of diagnostic services not addressed or explained in the medical record
- Intravenous fluids or drugs given on the day of discharge (excludes the ones that keep veins open, antibiotics, chemotherapy, or total parenteral nutrition)
- Purulent or bloody drainage of postoperative wound within 24 hours before discharge

Deaths
- During or after elective surgery
- After return to intensive care unit, coronary care, or special care unit within 24 hours of being transferred out
- Other unexpected death

Nosocomial infections
- Temperature increase of more than 2°F more than 72 hours from admission
- Indication of infection after an invasive procedure (e.g., suctioning, catheter insertion, tube feedings, surgery)

Unscheduled return to surgery within same admission for same condition as previous sur-gery or to correct operative problem (excludes staged procedures)

Trauma suffered in the hospital
- Unplanned removal or repair of a normal organ (i.e., removal or repair not addressed in operative consent)
- Fall with injury or untoward effect (including but not limited to fracture, dislocation, concussion, laceration)
- Life-threatening complications of anesthesia
- Life-threatening transfusion error or reaction
- Hospital-acquired decubitus ulcer
- Care resulting in serious or life-threatening complications not related to admitting signs and symptoms, including but not limited to neurological, endocrine, cardiovascular, renal, or respiratory body systems (e.g., resulting in dialysis, unplanned transfer to special care unit, lengthened hospital stay)
- Major adverse drug reaction or medication error with serious potential for harm or resulting in special measures to correct (e.g., intubation, cardiopulmonary resuscitation, gastric lavage), including but not limited to the following:
  1. Incorrect antibiotic ordered by physician (e.g., inconsistent with diagnostic studies or patient's history of drug allergy)
  2. No diagnostic study to confirm which drug is correct to administer (e.g., culture and sensitivity)
  3. Serum drug levels not measured as needed
  4. Diagnostic studies or other measures for side effects not performed as needed (e.g., blood urea nitrogen, creatinine, intake and output)

Source: Reprinted from Health Care Financing Administration, 1986.

Exhibit 30–2 Examples of Inpatient Diagnoses That May Indicate Inadequate or Improper Outpatient Care

- Cellulitis (extremities)
- Dehydration of child younger than 2 years who has severe diarrhea
- Diabetic coma—ketoacidosis
- Essential hypertension
- Gangrene (angiosclerotic, extremities)
- Hemorrhage secondary to anticoagulant therapy
- Hypokalemia secondary to potassium-depleting diuretic
- Low-birthweight infant (premature, < 2,500 g)
- Malunion or nonunion of fracture (extremities)
- Perforated or hemorrhaging ulcer (duodenal, gastric)
- Pregnancy-induced hypertension (preeclampsia, eclampsia, toxemia)
- Pulmonary embolism (admitting diagnosis)
- Readmission of same condition within 14 days
- Ruptured appendix
- Septicemia (admitting diagnosis)
- Status asthmaticus
- Urinary tract infection (bacturia, pyuria)

Courtesy of Blue Cross and Blue Shield Association, Chicago, Illinois.

outcomes measures are purported to reflect the performance of the entire system of care and service processes, they often offer little insight into the causes of poor performance.

Despite the limitations of current outcomes assessment, most MCOs have systems in place to screen for adverse events. These screening criteria are often evaluated during the utilization review process to detect sentinel events. Some of these same measures are being applied to the peer review process within the MCO.

Peer Review and Appropriateness Evaluation

In addition to Donabedian's three quality criteria, peer review and appropriateness review have been key components of the traditional quality assurance model. Peer review and appropriateness of care are central to the current managed care debate.

Peer Review

Peer review involves a comparison of an individual provider's practice either with practice by the provider's peers or with an acceptable standard of care. These standards may be developed within the MCO (e.g., practice guidelines), be described by national professional associations, or be required by a regulatory or legislative agency. Cases for peer review are identified ei-

ther as outliers to specific indicators or through audits of medical records. Peer review has traditionally been used as an informal educational tool. It is typified by morbidity and mortality conferences currently in existence.

Peer review has its limitations. First, opportunities for improvement may be missed by a paradigm that rests on conformance with standards. Deming emphasized that meeting specifications does not result in constant improvement but rather ensures the status quo.[4] Second, peer review is limited by the scope of the indicators or processes under review and is traditionally driven by sentinel events.

In the current environment of reform, more emphasis is being placed on the what, the how, and the who of clinical decision making to approve or deny coverage. An integral component of a modern quality management program is the evaluation of consistency of decision making by both MCO physicians and case managers. Interrater reliability audits are useful tools to be added to an MCO's internal peer review process to monitor consistency of decision making and application of criteria.

Appropriateness Evaluation

Appropriateness evaluation reviews the extent to which the MCO provides timely, necessary care at the right level of service. Appropriateness review frequently occurs before an elective clinical event (admission or procedure). Procedures or admissions most frequently selected for appropriateness review include those for which there is a wide variation of opinion as to their usefulness or effectiveness and those that have been notably expensive. Examples of procedures frequently selected for appropriateness review include hysterectomy, coronary artery bypass surgery, and laminectomy. The proposed indication for the event is compared with a list of approved indications obtained from a professional society or a specialty vendor or designed by the MCO itself. Appropriateness review is intended to identify and minimize areas of overutilization. Optimum care management systems are applying appropriateness criteria to assess the potential underutilization of needed services.

COMPONENTS OF A QUALITY MANAGEMENT PROGRAM

Donabedian's three criteria for quality assessment serve as a useful foundation for a quality management program. The traditional quality assurance model can be made better, however, with an infusion of systems thinking, customer focus, and knowledge to inform improvement.

First, systems thinking recognizes that processes are interrelated. It offers a method for structural design, assessment, and management of performance with a clear aim and shared purpose, permitting payers and providers to form a connected, efficient network. A disconnected network will eventually engage in contradictory and inefficient behaviors. Organizational goals can be achieved first by identifying customer needs, finding the organization's central shared purpose, and expanding the shared purpose across the integrated delivery system. When MCOs and provider groups have a shared purpose and shared financial risk, inappropriate care and service denials can be reduced and coordination of care can be improved.

In previous versions of this chapter, customer focus was identified as the cornerstone of a modern quality management program. An organization that embraces this philosophy as part of its strategic vision is well suited to address the

needs of rising consumerism. Regulators and accreditors without explicit knowledge of what the customer (member, purchaser, provider) needed drove the traditional quality assurance model, in part. The modern quality management program identifies key customers, anticipates customer needs, measures how effectively those needs are met, and improves processes to meet those needs.

Finally, an enhancement of the traditional quality assurance model is knowledge to inform improvement. Improvement involves measurement and change management. According to Moen and Nolan, three fundamental questions can be used as guides for improvement efforts:

1. What are you trying to accomplish? Information gained from understanding customer needs, the current process and outcome performance, and expected performance will assist the MCO in answering this question.
2. How will you know that a change is an improvement? Establishing performance expectations before implementing an improvement activity assists the MCO in understanding whether a change is an improvement and minimizes any potential confusion between measures of utilization and indicators of quality.
3. What changes can be made that will result in an improvement?[5]

To develop tests and implement changes, the plan-do-study-act (PDSA) cycle is used as a framework for an efficient trial and learning model. The term "study" is used in the third cycle to emphasize this phase's primary purpose: to gain knowledge. Increased knowledge leads to a better prediction of whether a change in a current process will result in an improvement.[6]

According to Langley and Nolan, to be considered a PDSA cycle, the following aspects of the activity should be identifiable. First, the activity was planned and includes a strategy to collect data. Second, a plan was attempted. Third, time was set aside to analyze the data and study the results. Finally, action was rationally based on what was learned.[7] For example, a health plan experimenting with the most effective means to ensure an adequate response rate on a self-reported health risk assessment deployed two strategies. In one, a telephone call was placed to the member; in the other, a written survey was mailed. Response rates were collected for both methods to determine which yielded more favorable rates. It was found that telephone calls yielded a higher response rate, so this was the strategy deployed.

Improvement strategies do not necessarily have to involve sweeping changes. Small, incremental improvements are often more sustainable over time.

A PROCESS MODEL FOR A MODERN QUALITY MANAGEMENT PROGRAM

This section discusses the key steps in developing a modern quality management program that is based on the fundamentals of managed care and responsive to the changing marketplace.

Understand Customer Need

Understanding customer need (Figure 30–1) is the first step of all quality management programs. Juran and Gyrna describe a customer as anyone who is affected by a product or process.[8] Three categories of customers are external customers, internal customers, and suppliers. External customers of an MCO include members or benefactors and purchasers. Internal customers include the departments and services within the MCO, such as claims processing and member education, as well as the health care professionals themselves. Customer needs may be clear or disguised, rational or less than rational. These needs must be discovered and served.[9] Negotiating and balancing the needs of these diverse and sometimes conflicting customer groups is a challenge for MCOs, as it is for any organization.

Methods to understand customer need are as diverse as the customer groups. Customer complaints are a usual signal of a quality problem. Low levels of complaints, however, do not necessarily mean high satisfaction. Frequently, dissatisfied customers will purchase services else-

Figure 30–1 Continuous Improvement Process—Understand Customer Need.

where without ever registering a complaint. Most MCOs have a formal process to survey their membership for satisfaction with care or services (Exhibit 30–3), but this may not be adequate in an era of patient protection. MCOs need to carefully examine their internal policies and processes that directly affect members.

Exhibit 30–3 Examples of Satisfaction Surveys*

How would you rate:	Excellent	Very Good	Good	Fair	Poor
The thoroughness and technical skills of the:					
Attending doctor					
Nursing staff					
Consulting doctors					
Other personnel (lab, x-ray, etc.)					
The friendliness and compassion of the:					
Attending doctor					
Nursing staff					
Consulting doctors					
Other personnel (lab, x-ray, etc.)					
The explanations, instructions, and responses to questions by the:					
Attending doctor					
Nursing staff					
Consulting doctors					
Other personnel (lab, x-ray, etc.)					
Admission process (timeliness, friendliness, convenience)					
Explanation of your rights as a patient					
Discharge instructions and arrangements					
Food quality and service					
Appearance and cleanliness of the hospital					
Overall quality of care provided by the attending doctor					
Overall rating of this hospital					
Satisfaction with the outcome of your procedure (if applicable)					

Would you recommend this hospital to a friend or loved one?	❑ Yes	❑ No
Would you recommend your attending doctor to a friend or loved one?	❑ Yes	❑ No

© U.S. Quality Algorithms (USQA), 1991

How would you rate each of the following: Excellent ◄————————► Poor   No Opinion

10   9   8   7   6   5   4   3   2   1   0

Nursing Care
Emergency Room Services
Laboratory Department
Quality Assurance/Improvement Program
Utilization Review Department
Social Services/Discharge Planning
Medical Records
Bed availability
Patient satisfaction with the hospital

Please rate the following clinical departments: Excellent ◄————————► Poor   No Opinion

10   9   8   7   6   5   4   3   2   1   0

OB/GYN
General Surgery
Orthopaedics
Urology
Cardiology
ENT
Other _____
Other _____

Would you refer a family member to this hospital?   ❑ Yes   ❑ No   © U.S. Quality Algorithms (USQA), 1991

* This example includes selected questions from USQA's survey of members and USQA's survey of physicians.

Source: © Journal on Quality Improvement. Oakbrook Terrace, IL: Joint Commission on Accreditation of Healthcare Organizations, 1993, p. 377. Reprinted with permission.

Front-end member services functions need to be evaluated for ease of access to care and services and responsiveness to member needs. Medical management operations must evaluate the appropriateness and consistency of care decisions, particularly denials, and the degree to which care is coordinated.

Juran and Gyrna state that it is important to recognize that some customers are more important than others. It is typical that 80 percent of the total sales volume comes from about 20 percent of the customers; these are the vital few customers who command priority.[10] Within these key customer groups, there is a distribution of individual customers that also may have a hierarchy of importance, such as a government agency, a gold card purchaser account, or an academic teaching center. Explicit understanding of the needs of all the MCO customer groups will minimize situations in which one customer's needs are met to the exclusion of another's.

Identify Processes and Outcomes That Meet Customer Need

Identification of processes and outcomes that meet customer need is the next step of the continuous improvement process. How do customers view the MCO's quality? To begin with, they want to know whether the MCO meets their expectations. MCOs are expected to treat members who are ill and to maintain the health and functional capabilities of those who are not. To treat sick patients, MCOs first have to make it easy for them to access services and second must provide them with appropriate care. Purchasers and members value access and appropriateness.[11] Purchasers also value assessments of disease screening activities, service quality, and encounter outcomes to the extent that they support or embellish information about access and appropriateness.[12] Similarly, purchasers know that to maintain health and functional capacity, MCOs must support prevention of illness and management of health status. Therefore, the three key processes in this step are treating disease, managing health, and service quality.

Treating Disease

The treatment of disease is a broad topic and is addressed throughout this section (Chapters 16–34) as well as in greater detail in *Best Practices in Medical Management* (Aspen Publishers, 1998). This section will focus on those aspects of treating disease that are most germane to a quality management program.

Screening

Disease screening measures assess the MCO's performance in detecting the medical conditions of its membership at an asymptomatic, treatable stage. Familiar examples of disease screening include mammography, Pap smears, cholesterol screening, and sigmoidoscopy. Disease screening measures defined as number of screenings for every x members are easy for consumers to understand. There are some problems with screening, however. There are controversies about the timing of disease screening. In addition, the evidence that screening procedures are useful and cost-effective is weak. Nevertheless, screening processes are likely to remain important to purchasers.

In the future, consumers and purchasers may consider outcomes of screening more important than screening rates. After all, screening rates do not explain whether the patient benefited from early detection. For example, effectiveness in screening breast cancer may someday involve two outcome measures—the stage of breast cancer at diagnosis and the 5-year mortality rate for breast cancer—rather than only mammography rates over time.

Encounter Outcomes

Encounter outcome measures evaluate the results of specific clinical encounters, such as hospitalizations or office visits. Included in this category are the traditional assessments of mortality, readmission rates, adverse events, provider empathy, and satisfaction. Traditionally, small sample sizes, case mix adjustment issues, and unreliable data collection methods have confounded encounter outcome measures.

These problems have made it difficult to compare data across systems or even within an MCO over time. Purchasers are likely to continue asking for encounter outcomes for high-volume clinical conditions. Because of the methodological issues mentioned, however, purchasers are likely to set relatively low performance standards in these areas. Approaches to using this information to overcome the limitations discussed here are found in Chapter 32.

Managing Health

Prevention/Wellness. The next set of key processes is associated with prevention of illness. Prevention activities are designed to keep the membership free of disease. Examples of prevention programs include smoking cessation, nutritional counseling, and stress reduction. Measures of prevention include the percentage of eligible patients enrolled in one of the above programs, immunization rates, and first trimester prenatal care visit rates. Such prevention programs assess process performance. As discussed earlier, the effectiveness of such programs is questionable without a study of outcomes. High disenrollment rates make it hard for MCOs to realize long-term benefits from prevention programs. At least in the short term, it appears that consistently poor performance in this area would dampen a purchaser's enthusiasm for a particular MCO.

Member Health Status. The evaluation of a member's health status may include assessment of functioning in physiological terms (e.g., blood pressure, laboratory tests), physical terms (e.g., activities of daily living), mental or psychological terms (e.g., cognitive skill, affective interaction), social terms (e.g., ability to engage in work), and other health-related quality of life areas (e.g., pain, energy, sleep, sex).[13] Two purposes are served by health status evaluations. First, members at risk who need services can be identified before a catastrophic event. Second, a member's health status assessment can serve as an outcome measure for care or treatment received. The recent popularity of health status assessment stems from two ideas. The first is that members' perceptions of their health are both important and easy to obtain.[14] The second is that health systems should be accountable not only for treating disease and managing health but for enhancing members' well-being as well.

Although it is believed that purchasers will rely heavily on member health status measures in their assessments of MCO quality, the Health Care Advisory Board recently articulated a persuasive countervailing opinion. According to the Advisory Board, health status data are not likely to play a prominent role in MCO selection. The Advisory Board called attention to two facts in presenting its argument. First, member health status is influenced by factors beyond the control of the MCO, including genetic predisposition to illness, sociodemographic factors, diet and exercise, and so forth. Second, most systems exhibit member turnover rates of 10 percent or higher, and this makes it difficult to link health status to activities in any one system. According to the Advisory Board, purchasers are unlikely to hold MCOs accountable for (much less make a decisive negotiating decision in light of) the health status of their members.[15] Only time will tell how much influence member health status measures will have.

Service Quality

Service quality measures evaluate the timeliness, responsiveness, and courtesy with which the MCO serves its members. The spectrum of service quality spans key managed care functions such as member education, enrollment, complaint resolution, and appeals/grievance settlement. Consumers expect timely, accurate, and respectful responses to their requests by knowledgeable individuals. These attributes are of critical importance to MCO members in the age of rising consumerism.

Assess Performance Compared with Professional or "Best-of-Class" Standards

The third step of the continuous improvement process is assessing the MCO's performance compared with a professional or "best-of-class" standard. The modern quality management program includes appropriateness evaluation and peer review as well as benchmarking and outcomes assessment.

Appropriateness Evaluation

As discussed above, appropriateness indicators evaluate the extent to which the MCO provides necessary care and does not provide unnecessary care in the service location best suited for quality and cost efficiency. Purchasers understand that they cannot obtain good value from an MCO unless it provides appropriate services, so appropriateness indicators are important.

Unfortunately, appropriateness assessment has been dogged by methodological problems, such as adjusting the data for case mix (discussed later) and the surprising lack of data from controlled trials that would define appropriate care in the first place. This issue affects the evaluation of both overutilization and underutilization of services.

In response to these challenges, the MCO can do two things. First, the MCO can identify minimum performance standards for high-cost diagnoses and use them to select processes having excess utilization. Second, the MCO can demonstrate evidence of consistent success and/or an improvement trend in clinical appropriateness indicators. If these two approaches are employed, purchasers seem inclined to offer MCOs some flexibility in the short run even if some isolated indicators suggest that there may be quality problems.

Peer Review

As discussed previously, peer review involves a comparison of an individual provider's practice against an accepted standard of care. A key difference between peer review in a traditional quality assurance model and peer review in a modern quality management model is the topic of comparison.

Benchmarking

A third method of assessing an MCO's performance is benchmarking. Robert Camp of Xerox (Rochester, New York) popularized benchmarking over the last 20 years. Camp and Tweet define benchmarking as "the continuous process of measuring products, services and practices against the company's toughest competitors or those companies renowned as industry leaders."[16(p.229)] Two types of benchmarking may be used by MCOs. First, internal benchmarking identifies internal functions to serve as pilot sites for comparison. This type of benchmarking is particularly useful in newly integrated delivery systems with multiple, diverse component entities.[17] The second type of benchmarking is external or competitive benchmarking. Competitive benchmarking is the comparison of work processes with those of the best competitor and reveals which performance measure levels can be surpassed.[18] The benchmarking process can be applied to service and clinical processes to assess current performance.

Outcomes Assessment

A fourth method is outcomes assessment. An outcomes assessment may be performed on the MCO's 10 highest-volume or highest-cost diagnoses or procedure groups. An outcomes assessment permits the MCO to assess its own performance over time and to identify variation within the MCO. Davies and colleagues have outlined three core aspects of an outcomes assessment:

1. Outcomes measurements are "point-in-time" observations.
2. Outcomes monitoring includes repeated measurements over time, which permit causal inferences to be drawn about the observed outcomes.
3. Outcomes management is the application of the information and knowledge gained from outcome assessment to achieve optimal outcomes through improved decision making and delivery.[19(p.8)]

The purpose of an outcomes assessment is to provide a quantitative comparison of treatment programs, to map the typical course of a chronic disease across a continuum, or to identify variations in the outcome of care as potential markers of process variation.[20]

Define Indicators To Measure Performance

Defining indicators to measure performance is the fourth step of the continuous improvement process. The MCO may apply the quality criteria (structure, process, and outcome), as discussed for the traditional quality assurance model. In addition, it is useful for MCOs to evaluate their processes and outcomes by populations of customers served. The MCO quality management matrix (Figure 30–2) is a diagram of how this may occur. A key issue faced by MCOs in indicator definition and analysis is case mix adjustment.

Case mix adjustment is the process of correcting data for variations in illness or wellness in patient populations. It is a statistical model that takes into account specific attributes of a patient population (e.g., age, sex, severity of illness, chronic health status) that are beyond the control of the MCO or health provider.[21] This adjustment is particularly important in comparative analyses of providers or MCOs.

Case mix adjustment permits fair comparisons of same-population groups because it accounts for preexisting phenomena that may affect the outcome of care. Potentially required variables in a useful risk adjustment system include the following:

- demographic factors
- diagnostic information
- patient-derived health status
- claims-derived health status
- prior use of all services
- prior use of nonelective hospitalization
- prior use of medical procedures
- prior or current use of pharmaceuticals[22]

Issues of case mix affect the analysis of both inpatient and outpatient care. The problem is more serious for some performance measures

Population \ Key Function	Treatment of Disease				Managing Health		
	Access	Appropriateness	Screening	Encounter Outcomes	Prevention	Health Status	Service Quality
Primary Care	# of primary care physicians with open panels # of days for routine physical		Mammography Cholesterol		Childhood immunization Adult immunization		Member satisfaction
Senior Care		% of seniors with > 7 prescriptions					
Specialty Care							
High-Risk Obstetric Care							
Other High-Volume or Special Need Population							

Figure 30–2 Quality Management Matrix. *Source:* Adapted from N. Goldfield. Case Mix, Risk Adjustment, Reinsurance, and Health Reform. *Managed Care Quarterly*, Vol. 2, No. 3, p. iv. © 1994, Aspen Publishers, Inc.

than for others, however. Case mix is important for clinically oriented indicators such as appropriateness and encounter outcomes. It also has a significant impact on assessments of health status, resource use, and member satisfaction. Case mix is not nearly as important for measures of access and prevention, and thus these measures should be considered for physician profiles and report cards. The topic of case mix adjustment exceeds the scope of this chapter; Chapter 32 provides a detailed discussion of this issue.

Establish Performance Expectations

Establishing performance expectations is the fifth step of the continuous improvement process. Performance expectations are defined by understanding customer needs (step 1), evaluating the performance of the processes and outcomes designed to meet those needs (step 2), and comparing performance against "best-of-class" standards either internal or external to the MCO (step 3).

Purchasers have had an influence on establishing performance expectations. In 1990, Digital Corporation (now owned by Compaq Corporation) identified priority areas where quality improvement efforts might promote better outcomes. Digital began this effort by developing health maintenance organization (HMO) standards and by setting expectations in the areas of utilization management, access, quality assurance, mental health services, data capabilities, and financial performance.[23] Digital examined its health care costs and used weightings that drew on multiple data sources to identify priority areas to be considered by the participating plans. Clinical indicators selected for performance measurement and improvement included mental health inpatient readmissions and inpatient days per patient, Caesarean section rates, prenatal care in the first trimester, screening mammography rates, asthma inpatient admissions, and blood pressure screenings. The results from these measurements were not meant to be used punitively but rather enabled Digital to gauge the participating managed care plans in terms of their success in managing specific aspects of health care.

Monitor Performance and Compare with Expectations

The sixth step is the monitoring of performance and comparison with expectations. The frequency of monitoring is determined by the indicators the MCO has selected to measure performance. An MCO can compare its own performance during different periods or compare its performance to that of other MCOs if the same indicator definitions are used.

Provide Feedback to Providers and Customers

The seventh step of the continuous improvement process is providing feedback. Two methods of feedback are discussed here: profiling, which assesses the performance of individual providers; and report cards, which assess overall MCO performance.

Profiling

Profiling focuses on the patterns of an individual provider's care rather than that provider's specific clinical decisions (see also Chapter 32). The practice pattern of an individual provider hospital or physician is expressed as a rate or a measure of resource use during a defined period and for a defined population.[24] The resulting profile can then be compared against a peer group or a standard. MCOs are using profiling to measure provider performance, to guide quality improvement efforts, and to select providers for managed care networks.[25]

The Physician Payment Review Commission (PPRC) has suggested several guidelines for effective physician profiling.[26] According to the PPRC, profiles first must be analyzed for a well-defined population. Second, they must include a sufficient number of observations to ensure that differences are not due to chance. Third, they should include adjustments for case mix. Finally, profiles must be analyzed for a small enough organizational unit that the parties involved can be responsible for the results and take the necessary courses of action for improvement. A successful profiling system defines an episode of care, accounts for severity of illness and comorbidities, and identifies all the resources used per episode of care.[27] Most profiling systems rely heavily on standard billing information, such as diagnosis-related groups, categories in the tenth revision of the International Classification of Diseases, and Current Procedural Terminology codes.

Examples of measures used in provider profiling include average wait time to schedule a routine physical, number of hospital admissions, number of referrals out of network, number of emergency department visits, member satisfaction, percentage compliance with the MCO's clinical practice guidelines, and, if applicable, the percentage of children receiving appropriate immunizations and the Caesarean section rate. As noted earlier, profiling is discussed in detail in Chapter 32.

Report Cards

Report cards have become a popular method of conveying performance within an individual MCO with multiple geographic sites or across many diverse MCOs. The purpose of a report card is to provide customers (purchasers and consumers) with comparable quality and cost information in a common language to help them select a health plan. Purchasers have formed groups across the country to facilitate the development of a standardized approach to health plan performance measurement. For example, in 1993, 27 corporate and government purchasers of health care formed the Massachusetts Health Care Purchaser Group. The group challenged the health plans in Massachusetts to submit data on six clinical indicators: mammography screening rate, hypertension screening rate, asthma admission rate, prenatal care rate, Caesarean section rate, and mental health readmission rate (Exhibit 30–4).[28] Each health plan was compared with the clinically significant average range, and a consumer-friendly pie chart graphic was used to summarize performance.

Exhibit 30–4 Massachusetts Health Care Purchaser Group Clinical Indicators

Mammography Screening Rate: Percentage of members aged 52–64 who were continuously enrolled in the plan during 1991 and 1992 who received mammograms.

Hypertension Screening Rate: Percentage of members aged 52–64 who were continuously enrolled in the plan in 1991 and 1992 who were screened for high blood pressure.

Asthma Admission Rate: The number of hospital admissions for asthmatics of both sexes between the ages of 1 and 19 and ages 20 and 64 divided by the number of enrollees in the plan of the same age cohorts over a 1-year period.

Prenatal Care Rate: The percentage of pregnancies among women who delivered babies and who were continuously enrolled for 7 months in 1992 for which prenatal care was received during the first trimester of pregnancy.

Caesarean Section Rate: The percentage of all deliveries in 1992 that were performed by Caesarean section.

Mental Health Readmission Rate: Males and females aged 18–64 years continuously enrolled in a given health plan for the previous 2 years, and hospitalized with a discharge date in the second year for psychiatric care. There were two measures: the average number of individual hospital admissions per patient, and the average number of mental health hospital days per patient for all hospital admissions.

Source: © *Journal on Quality Improvement.* Oakbrook Terrace, IL: Joint Commission on Accreditation of Healthcare Organizations, 1995, p. 169. Reprinted with permission.

The report card concept is equally valuable when applied to internal customers of the MCO. Key quality measures can be tracked, trends can be identified, and the results can be utilized for strategic quality planning and to assess the effectiveness of improvement efforts.

The benefits of the report card movement include the stimulus for MCOs to build the capacity to produce performance information and strengthen data quality. Public disclosure of performance information also lends itself to plan, provider, and hospital accountability. The main limitation of the report card movement continues to be measurement. Although the NCQA and Health Plan Employer Data and Information Set have made moves to standardize measurement, there continues to be variation in measurement, coding, and clinical classification. Additionally, there is variation in the administrative source data sets that plans use to obtain their measurements. Possible improvements include risk adjustment and a broader clinical focus. Finally, no conclusion can be drawn about processes or outcomes that are not assessed by the report card measurements.

Implement Improvements

The eighth step of the continuous improvement process is implementation of improvements. The PDSA cycle is a vehicle for learning and acting. According to Langley and Nolan, PDSA can be used to build knowledge about a process, to test a change, or to implement a change.[29] Current strategies employed by MCOs as tools to improve health care delivery processes and outcomes are practice guidelines, quality improvement teams, and consumer education.

Practice Guidelines

Clinical practice guidelines are systematically developed statements to assist practitioners and patients in making decisions about appropriate health care for specific clinical circumstances. Clinical guidelines may inform a disease management program or be applied separately. Guidelines offer an opportunity to improve health care delivery processes by reducing unwanted variation and can also be viewed as restrictive when applied to care or service denials. An appointed committee of the Institute of Medicine recommended the following attributes of guideline design:

- *Validity.* Practice guidelines are deemed valid if they lead to the health and cost outcomes projected for them.
- *Reliability/reproducibility.* If given the same evidence and development methods, another set of experts would come up with the same recommendations. The guidelines are interpreted and applied consistently across providers.
- *Clinical applicability.* Guidelines should apply to a clearly defined patient population.
- *Clinical flexibility.* Guidelines should recognize the generally anticipated exceptions to the recommendations proposed.
- *Multidisciplinary process.* Representatives of key disciplines involved in the process of care should participate in the guideline development process.
- *Scheduled review.* Guideline evaluation should be planned in advance and occur at a frequency that reflects the evolution of clinical evidence for the guideline topic.
- *Documentation.* Detailed summaries of the guideline development process should be maintained that reflect the procedures followed, the participants involved, the evidence and analytical methods employed, and the assumptions and rationales accepted.[30]

In addition to a development process, guideline programs have an implementation process. The first step in designing an implementation strategy for clinical guidelines is to identify the forces driving and restraining clinical practice change.[31] Thus, an MCO may want to convene a group of local content experts along with its own medical leadership to initiate guideline planning and adoption. An effective implementation team strengthens the driving forces for the guideline and weakens the restraining forces for a given clinical practice change. To implement guidelines as an improvement strategy, performance must be measured on two levels. First, the gap between prior and optimal practice is measured to assess the degree of implementation. Second, feedback may be given to providers to reinforce the change in clinical practice. As an example, the following is a summary of United HealthCare's guideline implementation process:

1. Prioritize your objectives. *Select guidelines that*
   * are likely to be accepted by physicians
   * have a cost impact for the health plan
   * affect a quality issue for patients
   * affect a large population
   * fulfill a regulatory issue
2. Document the need to change.
3. Look for guideline credibility.
4. Get the word out.
5. Use timely feedback to physicians.
6. Remember, you are dealing with a system.[32]

Practice guidelines are not without limitations. Studies have shown that traditional methods of guideline dissemination have not resulted in significant changes in practice.[33,34] Frequently, guidelines are not designed to be implemented directly into practice. This has a particular impact in preferred provider organizations (PPOs) and independent practice associations (IPAs), where there are multiple and varied processes. An MCO can facilitate the implementation of guidelines through the corresponding development of algorithms, summaries, laminated cards, medical record tools, and reminder systems. Second, as mentioned earlier in this chapter, meeting specifications does not necessarily result in constant improvement but rather may maintain the status quo.[35] Guidelines should be designed with flexibility to encourage improvement and innovation. Accreditation agencies (e.g., NCQA) and proposed legislation are increasingly requiring guidelines to be flexible and allow for the unique health needs of individuals.

Clinical pathways and protocols are discussed in detail in Chapter 29.

Quality Improvement Teams

A second tool employed by MCOs to facilitate improvement of health care delivery is the quality improvement team. MCOs are complex organizations with many types of employees and locations. To achieve results, quality management programs must be supported by employees with diverse talents and skills. Given the variety of network configurations (e.g., staff model HMO, PPO, IPA), there must be a single method to incorporate provider input from a variety of perspectives. Quality improvement teams offer an alternative in an environment where administrative expense must be controlled and minimized. Teams outperform individuals acting alone or in larger organizational groupings, especially when performance requires many different types of skills and experiences.[36]

There are several well-known phenomena that explain why teams perform well. First, the broad skill mix and know-how help the team respond to multifaceted challenges, such as innovations, quality, and customer service. Second, in developing clear goals and approaches to problem solving, teams can support real-time resolution and initiative. Finally, teams provide a unique social dimension that enhances the economic and administrative aspects of work. By surmounting barriers to collective performance, team members build trust and confidence in each other's capabilities. This supports the pursuit of team purpose above and beyond individual or functional agendas.[37]

How can the team concept be applied to quality management in an MCO? Examples include a team consisting of MCO leaders, purchasers, members, and providers setting the evaluation and improvement agendas for the MCO by prioritizing goals. Alternately, a cross-functional team might evaluate the disease- or population-specific needs of a member group and test interventions, such as practice guidelines, for care improvement. Finally, a team could form to design an MCO's strategy to meet accreditation requirements. Teams can be chartered to address most issues faced by an MCO as long as an explicit purpose and a defined time frame for completion have been identified.

Consumer Education

Many MCOs' quality management programs include evaluation of the effectiveness of consumer education. Consumer education is targeted at beneficiaries so that they can become effective health care consumers and participate in meeting the aforementioned needs of treating disease and managing health. Examples of consumer education utilized by MCOs include telephone resource lines, health risk appraisals, workplace-based consumer education programs, and consumer health education materials. Many MCOs have developed and provide members with self-care guidelines for preventing illness and treating common complaints at the time of enrollment. These topics are also discussed in Chapter 17.

Setting the Improvement Agenda

The MCO must evaluate whether the improvements actually made a change and met customer need. If not, the cycle begins again with step 1. If improvements did occur and customer needs were met, the cycle can begin again for new or unaddressed customer needs.

How can an MCO design such a cycle? MCOs have limited resources with which to assess and improve performance, and strategic decisions must be made to target resources effectively. *An MCO's leadership group may begin the cycle of improvement by applying the following criteria:*

1. Identify which customer need is being addressed by the proposed project.
2. Evaluate the strength of the evidence for the need to improve.
3. Assess the probability that there will be a measurable impact.
4. Determine the likelihood of success.
5. Identify the immediacy of impact in meeting the customer's need.

CONCLUSION

Legislators and politicians are now acting as the voice for consumers in demanding freedom of choice and access to treatment. Purchasers of health care continue to demand quality at a reasonable price. To address these needs, a quality management program in a managed care setting must be designed for complex delivery systems and diverse customer groups. Success in managing cost and optimizing health outcomes begins with an understanding of customer needs, assessment of performance to meet those needs, and continuous improvement. Attention focused on the provision of appropriate care in an appropriate setting will continue to shape the quality resource programs in MCOs. The definition of "appropriate" and the medical decision-making process within MCOs will be under increasing scrutiny. MCOs with a clear understanding of their customers, responsive customer service programs, consistent medical decision making based on clinical facts and scientific evidence, and a philosophy of continuous improvement will have a quality management program responsive to the needs of the day.

REFERENCES

1. A. Donabedian, Exploration in Quality Assessment and Monitoring: The Definition of Quality and Approaches to Its Assessment, Vol. 1 (Ann Arbor, MI: Health Administration Press, 1980).

2. S.M. Shortell and J.P. LoGerfo, Hospital Medical Staff Organization and Quality of Care: Results from Myocardial Infarction and Appendectomy, *Medical Care* 19 (1981): 1041–1056.

3. G.J. Langley et al., The Foundation of Improvement, *Quality Progress* 27 (1994): 81–86.

4. M. Walton, Improve Constantly and Forever the System of Production and Service, in *The Deming Management Method* (New York: Putnam, 1986), 66–67.

5. R.D. Moen and T.W. Nolan, Process Improvement, *Quality Progress* 20 (1987): 62–68.

6. G.J. Langley et al., The Foundation of Improvement, 81–86.

7. G.J. Langley et al., The Foundation of Improvement, 81–86.

8. J. Juran and F. Gyrna, Understanding Customer Need, in *Quality Planning and Analysis,* 3rd ed. (New York: McGraw-Hill, 1993), 240–252.

9. Juran and Gyrna, Understanding Customer Need, 241.

10. Juran and Gyrna, Understanding Customer Need, 241.

11. Health Care Advisory Board, *Next Generation of Outcomes Tracking* (Washington, DC: 1994).

12. Health Care Advisory Board, *Next Generation of Outcomes Tracking.*

13. P.B. Batalden et al., Linking Outcomes Measurement to Continual Improvement: The Serial "V" Way of Thinking about Improving Clinical Care, *Joint Commission Journal on Quality Improvement* 20 (1994): 167–180.

14. E.C. Nelson et al., Patient-Based Quality Measurement Systems, *Quality Management in Health Care* 2 (1993): 18–30.

15. Health Care Advisory Board, *Next Generation of Outcomes Tracking.*

16. R.L. Camp and A.G. Tweet, Benchmarking Applied to Health Care, *Joint Commission Journal on Quality Improvement* 20 (1994): 229–238.

17. Camp and Tweet, Benchmarking Applied to Health Care, 230.

18. Camp and Tweet, Benchmarking Applied to Health Care, 230.

19. A.R. Davies et al., Outcomes Assessment in Clinical Settings: A Consensus Statement on Principles and Best Practices in Project Management, *Joint Commission Journal on Quality Improvement* 20 (1994): 6–16.

20. Davies et al., Outcomes Assessment in Clinical Settings, 11.

21. M. Pine and D.L. Harper, Designing and Using Case Mix Indices, *Managed Care Quarterly* 2 (1994): 1–11.

22. N. Goldfield, Case Mix, Risk Adjustment, Reinsurance, and Health Reform, *Managed Care Quarterly* 2 (1994): iv.

23. M.A. Bloomberg et al., Development of Indicators for Performance Measurement and Improvement: An HMO/Purchaser Collaborative Effort, *Joint Commission Journal on Quality Improvement* 19 (1993): 586–595.

24. P.R. Lee et al., Managed Care: Provider Profiling, *Journal of Insurance Medicine* 24 (1992): 179–181.

25. L.M. Walker, Can a Computer Tell How Good a Doctor You Are? *Medical Economics* 71 (1994): 136–147.

26. Physician Payment Review Commission (PPRC), *Conference on Profiling* (Washington, DC: 1992).

27. Walker, Can a Computer Tell? 138.

28. H. Jordan et al., Reporting and Using Health Plan Performance Information in Massachusetts, *Joint Commission Journal on Quality Improvement* 21 (1995): 167–177.

29. G.J. Langley et al., The Foundation of Improvement, 81–86.

30. Institute of Medicine, Committee to Advise the Public Health Service on Clinical Practice Guidelines, *Clinical Practice Guidelines: Directions for a New Program* (Washington, DC: National Academy Press, 1990).

31. M.R. Handley et al., An Evidence-Based Approach to Evaluating and Improving Clinical Practice: Implementing Practice Guidelines, *HMO Practice* 8 (1994): 75–83.

32. L.N. Newcomber, Six Pointers for Implementing Guidelines, *Healthcare Forum Journal,* July/August 1994, 31–33.

33. J. Kosecoff et al., Effects of a National Institutes of Health Consensus Development Program on Physician Practice, *Journal of the American Medical Association* 258 (1987): 2708–2713.

34. J. Lomas et al., Do Practice Guidelines Guide Practice: The Effect of a Consensus Statement on the Practice of Physicians, *New England Journal of Medicine* 321 (1989): 1306–1311.

35. Walton, Improve Constantly and Forever, 67.

36. J.R. Katzenbach and D.K. Smith, *The Wisdom of Teams. Creating the High Performance Organization* (Boston, MA: Harvard University Press, 1993).

37. Katzenbach and Smith, *The Wisdom of Teams.*

SUGGESTED READING

Couch, J.B., ed. 1991. *Health Care Quality Management for the 21st Century.* Tampa, FL: American College of Medical Quality and the American College of Physician Executives.

The Deming Management Method. 1986. New York: Putnam.

Goldfield, N., et al. 1992. *Measuring and Managing Health Care Quality: Procedures, Techniques, and Protocols.* Gaithersburg, MD: Aspen Publishers.

Langley, G.J., et al. 1996. *The Improvement Guide. A Practical Approach to Enhancing Organizational Performance.* San Francisco: Jossey-Bass Publishers.

Senge, P. 1993. *The Fifth Discipline: The Art and Practice of the Learning Organization* (New York: Currency Doubleday).

Senge, P., and Kleiner, A. 1994. *The Fifth Discipline Fieldbook* (New York: Currency Doubleday).

Youngs, M.T. and Wingerson, L. 1995. *The 1996 Medical Outcomes and Guidelines Sourcebook.* New York: Faulkner & Gray

Eye on Improvement. Institute for Healthcare Improvement, P.O. Box 38100, Cleveland, OH 44138–0100.

Joint Commission Journal on Quality Improvement. Joint Commission on Accreditation of Healthcare Organizations, One Renaissance Boulevard, Oakbrook Terrace, IL 60181.

Quality Management in Health Care. Aspen Publishers, Inc., 200 Orchard Ridge Drive, Suite 200, Gaithersburg, MD 20878.

CHAPTER 31

Measuring and Managing of Clinical Outcomes

Michael Pine

The success of any organization that purports to manage the delivery of health care, regardless of that organization's structure or the services it provides, ultimately must be determined by how often and how well its goals are achieved.

Unfortunately, "outcomes research" has failed to provide simple answers to apparently straightforward questions about the goals of health care. Even the most basic outcomes studies require: (1) a clearly defined input, such as patients' characteristics and conditions when care begins; (2) one or more processes that can transform the input to achieve the desired outcome; and (3) a cause-and-effect relationship between at least one of these processes and the outcome of interest (see Figure 31–1). Measuring "outcomes" without specifying inputs and processes will yield only misinformation and misunderstanding.

An outcome cannot be measured until the patient's initial status is defined and all factors that may influence that outcome are delineated. If these requirements are fulfilled properly, the

measurement of clinical outcomes can be a powerful tool in clinical management.

DOMAINS OF CLINICAL OUTCOMES MEASUREMENT

Information about clinical outcomes spans (1) clinical status, (2) physical function, (3) social function, and (4) feelings and perceptions (see Figure 31–2). Although outcomes in any one domain may be related to outcomes in another, each domain provides unique, important insights into clinical performance.

Each domain has a distinctive set of outcome measures. Clinical status can be characterized either by objective clinical measures or by the judgment of trained clinicians. Physical function can be measured objectively or patients can report it on the basis of objective criteria. Social function can be assessed by applying objective criteria to data derived from patients' reports. Finally, feelings and perceptions related to a patient's condition (e.g., pain, anxiety) or to a patient's care (e.g., satisfaction, perceived competence of clinical staff) are gathered directly through surveys and questionnaires. A comprehensive assessment of clinical performance should consider both desired outcomes and adverse outcomes in all four domains.

GOALS OF CLINICAL OUTCOMES MEASUREMENT

Much fanfare is attached to the transformation of data into information, but information alone is

Michael Pine, MD, MBA, is President of Michael Pine and Associates and a Research Associate in the cardiology section at the University of Chicago. He is a board-certified cardiologist and has served on the medical faculties of Harvard, the University of California, and the University of Cincinnati. Since founding his consulting firm in 1988, Pine has helped purchasers, providers, coalitions, insurers, professional associations, and others to measure clinical outcomes and manage and improve the clinical quality of care.

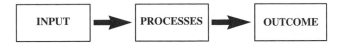

Figure 31–1 Characterization of Outcomes. Courtesy of Michael Pine and Associates, Inc., 1998, Chicago, Illinois.

no more valuable than raw data unless it can be applied. Information about clinical outcomes can be applied to (1) selecting individuals and organizations to provide health care services and (2) improving health care services, either to achieve better outcomes (i.e., improve effectiveness) or to achieve comparable outcomes while consuming fewer resources (i.e., improve efficiency). The first application requires only the assessment of performance (i.e., external monitoring). The second requires both external monitoring and a detailed understanding of how processes of care are linked to observed outcomes (i.e., internal monitoring).

Both applications require using information about clinical performance to make informed decisions and take appropriate actions (see Figure 31–3). However, even correct information about clinical outcomes does not guarantee truly informed decisions. Often such information can be interpreted in more than one way, and each possible interpretation may support a different

decision. For example, external monitoring may show conclusively that patients treated at Clinic A have uniformly better outcomes than patients treated at Clinic B. But this superiority may be due solely to Clinic A's success in treating elderly patients with cardiopulmonary diseases. In this instance, a young patient with limited resources and a gastrointestinal disorder would not be better off paying a premium for "superior" care at Clinic A. Or internal monitoring may prove that patients treated with novobiocin recover from pneumonia twice as fast as patients receiving conventional treatment. However, if 10 percent of patients receiving novobiocin for pneumonia develop fatal dysrhythmias during therapy, clinicians seeking a more rapid therapeutic response would be well-advised to consider a less risky alternative.

For information about clinical outcomes to be useful, it must adequately support decisions by patients, purchasers, providers, practitioners, and other participants in the process of health care delivery. Decision makers must be able to draw correct conclusions that pertain directly to realistic options under consideration. Conclusions, not information, are the yardsticks by which performance monitoring ultimately must be judged.

In sum, whether for external or for internal monitoring, (1) valid data must be transformed into accurate information, (2) accurate information must be used to draw correct conclusions, (3) correct conclusions must be used to make wise decisions, (4) wise decisions must guide effective action, and (5) effective action must produce demonstrable, desired results. Any interruption in the chain of events illustrated in Figure 31–3 greatly diminishes the usefulness of all preceding steps and makes all subsequent steps extremely perilous.

Figure 31–2 Domains of Clinical Outcomes Measurement. Courtesy of Michael Pine and Associates, Inc., 1998, Chicago, Illinois.

Figure 31–3 Linking Data to Action. Courtesy of Healthcare Quality Insights, Inc., 1997.

MEASURING COMPARATIVE RISK-ADJUSTED CLINICAL OUTCOMES

Obtaining accurate and relevant measurements of patient outcomes can be made considerably more manageable by dividing the task into discrete steps. Careful completion of each step will ensure that final results reflect actual clinical performance and can be used by decision makers.

The following six steps are recommended:

1. Clearly distinguish clinical outcomes from processes of care and select specific outcomes of interest.
2. Craft outcome measures and clinical indicators and identify potential risk factors that may influence comparative performance.
3. Define and collect data elements required to perform analyses.
4. Develop risk-adjustment models for each clinical indicator.
5. Compare risk-adjusted clinical outcomes.
6. Evaluate comparative performance based on analytic findings.

Step 1: Distinguish Clinical Outcomes from Processes and Select Outcomes To Be Measured

Although the distinction between *clinical outcomes* and *processes of care* seems self-evident, the two are easily confused in practice. When asked to select outcomes that can be used to assess the quality of clinical care, clinicians often list actions they consider important instead of results they desire to achieve. For instance, they will propose as a measure of quality the use of angiotensin-converting enzyme (ACE) inhibitors to treat patients with severe congestive heart failure, rather than delineate the clinical, functional, and cognitive changes associated with successful treatment of this condition. Such changes would be reduction in objective findings of clinical pulmonary congestion, increased ability to climb stairs, patient's return to work, and reduction in dyspnea.

Outcomes of care always center on the patient, not on the care. They are the reasons why care is rendered. They can be derived from lists of diagnostic and therapeutic actions by asking, "What would happen to the patient if each action on the list were omitted or were performed incorrectly?"

Medical judgment about clinical outcomes is extremely consistent and stable. In contrast, disagreements about best practices occur frequently, and clinical guidelines often evolve fairly rapidly. Therefore, outcomes are preferable to processes as a yardstick for initial screening of clinical performance.

Global outcomes generally will provide a better overview of clinical quality than will their more narrowly defined equivalents. Some examples are:

- occurrence of any complication that prolonged hospitalization, rather than the development of acute renal failure in particular
- admission to a hospital within 48 hours of discharge from ambulatory surgery, rather than hypotension during administration of anesthesia for such surgery
- unscheduled delivery of a premature infant in the second or third trimester, rather than the development of eclampsia
- deterioration in self-reported physical function, rather than reduction in a single measure of range of motion
- total annual cost of caring for pediatric asthmatic patients, rather than total annual cost of medications for those patients
- dissatisfaction with care provided by a health plan, rather than dissatisfaction with the plan's billing practices

Cost-effective monitoring of clinical outcomes, like cost-effective monitoring of financial performance, begins with general measures. It resorts to detailed analyses only when initial findings suggest that additional study is required.

Step 2: Craft Outcome Measures and Clinical Indicators and Identify Potential Risk Factors

Outcome measures must be crafted to reflect validly the actual clinical status of patients receiving care. These measures must be defined precisely and must not be influenced unduly by variations in how data are obtained. The exact timing and method of assessment often must be specified because systematic differences in reporting can be mistaken easily for systematic differences in performance. For example, inpatient mortality, mortality within 30 days of admission, and mortality within one year of diagnosis all are reasonable measures of mortality, but information obtained using one of these measures cannot be compared directly to information obtained using another. Similarly, general satisfaction information obtained by a 20-question phone survey of a random sample of clinic patients cannot be compared directly to results of a two-question survey mailed to all patients leaving the clinic.

Also, reporting biases must be minimized. Although systematic differences in what is reported and how it is reported may "average out" in estimates of overall results, they will not average out when performances are compared. For example, the average rate of wound infection after abdominal surgery may be estimated correctly at 3.2 percent, despite systematic reporting biases by a group of surgeons who underreport their infection rate by 1.0 percent and by a group of surgeons who overreport their rate by 1.0 percent. However, if Surgeon A and Surgeon B have actually similar rates of wound infections, but Surgeon A reports his rate as 2.2 percent and Surgeon B reports his rate as 4.2 percent, a naive observer would conclude that Surgeon B has almost twice Surgeon A's rate of wound infections.

In crafting measures of clinical outcomes, clinical events that can be classified as processes rather than as outcomes of care may be used as surrogates for actual clinical outcomes that cannot be measured directly in a valid, consistent fashion. For instance, hospitalization of a patient with asthma is a treatment decision, part of the process of care. But it is also a marker for unsuccessful outpatient management of asthma (i.e., a clinical outcome measure) in that the patient's condition deteriorated seriously enough to require hospital care.

Clinical performances can be compared only when measures are applied to well-defined populations of patients. A *clinical indicator* specifies both the measure to be applied and the population to which it is applicable. The measure generally provides information contained in the numerator of a fraction (e.g., the number of inpatient deaths, the total cost of treatment). The population studied generally provides information contained in the denominator (e.g., the number of patients hospitalized, the number of patients treated).

Single measures can be used to create multiple indicators. For instance, a specific measure of adverse outcomes can be applied to men, women, men with blue eyes, women with gray eyes, unmarried men between the ages of 40 and 65, and divorced women between the ages of 25 and 27. However, these divisions of the patient population may not be particularly relevant to clinical performance. Therefore, in assessing systems designed to compare clinical performance, it is best to consider individual measures rather than individual indicators.

If each patient in the population to be studied has the same probability of achieving each possible outcome, then all data elements required for the assessment of comparative clinical performance have been defined. However, different patients usually differ in their likelihood of achieving one or more of the outcomes being measured. These differences can be related to differences in patients' characteristics and conditions when care begins (i.e., to different inputs). To compensate for these differences, it is necessary to identify measurable potential risk factors that can be used to predict each patient's outcome given uniform care. Like outcome measures, risk factors must be defined clearly and must not be influenced unduly by vagaries in

data acquisition. Risk factors must be present before delivery of the care being evaluated. Data needed to define outcome indicators and data required to define risk factors comprise the analytic data set that must be acquired in order to use risk-adjusted outcomes to evaluate clinical performance.

Step 3: Specify and Collect Data Elements

The nature and quality of data used to compare risk-adjusted clinical outcomes are crucial to the validity and relevance of conclusions drawn from these analyses. Clear data specifications must be prepared and followed in order to obtain fair comparisons. A data element may be obtained from any one of several acceptable sources, but the comparability of data from different sources must be evaluated carefully before these data are analyzed. The topics of sources of data and data collection are also discussed in the context of the use of data for medical management and profiling in Chapter 32.

Currently, billing data are readily available in electronic form, and ambulatory Health Care Financing Administration (HCFA) 1500 formats and hospital UB-92 forms are relatively well-standardized. However, HCFA 1500 reports often fail to list many important, active clinical diagnoses, and secondary diagnostic codes used in UB-92 reports do not distinguish between comorbidities present on admission (i.e., potential risk factors) and complications that developed during hospitalization (i.e., potential adverse outcomes of care). This latter problem can be corrected by linking each secondary diagnostic code to a field that specifies whether the diagnosis was present on admission or was acquired during hospitalization. This approach was reported first in 1991 by the Mayo Clinic, which found that obtaining these data consumed less than two minutes per medical record. Moreover, the rate of agreement among coders was 87 percent. Routine submission of this information has been required in New York state since 1993 and in California since 1996.

More detailed hospital charge master databases also are available in electronic form and can provide a wealth of important information. However, the structure of these databases varies among facilities, and painstaking mapping must be performed in order to obtain comparable information.

Many other operational databases (e.g., laboratory, pharmacy) can be accessed to obtain information about outcomes and risk factors, but linking these databases and obtaining comparable data from multiple facilities are far more difficult in practice than in theory. For all the rhetoric and hype surrounding "the electronic medical record," medical record systems remain extremely primitive and disjointed. Even when electronic linkage is achieved, incompatibly defined data often prevent valid comparisons.

The most direct method of collecting data elements required to evaluate comparative risk-adjusted clinical outcomes is to create a customized database and either to obtain required data elements directly from caregivers or to abstract them directly from medical records. Incorporating data collection for outcomes analyses into the process of documenting clinical care is appealing but has proven difficult to implement for more than a few conditions at relatively few institutions. On the other hand, abstraction of medical records is an effective but extremely costly method of obtaining data for comparative analyses of clinical outcomes.

In sum, ideal sources of data to support comparative analyses of risk-adjusted clinical outcomes are not available at present. However, promising new methods of reducing the cost of data collection without compromising the validity or relevance of analytic conclusions are under development.

Step 4: Develop Risk-Adjustment Models for Each Clinical Indicator

Rarely, if ever, is a population of patients so homogeneous that individuals do not differ in their probability of experiencing a particular outcome. Therefore, some adjustment must be made for these differences in "severity of illness." Otherwise, differences in performance that really are due to variations in patients' risks (i.e., differences in case mix) may be interpreted falsely as differences in quality of care. Risk adjustment approaches are discussed in Chapter 32.

For instance, measurements that appear to show different levels of care at two different hospitals may not explain that one hospital tended to treat much sicker patients or patients more likely to be at risk of developing a particular complication. Simply put, risk-adjustment models are algorithms or equations that express the intrinsic risk (or severity) of a given patient or group of patients, based on specific descriptors of each patient's characteristics and condition prior to receiving care.

It is important to note that risk is outcome-specific as well as patient-specific. For instance, a patient undergoing emergency surgery may have a high probability of dying but a low probability of a postoperative wound infection. Another patient undergoing the same surgical procedure may have a low probability of dying but a high probability of a postoperative infection. And both patients may have moderate probabilities of substantial postoperative physical impairment. Therefore, severity systems that give each patient a single score for burden of illness are poor risk-adjustment tools. Instead, a complete risk profile should be created for each patient by computing an individual predicted value for each outcome of interest.

Complete dependence upon expert judgment to classify patients' risks has proven to be extremely problematic. Instead, expert judgment is best directed toward the identification of potential risk factors (see Step 2) and toward review of empirically derived risk-adjustment algorithms or equations for clinical credibility. Final selection of predictive data elements and assignment of relative weights are performed best by applying statistical techniques to a large database drawn from multiple providers that serve diverse populations of patients.

Many different statistical techniques can be used to develop valid risk-adjustment models, but all have the same general approach and underlying assumptions. First, data must be evaluated carefully to ensure that they are internally consistent and relatively free of errors. Assuming that measurement errors are negligible, each patient's outcome will be dependent upon three factors (see Figure 31–4): (1) those specific to each individual patient prior to the delivery of care (i.e., patient-specific factors), (2) those specific to the quality of the care provided (i.e., provider-specific factors), and (3) those due to chance alone (i.e., random variation not attributable to any identifiable factor).

The influence of random variation can be reduced by limiting a risk-adjustment model only to those risk factors that have a statistically significant relationship to the outcome of interest. And because many different providers and institutions contribute to the database used in creating the model, the influence of differences in quality of care is reduced greatly. This permits the analyst to relate patient-specific factors directly to observed outcomes and to use the available data to assign a relative weight to each risk factor selected for inclusion in the model. Thus, as shown in Figure 31–5, residual random variation and provider-specific factors can be minimized, and risk factors and weights reflect mainly intrinsic patient-specific characteristics that alter the probability that a specific outcome will occur.

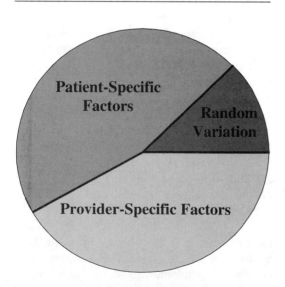

Figure 31–4 Factors Affecting Each Measured Outcome. Courtesy of Michael Pine and Associates, Inc., 1998, Chicago, Illinois.

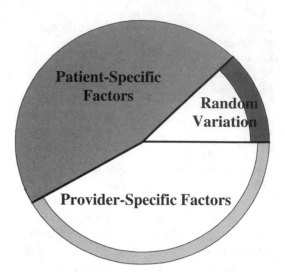

Figure 31–5 Residual Factors Affecting Risk-Adjustment Models. Courtesy of Michael Pine and Associates, Inc., 1998, Chicago, Illinois.

Step 5: Compare Risk-Adjusted Clinical Outcomes

When combined with risk-adjustment models derived as in Step 4, clinical outcome measures can be converted into valid, relevant indices of clinical performance. Observed and predicted values for a clinical measure are available for each patient to whom the measure was applied. Therefore, clinical performance can be assessed for different combinations of patients (i.e., reporting categories), regardless of how these patients were assigned to risk-adjustment models (i.e., to analytic categories). This flexibility permits analysts to create new clinical indicators (in contrast to measures) at will and to explore issues and concerns that arise after initial measurements and risk-adjustment models are developed.

Each measured outcome has four basic components: (1) intrinsic patient-specific risk, (2) quality of care provided, (3) random variation, and (4) bias introduced by systematic errors in measurement. Figure 31–6 illustrates their relationship as a simple sum.

Because patients' outcomes can be observed directly, they are far easier to measure directly

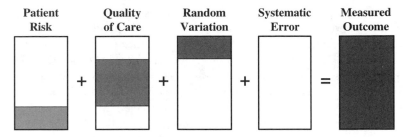

Figure 31–6 Basic Components of Measured Outcome. Courtesy of Michael Pine and Associates, Inc., 1998, Chicago, Illinois.

than is quality of care (i.e., the providers' contribution of patient outcomes). Patients' risks can be calculated by measuring relevant risk factors and computing predicted values using risk-adjustment models derived as in Step 4. Allowance can be made statistically for random variation, and systematic errors can be minimized by careful data acquisition and analysis. As quality of care remains the only unknown component, it is possible to estimate its contribution to measured clinical outcome by subtracting patient risk, random variation, and systematic error from both sides of the outcomes equation described above. This yields a new equation (shown in Figure 31–7) in which quality of care equals patients' measured outcomes minus systematic error (here assumed to be zero) minus patient-specific risk (computed using an appropriate risk-adjustment model) minus random variation (estimated using statistical formulae).

In the equation illustrated in Figure 31 7, quantities are assumed to be absolute values. However,

a patient's risk (i.e., the probability that the patient, given standard care, will experience a particular outcome) is not absolute, because it depends upon the arbitrary selection of one of a large number of reasonable standards of care. Often the standard selected is the average of all patients analyzed (i.e., for the entire group of patients, the observed outcome is equal to the predicted outcome). Alternatively, a risk-adjustment model can be calibrated using a reference set of patients, and that reference then can be used to define a standard of care. The selection of a standard of care does not affect the choice of risk factors or the relative weights assigned to them, nor does it affect the relative performance of organizations or providers being evaluated. However, it does affect the designation of an organization or provider as better than, comparable to, or worse than average. If low standards are selected, everyone being evaluated may be above "average," while if high standards are used, everyone being evaluated may fail to achieve "average" levels of performance.

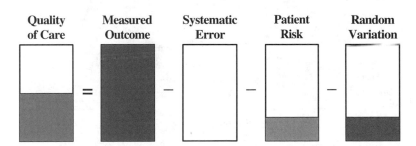

Figure 31–7 Computation To Derive Quality of Care. Courtesy of Michael Pine and Associates, Inc., 1998, Chicago, Illinois.

Once a standard of care has been selected and used to calibrate an appropriate risk-adjustment model, risk-adjusted outcomes for a group of organizations or providers can be compared. Figure 31–8 illustrates one such comparison for adverse outcomes in patients undergoing nonsurgical coronary revascularization. This illustration shows all the components in the quality equation: (1) observed rates, (2) predicted rates, and (3) ranges associated with specified levels of confidence that differences between observed and predicted rates are not due solely to chance. (For purposes of these reports, systematic error is assumed to be negligible.) Differences in case mix among providers (i.e., the relative riskiness of patients treated by different organizations or providers) are reflected in dif-

ferences in predicted values. The difference between each provider's observed and predicted values reflects the degree to which its actual performance was better or worse than standard care.

Three sets of confidence limits mark the intervals within which differences between observed and predicted values should be considered statistically insignificant (i.e., consistent with chance variation alone). A difference outside the smallest confidence interval will occur by chance alone less than 5 percent of the time; a difference outside the largest confidence interval will occur by chance alone less than 0.1 percent of the time. Managers can base their decisions on more or less demanding confidence limits, depending upon the relative importance of the decision. Requiring higher degrees of confidence reduces

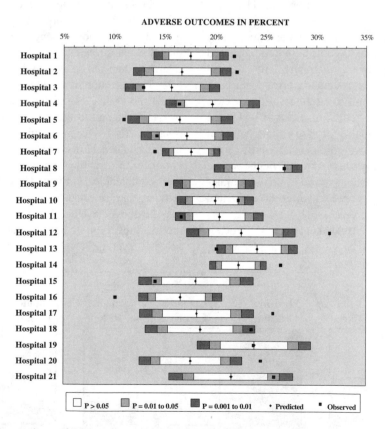

Figure 31–8 Comparison of Risk-Adjusted Adverse Outcome Rates for Patients Undergoing Nonsurgical Coronary Revascularization at 21 Hospitals in the Nationwide Cardiac Alliance. Courtesy of Healthcare Quality Insights, Inc., 1997.

the likelihood that a difference due solely to chance will be mistaken for a difference in quality of care.

The influence of random variation always can be reduced by increasing the number of measurements for each organization or provider. However, sample size often can be increased only by making studied populations more heterogeneous or by increasing the time period in which data are collected. Sample sizes used in reports of comparative risk-adjusted outcomes represent compromises between the desire to reduce the influence of random variation and the desire to obtain information about homogeneous groups of patients in relatively short periods of time.

Confidence limits provide information about *statistical significance* (i.e., the probability that a difference between observed and predicted values is due solely to chance variation). However, they do not provide comparable information about clinical or operational *importance* (i.e., whether the difference between observed and predicted values is large enough to be considered in decision making). In Figure 31–8 confidence intervals are relatively wide, and all statistically significant differences in performance also are clinically important. However, when confidence intervals are relatively narrow, some statistically significant differences may be considered neither clinically nor operationally important.

When comparing large numbers of organizations or providers, it is important to remember that as the number of comparisons increases, so does the likelihood that one or more organizations or providers will be identified as outliers (i.e., as having differences between observed and predicted values that exceed the confidence interval selected for the comparison). For instance, if a confidence limit of 5 percent is selected, there will be less than one chance in 20 that a single determination will incorrectly attribute a chance difference to a difference in quality of care. However, if 20 determinations are considered, there are almost two chances in three that at least one organization or provider will be an outlier by chance alone. If 50 determinations are considered, the likelihood is greater than 90 percent that at least one organization or

provider will be an outlier by chance alone. Therefore, when considering multiple comparisons, it is important to determine whether the distribution of differences between observed and predicted values is significantly greater than the distribution that ordinarily might occur by chance alone. If statistical tests indicate that this distribution is consistent with chance variation alone, no single difference should be viewed as definitively superior or inferior performance.

Step 6: Evaluate Performance Based on Analytic Findings

An important statistically significant difference between observed and predicted values for a clinical indicator measured for a single organization or provider may be due to one or more or the following: (1) flaws in the process of risk adjustment, (2) other systematic errors in measurement or analysis that bias results in favor of or against an organization or provider, (3) random variation not accounted for by established confidence limits, and (4) real differences between the organization or provider and the reference standard in the quality of care provided.

Risk-adjustment models may not compensate completely for differences in case mix. They may either omit or underestimate the importance of one or more patient-specific risk factors (e.g., poorly controlled diabetes mellitus, severe dementia). When this occurs, as Figure 31–9 illustrates, some of the difference between observed and predicted outcomes that should have been attributed to intrinsic patient-specific risk will be attributed instead to quality of care.

Another problem is created when risk factors reflect the intermediate results of the care a patient receives rather than the patient's actual status when care began (e.g., pulmonary edema resulting from too vigorous administration of intravenous fluids, a cerebrovascular accident first noted after a carotid endarterectomy). In this case, as Figure 31–10 shows, some of the difference between observed and predicted outcomes that should have been attributed to quality of care will be attributed instead to intrinsic patient-specific risk.

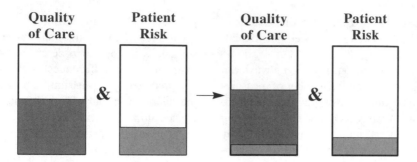

Figure 31–9 Misattribution of Patient Risk to Quality of Care. Courtesy of Michael Pine and Associates, Inc., 1998, Chicago, Illinois.

Both types of errors will result in some organizations or providers appearing to perform better and some appearing to perform worse than they would without these errors.

Systematic errors in measurement or analysis can distort some of the effect of quality of care by introducing some degree of positive or negative bias, as Figure 31–11 illustrates. For example, one provider or organization may report minor wound infections as complications while another may report only wound infections that delay discharge. One facility may treat every patient with hemophilia in the entire community, making it impossible to develop fair comparative standards for outcomes involving these patients. Or low-risk patients may have better risk-adjusted results than high-risk patients, so that facilities that primarily treat low-risk patients are favored systematically. In contrast to random errors, systematic errors cannot be reduced by increasing the number of cases. Nor are there routine tests that will automatically detect the presence of all possible systematic errors. Systematic errors can be avoided only by carefully designing and critically evaluating studies of comparative risk-adjusted clinical outcomes.

Whatever confidence limits are selected, the difference between observed and predicted outcomes will be due, at least in part, to chance variation, as Figure 31–12 illustrates. The influence of chance variation can be reduced by requiring higher degrees of confidence. However, this will increase the possibility of attributing to chance some differences that really reflect differences in quality of care.

Figure 31–10 Misattribution of Quality of Care to Patient Risk. Courtesy of Michael Pine and Associates, Inc., 1998, Chicago, Illinois.

Figure 31–11 Effect of Systematic Error on Measured Quality of Care. Courtesy of Michael Pine and Associates, Inc., 1998, Chicago, Illinois.

Larger volumes of cases will reduce the relative magnitude of chance variation. However, increasing the number of cases generally requires making groups of patients more heterogeneous or lengthening the period of data collection. This makes it more difficult to draw clinical and operational conclusions from analytic reports.

In sum, the ideal equation illustrated in Figure 31–7 must be revised to incorporate all the errors that can enter into computations of clinical performance based on risk-adjusted outcomes. As Figure 31–13 shows, the effects of intrinsic patient-specific risk and quality of care can be confused, and random variation and uncorrected systematic errors can distort estimates of quality of care. These errors never can be eliminated entirely, but they can be minimized by careful de-

sign and execution of comparative studies of risk-adjusted clinical outcomes.

If important, statistically significant differences between observed and predicted outcomes remain even after allowance for possible sources of error, the differences can be attributed to differences in quality of care. Almost invariably, however, further analysis and interpretation are required to support effective decision making.

USING DATA ON RISK-ADJUSTED COSTS TO CRAFT MEASURES OF CLINICAL PERFORMANCE

Clinical outcomes must be measured consistently to ensure valid comparisons of performance among providers or organizations. How-

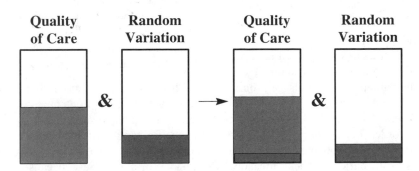

Figure 31–12 Effect of Random Variation on Measured Quality of Care. Courtesy of Michael Pine and Associates, Inc., 1998, Chicago, Illinois.

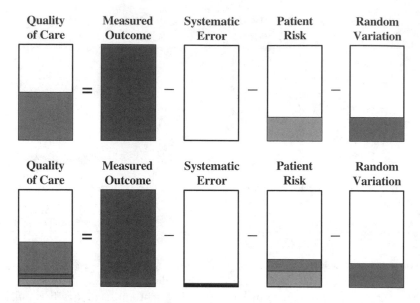

Figure 31–13 Effect of Multiple Errors on Measured Quality of Care. Courtesy of Michael Pine and Associates, Inc., 1998, Chicago, Illinois.

---

ever, descriptive and diagnostic data are extremely sensitive to differences in how they are observed and reported by different individuals. This is true especially when many people are involved in recording or collecting data and when they have not received consistent training and evaluation of their data quality.

Objective data also may be biased if they are not obtained consistently. For instance, positive findings may be missed when tests are not performed. Just the fact that a test is ordered, even though results are normal, may indicate increased risk of an adverse outcome. Ideally, therefore, assessments of risk-adjusted clinical outcomes should be based on uniformly collected objective measures as are used in expensive cooperative clinical research studies.

Because such an approach would be prohibitively expensive, valid measures of clinical outcomes must be created from data that can be acquired and recorded in the course of ordinary clinical care or that can be obtained directly and economically from patients. These measures need not correspond directly with measures used in clinical practice. However, they must (1) re-

flect patient outcomes accurately and (2) reflect clinical performance consistently.

One method of creating acceptable outcome measures from flawed data is as follows:

1. Screen patients using a crude indicator of an outcome of interest.
2. Based on initial findings, apply methods of statistical process control to a readily available, objective measure associated with the outcome of interest.
3. From this measure, create a new indicator that can be calibrated and applied consistently to individual providers or organizations.
4. Use the new indicator as a surrogate for the outcome of interest.

This method can be used, for example, to obtain rates of adverse outcomes (i.e., complications) during an episode of care associated with a specific condition or procedure. Rates of reported nonfatal complications are extremely unreliable for this purpose, because systematic biases in identifying, recording, and reporting complications may easily halve or double such rates. On the other hand, objective data about the cost of care are readily available, and unusually high risk-adjusted costs are a reasonable surrogate for clinical complications. Therefore, risk-adjusted costs that are unusually high compared with predicted values for an individual provider or organization can reflect accurately and consistently the occurrence of important clinical complications.

An illustration of an application of this method follows. Of 1,000 episodes of nonsurgical coronary revascularization managed by the "Quickfix Cardiovascular Center," 342 had procedure-related complications that occurred during the procedure or during one year of follow-up care. Standardized (i.e., risk-adjusted) costs for these episodes were computed by (1) dividing observed by predicted values and (2) multiplying this ratio by the median predicted routine cost of these episodes (i.e., the cost predicted in the absence of complications).

Next, a control chart was constructed for standardized costs for the 658 episodes without re-

ported complications. Standardized costs that exceeded a three-standard-deviation upper control limit were removed from the data set, and control limits were recomputed. This process was repeated until all standardized costs in the data set were less than the upper control limit of three standard deviations computed from that data set.

In the control chart for Quickfix Cardiovascular Center shown in Figure 31–14, the three episodes with excessive costs that were removed from the data set are shown as squares and labeled "Excessive Cost." Control limits are based on the 655 costs shown as diamonds and labeled "Normal Cost."

The final upper control limit derived as explained above was used to identify outliers from among the 342 episodes of nonsurgical coronary revascularization with reported complications. The results are shown in Figure 31–15. Compared to episodes without reported complications, a much higher proportion of episodes with reported complications had excessive costs

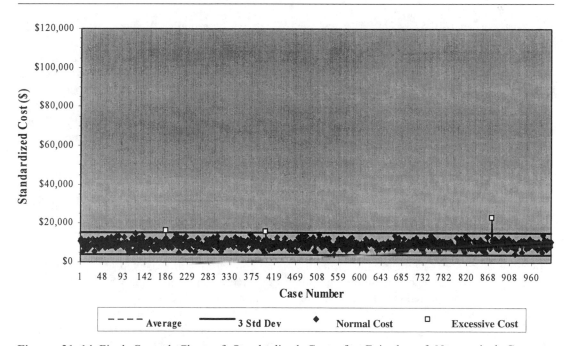

Figure 31–14 Final Control Chart of Standardized Costs for Episodes of Nonsurgical Coronary Revascularization without Reported Complications at Quickfix Cardiovascular Center. Copyright © 1998, Michael Pine and Associates, Inc.

Figure 31–15 Control Chart of Standardized Costs for Episodes of Nonsurgical Coronary Revascularization with Reported Complications at Quickfix Cardiovascular Center. Copyright © 1998, Michael Pine and Associates, Inc.

(48.2 percent versus 0.5 percent). The low rate of adverse outcomes in episodes without reported complications and the substantially higher rate of adverse outcomes in episodes with reported complications both are consistent with high data integrity.

USING ADVERSE OUTCOME RATES TO REDUCE COSTS

Comparisons of observed to predicted costs for episodes of care are useful not only in objectively identifying adverse outcomes, but also in dissecting total costs into more manageable components.

Routine costs are costs incurred in caring for patients who have no important clinical complications. They may be reduced by developing protocols to guide standard clinical practice and by effective case management. For a specified episode managed by a group practice, the ratio of observed to predicted costs for routine episodes (i.e., episodes without adverse outcomes)

defines the group's efficiency for that episode. For episodes associated with adverse outcomes, the cost of the routine component of care can be calculated by multiplying the predicted routine cost by this ratio. Total routine costs for the specified episode for the practice are the sum of all routine costs. This value can be compared with a predicted value based on routine costs for a comparative standard.

The cost of adverse outcomes is the difference between total costs and routine costs. It is the product of the percentage of adverse outcomes and the average excess cost of each adverse outcome. Both the rate of adverse outcomes and the average excess cost of each adverse outcome can be compared with predicted values that reflect the average performance of group practices treating similar patients.

The power of using these data to guide efforts to improve profitability is demonstrated in Figure 31–16. This figure shows the results of further analyses of data presented in Figures 31–14 and 31–15 for 1,000 episodes of nonsurgical

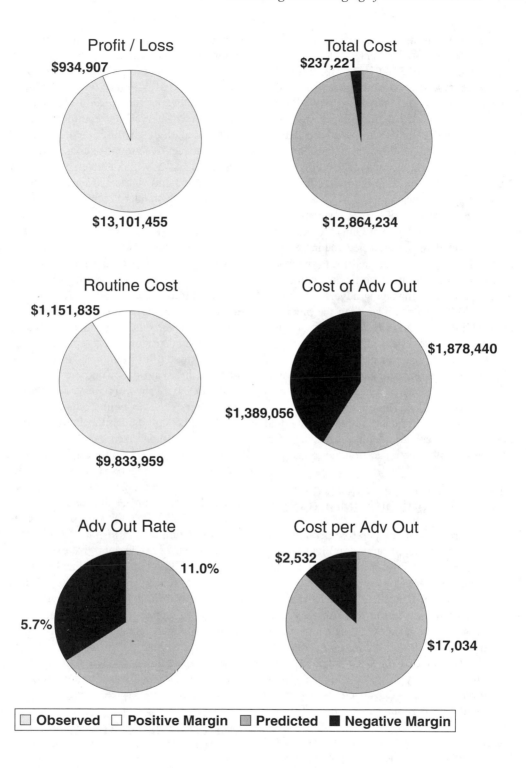

Figure 31–16 Variance Analysis of Components of Total Cost of Episodes of Nonsurgical Coronary Revascularization at Quickfix Cardiovascular Center. Copyright © 1998, Michael Pine and Associates, Inc.

coronary revascularization managed by the Quickfix Cardiovascular Center.

A total revenue of $14,036,362 for this product line generated an operating margin of 6.7 percent. However, an analysis of risk-adjusted total costs revealed that this margin was 20.2 percent lower than it would have been if total costs had not been 1.8 percent higher than predicted. Under these circumstances, aggressive case management and efforts to identify avoidable costs appear reasonable.

However, actual routine costs for nonsurgical coronary revascularization at Quickfix were 10.5 percent lower than the predicted routine cost of nearly $10,985,794. Poor cost performance at Quickfix resulted, not from inefficient routine care but from a cost of managing adverse outcomes that was 73.9 percent higher than the predicted cost of $1,878,440. These avoidable costs, in turn, were attributable to an adverse outcome rate that was 51.4 percent higher than the predicted rate of 11.0 percent. The cost per patient with an adverse outcome was 14.9 percent higher than the predicted cost of $17,034. Thus, in this instance, concentrating on clinical quality improvement could achieve far greater increases in profitability than could further efforts to reduce routine costs.

USING CONTROL CHARTS TO GET A DYNAMIC VIEW OF PERFORMANCE

Periodic reports of comparative risk-adjusted clinical outcomes (as illustrated in Figure 31–8) can provide useful information about performance. However, most practitioners or providers will not benefit much from increasing the frequency of these reports because they treat relatively few patients in each diagnostic or procedural category. Small numbers increase the relative importance of random variation, resulting in unacceptably large confidence limits. Therefore, it is advisable to compare performance with external standards relatively infrequently (e.g., annually or semiannually) and to look for trends by creating control charts for standardized (i.e., risk-adjusted) outcomes.

For discrete indicators such as mortality or adverse outcomes, the ratio of observed to pre-

dicted values can be charted over intervals that begin immediately after an event occurs and end with a subsequent event. The number of events in each interval will vary with the relative frequency of events and the algorithm used to terminate each interval. For continuous indicators such as length of stay or cost, standardized values for successive groups of consecutive routine cases (i.e., cases without adverse outcomes) can be averaged and charted. Control limits can be derived using standard techniques of statistical process control.

Figures 31–17, 31–18, and 31–19 were produced from the same data set of risk-adjusted adverse outcome rates and lengths of stay for 393 patient hospitalized with pulmonary diseases. Only the dates of admission were altered to create different patterns of risk-adjusted outcomes at the three facilities used in this example. Thus, annual performance reports for the 393 patients treated for pulmonary diseases at each of these three hospitals would be identical.

Figure 31–17 shows no identifiable trends and no outliers (i.e., no points outside the control limits) either for standardized adverse outcome rates or for standardized lengths of stay for pulmonary patients at "Sample Memorial Hospital." In contrast, Figure 31–18 shows a precipitous fall in standardized adverse outcome rates and a slow but unmistakable decline in standardized lengths of stay for pulmonary patients at "Neway Community Hospital." Finally, Figure 31–19 shows a single point that exceeds the upper control limit for standardized adverse outcome rates and a single point that exceeds the upper control limit for standardized lengths of stay for pulmonary patients at "BadTime Academic Medical Center." These outliers are not associated with any identifiable trend. Both occurred during the second two months of the year when "Dr. Careless" was the attending physician on the pulmonary service.

RELATING CLINICAL OUTCOMES TO PROCESSES OF CARE

As clinical outcomes cannot be managed directly, they must be linked to processes of care

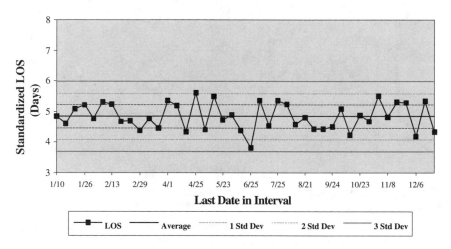

Figure 31–17 Dynamic View of Rates of Adverse Outcomes and Lengths of Stay for Pulmonary Diseases at Sample Memorial Hospital. Courtesy of Healthcare Quality Insights, Inc., 1997.

that can be managed to maintain or improve related outcomes. A complete review of methods of linking processes of care to risk-adjusted outcomes is beyond the scope of this chapter, but a description of one such method may be helpful.

Insights into underlying causes of superior or unsatisfactory performance can be gained by comparing the distribution and timing of initial complications of clinical care to risk-adjusted reference standards. The effect of reporting biases on analytic findings can be reduced by lim-

iting this analysis to cases with important adverse outcomes. Concentration on initial events rather than on later sequelae can detect potential root causes rather than complicating factors. These analyses are particularly useful in identifying (1) isolated problem areas when overall performance is average or above average and (2) isolated areas of excellence when overall performance is average or below average.

For example, "Cutemup Regional Medical Center's" observed mortality rate for coronary ar-

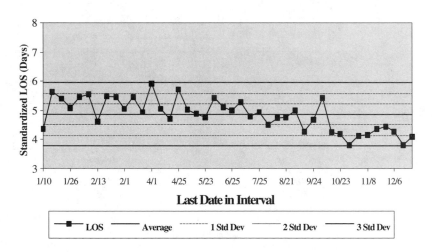

Figure 31–18 Dynamic View of Rates of Adverse Outcomes and Lengths of Stay for Pulmonary Diseases at Neway Community Hospital. Courtesy of Healthcare Quality Insights, Inc., 1997.

tery bypass graft surgery is more than one-third higher than predicted. Figure 31–20 shows that this excess mortality is associated with initial cardiopulmonary complications, many of which are associated with the surgical procedure itself. Figure 31–21 demonstrates that excess mortality is associated almost entirely with initial complications that occur within a day of operation. With these findings, attention can be directed to potential problems in judgment and technique associated with operative and early postoperative clinical management. More extensive discussions of the wide array of methods available to guide pro-

cess improvement by relating processes of care to clinical outcomes are available in other texts.* These methods are ideally suited to solving problems like those of Quickfix Cardiovascular Cen-

*For more extensive discussions of the wide array of methods available to guide process improvement by relating processes of care to clinical outcomes, see Peter R. Kongstvedt and David P. Plocher, *Best Practices in Medical Management* (Gaithersburg, MD: Aspen Publishers, Inc., 1998) and N. Goldfield, M. Pine, and J. Pine, *Measuring and Managing Health Care Quality: Procedures, Techniques, and Protocols* (Gaithersburg, MD: Aspen Publishers, Inc., 1999).

Figure 31–19 Dynamic View of Rates of Adverse Outcomes and Lengths of Stay for Pulmonary Diseases at BadTime Academic Medical Center. Courtesy of Healthcare Quality Insights, Inc., 1997.

ter, described earlier. Together they can suggest and support hypotheses for improving clinical outcomes by altering specific processes of care. They are a powerful supplement to clinical and managerial insight and judgment, to standard methods of statistical quality control and process improvement, and to more familiar methods of clinical investigation.

MONITORING CLINICAL OUTCOMES OF AMBULATORY CARE

Ideally, the principles and methods described in this chapter should apply directly to outpatient care. However, several practical problems have restrained the diffusion of this technology from the inpatient environment.

First, few objective data are collected routinely during outpatient encounters. This makes proper classification of patients difficult, if not impossible. Diagnostic information often is incomplete and is far more likely to be inaccurate than is diagnostic information for hospitalized patients. Important chronic conditions may pass unnoticed or unnoted during relatively brief ambulatory encounters for self-limited acute medical problems. When a chronic condition is noted, little information may be recorded about its du-

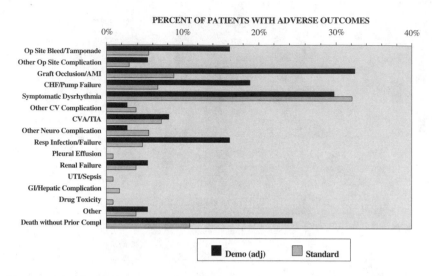

Figure 31–20 Comparison of Adjusted Proportions of Specific Initial Complications among Inpatients Who Died During or after CABG Surgery at Cutemup Regional Medical Center and at All Hospitals in the HealthyHeart Cardiac Alliance. Courtesy of Michael Pine and Associates, Inc., 1998, Chicago, Illinois.

ration, extent, or progression. Current ambulatory care classification systems either gloss over these problems, creating groupings that are clinically suspect, or require such extensive documentation that only the most enthusiastic, resource-rich organizations can use them. Consequently, until more cost-effective methods are developed for classifying patients accurately, differences in

measured performance are as likely to be due to systematic differences in documentation and classification as to systematic differences in the quality of ambulatory care.

Second, important changes in health status often unfold slowly, while dramatic, rapid changes that precipitate many ambulatory encounters often are self-limited and transient. Incomplete

Figure 31–21 Comparison of Times of Occurrence of Initial Complications among Inpatients Who Died During or after CABG Surgery at Cutemup Regional Medical Center and at All Hospitals in the HealthyHeart Cardiac Alliance. Courtesy of Michael Pine and Associates, Inc., 1998, Chicago, Illinois.

long-term follow-up can introduce systematic biases that invalidate comparisons of alternative providers or patterns of care. Unfocused measures of general health status may fail to uncover important differences in condition-specific outcomes or may reveal differences but give no insights into their underlying cause. On the other hand, condition-specific measures can be misapplied when diagnoses are incomplete or incorrect. This creates problems in numerous cases in which multiple chronic conditions coexist. Therefore, problems with interpreting apparent differences in performance and properly relating these differences to actionable alternatives remain important barriers to the widespread adoption of outcomes monitoring in ambulatory settings.

Finally, multiple sources of data generally are required to track outcomes related to ambulatory care and to create and apply appropriate risk-adjustment models. Numerous technical difficulties and considerable expense are associated with collecting, integrating, managing, and analyzing a vast array of data from multiple sources. In a cost-conscious environment that emphasizes the provision of health care services rather than their assessment, there is a strong tendency to accept sloppy, misleading evaluations rather than to commit the resources needed to develop cost-effective systems that ensure the accuracy and relevance of analytic findings.

If monitoring risk-adjusted clinical outcomes in acute care settings is in its infancy, monitoring risk-adjusted clinical outcomes in outpatient settings has yet to be born. However, patient-derived information about functional status is applicable to the ambulatory environment, and the use of data about cost to create objective surrogates for adverse clinical outcomes can facilitate valid investigations of comparative clinical performance in ambulatory settings. By focusing on several areas of outpatient care that are particularly well suited to developmental work, analysts can begin to provide useful information to both purchasers and providers of care.

First, important chronic conditions can be identified and tracked using objective markers rather than inconstant diagnostic assignment. For instance, in the Health Plan Employer Data

Information Set (HEDIS; see Chapter 35), treatment with insulin or oral hypoglycemic agents is used as a marker for diabetes mellitus. This technique parallels the use of prolonged risk-adjusted length of stay as a marker for important hospital-acquired complications. It will not identify all patients in a category (e.g., with diabetes), but it will identify a relatively uniform subset of such patients. Similarly, alterations in patterns of care can be identified and used to mark important outcomes of ambulatory care. To use such alterations successfully as a proxy for ambulatory outcomes, actual baseline patterns must be characterized for individual practitioners. The use of universal external standards is inappropriate for proxy measurement.

Second, patients can be selected for study based on the occurrence of particular adverse outcomes rather than on diagnoses or findings at the onset of an episode or course of ambulatory care. Evaluations of care in these instances must be interpreted cautiously, because analytic techniques required to draw useful conclusions from these patients differ markedly from standard methods described earlier in this chapter.

Third, measures of adherence to well-substantiated standards of care can substitute for measures of outcomes where scientific evidence linking processes to outcomes is extremely strong. The benefits of adherence to standards occur only after considerable time has elapsed. A compendium of such practice standards is available in the *Guide to Clinical Preventive Services* (second edition, 1996), which is prepared by the U.S. Preventive Services Task Force. Recommendations rated "A" (for good evidence supporting intervention) are the best candidates for incorporation in process-based performance measures.

When relying on process-based measures, it is important to acknowledge circumstances in which processes must be altered (e.g., failure to perform periodic Pap smears after total hysterectomy for benign disease), or in which adherence to standards is more difficult due to factors beyond the provider's control (e.g., administration of vaccines to patients who may be allergic to eggs). These cases either can be excluded from analyses (which limits the applicability of findings) or allowed for in risk adjustment.

Finally, ambulatory care following acute episodes or interventions can be evaluated using methods described in this chapter. For instance, care following discharge from a hospital or following ambulatory surgical procedures can be evaluated after calculating the patient's risks at the conclusion of the acute care intervention. Similarly, patients entering formal rehabilitation programs are good candidates for external monitoring of risk-adjusted clinical outcomes. In these situations, data for risk-adjustment are more readily available because an acute intervention requires more intensive clinical monitoring than generally is needed in routine ambulatory settings.

Growing concerns with the quality of ambulatory care have fueled demand for plausible systems to monitor outcomes attributable to outpatient management. However, it is important to remember that plausible information may be neither accurate nor valid. To ignore methodological barriers and limitations is to court disaster. Invalid conclusions can result in poor policy, poor management, and poor practice, ultimately undermining the credibility of outcomes monitoring in general. The goal of comprehensive monitoring of risk-adjusted outcomes of ambulatory care can be achieved only by investing carefully in limited solutions that can serve as prototypes for expanded development and applications.

CONCLUSION

Clinical outcomes measurement (i.e., external monitoring) can give valuable guidance to patients, purchasers, and providers of health care. Internal monitoring in conjunction with clinical process control and improvement can improve the effectiveness and efficiency of clinical care and can provide a competitive edge for providers and organizations that utilize them successfully. However, casual or poorly designed clinical outcomes measurement and management can demonstrate quickly the wisdom behind the old adage: "It isn't what you don't know that hurts you; it's what you know that isn't so." On the other hand, well-designed and well-executed programs can supply otherwise unobtainable insights into an organization's performance as it really is. Used properly, these programs embody the true spirit and purpose of managed care.

CHAPTER 32

Using Data and Provider Profiling in Medical Management

Peter R. Kongstvedt, Norbert I. Goldfield, and David W. Plocher

INTRODUCTION

Of all the activities involved in managing health care, the use of data and information for purposes of medical management, and particularly for provider profiling, continues to take on ever increasing importance. The ability of medical managers to intelligently use data and information to better manage the health care delivery system has been a key factor distinguishing those plans that truly excel from those plans that are, at best, adequate performers. This ability to use data and information is only expected to increase rapidly, especially as electronic commerce (e-commerce; see Chapter 37) achieves its rapid growth. Through e-commerce, more data become available, transmission of data and information becomes more rapid and more widespread (via the Internet, in particular), and demands for useful information increase in all sectors of the industry.

This is not to say that the other management activities have lesser merit. Just the opposite; the use of data allows those activities to be carried out more effectively. However, it is important to bear in mind that information is not magic. Data and information are merely powerful tools for the medical manager to carry out necessary functions.

The initial focus of many medical reporting activities has historically been inpatient care. Due to the cost of inpatient care, managing hospital utilization remains a prominent and useful part of the overall management of utilization (as

Norbert I. Goldfield, MD, is Medical Director for 3M Health Information Systems. He has worked on a number of projects including the development of the outpatient prospective payment system recently passed by Congress, the development of risk adjusters for capitation payment/retrospective analyses of episodes, the refinement of severity adjusted DRGs and new methods of measuring quality of care. He is editor of *The Journal of Ambulatory Care Management*. The second edition of *Physician Profiling and Risk Adjustment* is his most recent book.

David W. Plocher, MD, is a Partner in Ernst & Young's Health Care Consulting Practice and has 18 years of experience in the managed care field. His early areas of expertise include national point-of-service program administration and the development of the centers of excellence product known as "Institutes of Quality." More recently, he has designed and implemented integrated delivery systems and advanced care management programs. In addition, he has worked on quality audits and accreditation with both the Joint Commission for Accreditation of Healthcare Organizations and the National Committee for Quality Assurance.

discussed below and in Chapter 18). A hospital case is usually easily definable (except for transferred or readmitted ones), and the physicians delivering care are usually identifiable. Beyond basic utilization reports, basic hospital care profiling (adjusted for case mix and severity, without which the relevance of the entire discussion on hospitals is diminished) combined with feedback to physicians and active intervention has been shown to effectively reduce length of stay[1] and decrease exposure to potential dangers in the hospital setting, such as medication errors.[2]

Recent activity has shifted to consider outpatient procedural and office-based care as well, recognizing that care occurs across a continuum, rather than in isolated episodes. This is of greater interest by acquiring statistical power through meaningful sample sizes per practitioner, as more data points occur outside of the acute hospitalizations. The key question here is the unit of analysis. With respect to outpatient services, one can examine care at the individual visit level or across ambulatory visits into episodes. For each of these independent variables, there is a host of dependent variables that one can examine; they are summarized below. From a disease management perspective, ideally one would like to look across the continuum of care, but the collection of this type of data is often complex and impractical. Thus it is sometimes better to examine and act upon the parts of the episode for which data are frequently available and have a direct bearing on both quality and cost, as discussed later in this chapter.

Provider profiling as a specific topic is the focused subject of the latter portion of this chapter. Profiling means the identification, collection, collation, and analysis of data to develop provider-specific characterization of their performance. As used in this chapter, *providers* can be any type of provider of health services, including physicians, hospitals, and managed care organizations (MCOs). Done correctly, provider profiling represents an important part of quality improvement and the external documentation of the positive impact of managed care on the population.

Of particular importance in this chapter is the issue of confidentiality of data and information.

While it appears obvious that confidentiality should be maintained, this requirement has escalated with the passage of the Health Insurance Portability and Accountability Act of 1996 (HIPAA). A detailed discussion of this act is provided in Chapter 67. Due to its pervasive scope, HIPAA is also referenced in several other chapters (especially Chapter 35). A summary of requirements for confidentiality and security of data that contain clinical information is provided later in this chapter. The reader is cautioned to be thoroughly familiar with these confidentiality and security requirements as they apply to the subject of data and information in medical management.

USE OF DATA AND INFORMATION IN MEDICAL MANAGEMENT

Data Elements and Reports: General User Needs

There are certain general requirements that must be met in order to make data more useful to end users. Raw data have no immediate value to the typical manager. Users must be able to access usable data as directly as possible. If a manager must stand in line to supplicate the guardians of the management information systems (MIS) in order to extract critical information, opportunities will be lost. Access must be as timely, and as easy to use, as possible. The ability of managers to have considerable flexibility with data is also desirable. If a manager must accept a hard-coded report and cannot cut the data in another fashion without a lot of wasted time and coding expense, then that manager will be trapped into managing only with whatever information the programmers have permitted.

Ability To Use System Data with Other Tools

It is important that managers be able to obtain data from the system and use those data with other analytic tools. Advanced statistical analysis programs can be useful to the medical department when performing practice profiling (discussed below) or other trend analysis, and there are several third-party software programs that require such data transfer. The ability to export or download data into other programs, such as spreadsheets or database programs in personal computers, is also desirable. The ability to securely transmit analyzed data to physicians' offices via the Internet is a feature that will rapidly gain importance with the acceleration of e-commerce.

Format

How reports are formatted is a matter of taste (for the user, *not* for the MIS department producing the report!) and the MIS department's ability to produce the requested format. The easiest type of report for MIS to produce is one that tabulates columns of numbers. That is also usually the type most deadly to a busy manager. An already overburdened medical director has better things to do than sift through 20 pages of printout looking at raw numbers of referrals for each physician to get an idea of the referral rate. The best types of report formats for plan medical managers usually are ones that can fit onto one or two 8" x 11" sheets of paper. Those reports should summarize the important data, indicate the outliers and deviations from the norm (or from preset standards), and indicate whether the manager will need to seek more detail. If managers need the raw data, they can always ask for them. For example, a two-page report giving the overall referral rate for the plan and the annualized referral rate for each primary care physician (PCP) for the month and the year to date may be sufficient by itself. If there are PCPs who are grossly over the norm, the medical director can then ask for the detail behind the report.

Graphic reports are useful for conveying large amounts of information quickly to busy managers. This is particularly true when one is presenting data to managers and providers who are not used to looking at reports. Unfortunately, most mainframe computer systems and even some dedicated medical management software programs are not set up to produce graphic reports, so that data must be entered (or downloaded and then imported) into a personal computer before the graphs can be produced. This is a cumbersome process and not amenable to mass produc-

tion. As computers and software become more sophisticated and the use of the data warehouse (see Chapter 35) and reporting tools becomes common, production of graphic reports will also become more common.

The message here is that reports for busy managers should be concise, readable, and easily interpreted and allow the manager to request further detail as needed. One common problem is overkill with detail. Judging by the ceiling-high stacks of computer printouts, reports in some plans must be valued by weight. It is easy to believe that the more data and detail the better. When that happens, you get the classic problem of not seeing the forest for the trees, with the manager spending more time grinding through reports than managing. Computers are wonderful tools, but they can smother you with data. Know what to ask for and when to ask for it.

Routine and Ad Hoc Reports

To manage information wisely, one needs to decide which reports will be wanted on a routine basis and which will be ordered on an ad hoc basis. For example, in a stable open-panel plan, it is unnecessary for the medical director to receive a monthly report listing the recruiting activity or membership for each participating physician. That information, if it is needed, could be provided once per quarter. On the other hand, the medical director or associate medical director will usually want a hospital report on a daily basis.

The basic rule of thumb is to ask for routine reports for those functions that require constant management and will provide sufficient data to spot trends and aberrations. Routine reports should allow the manager to decide when to focus on specific areas for further investigation. For example, watching the trend in specialty costs could reveal an upswing that would result in a request for detail about utilization by a particular specialty. That, in turn, could lead to a need to look at utilization by individual providers in that single specialty. Save the highly detailed reports for infrequent intervals or ad hoc requests. Time spent deciphering cryptic reports is time spent not managing.

Making Sure One Has Clean Data

Hospitals and MCOs receive and are repositories for many sources of data. At present, it is likely that medical groups harvesting data will have an outside group processing their data, although that could change in the future as larger medical groups internalize such functions. Such data are subject to a great deal of editing and are fraught with potential problems that can lead to poor accuracy and integrity. The old maxim of garbage in and garbage out definitely applies to the data collection and information process. The data included in a medical management report or a provider profile are only as good as the effort the physician and other members of the health care team have made in completing the required data entry. It is as easy to collect data that produce bad results as it is the opposite. Potential problems with integrity of cost and quality data include (but certainly are not limited to):

- bad data (that is, incorrect or grossly inaccurate data)
- managing physician not correctly identified
- specialist category not consistently identified
- practice does not match specialist category
- parameter is not practical to measure
- no adjustment for illness severity
- no statistical significance testing

These considerations are among the most basic in the data harvesting process. Errors are common, especially in data that require manual entry (that is, data entered via keystrokes); such errors must be prevented when possible and identified and corrected when present. In some plans, especially large, older insurance companies still depending on legacy software systems, the database may not even use all the available information.

Data must also be valid. They must actually mean what you think they mean. Even when there is great attention to diagnostic coding, the reason for the visit may or may not be related to everything that gets done (for example, a patient is seen with the diagnosis of hypertension but also gets a hearing test), or the diagnostic code may not be the same as the underlying disease (for example, a patient is seen for an upper respiratory infection, but the relevant diagnosis is emphysema). In addition to coding validity, it is important to validate data against other potential sources of the same data. For example, physician identification data may be kept in two separate databases, which may not match. It is also common for providers to have different identifiers depending on what office they are practicing in, what group they are with, and so forth. For example, a physician may work with a medical group on certain days, but have a solo practice on other days. This last problem will eventually be resolved through the introduction of the National Provider Identification Numbers (NPIs), as noted below.

The measures must be meaningful. It is of no value (other than academic) to measure things that have no real impact on the plan's ability to manage the system or a physician's ability to practice effectively. Even worse, there is potential harm in producing reports that purport to mean one thing but really mean another.

The sample size must be adequate. Measuring encounters or referral statistics by physician is of little value if a physician has only 20 members in the panel. Even large databases may fall prey to this problem if the claims and clinical data are spread over too large a provider base so that there are insufficient data for any given provider. Even when there are sufficient outpatient data for participating PCPs, there frequently are insufficient data regarding inpatient admissions to be meaningful, even in large insurance claims databases.[3,4]

The issue of adequate sample size is significant. The ideal sample size depends on what the information will be used for. If the information is to be released to the public, the standard has to pass a much higher test compared to internal release of information. Merging across diseases (such as hospitalizations) is almost always necessary, as it is almost never the case that a physician has sufficient patients with any one diagnosis. It is important, after one has adjusted for severity of illness (discussed below), to combine diseases at appropriate levels of severity. Thus a patient hospitalized for an acute myocardial infarction (AMI, or MI), which has a high risk of mortality, cannot be simply added with uncomplicated pneumonia patients. This represents a complex task and is done using specialized software. It is important to understand whether and how the commercial software is designed to handle severity adjustment and risk of mortality adjustment account for this issue and what algorithms are used for merging data. A similar issue exists in software packages that purport to profile across an episode of illness. Software evaluation and selection are discussed later in this chapter.

The data must encompass an adequate time period. Simple snapshots in time do not reveal the true picture. This is particularly important when looking at total health care resource consumption of patients, and even more important when trying to determine whether a provider's behavior is consistent. Analyses that encompass long periods of time need to be viewed with the knowledge that practice patterns and behavior change over time, and that must be taken into account when comparing long time periods to short ones for the same types of episodes.

It is not unusual for data to come from multiple sources. Linking these data represents one of the biggest challenges for anyone attempting to produce useful provider profiles. A health plan may use more than one system to administer different activities (for example, enrollment and billing on one system, general ledger on another, utilization management on another, claims on still another). Some older and larger plans often use more than one system to carry out the same functions (for example, it may run two or three different claims processing systems), and some large companies use separate systems at each local plan level. Merging data from external sources such as a pharmacy benefits management company (see Chapter 24) or reference laboratory has also proven to be challenging. It is also possible that multiple plans, or a combination of a plan and a provider system, such as an integrated delivery system (IDS; see Chapter 4), will desire to combine data in order to improve the robustness of the database. In all such cases, the data must be integrated into a common database, again, facing the problems of conformance in meaning. This leads to a requirement to standardize a format for use in data analyses. The only other option when faced with multiple systems is to use only a subset of data from a single system, but that is a poor alternative.

Data must be consistent and mean the same thing from provider to provider. For example, one provider may code differently from other providers for the same procedure, and a hospital may code an event differently from the attending physician. Diagnostic coding is particularly problematic when analyzing data from physician outpatient reports. Because diagnostic coding is not important in determining what a physician is paid (except for those claims systems that match diagnostic code to procedure code), there is a great deal of laxity in diagnostic coding for office visits. Procedure coding tends to be more accurate because there is a direct relationship between what a provider codes as having been performed and what the provider gets paid (except in capitated systems). Accuracy, however, does not rule out creative coding, common upcoding, or even fraud, resulting in deliberate coding inconsistencies. For example, one surgeon may bill for a total hysterectomy, whereas another surgeon performing the same procedure may bill for an exploratory laparotomy, removal of the uterus, removal of the ovaries, and lysis of adhesions, all of which generate a fee. The need for consistency may mean having to change or otherwise modify data to force conformance of meaning.

PATIENT DATA CONFIDENTIALITY

There have always been requirements on providers and MCOs to protect the confidentiality of patient information. Those requirements have been variable from state to state to some degree. That has recently changed with the passage of HIPAA, which creates a stringent minimum set of privacy and security standards, though states remain free to impose even greater stringency. Privacy and confidentiality regulations are a substantial portion of HIPAA, though at the time of publication, final delineation and application of some of those regulations were still being re-solved. In addition to privacy and security standards, the implementing regulations for electronic business transactions also include detailed technical specifications based on ANSI X.12 N transaction data standards for both the data fields contained in a transaction and for the electronic format for transmitting a transaction and also mandates the use of standard procedure and diagnostic codes; these are discussed in Chapter 35.

As illustrated in Exhibit 32–1, adapted from Chapter 67, HIPAA focuses on requirements to maintain the physical security of health information. The legislation applies to any person or organization that maintains or transmits electronic health information. HIPAA outlines standards for maintaining reasonable and appropriate administrative, technical, and physical safeguards. The safeguards aim to protect the physical security and integrity of personal health information

Exhibit 32–1 HIPAA Requirements Regarding Health Information

The health care industry business transactions set forth in HIPAA include:

- *Health claims or equivalent encounter information*—a transaction used to submit health care claim billing information, encounter information, or both, from health care providers to health plans.
- *Health claims attachments*—a transaction used to transmit health care service information, such as subscriber, patient, demographic, diagnosis, or treatment data for the purpose of a request for review, certification, notification, or reporting the outcome of a health care services review.
- *Enrollment and disenrollment in a health plan*—a transaction used to establish communication between the sponsor of a health benefit and the health plan. It provides enrollment data, such as on the subscriber and dependents, as well as information on employers and health care providers. The "sponsor" is the backer of the coverage, benefit, or product. A sponsor can be an employer, union, government agency, association, or insurance company. The health plan refers to an entity that pays claims, administers the insurance product or benefit, or both.
- *Eligibility for a health plan*—a transaction used to inquire about the eligibility, coverage, or benefits associated with a benefit plan, employer, plan sponsor, subscriber, or a dependent under the subscriber's policy. It also can be used to communicate information about, or changes in, eligibility, coverage, or benefits—informa-

tion from sources such as insurers, sponsors, and health plans, that is sent to recipients such as physicians, hospitals, third-party administrators, and government agencies.

- *Health care payment and remittance advice*—a transaction used by a health plan to make a payment to a health care provider, to send an explanation of benefits or a remittance advice to a health care provider, or to send both payment and data to a health care provider.
- *Health plan premium payments*—a transaction used by employers, employees, unions, associations, or other entities to make and keep track of payments of health plan premiums to health insurers.
- *First report of injury*—a transaction used to report information about an injury, illness, or incident to entities interested in the information for statistical, legal, claims, and risk management purposes.
- *Health claim status*—a transaction used by health care providers and recipients of health care products or services to request from a health plan the status of a health care claim or encounter.
- *Referral certification and authorization*—a transaction used to transmit health care service referral information among health care providers, health care providers furnishing services, and health plans. It may also be used to obtain authorization for certain health care services from a health plan.

Source: Reprinted from "Health Insurance Reform: Standards for Electronic Transaction; National Standard Health Care Provider Identifier; Proposed Rules," PP 25278-79. Adapted from Chapter 67, courtesy of HIAA, *Federal Register*, May 7, 1998.

from threats, hazards, or unauthorized uses. HIPAA prohibits wrongful disclosures of individually identifiable health information and proscribes penalties for violations. Unlike the other parts of the administrative simplification title, however, the confidentiality provisions do not supersede all state laws about privacy of health information; a state may implement stricter, but not less strict, regulations. Table 32–1 further illustrates some of the applicable data security standards, which fall into three categories: administrative procedures, physical safeguards, and technical security issues.

HIPAA allows data to be used for medical management, including managing utilization and quality. It also allows for the use of

Table 32–1 HIPAA Data Privacy Requirement

Category	Requirement
Administrative procedures	• a certification review (HHS must decide if this will be either an internal or external certification) • chain of trust partner agreements that signify that contractors or partners are security compliant • policies and procedures for processing records (including security standards) • access authorization, establishment, and modification policies • internal audit of MIS security • personnel authorization and security process • MIS security configuration management procedures • security incident procedures • security management process (includes a risk analysis, risk management, sanction policy, and a security policy) • termination process for internal and external users • security training
Physical safeguards	• assigned security responsibility • media controls over receipt and removal of hardware and software • physical access controls • workstation policies • secure workstations • security awareness training
Technical security issues	• access controls, including procedures for emergency access and one of the following: context-based access, role-based access, or user-based access • audit controls to record and examine system activity • authorization control over the use and disclosure of health information either by role-based access or user-based access • data authentication to prove data have not been altered or destroyed illegally by use of check sum, double keying, message authentication, or digital signature • entity authentication—verify entity is who they say they are by use of automatic logoff and unique user identification plus one of the following: biometric ID system; a password system; or a PIN, telephone call back, or a physical device system

Courtesy of Ernst & Young LLP, 2000, Washington, DC.

"blinded" data—aggregate data for purposes of producing population-level reports—as long as there is no way for someone to use those data to track back to an individual patient. Special protections are provided for mental health records. There are also situations where specific permission to use the data must be obtained from the patient (for example, providing that information to an employer or to anyone that is not involved in the provision or direct management of the patient's medical care). HIPAA expressly prohibits the sale of patient-identifiable data for any marketing or sales purpose.

At the time this is being written, the proposed regulations on privacy have been issued and are undergoing final revision, so the reader must review the final regulations and not rely on any of the summaries provided here. By starting at www.hcfa.gov, the reader will be able to navigate to all relevant material on HIPAA, including privacy and security regulations, as well as other aspects, such as the NPI, new databanks, and so forth.

Based on the above, it is clear that the use of data for medical management purposes requires a high degree of attention to policy and procedure to protect the confidentiality of the data. Methods to produce reports must take these confidentiality requirements into account. Nevertheless, these confidentiality requirements, while creating high standards, do not prevent medical managers from using data.

DATA ELEMENTS AND THE APPLICATION OF REPORTS

General Sources of Data

Data elements can be drawn from a variety of sources, such as claims and encounter data from the main system, data from medical management software, and patient-derived information. Examples of common data derived from the plan's operational systems might include demographics, encounter rates, referral rates, admission rates, pharmaceutical use, and so forth. Clinical data are derived from sources other than the plan's operational systems (for example,

medical records abstracting); these might include outcomes data (see Chapter 31), quality data (see Chapter 30), and so forth. It is important to understand the sources of data and the limiting factors that those sources place on the utility of data in medical management.

Specifically regarding profiling, the following data elements are generally necessary:

- Unique patient identifier (scrambled for patient confidentiality)
- Diagnostic information—typically provided using codes from the International Classification of Diseases, Ninth Edition, Clinical Modification (ICD-9-CM), which will soon be replaced by ICD-10
- Procedural information—derived from volume III of ICD-9-CM, current procedural terminology (CPT) and HCFA Common Procedure Coding System (HCPCS) codes. In addition, identifying information relative to the name of the pharmaceutical used is often present.
- Level of service information—such as that provided by evaluation and management CPT codes
- Charges from services ordered by the physician or health care facility
- Results of information derived from additional studies—such as patient satisfaction and measurement of patient health status.
- Unique provider identifier. Universal Provider Identification Numbers (UPIN) codes for physicians, as used by the Health Care Financing Administration (HCFA), are not necessarily unique. The UPIN code will be replaced by a new numbering convention, the NPI in 2002 (2003 for smaller health plans and payer organizations), though that time line could slip. The new NPI is discussed in Chapter 35.

Expanding the provider profile to encompass episodes of illness is an important development in this discipline. This is a complex undertaking from every perspective, but two issues in particular merit emphasis. In this case, there is an absolute need for a valid patient identifier that will allow linkage of various outpatient and inpatient encounters; and a master member index (MMI) that identifies in a reliable manner each patient receiving care from a particular physician. To put it simply, such an MMI would be able to ferret out whether or not John Smith is the same individual as John D. Smith. The MMI issue is a significant one for capitated medical groups, as they often do not have access to a complete listing of all their covered members, or they have this information in a format that is not useable for analytic purposes (for example, a paper printout of members). As noted earlier, such patient identifiers and a MMI must conform to security and privacy requirements.

Especially when one is looking at quality of care, the data elements chosen for a profile need to be clinically and scientifically acceptable. To quote a recent Massachusetts Medical Society report on physician profiling, the data elements chosen need to have:

- content validity
- face validity
- clinical practicality
- consensus validity
- demonstrated safety and effectiveness
- transportability
- an updating process [5]

Claims-Based Data

With respect to the much maligned claims data, there is substantial experience with the use of inpatient claims data for physician and institutional profiling.[6] There are several advantages to the use of inpatient claims data for quality improvement and utilization management purposes:

- With the implementation of diagnosis-related groups (DRGs), there is an extended period of experience with inpatient coding.[7]
- As there are significant financial issues at stake for the hospital, there typically is a considerable effort to code as accurately as possible.[8]
- For enrollees with a chronic illness—individuals with the highest likelihood of interaction with the health care system—information pertaining to the quality of hospital care is likely to be important. This has be-

come all the more important with the recent decision by HCFA to use inpatient diagnoses as the initial risk adjuster for capitation rates (see Chapter 55 on Medicare managed care).

- Most simplistically, a significant portion of a managed care plan's expenditures comes from a relatively small number of enrollees.
- For at least one important aspect of quality within a hospital, mortality, the information is reliably coded and is of great importance to all consumers interested in physician profiles. Mortality, though, represents a very small set of events, and morbidity must also be measured.
- For many physicians, there are an insufficient number of patients for whom one can examine issues pertaining to either quality and or utilization.[9] When that is not possible, there are statistical methods to aggregate clinically dissimilar patients into categories, which have been adjusted for complexity.

While still sometimes criticized, claims-based data have been widely used for quality improvement purposes.[10] The Maine Medical Assessment Project has extensively utilized inpatient claims data for the purpose of developing physician-specific profiles.[11] These profiles are then released directly to the physician. This project has had a significant impact on medical practice, not only because of the rigorous scientific nature of data elements used within the physician profiles but, just as importantly, the release process of the profiles. That is, the physician profiles are not only released for internal purposes only, but senior physicians have provided extensive follow-up to the physicians involved in this profile effort.

Controversy still exists with respect to the validity of using claims-based data for quality improvement purposes. Recently published literature has begun to address this controversy, which has until now consisted more of noise than understanding. Chen and colleagues at Yale University determined that at least one methodology—that used in the creation of the *U.S.*

News and World Report Quality Ranking—correlated with outcomes and processes of care for the one condition examined, AMI.[12] On the other hand, Iezzoni and colleagues also determined that complication rates derived from claims data do not correlate with quality of care information abstracted from the medical record.[13] MCOs should be cognizant of the inadequacy of hospital complication rates that rely on claims data. Several entities, such as the state of California, are working to improve the validity of claims data by collecting data that indicate whether or not a secondary diagnosis was present on admission.

With respect to visit-based ambulatory care claims data, profiling can provide information pertaining to utilization of services (provided that procedures are not a significant part of the case mix adjustment that is used to account for differences in illness severity of the patient).[14] So long as the objective is clearly specified, profiling can also provide information pertaining to quality of care provided to enrollees. Thus the following types of information obtained from visit-based ambulatory claims data are useful for physician profiles for quality monitoring purposes:

- presence or absence of a particular procedure (such as a vaccination or mammogram for preventive services or a retina examination for a diabetic patient), the performance of which typically indicates that quality care has been provided for that particular condition
- utilization of inappropriate site of care (such as the emergency department for an asthmatic), which, if repeated continuously, may indicate an opportunity for improvement.[15]

According to a recent review of claims data used for physician report cards: "Despite their imperfections, claims data can be extremely useful probes to improve utilization, target continuing medical education, help manage complex patients, identify underserved patients and detect misprescribing, as well as fraud and abuse."[16] The author goes on to indicate that there is little training available for physicians to accurately and reliably code with ICD-9-CM and CPT-4. While training programs are important, accurate coding will emerge only when physicians have an incentive to code accurately. For example, one of the authors of this chapter has seen a marked increase in physician interest in accurate coding when the physicians are committed to and trusting of inpatient risk adjustment methodologies that a hospital, together with physician input, has decided to use for profiling purposes.

Relatively speaking, we remain at a primitive state of physician profiling, depending on claims data for episodes of illness. Yet, significant enhancements are currently available in the market (as discussed below under severity of illness for episodes), including the development of severity-adjusted disease-specific categories that:

- could be tracked over an episode of illness[17]
- begin at hospitalization (such as a myocardial infarction) and track mortality over a 90-day period of time
- identify procedure codes, which may represent a complication of care (for example, in a recently published paper, the Center for Health Economics Research identified the performance of a computerized tomography scan shortly after discharge for an endarterectomy as a possible indicator of a complication of care)[18]

Encounter-Based Data

The common use of the term *encounter* refers to an office visit and may be used by a health plan to describe patient visits in a capitated system in which no claim is generated; in some MCOs this is referred to, and treated as, a "no-pay" claim. This would appear, then, to be similar or identical to the use of claims data, but it is not. In a capitated system, there is less motivation to report the visit since it has no impact on reimbursement. A physician or medical group may choose to track those visits for its own internal management but may or may not make those data available to the health plan (or they may exist in a format unusable by the plan). Therefore, one must be cautious when equating encounter numbers in a capitated system to claims in a fee-for-service system.

Medical Records-Based Data

Medical records-based data include any information drawn from the medical record and any other pieces of paper or data files completed by a provider at the time of an encounter with a patient. Medical records-based information is data derived from encounters between the patient and the health care system. Typically, medical records-based data are derived from the MCO's medical management system or from data abstracted from the office or hospital medical record into a health data management tool. Some examples of this type of information might include:

- conformance with clinical care algorithms
- diagnostic and therapeutic resource use
- hospital nosocomial rates
- transfusion errors

Member Questionnaires

Two general types of information are typically drawn from enrollees: satisfaction and health status.[19] Exhibit 32–2 provides examples of different types of information drawn from enrollees. One of the authors of this chapter was involved in the development and use of a patient satisfaction questionnaire in a large staff model health maintenance organization (HMO). The results of this questionnaire were used as part of the salary increase for the staff model physicians. Of significant importance, the physicians themselves were involved in the development of the questionnaire. Many MCOs are using results of patient-derived information in their quality bonus plans (see Chapters 9 and 10). From a cost point of view, it should be emphasized that patient satisfaction questionnaires do not require large numbers of enrollees to produce statistically valid information.[20]

When using member surveys, there are several issues to bear in mind. The survey must be carried out with these principles:

- *Conducting the survey to measure an outcome:* health status, enrollee satisfaction with health care received, or other summary assessments
- *Establishing a baseline:* that is, the survey will be readministered in the future
- *Defining needs:* defining the gap between the ideal and current states
- *Collecting data on actual experiences:* for example, reports of actual waiting times for appointments
- *Collecting evaluations:* for example, ratings of satisfaction with waiting times for appointments
- *Measuring against established standards:* for example, are such goals as "patients will see a specialist within five days of being referred" being achieved?[21]

The last few years has seen the development of a large number of well-validated questionnaires

---

Exhibit 32-2 Differences between Ratings and Reports of Health and Health Care

	Ratings	Reports
Health	Rating of physical shape or condition (Excellent . . . Poor)	Able to participate in sports, strenuous activities (Yes/No)
Health Care	Rating of quality of doctors (Excellent . . . Poor)	Side effects of medication discussed? (Yes/No)

Source: Adapted from N. Goldfield and D. Nash, eds., *Providing Quality Care: The Challenge to Clinicians,* © 1989, American College of Physicians.

that measure a patient's health status.[22] The Foundation for Accountability (FACT), the National Committee for Quality Assurance (NCQA), and Joint Commission on Accreditation of Healthcare Organizations (Joint Commission), emphasize improving all three aspects of quality (structure, process, and outcomes).[23] See Chapter 44 for a discussion of these accreditation agencies.

Incorporation of Other Data

Many MCOs incorporate other data into a provider profile analysis. Claims and encounter data are important, as are data from hospital episodes, but there are additional sources of data as well. Credentialing data may be automated and referenced. Data from member services, such as complaints, transfer rates, or administrative problems, may be incorporated. As noted earlier, data from the quality management program (see Chapter 30) and member satisfaction are now included in the profiling reports and even compensation programs of advanced MCOs. *Examples of supplemental data incorporation include, but are not limited to:*

- *Clinical measures or data, such as:*
  — condition-specific functional status measures
  — laboratory or imaging result (that is, not only the blood sugar or hemoglobin A1C CPT-4 code, but the numeric result of the lab test compared to a desired level)
  — measures specific to Medicare and Medicaid.
- *Nonclinical measures or data, such as:*
  — designation of the imputed PCP (that is, for networks in which PCP assignment is not required, advanced profilers deduce by resource consumption pattern which provider is the PCP)
  — compliance with administrative priorities (for example, being able to communicate electronically with the MCO)

Publicly Available Hospital Data

For trends (where time is not critical) and assessment of validity of internally derived data, MCOs may want to order state data tapes containing hospital claims data. There are nearly 20 states that produce these data tapes. Most of them use severity adjustment, thus increasing the value and validity of the tape. Less detailed information is also available at the federal level, and general data may also be purchased, but these have more limited applicability for management purposes.

Data Warehousing

The concept of a data warehouse is discussed in Chapters 35 and 36. Briefly, a data warehouse is a collection of a broad set of data spanning a significant period of time, as well as a repository of information derived from those data. For example, a data warehouse would be used to collect and store data relevant to physician practice profiling, both raw data as well as information generated by subjecting those raw data to appropriate modification and the creation of computer-generated data sets. This allows for faster and less expensive access to data by whatever analytic systems a plan or medical group is using to generate medical management information. If the organization must run tapes or files for the myriad sources of data (for example, claims tapes, pharmacy tapes, eligibility files, provider files, and so forth) each time they want to perform an analysis, the cost, computer processing unit cycle use, and time lag all become barriers to use. Lack of a data warehouse also sharply reduces the ability to create ad hoc or specialized and focused reports. By being able to access the data in a data warehouse, efficiency is vastly improved and use of the data becomes more practical. The advantages of using a data warehouse have even been extolled in the popular media.[24]

GENERAL TYPES OF REPORTS

Plan Average

Plan average simply looks at the average performance for the entire plan. It is useful in that it will relate closely to the plan's financial performance. For example, if the plan is over budget in medical expense, a plan average report that reveals hospital admissions to be greatly over budget will allow management to focus on that first. It also allows for comparative data between plans that may have somewhat different types of arrangements for the delivery of care.

Plan average is limited because it is relatively insensitive to specific causes of problems. However, that can be an advantage in some circumstances. In plans that manage by trying to keep performance clustered around a norm, that norm can sometimes be one of mediocrity. If the plan average reports and the provider-specific reports tie closely (that is, there are no real outliers in performance), and if the plan is not doing as well as it should, then it is clear that there is a general problem, not a problem with a few recalcitrant providers or hospitals.

Plan average reports are frequently required by regulatory agencies and are also useful for reporting the overall performance of the plan to participating physicians, corporate owners of a health plan, or investors (in the case of for-profit plans) and the public. Plan average reports also function as the backdrop against which other reports are viewed. A plan with multiple lines of business, such as commercial, Medicare, and Medicaid, will likely create additional plan average reports that focus on each line of business: health centers, independent practice associations (IPAs), physician-hospital organizations (PHOs), management service organizations (MSOs), or geographically related centers.

The purpose of this focus is to provide mid-level or local managers with data for their own areas of responsibility. In many plans, especially large or geographically diverse ones, it is common to divide up responsibility into manageable units. The span of control in large or diverse plans can be a real problem. In closed panels, this often refers to a health center or a small number of geographically related health centers. In open panels, this usually refers to discrete multiple IPAs; subunits within the overall health plan, such as pools of physicians (POPs); or geographically divided territories. In plans that contract with IDSs, PHOs, or MSOs, it will be important to develop reports focused on each individual IDS.

Individual Physician

Most managed care plans produce physician profiles that focus on individual physicians. This may refer to PCPs who are functioning as gatekeepers or care coordinators, but may apply equally to open access HMOs, specialty physicians, or preferred provider organizations (PPOs). Virtually all the types of utilization reports discussed later in this chapter are amenable to focusing on individual physicians. Mentioned only briefly here, profiling is discussed in detail later in this chapter.

Physicians become understandably concerned about the plethora of reports that are produced about them. They feel that they are being judged by machines or by standards that fail to take into account any extenuating circumstances and that their fate will be decided on the basis of sterile reports. Realistically, the ability to report the behavior of individual physicians not only provides medical managers with a powerful tool, but it also provides physicians with a great source of both concern and potential help.

Special care must be taken when one is using physician-specific reports. The medical director must look behind the data of the report for the reasons for the reported performance. This is not to say that any behavior should be rationalized, and physicians are as adept as anyone in arguing that they are different and should not be held to the same standards as everyone else. Rather, this is to say that individual physician performance reports need to be used with attention to measures of statistical confidence and as a starting point in physician behavior change discussions.

Premium Source Group

These reports track utilization and other data by enrolled group. They most frequently apply to individual commercial groups (for example, Wendy's Wonderful World o' Widgets, Inc.), but can also apply to any group of enrollees whose premiums come from a common source (for example, Medicare or Medicaid). For those plans that use experience premium rating (see Chapter 49), this will be necessary to develop the actual cost experience. Even for those benefits plans that must be community rated, or for governmental (and nonnegotiable) rates, these data will tell you whether you have a problem with that group that may need to be addressed. Also, some large employers are demanding such data as a requisite for offering your plan to their employees. In the case of Medicare risk plans, reporting Health Plan Employer Data and Information Set (HEDIS) is mandatory, as well as compliance with Medicare's Quality Improvement System for Managed Care. The HEDIS data set is discussed in Chapters 35 and 44.

Hospital Reports

Routine hospital utilization management reports may be divided into two categories: the daily log and monthly summaries. Many plans now automate their utilization management systems. In addition to producing reports as discussed below, these systems allow for on-line access to far more information than would be practical on a printed report.

Daily Log

For optimal management of utilization, it is almost a requirement for a managed care plan to produce a daily hospital log. This document serves as a working tool for the utilization management nurse and the medical director in managing institutional utilization. Its design should be directed toward providing the necessary information to actively manage cases that are current or prospective. Data should be able to be sorted by whatever management criteria make sense. For example, each hospital's census is reported separately so that the utilization review nurse can use it when making hospital rounds, or the log may be sorted by geographic region, IPA, IDS, or health center for regional medical directors to use. Example elements of a useful daily hospital log are illustrated in Exhibit 32–3.

Monthly Summary

A monthly summary report of hospital utilization should also be produced. This differs somewhat from the daily log because it is used to identify patterns for overall management rather than to serve as a mechanism for performing concurrent utilization review. A monthly report might include the data illustrated in Exhibit 32–4 for both the month ended and the year to date.

Exhibit 32–3 Daily Hospital Log Elements

Minimum Data Elements
- Current census
  — name of hospital
  — hospital
  — diagnosis and procedures
  — PCP
  — admitting physician
  — consultants or specialists
  — admission date
  — length of stay to date
  — free text narrative with clinical information
  — in-network compared to out-of-network status
- Hospital statistics
  — days per 1,000 today
  — days per 1,000 month to date
- Prospective admits and outpatient surgeries

Additional Useful Data Elements
- Service type (as part of current census)
  — medicine
  — surgery
  — pediatrics
  — gynecologic surgery
  — obstetrics
  — mental health
  — chemical dependency
  — intensive care unit/cardiac care unit
  — neonatal intensive care unit
  — rehabilitation
  — outpatient surgery
- Estimated length of stay or maximum length of stay
- Admissions and discharges today and month to date
- Authorization or denial status
- Catastrophic case report
- Line of business code
  — commercial
  — Medicare
  — Medicaid
  — self-insured versus fully insured
  — special accounts

Specialty-Focused Hospital-Based Reports

Any or all of the above reports can be created so that they focus on physicians of a single specialty for hospital-based care. A common ex-

Exhibit 32–4 Sample Data Elements for a Monthly Summary of Hospital Utilization*

- Plan statistics
  — days per 1,000
  — admissions per 1,000
  — average length of stay
  — average per diem cost
  — average per case (per admission) cost
  — emergency department visits and average cost
- Hospital- and provider-specific statistics
  — days per 1,000
  — admissions per 1,000
  — average length of stay
  — average per diem cost
  — average per case (per admission) cost
  — emergency department visits and average cost
- Statistics by service type (see Exhibit 16–2)
  — days per 1,000
  — admissions per 1,000
  — average length of stay
  — average per diem cost
  — average per case (per admission) cost
- Retrospective authorizations
- Pended cases for review
- In-network compared to out-of-network statistics
- Number and percentage of denied days

*The plan will want to produce these statistics not only for the entire plan, but for major lines of business as well (that is, commercial, Medicare, Medicaid, self-insured versus fully insured, and so forth).

ample is cardiovascular surgery, but the concept applies to other specialties as well. In general, this has the most utility when medical managers are focusing on that particular specialty for contracting issues, quality issues, or cost issues.

Several medical specialty societies (e.g., urology, cardiovascular surgery) have also ventured into the field of physician profiles for specific hospital-based surgical procedures. Unfortunately, many of these efforts are proprietary and the developers have not opened the logic for scrutiny by independent researchers. While it is thus difficult at the present time to evaluate the reliability and validity of these medical specialty society efforts, it is likely that such efforts will increase in importance. If the members of a specialty society are supportive of such efforts, it is likely that, over time and after considerable internal development, these physician profiles will be publicly released.

Outpatient Utilization

Although daily reports are generally necessary for managing hospital utilization, in only the most tightly managed health plans or IDSs will that be done for managing referral or outpatient utilization. Practically speaking, referral and outpatient utilization management is best done by using monthly reports, both routine and ad hoc. Reports should include data both for the month ended and for the year to date. Data may also be reported by month on a 12-month rolling basis. Data for such reports might include elements as illustrated in Exhibit 32–5, depending on the needs of medical management.

Categories of outpatient or ambulatory care may be divided into several components, each with its own unique characteristics. The office visit for primary care, including any testing or procedures, is one such category, as is the related category of the office visit for specialty care. Ambulatory procedures are a different matter, as is the setting for the procedure. The identical procedure may be performed in a physician's office, an ambulatory care center, or the outpatient department of a hospital. Some plans have addressed the issue of ambulatory care, especially outpatient procedures, by using statistical groupings.

As has been mentioned earlier, these types of reports are usually used on an ad hoc basis. For example, if total expenses for cardiology appear to be high, medical managers could investigate further by requesting reports that show who is ordering the referrals, what ancillary testing is being done, who the specialists are that are seeing the patients, how much they are charging, and so forth.

Open Access Plans

Open access systems, or systems that do not use a primary care gatekeeper model, present

Exhibit 32–5 Sample Data for a Monthly Summary of Outpatient Utilization*

- *Primary care enounter rates*
  - visits per 1,000 members per year
  - visits per member per year (annualized)
  - percentage of new visits
  - revisit interval rates (to look for churning)
- *Preventive care*—use HEDIS data
- *Laboratory/pathology utilization per visit*
- *Radiology utilization per visit*
  - total
  - focused (for example, magnetic resonance imaging)
- *Prescriptions*
  - prescriptions per visit or prescriptions per member per year
  - average cost per prescription
  - percentage generic
  - formulary compliance
- *Referral utilization*
  - referral rate per 100 primary care visits or per 1,000 members per year
  - comparison of PCP referral rate to peer group
  - initial referrals only compared to total referral visits
  - cost per referral by PCP, plan average, and specialty
  - number of visits and cost by specialty
    - top specialty referrals for each PCP
    - average cost per visit
    - per member per month cost by specialty

- *Out-of-network specialty care in POS plans*
  - percentage of total specialty care
  - cost
  - specialty and utilization categories
- *Ambulatory procedures*
  - by ambulatory patient groups
  - by ambulatory care groups and ambulatory diagnosis groups
  - by diagnostic or procedure code
- *Ancillary care*
  - physical therapy and other rehabilitation therapies
  - podiatry
  - eye care
  - oral surgery
  - other
- *Other HEDIS ambulatory reports*

*The plan will want to produce these statistics not only for the entire plan, but for major lines of business as well (that is, commercial, Medicare, Medicaid, self-insured versus fully insured, and so forth).

special problems in monitoring utilization. In a PPO (see also Chapter 3) or managed indemnity plan, there will be no physician-specific membership base to use as a denominator. In HMOs that allow open access to specialists or allow specialists to self-authorize revisits or secondarily to authorize referrals to other specialists, one cannot measure specialist utilization against a fixed membership base associated with particular PCPs. Some open access HMOs do indeed capitate specialists or employ contact capitation (see Chapter 11), which creates the appearance of a fixed membership base, but that is not common at this time.

In these situations, one must use both less precise methods of measuring utilization of referral services and specialist utilization (for example, specialist visits or procedures per 1,000 members), and more advanced physician profiling, as discussed below. Reports should focus on those areas under control of the specialist, as well as primary care. Examples of typical data elements are illustrated in Exhibit 32–6. These data are not considered advanced physician profiling and can only be used in general terms. In order to make an open access plan perform well, it is necessary to use the more sophisticated profiling methods discussed in the rest of this chapter.

Exhibit 32–6 Sample Data for an Open Access Model Plan

Outpatient Services
- average number of visits per member per year
- average number of visits per member per year to each specialty
- diagnostic utilization per visit
  — laboratory
  — radiology and imaging
  — other
- average cost per visit
- procedures per 1,000 visits per year (annualized)
  — aggregate
  — by procedure for top 10, by specialty type
  — by individual specialist
- average cost per episode (as defined for each sentinal diagnosis) over a defined time period, including charges not directly billed by provider

Inpatient Services
- average total cost per case, including charges not billed by provider, for hospitalized cases
- average length of stay for defined procedures
- average rate of performance of a procedure, such as:
  — Caesarean section rate
  — hysterectomy rate
  — transurethral prostatectomy rate
  — cardiac procedures
- readmission rate or complication rate
- use of resources before and after the hospitalization

PROVIDER PROFILING

Provider or practice profiles have a variety of uses. Examples include producing feedback reports to help the providers modify their own behavior, recruiting providers into the network, and choosing which providers are not the right fit with the organization's managed care philosophy and goals (whether the organization is an organized medical group, MCO, IDS, POP, or IPA; the term *MCO* will be used to refer to any and all of these types of organizations). Other uses include supporting performance-based reimbursement systems, determining specialists to whom the MCO will send certain types of cases, detecting fraud and abuse, determining how to focus the utilization management program, supporting quality management, and performing financial modeling.

With respect to quality improvement, there are two types of variables one can profile: those that have a direct relation to costs and those that, while over the long term will possibly lead to decreased costs, have a closer relationship to our traditional understanding of quality. An example of the first type would be the variation in use of coronary artery bypass graft (CABG) for patients with angina, while mammography rates represent an example of the second category. From a quality of care perspective, both types of variables are of equal value, and both should be used.

Unfortunately, so many meaningless profiles have been developed that physicians have become understandably suspicious of their intent. That is, rather than integrating quality with efficiency, many provider profiles today are simply economic reports. Profile implementation focused on quality improvement is always challenging, but is necessary to combine that with profiles that focus on economic issues.

Also bear in mind that one cannot simply hand out the profile and expect change to occur. While there are some reports in the literature stating that simply disseminating profile reports results in change, there is more evidence that profile reports, as important and powerful as they are, are but one tool out of several when working with physicians to examine and change practice patterns and habits. This topic is discussed further in Chapter 33.

When designing provider profiling reports, the following principles should be kept in mind:

- identify high volume and costly clinical areas to profile
- involve appropriate internal and external customers in the development and implementation of the profile

- involve the providers in the development and implementation of the profile
- compare results with published performance (external versus internal norms)
- report performance using a uniform clinical data set
- when possible, employ an external data source for independent validation of the provider's data
- consider on-site verification of data from the provider's information system
- present comparative performance using clinically relevant risk stratification
- require measures of statistical significance
- revise performance measurements using formal severity adjustment instruments

These principles will be explored further in this chapter.

Customers and Users of Provider Profiles

There are many customers or users of provider profiles. Identification of these customers and paying attention to their needs when developing and implementing the profile are important to success. Profiles are not inexpensive in both time and money. Profile customers include:

- *Managed care organizations:* All levels (provider relations, medical directors, and so on).
- *Enrollees:* While enrollees are the ultimate customer, we are still in the process of developing profiles and approaches to their effective dissemination to enrollees.[25]
- *Employers:* With notable exceptions, most employers are still less interested in quality than they are in cost control. Thus the hook to get employers interested in quality is the use of tools and approaches that integrate cost control with quality.
- *Providers:* Perhaps, for today, providers are the most important customer of all. Most providers are interested in change if methods to measure performance are well grounded in scientific evidence or professional consensus.[26]

Public versus Internal Disclosure of Provider Profiles

A key flashpoint of debate is internal versus external disclosure of provider profiles. By way of example, there are nearly 20 states that produce publicly available profiles of hospital services. MCOs are beginning to use this information in their feedback loop to hospitals. The report format itself is an important aspect of the development process. For example, the state of Florida, which has released hospital-specific mortality and severity of illness rates for several years, has established wide confidence intervals and designed a format that places a great emphasis on information and deliberately underemphasizes identification of poor or excellent performers. This approach improves the acceptance and utility of the report, while lowering the potential for sensationalism. Pennsylvania has undertaken similar efforts in producing reports on hospitals, taking into account severity adjustments. See Exhibit 32–7 for a generic sample of such a report.

There is at least one major difference in the characteristics desired of physician profiles when used for internal purposes (for example, private and confidential to the physician) versus when used for external purposes: the threshold of statistical and clinical validity. The threshold does not need to be as high when, for example, physician profiles are used for internal quality improvement activities.

Physicians have a legitimate concern when they assert that external release of their profiles needs to be held to a higher standard. While public disclosure of comparative information is well established for MCOs and hospitals, there is little experience with public release of physician-specific information. There is a large difference between releasing information pertaining to a hospital with thousands of employees and a high number of measurable events, and releasing information pertaining to one physician or a small group of physicians. Yet physicians cannot burrow their heads into the sand and simply claim that currently available information is not scientifically valid. That position is not only inadequate in today's marketplace of ideas, but it

Exhibit 32–7 Hospital Comparative Report

Hospital	Total Discharges	Average Charges		Average Length of Stay		Mortality	
		Observed	*Expected*	*Observed*	*Expected*	*Observed*	*Expected*
A	1,061	8,000	8,700	4.26	4.64	2.73%	3.51%
B	870	10,300	9,600	4.35	4.63	3.22%	2.92%
C	1,663	9,300	9,700	4	5	3.61%	4.17%
D	593	10,900	9,300	4.91	4.76	3.20%	4.27%

Source: Reprinted from *1996 Guide to Hospitals in Florida,* Agency for Healthcare Administration, State of Florida.

denies consumers information that would allow them to make better choices and better manage their own care.

The NCQA uses HEDIS information to evaluate MCOs and makes this information available through its *Quality Compass* publication. The Pacific Business Group on Health has also made an effort to use this HEDIS data set to evaluate medical groups that contract with MCOs and plans to release this information to the public.[27] There are also several Internet websites that provide information from multiple sources, ranking MCOs, hospitals, and physicians.[28]

More recently, there have been some health plans and employers that have produced and released physician practice quality and service profiles to their members or employees and have reported a shifting in enrollment into practices that were reported as "best practices."[29] This is a significant step forward in the development of physician profiles for external or public release. Its importance derives from the fact that many physicians, particularly on the West Coast, are not solo practitioners or members of small medical groups; they are members of large medical groups that contract with HMOs for the entire risk and are the key providers of medical care.

DESIRED CHARACTERISTICS OF PROVIDER PROFILES

Provider profiles should share these characteristics, as discussed below:

- accurately identify the provider in the profile

- accurately identify the specialty of the provider
- help to improve the process and outcome of care, both dollar and quality outcomes
- have a firm basis in scientific literature and professional consensus
- meet certain statistical thresholds of validity and reliability
- compare the provider to a norm
- cost the minimum amount possible to produce
- respect patient confidentiality and, if obtaining information from the medical record or using patient-derived information, obtain patient consent

Accurate Identification of the Provider

As noted earlier, the accurate identification of the provider is not always easy or straightforward. Problems of multiple databases, the use of multiple identifiers, inconsistent data, poor linkages between provider codes and clinical information, and so forth make this a challenge. At present, the use of the NPI will address this issue in future years, but will not even begin until 2002 at the earliest. Unless an MCO uses a single master provider identification file, and has taken great care to ensure nonduplication of provider identification data, it will require a significant amount of attention to address this. In addition, profiling software must employ algorithms to ensure that data about cost, utilization, and quality are linked to the appropriate provider(s).

There are increased efforts to link hospital and physician payment for services provided in the hospital, since these data are usually not coming from the same sources. In other words, physician claims or encounters are entered into the system via both claims and the medical management system, while hospital data are likewise entered, but independently from the physician data. And none of these sets of data are automatically linked in most information systems.

In hospital care, accurate identification of the "responsible" physician is not always clear. For example, the physician of "record" for hospital administrative purposes may not be the same as the physician who actually cares for the patient. For MCOs engaging in, for example, capitation for the entire hospital portion of care, it is necessary for them to work with the hospital and its affiliated physicians (both hospitalists [see Chapter 18] and independent practitioners) to establish clear procedures on this thorny question. While it may not be immediately clear to MCOs why they need to get involved in this level of detail, without a clear understanding of this issue accurate profiles for hospitalization care will be impossible. In addition, several MCOs are now able to provide profiles of hospitalizations for a procedure (CABG, for example) that includes 90 days postdischarge. These are much more valuable profiles from both a cost and quality perspective.

An additional problem concerns providers who behave as though they are in a group but are not legally connected and do not appear as a group in the MCO's provider file. An example would be two physicians who share an office, share after-hours on-call responsiblities, and see each other's patients, but who are actually independent of each other. The reason that this is important in managed care is that, if the MCO contracts with one but not the other, the member may wind up seeing the nonparticipating physician and be subject to balance billing. Even if the physicians agree not to balance bill, the MCO still may not actually want the other physician in the network, even on an occasional basis. Related to the above is the ability to detect linkages between practices or ancillary services. Examples include orthopedists who own physical therapy practices or neurologists who have a proprietary interest in a magnetic resonance imaging center.

Accurate Identification of the Specialty Type

The specialty of the physician is not always clear. Most MCOs have provider files that indicate what specialty type a physician has self-indicated, but it is surprising how often that information does not match up with specialty indicators in the claims file. Of course, MCOs that perform comprehensive verification of board specialty status as part of the credentialing process (see Chapter 7) will have more accurate data than MCOs that depend on self-reporting by physicians. Ironically, the creation of the NPI will exacerbate this problem, since by (HIPAA) definition the NPI will contain no inbedded intelligence, such as specialty-specific indicators.

The problem of provider specialty definition is particularly acute when looking at primary care. Many board-certified medical specialists actually spend a considerable amount of time performing primary care, whereas others spend the majority of their time practicing true specialty medicine. This has great implications for how an MCO will evaluate performance of specialists as well as PCPs when comparisons to peers are used (a common practice). A related issue is determining which physicians will be considered specialists at all because the MCO may not want to send referrals to a specialist who is not particularly active in his or her designated specialty. Even within a single specialty there will be differences in how "specialized" a specialist is. For example, a specialist may have a majority of primary care patients or may not care for patients in the intensive care unit (ICU). Therefore, the MCO or IDS will want to look at the degree to which a physician is truly a specialist in his or her mix of routine and complex cases.

Even when the issue of specialty definition is resolved, there remains the problem that no two practices are exactly alike. As an example, some general internists perform flexible sigmoidoscopies and some do not. If one looks only at charge patterns, the internist who performs the procedure will look more expensive compared to the internist who does not, but that analysis will fail to pick up the fact that the internist who does not perform flexible sigmoidoscopies instead refers them all to a gastroenterologist who charges more than the first internist (in addition, the first internist could be overutilizing the procedure or the second internist could be failing to provide this common preventive care activity, but those are separate types of analysis). The same problem arises outside of primary care medicine. For example, when neurosurgeons are assumed to be a homogeneous group, accurate profiling cannot be done when one neurosurgeon works only on atrioventricular (AV) malformations, another on brain tumors, and so on. This problem extends to related procedures, such as whether neurosurgeons or vascular surgeons perform carotid endarterectomies or whether neurosurgeons or orthopaedists perform various types of spine fusions.

Improve Process and Outcome Using Scientific Criteria

It is important to not only be certain that quality of care variables have relevance for either process or outcomes of care, but that there also be scientific and professional consensus that the variables are worth examining. Generally speaking, this can be done in one of four ways:

- Accrediting organizations, such as NCQA, have increasingly put their screening items through a rigorous evaluation process.
- There are several proprietary software packages from reputable developers that include guidelines or quality of care criteria.
- Most will use professional literature, including peer-reviewed journals or trusted locations on the Internet, such as the website hosted by the Agency for Health Care Policy and Research, *www.guideline.gov*.
- Self-development is always an option, but development of reliable and valid quality of

care criteria always takes more time than one expects.

Need for Statistics

Appropriate statistical techniques are required for both quality of care and efficiency criteria. Without their use, one can easily be misled by noise into arriving at a mistaken conclusion. Most stand-alone software packages have statistical tests embedded. If one is obtaining reports from the MIS department, it is important to ask for the addition of statistical tests, especially when faced with decisions pertaining to network determination. Reports should include basic measures of confidence, such as standard deviations or p values.

From a design point of view, it is likely that there will be enough data over time to profile a provider using statistical process control (SPC). "SPC consists of a set of powerful techniques to ensure the continued stability of any process and to detect the presence of sources of instability."[30] One can develop control charts or simpler reports if one is not able to use SPC for a wide variety of independent variables using claims data such as:

- daily hospital log
- length of stay
- cost of care (by type of cost; claims forms are divided into approximately 20 departmental categories ranging from pharmaceutical to medical supply to ICUs)

Compare the Provider to a Norm

Practice profiles are of no use unless the results are compared to some type of standard. There are certain problems inherent with comparisons in provider profiling. All these problems are resolvable, but medical managers need to be aware of them before embarking on profiling. Comparison against norms is necessary, but it is fraught with potential difficulties, chief of which is defining the norm. There are, broadly speaking, two types of norms: internal (that is, one's own norms if one has enough enrollees or patients) and comparative norms (using external data).

The usual ways of comparing profiling results are to provide data for each individual practice in comparison to one or more of the following internal norms discussed earlier:

- **Total MCO average results.** This standard is simply the average for the entire MCO and is the crudest method of comparison.
- **IPA, POP, or IDS.** A variation of MCO average, this compares the practice only to other practices within a set of providers smaller than the entire network. This approach may be combined with multiple other approaches when an MCO contracts through organized provider systems. Another variation on this is geography, even in the absence of organized provider groups.
- **Specialty specific or peer group.** This compares each practice only to its own specialty (for example, internists are only compared to other internists).
- **Peer group, adjusted for age, sex, and case-mix/severity of illness.** This is the most complicated approach, as noted earlier, but provides the most meaningful comparative data.
- **Budget.** This compares the profile to budgeted utilization and cost, a necessary activity when providers are accepting full or substantial risk for medical expenses.
- **Advanced and statistically based comparisons.** This is coupled with confidence intervals so that a provider will know whether the difference versus the peer group is statistically significant.

Examples of comparative norms include hospital charges or costs; mortality; group practice charges; certain outcomes, such as hospital admission rates; and parameters of greatest interest to MCOs, such as utilization rates (for example, referral rates, prescribing behavior, and so forth), immunization, mammography, or other HEDIS rates. Some of these norms, such as hospital charges and mortality, may be augmented through public use state data tapes. Occasionally, state data tapes (such as in Florida, California, Pennsylvania, and Texas) are adjusted using a reputable severity adjustment tool. More often

than not, the state data tape is either not available or, if it is, no risk adjustment is performed. Normative data sets may be internally generated if the MCO is large or part of an alliance that pools similar data. Data sets tailored to the needs of a specific organization are also available for purchase from reputable commercial organizations.

Cost the Minimum Amount To Produce

The specifics of provider profiling costs will not be quantified for the purpose of this chapter. That is, costs are often confidential and are always changing. The concept here is an emphasis on cost minimization, as certain features of profiling are nearing commodity status. The chief financial officer (CFO) cannot be guaranteed a precise return on investment for the costs incurred and must accept them as a necessary, additional cost of doing business better. "Better" means the value added through data-driven prioritization of medical management and other management initiatives, summarized above as the purposes and benefits of profiling.

THE NEED TO ADJUST FOR SEVERITY OF ILLNESS

Case mix and severity are always issues of contention when profiling providers. Providers with costly profiles will always complain that they have the sickest patients. Even if the medical director feels that this really represents whining, when performing profiling the issue of severity *must* be addressed.

At this point, a caution to the reader is required: **Do not** develop your own severity of illness adjustment. Researchers have spent years developing the ones that are summarized below. The cost for licensing the software is substantially less than the cost it would take to develop a home-grown and possibly inadequate system, which would then have to undergo years of independent testing for external validation, prior to achieving the common language status enjoyed by the incumbents.

Practices have differences in the age and sex make-up of their patient panel, which must be considered. These two sets of variables have been the traditional methods that served as a proxy for severity and case mix adjustments. Age and sex are intuitively useful, and capitation payments are routinely modified based on these two parameters. The basic and valid argument is that utilization is predictable based on age and sex, using actuarial tables. While this is true for any large population of individuals (such as what a large insurance company would use to set rates), it provides little real value to any individual physician's expected utilization profile, since, when the numbers are small, chance has more of an influence than do population-based statistics.*

Geographic differences may also account for some differences in utilization. This certainly occurs when comparing community to community (as discussed and illustrated in Chapter 18). It is likewise common to see differences between rural and urban levels of utilization. As noted above, these trends, whether or not they make empirical sense, are useful when observing population-based numbers, but they retain little relevance when looking at small numbers of events (for example, covered lives, surgical procedures, and so forth). Unlike age and sex, it is legitimate to decide whether or not to include an adjustment for geographic location when crafting profiles. It is more likely to be useful when looking at large numbers of providers or patients that share the same geographic location; it is less likely to be useful if applied to individual providers based on ZIP code on a one-by-one basis. Noting that one of the purposes of severity adjustment is to better explain differences in utilization, other potential contributors to variation in resource consumption not explored in this chapter are level of education, level of financial income, ethnicity, marital status, and social isolation.

When confronted with the need to examine quality of care and utilization of services, most physicians immediately register the "my-patients-are-sicker" complaint. If possible, *severity* is even more misunderstood than the term *quality improvement*. The following is a summary of the terms that are often thrown about as different parties try to communicate with each other and make decisions on the my-patients-are-sicker issue.

- **Severity of illness** refers to the relative levels of loss of function. At a minimum, this function can be measured in physiologic terms and the ability to perform activities of daily living.
- **Treatment difficulty** **refers** to the patient management problems that a particular illness presents to the health care provider.
- **Resource intensity** or **severity of service** refers to the relative volume and types of diagnostic, therapeutic, and bed services used in the management of a particular illness.

In the final analysis, however, one must take the approach that case mix adjustments for purposes of quality improvement or utilization management represents the first step and the first step only in the quality improvement process. Provider profiles adjusted for case mix taken at one pinpoint in time should never be used to make final decisions regarding a physician's medical practice. A second step involves the choice of one of several technologies, either claims based or nonclaims based, for case mix adjustment. While current case mix adjustment technologies have significant limitations, they are far superior to that which existed even five years ago, and they continue to evolve. Examination and verification includes posing the types of questions to both the purchaser and software developer that are summarized in Exhibit 32–8.

Severity of illness can be addressed only if one asks, "What is the focus of the analysis?" That is, does the profiling analyze:

- ambulatory visits?
- inpatient episodes excluding the intensive care unit?
- episodes of illness across ambulatory and inpatient episodes?

---

*This is sometimes referred to as the "Rule of Small Numbers"—that is, when there are few events to measure, then chance is more influential than are predictions on large numbers of events.

Exhibit 32–8 Questions To Consider When Choosing an Ambulatory Case Mix System

Clinical
- Are the base units expressed in clinical terms easily understood and supported by health care professionals?
- Are the base units driven by *International Classification of Diseases,* Ninth Edition, Clinical Modification (ICD-9-CM) or *Current Procedural Terminology,* Fourth Edition (CPT-4), or both?
- Does a mapper exist to trace codes utilizing the code system currently in use in your system?
- If you are looking at episodes, is the unit of analysis the total episode of care (inpatient and outpatient) or are outpatient services only considered?
- Can case examples of the use of the system be provided?
- Does the episode-of-illness system distinguish complications from comorbidities, and, if so, how does it do this?
- Is the episode-of-illness system best used for primary care physicians or specialists or both?

Statistical
- What is the predictive capability of the case mix adjustment?
- How are outliers treated? It should be pointed out that the more outliers are removed, the more the statistics will improve at the expense of explaining the entire ambulatory care contact.
- Is it an ICD-9 code-driven system?
- Is a valid method for assigning an ICD-9 code to encounters with missing and nonspecific ICD-9 codes available?

- Is the unit of analysis the total episode of care (that is, links all ambulatory, outpatient, inpatient, and prescription drugs)?
- Does it have a large number of diagnostic groupings (that is, medical conditions)?
- Does it place all available encounter and claims data for each patient into at least one episode of care?
- Is an episode duration defined by the maximum number of days between contact with a physician (that is, window period)?
- For multiple concurrent episodes, is an encounter placed into only one episode (for example, one lab is placed into one and only one episode)?
- Do episodes have an adjustment for comorbidities, severity of illness, and patient age?
- Is the predictive ability of the episode adjustments very high?
- To reduce fragmentation of episodes, are two years of encounter data required?
- Can pattern-of-treatment results for treating specific medical conditions easily be compared across networks and physicians?
- Are the following uses supported?
  — global patterns-of-treatment profiling
  — prescription drug performance/risk
  — clinical guideline development
  — outcomes research
  — physician compensation
  — high-cost patient risk management
  — medical capitation performance/risk
  — workers' compensation performance/risk
  — chronic disease management
  — Health Plan Employer Data and Information Set reporting

Source: Adapted from Norbert Goldfield, Episodes of Illness: Introduction, in *Physician Profiling and Risk Adjustment, Second Edition,* Norbert Goldfield, ed., p. 481, © 1999, Aspen Publishers, Inc.

- nursing homes, rehabilitation facilities, and home care?
- intensive care units?

Ambulatory Visits

There are two classification systems developed and used in the profiling of individual ambulatory visits or encounters: ambulatory patient groups (APGs) and ambulatory payment classifications (APCs). APGs were developed as a forerunner and are quite similar to APCs. Both are in the public domain. The APCs are to be implemented by HCFA for outpatient prospective payment in hospital outpatient departments and ambulatory surgery centers for Medicare patients. APGs are already used by a variety of payers (for example, Medicaid and several Blue Cross Blue Shield plans) A number of companies produce mainframe and desktop versions of soft-

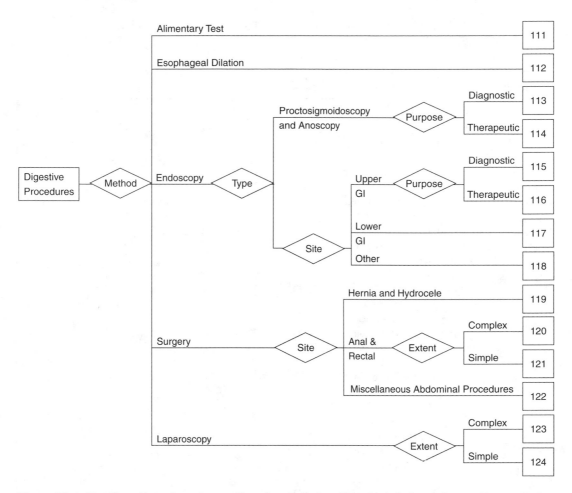

Figure 32–1 Significant Procedure. *Source:* Data from R.F. Averill et al., *Ambulatory Patient Groups, Definitions Manual, Version 2.0,* Health Care Financing Administration, Office of Research and Demonstrations, and 3M Information Systems.

ware for these classification systems. Figure 32–1 provides an example of significant digestive procedures for version 2.0 of the APGs. From a cost and quality perspective, one could, for example, profile providers or MCOs by:

- frequency of the performance of these procedures
- performance of minor procedures (such as laboratory tests) for each of these procedures
- satisfaction or other patient derived outcome for any desired APG categories
- profit or loss for specific APGs and APCs

Exhibits 32–9 and 32–10 provide examples of such reports.

Inpatient Episodes

As of 1999 a number of case mix classification systems were available for provider profiling of inpatient care*:

- HCFA DRGs are public domain but are *not* severity adjusted. One needs to profile at an

---

*The authors cannot guarantee that these names will remain current; they are provided as a "snapshot" of 1999.

Exhibit 32–9 Expected Profit or Loss Statement: Outpatient Cardiovascular Product Line

APG/APC Category	Description	Type	Count	Paid Amount ($)	Total Cost ($)	Profit or Loss	Percent Profit or Loss
71	Exercise tolerance tests	SP	1,056	160	150	10	6.67
72	Echocardiography	SP	969	210	224	–14	–6.25
74	Cardiac electrophysio-logic tests	SP	4	1,250	1,524	–274	–17.98
75	Placement of transvenous catheter	SP	32	780	881	–101	–11.46
76	Diagnostic cardiac catheter	SP	224	1,310	1,940	–630	–32.47
77	Angioplasty and trans-catheter procedure	SP	7	1,250	1,321	–71	–5.27
571	Congestive heart failure and ischemic heart disease	MED	295	180	203	–23	–11.33
572	Hypertension	MED	1,278	67	87	–20	–22.99
573	Chest pain with cardiac enzymes to rule out myocardial infarction	MED	172	390	333	57	17.12
574	Chest pain with cardiac enzymes to rule out myocardial infarction	MED	534	220	197	23	11.68
575	Simple cardiovascular disease except CHF, ischemic heart disease, and hypertension	MED	692	90	114	–24	–21.05
576	Complex cardiovascular disease except CHF, ischemic heart disease, and hypertension	MED	248	160	200	–40	–20.00

Courtesy of 3M Health Information Systems, Wallingford, Connecticut.

Exhibit 32–10 Sample Report: Costs by Provider Service

Surgeon	Number of Cases	Average Procedure (minutes)	Labor	Supplies	Drugs	Equipment	Anesthesia, Drugs, and Supplies	Total
Smith, John	110	75.21	$608.75	$208.35	$60.74	$195.60	$182.60	$1,256.04
Jones, Alice	85	82.09	$664.47	$222.49	$55.43	$200.58	$199.43	$1,342.40
Frank, Bret	60	64.52	$522.21	$254.76	$43.76	$226.91	$226.11	$1,273.75
Kelly, Steve	14	84.80	$686.37	$199.76	$66.72	$266.40	$204.62	$1,423.87
Average		75.50	$611.09	$222.72	$55.59	$207.84	$198.77	$1,296.01

Courtesy of 3M Health Information Systems, Wallingford, Connecticut.

institutional level using HCFA DRGs to know the overall financial performance. However, the reasons for that performance cannot be ascertained without using one of the systems described below.

- APR-DRGs (3M/HIS Inc.) are proprietary, use claims data, and are the most widely used severity adjustment in the United States. Two dependent variables are available: severity of illness and intensity of service and mortality.
- Acuity Index Method (Iameter Inc.) is proprietary and uses claims data. Charges are the dependent variables.
- Caduceus (Care Management Sciences Inc., Philadelphia, Pa.) is proprietary and uses claims data. A variety of dependent variables are available.
- Disease Staging is proprietary (Medstat Inc., Ann Arbor, Michigan) and uses claims data. A variety of dependent variables are available.
- Medisgroups is proprietary and uses both claims data and information drawn from the medical record. It is used primarily in Pennsylvania for state reporting purposes.
- Michael Pine and Associates have developed customized and proprietary, risk adjustment tools.

A number of intermediary vendors aggregate severity adjusted data from either their own customers or from public use data tapes to produce comparative data. These include not-for-profit alliances and proprietary companies. A practical issue the user needs to decide is whether to hold and manipulate the data in-house and thus have greater flexibility in creating one's own reports or to send the data to a third party and receive reports from that intermediary. Thus, for example, with respect to the APR-DRGs, users can license a work station that provides both standard and ad hoc reports, but they still must load in their data, or they can work with a third-party vendor that processes the data and provides canned or, at a higher price, tailored reports. The choice is made based on economic issues, internal capabilities, and the need to manipulate the data on a frequent basis.

There are several theoretical issues that the medical director of an MCO or large provider system should understand. One of the most contentious is the inclusion of complications versus comorbidities in the logic of the risk adjustment. For example, with specific respect to myocardial infarction, many secondary diagnoses present on admission after an MI likely represent comorbidities or sequelae of the MI. Thus if a patient develops complete AV blockage on the second day of admission, it is likely that this secondary diagnosis represents a comorbidity or sequelae of the MI and not an *avoidable* complication of an MI. One could extend this analysis to a large number of other secondary diagnoses—with specific respect to MI. The state of California has been a leader in providing a middle ground, by collecting data on whether the secondary diagnosis was present on admission.[31] Such knowledge would allow the calculation of separate indices for all codes, rather than only those codes present on admission. This issue extends itself to episodes of illness.

Several articles have appeared recently highlighting the importance of severity adjustment in negotiations between MCOs and hospitals. The following excerpt describes the importance of risk adjustment both from a financial and clinical care perspective.

> An MCO with significant volume approached the hospital requesting a reduction in rates. Specifically, the company had targeted this reduction to an amount that they perceived was the rate being offered by our hospital to other MCOs. Quantification of differences in the relative costliness of a specific hospital's case mix is computed using case mix indices; relative weights had to be calculated An example for just one condition, congestive heart failure, is provided in Exhibit 32–11. Aggregating these weights across all patients revealed that the managed care plan's weighted average severity index was 1.048, whereas the average for the other plans was .88 (not shown). This difference translated into a 19.1% differ-

Exhibit 32–11 All Patient Refined DRG Severity Index for Congestive Heart Failure (APR-DRG 127)

	Cases	Percent of Total	Relative Weight
No/minor severity	86	17.6	.6674
Moderate severity	232	47.4	.8562
Major severity	112	22.9	1.2167
Extreme severity	59	12.1	2.0645
Total APR-DRG 127	489	100	1.0514

Source: Adapted from P. Jones and G. Strudgeon, Logic and Applications of the All Patient Refined DRGs: The Greater Southeast Community Hospital Experience, in *Physician Profiling and Risk Adjustment,* N. Goldfield, ed., p. 367, © 1999, Aspen Publishers, Inc.

ence in resource intensity, which was acknowledged by the company as significant. Yet, even though negotiations concluded with new rates that reflected the historical case intensity of the plan's patient population, we knew there were significant differences in treatment patterns. Thus, Figure 32–2

reveals that losses for the hospital predominated among severely ill individuals with congestive heart failure, indicating that a high cost case management program might be very efficacious for our institution. In addition, Exhibit 32–12 indicates that there are significant differences in physician practice patterns in the treatment of congestive heart failure with (not shown) similar mortality rates, indicating that implementation of a congestive heart failure guideline might be useful.[32]

Episodes of Illness

Measuring episodes of illness represents the new frontier of profiling and case mix. It finally will allow researchers and providers alike to examine care provided across a continuum of care. We will not be able to argue anymore, for example, that we cannot measure the risk-adjusted mortality and resource consumption for:

- diabetics for a year's period of time
- patients who have suffered an MI and undergo not only hospitalization but 90 days of posthospitalization treatment

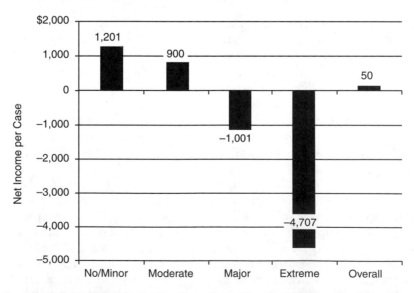

Figure 32–2 Severity Adjusted Net Income Per Case, Congestive Heart Failure Total New Income $54,558. Courtesy of 3M Health Information Systems, Wallingford, Connecticut.

Exhibit 32–12 Select Ancillary Cost Analysis To Support PHO Case Mix and Severity Adjusted 1992 and 1993 Discharges

	Least Efficient		Most Efficient
	Cases	Cost	Cost
APR-DRG 127, CHF			
Severity 1	25	$7,400	$5,950
Severity 2	36	8,670	6,770
Severity 3	26	18,390	11,540
Actual		→11,120	7,950
Expected Cost		→	
Variance		→	($3,240)

Note: 34 and 23 percent of the cases are age > 74 for the most efficient and least efficient practices.

Courtesy of 3M Health Information Systems, Wallingford, Connecticut.

- specific pneumonias, whether the care was provided on an inpatient or outpatient basis

Episodes of care are defined as time-related intervals that have meaning to the behavior you are trying to measure. Episodes may vary considerably both by clinical condition and by the provider type that is being measured. In the case of obstetrics, obvious measures such as Caesarean section rate are important but will not reveal the full picture. Looking at the entire prenatal and postnatal episode may reveal significant differences in the use of ultrasound and other diagnostics, differences in early detection and prevention of complications, or perhaps a great deal of unbundled claims during the prenatal period. In the case of some medical conditions, the episode may extend over the course of years or have no endpoint short of the patient's death (or, in the case of an MCO, disenrollment, at which point data are no longer available).

Furthermore, it is possible for patients with multiple medical conditions to have overlapping episodes of care, making it more difficult to sort out what resources are being used for what episode. Several of the proprietary software programs attempt to deal with this issue by, for example, identifying patients with both congestive heart failure (CHF) and diabetes and separating this group of patients from those who only have CHF.

Related to the issue of episode is the problem noted earlier, of identifying which provider is actually responsible for the patient's care. As an example, an internist or a diabetologist may be responsible for the care of a diabetic but may have little responsibility for managing that patient's broken leg, other than to refer the patient to a good orthopaedist. Identification of the responsible physician is also difficult regarding hospitalized patients; it is not uncommon for the admitting physician not to be the attending physician, especially when surgery is involved.

The hallmark of episode definition is the ability to link up all the health care resources into a defined event. This may mean diagnostic services (for example, laboratory or imaging), therapeutic services (for example, physical therapy), drugs, consultations, outpatient visits, and inpatient visits. In other words, it must be a patient-based analysis rather than a provider-based one; the analysis of the behavior of providers is a product of examining what happens to their patients. As summarized below, various vendors have constructed proprietary groups for the purpose of simplifying episode development.

There are two purposes for profiling data collected over an episode of illness:

- to prospectively predict costs for the coming year, as this information is useful to adjust capitation rates
- to retrospectively profile for purposes of comparing actual versus expected costs or actual versus expected performance on a variety of quality of care indicators.

Exhibit 32–13 provides a list of currently available episode of illness systems, along with references to informative articles on the systems.

Exhibit 32–14 provides a sample of a data report on diabetes—*severity adjusted*. While the dollars displayed are next year's predicted expenditures, the same type of report can be produced for last year's expenditures (see Exhibit 32–15). One can imagine that such information is useful for disease management programs. Each level of severity can be arrayed against other variables, such as complications or visits to the emergency department.

Exhibit 32–13 Episode-of-Illness Profiling Systems

Payment Purposes
- Ambulatory Care Groups (ACGs)[1]
- Diagnostic Cost Groups (DCGs)[2]
- Hierarchical Cost Groups (HCGs)[3]
- Episode Grouper[4]
- The Disability Payment System (DPS)[5]

Profiling Purposes
- Episode Treatment Groups (ETGs)
- Episode Grouper
- Diagnosis Episode Clusters (DECs)[6]

[1] J. Wiener, et al., "Ambulatory Care Groups: A Categorization of Diagnoses for Research and Management," *Health Services Research* 26, no. 1 (1991): 53–74.

[2] A. Ash, et al., "Adjusting Medicare Capitation Payments Using Prior Hospitalization Data," *Health Care Financing Review* 10, no. 4 (1989): 17–29.

[3] R.P. Ellis et al., Diagnostic Cost Group (DCG) and Hierarchical Cost Conditions (HCC) Models for Medicare Risk Adjustment. (Prepared for the Health Care Financing Administration, Contract No. 500-92-0020), Washington, DC; April, 1996.

[4] R. Averill, et al., "The Episode Classification System Project," *Journal of Ambulatory Care Management,* forthcoming.

[5] R. Kronick, et al., "Diagnostic Risk Adjustment for Medicaid: The Disability Payment System," *Health Care Financing Review* 17, no. 3 (1996): 7–33.

[6] D. Cave and E. Geehr, "Analyzing Patterns of Treatment Data To Provide Feedback to Physicians," *Medical Interface,* July 1994, 125.

Source: Adapted from Norbert Goldfield, Episodes of Illness: Introduction, in *Physician Profiling and Risk Adjustment, Second Edition,* Norbert Goldfield, ed., p. 480, © 1999, Aspen Publishers, Inc.

Exhibit 32–14 Next Year's Expenditures for Diabetics—Severity Adjusted

Diabetes Level 1	$3,693
Diabetes Level 2	$4,514
Diabetes Level 3	$5,794
Diabetes Level 4	$7,418

Source: Reprinted from Final Report for CRG Contract for the U.S. Department of Commerce, Washington, D.C.

Nursing Homes, Rehabilitation Facilities, and Home Care

The numerous proposals and enacted federal legislation to pay for these services on a prospective basis have heightened the importance of case mix measures, all of which are severity adjusted. MCOs will increasingly need to become familiar with these case mix measures as disease management programs begin to more frequently use these types of facilities. Descriptions of the two most commonly used case mix measures follow.

- *Resource utilization groups (RUGs)* have the least severity adjustment built into the system. They are currently used in the prospective payment for nursing homes.[33]
- *Functional independence measure (FIM)* and the *Patient Evaluation and Conference System (PECS)* are used primarily in rehabilitation facilities. Both have excellent severity adjustment measures built into the system. Recently, the Function Resource Groups (FRGs) were developed, using the FIM, for prospective payment.[34] The Outcome and Assessment Information Set (OASIS) has been developed as both a quality of care and payment tool for home care services.

Intensive Care Units

While typically beyond the purview of the MCO, directors of medical centers will likely want to know the resource consumption and outcomes within the ICU of their, for example,

Exhibit 32–15 Diabetes Mellitus: Cost and Quality

CRG DM	Outpatient Laboratory		Mortality APR-DRGs			Complications		Average APR-DRG Charges		Hospitalization	
	Actual	Expected	Actual	Expected		Actual	Expected	Actual	Expected	Actual	Expected
Level 1	0.39	0.25	0.12	0.13	EDCs	4	7				
					APG	3	2				
					APR	4	3	$3,700	$4,106	1.4	0.5
Level 2	0.47	0.39	0.25	0.19	EDC	2	9				
					APG	3	4				
					APR	4	6	4,700	5,757	2.8	1.2
Level 3	0.40	0.59	4.85	2.26	EDC	6	12				
					APG	9	6				
					APR	12	11	12,537	9,085	3.1	3.5
Level 4	0.30	0.75	25.13	17.27	EDC	12	18				
					APG	14	9				
					APR	29	17	33,445	21,695	6.8	9.6

Courtesy of 3M Health Systems, Wallingford, Connecticut.

CHF or transplant patients. The most commonly used case mix measures:

- Acute Physiology and Chronic Health Evaluation (APACHE)[35]
- (MPM)[36]
- (SAPS)[37]

A discussion of these systems is beyond the scope of this chapter, as most users are not engaged in this level of detailed analysis. However references are provided for the interested reader.

SELECTION OF A PROFILING VENDOR

Unless an MCO has an extraordinary information system, it will be required to purchase or license services from an outside vendor of profiling systems. In terms of software, there are an increasing number of software products that provide assistance to the health care professional engaged in profiling activities. Broadly speaking, there are three types of products:

- Database or data management tools that allow one to collect information and report that information in useful formats. These are sophisticated (from an informatics perspective) empty shells.
- Tools that interface with data management and provide "clinical logic," which points the health professional in particular avenues of investigation of either cost or quality.
- Risk adjustment systems that provide the user with the assurance that apples are being compared with apples. This issue has been discussed above in detail.

There is no need to have all three features in one piece of software. In fact, the key determining factor is whether or not each piece of software is designed in such a way that it can easily interface with other types of software. As illustrated in Exhibit 32–16, there are several distinguishing features that one looks at to aid in the selection of a system.

Exhibit 32–17 provides a more detailed overview of features typically contained in the inventory of the typical service offering of leading vendors who perform physician profiling.

The reader should note that Exhibit 32–17 combines three different elements: the classification systems, information system (IS) platforms, and applications. There will be a somewhat different perspective on each of these three elements depending on the role of the reviewer (for example, the IS director will look at platforms while others may focus on classifications systems or the ease of usability of the application). A brief discussion of some selected points noted in Exhibit 32–17 follows.

- *Validated methodology.* Methodologies used for severity adjustment and episode construction are more trusted by new users if they have already been evaluated for predictive validity and reliability by the peer reviewed literature and multiple installations.
- *Multiple products for HMO, Point of Service (POS), Medicare, Medicaid.* While profiling in the "lock-in" or 100:0 plan HMO environment is usually straightforward, POS products add new complexity. Whether referred by the PCP with or without the MCO's approval or if self-referred by the member, resource consumption out of network and in-service area or out-of-service area, strains the information collection completeness and timeliness. Metrics for Medicare must include influenza vaccination adherence rates, pneumonia and CHF readmissions, and additional items beyond HEDIS requirements. Medicaid populations must build profiles that address maternities with high risk, asthma, HIV-AIDS, care for substance abuse, and care for the elderly, blind, and disabled.
- *Comprehensible by average PC user.* Customers for profiling software and services may settle for shipping a claim tape to the vendor and waiting for a report. However, the recent users are asking for the option to have a terminal on their own bench and training to design ad hoc reports for customized circumstances in real time. They prefer the visual relief provided by a graphical user interface and deplore tabular data. They want to be self-managing. There

Exhibit 32–16 Distinguishing Features and Selection Criteria To Use When Evaluating Physician Profiling Vendors

Sound Clinical Methodology
- independently validated in peer reviewed literature with acceptable R2
- applicable to primary and specialty care physicians
- intuitive and easy to explain to practicing providers
- industry standard "universal language" (for example, standard definitions of episodes)
- ability to incorporate inpatient and outpatient care into episodes of care
- sound statistical methodologies

Reporting Comprehensiveness
- all data incorporated (ICD-9, CPT, NDC, HCPCS, local codes, NY DRGs)
- all places of services captured
- ability to incorporate user defined fields
- ability to incorporate external benchmarks

Reporting Flexibility and Presentation
- ability to report by individual provider, specialty, risk pools, or other user defined group
- analysis variability to include billed, paid, allowed amounts, relative value units, rates per 1,000, per member per month
- ability to complete clinical performance reporting
- ability to vary reporting period and trend data
- ability to drill down to claim level detail
- ability to report by product lines (Medicare, Medicaid, commercial) or aggregate products
- indicates statistical significance for comparisons
- ability to severity adjust at patient level
- ability to integrate with existing legacy systems/programs for reporting flexibility
- graphic presentation
- actionable reports
- summary level report available with ability to add detail pages

System Platform/Training and Support
- platform and Technical Requirement compatibility
- technical and clinical training and support available
- data cleansing process

Courtesy of Ernst & Young LLP, 2000, Washington, DC.

are several work stations that provide this facility to the average PC user.

- **Carve-out accommodated.** As MCOs have separate agreements with subcapitated programs (managed behavioral health, chiropractic, pharmaceuticals, lab, and so on), the better profilers are equilibrating their report packages to ensure apples-to-apples comparisons. Although important throughout this chapter, profiling from within any capitated entity (especially physician group) will not be possible if encounter CPT-4 data are not submitted, such that MCOs have had to develop reward programs for completeness-of-capture for encounter information. In addition, pharmaceutical information should get to the level of drug name, dose, and route of administration.

- **Prioritization of services for focused review.** Briefly mentioned earlier in this chapter, this capability represents an essential management tool for MCO utilization management departments. They do not want to hassle righteous physicians. They want to reduce the overhead attached to operating these oversight activities dedicated to micromanagement. They would prefer not having to do old-fashioned "utilization review" at all. The better profilers arm them with information to perform this targeting.

- **HEDIS production and other accreditation requirements.** Profiling vendors vary in their willingness to produce the administrative data portion of HEDIS reports (see Chapters 35 and 44 for HEDIS data requirements). Conservative vendors argue

Exhibit 32–17 Typical Service Offering of Leading Physician Profiling Vendors

Tool

1.0 Inputs:
1.1 Standard Data Inputs:
1.1a Medical claims
1.1b Encounters
1.1c Membership (subscriber & dependent level)
1.1d Provider claims with group level and individual physician identifiers along with specialty
1.1e Pharmacy claims (including formulary and generic indicators)
1.1f Referrals authorizations
1.1h Lab/radiology results
1.1i Medical records
1.1j Little or no reliance on nonstandard vendor-specific output

1.2 User Defined Inputs:
1.2a Credentialing and site visits
1.2b Satisfaction survey results
1.2c Outcomes (that is, health status survey information, preventive screening information)
1.2d Site visit and chart audit results (from medical record reviews)
1.2e Complaint rates
1.2f Billing practice audit results

2.0 Formatting/Data Mapping:
2.1 Map data from multiple operational systems (claims UR, administration, pharmacy, enrollment, or membership)
2.2 Map data from multiple external systems (that is, three different claim systems)
2.3 Integrate external reference files (external benchmarks)
2.4 Standardize formats across multiple sources (internal and external)
2.5 Reference tables to match codes to descriptions (provider name, diagnosis, procedures)
2.6 Vendor-defined case types (that is, high cost user, chronic condition, and so on)
2.7 User defined case types
2.8 Medical service unit costs (for capitated services)
2.9 Relative value units

3.0 Adjustment Tools:
3.1 Age/gender adjustment

3.2 Inpatient case mix adjustment method:
3.2a Based on DRGs
3.2b Based on other methodology
3.2c Based on proprietary methodology (see examples in chapter text)
3.2d Based on user-defined methodology
3.3 Outpatient case mix adjustment method:
3.3a Based on APGs, APCs
3.3b Based on other methodology
3.3c Based on proprietary methodology (see examples in chapter text)
3.3d Based on user-defined methodology
3.3e Ability to develop episodes of care and method for linking case events
3.4 Exclusion of outliers:
3.4a Vendor defined
3.4b Different thresholds by specialty or based on other criteria
3.4c User defined
3.5 Comparison Standards/Norms
3.5a Vendor methodology to create client-specific practice norms
3.5b User defined methodology to create client-specific practice norms
3.5c Menu/parameter driven ad hoc query tool
3.5d Programmer level ad hoc query tool
3.5e Export spreadsheet/graphics/work processing software
3.6 Statistical capability within the product:
3.6a Measures of central tendency (mean, mode, and so on)
3.6b Significance tests
3.7c Regression
3.7d Other techniques (specify)

4.0 Pre-formatted Reports/Views:
4.1 Reports by product lines (Medicare, Medicaid, POS, HMO, PPO)
4.2 Financial reports:
4.2a Medical budgeting (by standard categories—medicine, surgery, OB/GYN, MH/CD)
4.2b Rating/Underwriting
4.3 Hospital:
4.3a Financial
4.3b Utilization (that is, service use per members)
4.3c Quality

continues

Exhibit 32–17 continued

4.4 Physician (Individual with specialty norms):
4.4a Financial
4.4b Utilization
4.4c Quality
4.4d Clinical practice management
4.5 Risk group (by practice, IDS, planwide):
4.5a Financial
4.5b Utilization
4.5c Quality
4.6 Across sites/places of care:
4.6a Utilization
4.6b Quality
4.6c Referred, self-referral, referred out of network rates
4.7 Employer Reporting:
4.7a Vendor defined
4.7b HEDIS formats (planwide, by product line, by IDS, by practice)
4.7c Quality/outcomes indicators
4.8 Standard report features including graphic capability:
4.8a Executive level reports
4.8b Management level reports
4.8c Transaction level reports
4.8d Drill down capability between reports and levels
4.8e Vendor defined parameter for exception/ outlier reports
4.8f User defined parameter for exception/ outlier reports
4.8g Trend analysis
4.8h Actual versus budgeted
4.8i Actual versus expected ratio based on statistical norm
4.8j Actual versus expected based on clinical norms
4.8k User defined changes in the sort order
4.8l User defined changes in populations (different providers, diagnoses, and so on)
4.8m Routines for ranking variations (providers, employer groups, diagnoses)
4.8n Vendor-defined exclusion criteria (other than outliers)
4.8o User-defined exclusion criteria (other than outliers)
4.9 Precalculated descriptive statistics:
4.9a Utilization rates
4.9b Unit costs for medical services
4.9c Per member per month
4.9d Expected versus actual
4.10 Modeling capability:
4.10a Alternate benefit design
4.10b Alternate payment/reimbursement methodology
4.10c User customization of standard reports/ views
4.10d Standard graphs as companion to standard reports
4.10e User customization of graphs
4.10f Presentation quality output for external distribution
4.10g Production report capability

5.0 System Operational Features
5.1 System security
5.2 Licensing agreement details regarding use by affiliated provider groups
5.3 Interface ease (for graphic packages)
5.4 Analytic/interpretive support
5.5 Technical support
5.6 Training/user documentation—retraining for updates and user groups
5.7 Data dictionary
5.8 Help desk availability and hours or operation

6.0 Corporation Specifics
6.1 Years in business
6.2 Revenue/earnings growth
6.3 Number of employees in company
6.4 Employees dedicated to technical support
6.5 Current client count
6.6 Current installations and average time for installation
6.7 Data format

7.0 Technical Architecture
7.1 Operating platform
7.2 Frequency of updates (include the most recent update dates)
7.3 Service bureau capabilities
7.4 System hardware needs (specify)
7.5 Turnaround time for data processing
7.6 On-line capability with remote access connectivity

Courtesy of Ernst & Young LLP, 2000, Washington, DC.

that claim data integrity is unknown, such that the electronic production of such a report is unreliable. Other vendors dedicate energy to claim tape edits and "cleansing" processes, whereby a level of confidence is achieved. The user can learn portions of this track record where a vendor has produced a HEDIS report that was externally audited.

- *Statistical packages.* Simple averages or colorful pie graphs are not adequate today. Tests of statistical power expressing significance using *p* values and confidence intervals using standard deviation are essential.
- *Easy-to-use interfaces.* This is critical if a user wants to import data from other sources or to integrate plan data with, for example, software that will help build a clinical guideline.

THE FUTURE OF DATA USE

The future of data use in medical management and provider profiling can be expected to increase far more rapidly than has occurred to date. With the increasing presence of e-commerce (see Chapter 37), technology that allows for cheaper and faster storage and processing, and increasing sophistication in applications, there will be uses of data that are either now only just being realized, have not even been conceived of at the time of publication, or have been conceived but are unknown to the authors.

To get a sense of immediate future uses, it is useful to look at some examples of advanced applications of data and information that are being implemented by some organizations at the time of publication, but are not yet widespread. These examples include the following.

- A large MCO is utilizing a clinical data warehouse for studying medical cases. The system stratifies the member population into groups that can benefit from outreach programs and case management, and measures effectiveness and outcomes of quality improvement programs.
- A large MCO partnered with a vendor to develop a data warehouse housing both op-

erational and medical information. They plan to use the data warehouse to identify profitability of business, operational improvement opportunities, and improve quality of care.
- A major vendor is using a centralized data repository that integrates financial and patient encounter data into a single location. This solution also includes an electronic medical record that supports inpatient and outpatient care delivery and drives financial and administrative systems.
- A large MCO has developed a long-range plan to link its disease management database with clinical records to track medical outcomes.
- A large MCO provides computerized patient profiles, with red-print flagging tests or procedures that are due according to treatment guidelines to assist physicians in treating patients with coronary artery disease.
- A large MCO is implementing a national clinical information system bringing clinical knowledge to individual physicians at the most important moment when encountering a patient and in a manner that supports the best clinical decisions.
- A large MCO has developed a disease management program that is entirely supported by an on-line library of clinical guidelines and other forms of decision support powered by the organization's clinical intranet.

The future of provider profiling can be analyzed from two perspectives: the push for external release and the integration of disparate types of information leading to a significant reduction in costs and simultaneous increase in validity for increasingly sophisticated physician profiles. With respect to the latter, it is clear that increasingly sophisticated, yet inexpensive provider profiles will be available. We are on the threshold of a revolution in lifting the electronic and organizational barriers to inexpensively linking salient elements for physician profiling. With respect to hospital-based care, many hospital-based systems will be able to link clinical and administrative data in the near future, significantly increasing the power of the profiles for hospital-based services. Health care organizations are expending significant resources in an effort to link hospital and ambulatory care data. In the short (or already existing) term, advances in this area will result in:

- A link between specific pharmaceutical and severity adjusted claims data. This will increase the clinical validity of, for example, examining outcomes of care for diabetics. These databases are available now.
- A link with outpatient laboratory values. For example, this will provide further clinical validity for the analysis of outcomes for diabetics. The value of a hemoglobin A1C is an example of an excellent outcome-dependent variable in the follow-up of diabetes.
- A link between patient health status and claims-based, laboratory, and pharmaceutical information.

The challenge will be implementation, which is still difficult. Policy makers will need to pay attention to the following types of issues:

- Acceptance by individual physicians and other consumers of the report card. Acceptance includes not only participation in the development of the profile but also an inbuilt quality improvement process to use the profiles effectively. This applies to all consumers of the profile, not just physicians. Though profiles and information are now being made available to consumers, we still understand very little about how consumers can best use these profiles.[38]
- Protection of patient confidentiality through existing and future regulation,

without eliminating the ability of medical management to improve quality and manage cost appropriately.
- The development and implementation of new statistical and profiling techniques to enhance the validity of the physician profiles.[39]

In the meantime, however, we need to have strategies in place for current efforts to promote valid and reliable provider profiling. Such strategies on provider profiling need to address the need to constructively deal with issues of patient confidentiality, a research agenda on provider profiling, and internal and external release of information.

CONCLUSION

Profiling has become a necessary tool for any medical manager or provider in order to compare performance and results against both peers and expected results. While this is often seen as threatening (and has sometimes been used that way), it can also provide useful data to allow a physician (or other provider) to improve performance. Profiling is far more complex than simply taking snapshots of individual activities of a provider, and, in fact, that type of profiling is of little value. Profiling must be performed from the perspective of what happens to the patient, it must incorporate adjustments for severity and case mix (as well as age and sex), and it must be meaningful and useful to the medical managers and the providers themselves. Ultimately, profiling must also be meaningful and useful to consumers as well. Profiling is a continually evolving tool that will become ever more effective.

REFERENCES AND NOTES

1. G. Bennett, W. McKee, and L. Kilberg, Case Study in Physician Profiling, *Managed Care Quarterly* 2, no. 4 (1994): 60–70.
2. R.S. Evans, S.L. Pestotnik, D.C. Classen, et al., A Computer-Assisted Management Program for Antibiotics and Other Anti-Infective Agents, *New England Journal of Medicine* 22, no. 338 (January 1998): 232–38.
3. R.D. Lasker, D.W. Shapiro, and A.M. Tucker, Realizing the Potential of Practice Pattern Profiling, *Inquiry* 29 (1992): 287–97.
4. R. Nathanson, M. Noether, and R.J. Ozminkowski, Using Claims Data To Select Primary Care Physicians for a Managed Care Network, *Managed Care Quarterly* 1994; 2, no. 4: 50–59.

5. W.B. Stason, B. Auerbach, M. Bloomberg, et al., *Principles for Profiling Physician Performance,* Massachusetts Medical Society, 1999.

6. N. Goldfield, *Provider Profiling and Risk Adjustment,* 2d ed. (Gaithersburg, MD: Aspen Publishers, Inc., 1999).

7. R.F. Coulam and G.L. Gauler, Medicare's Prospective Payment System: A Critical Appraisal, *Health Care Financing Review,* annual supplement 13 (1997): 45–76.

8. L.B. Russell and C.L. Manning, The Effect of Prospective Payment on Medicare Expenditures, *New England Journal of Medicine* 320, no. 7 (1989): 439–444.

9. T.P. Hofer, R.A. Hayword, S. Greenfield, et al., The Unreliability of Individual Physician "Report Cards" for Assessing the Costs and Quality of Care of a Chronic Disease, *JAMA* 281: 2098–105.

10. Goldfield, *Physician Profiling and Risk Adjustment.*

11. E.J. Schneiter, R.B. Keller, and D. Wennberg, Physician Partnering in Maine: An Update from the Maine Medical Assessment Foundation, *Joint Commission Journal on Quality Improvement* 24, no. 10 (October 1998): 579–84.

12. J. Chen, M. Radford, Y. Wang, T.A. Marciniak, and H.M. Krumholz, Do America's Best Hospitals Perform Better for Acute Myocardial Infarction? *New England Journal of Medicine* 340, no. 4 (1999): 286–92.

13. L.I. Iezzoni, R.B. Davis, R.H. Palmer, et al., Does the Complications Screening Program Flag Cases with Process of Care Problems? Using Explicit Criteria To Judge Processes, *International Journal on Quality Health Care* 1, no. 2 (April 1999): 107–18.

14. N. Goldfield, A Quality Improvement Process for Ambulatory Prospective Payment, *Journal of Ambulatory Care Management* 16, no. 2 (1993): 50–60.

15. T.A. Lieu, C.P. Quesenberry, M.E. Sorel, et al., Computer-Based Models To Identify High-Risk Children with Asthma, part 1, *American Journal of Respiratory Critical Care Medicine* 157, no. 4 (April 1998): 1173–80.

16. P.E. Dans, Caveat Doctor: How To Analyze Claims-Based Report Cards, *Joint Commission Journal on Quality Improvement* 24, no. 1 (January 1998): 27–30.

17. A.F. Averill, N. Goldfield, and J. Eisenhandler, Development and Evaluation of Clinical Risk Groups (CRGs), National Institute of Standards and Technology, Advanced Technology Program under Cooperative Agreement, no. 70NANB5H1013.

18. J.B. Mitchell et al., Using Physician Claims To Identify Postoperative Complications of Carotid Endarterectomy, *Health Services Research* 31 (1996): 141–52.

19. N. Goldfield and D. Nash, eds., *Managing Quality of Care in a Cost-Focused Environment,* 3d ed. (Gaithersburg, MD: Aspen Publishers, Inc., and American College of Physician Executives, 1999).

20. J. McGhee et al., *Collecting Information from Health Care Consumers: A Resource Manual of Tested Questionnaires and Practical Advice* (Gaithersburg, Md.: Aspen Publishers, Inc., 1996).

21. McGhee et al., *Collecting Information.*

22. McGhee et al., *Collecting Information.*

23. Margaret O'Kane, The National Committee for Quality Assurance, in *Managing Quality of Care.*

24. Charles Ornstein, Aetna Puts Its Faith in Nationwide Database: Nation's Largest Insurer Creates a Repository for Health Histories, *San Diego Union-Tribune,* March 12, 1999.

25. N. Goldfield, C. Larson, D. Roblin, et al., The Content of Report Cards: Do Primary Care Physicians and Managed Care Medical Directors Know What Health Plan Members Think Is Important? *Joint Commission Journal on Quality Improvement* 25, no. 8 (1999): 422–33.

26. For a detailed review please see W.B. Stason, B. Auerbach, M. Bloomberg, et al., Principles for Profiling Physician Performance, Massachusetts Medical Society, 1999.

27. Pacific Business Group on Health, *www.healthscope.org.*

28. At the time of publication, some (but not all) examples of consumer-oriented websites that provide data, rankings, and high-level profiles of providers (including physicians) and MCOs can be found at: www.healthgrades.com, www.Patientwatch.com, www.AHN.com, and www.Healthcarereportcards.com. The authors make neither recommendations nor endorsements regarding any of these sites, nor can we ensure that they will even be at the same URL at any moment in time.

29. H. Larkin, Doctors Starting To Feel Report Cards' Impact, *American Medical News,* July 26, 1999.

30. R.B. Fetter, DRGs and Quality Management in Hospitals, in *Physician Profiling.*

31. Cal-APR-DRGs working draft, internal memo, California Health Care Association, Sacramento, Calif., 1999.

32. P. Jones and G. Strudgeon, Logic and Applications of the All-Patient-Refined DRGs: The Greater Southeast Community Hospital Experience, in *Physician Profiling.*

33. A MedPAC suggests modifications to SNF PPS system, new RUG III group may be an option. *Natl Rep Subacute Care* 7, no. 5 (March 10, 1999): 3–5.

34. R. Smith and C. Granger, Outcomes and Rehabilitation Care, in *Managing Quality of Care,* 586–627

35. A. Collins, MPM-2 and SAPS-2: A Review of Easy To Use Severity Systems, *Care of the Critically Ill* 11, no. 2 (1995): 73–76.

36. Collins, MPM-2 and SAPS-2.

37. D.T. Wong, P.M. Barrow, M. Gomez, and G.P. McGuire, A Comparison of the Acute Physiology and Chronic Health Evaluation (APACHE) II Score and the Trauma-Injury Severity Score (TRISS) for Outcome Assessment in Intensive Care Unit Trauma Patients, *Critical Care Medicine* 24, no. 10 (October 24, 1996): 1642–48.

38. Goldfield, Larson, Roblin, et al., The Content of Report Cards, pp. 422–33.

39. N. Goldfield, Current Challenges to Quality Improvement, in *Providing Quality Care.*

SUGGESTED READING

Betty, W.R., H.K. Hendricks, H.S. Ruchlin, and R.L. Braham. 1990. Physician Practice Profiles: A Valuable Information System for HMOs. *Medical Group Management* 37: 68–75.

Braham, R.L., and H.S. Ruchlin. 1987. Physician Practice Profiles: A Case Study of the Use of Audit and Feedback in an Ambulatory Care Group Practice. *Health Care Management Review* 12: 11–16.

Doubilet, P., M.C. Weinstein, and B.J. McNeil. 1986. Use and Misuse of the Term *Cost Effective* in Medicine. *New England Journal of Medicine* 314: 253–56.

Eisenberg, J.M. 1989. Clinical Economics: A Guide to the Economic Analysis of Clinical Practices. *Journal of the American Medical Association* 262: 2879–86.

Goldfield, N., C. Larson, D. Roblin, et al. 1999. The Content of Report Cards: Do Primary Care Physicians and Managed Care Medical Directors Know What Health Plan Members Think Is Important? *Joint Commission Journal on Quality Improvement* 25, no. 8: 422–33.

Goldfield, N. 1999. *Provider Profiling and Risk Adjustment*, 2d ed. Gaithersburg, MD: Aspen Publishers, Inc.

Goldfield, N., and D. Nash. 1999. *Managing Quality of Care,* 3d ed. Gaithersburg, MD: Aspen Publishers, Inc., and American College of Physicians.

Gotowka, T.D., M. Jackson, and D. Aquilina. 1993. Health Data Analysis and Reporting: Organization and System Strategies. *Managed Care Quarterly* 1, no. 3: 26–34.

Harris, J.S. 1991. Watching the Numbers: Basic Data for Health Care Management. *Journal of Occupational Medicine* 33: 275–78.

Hughes, R.G., and D.E. Lee. 1991. Using Data Describing Physician Inpatient Practice Patterns: Issues and Opportunities. *Health Care Management Review* 16: 33–40.

Iezzoni, L., M. Shwartz, A.S. Ash, J.S. Hughes, J. Daley, and Y.D. Mackierman. 1996. Severity Measurement Methods and Judging Hospital Death Rates for Pneumonia. *Medical Care* 34, no. 1 (January): 11–28.

McGhee J., et al. 1996. Collecting Information from Health Care Consumers: A Resource Manual of Tested Questionnaires and Practical Advice. Gaithersburg, MD: Aspen Publishers, Inc.

Nathanson, R., M. Noether, and R.J. Ozminkowski. 1994. Using Claims Data To Select Primary Care Physicians for a Managed Care Network. *Managed Care Quarterly* 2, no. 4: 50–59.

National Health Information LLC. 1999. *Physician Profiling and Performance: Changing Practice Patterns Under Managed Care.* Atlanta, GA.

Physician Payment Review Commission. 1992. Physician Payment Review Commission Conference on Profiling. Washington, DC.

Smith, N.S., and J.P. Weiner. 1994. Applying Population-Based Case Mix Adjustment in Managed Care: The Johns Hopkins Ambulatory Care Group System. *Managed Care Quarterly* 2, no. 3 (1999): 21–34.

Thomas, J.W., and M.L.F. Ashcraft. 1991. Measuring Severity of Illness: Six Severity Systems and Their Ability To Explain Cost Variations. *Inquiry* 28 (Spring): 39–55.

Weiner, J.P., B.H. Starfield, D.M. Steinwachs, and L.M. Mumford. 1991. Development and Application of a Population-Oriented Measure of Ambulatory Care Case-Mix. *Medical Care* 29, no. 5 (May): 452–72.

CHAPTER 33

Physician Behavior Change in Managed Health Care

Peter R. Kongstvedt

INTRODUCTION

The practice behavior of physicians in managed care organizations (MCOs) is one of the most important elements in managing cost, quality, and access. Although much talk occurs around the idea that this process begins by selecting and recruiting only those physicians who demonstrate good quality and cost-effective practice behavior, the reality is that there will be great heterogeneity of physician practice behaviors in the network. Marketing and delivery system or access needs dictate that adequate or even broad geographical coverage be present. The resultant large network will be made up of physicians with quite variable practice behaviors. It falls to medical managers to work with participating physicians to modify practice behaviors that are inconsistent with the goals of managed health care. The best contractual reimbursement arrangements in the industry have diminished value if there are poor utilization patterns, suboptimal quality, or a lack of cooperation with plan policies and procedures.

The purpose of this chapter is to discuss some of the issues and approaches involved in promoting change in the practice behavior of participating physicians as needed for good medical management. Financial incentives are a useful method of aligning financial and MCO goals but are not the subject of this chapter. Financial incentives appear to have some effect on overall utilization patterns, but financial incentives alone are inadequate for purposes of quality and cost management through practice behavior change. Financial incentives are simply tools to support the more important programs of medical management, as discussed throughout Part III, rather than as the primary approach to medical management. An in-depth discussion of reimbursement methods may be found in Chapters 8 through 11.

What follows is a discussion of at least some of the aspects of physician practice behavior, a discussion of methods to achieve change, and last a discussion of what approaches to take in those atypical situations in which a physician's practice behavior is irreconcilably incompatible with managed health care. As the reader proceeds through the chapter, he or she should bear in mind that physicians and medical directors are individuals, each with their own strengths and weaknesses, who will have unique abilities and responses around any of the approaches discussed here.

GENERAL ASPECTS OF PHYSICIAN PRACTICE BEHAVIOR

Physicians are highly intelligent, highly educated professionals who develop an inordinately large set of clinical practice behavior biases. This is due to many factors, including their initial training, the current environment of medical practice today, peer interactions, professional and commercial (i.e., nonclinical) literature, personal income, personal lifestyle needs, human nature, and the types of pressures now being brought to bear on them. None of these issues are unique to the medical profession, but their combination and depth make for a complex and often emotionally charged atmosphere in which practice behavior change must occur.

What follows are brief discussions of a few of the more important aspects of practice behavior. Medical and nonclinical managers in MCOs, medical groups, or integrated delivery systems (IDSs; see Chapter 4) need to be aware of these to better understand at least some of the dynamics involved in approaching practice behavior change.

General Environment

Over the last two decades, the environment in which physicians practice has been continually changing. It is important for medical managers and executives with responsibilities in medical management to recognize that as managed health care has evolved, so have physicians' practice behaviors. In the 1970s and 1980s, physicians were relatively unconcerned with cost issues, there was far less actual measurement of quality of care, and there were practice behaviors linked to the old fee-for-service incentives that contributed to high health care cost inflation.

By the late 1990s and into the 2000s, managed health care has become predominant, and physicians' practice behaviors have changed as a result. There are still pressures that drive medical costs up, such as shifting demographics of our population, advances in medical interventions, and drug costs. While still addressing these issues, there is now more attention to quality, physicians are more aware of cost considerations, and there is less need for some of the approaches to medical management required in the past. These evolutionary changes in the environment and physician practice behavior are not uniform across all parts of the country. There are differences in the degree and the substance of change. For example, attitudes and behaviors in Southern California are strikingly dissimilar to those

in Texas; but even in Texas, there has been considerable change.

Despite this evolution in practice behavior, the need to continually work with physicians to change practice behavior remains. It is the foci of needed changes that have shifted along with the environment. With managed health care's greater ability to measure quality and outcomes (see Chapters 30 and 31), as well as risk-adjusted practice profiling (see Chapter 32), there is now as much focus on quality and outcomes as on cost. Standard reporting instruments such as the Health Plan Employer Data and Information Set (see Chapters 35 and 44) report on preventive medical care, common chronic conditions and processes of care, and certain acute and preventable conditions, among other measures. These are measures that were not routinely collected in the past but are now widely available in MCOs and provide one example of goals for physician practice behavior change. Other common examples might include the use of beta-blockers in patients after acute myocardial infarction, the use of angiotensin-converting enzyme inhibitors in congestive heart failure patients, and the appropriate use of clinical guidelines.

The focus on cost still remains as important as ever. What has changed is that there is less need or desire to change practice behavior at the micromanagement level than there was in prior years when health care costs were on a rocket. Now, there is greater focus on overall patterns of practice behavior rather than individual events, although focus on individual events continues for high-cost, marginal value procedures or for services that are highly subject to interpretation of medical necessity. It would be inaccurate to say that all MCOs no longer focus on individual events, but the trend is there.

Although most physicians remain either relatively or very satisfied with their careers, the attitudes of physicians toward managed care are generally more negative than positive, particularly in locations with high levels of managed care penetration.[1,2] The news media, both general and medical, play up stories of unhappy physicians and their problems with managed care, giving an impression of widespread unhappiness.* Many physicians find practicing in a managed care environment stressful and perceive that certain aspects of managed care, particularly medical management, are intrusive.

Managed care has also placed downward pressure on incomes, although it is worth observing that physicians have actually maintained their incomes or experienced small income increases. This pressure has led some physician organizations to attempt to become labor unions to improve their negotiating power, an approach that is probably ineffective (see Chapter 63).

Physicians' abilities to maintain or even increase their incomes may be coming through changes they have made to adjust for the downward pressure on income from direct patient care. Examples of such changes include:[3]

- Reducing staff costs
- Increased productivity
- Reduced patient amenities
- Delay in the purchase of new equipment
- Joining larger practices
- Diversification of services to patients (e.g., dispensing pharmaceuticals, performing in-office testing)

It would be a mistake for the reader to conclude that physicians are miserable, trapped in professional bondage, and waiting for the day when they can flee from the practice of medicine. The nature of the news is to report negative stories, and even research literature can only answer the questions that a study asks (e.g., if one looks for dissatisfaction, one is likely to find it). The practice of medicine remains a sought-after professional goal, continues to enjoy high esteem in the public's eye, is able to provide a good income, and offers professional satisfaction through the care of patients.

_____

*One must accept the simple fact that it is in the self-interest of reporters and editors of popular media to report negative stories. A reporter for a national news publication once stated to this author that "We don't report safe airplane landings at La Guardia, either."

Medical Education

For medical students or physicians currently in training (residents or fellows), the formal medical education they receive has an impact on their attitudes about managed health care and their ability to succeed in a managed care environment. It is not only the clinical approach to patient care but also the socializing effect of medical education that has an impact.

The overall attitude of medical educators toward managed care is quite negative, and that attitude is strongly imparted to students and residents.[4] There are differences in attitudes on the basis of attributes such as specialty type (primary care residents are slightly more favorable, for example) or academic position occupied (chairs of subspecialty departments are more negative, for example). There is also some acknowledgment that managed health care does provide for greater continuity of care, and there are certain other positive attributes regarding clinical care, but the overall attitude is strongly negative.* Because it is during these periods of training that individuals are the most receptive to learning and changing, the creation of attitudinal biases is also likely to occur.

There has historically been great heterogeneity in attitudes and prior training in cost containment.[5] Despite the general negative attitudes on the part of medical educators, medical education and academic programs are not ignoring managed health care. Many medical schools and academic health centers, in addition to providing clinical care to patients who belong to MCOs, have developed specific training modules in managed care and have clinical preceptorships in practices with high volumes of managed care patients. Thus, there has been an increase in knowledge and understanding about managed

_____

*It should also be noted that most respondents in the study cited favored a single-payer system, with managed health care a distant second, and traditional fee-for-service an even more distant third in preference. Because most privately practicing physicians do not favor a single-payer system over the others, such attitudes appear mutable.

health care in medical students and residents, as well as some increased focus on training, but the variability remains quite high.[6-9] As physicians move out of the academic setting into private practice or employment, their attitudes evolve, as does their receptivity to change.

An in-depth discussion of academic medical centers and medical education in managed health care is found in Chapter 13.

Strong Autonomy and Control Needs

There is perhaps no more emotionally charged issue than autonomy and control. Although closely supervised during training, once they leave training and enter the world of private practice, physicians experience a high level of professional autonomy. As part of their training, physicians are taught to function in an autonomous way, to stand up for themselves, and to be the authority. It is difficult for them to accept a role in which another entity has control over their professional activities, whether it is managed care, peer review, or practice guidelines.[10,11] Because of that, physicians participating in MCOs often feel antagonistic when they perceive that their control has been lost or lessened.

In certain medical groups, there may be some element of supervision and influence or peer review, but generally this is a low-level activity. By definition, managed care introduces elements of management control into the arena of health care delivery, management that appears to, and in some cases does, reduce the physician's autonomy. Numerous studies regarding this topic have been conducted, with results supporting contentions on both sides of the equation. Those two contentions are that managed health care does indeed reduce the level of autonomy or that a physician's belief that his or her autonomy is restricted is not supported by reality. Issues such as precertification review and requirements for documentation, or at least reasoning for certain clinical decisions (e.g., if a physician wants to refer a patient for a procedure that the MCO considers to be either investigational or frequently subject to inappropriate use), are clear examples of a MCO intruding on the

decision-making process of a physician. On the other hand, a high percentage of all clinical encounters with patients enrolled in a MCO will not result in any type of impediment to action or even prenotification.

Over the past 10 years, there has been an increase in the percentage of a typical physician's practice that is subject to some form of external control. Health maintenance organizations (HMOs), point-of-service (POS) plans, preferred provider organizations (PPOs), indemnity plans with managed care elements (e.g., preadmission authorization requirements), Medicare, and Medicaid are all programs that have been increasing their control over medical practice as health care costs have risen. The degree of control will vary considerably, depending on the type of program involved, but managed health care, particularly in tightly managed HMOs, currently exerts the greatest degree of external control outside of medical residency training. The greater the degree of external control, the greater the danger of overt or covert resistance to medical management or benefits interpretation. For example, in one small survey of internists, slightly more than half were willing to deceive the medical management function of an MCO to obtain authorization of services for their patients (it was not clear how often this actually occurred, though).[12] In another, larger survey, 39 percent of physicians reported that they had deliberately misled health insurance companies at least once regarding insurance coverage for a patient in order to secure coverage for care the physician perceived was needed; there was no association between this behavior and reimbursement methodology or physician income.[13]

Many of the issues discussed in the course of this chapter are pertinent to ameliorating some of the anxieties that arise in dealing with control issues. It is probably not unreasonable to point out that failure of the private sector and the physician community to control medical costs in the nation will lead to even greater interventions by nonphysicians charged with bringing medical costs under control. Enlisting the physician's help in achieving the plan's goals is possible by empowering the physicians within the system.

Control of Where Care Is Received

Virtually all managed care plans will have some controls over where members receive their care. In a simple PPO, that control will be confined to a differential in benefits that is based on whether a member uses participating hospitals and physicians. In a tightly managed HMO, the plan will cover only the use of participating providers, and even then only for certain services. For example, the HMO may have an exclusive contract for mammography; even though all the participating hospitals have the ability to perform mammography, only one provider will be allowed to do it and get paid.

If a plan intends to have a highly restricted panel of participating providers, it is sometimes helpful to elicit the opinions of those physicians already on the panel, even though the final decision will still rest with the plan. For example, if the decision has been made to use only two or three orthopedic groups to provide services, the primary care physicians could be canvassed for nominations of groups to approach. The plan should clearly state that it is not having a majority rule vote but is looking for input on who to approach; the final selection will be based on a combination of the plan's regular credentialing process, the group's willingness to cooperate with plan policies and procedures, and cost.

The larger the health plan, the less ability to solicit and act on such physician input, but, paradoxically, the less need there is to do it because large plans also have large networks. In the case of MCOs that are part of a national company or that are very large regional plans, it is common for the MCO to contract with a narrow group of providers for management of specific clinical conditions (e.g., diabetes) as part of the disease management program (see Chapter 23). In such carve-out arrangements, input from the network physicians may be sought, but that is not the norm, and the MCO must determine that the carve-out clinical manager will provide high quality and service. This illustrates that there will be many times when soliciting the input from network physicians will not be practical, but medical managers should be alert to those opportunities when input can be useful and applied.

Control of Patient Care

Much more volatile than the preceding, control of patient care is a real hot button with most physicians. This control can range from the prospective authorization for elective admissions that is found in most plans to the mandatory preauthorization of all nonprimary care services that is found in most HMOs. The greater the degree of plan involvement in clinical decision making, the greater the chances of antagonism between physicians and plan managers, but also the greater the degree of medical cost control.

Because this management of medical services is the hallmark of managed care, it is neither possible nor desirable to eliminate it. How that control is exercised, though, will have a great effect on its acceptance and success. If the plan intervenes in a heavy-handed manner or in a way that appears to the physicians to be arbitrary, there will be problems. If interventions are done with an element of understanding and respect, there should be greater cooperation.

Many of the approaches described in later sections of this chapter are particularly important here. Frequent and regular contact, both positive and negative, will help a great deal. Discussing cases, and suggesting and soliciting alternatives for case management will yield better results than issuing demands for improvement.

Control of Quality

The most common objection that physicians will actually voice about managed care is that it reduces the quality of care. Even if that argument is sometimes a smoke screen for purely economic concerns, the issue is still a valid one. Any health plan that requires the use of a restricted network of providers and has an authorization system must be able to demonstrate that it is not reducing the quality of care delivered.

There is no consistent evidence that managed care systematically results in inferior care. The medical research literature does consistently demonstrate that managed health care provides equal and sometimes superior care than does unmanaged fee-for-service (see also Chapter 6).[14–37] Despite the scarcity of evidence that managed care is inferior, concerns about poor quality of care persist in most physicians' minds.

The best approach here is to place responsibility for participating with the plan's quality management (QM) program squarely with the physicians themselves. It is vital to have a properly constructed QM program so that physician participation is meaningful; this refers not only to survey types of studies but also to the creation of meaningful changes across the network to improve quality. A solid QM program allows the physicians to feel that the plan genuinely does have an interest in quality and should allow for some pride in participation. A more detailed discussion of QM programs is found in Chapter 30.

Role Conflict

It is often stated that physicians are trained to be the patient's advocate. This is partially true, but that notion presupposes a system in which a patient, like a plaintiff or defendant in a lawsuit, needs an advocate. In fact, physicians are trained to be the patient's caregiver, that is, the coordinator and deliverer of medical care.

An often-heard statement may be paraphrased as: "We must give the patient everything they need." Superficially, this statement gives the appearance of a black-and-white difference, a dichotomy. In truth, this issue is one of gradation or degree. To take to a ludicrous degree the notion of giving a patient everything he or she needs, a physician would have only one patient, whom he or she would follow around 24 hours per day, never charging for care, and even giving that patient all the physician's worldly goods. The real world requires physicians to "ration" care by scheduling appointments during working hours, to charge for their services, to share after-hours call, and so forth.

Managed health care, when performed properly, is focused on reducing cost while maintaining or improving quality of care, and by so doing, is aimed at meeting the patient's needs, not necessarily all expressed desires by the physicians or the patients. The issue of advocacy arises when a physician feels that the needs of the plan and the needs of the patient are in conflict.[38] When that happens, the physician feels genuinely torn between being the patient's advocate and the plan's advocate. This most frequently comes up when patients request or demand a service that is not really necessary or is medically marginal. Physicians feel on the spot if they must deny the service, putting themselves in a role in conflict with their patients: "Just whose side are you on, anyway?" This is a difficult situation that is handled better by some physicians than others.[39]

Plan managers need to acknowledge this conflict, even though this conflict occurs less frequently in reality than in perception. Because of poor understanding of the insurance function (discussed later), the conflict may come up when the physician feels a service is medically necessary when, in fact, it is not a covered benefit. In some cases, there is poor understanding of the difference between what is actually medically necessary and what is essentially a convenience. The health plan is not in the business of denying truly needed services, assuming that they are covered under the schedule of benefits; denial of such services would be ethically unacceptable and financially foolish.

What the health plan is in the business of doing is providing health benefits within a constrained financial system; i.e., constrained by available premium dollars or payments by Medicare or Medicaid. The physician is charged with conserving the resources, primarily economic, of the plan to ensure availability of those resources to those who truly need them. It is the physician who will best be able to determine what is really needed and what is really not, and that will help provide more appropriate allocation of those resources. The plan's utilization management efforts are (or should be) aimed at aiding the physician in carrying out that function.

Poor Understanding of the Insurance Function of the Plan

As mentioned earlier, some of the problems of role conflict stem from a poor understanding of the insurance aspect of the plan. HMOs in particular are marketed as offering comprehensive benefits, even though there are clearly certain exclusions and limitations, just as there are for any form of health care coverage. Physicians and members often do not differentiate between what is medically necessary and what is a covered benefit.

Every plan has certain exclusions and limitations of coverage. For example, a member may require 3 months of skilled nursing care, but the plan covers only 30 days. Plan management may make exceptions to the exclusions and limitations policy, but that should be done only rarely and after much thought. In some cases it will be clearly cost-effective to do so (e.g., providing 30 days of home durable medical equipment to avoid a hospitalization). In other cases it will not be. If frequent exceptions are made, it can lead to an open-ended commitment to provide lifetime noncovered services, a commitment that the plan cannot afford if it is to remain in business.

A more difficult example is an experimental transplant procedure. In most cases experimental or investigational treatments are not covered benefits under the plan's schedule of benefits. This becomes emotionally charged when the patient has a fatal condition and the investigational treatment is held out as their only hope for survival. Often decided by the courts rather than by medical evidence, this is an area in which the physicians, the press, and pretty much the entire world will excoriate an MCO for "withholding life-saving care in order to make a profit." Legislation in many states, and to some degree at the federal level, has created requirements for coverage of certain treatments, but this has generally been on the basis of politics rather than scientific evidence. At the time of publication, there is debate in Congress that would require a health plan to cover an investigational treatment if it is part of a research protocol or formal study. Regardless of the specifics, dealing with coverage for investigational procedures requires extraordinarily high competencies in communications between the plan's medical management (which includes personal involvement by the medical director), the physicians, the member, and the member's family.

Helping a physician understand the insurance nature of the plan and that there are limitations to coverage is a wise investment on the part of the plan managers. In some cases, it may help the physician if the plan takes on the role of communicating a negative message; in other words, plan management contacts the member in such cases to reinforce that it is a contract (i.e., schedule of benefits) issue and not a matter of the physician being callous and hard hearted.

Recent state (and possibly federal) legislation regarding mandatory external appeals for denied services may come into play here. Mandatory appeals are supposed to be for issues of medical necessity and appropriateness, not for changing the schedule of benefits. The plan will need to separate the two issues.

Bad Habits

Physicians, like all of us, have habits and patterns in their lives. Habits also extend to clinical practices that are not cost-effective but are difficult to change. One example would be the practice of not seeing patients or making rounds on Wednesdays; the physician's partner may not feel comfortable discharging a partner's patient, so the stay is lengthened by an extra day. Another example is a physician who keeps a routine, uncomplicated surgical case in longer than necessary, stating "That's the way I've always done it, and who are you to question me?"

This problem is a touchy one. It is usually poor form bluntly to accuse a physician of bad practice habits. The frontal assault is often met with the indignant question, "Are you questioning my judgment?" The medical manager is not (or should not be), of course; he or she is questioning a bad habit.

It is preferable to help lead physicians to the appropriate conclusion themselves. By discussing the issue objectively, presenting supporting information, and asking physicians to examine critically the difference in practice behavior, many physicians will arrive at the conclusion that their old habits must change. By allowing physicians gracefully and quietly to make the change, there is less risk of creating the need for a rigid defensive posture on their part, and it also allows for greater acceptance of a new practice behavior.

In some cases, this approach will not work. If calm and rational discussions fail to effect a change, firmer action may be needed, as discussed later in this chapter. Physicians may change a habit, but not necessarily accept that the behavior *is* a habit, resulting in grudging compliance; in that circumstance, the physician may tell the patient that the health plan is making him or her do it against his or her judgment. In most cases, this type of grumbling will go away after a short while. If it does not, the medical director must counsel these physicians about appropriate behavior in this litigious era. If there is an adverse outcome, even though it had nothing to do with the changed practice pattern, the chances of a lawsuit are probably heightened if those types of comments have been made. Despite recent laws passed in several states that encourage plaintiffs to sue MCOs for malpractice, a physician should not mistakenly believe his or her chances of not being dragged through that same lawsuit are improved. If genuine malpractice has occurred, then appropriate managerial and legal steps should be taken and the patient's problems attended to. If, however, malpractice has not occurred, it is neither in the interest of the physician nor the plan to engage in the types of communications that would encourage baseless legal action.

Poor Understanding of Economics

Even though physicians and their business managers are becoming more sophisticated about managed care, there is still a surprising lack of understanding of the economics, especially in capitated or other performance-based reimbursement systems as discussed in Chapters 8 and 11. There may be little understanding of withholds and incentive pools, or physicians may feel so distant from those incentives that there is little or no effect on behavior.

It is worthwhile to have continual communications and re-education about the economics of the plan as it relates to the physician's income. Plan management should always be aware of the whole dollars involved in compensating physicians. A small number, such as an $11.25 per member per month capitation payment, may seem like funny money to a physician, but if that

$11.25 per member per month really means $40,000 per year, that has a considerable impact on the financial position of a practice.

On the reverse side, a physician, medical group, or IDS that has accepted a considerable degree of financial risk for medical costs may have little or no understanding of how cash flows and liability accrues in a managed care system, and thus find themselves in serious financial trouble (see Chapter 47 for a discussion of financial management issues). The most common problem is failing to understand that under capitation, cash comes in immediately, whereas costs trail, leading the providers to underestimate the true financial liability they face. In addition to ensuring that these providers are using good medical management methods, are capturing data, providing quality service, and so forth, it is important for plan managers to regularly re-educate the group or IDS on financial management in managed care.

Related to all of this is the need for accurate and timely feedback to the physicians about their economic status on the basis of payments and utilization. Inaccurate feedback is far worse than no feedback at all. The subject of physician profiling and the use of data in medical management is found in Chapter 32 and is not repeated here. Unlike profiling reports that look at practice patterns, which are necessary for medical management, the ability to produce reports to the physicians on their financial status and other business-related functions is valuable. In some cases, the data may not be available to the MCO because of the IDS or medical group performing many of the administrative functions, but that is a state of affairs that the MCO must make every effort to change. If the plan does not have accurate data itself, then it has no hope of addressing the issues raised here.

Poor Differentiation among Competing Plans

Considerable difficulty arises when there is little or no differentiation among competing plans. In many markets, the benefits may be the same and the provider network may be similar or the same; the only difference is the premium rates (which then take on the ominous characteristics of a commodity market). This is particularly the case in Medicare + Choice markets in which the federal government sets standards and the MCOs provide added benefits that are essentially alike from plan to plan (to avoid adverse selection); Medicare is a pure retail market in most cases, so differentiation on the basis of employers does not occur, and members may easily move from plan to plan.

The problem increases when each plan has different internal policies and procedures with which the physicians and their office staff must comply. If a physician is contracting with three or more plans, the frustration involved with trying to remember which one wants what can be quite high. This is exacerbated when the same patient changes to a different managed care plan. For example, on Friday Mr. Jones was with the ABC Health Plan, but when he came in for his return appointment on Monday he had switched to the XYZ Health Plan; the office staff did not take notice, which resulted in claims or authorization denials and late payments from the new MCO. This can be a real morale problem with the physician's office staff as well. When frustration rises, compliance falls.

There are several ways to approach this problem. One way is by increased attention and service to the physicians and their office staff. Frequent and timely communications help, and the more such communications are done in person, the better. Newsletters have a way of appearing on the bottom of the parakeet cage without getting read. Some physicians have ready access to e-mail, but that is inconsistent and the physician may access e-mail at home rather than the office, and not transmit the information to his or her office staff. Furthermore, privacy and security concerns exist with e-mail, thus restricting its use in any event.

In this area, nonmonetary issues can have as much impact as monetary ones. Examples include difficult-to-use forms that require unnecessary writing; frequent busy signals, long hold times, or lack of response on service lines; and inconsistencies in responses to questions. It can-

not be overstressed that prompt and courteous responsiveness to questions and concerns is required. The plan managers or service representatives do not have to give the answer that they think physicians will want to hear, but they do have to give an answer or response that is consistent, clear, and reasonably fair.

Electronic commerce (e-commerce; see Chapter 37) will address many of these problems as it becomes more widely used by physicians. The ability to automate and conduct by way of the Internet many necessary functions such as checking member eligibility, sending claims, sending or obtaining referrals or authorizations, and checking the status of submitted claims, will go far in reducing the aggravations created by administrative requirements. Because of data and transaction standards mandated in the Health Insurance Portability and Accountability Act of 1996 (HIPAA, see Chapters 35, 36, and 67), the potential ease of e-commerce will increase, although there will clearly be some difficult transition issues as this portion of HIPAA is put into effect beginning in 2002.

GENERAL APPROACHES TO CHANGING BEHAVIOR

Translating Goals and Objectives

One useful way of looking at communications between plan management and physicians is to consider the concept of translation. It is easy to overlook the fact that managers and physicians may have radically different ways of viewing matters relating to the delivery of health care services to plan members. For example, the area of cost containment is rife with possibilities for opposing views. Physicians frequently look on cost containment measures as unnecessary intrusions into their domain, whereas nonphysician managers view the same measures as the only way to control headstrong physicians. Translating the goal of cost containment into terms that are both understandable and acceptable to both parties will go far toward obtaining cooperation and acceptance. To ensure that the economic resources will be available to compensate providers and to make services available at all to patients, cost containment must take place.

Rewards Are More Effective Than Sanctions

A tenet of behavior modification theory is that positive interactions or rewards are more effective for achieving long-term changes in behavior than are negative interactions or sanctions. Physicians will have a more positive response to approaches that involve education and peer-influenced interventions than they will to approaches that rely heavily on rules and regulations.[40] It is not good policy for managers to impose their will on others in a heavy-handed manner that might be viewed as arbitrary actions. In some cases it is necessary to be directive, but if it is done as a matter of course, cooperation by the physicians will be poor if they cooperate at all. In the worst case, heavy-handed dictates can lead to widespread dissatisfaction and defection from the network. Even without such attrition, overt cooperation may occur, but covert resistance undoes any progress made, and physician dissatisfaction creates a plethora of other problems. As stated in the beginning of this chapter, physicians (even in closed panel operations or medical groups) behave with a great deal of autonomy and power (much of which is necessary to deliver effective medical care) and cannot effectively be treated as though they are employees or nonprofessional service contractors.

In the context of this discussion, rewards refer primarily to forms of positive feedback and communication about good performance. Clearly, good case management should yield economic rewards as well, but positive feedback from plan management will be a reward system all its own. Other rewards could include accredited continuing education seminars about managed care, small gifts or acknowledgments for good work, and so forth.* Economic rewards for

non-utilization-based performance and behavior are found in Chapter 10.

Although it is unrealistic to expect that every physician will embrace every policy and procedure the plan has, the odds of cooperation will increase when the interactions between the physician and the plan are more positive than negative. This is not to be confused with capitulation on necessary policies and procedures: There were once plenty of "physician-friendly" health plans that are now little more than smoking rubble. Rather, this is to emphasize that too heavy a hand will eventually cause problems.

Be Involved

It is shocking how often managers of health plans fail to maintain an active involvement with the participating physicians. Often the only communications from the MCO to the physicians are occasional newsletters or memos, claims denials, and calls from the utilization management department harassing the physicians about hospital cases. Those types of interactions tend not to add to the luster of plan management in the physicians' eyes.

Frequent and regular contact, either through scheduled meetings, personal visits, or telephone calls, will help create an environment for positive change. If the only time physicians hear from the plan is when there is a problem, they will try to avoid contact in the future and will be inclined to have decreased responsiveness to the plan's needs. When communicating about utilization or quality issues, offer advice, suggestions, and alternatives, not just demands to change something. Ask intelligent questions about the clinical issues at hand, and solicit advice about alternative ways to provide the care. Work to get to the point at which physicians will be asking themselves the same questions the medical director would ask, without the medical director having to ask them.

Involvement is a two-way proposition. It is fair and reasonable to expect some network physicians to participate in plan committees to help set medical policy, monitor and manage clinical quality, and so forth. Network physicians should

---

*Good examples of the use of tchotchkes, albeit in an inflated manner not possible by an MCO, are found in the way the pharmaceutical industry showers physicians with a mind-boggling array of gifts, doodads, and stuff that litters up all corners of the typical physician's office.

also be involved in many aspects of utilization management. For purposes of broad behavior changes applicable to the entire network, physicians will participate and "buy in" to a process that is fair, iterative, and accurate, and they will contribute strongly to helping create change.[41] Soliciting active participation in such functions helps promote a sense of ownership on the part of the involved physicians and will clearly provide the plan with valuable input. The plan also should compensate those physicians for time spent on such activities by means of an honorarium.

PROGRAMMATIC APPROACHES TO CHANGING PHYSICIAN BEHAVIOR

Formal Continuing Medical Education

Formal continuing medical education (CME) is the provision of additional clinical training or medically oriented information through seminars, conferences, home-study, and so forth. The hallmark of CME is that it provides CME credits by virtue of the accreditation of the sponsoring body. This method of information dissemination, although traditionally the most prevalent, has mixed effectiveness at best when it comes to changing behavior. Review studies of the medical literature have found little evidence that traditional CME changed patient outcomes or changed behavior.[42–46] There is some evidence that changes in behavior will occur when the curriculum is *designed* to change specific types of behavior; for example, by creating in the CME program a strong focus on change.[47] Other useful adjuncts to CME include academic detailing (i.e., one-on-one education focused on specific issues), reminders (i.e., specific reminders at the time of a patient visit), and the influence of opinion leaders.[48] The addition of more intensive and personalized interventions such as the ability to practice new skills (an intervention more useful for learning procedures than for changing practice behavior) or a high level of individual interactivity may also effect some level of change in the setting of a CME program.[49]

On the basis of this evidence, formal CME may be a useful tool for disseminating clinical information and may be a useful adjunct to other approaches to changing physician behavior in general. However, formal didactic CME alone is not a useful tool for changing physician practice behavior when compared with other available methods.

Data and Feedback

As has been mentioned in other chapters, particularly Chapters 30, 31, and 32, data regarding quality, utilization, and cost are an integral part of a managed care plan. The value of data is not restricted to plan managers; data are equally important to individual physicians. If the only data physicians get are letters at the end of the year informing them that all of their withhold is used up, they can credibly argue that they were blindsided because, in fact, they were. Providing regular and accurate data about an individual physician's performance from a quality, utilization, and (for risk/bonus models) an economic standpoint is important for changing behavior. Most physicians will want to perform well, but can do so only when they can judge their own performance against that of their peers or against expectations.

The research literature is actually mixed in its support for feedback as a means of changing behavior, although a small majority of the research data are positive. There are studies reporting significant reductions in utilization and costs in response to feedback about individual physician behavior.[50–58] There are, however, other studies that report no effect from information feedback, report that feedback has little lasting effect unless continuously reinforced, or are at best ambiguous regarding the role of feedback.[59–65]

When reviewing the possible reasons for feedback being shown to be effective or ineffective (at least over the long term), it is possible to conjecture on some conditions that improve the effectiveness of feedback. These conjectures, although not studied in the research literature, are valid from the standpoint of industry experience.

- Physicians must believe that their behavior needs to change, whether for clinical reasons, economic reasons, or simply to remain part of the participating panel in the plan; if physicians do not believe that they need to change, then feedback provides little value.

- Feedback must be credible; in other words, the data must be seen as taking into account such things as severity of illness for patient-related practice profiling.
- Feedback must be consistent and usable; in other words, a physician must clearly understand the data in the report and be able to use that information in a concrete way and to be able to keep using it to measure his or her own performance.
- Feedback needs to be closely related to what a physician is doing at the time; in other words, feedback about behavior that is remote in time or infrequent is less likely to be acted on.
- Feedback must be regular to sustain changed behavior; feedback that is sporadic or unsustained will result in behavior changes returning to the condition before the feedback caused any change to begin with (assuming that any change took place at all).
- Feedback that is linked to economic performance may be more likely to produce substantial change than is feedback that is not so linked; in other words, feedback about utilization or nonutilization measures that are tied to compensation has more potential for use by the physician than data that do not have such a linkage.

Practice Guidelines and Clinical Protocols

Practice guidelines and clinical protocols refer to codified approaches to medical care. Guidelines may be for both diagnostic and therapeutic modalities, and they may be used to guide physicians in the care of patients with defined diseases or symptoms, or as surveillance tools to monitor practice on a retrospective basis. Clinical pathways or protocols are discussed in great detail in Chapter 29, and the reader is urged to review that chapter. It should also be noted here that not all clinical guidelines and protocols for the same clinical condition are alike. In one recent study, it was reported that guidelines published in peer-reviewed medical literature did not adhere well to published methodological standards,[66] although it is not clear whether this represents a barrier to the practical usefulness of the guidelines.

Some physicians have an initial negative reaction to practice guidelines: they believe that guidelines make for cookbook medicine[67,68] or that guidelines represent a high risk in the event of a malpractice lawsuit because guidelines provide a template against which all actions will be judged. Practice guidelines actually have been used to support both lack of negligence and negligence in malpractice cases.[69] Broadly speaking, though, practice guidelines and protocols do not appear to be related to malpractice awards, although other factors have a loose association with the incidence of malpractice lawsuits.[70–73] Even when practice guidelines or protocols are present, in most cases expert witnesses set the "standards" of care, not necessarily written protocols.[74] In all events, courts have consistently upheld the notion that the physician is ultimately responsible for treatment and for the exercise of clinical judgment, regardless of the existence of a protocol.

Implementing practice guidelines is not always easy, particularly in an open panel setting. There is frequent lack of enthusiasm on the part of the physicians, and the plan's ability actually to monitor the guidelines is limited. Generally, the plan's QM process is best able to monitor the use of guidelines (see Chapter 30), although there may be some ability to use the medical management software support systems, or even the claims system, to provide the necessary data.

There is some evidence that simple publication of practice guidelines alone may predispose physicians to consider changing their behavior, but that such guidelines by themselves are unlikely to effect rapid change.[75,76] When such protocols are accompanied by direct presentations by opinion leaders, so-called academic detailing, then changes are more sustained.[77] There are multiple other interventions that have been reported to improve compliance with the guidelines,[78] but it is difficult to isolate specific techniques to increase compliance.[79] As discussed in Chapter 29, clinical pathways that are developed by the physicians who will then use those pathways, especially in the inpatient setting, are most likely to have significant effects.

Small Group Programs

There is good evidence that educating physicians in a highly interactive, small group setting can produce positive changes in behavior, including improved outcomes and lower utilization. Several authors of studies about interactive, small group physician education believe that the effectiveness is explained by theories of self-regulation.[80–82] These small group seminars or educational sessions are frequently focused on specific clinical conditions; for example, asthma,[83] hypertension,[84] hysterectomy,[85] pelvic pain and/or abnormal uterine bleeding,[86] sciatica,[87] and spinal stenosis.[88] The same approach has been studied in physician practice behavior for chronic conditions in general (including the creation of physician-patient "partnerships")[89] and for test-ordering behavior.[90]

Well-regarded academic or community physicians are most appropriate for conducting these types of highly interactive small group seminars or educational sessions. Because of potential concerns of conflict of interest, medical managers from the MCO are not in a good position to conduct such seminars unless the program is based on data and feedback that only the MCO has. The investment required to conduct these programs is potentially sizable, so it is important for an MCO to leverage its resources to improve the likelihood of a positive outcome. Probably the best approach is for an MCO to provide educational supporting grants to an academic center or tertiary health system to conduct the program. Supporting grants may be restricted to seminars focusing on improving quality and utilization, although the MCO should not attempt to dictate the educational content. Although only superficially related to formal CME, such sessions should still provide for CME credit.

ADDRESSING NONCOMPLIANCE BY INDIVIDUAL PHYSICIANS

There are no programmatic approaches to changing practice behavior that will have a positive impact on every single physician in the network. Many variables such as geographical location, local practice attitudes, the training a physician has received, economic or financial conditions, availability and acceptability of data and information, and personality will have effects on the degree of success medical managers will achieve. The design of the benefits products that the MCO is selling and administering in the marketplace will also have an effect, with those plans that are more restrictive (e.g., a "pure" HMO) having greater need and ability to address practice behavior change compared with relatively loosely managed plans (e.g., a PPO). But in all events, there will be variability in the degrees or amount of positive changes that each individual physician makes. In some cases, there will be so little positive change that medical managers must undertake an approach focused on an individual physician.

The amount of investment in medical management an MCO makes is directly related to the types of approaches that are possible to use for changing behavior. Those MCOs that make little investment in medical management will rely more on data dissemination and rules, whereas MCOs that make heavier investments in medical management will use the broader array of available options. Loosely managed MCOs may choose to not deal with individual physician behavior at all, whereas HMOs are far more likely to do so. MCOs with very large networks will need to focus on those physicians that are significantly out of conformance, whereas MCOs with smaller networks can take the approach of working with a higher percentage of individual physicians. Of course, the degree to which medical managers are able to focus on individual physicians will at least in part depend on available resources such as personnel (especially medical directors), valid data, and time.

Positive feedback is a powerful long-term approach.* It is an effective tool for change that

---

* The use of the term "positive feedback" here is different than when using the term "feedback" regarding data. Although both forms of feedback provide information to the provider regarding performance, data feedback is objective, whereas positive feedback in the context of this section refers to subjective information from plan managers.

most managers fail to use to any great degree and in fact is quite uncommon in medical management. Positive feedback does not refer to mindless or misleading praise but rather to letting a physician know when things are done well. Most managers get so involved in firefighting that they tend to neglect sending positive messages to those providers who are managing well. In the absence of such messages, providers have to figure out for themselves what they are doing right, although the plan will usually tell them what they are doing wrong. This is certainly a missed opportunity.

Stepwise Approach to Changing Behavior in Individual Physicians

Changing behavior in individual providers requires a stepwise approach. The first and most common step is collegial discussion. Discussing cases and utilization patterns in a nonthreatening way, colleague to colleague, is generally an effective method of bringing about change. In most cases, this is adequate and no further steps are necessary.

Persuasion is also commonly used. Somewhat stronger than collegial discussion, persuasion refers to plan managers persuading providers to act in ways that the providers may not initially choose themselves. For example, if a patient requires intravenous antibiotics for a chronic infection but is generally doing well, that patient is a candidate for home intravenous therapy. Some physicians will resist discharging the patient to home therapy because it is inconvenient to follow the case; keeping the patient in the hospital is a lot easier in terms of rounding. The physician must then be persuaded to discharge the patient because of the cost-effectiveness of home therapy.

Firm direction of plan policies, procedures, and requirements (i.e., the "rules and regulations") is the next step after persuasion. If a physician refuses to cooperate with the plan to deliver care cost-effectively and discussions and persuasion have failed, a medical director may be required to give a physician firm direction, reminding him or her of the contractual agreement to cooperate with plan policies and procedures. Behind firm direction is the implied threat of refusal to pay for ser-

vices or even more severe sanctions. It is clearly a display of power and should not be done with a heavy hand. When giving firm direction, it is best to not be drawn into long and unresolvable arguments. Presumably the discussions and even the arguments have already occurred, so it is pointless to keep rehashing them. This is sometimes called a broken record type of response because, rather than respond to old arguments, the medical director always gives the same response: firm direction. Medical managers should reserve this approach to behavior change to those instances when the approaches discussed earlier are ineffective. Inexperienced managers, or managers who are overwhelmed with work and have no time or resources, may use this as a first step; that may be effective, but it will come at the cost of physician dissatisfaction with the plan.

One last thought in this section: Avoid global responses to individual problems. When managers are uncomfortable confronting individual physicians about problems in behavior, a dysfunctional response is to make a global change in policy or procedure because of the actions of one or two physicians. That type of response frequently has the effect of alienating all the other physicians who have been working positively with the plan, while failing to change the behavior of the problem providers. If a policy change is required, make it. If the problem is really just with a few individuals, however, deal with them and do not harass the rest of the panel.

Discipline and Sanctions

This section discusses the most serious form of behavior modification. Sanctions or threats of sanctions are only applied when the problem is so serious that action must be taken and the provider fails to cooperate to improve the situation.* Any disciplinary action, especially one

---

*In some cases, the provider may be willing to cooperate, but the offense is so serious that sanctions must be taken anyway; for example, a serious problem in quality of care such as malpractice resulting in death or serious morbidity and that the medical director has reason to believe may represent an ongoing danger to patients.

that leads to termination or even the threat of termination, should only be undertaken because the other approaches have failed. In addition to the significant emotional trauma and potential financial consequences to the provider, the sanctioning process has legal overtones that must be kept in mind.

Plan management may initiate disciplinary actions short of a formal sanctioning process. In most cases, such discipline is also helpful in creating documentation of chronic problems or failure to cooperate. Discipline may involve verbal warnings or letters; in either case, the thrust of the action is to document the offensive behavior and to describe the consequences of failure to cooperate.

One example of verbal discipline is sometimes called ticketing. It is called that because it is similar to getting a ticket from a traffic cop. This is a verbal reprimand about a specific behavior; the behavior and corrective action are described, as are the consequences of failure to carry out the corrective action. Much like the firm direction described previously, the manager refuses to get into an argument at that time and requires the offending provider to make an appointment at a future date to discuss the issue (similar to a court date). This allows tempers to cool off a bit and ensures that the disciplinary message does not get muddied up with other issues. When a manager issues a ticket, there should be a document placed in a file that describes what transpired. Ticketing is a viable approach when significant time and energy have already been expended to no effect and should not be used unless the more collegial approaches have been exhausted.

A more formal approach is an actual disciplinary letter. Like a ticket, the letter describes the offending behavior and the required corrective action and invites the provider to make an appointment to discuss the issue. In the case of a verbal ticket or a disciplinary letter, the consequence of failure to change errant ways is initiation of the formal sanctioning process.

Formal sanctioning has potentially serious legal overtones. Due process, or a policy regarding rights and responsibilities of both parties, is a requirement for an effective sanctioning procedure, at least when one is sanctioning for reasons

of quality. The Health Care Quality Improvement Act of 1986 (HCQIA) has formalized due process in the sanctioning procedure as it relates to quality, and the MCO must adhere to the prescribed steps, actions, and physician rights to maintain protection from antitrust action. Although this Act was primarily aimed at hospital peer review activities, HMOs are specifically mentioned, and other forms of managed care are potentially subject to it as well.[91]

Following the requirements of the HCQIA regarding due process is cumbersome and is obviously the final step before removing a physician from the panel for reasons of poor quality care. Termination of a provider for reasons of quality is a serious charge and has a negative impact on a physician. Because it is such a drastic step, compliance with the HCQIA, including the reporting requirements, is the best protection the plan has against a legal action.

It should be emphasized that the HCQIA is in regard to peer review activities resulting in actions against physicians for quality problems. If a physician fails to cooperate with contractually agreed-to plan policies and procedures, the plan may have reason to terminate the contract with the physician "for cause." Even in that case, it may be wise to have a due process policy that allows for formal steps to be taken in the event that the plan contemplates termination. Presentation of facts to a medical advisory committee made up of physicians who are not in direct economic competition with the involved physician provides a backup to plan management. Such a committee may be able to effect changes by the physician where the medical director may not. Finally, the backing of a committee underscores that severe sanctions are not arbitrary but are the result of failure on the part of the physician, not plan management.

Situations may arise in which a physician's utilization performance is such that there is a clear mismatch with managed care practice philosophy. The quality of the physician's medical care may be adequate, and there even may have been no gross lack of cooperation with plan policies and procedures, but the physician simply practices medicine in such a style that medical resources are heavily and inappropriately overutilized. In such cases, the medical director must assess whether the physician can change his or her behavior. Assuming that the medical director concludes that the provider in question cannot change (or change sufficiently) and has failed to change despite warnings and feedback, the plan may choose to terminate the relationship solely on the basis of contractual terms that allow either party to terminate without cause when adequate notice is given (see Chapter 62 for discussion about provider contracting).

When the plan departicipates a physician in this way, it is not always subject to a due process type of review. The reason is that the separation is based on practice style and fit, not accusations of rule breaking or poor quality. Terminating physicians in this manner has the potential for creating adverse relations in the network if there is the perception that the plan is acting arbitrarily and without reason. Even without the need for a due process approach in these situations, such steps are drastic and should not be done frequently or lightly.

Many states have legislated due process requirements for physician termination from an MCO network. In many of these state laws, due process is required when an MCO desires to terminate a participating provider for any reason at all, whether for cause or because of serious and irreconcilable differences in practice behavior in a managed health care environment, or even because the provider does so little business with the plan that it is not worth either party's time or effort to maintain the relationship. Because of the rapidly changing and unstable nature of state legislation, it is impossible to provide detail on this issue. The reader is referred to Chapter 69

for a discussion of state regulation of managed health care, although the specific requirements (if they exist) in any state must be ascertained by the reader.

CONCLUSION

Changing physician behavior is central to the success of any managed health care plan. Physicians are unique with their strong need for autonomy and control, potential for role conflicts, uneven understanding of the economics or insurance functions of managed care, and ingrained practice habits. Plan managers can exacerbate the difficulties in changing physician behavior by failing to be responsive and consistent, failing to differentiate their plan from other plans, failing to provide positive feedback, failing to address specific problems with providers early, and failing to take a stepwise approach to managing change.

Systematic approaches to changing physician behavior can be successfully used for many aspects of practice. Continuing education, small group seminars, creation and dissemination of practice protocols, and data feedback are all useful techniques.

When reasonable efforts to obtain necessary and important physician practice behavior change are unsuccessful, discipline and sanctions may be required. Due process must be followed before termination for poor quality, and it may be useful in other settings as well. In the final analysis, it is the plan's responsibility to make the effort to effect changes in provider behavior that will benefit all the parties concerned, and it is the plan's responsibility to take action when necessary.

REFERENCES AND NOTES

1. J.P. Kassirer, Doctor Discontent, *New England Journal of Medicine* 339 (1998): 21, 1538–1541.

2. K. Donelan et al., The New Medical Marketplace: Physicians' Views, *Health Affairs (Millwood)* September–October; 16 (1997) 5, 139–148.

3. Socioeconomic Monitoring System of the American Medical Association, *http://www.ama-assn.org/advocacy/healthpolicy*.

4. S.R. Simon et al., Views of Managed Care—A Survey of Students, Residents, Faculty, and Deans at Medical Schools in the United States, *New England Journal of Medicine* 340 (1999): 928–936.

5. H.L. Greene et al., Physician Attitudes Toward Cost Containment: The Missing Piece of the Puzzle. *Archives of Internal Medicine,* 149 (1989): 1966–1968.

6. M.S. Wilkes, S.A. Skootsky, S. Slavin, C.S. Hodgson,

and L. Wilkerson, Entering First-Year Medical Students' Attitudes Toward Managed Care, *Academic Medicine* 69 (1994): 307–309.

7. J. Veloski, B. Barzansky, D.B. Nash, S. Bastacky, and D.P. Stevens, Medical Student Education in Managed Care Settings: Beyond HMOs, *Journal of the American Medical Association* 276 (1996): 667–671.

8. H.D. Nelson, A.M. Matthews, G.R. Patrizio, and T.G. Cooney, Managed Care, Attitudes, and Career Choices of Internal Medicine Residents, *Journal of General Internal Medicine* 13 (1998): 39–42.

9. R. Ramsbottom-Lucier, J. Pregler, and A.G. Gomez, Challenges in Medical Education: Training Physicians to Work Collaboratively, *Journal of General Internal Medicine* 14 (1999): Suppl 1, S21–25.

10. S.J. O'Connor and J.A. Lanning, The End of Autonomy? Reflections on the Postprofessional Physician, *Health Care Management Review* 17 (1992): 1, 63–72.

11. J.W. Salmon, W. White, and J. Feinglass, The Futures of Physicians: Agency and Autonomy Reconsidered, *Theoretical Medicine* 11 (1990): 261–274.

12. V. Freeman, *Archives of Internal Medicine* 159 (1999): 2263–2270.

13. M.K. Wynia, D.S. Cummins, J.B. Van Geest, and I.B. Wilson. Physician Manipulation of Reimbursement Rules for Patients. *Journal of the American Medical Association* 283 (2000): 1858–1865.

14. J.E. Ware et al., Comparison of Health Outcomes at a Health Maintenance Organization with Those of FFS Care, *Lancet* (1986): 1017–1022.

15. I.S. Udvarhelyi et al., Comparison of the Quality of Ambulatory Care for FFS and Prepaid Patients, *Annals of Internal Medicine* 115 (1991): 394–400.

16. E.M. Sloss et al., Effect of a Health Maintenance Organization on Physiologic Health, *Annals of Internal Medicine* 106 (1987): 130–138.

17. C.M. Clancy and B.E. Hillner, Physicians as Gatekeepers—The Impact of Financial Incentives, *Archives of Internal Medicine* 149 (1989): 917–920.

18. N. Lurie, J. Christianson, M. Finch, and I. Moscovice, The Effects of Capitation on Health and Functional Status of the Medicaid Elderly: A Randomized Trial, *Annals of Internal Medicine* 120 (1994): 506–511.

19. P. Braveman et al., Insurance-Related Differences in the Risk of Ruptured Appendix, *New England Journal of Medicine* 331 (1994): 7, 444–449.

20. A. Relman, Medical Insurance and Health: What About Managed Care? *New England Journal of Medicine* 331 (1994): 7, 471–472.

21. J.P. Murray, S. Greenfield, S.H. Kaplan, and E.M. Yano, Ambulatory Testing for Capitation and FFS Patients in the Same Practice Setting: Relationship to Outcomes, *Medical Care* 30 (1992): 3, 252–261.

22. D.R. Adams et al., The Impact of Financial Incentives on Quality of Health Care, *The Milbank Quarterly* 76, 4 (1999).

23. R.H. Brook, Managed Care Is Not the Problem, Quality Is. *Journal of the American Medical Association* 278 (1997): 1612–1614.

24. L.C. Baker and J.C. Cantor, Physician Satisfaction Under Managed Care. *Health Affairs Supplement* (1993): 258–270.

25. M.D. Weiss, Capitation Can Be Beneficial to Providers and Patients, *Maryland Medical Journal* 46 (1997): 4, 170–171.

26. R.H. Miller and H.S. Luft, Does Managed Care Lead to Better or Worse Quality of Care? *Health Affairs,* September–October 1997.

27. J. Seidman et al., Review of Studies That Compare the Quality of Cardiovascular Care in HMO Verses Non-HMO Settings. *Medical Care* 36 (1998): 1607.

28. R. Bruno and B. Gilbert, In California, Medi-Cal Managed Care Is Superior to Medi-Cal Fee-for-Service. *Managed Care Quarterly* 6 (1998): 4, 7–14.

29. H. Whitmore, Comparing Outcomes in Managed Care, *HMO Magazine,* January–February (1996): 75.

30. F.J. Hellinger, The Effect of Managed Care on Quality, *Archives of Internal Medicine,* 27 April 1998.

31. D.M. Berwick, Quality of Health Care, V: Payment by Capitation and the Quality of Care. *New England Journal of Medicine* 335 (1996): 1227–1231.

32. G. Riely et al., Stage of Cancer at Diagnosis for Medicare HMO and Fee-for-Service Enrollees. *American Journal of Public Health,* October 1994.

33. D. Carlisle et al., HMO vs. Fee-for-Service Care of Older Persons with Acute Myocardial Infarction. *American Journal of Public Health,* December 1992.

34. P. Braveman et al., Insurance Related Differences in the Risk of Ruptured Appendix, *New England Journal of Medicine,* 18 August (1994): 447–448.

35. T. Carey et al., The Outcomes and Costs of Care for Acute Low Back Pain among Patients Seen by Primary Care Practitioners, Chiropractics, and Orthopedic Surgeons, *New England Journal of Medicine* 5, October (1995): 914–916.

36. E.H. Yelin et al., Health Care Utilization and Outcomes Among Persons with Rheumatoid Arthritis in Fee-for-service and Prepaid Group Practice Settings. *Journal of the American Medical Association* 2, October 1996.

37. Collaborating with Managed Care Organizations for Mammogram Screening and Rescreening. *Centers for Disease Control* 1997.

38. E.J. Emanuel and N.N. Dubler, Preserving the Physician-Patient Relationship in the Era of Managed Care. *Journal of the American Medical Association* 273 (1995): 4, 323–329.

39. R.O. Anderson, How Do You Manage the Demanding (Difficult) Patient? *HMO Practice* 4 (1990): 15–16.

40. T.V. Williams, A.M. Zaslavsky, and P.D. Cleary, Physician Experiences with, and Ratings of, Managed Care Organizations in Massachusetts, *Medical Care* 37 (1999): 589–600.

41. R.B. Keller, D.E. Wennberg, and D.N. Soule, Changing Physician Behavior: The Maine Medical Assessment Foundation, *Quality Management in Health Care* 5 (1997): 4, 1–11.

42. J. Heale et al., A Randomized Controlled Trial Assessing the Impact of Problem-Based versus Didactic Teaching Methods in CME, *Proceedings of the Conference on Research in Medical Education of the Association of the American Medical College* 27 (1988): 72–77.

43. W.S. Browner et al., Physician Management of Hypercholesterolemia: A Randomized Trial of Continuing Medical Education. *Western Journal of Medicine* 161 (1994): 572–578.

44. J.P. Boissel et al., Education Program for General Practitioners on Breast and Cervical Cancer Screening: A Randomized Trial. *Reviews in Epidemiology Sante Publique* 43 (1995): 541–547.

45. D.A. Davis, M.A. Thomson, A.D. Oxman, and R.B. Haynes, Evidence for the Effectiveness of CME: A Review of 50 Randomized Controlled Trials, *Journal of the American Medical Association* 268 (1992): 1111–1117.

46. D. Davis et al., Impact of Formal Continuing Medical Education: Do Conferences, Workshops, Rounds, and Other Traditional Continuing Education Activities Change Physician Behavior or Health Care Outcomes? *Journal of the American Medical Association* 282 (1999): 867–874.

47. C.W. White, M.A. Albanese, D.D. Brown, and R.M. Caplan, The Effectiveness of Continuing Medical Education in Changing the Behavior of Physicians Caring for Patients with Acute Myocardial Infarction: a Controlled Randomized Trial, *Annals of Internal Medicine* 102 (1985): 686–692.

48. D.A. Davis, M.A. Thomson, A.D. Oxman, and R.B. Haynes, Changing Physician Performance: A Systematic Review of the Effect of Continuing Medical Education Strategies, *Journal of the American Medical Association* 274 (1995): 9, 700–706.

49. Davis, Thomson, Oxman, and Haynes, Changing Physician Performance, 700–706.

50. S.A. Myers and N. Gleicher, A Successful Program to Lower Cesarean Section Rates, *New England Journal of Medicine* 319 (1989): 1511–1516.

51. J.E. Wennberg, L. Blowers, R. Parker, and A.M. Gittelsohn, Changes in Tonsillectomy Rates Associated with Feedback and Review, *Pediatrics* 59 (1977): 821–826.

52. L.M. Frazier et al., Academia and Clinic: Can Physician Education Lower the Cost of Prescription Drugs? A Prospective, Controlled Trial, *Annals of Internal Medicine* 15 (1991): 116–121.

53. K.I. Marton, V. Tul, and H.C. Sox, Modifying Test-Ordering Behavior in the Outpatient Medical Clinic, *Archives of Internal Medicine* 145 (1985): 816–821.

54. D.M. Berwick and K.L. Coltin, Feedback Reduces Test Use in a Health Maintenance Organization, *Journal of the American Medical Association* 255 (1986): 1450–1454.

55. J.E. Billi et al., The Effects of a Cost-Education Program on Hospital Charges. *Journal of General Internal Medicine* 2 (1987): 306–311.

56. J.E. Billi et al., The Effects of a Low-Cost Intervention Program on Hospital Costs, *Journal of General Internal Medicine* 7 (1992): 411–416.

57. L.M. Manheim et al., Training House Officers To Be Cost Conscious: Effects of an Educational Intervention on Charges and Length of Stay, *Medical Care* 28 (1990): 29–42.

58. E. Zablocki, Sharing Data with Physicians, in Changing Physician Practice Patterns: Strategies for Success in a Capitated Health Care System. Aspen Executive Reports (Gaithersburg, MD: Aspen Publishers, 1995).

59. F.J. Dyck et al., Effect of Surveillance on the Number of Hysterectomies in the Province of Saskatchewan, *New England Journal of Medicine* 296 (1977): 1326–1328.

60. J. Lomas et al., Opinion Leaders vs. Audits and Feedback To Implement Practice Guidelines: Delivery after Previous Cesarean Section, *Journal of the American Medical Association* 265 (1991): 2202–2207.

61. Failure of Information as an Intervention To Modify Clinical Management: A Time-Series Trial in Patients with Acute Chest Pain, *Annals of Internal Medicine* 122 (1995): 434–437.

62. P. Axt-Adam, J.C. van der Wouden, and E. van der Does, Influencing Behavior of Physicians Ordering Laboratory Tests: A Literature Study, *Medical Care* 31 (1993): 9, 784–794.

63. T.A. Parrino, The Nonvalue of Retrospective Peer Comparison Feedback in Containing Hospital Antibiotic Costs, *American Journal of Medicine* 86 (1989): 442–448.

64. S.B. Soumerai, T.J. McLaughlin, and J. Avorn, Improving Drug Prescribing in Primary Care: A Critical Analysis of the Experimental Literature, *Milbank Quarterly* 67 (1989): 268–317.

65. A.R. Martin et al., A Trial of Two Strategies To Modify the Test-Ordering Behavior of Medical Residents, *New England Journal of Medicine* 303 (1980): 1330–1336.

66. T.M. Shanayfelt, M.F. Mayo-Smith, and J. Rothwangl, Are Guidelines Following Guidelines? The Methodological Quality of Clinical Practice Guidelines in the Peer-Reviewed Medical Literature. *Journal of the American Medical Association* 281 (1999): 1900–1905.

67. O. Costantini, K.K. Papp, J. Como, J. Aucott, M.D. Carlson, and D.C. Aron, Attitudes of Faculty, Housestaff, and Medical Students Toward Clinical Practice Guidelines, *Academic Medicine* 74 (1999): 10, 1138–1143.

68. S.H. Woolf, Practice Guidelines: A New Reality in Medicine III: Impact on Patient Care, *Archives of Internal Medicine* 153 (1993): 23, 2646–2655.

69. A.L. Hyams, J.A. Brandenburg, S.R. Lipsitz, D.W. Shapiro, and T.A. Brennan, Practice Guidelines and Malpractice Litigation: A Two-Way Street, *Annals of Internal Medicine* 122 (1995): 6, 450–455.

70. T.A. Brennan, C.M. Sox, and H.R. Burstin, Relation between Negligent Adverse Events and the Outcomes of Medical-Malpractice Litigation, *New England Journal of Medicine* 335 (1996): 1963–1967.

71. A.R. Localio et al., Relation between Malpractice Claims and Adverse Events Due to Negligence: Results of the Harvard Medical Practice Study III, *New England Journal of Medicine* 325 (1991): 245–251.

72. M.I. Taragin, L.R. Willett, A.P. Wilczek, R. Trout, and J.L. Carson, The Influence of Standard of Care and Severity of Injury on the Resolution of Medical Malpractice Claims, *Annals of Internal Medicine* 117 (1992): 9, 780–784.

73. M.I. Taragin, A.P. Wilczek, M.E. Karns, R. Trout, and J.L. Carson, Physician Demographics and the Risk of Medical Malpractice, *American Journal of Medicine* 93 (1992): 5, 537–542.

74. G.J. Gittler and E.J. Goldstein, The Standard of Care Is Not So Standard, *Clinical Infectious Diseases* 24 (1997): 2, 254–257.

75. J. Kosecoff et al., Effects of the National Institutes of Health Consensus Development Program on Physician Practice, *Journal of the American Medical Association* 258 (1987): 2708–2713.

76. J. Lomas et al., Do Practice Guidelines Guide Practice? The Effect of a Consensus Statement on the Practice of Physicians, *New England Journal of Medicine* 321 (1989): 1306–1311.

77. S.B. Soumersai and J. Avorn, Principles of Educational Outreach ("Academic Detailing") To Improve Clinical Decision Making, *Journal of the American Medical Association* 263 (1990): 549–556.

78. D.H. Anderson (Ed.), *Changing Physician Behavior Through Practice Guidelines: The Zitter Group's 1996 Implementing Practice Guidelines Seminar Proceedings.* Santa Barbara, CA: Cor Healthcare Resources, 1996).

79. A.G. Ellrodt, L. Conner, M. Riedinger, and S. Weingarten, Measuring and Improving Physician Compliance with Clinical Practice Guidelines: A Controlled Intervention Trial, *Annals of Internal Medicine* 122 (1995): 277–282.

80. A. Bandura, *Social Foundations of Thought and Action.* (Englewood Cliffs, NJ: Prentice-Hall, 1986).

81. N. Clark and B.J. Zimmerman, A Social Cognitive View of Self-Regulated Learning about Health. *Health Education Research* 5 (1990): 371–379.

82. N.M. Clark et al., Impact of Education for Physicians on Patient Outcomes. *Pediatrics* 101 (1998): 831–836.

83. Clark et al., Impact of Education for Physicians on Patient Outcomes, 831–836.

84. T.S. Inui, E.L. Yourtee, and J.W. Williamson, Improving Outcomes in Hypertension after Physician Tutorials, *Annals of Internal Medicine* 84 (1976): 646–651.

85. K.J. Carlson et al., The Maine Women's Health Study I: Outcomes of Hysterectomy, *Obstetrics and Gynecology* 83 (1994): 556–565.

86. K.J. Carlson et al., The Maine Women's Health Study II: Outcomes of Non-surgical Management of Leiomyomas, Abnormal Bleeding, and Chronic Pelvic Pain, *Obstetrics and Gynecology* 83 (1994): 566–572.

87. S.J. Atlas et al., The Maine Lumbar Spine Study II: One Year Outcomes of Surgical and Non-surgical Treatment of Sciatica, *Spine* 21 (1996): 1777–1786.

88. S.J. Atlas et al., The Maine Lumbar Spine Study II: One Year Outcomes of Surgical and Non-surgical Treatment of Lumbar Spinal Stenosis, *Spine* 21 (1996): 1787–1795.

89. N.M. Clark et al., Physician-Patient Partnership in Managing Chronic Illness, *Academic Medicine* 70 (1995): 957–959.

90. J.S. Spiegal, M.F. Shapiro, B. Berman, and S. Greenfield, Changing Physician Test Ordering in a University Hospital: An Intervention of Physician Participation, Explicit Criteria, and Feedback, *Archives of Internal Medicine* 149 (1989): 549–553.

91. Healthcare Quality Improvement Act of 1986. 45 US Code §11101–11152. Sec 412, Standards for Professional Review Actions.

CHAPTER 34

Member Behavior Change

Nancy W. Spangler

INTRODUCTION

In recent decades, most people in the United States have blindly placed their trust in the miracles of the medical system. They have been content to be taken care of and have "followed doctor's orders" obediently. *With the advent of managed care, however, patients are now being asked to:*

- be proactive in preventing disease and disability
- become involved in health care decision making
- take part in actively managing chronic conditions
- interact effectively with providers

All these expectations require a significant change in attitudes about health. Achieving greater active participation from and assigning greater responsibility to people previously con-

---

Nancy W. Spangler is President of Spangler Associates, a Kansas City consulting company that specializes in health promotion, demand management, and patient education. She brings over 20 years of health care experience to the enhancement of patient behavior change. Previously, she was a corporate health promotion specialist for Saint Luke's Health System in Kansas City, and she has worked with the consulting group Wendy Fink Associates in the Boston area.

This chapter is adapted from Chapter 40, of the same name, in *Best Practices in Medical Management,* P. Kongstvedt and D. Plocher, eds. (Gaithersburg, MD: Aspen Publishers, Inc., 1998).

ditioned to be passive recipients of care is no easy task. This chapter explores some of the major constructs and theories of behavior change and adult learning and how they apply to such areas as health risk reduction, demand management, disease management, compliance, and community health initiatives. Examples of and rationales for some of the strategies being used by managed care organizations (MCOs) to affect patient behavior will be provided. The reader is also encouraged to review Chapters 17 and 23 because of the close relationship between those topics and material discussed here.

THEY KNOW BETTER, SO WHY DON'T THEY JUST STOP?

Watch any old movie from the 1940s and notice the amount of cigarette smoking. While intending to appear sophisticated and refined, the actors (probably) did not know at the time the negative effect of all that smoking on their health. In today's movies, characters light up much less often. When they do, it is more likely to indicate shadiness than to indicate refinement. With today's knowledge about the hazards of smoking, large numbers of people attempt to quit. Smoking has declined since the 1960s, yet a large portion of the U.S. population continues to smoke. If they consciously acknowledge that they would be better off if they did not smoke, overeat, abuse alcohol, or drive without seat belts, why do they continue these self-defeating behaviors? Why not just stop? This is a question asked by many professionals in fields from adult education to health psychology, primary care to health promotion. The answer appears far from simple. Attempting to change the behavior of human beings can be complex and problematic.

Readiness To Change

According to Prochaska and DiClemente, originators of the transtheoretical theory (also known as the stages of change model), simple knowledge that one *should* change a certain behavior will not necessarily cause a person to initiate or sustain a change.[1] The following example is familiar to many. After nagging your smoking patient (or loved one) to stop, and providing yet more information on nicotine patches and other quitting strategies, you are met not with the typical disinterested stare and nod, but with outright belligerence and anger. Your response? A mental note to yourself not to bring up the subject again. After all, you do not want the patient to stop coming to you altogether. (In the case of a loved one, you opt for harmony rather than another argument.) Unfortunately, the message your patient hears in your silence about the behavior in succeeding visits is:

"Smoking must not be all that important. My doctor doesn't even mention it any more."

Prochaska and DiClemente point out that efforts to change patient behaviors focus most of their resources in techniques appropriate for those in an active state of change, although fewer than 20 percent of people in a target population are prepared for action at any given time. The remainder are in one of several other stages of readiness to change. Figure 34–1 depicts an adaptation of Prochaska's model to illustrate the cyclical nature of change and the type of support that will be most effective in moving people toward action. Table 34–1 provides additional description of these phases or events.

Cycling between the stages is common, and successful termination (ending the cycle of change in permanent maintenance) typically requires numerous attempts to change. Tailoring the health professional's response to individuals based on their stage may be helpful in moving patients through the change cycle. As in the previous example with the smoking patient, a threatening approach or suggestion of tools and techniques will likely elicit resistance and defensiveness from a person who is not yet contemplating change in that behavior, while a matter of

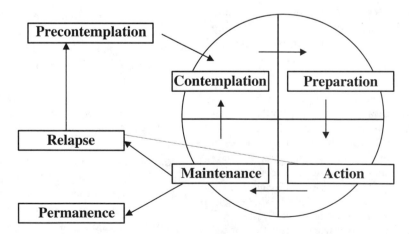

Figure 34–1 Stages of Change Model. *Source:* J. Prochaska and C. DiClemente, Stages and Processes of Self-Change of Smoking: Toward an Integrative Model of Change, *Journal of Consulting and Clinical Psychology,* Vol. 51, pp. 390–95, Copyright © 1983 by the American Psychological Association. Adapted with permission.

Table 34–1 Patient Approaches Based on Stage of Readiness To Change

Stage	Patient Characteristics	Tailored Response Needed
Precontemplation	Unaware of the need to change; unwilling or too discouraged to try, at least within the next six months; may be defensive.	Consciousness raising to increase patients' awareness of the negative consequences of the behavior and the inaccuracy of their denial or other defenses; nonjudgmental information.
Contemplation	Self-reflection; open to information; asking more questions; evaluating options for change, and weighing the pros and cons; ambivalence about next steps. Seriously considering change in next six months.	Emotional arousal; assistance in evaluating the pros and cons of change and ways to reduce the cons; provision of information; identification of supportive tools and resources.
Preparation	Determined to take action within next 30 days; sense of confidence and commitment.	Gain commitment to action; assist in setting attainable goals and dates for achieving them; praise incremental efforts; help with skill development; encourage support seeking.
Action	Overt change in behavior; attempts at reaching new goals; skill development.	Encourage rewards for achieving goals; assist in thinking through potential relapse situations and how to avoid; explore irrational self-talk ("I can't, I must") and encourage counterthinking; continue to reinforce social support.
Maintenance	Action sustained for six months or more; potential overconfidence may lead to slips in behavior if patients let up their guard.	Reinforce likelihood of slips and erosion of resolve; reduce self-blame for lapses and encourage sticking with plan; remind of achievements.

Source: Reprinted from N. Spangler, Member Behavior Change, in *Best Practices in Medical Management*, P.R. Kongstvedt, D.W. Plocher, eds., p. 551, © 1998, Aspen Publishers, Inc.

fact, nonjudgmental approach, advising the patient to quit and repeating the consequences of the behavior at *each* visit, may invoke a less emotional response and, over time, move the patient toward contemplating life as a nonsmoker. Thus, the health professionals' "success" (both in terms of patient health and the professionals' abilities to help) must be measured not only by the end behavior, but by incremental movements toward the goal.

For many health professionals, working with patients who are in the precontemplation stage can be frustrating. Some patients are simply un-

aware of the value of changing their behaviors. A discussion of social marketing to increase knowledge and motivation will follow later in this chapter. For many others, however, one can often sense an attitude of resignation, a "why bother?" mindset. What are some factors that could contribute to lingering in this stage of precontemplation?

Effect of Beliefs

Bandura's theory of self-efficacy suggests that a person's goal-directed behavior toward changing a health habit is based on two expectancies held by the individual:

- *Outcome expectancy*—a belief that a particular behavior will result in a desired outcome (e.g., that exercise could help one lose weight)
- *Efficacy expectancy*—a belief that the individual is capable of performing the behavior (e.g., that he or she could learn the necessary skills and overcome whatever barriers might get in the way)

Thus, self-efficacy can be said to be based on a sense of control over one's abilities and one's environment. Without a sense of self-efficacy, a person is unlikely to contemplate changes that require risking failure.[2]

Additional Theories

Seligman's work has examined how our early experiences may play a part in how we develop a sense of control and ability to cope. Seligman's theory of learned helplessness was established through experiments by his student, Madelon Visintainer, where rats were placed in highly stressful situations with no means of escape. Initial goal-directed escape behaviors of the active, aroused rats included multiple attempts at problem-solving behaviors to gain access to an escape route. As these attempts failed, the rats grew angry, agitated, and vocal. With repeated attempts at unsuccessfully controlling their circumstances, however, the rats reduced their attempts at escape and fell into a passive state of helplessness, comparable to human depression. This learned helplessness, due to the blockage of goal-directed behavior, also was found to compromise immune system function. The comparison rats who were allowed to experience success over their circumstances were better able to reject tumor growth than those who experienced early helplessness. The rat's "childhood" mastery experience served as an immunization against cancer.[3]

Seligman's subsequent work has been directed toward factors that modulate a sense of learned helplessness in people's lives. He has postulated that a sense of optimism can also be learned and that this optimism can positively affect health outcomes as described. According to Seligman, optimistic people can develop:

- a stronger immune system
- a belief in their abilities to stick with health regimens and seek medical care
- an ability to cope with change and negative life events
- stronger systems of social support

Much of the direction of Seligman and his colleagues was inspired by the work of Langer and Rodin, whose research looked at issues of personal control.[4] In their studies, individuals in nursing homes were given greater control over decisions about their day-to-day lives (meals, activities, room arrangement, etc.) and some responsibility (plants that they were assigned to care for). After 18 months, levels of activity, alertness, and general well-being improved in the group with greater control and got worse in those who were not similarly empowered. In addition, lower levels of mortality were found in the group with enhanced control. This body of work suggests that as we age, control becomes of special significance, because older people may be viewed as less competent and may be assisted with tasks that they had previously accomplished independently. The resulting sense of limited self-efficacy, perceived lack of control, and helplessness may hasten a decline in physical and emotional functioning.

In applying such work to human children, we can see that exposure to traumatic life circumstances they are unable to control, such as divorce, alcoholic or abusive parents, and danger in inner cities, could create a pervasive sense of helplessness. In fact, Wallerstein postulates that this resulting generalized powerlessness, or lack of control over living conditions, employment opportunities, social status, and so on, should receive greater attention as a risk factor for many diseases. Interventions that build up community empowerment may, thus, result in an improved collective sense of control and ability that contributes to improved population health status, as shown in Figure 34–2.[5]

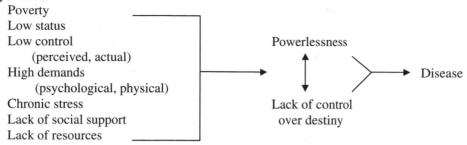

Figure 34–2 Disease as Related to Powerlessness. *Source:* Reprinted with permission from N. Wallerstein, Powerlessness, Empowerment, and Health: Implications for Health Promotion Programs, *American Journal of Health Promotion,* Vol. 6, pp. 197–205, © 1992.

MODELS FOR AFFECTING PATIENT BEHAVIORS

If poor health results from the factors described above, what accounts for the fact that some people *do* make changes in their lives, become optimistic, or begin to take charge of their health? Prochaska and colleagues suggest that in moving from precontemplation to action an individual comes to perceive that the "pros" of changing outweigh the "cons," or the benefits outweigh the barriers.[6] As summarized in Figure 34–1, the processes used in moving toward change may include consciousness raising, emotional arousal, self-evaluation, commitment, rewards, and helping relationships. What intervention models can be used by organizations to support this change?

System-Based Models

MCOs (and organized medical care delivery systems, a subset of MCOs) are ideally positioned to have an effect on health attitudes and behaviors because of their access to patient populations and their ability to systematically measure improvement in health status. In addition, unique approaches to communicating with patients in a controlled fashion may be attempted by MCOs with adequate contact database systems. Health promotion, demand management, and disease management can reach new heights with "social marketing," an approach currently uncommon in health care, to raise health consciousness and create conditions for self-evaluation and decision making in targeted populations. Kotler and Roberto define social marketing as "a strategy for changing behavior. It combines the best elements of the traditional approaches to social change in an integrated planning and action framework and utilizes advances in communication technology and marketing skills.... The goal is to advance a social cause, idea, or behavior."[7]

While most MCOs have used public relations campaigns to promote issues such as immunizations and healthy lifestyles, few have become highly sophisticated in the marketing techniques used by many businesses. Corporations such as Nike or Philip Morris have not affected buying behaviors of the American public by mailing out photocopied fliers to interested consumers who call for information, a primary promotional technique for many health education departments on a shoestring budget. On the other extreme, many MCOs are currently bombarding their members indiscriminately with printed material; the overwhelmed members tire of searching for what might be meaningful in the sea of information.

Techniques that will increase effect on behavior include:

- segmenting the target audience according to geographic, demographic, or psychographic variables

- "product" and brand name testing
- positioning research to determine perceptions of target audiences
- "product packaging," communications testing, and postcommunication recall testing
- test marketing for adoption behavior, and research on and selection of distribution channels

Use of computer-tailored communications has great promise for affecting behavior. Strecher et al. found that using patients' perceived benefits of and barriers to quitting smoking in creating a highly personal letter recommending that they quit had a significantly greater effect on quit rates than a generic letter.[8] Such techniques can better target the individual's personal beliefs and attitudes and improve persuasiveness.

Community Systems

To reach improved levels of population health, health professionals must become better at viewing member care from a systems view. In this view, one part of a system rarely changes in isolation. A family member will be more successful in changing eating habits if the whole family changes. One family will be more successful if the entire community begins adopting healthier habits of exercising, relating positively to one another, reducing smoking, and so on. A common rationale among MCOs seems to be to invest in programs that will produce an effect within 2 years. "Why invest in patients who will likely be in someone else's plan before there is a return on our investment?" some executives have been heard to ask (or imputed to be thinking, based on their actions). This is not systems thinking.

With a systems view, *all* MCOs in a community work collaboratively in issues of health improvement. Media campaigns are created with sufficient power and persuasion to raise the population's consciousness on targeted issues, and larger numbers of people are moved toward action. MCOs can contribute jointly to analyses of cultural incentives for particular behaviors,

such as teen pregnancy, alcohol use, or high-risk behaviors, and in strategies to address those issues. Community programs to improve personal safety, transportation, job availability, and neighborhood pride and social support should be supported politically, financially, and through broad involvement by major health organizations serving the community. People *do* change when their attitudes and opinions are influenced. In fact, people will do amazing things, both positive and negative, when they *believe* they can and should. Just as the rudder of a ship is powerful in changing the ship's direction, so can MCOs become powerful in positively changing the behavior of a community and reap the rewards over the long term.

Patient-Provider Models

Direct interaction between the patient and physician or other clinician can also be very effective in encouraging changes in health behaviors. According to Greenfield, DiMatteo, and others, efforts at improving patient–physician communication and enhancing the patient's sense of control through participation in treatment decisions can result in

- improved *adherence* to medication and other treatment regimens[9]
- improved *health outcomes*, such as blood pressure and blood sugar control[10]
- enhanced *patient satisfaction*[11]

When written information about the patient's medical condition was provided and patients were coached in behavioral strategies (such as asking questions of the provider, negotiating treatment options, and decreasing anxiety and feelings of intimidation), the group's functional status and other health measures improved.

Most patients respect their physician's knowledge and value information they receive from him or her highly. Therefore, the role of the physician in changing behavior cannot be overemphasized. Unfortunately, increased pressures for providers to help cut costs by seeing more patients in less time have made many providers feel reluctant or unable to educate or counsel patients as they might have done in the past. Few physicians are well prepared in counseling techniques during medical training, and many report feeling ill equipped for these tasks. Furthermore, most physicians tend to be pessimistic about their patients' abilities to change even when they do discuss lifestyle issues with patients. Numerous studies, however, document the effectiveness of repeated advice and brief behavior counseling in such areas as alcohol abuse, smoking, obesity, and lack of physical activity.

The physician recommendation or brief intervention is more likely to motivate the patient toward greater readiness to change, gaining their commitment and offering them hope that others just like them have made similar changes, than in teaching them the actual skills for change. Teaching skills demands more time than an office visit could allow, but motivating, gaining commitments, and offering hope can be brief, but powerful, considering that an estimated 70 percent of adults visit their physician yearly. And, while a limited number of people actually enroll in formal behavior change programs, many will attempt a change on their own. (It is estimated that 95 percent of smokers who quit do so on their own without participating in a group program. Most people will make several, if not many, attempts at quitting before they finally quit for good.)[12] Fiore recommends assessment of smoking status as the "fifth vital sign."[13] In other words, by asking every patient about their smoking status and documenting it at every visit (as is standard practice for vital signs such as blood pressure and weight), physicians can ensure that all smokers are identified and routinely advised to quit. Exhibit 34–1 lists ways in which physicians can personalize reasons to quit smoking.

The "4 A's" method was developed by the National Cancer Institute for physicians to follow for enhancing smoking cessation, but it can be applied to other issues in health promotion and disease management as well.[14] It consists of these tasks:

1. *Ask* about smoking status at every visit. If patients smoke, ask how much, how soon

Exhibit 34–1 Personalizing the Reasons To Quit Smoking

New smokers
- Easier to quit now

Long-term smokers
- Reduce risks for cancer and heart disease
- Be able to enjoy retirement and grandchildren

Smokers with a positive family history
- Reduce risks for cancer or heart disease

Asymptomatic adults
- Reduce risks for heart disease, cancer, emphysema
- Cost
- Wrinkles
- Inconvenience
- Bad breath
- Socially unacceptable

Pregnant women
- Miscarriage
- Low-birthweight infant
- Fetal death

Symptomatic adults
- Respiratory infections, cough
- Dyspnea
- Claudication
- Esophagitis
- Sore throats
- Ulcers
- Osteoporosis
- Gum disease

Teenagers
- Bad breath
- Cost
- Cough
- Respiratory infections
- Sore throats
- Effect on sports
- Life controlled by cigarettes

All smokers
- Cost
- Ability to exercise
- Sense of well-being
- Health

Source: Adapted with permission from C.G. Husten and M.W. Manley, How To Help Your Patients Stop Smoking, *American Family Physician,* © 1990, American Academy of Family Physicians.

after waking, if they have ever tried to stop before, and if they are currently interested in stopping.

2. *Advise* all smoking patients to quit. Personalize reasons according to the individual.

3. *Assist* patients in stopping. If patients express interest, help them set a quit date, provide self-help materials, and discuss nicotine replacement therapies. If patients resist, simply let them know that when they eventually become ready, support will be available.

4. *Arrange* follow-up visits. Since relapse (for any behavior change) is common in the first two weeks, a follow-up visit within one to two weeks of the selected quit date is recommended. If the patient has lapsed, circumstances for the lapse should be discussed and strategies for the next attempt determined.

Stepped Model

To reach optimal effect of behavior-change interventions, the stepped care and matching model advanced by Abrams et al. also serves as an excellent guide for delivering the appropriate level of intervention.[15] The authors acknowledge that intensive clinician intervention can be highly effective, yet may not be necessary for all patients and can be costly and difficult to access for many. While health education approaches of self-help pamphlets and posters have a wider reach, their effectiveness is lower. Even so, following this stepped model, by tailoring interventions according to such factors as the patient's motivational level, level of nicotine dependence, co-morbidities, and number of previous attempts to change, a larger total effect can be achieved. For example, smokers who are ready to quit, are not heavily addicted, and have made no previous attempts to quit would first be given low-cost self-help materials and encouragement to attempt to quit on their own.

If these smokers' attempts to quit are unsuccessful independently, the approach would move to brief counseling with follow up (e.g., by telephone). If smokers are still unsuccessful, intensive clinical treatment with a specialist highly experienced in behavior change would take place. This stepped-up model protects individuals from a sense of failure by assuring them that there is another novel approach "if at first they don't succeed"; the model does not re-cycle through the same old approaches. It also reserves the time of highly trained specialists for those who truly need it while broadening the effect of the total intervention.

Dealing with Relapse

Success in sustaining change may be predicted in the way the individual reacts to a momentary lapse or recurrence of a previous unhealthy behavior. As Marlatt and Gordon describe, if individuals attribute lapses to a global failure of their personal and moral character (observed through such statements as, "I'm just basically weak, no wonder I blew it."), this negative emotional state can create a mindset that makes it likely for the individual to relapse completely.[16] If, however, the individual can be assisted to view the lapse as an isolated mistake and not a *pattern* of failure, to learn from the lapse, to prepare cognitively for similar situations in the future, and to set a new date, the person is much more likely to try again and stay on track. The encouragement of the physician here again cannot be overstated. These thinking styles begin early and contribute to many patterns of life behaviors.

Relapse can also be looked at through concepts in cognitive neuroscience. When a person is learning any new motor pattern, a multitude of cortical pathways in the brain are used initially. After many repetitions, however, the movements become automatic and are managed by brain centers other than the initial cortical connections. For example, when first learning to drive, people consciously think about where to place their feet, how quickly to press the gas pedal when entering traffic, and so on. Years later, drivers can reach their destinations without giving much thought to how they got there. Operating an automobile has become a "no brainer."

Similarly, when first consciously attempting to change a health behavior, people are highly vigilant and attentive to their task. Many cortical subsystems are activated, and multiple synaptic connections are utilized. Memory traces, or engrams, are encoded and become strengthened with each repetition of the new behavior. This analogy from Kosslyn and Koenig is illustrative of this concept:

> During the initial phases of memory encoding, it is as if one is preserving the shape of a letter by walking a particular route on a lawn. The pattern is dynamic, and is only evident in the way one moves. After a period of time, however, the grass will wear through, creating a dirt pathway. At that point, one can stop walking; the information is preserved structurally.[17]

The analogy suggests that as one performs a new behavior, over time, and with many repetitions, the memory traces and neural pathways become stronger, as in wearing down a path. Yet if one stops the behavior before the grass has worn through, so to speak, the likelihood of relapse remains higher. If people try to "get back on the right path," the traces of their former steps remain, making it easier to stay on track with each successive attempt.[18] These authors also offer a neurological rationale for using imagery for relapse prevention. Brain scans of patients asked to simply imagine they are moving objects have documented the same neural activity in the motor cortex of the frontal and parietal lobes as patients who actually moved the objects. Thus, patients' mental preparations for situations that could be tempting are likely to involve the same neural subsystems that patients would use if they were in that situation; memory traces for positive coping skills can begin developing in advance.

Worksite Models

Progressive MCOs work in partnership with their purchasers when they realize the advantages inherent in offering health promotion and rehabilitation programs at the work site. These include:

1. Policies, such as limitations on smoking, and environmental support, such as availability of healthy foods, flextime, and adequate work spaces, create opportunities for healthy practices.
2. Support from peers to help increase readiness to change and reinforce maintenance.
3. Incentives, whether direct financial incentives, tangibles (T-shirts, fitness equipment, gift certificates, etc.), reward days off, or social recognition.
4. Employee assistance programs to help employees deal with the emotional issues that frequently affect health.
5. Early return-to-work programs and on-site rehabilitation following injuries; this promotes a sense of ability rather than disability and keeps workers accustomed to their work routine and connected to vital social support systems.
6. On-site support staff for individual coaching, periodic tracking of health status, and group education.

Providing programs at employer sites enables MCOs to use the employer's internal marketing approaches to advertise programs and reach a more "captive" audience. While the U.S. workplace is a melting pot of cultures, workplace programs can reduce some of the variables that make teaching group programs at clinics very difficult, such as vast differences in age, language, and health status. In addition, workplace programs eliminate problems in taking time off work and obtaining transportation. Access to corporate training departments will frequently allow use of advanced teaching approaches ideal for adult learning.

According to Knowles, adult learning differs vastly from children's learning.[19] Adults learn best when

- they feel respected
- new learning is related to their own life experiences
- new learning has immediate usefulness to them
- they are allowed to *do,* or discover concepts actively (we remember 20 percent of what

we hear, 40 percent of what we hear and see, and 80 percent of what we hear, see, and do)

Knowles also addresses readiness to learn, suggesting that movement from one stage of life to another—getting married, having children, losing a loved one—can trigger a "need-to-know" situation. For example, until one has children, there is little motivation to learn about parenting skills, discipline methods, or childhood immunizations. Engaging employees in "diagnostic experiences" where they can assess where they are now (as through the use of health risk appraisals; see above) and receive support to determine where they want to go (through worksite health promotion staff or telephone "coaches"; see Chapter 6) can provide opportunities for valuable learning.

TOOLS FOR ENHANCING CHANGE

With patients in various stages of readiness and with many types of health behaviors, developing strategies to support change can be challenging. The following are some examples of approaches that are in use. As the high interest in behavior change generates research over the next decade, health professionals' level of sophistication and the effectiveness of tools will increase significantly.

Communications

As mentioned in previous sections, communication techniques employed to help patients understand the consequences of their current behavior and to see the possibilities of changing it can be helpful in moving people from "just thinking about it" to "doing something about it." Broad, highly visible campaigns around targeted health topics can be implemented for this purpose. Table 34–2 shows various uses of media for communicating information, contrasting the qualities and abilities of each.

In addition to selecting media carefully, targeting information to critical life stages is recommended (for example, a birthday card to women on their fortieth birthday to encourage a mammo-

gram or information given to parents of 4-year-olds to encourage continued immunization).

Reinforcers

For individuals who are in a preparation or action stage of change, there are a number of ways that desired behaviors can be supported and reinforced.

Tracking Methods

Tools that assist the patient in tracking behaviors (such as number of cigarettes smoked and time of day, amount and perceived level of exertion when exercising, types and amounts of foods consumed and feelings of satisfaction after eating) are effective ways to increase awareness about behaviors. They assist in setting goals and identifying barriers, actively involve the patient in the change process, and reinforce progress. In many cases, it is best to track the *behavior* (eating pattern), rather than the *result* (actual daily weight), because the behavior is more in the control of the patient and is easier to reinforce for a sense of self-efficacy. Such tools as blood pressure wallet cards and personal medical records for referring to during interactions with providers can also stimulate a greater sense of individual responsibility, particularly if the patient is encouraged by the provider to use the materials.

Action Plans and Contracts

Written plans and contracts serve several purposes (an example is provided in Exhibit 34–2). By thinking through goals, patients personalize the approach, planning the series of steps needed. Preparing ahead equips them for inevitable barriers and solutions. Signing the plan with another person (physician, medical assistant, program facilitator, family member) serves as a public announcement, a declaration of the intention to change, and an expectation that the cosigner will follow up with patients on their progress. In addition, the physical act of writing the goals, rather than just thinking about them, uses additional neural subsystems and develops a visual memory trace, possibly reinforcing success, as mentioned earlier.

Table 34–2 Comparative Value of Media for Health Communication and Education

Type	High Emotional Appeal, Persuasive	Able To Convey Detailed or Complicated Information	Easy To Personalize	Low Cost	Life-long
Print materials					
• Newspaper advertisements	xxx	x		xx	
• Newsletters	x	xx	x	xx	x
• Magazine articles	xx	xxx			xx
• Pamphlets	x	xx	x	xxx	xxx
• Postcards	xx		xxx	xxx	x
• Books	x	xxx		xx	xxx
Billboards	xxxx				
Television advertisements or programs	xxxx				
Radio advertisements	xxx	x			
Audiotapes	xx	xx	x	x	xx
Videotapes	xxx	x			x
Telephone contacts	xx	xx	xxx	xx	x
Interactive CDs	xx	xx	x		x

Key: (blank indicates minimal application)
x = low suitability
xx = medium to low suitability
xxx = medium to high suitability
xxxx = high suitability
Source: Reprinted from N. Spangler, Member Behavior Change, in *Best Practices in Medical Management*, P.R. Kongstvedt, D.W. Plocher, eds., p. 559, © 1998, Aspen Publishers, Inc.

Reminder Systems

Tools for reminding patients of desired behaviors can take many forms. Pill boxes allowing patients to separate their various pills for the day in small compartments are helpful, as are pill containers that can be clipped to the toothbrush, serving as a reminder for adherence to medications. Written reminders for exercise sessions recorded in the patient's weekly calendar can help reduce the perceived barrier of "not enough time."

Incentives and Rewards

Patients should be encouraged to establish personal rewards for achieving goals as part of the action plan/contract process. Rewards should be set for each progressive step toward the goal to reinforce a perception of momentum. As with tracking, the reward should be based on completing specific behaviors rather than achieving specific physiologic outcomes. Rewards may be tangible items the patient might be preparing to buy but can postpone the purchase of, or they can be gifts of time to be spent in a unique way, such as browsing in a museum or attending a sporting event. Work sites have successfully used rewards and recognition to reinforce behaviors. This setting is ideal for promoting good-natured competitions and lotteries for targeted behaviors (e.g., all participants who record the type and amount of physical activity engaged in over a period of weeks may receive a chance to win a gift certificate toward exercise clothing or equipment).

Exhibit 34–2 Sample Action Plan

Name _____

Member ID# _____

Your Action Plan for _____

(Insert goal you chose on enrollment form)

Specific objectives and dates for achieving them:

_____

_____

Success strategies for reaching goal:

_____

_____

Roadblocks that might get in my way and how I will deal with them:

_____

_____

Additional information or support I need:

_____

_____

My reward and when I will give it to myself:

_____

_____

Return original with enrollment form. Keep copy for your records.

Courtesy of Humana, Inc., Process Model for Human CHIP Program, 1996, Kansas City, Missouri.

Social Support

Coaching

Whether completed face-to-face or by phone, coaching to assist patients in setting progressive goals, identifying barriers, recovering quickly from lapses, and preparing cognitively for future problems has been used successfully in areas of lifestyle change and medication adherence. This type of intervention has been effective both with patients who have expressed an interest in changing, as well as with "nonvolunteer" smokers. Just setting up the expectation that the coach will be following up with them can be reinforcing for some patients. Coaches should be well trained in motivational counseling techniques that enhance empathy and support self-efficacy. These include exploring resistance in a non-threatening way, asking open-ended questions, reflective listening (responding to the speaker with a clarification of what you heard), and eliciting concerns and fears. Coaches should also be trained in sensitivity to cultural and emotional issues that may be at the root of many behaviors.

Enlisting Support

Family members can be enlisted to actively support patients' revised behavior. Their inclusion is especially important when the changes will affect them as well (such as changes in diet or in ways of communicating to better manage stress). Support groups abound for many conditions and interests. Most are directed by lay leaders, and many have been highly successful in helping patients maintain changed behavior.

FROM THEORY INTO PRACTICE: HUMANA'S CHIP PROGRAM

This section presents an example of a program that turned these concepts into action. Discussions between Kansas City administrators of the MCO Humana and the pharmaceutical company Hoechst Marion Roussel about improving care for patients with cardiovascular health problems led to a partnership in patient education between the two organizations. The program, called the Cardiovascular Health Improvement Process, or CHIP, was developed in 1995 and implemented in 1996. Patients with hypertension were selected for the CHIP intervention due to the prevalence of hypertension within the Humana population and the potential reduction in cardiovascular complications that could be achieved with hypertensive management through lifestyle change and medication compliance.

With Prochaska and DiClemente's stages of change model in mind (see "Readiness To Change," above), hypertensive members were subdivided according to their response to an ini-

tial mailing (Figure 34–3). The level of intervention was determined by the member's expressed commitment to change. The groups were labeled as follows:

1. *Participants* showed they were *contemplating* change by participating in the cardiac risk check (CRC), a computerized assessment of risks for cardiovascular disease. They received encouragement, first through a reminder postcard, then through a video, to commit to change by enrolling in the CHIP program.

2. *Enrollees,* or patients who indicated *active* readiness for a lifestyle change by completing the CRC *and* enrolling (i.e., selecting a particular area of lifestyle change or medication compliance and setting specific goals to work on), were provided intervention. The intervention consisted of printed booklets specific to the lifestyle area selected and a customized CHIP newsletter providing information on behavior change, lifestyle, and medications. Other interventions, including telephone support, were also explored, but print interventions were selected as the focus for the first phase. Materials were developed for all participants and enrollees to encourage self-monitoring of blood pressure, medications, and health status and to enhance effective interaction with providers.

3. *Nonresponders* were those members who did not respond after several invitation reminders to participate. This group was thought to include many "precontemplators" who were not ready to begin a change process. Nonresponders were contacted in six months, provided information on the benefits of hypertension management, and invited again to participate.

In addition to the printed mailings to patients, meetings were held with Humana's Kansas City area physicians to describe the program and to discuss newly developed guidelines for treating hypertensive patients. The guidelines, based on recommendations in the Fifth Report of the Joint National Committee on Prevention, Detection,

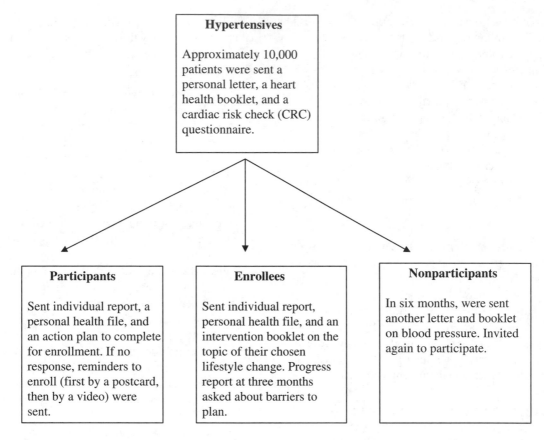

Figure 34–3 Process Model for Humana CHIP Program. Courtesy of Humana, Inc., 1996, Kansas City, Missouri.

Evaluation, and Treatment of High Blood Pressure, placed a heavy emphasis on lifestyle modifications both prior to and in conjunction with drug therapy for hypertension management.[20]

Program Effect

Telephone interview research provided by Hoechst Marion Roussel in October 1997 elicited valuable information regarding patients' opinions of the CHIP program, process, and materials. One hundred patients from each of the three groups were contacted.

Patient Changes

Overall, 56 percent of patients reported making positive lifestyle changes after receiving the CHIP information, with the largest response being from those who made a formal commitment to change and developed a written plan of action (84 percent of enrollees, 60 percent of participants, 24 percent of nonparticipants). Of those who made changes, 70 percent maintained them for 6 months or more, a time period considered significant for behavior maintenance. Changes included:

- chose more healthful foods—78 percent
- increased activity levels—53 percent
- looked more at food labels—36 percent
- read more about high blood pressure—30 percent
- became more aware of triggers (e.g., for smoking/stress/eating)—26 percent
- made more attempts to manage stress—24 percent
- used reminders for medications—23 percent
- asked physician more questions—21 percent
- reduced or quit smoking—8 percent

While hypertension is generally considered to be an "older person's disease," younger patients were more likely to make a behavior change. Age breakouts were:

- 20–39 year olds—67 percent
- 40–59 year olds—74 percent
- 60–79 year olds—57 percent
- 80+ year olds—43 percent

Participation Information

The main reasons given for not participating in CHIP included:

- patient did not recall receiving the information—56 percent
- patient thought he or she *did* return the questionnaire—11 percent
- forgot—7 percent
- just not a priority right now—7 percent

Main reasons for not enrolling included:

- did not recall the enrollment information—29 percent
- did not want to commit to a "program"—24 percent
- not a priority—16 percent
- did not want to complete the action plan required for enrolling—14 percent

Of those who did enroll, 58 percent reported that the goal-setting process was very helpful. Interestingly, a large percent (92 percent) of African-American enrollees found this process very helpful.

Materials

Responses to all of the CHIP materials were favorable, and most patients (64 percent) said they would like to continue to receive information about high blood pressure, medications, and healthy lifestyles (59 percent of nonparticipants, 60 percent of participants, 73 percent of enrollees, 76 percent of African Americans, 60 percent of Caucasians).

Favored formats for intervention include:

- mailed materials—85 percent (This strong response supports the decision to use print intervention as the primary vehicle for patient education in projects like CHIP.)
- videotapes—26 percent
- appointments with health professional—15 percent
- telephone support—12 percent
- group classes—6 percent
- Internet programs—6 percent

Effect on Opinion

Many patients (72 percent) reported that programs like CHIP affect their opinion of Humana in a very favorable way. Clearly, patients have valued CHIP and are eager for the health information and support the plan provides through such programs.

CONCLUSION

Patient behavior change may well be the next frontier in modern medicine. While not an easy task, improving patient adherence to lifestyle modifications, drug therapy regimens, and other treatment goals can enable managed care organizations to reduce costs and improve the quality of care. Efforts at applying current theories of behavior change as well as support of research to expand our body of knowledge in this area will become increasingly important in the near future.

REFERENCES AND NOTES

1. J. Prochaska and C. DiClemente, Stages and Processes of Self-Change of Smoking: Toward an Integrative Model of Change, *Journal of Consulting and Clinical Psychology* 51 (1983): 390–95; J. Prochaska and C. DiClemente, Towards a Comprehensive Model of Change, in *Treating Addictive Disorders: Processes of Change,* W.R. Miller and N. Heather, eds. (New York: Plenum Press, 1986), 3–27.

2. A. Bandura, *Principles of Behavior Modification* (New York: Holt, Rinehart, and Winston, 1969).

3. M. Seligman and M. Visintainer, Tumor Rejection and Early Experience of Uncontrollable Shock in the Rat, in *Affect, Conditioning, and Cognition: Essays on the Determinants of Behavior,* F.R. Brush and J.B. Overmier, eds. (Hillsdale, NJ: Erlbaum, 1985), 203–10.

4. E.J. Langer and J. Rodin, Effects of Choice and Enhanced Personal Responsibility for the Aged: A Field Experiment in an Institutional Setting, *Journal of Personality and Social Psychology* 34 (1982): 437–39; J. Rodin, Effects of the Sense of Control, *Science* 233 (1986): 1271–76.

5. N. Wallerstein, Powerlessness, Empowerment, and Health: Implications for Health Promotion Programs, *American Journal of Health Promotion* 6 (1992): 197–205.

6. Bandura, *Principles of Behavior Modification.*

7. P. Kotler and E. Roberto, *Social Marketing: Strategies for Changing Public Behavior* (New York: Free Press, 1989), 24.

8. V. Strecher, M. Kreuter, D. Den Boer, et al., The Effects of Computer-Tailored Smoking Cessation Messages in Family Practice Settings, *Journal of Family Practice* 39 (1994): 262–70.

9. S. Greenfield, S. Kaplan, J. Ware, et al., Patient's Participation in Medical Care: Effects on Blood Sugar and Quality of Life in Diabetes, *Journal of General Internal Medicine* 3 (1988): 448–57.

10. Ibid.

11. R. DiMatteo et al. The Significance of Patients' Perceptions of Physician Conduct: A Study of Patient Satisfaction in a Family Practice Center, *Community Health* 6 (1980): 18–34.

12. C.T. Orleans, Understanding and Promoting Smoking Cessation: Overview and Guidelines for Physician Intervention, *Annual Review of Medicine* 142, no. 1 (1985): 52–57.

13. M. Fiore, The New Vital Sign: Assessing and Documenting Smoking Status, *JAMA* 266, no. 22 (1991): 3183–84.

14. T.J. Glynn and M.W. Manley, *How To Help Your Patients Stop Smoking: A National Cancer Institute Manual for Physicians.* National Institutes of Health Publication no. 90–3064. Bethesda, MD: U.S. Department of Health and Human Services, Public Health Service, National Institutes of Health, National Cancer Institute, 1990.

15. D.B. Abrams, C.T. Orleans, R.S. Niaura, et al., Integrating Individual and Public Health Perspectives for Treatment of Tobacco Dependence under Managed Health Care: A Combined Stepped-Care and Matching Model, *Annals of Behavioral Medicine* 18, no. 4 (1996): 290–304.

16. G.A. Marlatt and J.R. Gordon, eds., *Relapse Prevention* (New York: Guilford Press, 1985).

17. S.M. Kosslyn and O. Koenig, *Wet Mind: The New Cognitive Neuroscience* (New York: Free Press, 1992), 351.

18. Ibid.

19. M. Knowles, *The Adult Learner: A Neglected Species* (Houston, TX: Gulf, 1978).

20. Joint National Committee on Detection, Evaluation, and Treatment of High Blood Pressure, The Fifth Report on the Joint National Committee on Detection, Evaluation, and Treatment of High Blood Pressure, *Archives of Internal Medicine* 153 (1993): 153–83.

SUGGESTED READING

Gerteis, M., Edgman-Levitan, S., and Daley, J., eds. 1993. *Through the Patient's Eyes: Understanding and Promoting Patient-Centered Care.* San Francisco: Jossey-Bass.

Lorig, K., Holman, H., Sobel, D., and Gonzalez, V. 1994. *Living a Healthy Life with Chronic Conditions: Self Management of Heart Disease, Arthritis, Stroke, Diabetes, Asthma, Bronchitis, Emphysema and Others.* Palo Alto, CA: Bull Publishing Co.

Meichenbaum, D., and Turk, D. 1987. *Facilitating Treatment Adherence: A Practitioner's Guidebook.* New York: Plenum Press.

Miller, W., and Rollnick, S. 1991. *Motivational Interviewing: Preparing People To Change Addictive Behavior.* New York: Guilford Press.

Prochaska, J., Norcross, J., and DiClemente, C. 1994. *Changing for Good.* New York: Avon Books.

Seligman, M. 1990. *Learned Optimism.* New York: Alfred A. Knopf.

Snyder, C. 1994. *The Psychology of Hope: You Can Get There from Here.* New York: Free Press.

Vella, J. 1994. Learning to Listen, Learning to Teach: The Power of Dialogue in Educating Adults. San Francisco: Jossey-Bass.

PART IV

Operational Marketing and Management

"We could manage this matter to a T."

Sterne
Tristram Shandy, bk. II, ch. 5, [1760]

CHAPTER 35

Information Systems in Managed Health Care Plans

James S. Slubowski

INTRODUCTION

Managed care organizations (MCOs)* or health plans are keenly dependent on technology and information to service their customers, including providers, the government, employers, agents, and members. MCOs do not produce a product; rather, they deliver a gamut of services. The delivery of these services must be timely, cost-effective, and actionable. MCOs are now expected to offer electronic on-line servicing and respond to frequent requests for information. Making the best use of information technology can help a health plan succeed.

To survive, health plans must ensure they are operating as efficiently as possible. Technology is a key enabler for automation. Health plans have most recently focused on automation of

James S. Slubowski is Vice President, Information Services, at Priority Health in Grand Rapids, Michigan. He is responsible for the strategic vision and implementation of information systems and technology that support the health plan and health system strategic and operational requirements. Prior to joining Priority Health, he served as a Manager in the health care consulting practice of Ernst & Young and served in various leadership positions within managed care services and information services of Henry Ford Health System.

*The term "MCO" will be used to refer to several different types of managed care plans, such as health maintenance organizations, preferred provider organizations, and point-of-service plans. When necessary, distinctions will be made between these types of plans.

core business functions such as claim payment, enrollment, and premium billing. With the exploding costs of new medical technologies, pharmaceuticals, and medical services, the health plan must expand its focus to health management of its membership. To put this financial issue into perspective, the country's total health expenditures reached $767 billion in 1991, an increase of 9.6 percent from the previous year. By 1997, that figure was $1.1 trillion. The federal government predicts that expenditures will double by 2007.[1]

The next generation of health plans will focus not only on cost controls but on overall health status because of pressure from consumers. New health plan program features will include consumer and provider education, disease and demand management, and self-care and wellness initiatives. To manage health risk, leading organizations will need to (1) expand their ability to capture, measure, and track individual health status information beyond the narrow demographic information captured today; (2) expand the ability to identify health risk factors at the member level through intelligent mining of health demographics as well as claims/encounters; and (3) expand the ability to assess and measure the outcomes associated with preventative health initiatives as well as clinical treatments.[2]

This chapter will review the key health plan information systems required to run the day-to-day operations along with the systems that will add new value to the health plan's customer relationships, thus moving the health plan into the next generation. Additionally, this chapter will review the information services department organizational structure required to support and advance the new breed of health plan. Chapters 36 (regarding information systems in provider systems) and 37 (regarding electronic commerce) are also relevant to this topic, and readers are encouraged to review them.

CORE MANAGED CARE INFORMATION SYSTEM

To support the day-to-day functions of the plan, a core managed care information system is needed. The data captured will also support the health plan's responsibility for analysis and reporting. This next section will provide a general strategy and overview of the components of the infrastructure system.

In today's market, although most vendors will claim that they have the complete functionality to run the entire health plan's operations, a single solution is truly not available. Vendors who claim they have complete functionality often offer some type of service in each area but do not have thorough solutions for each area (e.g., provider credentialing). Frequently, health plans will adopt a "best of breed" software solution approach. In other words, instead of the product modules, superior software solutions will be used with the core managed care product. For example, a third-party financial or enterprise resource planning system (e.g., Lawson or PeopleSoft) will be interfaced with the managed care system to support the general ledger, accounts payable, accounts receivable, and purchasing requirements of the health plan.

There are a handful of top managed care system vendors that have significant penetration in the marketplace today. Even fewer are vendors with fully developed and time-proven client/server solutions (in other words, a graphical desktop interface coupled with database and application servers connected on a network) with effective user workflow screens. Client/server solutions have been slowly adopted by health plans in a wait-and-see approach. According to some consultants, the main area where these cli-

ent/server solutions have not lived up to expectations is claim processing. A transaction-intensive function like claim processing requires a level of scalability that needs to be proven by the vendor.[3]

A managed care information system should be relied on for the following core operational competencies: (1) claim payment; (2) enrollment; (3) premium billing; and (4) provider reimbursement (e.g., capitation).

Claim Payment

Claim processing/pricing is the core feature of all managed care systems. Systems will accept a variety of claim forms, such as the HCFA 1450 for hospital charges and 1500 for professional services and dental. A claim can be entered either manually or through an electronic data feed (see the discussion on electronic data interchange).

Key data elements captured during the claim entry process include

- member identification
- provider identification
- date of service(s)
- procedure code(s)
- diagnosis code(s)
- place of service code(s)
- type of service code(s)
- quantity

After the claim is entered, it will go through a process of adjudication, which validates the claim information and approves or denies payment for the service or product. This adjudication process relies on tables and approval rules established by the health plan and directly and appropriately aligned with the member's benefit package and provider reimbursement contract information. Claim systems allow for both real-time and batch adjudication processing. Batch adjudication allows for data entry of claim information either by less highly paid staff or by an electronic data feed referred to as electronic data interchange. On a cycle determined by the system administrator, the system will process each batch through the adjudication review process and send the information directly to the accounts payable system if approved or will hold (usually referred to as "pend") the claim for review by an examiner. If the claim is pended, a claim examiner must manually open it to review the status and determine if the system properly adjudicated and then deny the claim or override the pend code and pay the claim.

Adjudication rules within the claim system can be extensive or minimal. Checks for age, gender, eligibility, authorizations (see also the discussion of care management), accumulators, benefit maximums, special holds, and so forth can be taken into account as the system determines if and how the claims should be paid. These rules are determined by the individual health plan.

Claim modules will allow for integrated medical editing, either real-time or through batch processing, which checks all physician-generated claims for coding errors. This claim review process looks at the appropriateness of billing versus the reimbursement policies, and the cost of claims. Savings, realized through claim denials, are experienced from daily claim review, historical claim analysis, multiple procedure hierarchy, and correct use of claim modifiers. The claim review evaluates the common practice of bundling or unbundling of submitted charges in a clinically and professionally responsible way. For example, it verifies if the services were already reimbursed as part of an earlier billing (e.g., postoperative office visit). Third-party software can be licensed to interface with the claim system to validate provider billing "appropriateness." If the claim meets any of the criteria, it is held for manual review. This feature can result in average savings of 3 to 8 percent of submitted charges

For utilization and health management reporting, the claim modules will accept encounter information, which is claim experience data for capitated members. The claim system will recognize the data as an encounter and will not generate a transaction (check request) to the accounts payable system. The encounter information is written to the system database tables as if it were a payable claim, though the system treats it as already paid.

Operational reports that the core module will generate include

- pended claims
- claim examiner productivity
- claims missing authorizations
- various claim activity reports

Managed care systems that are client/server based (see earlier definition) contain screens allowing "heads-down" data entry function. This is used by staff entering high volumes of data such as claims or enrollment forms. Graphical user interface screens within a claims system are generally found to be a hindrance for high-volume data entry work, so many systems offer both text and graphical options.

The ideal situation is this: claims are received electronically, they are automatically adjudicated by the system, and a record is sent to the accounts payable system for a check to be mailed or an electronic payment transfer to occur. In this situation, there is little or no manual intervention required, thus reducing labor expense.

The claims management process is discussed further in Chapter 38.

Enrollment

Providers, employer groups, and members must be set up within the system for the core system processes to function. The enrollment modules will track new records and updates to the existing records, along with terminations. In the enrollment module, records are never deleted since they are used for future reporting or processing of retroactivity (e.g., claim received after the member's coverage terminated but for services while the member was active).

Provider Enrollment

The provider enrollment modules of managed care software systems will capture enough information about providers to ensure that their claims will be paid properly. Information captured about the provider includes name, address, clinic, and telephone and fax numbers as well as reimbursement information such as capitation, fee schedule assignment, or withhold percentages. Providers will also be associated with one or more product offerings, such as health maintenance organization (HMO), preferred provider organization, point of service, or indemnity insurance. The provider enrollment function also captures the provider's tax identification number (for the generation of 1099s for tax purposes) and risk group affiliation. Hospitals, professional providers, and equipment suppliers and possibly pharmacies are enrolled within this module to allow appropriate adjudication of claims received from these entities.

Some managed care system vendors are expanding the provider enrollment modules to support credentialing; however, be very cautious. This is an area in which a third-party solution may better suit the health plan. The credentialing process has very specific data needs and is very different from the provider reimbursement process. Based on the approach adopted within the health plan, a provider database "source of truth" will need to be identified. That system will then be used for provider information data feeds to other systems. Maintaining provider information is a laborious task within all health plans since many provider databases generally exist. Without identifying and maintaining a single, ultimate provider database, doing a relatively simple task such as producing a provider directory can become very difficult. Since managed care systems are designed to pay claims, provider enrollment modules mainly focus on data collection to support the claim payment process and not necessarily the credentialing process; however, new managed care system releases are offering more features to support credentialing. Specific credential data elements include medical license information, malpractice data, and schooling in addition to pertinent member-requested information such as gender, age, languages spoken, and so forth. These elements are discussed in Chapter 7.

Employer Group Enrollment

Employer group enrollment establishes the employer within the system. Basic demographic information is captured along with the appropriate product and benefit package that the group has agreed to offer its employees through the health plan. Employer group information is important so the health plan can bill for coverage premiums, referred to as premium billing.

Member Enrollment

Member enrollment is the largest enrollment portion of all three. Basic demographic information is captured along with the appropriate employer group, if applicable; the product; and the benefit package. If the product is managed, a primary care provider will need to be selected so the authorization system and claim systems can properly adjudicate the claims. At the time the member is enrolled, the spouse and family data will be linked to the member's account, referred to as the contract. To minimize financial loss to the plan, it is critical to capture other party liability (OPL) information, including the coordination of benefits (COB) information if another payer is liable either primarily or secondarily. OPL and COB are discussed in detail in Chapter 39. For products requiring a primary care physician (PCP) assignment, an operational report is included to identify members without a PCP assignment.

Once all the member information is entered either manually or electronically, member rosters and identification (ID) cards can be produced. Most managed care software products have the ability to generate ID cards either by contract or by employer.

The membership module will allow for retroactivity—allowing the member to be added on one day with an earlier enrollment date. This is a frequent occurrence. When retroactivity occurs, claim payment, provider reimbursement, and premium billings need to be adjusted accordingly in the next billing or accounts payable cycle. Retroactivity is generally limited to 90 days prior. More than 90 days, and reconciliation with claim payment, provider reimbursement, and premium billing would be extremely difficult.

Premium Billing

The primary source of income for a health plan is premium billing of individuals, purchaser or employer groups, and the government. The system will determine who is eligible for the coming month, the benefit package level, and spouse/dependent information. The information is summarized, listing number of contracts at each level and premium amount negotiated when the purchaser signed with the health plan. A detailed list of policyholder names is also available to assist the purchaser in reconciling the bill. Premium billing is performed for the following month, and an accounts receivable record is generated.

Within this module, broker or agent commissions are calculated based on the commission rate and active membership. Commission rates may be a percent of premiums, a per member fee, or a flat fee and are agreed upon at the onset of the broker relationship with the health plan. An accounts payable record is generated for the broker or agent on a predetermined basis.

Premium rates are determined by the underwriting department based on service industry code information and group size. Rates are further calculated based on policyholder family size. Rating and underwriting are discussed in great detail in Chapters 49 through 52.

Operational reports created by the premium billing module include

- billing status
- accounts receivable aging
- billing summary

Provider Reimbursement

The key output for claim processing is provider reimbursement and support of managed care reporting. Managed care information systems support different forms of provider reimbursement, including capitation, fee-for-service with a withhold, and a combination of both (see Chapters 8 through 11 for discussion of reimbursement in MCOs). It should be noted here, as has been noted in Chapter 8, that those responsible for provider contracting sometimes agree to a form of reimbursement that, while logical or rational, is not supportable by the existing information systems without considerable programming or "work-around" solutions. In such cases,

the administrative cost of administering reimbursement becomes high as the value of automation is decreased. Not to belabor the obvious, but it is incumbent on those in network contracting to communicate with those in information systems, and vice versa.

The provider reimbursement module will incorporate information captured in the provider and member enrollment modules to determine the appropriate reimbursement. Capitation payments can be based on a number of items, such as active membership, age, gender, copayment, county code, and services included within the capitation. With the capitation check distribution, the system should produce a member roster for the provider so the capitation payment can be reconciled and the provider can be aware of the members within the panel. As will be discussed later, this is also something that may be done electronically.

For services that are not capitated, fee-for-service payments with or without a withhold are made based on the provider's contract. The appropriate fee schedule is chosen within the system, and the payment is calculated. An explanation of payment (EOP) or remittance advice (RA) is included and demonstrates what claims were paid with the check. Providers can then use the EOP to close the open accounts receivable records within their billing systems. Depending on contractual arrangements, a withhold may be imposed that holds a specified amount of payment. Depending on the cycle, which is generated annually, the provider utilization is compared against budget, and the withhold is then distributed in whole, in part, or not at all. In the third case, the withhold is consumed fully by the health plan to cover the medical loss.

In a common form of capitation, a fund settlement process is calculated annually. It compares utilization against the funds funded by the number of members, PCP selection, and risk group selection. At that time, the membership utilization assigned to the risk group is analyzed and compared to predetermined allocations based on the health plan's reimbursement model and membership size. If the utilization is lower than the budget, the surplus is released to the risk group and/or provider. If the utilization exceeds the budget, then no money is distributed to the provider. The provider's withhold is used to supplement any additional loss. Unless a global capitation payment is in place, the provider's risk is generally limited to the amount of withhold, and the health plan's risk is typically limitless. To support this process, the managed care information system must appropriately tag the claim to the proper fund, primary care provider, and risk group for the annual fund settlement process to be calculated. Moreover, the managed care system must be able to support the establishment of the funds along with the building of the fund based on monthly membership activity. A few managed care systems provide a real-time status to the fund based on utilization and funding experienced to date.

ELECTRONIC DATA INTERCHANGE

Electronic data interchange (EDI) offers great opportunities for MCOs. It can assist with automation and lower the administrative ratio. EDI allows the health plan to streamline its internal processes and improve its service levels for claim payment and enrollment. In the case of claims, manual data entry is eliminated and the claim information is entered sooner; as a result, the claim payment cycle is shortened, and providers are paid faster. Some of these transactions will be regulated, and, in some cases, health plans can develop proprietary interfaces to support the unique needs of their customers.

The health care community is now rallying around a set of data transmission standards, the ANSI X.12 version 4010 standards. Managed care system vendors can develop interfaces for these standards, thus minimizing the plans' need to develop interfaces of their own. The Health Insurance Portability and Accountability Act (HIPAA; see also Chapter 67) that passed in late 1996 is enforcing this standard for health care institutions but not employer groups. In early 2000, the standards were expected to be approved with full operational implementation within 2 years for large plans and 3 years for small plans with fewer than 25,000 members.

Most institutions and vendors are developing internal standards to support these ANSI guidelines. The most popular and eagerly awaited interfaces include the following:

- 834 for enrollment (including adds, updates, and terminations)
- 837 for claims
- 270, 271, and 271R for eligibility inquiry request, eligibility reply, and eligibility roster, respectively
- 835 for RA (or EOP)
- 278 for referral and authorization
- 276 and 277 for claim inquiry request and claim status reply, respectively
- 820 for premium payment

Health plans benefit greatly from EDI transactions for obvious reasons. First, the need for hired staff is lessened when the information does not need to be entered manually. Second, accuracy increases since data entry allows for human error. Third, internal processes can be shortened, thereby speeding the process of releasing payment, generating ID cards, and so forth. In addition, most employers are now expecting the health plan to be able to fully process electronic files. Employers expect to see higher quality, faster turnaround, and greater efficiencies without premium increases. The financial benefits of EDI can be substantial. For example, the cost for data entry, imaging, and filing of a hospital insurance claim can drop to $0.25 compared to $1.25 for a paper claim.[4]

Without industrywide standards for consistency, EDI could be a costly and laborious task for the health plans. This is becoming true for enrollment and eligibility for employer groups. As mentioned earlier, the HIPAA requirements do not include mandates for employers. As a result, most employers will send the enrollment file in a format convenient to them, not the X.12 format, expecting the health plan to conform. This means that the health plan must develop and maintain custom interfaces for each employer, which requires high-cost technical staff. For example, most employers will use their human resources information systems to generate enrollment files for the health plan. Human resources systems manage many portions of employee benefits, including health care coverage. Any change to the employee's record in the employer's human resources system could result in a record being sent to the health plan. The health plan's enrollment system must then be sophisticated enough to detect if the change is pertinent to the health plan. These "edits" must be uniquely programmed for each employer that exchanges files with the health plan.

Many companies called clearinghouses have been established over the years to help health plans, providers, and employers with their EDI transmissions. The clearinghouse has relationships with many practice management system vendors and providers. The providers submit their claims electronically to the clearinghouse for distribution to the appropriate payer. Clearinghouses provide value-added services such as claim editing and reformatting. The provider who submits claims and the health plan who receives claims pay a per claim fee to the clearinghouse that could range from $0.25 to $1.00.

Electronic interfaces can be customized by the health plan to offer unique services to its customers. The health plan is well placed to share information about a population since it receives information about utilization that occurs within or outside of the network. Utilization can involve medical services, drugs, or products such as durable medical equipment. This information can be analyzed for potential high utilization or simply as a notice to the PCP. If the provider is using a computerized medical record (see Chapter 36), electronic information or "notices" can be transmitted to the provider by the health plan. Information could include out-of-network admissions; emergency room encounters; disease management member registries along with high-, medium-, and low-risk indicators; utilization reports; and member rosters. Upon signing onto the computerized medical record, providers could access a profile of their managed care population.

Another option includes an electronic file of member eligibility transmitted from the health plan to the provider so the information can be incorporated within the provider's practice management systems (e.g., appointment scheduling, registration, admitting, contract administration). This allows health insurance status and copayment information to be verified by one system while the member is present for service at a provider's office. This supports providers by streamlining their clinical processes and improving cash collections.

Claim Scanning and Imaging

To further support the claim processing team and improve the health plan's efficiency, scanning and imaging technology can be used with many paper data entry–intensive processes. A scanner supported by an optical character recognition (OCR) application can interpret alphanumeric characters on paper documents and write this information to an electronic file. The accuracy of OCR has improved greatly over the past few years. Paper claims received at the health plan can be scanned with the data transferred to an electronic file formatted to the managed care system's preference (typically the X.12 standard). The file is read into the system automatically, just like any other EDI file that the plan would receive directly from a provider or clearinghouse. The document image is also stored so it can be easily retrieved and referenced when needed, thus eliminating the need for microfiche or paper files. Some organizations have found that this system increased the number of claims entered per hour threefold to fivefold. The process requires a scanner, an OCR application, a network server, workstations, and an electronic image storage device.

PRIVACY AND CONFIDENTIALITY UNDER HIPAA

HIPAA privacy and confidentiality regulations are, as of 1999, still in the phase of public commentary. The reader is urged to review the final regulations and not rely on any of the summaries provided here. By starting at www.hcfa.gov, the reader will be able to find all relevant material on HIPAA, including privacy and security regulations, the provider identification number, new databanks, and so forth.

Despite the relative uncertainty about certain aspects of these regulations, there are requirements in HIPAA that are worth describing here. As illustrated in Exhibit 35–1, adapted from Chapter 67, HIPAA focuses on requirements to maintain the physical security of health information and also apply to any person or organization that maintains or transmits electronic health information and it outlines standards for maintaining reasonable and appropriate administrative, technical, and physical safeguards. The safeguards aim to protect the physical security and integrity of personal health information from threats, hazards, or unauthorized uses. HIPAA prohibits wrongful disclosures of individually identifiable health information, and penalties for violations are described in the act. Unlike the other parts of the administrative simplification title, however, the confidential-

Exhibit 35–1 Some Health Care Industry Business Transactions Set Forth in HIPAA

- Health claims or equivalent encounter information—a transaction used to submit health care claim billing information, encounter information, or both, from health care providers to health plans.
- Health claims attachments—a transaction used to transmit health care service information, such as subscriber, patient, demographic, diagnosis, or treatment data, for the purpose of a request for review, certification, notification, or report of the outcome of a health care services review.
- Enrollment and disenrollment in a health plan—a transaction used to establish communication between the sponsor of a health benefit and the health plan. It provides enrollment data, such as data on the subscriber and dependents, as well as information on employers and health care providers. The sponsor is the backer of the coverage, benefit, or product. A sponsor can be an employer, union, government agency, association, or insurance company. The health plan is the entity that pays claims, administers the insurance product or benefit, or both.
- Eligibility for a health plan—a transaction used to inquire about the eligibility, coverage, or benefits associated with a benefit plan, employer, plan sponsor, subscriber, or a dependent under the subscriber's policy. It also can be used to communicate information about, or changes in, eligibility, coverage, or benefits—information from sources such as insurers, sponsors, and health plans that is sent to recipients such as physicians, hospitals, third-party administrators, and government agencies.
- Health care payment and remittance advice—a transaction used by a health plan to make a payment to a health care provider, or to send an explanation of benefits or a remittance advice to a health care provider, or to send both payment and data to a health care provider.
- Health plan premium payments—a transaction used by employers, employees, unions, associations, or other entities to make and keep track of payments of health plan premiums to health insurers.
- First report of injury—a transaction used to report information about an injury, illness, or incident to entities interested in the information for statistical, legal, claims, and risk management purposes.
- Health claim status—a transaction used by health care providers and recipients of health care products or services to request from a health plan the status of a health care claim or encounter.
- Referral certification and authorization—a transaction used to transmit health care service referral information among health care providers, health care providers furnishing services, and health plans. It may also be used to obtain authorization for certain health care services from a health plan.

Source: Reprinted from *Federal Register,* May 7, 1998. "Health Insurance Reform: Standards for Electronic Transaction; National Standard Health Provider Identifier; Proposed Rules," pp. 25278–79. Adapted from Chapter 67, courtesy of HIPAA.

ity provisions do not supersede all state laws about privacy of health information; a state may implement stricter, but not less strict, regulations.

Table 35–1, adapted from Chapter 32, further illustrates some of the applicable data security standards, which fall into three categories: administrative procedures, physical safeguards, and technical security.

HIPAA is clear in allowing data to be used for payment of claims, billing, and medical management, including managing utilization and quality. It also allows for the use of "blinded" data, aggregate data used for population-level reports, as long as there is no way for someone to use those data to track back to an individual patient. There are also situations where specific permission to use the data must be obtained from the patient (e.g., providing that information to an employer or to anyone that is not involved in the provision or direct management of the patient's

Table 35–1 HIPAA Data Privacy Requirements

Category	Requirement
Administrative procedures	• Certification review (the Department of Health and Human Services must decide if this will be either an internal or an external certification) • Chain of trust partner agreements that signify that contractors or partners are security compliant • Policies and procedures for processing records (including security standards) • Access authorization, establishment, and modification policies • Internal audit of management information systems (MIS) security • Personnel authorization and security process • MIS security configuration management procedures • Security incident procedures • Security management process (includes a risk analysis, risk management, a sanction policy, and a security policy) • Termination process for internal and external users • Security training
Physical safeguards	• Assigned security responsibility • Media controls over receipt and removal of hardware and software • Physical access controls • Workstation policies • Secure workstations • Security awareness training
Technical security	• Access controls, including procedures for emergency access and one of the following: context-based access, role-based access, or user-based access • Audit controls to record and examine system activity • Authorization control over the use and disclosure of health information either by role-based access or user-based access • Data authentication to prove data has not been altered or destroyed illegally by use of check sum, double keying, message authentication, or digital signature • Entity authentication to verify that entities are who they say they are by use of automatic logoff and unique user identification plus one of the following: biometric ID system, a password system, a personal identification number, telephone call back, or a physical device system

Courtesy of Ernst & Young LLP; adapted from Chapter 32.

medical care). HIPAA expressly prohibits the sale of patient-identifiable data for any marketing or sales purpose.

Another way to look at this is that there is a corporate compliance function required under HIPAA and involving the following components:

- designation of a privacy official who will be responsible for the development and implementation of the privacy policies and procedures
- training for all members of the workforce who obtain protected health information (PHI), including an attestation every three years that the employee will honor the covered entity's privacy policies
- administrative, technical, and physical safeguards to protect the privacy of PHI, including procedures for verifying the identity and authority of requestors of information
- detailed specifications of what must be documented to ensure compliance with the regulation

VALUE-ADDED SERVICES—THE NEXT GENERATION

This next section will discuss expanded or new services that health plans can offer to their customers. These services will increase customer satisfaction while changing the focus to health management. Services like the ones mentioned will give a health plan an advantage over its competitors.

Internet Technology Services

Providers, employers, agents, and members now expect that many health plan services will be available on line. Employers are asking for access to the health plan's systems to perform certain tasks within their human resources department such as individual enrollment for newborns, disenrollments, and PCP changes. Providers are requesting on-line access to better treat their patients with quicker responses and fewer calls to the health plan. The health plan

has two choices: either allow direct access to the individual health plan systems or develop an interface system for predetermined functions such as enrollment.

Since a health plan may have many systems running, the preferred approach is to develop an interface system that is securely accessible via the Internet or through an extranet. Web-based interface systems offer many benefits. (Chapter 37 discusses electronic commerce in depth.) Access can be granted to many customers through established technologies, training can be conducted for just one web-based system (versus training for each back-end system), and services can be controlled easily (since some managed care systems cannot limit security to a certain member or function). A web-based solution can offer a useful option to both the customer and the health plan. Each service will need to be evaluated for feasibility as well as security and confidentiality issues.

With providers, employers, and members eager to get information on line, *health plans should design their web sites to be the launching point for on-line information or services such as:*

- health plan marketing information
- member handbooks
- provider directories listing providers by product, ZIP code, specialty, languages spoken, gender, and so forth
- member eligibility information
- member rosters
- claim status information
- enrollment (new and updates)
- PCP changes
- questions (sent to the plan via e-mail)
- clinical guidelines
- referral and authorization submission and status information
- links to other sites with wellness and healthy living information
- pharmacy formulary (by specific drug or therapeutic class)
- agent and broker rates
- report distribution and decision support

The greater the health plan's web capabilities, the greater the plan's potential competitive advantage. Web services help a plan demonstrate its commitment to providing better and more cost-effective services. Health plans should aim to have "one-stop shopping" sites where users can find links to other health information sites (e.g., health systems, the National Committee on Quality Assurance [NCQA]).

To satisfy the consumer, leading health plan organizations will need to:

1. expand the ability to deliver multiple health plan options and integrate multiple health resource networks while enhancing consumer access to these resources
2. expand the ability to select and distribute information and education that is tailored to specific consumers and their health profiles
3. expand the ability to deliver integrated service to the consumer that is individualized and enabling rather than limiting[5]

The Internet and web technologies can be leveraged to support these expanded consumer demands.

Customer Services—Contact Management and Intranets

Health plans offer services, not products, so exceptional customer service is critical to their success. NCQA accreditation requires that health plans track contacts (calls, letters, and in-person visits), issues, resolution, and turnaround times. The plan must demonstrate its continuous commitment to addressing member and provider issues by utilizing this contact and resolution data. To do so, a health plan must engage a contact tracking solution. Data to be captured should include the reason for the call, the date of the call, and solutions to the issue with a resolution date (a detailed list of potential data to capture for this service may be found in Chapter 40). Also, the contact tracking system should allow a contact record to be forwarded to another person or team for resolution if the customer service representative is unable to resolve the issue. Needless to say, the contact tracking tool is extensively, if not exclusively, used by the customer service department for its day-to-day op-

erations. Many managed care systems contain a call tracking module, but the individual health plan must determine if that module will meet the plan's needs. Call tracking solutions are generally not the core competency of a managed care system, so a third-party or internally developed solution may be needed. Many of these applications are now being referred to as customer relationship management systems.

Reports from the contact system are vital. Customer service departments must religiously review reports of open contacts to ensure that they are being processed. Issues that arise frequently must be investigated to determine if they can be prevented or if additional education, either for the health plan or its customers, is needed on a specific topic. Resolution time reports should be analyzed to determine if the cycle time can be shortened, if not eliminated. Satisfaction surveys indicate that if issues are not resolved within 24 hours, customers feel dissatisfied with the health plan.

To properly serve the customer service team, the contact tracking module must be easy to use, quick to capture information, and self-contained. If the customer service representative must jump to many other systems for information and reenter member, provider, or employer data, the process will become laborious and time-consuming, thus disappointing the customers by adding time to the call. Eligibility, claims inquiry, and authorization/referral inquiry information must be contained within the product for quick reference.

Internally developed intranet web-based systems complement customer service and other health plan processes by providing electronic policy or reference information that is up-to-date and easily obtained. Distribution of reference material to the health plan staff is much easier when using an intranet (rather than making paper copies). *Health plan intranet resources can include:*

- summary plan descriptions for each enrolled group
- certificates of coverage
- member handbooks
- medical policies

- clinical guidelines
- key performance indicators
- departmental policies (claims, enrollment, premium billing)

Intranet web-based solutions and contact tracking systems can assist the health plan in providing excellent customer service that is quick and efficient.

Medical Management Information Systems

The largest opportunity to improve health care utilization, quality, and cost is through proactive and intensive medical or care management. The medical expense is the single largest expense managed by the health plan, typically averaging 80 percent to 90 percent of premiums received. In addition to helping contain costs, the medical management system can help the health plan to focus on proactive health management.

A health plan's medical department needs an information system to help with case, referral, and disease management. Contained within the medical management system will be health plan members' utilization data based on claims and clinical information. The medical management system goes beyond the claim payment system (or administrative data, as it is sometimes called) for member utilization and case profiling since it allows the medical department staff to enter clinical information—information that could not be obtained from a claim.

The medical management system allows the medical team to build a case either through an event such as an admission or through proactive management such as disease management or a member registry. The system allows the user to capture a predefined set of clinical information (e.g., blood pressure, peak flow meter readings) and ensures that a certain protocol of intervention or activity is followed by the health plan's case manager or disease management nurses. Intervention dates can be set to notify users of key intervention points for themselves or others on the team. Clinical cases can be forwarded to the medical director for review and approval.

Referral and authorization management is another key component of a care management sys-

tem. Interfaces between the managed care system and the care management system will be needed so referral and authorization data can be available for appropriate claim payment. Membership, provider, and claim data are fed into the care management system from the managed care system.

A care management system will create a paperless environment for the medical department, which is typically a paper-intensive department. Laptop computers with remote databases can be utilized for case managers performing concurrent reviews at network hospitals. Ideally, medical management systems allow for true integration within an integrated delivery system since both the delegated entity and the plan can use a similar system for medical management. Lastly, the medical management system allows the health plan to capture true clinical information to supplement the claim information to support the medical department processes and for future analysis and reporting. For example, clinical information is critical to enhancing the plan's ability to stratify patients based on disease severity, as discussed in detail in Chapter 32.

Decision Support Services

The importance and dependency on information has grown significantly because information can influence behavior, especially with care delivery. Health plans are in a unique and beneficial position since they can supply information about the continuum of care based on administrative and clinical information. This information can be used by providers to be proactive in member care. For example, a physician can be notified by the health plan that his or her member was admitted or had an emergency encounter out of the service area (the health plan must be notified typically with 48 hours of one of these events). This prompt notification offers many advantages to the provider, such as the opportunity to contact the member and coordinate any additional care if needed. Another example is a patient listing (or registry) of members by disease state so the provider can devote time to the appropriate population for disease state management initiatives. Health plan information systems can truly aid the delivery of managed care and member health by providing timely, complete information to the provider.

Concurrently, employers' interest in helping with health management is increasing. Employers are interested in promoting wellness within their organization to reduce utilization and health care costs. As a result, they are requesting assistance from health plans either through population profiles (e.g., profiles of member obesity and smoking habits) or through member assessments and health risk appraisals. Survey data obtained through health risk appraisals coupled with claim experience data can successfully identify a high-risk population needing provider intervention. (There are some limitations on the amount of detailed data that can be shared with an employer.) In a world with advanced technology and longer life spans, employers, providers, and health plans must partner to ensure that appropriate, high-quality, and cost-effective health care is delivered.

The health plan's greatest strength is the ability to influence provider behavior based on detailed experience and cost data formed from claim (both medical and drug), membership, and clinical information. With the data manipulated through third-party algorithms, utilization or health predictions can be made. The health plan's enrollment and utilization information allows the member to be identified by the provider—possibly prior to becoming a patient. By proactively analyzing the member's utilization, health plans can provide their greatest assistance to providers by ensuring that people remain healthy and appropriately utilize their health benefits.

Data Sets, Enhancers, Data Warehouses and Reporting

By utilizing the information captured within all of the systems mentioned in this "Value-Added Services—The Next Generation" section, health plans can leverage a series of data sets for analytical purposes and create a continuum of care. *The relevant data sets include:*

- medical claims—within network and out of network
- preauthorizations and specialty referrals
- prescription drug claims
- durable medical equipment claims
- home care, skilled nursing, and behavioral health claims
- medical management data, including non–claims-captured information such as vital signs
- pathology and radiology result data based on special partnerships
- health risk appraisals

This information is captured by the core managed care information system and other systems utilized by the health plan. It is generally extracted to a data warehouse environment that is solely dedicated to financial, utilization, and outcomes analysis and reporting. This allows the health plan to easily analyze and report on this information while ensuring that production functions such as claims and enrollment are not impacted by intensive reporting. The data warehouse can support both production report queries and ad hoc queries; for health plans, the data warehouse must support both. Although routine information is important, quick analytical support is needed to immediately analyze practice pattern changes or newly enrolled groups.

In addition to storing the information in a separate environment, the health plan can develop or purchase data "enhancers" that add new characteristics to the claims records to aid the analytical process. These third-party solutions can enhance the data so that certain utilization trends or health risks of the defined population can be predicted. Discussed in detail in Chapter 32, enhancers might include:

- episode of care
- event (e.g., inpatient event, obstetrical event, emergency event, outpatient event)
- diagnosis-related groups (DRGs)
- diagnostic categories
- case severity indicators
- therapeutic drug classes
- unique specialty classes

In determining how the data warehouse and reporting environment should be designed, it is critical to engage a multidisciplinary team within the health plan. Users of the data warehouse must trust the data and understand how data pieces fit together. A provider reporting committee and medical information committee can assist with the design and attributes of the data warehouse along with the design of provider reports.

The data warehouse can be leveraged to produce the following reports for use by the health plan, provider, and employer:

- capitation fund status reports
- reports on medical utilization (e.g., inpatient, outpatient, specialty referrals)
- provider profiling that utilizes a common denominator such as episode of care
- specialty profiling
- hospital profiling
- physician key indicator reports
- registries—member listings based on predefined present or nonpresent medical indicators, predictive and stratified
- drug utilization profiling, including alternate prescribing opportunities
- group utilization reports: employer demographics, medical and pharmacy utilization, inpatient analysis, and expenses by relationship to policyholder with comparisons to the health plan and the group's industry
- Health Employer Data and Information Set (HEDIS) reporting for NCQA accreditation

With this combination of data enhancers and reports, data can truly be converted into accurate information that a provider can utilize.

HEDIS

Another value-added service that the health plan can provide is the HEDIS reports. HEDIS was developed by the NCQA to respond to employer groups who wanted to understand the value of their health care dollars. HEDIS has been adopted for use by public purchasers, regulators, and consumers to understand and rate the health plan's overall value and quality. HEDIS is now being used as part of quality, health management systems, provider profiling, purchaser requests, NCQA accreditation, and consumer report cards. At one time, creating HEDIS reports was a mandate for NCQA accreditation. Now, the actual scores are accounting for 25 percent of the health plans' overall NCQA rating. The ratings are excellent, commendable, accredited, provisional, and denied.

HEDIS specifications are updated annually by NCQA with results due to NCQA in June of every year. *HEDIS 2000 contains 56 measures across eight domains of care, which are:*

1. effectiveness of care
2. access/availability of care
3. satisfaction with the experience of care
4. health plan stability
5. use of services
6. cost of care
7. informed health care choices
8. health plan descriptive information

As mentioned earlier, health plans are required to update their process to accurately calculate the measures based on the latest HEDIS version. HEDIS 2000 measures, the most recent release at the time of publication, are listed in Table 35–2. *Differences between HEDIS 1999 and HEDIS 2000 include the following:*

- The retired measure of Eye Exams for People with Diabetes is replaced by the Eye Exams numerator in the Comprehensive Diabetes Care measure.
- There are new measures that address effectiveness of care for Chlamydia Screening in Women (first year), Controlling High Blood Pressure (first year), and Use of Appropriate Medications for People with Asthma (first year).
- Gaps in continuous enrollment are allowed.
- There are measures using pharmacy data.
- Systematic sampling will incorporate changes such as date of birth being added to the sort and new/updated formulas.
- Patient self-reported data must be documented in the medical record.
- Internally built administrative databases may be used.

Table 35–2 HEDIS 2000 List of Measures

HEDIS 2000 Measures	Applicable To		
	Medicaid	Commercial	Medicare
Effectiveness of Care			
Childhood Immunization Status	X	X	
Adolescent Immunization Status	X	X	
Breast Cancer Screening	X	X	X
Cervical Cancer Screening	X	X	
Chlamydia Screening in Women (First Year)	X	X	
Prenatal Care in the First Trimester	X	X	
Check-Ups After Delivery	X	X	
Controlling High Blood Pressure (First Year)	X	X	X
Beta Blocker Treatment After a Heart Attack	X	X	X
Cholesterol Management After Acute Cardiovascular Events	X	X	X
Comprehensive Diabetes Care	X	X	X
Use of Appropriate Medications for People with Asthma (First Year)	X	X	
Follow-up After Hospitalization for Mental Illness	X	X	X
Antidepressant Medication Management	X	X	X
Advising Smokers to Quit	X	X	X
Flu Shots for Older Adults			X
Medicare Health Outcomes Survey			X
Access/Availability of Care			
Adults' Access to Preventive/Ambulatory Health Services	X	X	X
Childrens' Access to Primary Care Practitioners	X	X	
Initiation of Prenatal Care	X		
Annual Dental Visit	X		
Availability of Language Interpretation Services	X	X	X
Satisfaction with the Experience of Care			
HEDIS/CAHPS™ 2.0H, Adult	X	X	
HEDIS/CAHPS™ 2.0H, Child	X	X	
Health Plan Stability			
Disenrollment		X	X
Practitioner Turnover	X	X	X
Years in Business/Total Membership	X	X	X
Indicators of Financial Stability	X	X	X
Use of Services			
Frequency of Ongoing Prenatal Care	X		
Well-Child Visits in the First 15 Months of Life	X	X	
Well-Child Visits in the Third, Fourth, Fifth, and Sixth Year of Life	X	X	
Adolescent Well-Care Visit	X	X	
Frequency of Selected Procedures	X	X	X
Inpatient Utilization: General Hospital/Acute Care	X	X	X
Ambulatory Care	X	X	X
Inpatient Utilization: Non-Acute Care	X	X	X

continues

Table 35–2 Continued

HEDIS 2000 Measures	Applicable To		
	Medicaid	Commercial	Medicare
Discharge and Average Length of Stay Maternity Care	X	X	
Cesarean Section	X	X	
Vaginal Birth After Cesarean Rate (VBAC Rate)	X	X	
Births and Average Length of Stay, Newborns	X	X	
Mental Health Utilization: Inpatient Discharges and Average Length of Stay	X	X	X
Mental Health Utilization: Percentage of Members Receiving Services	X	X	X
Chemical Dependency Utilization: Inpatient Discharges and Average Length of Stay	X	X	X
Chemical Dependency Utilization: Percentage of Members Receiving Services	X	X	X
Outpatient Drug Utilization	X	X	X
Cost of Care			
Rate Trends	X	X	X
High-Occurrence/High-Cost DRGs		X	X
Informed Health Care Choices			
Management of Menopause (First Year)		X	
Health Plan Descriptive Information			
Board Certification/Residency Completion	X	X	X
Practitioner Compensation	X	X	X
Arrangements with Public Health, Educational, and Social Service Organizations	X	X	X
Total Enrollment by Percentage	X	X	X
Enrollment by Product Line (Member Years/Member Months)	X	X	X
Unduplicated Count of Medicaid Members	X		
Cultural Diversity of Medicaid Membership	X		
Weeks of Pregnancy at Time of Enrollment in the MCO	X		

Note: CAHPS = Consumer Assessment of Health Plans
Courtesy of National Committee for Quality Assurance.

Starting with HEDIS 1999, NCQA requires that information be audited by a certified third-party audit firm in order for the information to be published. Data will not be accepted unless a satisfactory report is delivered by the auditor. The audit process includes review of system documentation, review of specifications and source code, on-site process review, and audits of the medical record review process. The HEDIS report is al-ways for the previous year's data. For example, HEDIS 2000 is for 1999 information, which allows for closure of the claims run-out period.

The information services team plays a critical role in the development of the HEDIS report since the majority of measures are produced using administrative and clinical data stored in the health plan's core information systems. Another option includes outsourcing the HEDIS report to one of many third-party companies by extracting the data off of the core systems. Creating the HEDIS measures is a task that should not be taken lightly by the health plan. It is a project that requires multidisciplinary teams to develop the methodologies, produce the results, validate the data, perform possible medical record reviews, and participate in the auditor review. Health plan data used to produce the HEDIS reports include:

- medical claims
- pharmacy claims
- clinical data (e.g., delivery date, prematurity status) stored in care management systems
- financial system indicators
- member and provider surveys
- credentialing

Certain measures cannot be fully determined by administrative data (e.g., claims), so a sampling is performed and medical record audits are done to determine the actual measure. These measures are referred to as "hybrid measures."

INFORMATION SERVICES DEPARTMENT

As discussed above, good information systems help to make a health plan competitive, leading it to the next generation of automation, servicing, and health management. Equally important is the information services department, whose staff members implement these systems.

Health plan information services teams (see Figure 35–1 for a sample organizational chart) are much like those in most industries: There is a software engineering team of developers and a technical services team to ensure that the technology infrastructure continues running and can expand. But there are some ways that health plans' information services departments may be different from other organizations' information services departments.

- There must be a chief information officer (CIO) who reports directly to the chief executive officer (CEO) and is a member of the executive management team. As discussed earlier, health plans deliver services, not

Figure 35–1 Organizational Structure of an Information Services Department

products, and those services depend on technology. Information system demands are great and must be balanced to ensure the plan's success. Also, the CIO must ensure that information is captured and available for analysis and reporting to assist in the management of the medical loss ratio. The CIO could also be called the chief automation officer because he or she ensures that all processes are automated as much as possible to improve service and lower the administrative expense ratio. The CIO must also ensure that services are meeting and exceeding the expectations of the providers, purchasers, and, most important, consumers. With a CIO who reports to the CEO and with the executive management team, technology solutions will be given serious enough consideration to ensure that the business will grow and succeed. Lastly, the CIO must ensure that the information services department remains focused on its immediate tasks. Information services departments can be easily pulled in many different directions. Focus ensures project completion, so annual project planning is vital.

- Information services departments must receive help from business analysts to ensure that the departments have a full understanding of the health plan's operations. Most systems are installed with the expectations that data will need to be analyzed either for efficiency gains or outcomes. Business analysts are typically individuals who have strong proficiency with systems and have worked in various roles throughout the health plan or a health system.
- Having a team dedicated to the design and development of the data warehouse and reporting is vital. Typically called the information center (IC), this team understands the business of managed care as well as its implications for technology. The mission of the IC is to assist the health plan in developing, using, and analyzing information better. The IC works extensively with other health plan departments (e.g., medical, provider network

support, marketing) to help discern their informational needs. Because members of the IC have knowledge of information technology, they can apply their knowledge and create innovative solutions to the needs presented. Using decision support tools (and other tools), the IC responds to requests that are one-time only and ad hoc in nature and assists in the development and roll out of production reports. The duties of the IC, therefore, include evaluating and selecting decision support tools, using those tools to produce reports, setting up decision support tools for external users, training staff on how to use the tools, and following up to ensure that the tools are meeting staff members' needs.

- Because of the many data interfaces that the plan will need to support, there will need to be a team dedicated to EDI. This team will design and oversee the information flow into and out of the health plan.

Lastly, members of the information services department must consider themselves technology solution leaders. Just as important, they must recognize their internal users as customers. They must establish their core purpose as ensuring the health plan remains successful, improves its service levels, expands its membership, and remains financially self-sustaining. Exhibit 35–2 lists one information services department's core purpose and activities.

CONCLUSION

Health plan information technology expense budgets increased approximately 40 percent from 1995 to 1997 to $3.75 per member per month.[6] This is relatively good news since health care has a history of lagging in appropriate support for information technology initiatives to stay ahead with operational efficiencies and consumer needs. As this chapter discussed, health plans are very dependent on information systems and technology to become more efficient, improve customer service, and lower both medical and administrative expense ratios. As health plans expand

Exhibit 35–2 Example of Information Services Department Core Purpose and Activities

Our information services department wants to help ensure that Priority Health remains the preeminent health plan in Michigan. To this end, we will commit to the following core purpose and activities.

Core Purpose

We will provide innovative technical solutions to complement the dynamics of managed care.

Core Activities

We will continuously maintain and improve the information technology within Priority Health.

- We will provide the hardware, software, and networking tools to facilitate data collection, processing, and storage.
- We will remain knowledgeable about the latest technology and proactive in recommending its implementation.
- We will strive to be the technology solution provider of choice.

We will empower our customers to turn data into information.

- We will provide retrieval tools to help customers gain access to data, enabling them to solve problems on their own.
- We will provide communication, training, and educational services to help customers use data more effectively.

We will collaborate with our customers to meet the organization's needs.

- We will continually monitor our project priorities and resources to adjust to the organization's needs.
- We will publish tactical plans and project status reports to include the entire organization in the stewardship of its information technology investments.
- We will build flexibility and responsiveness into our departmental "entry points" so that we can effectively resolve problems and respond to projects in a timely manner.
- We will offer options to aid our customers with problem resolution.

We will empower ourselves to be successful.

- We will develop our employees' core competencies to meet current demands of the organization.
- We will provide opportunities and encourage our team members to expand their business and technical skills and explore new technologies to retain highly skilled talent.
- We will remain committed to working as a team to service our customers, because we will achieve the most success by working together.

---

their medical informatics capabilities and services, the next generation of health management can be achieved. Leveraging web-based solutions to serve providers, purchasers, and consumers, health plans will have a competitive advantage and strong customer loyalty. Information systems are a key enabler to advance the health plan and turn data into actionable information. The true health plan leader will fully embrace information systems and technology.

REFERENCES

1. P. Wehrwein, *Follow the Shrinking Managed Care Savings* (Trenton, NJ: Stezzi Communications, 1999).
2. R.L. Schaich, IT Implications of the Next Generation of Managed Care, *Health Management Technology* (January 1998): 1–4.
3. J.A. Gilbert, HMOs Slow to Embrace Client/Server Systems, *Health Data Management* (July 1998): 34–38.
4. D. Pedersen, *The Inevitability of E-commerce* (Trenton, NJ: Stezzi Communications, 1999).
5. Schaich, IT Implications, 1–4.
6. The Gartner Group, *IT Strategic and Budgeting Trends in HMOs* (Stamford, CT, 1998).

Information Systems and Electronic Commerce for Provider Systems in Managed Health Care

Robert G. Reese and Rick Majzun

INTRODUCTION: MAJOR ISSUES FACING HEALTH CARE PROVIDER ORGANIZATIONS IN THE YEAR 2000

As health care provider organizations begin the 21st century, they are faced with a variety of internal and external challenges. To succeed in

---

Robert G. Reese is a Partner in the National Health Practice at Ernst & Young LLP specializing in information technology, performance improvement, and strategic planning related to the health care industry. Bob has led large scale application system implementations in a variety of health care settings. He has been involved in providing technology services for the past 17 years to a variety of institutions. His prior experience includes creation and operation of large scale information system infrastructures in the health, communications, and services industries. His experience in developing strategic relationships for clients with vendors has led to a variety of successful client relationships. Current responsibilities include development of broad strategic initiatives for integrated delivery networks in leveraging their technology infrastructure.

Rick Majzun is a Regional Practice Director for the BJC Medical Group in St. Louis, Missouri, responsible for providing leadership for approximately 20 primary care and multispecialty physician offices. Before joining BJC, Rick was a Senior Consultant in Ernst and Young's Health Care Practice, specializing in providing strategic and operational consulting services in the area of information technology. Previous experience includes four years in inpatient and ambulatory operations with the Henry Ford Health System and two years as an evening administrator at Barnes Hospital.

this dynamic environment, leading organizations are using information technology to improve their ability to be clinically effective and financially efficient. With the growth of managed care contracting, disease management, and the need for greater public accountability, low-cost health care providers who can quickly and efficiently share information will have a distinct advantage. Health care provider organizations and integrated delivery systems have already begun to transition themselves toward reduced cost by leveraging new technologies and providing value through information management among physicians and patients and between payers and providers. As the health care industry begins the new millennium, several key facts present themselves as particularly relevant. Those key facts are discussed as follows. Chapters 35 (regarding information systems [IS] in managed care organizations) and 37 (regarding electronic commerce) are also relevant to this topic, and the reader is encouraged to review them.

HEALTH CARE IS A BUSINESS IN AN INFORMATION ECONOMY

Although the health care industry has learned many lessons from the manufacturing sector, and increasingly the service sector, health care takes place in an information economy. Few industries can benefit from information technology in a more meaningful way. Unfortunately, the rate of investment is significantly behind those made in general industry. The typical health care organization spends approximately 2 percent of its capital budget on information technology compared with an average of 10 percent in all other industries.[1] As a result of minimal investment, information technologies in many hospitals can be characterized as disjointed service-specific applications with little internal or external connectivity. On a positive note, this low level of investment is quickly changing, as evidenced by the 1999 Health Information Management Systems Society (HIMSS) survey. In that survey, 71 percent of the chief information officers (CIOs) who responded indicated that their IS budgets were growing. This fact is especially remarkable when one considers the differential impact information technology can have in improving the quality of patient care—not solely in saving dollars but in saving lives.

HEALTH CARE PROVIDER ORGANIZATIONS ARE BUILDING THE INFORMATION INFRASTRUCTURE FOR A NEW ERA IN HEALTH CARE

The dollars health care organizations are spending on information technology represent a capital investment similar to those our predecessors made in railways and telephone lines and will not be dissimilar in their effect on society. The widespread introduction of information technology will truly change the way medical care is provided in this country by serving as the infrastructure for the health care system of the next century. This improved infrastructure will accelerate the introduction of findings of genetic research into daily practice, the conversion of disease from an event into a process, and the rapid translation of clinical trials into protocols of care.

PRESSURES ON BOTH THE COST AND REVENUE SIDES OF THE EQUATION ARE INCREASING

Health care provider organizations are increasingly dependent on the government for most patient revenue as illustrated in Table 36–1.

Table 36–1 Who Pays for Health Care?

	1960	1990	1997
Out of pocket	55	24	19
Government	22	39	45
Private insurance	23	37	36

Source: Copyright 1999, *USA Today.* Reprinted with permission.

Largely as a result of the Balanced Budget Act of 1997, provider organizations are seeing reimbursement levels decrease. For example, Medicare payments to hospitals will be cut by $71.2 billion from 1998 to 2002—an overall reduction of 10.5 percent.[2] These reductions encompass Medicare payments for inpatient care by the prospective payment system (PPS), outpatient services, home health services, as well as PPS-exempt services. Cost pressures from other third-party payers, including managed care organizations, continue to increase, forcing the need for immediate improvement in operational efficiency.

At the same time that organizations are feeling this balance sheet pressure, they are being pressured by consumers and employer groups to drastically improve the quality of patient care and customer service. Strategic investments in information technology will enable health care provider organizations to withstand the pressures previously discussed and to achieve these improvements. Information technology allows an organization to differentiate itself in the market by performance on various cost, quality, and service measurements. Examples of these technologies are illustrated in Table 36–2.

INFORMATION TECHNOLOGY SHOULD SUPPORT BUSINESS STRATEGY AND MARKET NEED

Today, health care organizations better understand the ability of technology-enabled systems to lower their operating costs and manage the entire enterprise. Technology-enabled systems are now viewed as an investment in the future of

Table 36–2 Technology Can Reduce Cost While Improving Quality and Service

Measurement	System	Benefits
Cost	Technology-enabled supply chain management	Stronger inventory flow, better cash management
Quality	Pharmacy decision support systems	Reduced medication interactions, overdoses, and other errors
Service	Automated call directors	Increased operational efficiency leading to shorter hold times for patients

the enterprise rather than an expense. As a result, many health care organizations are exploring the most efficient means of building and supporting technology-enabled systems throughout their enterprises.

Over the past several years, information services departments have devoted a great deal of attention and capital to resolving the year 2000 (Y2K) issue. Having successfully navigated this issue, health care provider organizations are again turning their attention to a variety of information technology solutions, as noted in Table 36–3.

Technology such as enterprise resource planning systems, which facilitate efficiencies in large, complex organizations, and computer-based patient records, which enable providers to care for individuals more effectively and populations more efficiently, will be among the most popular of applications.

Table 36–3 Information Technology Priorities of Health Care Provider Organizations

Issue	% of Respondents Selecting
Year 2000 (Y2K) conversion	44
Integrating systems in a multivendor environment	16
Implementing a computer-based patient record (CPR)	12
Recruiting and retaining high-quality IT staff	7

Source: Reprinted by permission of *10th Annual HIMSS Leadership Survey* sponsored by International Business Machines Corporation.

INTERCONNECTIVITY

The term *interconnectivity* refers to an enterprise's ability to allow multiple, disparate systems to share information from department to department, from the hospital to other entities in the enterprise, and from the enterprise to the insurance company or employer. The opportunities are significant.

Some in the health care IS industry have noted that the lack of spending in health care information technology has resulted in the technical and financial impossibility of acquiring a single system solution to meet all of a health care provider organization's needs. One study noted: "Given the multitude of competing interests, a single, monolithic IS is a virtual impossibility in the near future."[3] Therefore, methods for integrating disparate systems are essential to develop effective enterprise-wide solutions.

System interconnectivity is occurring within institutions through system integration and between provider institutions and payers through electronic eligibility verification, authorizations, claim submission, and remittance advice receipts. In addition, interconnectivity exists between health care provider organizations and banks through electronic reimbursement (electronic funds transmission [EFT]) and between hospitals and suppliers through electronic inventory management. In health care today, interconnectivities that occur among health care applications are primarily financial in nature (e.g., submitting a claim for payment, transferring funds electronically, and sending automated remittance advice to providers).

Managed care organizations have already seen significant advances in interconnectivity with the development of patient eligibility and provider referrals. As the health care industry emerges into the information age, interconnectivity will include the exchange of financial and clinical information within and external to the enterprise and the full support of a computer-based patient record.

DATA REPOSITORIES OR WAREHOUSES: THE BACKBONE OF THE ORGANIZATION'S CLINICAL AND FINANCIAL SYSTEMS

Enterprise-wide data repositories (also referred to as data warehouses) are relational databases that bring together snapshots of transactional data from multiple systems to provide a single source of data for executive decision making, customer management, patient care, and end-user applications. According to Inmon,[4] a data repository or warehouse is a collection of data in support of management's decisions. The data are subject oriented rather than application oriented; integrated or transformed into a consistent format; nonvolatile, meaning that the snapshot never changes; and time variant, with snapshots over a period of five years or more.

Health care provider organizations have historically led the way in developing large repositories of encounter data. In the early 1980s, health systems, specifically those linked with health care–focused teaching institutions, began to analyze the data contained in these repositories to improve their negotiating position with payer organizations and employers. At that time, computer hardware was not capable of sufficiently managing the huge volumes of data contained in a repository. As technology advanced, organizations began to review more broadly the large-scale data repositories of clinically related services.

Although still in its infancy stages, data warehousing is becoming more popular. The Gartner Group has predicted that more than 90 percent of all information processing organizations will implement this technology by the end of the year 2000, and some industry analysts believe that its implementation is a key success factor for competing in the managed care environment.[5] The implementation of central data repositories is considered a key success factor primarily because data warehousing supports business process redesign and has been, in many cases, the first step in the reengineering process.

Data within a repository are stored according to the structure of the database model, either central or relational. Central databases are characterized by centralized control through a single hardware platform with a database management system serving both operations and enterprise decision support. With central databases, end-user functional needs are more difficult to meet. This is especially apparent when the community physician user group and other user groups are not using the same central hardware platform. Relational databases, although efficient in enabling storage and extraction functions, do not meet enterprise decision support needs for analysis and comparisons because decision support functions frequently involve complex queries and comparisons of cross-tabulated data.

Development of the data warehouse often occurs in opposite sequence to the standard systems development life cycle: implementation followed by data integration, testing, programming, design of the decision support system, analysis, and requirements definition. For this reason, cost justification is difficult because benefits are not understood at the outset. Historically, benefits of established data warehouse implementations have been measured in terms of differentiation of product/services with increases in market share, improved production efficiency as evidenced by increased revenue per unit cost, and improved management through a better understanding of the profitability of products and services. Data warehousing supports online transaction processing, online analytical processing, enterprise decision support, executive IS, business process redesign, legacy refurbishment, clinical workstation development, clinical decision support, distributed processing, and client-server implementation. Although distributed client-server standards-based environments are supported fully by many data warehouse vendors, specific characteristics such as management preferences, technology infrastructures, products and services, and market volatility make each data warehouse organizationally specific. Individual organizational characteristics and long-term strategic plans will drive the structure of the storage of information within the database because each type of database is suited to meet different needs.

ENTERPRISE-WIDE INFORMATION SYSTEMS

Administrators have typically used information technology to manage the financial, distribution, and operational functions of organizations. As the pace of mergers and acquisitions has quickened, many health care provider organizations are finding themselves with complex, disparate systems that are unable to communicate. Often the better solution to integration is replacement of legacy systems with enterprise-wide resource planning systems (ERPs), which are far-reaching in their benefits.

Although recent developments in web technology have reduced the cost and risk of implementing ERP packages, these systems can be complex and costly to install. An organization can follow several best practices to reduce the cycle time of the implementation of these systems—thus achieving a quicker return on investment. These practices include:

- clear business vision and strategy
- a structured work plan that defines the roles of client, vendor, systems integrator, and consultant team members

- a structured development life cycle, with clearly delineated milestones through the project
- a preconfigured application package near-ready for use by the health care provider organization, with modifications made to reflect the organization's individual IS needs

The key to successful implementation of any system is the identification of key organizational sponsors and stakeholders who can lead decision making to timely consensus and create alignment of varying views and organizational behaviors. Implementing an ERP solution can mean fundamentally changing business processes that have an impact on organizational culture. Therefore, the approach must be built around strong change management methods and a fused technical implementation plan. Organizations that establish a tight linkage with their business strategy/vision and ERP design have realized the benefits of an ERP system and have achieved the greatest operational and financial impacts. An example is provided in Exhibit 36–1.

USE OF INFORMATION TECHNOLOGY IN MANAGING CARE

Accelerating the proper and judicious use of information technology to improve the quality

---

Exhibit 36–1 An Example of Interconnectivity: Supply Chain Management Systems

Of the many enterprise systems available, one that has among the most promise for an organization is a technology-enabled supply chain management system. These systems have been used to transfer highly manual, labor-intensive, difficult-to-use systems into user-friendly automated systems. Through implementation of these systems, health care provider organizations can achieve operational cost savings in materials management through technology enablers, including:

- Product standardization, compliance, supplier management

- Stronger inventory flow, JIT, stockless programs
- More efficient material handling
- Improved timing and effectiveness of management information
- Improved workflow, efficiency of transaction handling
- Reduced lost payable discounts
- Implement an integrated solution to support systemwide requirements for facilities that are spread over large geographical areas

Courtesy of Ernst & Young LLP, 2000, Washington, DC.

of care—with a concomitant decrease in cost— presents administrators with the greatest possible chance to truly affect the health of their patient populations. At one level, information technology can assist in the stratification of patients by risk category; at another level, it can help to implement strategies to improve the health of each member. To be successfully adopted, information technology must allow providing the best quality of medical care to be the path of least resistance for physicians, and administrators who work at different "points of care" will implement these tactics differently, as illustrated in Table 36–4.

COMPUTERIZED MEDICAL RECORDS

It is our opinion that the tool that by far presents the health care industry with the greatest opportunity to manage care is the electronic medical record. A common, enterprise-wide medical record supports the concept of data integration. Immediate, accurate information is vital to controlling operating costs. By developing one common computerized medical record, the ability to reduce unnecessary, duplicative procedures is significantly enhanced, paper flow is reduced, the number of lost documents is reduced, and more accurate and reliable treatment is administered. Because a patient's history and medical information can be accessed at any time in an organized, legible format, the computerized medical record can also help clinical staff provide better care to the patient. Unnecessary tests resulting from unavailable patient records are eliminated.

According to an Institute of Medicine report,[6] a computerized medical record should do the following:

- record and organize clinically all transactions, encounters, and events
- streamline and guide the business of the caregiver or caregiving team
- add substantively to the body of medical knowledge
- support population and epidemiological studies

The report defined the computer-based patient record as an "electronic record that resides in a system specifically designed to support users through availability of complete and accurate data, practitioner reminders and alerts, clinical decision support systems, links to bodies of medical knowledge, and other aids."[7] The report also noted that a patient's medical record is unavailable 30 percent of the time during clinical evaluation and that 11 percent of laboratory tests

---

Table 36–4 The Use of Information Technology Along the Continuum of Health

Category	Information Technology–Based Quality Improvement Tactic
The generally well	Automated reminders that specific patients are due for scheduled activities (e.g., Pap smears, mammograms, prostate-specific antigen [PSA] testing)
Those with risk factors for decreasing health	Automated reminders using health plan data that specific patients aren't on certain drugs but should be (e.g., beta-blockers, cholesterol-lowering medications)
The chronically ill	Implementation of care management systems that provide notification of acute onset of chronic conditions (e.g., notification of all asthmatics requiring emergency department treatment)
The acutely ill	Information technology in pharmacy can be leveraged to assist decision making and change behavior (e.g., automated reminders, warnings of adverse medication reactions, and computerized guidelines)

Courtesy of Ernst & Young LLP, 2000, Washington, DC.

are reordered because the first test results are lost. According to Kenneth McCarty, director of the Pittsburgh Cancer Institute's (PCI's) Endocrine Laboratories, "Participating physicians could access necessary patient records instantly, regardless of where and when the clinical and laboratory information was generated."[8] By connecting with the networking infrastructure at PCI, community physicians can analyze the various diagnostic and treatment alternatives available to their patients and can readily access experts. An alarms-and-alerts subsystem of the network will notify health care professionals when they have not entered all the information necessary for each patient or when they need to order additional procedures.

Clinical systems like these are crucial for systems wishing to establish themselves as the market leaders of the future. Although only 11 percent of health care provider organizations have implemented fully operational computer-based patient records, 32 percent have begun the process and another 25 percent have developed an implementation plan.[9] These information systems provide information and analysis, and will be leveraged using web-based linkages to accelerate the translation of research from bench to bedside. In turn, this will reduce the risk inherent in medical care. Information systems are effective in improving the quality of care because they reduce risk for individual patients, for patient groups, and in individual physician decision making.

These changes are requiring not only a revamped physician role but a drastically different role for health care provider organizations as well. One of the primary responsibilities will be to produce and provide information that physicians can interpret into improved clinical practice. To be effective, a clinical information system must deliver the necessary information to physicians at the point of care, and it must challenge and enhance their decisions. It is the responsibility of a health care provider organization to work with its physicians who lack experience using information technology to achieve the end benefit of an improved quality of care.

CLINICAL DECISION SUPPORT SYSTEMS

An area of high potential for knowledge management is that of ongoing physician education. The rise of a medically literate public and technologies such as the Internet have drastically changed the role of the physician. In the past, knowledge of medicine was the exclusive domain of the physician. Today, through the use of information technology, patients have access to the latest clinical information. Current popular arguments hold as their tenets that it is unacceptable for a patient to be the one to provide a busy physician with new clinical knowledge, that a patient is not truly able to comprehend medical information found on the Internet, and that the information found does not always withstand the rigors of science. Although these arguments hold limited merit, the fact is that the Internet has forced a change in the role of the physician. Physicians now are the sole interpreters—but no longer the sole holders and distributors—of information readily available to anyone with Internet access. It is important to note that health care provider organizations do not have to be content providers. Effort would be better spent in providing linkages to existing expert content.

Collective knowledge provided by information technology, combined with individual clinical judgment—and only overruled in the face of contrary evidence—will be the way care will be delivered in the future and can be facilitated through the use of desktop linkages. It is imperative that these systems be "push" systems to the greatest extent possible to minimize the time a physician needs to take to seek advice.

Health care provider organizations should invest resources in systems that support the practice of medicine from a standard general method, with individual specific deviations made on the basis of the individual characteristics pertaining to the patient, not of the physician. Information technology should be leveraged to establish and implement nationally established protocols of care, resulting in an overall redesign of the care process.

KNOWLEDGE MANAGEMENT SYSTEMS

In a service-oriented, knowledge-intensive industry like health care, intellectual capital is the critical resource for success. Knowledge management is the strategic use of information to improve effectiveness for organizations and for individuals.[10] It is the tool leading health care organizations use in proactively planning and managing the process for leveraging information and employee knowledge to achieve a competitive advantage through innovation; efficiency; and faster, better decision making. Processes for creating, sharing, deploying, and measuring knowledge exist within every enterprise and have a profound effect on the decisions and actions we take. Systems that promote the sharing of knowledge between colleagues serve to increase the overall competence of the organization. When this knowledge is shared with patients/members/customers, relationships improve. Identifying and enhancing the processes to promote knowledge sharing will enhance overall organizational effectiveness.

The benefits of knowledge management include:

- *Innovation and growth:* A knowledge strategy focuses on the potential for professionals to increase capabilities (and revenue growth) through enhanced communication between colleagues with disparate perspectives; creativity is latent but can be tapped.
- *More with less:* Knowledge management leverages resources to *reduce costs while also improving quality.* A deliberate strategy of capturing, sharing, and deploying knowledge; of measuring outcomes; and of learning quickly will permit us to do more with less and do it better. Clinical guidelines and standardized information technology tools are examples of knowledge that leverage resources to enhance quality and effectiveness. By capturing and sharing "best practices," the enterprise improves its ability to manage patient care.
- *Reduce cycle time by finding knowledge quickly:* Health care must provide profes-

sionals with rapid access to the full repository of available knowledge. Physicians should have access to tools that provide real-time clinical knowledge, learning-on-demand, and instant access to critical expertise. The architecture and technology to enable this is available through a variety of sources, notably among them established Internet sites.

- *Enhancing competence:* Knowledge management focuses on sharing knowledge to increase competence and promote innovation. There is enormous potential to create new levels of effectiveness through widespread and rapid learning. Technology enablers and organizational incentives can promote faster, easier consultations, education, shared diagnosis, and treatment findings; hence leveraging collective wisdom to achieve business and clinical strategies.[11]

At its core, a knowledge management strategy focuses on the challenges of capturing, filtering, and sharing critical knowledge as it is applied to generate outcomes. As a knowledge-intensive service arena, the health care industry is poised to become an early beneficiary of the creative, cost-conscious, and outcomes-oriented focus of knowledge management.

Information technology executives in health care provider organizations will need to support this evolving field with enabling technologies. More importantly, they can play a leading role in its development. Knowledge management focuses on gaining knowledge from experience and on the judicious application of that knowledge to fulfill the mission of the organization. These activities are executed by marrying technology, organizational structures, and business strategies with a focus on outcomes. Critical in this endeavor is the enhancement of all systems (human, structural, and technological) for acquiring, storing, and using knowledge.

The collective knowledge of an organization, its intellectual capital, is embodied in the personal skills, experience, and brain power of its employees and in its processes, policies, electronic databases, and other information repositories. Knowledge sharing should be an integral part of an organization's culture, and the information technology department must provide the infrastructure to facilitate knowledge transfer across an enterprise. It is key that one individual, usually the CIO, be responsible for ensuring that these systems are developed and implemented to better support the delivery of patient care.

A health care provider organization can use several tools to ensure that all employees are able to tap into the collective knowledge of the organization. For example, many organizations seeking to improve operational efficiency and managerial effectiveness have begun the use of intranets. An intranet is best defined as a secure "internal internet." Use of an intranet allows a health care provider organization to more easily share financial, clinical, and operational information with a wider variety of internal users.

DATA PRIVACY AND SECURITY

As a result of the Health Insurance Portability and Accountability Act of 1996 (HIPAA; see Chapter 67), a large number of new measures that affect data and IS have been created. These new requirements have not been finalized at the time this chapter was written, but the basic requirements are unlikely to change. These include a new National Provider Identification Number (NPID), new form of PayerID, the required use of certain ANSI X.12N standards, and many security and privacy policies and procedures. Rather than reduplicate a discussion of these requirements, the reader is referred to Chapters 35 and 67 for more detailed discussion. Also, the reader is strongly urged to access Health Care Financing Administration's website at www.hcfa.gov for detailed information on the final regulations.

ELECTRONIC COMMERCE

The Internet has revolutionized commerce in the United States and around the globe. The pace at which the Internet has become a mass medium is unprecedented, reaching a market penetration of 50 million users in less than five years (see Figure 36–1). The value of the Internet as a business tool

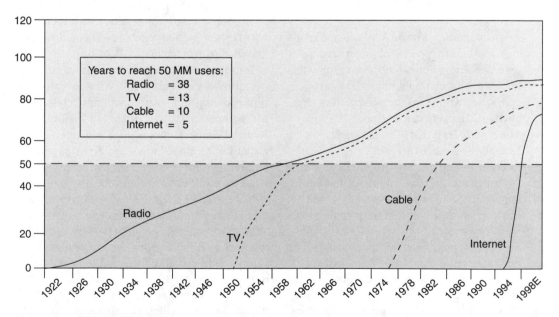

*The pace at which the Internet has become a mass medium is unprecedented, reaching a market penetration of 50 million users in less than five years.

Figure 36–1 The Growth Rate of Mass Media. *Source:* Data from Morgan Stanley Technology Research Estimate, Morgan Stanley Dean Witter and Ernst & Young.

must not be underestimated by provider organizations. The Internet is changing the way business is done as it accomplishes the following:

- blurs geographical boundaries
- creates more efficient markets
- reconstructs value chains
- promotes networks of affiliation
- favors customer-centric offerings
- compresses cycle times
- enables unbounded competition
- values knowledge/trust as scarce

Each of these accomplishments is further illustrated in Exhibit 36–2.

The term commonly used for conducting business using the Internet is e-commerce (for electronic commerce; see also Chapters 35 and 37). E-commerce can be defined as the infrastructure, processes, and business models that allow enterprises to develop, operate efficiently, grow, and diversify in a fully connected world.[12] The health care industry has lagged behind other industries in e-commerce change; the Gartner Group notes as much as a 10-year lag between banking and health. Nevertheless, health care is progressing, primarily because of consumer demands.

Consumers have been provided with knowledge and understanding of how to integrate e-commerce into their lives by banking and other cutting-edge industries. Increasingly, consumer interactions are taking place over the Internet, with a doubling of global use of the World Wide Web (the web) occurring every 100 days.[13] Increasingly sophisticated consumers are beginning to demand the same levels of online performance from health care provider organizations that they demand from other businesses with which they interact. As they become accustomed to solving problems online by using e-commerce solutions provided by retailers, grocery stores, and other businesses, pressure will increase on provider organizations to match this level of online service. As illustrated in Table 36–5, according to the 1999 Healthcare Informatics Pulse Survey, financial managers at health care provider organizations believe that e-commerce will increase in the next 12 months with the groups indicated.

There are three main types of e-commerce, examples of which are shown in Figure 36–2:

Table 36–5 Rapid Growth in E-commerce Predicted

Group	Will Increase Use of eBusiness with Health Care Organizations
Providers	71%
Payers	82%
Patients/members	51%
Suppliers	71%
Other business partners	69%

Courtesy of 1999 Healthcare Informatics, Pulse Survey 1999, Minneapolis, Minnesota.

- B2C: Business to Consumer (Consumer can be defined as patient, physician, payer, or other stakeholder.)
- B2B: Business to Business (See supply chain example.)
- B2E: Business to Employees (See intranet example.)

Traditional health care providers have responded by creating websites that offer patients and physicians general information, as illustrated in Figures 36–3 and 36–4. Although many providers are focusing on B2C, the Gartner Group predicts that B2B e-commerce revenue will be 1000 percent of B2C e-commerce by 2002. This represents an enormous opportunity for providers looking to reduce their operating costs, notably in the area of supply chain operations. It will be important for health care provider organizations to focus on those e-commerce activities that offer them both short-term and long-term value. Although having a presence on the Internet is valuable, it is simply a business card, unless technologies are leveraged that invite a patient to use the site for a variety of purposes (see Figure 36–5 for examples). Although health care provider organizations might be inclined to attempt to be all things to all users, providing patients with links to existing complementary sites is often a good use of capital.

Several national name brand providers have leveraged their brand names and established themselves as highly credible information sites for patients and providers. Examples at the time of

Exhibit 36–2 The Internet Redefines Traditional Business Rules

1. **Blurs Geographical Boundaries**
Time and geographical proximity become less important.
- As the cost of communications decreases, distance becomes increasingly irrelevant.
- Even the smallest companies can now sell products and provide services worldwide.
- Businesses are able to source materials and labor regardless of distance and political boundaries.
- Governments have not yet adopted the legal and regulatory implications.

2. **Creates More Efficient Markets**
As economic search costs decrease, customers become all powerful.
- The Internet helps customers find what they want, when they want it, at the very best price.
- Customer power is increasing, relative to sellers because of better access to information and a greater choice of suppliers.

3. **Reconstructs Value Chains**
Restructures supply and demand chains to maximize efficiency and value.
- Some companies are building direct connections to their end customers, bypassing traditional channels:
  — Greater efficiency and lower prices
  — Enables supplier to learn more about customer needs and build deeper relationships

4. **Promotes Networks of Affiliation**
People and organizations form around common interests and objectives.
- Ubiquitous Internet connectivity
- Enables the formation of communities around interests and affiliations

5. **Favors Customer-Centric Offerings**
Companies are tailoring offerings to individual customer preferences.
- Content providers among the first to offer individualized products, such as WSJ Interactive and My Yahoo!

- A broad range of competitors are personalizing customer interactions:
  — "One-to-one marketing" or "mass customization"
  — Both purchasing and customer service processes
- Over time, the Internet will enable more real-time customization of physical goods.

6. **Compresses Cycle Times**
The pace of change increases as everything becomes connected.
- Information and innovation spread rapidly through growing networks of people and organizations.
- Transaction and product development cycles are reduced through the use of electronic networks.
- Customers increasingly expect "real-time" interactions with businesses.

7. **Enables Unbounded Competition**
Proliferation of entrants because of discontinuities and lower entry barriers.
- New business models are emerging that leverage the changing rules of the competitive environment.
- The result is more formidable for new competitors than in any other time in modern history.
- Internet discontinuities are attracting entrepreneurs and financial capital.

8. **Values Knowledge/Trust As Scarce**
Managing intellectual capital/trust/brand has become a major source of competitive advantage.
- Businesses are seeking to deploy intranets/extranets and information analysis and management applications to
  — Improve knowledge creation, capture, and retention
  — Enhance innovation, communication, and collaboration among employees and business partners

Courtesy of Ernst & Young LLP, 2000, Washington, DC.

publication include sites sponsored by the Mayo Clinic, Intellihealth, and the Cleveland Clinic; these are viewed as sites of leading expert opinion because of name recognition and have acquired a significant "first-to-market" advantage.

A variety of web-based companies have begun to establish themselves as entry points for consumers wishing to gain health information over the Internet; examples at the time of publication include www.webmd.com, www.

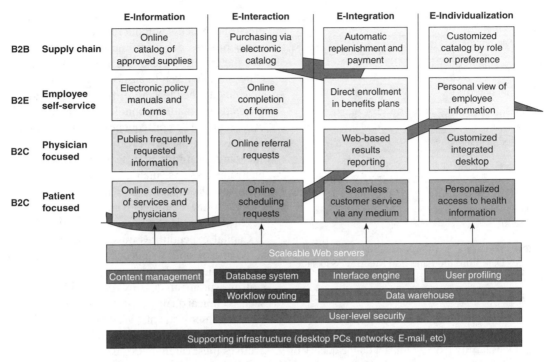

Figure 36–2 Types of E-Commerce Activities. Courtesy of Ernst & Young LLP, 2000, Washington, DC.

intellihealth.com, and www.drkoop.com. These companies, in partnership with major portals such as AOL, Yahoo, Lycos, and media companies such as CBS, CNN, and ABC, have already claimed the health portal opportunity. Portals

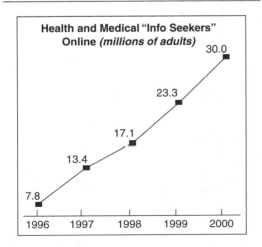

Figure 36–3 Rapid Growth in Use of Internet to Find Health Information. Courtesy of Ernst & Young LLP, 2000, Washington, DC.

such as these provide a good reference point for organizations seeking to design their own websites and represent potential content partners as well.

Provider organizations in the process of developing their e-commerce strategy or reassessing their existing strategy should be able to satisfactorily answer the questions listed in Exhibit 36–3.

CAPITAL BUDGETING FOR INFORMATION TECHNOLOGY

Building this infrastructure will require a great deal of capital investment. It is important to remember that information technology is only a tool, just as bricks and mortar are tools, and the use of any tool needs to be well planned. Simply accelerating the same decision process does not always lead to a superior decision. Before making a capital decision, an administrator should consider the following questions:

• Does this decision make internal operations more efficient in a quantifiable manner?

Figure 36–4 Type of Information Sought by Patients. *Source:* Data from the American Medical Association and Medical Media & Marketing.

- Does it provide us with the opportunity to capture new revenue streams?
- Does it truly have an impact on the quality of the patient care our organization provides?
- Does this technology demonstrate differentiated value in improving the quality of our patients' lives?
- Does it improve our ability to manage care at the individual and population levels?
- Which of the following needs of major stakeholders does this technology meet (see Table 36–6)?

It is important to remember that adding an electronic process without replacing the existing paper process does not improve the efficiency and the effectiveness of the health care system. Care must be taken to ensure that the significant investments health care provider organizations make in information technology result in significant results. The consequences of failure in this objective can be severe. Errors in this capital spending on information technology have serious ramifications, including the possibility of bond rating downgrades. The issues presented by the current reality led to an all time high number of downgrades by Moody's in 1999.[14]

Capital expenditures must be carefully measured in their ability to accelerate a strong return on investment, as determined by traditional financial measurements and by value-added metrics such as clinical quality, customer service, and productivity improvements. When making decisions on how to best use limited capital, health care executives must carefully evaluate the technology's overall benefit. An organization must also be realistic about its ability to successfully implement the technology to drive value for its key stakeholders. The ability to implement—with or without vendor partnership—large, complex information systems will become a core competency for health care provider organizations in the near future. As can be seen in Table 36–7, a number of potential obstacles exist to successfully implementing a new

---

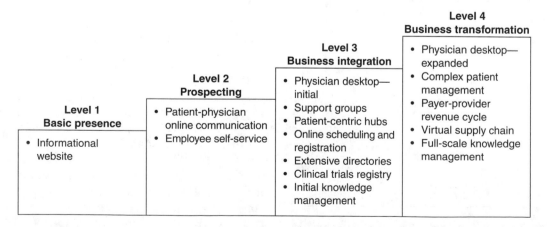

Figure 36–5 Stages of E-Commerce Activity. Courtesy of Ernst & Young LLP, 2000, Washington, DC.

Exhibit 36–3 Key Questions Health Care Provider Organizations Should Ask Themselves in Planning Their E-commerce Strategies

1. Can electronic commerce provide sustainable *competitive advantage* by offering easier access to customers, employees, suppliers, and business partners?
2. How does the organization's e-commerce strategy relate to overall *business, marketing, and branding strategies*?
3. Can electronic commerce significantly *reduce cost* and *drive profitable growth*?
4. What are the *major threats* posed by e-commerce and competitor/customer actions?
5. What are the *expected returns* on investments in electronic commerce?
6. Can the organization obtain *competitive flexibility* and be in a position to respond rapidly as new market opportunities develop?
7. What are the effects of the e-commerce strategy on *time to market and new product development*?
8. What are our *major capability gaps* (technology, skills, organization, process, etc.)?

Source: Courtesy of Ernst & Young LLP, 2000, Washington, DC.

information system (IS). In addition, implementing any system will require organizational change, and it is important not to underestimate the power of human resistance to change.

ORGANIZATIONAL STRUCTURE OF INFORMATION TECHNOLOGY DEPARTMENTS

To best support the delivery/managing of care in health care provider organizations, the IS department must be structured in a manner that makes it responsive not only to an organization's current needs, but challenges it to operate in an anticipatory mode as well.

General Organization Structure and Reporting Relationships

Organizational structure and reporting relationships are vital to the successful management of the IS operations within the health care provider organization. A CIO is necessary to oversee the use of information technology across the entire organization and to represent IS operations on the enterprise's strategic planning committee. The CIO's main responsibility is to align the IS operations with the strategic direction of the organization and to ensure that targeted efficiencies are achieved.

According to the 1999 Healthcare Informatics Pulse Survey, 42 percent of IS departments report to the chief financial officer of the organization. This percentage is expected to decrease as information technology departments are redefined not as a support function for finance but as a key stand-alone operational function. As such, the department should be structured in a manner that ensures that it supports both overall business strategy and clinical and business processes.

CLIENT RELATIONSHIPS

The IS department generally has more customers than any other department within a health care provider organization. Its customers and clients include every staff member who uses the IS and every staff member who uses the data (reports and so forth) produced by the IS. All the constituencies may make requests to the IS department about the format and content of reports, the format and content of user workstation screens, and application errors. This flexibility places a significant responsibility on the department to manage its staff and prioritize user requests.

One of the goals of a progressive IS organization is to help users become more proactive, responsible, and accountable for identifying systems needs and assisting with implementations. To meet the daily and long-term needs of users, as well as patients, an effective IS department must develop an enterprise-wide user support philosophy.

Client Support Philosophy

In the past, most IS departments have operated in a reactive mode with respect to client end-user requests for application enhancements and/or sup-

Table 36–6 What Major Stakeholders of a Health Care Organization Need from Information Technology

Major Stakeholders	What Information Do They Need or Want?	What Tool Will They Use to Access It?
Patients	Specific information to assist in making personal decisions regarding patient care General health and wellness information Information regarding billing statements Logistical information: directions, maps, test directions	*Traditional* Face-to-face Telephone Mail *Future* E-mail Secure Internet site
Providers and support staff	Clinical information regarding a specific patient • Access in the hospital • Access in the office • Access at home Online order entry for laboratory, radiology, and pharmacy Up-to-date decision support for the treatment of various diseases and conditions Real-time assistance in managing chronically ill patients	*Traditional* Paper chart Reference texts *Future* Web-based CPR In-home monitoring devices Online decision-making systems Real-time information regarding clinical advances
Employees	Employee services • Retirement/benefits management • Job openings • Online education and training Knowledge management tools • Internal best practices Policy and procedure manuals	*Traditional* Human resources department Informal networks *Future* Intranet Internet
Payers • Government • Third-party payers • Industry • Small businesses • Employer groups • Self-insured	Organizational performance information • Cost information • Case management • Performance on disease management indicators Financial partnerships • Electronic data exchange • Direct contracting • Auction/barter systems • Electronic bill remittance	*Traditional* Mail Limited EDI capabilities Clearinghouses *Future* Directly connected extranets
Suppliers	Relationship management • Online catalogs • Online purchasing ability • Online order tracking • JIT inventory systems	*Traditional* Paper-based Telephone and personal interaction *Future* Extranets Internet

Source: Courtesy of Ernst & Young LLP, 2000, Washington, DC.

Table 36–7 Barriers to Successful IT Implementation

Barrier	% of Respondents Selecting
Recruiting and retaining high quality IT staff	23
Lack of adequate financial support/budget for IT	16
Difficulty in proving IT quantifiable benefits	15

Source: Reprinted with permission from *10th Annual HIMSS Leadership Survey.* Sponsored by International Business Machines Corporation.

port. Often, the end-user would have to track down an individual within the IS division to issue a request. The schedule of the IS department would often determine the priority level of the request. IS would then react to the request by developing and implementing a solution. Most commonly, the solution would address only the immediate request and not the long-term impact as time became a limiting factor and more requests were being made. In this scenario, the end-user had little input into how the IS department prioritized or completed user requests, and users often became disillusioned and frustrated. In an effort to provide quality community service today, health care provider organizations are implementing quality initiatives throughout their organizations. Effective IS services, whether owned or outsourced, are beginning to develop service level agreements, customer teams, and user satisfaction surveys to provide the level of service expected by their customers.

Service Level Agreements

Under the direction of the CIO, the IS strategic planning committee should develop service level agreements that clearly define the expected level of service that IS operations are to provide to their customers and a recourse for scenarios where the level of service falls short. Service level agreements, also known as guiding prin-

ciples, serve as boundaries regarding expectations, roles, and responsibilities for senior management, the user community, and the IS department. The agreement should address such areas as expectations of support provided by each party, the working relationships among the three parties, how IS-related projects are coordinated from project initiation through postimplementation, and benefits realization. The agreement should also drive the philosophy of the customer teams and satisfaction surveys.

Customer Teams

Today, health care provider organizations are assigning teams to work with each constituency. These teams develop an understanding of the business issues facing the customer and work with the customer to develop systems (people, processes, and technology) to improve an organization's ability to manage care. In this manner, proactive steps are being taken to improve operations and to reduce costs.

OUTSOURCING THE INFORMATION TECHNOLOGY FUNCTION

Although many readers may assume that information technology is an internally managed function, this is not always strictly the case. As a result of the expertise required to purchase, install, and manage IS operations within an organization, many health care companies choose to contract with outside vendors to provide the information technology to meet their needs. For some organizations, outsourcing all or part of their IS operations has significant potential to provide quality customer service while reducing operating costs. The central issue is to examine closely each function that the IS division performs, compare those functions with vendors' products and services, and identify areas that may benefit from outsourcing.

The level of outsourcing, as in other industries, can vary significantly from providing limited application support to providing complete IS staff and technology. Similarly, the types of organizations that provide outsourcing services range from consulting firms, to health care IS hardware and software vendors, to neighboring (noncompeting) or organizationally related health care organizations with excess resources.

Options exist for organizations that wish to maintain greater control over information technology operations. As health care provider organizations realize the value of partnering with outside vendors to address noncore activities, they can expect to see benefits, including:

- access to industry best practices, which results in cost decreases over time as the organization is able to move toward "best-in-class" operations through process, technology, and organizational transformation
- predeveloped solutions that are specifically tailored to the needs of individual health care provider organizations, offering a much more rapid implementation and leading to a quicker return on investment

Outsourcing has (or can have) many benefits. The most notable benefit is when another company, whose service is its core competency, can provide the service in a more cost-effective and cost-efficient manner than can be achieved by providing the service in house. Outsourcing can allow an organization to focus on its core business while providing access to state-of-the-art technology and scarce resources. From a cost standpoint, it can preserve capital resources while reducing and providing for predictable operating costs. Some additional benefits include guaranteed levels of service, shared risk, and improved user satisfaction.

As in seen in Table 36–8, the number of organizations that outsource IT functions grew by 24 percent in 1999. Areas in information technology that commonly reap benefits from outsourcing are management, purchasing, hardware support and maintenance, employee training, specific application support, and application development. Outsourcing the purchasing function often leads to volume discounts, consistencies among purchased equipment, and better inventory tracking and control. Outsourcing other areas often improves quality while reducing nec-

Table 36–8 IT Outsourcing Continues To Increase

Outsourced Function	1998 (%)	1999 (%)
Applications support	11	14
PC support	11	13
Technical support	3	12
Website support	7	12

Source: Reprinted with permission from *10th Annual HIMSS Leadership Survey.* Sponsored by International Business Machines Corporation.

essary staffing levels. Again, each area being considered for outsourcing should be examined closely and weighed against the value of ownership of that area. Many of the outsourcing contracts over the past five years have involved some form of upfront payment by the vendor. Some of the payments provided cash for capital equipment acquired as part of the contract. In return, the vendor received a long-term annuity agreement. The term, usually 10 to 15 years, enabled the vendor to begin to expect a certain level of cash flow. It was this guaranteed cash flow that enabled many of the vendors to experience substantial increases in the value of their companies. Because the cost of technology (most notably hardware) has dropped dramatically, however, clients now realize that they are paying far more than the vendor's true cost plus margin. It is for this reason, along with other lesser issues, that many of the outsourcing agreements of the past are being renegotiated. Health care provider organizations should regard outsourcing as an option when deciding to focus on core services.

CONCLUSION: INFORMATION TECHNOLOGY WILL PLAY A KEY ROLE IN IMPROVING THE HEALTH CARE PROVIDER ORGANIZATION'S ABILITY TO MANAGE CARE

"Health care delivery systems need flexibility with empowered users to meet and surpass the competition in managed care entrainments. Ideally, enterprise data could be transformed into strategic information and implemented via package parameters. Clerical workers would be converted to knowledge workers, empowered with preconceived information that would be used during the operations of health care delivery."[15]

Health care in the 1990s was characterized by tremendous change, the need to reduce costs overall within the industry, and the development of new processes and methods to provide better patient care. In 1994, Wendy Herr, vice president of the Healthcare Financial Management Association, testified before the House Ways and Means Health Care Subcommittee. In urging Congress to adopt standard electronic patient and processing practices for health care, Herr advocated "the development of legislation to simplify health care administrative processes rather than waiting for a complete reform package."[16] Even without such legislation, health care provider organizations throughout the United States have been diligently working to streamline their processes and invent new ways to reduce operating costs while providing high-quality care to the patient.

Health care provider organizations will use information technology to link disparate parts of the enterprise, provide clinicians with the latest information, and increase operational efficiency. Information technology can be leveraged to bridge the gap between the health care system currently in place and the health care system patients need. The Internet will be but one technology vehicle to address the future needs of providers of care. Information technology will be the key to a health care provider organization's ability to thrive and compete successfully in the health care marketplace.

REFERENCES

1. M. Millenson, *Demanding Medical Excellence* (Chicago: The University of Chicago Press, 1997), 91.

2. *An Overview of the BBA*. Published on the Web at www.aha.org/bba/aboutbba.html

3. J.D. Ladd and R.G. Reese, Traveling the Information Superhighway, *Michigan Hospitals* 30(2) (1994), 189.

4. W. H. Inmon, *Building the Data Warehouse* (New York: Wiley, 1993).

5. R. E. Gilbreath, Health Care Data Repositories: Components and a Model, *Healthcare Information Management* 9 (1995).

6. Institute of Medicine, *The Computer-Based Patient Record: An Essential Technology for Health Care* (Institute of Medicine, 1991).

7. Institute of Medicine, *The Computer-Based Patient Record*.

8. Ladd and Reese, Traveling the Information Superhighway, 131

9. 10th Annual HIMSS Leadership Survey Sponsored by IBM. Published on the web at http://www.himss.org/survey/.

10. J. Fitchett, Knowledge Management in Health Care. *Advance*: January 1998.

11. J. Fitchett, Knowledge Management in Health Care. *Advance*: January 1998.

12. E. Purchase and M. West, *Electronic Commerce Platforms and Applications* (Gartner Group, 1999), 1.

13. ECommerce is the force. Kennedy Global IT Consulting Report. June 1999.

14. Credit Deterioration Continues for U.S. Not-for-Profit Hospitals. *Moody's Second Quarter 1999 Update*, 3.

15. Reynolds, Informatting the IDS, 98.

16. Ladd and Reese, Traveling the Information Superhighway.

SUGGESTED READING

Majzun, R., and Clarke, K. 1999. Can Information Technology Save Health Care Quality? *Group Practice Journal*, May, 13–17.

Solovy, A., and Serb, C. 1999. Health Care's 100 Most Wired. *Hospitals and Health Networks*, February, 43–51.

Taylor, C. The eVolution of Healthcare. Industry white paper published on the web at www.eoffering.com.

CHAPTER 37

Electronic Commerce in Managed Health Care

Britton L. Pim and Sean D. Kenny

Electronic commerce (e-commerce) is dramatically changing the way businesses interact with customers, with other businesses, and even internally within a business's own operations. E-commerce is redesigning many of the fundamental business processes. E-commerce is defined as any automated exchange of goods or information. Although e-commerce is more than just those exchanges enabled by the Internet, the prolific growth in the use of the Internet (see Figure 37–1) represents the single largest contributing factor to the phenomenal growth of e-commerce.

The Internet is the most revolutionary information tool to come along since radio and television. In the four short years since the Internet first came

Britton Pim is a Manager in Ernst & Young's Health Consulting Practice. Within health care his focus has been on managed care. More recently, he has spent considerable time assisting clients understand the implications of e-commerce on managed care organizations. Before joining Ernst & Young LLP, he was an Internal Auditor for Blue Cross and Blue Shield of Ohio.

Sean Kenny is the National Director of Managed Care Consulting for Ernst & Young.

The authors wish to acknowledge Lee Clark, a Consultant for Ernst & Young LLP and John Iozzia, a Senior Consultant for Ernst & Young LLP. Craig Fagin, Ernst & Young LLP Senior Consultant; Rachel Hall, Ernst & Young LLP Senior Manager; Mary Edwards, Ernst & Young LLP Partner; and George Van Antwerp, Director of Alliances, Firepond also contributed their time to review and advise on parts of this chapter.

into widespread commercial and consumer use, it has fundamentally altered the way we communicate and transact business. The Internet has significantly lowered the costs of transmitting information within and between firms, resulting in efficiency and productivity improvements. As a result, the technology analysis firm Forrester predicts that Internet-based e-commerce will exceed $1.3 trillion in 2003.[1]

E-COMMERCE IN HEALTH CARE

Health care represents the single largest sector of the U.S. economy, $1 trillion, or 14 percent of the gross domestic product (GDP). To quote Caren Taylor in *The E*Volution of Health Care*: "While the Internet has transformed other sectors of the economy more rapidly, the health care industry, a perennial laggard when it comes to adopting new information technologies, has only recently joint the Internet Bandwagon."[2] The dynamics of the health care sector make it an ideal candidate for e-commerce. It has been estimated that nearly $250 billion in health care spending can be attributed to redundant and unnecessary services and administration. E-commerce represents one avenue through which these excessive costs can be controlled. E*OFFERING believes that by 2003, the value of the eHealth market will exceed $205 billion.[3] Today, that market is relatively untapped. However, managed care organizations (MCOs) face several key trends that will drive the industry to embrace e-commerce.

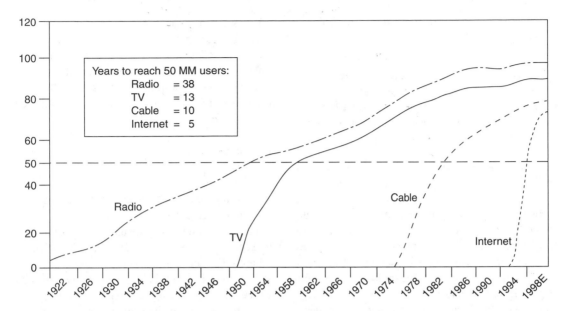

Figure 37–1 Growth of Acceptance of Internet Use. *Source:* Data from Morgan Stanley Technology Research Estimate, Morgan Stanley Dean Witter, and Ernst & Young.

The Health Insurance Portability and Accountability Act of 1996 (HIPAA) Mandate Will Catalyze Explosive Growth of Internet-Based Business-to-Business e-commerce

At present, most non-Medicare/Medicaid electronic claims are processed by clearinghouses, which transform claims from provider formats into a myriad of proprietary payer formats. But the Department of Health and Human Services (DHHS) standards for health care administrative and financial transactions will eliminate proprietary data field definitions for the most important data and perhaps eliminate the need for this function.[4] In addition, the Internet is the ideal choice for aggregating and delivering transactions from many sources to many destinations. The reader is strongly urged to read Chapters 35 and 67 for more discussion of HIPAA because this law has a major impact on how e-commerce will need to be carried out in health care.

Premium Compression in Health Plans Will Continue To Press toward Price Parity, Leaving Service and Quality as the Main Differentiators

Market forces have recently allowed health plans to increase premiums, but market pressures will also continue to exert downward pressure on premiums. To deal with this pressure, MCOs are turning to technology to improve administrative efficiency and enhance connectivity with providers, employers, and members. Health plans that are able to demonstrate quality customer service through faster, effective, and efficient response to customer calls and resolution of issues will have a competitive advantage in the market. In addition, there is an opportunity for plans to use connectivity and the concepts of mass customization to revolutionize the management of care to lower medical costs through case and disease management, patient education and outreach, and other forms of medical care management. The reader is referred to all of Part

III for discussions on many medical management activities.

The Rise in Empowered, Technologically Savvy Consumers and Providers Is Forcing Payers To Take a Closer Look at the Internet and Reach Their Customers through New Distribution Channels

Customers are demanding to be educated and effective advocates for their own health care. Members of health maintenance organizations (HMOs) and other managed care plans demand to be able to select and change their primary care physician (PCP; see Chapter 7). It is estimated that by 2003, more than 20 percent of all consumers will use Internet technology to do their own clinical research and communicate with providers. In addition, the Internet is increasing physician use of technology. The method and delivery of care is expected to change based on the reach and "mass customization" capabilities provided by e-commerce and new technologies. The physician's office will no longer be the primary hub; more and more care will become virtual and connected such that the patient may never leave the home for a diagnosis to be reached, care ordered, drugs delivered, and recovery to begin. Even the way in which payments are determined and funds moved will change.

Capital Markets Have Begun To Ask Publicly Held MCOs about Their e-commerce Strategies

Having recognized the significance of e-commerce, equities and debt analysts have begun to give serious consideration to MCOs' e-commerce capabilities and strategies when determining stock valuations and bond ratings.

E-COMMERCE TECHNOLOGIES

The Internet is largely responsible for the tremendous growth in e-commerce. However, e-commerce is not limited to the Internet. E-commerce is any electronic means through which businesses and consumers interact or transact business. With that in mind, other technologies such as electronic data interchange (EDI), electronic funds transfer (EFT), and interactive voice response (IVR) represent additional, viable e-commerce solutions. The section that follows describes the most common e-commerce technologies in more detail.

Internet/Intranet

The Internet

The Internet, or the "Net" as it is commonly known, is a global arrangement of computer networks designed to provide users with the ability to access and exchange information with any other online computer (subject to security restrictions). Originally conceived by the Advanced Research Projects Agency (ARPA) in 1969 to provide university research facilities with the means to electronically communicate, the Internet has evolved into a self-sustaining public facility accessible to hundreds of millions of people worldwide.

In 1995, the Federal Networking Council (FNC) passed a resolution defining the term Internet. This definition was developed in consultation with the leadership of the Internet and intellectual property rights (IPR) communities. That definition is as follows:

"Internet" refers to the global information system that:

> (i) Is logically linked together by a globally unique address space based on the Internet Protocol (IP) or its subsequent extensions/follow-ons;
>
> (ii) Is able to support communications using the Transmission Control Protocol/Internet Protocol (TCP/IP) standards or its subsequent extensions/follow-ons and/or other IP-compatible protocols; and
>
> (iii) Provides, uses, or makes accessible, either publicly or privately, high-level services layered on the communications and related infrastructure described herein.

Communicating via the Internet has become an increasingly mainstream way for people to exchange ideas. Electronic mail (e-mail) is the most widely used application of the Internet and facilitates the expeditious exchange of written transactions. Other developments in Internet communications include internet relay chat, which allows real-time online "chat" sessions and, more recently, the emergence of new hardware and software that allow real-time voice and video conferencing over the Net.

The World Wide Web, or the "Web," has become the most widely used part of the Internet. With a Web browser, users can access millions of pages of information contained within various websites. As the Web becomes more pervasive in our society, businesses and individual users alike will increasingly find ways to incorporate the Web into day-to-day activities, such as currently exist for online banking and purchasing.

Intranet

As defined by the Gartner Group, Intranets represent a deployment model based on the adoption, adaptation, and integration of Internet-derived technologies and communications protocols for use in internal information systems. An intranet is a network that uses common Internet-based technology but that is internal to a specific organizational structure and is secured from, or disconnected from, the global Internet, typically by means of a "firewall."[5]

Deployment of intranets within companies, especially technology-driven enterprises, has steadily increased. The most common use of a company intranet is Web publishing. Web publishing presents companies with a low-cost way to provide employees with useful, current information covering a broad range of topics, such as company newsletters and employee benefit information. Intranets also facilitate the use of various collaborative applications. E-mail, discussion groups, chat rooms, and audio/video conferencing are examples of such applications.

Enterprises have also begun to use Intranets to support internal software development and deployment of packages for line of business applications. This may include anything from cus-

tomer or employee self-service packages to deployment of mission-critical applications.

Although Intranets provide many benefits, their fiscal returns are not easily quantified. Companies often encounter difficulty when attempting to measure the return on Intranet implementations because many initiatives are not intended to generate revenue. Examples of such nonrevenue-generating gains are improved employee satisfaction, information sharing, and decision making.

Interactive Voice Response (IVR)/Voice Response Unit (VRU)

IVR or voice response unit (VRU) is a set of technologies that enable callers to use a set of voice or touch-tone commands to navigate and execute commands from a computer-based menu system (automated attendants may be included in an IVR or voice mail system to provide stand-alone, automated functionality). IVR/VRU systems can be connected to customer service and support systems, such as help desks and clinical health information or triage systems that provide front-line support with back-end linkage for customer interaction.[6]

There are four types of IVR/VRU applications: informational, transactional, prescreening, and personalized. Over the next five years, most applications will continue to be informational and transactional. Prescreening and personalized applications will constitute only 15 percent and 5 percent, respectively. The following is a description of each of the four types of IVR/VRU applications.[7]

Informational IVR Applications

Informational IVR applications provide callers with basic information, such as credit card account information (i.e., balances, last payment). Informational applications are the easiest types to implement and are the most common.

Transactional IVR Applications

Transactional IVR applications are scripts that promote interaction with the callers by asking questions and allowing the caller to respond by voice or touch-tone. Once a reply has been entered, the system can then process the response and react accordingly. Examples of such applications include banking transactions (such as stop payments or balance transfers), requesting specific merchandise catalogs, ordering refills of maintenance prescriptions, enrolling in a health plan, choosing a PCP, or verifying the status of a claim. Transactional applications can be used in conjunction with informational applications.

Prescreening IVR Applications

Prescreening IVR application scripts can identify the caller and then provide the caller with menu options applicable only to him or her. An example of such an application could be when a credit card company would provide a caller with the option to increase his or her account spending limit. This option would be provided only if the caller satisfied a predetermined set of rules to determine creditworthiness. Although prescreening applications are not very common today, as scripting technologies improve and companies seek to increase IVR use, deployment of these applications will increase.

Personalized IVR Applications

Personalized IVR applications use a caller's preferences to create a personalized script. These scripts vary in sophistication and may be placed in one of three categories:

- The simplest method is a combination of prescreening and personalization. With this method, the organization develops a number of scripts and then presents the predefined "customized" script to the different calling groups on the basis of different criteria.
- A second approach allows customers to define their own scripts, as well as the order in which the IVR options are presented.
- The most advanced and challenging approach involves the IVR compiling a script while the caller is on the line. In this case, the IVR assesses the value of the caller to the institution, determines relevant options, and then presents them to the caller.

When scripts are well designed and properly implemented, IVR systems are powerful self-service tools. However, IVR/VRU systems do not provide solutions to all business situations. In certain situations, these systems will fail to support the business objectives. Such situations may include high-value customers, who demand personalized service; high-value transactions; and complex informational transactions where the client desires direct agent expertise.

Imaging and Optical Character Recognition

Document imaging is the online storage, retrieval, and management of electronic images of documents. The primary method of capturing images is by scanning paper documents. Optical character recognition (OCR) refers to software that is able to convert information from the scanned-in paper document into electronic data (e.g., convert printed text into the correct computer characters). Documents can then be shared by all users on a network and routed by computer according to assigned work flows.[8]

The need for reducing costs has prompted many MCOs to invest in imaging and workflow technologies. Once implemented, these systems will streamline processes, gain access to electronic or scanned paper information, and reduce administrative costs.

Imaging and workflow systems are composed of integrated hardware and software that manage the massive amounts of information MCOs handle and process every day. They facilitate quicker, more efficient employee performance without wasting resources on huge amounts of paper documents. Organizations that expect to rely heavily on OCR for a high volume type of transaction from a defined population (e.g., paper claims from physicians) may use forms that are printed in red "drop out" ink, so that the OCR software eliminates anything in red, thereby decreasing errors based on characters written in such a way as to cause the form itself to interfere with the ability to recognize a character. In all OCR systems, there will be a small number of forms that the OCR software cannot interpret, and manual intervention is then required; the number of manual interventions, however, is enormously reduced compared with wholly manual data entry of paper forms.

As it pertains to MCOs, document imaging/management offers several benefits.[9] The following are examples of such benefits.

Enrollment

Document imaging/management allows enrollment forms to be scanned and the information to be read electronically from the images and turned into discrete data fields, allowing immediate response to questions regarding enrollment status; electronic queues can be created to flag forms with incomplete or inaccurate information; any enrollment form can be accessed for updating.

Claims

Document imaging/management automates most of the data entry process and reduces turnaround time for medical claim forms; cuts the operating expenses of the manual claims-logging process; increases claims processing and enables better customer service; integrates with the host adjudication system; and increases data accuracy with a single entry, increasing both precision and speed.

Customer Service

Document imaging/management makes scanned documents available for immediate response to customer inquiries, allowing customers to receive answers to their questions the first time they call; eliminates lengthy searches for lost or misfiled documents; logs routing and management of issues in the system; manages all forms of information—paper documents, faxes, e-mail, and electronic claims (EDI)

Medical Review

Document imaging/management combines documents and medical images into a single presentation designed for clinicians and allows clinicians to electronically sign scanned documents.

Electronic Funds Transfer

Before the 1970s, the paper check was the primary means of payment for products and services. As business grew, this form of payment became more labor intensive and expensive, driving organizations to seek relief from the mounting cost.

In the early 1970s the automated clearing-house (ACH) network was developed to facilitate the transfer of funds between financial institutions. Previously a paper check from the purchaser was verified by the host financial institution, and the funds were physically routed to the financial institution of the vendor. This process would be more complicated if the financial institutions resided in different federal reserve districts. In the manual environment, a check is handled many times and can remain in the work queue for several days. It may even become lost, thus preventing prompt payment. The revenue cycle for an organization is greatly impacted in a manual environment.

The ACH network was developed to facilitate EFT between financial institutions. The role of the ACH is to act as the "clearinghouse" of debits and credits of funds as they are moved between institutions. This network began as a series of regional networks that were joined by agreeing on common payment protocols and standards. The National Automate Clearing House Association (NACHA) oversees these protocols and standards for the regional ACHs. The first use of ACH/EFT technology was for payroll payments to employees. Rather than cut an actual check, the employer would gather information about the employee's financial institution and arrange to have funds transferred electronically each pay period. This eliminated excessive paper cost and check-handling cost.

Shortly thereafter, the federal government adopted the ACH/EFT technology for payment of Social Security benefits. The recipient would be required to provide information about his or her financial institution. Payments would be made directly to the recipient by EFT.

The use of ACH/EFT in the private sector lagged behind the federal government for several years. However, the NACHA embarked on several national campaigns to encourage individuals to participate in direct-deposit programs. At present more than 50 percent of employees are enrolled in direct-deposit programs; this figure is predicted to continue to rise over the next few years.[10]

The benefits of ACH/EFT include lower transaction costs, increased speed of transaction, and less handling of checks. On average, by shifting to EFT-type transactions, firms can save more than 60 percent over the cost of a traditional paper-based transaction.[11] In addition, the electronic medium accelerates the flow of cash, improving revenue cycles and providing more working capital. Last, because an ACH processes electronic debits and credits, there is a decreased chance that a payment will be lost or entered into the system incorrectly.

Currently at hand is the issue of increasing the penetration of this technology. ACH/EFT is particularly useful for high-volume, low-dollar transactions that occur on a regular basis. Provider claims and capitation payments are ideal candidates for EFT.

Electronic Data Interchange

Before the advent of electronic technology, business transactions were, by necessity, carried out manually. As computer technology improved, businesses leveraged this technology to improve the efficiency and effectiveness of business transactions. EDI was a key technology used in transforming business processes.

EDI technology allows an organization to do more than just share information; it enables an organization to engage in transactions with its partners with increased efficiency and effectiveness. EDI surpasses simple electronic mail capabilities in that its primary functionality enables automated transactions such as order fulfillment or inventory management.

To engage in EDI, organizations must first come together to agree on the common standard by which the transactions will occur. Once the physical network is established, EDI translates the initiator's transaction information into that standardized electronic format and transmits the information electronically. Carriers, called value added networks (VANs), develop and own the networks on which the information is transmitted. This encoded information is received by the recipient, where it is translated into the recipient's format and acted on.

The advantages of EDI reside in its speed, its ability to reduce data entry errors, its reduction of paper and administrative overhead costs, and the manner in which it brings business partners closer together. First, the electronic medium allows transactions to move more quickly than if they were done by hand. This translates into reduced product life cycle times, compressed revenue collection times, and improved customer service times, all of which have significant financial implications. Because transactional data are touched by fewer hands in the EDI environment, there is a greater degree of data integrity and a decreased chance that data will be entered incorrectly. This reduces time spent correcting errors that may occur in a manual environment. The electronic medium eliminates the need for paper and head count to move the paper, reducing operational expenses. Finally, because business partners must agree on a common standard, this brings the business closer to its suppliers and customers, resulting in improved relations that benefit both organizations.

There are several disadvantages of EDI technology. First, electronic transmission standards do not typically translate across industry lines, thus preventing an organization from being able to develop connections to other organizations outside the industry. Moreover, it is cost prohibitive for smaller organizations to purchase the requisite EDI network hardware to engage in this type of transaction with larger organizations. In order for a small organization to use EDI, an intermediary must be used (e.g., an electronic claims company that collects a paper bill from physicians and converts the data into an electronic format for transmission to a payer). This intermediary obviously adds to the cost although, on a net basis, the cost of transactions may still be reduced compared with paper-based transactions.

The closed nature of the EDI network environment can severely limit the access an organization may have to potential markets, suppliers, and partners. The future of EDI will depend on its integration with Internet technology, which has become more ubiquitous and more easily accessed by a wider market.

E-commerce Technologies Conclusion

Today, the technologies described in this section are distinct technologies that each offer different advantages or disadvantages given different applications. IVR, for instance, works well for checking the status of a claim but would not be an efficient solution for entering large volumes of claims. However, as future technical developments are made at a faster and faster pace, the line between these technologies will

begin to fade. For example, many industry experts note that telephone calls by way of the Internet are becoming commonplace.

E-COMMERCE FUNCTIONALITY

Today, the question for MCOs is not whether they embrace e-commerce or not, but rather, to what degree they embrace e-commerce. E-commerce provides an effective means to enable many MCOs' current business processes. A broad array of managed care transactions even today can be completed by means of the Internet, as described in Table 37–1, adapted from a 1999 Ernst &Young payer e-commerce study. The data in that study reveal that most payers as of 1999 had tackled the static (or look-up) category; many had moved into delivering interactive functionality, and only a few had even attempted to deliver semi-

---

Table 37–1 Categories of Internet Transactions by MCOs—1999

Static	Interactive	Semi-Integrated	Integrated Processing
• Basic health/wellness information • Formulary • Basic product descriptions • Practice guidelines • Provider listings	• Basic health assessment • Provider directories with sorting by attributes, and map creation • PCP change • Basic member changes (address) • Request new ID • Rx refill ordering	• Benefits inquiry • Claim status inquiry • Eligibility inquiry • Online enrollment for existing accounts • Initial PCP selection • Capture of referral authorizations • Account claim, cost, and utilization reports	• Employer-based eligibility maintenance • Online product selection, sales, and enrollment of new business • Online proposal generation and quotes • Online ability to provide underwriting, pricing, and installation of new groups • Authorizations and precertifications based on rules-based algorithms • Direct claims submissions • EFT and electronic EOBs to providers and consumers

Courtesy of Ernst & Young LLP, 2000, Washington, DC.

integrated functionality.[12] These categories are described further in the following.

The reader will note that the areas of claims submission and EFT, listed under the category of integrated processing, are currently undertaken by means of EDI using proprietary VANs rather than by means of the Internet. However, at the time of publication, several new Internet companies began to move into that market space to perform those functions as an intermediary between payers, providers, and consumers. As with many Internet startups (collectively referred to as "dot coms"), full and actual functionality has yet to follow the promise. A key reason for this is the need to integrate with legacy applications—what matters is not how quickly the intermediary can drop information at the plan's doorstep, but how quickly the information exchange can be fully completed through the legacy environment such that the next information provided by the site is already updated with the last information. For instance, if a member selects a PCP by means of an Internet site, that change must also update the legacy system such that the provider sees that patient on his or her list view, and the operational areas of the health plan (e.g., claims, enrollment) also see the updated information as soon as it is entered.

The use of these new intermediary companies is by no means a clear direction for health plans or providers to take. The presence of an intermediary is always something that any business must evaluate for the benefits versus the risk of having another company between itself and its constituencies (e.g., between a health plan and the physicians, the members, or the customers). Some plans will choose to develop capabilities that make it easy for all constituents to access all appropriate functions directly by way of the Internet. On the other hand, many physicians will be inclined to deal only with one company that in turn will interface with the variety of health plans and governmental programs. With the advent of the new American National Standards Institute (ASNI) standards noted earlier, this issue becomes more complex, but also enables an intermediary to more easily provide uniform data exchange with a variety of health plans.

In all events, if a health plan is unable to effectively carry out e-commerce, the use of an intermediary can make sense (assuming that the intermediary is not selling vaporware, and can actually do what it says). When working with such companies, the question looming for plans, and to a lesser degree providers, is how to take advantage of what these intermediaries can offer in the way of user-friendly portals by integrating and interfacing with legacy environments.

Static

The simplest category of e-commerce functionality for MCOs to deliver is the static category. In this category, MCOs are just making information available to Internet site visitors. This information includes general company and product information, basic health and wellness information, a listing of participating providers, or a drug formulary. At this stage, MCOs are not able to transact business by means of any electronic means. Most MCOs have effectively tackled this level of functionality. Having an Internet site is an expectation of the market, not a differentiator for the market. It is therefore quickly becoming the lowest common denominator in the e-commerce marketplace.

Interactive

As MCOs look to deliver interactive functionality, they develop the ability for some constituents to complete transactions in some self-service manner. A common example of a function midway between static and interactive would be a provider directory that allows a member to search and select providers using a variety of attributes (e.g., specialty, location, language, and so forth) and be able to have a map to that physician's office created based on whatever address the member chooses to start from (usually home).

Other examples of interactive functionality include online PCP changes, basic member changes, or ordering a replacement ID card. Very often, at this stage MCOs have manual back-end processes in place to complete what they hope the consumer will perceive as electronic transactions. The early benefits of this stage are that an MCO can give the outward appearance that it has begun to develop e-commerce capabilities. The downside of this stage is that MCOs will not receive the cost-savings benefits that are available from true e-commerce. In addition, they run the risk of creating an expectation with consumers of real-time response when in fact there has been no significant change to response times for any of the functions. When organizations reach the Web, the expectations of the consumer are raised—they expect fast response, communication capabilities, customized response, and an ability to complete a transaction.

Semi-Integrated

As MCOs start to deliver semi-integrated functionality, external stakeholders, as well as the MCO itself, start to realize the potential benefits of true e-commerce. The unique feature that semi-integrated functionality has over static or interactive functionality is that front-end applications that interface with external stakeholders are integrated with back-end transaction systems and data stores. Members and providers have more self-service options available. This is a benefit to them because they, very often, can accomplish what is necessary without ever having to talk to a call representative. Furthermore, they can do these things at times that are convenient for them, not just during the hours in which the call center is open. This is a benefit to the health plan because it cuts down on the volume of inbound live calls and the labor and time required to generate requested information. The most common examples of this include the ability to determine the status of a claim, submission and status of authorizations, and eligibility determinations.

Integrated

The biggest difference between integrated and semi-integrated is the functionality and volume of transactions. In semi-integrated, the enabled functions are inquiry-type functions for the most part. Only by moving into the integrated stage can MCOs really achieve the full benefits of true e-commerce. In the integrated stage, MCOs look to e-commerce–enabling technologies to complete large-volume transactions such as enrollment and eligibility maintenance, claims processing, and claims and capitation payments. In addition, the ability to achieve real-time reach during the care continuum is achieved. For instance, referrals are done in real time, with automated approval and notification to the specialist, online scheduling for the specialist, and exchange of medical notes and records between referring physician and specialist.

Note that for purposes of discussing e-commerce, we are referring to these transactions as occurring through the Internet, not through proprietary systems described earlier. This requires standards applicable to a broad constituency, as discussed later. Table 37–2 illustrates examples of managed care e-commerce functionality by external constituent.

EXTERNAL IMPACT

To fully understand the impact e-commerce will have on MCOs, it is useful to examine the impact e-commerce will have on an MCO's external constituents. This recognizes that as e-commerce evolves, the divisions between internal and external constituents blur; but for purposes of this discussion, they are addressed separately.

Employers

Implementation of e-commerce–enabling technologies will empower employers in the Internet-connected economy. The benefits for the employer include ease of access to information, immediate bill presentation and payment, online utilization and cost reporting, and eligibility maintenance. Employers can immediately update their eligibility information and delete the names of employees that will not be covered in the future to ensure accurate billing. They will be able to maintain current provider directories for locations throughout the country. Employers

Table 37–2 Categories of Managed Care E-Commerce by External Constituent

Employer	Member	Providers	Broker/Producer
• Online utilization and cost reporting • Electronic bill presentation and payment • Verify/change employee/dependent eligibility • Ability to print customized directories • Review claims status online	• Provider information online (maps, directions, ability to change PCPs) • Online eligibility and benefits • Online claim status • Online ID cards • Online inquiries • Profile-based information delivery • Proactive disease management	• Online authorization and precertification • Online referrals • Online claim submission • Electronic capitation payments and reports • Online eligibility and benefits • Online formulary • Link to online pharmacy for real-time shipment of drugs	• Online product information • Online underwriting and pricing for standard products • Electronic proposal preparation and delivery • Internet lead generation • Direct sales to consumers

Courtesy of Ernst & Young LLP, 2000, Washington, DC.

and insurers are developing Internet sites where employees can immediately access the provider panel and gain information about coverage through e-mail or a frequently asked questions site. Detailed information on the nature of medical costs will enable the employer to institute programs of prevention and better predict utilization patterns. Enrollment forms will be online, reducing the chance for error in desired coverage and deductions from employee compensation. All these benefits can reduce human resources staff and save cost for the employer.

Members

The member's benefits are numerous and cross multiple spectrums. A member can gain information online about his or her physician, including maps, directions, physician education histories, and other relevant physician information 24 hours a day. Members will not be limited to customer service hours or wait times for assistance. Patients through an effective managed care Internet site can verify eligibility, change PCPs, educate themselves regarding benefits, and determine claim and referral status. Members are also able to order prescription drugs

online from local pharmacies or mail-order firms. Members have access to relevant clinical information and may be directed in the management of their specific medical problems.

Providers

Providers benefit from effective use of the Internet. Examples include reduced staff and time necessary for submitting and verifying referrals to providers of clinical services. They will have a direct link to pharmacies and online formularies for simplifying ordering prescriptions and refills. Online authorization and precertification by the insurer allows the provider to gain immediate information regarding the patient's authorization status for services. The provider has the ability to obtain information on patients' benefits and their eligibility for receiving benefits on an in-network or out-of-network basis, or even if the patient is eligible for coverage at all (a nontrivial issue for all providers). Access to information on patient copayments and deductibles also simplifies the payment process. It can also be possible to link to other types of transactions; for example, accessing Internet banking (e.g., by means of a commercial credit card) to combine the collection of the member's copayment with the submission of the claim to the health plan.

Brokers/Producers

Brokers can use the Internet to improve their delivery, speed, and access to information. Common uses pertain to proposal generation and pricing of products. Brokers can quickly send information to alternative insurers to obtain quotes in a virtual online auction. The bids and necessary underwriting for revised quotes can easily be refined on the basis of employer preferences through use of the Internet. Plans will offer more alternatives for coverage of health, life, dental, disability, vision, long-term care, medical reimbursement, and dependent care. Other impacts are the ability to quickly transition employees between plans and explain programs to employees for more appropriate enrollment.

Last, a small but increasing number of brokers operate solely by means of the Internet and never have face-to-face interactions with customers. In this model, the underwriting and product offering processes are highly automated. Depending on how state and federal laws are promulgated in years to come, this type of health coverage distribution channel for individuals and small businesses could become a significant segment of the market.

INTERNAL E-COMMERCE OPPORTUNITIES

All the aforementioned functionality has been focused on external constituents, for example, employers, members, and providers. Internally, MCOs can use e-commerce–enabling technologies to improve operations as well. Knowledge management represents one of the most significant internal opportunities to use e-commerce–enabling technologies. Knowledge management is the efficient capture, indexing, electronic storage, and easy retrieval of an organization's information for effective future reuse.

As an example of a type of knowledge management that is both internal and external, customer proposal responses represent an ideal opportunity for knowledge management. Once an MCO has prepared a proposal for an employer group, it should be cataloged and saved electronically for future use. Then, in the future, when the MCO is presented with another proposal opportunity, rather than expending the effort to re-create a response from scratch, it can pull from existing responses to quickly create a response that is commensurate with the existing proposal needs. This decreases the effort necessary to produce proposal responses and also allows for responses that are more consistent over time.

Policy and procedure manuals represent a highly important knowledge management opportunity for MCOs. The task of keeping current, printed versions of policy and procedure manuals for claims processors, for example, is extremely arduous for any MCO. However, if this information were published online using Intranet technology (including easy links from claims systems to the relevant policies), claims processors would have easy access to the most current and up-to-date versions.

Proposals and policy and procedure manuals represent only two common knowledge management opportunities for MCOs. Provider contracts, medical protocols, disease management, and enrollment collateral are just a few of the many other knowledge management opportunities. All these and others could be stored electronically, to allow MCO employees Intranet access for future reuse. Once they are available online for employees, it is a short leap to extending the information to the external customer for self-service purposes.

An example of a more advanced use of internal e-commerce is in underwriting and rating of accounts (see Chapters 48 through 51). The usual process of moving a new or renewal case through underwriting and rating is time consuming and an often frustrating step in an MCO's sales process. Varying degrees of automation may improve efficiencies somewhat, but a fully functional Intranet capability would allow field sales personnel (and external brokers and agents through the Internet, as noted earlier) to input data and group information and generate an automated underwriting and pricing response; this could even be done by means of a dial-up from the salesperson's laptop computer while on site at the account. This type of functionality requires that standardized products be offered, even if there are a large number of potential combinations of copayments, benefits riders, and so forth. It also requires that all necessary data be input before an automated quote is generated. Last, if the sale is successful, the group could be installed right on the spot by means of the same dial-up capabilities.

Future e-commerce Opportunities

All the external and internal e-commerce opportunities discussed thus far have in one way or another been to enable current MCO business processes. Because of the dramatic impact that e-commerce and, more specifically the Internet, will have on our economy, new business opportunities may exist that never could have been considered before. A few MCOs have started to experiment with new business models to reflect the new dynamics of our evolving economy.

Rapid advancement in Internet technologies is responsible for creating the opportunity for these new business models. One of the most notable advancements is the development of a new Internet programming language called the extensible markup language (XML). Hyper-text markup language (HTML) allowed Web page designers to create appealing layouts for Web pages. The problem with HTML and other early Internet programming languages was that they were not particularly versatile. XML on the other hand is extremely powerful. XML can be used to send data from one computer to another computer by means of the Internet. When the second computer receives the data from the first, because of the nature of XML, it knows exactly what the data are because they arrive in a predefined standard format. HTML is not an especially efficient language for transmitting claims by way of the Internet, but this is an excellent application to use XML. Other industries such as the financial services industry have found numerous opportunities to use XML, not the least

of which is the consumer's ability to use credit card information to purchase goods and services and to conduct banking and investing by means of the Internet.

At this point, new business models for MCOs have fallen into one of two categories. The first is data or information management-related opportunities and the second is medical or care delivery-related opportunities.

Several MCOs have decided to take advantage of economical e-commerce technologies to develop business models around data or information management. Although many examples of data or information management business models have surfaced, two of the most common are online medical insurance brokers as noted earlier and managed care transaction clearinghouses. Early evidence shows that the Internet is an effective tool for buying and selling insurance. A few smaller MCOs have moved from the familiar role of medical management, claims processing, and the like to a role where they bring employer groups and individual members together with larger MCOs. These larger MCOs have greater economies of scale when it comes to such functions as claims processing, provider contracting, or medical management. Essentially, these smaller plans have developed Internet-based tools to collect insurance needs and requirements from a variety of constituents and then work with a larger health plan for the actual coverage. A special note is worthwhile here: under HIPAA, it is illegal to use confidential information (e.g., enrollment data or health status data) for purposes of sales and marketing other than in well-defined circumstances involving an MCO's own membership. Therefore, it is incumbent on any organization to be familiar with HIPAA restrictions on this type of activity.

A second data or information management opportunity is to act as a transaction clearinghouse. MCOs have been slow to develop the e-commerce solutions that would allow them to communicate and conduct transactions directly with all contracted providers by means of the Internet. This is understandable, given the large number of providers that an MCO transacts business with in a given year. Each provider is likely to have different requirements and abilities, providers rarely serve patients from just one health plan, and there are as many practice management software systems as there are providers.[13]

Therefore, a provider is not likely to adopt an Internet-based solution from one MCO that does not work for another MCO. Without an open source set of standards and widely available software, this is a role that some transaction clearinghouses have started to fill. They have developed Internet-based solutions to which providers can send all transactions, for example, claims submissions, referrals, and eligibility confirmations. The clearinghouse accepts these transactions in whatever format they arrive, translates them, and sends them on to the appropriate MCO in the appropriate format, for a fee. This is just one example where a clearinghouse type of solution is effective and efficient. It could also be used to send employer group enrollment data to multiple MCOs. Another possible direction could occur if open standards do evolve, and cheap and reliable high-speed Internet access becomes ubiquitous. In that case, physicians might find that their new practice management software can conduct business directly with the MCO. This is very much the same business model as the independent intermediary "dot com" companies discussed earlier.

The other category of new business models with which MCOs have started to experiment is medical or care delivery related. Because of such developments as XML, early evidence has also shown that the Internet provides an efficient, economical, and secure way to transmit clinical data. This opens up a world of opportunities not available before. A few MCOs have started to pilot a variety of new Internet-based health care delivery-related solutions.

One medical application for new e-commerce technologies is telemedicine. XML, for example, allows a radiologist to read a computed tomography scan and diagnose a patient's condition from virtually anywhere. A patient in a rural town can be scanned, and the image can be transmitted by means of the Internet and reviewed by a specialist using a home personal computer (with a very high-resolution monitor,

of course) several states away. On a more prosaic basis, it is now common for radiologists to use such telemedicine capabilities to read radiological images remotely when on call or to cover a wide group of hospitals from a central location. Another care delivery example is the use of remote personal clinical devices that periodically connect to a larger system to monitor a patient's condition and even provide feedback, as well as providing data to the patient's physician.

CHALLENGES

MCOs face several key challenges as they move to adopt e-commerce–enabling technologies. A multitude of pressures are pushing MCOs to embrace e-commerce. But contemporaneously, MCOs will face several challenges as they start to move more aggressively into the e-commerce marketplace. Examples of such challenges follow, with the understanding that these represent examples that are current as of early 2000; in Internet time, that's a bygone era by the time this chapter is read.[14]

- *There is no clear leader in the managed care e-commerce marketplace.* The absence of a clear managed care leader, in some respects, discourages other payers from rapidly moving toward fully integrated e-commerce managed care functionality.
- *There are virtually no Internet-based managed care transaction standards.* This lack of standards significantly prohibits wide-scale adoption of fully integrated e-commerce managed care functionality. The HIPAA-required use of the ANSI X.12.N standards as noted earlier is a good move in this direction but is applicable to any form of EDI and not focused on the Internet; in addition, those standards are not sufficiently comprehensive to support all of the e-commerce requirements for the rapidly evolving market.
- *Most managed care organizations are not able to measure the financial impact of e-commerce on operations, as yet.* Many MCOs are reluctant to make the significant

information technology investment with a clear understanding for the financial payback.

- *Security issues and regulatory requirements represent significant barriers to true e-commerce for managed care.* Most consumers are concerned that health information transmitted by means of the Internet will not be private and secure. Legislation such as HIPAA requires security and privacy policies and procedures that are not yet fully developed but will be defined by the time this book is published and will be implemented on a mandatory basis over the next several years.

- *Nearly all MCOs have an extensive collection of back-end legacy systems.* Initial efforts at integration with these back-end processing systems have proven to be cumbersome. Some MCOs are replacing these legacy systems and will thus gain improved e-commerce potential, but many other MCOs, particularly large companies, cannot easily eliminate such legacy systems (of which there are usually several) and must develop solutions to connect e-commerce capabilities to those systems.

- *There is widespread exposure of bad data and poor systems integration.* With more traditional business approaches, companies are able to insulate customers and suppliers from poor data and back-office technology inefficiencies. When going "online," companies risk exposing their internal weaknesses to a multitude of external stakeholders.

- *There is national presence versus geographical depth.* Many large MCOs have either broad national presence with little geographical depth or significant geographical depth and little national presence. This industry dynamic leads to very different e-commerce approaches.

CRITICAL SUCCESS FACTORS

To mitigate the challenges mentioned in the previous section, there are a number of critical success factors. MCOs looking to make the foray into e-commerce should recognize these factors.

Adopt the e-commerce Mindset

To be successful in this new business marketplace, the MCOs' most senior level executives need to be committed to e-commerce. They need to be prepared to demonstrate this commitment on a regular and ongoing business. This support starts by building the requisite skill sets within their own organizations. MCOs need to have trained, knowledgeable resources that understand the implications of e-commerce because of such things as security and privacy concerns, compliance with laws and regulations, and legacy system integration. This is not a strategic initiative to be fully delegated to the information systems function—representatives from all aspects of the business must be involved.

Accept That e-commerce Strategy Development Will Be Continuous

MCO executives must recognize the rapid increase in the pace of change (so-called Internet time, as mentioned earlier). Consequently, business strategy, which has not been static for decades, will require even greater adaptability and must be ongoing. MCOs must evaluate new opportunities on the basis of constantly evolving information. The new opportunities should be evaluated on their ability to add value and differentiate. MCOs must create a culture that is flexible, follows an accelerated decision-making process, and can adapt to changing directions without hesitation. And the MCO must be able to execute the strategies quickly, efficiently, and with required functionality.

Adopt a Rapid, Iterative Design, Development, and Implementation Approach

In response to continuous strategy development, MCOs must adopt a rapid, iterative design, development, and implementation approach. No longer can organizations expect 12+

month implementation schedules. Organizations need to deliver incremental e-commerce functionality in short intervals, three months or less. The benefits of this short interval approach are that it allows organizations to learn from early success and to pilot new opportunities with little overall risk to the organization.

Build a Sound Technical Infrastructure

Last, integrated e-commerce will require a sound technical infrastructure. Individual e-commerce solutions should be developed on a foundation that is scalable, allows for legacy system integration, and mitigates security and privacy concerns.

CONCLUSION

E-commerce represents the single largest opportunity to hit MCOs in many years. Spurred by the tremendous growth in the use of the Internet, e-commerce actually encompasses a wide array of technologies, for example, IVR and EDI. Today these technologies are separate and distinct from each other, but soon the differences will be nearly indistinguishable to all but the most knowledgeable information technology individuals. In concert with the tremendous growth in the Internet, several other trends will push MCOs to embrace e-commerce. These trends include HIPAA mandates, price compression, consumer market demand, and capital market pressures. The e-commerce opportunities available to MCOs are nearly limitless but can loosely be defined to fit into one of four categories: static, interactive, semi-integrated, and integrated. As MCOs begin to foray into e-commerce, they will face some significant challenges. However, by implementing an approach that incorporates adopting an e-commerce mindset and accepting that strategy development will be continuous, relies on iterative development, and rests on a sound technical infrastructure, MCOs will increase their chances of success in this new business marketplace.

REFERENCES AND NOTES

1. S. Bell et al., "Resizing On-Line Business Trends," *The Forrester Report*, November 1998.
2. C. Taylor, The E*Volution of Health Care, *E*Offering*, July 27, 1999.
3. C. Taylor, The E*Volution of Health Care.
4. http://www.wpc-edi.com/hipaa/ and http://www.ansi.org/.
5. D. Plummer, *Intranets, Extranets and the Internet: Different Names; Same Game*, Gartner Group, October 24, 1996.
6. J. Blair, R. Caspmatp, R. Egan, K. Kleinberg, and A. Schoeller, *Six Enabling Technologies for Healthcare, Ready When You Are*? Gartner Group, November 18, 1998.
7. D. Fluss, *Press 1 for the Future of IVR Application Development*, Gartner Group, January 6, 1999.
8. J. Carr, *Benefits of Document Imaging/Management Technologies*, Gartner Group, May 28, 1997.
9. J. Galimi, *Selection Criteria for Imaging and Workflow Systems*, Gartner Group, June 8, 1999.
10. V. Wheatman, *Financial EDI: Getting from Here to There*, Gartner Group, April 25, 1994.
11. Wheatman, *Financial EDI: Getting from Here to There*.
12. The term "Internet speed" refers to the stunningly rapid change that occurs in Internet-based business and transaction capabilities. It is fully expected that health plans' capabilities in Internet-based e-commerce will have evolved rapidly no matter when the reader is looking at this. In other words, you can quite safely assume that most health plans have dramatically increased their e-commerce capabilities since the data presented in Table 37–1 were collected. In fact, it is likely that newer data are available right now, so point your browser to http://www.ey.com and navigate your way to the managed care publications and take a look!
13. By the time this book is in the reader's hands, we will have passed into the year 2000, and it is quite likely that many of the older management practice software systems turned their host computers into toasters.
14. By the time this book is several years old, these examples will even be downright quaint but still charming because of the now (or then?)-preposterous notion that these examples could even be *considered* challenges.

CHAPTER 38

Claims and Benefits Administration

Robin L. McElfatrick and Robert S. Eichler

INTRODUCTION

The claims and benefits administration department is literally where the buck stops, or goes, within a managed care organization (MCO). When all else is said and done in terms of other corporate functions (sales, enrollment, utilization management [UM], etc.), the bottom line is that

---

Robin L. McElfatrick, Vice President of Scheur Management Group, Inc., has spent a decade in managed care consulting after having worked in a variety of positions for both an indemnity plan and an HMO. She provides consulting services to a diverse set of managed care organizations and specializes in the areas of medical management, claims, other party liability, enrollment, billing and collection, customer services, and management information systems. Within her areas of specialty, consulting engagements have spanned operations design and development for new organizations, problem identification and resolution for established organizations, claims functional analyses and audits, program-specific development (Medicare and Medicaid), and plan liquidation management.

Robert S. Eichler, Vice President of Scheur Management Group, Inc., is a founding member of the consulting firm. He specializes in evaluating health care management information systems (MIS), operational auditing and re-engineering, system conversions, systems/product linkages, development of business rules, system requirements and functional work flows, with emphasis on MIS, claims, enrollment, billing, provider credentialing, and customer services departments. He has assisted managed care and hospital association clients in system strategy, as well as providing claims and other party liability audits and functional analyses.

somewhere between 75 percent and 93 percent of all premium dollars are paid out for medical care in capitation and claims payments combined. The effectiveness of the claims department can literally either make or break the company. It is precisely this point that provides MCOs with the impetus to pay close attention to their claims and benefits administration responsibilities.

Claims and benefits administration is not an independent function that gathers, records, and manages all the information necessary to do its job effectively. Instead, claims is part of an integrated organization and process that is actually downstream of and dependent upon many other functions and departments within the MCO.

Historically, within indemnity insurance, and even in most MCOs, claims and benefits administration functions were viewed (and positioned) as back-room operations. Little attention was given to their positioning within the organization, their internal structures, and even their physical settings. In today's MCOs the realization of the importance of the claims and benefits administration function has meant an elevation of its status. Claims and benefits administration is now viewed as being equally important as other core organizational functions, such as medical management and finance.

Throughout this chapter, we attempt to place equal focus on management and operations tasks to assist readers in establishing new claims and benefits administration functions or in evaluating existing ones. The subject of other party liability (OPL) is discussed separately in Chapter 39.

CLAIMS: POSITIONING, PURPOSE, AND OPPORTUNITIES

To understand the purpose of and opportunities presented by claims and benefits administration functions, one must understand this area's positioning within the organization.

Positioning

Claims and benefits administration is really a "middleman" between various internal and external groups. Claims administration comes between sales and enrollment and group accounts when providing benefits coverage. It also comes between the providers and customer service when processing claims and providing reimbursement for those services. You will, no doubt, know of many other examples where the claims process assumes a middleman position.

In examining the strategic positioning of claims and benefits administration, it is fair to say that the function lies at the last point in the flow of organizational activities where the company has an opportunity to "make it right" (the first time around) with the provider and/or member customer. Other than sales and enrollment functions, where the MCO faces employer and member customers and has a chance to make positive first impressions, conduct of the claims and benefits administration process frequently presents the first real occasion for the MCO to demonstrate its ability to deliver on its service promise. Groups, members, and providers expect prompt and accurate payment of claims. It is often these first demonstrations of service abilities that form the basis of the purchasers', members', and participating providers' lasting opinions about an MCO's performance.

Many MCOs get caught up in internal conflict and argument over what went wrong, why, and who is to blame when claims and benefits administration functions are performed less than optimally. When asked to explain or account for high backlog or claims error rates in claims production, frustrated claims examiners, supervisors, and managers typically respond with such statements as: "If only the enrollment records were timely and accurate, I'd be able to get these claims out faster." "How can I process a claim when the authorization is never in the system when I need it?" "If given more automation through systems support, the claims shop would make fewer errors." Although all these conditions may be true at times, they are internal issues that customers could care less about. When claims decisions are delayed or payments are inaccurate, the customer forms one opinion: this MCO cannot deliver on the promises it makes.

Rather than get caught in the quagmire of backpedaling to correct customers' dissatisfaction with claims service, the MCO must employ preemptive strategies and tactics to ensure a successful claims and benefits administration operation.

Purpose

The first step in ensuring the success of the claims and benefits administration process is to define clearly and agree on its purpose both within the department and between the department and other corporate areas or functions. Claims and benefits administration fulfills the following five basic purposes for the MCO and its customers.

Plan Contract Administration

MCOs have several different contracts with many types of individuals or entities. Claims and benefits administration is concerned with meeting relevant contractual obligations that the MCO has made to groups, members, and providers. Claims-related contractual obligations include benefits (see below), processing time frames, reimbursement methodologies and amounts, appeal mechanisms, and grievance procedures. To meet these obligations, claims and benefits administration must establish and maintain adequate work flow and control procedures to ensure timely and appropriate processing of claims, appeals, and grievances and must coordinate with and rely on assistance from other areas within the MCO. Reimbursement methodologies and amounts are translated into pricing fee schedules and guidelines that should be automated to ensure consistency in and timeliness of application.

Benefits Administration

For each group and individual contract, claims and benefits administration is responsible for ensuring coverage for the defined benefits program. Contracts typically describe benefits for eligible members in general terms and by category of care and include benefit limitations, member cost-sharing obligations, and exclusions. To administer contractually provided benefits, claims and benefits administration must translate the more generally described benefits into specific coverage issues, to the point of defining what is covered (or excluded) by *Current Procedural Terminology,* fourth edition (CPT-4) or Health Care Financing Administration Common Procedural Coding System (HCPCS) procedure codes. The task of translating coverage issues into specific procedure codes is often tedious but is absolutely necessary if claims are to be processed accurately and on time. As an example, if the benefit description includes coverage for durable medical equipment (DME), including repairs, when medically necessary and appropriate, are all types of wheelchairs covered? Do repairs include routine service? Member cost sharing via coinsurance, copayments, and deductibles requires specific interpretation to be applied correctly at the claim line-item level.

Medical Management Policy Administration

A common overriding premise in an MCO benefits program is that covered services must also be medically necessary and appropriate. Medical necessity and appropriateness is a concept that is administered on a claim- or case-specific basis given individual clinical circumstances. The most frequently occurring examples of medical necessity and appropriateness decisions are those that are made before the provision of care. In these circumstances the MCO establishes, contractually and with its providers, the types of services and procedures that require prior approval by MCO medical management staff. Prior approval is translated into referral authorizations and precertifications,

which serve as instructions to the claims and benefits administration staff in handling subsequent claims. The second most frequently occurring case of medical policy administration is when the claims and benefits administration department coordinates with medical management to define those types of cases that must receive clinical review for coverage determination and those that can be processed by claims staff given specific guidelines and procedures.

Member and Provider Service

Although most MCOs maintain separate member and provider service functions, the core of what the claims and benefits administration department does is provide service to these customers. Claims and benefits administration fulfills a large percentage of the total service promise that the MCO has sold. When claims are processed incorrectly or late, providers' cash flow is affected, which can (although typically prohibited in MCO-provider contracts) result in balance billing to members. At a minimum, providers and members are pitted against each other when MCO claims functions do not run smoothly. The member and provider services departments rely on claims and benefits administration staff to solve claims questions. No matter how well trained the staff, they will never understand, and cannot reasonably be expected to understand, all the nuances of claims adjudication.

Liability Protection

By virtue of its contractual obligations, the MCO holds itself out as responsible for coverage of defined benefits in the types, quantities, time frames, and reimbursement amounts specified. Anything less creates an unnecessary liability for the organization. All claims errors, whether they result in overpayment or underpayment, present additional and unnecessary financial liability to the MCO. Overpayments, which are often, but not always, detected or reported, inflate medical expense at worst (if undetected or unreported) and increase administrative expense at best (if adjusted). Underpayments, which are almost always reported, require adjustment and additional payment, thereby increasing administrative expense. Some state regulatory agencies or legislative bodies impose fines on MCOs that do not meet defined claims processing time frames. The third area of liability risk that a claims and benefits administration operation may impose on an MCO is related to the timeliness of claims decisions and payments. In the last decade there has been precedent in several areas of the country for compensatory, and even punitive, damage awarded to members of MCOs who have held that delayed coverage and/or payment decisions resulted in roadblocks to needed medical care.

Opportunities

Even with all the obligations and risks inherent in the act of processing a claim, and with all the difficulties implicit in the positioning of the claims operation, claims and benefits administration presents a situation rich in opportunities. The first opportunity is the prospect of providing excellent service to provider and member customers. The challenge to MCOs is to operate by design versus chance when organizing, staffing, managing, and coordinating the necessary resources and activities to effect optimum claims and benefits administration operations. No less attention and no fewer resources should be committed to this function than to any other function within the MCO.

There is also the opportunity to establish and maintain effective relationships with corporate colleagues. To do its job well, the claims and benefits administration department must coordinate with and develop constructive working relationships with virtually every other function within the organization. It is the responsibility of management in all organizational areas to ensure, directly or through delegation, that the necessary integrated policies, procedures, information, and work flows exist to enable the claims operation to run effectively.

Because of the relative positioning of claims and benefits administration within the MCO (i.e., downstream of most other corporate functions and middleman for others), the opportunity exists within claims to identify weak spots in

both precedent and subsequent processes. Although one may consider this a tenuous position to be in, if handled judiciously and in politically appropriate ways, reporting issues and working with colleagues to resolve problems in other areas can be significant assets to the corporation.

The various tasks associated with claims and benefits administration often require review of contracts and other corporate documents for clarification and guidance. In doing so, the staff have an opportunity to observe any extant inconsistencies between documents and/or loopholes in particular documents. Left unresolved, these issues can create confusion and ambiguity for customers and unnecessary liability for the MCO.

The outcome of the claims and benefits administration process is the creation and maintenance of a total rendered care database. This database is the source of information for innumerable, important corporate functions and activities. For example, claims and encounter data are used for quality assurance (QA) and quality improvement studies, the development and reporting of utilization statistics, and the development of capitation and premium rates. All these activities rely on the completeness, accuracy, and timeliness of the database, again an opportunity for claims and benefits administration.

ORGANIZATIONAL STRUCTURE AND STAFFING

Positioning within the Company

The claims function within an MCO holds a unique position in that it can be viewed alternatively as a primarily financial or operational function. Add to this equation claims processing's heavy reliance upon, and contribution to, the definition of management information system (MIS) requirements (see Chapters 35 and 36), and strong arguments may be made for placing claims processing under the control of finance, operations, or MIS. In spite of the financial focus (i.e., that claims processing is, in effect, a highly complex accounts payable function), it is precisely the degree of operational complexity that places it more effectively under the auspices of operations. The financial components of claims work—the generation of checks, the recovery of overpayments due to OPL, retroactive terminations, claims processing adjustments, and so forth—can be controlled effectively through direct coordination with appropriate contacts in the finance area. Similarly, despite the high degree of MIS involvement, both claims and MIS functions have substantial areas of responsibility that require specialized expertise that is not interdependent. Claims, for example, combines significant operational flow and areas of intelligent intervention (clinical expertise, reinsurance, and OPL recovery operations) that, although requiring system support, to date extend beyond the ability to codify decision-making processes. MIS, too, has responsibilities (technical and plant operations and other functional areas requiring significant MIS support) that extend beyond the focus of claims functions. Therefore, these two functions, although codependent, if combined do not contribute to efficient or effective plan management.

More effectively, claims is under the direction of a director or vice president on equal footing with the directors of MIS, finance, medical management, and so forth. This organizational structure appears to be more effective than one in which a claims manager reports to finance or MIS because it gives the claims function the importance it needs within the organization.

Organization within Claims

The director or vice president of claims is the planner, coordinator (with other areas), and strategist; he or she is knowledgeable about all aspects of the organization and knows contracts and local legislative and regulatory requirements. A sample job description is included in Table 38–1, and a sample organizational chart is shown in Figure 38–1. Reporting to the director, the manager has direct control over line operations. The manager is responsible for designing, monitoring, and managing work flow; maintaining procedural documentation; conducting staff

training and development; and resolving claim-specific and work flow problems. Other positions within claims include a number of supervisors (depending on the size of the shop and the span of management) reporting to the manager and a hierarchy of examiners (junior and senior).

Supervisors may be organized to encompass responsibility for equivalent, comprehensive processing steps for all claims within a line of business or for particular customers, or they may be designated as responsible for specific functional areas (e.g., clerical support staff, data entry, pended claims resolution, OPL claims, QA, and so forth). Typically, designation as an examiner reflects experience and authority. Additionally, the examiner level may indicate expertise in a particular specialized claim type by line of business (e.g., Medicare claims), by function (e.g., training, OPL, or QA), or by complexity of provider contract (particularly if contract terms cannot be supported by MIS). Finally, claims operations include a number of clerical support personnel: secretary(ies) to the director, manager, and supervisors as well as mail room support for the activities of incoming document control, imaging (if performed), and sorting and support for file room document storage and retrieval.

The various choices for structuring the claims department carry implications for smooth work flow through the department. In small plans the ability to define specialized units within claims is contraindicated by the necessity for cross-training to provide coverage for absenteeism. In larger plans management will have the luxury of designing the organizational structure according to functional requirements and corporate strategy (e.g., customer-driven units in combination with similar alignment through marketing, enrollment, benefits and medical management, and customer service). More often, the organizational structure of the department may be driven by MIS deficiencies. For example, if the system cannot support differentiated benefits and product rules, claims units may be divided by line of business or employer group so that examiner knowledge and proficiency may compensate during claims processing. Likewise, if the complexity of provider pricing arrangements is not

Table 38–1 Sample Job Descriptions

Title/Goal	Tasks Required	Experience
Claims Director: Plans and strategizes claims operational support of business lines, groups, products, and contracts. Knowledgeable about all aspects of the organization.	Coordinates (with other areas within the company and with peer companies) and develops interdepartmental operational strategies. Develops and monitors annual budget. Through auditing and internal reporting, proactively identifies negative or positive trends and develops recommendations for change. Establishes and maintains cost-effective and high-quality relationships with contracted vendors for OPL, equipment maintenance, third party claims coding, or procedure review vendors. Maintains current industry knowledge through association memberships, annual meetings, etc. Payment authority up to $XXX.	Thorough knowledge of contracts, laws, and regulations relating to managed care claims processing and related functions. Demonstrated management ability to budget and administer a claims program. Master's degree in health care administration preferred. Equivalent experience acceptable.
Claims Manager: Plans and manages the activities of the claims administration department to ensure the achievement of stated department and plan goals and objectives.	Oversees all activities related to claims processing. Establishes standards of performance for each unit, including training, policies and procedures, auditing, and other performance measurement techniques. Evaluates and monitors staff performance with respect to complaint handling and resolution. Develops and implements cost control measures. Identifies areas for improvement in communication, benefit structure, and plan administration. Resolves high level problems related to claims, eligibility, or benefits. Payment authority up to $XXX.	Knowledge of laws and regulations relating to managed care claims processing and related functions. Knowledge of managed care computer systems, features, and reporting. Knowledgeable about employment practices, budgeting, and general management functions. Demonstrated management ability to coach, train, and administer a claims program. Bachelor's degree preferred. Equivalent experience acceptable.
Claims Supervisor: Plans and supervises the activities of subunits within the claims department to ensure that department, plan, and regulatory requirements are met for output, quality, timeliness, and service.	Supervises employees' daily activities, delegates work, and trains and coaches employees regularly regarding performance. Resolves problems related to claims, eligibility, or benefits. Provides necessary information to related plan units and their systems. Prepares materials for the grievance committee. Reviews and releases claims up to $XXX. Prepares routine reports for the manager on productivity, error rates, complaint rates, financial recordkeeping, and other activities.	Thorough knowledge of claims processing regulations, systems, and procedures, preferably in a managed care setting. Demonstrated supervisory background and experience. Ability to work with computer programs to perform analysis and word processing. Education and experience equivalent to 2 years of college education, 3–5 years of claims processing adjudication experience, preferably in a managed care setting.

continues

Table 38–1 continued

Title/Goal	Tasks Required	Experience
Claims Examiner: Reviews and pays health claims up to a certain complexity level.	Pays claims within authorization limits according to established quality and service standards. Determines eligibility of members, acceptability of evidence submitted, and necessity for additional information or review. Resolves issues before claims payment to avoid readjudication. Refers complex claims or claims falling out of standard procedure guidelines to senior examiner or supervisor. Provides routine reporting of work volume and productivity as required by the supervisor. Analyzes all relevant materials for the processing of claims up to $XXX.	High school education. Minimum of 1–3 years of claims processing experience in an environment of multiple plan benefits and provider contracts.

supported by automation, claims may default to designated units by provider type.

The critical element in structuring an effective work flow through the organizational structure is determining communication requirements among and between the units and designing efficient methods for claims to cross organizational structural boundaries without the respective units succumbing to finger pointing for lost or substandard work. Figures 38–2 and 38–3 show the impact of organizational structure on work flow.

Staffing

Table 38–2 provides a guideline for administrative, examiner, and clerical full-time equivalent

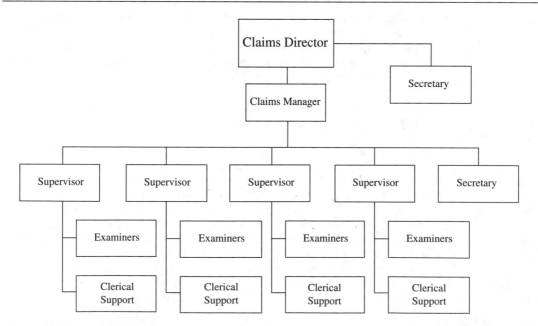

Figure 38–1 Claims Department Organizational Structure

Figure 38–2 Impact of Organizational Structure on Work Flow: Supervisory Units Organized by Function

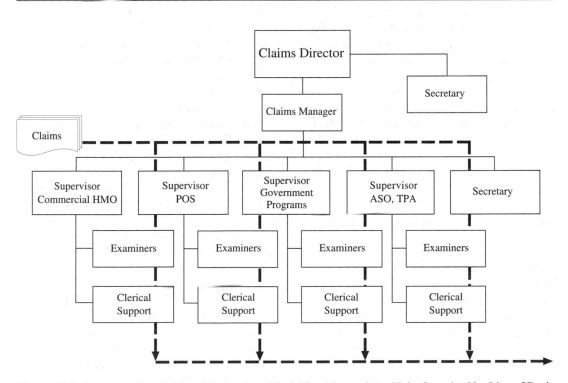

Figure 38–3 Impact of Organizational Structure on Work Flow: Supervisory Units Organized by Line of Business or Customer-Driven Unit. HMO, health maintenance organization; POS, point of service; ASO, administrative services only; TPA, third party administrator.

Table 38–2 Claims Staffing Ratios by Health Maintenance Organization Model and Membership: Average Ratio of Staff to Members

Model/Membership	Total Staff	Analysts	Clerks
Model			
Staff	1:4,711	1:18,958	1:22,164
Group	1:3,697	1:20,176	1:17,305
Independent practice association	1:4,899	1:12,465	1:21,808
Membership			
< 25,000	1:3,135	1:6,483	1:8,000
25–50,000	1:4,653	1:13,518	1:17,166
51–100,000	1:4,630	1:13,549	1:21,498
101–200,000	1:4,237	1:24,731	1:25,561
> 200,000	1:7,938	1:19,085	1:38,867

Source: Reprinted with permission from Average Ratio Claims Average Staffing Ratio of Employees to Members, *Warren Surveys 1999 Managed Care Staffing Ratio Update,* pp. 53, 55, 57. For further information call Warren Surveys (815) 877-8794.

(FTE) employees based upon the delivery model and the number of members enrolled in the plan. The table is only a starting point, however, for establishing staffing levels. It is important to include in any staffing equation the number and complexity of products serviced, the number and complexity of reimbursement methodologies used, and the degree and quality of automated support that may be brought to bear upon the claims adjudication process. A high degree of complexity in any of these areas or a lack of system support for these or any adjudication, and pricing functions will require a greater number of FTEs. Table 38–1 provides general guidelines for claims staff tasks and required expertise.

CLAIMS OPERATIONS MANAGEMENT

For claims and benefits administration, operations management means the base resources, methods, processes, procedures, and systems employed to form the foundation of a successful department. Since there is no magic formula for arriving at the exact best configuration of these elements for each MCO, each component is a direct contributor to overall success or failure. Careful planning, implementation, and maintenance of each of these operational factors are essential to claims and benefits administration.

Inventory Control

To control inventory, there must first be agreement as to just what inventory is. *Webster's Dictionary* defines *inventory* as a "detailed, often descriptive, list of articles, giving the code number, quantity and value of each." The key words here are *detailed, articles* (claims and encounters), *code number* (type of claim), and *quantity and value of each.*

Most businesses rely on inventory control as a means of managing and accounting for assets. In an MCO, cash obtained through premium revenue is the primary source of assets; capitation and claims expense are the primary sources of liabilities. Claims and benefits administration must effectively control its inventory in support of corporate management of assets and liabilities. The inventory control responsibility includes a definition of inventory, what an acceptable level is, how to evaluate current inventory, how to control it (including retrieval as necessary), and how to report on it.

Mechanisms for inventory control include clearly written procedures (including definitions, categories, methods, etc.), a sound inventory process that occurs at reasonable intervals, ways to record receipts on a timely basis and to monitor the movement of those receipts throughout the process, automation support, work flow simplicity, and assigned responsibility and authority for controlling inventory. Basic principles, or rules, of inventory management include the following:

- All receipts need to be logged in to the mainframe claims processing system within a day or two of their receipt.
- When claims are transferred (permanently or temporarily) to another department, they need to be noted as a transferal. If a claim (or copy of a claim) goes to another department, there should be an agreed-upon time frame for the return of that transaction, and that time frame should be monitored actively.
- Work to be done should be stored centrally to the extent possible; file integrity must be maintained to ensure that work to be done is not misplaced.
- Control and recording mechanisms should be checked periodically to make sure they are still effective and accurate.

The essence of inventory control is accounting for all units of work on hand by category of work/transaction, defining where these transactions are in terms of their processing, and verifying the validity of ongoing counting. Basically all units of work on hand get counted. All claims and transactions, no matter what their form, get counted: paper, electronic, or tape submissions; encounters (sometimes called statistical claims); pended (on hold) or suspended claims (placed on hold automatically by one or more systems edits); requests for adjustments; and authorizations and referrals (if done in your claims shop). There may be other transactions as well (e.g., member-submitted claims, laboratory billings that come in on computer printouts, and telephone and written inquiries)

You may ask: Why count everything if claims and encounters are our main responsibility? The answer is that a complete and detailed inventory will tell you much more than what you have on hand. It is a measure of productivity. You can see how well your current work flow facilitates movement of claims and other transactions through your department. You can test staffing levels, task allocation, and grouping of tasks. You can identify problems, such as bottlenecks in the flow, aged claims in suspense/pend status, illogical groupings of tasks, and counting problems.

For each work unit, you want to know type and processing stage:

- *electronic receipts:* in preparation, received but untouched, or received and processed (again, by type of claim)
- *paper claims/encounters:* in preparation (in the mail room), to be processed (on the shelf/desk to be done), to be entered (if done by operations rather than claims examiners), or processed
- *suspended/pended transactions* (electronic or paper; claims or encounters): by suspense/pend status (why pended/suspended), pend/suspense age (how long in that status), and if resolved
- *authorizations and referrals* (if entered within claims): by processing stage and type

A key principle in the management of inventory is front-end control. Under this principle, everything—be it new receipts that come into the department or documents returned from internal or external sources—is date stamped, counted, categorized, batched, and recorded at the point of receipt. Batches are rational units, groupings of work that can be done in reasonable periods of time (e.g., claims to be processed in batches of 50). The practice of front-end control enables management to ensure that all units of work are accounted for from the minute they are received within the department.

In addition to required definitions and principles, inventory control can be aided significantly through automation support. Electronic data interchange (EDI) enables MCOs to receive claims electronically, thereby negating the need to count in, batch, and store receipts manually until they are processed. Although there needs to be a reconciliation procedure between what the biller submitted electronically and what the MCO received, electronically received transactions should, for the most part, be capable of being controlled and processed automatically.

The ability to log transactions into the claims processing system as they are received but before they are processed is critical. Computerized logs, on the mainframe or in personal computer applications, are important to track movement of claims into and out of the department before they are finalized. The claims processing system should be able to support predetermined age and status assignment categories for claims as they move along the various processing stages. This is particularly true for suspended/pended claims.

Reporting can also be significantly supported through automation. These reports need to be thorough yet usable. Certain automation aids, such as optical character recognition, can cut certain inventory control steps considerably and ensure a greater level of accuracy.

The last significant area of automation support for inventory control is document filming, archiving, and retrieval. Microfilming and optical digital imaging are the most commonly used forms of document imaging at present. Although a surprisingly large number of claims and benefits administration operations still maintain hard copy claims files for retrieval, unless there is a relatively small membership in the MCO and/or the MCO is new, automated forms of imaging and retrieval are much more efficient for claims operations. One of the pitfalls of digital imaging processes is the false pretense that by imaging claims the plan has controlled its incoming inventory. Imaging, whether by microfiche, microfilm, or digital storage, addresses a number of important issues: claims documents are less likely to be lost, and claims may be accessed by, or copied to, various people in the organization simultaneously. Imaging, however, does not guarantee that claims are counted (by type and value), nor does it guarantee that the claims will be entered into the claims processing system any faster than if they had remained in paper format. The authors have observed a number of claims shops where managers and directors mistakenly believed that by imaging claims within a day of their receipt there was no claims inventory. Backlogged claims, because they could not be seen, were no longer acknowledged and understood to be a problem.

One advantage of digital imaging over microfiche or film is that many of the imaging programs include work flow management. This functionality provides for maintaining work flow queues, which may be assigned to various departments, units, or individuals. It also provides automated support for inventory management—system-generated counts of claims—but requires a clear understanding and management of multiple intangible, virtual, work queues. Digital imaging of claims also adds another step to front-end control: the images must be indexed in order to be accessed. The indexing process requires review of the image on-screen and entering at least basic claims information, such as service date, provider, member, and charged value. Such entry of index elements may be redundant to data entry into the claims processing system. A second advantage of some imaging systems over microfiche or film is that many include an optical character recognition (OCR) or intelligent character recognition (ICR) component. OCR software recognizes the images on standard claims forms and translates them into data elements for indexing and data entry purposes. Images where the OCR software is less than certain of its translation must be reviewed on-line for verification and correction in a process known as *vertexing*.

Once the steps of digital imaging are complete, the claims still require entry into the claims processing system. There are a variety of approaches to this step, ranging from on-line entry (where the operator refers to the image on-screen rather than to a paper on the desk), to automated placement of the OCR data elements into a file format that the claims processing system reads as if it were an EDI input file. The method used will depend upon MIS technical expertise and system capability and requires operational understanding and management of the various processing points that will need to be included in front-end inventory and control.

An outcome of inventory control is productivity measurement. By virtue of the fact that inventory management includes a running count of what came into and went out of the department, it necessarily captures and records individual and departmental productivity counts. Accounting for and managing pended/suspended claims is also an integral part of inventory control. Because pended/suspended transactions usually represent the largest single category of aged claims, it is necessary to track their location, status, and age within each location and status at all times. Aggregate pended/suspended counts are routinely tracked and reported in inventory processes.

To keep ongoing inventory counts and control, it is necessary to create a starting point with a physical inventory of all work on hand and to proceed from that point with daily counts of receipts, productivity, and remaining inventory. Daily counts are produced in two forms—individual and departmental—and rely on ongoing counting measures between physical inventories. For each job function within the claims and benefits administration department, a daily count sheet is filled out and collected for tabulation into a departmental total. Daily count sheets should be simple for easy completion and should capture units of work received by type; transactions completed by type; transactions pended, suspended, or remaining on the desk by type; and date of receipt of the oldest claim and the oldest encounter on the desk. Weekly reporting consists of a summary of daily counts. See Exhibit 38–1 for a sample claims and benefits administration productivity/inventory report.

There are two basic levels of claims reporting: departmental reporting and plan reporting. Departmental reporting is detailed and specific; it encompasses all the information you need to manage your shop. It should cover, at a minimum, all claims/encounter productivity and inventory (beginning, received, processed, and ending) by work unit and type of claim/encounter, nonclaim inventory and production (adjustments, internal inquiries, authorizations, and referrals; if applicable, written and telephone inquiries from providers and members; and walk-ins if they are handled by claims), number of weeks' work on hand (volume divided by average weekly production), oldest claim to be worked and date being worked (for new receipts), and a comments or notes section for

things such as resource expenditure (total hours worked, regular and overtime), systems availability (any significant downtime), unavailability of staff (due to holidays, absenteeism, training/seminar time, etc.), or any other reasons for variances in normal productivity and inventory.

Claims reports for others in the MCO are generally less detailed and focus on the main work responsibilities of the department and their status. Plan reporting of claims and benefits administration inventory and productivity is usually limited to total production and inventory by work unit and type of claim/encounter, number of weeks' work on hand, oldest claim to be worked, and special inventory issues, such as certain types of claims that are being given priority or explanations of major variances.

To maintain an accurate count of all work on hand, it is necessary to perform a physical inventory on a periodic basis. With a physical inventory, all units of work are counted by work unit, type of transaction, and stage in processing. As the work is counted, the batches are labeled to avoid recounting. All work is then tallied. The results of the physical inventory are then compared with the count balances that are run from week to week (again, by type of claim/work unit and processing stage). The physical inventory counts, by category, are then reconciled to the weekly running counts. Reasons for possible discrepancies are then identified. Some common culprits are live claims sent to other departments, claims done at home (cottage industry), claims buried on someone's desk, and erroneous batch labeling. Sometimes a partial inventory is called for. A good example is pended/suspended claims reported by the system that cannot be accounted for in live claims.

Pended Claims Management

Pended/suspended claims typically account for the largest portion of a claims and benefits administration department's problem cases. Although the terms *pend* and *suspend* are often used synonymously, some MCOs differentiate between pends (claims that examiners place on hold) and suspends (those that are placed on

Exhibit 38–1 Sample Claims Productivity/Inventory Report

Unit	Inventory	IP	OP	1500	ENCS	OTHER	TOTAL
MAIL/PREP DATE OF OLDEST WORK _____	BEGINNING						
	RECEIVED						
	PROCESSED						
	ENDING						
TAPE & ELECTRONIC RECEIPTS							
EXAMINERS DATE OF OLDEST WORK _____	BEGINNING						
	RECEIVED						
	PROCESSED						
	ENDING						
DATA ENTRY DATE OF OLDEST WORK _____	BEGINNING						
	RECEIVED						
	PROCESSED						
	ENDING						
SUSPENSE DATE OF OLDEST WORK _____	BEGINNING						
	RECEIVED						
	PROCESSED						
	ENDING						

OTHER WORK: PRODUCTIVITY AND INVENTORY

	AUTH/CERTS	REFERRALS	INTERNAL QS	EXTERNAL QS
BEGINNING				
RECEIVED				
PROCESSED				
ENDING				

TOTALS	BEGINNING	RECEIVED	PROCESSED	ENDING
CLAIMS	_____	_____	_____	_____
ENCOUNTERS	_____	_____	_____	_____
AUTH/REF	_____	_____	_____	_____
INQUIRIES	_____	_____	_____	_____

hold automatically by one or more systems edits). In this discussion, both types of transactions are addressed.

The volume of pended/suspended claims is directly linked to the accuracy and completeness of predecessor functions (e.g., enrollment, provider relations, utilization management, etc.) and the number, type, and logic of edits that are defined in the claims module (and any related "side-car" modules, such as rebundlers, software programs that roll up and reprice fragmented bills as well as apply industry-standard claims adjudication conventions) of the computer system. Computerized edits may be set to force on-line examiner resolution, suspend claims that fail criteria for examiner intervention, or adjudicate automatically based on predetermined and preprogrammed guidelines. Electronically submitted claims that do not pass system edits will necessarily result in suspension or system resolution. A distressingly common reason for pended/suspended claims occurs in point of service benefits plans (see Chapter 3), where an electronically submitted claim arrives before a paper-based authorization form (see Chapter 19 for a discussion of authorization systems). Claims may be pended/suspended for a variety of reasons, including some of the most common reasons, as described in Table 38–3.

The management of pended/suspended claims requires constant vigilance on the part of claims staff. The first consideration is careful planning for and understanding of the rules that will be applied to the claims adjudication process manually, by the computer system, and in combination. Not only must claims and benefits administration staff understand the circumstances that will cause claims to be pended/suspended, but staff in other areas whose functions manage data that are accessed in claims adjudication must also understand their impact on the process. Claims rules should be developed and administered based on a combination of program requirements (contract issues, regulations, etc.) and standard industry practices.

The second key to pended/suspended claims management is the predetermination of guidelines and procedures for addressing pend/suspend situations when they occur. For every category of pended/suspended claims, there should be documented policy and procedure to address which department (and individual) will provide the necessary information/decision needed to resolve the issue, what information/documentation will be needed by that individual, the procedure and time frame for conveying information/documentation to the decision maker, the time frame for response, how decisions are conveyed back to the claims department or individual staff member (for cases resolved within claims), the time frame and responsibility for completing the pended/suspended claim within the computer system, and a process (with contact person) to follow when predetermined guidelines and procedures do not work. One of the best ways of developing such policy and procedure is to sit down with staff in the supporting areas to review the reasons for pended/suspended claims and agree on what exactly will occur for each type of transaction.

The last, but certainly not the least important, factor in pended/suspended claims management is a satisfactory tracking and monitoring mechanism. The ideal process begins with an adequate pended/suspended claims and encounter report. A computer-generated report should be produced at routine intervals (and be available on an ad hoc basis) and should include, at minimum, member name, member identification number, claim number, date of receipt, date pended/suspended, provider name/number, dates of service (from and to), total charge, pend/suspend reason (code and explanation), number of days in status, and examiner. The report should be sorted in pend/suspend reason order so that all the same and grouped pend/suspend reasons are printed together in a subsection. Next, it is crucial to designate an individual to be responsible for reviewing the report on a routine basis (usually weekly), distributing its various sections, and following up with the appropriate MCO staff on individual claims that are nearing or have exceeded their predetermined pend/suspend reason aging factor. The individual who reviews and manages this report must be empowered to work with others (inside and outside claims and benefits administration) to resolve claims/encoun-

Table 38–3 Reasons for Claims Being Pended/Suspended

Issue	Description
Eligibility	Member eligibility not found, date(s) of service before or after eligibility effective dates, claim date(s) of service within preexisting condition period, member primary with alternate insurance carrier (the MCO would be secondarily liable for this dependent member in the presence of alternate insurance), student eligibility in question, group premium in arrears, and/or individual premium in arrears.
Provider	Provider not in system, member not assigned to this primary care provider, provider's claims flagged for suspense, provider suspended/terminated, provider not approved for this procedure, provider not eligible for date(s) of service, and provider not a member of billing group.
Utilization management (UM)	Precertification required but not in system (no match), referral authorization required but not in system (no match), claim exceeds limits of precertification or referral authorization, claim does not match with provider in referral authorization or precertification, specified field(s) of information missing from referral authorization or precertification (number of visits/days, admission date), and procedure flagged for UM review.
Claims line item	*Validity edits:* Date(s) of service after claim receipt or current date and invalid information (dates of service, type of service, place of service, procedure/modifier code, diagnosis code, units of service, and/or charge). *Consistency edits:* Procedure–place inconsistency, procedure–type inconsistency, place–type inconsistency, procedure–gender inconsistency, diagnosis–gender inconsistency, and procedure–member age inconsistency. *Claims rules edits:* Claim dates of service past filing limit, submitted/allowed charges require supervisory review, procedure allowed charge exceeds predetermined maximum (supervisory/UM review required), possible subrogation or workers' compensation, related surgical procedures, no price in fee schedule, billed care in surgical follow-up (same provider), duplicate suspect, second lifetime procedure reported, bilateral procedure for unilateral diagnosis, unbundling (fragmented charges), concurrent care, cosmetic procedure (requires medical record), new patient procedure with established patient, assistant surgery by same provider, obsolete procedure, and selected procedures reported on same date of service.

ters on a timely basis and to recommend modifications to related policy and procedure.

Task Allocation and Work Distribution

It is helpful while claims work flow is being designed to consider the variety of tasks in which the claims department engages. In addition to processing claims, the department is responsible for answering correspondence, correcting prior claims processing errors (adjustments), assembling information to support appeals and grievance processes, reducing liability through administrative procedures such as OPL and reinsurance claims submission (see Chapter 53 for a discussion of reinsurance). The department also engages in activities to monitor and continually improve the quality of its work, provide training to its staff, identify fraud, and contribute to special studies regarding utilization or payment patterns. The claims department may be responsible for the configuration of the system to maintain benefits logic and provider contract pricing arrangements. Some of these tasks combine with the overall flow of claims through the department, some are specialized subroutines within the claims process, and others are separate from the main flow of claims payment. By defining the tasks, mapping their flow(s) in the context of the claims process, and determining the volume of work attributable to each task, department management will recognize those tasks requiring dedicated, specialized staff.

Claims themselves can be categorized to determine the most appropriate staff assignment. Generally, claims categorized by type identify an implied level of processing difficulty. Typical definitional categories, in order of increasing complexity, are office visit, laboratory, radiology, surgical, ancillary, and hospital (outpatient and inpatient). Finally, there are a variety of specialized facility claims, such as those for nursing homes, drug and alcohol detoxification centers, and mental health clinics. Categorization by complexity allows management to assign staff to tasks according to skill level. Secondarily, such claim delineations tend to mirror dollar value ranges, which is another control mechanism for authorizing more highly skilled examiners with authority to pay claims up to higher dollar thresholds. Mail room procedures can include sorting claims by type to accomplish appropriate work allocation among examiners of various skill levels.

Because one of claims' responsibilities is to record all utilization rendered to eligible members, it becomes the claims department's task to enter encounters as well as pay claims. Encounters, or statistical claims, are bills for services where reimbursement is made by virtue of salary (staff model health maintenance organizations) or capitation payment. Statistical claims, because they have no inherent financial impact

upon the plan, may be assigned to less highly skilled examiners. This presupposes that mail room sorting procedures can identify and separate encounters from payable claims. Increasingly complex provider reimbursement arrangements, which reimburse a provider alternatively by capitation or fee basis depending upon the place of service and the service provided, are making it more difficult to identify encounters from claims at this preliminary stage.

Correspondence that is easily identifiable as not an acceptable bill format should be separated from claims in the mail room and given over to staff assigned to researching and responding to correspondence issues. Correspondence will include requests for information, response forms to OPL questionnaires, letters initiating the formal appeal process, and so forth. Some types and volumes of mail receipts merit identification and forwarding to additional, specialized examiners (OPL is a prime example). Inventory and turnaround time (TAT) control mechanisms should be in place to ensure resolution of correspondence issues, just as they are for claims.

The requirement for a claim adjustment may enter the claims area from a number of sources and in a variety of formats. Management should consider a formal policy for identifying valid adjustment requests. Some requests will arrive in the mail and therefore deserve consideration for their impact upon mail room flow and tasks. These could be in the form of correspondence or returned checks. More highly skilled examiners usually make claim adjustments. Even so, claim adjustment specialists should not be sequestered. Claims requiring adjustment constitute an important feedback mechanism for claim process quality, and they create their own information flow back to the department. Claim adjustments, categorized by type of adjustment, provider requiring adjustment, and processor responsible for the initial process, may indicate the need for system configuration review, revision of operational policy, or staff training.

Once the task categories are identified and their proportional volumes determined, tasks may be grouped logically according to a number of parameters to determine the appropriate assignment allocation according to plan staffing resources. Table 38–4 shows how various tasks can be allocated according to logical position with respect to claims processing as well as required skills.

Claims processes are controlled straightforwardly enough by monitoring input and output measures. Control of ancillary tasks may be accomplished through similar means focused on the input and output of the subtask. Claims and pended claims control standards and measures are discussed in separate sections of this chapter. The control of logically separate tasks can be accomplished by establishing, for each task, initiating events, interim milestones achievable through the application of measurable tasks, and recognizable goals. For example, the initiating event for reinsurance claim submission is the acquisition of a single claim, or an aggregate number of claims, whose total value reaches a threshold over which the reinsurer is liable for the cost of the claim. Identification of reinsurance situations will require a combination of examiner or system notification of single claims over the reinsurance amount threshold and continual monitoring of claims and authorization history to

identify claim combinations that meet the threshold. Interim tasks involve preparing the claim with its supporting documentation, submitting the claim, tracking the receivable amount, and working with the reinsurance claim examiner to resolve any issues. The goal is reached when the reinsurance check has been received, deposited, and appropriately recorded.

Monitoring of task allocations is an ongoing process. Any of a number of events can affect the volume of work that makes up a task, including enrollment of large groups, deployment of new products or business lines, improved systems support, more expert staff, and so forth. It is therefore important not only to obtain and review snapshots of work productivity but also to evaluate trends identified by a series of such measures.

Work Flow

Work flow design of claims processing considers the processing points for claims from receipt by the organization through adjudication to final disposition and storage. Note that the initi-

Table 38–4 Task Allocation

Required Skill Set	Examiner (by Skill Level)	Research/ Analyst	Investigative/ Personal Contact
Part of claims flow			
Encounters, claims	X		
Specialized subset of claims flow			
Correspondence review		X	X
Information development for various pend types		X	X
OPL		X	X
Separate from claims flow			
Adjustments, training	X	X	
Reinsurance claim submission		X	
System configuration		X	
Processing returned checks		X	
Special studies		X	
Appeals, grievance support development		X	X

ating event is receipt by the organization, not simply receipt by the claims department within the organization. Statutory requirements and the plan's own processing standards stipulate claims processing within a certain time period of their having been received irrespective of their entry date into a controlling automated information system. The plan is compelled to implement and document inventory control mechanisms, manually if necessary, to identify and track claims from the moment the organization receives them.

Work flow design should combine inventory control functions with processing functions so that claims processing is as efficient as possible. As an example, if hard copy claims are sorted in the mail room, they may as well be counted there simultaneously for the purpose of inventory control. As they are counted, they should be batched and placed for data entry or claims examiner retrieval. Design the work flow so that claims picked up for one purpose are not replaced in the identical stage of processing but move toward the next processing step. Handle transactions as few times as possible while maintaining and documenting inventory control points.

Claims processing is akin to assembly-line production: Each logical step of adjudication requires certain readily available information in the same way that production assembly requires component parts. As claims are entered into an information system for processing, the system provides much of the necessary information pertaining to claim adjudication. Depending upon the system, certain information may only be available to claims examiners via reference works, claim guidelines, or communications with other plan areas. Clearly, the facility with which claims examiners access and retrieve additional information pertaining to claim adjudication directly affects productivity and accuracy. A corollary to the production model view of claims is that other plan departments involved in resolving pended claims are part of the claims production line. It may be necessary to reinforce the requirement for timely resolution of claims-related questions from plan departments that are not usually attuned to production-oriented work management.

Claims work flow should be reevaluated periodically. In addition to major events that affect work flow design, such as system development or conversion, new product deployment, or different pricing arrangements, management should be aware of innovative desk procedures that either embellish upon or stray from published operational documentation. Where desk procedures improve upon existing work flow, they should be incorporated into claims documentation. In some cases, individual desk flows may run contrary to established guidelines or negatively affect the process farther down the assembly line. In these cases, corrective action should be taken.

In addition to the effects of organizational structure upon work flow mentioned in the preceding section, claims work flow follows one of two principle designs: on-line adjudication or batch adjudication. Although electronic claims submission usually presupposes batch adjudication, the processing method and claims submission format are distinct events and are considered separately here. In on-line adjudication, examiners entering claim information into the system follow all adjudication steps, attempting to bring the claim to final disposition (either payment or denial). In some instances, the examiner may have to pend a claim while additional information is requested of the provider or member or for review in another area, such as medical management or OPL. In batch processing, the system performs minimal verification steps upon the data as they are entered to ensure that the claim meets minimal data requirements defining a valid claim. Such system verification of data format, syntax, and validity is generally referred to as *edits*. Later, system operations staff initiate a computer program that performs all adjudication steps on a batch of claims. Many claims, with valid data elements, involving adjudication and pricing criteria that can be codified within the system are brought to final disposition without human intervention. Claims requiring decisions that cannot have been programmed or configured into the system are suspended, for claims examiner intervention, research, and resolution.

Both methods, on-line and batch adjudication, have inherent merits and problems. The batch method is appealing because data entry tasks are allocated to employees of an appropriate, lesser, skill level rather than to more expensive claims examiners. Once entered, many claims are adjudicated (pass through) without more costly claims examiner intervention. A typical target is an 80 percent or better pass-through rate. To the detriment of batch processing, data entry clerks who are less skilled in identifying unreasonable looking data may not make simple adjustments to the data as they are entered that would permit a better pass-through rate. Claims, once pended, may require extra time-consuming steps of retrieval of the hard copy for additional information not contained in the system that contributes to an examiner's ability to process a claim. Claims managers must be comfortable managing the virtual flow of reported pends as opposed to the more tangible flow of claims through a department in on-line processing. The decision to use on-line or batch processing is generally dictated by the combined effects of system capability and management predisposition.

Electronic Claims Submission

Electronic claims submission (ECS), or the electronic data interchange of claims, reduces claims data entry tasks. Electronically submitted provider claims may also require the plan to engage in batch claim processing in the event that the data come in from a claims clearinghouse in batch form (which is most common in routine EDI). For those plans that are accustomed to resolving claims in real time with on-line edits, this will result in maintaining and managing two operational flows: one for manual data entry claims processed to completion on-line, and a batch review and resolution of the previous day's pend report based on manual claims that pended, as well as electronic claims that failed to process.

Where the claims processing system's batch process is underdeveloped, newer technology permits the translation of EDI claims files into data elements that are automatically input into real-time sessions of the claims processing system. This maintains the benefits of reducing data entry and ensures that all claims are processed according to the same software code. This approach will require programming expertise from MIS and adjustments to inventory and work flow management from operations.

Since the previous edition of this text, we have witnessed the exponential growth of the Internet and web-based technology. This is generally referred to as electronic commerce, or e-commerce for short. While such technology holds the potential for more direct electronic connection from health care providers to payers, at the time of publication use of the Internet for ECS is hampered by incomplete or competing data standards and lack of appropriate security for the transmission of claims, which include clinical information. Methodology, standards, and pricing structures of e-commerce claims submissions will likely change quickly in the next few years, affected by advances in technology and the Internet and the development and adoption of industry standards. Security issues as well as administrative simplification requirements also arise in e-commerce by the implementation of regulations such as the Health Insurance Portability and Accountability Act (HIPAA; see Chapter 67). See Chapter 37 for a broader discussion of e-commerce in managed health care.

Current EDI business practice is for a payer to engage the services of an EDI clearinghouse, referred to as an automated clearinghouse (ACH), which may work directly with providers and through a series of other EDI transmission vendors to secure claims from providers to deliver them to payers. Such ACHs not only transfer the claims from provider to payer(s), but they retain some information to identify and return incomplete or unacceptable claims to the providers and reformat information to meet the payer's claim system's capability for EDI receipt. For this service the ACH charges the payer a per-claim fee for successfully submitted claims. This pricing structure places an additional burden on the payer to identify claims improperly received—technical errors in the file as well as issues of ineligibility—and reject them back through the ACH rather than directly to the submitting provider. Increased opportunity to take advantage of information technology will require both additional systems expertise and operational knowledge and management. The National Automated Clearing House Association oversees the protocols and standards for the regional ACHs.

PRODUCTIVITY

Although some believe that performance standards are archaic, unnecessary, and stifling when it comes to creativity, the largest part of the responsibility of claims and benefits administration is production oriented: processing claims accurately and on time. For this reason, productivity must be closely monitored and managed. Productivity management starts with the establishment of goals. *Before goals can be established, several things must be considered:*

1. *What is the nature of the work to be accomplished?*
   - volumes of claims, encounters, and other work units
   - types of work units and their relative degree of complexity (e.g., encounters versus hospital claims)
   - fluctuations in volumes and mix by season and over time
   - completeness of receipts
2. *Who will accomplish the work?*
   - FTEs
   - areas of expertise and task allocation
   - experience, training, and cross-training
   - current productivity by type of work unit
3. *What tools and other resources are available to support the work effort?*
   - management and supervision
   - policy and procedure
   - work flow
   - degree of automation
   - assistance from other departments (e.g., utilization management, provider relations, and enrollment)

Once these areas of information are identified and analyzed, it is time to observe the current processes and time frames for producing (completing) the various units of work within the claims and benefits administration department. What this requires is actual observation, over time, of the completion of each work unit type, collection of information about the observation processes and results (units of work completed, interruptions and delays, etc.), projection of productivity over the period of a work day, and consideration and allowance for normal downtime (time away from desk, interruptions, etc.).

For example, if you are trying to determine a reasonable productivity goal for processing hospital claims, you will want to observe a trained and established claims examiner processing hospital claims in the typical way under typical circumstances. Because one period of observation of one claims examiner cannot reasonably be used to establish productivity goals for the processing of hospital claims overall, it will be necessary to conduct several observations, preferably of two or three claims examiners.

To illustrate the degree of variability that the above-described factors can have on productivity, consider a temporary claims agency employee who was asked to quantify claims productivity in the various temporary assignment environments where he had worked most recently (Exhibit 38–2). The individual was asked to describe the claims processing environment of six MCO assignments, to indicate whether productivity standards had been established and to quantify his productivity (mixed claim types). Keep in mind that claims examiners from a good temporary agency, once oriented, can typically achieve higher productivity than full-time permanent employees because temporary staff are not subject to the same level of interruption as employees.

It is clear from Exhibit 38–2 that productivity varies greatly depending on whether claims are prescreened, the degree of adjudication automation, the number of claims entry screens, and the number of work hours in a day. What we cannot determine from this illustration is the degree to which productivity was affected by other factors, such as volume and type of work units, completeness of receipts, policy and procedure, and support by other departments.

730   THE MANAGED HEALTH CARE HANDBOOK

Exhibit 38–2 Variability of Claims Productivity Based on Processing Environment

---

Temporary Assignment 1

System:	large commercial
Number of claims screens:	3
Estimated automation:	90%
Productivity standard:	13.3/hour, 100/7.5-hour day

Comments: Claims had not been prescreened, standard deemed too low, examiner indicated that a reasonable standard would have been 16/hour, 120/7.5-hour day.

Temporary Assignment 2

System:	large commercial
Number of claims screens:	4
Estimated automation:	60%
Productivity standard:	none set

Comments: Claims had not been prescreened, two-computer system in use (claims prescreened in one and processed in the second), examiner indicated that a reasonable standard would have been 11.25/hour, 90/8-hour day.

Temporary Assignment 3

System:	large commercial
Number of claims screens:	2
Estimated automation:	40%
Productivity standard:	20/hour, 150/7.5-hour day

Comments: Claims had been prescreened, standard was not met by permanent or temporary employees because of "systems problems," examiner indicated that a reasonable standard would have been 13.3/hour, 100/7.5-hour day.

Temporary Assignment 4

System:	"home grown"
Number of claims screens:	2
Estimated automation:	none (manual)
Productivity standard:	15/hour, 120/8-hour day

Comments: Claims had not been prescreened, manually adjudicated claims were entered via two claims screens, examiner indicated that standard was reasonable.

Temporary Assignment 5

System:	"home grown"
Number of claims screens:	2
Estimated automation:	none (manual)
Productivity standard:	12.5/hour, 100/8-hour day

Comments: Claims had not been prescreened, manually adjudicated claims were entered via two claims screens, examiner indicated that standard was reasonable.

Temporary Assignment 6

System:	"home grown"
Number of claims screens:	6
Estimated automation:	80%
Productivity standard:	12.5/hour, 100/8-hour day

Comments: Claims had not been prescreened, standard deemed too high, examiner indicated that a reasonable standard would have been 10/hour, 80/8-hour day.

Productivity and, therefore, the productivity standard also vary depending on whether the individual is a new or established claims examiner. Productivity standards are typically set at a lower level for new examiners for a set period of time after a training process has been completed. The idea behind this temporarily lowered productivity standard is to allow a relatively new employee time to concentrate on quality while gradually building productivity to desired levels. It is often the case that a new employee will be given the easier types of transactions (e.g., encounters and specialty referrals) to process initially and be allowed to progress at a reasonable pace toward processing the more complicated transactions (ancillary and hospital claims).

Monitoring performance in relation to productivity goals is essential. The reasons to monitor performance to goals are obvious in some respects and not so obvious in others. Obvious reasons include gaining an objective measure of individual performance (for employee evaluations and merit increases) and a tool to use in managing departmental inventory levels and staffing. The more inconspicuous reasons for monitoring performance in relation to productivity goals, on an aggregate level and at an individual level, are as follows:

- Overall low productivity can signal one problem or a combination of problems: standards are unreasonably high, systems and/or other support resources are inadequate, departmental morale is low, outside interruptions are detracting from processing time, and the like.

- Overall high productivity, assuming that it is significantly higher than standards on a consistent basis, usually indicates that the standards are artificially low and need to be reevaluated.
- Individual low productivity can often be attributed to inadequate training, lack of understanding (of standards, policies, procedures, etc.), poor work habits, personal problems, or just plain poor performance.
- Individual high performance, assuming that it is significantly higher than standards on a consistent basis, usually signals a "star" performer but can also mark an individual who is capable of, and should be, handling more complicated work. Although quite unusual, an occasional star performer has been known to have manipulated work so as to get the easiest transactions by type or within type.

Standards are obviously needed to plan and manage the work of the claims and benefits administration function, but they are also necessary to monitor performance in relation to standards as a mechanism by which to identify and resolve problems. Any significant variation in productivity that is not attributable to a known cause (e.g., system downtime or absenteeism) should be evaluated immediately. Part of the evaluation process includes asking departmental staff why they think productivity is off the standard(s). As problems arise, signaled by variations in productivity, their root causes need to be identified and addressed.

TURN AROUND TIME

In its most general sense, turn around time, or TAT, is the measure of the claims and benefits administration department's responsiveness to its provider and member clients. It is expressed in calendar days and measures the time from receipt of a claim to final disposition (payment or denial and notification). TAT also measures the time frames for all the points between claim date of receipt and date of final disposition (e.g., date of receipt to date of system entry). The act of establishing goals for and recording and tracking TAT yields a tool with which to monitor and manage the timeliness of claims processing. Receipt to final disposition TAT goals are established based on certain relevant considerations:

- *contractual and regulatory requirements:* those commitments defined in MCO provider agreements and/or established by state legislation or regulatory mandate (e.g., Medicare and Medicaid)
- *provider billing cycles:* local billing practices, especially of large provider groups and/or high-volume billers, the idea being to manage TAT to minimize duplicate claims submission
- *competitor practice:* maintaining a par with local competitors in the timeliness of claims payments to remain attractive to contracting providers
- *MCO cash flow:* the balancing of TAT with cash flow to meet all other TAT requirements without releasing payments too early

In establishing TAT goals, consideration is also given to the types of claims (or units of work) that are handled. For example, encounters (or statistical claims) record patient care but do not result in provider payment. The TAT goal for encounters can be longer than for nonstatistical claims, but encounters should be processed on a regular basis to provide necessary rendered care data to MCO management. The TAT goal for clean claims (those submitted with all information required for adjudication) is typically lower than for nonclean claims. Even the Health Care Financing Administration (HCFA) recognizes the difference between these two categories of claims and requires that Medicare managed care contractors process clean claims faster than other claims.

To ensure the timely processing of claims overall, incremental TAT goals are assigned to the various points at which a claim may be stopped temporarily during processing. Date of receipt to date of systems entry is an important incremental TAT because it establishes front-end control of each transaction. The ideal goal for TAT from date of receipt to date of entry is one to two days. Pended/suspended claims are assigned TATs per pend/suspend reason to ensure that the issues causing the pend/suspend are addressed promptly. When pended/suspended claims require the intervention of areas other than claims and benefits administration, pend type-specific TATs are agreed upon between claims and the various other support areas (e.g., enrollment, medical management, provider relations). Reasonable TATs are also assigned to claims requiring development for additional information and those requiring OPL (coordination of benefits, subrogation, and workers' compensation) investigation.

Ongoing tracking and monitoring of TATs are imperative to manage the claims and benefits administration function effectively. There are several tools that the claims manager should have at his or her disposal for tracking and monitoring claims TATs:

- *pended/suspended claims report:* a listing, by category of pend/suspend in oldest (from date of receipt) first descending order within category, of all pended/suspended claims (document control number, member name and number, provider name and number, dollars charged, pend/suspend reason, age in house, and age in pend/suspend status)
- *claim status by date of receipt:* a listing by date of receipt (expressed in ranges; e.g., received within 1 to 10 days, received within 11 to 20 days, etc.) of total claims (number, charged dollars, and paid dollars) and claims by processing status (to be paid, in process, in review, and denied)
- *paid claims report:* a listing of the detail (member, provider, diagnosis, date of service, received date, processed date, charge, cost sharing, paid amount, etc.) of all claims by type of claim (e.g., facility or professional, and potentially more detailed categories within these two general types) that have completed processing (to final disposition) as of the current date and for a

specified preceding time period, including summary totals
- *check register:* a listing, sorted by MCO-specified provider number and provider name, of all claims to be paid in the next check run, including the number of claims and the aggregate amount to be paid
- *lag claims report:* a listing within date category (e.g., in 15- or 30-day increments, 1 to 15 days from date of service, 16 to 30 days from date of service, 31 to 45 days from date of service, etc.) of claims that shows the time between date of service and receipt and the length of time between date of service and payment

Monitoring of encounter and claim TATs is an ongoing and continual process that involves routine review of reports to determine whether overall and incremental TATs are being met and, if not, to determine where the bottlenecks are. Once bottlenecks are identified, they must be addressed immediately. Problems may include insufficient staffing and task allocation for front-end control, systems adjudication and edit logic problems, delays in resolving pended/suspended claims, delays in check runs, and the like. It is the claims and benefits administration manager's job to qualify and quantify each issue and bring about its resolution.

STAFF TRAINING AND DEVELOPMENT

Staff training and development are as necessary to claims and benefits administration as they are to any other department/function within the MCO. In staffing a managed care claims and benefits administration department, it is essential to hire experienced claims examiners, preferably those with experience in managed care claims adjudication. Some MCOs make the mistake of believing that an indemnity claims examiner can make an automatic transition to managed care claims processing with little or no training. The differences between indemnity and managed care programs, especially in the areas of provider network service delivery and medical management, make the two types of claims processing decidedly different.

As new staff come into the department, the ideal training situation involves MCO orientation and 3 to 8 weeks of classroom training (depending on skills and experience upon hire) with a subsequent on-the-job training probationary period, during which time the new employee has close supervision and a 100 percent quality check of his or her work. Regardless of the format and length of training, there is a plethora of information and skills that claims and benefits administration staff must have. Table 38–5 lists those information and skill needs.

If you are taking over an existing claims and benefits administration department and are not quite sure of the adequacy of staff training and development to date, a self-assessment can assist

Table 38–5 Claims Information and Skill Needs

Information/Skills Area	Description
Overall knowledge of MCO	Organizational structure, corporate mission and goals, group account information, membership information, products offered, service area, corporate groups/committees, history of MCO, major competitors, medical management philosophy, center locations and hours (staff model), physician staff (staff model), contracting provider network, reimbursement mechanisms and methods, major functions of all departments, regulatory parameters, MCO marketing practices
Claims functional knowledge/skills	Enrollment regulations and guidelines, medical underwriting (if applicable), coding schema (ICD-9-CM diagnosis and procedure, CPT-4, and HCPCS), medical terminology, benefit programs (covered, denied, and limited benefits; cost sharing applications), claims department work flow and task allocation, claims mail handling, document filing and retrieval, claims filing limitations and TATs, inventory control mechanisms, referral and precertification processes, medical necessity and appropriateness guidelines, pended claims resolution and management procedures, OPL processing, suspect duplicate claims processing, out-of-area claims processing, member claims processing, claims quality standards and review process, productivity standards and performance measurement, adjustment processing, responding to claims status/disposition questions, claims development (for additional information) process, benefit interpretation process, check and explanation of benefits/remittance production and schedule, claims appeals process, overpayment and refund processing, computer system knowledge (claims processing screens, provider inquiry, claims history, enrollment inquiry, pricing file inquiry, computer edits, all code files, referral and precertification screens, pend/suspense resolution screens, adjustment screens, etc.), all other claims policies and procedures
Knowledge of and coordination with other areas/functions	Enrollment and billing, provider relations and contracting, utilization management, quality improvement, finance, legal, member services, internal auditing, etc.
General skills	Letter writing, telephone techniques, handling irate callers, problem solving, computer skills, personal computer skills, stress management, research skills, time management, dealing with conflict

in determining training and development needs. An easy way to conduct a self-assessment of training and development needs is to design a survey instrument to be completed by each employee. The instrument should be designed to provide an easy method for respondents to define their total training and development needs related to general skills, knowledge of the MCO, and functional/technical and interface knowledge about other key departments. Such a survey is typically presented to employees during a departmental meeting, where an explanation of the purpose of the project as well as a review of the instrument itself can be provided.

Once surveys are completed, group responses of employees with similar job functions are tabulated. This method reduces skewing that would occur if all responses, regardless of job-specific knowledge required, were grouped together. For example, all responses may be grouped for tabulating and analyzing training needs on general skills and overall MCO knowledge. Responses of clerical workers, however, should not be grouped with those of more technical respondents when training needs associated with claims adjudication processes are tabulated.

An analysis of tabulated survey results should be conducted in concert with a review of claims QA results (i.e., the nature and volume of errors detected during routine claims quality assessments). Using these two sources of information, a training and development program can be formulated with reasonable assurance that it will meet individual and departmental needs while addressing issues on a priority basis.

Although the exact nature of and resources for training will vary depending on the age, level of experience, and size of the claims department, the following are some tips for developing and conducting effective training and development sessions:

- Begin training on those issues that will effect the greatest improvement in claims payment errors and development of the rendered care database.
- Focus initial training on those individuals with the greatest rate of self-reported need and those with the highest related error rates.

- To ensure consistency of training among the smaller groups, standard materials should be prepared and used. Materials should include documented policies and procedures, live claims samples, relevant forms, anonymous quality review results, prints of claims system screens, and so forth.
- Active participation as well as question-and-answer sessions should be employed, with results being documented and disseminated. Depending on availability of equipment, videotaping of sessions may also be helpful.
- Feedback mechanisms to evaluate the effectiveness of training should be developed and used for all sessions.
- After training, claims QA examiners should focus on newly presented materials and how well they are applied in the production environment. Feedback and remedial training should be conducted as necessary.
- The outcome of training sessions should result in a package of materials suitable for use in training new employees and for use as a procedure/reference manual for existing employees.
- Coding schemes and medical terminology are most effectively taught using commercially available training tools and packages. Training needs in the area of general skills are probably best met though personal development plans by employees.

Staff training and development should also include consideration of cross-training and job enrichment. On an individual employee basis, a manager or supervisor should determine, along with input from the employee, a plan for increasing job skills and experience. Those employees who are able, willing, and ready (as determined by quality and productivity performance levels) for cross-training and additional or increasingly complex responsibilities should be given those opportunities. Outside courses and special seminars (through universities, professional and trade organizations, software manufacturers and distributors, etc.) should also be used as resources to meet training and development needs.

QUALITY

Quality is the measure of the accuracy and completeness of the product of the claims and benefits administration process. Quality cannot be neglected in favor of productivity; the two go hand in hand. The overall goal of claims QA is to assist in effecting continuous quality improvement of departmental work. There is also an individual performance component of claims QA, and by measuring and evaluating individual quality, retraining, coaching, and counseling needs can be identified. The key is to use claims QA as a tool to ensure quality performance rather than as a stick to apply to individuals who make errors.

The first step in ensuring a quality process is to develop standards. There are three measures of claims quality. *Overall accuracy* is the percentage of claims paid correctly in every respect, with no errors. *Payment accuracy* is the proportion of claims for which the payment amount is correct but other processing errors are identified (incorrect payee, match to wrong authorization, etc.). *Financial accuracy* is determined by dividing the sum of all overpayment plus underpayment amounts by the total amount paid. Table 38–6 shows typical industry standards for the three types of claims quality (accuracy) measures.

As you can see by the industry standards, financial errors are weighted more heavily than procedural errors. In the case of an acceptable level of financial errors, where only 1 percent of claims dollars are paid erroneously, that 1 percentage point can translate into hundreds of thousands of dollars in error over the course of a year for a relatively large claims shop.

The next step in developing a QA process for claims is to identify auditing criteria, that is, what specific fields in the claim and associated records (e.g., eligibility, referral authorization, etc.) will be audited, what will be acceptable as accurate, and what will be considered an error. There are basically three major issues to be considered in performing an audit:

1. *Was the claimant eligible at the date of service?* There is little room for dispute on this particular question.
2. *What was the provider's status and payment arrangement?* This refers to whether the provider was a contract or noncontract provider as well as whether contractual reimbursement obligations were followed accurately. This is also relatively straightforward.
3. *Were written MCO policies, procedures, and guidelines followed when the claim was adjudicated?* This does not mean that the policies, procedures, and guidelines represent acceptable levels of control. It merely is meant to indicate whether the organization complies with its own rules, however appropriate or inappropriate they are. *Examples of this criterion as it would be applied include the following:*
   - Were the services authorized or referred by a plan primary care physician (PCP) or participating physician?
   - Were contractual obligations with respect to benefits, exclusions, limitations, and conditions appropriately applied?
   - Was the paid amount accurate, including any copayments, deductibles, and so forth?
   - Was the coding accurate? Put another way, were all the data elements translated and entered into the computer system in such a way as to create an accurate and appropriate record of rendered care?
   - Was the right person paid?

All these items should be noted on a claims QA worksheet. With this information in hand, a representative sample of each claims examiner's work is reviewed on a routine basis, and accuracy and error types and numbers are recorded.

Table 38–6 Industry Standards for Claims Quality

Accuracy Category	Industry Standards		
	Acceptable	Good	Excellent
Overall	90.0	95.0	98.0
Payment	95.0	97.0	99.0
Financial	99.0	99.3	99.6

The flow of the actual quality review process may go accordingly:

1. Every morning, or at some predetermined interval, the reviewer gets the report of the previous day's productivity by examiner. Conversely, it may be easier to do the quality review at the point of the examiner completing a batch of work.
2. The reviewer then manually and randomly selects X claims for every examiner (claims/encounters can be paid [processed] or pended/suspended).
3. The reviewer audits each claim (against the checklist) and checks it in the system (he or she will need to access enrollment records, preauthorization and precertification records, and claims/encounter screens). Comparison of actual reimbursement to original provider contract is also needed.
4. The reviewer completes the claims QA worksheet. The claim form and printouts of enrollment records, preauthorization and precertification records, and claims/encounter screens are kept for those claims where the reviewer identifies a potential error.
5. The reviewer meets with every claims examiner to review:
   • the QA worksheet only where there is no potential error
   • the QA worksheet plus copy(ies) of claim documentation, if there is one or more suspected errors
6. The reviewer and the examiner reach consensus on whether a suspected error is, in fact, an error. Here it is important also to reach agreement on the cause of the error.
7. Confirmed errors should be corrected in the system by the examiner that day, with confirmation of the fix (by the reviewer) being documented on the QA worksheet. The reviewer will typically instruct the examiner (on the QA worksheet) as to the adjustment to be made. Certain errors may not get adjusted; it is up to the judgment of the reviewer.
8. If the reviewer and the examiner cannot reach consensus on whether a particular issue is an error, the claims manager or supervisor should be the tie breaker.
9. Actual errors are recorded in a log for the individual and in aggregate for the department. For verified errors that are not attributable to claims examiners (e.g., systems configuration problems, provider contracts incorrectly loaded), it is incumbent upon the QA reviewer to facilitate a solution to the core problem.

Before the actual audit is instituted on a routine basis, it is important to discuss the process with departmental staff. Review and discuss standards and calculations to evaluate performance against standards. Determine your short-term and long-term goals regarding standards. You may want to shoot for good performance for the first few months and for excellent performance thereafter. Discuss how quality standards and measurement will be applied to new staff versus seasoned staff. New employees may require 100 percent claims review, whereas 10 percent review for established examiners may be sufficient. Also, the standards themselves may be somewhat relaxed for an initial training period.

Discuss and determine how significant problems (errors) will be resolved. If everyone is making the same types of errors, is more training indicated? Do policies need clarification? Coordination with other areas for changes in interdepartmental procedures may be indicated. Raise the subject of claims quality as a performance measure whereby repeated/voluminous errors (given clear policy and adequate training) can and should be used as a measure of individual performance. Although this is not the overall purpose for claims QA, there must be some objective way to measure the quality of individual performance. Also discuss with staff how the process will help the department and the organization (e.g., as a continuous process for improvement; to identify areas for policy and procedure clarification, retraining, and so forth; to let the rest of the organization know the quality of the claims department's product; and to identify problems upstream and downstream of claims).

Start the claims QA process and report results intradepartmentally for the first few reporting periods. This will give everyone a chance to experience the process, work out the kinks, and make any refinements that are indicated. Set a target date for reporting departmental quality to the organization as a whole. Anyone in the program (reviewers and the reviewed) should feel comfortable with raising issues (problems, enhancements, etc.) at any time. Review program results periodically, perhaps every quarter, to determine whether quality has improved and is at the desired level, what improvements in policy and procedure (intra- and interdepartmentally) have occurred as the result of the program, and what program changes, if any, are indicated.

As the results of quality reviews are known and the financial impact is calculated, claims management is in a position to determine what steps should be taken operationally, procedurally, and in terms of resources. In many cases, claims audits result in the promulgation or tightening of policies, procedures, and guidelines. The results may also spur management to consider dedicating additional staffing or technology resources or to focus more closely on a particular identified problem area, such as claims backlog, poor coordination of benefits performance, or unclear precertification or referral authorization instructions.

POLICY AND PROCEDURE

Policy and procedure are the mainstay of the claims and benefits administration department. Policy statements are different from procedures in that they provide direction as to what is to occur and why. Procedures define, specifically, the steps involved in carrying out policy, the responsible person or department, and the required time frames. As an example, a policy statement may say that clean claims are to be processed within 30 calendar days of their receipt, but the related procedures would specify the steps to be taken in processing a claim, who is responsible for each step, and the time frame for processing.

Procedures will also provide specific instructions for defined exceptions. The combination of policy statements and procedures provides a complete set of instructions for the given topic.

Without appropriate policy and procedure as supports, the claims department can anticipate delayed, erroneous, and inconsistent claim decisions. All too often, claims guidelines exist, but in the form of a variety of memoranda, charts, "cheat sheets," and notes based on verbal instructions. Those documents that do exist often speak mostly to the mechanics of getting the claims processed rather than the application of managed care principles. A comprehensive policy and procedure database, including administrative, coordinative, and medical-operational policies and procedures, is required to provide staff with the direction needed to ensure an accurate, timely, and consistent work product. In smaller plans, this is likely to be in the form of a manual that is easy to access by the claims examiners. In other plans this function is automated, and the information is available on the examiner's terminal, with easy access.

There are basically three types of claims policies and procedures: administrative, coordinative, and medical-operational. Administrative policies and procedures instruct staff on processes internal to the claims department, including such things as work flow, TAT, inventory and productivity reporting, claims adjustments, and work distribution. Coordinative policies and procedures address the ways in which claims staff interact with other departments/functions to acquire information or decisions necessary to complete processing of claims. An example of a coordinative policy and procedure is a description of the kinds of cases and methods used between claims and enrollment when eligibility issues delay the processing of a claim. Medical-operational policy consists primarily of internal guidelines and instructions used in MCO authorization of care and in adjudication of associated claims. The purpose of developing such policy is to ensure that coverage of services is provided within the context of what is medically necessary and appropriate, what is reasonable in terms of billing practice, and what is provided for in terms of the purchased benefit plan(s). Guidelines for adjudicating claims for related surgical procedures and "incident to" billings are examples of medical-operational policy and procedure. Table 38–7 provides a list of the most frequently seen claims policies and procedures by type.

As you can see, there is a large number of policies and procedures required for claims and benefits administration, which may seem daunt-

Table 38–7 Claims Policies and Procedures by Type

Type	Description
Administrative	Adjustments; appeals and grievances; application of copayments, coinsurances, and out-of-pocket maximums; authority limits; claims codes; claim forms and documentation; claim definition and TAT requirements; claims QA; coding schemes used; computer screens; confidentiality; duplicate suspect processing; flowcharts and procedures; level of care coding; manual pricing; OPL; overpayment recovery; pended claims procedures and management; plan information; and terms and definitions
Coordinative	Alternate insurance information updates, authorization matching, benefit interpretation, claim check reconciliation, eligibility updates, grievances, group eligibility, incurred but not reported tracking, medical review, member eligibility, member services interfaces (questions, adjustments, OPL information), OPL information from utilization management, pended claims interfaces, providers' claims inquiries, provider flagged, provider not on file, refund processing, reinsurance processing, and unfunded claims liability
Medical–operational	Allergy testing, injections, and serum; ambulance transportation services; ambulatory surgery; anesthesia services; authorizations (referral, precertification, case management, concurrent review, treatment plan); benefits, exclusions, and limitations; bilateral procedures; cardiac procedures; concurrent inpatient care; cosmetic and discretionary services/procedures; cosurgeons; diagnostic studies; dialysis; DME; emergency care; endoscopic procedures; experimental/investigative services and procedures; global fee surgery; home infusion; home health care; hospice care; immunizations and other injections; incidental services and supplies; individual consideration procedures and services; inpatient preoperative and postoperative care; medical–surgical supplies; mental health and substance abuse services; minor surgery and medical care by same physician; multiple intensive care unit visits; mutually exclusive procedures; observation beds; obsolete procedures; obstetrical services–global fees; occupational therapy; out-of-area care; orthotics and prosthetics; physical therapy; physician assistants, certified nurse anesthetists, and nurse practitioners; podiatry services; preadmission testing; preexisting conditions; procedures with diagnosis restrictions; providers under supervision; rehabilitation services; related and unrelated multiple surgeries; repeat initial inpatient examinations; repeat new patient code procedures; risk management; speech therapy; skilled nursing facility care; specialist-to-specialist referrals; sterilization/reversal and fertility services; surgical assistants; temporomandibular joint dysfunction; transplants; unbundled services/procedures; and urgent care

ing to a new claims shop. The numerous required medical-operational policies and procedures may only be developed through collaboration between claims and medical management because they require clinical knowledge for medical necessity and appropriateness. A claims rebundling software package will apply many standard medical necessity and appropriateness guidelines to claims, thereby lessening the degree of required manual adjudication. Additionally, many other types of claims guidelines can be applied through user-defined computer system edits (e.g., procedure/gender, age/procedure, diagnosis/procedure, and procedure/frequency edits). Policies and procedures that require coordination between claims and the various different functional areas (e.g., enrollment, member services, provider relations, MIS, etc.) should also be developed jointly. Information/guidelines for many of the policy and procedure items noted should come primarily from other areas of the organization, with claims adding relevant policy and procedure language (e.g., enrollment guidelines).

A standard format is recommended, as is consistency in who approves and signs off on policy and procedure. Within the standard format, there should be a note of which lines of business or products are affected by each policy and procedure. One recommended format includes the following:

- *policy header information:* policy name and number, effective date of policy, new or revised (if revised, the name, number, and date of the superseded policy), products/groups affected, and approved by (chief operating officer, chief executive officer, finance, medical director, and perhaps others, depending on the nature of the policy)
- *body of policy:* statement(s) of MCO policy; rationale for the policy (definitions, reasons for the MCO's decision, explanations of the intent of the policy, description of new technologies, etc.) and operational instructions and implications (specific guidelines on how to deal with cases covered by this policy; includes specific cir-

cumstances under which services will be authorized/covered and detail at the level of diagnosis and procedure codes)

COORDINATION WITH OTHER DEPARTMENTS/FUNCTIONS

To do its job effectively, the claims and benefits administration department must establish and maintain positive working relationships with many other departments/functions within the MCO. Most of these departments/functions are upstream of claims and provide critical information to enable adjudication of claims; some are downstream of and rely on information from claims. When any of these relationships weakens or breaks down, the claims adjudication process is obfuscated and, most often, delayed. It is the claims manager's responsibility to effect and preserve affiliations with all corporate colleagues and to facilitate the necessary coordination with claims and benefits administration.

For each area or department with which claims must coordinate, the terms of a mutually beneficial relationship must be negotiated, and specific procedures must be developed, agreed upon, implemented, and monitored. One way to start is to identify information and process needs for each area of coordination and from there to develop procedures and standards. Exhibit 38–3 describes procedures/guidelines, standards, information exchange, and desired outcomes for five of the major claims functions.

When procedures/guidelines and standards are developed between claims and its various corporate colleagues, there must also be monitoring and feedback mechanisms to evaluate the effectiveness of the coordination and to fix problems once they arise. Good working relationships are based on mutual understanding and trust, accountability for specific procedures and standards, frequent feedback, and open communication.

SYSTEMS SUPPORT

Claims processing relies heavily upon MIS capability and contributes to the definition of MIS requirements. System application design

Exhibit 38–3 Claims Coordination with Other Departments: Accountability and Goals

---

Enrollment and Billing
- *Procedures/guidelines:* Eligibility, medical underwriting or waiting period stipulations, unpaid premium (withholding claims payment), identification and maintenance of alternate insurance information, identifying and billing for paid services after termination (retroactive)
- *Standards:* Timeliness of eligibility verification, TAT for responses on problem cases, time frame for retroactive terminations (how far back)
- *Information exchange:* Updated name and address, alternate carrier information (new or updated), and incurred care (retroactive eligibility requests)
- *Desired outcomes:* Routine communication and problem-solving methods, compliance with enrollment and underwriting regulations, limited adjustments (especially if they are based on lack of information), and no overpayments

Provider Relations
- *Procedures/guidelines:* Provider not on file, provider flagged, resolving claims questions, required claims adjustments
- *Standards:* Information required for questions, TAT for responses from claims, TAT for responses from provider relations
- *Information exchange:* Open communication about claims inventory/backlogs, information about billing anomalies
- *Desired outcomes:* Accurate and timely provider claim processing, accurate submission of claims by providers, feedback on the quality of the claims operation

Utilization Management
- *Procedures/guidelines:* Matching claims to referral authorization records, matching claims to precertification records, claims requiring medical review, procedures without prices, medical necessity and appropriateness, claims without authorizations/precertifications, experimental procedures
- *Standards:* TAT for establishing authorization and precertification records, TAT for medical review/special pricing, TAT for updating authorizations and precertifications, identifying and recording potential OPL
- *Information exchange:* Utilization anomalies, information to update authorization and precertification records, claims information related to managed cases
- *Desired outcomes:* Appropriate payments (based on medical necessity and appropriateness), enable medical review (when indicated), collaboration on development of medical/operational policy and procedure, assist finance in estimating incurred but not reported costs

Member Services
- *Procedures/guidelines:* Resolving claims questions, required claims adjustments, updating member information
- *Standards:* Information required for questions, TAT for responses from claims, TAT for claims adjustments
- *Information exchange:* Additional claim information, alternate carrier information, OPL information
- *Desired outcomes:* Timely and satisfactory resolution of members' claims questions/issues, knowledgeable representatives who can answer most questions, minimal disruption to productivity (due to unnecessary inquiries and adjustments), feedback on the quality of the claims operation

Finance
- *Procedures/guidelines:* Claims adjustments due to refunds/adjustments and check register audit and reconciliation
- *Standards:* TAT for refunds/adjustments, TAT for check register audit and reconciliation
- *Information exchange:* Changed payees and check register anomalies
- *Desired outcomes:* Correct and timely payments, minimal claims adjustments, accurate claims records

rests on two pillars. The first is the design of the data structures, or files, that record information. The second is the application's ability to manipulate the information in ways that serve the user in performing operational tasks.

Minimum requirements of an automated system begin with the definition and presence of data elements necessary to process claims. This function of the system is essentially that of an electronic filing cabinet. Within the model of claims as an assembly-line production environment, the system should, at a minimum, provide required data elements for examiner review and decision during claim adjudication. The technological aspects of the data structures are of concern to the technologists, affecting system response time and the accumulation of data elements in structures that support data integrity, security, auditability, and intelligent reporting. The claims department user, however, considers the level of system support available to claims processing by identifying data elements included in the database that contribute to efficient claims adjudication and those critical elements that are absent. In addition to demographic, medical, and payment information about each claim, the system should provide eligibility information about the member, benefits information, participatory status and contracting information about the provider, and a record of any events of medical management activities that affect final claim disposition or payment amount. A comprehensive list of the data elements and business rules that should be available within the system are included in Table 38–8.

The second parameter defining the minimum level of system support for claims processing is the extent to which it supports operational tasks. This aspect of system support can be divided into two major functions: the application of logic to assist with adjudication and general ease of use. Application logic in support of adjudication can be divided into two categories: validity edits during data entry that ensure proper data type and format, and the more involved logic that performs adjudication and pricing steps. The steps described in detail in the next section provide a map of claims processing decisions that must be followed, whether claims are processed with system support (on-line or in batch mode) or entirely manually. Steps of particular importance are eligibility verification, adjudication of the claim within the limitations of benefits, the ability to select and apply contract reimbursement methodology, the ability to apply medical management rules by matching claims to appropriate authorization records, and the ability to perform final pricing calculations.

System ease of use relates to the system's ability to present information in a manner that supports desk procedure tasks. Are claims entry screens organized to facilitate entry (number of screens to enter per claim, fields appropriate to claim type, navigation from screen to screen)? Particularly with respect to newer, graphical user interface (GUI) screens, can data entry be accomplished without removing the hands from the keyboard to the mouse? Are appropriate reference file look-ups available to assist with data entry (member and provider look-up, procedure and diagnosis codes, medical authorizations)? Does the system populate the claims record field with values identified and selected by the user during look-up? Can the user move from one record to another easily? If the user scrolls in one direction past the desired record, does the system scroll back? Is it possible to jump easily from reviewing a claim to reviewing an entirely different set of data (e.g., eligibility information such as group premium payments or medical management data such as an authorization record)? Does the system provide menus for navigation (for novice users) as well as support commands (for expert users who know exactly what they need to look for)?

To support customer service, claims adjustments, quality review, pended claims resolution, and other research, claim records ought to be able to be searched for and presented in several ways. Typical requirements include access by claim number (to work through a batch of claims or to retrieve claims listed in a pend report), alphabetically by provider (provider relations), alphabetically by member (case history), by date (member/customer service), and so forth. It should be possible to scroll through the informa-

Table 38–8 Claims System Information

Type	Elements
Group record	Account and subaccount identifiers, benefit plans purchased by accounts and subaccounts, eligibility period, premium payment status, eligibility rules (e.g., preexisting conditions, waiting periods, student age limitations)
Member record	Member identifiers, alternate carrier information, relationship to subscriber, group affiliation, PCP selection, member benefit accounting, eligibility period
Benefit record	Description of covered services and procedures, benefit limitations and maximums, benefit exclusions and benefit cost sharing at the CPT-4, HCPCS, and ICD-9-CM procedure code levels
Provider record	Contracted and credentialed network providers, reimbursement methodologies, eligible services, tax identifier, payment location, practice relationships and network affiliations, contract period, payment status, covering physicians, risk-sharing mechanisms
Price	A series of reimbursement tables: capitation (procedure specific), planwide fee schedules (procedure specific), provider-specific fee schedules (case rates, procedure-specific rates, per diems, percentage of charge, percentage of fee schedule), other plan- and/or provider-specific tables (resource-based relative value scale, relative value units, ambulatory patient groups, diagnosis-related groups), location-specific tables at the procedure level
Authorization record	Medical management parameters to define preapproved procedures, provider, number of services and time frame, case management identifier and to identify third party liability (TPL) potential
Code files	Place of service, type of service, procedure codes with modifiers, diagnosis codes (identify TPL potential), remittance and explanation of benefits codes (denials, limitations, reductions, cost sharing, etc.), pend reasons, adjustment reasons, processor codes
Claim rules	A series of tables that define benefit coverage issues, including medical necessity and appropriateness, validity and consistency edits (gender–procedure, age–procedure, place–procedure, provider/specialty–procedure, type–procedure, diagnosis–procedure, lifetime–procedure, etc.), rebundling rules, reinsurance amounts, duplicate parameters, processor limitations, claim to authorization record matching parameters, table of procedures that allow assistants
Accounts payable information	A table mapping procedure codes or ranges and/or type of service codes to financial revenue codes
Vendor record	A record that identifies the payee, including tax and discount information

tion easily, to search by various fields (e.g., to find a particular claim or claims for a particular member, group, or provider), and to locate claims occurring on a particular date. It is also important that customer service representatives, as well as claims examiners, be able to access this information in a relatively straightforward way, without having to wade through multiple screens of information or having to translate information from a code into English.

System ability to support claims processing contributes significantly to efficient and accurate claims processing. To the extent that the managed care system fails to support eligibility, product, line of business, medical management requirements, and payment arrangements, a plan will have to make up for system inadequacies through increased manual processing. Increased manual processing is a detriment to the claims process in two ways. First, work flows will be compounded to ensure that claims of a specific type are routed to examiners who are trained to handle them. Second, individual interpretation of adjudication rules is prone to misjudgment, and pricing is prone to calculation errors. Manual claims adjudication is slower, less accurate, and less consistent.

Systems involve increasingly complex configuration in direct proportion to the amount of flexibility they offer, such as varied eligibility rules, products, or benefits packages; different rules regarding necessity for referral or precertification authorization; and complex reimbursement methodology. Eligibility rules (e.g., preexisting conditions, waiting periods, and student age limitations) vary per group. Plan enrollment processes, which generally focus on entry of member data, need to include transmittal of eligibility rules to claims. Likewise, the benefits that make up a product must be loaded into the system. Any new product development or revision of benefits to suit a particular employer group must be transmitted to claims for codification into the supporting system. The effort required to interpret benefits is often underestimated. Covered and excluded benefits must be listed not generically by type, as they are in marketing materials and member contracts, but as specific procedures or ranges that will cause claim payment or denial. Claims should solicit medical management direction while codifying benefits as well for those procedures, such as reconstructive surgery, where coverage depends upon medical necessity. Additionally, medical management and claims must work together to determine the parameters for claim and authorization record matches. The reimbursement methodologies stipulated in provider contracts must also be codified in the system. Again, as with benefits, definitions of reimbursements according to procedure type and location must be translated into specific procedure codes and place of service types to support automated claim adjudication.

Successful system support of claims adjudication relies upon correct and timely system configuration. Irrespective of the company area that controls the information in related subsystems, it becomes claims' responsibility to ensure the correct implementation of configuration parameters—the controlling logic rules that support claims processing. More than translating business rules into system parameters and logic, maintenance of system configuration requires timely acquisition of clear and specific business rules from other areas in the company in mutually acceptable formats.

As a corollary to requiring timely and precisely stated information from other company areas, system codification requires management sign-off from those areas that parameters have been loaded properly.

Administration of system configuration is a distinct function within claims, one that requires prompt turnaround, accurate coding, and its own QA controls. Correct configuration substantially increases claims accuracy, timeliness, and consistency, all of which contribute to provider and member satisfaction with plan service.

CLAIMS BUSINESS FUNCTIONS

Whether your claims process is fully or partially automated or entirely manual, the following business functions contribute to the adjudication of any particular claim. To accommodate many of these steps and processes, information from other areas within the organization must be gleaned and codified into the computer system to serve as guidelines in the adjudication of claims. It is important to note that these steps and processes must be continually evaluated and updated because they rely on information and guidelines that are subject to change over time. The accompanying flowchart (Figure 38–4) depicts the entire flow of claims processing starting with preparation.

Determination of Liability

The first step in claim adjudication determines the plan's liability based on the contractual relationship between the plan and the pa-

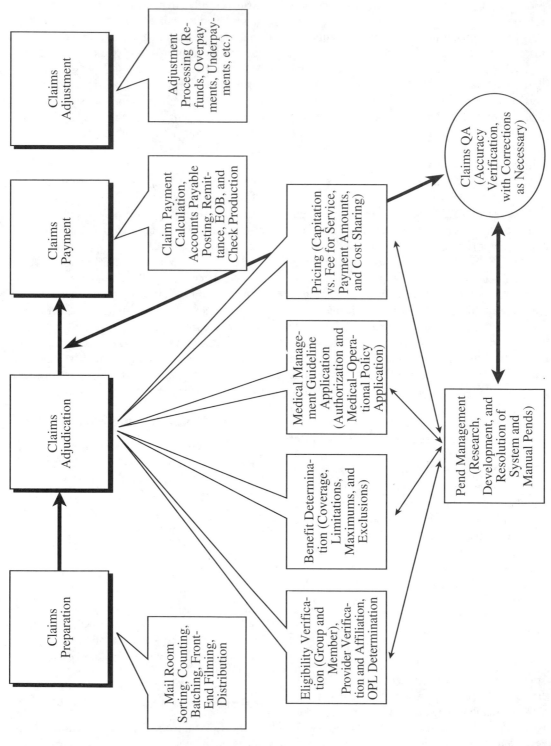

Figure 38–4 Claims processing flow. EOB, explanation of benefits.

tient. Membership eligibility steps determine the relationship of the member to the contract holder (direct contract or dependent membership), compare the service date(s) for the claim with the effective dates of the policy, and evaluate whether the member has coverage through another group health plan that could be responsible for the primary payment of the claim under the terms of coordination of benefits. Based on the member's eligibility status through a particular employer group account, further conditions of eligibility are determined. If group premiums are in arrears for the period in which the service date of the claim occurs, there may be cause to withhold payment. Group-specific rules regarding age cut-offs for dependent members may apply. Proof of full-time student status in an accredited continuing education program may be required. Through the establishment of eligibility as a member of an employer group, the particular product and its specific list of benefits may be retrieved. Benefits, in addition to listing covered and excluded services, list member contribution amounts applicable toward claim payment (copayments, coinsurance, and deductibles). Member annual and lifetime benefits limits may limit the plan's liability with respect to the particular claim. Out-of-pocket limitations may curtail the member's responsibility for copayments if they have already been met. Depending upon the health care product, the amount of the plan's liability for the rendered services may differ based on the member's adherence to medical management policies. The member's relationship to the provider of services is reviewed to determine whether the provider is the member's PCP, a specialist within the network to whom the member was referred by his or her PCP, or an out-of-network provider. The combination of information obtained from the member and group records begins to shape a picture of the proportionate shares of plan and member liability. Additional information regarding adherence to medical management guidelines will be found in a matching authorization record (if any). Final pricing will necessarily take into account the plan's contractual arrangement with the provider.

Benefit Administration

Although benefits are defined in evidence of coverage documents and are summarized in benefits brochures provided by the MCO, many instances will arise where an interpretation must be issued to state more specifically what the MCO's position is regarding coverage for specific services. With the introduction of new benefits packages where more than just copayments are modified, interpretation activities will intensify. It must be remembered that every benefit is covered only within the context of medical necessity and medical appropriateness as determined by the MCO and within the rules regarding eligibility, use of the participating delivery system, and so forth.

Benefits interpretations involve decisions of what the MCO will and will not cover from an insurance perspective. This function is not to be confused with medical policy determinations, which involve decisions regarding the conditions under which the MCO will consider services medically necessary and/or nonexperimental in nature.

The process of interpreting benefits within an MCO must be a managed, monitored, and documented activity for several reasons:

- Once a benefit has been interpreted, the interpretation must be consistently applied and consistently communicated whenever the same issue is raised (by marketing, member services, provider relations, or elsewhere).
- Benefit determinations can have an impact on all operating areas, from finance (because of the costs associated with the benefit) to claims (which must pay in accordance with the interpretation) and all other operating areas.
- The degree to which an interpretation meets needs may vary from operating area to operating area. For example, marketing needs for coverage of a benefit may not be consistent with good medical practice or with product pricing. As a consequence, decisions may have to balance competing demands.

The interpretation of benefits within the MCO should be a centralized function and must also be responsive to the need to resolve interpretation issues in a timely and well-considered fashion. An executive-level committee is the typical vehicle for interpreting benefits within an MCO. The committee may consist of the chief executive officer/chief operating officer, the director of health services or medical director, one representative from claims, and one representative from the marketing department. The committee convenes on an ad hoc basis as issues arise for interpretation. Participation from the Finance Department may be included for purposes of determining financial impact of benefit interpretations. The committee should hold itself to a TAT standard for rendering benefit interpretation decisions.

Determinations will frequently require research regarding the exact nature of a procedure or service as well as clinical circumstances and considerations. Such determinations may require a joint effort involving both a benefits interpretation and a medical policy decision.

When benefits interpretation decisions are reached by the committee, they should be documented in a standard format and provided to all staff who need to have such information (e.g., claims, member services, health services, provider relations, etc.). Many MCOs maintain benefit interpretation manuals for this purpose.

Information to members, providers, and groups regarding covered benefits must be both accurate and consistent. Failure to provide accurate information may wrongfully deny a member needed services or may obligate the MCO to provide services that were not contemplated in the development of premiums/rates. When an MCO employee is asked a question regarding coverage of services, procedures, supplies, and the like, responses must be based word-for-word on one of two sources:

1. The first response provided should be an exact presentation of the applicable evidence of coverage language and must include a search for covered benefits and a search for any exclusions or limitations. It must further include a common warning regarding the medical necessity of all MCO covered services.

2. If the exact evidence of coverage language does not answer the question, the benefits interpretation manual should be searched to determine whether an interpretation has been reached that satisfies the question, again with the medical necessity requirements being kept in mind.

If neither of these two sources answers the question, the question should be referred to the benefits interpretation committee. If a question needs to be referred either because the answer is not clear or because there appears not to have been an interpretation that addresses the question, a standard form may be used to convey the needed benefit interpretation and any supporting documentation to the committee. Although the committee should be responsive to requests for interpretation, the person posing the question should be clearly told that getting an answer may take several days.

The benefit interpretations themselves should be sufficiently detailed and specific to provide exact claims adjudication guidelines. For example, stating in a benefit interpretation that ambulance transportation is covered in full does not give a claims examiner enough detail to adjudicate a claim properly. The level of detail needed includes answers to the following questions: Is mileage, in addition to the transport charge, reimbursable? Is transportation between two hospital facilities covered? Is air ambulance covered? Is transportation from the hospital to home covered? If an ambulance is summoned but the patient refuses transportation, is the MCO financially responsible? Is medical necessity to be questioned (only certain diagnoses are coverable)? Is transportation from the hospital to a nursing home, or vice versa, covered? A benefit interpretation should address all these coverage issues thereby allowing the claims examiner to make an informed benefit coverage decision within the circumstantial and clinical contexts of any given claim.

Pricing

Pricing claims involves the determination of three things: the contractual reimbursement amount, member cost sharing, and OPL. The majority of claims are priced by the MCO's computer system based on established planwide and individual fee schedules, capitation tables, diagnosis-related group/ambulatory patient group tables, global fees, deductible and copayment tables, secondary payment calculation formulas, provider records, and vendor records. The key in a new MCO is to identify the individuals and departments responsible for these initial set-ups and to establish the means for ongoing maintenance of the various files and tables as existing provider agreements are updated and new arrangements are entered into. Benefit design changes and implementation of new products will also effect changes/additions to pricing information.

Although claims and benefits administration does not typically own or control the various fee schedules, tables, formulas, and provider/vendor records required to establish pricing rules and automate the process, the pricing component of claims adjudication relies on the timeliness and accuracy of these data to produce precise claims payments. For this reason, the astute claims manager understands all the inputs to claims pricing and maintains effective working relationships with those individuals responsible for provider contracting and associated computer systems set-up and maintenance. Although pricing files are not usually under the purview of claims and benefits administration, information about new contracts and changes to existing ones must be conveyed to claims on a routine and timely basis. The need for this information stems from claims QA requirements and the need, on occasion, to be able to price claims manually until the computer system parameters are established and implemented. Many audits have resulted in findings of erroneous claims payments due to inaccurate interpretation/set-up of computer pricing files.

In addition to the plan's MIS being able to cross-reference the fee schedules and payment mechanisms for purposes of processing claims, many MCOs also use a transmittal sheet to convey provider identification, payment, and payee information from contract administration to claims and benefits administration. The transmittal sheet is modeled after the various data requirements in the MCO computer system's provider, pricing, and vendor files. When sent to claims, the transmittal form either includes a copy of the signed contract or references the exact contract (and addenda) by name and number (which claims can then reference to sample contracts on file).

Member cost sharing through deductibles, copayments, and coinsurances (and circumscribed by out-of-pocket maximums) is also typically driven by computer system tables that are established initially and updated for new or modified benefit designs. As with pricing file information, the need for cost-sharing information stems from claims QA requirements and the need, on occasion, to be able to price claims manually.

Following are examples of cost-sharing provisions and how they are applied:

- *Physician office visits:* Only one copayment is assessed for each office visit regardless of the number and type of service performed and reported for that visit. The copayment need not be assessed only against evaluation and management CPT-4 codes. For example, if the only service reported is suture removal, any applicable copayment is assessed against the suture removal code.
- *Chiropractic services:* Copayment/coinsurance applies to all covered services rendered, including, but not limited to, manual manipulation of subluxation and radiology. Coinsurance applies to all services regardless of place of service.
- *Inpatient admission:* Deductible is waived for a second admission resulting from a transfer from one acute care facility to another (look for a transfer code in the discharge disposition field of the UB-92). Emergency department copayment is waived when the visit results in an inpatient admission. When there is a readmission for the same condition any applicable inpatient admission deductible is assessed against the second admission.

- *Female and male sterilization:* The copayment applies to each of these surgical procedures and is always assessed against the professional fee.
- *DME and prosthetics:* The DME and prosthetic out-of-pocket maximum is calculated per benefit year; copayment/coinsurance applies to all DME and prosthetics charges.
- *Out-of-pocket maximums:* The individual and family out-of-pocket maximums apply per benefit year and include the member cost sharing (deductible, copayment, and coinsurance) portion of covered services.

OPL also affects claims pricing. For coordination of benefits when your MCO is secondary, the payment on a claim is generally reduced to the difference between the primary plan's payment and the usual and customary charge for the services in question. Depending on the specific state's regulations concerning workers' compensation and any arrangement that the MCO may have made with the workers' compensation carrier, your MCO will either price and pay claims as if it were fully liable (and recoverable through the workers' compensation carrier) or deny services that are confirmed as being coverable by workers' compensation (see Chapter 61). Subrogation cases, because they are typically carried out over an extended period, usually result in initial full claims payment by the MCO with liens applied to whatever monies may be gleaned through settlement or court award. It should be noted that each state has its own regulations for OPL, and their effects on claims pricing will differ depending on their content. See Chapter 39 for more details.

Customer Service

Because one of the five basic functions of claims and benefits administration is to provide, by way of claims processing, service to both member and provider customers, it is important for the department to interact with and get feedback from those departments whose sole purpose is customer contact (see Chapter 40). As a measure of overall performance, the claims department should track claims-related inquiries, complaints, and grievances from both members and providers. The primary way to do this is through review of reports provided by member services and provider relations. When specific categories of claims-related questions/complaints occur in any significant volume over a period of time, it is incumbent on claims and benefits administration to determine the cause(s) of the problem(s) and to work within the department and with member service/provider relations personnel to resolve the issues. The relationships between claims and these departments should be such that:

- claims management periodically sits in on member services and provider relations staff meetings, and vice versa
- claims management is designated as a review point for grievances
- provider relations, on behalf of claims, returns to a particular provider for correction a complete batch of claims submitted incorrectly
- claims staff give priority to resolving predefined, specific claims issues related to member/provider complaints
- claims staff occasionally accompany provider relations staff on site visits to providers' locations to provide orientation on claims submission or to resolve voluminous claims-related issues
- member services staff collect and report to claims updated alternate carrier information about individual members

Claims should also provide management of these two departments, among others, with routine inventory, productivity, and quality statistics. Maintaining effective relationships with member services and provider relations is essential.

Adjustments

There are two types of adjustments: clinical/clerical, which may involve spelling errors, coding errors, and omissions; and financial. Clinical/clerical adjustments make changes that do not affect payment but rectify inaccurately recorded utilization information. These are important for providing accurate information to support the analysis of the plan's utilization patterns to estimate future liability (see Chapter 47), support physician profiling (see Chapter 32), and support appeals and grievance processes (see Chapter 40). Financial adjustments involve claim corrections for payment errors (wrong payee or wrong amount) and may or may not involve clinical adjustments as well. The two usually are intertwined, as when the wrong number of units, visits, or days affects both clinical information and payment calculation.

Adjustments are triggered by returned checks, customer/provider service calls, and a variety of other transactions. Methods for achieving adjustments differ from system to system. Effectively, the original claim information is nullified by the creation of a reversal claim record. Subsequently, the correct claim is entered. This methodology provides for the ability to recreate a snapshot of prior months' activities, as well as year-to-date information. Difficulties arise when corrective claims are entered after the prior period's finances have been closed out.

Management will want to maintain information about and routinely analyze the types of claims that are susceptible to readjustment, categories of adjustment, and processors responsible for erroneous claims. The adjustment process itself is subject to QA, along with all other claims transactions, to ensure it is done correctly. Claims adjustments, rather than being a reactive step to correct processing errors, can then be used proactively to identify system configuration errors, benefits design ambiguities, and processor training issues.

Management Reporting

Claims operations management reporting is required internally for claims and benefits administration, within the operations division and companywide. The term *claims operations management reporting* refers to standard information about inventory, productivity, and quality. Intra-departmentally, it will be necessary to have, on a daily basis, individual claims exam-

iner and aggregated departmental reports of inventory and productivity.

Departmental reporting starts with the mail room function, wherein, on a daily basis, total receipts are sorted (by type and category), recorded, and totaled. The exact format of a claims mail room daily count sheet will depend on the degree of sorting that is done. For example, depending on task allocation within the claims shop, some claims mail room functions may sort paper claim submissions into inpatient UB-92s, outpatient UB-92s, encounter HCFA-1500s, specialist HCFA-1500s, ancillary HCFA-1500s, and member-submitted claims; other shops might simply sort by UB-92s and HCFA-1500s. Additional types of receipts may include correspondence, explanations of benefits, explanations of Medicare benefits, medical records, duplicate coverage inquiry responses (for coordination of benefits), refund checks, and other miscellaneous documents. In any event, a daily count of all receipts into the department is completed by mail room staff and forwarded to the claims manager or supervisor.

The second departmental report is an individual count sheet for each person contributing to daily productivity. On this daily report there is a count of beginning desk inventory (claims/encounters), receipts, spit claims, pended/suspended transactions, processed work (including transactions released from pending/suspension and completed), and ending desk inventory. For those individuals who are responsible for the majority of the daily production (i.e., claims examiners or resolution analysts, depending on task allocation and job title), the daily inventory and productivity report also includes a section for comments about extraordinary circumstances. These are circumstances that detract from an examiner's ability to produce fully, such as system downtime or slowness, training time, and the like.

The statistics on these individual reports are combined with other information to produce a daily departmental inventory and productivity report. Other information that will be shown on a daily departmental inventory and productivity report includes oldest date of receipt in house by type of claim and information about electronic receipts, productivity, and inventory.

These daily reports are consolidated into a weekly inventory and productivity report for internal departmental purposes and then into a monthly report that is shared with operations management and claims' other corporate colleagues. The weekly and monthly reports are similar to daily reports except that they provide a snapshot of a week's or month's activity (versus a day's). These manually produced reports provide a running count of receipts, production, and inventory by category of work; are compared on a routine basis with physical inventory counts and system-produced reports; and are reconciled. An accurate count of inventory must include all work to be done, not just those transactions that have been entered into the computer system. Also, it is customary for inventory descriptions to differentiate not only among categories of work on hand but also within categories among the various stages of incomplete work (on the shelf, logged, and pended).

Weekly consolidation of all claims' inventory and production reporting is critical to ongoing inventory control because it enables management to identify quickly and manage variation in workload among units. This type of evaluation, coupled with redeployment of resources (based on workload, by unit), allows the department to maintain some parity in the age of work on hand, ensuring that oldest claims are worked first.

Claims business function reporting refers to the ability to determine and report on, at any given point in time, key statistics such as percentage of paid and denied claims, lag time and outstanding claims liability, and OPL savings for input to other MCO management functions. The following statistics must be routinely tracked and monitored by claims management:

- monthly and annual receipts (numbers and dollars)
- average number of claims on hand (numbers and dollars)
- average productivity (by examiner and in aggregate, daily and weekly)
- weeks' work on hand (volume divided by average weekly productivity)

- claims pended/suspended by type of pend/suspend and in total (number, percentage, and dollars)
- denied claims (number, percentage, and dollars)
- average claims per member
- OPL savings (coordination of benefits, subrogation, and workers' compensation) by avoidance, diversion, and recovery

Not only does this information provide valuable input to other management functions, but it also assists in the effective management of the claims and benefits administration function (e.g., anticipating and planning for reduction of backlogs, staffing projection, performance management, etc.).

Claims Business Function Reporting

In addition to reporting on the status of claims work flow and inventory, a second set of claims reports focuses on the analysis of the way the business is conducted. Utilization reports are used to manage, on an individual case basis and in aggregate, the cost of health care, which is the overwhelming expense category for any health care concern. Analysis of these kinds of reports provides a forecast for liability trends and informs the plan of corrective policy and operational steps that may be taken. Examples of this type of report include paid claims versus denied claims and claims lag to anticipate incurred but not reported (IBNR) costs. Claims and encounter reports may be evaluated to monitor the adequacy of capitation, to serve as the basis for reevaluation and renegotiation of capitation rates, and to determine those types of care that can be better managed through capitation (versus fee-for-service) arrangements.

On an individual provider basis, these reports will be used to profile practice patterns and serve as a tool to ensure, over time, the appropriate and medically necessary use of health care resources. Utilization data serve as an indicator of product and pricing needs to remain viable in the long term while providing necessary benefits and coverage to the membership base.

Reports extracted from the paid (or processed) claims file may also be used to modify existing benefits packages to the extent that reported services serve as indicators of actual utilization versus covered services. Medical management, specifically the quality management (QM) function, uses the claims database as a source for claims-based studies regarding quality of care and adherence to practice protocols, preventive health service guidelines, and other clinical standards. The QM function also uses the claims database as a repository from which to select sample cases for special studies (e.g., all members with a reported diagnosis of diabetes mellitus) and to identify aberrant clinical practices. As previously mentioned, finance routinely makes use of many reports that use as their basis the claims history file.

OTHER ISSUES

This section addresses issues that organizations consider with respect to claims, often reactively. Common claims problems, unaddressed, may have a seemingly disproportionate impact upon an organization's operational and financial stability. Once such problems have become entrenched in the corporate infrastructure they become increasingly difficult to resolve. Some plans have turned successfully to outsourcing claims administration. Valid reasons for doing so, and various options regarding what portions of claims processing to outsource, are addressed below.

Common Claims and Benefits Administration Problems

Since claims and benefits administration is such a multifaceted and complex task, it is subject to many pitfalls. Some of the most commonly seen problems are described here along with their ramifications. It is hoped that by bringing these issues to the reader's attention, they can be recognized and preemptively avoided.

Claims Backlog

A sustained claims backlog translates into provider dissatisfaction with possible degrada-

tion of the network, potential balance billing of members, stresses on internal operations (member and provider services), increased duplicate billings (therefore, increased claims volume), noncompliance with state or federal turnaround time regulation, potential undetected increases in the medical expense trend, and the inability to accurately accrue for claims expense. This situation presages a potential disaster for an MCO. Any claims backlog should be resolved quickly and effectively to avoid irreparable damage to the MCO. The resolution should include the development, documentation, and management of an inventory reduction plan.

Inadequate Front-End Control

Inadequate front-end control refers to not entering claims into the computer system, at least in skeletal form, within two days of their receipt. At a minimum, claims control information should include a claim number, member and provider identification, date of service, and a total charge for each claim. Electronic input of claims data via OCR, tape, or other electronic transmissions eliminates the need for manual front-end control, but there are still many shops where paper claims sit on shelves untouched, marked as "work to be done." When this occurs, provider and member services functions cannot be performed adequately, the likelihood of increased duplicate claims receipts increases, and MCOs founder in their attempts to accurately predict IBNR claims expense, as discussed in Chapter 46.

Inadequate Pended Claims Management

The management of pended claims, although critical to turnaround time, is often decentralized (relegated to each claims examiner), informal (no turnaround time standards per pend reason), and/or allocated to the "when we have a minute" time frame. In fact, management and timely resolution of pended claims is every bit as important, and perhaps more so, than initial processing. Pended claims are older than new inventory, often are caught in "problem" pockets, and usually require intra- and/or interdepartmental coordination to resolve. Beside the obvious impacts of claims delays, with associated increases in member and provider complaints, increased volumes of pended claims disrupt the normal balance of simple-to-complex claims and stress the relationships between claims and supporting departments.

Outdated Structure/Task Allocation (Misaligned with New Business Needs)

Shifts in membership concentration, changes in provider reimbursement mechanisms, and new lines of business and alterations in an MCO's relationships with its participating providers are among the most prevalent reasons why claims shops must routinely monitor and update organizational structures and task allocation. For example, Medicare beneficiaries are higher utilizers of inpatient care than commercial members. If claims is organized by claim type and new or increased Medicare membership is anticipated, staffing reallocations or possibly additions will likely be required. Such reallocations are not always quickly made, as they often require additional training. As another example, the provision of health care through a risk-assuming preferred provider network may signal a decrease in claim volumes. A proactive administrator will continuously review changes in membership and provider relationships to predict and plan for needed changes in organizational structure and task allocation. When these factors are not synchronized with claims processing needs, backlogs and errors will doubtless ensue.

Supporting Data File Integrity Problems

There are several key MCO data files, the timely and accurate maintenance of which are critical to effective claims and benefit administration. Key data files include: membership file (including alternate insurance information), provider file, pricing files, and code files. When these files are corrupt and/or outdated, or there are multiple such files that do not match each other, claims errors and increased pends result. Most MCOs designate a "user owner" for each of the key data files and it is the responsibility of

these individuals to assure that file information is accurate, nonduplicative, and timely. In support of these endeavors, others within the MCO are responsible for providing corrective/updated information, as received, to the user owners, who then must take immediate action in correcting file records. Among the most common reasons for claims pends are "member eligibility" and "provider not on file." Claims payment errors frequently result when inadequate provider file maintenance yields multiple records for the same provider, often due simply to variance in data entry protocol (this same problem affects provider profiling, as discussed in Chapter 32). Pricing file errors cause payment mistakes. Outdated code files cause increased pends, payment errors, and inaccurate claims history.

Benefits Configuration Problems

All too frequently the way that benefit rules are set up in an MCO's computer system results in claims errors and pends. Set-up errors are critical because they affect every claim that coincides with a particular automated benefit rule; human errors occur more randomly and, hopefully, with less regularity. Some of the most constantly observed benefit set-up mistakes are incomplete codes or code ranges, erroneous copayment application, and outdated code rules (not updated annually with standard code files). An astute claims examiner can easily recognize benefit set-up problems; the same is true for claims training and quality control staff. When errors are found, it is imperative that they are communicated and corrected immediately to avoid continued pends and mispayments.

Informal Benefits Interpretation

Anyone who has ever processed a claim, or managed the function, knows that benefit summaries, evidence of coverage documents, and group or individual contracts do not provide the level of detail necessary to determine benefit eligibility for every service reported on every claim. Since services are reported at code level detail, using standard coding schema (CPT-4, HCPCS, DRG, APG, etc.), it is unrealistic to believe that any written benefits description will ever anticipate and specify coverage guidelines for all of the many thousands of code choices. For this reason it is necessary for MCOs to have a formalized and rational approach to benefits interpretation. Absent this integral part of benefits administration, MCOs likely will make inconsistent and/or incorrect benefits decisions and, as the result, will face increased member and provider appeals, increased claims adjustments, and possible litigation.

Utilization Management–Claims Clash

Claims and utilization management are integrally linked in that UM provides instructions required by claims to effectively complete adjudication tasks. While prudence may suggest that the relationship between the two functions is inherently interdependent, it is not atypical to see rifts. A common UM complaint is that "claims doesn't pay according to the instructions on authorizations and precertifications." Just as typical is the criticism, by claims, that "UM doesn't enter authorizations on time and when they do their instructions are unclear, incomplete, and/or hard to decipher." To avoid, or at least mitigate, ineffective coordination between UM and claims, the guidelines within which they will coordinate must be established, monitored, and updated on an as-needed basis. To assure that UM instructions are followed in the adjudication of claims, the two areas should jointly develop an audit mechanism that routinely determines the accuracy with which UM instructions are used. The consequences of ineffective coordination include: delayed claims, increased pended claims volumes, inappropriately paid or denied claims, increased claims expense, increased appeals and adjustment volumes, and dissatisfied provider and member customers. The advent of newer UM software support systems is helping to resolve these coordination problems since these systems often have the ability to pass data directly to the claims system, as well as draw data from it.

Outsourcing Claims Processing

There are circumstances under which it is desirable, even necessary, for an MCO to outsource the processing of claims. These circumstances may occur at initial MCO set-up or after an organization is operational. Outsourcing can take several forms: for some or all aspects of claims administration, for some or all types of claims, permanently or on a temporary basis, and with a single or multiple vendors. What is most important is that the MCO keep outsourcing in mind as an option and, when exploring the option, employ a systematic approach to decision making.

Indications for outsourcing, or circumstances where it may be desirable, include:

1. *At initial MCO set-up:*
   - local, experienced staff cannot be found
   - MCO staff lacks the expertise to process one or more types of claims
   - MCO finds it too costly to set up its own claims department
   - MCO is outsourcing its total systems needs (or renting, time-sharing) and the systems vendor provides TPA services
   - initial membership projections do not allow the MCO to get to "critical mass" within one to two years to make inside claims administration cost effective

2. *Postoperational:*
   - claims performance is poor (accuracy, TAT, management control) and the MCO is in jeopardy (with state regulators, HCFA, large group accounts, etc.)
   - MCO has experienced a chronic claims backlog
   - high staff turnover in the claims department
   - regulatory complaints regarding claims performance (TAT, accuracy, and so forth) are voluminous
   - MCO incurs large membership growth (due to purchase of business, incoming large group accounts, etc.) in a short time frame
   - MCO acquires additional business/licensure/geographic expansion in disparate location(s)
   - MCO's computer system is "wearing out" (e.g., throughput problems, inadequate functionality or scalability, outdated or orphaned technology)

- MCO is in the process of evaluating computer systems for conversion and during implementation may look to the vendor to provide claims processing, at least on a temporary basis

Outsourcing claims is also an option in the context of the MCO's contracts with provider organizations; that is, when provider groups (typically integrated delivery systems or organized health systems, referred to generally as IDSs; see Chapter 4) are capitated by the MCO, the arrangement may or may not include adjudication and payment of claims by the IDSs. Another form of outsourcing is where "carve-out" benefits (e.g., pharmacy and mental health/substance abuse) are managed outside of the MCO by a contracted vendor. These carve-out vendors most often process benefit-related claims. For risk-taking providers and carve-out vendors who process claims, integrating their claims data into the MCO's health care utilization database is a fundamental issue.

When considering outsourcing, remember that all or portions of claims administration responsibility may be outsourced. For example, some firms specialize only in data entry and can provide electronic versions of claims, which are then loaded into the MCO's computer system for editing and adjudication. In this case, the MCO's claims examiners resolve only those transactions that could not be entered by the vendor, those that did not pass initial MCO edits, and those that pend during the adjudication process.

Other firms provide full claims entry, adjudication, and payment services through interfacing with the MCO's supporting data files. Carve-out vendors typically provide full processing services for their specific claim types.

Whether outsourcing all or any portion of claims and benefits administration, the MCO cannot abrogate its responsibility for the accuracy and timeliness of claims and benefits administration functions and data. Its constituents (members, providers, and regulators) look to the MCO to provide and effectively administer the health care benefits that have been purchased.

CONCLUSION

Claims, medical management, enrollment, and billing together form the core of plan operations and control. Those plans that dedicate resources to marketing, product development, customer service, and other activities to the exclusion of claims operations run the risk of failing to deliver to plan customers what they have purchased or contracted to receive. Claims is where the plan has a direct relationship with all its customers (providers, members, and groups) and where all preceding relationships and information come together. Additionally, the plan relies on information created in the process of adjudicating claims to understand and manage many other aspects of its business. The quality of claims and benefits administration significantly determines the plan's overall success.

CHAPTER 39

Other Party Liability and Coordination of Benefits

Barry S. Scheur, Robin L. McElfatrick, and Robert S. Eichler

With one exception, the claims processing function reports cost but does not control cost. Control of cost is exercised through medical management, provider contracting, and other means. Only a properly structured claims process, however, can provide the data that will permit the plan to control cost. The exception is other party liability (OPL). In the case of OPL, the claims process controls cost by obtaining reductions in the net cost of medical services provided through the avoidance, diversion, or recovery of costs that should be borne by other parties. OPL is an integral part of the claims management process and depends upon the effective conduct of claims processing.

Although traditionally indemnity plans have reported OPL savings as a percentage of premium, health maintenance organizations (HMOs) typically report such savings in the same manner as other financial factors: as a per member per month (PMPM) value. Alternatively, HMOs may report OPL savings as a percentage of net paid claims amount. An aggressive OPL program, for an organization in a metropolitan area where double-income families are the norm and in a jurisdiction that permits

Barry S. Scheur, JD, is the Founder and President of Scheur Management Group, Inc., a health care management and consulting firm in Newton, Massachusetts, specializing in the conceptualization and implementation of innovative and effective managed care solutions. He writes and lectures extensively on the operational and futuristic trends in the provision of health care, as well as on innovative marketing strategies, the vital importance of customer service, and the newest challenges in the Medicaid and Medicare arenas. Scheur's advice and counsel have been sought by hundreds of HMOs, physician groups, hospitals, insurance companies, and major employers.

Robin L. McElfatrick, Vice President of Scheur Management Group, Inc., has spent a decade in managed care consulting after having worked in a variety of positions for both an indemnity plan and an HMO. She provides consulting services to a diverse set of managed care organizations and specializes in the areas of medical management, claims, other party liabil-

ity, enrollment, billing and collection, customer services, and management information systems (MIS). Her consulting engagements have spanned operations design and development for new organizations, problem identification and resolution for established organizations, claims functional analyses and audits, program-specific development (Medicare and Medicaid), and plan liquidation management.

Robert S. Eichler, Vice President of Scheur Management Group, Inc., is a founding member of the consulting firm. He specializes in evaluating health care MIS, operational auditing and re-engineering, system conversions, systems/product linkages, development of business rules, system requirements and functional workflows, with emphasis on MIS, claims, enrollment, billing and collection, provider credentialing, and customer services departments. He has assisted managed care and hospital association clients in system strategy and provided claims and other party liability audits and functional analyses.

subrogation, can expect to save from $3.50 to $4.50 PMPM (in 1999 dollars), or roughly 3.5 percent to 4.5 percent of net paid claims.

DEFINITIONS

OPL may be categorized by two factors: the manner in which costs that may be avoided are identified; and in the processes, operational and legal, by which to effect the cost reduction. Plans often lump all categories under one definitional term (usually, inaccurately, coordination of benefits—COB) and suffer the financial consequences of reduced savings from these activities because the differentiating operational nuances are also lumped together. The following definitions clarify the distinctions between the two categories of OPL. Whether or not the exact terminology presented here is adopted in a particular plan, clear terminology consistently understood within the claims department and throughout the organization provides a foundation for effective OPL activities.

OPL activities usually encompass three kinds of mechanisms by which the costs of health care delivery that should be paid by someone other than the plan are avoided by the plan or are diverted to or recovered from an alternative payer: COB, third-party recovery (TPR), and nonplan liability. COB and TPR are usually grouped under the heading of insurance and liability recovery or OPL. The three mechanisms are operationally handled in quite different ways.

Coordination of Benefits

COB is an administrative process whereby plans coordinate the reimbursement of health care services for members covered by two or more plans. If a patient has costs that are payable by the plan under the certificate of benefits that applies to the patient as a member of the plan, and some or all of the costs may also be payable by another health insurance coverage held by the patient, then the respective primary and secondary payment obligations of the two coverages are determined by the Order of Benefits Determination (OOBD) Rules contained in the Na-

tional Association of Insurance Commissioners (NAIC) Model COB Regulation, as interpreted and adopted by the various states. Generally, the OOBD rules among commercial plans specify that a plan is primary for its own subscribers, secondary for the spouse of its subscriber, and for children of married, non-separated parents, the plan of the parent whose birthday falls earlier in the year is primary. For children of separated or divorced parents, either a court order will stipulate responsibility for health coverage, or in the absence of a court decree, the plan of the natural parent with custody is primary, the plan of the spouse of the natural parent with custody is secondary, and the plan of the natural parent without custody is third. Plans covering a subscriber through active employment are primary to plans covering the subscriber as a retiree. Finally, as a tie-breaker, plans that have been in effect longer are primary over plans in effect for a shorter period of time. These rules must comply with the regulation as adopted within the jurisdiction where the plan operates. Primary means that the carrier is responsible for costs of the claim up to the benefit limit of the coverage. Secondary means that the carrier is responsible for any unpaid balance of the total allowable expenses, up to what it would have paid if it had been primary within the claim determination period. COB applies to group health benefits and, in some jurisdictions, to nongroup (or direct pay) health benefits. The definition also applies to the health care portion of automobile insurance. Auto insurance may be primary or secondary to the plan, depending on state regulations and specific auto insurance contracts. Personal injury protection may likewise be primary or secondary to the plan.

COB is the process of applying the NAIC rules to determine the costs for which the plan is primarily responsible and the costs for which the plan would be in a secondary position if applicable alternative coverage exists. If the plan is secondary for any costs, COB is the process of discovering whether any applicable alternative coverage is (or may be) in effect. If applicable alternative coverage is (or may be) in effect and the plan is secondary, COB is the process of avoiding those costs for which another carrier is known to be liable by denying the claim, diverting those costs for which the plan is secondary to the alternative carrier (if the costs have not already been paid by the plan), or recovering those costs for which the plan is secondary to the alternative carrier. Medicare and Medicaid coordination is a special case of COB, where the alternative coverage is provided by a government plan.

The definition of COB also applies to Medicare and Medicaid, although the order of benefits determination—which plan is primary and which secondary—differs from that of coordination between commercial plans. The trend we have witnessed is that Medicare more frequently is positioned in the secondary payer role, after other coverage such as employer group health plans, no-fault insurance, automobile medical insurance, liability insurance, and workers' compensation. The OOBD rules that apply to Medicare will continue to change over time, according to stipulations within the Balanced Budget Act (BBA) of 1996 and other regulations, as they become effective. At the time of publication, Medicare OOBD may be summarized as follows: If the member is still actively employed or the spouse of an active employee, Medicare is usually secondary to the commercial coverage, contingent upon the employer group size. The single exception to this is for patients with end-stage renal disease, where Medicare is primary after a 30-month period. If the member is eligible based on disability, Medicare is primary. If the member is retired, the commercial plan is primary from age 65 to 70, and Medicare becomes primary at age 70. Again, group size may be a determining factor for whether coverage is primary or secondary, and these age limitations are set to change over the next decade. Medicaid, a joint federal- and state-funded program administered by each state, is generally the payer of last resort, standing secondary to all other payment sources.

The term *avoidance* applies when the plan is made aware before paying the claim that another party is responsible and simply denies part or all of the claim, forwarding it to the correctly liable party for payment. The term *diversion* applies when the plan pends a claim for COB determina-

tion and does not pay it until the COB process is performed. These two processes are commonly referred to as "pursue and pay" or "chase and pay." The term *recovery* applies when the plan pays the entire claim and then performs the COB process in an effort to recover that portion of the costs of the claim for which the plan is in a secondary position under the NAIC rules. This process is commonly referred to as "pay and pursue" or "pay and chase."

Third-Party Recovery (Subrogation)

Subrogation is a legal process whereby the plan may seek reimbursement—from its members or a third party that is legally responsible (at fault) for claims arising from a negligent act or omission—by standing legally in place of its members in pursuit of that recovery. TPR encompasses accident, malpractice, and other negligence and omission events. Workers' compensation is a special case of TPR (see Chapter 61). Case identification methods include medical record notations, examination of specific diagnoses that are often accident related, and others. In some states, such as Virginia, the legal process of subrogation is prohibited. In other states, such as California, although subrogation is prohibited, the organization is permitted to recover TPR savings where two criteria are met: the member recovered monies in a tort case where a portion of the damages was afforded for the costs of medical care provided by the plan, and the organization has obtained the member's prior consent. Such stipulations will both complicate the operational steps required to secure TPR recovery and limit a plan's overall TPR program effectiveness. TPR operations must identify which situations merit investigation for possible third-party liability, conduct the investigation, make the determination, and pursue reimbursement when appropriate.

TPR issues typically take a considerable time to resolve. In almost every case the claim is paid before the process is initiated; the process is therefore usually "pay and pursue." Funds reimbursed for medical costs on TPR claims are recoveries.

Nonplan Liability

Nonplan liability claims are claims that the plan is not responsible for paying because the services are not covered under the applicable statement of benefits or under plan policy as defined in the applicable member handbook. ***Common occurrences include:***

- services provided to members before plan coverage applies or after plan coverage has terminated
- claims improperly billed to the plan on which the plan takes an adjustment from the provider
- claims with incorrect billing amounts that were paid and the error was discovered later
- costs not covered under the member's contract or for which required approval has not been obtained

These situations are commonly confused with COB. The distinction to be made is that if the cost is not a covered cost, then there is no plan liability to pay the cost; hence there is no subsequent determination to be made of the plan's primary or secondary liability for any portion of the cost. Nonplan liability claims are not, strictly speaking, OPL and are not addressed further in this section.

CONTRACTUAL SUPPORT/ REQUIREMENTS

COB and TPR, like nonplan liability claims, rely upon legally binding contractual language in a number of plan documents: group certificate of coverage, subscriber agreement or certificate of coverage, plan summary documents, and provider agreements. Plan summary documents and group and subscriber agreements secure the plan's right to limit or reduce benefits due to COB and TPR, and secure the plan's rights to pursue these activities. Provider agreement language delineates the administrative responsibilities of providers and the plan with respect to OPL operations and the right of recovery. Subscriber application forms should also contain a statement regarding the plan's right to receive and release information pertaining to these functions over the subscriber's signature. The impetus behind contractually binding language supportive of COB and TPR is that, without it, the plan has no legal footing for reducing liabilities through either of these activities. The legal consequences of inadequate or inconsistent definitional language in plan contractual documents will be discussed in a later section.

Group and Subscriber Agreements

The language in the group and subscriber agreements should conform to state regulations (if any) regarding COB and subrogation. Most states have adopted some form of the NAIC Model COB Regulation and promulgate sample language. Although in many instances COB and TPR are handled within the same section in plan contracts, the distinctive legal basis for their respective operations merits separate contract sections. At a minimum, the COB section should include the following subsections: definitions, order of benefits determination rules, effect on benefits, right to receive and release information, responsibility and cooperation of members, and right of recovery.

Definitions include the following:

- identification and description of a plan for purposes of coordinating benefits among plans
- total allowable expense as any health benefit for which the member is covered, at least in part, by at least one of the coordinating plans
- a claim determination period as the time frame encompassing incurred claims within which the total allowable expense is applied for coordination purposes (generally one calendar year)
- order of benefits determination rules, which identify which plan is to be primary and which secondary for a particular member in a given set of circumstances
- effect on benefits, which describes the reduction of benefits when the plan is second-

ary with respect to another plan and the notion that benefits may be rendered as either services provided or reimbursement for services

- right to receive and release information, which secures the plan's right to communicate whatever information, medical or administrative, it deems necessary to other parties to carry out the COB function
- responsibility and cooperation of members, which binds the member to comply with plan requests for information, signatures on forms or statements, and so forth for the plan to exercise its COB right (the plan may include some teeth in its COB provision here, stating noncompliance as grounds for claim denial and/or member termination)
- right of recovery, which secures the plan's right to recover money from any involved party for reimbursement of benefits provided by the plan as primary where it subsequently discovered it should have been secondary

It is particularly important to define a total allowable expense in such a way as to encompass the provision of services, the typical benefit within a managed care setting, as a benefit paid. Furthermore, the NAIC Model COB Regulation permits the allowable expense to be defined as the reasonable and customary cost of services provided irrespective of any particular provider reimbursement arrangement. A commonly misunderstood concept is the member credit bank, or credit reserve amount, as it applies to COB. Although these terms are generally known, they are rarely seen within state COB regulations or model language or in plan agreements and are not present at all in the NAIC Model COB Regulation. Hence plans often assume that they are not required to implement member-specific tracking of COB savings. The concept and obligation of a member bank are built into COB by virtue of defining the total allowable expense within the context of a claim determination period. Where savings have been accrued on behalf of a particular member for claims at one time in the period, such savings are available to

pay other claims in the period on behalf of that member, where the combination of benefits from coordinating plans does not meet providers' usual and customary charges. The challenges in drafting effective, legally binding COB language include attaining appropriate readability scores as well as reducing the member perception that COB reduces the quality of services or benefits expected of the plan. Effective language in plan marketing materials may assuage this effect.

TPR subsections should include definitions, right of subrogation or recovery (in accordance with state regulations regarding subrogation), effect on benefits, right to receive and release information, responsibility and cooperation of members, and right of recovery. These subsections are comparable with those describing COB, differentiating the administrative basis for COB from the liability foundation of TPR.

Provider Agreements

COB and subrogation language should be included in provider agreements for two purposes: to establish the operational responsibilities of each of the parties with respect to identifying and transmitting COB information, and to establish and secure the right of ownership of COB and subrogation savings and recovery dollars. Particularly in a managed care setting where providers have accepted some level of risk by virtue of reimbursement arrangements based on other than episode of care, providers will contend that, with reduced reimbursement arrangements, they should be able to recapture reimbursement through OPL activities. The intent of the typical hold-harmless clause is at stake here: May the provider bill the balance of a claim where it is known that a secondary insurer, not the member, will pay? The plan, on the other hand, has actuarial calculations as the foundation of its reimbursement arrangements, calculations that presumably take into account the fact that the plan's net payable liability is reduced by virtue of OPL. The plan also has, on its side, the NAIC Model COB Regulation definition of a plan as excluding providers of health care. COB is a function specifically performable by and among health plans. The NAIC model does not address COB in a capitated reimbursement environment.

A healthy approach acknowledges that, without providers' assistance in identifying and transmitting OPL information to the plan, the plan's net reduction due to OPL activities suffers. The far-thinking plan will structure provider agreements to include and reward provider responsibilities with respect to OPL information gathering and transmittal with specific monetary guarantees. Compensation could include allocation of a savings pool or outright payment, to a maximum, of either a percentage of the claim value or a fixed amount for a newly identified OPL of which the plan had no prior knowledge. Contract language that addresses these issues fairly and comprehensively lays the groundwork for effective operations and obviates misunderstandings regarding reimbursement.

See Chapter 62 for further discussion of provider agreements.

LEGAL ISSUES BASED ON CASE LAW

The clarity and specificity of a plan's subrogation rights, as defined in both plan summary documents and certificates of agreement, directly controls the extent to which a plan may pursue and recover claims. As a legal process, successful subrogation depends not only upon adherence to statute and regulations, but will be affected by case law precedent. Conflicting case law exists regarding use of summary plan document language, or subscriber or group agreement (contract) language. Conflicting case law exists regarding a plan's right to recover based upon plan's actual costs or the reasonable value of the services provided. Case law supports plan pursuit of subrogation recoveries to the full extent of costs—even beyond the member's recovery amount—if it can be shown that the member impeded the plan's rights, and if recovery rights were upheld by clear subrogation language in plan documents. Conflicting case law exists regarding the plan's responsibility to reimburse the member's attorneys, where it might be shown that the member's attorneys performed a

service for the plan by investigating the circumstances, constructing the case value, researching law, and arguing the case. There is no ambiguity regarding the requirement that some language be present in order to retain and exercise subrogation rights. The authors are aware of at least one case (settled before trial) where a plan not only forfeited the costs of medical care, but faced breach of contract and annoyance and inconvenience damages for pursuing subrogation with no supporting language in the subscriber agreement. It is not sufficient for subrogation language to appear only in the handbook; it should be in the contracts as well to uphold a plan's subrogation rights.

A few examples should suffice to illustrate the complexity and inconsistency of case law pertaining to subrogation. In *John Deere Health Benefit Plan v. Chubb,* 1999 U.S. Dist. Kan., Feb. 17, 1999, the court enforced the subrogation clause in the summary plan description—discrepant and more limiting than the language in the contract—permitting the plan to seek reimbursement only from third-party tortfeasors.[1] In this case, the plan was simply prohibited from collecting monies it had spent on medical care, because they were already retained by the member and summary language did not establish the plan's right to pursue recovery from its own members.

In spite of the specificity with which regulators and courts require consistent and clear subrogation language in plan documents, there is a great deal of latitude—or ambiguity—with respect to the value of the recovery amount. In the case of *Ince v. Aetna Health Management Inc.,* 8th Cir., No. 98–1718, April 9, 1999, the court ruled that "the plan was entitled to recover the fair value of services rendered and was not limited to cash expenditures made."[2] Part of the direction of the court appears to be based on the presence of clear language in the subrogation provision in the plan documents. To the contrary, in a case settled before proceeding to trial, a plan capitulated to damages as well as actual costs to its members' class-action suit alleging that the plan was seeking recovery based on provider charges rather than its actual costs. The issues in this case included inconsistent subrogation language and inconsistency in policy over time. The muddled and contradicting language between group and member agreements, member materials, correspondence, and forms eroded the plan's ability to recover in a legally defensible manner. At question were the bases for the value to be recovered and from whom.

As this particular case did not go to trial, it does not set a precedent, but it should stand as a warning signal to the level of aggressiveness permissible in pursuit of subrogation recoveries. Aggressiveness here means both any discrepancy between plan costs and the basis for recoverable amounts, and inconsistency in language between the subscriber agreement and all other materials, letters, and forms used in the course of subrogation pursuit. More importantly, these examples serve as a reminder that pursuit of subrogation is a legal process requiring consistent and precise language and legal review to ensure the plan's rights are sustainable. Finally, the inconsistency of case law reflects the range of potential outcomes as based upon different jurisdictional statutes and regulations, as well as upon inconsistent interpretation between state and federal level. Plans should obtain a clear understanding of regulatory requirements and case law precedents in the jurisdictions of their delivery areas. Plan subrogation language should be drafted within this legal context.

ORGANIZATIONAL PLACEMENT (WITH DEDICATED STAFF)

COB and subrogation activities are closely integrated yet distinct from the mainstream of claims processing. To some degree, decisions relating to organizational structure depend upon the level and sophistication of claims transaction information system support. With appropriate automation, claims examiners may perform routine processing of OPL claims where alternative coverage has already been identified. Even in these most sophisticated shops, however, the labor-intensive and manual tasks of identifying new potential cases and investigating alternative coverage via phone and mail require and deserve

dedicated staff. If the claims-processing automation does not include appropriate adjudication of COB secondary payments, calculation of savings, and retention and management of member credit reserve amounts, then these functions also fall within the purview of dedicated OPL staff. In larger plans (generally, those with more than 50,000 members), a second division of labor occurs between COB and TPR tasks. Although both activities share comparable investigative tasks to disclose either the existence of alternative group coverage or the potential for subrogation, resultant COB activities involve administrative duties relating to data management of alternative coverage information and specialized claim adjudication. TPR activities focus instead on paralegal type activities: establishing and updating lien amounts and negotiating settlement amounts with often adverse attorneys.

The specialized and dedicated team of OPL analysts may work under a supervisor or manager reporting to the claims director. In some instances the OPL unit is set on par with the claims department, reporting directly to a director of operations or finance. Either design recognizes the highly specialized skills required to perform a set of tasks distinct from the routine claims adjudication process. Furthermore, it recognizes and encourages implementation of incentives based on effective work whose goal is reduced liability (value of claims processed) as opposed to routine claims processing with its incentives for productivity (volume of claims processed).

COB: BASIC PROCEDURE DEFINED

In its most simplistic form, effective COB comprises two operational flows: information regarding members with other coverage is discovered and retained, and such information is brought to bear upon claims during adjudication. The first flow involves staff from across almost all plan departments. Marketing and sales staff encourage prospects to include alternative coverage information on plan applications. Enrollment should reinforce the requirement for this information by rejecting as incomplete any applications without COB information. Provider relations staff may be privy to COB information contained in medical charts. Medical management staff can routinely ask regarding alternative coverage or ask whether the occurrence of an accident is the initiating factor behind the requirement for care. The customer services area uses customer contact as an opportunity to discover subrogation potential and forwards such information to OPL staff routinely. Also, customer services staff will respond to general COB and subrogation questions and will forward questions regarding complicated cases or aspects of cases to OPL staff for research and response. Claims examiners may recognize COB- or TPR-related information on claims forms (e.g., check boxes regarding accidents or other payment sources), or explanations of benefits paid may be included with the bills. In any event, the plan must structure the conduits for such information so that it can be applied at the time of claim payment. Generally, the information should accumulate to a central repository to ensure its consistency and obviate any redundancy. The OPL unit is responsible for maintaining this database, including investigating incomplete information. The OPL unit is also responsible for the second flow: applying alternative coverage knowledge to claims.

In point of fact, the two operations are intertwined. Rarely does a plan acquire COB information on more than 5 percent of its membership from up-front gathering mechanisms such as enrollment applications. Conversely, even if it did acquire COB information before a claim submission, there is little likelihood that each of the members researched would submit claims before the information was out of date and therefore inaccurate. A more productive method of working is to apply the order of benefit determination rules to claims as they are submitted to determine if, in the presence of other coverage, the plan would be secondary. A statistical analysis of claims data usually shows this to be the case for most of a plan's dependent-member claims. The potential for COB could be anywhere from 25 percent of claims to 60 percent or more. Restated, between 25 percent and 60 percent of claims are likely to be for dependent

members for whom a plan will be secondary if other coverage exists for these members. According to the Order of Benefits Determination rules, potential COB claims include claims for spouses and for children where the spouse's birthday falls earlier in the year than that of the plan's subscriber. The volume of claims to be investigated for other COB coverage is usually reduced by ignoring claims under a certain dollar amount. The NAIC Model COB Regulation stipulates that COB should be performed for all claims except those under $50. The plan should analyze its paid claim data to determine a reasonable dollar threshold under which to ignore investigations for new COB.

Investigative efforts are then applied to these claims' members to determine the existence of other coverage. Not all potential COB claims (claims for dependent members) result in COB savings. Factors that contribute to reduced COB include situations in which one spouse does not work and, when both spouses work, one does not receive health benefits through his or her employer. Upon verification of the existence of other coverage, if the claim has been pended during this investigative process ("pursue and pay"), then the claim may be diverted to the appropriate carrier. A duplicate coverage inquiry (DCI) is the process and document used to contact another plan thought to be primary for the claim and member in question. The process and document seek to determine the exact liability status of the alternative plan and the already made or intended payment for the services in question. The plan would initiate recovery efforts for such paid claims.

Although these tasks can be performed on a manual basis, they are executed much more efficiently and require fewer human resources when supported by computer systems. Information system support can usually identify claims where alternative coverage information is known, but the authors have not witnessed any system capable of identifying and pending claims in the absence of known COB information where, as a result of the dependent relationship of the member to the subscriber, the plan would be secondary if there were other coverage.

SUBROGATION: BASIC PROCEDURE DEFINED

Subrogation operations begin with identification of cases for investigation using a combination of automated screening of the claim, referral/authorization records for selected diagnoses, and input from various other sources of provider/member/attorney contact (claims, provider relations, medical services, etc.). Suspected cases, once identified, will be pended (temporarily) for investigation. Subsequent tasks include written correspondence and telephone investigation (with members, employers, attorneys, providers, and third parties) as a means to follow up on any additional information needed. Upon the confirmation of a case, OPL staff release the associated claims from pending status to pay them. Staff determine which cases will be handled in house and which will be referred to outside entities. The decisions on the type of cases to be handled in house versus outside entities will be reevaluated periodically based on case volume, number of cases going to litigation, and any changes in the laws governing TPR. For those suspected subrogation cases to be handled in house, staff will contact the member to determine whether a claim has been made and whether an attorney has been hired. Initial correspondence to the member and the member's attorney (if one has been retained):

- explains the plan's recovery rights and need for information;
- includes a questionnaire to solicit necessary information about the accident or injury;
- provides a standard form, for the member's signature, that acknowledges the plan's recovery rights, confirms the member's responsibility to provide information, and assigns payment to the plan;
- gives notice of the plan's lien; and
- provides copies of related bills (claims).

Subsequent to establishing a case, examiners notify all parties periodically of the plan's subrogation interest in the settlement. As a standard, the following parties will be notified: the member, the third party (if applicable), all insurance carriers involved, and all attorneys involved (plaintiff and defendant). After these initial contacts, and on a periodic basis (every 30 to 60 days), examiners request a status report from attorneys and insurers, update lien amounts, and check court files to determine whether a lawsuit has been filed and to monitor the lawsuit once it has been filed. The defined tasks presume the development of internal tracking reports to provide information about the amount and age of outstanding liens and to flag cases for the next follow-up steps.

In settlement of cases, OPL staff (or corporate counsel for selected cases) follow all relevant laws, principles, and regulations, including reasonableness, in the pursuit of plan expense recoveries. Settlement applies to the member's acceptance of a recovery amount from the third party (or his or her liability insurer) or the plan's acceptance of all or a portion of the monies due it for the cost of claims expense incurred for a specific subrogation event.

The procedures for identifying, managing, and settling workers' compensation claims are similar to those of general subrogation cases, of which workers' compensation is a subset. These cases have the additional research resource of state employment agencies or boards that consolidate and coordinate workers' compensation claims. See Chapter 61 for further discussion of workers' compensation.

ACCOUNTING FOR OPL

Financial management, discussed in Chapter 47, requires a method of accounting for OPL. The OPL staff are responsible for realizing savings as the result of discovery and investigation activities; savings are retained and tracked in concert and cooperation with claims and encounter processing staff, corporate legal counsel, corporate finance, providers, and other insurers. Mechanisms and communications links between claims and insurance and liability recovery staff are necessary to pend potentially duplicative payments and to adjudicate and release claims for secondary liability. Complete claims and encounter detail must be available to the OPL staff to produce a "bill" to the alternative carrier or provider if a duplicative payment has already been made and must be recovered. Providers must understand their roles and be contractually liable to return plan payments that are duplicative of alternative carrier remittances. Offsetting or withholding, an alternative to COB recovery, requires communication and cooperation between OPL, accounting staff, and providers.

"Pursue and pay" presupposes the acceptance, philosophically, that costs avoided, diverted, or recovered through COB and TPR programs are not revenue but rather reduced claims liability. Furthermore, reduced claims liability via accrual must be considered at least as valuable as a recovery. If one contemplates a comparison of the administrative expenses associated with "pay and pursue" and "pursue and pay" programs, an additional impact can be seen. Savings achieved through recoveries (cash receipts) require claims adjustments as well as accounting adjustments. When savings result from diversion, claims are readjudicated before final payment rather than being paid and later adjusted. The plan not only reduces administrative costs but realizes the immediate cash flow advantage of reduced claims payment. When diversions and avoidances are accounted for, the claims expense reduction is booked based on the actual amount of savings as they occur. Recoveries require an accrual of the estimated amount of recovery and the reversal or adjustment of that accrual when the cash is received.

Accounting for Diversions

Unlike "pay and pursue," which reaps its cost reduction benefits by way of cash receipts (recoveries), "pursue and pay" accrues savings via avoidance and diversion. Within the "pursue and pay" context, there are still, albeit minimal, cash receipts resulting from recoupment of erroneously paid Medicare claims, retroactive enrollment (the plan or alternative carrier) causing duplicate carrier payment, or cases where the plan simply exercises its judgment to pay a claim before concluding the investigation. This may be particularly true with long-term subrogation cases. For the most part, "pursue and pay" is considered an alternative COB process.

Upon conversion to a "pursue and pay" accrual system, a plan will experience almost immediate reduction in cash receipts. In the short term, administrative expense will increase as a result of additional case volumes and new operational procedures. This should be more than offset by reduced claims liability and, ultimately, an additional reduction in administrative expense because far fewer claims will require adjustment.

There are several financial accounting guidelines and procedures that must be established to ensure accurate accrual processing. They include the development of an accounting system to record accruals as a suspect or positively identified claim is released from its pend status. The information system should be investigated to determine whether it has the capability to perform the requisite accounting functions. If not, manual procedures will need to be implemented to perform this function. Savings will need to be recorded and reported by individual member; category of savings—avoidance (accrual), diversion (accrual), and, for the exception, recovery (cash receipt); type of accrual or cash receipt (COB, workers' compensation, subrogation); individual account and established account groupings; and line of business (commercial, Medicare).

The accounting process should be capable of relating accruals and recoveries to incurred but not reported (IBNR) costs and lessening the IBNR by the sum of the values of savings and recoveries. This may need to be accomplished manually through the use of specified reports produced by the automated accounting system. There should be a mechanism for the automated system to transfer accrued savings and recoveries from one employer account to another when a member is covered under two separate risk group accounts. Finally, financial accounting for COB includes the ability to establish and maintain a benefits reserve bank account on each member for whom savings or recoveries are booked. Amounts on credit in the reserve bank will be applied to a plan's secondary COB payments when benefits for a specified claim have been exhausted. The automated accrual system must provide accurate data on such transactions to the claims payment system. On a calendar year-end basis, these accounts will require zero balancing of unused savings.

A critical issue in establishing a financial accounting system for OPL is the development and implementation of a standard definition and calculation method for accruals. Claims, legal, and finance personnel must all operate with the same knowledge and understanding. By definition, the savings for an avoidance or diversion (accrual) is the amount that the plan would have paid had it been primary payer minus any amount that it will pay or has paid as secondary payer or from the credit reserve bank. Hospital discounts and differentials should be applied before accruals are calculated for claims. When the alternative, primary carrier is billed via DCI, however, it is the total allowable expense or, in this case, the provider's charge(s) that is requested as payable.

When savings are realized vis-à-vis recoveries (cash receipts), it is the exact amount of money recovered that is booked as savings. This amount does not affect the claims payment amount to the provider. An illustrative example is given in Exhibit 39–1. Here, the plan's secondary payment is made within the terms of total allowable expense as any claim at least a portion of which is covered under at least one of the plans covering the patient for whom the claim is made. The secondary payment, when added to the primary payment, is attempting to total to the usual and customary charges for the service(s) rendered. The amount charged in these examples is presumed to be a usual and customary charge. The plan is liable, as a secondary payer, up to the amount it would have paid as primary. The savings are calculated as the remainder of what the plan would have paid as primary less its secondary payment.

The alternative payer primary payment in the second example in Exhibit 39–1 is set at such an extreme minimal amount for illustrative purposes. There are times (e.g., mental health benefits) when the primary payer's deductible amount and/or benefit amount result in a payment allotment similar in principle to this example, where the total benefits available from

Exhibit 39–1 Savings Accounting Examples

Example 1: Total Allowable Benefits		
Charge:	$100.00	
Plan benefit:	$96.00	
Alternative primary payment:	$64.00	(Assumption: indemnity applies small deductible, pays 80% of remainder)
Plan secondary payment:	$36.99	
Plan COB savings:	$60.00	

Example 2: With a Credit Reserve		
Previous bank amount:		$3,000.00
Charge:	$100.00	
Plan benefit:	$60.00	
Alternative primary payment:	$1.00	
Plan secondary payment:	$99.00	
Plan COB savings:	−39.00	
New bank amount:		$2,961.00

the two plans covering a particular member are still less than the charged amount. Again, the total of the two plan payments attempts to reach the usual and customary charge. The assumption here is that we have experienced a savings of $3,000 within the year for this particular member. The savings are then available to pay for subsequent claims where the sum of an alternative primary payment plus the plan's primary payment would not come up to the usual and customary changes. The previous bank amount of $3,000 is reduced by $39 to permit the plan secondary payment of $99; $99 is paid so that it, together with the primary payment, reimburses the usual and customary $100 charge for the services. The plan's payment limit is always what it would have paid as primary plus any available credit reserve amount accrued for this particular patient. If there were no positive bank amount for this member from which to draw, the maximum of the plan's secondary payment is the allowed amount, in this example $60. The credit reserve or bank amount is zero balanced at the beginning of each claim determination period.

Accounting for Recoveries

Conversion to an accrual system, although requiring new or modified accounting procedures, will also require maintenance of the existing cash recovery accounting process. Allowed charges, savings, and payment amounts will need to be calculated and recorded differently depending on whether the accrual or cash receipt method of savings has been applied. In general, the accrual method will most often apply to COB savings, and the cash receipt method will most often be used in subrogation. Guidelines for accounting for recoveries should be developed along the following lines: as reductions to claims expense if realized within X months and during the same calendar year as the date on which the claim(s) was paid and as revenue if realized beyond these limits.

To account for OPL, the finance department will need to develop processes for:

- communicating savings and agreement on posting practices
- achieving a common understanding of bank credit reserve and reasonable cash value and their applications
- developing and implementing procedures between finance and OPL to reconcile booked and reported savings
- arriving at a common understanding of the effects of accruals and recoveries on IBNR

OPL POLICY ISSUES

Effective OPL requires proactive, assertive behavior in the pursuit of all OPL. This philosophical approach to claims liability requires innovative cooperation and responsible behavior on the part of subscribers, providers, employers, and other carriers. Success can only be accomplished when policy issues are identified and resolved, effects on constituents are anticipated, and rules and expectations are developed and communicated to everyone.

The key policy decision, upon which others are contingent, is whether to establish "pay and pursue" or "pursue and pay" as the principal foundation for COB. Given a positive response to this issue, *the following policy considerations must be addressed:*

- To what degree and in what ways will subscribers be held to their contractual obligations to provide alternative carrier information? Will claims be denied for failure to respond to questionnaires or inquiries, and, if so, at what point in OPL processing?
- Will providers be expected to bill and receive payment from known or newly identified alternative carriers before billing the plan? Will the plan deny claims when this procedure is not followed?
- How will employers be expected to participate in the OPL program? Will the plan expect employers periodically to canvass employees for alternative carrier information? Will employers be required to provide case-specific information for COB, subrogation, and workers' compensation claims? What actions, if any, will be taken by the plan for lack of cooperation?
- How does the plan intend to develop and implement a benefit credit reserve?

Operational policies to be decided upon include the following:

- What is an acceptable claims payment delay time for OPL processing?
- Considering the need to maintain data integrity, who will adjust or readjudicate claims?
- What controls are necessary?
- At what point in OPL processing are cases closed?
- Are claims paid or denied if not successfully concluded?
- What incentive options are most likely to produce the desired results?
- Who, internally and externally, should be included in an incentive program? If adopted, what overriding principles are to be used in the administration of an incentive program?

OPL IN A CAPITATED ENVIRONMENT

The capitation issue has not been adequately addressed by the NAIC in its most recent version of the model COB regulation. Nevertheless, an approach to COB and TPR can be constructed that will meet several criteria. The COB program should be perceived as favorable by sponsoring participants in terms of compensation. It should retain a legal basis under the diversion of claims to alternative primary carriers according to the NAIC Model COB Regulation and have the potential for yielding significant savings and recoveries from this often overlooked source of revenue.

The NAIC model defines two terms that are specifically applicable in approaching the capitation question. The term *plan* means, in its major context, an organization providing benefits or services to enrollees on a group basis. Many insurers and state regulators have considered HMO plans to fall within this definition, but the revisions to the NAIC Model COB Regulation in 1985 clearly indicated that an HMO is, for the purposes of COB, to be considered a plan. It is the plan that is permitted under the NAIC model to coordinate benefits. It should be noted that no reference is made to the ability of the provider or institution to coordinate benefits with those of a carrier or other form of plan. Because the COB process envisioned by the NAIC model guarantees payment to the providers and/or facilities regardless of whether benefits or services are provided by one or more plans, neither a provider nor a facility is strictly entitled to engage in direct COB.

The second definition of relevance concerns what is meant by the term *benefits*. In an HMO setting, benefits are usually provided in the form of direct services rather than merely, as to carriers, facilitating the payment for such services. In such a situation, the NAIC model also clearly indicates that, where benefits are provided in the form of services, the plan that is coordinating is entitled, if applicable, to be credited with or reimbursed the reasonable cash value of the services provided or arranged. This means that the coordinating plan would be entitled to any reduction in costs occasioned by its voluntary determination to coordinate benefits.

The underlying assumption about capitation rates is that it is understood that the providers are capitated with a pre-budgeted amount for COB and TPR being built into those rates. In other words, the capitation formulas have been derived on the basis that a plan is entitled to all proceeds (consistent with the language of the NAIC model) reimbursed or diverted as a result of COB or TPR. In one sense, a provider (physician or hospital) receiving capitation that then, on the basis of a denied claim by one of the plans, bills and collects from another carrier for services provided or arranged through that plan is actually collecting twice for the provision of the identical service. This clearly was not intended as part of the capitation process, nor does it fall within the spirit or letter of NAIC Model COB Regulation. It cannot be forgotten, however, that much of the COB and TPR information upon which a plan relies is furnished through providers and participating hospitals. Therefore, the following process is being proposed that will both satisfy the underlying purpose of COB and TPR and reward providers and facilities and their respective staffs for their cooperation in making this program as effective as possible.

The Capitation Process: Physicians

The plan's negotiated agreement with physician providers should explicitly acknowledge that physician capitation contains an amount that has been budgeted to include COB and TPR savings/diversions (amount paid by another) arising out of professional services provided by physicians. The participating physicians will agree, either contractually or implicitly, to cooperate with the plan to maximize revenues derived from the COB and TPR process. This will include the gathering of information about other coverage by office staff and the refraining from billing by individual physicians for services for which the COB and TPR component has been built into the provider's capitation. At the end of each mutually agreed-upon period, the amount of actual COB and TPR recoveries and diversions achieved by the plan will be compared with the amount budgeted for that period of time. A formula should be derived splitting any excess amounts in an equitable manner between the plan and the capitated physician(s). Any deficit from amounts budgeted will be borne by the plan.

The Capitation Process: Hospitals

The concept of paying a hospital an incentive for assisting a carrier in diverting COB claims away from itself is one utilized by a number of commercial carriers. Carriers in a number of states have an arrangement with hospitals by which the carrier pays the hospital the lesser of a fixed amount or a percentage of the value of the diverted COB claim when the hospital provides information about other coverage not previously existing in the carrier's database. A bonus payment mechanism could be worked out for hospitals that assist in providing managed care plans with undetected COB or TPR information. As an alternative, a similar risk-sharing arrangement as utilized for the physician providers could be applied in the case of hospitals. Both approaches—award sharing vis-à-vis budget and direct bonus payments—should be presented to each facility with which a managed care plan interacts.

Although the rules governing TPR are different (the plan is attempting to shift all costs arising out of an accident or injury to another party), the same budgeting, reward mechanism, and bonus program could be applied. Generally, TPR claims amount to a smaller percentage of revenue or PMPM income than those for COB. The plan budget for COB/TPR amounts could be subdivided into their two respective categories with various incentive mechanisms determined separately.

OUTSOURCING OPL

Like claims processing, OPL is a viable candidate for outsourcing. In considering this possibility, the plan must first determine what portions of OPL can be effectively outsourced. There are some vendors who purport to be able to carve out and manage COB for their customers, although the authors have not yet seen this successfully accomplished. Further, COB is more of an administrative process that is closely integrated, in terms of data support and time frame, with plan eligibility and claims and benefits administration tasks. For this reason we believe it to be a process more effectively and appropriately handled within the plan. TPR is, however, done quite routinely by outsourcing vendors, many of which have demonstrated significant expertise and savings results. The remainder of this section is devoted to considerations regarding the outsourcing of TPR.

Indications for outsourcing TPR may include:

- lack of experienced staff to conduct the process
- no access to legal counsel for case consultation
- the plan finds it too costly to set up the administrative function internally
- recovery results have been minimal for plans that have managed their own TPR
- no automated screening capability to identify potential cases
- the plan operates in multiple states, with differing TPR rules, rendering the TPR process overly complicated

Plans will need to carefully evaluate each vendor's capabilities when considering outsourcing TPR. In addition to the normal "due diligence" checking (for example, topic and legislative knowledge, financial stability, capacity for additional work, history of satisfied clients, successful recovery rates, acceptable contractual terms, and so forth), plans will want to pay particular attention to certain issues:

- ***Legal principles:*** Does the vendor appropriately apply standard legal principles to the initiation and investigation of cases (primary/contributory/comparative negligence, last clear chance, assumption of risk, promissory estoppel, principal-agent relationship, privacy, antiharassment, statute of limitations, service of process, third-party beneficiary, etc.)?
- ***Case identification:*** Exactly how does the vendor identify potential cases? Are all

claims, encounters, and referrals/authorizations screened by diagnosis and procedure code? How are self-report cases integrated? Are code screening lists extensive and kept current; for example, do they include diagnoses for the less obvious potential cases, like food and chemical poisoning, not just accidents and injuries? Is there a dollar limit under which investigation will not automatically occur? If so, is it reasonable (and flexible) given the plan's claims charges?

- *Case initiation and management:* How are cases initiated and investigated (automated questionnaires based on a positive screening result)? Does the vendor rely solely on written inquiries or is phone investigation also used? Does the vendor automatically follow up on no response questionnaires, in a reasonable time frame? Once it is determined that there is a case, does the vendor quickly determine whether an attorney is involved, then notify all parties of the plan's subrogation lien? How and with what frequency does the vendor assure that liens are kept up to date?

- *Litigation and compromise:* How does the vendor deal with litigation? What are the vendor's criteria for initiating litigation? How competent and adequate is the vendor's legal staff? What levels of staff (paralegal, attorney, etc.) are dedicated and to what processes? What is the plan's involvement in the process? Is there the facility, on a case-specific basis, for the plan to make the final decision as to whether a case is litigated? Are cases adequately prepared for court? What is the vendor's track record in litigation? What percentage of cases are litigated? How does the vendor deal with case compromise? Is there a reasonable set of considerations before reaching a compromise (amount of lien, liability issues involved, length of time to establish lien, amount of unpaid bills to be paid by plaintiff, waiver of attorney fees, and so forth)? Who is involved in making compromise

decisions? Is there a group or team, including a plan representative, that evaluates and decides on compromise offers prior to acceptance? Are there dollar limits to the amount of compromise (write-off) that drive who makes the decision? What is the vendor's track record with regard to compromise (number and percent of cases compromised, write-off amounts, etc.)?

- *Vendor-plan interface and reporting:* How does the vendor interface with the plan and how easy will the interface be? Does the vendor accept, on a scheduled, routine basis and in a format that is easy for the plan to provide, output from referral/authorization, pended/suspended and paid claims files for investigation and lien update? Does the vendor accept responsibility for reformatting plan provided files? What routine and ad hoc reporting will the plan receive? Will the vendor provide monthly reports of lien amounts (by age of receivable) and savings? Will the plan have some flexibility in requesting account and product-specific reports as well as in aggregate?

- *Vendor fees and recovery remittance:* What is the basis for the vendor's fees? Are they based solely on a percentage of recovery, with no added fees? Are they within the industry-standard percentage (25 percent to 33 percent)? How does the vendor remit savings to the plan? Is remittance on a routine (monthly) schedule, with appropriate documentation to record recoveries in the general ledger?

- *Retrospective recovery:* Is the vendor willing to undertake a retrospective recovery effort as well as to implement an ongoing process? If so, what will the process and fees be (are they reasonable)?

CONCLUSION

All the functions, processes, and relationships described in this chapter depend on senior management support. The function of senior management as it relates to an OPL operation is to engender corporate understanding and support of the OPL effort and to provide the necessary policy and resources with which to succeed. ***Resource support includes:***

- competent and adequate OPL staff
- direct access to corporate legal counsel when necessary
- systems availability and support
- commitment to assistance in discovery, including data capture documents and procedures to convey such data on a timely and regular basis
- contractual support for plan rights to coordinate benefits and subrogate
- availability of all utilization data (claims, encounters, and referrals)
- the ability to replicate claims/referrals efficiently and to produce fee-for-service-equivalent bills for any capitated care.

Policy support includes:

- identification and corporatewide adoption of common terms and definitions
- adoption and practice of the NAIC model (as promulgated by state[s] within which the plan operates), including, but not limited to, total allowable expense and its implications, benefit credit reserve, and order of benefits determination

- adoption and practice of state legislation and regulation regarding the plan's right to subrogate and collect from third parties
- "pay and pursue" versus "pursue and pay" for COB
- whether to deny claims payment absent response to investigation activities.

OPL activities are a complex process. Coordinated and consistent policy establishes and maintains an effective operational engine that identifies, researches, and adjudicates OPL claims. Additionally, policy builds the proper incentives to encourage the disclosure of other coverage or subrogation information. Such policies reach throughout the plan and extend beyond to providers, members, and group customers. The most common flaws in OPL programs are:

- member disincentives for disclosure (perception that benefits will be reduced or denied)
- provider disincentives for contributing to the process (i.e., additional administrative tasks resulting in lowered reimbursement)
- staff disincentives (i.e., promotion of the number of cases processed rather than valuing effective procedures that contribute to the plan's OPL financial goals).

A well run OPL program will provide a significant contribution to the overall operational and fiscal health of any managed care organization.

REFERENCES AND NOTES

1. If Subrogation Provision in SPD and Plan Document Conflict, Unambiguous SPD Language Controls, *Coordination of Benefits Handbook,* Quarterly Bulletin 7, 3 (July 1999), p. 5.

2. Subrogation Can Be Based on Reasonable Value of Services, Not Amounts Paid to Health Providers, *Coordination of Benefits Handbook,* Quarterly Bulletin 7, 3 (July 1999), p. 1.

SUGGESTED READING

Coordination of Benefits Handbook. 1999. Thompson Publishing Group, Inc., Washington, DC.

Scheur, B. 1987. "Why COB Plans Fail—And How To Make Them Work" *Managed Care Advisor* (1), 7, published by the Peabody Group.

CHAPTER 40

Member Services and Consumer Affairs

Peter R. Kongstvedt

All managed health care plans need a member services, customer services, or consumer affairs function. For purposes of discussion, the term "member services" will be used synonymously with the terms "customer services" and "consumer affairs." Member services are not to be confused with membership services; the latter term is sometimes used to describe the operational area responsible for processing enrollment applications and sending out membership cards and evidence of coverage documents. Member services, in the context of this chapter, refers to the department responsible for providing information to the members (either broadly to the entire membership or to individuals by request), helping members with any problems, handling member grievances and complaints, tracking and reporting patterns of problems encountered, and enhancing the relationship between the members of the plan and the plan itself. Each of these operational functions is described later in this chapter.

Managed care organizations (MCOs) are far more complicated than simple indemnity insurance plans (as though those are simple!). Members of health maintenance organizations (HMOs) or point-of-service (POS) plans are required to choose a primary care physician (PCP), to follow rules for accessing health care (e.g., obtaining an authorization from their PCP for referral services), to understand complex benefits structures, and so forth. HMOs are complicated enough; POS plans are even more complicated and have different levels of coverage

depending on how the member accessed services (intentionally or not). Preferred provider organizations (PPOs) that do not use a PCP-type model are less complicated but still require this function. See Chapter 3 for a description of these types of plans.

The central point is that plans that manage access to care through the use of a restricted provider panel and an authorization system need to have a system to help members understand how to use the plan, a system to resolve member's problems or questions, a system to monitor and track the nature of member contacts, and a mechanism for members to express dissatisfaction with their care because members have less ability simply to change providers. Likewise, plans that have the ability to deny or reduce coverage for nonauthorized services need a mechanism for members to seek review of claims that have been denied or covered at a lower than expected level of benefits. Managed care or not, any plan that provides for the financing of health care must have a system to manage member problems with those payments. Last, the plan must have a mechanism for members to get help addressing routine business issues such as change of address, issuance of identification cards, and so forth.

When a plan has delegated a large measure of responsibility to an integrated delivery system (IDS; see Chapter 4), special attention needs to be taken as to how member services will function. The IDS will have a higher than normal level of control over all aspects of the medical encounter, including access to care, the authorization system, availability of providers, and so forth. In some cases, the IDS will actually perform many traditional member services functions. It is important that there be consistency between the plan and the IDS and that there be clear distinctions about the responsibilities of the plan and the IDS. It is preferable for the plan to perform all member services functions, but if the IDS is to perform some of them, then it is necessary that the plan receive accurate and timely data from the IDS member services department. It is equally important for the plan to share its member services data with the IDS.

When looking at the actual interactions that any member has with an MCO, a significant number of them will be administrative or procedural; for example, getting an identification (ID) card or a benefits booklet explaining how the plan works. Interactions with providers are also a crucial element of a member's overall satisfaction with the MCO. Provision of information to members, for administrative type of information (e.g., benefits, participating providers, and so forth) to health education or community types of information, is also an important element of plan-member relations. Although member services cannot be responsible for the first issuance of an ID card or the ability of a member to get an appointment with a physician (at least not at first), it is this department that is responsible for the overall satisfaction of the membership, including resolving problems that occur in these other areas.

Each functional area of an MCO is responsible for its own operational quality, just as each provider is responsible for how he or she provides medical services to the members. But it is member services that is responsible for resolving problems when they arise, analyzing trends and data to help determine the causes of problems, managing the formal grievance and complaint process, and providing the added value of "high touch" that a successful MCO needs to have. In one 1999 survey of consumer attitudes regarding managed health care, it was determined that although 87 percent of employees with health insurance are covered by managed care, only 29 percent of all Americans base their opinion of managed care on their own, first-hand experience, slightly over 29 percent base their opinion on what they have seen or heard in the media, 23 percent base it on what they have learned from family and friends, and the rest say they do not know how they came about their information.[1] In other words, the value of member satisfaction will be magnified by interactions between members and their friends and family (e.g., "My plan really treats you well—you should sign up with them.") and will have an impact on how the member perceives media stories (e.g., "My plan treats me better than that!").

PROVISION OF GENERAL INFORMATION

The provision of general information to members is one of the key aspects of member services. This is differentiated from the function of responding to individual inquiries about problems or the need to interact with the plan for some reason (e.g., PCP selection, ID card corrections, and so forth). Such information may be broadly disseminated to the entire membership by means of one or more of the following routes:[2]

- mass mailings
- the plan newsletter
- group information sessions
- the MCO's website
- electronic kiosks at the work site or other high traffic areas (e.g., at a shopping mall)
- one-on-one individual sessions
- toll-free telephone service

Figure 40–1 describes the most common types of information provided to current and prospective enrollees. Exhibit 40–1 provides a good example of one national managed care company's member rights and responsibilities, a document made available to all members.

Training and Staffing

The amount of training required of member services representatives before they are allowed to interact with members varies from plan to

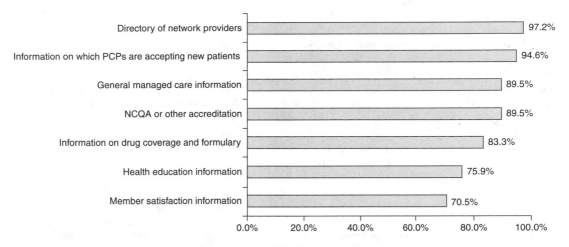

Figure 40–1 Information Services Most Commonly Provided to Current and Prospective Enrollees. *Source:* Reprinted with permission from *The InterStudy Competitive Edge Part: HMO Industry Report 9.1,* © 1999, InterStudy publications.

Exhibit 40–1 Aetna U.S. Healthcare Member Rights and Responsibilities

As a member, you have a right to:

- Get up-to-date information about the physicians and hospitals who participate in the plan.
- Obtain primary and preventive care from the PCP you chose from the plan's network for covered services.
- Change the PCP you selected to another available PCP who participates in the plan.
- Obtain covered medically necessary care from participating specialists, hospitals, and other providers.
- Be referred to participating specialists who are experienced in treating your chronic illness for covered benefits.
- Be told by your physicians how to schedule appointments and get health care during and after office hours.
- Be told how to get in touch with your PCP or a back-up physician 24 hours a day, every day.
- Call 911 (or any available area emergency response service). Go to the nearest emergency facility in a situation that might be life- or limb-threatening.
- Be treated with respect for your privacy and dignity.
- Have your medical records kept private, except when required by law or with your approval.

- Help your physician make decisions about your health care.
- Have a doctor decide when coverage for treatment should be denied.
- Discuss with your physician your condition and all care alternatives, including potential risks and benefits, even if a care option is not covered.
- Know that your physician cannot be penalized for filing a complaint or appeal.
- Know how your plan decides what services are covered.
- Know how the plan pays your physicians.
- Get up-to-date information about the services covered or not covered by your plan, and any applicable limitations or exclusions.
- Get information about copayments and fees you must pay.
- Be told how to file a complaint, grievance, or appeal with the plan.
- Receive a prompt reply when you ask the plan questions or request information.
- Have your physician's help in decisions about the need for services and in the grievance process.
- Suggest changes in the plan's policies and services.

continues

Exhibit 40–1 continued

As a member, you have the responsibility to:
- Choose a PCP from the plan's network and form an ongoing patient-physician relationship.
- Help your physician make decisions about your health care.
- Tell your PCP if you do not understand the treatment you receive and ask if you do not understand how to care for your illness.
- Follow the directions and advice you and your physicians have agreed upon.
- Tell your physician promptly when you have unexpected problems or symptoms.
- Consult with your PCP for non-emergency referrals to specialists or hospital care for covered benefits.
- See the specialists to whom your PCP refers you.
- Make sure you have the appropriate prior authorization for certain services, including inpatient hospitalization and out-of-network treatment.
- Understand that participating physicians and other health care providers who care for you are not employees of Aetna U.S. Healthcare and that Aetna U.S. Healthcare does not control them.
- Show your member ID card to providers before receiving care from them.
- Pay the copayments required by your plan.
- Call Member Services about your plan if you do not understand how to use your benefits.
- Promptly follow your plan's grievance procedures if you believe you need to submit a grievance.
- Give correct and complete information to physicians and other health care providers who care for you.
- Treat physicians and all providers, their staffs, and the staff of the plan with respect.
- Advise Aetna U.S. Healthcare about other medical insurance coverage you or your family members may have.
- Not be involved in dishonest activity directed to the plan or any provider.
- Read and understand your plan and benefits. Know the copayments and what services are covered and what services are not covered.
- Ask your treating physician about all treatment options and the physician's compensation arrangement with Aetna U.S. Healthcare.

You may have additional rights and responsibilities depending upon the state law applicable to your plan.

Source: Aetna/USHealthcare, 1999. www.aetnaushc.com/products/member_disclosure_hmo.html. Reprinted with permission.

---

plan. It is common for large MCOs to require new representatives to spend 20 to 30 working days in training before they begin actually interfacing with members,[3] and even then the first few weeks are monitored by the supervisor. Ongoing training averages 1 to 2 weeks per year in aggregate.[4] Smaller or less complicated plans generally require less training. It is a clear mistake to skimp on training because how the member services representative performs will have a direct impact on member satisfaction and perhaps on the legal risk profile of the plan. Remember: Every interaction a member has with the plan will either reaffirm the decision to join or cause the member to wonder whether he or she made a mistake; that goes for member services and medical encounters.

Staffing this department is a function of both the scope of responsibilities of the representatives and the complexity of the plan. In the Ernst & Young study cited previously, the mean staffing ratio was 1 full-time equivalent (FTE) member representative per 5,000 enrollees. For highly complex plans with significant growth, complicated products such as POS, and active outreach (discussed later), staffing ratios may be as generous as 1 FTE for every 3,500 members. Plans with benefits designs that are simple and consistent, that have stable membership levels, a high level of self-service capabilities (discussed later), and generally have good service levels may staff at a ratio of 1 FTE for every 7,500 members, although that would be tight staffing in most plans.

The degree that a plan can automate support for certain routine customer calls will have a substantial effect on staffing ratios as well and will clearly improve responsiveness in the eyes of the member. If the member services representative is required to manually look up information such as benefits (base plan and riders), claims history, the provider directory, and so forth, that will reduce efficiency and the member's satisfaction with the interaction. In addition, if the member services representative is required to access multiple, awkward screens, many of which may actually add no value to the transaction, the work required will be disproportionately high. Automation will also help the member services representative resolve the problem or issue on that first call, thereby lowering the amount of required follow-up work and administrative cost.

It is common in large plans to organize the department into dedicated service units. Such units are responsible for a limited number of accounts, particularly if those accounts are large. In that way, the representatives working in the unit are better able to be familiar with a limited set of benefits issues, to gain knowledge about particular problems unique to an account, and to be more responsive to the accounts. Dedicated service units are sometimes required of MCOs by large employers.

Accessing Member Services by Individual Members

Mail and Paper-Based Communication

Even though most of the individual member activity in member services takes place by the telephone (discussed later), mail and paper communication remains highly important and must be managed properly. It is common that inbound mail correspondence will take place in the context of formal complaints or grievances (discussed later in this chapter) as part of a documentation effort by the individual initiating the correspondence, although it can occur in the normal course of communications from those members who simply prefer to use the mail rather than another means of communication.

All inbound correspondence must be logged and tracked, policies and procedures must be in place regarding the routing of correspondence, and master files need to be kept of both incoming and outgoing correspondence. In a small plan, this is usually done with the actual paper documents; large plans frequently use imaging technology to store the massive amounts of paper documents, the originals of which may be then stored off site for a number of years. It is important to ensure that paper correspondence receives the same attention that telephone calls do, with time standards for response.

All MCOs use mail and paper-based correspondence for outbound communications. This is required for any form of communication that takes place on a plan-wide or other large scale (e.g., to all members of an enrolled group). It is also used by the plan for documentation purposes when communicating important changes or notices to the members, such as a change in the pharmacy network or a change in policy coverage determinations.

On an individual member level, outbound mail correspondence will always be used for formal communications and documentation of the complaint or grievance process discussed later in this chapter. Outbound mail is also used to reply to inbound mail from members, although that may serve as a supplement to telephone communications.

Telephone Communications

The greatest volume of interactions between an MCO and its members will occur by means of the telephone, excluding routine mailings such as the issuance of identification cards, member newsletters, and other nonindividualized forms of communications. Several aspects to telephone communications must be looked at by any plan, and these are discussed as follows.

Types of Telephone Communications. Traditional telephone lines must be adequate in number and must be properly automated in function, depending on plan size; for example, automatic call distribution and sequencing. These are the functions of the MCO's telephone system, generally referred to as a PBX. For historical reasons, even though this system is actually a specialized computer, it is referred to as a "switch."* It is common for large MCOs to have more than one switch and for some of the switches to be specialized for use by plan functional areas. Because the switch is really a computer that is open to the telephone systems of the entire world, intense and specialized security precautions are required but are beyond the scope of this chapter.

Virtually all MCOs (98.4 percent as of 1999,[6] for those readers who like precise numbers) use a toll-free line for use by members. The use of direct inward dialing (DID) is used by some MCOs and relieves a member from having to grind through several automated telephone menus. This means that the member's identification card or member handbook lists different numbers for different needs. For example, a plan may have a dedicated, direct inward dial-in line for members to select a new PCP, or to obtain a new identification card, or to resolve a problem. Other plans take the route of having one single member services telephone number, and the member then will be directed by an interactive voice response unit (IVR) or may be connected immediately to a service representative who will then deal with whatever issue the member has.

However the member accesses the MCO by telephone, the first point of action occurs with the use of an automated call distributor (ACD). This is a device or switch that automatically routes calls on the basis of programmed distribution instructions. There may be two levels of ACD use in a plan. The first is to serve as the initial automated answering system ("Hello. You have reached the member services department of Harry's House-o-Health"), which will

then send the call on (directly or to an IVR as discussed later), as well as serve to provide wait instructions and background content for those members put on hold. The second function is to distribute calls on the basis of operator availability; in other words, spread the workload and maximize the speed to answer.

The IVR is a system that provides the caller with a menu or several menus to choose from to direct the call to the most appropriate department. The member responds to questions from the IVR by pressing the appropriate key on the telephone or, increasingly, by simply saying the number aloud into the telephone.

As an example of an IVR system, the member's call would be answered by the automated system. The member is instructed to: "Press or say 1 if your call is about a claim, press or say 2 if your call is about an identification card, press or say 3 if your call is about selecting or changing your primary care physician, press or say 4 if you are requesting information, press or say 5 if…" and so forth. Some plans nest the menus as well; for example, after the member presses 1 because their call is about a claim, the menu may then instruct them to "Press or say 1 if your call is about an unpaid claim, press or say 2 if your call is about an incorrectly paid claim, press or say 3 if your call is to inquire about the status of a submitted claim, press or say 4 if you wish to receive a claim form, press or say 5 if…" and so forth. A few plans may even add a third nested level of menus, but that strikes this author as fiendishly complicated for members who are simply trying to get their issues resolved.

IVR systems may also provide for member self-service. This refers to providing the member with a form of service that does not require the intervention of a member services representative. Examples of these would include requesting a new identification card to be mailed, providing fax-back information (e.g., a listing of all participating PCPs in the member's ZIP code or within 5 miles of their ZIP code; or other provider listings), providing a copy of certain plan policies and procedures (e.g., how the member may receive benefits for alternative medicine), allowing the member to find out the status of a

---

*This is because in the precomputer days, it actually was a mechanical switch that opened and closed connections. A charming holdover of a term into the computer age.

claim in process, determine the status of an authorization for services, or other information.

Self-service IVR is also being increasingly used for enrollment purposes.* In this use, the member responds to the IVR questions by entering information by use of the telephone, not just responding to simple Boolean-type questions. This type of self-service generally requires that the MCO receives a base level of information from the enrolled group (i.e., the employer) ahead of time, so that the subscriber calling in (i.e., the member who is the individual actually receiving the benefit from the employer) is able to identify himself or herself by way of an identification number. The enrollment system then collects responses regarding the type of benefit plan the subscriber wants, the PCP each family member wants (by using a directory of PCPs in which numbers are associated with each PCP),

and so forth. Additional nonhealth benefits may also be enrolled this way, but often this occurs through a party other than the MCO, such as a benefits consulting firm or an outsourced human resources administrator. The advantages of using this type of IVR are obvious: faster data entry, increased accuracy (the IVR simply requires reentry of incorrect data, and also reads back the choices in plain language before asking the subscriber to confirm those choices), and lower costs.

The amount of IVR use is illustrated in Figure 40–2, using 1997 and 1998 data from 19 large MCOs covering 26 million lives.[6]

In MCOs with newer and more sophisticated information systems, the member services representative receives the member's (nonmedical) records and other data on the terminal screen at the same time the call is coming through. This is done by means of the switch's ability to recognize the calling number, either by Caller ID or the MCO's own database of numbers, as well as an ability for the system to remember prior calls. Although this provides the member services representative with the ability to greet the caller by

---

*Although the introduction of this chapter made clear that membership and enrollment services are not part of the scope of discussion, it is most appropriate to discuss this capability here because it is in the context of overall self-service provision of member services.

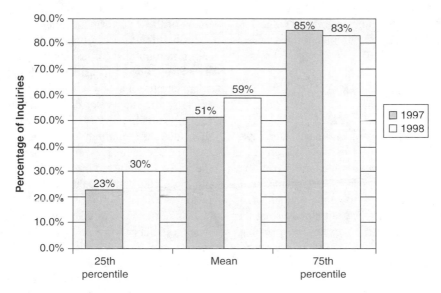

Figure 40–2 Range of Use of IVR by 19 Large MCOs. *Source:* Ernst & Young LLP Proprietary Managed Care Benchmarking Study, 1997–1999, Washington, DC.

name, there is no way to ensure that the caller is actually who the system identifies him or her as, and so the representative must still ask the name of the caller and generally some form of confirmation (e.g., their address). Once such identification is clear, the representative has the ability to address the caller's needs or questions rapidly because the information is already available, including, of course, notes from prior calls.

The last major type of telephone communications is the outbound, predictive dialer. This is a system in which the call center's switch is programmed to make calls to members on a proactive basis. The most common use for this in a MCO's member services department is outreach to new members, discussed later. Another common use of this capability is for follow-up on a member's call; in other words, the MCO representative calls the member to make sure that their issues or needs have been met. The effect on member satisfaction is quite positive. Other uses of outbound predictive dialing exist, particularly in the clinical arena. Examples would include regular follow-up calls to patients with serious chronic diseases (see Chapter 23) or reminders to members to use preventive services (e.g., calling women who have no record of a mammogram when they are of an age at which screening mammograms are recommended). When using this for clinically-related calls, data privacy and security requirements must be adhered to (see Chapter 67).

Performance Standards for Telephone Communications

Member services departments have responsiveness requirements as part of their performance standards. Such standards generally revolve around a few simple measures. Performance standards must be tailored to meet the standards that the *members* would expect, not simply what the plan chooses to measure. For example, a plan may measure telephone responsiveness by measuring how long it takes an operator to answer once that operator receives the call; such a measurement would fail to capture the fact that the member had to wade through seven menus of an IVR to get there, resulting in 3 minutes of frustration by the member.

Telephone responsiveness is usually measured by how many times the telephone rings on average or the elapsed time (in seconds) before it is answered by a representative and what percentage of calls are abandoned before they are ever answered. For example, a plan may have a goal of less than 2 percent of callers hanging up because their call did not get through, and 80 percent of all calls are answered in 20 seconds or less. Timeliness of response is also measured against goals. Examples include the percentage of calls that are resolved on the spot (i.e., no follow-up is required); for example, 90 percent of calls require no follow-up. For problems or questions that require follow-up, there are goals for how long that takes (e.g., 90 percent of outstanding inquiries or problems are resolved within 14 days and 98 percent within 28 days). Similar standards apply to written correspondence.

Productivity may be measured by tracking the number of contacts per day or per hour, the length of time each contact takes to complete, and the percentage of contacts that are resolved on the first call.

Data in Table 40–1, from the Ernst & Young study referenced several times in this chapter, provide examples of actual measurements of many of these performance metrics.[7]

Individual service representatives are usually monitored not just for productivity but for quality as well. Quality is usually monitored through silent monitoring of the calls themselves. This refers to the supervisor or manager listening to random calls for each service representative and then making a qualitative judgment about how well the service representative handled the call; the answering system informs the member calling in that the call may be monitored for quality purposes.

It is not enough to take and give information when a member has a problem or complaint; the representative must apply communication techniques developed for customer service to be optimally effective.[8] Some plans routinely send follow-up questionnaires to members after the member services inquiry or complaint is resolved

Table 40–1 Examples of Member Services Representatives Telephone Performance Measures

Measure	25th Percentile	Mean	75th Percentile
Calls per member service FTE	7,300	7,900	8,900
Percent of calls answered manually in 30 seconds or less	56%	66%	76%
Average call talk time (minutes)	3.0	3.7	4.2
Average speed to answer (seconds)	19.3	33.9	31.3
Abandonment rate	3%	6%	7%
Percent of calls resolved on 1st call	53%	64%	84%
Average resolution time (minutes)	4.7	5.8	6.5

Source: Ernst & Young LLP Proprietary Managed Care Benchmarking Study, 1997–1999, Washington, DC.

to solicit feedback on the process, as well as to reinforce the notion that the member is important.[9]

Electronic Communication

Many MCOs allow members access to certain functions through the Internet. Examples of common functions in most plans include the ability to access provider directories, benefits and coverage documentation, printable forms (e.g., claims forms), and other information. It is also common to provide a low-grade type of interactivity such as the ability to print out a map and directions to a selected provider.

Beyond such static lookup functions, the use of the Internet is rapidly taking shape. It is becoming common for MCOs to provide functions through the Internet such as enrollment, changing PCPs, issuance of a new or replacement ID card, lookup of the status of a claim, and other information. Electronic mail (e-mail) is also becoming more common, although some plans discourage it (or even do not provide for it) because of concern that e-mail is usually used by consumers in a nonsecure way, exposing the consumer to a possible breach of privacy. Other plans provide for e-mail by use of secure servers that do not use the standard Internet e-mail protocols but rather depend on secure communications just like other types of secure data transmission.

Many of the interactions between members and MCOs that take place electronically are subject to the privacy and security provisions of the Health Insurance Portability and Accountability Act of 1996 (HIPAA) that are discussed in Chapter 67. Therefore, the ability to encrypt data and to provide for the assurance that only the member is able to electronically access confidential data about him- or herself is required.

The growth of electronic commerce (e-commerce) is so rapid and the scope is becoming so expansive that it is not of any value to provide an exhibit or table of common member services e-commerce functions. Any such exhibit will be outdated well before this book even becomes available in the market. The reader is therefore advised to turn to current sources of information about the use of e-commerce in this area. Such sources include professional analyst's publications or journals that focus on this issue. The topic of e-commerce in general (including consumer issues) is discussed in Chapter 37.

Service and Help

Member services is responsible for helping members use the plan and for disseminating information broadly to the membership. For example, new members commonly have less than complete (or even no) understanding of how the plan operates, how to access care, how to obtain authorization for specialty services (in a PCP case manager–type plan), and so forth. These are services to members as opposed to complaint and concern resolution, which is discussed later. Although the broad types of services are generally the same across product lines, plans often find differing levels of need for each of these types of services in the commercial, Medicare, and Medicaid markets.

Special Considerations in the Provision of Member Services

There are some special considerations that must be considered in the provision of member services to individual members. The two that are the most important for this discussion are the hours that member services are available to members and the ability to communicate in languages other than English.

Hours of Availability. Availability is the most obvious issue to consider. Although 24 hour per day, 7 days per week (referred to as 24/7) is ideal, it will not be cost justified for all but the largest plans and not necessarily even then. More appropriate are extended hours on weekdays and availability on weekends. The size and geographical distribution of the MCO will play a role in determining the maximum hours that member services will be available. In one recent study, 37 percent of MCOs had hours after normal office hours on weekdays, and 22 percent had hours during the weekend.[10] During hours when no representative is available, the call should forwarded to a voicemail system that will be picked up first thing the next business day; the use of an IVR to direct the voicemail to the appropriate location is important for the sake of efficiency.

For any calls received during periods when the member services department is not open, it is not only necessary to provide for a voicemail message but the answering message must make clear that if the call is in reference to a clinical problem or medical emergency, the member should contact the physician or, in the case of a medical emergency, seek medical help directly.

In some MCOs, after-hours calls may be routed to a 24/7 nurse advice line (see Chapter 18) based on an initial choice the member makes through the IVR; for example: "If you are call-

ing with a clinical or medical problem, please press or say 1, or stay on the line. If your call is in reference to any other nonmedical problem and you would like to leave a message, please press or say 2." The calls are then forwarded to the nurse advice line for action. It is better for some inappropriate calls to go to the nurse advice line than for a medical problem to go unaddressed. In MCOs that use this approach, it is preferable for the nurse advice line organization (often an outside company that the MCO has contracted with) to have direct access to the MCO's systems and information and to be able to input information for action and follow-up by the plan's member services department when it reopens.

Automated self-service should be available at all times. Such services may be available through the telephone system or the Internet, as described later in this chapter.

Non-English Communications. The ability to communicate with members in languages other than English is becoming increasingly important, particularly in large urban areas with large immigrant populations. In those areas with high concentrations of individuals speaking a particular language other than English (e.g., Spanish), the MCO will often use member services representatives who speak that language. For languages that are not necessarily in high concentration, or in smaller plans, it is common for the multilingual services to be provided through externally contracted interpreter services.

In one large survey, 88 percent of MCOs offer interpreter services; and 84 percent of MCOs that offer interpreter services do so for Spanish-speaking members; 42 percent of those same MCOs offer no languages other than Spanish on a routine basis.[11] Other languages offered far less commonly include:[12]

- Vietnamese—14.9 percent
- Chinese (Mandarin or Cantonese)—11.1 percent
- Russian—7.6 percent
- French—6.3 percent
- Japanese—5.2 percent

- for each other languages, fewer than 5 percent of MCOs offer services

Table 40–2 illustrates multilingual services commonly provided by MCOs.

Types of Member-Specific Services

Table 40–3 provides a listing of the most common reasons individual members contact member services.

Claims Issues. Claims issues are the leading reason a member will call the plan. There are several aspects to claims that may prompt the call, such as denial of payment, incorrect payment, delay of payment, or other errors such as payment to the wrong provider or overpayment. Problems with claims payments will also be a major source of calls into the provider relations or network management area, and the cost of reworking a claim is grossly higher than the cost of processing the claim correctly in the first place (see Chapters 19 and 38 for discussion of authorization systems and claims payment systems, respectively). It is no exaggeration to say that incorrectly processed claims account for a disproportionately high amount of administrative cost and dissatisfaction by members and providers.

There are myriad causes for claims to be processed incorrectly. Some of these causes are internal, some external. Examples of internal causes are key entry transpositions (for manually entered claims), incorrect identification of provider, incorrect medical policy application, and double payment. Examples of external causes include incorrect coding by the provider, illegible paper claims, incorrect identification of the member/patient, failure to actually file the claim, and duplicate claims filings that categorize the duplicate as a new claim (i.e., even paying the first claim leaves the duplicate claim marked as unpaid). Causes that include both internal and external include claims being submitted electronically but authorizations being submitted on paper (allowing the claim to be processed immediately as though it were not authorized), lack of communication about changes in policy, disputes about the application of medical necessity, inconsistent interpretations of medical policy and benefits policy, and issues surrounding coordination of benefits and other party liability.

Beyond any required reengineering to eliminate regular causes of claims errors, the member

Table 40–2 Availability of Multilingual Services

Service	Percentage of MCOs Providing the Service
Staff to answer questions	81.6%
Translation services	81.0%
Non-English printed materials	79.3%
Accompany member to appointment	8.3%

Courtesy of AAHP Annual Industry Survey, 1998, American Association of Health Plans, Washington, DC.

Table 40–3 Most Common Reasons for Member Inquiries By Percentage of Total Inquires

Measure	25th Percentile	Mean	75th Percentile
Claims	27%	36%	47%
Enrollment issues	10%	16%	21%
Benefits	13%	18%	22%
Provider network/access issues	2%	6%	8%
Appeals of denials of payment	14%	25%	35%
Other reasons	1%	25%	26%

Courtesy of Ernst & Young LLP Proprietary Managed Care Benchmarking Study, 1997–1999, Washington, DC.

services department is that part of the MCO that must resolve the problem on the member's behalf, whereas provider or network management may do so on behalf of the provider. Which department is primarily responsible for resolution will depend on who initiated the inquiry and where the cause of the problem lies.

For member services to resolve claims problems efficiently, several factors are important to consider. First is the ability of the representative to access information easily and rapidly. MCOs with more advanced information systems are able to provide representatives with quick access to claims status screens, demographic information, provider information, medical policy information, and utilization management information. In most legacy systems, and even in some current systems, this is done through multiple screens that are reached through menu selection by pressing certain keys. The fewer screens and menus the representative must go through to find necessary information, the better. Those MCOs that are still struggling with multiple systems supporting multiple products will have the most difficult time with this, and in that case, short of replacing the old systems with a single new one, the MCO may need to consider "frontware" that will perform the interface with the old systems, allowing the member services representative to access information more easily. Newer systems generally use a graphical user interface that allows the representative to use combinations of the keyboard and mouse to rapidly access information.

It is not enough to access information, though. The representative must also be able to do something about it. This means that the management of the MCO must set policies about levels of intervention that various types of member services representatives may have. For example, all representatives may be allowed to process enrollment and ID card changes and to correct information that was entered or submitted incorrectly in the first place, allowing the regular processing to then occur. To make a substantial change in a claim payment may require a higher level of representative—one with more experience and training. For example, the ability to override a claim denial on the basis of information the member provides during the course of a telephone call. This ability to override the claims process must be available within the member services department, but not necessarily to all representatives, and clearly not to an unlimited degree. For example, any claims override greater than $500 may need to be approved by the medical director. In all cases, such overrides must be tracked and patterns analyzed to reduce their occurrence.

In the case of self-funded benefits plans, it is not unusual for the client (i.e., the company that is self-funded and has contracted with the MCO for benefits administration) to set a general tone of the latitude provided to the member services department. For example, a company may want the representatives to be able to override any claim dispute less than $1,000. If this is the case, then as noted earlier, it is reasonable for those member services representatives responsible for that company to be organized into a separate unit.

The reader is referred to Chapter 38 for information about claims management and Chapter 39 for information about other party liability. Determining the root cause of a pattern of incorrectly processed claims is worth every effort to identify the cause and change the processes and procedures to eliminate it.

Appeals and Denials of Payment. This is a subset of the claims problems discussed previously. As noted earlier, there is often a level of claim cost that determines whether the member services representative is able to resolve the issue in an autonomous way; and there may be different levels of override authority for different levels of member services representatives on the basis of experience and training. This is not to imply that representatives can or should override any denied claim just because a member calls in. Rather, this means that good judgment will be applied. For example, a member may be new to the plan and make a simple mistake such as going to a nonparticipating provider for an authorized referral, or a new member in a POS plan forgets (or fails) to get a PCP authorization for the referral; in these cases, the member services representative may make the judgment that the goodwill generated by overriding the claim denial (or lower payment, in the case of the POS plan) is worth more in enhanced member satisfaction and retention than the monetary value of denying the claim.

In more serious cases of claim payment disputes, the plan must have a more formal mechanism for the member to appeal the payment denial (the same issue applies for provider appeals of payment denials, as discussed in Chapter 18). This form of appeal or grievance is discussed separately later in this chapter because it is part of the broader discussion of complaints and grievances.

Enrollment Issues and Identification Cards. This is a generally straightforward type of service in which the member needs to correct an enrollment error or make a change to the coverage status. Although this chapter does not address the basic issues of entering enrollment information and issuing identification cards, it is inevitable that some members will have problems with their cards, and then member services will need to resolve those problems.

Common reasons for calls include lost cards, cards that were sent to the wrong address, incorrect information on the card, the member's (or a dependent's) name being misspelled, or change of address. Changes in enrollment status may be required because of change of status; for example, adding a new dependent such as a newborn or a newly adopted child or a change in marital status. In all these cases, the enrollment information must be updated and a new ID card(s) issued.

This type of service is increasingly becoming an automated self-service function as described earlier in this chapter.

Primary Care Physician Selection and Network Access. In plans that use PCPs to access care, member services will frequently be called on to help members select a PCP. This may occur because the member failed to select a PCP in the first place, particularly in a POS plan in which the member has no intention of using the HMO part of the plan. Even in POS, it is best to require the member to select a PCP because it is not known whether the member will change his

or her mind later and because the plan really does want to encourage the member to use the managed care system. The ability of a member to choose his or her personal physician is correlated with higher member satisfaction, so extra efforts to enable this are worth making.[13]

Another reason that a member may need to select a new PCP is if a participating PCP leaves the network for any reason; or if the PCP's practice closes because it is full but that information did not get into the most recent provider directory or even the plan's Website provider directory; or the member did not realize that a tiny, superscript asterisk meant that the practice was closed. Keeping the provider directory up to date is a difficult proposition because it is not practical to issue new directories on a frequent basis to members and to the providers themselves. The Internet, by way of the Web, provides the most practical solution to this, but not all members (and potential enrollees) have Internet access. Therefore, it is still too common for a member to select a PCP who is no longer accepting new patients. In all cases, the way the plan denotes that a practice is closed may not be as obvious to a member as it is to the plan personnel that came up with it.

One other common reason for change is that the member and the PCP simply are not the right match for each other, and the member is requesting a change to another PCP. This often occurs when a member is new to the system, and it occurs particularly often when managed care is installed as a replacement for all other insurance (as with most POS plans), thus requiring new members who never wanted to go into a managed care plan to select a PCP.

In any event, member services is generally responsible for helping the members with this issue. Many plans have more information about PCPs available to the member services representative than is available in the directory, and representatives may be able to help the member select a PCP on the basis of special information such as languages spoken, training, and hours available. Some plans, especially closed panel plans, have highly informative physician directories available for this purpose that they make available to members by way of the plan's website or may even mail to a subscriber on request. In the case of Web-based physician directories, the ability to sort on the basis of such selection criteria is valuable and increasingly common and often accompanied by the ability to change PCP status online. The member may also wish to obtain more detailed information about specialty physicians to have an informed choice of what specialist he or she sees (either through PCP authorized referral or self-referral, depending on the benefits plan).

Outreach

An outreach program can be of great benefit in preventing member complaints and problems. An outreach program is one that proactively contacts new members and discusses the way the plan works. By reaching out and letting members know how the authorization system works, how to obtain services, what the benefits are, and so forth, the plan can reduce confusion.

Virtually all HMOs, as well as other types of plans, mail an information pack to new members. This pack typically includes not only the new identification card but also descriptive language about how to use the plan, access care, how the authorization system works, information about coordination of benefits (see Chapter 39), how to access urgent or emergency care, an updated provider directory (possibly with maps in the case of a closed panel), and a description of how the pharmacy benefit works (see Chapter 24) if the member has such a benefit. Some plans may also include a copy of the benefits description and even possibly the group master contract or legal schedule of benefits. Some plans also include a "Member Bill of Rights" outlining the member's rights and responsibilities. Closed panels, medical groups in open panel plans, and IDSs may also include hours of operation and telephone numbers for their health centers. The various telephone numbers, mailing addresses, and website addresses are also provided.

Many plans accomplish a more aggressive and effective outreach program by conducting a telephone-based outreach program. A telephonic outreach requires a carefully scripted approach during the contact. Development of

scripts allows the plan to use lesser trained personnel to carry out the program; when questions arise that are not easily answered from the script or when problems are identified, the member may be transferred to an experienced member services representative. This also gives the member a chance to ask questions about the plan, especially when those questions do not come up until the member has heard about the plan from the outreach personnel. It is worthwhile to bear in mind that for many members who do not access medical services frequently, this contact may be the most important one; and clearly it is in the plan's interest to retain such members. Outreach is most effective when carried out during both daytime and early evening hours to ensure that contact is made.

Telephone outreach is especially useful when the plan undergoes a large enrollment surge. The level of problems that members experience with a managed care plan is generally highest during the initial period of enrollment (because new members are still unfamiliar with the way the plan operates), and outreach can help ameliorate that issue. The sooner the members understand how to access the system, the sooner the burden on the plan to deal with complaints and grievances will diminish.

Similarly, certain populations of enrollees may benefit disproportionately from an outreach program. The Medicare + Choice members (see Chapters 55 and 56) are one such population. An excellent example of a Medicare-focused member outreach program was instituted by one national managed care company, in which not only did the plan reach out to new members, but it also assigned a "personal service specialist" to each Medicare enrollee.[14] The personal service specialist then became the person that the Medicare enrollee could call for any problem or issue, rather than simply calling member services and talking to whomever picked up the call. The service specialist also does the follow up with the member.

Data Collection and Analysis

The member services department should be responsible for collecting, collating, and analyzing data. Data may be considered in two broad categories: data regarding general levels of satisfaction and dissatisfaction, and data regarding medical and administrative problems.

Satisfaction Data

Satisfaction data may include surveys of current members, disenrollment surveys, telephone response time and waiting time studies (these may be done in conjunction with the quality management department, but they are essentially patient satisfaction studies), and surveys of clients and accounts (although marketing rather than member services may perform many of these studies).

Member surveys are particularly useful when done properly. Even when a managed care plan is the sole carrier in an account (e.g., a replacement POS plan), surveys help the plan evaluate service levels and ascertain what issues are important to the members. Surveys may be focused on a few issues that the plan wants to study, or they may be broad and comprehensive. There are many examples of surveys that may be tailored for any particular use.[15]

In an environment where members have multiple choices for their health care coverage, member surveys will be geared toward issues that influence enrollment choices. It is easier and less expensive to retain a member than it is to sell a new one. Of special importance are those members who do not heavily use medical services because their premiums pay for the expenses of those members with high medical costs and because such members with low medical costs tend to disenroll more often than members who use services heavily.[16] Surveys designed to analyze what makes those low-utilizing members leave or stay (or join in the first place) can lead to the development of targeted member retention programs. Some plans develop direct mail campaigns that include giveaways or promote services available to low utilizers (e.g., health promotion) to have those members place a sense of value on their membership in the plan. It must be noted here, though, that under HIPAA (noted earlier and discussed in detail in Chapter 67), it is not permissible to specifically identify those

members by name for purposes of sales, nor may utilization or health data be made available on a member-identifiable basis to the sales and marketing department.

There are two forms of member satisfaction surveys that an MCO may be required to conduct, rather than conducting them on a voluntary basis. The first of these is the Consumer Assessment of Health Plans Survey (CAHPS; see Chapters 55 and 56) that is required of all Medicare+Choice plans. CAHPS data are made available to consumers several ways, with the government's goal of educating consumers so that they may make informed choices. Data on each health plan's beneficiary satisfaction (including CAHPS data), measurements from the Health Plan Employer Data Information Set (HEDIS), cost and benefits, and percentage of board-certified providers are available on the agency's website at www. Medicare.gov, through the agency's call-in center, and in the "Medicare & You" handbook that Medicare distributes to Medicare eligibles.

The second potentially required survey is HEDIS, developed and issued by the National Committee for Quality Assurance (NCQA; see Chapter 44). HEDIS contains many member satisfaction measures in addition to its other measures (see Chapter 35 for a listing of the HEDIS 2000 measures). HEDIS is required for Medicare+Choice plans, as well as by most large employer groups (i.e., commercial customers). There is also a crosswalk or mapping table to allow HEDIS and CAHPS data to be crosswalked between each survey (see Chapter 55 for a brief mention of Medicare's rationale for using a separate survey, i.e., CAHPS). HEDIS data on all participating health plans are available for purchase from NCQA (www.ncqa.org) under the publication title "Quality Compass." As of 1999, HEDIS data were collected on 247 organizations representing 410 separate health plans, and covering 70 million lives and more than 400 managed care products.[17]

Both CAHPs and HEDIS have standards defining how many members must be surveyed, what they must be surveyed about at a minimum, and how often such surveys must be undertaken. In the case of Medicare+Choice plans, there is an additional requirement for member surveys in the event that the MCO places physicians at "significant financial risk" as defined by Medicare; this is discussed in detail in Chapter 8.

Last, it is becoming increasingly common for companies outside of direct involvement in the MCO or enrollee group to perform member satisfaction surveys and to make such information available either to the public at large or on a paid basis to clients. An example of the former is the Pacific Business Group on Health, which provides information on California health plans to any consumer who accesses their website at www.pbgh.org or their comparative directory at www.healthscope.org. An example of a proprietary company that provides highly detailed and specific consumer satisfaction data for MCOs and health providers in specific markets is the Sachs Group, at www.sachs.com.*

Trends Analysis

Problems that are brought to the plan's attention not only require resolution but need to be analyzed to look for trends. If a problem is sporadic or random, there may be little required other than helping the individual member as needed. If problems are widespread or stem from something that is likely to cause continual problems, the plan must act to resolve the problems at the source. Such resolution may mean changing a policy or procedure, improving education materials to the members, dealing with a difficult provider, or any number of events. The point is that plan management will not know of chronic problems if the data are not analyzed.

Many plans now automate their member services tracking systems. Such automation not only serves to help member services track and manage individual problems but also serves as a method to collect and collate data. Each member contact with the plan is entered into the computerized tracking system and assigned a category

(or multiple categories if necessary); issues involving providers are generally tracked not only by category but by provider as well. Repeat or follow-up calls are also tracked but usually still count as only one problem or inquiry.

Producing regular reports summarizing frequency of each category, as well as frequency of problems or complaints by provider (along with monitoring of the rate at which members transfer out of a provider's practice), allows management to focus attention appropriately. An example of the types of categories that a plan may track is given in Exhibit 40–2. This example applies primarily to HMOs or POS plans and is by no means exhaustive; conversely, it is unlikely that a plan would use all these categories. In fact, if the plan uses too fine a division of reasons, it may be unable to obtain any statistically significant amounts of data.

Proactive Approaches to Member Services

Most member services departments become complaint departments. When that happens, the plan not only loses a valuable source of member satisfaction but runs the risk of burning out the personnel in the department. It is emotionally draining to listen to complaints all day. Even the satisfaction of successfully resolving most complaints can be inadequate if there is nothing else the plan is doing to address satisfaction. This leads to higher personnel turnover rates in this department than in most other areas of the MCO. In the Ernst & Young study cited earlier, annual turnover rates for this function varied between 18 and 25 percent, with a mean of 22 percent.[18]

In addition to analyzing the sources of dissatisfaction and complaints to resolve problems at the source, many member services departments are responsible for other, proactive programs. Some examples of such programs are briefly described in the following.

Member Education Programs

Member education may be clinically oriented or administratively oriented. The latter topic occurs most commonly during new member orien-

*As with all Internet addresses, there is no assurance that these Website URLs will remain current at the time the reader accesses them. However, these two organizations have a long and relatively stable history, so the odds are good.

Exhibit 40–2 Examples of Categories for a Member Contact Tracking System

Enrollment issues
Selecting a PCP
  Practice closed
  Never selected
  Special needs
Changing PCP
  Dissatisfied with PCP
  PCP no longer participating in plan
  Geographical reasons
ID card(s)
  Never received
  Errors on card
  Change in information
  Lost card
Change in enrollment status
  New dependent
  Delete dependent
  Student of disabled dependent verification
Change in address
  Subscriber
  Dependent(s)
Need evidence of coverage or other
  documentation
Need new directory of providers
Benefits issues
Questions
  Physician services
    Primary care
    Specialty care
  Hospital or institutional services
  Emergency services
  Ancillary services
    Pharmacy
    Other
  Point-of-service benefits questions
Complaints
  Copayment or coinsurance levels
  Limitations on coverage
  Did not know benefits levels
Claims issues
In-network
  Claims denied (HMO)
  Claim cascaded to lower level of benefits
    (POS)
  Unpaid claim
    Provider submitted
    Member submitted
  Received bill from provider

Coordination of benefits
Subrogation/other party liability
Out-of-network
  Claims denied (HMO)
  Claim cascaded to lower level of benefits
    (POS)
  Unpaid claim
    Provider submitted
    Member submitted
  Received bill from provider
  Coordination of benefits
  Subrogation/other party liability
Plan policies and procedures
Authorization system for specialty care
Precertification system for institutional care
Second opinion procedures
Copayments and coinsurance
Unable to understand printed materials or
  instructions
Complaint and grievance procedures
Plan administration
Personnel rude or unhelpful
Incorrect or inappropriate information given
Telephone responsiveness problems
  On hold
  Unanswered calls
  Call not returned
Complaints or grievances not addressed
  satisfactorily
Access to care
Unable to get an appointment
Too long before appointment scheduled
Office hours not convenient
Waiting time too long in office
Problems accessing care after hours
Too far to travel to get care
No public transportation
Calls not returned
Physician issues
Unpleasant or rude behavior
Unprofessional or inappropriate behavior
Does not spend adequate time with member
Does not provide adequate information
  Medical
  Financial
  Administrative (e.g., referral process)
Lack of compliance with use of plan network
Lack of compliance with authorization policies

continues

Exhibit 40–2 continued

Does not speak member's language	Unsafe or ill-equipped
Speaks negatively about the plan	Lack of adequate parking
Perceived appropriateness and quality of care	**Institutional care issues**
Delayed treatment	Perceived poor care in hospital
Inappropriate denial of treatment	Discharged too soon
Inappropriate denial of referral	Hospital or facility staff behavior
Unnecessary treatment	Rude or unpleasant behavior
Incorrect diagnosis or treatment	Unprofessional or inappropriate behavior
Lack of follow-up	Spoke negatively about the plan
Physician visit	Facility unclean or unpleasant
Diagnostic tests	Facility unsafe or ill-equipped
Medical office facility issues	Problems with admission or discharge process
Lack of privacy	Other administrative errors
Unclean or unpleasant	

tation meetings or seminars. New members are educated on how best to use the health plan, questions are answered, and so forth.

Health education is usually the responsibility of the medical management function of the plan, but it is common for member services to be involved and, in some cases, even be primarily responsible. The two broad categories of health education are general preventive educational services, and disease-specific or condition-specific education. These programs are often accompanied by medical self-help literature, interactive videos, and other consumer-oriented information.

Examples of general health promotion would include smoking cessation, weight control, and stress management. Examples of health education aimed at specific medical conditions would be programs focused on diabetes, congestive heart failure, angina pectoris, and pregnancy. The actual content of these programs may be provided by the medical department or an outside contractor, but it is member services that organizes the programs and manages communications with the members.

Member Suggestions and Recommendations

Soliciting member suggestions and recommendations is valuable. This may be done along with member surveys, or the plan may solicit suggestions through response cards in physi-

cians' offices, in the member newsletter, or on the Internet. There are times when the members will have ways of viewing the plan that provide valuable insight to managers. Although not all the suggestions may be practical, they may at least illuminate trouble spots that need attention of some sort.

Special Services, Affiliations, and Health Promotion Activities

Managed care plans frequently develop affiliations with health clubs and other types of health-related organizations. This usually takes the form of discounts on membership to health clubs, discounts on purchases of health-related products such as safety equipment or home medical equipment, and discounts on medical self-help products such as books or computer programs. This serves to underscore the emphasis on prevention and health maintenance, allows for differentiation with competitors, and provides value-added service to the member. Access to or sponsorship of various health promotion activities (e.g., support for community smoke-out programs) falls into the same category.

Member Complaints and Grievances

Complaints Compared with Grievances

Complaints by members may be generally defined as episodes of dissatisfaction that the member brings to the attention of the plan; they differ from grievances in that grievances are formal complaints, formally demanding resolution by the plan. Complaints differ from routine problems that members encounter (even though those problems certainly may cause dissatisfaction) in that the routine problems are resolved by the member services department as a function of day-to-day operations. MCOs generally categorize something as a complaint if it is not an easily resolvable problem (e.g., an incorrect ID card or a small claim problem resolved by member services) or if the attempt at resolution by member services fails to satisfy a member who then continues to express dissatisfaction.

A routine problem can evolve into a complaint if the member continues to follow up with the plan with the intent of pursuing either a different outcome or some other action on the part of the plan. Complaints that are not resolved to the satisfaction of the member may evolve into formal grievances. It is clearly in the best interest of the plan to try and resolve problems and complaints before they become formal grievances because there are greater legal implications and member satisfaction issues involved with grievances. Table 40–4 provides data from the Ernst & Young study referenced several times in this chapter comparing the numbers of member inquiries (which include routine problems as noted above), complaints, and grievances. Table 40–4 also notes the routine time to resolve complaints and grievances.

Resolution of complaints is usually informal, although the plan should have a clear policy for investigating complaints and responding to members. Despite the informal nature of complaint resolution, it is extremely important for the member services department, or in fact any staff member, to document carefully every contact with a member when the member expresses any dissatisfaction. For complaints, the member services representative should keep a log of even casual telephone calls from members, as well as notes of any conversations with members while he or she is trying to resolve complaints. Concise and thorough records may prove quite valuable if the complaint turns into a formal grievance. Such documentation also helps in data analysis, as discussed later in this chapter.

Grievance resolution is distinctly formal. State and federal regulations require HMOs to have clearly delineated member grievance procedures, to inform members of those procedures, and to abide by them. Clearly defined grievance and appeals procedures are usually required in insurance and self-funded plans, as well as in Medicare+Choice and Medicaid plans (see Chapters 55, 57, 66, and 69). As of 1999, members usually were contractually prohibited from filing a lawsuit over benefits denial until they had gone through the plan's grievance procedure; however, that requirement has been abolished in some states (see Chapter 69) and is under debate at the federal level at the time of publication. If a plan fails to inform a member of grievance rights or fails to abide by the grievance procedure, the plan has a clear potential for liability. Suggested steps in formal grievance resolution follow later in this chapter.

Table 40–4 Inquiries, Complaints, and Grievances

Measure	25th Percentile	Mean	75th Percentile
Inquiries per 1000 MPM	133	150	142
Total complaints per 1,000 MPM	0.34	0.40	0.49
Total grievances per 1,000 MPM	0.16	0.32	0.43
Average complaint resolution time (days)	15.8	20.5	30.0
Average grievance resolution time (days)	29.9	39.3	44.1

MPM = members per month.
Courtesy of Ernst & Young LLP Proprietary Managed Care Benchmarking Study, 1997–1999, Washington, DC.

Claims Problems Compared with Service Problems

Member complaints and grievances fall into two basic categories: claims problems and service problems. Service problems fall into two basic categories as well: medical service and administrative service.

Claims Problems. Claims problems generally occur when the member seeks coverage for a service that is not covered under the schedule of benefits, is not considered medically necessary, is from a provider not in the MCO's network, or when the member had services rendered without authorization and the plan denied or reduced coverage. The routine handling of claims problems by member services has been discussed earlier. The focus here is on claims payment complaints and grievances that have not been resolved at the initial contact stage.

In the first two situations, the plan must rely on both the schedule of benefits and determinations of medical necessity by the medical department. In the case of the member seeking coverage for services from a nonparticipating provider, the medical director must determine whether the same service is available from a participating provider and it is reasonable for the member to use the in-network provider. In the case of denial or reduction in payment of claims already incurred, the issue of plan policy and procedure is also present because this situation usually arises from cold claims received without prior PCP or case manager authorization.

For prospective denial or reduction of coverage, the plan should respond to the member with the exact contractual language on which it bases its denial of coverage. There also needs to be a mechanism in place for second opinions or external review of the medical director's opinion in those cases in which there is a dispute over medical necessity. This mechanism for a second opinion may be internal or external and is described later. The medical director must be careful not to confuse the issue of medical necessity with that of covered benefits: There may be times when a service can be considered medi-

cally necessary but the plan does not cover it under the schedule of benefits. That being said, there are also situations in which the treating physician or the member interprets a medical service as being covered under the schedule of benefits, while the medical director does not; such situations are handled procedurally the same as a disagreement over medical necessity unless the interpretation issue is so obvious that it is more appropriate for it to be handled solely by the plan's legal counsel (see Chapter 64).

Cases involving denial or reduction in coverage for services already incurred are a bit more complex. The claims department of the plan will receive a claim without an authorization for services. As discussed in detail in Chapter 38, the plan must have clear policies and procedures for processing such claims. In the case of an HMO without any benefits for out-of-network services, the plan may pend or hold the claims to investigate whether an authorization actually does exist (or should have been given). If an authorization for services ultimately is given, the claim is paid; if no authorization is forthcoming, the claim is denied. The plan may occasionally wish to pay the claim even without an authorization in certain circumstances, such as a genuine emergency, an urgent problem out of the area, or a first mistake by a new member, all of which were noted earlier in this chapter.

In POS plans an unauthorized claim is not denied (assuming it is covered under the schedule of benefits), but the coverage is substantially reduced. As discussed in Chapter 19, it is not always clear when a service was actually authorized and when the member chose to self-refer. The plan must have very clear policies to deal with these claims because it is impractical to pend every unauthorized claim since POS is predicated on a certain level of out-of-network use.

In those instances in which the claim is ultimately denied or coverage is reduced, members need an appeal mechanism. It is conceivable that the plan's claims payment policies will not envision every contingency, that the claims investigation mechanism will not always be accurate, or that there may be mitigating circumstances involved. There may be a genuine conflict of opinion over whether the member followed plan policies or over issues such as medical necessity. In the case of denial of a claim, the member needs to be informed of appeal rights; whether such information is required when one is processing POS claims is not clear, but most plans do not automatically do so under the assumption that nonauthorized claims are a result of voluntary self-referral by the member and that coverage has not been denied but only paid at the out-of-network level; information about appeal rights is provided to the member on request, however.

Last, it is important for plan management to continually analyze the reasons for claims disputes and appeals (discussed below) and look for patterns. It is common to find certain identifiable causes of these problems. For example, there may be a particular medical group that is not providing adequate after-hours access, or there may be a flaw in the claims processing logic, or there may be a significant change in what is considered accepted and rational medical practice that is not yet reflected in the claims processing logic. When such patterns are identified, remediating the root cause results in lowered disputes and complaints.

External Review of Appeals of Medical Necessity Decisions. As noted previously, there must be mechanisms in place to obtain a second opinion of a disputed issue of medical necessity in the event that the treating physician and the medical director cannot come to agreement. First of all, if for some reason the denial of coverage has reached the point of dispute and the medical director has not become personally involved, such involvement must occur immediately. Failure of the plan's medical director to be an active participant in this process is unacceptable.

There are both informal and formal approaches to obtaining a second opinion or an external review of a dispute over medical necessity (or the more rare occurrence of a disagreement over the interpretation of what the covered benefit actually is; such situations are often more appropriately managed by the plan's legal department). An informal review process may be

as simple as the medical director asking one of the plan's participating physicians in the appropriate specialty to review the case. Such physicians are usually members of a panel of physicians willing to act in this capacity and are appropriately compensated for their time, as well as being provided indemnification by the plan for their medical management activities. The opinion of the reviewing physician is not necessarily binding but rather advisory to the medical director.

Related to the preceding, many plans have formal peer review committees that provide advice and counsel to the medical director for such cases, but rather than occurring ad hoc, this committee meets on a regularly scheduled basis and considers multiple cases. Minutes are kept but are subject to confidentiality provisions. The membership of this committee usually spans the spectrum of specialties, with a core group of physicians making up the permanent peer review committee and a larger group of subspecialists making up an ad hoc group of physicians who participate only when there are cases to review that are appropriate to their specialty.

A formal external appeal mechanism is now required of MCOs by many states (although this applies only to insured groups, not self-funded groups; see Chapters 66 and 69) and is also required for certification by NCQA (see Chapter 44) and for Medicare+Choice plans (see Chapter 55). There is active consideration at the federal level for such a program at the time of publication, and has a high likelihood of passage, so readers are advised to seek out the status of this on their own. In the event that there is federal legislation mandating external appeals, the usual pattern of such legislation is to mandate a minimum requirement but allow each individual state to impose more stringent requirements should the state so choose.

Regardless of state, federal, or accreditation agency requirements, many MCOs have developed voluntary external appeals programs. Their reasoning is sound: this is something that consumers and physicians want, it is a good form of risk-management (see Chapter 45), it potentially lowers the MCO's exposure to lawsuits, and it provides a good and impartial (it is hoped) mechanism for review of the plan's most serious disputes. In any event, use of an external appeals programs remains low, generally less than 1 percent of the MCO's total membership. How often an external appeals process will be used is influenced by many factors, including how well the internal review process works, how well member services is able to communicate with the member, how well members understand the availability of the program and how to access it, and the willingness of an MCO to settle a dispute rather than subject it to the external review program.

Because there is quite a bit of flexibility in how external appeal programs operate, what follows are brief descriptions of some of the basic structural and procedural issues that must be addressed.

- *Determination of who is eligible for the external appeals program.* This refers to certain requirements (other than state and federally mandated programs as noted earlier) that must be met for a member to even access the external appeals program. For example, in many state and voluntary (i.e., nonmandated) programs, there is a financial threshold that must be met, such as the cost of the disputed service being in excess of $500. In some cases, members of self-funded plans regulated under ERISA (see Chapter 66) may not be eligible for a mandated program, although ERISA does have its own appeal requirements, which will be described in a later section. The appeals system may also be limited to medical necessity and not to interpretation of covered services. It is also common for the member to be required to work through the plan's internal appeal process (discussed later in this chapter) before he or she can demand the external review, but that is not uniform from state to state either.
- *Payment for the appeals process must be clear.* This refers to who pays what for this service. The MCO generally pays most of the cost (e.g., in some cases this cost is estimated at approximately $500 per review), but some states require the member to pay a

nominal fee such as $50 (which is refunded if the appeal is successful).
- *The external appeal body is identified.* This is something that has already been done as part of setting up the appeals mechanism. The reason for mentioning it here is that there may be different appeal organizations under different circumstances. For example, the external appeals organization for Medicare beneficiaries as of the time of publication is the Center for Health Dispute Resolution in Pittsford, New York, which provides binding opinions in disputes. There is likely to be a different organization or panel for non-Medicare members. In many cases, formal physician groups or companies have been formed solely to provide this service, and the MCO contracts with that organization. Some states require that the physicians performing the external review be licensed in the state where the member receives services, whereas other states are silent to this issue and allow for national review organizations to perform this service. Some states require regular certification of the appeals body. Some states mandate that all appeals be reviewed by one single organization and not by an organization selected by the MCO. Most states also provide for immunity from prosecution to the physicians participating in the appeals process, but in those states that do not, either the MCO or the appeals review organization itself must obtain appropriate insurance and indemnification from the parties to the appeals process.
- *An expedited appeals process must be in place.* An expedited appeals process is required for emergency cases or cases in which there is great clinical urgency (this is discussed in Chapters 18 and 64 as well). As an example, Medicare requires Medicare+ Choice HMOs to review members' appeals of coverage denials or termination of care in urgent situations within 72 hours of the request. For the sake of good clinical decision making, as well as risk management,

the MCO should create an expedited review process for certain situations that takes no longer than 24 hours.

- *How information is provided to the external appeals organization.* This refers to two structural concepts: the provision of written documentation and the ability of individuals to be physically present to provide information and to argue their case. In all cases, the full medical record needs to be provided to the review organization, as well as all of the MCO's medical management records pertinent to the case at hand, and appropriate permissions as well as maintenance of privacy of protected health information must be maintained. Documentation of plan medical policies may also be provided, but that may not always be necessary because this process is not one of benefits definition. The member or the member's treating physician may also add material to the medical record, and copies are provided to the plan's medical director. If there is a formal hearing, it must be clear who may attend that session. This is not as obvious an issue as it may first appear. If all parties appear at the same time, the potential for arguments between the parties is great and will significantly impede progress. Whether the member is allowed to have an attorney present is also a major issue because the presence of an attorney transforms the process into one more like a judicial hearing than a review of medical necessity and appropriateness. The entire process may take place solely through the review of medical records and written material. However, the appeals organization may want first-hand input, so there may need to be a policy in place that allows for such dialogues to take place, but in a nonconfrontational venue.
- *The timeline for the appeal process must be defined and clearly understood by all parties.* Similar to the formal grievance procedure discussed later in this chapter, there must be a clear timeline for the specific events that occur in the external appeals process. States that require external appeal mechanisms are not uniform in their time requirements. There is usually a time limit on when a member is still able to file for an external review or appeal, and this may vary from 3 months up to a year. State-mandated time requirements to achieve resolution may vary from 10 to 120 days, with 30 or 45 days being the most common. These timelines refer to nonurgent appeals cases, which are discussed later.
- *The process itself must be clearly understood and communicated.* Much like the issue of timelines, it is important to have a formal process in place to ensure that all necessary and appropriate steps are taken, documentation maintained, and requirements met. It is best for a single individual from the MCO to function as the appeals case manager through all steps of the process. If there are managerial "handoffs" taking place, the likelihood of mistakes occurring or procedures not being followed is great. Plan staff that manage this function, even if they are part of the member services organization, should be dedicated to it and not assigned on an as-needed basis (although because of the low volume of external appeals, that individual will also have other responsibilities). The ability of this individual to gain a deeper understanding of the issues may provide added insight to the medical director before the process proceeds to the final review.

Service Problems. Service problems include medical service and administrative service problems. Medical service problems could include a member's inability to get an appointment, rude treatment, lack of physicians located near where the member lives, difficulty getting a needed referral (difficult at least in the opinion of the member), and, most serious, problems with quality of care. Administrative problems could include incorrect identification cards, not getting a card at all, poor responsiveness to previous inquiries, not answering the telephone, and lack of documentation or education materials.

Member services personnel need to investigate service complaints and to get a response to the member. Most of these are routine problems that are easily resolved as discussed earlier in this chapter. When the complaint alleges quality of care problems, the medical director needs to be notified. If investigation reveals a genuine quality of care problem, the matter requires referral to the quality assurance committee or peer review committee (see Chapter 30). In most cases, the real problem may be one of communication or of a member demanding a service that the physician believes is unnecessary. In those cases, the member services representative needs to communicate back to the member the results of the investigation or to clarify plan policy regarding coverage.

In all cases of service problems, the key to success is communication. If member services communicates clearly and promptly to all parties, many problems can be cleared up. Such communication must not be confrontational or accusatory. It is important for member services always to keep in mind that there are at least two ways of looking at any one situation and that there is rarely a clear-cut right or wrong.

Formal Grievance Procedure

As indicated earlier, MCOs are required to have a formal grievance procedure, and the responsibility for implementing it falls to the member services department. State regulations and federal regulations for Medicare+Choice plans, as well as appeal rights in self-funded plans under ERISA, spell out the minimum requirements for the formal procedure. Such requirements may include timeliness of response, who will review the grievance, and what recourse the member has. Plans are also usually allowed to have a limitation on how long a member has to file a grievance; for example, if a member fails to file a grievance within 90 days after the problem arises, he or she may lose the right under the plan's grievance procedure to file. State or federal laws may override such time restrictions, however. Each plan must review current applicable state and federal regulations to develop its grievance procedure. The formal grievance procedure must also be reviewed by the plan's legal counsel to evaluate its usefulness as a risk management function (see Chapter 45).

A general outline of a grievance procedure follows, based on the guidelines proposed by the federal Department of Labor for self-funded health plans under ERISA. Exhibit 40–3 provides the terms of the proposed appeal requirements, including time requirements.

Filing of Formal Grievance

Assuming that the plan has been unable to satisfactorily resolve a member complaint, the member must be informed of and afforded the opportunity to file a formal grievance. This is usually done with a form specific to that purpose. The form usually asks for essential information (e.g., name, membership number, parties involved) and a narrative of the problem. The form may also contain space for tracking the grievance and responses by other parties. The filing of a formal grievance is a result of the plan denying payment of a claim after review by the informal mechanisms discussed earlier in this chapter and the member wishing to appeal that decision.

Investigation of Grievance

Between the time that begins when the form is received and ends when the plan responds, the grievance needs to be investigated. This may include further interviews with the member, interviews with or written responses from other parties, and any other pertinent information that needs to be collected. The information is then reviewed, generally by a senior officer of the plan, a panel of internal or external reviewers, or by an outside reviewer. A qualified physician must be involved in the review process if the claim involves any aspect of clinical judgment. At the end of the review period, the plan responds to the member with its findings and resolution. The response includes the rights and responsibilities for the member to appeal the determination if the resolution is not satisfactory.

Exhibit 40–3 Department of Labor Consumer Proposed Appeal Rights in Health Plans Regulated under ERISA

The Department of Labor proposes the following:

- Make clear that a benefit denial includes adverse determinations under a utilization review program; denials of access to (or reimbursement for) medical services; denials of access to (or reimbursement for) specialists; and any decision that a service, treatment, drug, or other benefit is not medically necessary.
- Require that benefit claims and appeals involving urgent care be processed within a time frame appropriate to the medical emergency, but no more than 72 hours.
- With respect to nonurgent benefit claims, require that the plan either decide the claim or notify the claimant that the claim is incomplete within 15 days of receipt of the claim; claimants must then be afforded not less than 45 days to provide any information that the plan has indicated is necessary to complete

the claim; once the claim is complete, it must be decided within 15 days.
- Make clear that benefit denials must be accompanied by a clear statement of the claimant's right to appeal and of the appeal process.
- Require that, if a nonurgent claim is denied in whole or in part, the claimant must be afforded at least 180 days to appeal the claim and a decision on the appealed claim must be made within 30 days of receipt of the appeal by the plan.
- Require consultation with qualified medical professionals in deciding appeals involving medical judgments.
- Require that appealed claims must be reviewed *de novo* (review may not be limited to information and documents considered in the initial claims denial) and must be decided by a party other than the party who made the original claims determination.

Source: Reprinted from Department of Labor, January 2000, www.dot.gov/dol/pwba/.

As noted in Exhibit 40–3, the time frames associated with this phase are different for urgent versus nonurgent situations.

Appeal

The formal appeal process occurs as a result of the member exercising his or her right for further review. The member formally requests or files for such an appeal under the required time frames as illustrated in Exhibit 40–3 (although each state may have different time requirements for insured members).

The appeal review must be undertaken by individuals other than the ones who first made the adverse determination. In the case of a medical judgment issue, this appeal may occur by means of the external medical review process described earlier in this section or at the least with the input from an unbiased physician reviewer from the appropriate specialty. In cases in which external medical review is not required or appropriate, the process occurs on an administrative basis. This review may occur solely through the review of

pertinent records, including additional material submitted by the member or the treating physician. The case is reviewed according to required time frames, and the decision is communicated to the member, along with any additional information about what other options the member has available in the event the decision is still negative (those options may vary, depending on the type of benefits plan the member is covered under).

Many MCOs choose to convene a formal hearing for this type of appeal. The purpose of a formal hearing is to afford the member a chance to present his or her case in person to an unbiased individual or a panel of unbiased individuals. The hearing officer or the voting members of the hearing panel should not have participated in the earlier decisions as noted previously. Plan managers who have been involved before will surely participate but not as the hearing officer or as voting members.

It is common to use a panel for formal hearings. Panels may be made up of board members, providers (who are not involved with the member on a professional basis), lay members of the plan, or managers from the plan who do not participate in member services issues except for grievances. It is best to use a panel size of odd numbers, preferably five or seven, to prevent ties. There should be a panel chairperson to function as the hearing officer. If a single hearing officer is used, that individual could be a board member, the president or executive director of the MCO, or an independent person capable of understanding the issues (e.g., an attorney specializing in health care).

The hearing provides the member the opportunity to present the grievance and any additional pertinent information. The plan does likewise, usually by having the member services representative present the plan's case. The executive director and medical director may likewise present information.

It is a poor idea to ask the member's provider to appear at the hearing in those cases in which the provider has been involved in the grievance. This carries the potential of disrupting the physician-patient relationship and of placing the provider in a no-win situation, and it can have implications for future legal action against the provider or plan. Any information from the member's provider should be presented by the medical director and accompanied by appropriate documentation.

A resolution of the grievance is rarely given to the member at the close of the hearing. When the hearing is over, the member is told that he or she will be informed of the results within the required time period. After the member and staff have left, the voting members of the panel discuss the case and reach a resolution. That resolution is communicated in writing to the member and any other pertinent parties, along with information that the member has the right of further appeal as appropriate, depending on the benefits plan he or she is covered under.

Arbitration

In some states, arbitration is allowed for cases involving insured plans. This may occur before or after appeal to the state agency (see later). In those states in which arbitration is allowed and if the plan wishes to pursue it (or if it is required), the plan would comply with the regulations regarding arbitration in terms of selection of the arbitrator(s) and form of the hearing.

Appeal to Government Agencies

In all cases, if the member is not satisfied with the results of the formal hearing, he or she has the right to appeal to the appropriate government agency.

Further appeal or the filing of a formal grievance with the appropriate state agency is available to members who are in commercial plans that are fully insured. Employees of state or municipal government (regardless if the municipal benefits plan is self-funded or fully insured) are also usually afforded appeal rights to state agencies. For commercially insured members, the state insurance department has jurisdiction. In cases in which the grievance involves quality of care, the health department may have jurisdiction. In either case, the state will have a formal process for filing such appeals and grievances, and each MCO must be familiar with these processes and requirements.

Federal employees, or those who are covered under the Office of Personnel Management (OPM), have the right of appeal to OPM. OPM specifically reserves the right in its contract with health plans to resolve and rule on grievances by members who are federal employees. Members who are covered under entitlement programs (Medicare and Medicaid) have the right to appeal to the respective government agency; for Medicare that means the Health Care Financing Administration and for Medicaid that refers to the state's human services (or welfare) department.

Lawsuits

Although not a part of a plan's grievance procedure, the last legal remedy for a disgruntled member is legal action. If the plan carefully follows its grievance procedure, the chances of a successful lawsuit against it are low. If the plan fails to follow proper policy and procedure, the chances become greater. In the environment that exists as 2000 begins, the rights of members to sue health plans is one of the most contentious issues under debate. Many states have enacted expanded rights for members to sue health plans, and debate is occurring at the federal level at the time of publication. Legal risks and actions are discussed further in Chapters 45, 64, 66, and 69.

CONCLUSION

Member services are a requirement of any managed care plan. The primary responsibilities of member services are to provide information to the membership in general, help guide members through the system, and help members resolve any problems or questions they may have. Member services must also track and analyze member problems and complaints so that management can act to correct problems at the source. Mechanisms to resolve complaints and grievances not only are required by law but make good business sense. Plan management should not be satisfied with a reactive member services function but should take a proactive approach as well.

REFERENCES AND NOTES

1. Employee Benefit Research Institute, Health Confidence Survey, September, 1999.
2. Interstudy Competitive Edge, HMO Industry Report 9.1. (St. Paul, MN: Interstudy Publications, 1999).
3. Ernst & Young LLP, Proprietary Managed Care Benchmarking Studies, 1997–1999, covering 19 large MCOs and 27 million covered lives.
4. Ernst & Young, Proprietary Managed Care Benchmarking Studies.
5. Interstudy Competetive Edge: HMO Industry Report 9.1.
6. Ernst & Young LLP, Proprietary Managed Care Benchmarking Studies.
7. Ernst & Young, Proprietary Managed Care Benchmarking Studies.
8. C. R. Bell, R. Zemke, Service breakdown: the road to recovery. *Managed Care Review* 76 (1987): 32–35.
9. S. W. Hall, Targeting Member Needs With Technology. *HMO Magazine,* July/August (1993): 55-56.
10. AAHP Annual Industry Survey. (Washington, DC: American Association of Health Plans, 1998).
11. Interstudy Competetive Edge: HMO Industry Report 9.1.
12. Interstudy Competitive Edge: HMO Industry Report 9.1.
13. J. Schmittdiel, J.V. Selby, K. Grumbach, C.P. Quesenberry, Choice of a Personal Physician and Patient Satisfaction in a Health Maintenance Organization. *JAMA* 278 (1997): 19, 1596–1599.
14. What Plans are Doing to Improve Customer Service. *Managed Care Week*, March 8 (1999): 6–7. The reference in the text is specifically to UnitedHealthcare of Alabama's Personal Service Program, but this program has also spread to many other UnitedHealthcare sites.
15. *A Guide to Patient Satisfaction Survey Instruments: Profiles of Patient Satisfaction Measurement Instruments and Their Use by Health Plans, Employers, Hospitals, and Insurers.* (Washington, DC: Atlantic Information Services).
16. W. Wrightson, J. Genuardi, S. Stephens, Demographic and Utilization Characteristics of HMO Disenrollees. *GHAA* Journal, Summer (1987): 23–42.
17. National Committee for Quality Assurance Website, January, 2000.
18. Ernst & Young LLP, Proprietary Managed Care Benchmarking Studies.

CHAPTER 41

Sales and Marketing in Managed Health Care Plans: The Process of Distribution

Gail Marcus and John C. Thomson

The marketing, sales, and distribution of managed health care products is one of the most complex processes in any business or industry today. This chapter's goal is to foster a better understanding of this aspect of the health care industry, the sophisticated environment it operates in, and the key players in the process and their needs. The focus will be on what the successful managed care organization (MCO) does to bring products and services to the marketplace.

WHAT MANAGED CARE ORGANIZATIONS DELIVER

The basic "product" of an MCO is a delivery system that brings together several components to offer consumers high-quality medical services at an affordable price. An MCO thus provides consumers affordable and manageable access to the complex medical system. At the same time, the MCO offers health care providers access to a steady stream of patients and revenue. The components of the delivery system include the following elements.

Gail Marcus, MBA, Senior Vice President, leads CIGNA HealthCare's product strategy and execution and is responsible for the middle market and large employer segments. She has a broad managed care background having managed the point of service, preferred provider, indemnity medical products, and several ancillary products, including stop loss, pharmacy, COBRA, flexible spending, and vision products.

Ms. Marcus has served as Controller of CIGNA Healthcare and has held several management assignments in other divisions at CIGNA.

John C. Thomson, MBA, is the Senior Vice President, Head of Disability Products, Aetna US Healthcare, Hartford, Connecticut. Prior to that, he was at Cigna. He has spent nine years in various positions within Special Risk Facilities focusing on marketing, underwriting and finance associated with casualty and property programs for Fortune 1000 employers. John has significant experience in risk retention and risk transfer programs both domestic U.S. and multinational in scope. In 1993, Mr. Thomson joined CIGNA Group Insurance. He specialized in managed disability programs, integrating Short-Term Disability and Long-Term Disability coverage and services.

- *Client/consumer service:* From the employer's point of view, single point of contact, a dedicated account service team, information on service trends within the organization, accurate and comprehensive statistical reporting, and alternative funding vehicles for the provision of the employee health benefit. From the employee's/consumer's perspective, a single point of contact, support in accessing care, maneuvering within the system, accurate response, one-call resolution of questions or problems, and technology in supporting consumers' needs. Additional perspectives on consumer and employer views of managed health care are also discussed in Chapters 40 and 42.

- *Product mix:* A depth and breadth of specific products to provide flexibility in plan design to meet the needs of different clients for choice, quality, and financing. The mix includes the key designs along the continuum of managed care: indemnity or managed indemnity, preferred provider organizations (PPOs), point of service (POS) plans, and health maintenance organizations (HMOs). These different forms of managed health care plans are described more fully in Chapter 3.

- *Provider networks:* Provide access to physicians, hospitals, specialists, and ancillary service organizations that are affiliated with the MCO and deliver health care to consumers in a given geographical area. The delivery of health care services needs to be consistent in terms of quality, and the network must be adequate in size to meet the access needs of the membership population. Detailed discussions of managed health care and the various types of providers in the delivery systems are discussed in Chapters 7, 11, 12, and 20, as well as throughout Part II.

- *Network capabilities:* For multisite organizations, these services need to be consistent in quality and cost in all areas where the company has employees. Some employers may require nationwide capabilities. Others may require the MCO's consistent quality and service only locally or in a few adjacent states.

- *Preventive programs:* Services focused on disease prevention and wellness, including programs for prenatal care, women's and men's health, childhood immunization, and senior's health. Preventive health services are discussed in detail in Chapter 17.

- *Care management:* Overall, long-term approaches to managing such chronic conditions as asthma, diabetes, and lower back problems. Care management for chronic diseases is discussed in Chapter 23.

- *Utilization management:* The application of effective and consistent methods, guidelines, and protocols in the delivery of health care to reduce unnecessary services while maintaining high-quality care and good access to desired medical services. The management of utilization and quality in managed health care is the focus of all of Part III.

- *Value-added products and services:* items that supplement and complement-basic medical service, such as medical and wellness information and 24-hour access to it, discount programs, and health care when away at school or traveling outside the local network.

- *Integrated services:* delivery of products related to basic health care, such as ancillary services (e.g., laboratory services); managed mental health and dental care; home health assistance and care; and supporting benefit programs such as disability insurance, which together offer consumers a single, seamless solution for health care needs and help clients better manage the "bottom line." Some of these types of integrated services are discussed in greater depth in Chapters 25–28, 60, and 61.

- *Quality:* accreditation and credentialing of health care providers; data on utilization and outcomes focused on indicative care, such as prenatal, child immunization, and

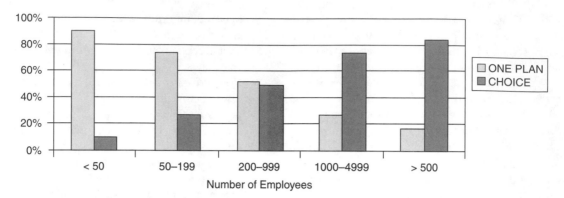

Figure 41–1 Employers Offering a Choice of Health Care Plans. *Source:* Data from Employers Offering a Choice of Health Care Plans, American Association of Health Plans, Barents Group LLC, 1997; KPMG Peat Marwick 1996 Survey of Employee Health Benefits.

women's health screening; and studies that address local results in those areas and support improvement in methods to raise the MCO's scores on quality measures. Quality management, the measurement and management of clinical outcomes, and the use of data in medical management are discussed in Chapters 30 to 32; accreditation of MCOs is the topic of Chapter 44.

CHALLENGES FACING MCOs

Delivering such a complex product poses many significant challenges to MCOs in today's diverse and changing health care marketplace. Some of the more important challenges are discussed as follows.

- *Meeting choice-based competition:* At present, consumer choice is a significant basis of competition among MCOs. A large percentage of employers now offer a choice among two or more MCO benefit plans, as illustrated in Figure 41–1. Individual consumers expect one MCO to offer a choice among different plan designs and platforms. The growth of two-income families has also created more choice because it provides consumers the option of choosing between the plans offered by each partner's employer.

The increasing focus on consumer choice means that the MCO marketing and sales process does not end when an employer commits to offering an MCO's benefits program. The decision by an employer to offer the MCO's program may be likened to a wholesale market (i.e., the employer's decision is that of purchasing for the entire company). With the high levels of consumer choice present in most client companies, a strong retail component is required as well. The marketing and sales organizations must analyze such demographics as educational levels, income, and geographical location to understand consumers' preferences and needs. Then the MCO must sell aggressively to the retail market—the consumers who exercise choice—and actively and continually recruit enrollees to achieve membership growth, and ultimately, the overall success of the MCO.

- *Increasing access to information:* The growing use of the Internet and electronic commerce (e-commerce; see also Chapter 37) is reshaping the way an MCO does business by changing the way it interacts with the various parties involved. Certain aspects of Internet-based data access and interchange (actually, not just Internet-based, but any form of electronic communications between affected parties in health care) are within the scope of the Health

Care Portability and Accountability Act (HIPAA) as discussed more fully in Chapters 35 and 67.[1] HIPAA defines strong requirements for the security and privacy of individually identifiable electronic health information. There are also mandates in HIPAA regarding electronic transaction codes and requirements and new standards for electronic identification of providers, MCOs, and employers. Although meeting the HIPAA mandates by 2002 (when they are expected to be in force) will represent a challenge for MCOs and providers alike, the administrative simplification afforded will enhance and promote e-commerce in the health industry.

- *Employees/consumers* will use the Internet to obtain information about the MCO selections open to them, about the providers affiliated with a particular MCO, and about specific issues of health management. For example, many MCOs have put their provider directories online (including detailed information about the physician such as specialty type, training, hours, ability to accept new patients, and so forth) and will generate a map to that location. It is also common for MCOs to make their drug formulary available online. Many offer E-mail or other types of inquiry services 24 hours a day, the ability to select a primary care physician online, the ability to request a new identification card to be generated and mailed, and even Internet-based access to the status of a medical claim in process. Thus, consumers can more quickly interact with their MCO and gain a great deal of information about services. Informed consumers are prone to "shop" more for a health plan and to demand more of it once they make a choice.

- *Employers* will also use the Internet to gather information to aid in the selection of MCO plans. They will also be able to access information and statistics about their employee populations' health care utilization and cost.[2] Other capabilities such as the ability to add or delete employees from the plan on a real-time basis; electronic billing, payment, and reconciliations; worksite wellness and prevention; and the ability to fine-tune their benefits plans are also near term functions that are or will be provided via e-commerce.

- *Providers* will use Internet-based services to obtain preauthorizations for procedures, submit claims, look up the status of submitted claims, receive payment through electronic funds transfer, reconcile billings, look up eligibility of members, and other capabilities as described elsewhere in other chapters.

- *Producer channels* (i.e., the brokers and sales personnel who interact directly with employers) will use it to deliver specifications for prospective new customers, access real-time underwriting and rating, fine tune benefits plans to balance cost and level of benefits, and even install new cases by means of e-commerce.

This increased access to information and functionality through the Internet may make it more challenging in the near term for an MCO to meet the needs of its various constituents. However, the Internet also offers new opportunities for reaching and interacting directly with these constituents and providing responsive, value-added services. Those MCOs that effectively use the Internet will be those that thrive in the next several years.

- *The quest for quality:* All participants in the health care delivery system are focused more than ever before on the issue of quality. To employers, quality means being able to satisfy employees' needs for quality care while effectively managing medical costs at the same time. For employees, quality means getting excellent care and service—value—from their managed care plan. For MCOs, meeting the challenge of quality means applying systems and resources to continually measure and improve quality throughout the network. Meeting the challenge of quality means dealing with issues of access to care, the provider network, and the consolidation of providers. A key concern here is that many consumers in their quest for choice want a broad range of providers, but the broader the network, the more difficult it is to manage its quality. Quality criteria often used by employers are illustrated in Exhibit 41–1.

The increasing emphasis on quality has driven the need for MCOs to obtain external validation from organizations such as the National Committee for Quality Assurance (NCQA) and the Joint Commission on Accreditation of Healthcare Organizations (Joint Commission). These organizations accredit health plans, hospitals, and other health care facilities—a "good housekeeping seal of approval" many clients and consumers look for when choosing a health plan. See Chapter 44 for detailed information about accreditation.

- *The importance of strategic sales goals:* The increasingly informed, competitive, quality-focused, and consumer-oriented marketplace means an MCO's sales and marketing organization needs more than ever to define and maintain its primary strategic focus. This primary focus may be to achieve growth by increasing revenues and building new business, to increase profitability, to increase repeat business, or to grow existing relationships. An MCO needs to know what industries match up with its delivery capabilities and how the managed care program addresses employee preferences in these industries. The challenge then is to set clear sales goals in line with the strategic objectives and focus on carrying them out in today's marketplace.

- *Regulatory pressure:* With managed care coming under increasing scrutiny by consumers and consumer advocates, as well as politicians, demand has grown for federal and state legislation regulating MCOs. Such issues as the length of hospital stay allowed after mastectomy or childbirth have already been addressed as add-on requirements under HIPAA. Increasing the rights of consumers to sue MCOs has also been targeted in the political process. Individual states have already passed a variety of measures affecting MCOs, as discussed in Chapter 69. Such regulation has the potential to impede an MCO's ability to manage quality and cost, and it presents a host of issues around marketing collateral material, as well as creating costs that will be passed along to consumers. But new laws

---

Exhibit 41–1 Employer Quality Measures

NCQA Accreditation	**Comparative Quality Information**	**MCO/Health Plan Initiatives**
Accreditation by the National Committee for Quality Assurance (NCQA). This accreditation process is conducted for the managed care operation through an exhaustive process that evaluates more than 50 measures of quality and performance. The end result is an accreditation decision recognizing their opinion of the quality and performance of an MCO.	Health Plan Employer Data and Information Set (HEDIS). This is a report card project sponsored by NCQA that compares MCO scores on achievement of clinical interventions for target preventive care objectives. These categories include mammography, prenatal care, and childhood immunization. Data on results are shared by the MCO on a voluntary basis.	This category includes initiatives undertaken by individual MCOs as part of their quality-of-care focus. • Provider credentialing • Provider profiling • Best practices library • Care management • Disease management • Customer advisory boards • Consumer satisfaction surveys

and regulations, whether state or federal, are a reality that an MCO must adapt to, and those laws and regulations will often affect aspects of the sales and marketing function. The continued change and promulgation of new laws and regulations is not expected to diminish in the near term, so continued vigilance of the regulatory landscape is required, and continued change in sales and marketing functions will also be necessary.

- **Consolidation:** Many MCOs are merging into larger entities to extend the organization's geographical reach, gain economy of scale, and increase its competitiveness on specific services or cost issues. Many hospitals and physicians are also joining to form larger integrated delivery systems (IDSs) for greater strength in negotiating contracts and reimbursement, although with variable levels of success as discussed in Chapter 4.

These new IDSs can provide consumers with increased access to quality care. However, they may form their own medical distribution systems that compete with MCOs. Moreover, many new provider organizations want to manage utilization, which may not necessarily meet the quality and cost objectives of the employer. The track record of IDSs in taking on global risk and managing utilization is mixed, and, as is discussed in Chapter 4, there have been some spectacular failures of provider organizations accepting global risk for medical expenses. This has led many MCOs to be wary of delegating this function, and many IDSs no longer seek it. The other effect, as discussed in Chapters 4 and 69, is that many states have increased their regulation and oversight of IDSs that accept global risk.

- **Increasing medical costs:** Over the last several years, medical costs have tended to go in cycles. In the late 1980s, costs were rising rapidly, which spurred the development of the managed care industry. Costs fell or stabilized for a time, then rose again in the early 1990s and plateaued or even dropped in the mid-1990s. In 1995, however, costs began to climb again, and they rose 4 to 5 percent in 1998. In 1999, costs were expected to rise from 5 to 7 percent. Medical cost trends are illustrated in Figure 41–2.

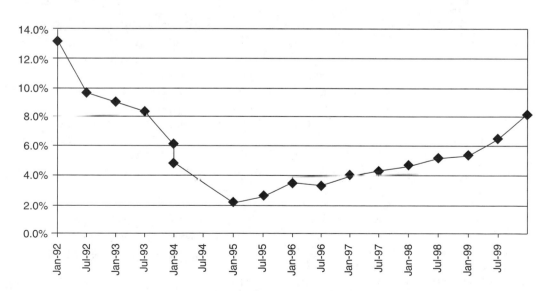

Figure 41–2 Medical Cost Trends. Courtesy of CIGNA, 2000, Avon, Connecticut.

Driving the cost issue are trends in inpatient, outpatient, and pharmacy services. Inpatient admissions account for approximately 21 percent of the total health care dollar and have shown the greatest total dollar increase in recent years. Outpatient costs have increased by 8 to 10 percent. MCOs often seek to lower costs by reducing inpatient admissions. When they do this, of course, they increase the number of outpatient encounters and procedures. This usually lowers cost overall, but not always. As noted in Chapter 12, reimbursement terms with hospitals for outpatient procedures may actually be higher than what would be paid under the inpatient terms. Even when these outpatient visits have a lower per unit cost, they may be too frequent or expensive to yield any reduction in medical costs overall.

Pharmacy costs alone account for 15 to 25 percent of the total health care dollar and have seen the highest percentage of increase over the past few years. Pharmacy costs are driven by many factors, including an increase in the total number of prescriptions written, an increase in the cost of the drugs coupled with the continued introduction of new and efficacious drugs, and the prescription-writing behavior of physicians who are placed under significant pressure by their patients as a result of direct-to-consumer advertising. The reader is referred to Chapter 24 for a detailed discussion of the management of the pharmacy benefit, including the effect of benefit design. The reader is also referred to Chapter 8 for a brief discussion of the effect of drug costs on some physician reimbursement methods, an issue relevant to the sales and marketing function of the plan because physician attitudes have an impact on consumers, and thus on marketing.

AN OVERVIEW OF THE MANAGED CARE MARKET

Managed care constitutes one of today's most complicated industries. Its size and potential alone are enormous. The number of HMO enrollment plans rose, from approximately 100 in 1980 to 700 in 1998. Today, 85 percent of insured Americans are enrolled in some form of a managed care plan, an increase of 30 percent over 1988.

To distribute its products effectively and reach all employer groups in such a large market, MCOs must segment their market. Traditionally, the size of the employer organization has largely determined how MCOs design products and approach the market. Each segment has different capability needs, while individual employers within a segment retain different perspectives on how to meet their employees' needs and fund their programs. Table 41–1 reflects the most current thinking on size segmentation.

Recently, MCO marketing professionals have questioned the long-standing belief that an organization's size can reliably predict the employer's choice of health plan. The assumption that "all employers with 50 or fewer employees behave like *this* when choosing a managed care company, while all those with more than 3,000 employees behave like *that*" no longer seems valid. Instead, many MCO marketers now believe that other variables are more likely to shape employers' decisions. These variables, which can cut across organizations of all sizes, include how committed the employer is to the concept of managed care, whether the company is multisite, the organization's geographical location or locations, and the maturity of the managed care market in each location.

In other words, capability requirements are likely to be similar throughout a segment, but how these capabilities are combined to meet the needs of individual employers depends on each one's specific concerns and philosophy. Understanding the key variables shaping an individual employer's choices is the key to MCO marketing. The closer an MCO aligns its products and marketing approaches with the variables at play in its different markets, the more likely it is to succeed.

KEY DECISION MAKERS AND INFLUENCERS IN THE MANAGED CARE DISTRIBUTION PROCESS

Marketing and distributing managed care plans is a complex, multitiered sale in which the MCO

Table 41–1 Market Size Segmentation and Characteristics

Market Segment	General Characteristics/Description
Small Employer	

Subsegments
  10 lives and less
  10–50 lives
	This segment represents the largest number of employer firms. These are true small businesses. This segment is regulatory driven and plan design tends to be simple with funding on a guaranteed cost basis.

Middle Market Employer	

Subsegments
  50–250 lives
  250–3,000 lives
	This represents the middle market where employers at the lower end tend to behave like small business. As the employee size increases, so does the employer's need for sophisticated services that are managed by a dedicated company individual who is responsible for the design and management of the benefit program. Multisite dimension appears. Benefit funding moves toward risk retention by the employer.

"National" Employer	
More than 3,000 lives	The "national employer" generally has many sites and diversity of needs. Choice of plan for large and national employers is typically experience rating or self-funding as the predominant funding design.

must appeal to four major groups of constituents: Distribution channels (brokers and consultants), employers, consumers (the end users of health care services), and providers. Each of these has unique concerns and needs. The successful MCO sales and marketing organization uses different thought processes with the different groups and develops strategies tailored to each.

Distribution Channels

There are some employers, primarily in the small group market segment, that an MCO will work with directly during the sales process. In most markets, though, this is not the case, with a large number of employers using brokers or consultants in helping to evaluate options and assist in the purchasing decision for health benefits plans. In fundamental but different ways, brokers and consultants represent or guide the employer's interests, needs, and requirements. They facilitate the design, marketing, and implementation process, and they most frequently initiate the discussion with the MCO about a prospective relationship or about managing an existing relationship. The relative positions of these distribution channels are illustrated in Figure 41–3.

Brokers and consultants may represent an MCO's primary source of business. In fact, 87 percent of employers use a distribution channel at some or all points in the purchase of a health benefits plan. The particular needs of brokers and consultants differ depending on the primary role they play and their method of compensation. Successful MCOs align their sales strategies and processes accordingly.

Brokers typically work with organizations that involve up to 1,000 lives. Brokers are required to be licensed by the state and usually must be specifically appointed by the MCO to sell the MCO's products. The level of interaction with the MCO depends on whether the broker views the health care program as a commodity or as a consultative solution for their client, the employer. Brokers frequently look for a streamlined and highly efficient sales process from the MCO.

A commission paid by the MCO compensates brokers or agents for brokerage services in most cases. Commissions are paid at the inception of the health benefits program, as well as at the time of program renewal. Commissions are also commonly paid as a percentage of the total premium each month by the MCO, and there are

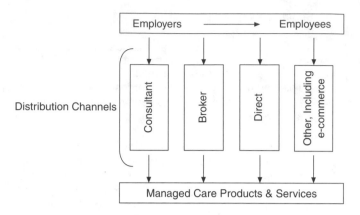

Figure 41–3 Distribution Channels

different regulations in the states regarding how the broker's fee is treated by the MCO in building the rates for insured products. In addition to receiving base commissions, brokers may also participate in incentive programs that reward growth, retention, or profitability.

Consultants seek to add value to an employer's benefit program. They generally work with organizations with more than 1,000 lives, which in most cases are self-funded rather than insured (see Chapter 66 for discussion of self-funding under the Employee Retirement Income Security Act). Although many consultants are freestanding operations, others are associated with large brokerage houses that are closely aligned with MCOs. To meet the needs of the employer, consultants expect MCO representatives to be value-added sales partners who can provide a wide breadth of flexible solutions to their clients' business problems. Consultants usually receive a fee from their clients, not from the MCO. This fee is often fixed and covers all professional services by the consultant.

Some employers do not use these distribution channels but instead deal directly with MCOs. Such situations require a specially trained sales organization that is prepared to invest a great deal of time in client contact. Managed care salespeople often regard distribution channels as obstacles complicating the sales process. But brokers and consultants can provide the client "hand-holding"

that a direct sale requires and that may not be the best use of the sales force's time.

External acquisition expenses, commissions, bonuses, and entertainment expenses must be monitored. The return on investment of these expenses is important to the success of the managed care enterprise. If external acquisition expenses are not yielding a positive result, then their use must be redirected.

Financial institutions have in the past been subject to a federal prohibition on banks affiliating, owning, or directly selling insurance. Some financial services organizations that were not banks have occasionally served as indirect distribution channels but focused on financial management types of products (e.g., variable life insurance). That is all now subject to change. The Gramm-Leach-Bliley Act, enacted in 1999, is highly complex and significant banking legislation, aimed at restructuring the financial system in the United States. The most significant change in this Act is to allow affiliations among banks, securities firms, and insurance companies. At the time of publication, there is little visible activity from this sector, but that is expected to change as banks and securities firms seek to enter into this market as part of their desire to serve as many needs as possible for their customers. How that will play out is not known at this time, nor is the potential for formal affiliations or even mergers between the banking and insurance industries. It holds the potential for creating significant new avenues for distribution of managed care products, as well as the potential to create new competition.

Marketing Strategy for Distribution Channels

An effective strategy for penetrating both types of distribution channels is based on:

- Developing strong, one-on-one relationships with individual brokers and consultants
- Understanding the distribution channel's specific orientation and basis of operations and tailoring the sales process to them
- Identifying those distribution channels that have access to employers who are attractive to the MCO, offer the highest financial return and potential, and partner with the MCO in cultivating relationships with those employers
- Providing incentive programs that motivate distribution channels to supply ongoing new business opportunities and retain established business

Strategies for the different distribution channels must be continually reevaluated and modified if conditions change. The marketing and sales executives must also understand which strategies are common to the type of distribution channel and which are specific to individual brokers or consulting firms.

Alternative Distribution

As the managed care industry evolves, new means of distribution are arising. Identifying those that are appropriate and managing them effectively constitute both an opportunity and a challenge for MCO marketing organizations.

As a central process for direct distribution, telemarketing or direct prospecting by the MCO has not been universally successful. Many employer decision makers are uncomfortable in a close one-on-one relationship with an MCO. As noted earlier, as many as 87 percent of employers with less than 1,000 employees use a broker or consultant.

Offering efficient, direct communication with employers and potential or existing health plan members, the Internet presents opportunities to enhance distribution initiatives on several fronts. It offers an alternative to telemarketing or direct prospecting, enabling the MCO to interact directly with prospective employer customers while avoiding the threat presented by strong face-to-face contact. At the same time, the employer is able to gather valuable information and brand messages and build a purchase preference for a professional and savvy MCO. In addition, consumers increasingly look to on-line sources to help them choose among the health care plans available to them.

The Internet is also changing the way brokers and consultants conduct business. Web sites offer an efficient way for them to obtain competitive pricing and proposals without direct contact with the managed care operation. Brokers are already marketing health care plans to small groups and individuals directly over the Internet. And the first on-line auction of group health insurance for large organizations was held in December 1999.

Employers

Once a broker or consultant has provided introduction and access to an organization, the MCO must sell to its second major constituency, the employer. In most organizations, this means selling not to one individual but to several different decision makers and influencers, such as the chief financial officer or comptroller, the benefits manager, the head of human resources, and the chief counsel.

In almost all organizations, a few basic needs drive the choice of health benefit plans. These basic needs include:

- Cost and financial suitability
- Compatibility with human resource objectives
- Network access that is appropriate to the employee population

- The assurance of quality care
- A choice among different plan designs
- Excellent local service
- A strong partner in health care coverage

Marketing Strategy Geared to Employers

These general needs can manifest themselves differently in different companies. The effective sales and marketing strategy focuses on understanding how general needs play out in a specific organization and then presenting appropriately customized managed care solutions. The relative importance of decision-making criteria will vary from employer to employer, and the value proposition must be tailored accordingly. For example, an employer with a clear, defined design/solution will most likely be unreceptive to a consultative stage. Hence, a fast-paced, transactional approach is probably more appropriate. Conversely, the employer with less defined requirements will probably expect and respond well to a consultative process.

One key to developing such solutions is to zero in on the needs of each decision maker or influencer with input into the choice of managed care plans. Although each individual and each organization is different, some patterns can be observed about the perspective and interests of executives from different functions. These observations can help guide the sales force's approach to the individuals and to the organization overall.

Employees or Consumers

Employers serve as the "gatekeepers" to health care for the third major constituency of MCOs, the employees and their family members covered under a health care plan who are the ultimate health care consumers. All consumers, including unions and union members, have become active influencers in the choice of health care benefit plans, making their needs and desires clear to employers. With the rise in two-income families and in the number of employers offering plans from more than one MCO, consumers are becoming ever more important as constituents and direct decision makers.

The increasingly powerful consumer constituency has changed over the last decade and today presents a new and different profile. Today's health care consumers tend to be:

- Self-reliant, taking more responsibility than in the past for their personal health and decisions about it
- Well educated, both academically and through the Internet, with a greater understanding of health care and the choices available to them
- More affluent than in previous decades and willing to pay more for higher-value products

As with employers, most of these consumers share certain basic needs for health care, which create criteria for their selections and choices. These criteria include:

- Convenient access to quality health care services
- Appropriate choices of plans (HMOs, POS, PPOs)
- Seeing their physician as a resource and their health plan as an administrator
- Low out-of-pocket expenses
- Easy-to-complete paperwork and less of it
- Fast and easy access to accurate service and information

Providers

The fourth group of constituents, providers *are* the MCO to the consumer. Providers are integral in the shaping of consumer satisfaction in health care. Research indicates that satisfied providers translate into satisfied consumers. Therefore, it is important for the MCO to negotiate win-win contracts and have effective network management, so that the MCO and the provider can work together to offer consumers high-quality, cost-effective health care. An adage of marketing in this industry is that the member makes a choice when selecting a health plan, and that every interaction thereafter either affirms or negates that choice; no form of interaction has more emotional content than that between the member and his or her physician.

THE MANAGED CARE SALES PROCESS

Identifying and selling to distribution channels, employers, and consumers in a specific managed care market add up to a rather complex sales process. An MCO's marketing department needs to work hand in hand with the sales force throughout this process, providing critical information and strategic support. Exhibit 41–2 outlines the major steps in the managed care sales process and sums up marketing's role in each step of the process.

- *Target opportunities:* The process starts with identifying potential new clients (prospects), renewal opportunities, and untapped distribution channels within a geographical area. Prospects are prioritized according to criteria supplied by underwriting, whereas channels are prioritized according to criteria developed locally. Marketing provides practical support to help the sales force quantify opportunities and identify prospects with the greatest potential. Collaboration among the underwriting, marketing, and sales functions will keep the distribution process focused and efficient.
- *Prospecting:* This process involves the contact activities to communicate the MCO's desire to establish a relationship with the targeted employer. This may be done on a direct basis or through a channel, depending on the selected distribution strategy.
- *Identify/analyze needs:* The sales force next obtains meetings with targeted prospects to learn about their organizations and identify needs the MCO can meet. Reviewing all available information and anticipating issues and questions before each meeting are essential. During the meeting, the sales representative learns about and responds to needs, provides information about the MCO's capabilities and how it can solve the prospect's needs, and, if appropriate, gets permission to make a formal presentation. The major outcome is a clear statement of needs understood by the employer, the channel, and the MCO. Marketing can provide background information on prospect organizations. Once the sales representative has completed a needs assessment, marketing helps translate those needs into a customized product solution.
- *Underwrite the risk:* Sales develops a sales strategy for a prospect, on the basis of such factors as the needs analysis, information about the competition, and feedback from the broker or consultant. Sales submits information to underwriting and other areas and collaborates with underwriting to ensure that any proposal optimizes the MCO's financial performance. At this stage, marketing can provide critical information to help underwriting assess the viability of the market or industry segment. For example, marketing might know that an industry, such as aerospace, is declining and laying people off in a particular geographical area, or that a specific company has just been awarded a major contract and will be expanding. There may be a certain level of creative or transactional tension at this point in the process, but this tension yields optimal solutions with optimal outcomes. Underwriting, which takes place outside of the sales and marketing organization, is discussed further in Chapters 49 to 52.
- *Prepare the proposal:* In preparing the proposal, sales gathers together all information and develops an approach tailored to the needs of the prospect. The proposal is used to both convey information about the MCO's capabilities as well as answer questions developed by the employee or the broker/consultant. As the proposal is being developed, sales maintains contact with the distribution channel and prospect; negotiates, if necessary, about such elements as rates and benefits design; learns about competing proposals; responds to any concerns or questions raised by the prospect; and seeks the broker's or consultant's recommendation. Marketing's expertise at this point helps sales shape and position the proposal to make sure the solution matches the prospect's needs and leverages the MCO's advantages over the

Exhibit 41–2 Marketing and the MCO Sales Process

Key Activities	Step	Marketing's Role
Target opportunities	• Identify prospects/channels • Prioritize and screen prospects/channels • Develop relationships with influencers • Develop a business action plan • Implement/track activities/results	• Helps sales identify and assess opportunities within geographical area/market segment • Helps keep sales operation focused and efficient

Prospecting	• Identify appropriate contact channels
	  —Via direct contact with prospect
	  —Via distribution channel
	• Contact prospective clients
		• Helps sales identify best means of contacting prospective clients
		• Helps sales select appropriate contact channels

Identify/analyze needs	• Meet with prospects • Conduct fact-finding/needs assessment • Translate needs into solutions • Document results • Formulate clear statement of needs	• Helps sales translate needs into appropriate product solutions
Underwrite the risk	• Develop preliminary sales strategy • Submit information to underwriting and other areas • Collaborate with underwriting • Track/record activity and decisions	• Helps underwriter assess viability of market • Helps sales develop quote and strategy
Prepare the proposal	• Identify key selling points that address established needs • Design customized solution • Maintain activities to promote sale	• Positions solution • Helps ensure solution structure matches client needs

Present the solution	• Plan presentation strategy
	• Develop customized presentation
	• Deliver presentation
		• Provides insight into
		  —Decision-making process
		  —Best way to present the solution

Close the account	• Respond to issues raised during presentation • Understand decision-making/implementation process • Ask for the business • Close the sale • Transition new client to implementation and account management team	• Provides insight into implementation process • Provides insight into roles • Helps sales obtain commitment • Creates and facilitates the value of brand awareness, which strengthens and underscores the specific employee offering
Consumer sale	• Directly contact employees at the direction of the employer • Create employee awareness of the MCO's features and benefits • Answer employee questions and address concerns • Provide additional information to employees as requested	• Helps create proactive approach to enrolling individual employees • Helps prepare consumer-focused advertising to use at the account • Helps prepare literature and consumer-focused information

competition. Keeping such a focus at this point will raise the efficiency of the sales force and make it more likely that the proposal will lead to a sale.

- *Present the solution:* At this point, sales makes a formal presentation of the final proposal, showing how the solution meets the prospect's specific needs and is superior to competition. Rehearsing and refining the presentation are essential parts of this step. Questions and concerns must be anticipated. If the needs analysis has been properly completed, the sales team can focus on demonstrating capabilities in addressing identified needs. Marketing provides key insights into the organization's decision process and helps develop a presentation that will engage the specific audience and meet its needs. The sales force's understanding of decision maker needs and preferences will keep the presentation keenly focused.

- *Close the account:* Once the solution has been presented and the prospect's questions and concerns addressed, sales seeks commitment from the prospect. Advancing the sale requires an understanding of the decision-making and implementation processes at the prospect's organization. Once sales have been successful, it will introduce the new client to an account management and implementation team. The sales lead must stay involved so that the new client can establish rapport with a new group of individuals representing the MCO without becoming concerned about their decision.

- *Consumer sale:* This is the "second sale" phase where the selected MCO must contact the employee population, at the direction of the employer. This contact may take several forms: advertising on site, direct mail or telephone, on-site enrollment meeting, or health fairs. The objective is to answer specific questions of the employee population and create awareness of the MCO's health plan, features, and ancillary benefits. In our current environment where offering employees choices among plans or

designs is growing in popularity, the MCO needs to adapt proactive behaviors to ensure the maximum level of participation is obtained vis-à-vis the competing plans.

Marketing continues to provide support during this final step, offering insight into the prospect's decision-making process and helping sales obtain commitment. Understanding the key decision makers, sponsors, and detractors—and their concerns—provides invaluable insight for the sales professional. Another aspect of marketing is the creation and promotion of brand awareness. Brand is the personality and position of a business enterprise, as known by the consuming public. Until recently, the insurance or health care industry has not had to concern itself with brand. Today, the choice among plans frequently offered by employers necessitates the focus on brand. The marketing unit of the MCO should understand these issues or retain the services of those who do. Brand will influence consumer behavior and enrollment.

The Role of Advertising

Most employers offer a choice among health care plans. Thus, it is critical that the MCO create brand awareness, familiarity, and preference of plans among consumers. In the MCO sales process, advertising's primary function is to create this brand awareness and familiarity. Advertising can also communicate more tactical information to consumers about such areas as the network, plan design, product offerings, new services, and industry recognition.

Different advertising messages are generally developed for consumer and employer. Employer messages usually focus on the MCO's strengths, such as costs, quality of service, ease of administration, and the range of products. Such areas help employers feel secure that they have made a good decision for their company. In most cases, advertising to employers is aligned with key decision-making time periods. These are either when employers are deciding which providers to offer to their employees or when employees are deciding which plan best suits their family's needs.

For employees or consumers, the MCO works with the advertising agency to direct the message to the audience that will be most receptive to messages about health care. This is usually the primary caregiver or guardian of the family's health—i.e., the person who makes appointments for the family and ensures that appropriate care is received. Because women often fill this role, many advertisers tend to target the woman in the household.

There are no established rules about which medium is best for advertising communications. In some cases a mix of media may be appropriate. Examples of media for advertising are as follows.

- *Television:* Because television offers both audio and visual communication, it is an effective vehicle to enhance the MCO's brand image or overall consumer message. It can help create a sense of trust and credibility for the MCO's brand. And television reaches a large audience and may be directed at consumers during enrollment periods. However, television advertising is very expensive and will generally be used only by large and financially strong MCOs seeking to build awareness and increase market share/penetration in a significant market.
- *Radio:* Although radio lacks television's visual component, it is also effective in reaching a broad audience. Radio can be particularly effective during select periods, such as open enrollment. It has the ability to reach specific demographic areas or local markets with a frequently repeated message. Radio advertising is considered to be quite cost-effective, particularly in markets where people may spend long periods listening to the radio, such as places where people commute long distances by car.
- *Print:* Print communication is essential for both consumer preenrollment and postenrollment phases. Advertising in publications can reach a targeted audience without the sizable investment required for television advertising. Moreover, print is tangible. It effectively conveys a specific message and can provide a "savable" reference for such items as terms and contract information.

Print advertising also includes collateral material—booklets, brochures, and handouts that explain such topics as specific health care programs or processes, contractual terms, or conditions. The MCO's brand message is woven into the collateral texts.

- *Outdoor:* Outdoor advertising on billboards gives intense and frequent exposure to the MCO's message. Such advertising is quite cost-effective, creating brand image and awareness through the dramatic impact of size and color. Billboards can be placed to target certain individuals—for example, commuters from a certain area or sport fan enthusiasts at a stadium.
- *Direct:* Direct mail can be a highly effective advertising medium. It has the ability to address particular issues in a personal and creative way while also focusing on a specific message.

The selection of advertising media depends on several criteria:

- What is the advertising goal (brand awareness or specific information)?
- Who is the target audience (consumers, employers, providers)?
- Which vehicles will best reach the target audience?
- Which vehicles are strongest in a specific geographical area?
- What is the available budget?
- What alternative media/vehicles are available?
- Which vehicle will best support the message?

HOW THE MANAGED CARE TEAM DELIVERS

Supplying the managed care product—health benefits and a delivery system that enables consumers to obtain high-quality medical services at an affordable price—requires the cooperation and coordination of many people from a wide variety of roles. These many roles can be divided into four major functions that together make up the managed care team: sales, marketing, service, and the health plans.

In the earlier days of managed care, these different functions tended to operate autonomously and interact relatively little. A more effective and efficient model is now being adopted by most MCOs, in which the functional areas work together toward the common goal of serving the client and consumer in a systematic approach, while achieving the appropriate financial results for the MCO. The current view is that success comes not from concentrating on the financial goal first and foremost, but from focusing first on meeting the needs of client and consumer. Satisfied customers are sustained and repeat customers, thereby generating profits.

The role each of these major functions plays in today's client-focused managed care delivery system is discussed as follows.

Sales

The *sales function*, as we have seen in the previous section, works with distribution channels and prospects to develop opportunities for bringing the managed care system to end users. This function supplies a good example of the changing MCO perspective. In the past, the sales function's main purpose was seen as generating revenue. In the newer view, the sales function's goal is defined as identifying potential distribution channels and clients and establishing, maintaining, and growing relationships with them. Sales provides a focused view of the external market, and the main mission of the sales force is to help employers and consumers obtain the health care services they need. Fulfilling that mission will, in turn, bring financial success to the MCO. Key areas within the sales function include the following.

- *New business development* focuses on finding and bringing in new clients.
- *Account management* takes over once an employer relationship has been established. This relationship is one of the most valuable assets the enterprise owns. The client or account manager has the responsibility for revenue growth, relationship expansion, financial results, and persistency results. The account manager is an advocate for the

delivery of superior customer service. Some specific actions an account manager should undertake include the following:
  — Complete program implementation and assess satisfaction
  — Establish and ensure attainment service standards
  — Manage customer expectations
  — Manage communication in a timely manner
  — Anticipate customer needs
  — Conduct in-term reviews
  — Implement a strategic account management plan
  — Identify additional product sales opportunities
  — Prepare the renewal strategy
  — Renew program and execute all strategies successfully
- *Consumer sales* are a specialized sales force dedicated to maximizing and retaining employee membership and participation within established client firms. This area also monitors consumer satisfaction. Dissatisfaction will result in disenrollment. Without such monitoring, the MCO membership base is eroded.

Marketing

Working closely with sales, *the marketing function* is organized to gain a high-level perspective on markets and market segments, to understand the general makeup of a geographical area, and to assess the health-care–related needs and preferences clients and consumers are likely to have. Marketing shares insights gained from this perspective with the sales force and helps develop strategies and tactical approaches for meeting the needs of specific clients. Marketing also creates brand awareness and client loyalty by communicating directly to clients and consumers. The following areas are major parts of the marketing function.

- *Marketing research* identifies vital information, statistics, and trends to help sales respond to opportunities and competitively position the MCO's products and services.

- *Field marketing* executes a consistent marketing strategy in all the MCO's local markets on the basis of national direction and local realities. Field marketing needs to provide local sales with tactical marketing support, assisting in the selection of market niches and targets.
- *Sales communications* creates materials the sales team uses to promote the MCO and inform distribution channels, clients, and members (as employees who sign up with an MCO are called) about the MCO's capabilities.
- *National advertising* creates brand awareness, contributes to consumer loyalty and member retention, and helps build ongoing relationships.
- *Consumer communications* provides the employer with materials, such as member newsletters and other publications, as well as e-commerce capabilities to help employees understand and access the MCO's services.

Service

The third key player within an MCO is the *consumer/client service function*, which focuses on meeting the daily service needs of the MCO's various constituencies—employers, employees/consumers, and providers. There are three major areas within client/consumer service.

- *Employer services* provide ongoing support for clients and respond to their needs, from presale activities throughout the installation of an account—funding, banking arrangements, preenrollment and enrollment, ID cards, etc.—and ongoing plan administration.
- *Member services* provide information and support to members (that is, employees or consumers), from preenrollment activities, through the enrollment process, and throughout their membership. Member services include technology, in the form of voice response systems and Internet sites that enhance consumers' access to service and information 24 hours a day. Member services are discussed further in Chapter 40.

- *Provider relations* serve as a liaison between the MCO and the physicians and other medical care providers within a network. Because providers are both clients of the MCO and its direct link to member satisfaction, provider relations personnel seek to build strong relationships with all providers by providing fast, accurate, and responsive service for claims payments, referrals, preadmission certification, and continued stay review. Dissatisfied providers translate into dissatisfied members because physicians may communicate their concerns and dissatisfaction to consumers. Relationship building and clear communications with providers are essential.

The Health Plan

The health plan is the fourth and perhaps most comprehensive factor in the managed care equation. The health plan is the means through which consumers have access to the high-quality, affordable medical care they expect and demand. A business or administrative entity of the MCO in a defined geographical area, the health plan includes the providers in the local network and the MCO's clinical and service employees who manage that network. A large regional or national MCO has many health plans serving different geographical areas. In today's competitive marketplace, each health plan must be accredited by a third-party organization (usually the NCQA) to satisfy the concerns of quality-conscious employers and consumers. There are four major components of a health plan.

- *The health plan staff* is headed by a medical director, a physician credentialed and employed by the MCO. Registered nurses interact with network physicians' offices to provide case and utilization management services and, in some MCOs, referral approval. The staff also includes care-quality personnel and service representatives.
- *Network physicians,* who deliver medical services to members, are often erroneously perceived as being the MCO itself. However, most physicians have contractual relationships with many MCOs. Physicians

are compensated either on a fee-for-service basis or by capitation fees and credentialed by the MCO, which uses data and metrics both to reward them and to improve their quality, cost, and performance.

- *Network hospitals* provide quality, cost-effective care for MCO members. Most hospitals are accredited (usually by the Joint Commission). Today, there is a growing trend for hospitals and providers to align to increase their bargaining power with MCOs.
- *Ancillary service providers* offer a range of medical services that support physician and hospital care. Examples of ancillaries with which MCOs contract include pharmacies, which are introducing programs to help manage quality and costs, physical therapists, and medical laboratories.

THE MANAGEMENT OF SALES AND MARKETING PROFESSIONALS

An MCO's marketing and sales professionals are responsible for:

- Identifying product and market opportunities (marketing)
- Tactical execution of business acquisition (sales)
- Maintaining and managing existing employer relationships and expanding them where possible (client/account managers)

Because these professionals are so critical to an MCO's success, how they are managed deserves some consideration. Sales professionals by their very nature are driven and competitive. They will benchmark their performance and evaluate themselves not only against their individual goals but also against their peers' performance. Recognition is frequently as important as compensation. All the competitive energy embodied in the sales and marketing force must be channeled and managed.

Goals must be established that are attainable yet challenging. Effective goals are based on the experience and capabilities of the individual and the opportunities within their assigned territory. Performance must be monitored consistently

and continually to provide a basis for evaluation and coaching. Collectively, the sales quotas must support the achievement of the MCO's revenue growth objectives.

All sales professionals need constructive feedback on performance. "Ride along" sessions are particularly effective for a sales manager to observe a sales representative in action. Constructive feedback based on observation is essential to keep sales professionals improving and motivated. Sometimes, however, sales professionals fail to improve to expected or acceptable levels, or they may be unable to maintain previous performance levels. The manager then needs to provide questions, observation, and feedback. If performance does not improve, an official performance management process should be initiated.

There is often a difference in temperament and approach between people suited for prospecting and initially contacting new business opportunities and those better suited to establishing and growing client relationships. It is not uncommon for sales professionals to be slotted into the wrong position. This mistake will be evident through missed objectives, negative attitudes, and nonproductive behavior. Sales professionals in the new business function must be highly motivated, resilient, and driven. If someone is more introverted and analytical, with moderate yet consistent energy, he or she may be a mismatch for the new business role but excellent in the account management position. Sometimes role rotation is all that is needed to create sales success for an individual.

The people balance of the sales and marketing force is difficult to achieve. How many accounts should one person be assigned, especially when the organization's employer portfolio is growing? The answer depends on several factors:

- The size of existing portfolio of the customer
- The desired growth rates or new sales targets
- The complexity of the MCO's programs
- The average number of employees per customer
- The length of the sales cycle
- The experience level of the sales force

- The distribution channels selected
- The sales resource development strategies (new hire training)
- The retention or persistency rate for existing customers
- The employer's experience or sophistication with managed care programs

Compensation

Sales and marketing professionals are compensated differently, depending on the behaviors that need to be incented and on the degree of risk, associated with variable market conditions, that the position entails.

New business sales professionals are compensated with a base salary, although it is usually a small percentage of their total compensation. In addition, they receive incentive compensation that rewards individual member sales, individual firm sales, or commission on the revenue generated.

Client or account managers have a base salary also. This may be higher than that of new business professionals, reflecting the account manager's reduced selling time. Their incentive compensation reflects their duties: profitable membership growth, membership retention, and sales compensation for additional products or sites sold to existing customers.

Compensation plans for both types of sales professionals may involve a comparison of results achieved versus quotas. Sales people who meet or exceed desired results may be eligible for "kickers" or bonus factors applied to base results and also for honors or recognition programs.

MCO marketing professionals are usually compensated with a base salary that is significantly higher than that of the sales professionals. Their salary reflects the internal nature of their position and the lack of selling responsibilities. They may also, though, be eligible for incentive compensation largely on the basis of the MCO enterprise's growth and profitability. Sales professionals can receive total compensation that significantly exceeds that of marketing professionals.

CONCLUSION

We have been considering how managed care plans are marketed and how MCOs bring their product—a delivery system for high-quality medical services at an affordable price—to employers and their employees, the consumers. We have seen that managed care companies are coming to view themselves as integrated organizations whose success will come from focusing on and meeting the varying needs of their key constituents—the brokers, consultants, and those employed professionals who bring MCOs together with their clients, the employers; the employer organizations that contract with MCOs; and the employees and their dependents who use the health care services. And we have looked at how the people and functional areas within MCOs work with their affiliated physicians and other medical care providers to bring the full range of care and services to the marketplace. This is a complex system with many functional areas that must interact effectively to achieve the performance goals of the MCO.

What we have seen, however, is a snapshot in time. Even as this chapter is being read, the managed care industry is growing, and the landscape it operates in is evolving daily. Government and citizen groups are continually scrutinizing the entire health care field, new competitors such as financial institutions loom on the horizon, and new laws and regulations are sure to mean more change in the years to come. The only things that are certain are that people will always need health care and that the managed care industry in one form or another will continue to seek new and better ways of providing it in a cost-effective, high-quality manner.

NOTES

1. Information that is strictly paper based is not currently addressed by HIPAA unless or until that information is converted into an electronic format.

2. Employers may not access information about individuals, however, because that is protected under the provisions of HIPAA.

CHAPTER 42

The Employer's View of Managed Health Care: Show Me the Value

Michael J. Taylor

Managed care is experiencing its toughest time since its early beginnings in the 1970s. As we begin the new millennium, managed care is getting more negative press and political attention than in the past 10 years combined. Much of this negative attention is focused on increasing costs, increasing employee dissatisfaction, and a real concern by major purchasers of managed care by both government and employers about where the value lies. This chapter focuses on how employers have gotten to this level of concern with managed care and how they are reacting. The final section of the chapter attempts to project these concerns and reactions into the future both short term and long term.

RECENT MANAGED CARE TRENDS AFFECTING EMPLOYERS

As described in detail in other chapters of this book, there are a number of key stakeholders involved in the complicated dynamic of health care delivery in the United States. They can be categorized as consumers, employers, providers, health plans, and the government. At present, the needs of these stakeholders are not aligned.

Market-driven forces and government policy shape the health care delivery dynamic. These two sets of forces have interacted in a variety of ways over the past 10 years. As explained in Chapter 1 of this book, managed care began with the strong influence of government policy through the Health Maintenance Organization (HMO) Act of 1973. In the 1990s, the market-driven influence took over. Now, both forces are exerting influence together.

The managed care trends affecting the employer stakeholder are the following:

*   *Restructuring*—Physicians have restructured into single- or multi-specialty groups and abandoned solo practice. Direct contracting and direct delivery by employers has challenged the existing delivery system structure. This trend makes it difficult to know how to define a delivery system, much less how to select and evaluate what delivery system is right for a particular employer.
*   *Competition*—As a result of restructuring and the growing numbers of for-profit, health care businesses, Wall Street and associated shareholders are becoming more influential with the provider and health plan stakeholders. These shareholders now focus on quarterly earnings reports. This trend forces the delivery systems to pro-

Michael J. Taylor is a Principal and National Managed Care Consultant in the Boston office of Towers Perrin. His expertise is in managed care delivery systems and consulting to large group purchasers of managed care benefits. He has 27 years of senior management experience in the managed care sector of the health care industry. He has been a Hospital Administrator, a Medical Group Administrator, and National Director of Network Development for a national insurance carrier in addition to his recent 10 years of employer consulting experience.

duce quick fixes and makes it hard for them to invest in long-term solutions. Health care delivery was used to a cycle time of at least one year and often two years. This increases competition within health care markets and across other industry sectors as the need for financial capital increases.

- *Consumerism*—One part backlash against managed care and one part "new deal" relationship between employers and employees, consumerism goes beyond employee choice. It calls into question the definition of the buyer of health care in employer-sponsored plans. As with other aspects of the economy, consumers have more knowledge about the health care product and in most cases want more control over how it is delivered and how value is determined.

- *Cost increases*—Cost-shifting strategies (from government to private payer and employer to employee) have almost run their course. Although cost increases were contained for a few years, factors like the aging of the population, who will demand more services and better organization of the providers who will resist discounting, will only escalate costs if unmanaged. The inability of managed care plans to control cost and medical use has to be addressed without cost shifting.

- *Quality*—This was mostly talk in the early days of managed care. However, the trend toward quality—real movement toward defining and measuring it—is growing. The increase in publicly reported quality measures, and the National Committee for Quality Assurance (NCQA), for accreditation process have supported this growth; accreditation is discussed in more depth in Chapter 44. The continued willingness of employers, employees, and delivery systems to invest in quality, in light of recent trends remains to be seen.

Although cost increases and restructuring are the trends most directly affecting all employers, there are others in addition to those identified previously that will drive change in the coming decade. These trends are reduction in available capital for health plans, the graying of America, and the effect of the Internet on how business is done and how care is delivered. These trends will be discussed in greater detail at the end of this chapter.

HOW THESE TRENDS IMPACT EMPLOYERS BOTH LARGE AND SMALL

The type of managed care delivery system and associated plan design and financing provided by employers is heavily dependent on the size of the employer. There are several reasons for this, but fundamentally it has to do with the amount of resource, financial and human, that is available to make purchase decisions and then manage health benefits, as illustrated in Table 42–1.

THE LARGE GROUP EMPLOYER: 5,000 LIVES PLUS

These employers are commonly multi-site. Self-funding is prevalent and plan performance is often monitored by the employer or more recently by an outsourced network manager. Nearly all large group employers have benefits staff, although the numbers of such staff have decreased in recent years. Almost all use benefits consultants to facilitate strategy and purchasing decisions.

Previously these employers drove the managed care market toward greater plan design flexibility, greater network access, and improved data reporting. This is changing as health plans suitable for these large employers merge and consolidate. A single large employer is losing leverage with the large multi-site health plans that now have millions of members. Many employers still use the strategy of a single plan administrator for preferred provider organization (PPO) and/or point-of-service (POS) programs, supplemented with HMOs in locations where strong, local HMOs are available. Other large group employers continue to look for the best vendor in each market and are coordinating management through a central administrative

Table 42–1 Employer Selection Process by Size of Employer

Employer Size	Plan Flexibility	Price	Sales Approach	Human Resources Staff	Self-Funding	Network Quality	Access	Reporting
Small (<50 employees)	1+	4+	Direct/agent/ brokers	No	No	3+	2+	0
Medium (50–500 employees)	2+	3+	Direct/agent/ brokers	No	Some	3+	2–3+	1+
Moderate (500–5,000 employees)	3+	3+	Broker/ consultant	Yes	Many	3–4+	3+	3+
Large (>5,000 employees)	4+	2+	Consultant	Yes	Most	3–4+	4+	4+

Ratings are made on a scale of 1+ to 4+. 1+ reflects issues of little importance, 4+ reflects issues of significant importance.
Courtesy of Towers Perrin, New York, New York.

organization or network manager. As prices moderated in 1995 to 1997, large employers focused on quality of care, member service, and network access. Performance guarantees and long-term contracts were focused on these areas. In 1999 with costs escalating rapidly, the focus was back on negotiating medical and administrative costs for short-term gains.

THE MODERATE GROUP EMPLOYER: 500–5,000 LIVES

These companies have seen the greatest reduction in benefits staffing. They are often multi-site with various separate businesses or divisions. They usually rely on benefit consultants or brokers for the purchasing decisions. They are more price sensitive than the larger employers but value network access and member service highly. Flexibility of plan design is important as is funding approach. Their leverage is decreasing as more national health plans use the cutoff of 5,000 lives for national account handling. This group is demanding in the area of

data reporting because they often have to allocate actual employee medical costs to the various divisions.

THE MEDIUM GROUP EMPLOYER: 50–500 LIVES

The purchasing habits of this group are variable. Price sensitivity is still significant, especially if drugs are part of the health plan benefit offering and not carved out. The nature of the employer is still local and network composition and access are important. Brokers remain the primary distribution chain. In recent years, the size requirement for self-funding has been lowered so more of this group are taking advantage of this. Some markets and states have encouraged self-funding through small group cooperatives. This trend is shown in Table 42–2. However, the recent, rapid increases in health care costs may reverse some of this trend. Some of the small business coalitions negotiating on behalf of these groups have gone out of business.

Table 42–2 Employees Covered by a Self-Insured Plan, by Plan Type, and Firm Size, 1993 and 1996

Plan Type and Firm Size	Percentage of Employees Covered by a Self-Insured Plan	
	1993	1996
All plans		
Overall small firms	34	35
Overall large firms	64	66
Conventional Plans		
Overall small firms	12	8
Overall large firms	46	67
HMO plans		
Overall small firms	N/A*	8
Overall large firms	N/A*	15
PPO Plans		
Overall small firms	13	16
Overall large firms	35	52
POS Plans		
Overall small firms	10	19
Overall large firms	59	68

Notes: HMO is health maintenance organization. PPO is preferred provider organization. POS is point of service.

*Information on HMO plans' self-insurance status is not available for years before 1996.

Source: Data from Health Insurance Association of America, 1988; and KPMG Peat Marwick, 1993 and 1996.

THE SMALL GROUP EMPLOYER: 0–50 LIVES

This group is nearly always purchasing based on price. Brokers and agents are the distribution channel. They used to purchase indemnity-type plans that have minimal coverage as a cost hedge or would use HMOs. However, that has been changing in recent years. They have migrated away from indemnity to PPOs and HMOs. Approximately 72 percent of small group employees are in some form of managed care. POS is fairly uncommon.[1]

One recent finding on small to medium group employers is revealing. In the 1990s, small to medium employers have become more likely to offer coverage to their employees, but their employees have been less likely to enroll. The net effect is a decline in the rate of employer-based health coverage for persons working at small to medium group employers. One factor behind this finding is the sharp increase in the size of the contributions required from small group workers. For example, a combination of premium increases and reduction in the proportion of premiums paid by employers caused the average monthly contribution for family coverage for workers in small firms to increase from $34 to $175 between 1988 and 1996.[2]

Many workers facing this increase will decline coverage, opting to limit coverage to their spouse's coverage, or may forgo coverage altogether. This has contributed to the increase in the number of uninsured (15 percent in 1979, 23 percent in 1995, 25 percent in 1999, and a projected 27 to 30 percent in 2005). In real numbers, uninsured Americans totaled 32.7 million in 1988 and 40.6 million in 1995 and 47 million in 1999.

Generally, the small to medium group employers still pay higher premiums relative to benefits. This is driven by underwriting rules that are disadvantageous for this group. This group also tends to be the last to get innovative products.

HOW EMPLOYERS PURCHASE VALUE (1988–1998)

Employers introduced health plans to better run their businesses. The health benefits helped keep employees actively at work; they provided a key, needed component of a valuable rewards package; and were a low-cost tax-effective way to deliver rewards.

In the early 1990s, employers drove the market toward certain interventions of managed care. These interventions included the use of carve-outs for behavioral health care and pharmacy benefit administration. These managed care interventions have been dealt with in earlier chapters. Another intervention involved the plan design modification of POS. POS in its purest form allows employees at the POS to decide whether to use the network provider through the use of a gatekeeper or to use any provider of their (out of network) choice. The in-network choice typically provides a higher level of benefit coverage than using any provider (out of network). Initially, this plan design modification involved different sizes of network and differing types of physician reimbursement. The POS network would be slightly larger than the HMO network to encourage greater in-network use. However, as the popularity of this plan design increased, many health plans have abandoned the different size networks and moved to a single network with different levels of medical management and a fee schedule physician reimbursement method for POS and PPO plan designs. The HMO plan retains primary care physician capitation and fee schedule reimbursement for specialists, although capitation for specialists is increasing. Physician reimbursement is dealt with in Chapters 8 through 11.

Employers also started moving pre-65 and post-65 retirees into managed care as a response to new federal accounting rules that required that they account for their retiree health liabilities in their financial statements. Savings for the employer are projected at $600 to $1,000 per person annually, mostly because the need for supplemental policies to fill gaps in Medicare coverage could be eliminated.[3]

Smaller employers also replaced single indemnity plans with managed care, typically PPO or HMO.

In concert with these managed care interventions, employers strengthened employee contribution strategies to focus membership and health care delivery into the most cost-efficient plans. They also required employees to contribute more toward the cost of care. Small group firms increased employee contribution for individual coverage from 18 to 35 percent and 34 to 44 percent for families from 1988 to 1996. Large group firms increased 13 to 22 percent for individual coverage and 29 to 30 percent for families during the same period.[4]

These interventions were quite successful and for a number of years, particularly 1995 through 1997, the annual health care trend for large employers was maintained at 3 to 6 percent.

The level of reported health care costs and cost movements varies widely within the large employer segment. As shown in Figure 42–1, about 48 percent of large employers surveyed by Towers Perrin reported 1999 cost increases exceeding 5 percent, whereas 52 percent reported cost increases of 5 percent or less.[5]

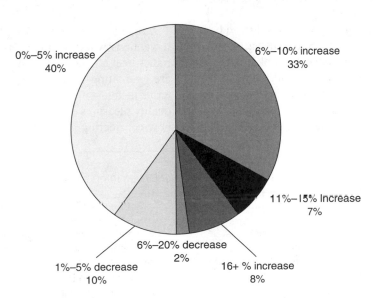

Figure 42–1 Breakdown of Reported 1999 Health Care Cost Movements (Active Employees). Courtesy of Towers Perrin, New York, New York.

Smaller employers saw a consistent trend that was higher and more variable across geographical markets, often averaging 6 to 10 percent.

These market driven interventions of 1988 to 1998 had certain advantages and disadvantages, as illustrated in Table 42–3.

During this period, employers defined value in a single way. Typically it was some variation of:

$$\frac{\text{Cost}}{\text{Quality}} = \text{Value}$$

Often, employee satisfaction was added to the equation as an additional denominator to quality

$$\frac{\text{Cost}}{\text{Quality} + \text{Employee satisfaction}} = \text{Value}$$

Although costs could be defined, it was much harder to define quality. The measures typically used for quality were those created by NCQA in the Health Plan Employer Data Information Set (HEDIS). They include childhood immunizations, mammography screening rates, and other diagnostic tests. A complete description of NCQA is found in Chapter 43, and descriptions of HEDIS are provided in Chapters 35 and 44. Employee satisfaction was frequently measured, but a variety of measuring tools and ratings make it almost impossible to compare across individual health plans.

Some pioneering employers tried to add employee productivity to the definition of value. However, the whole concept of linking occupational and nonoccupational health care delivery, often referred to as total health management, integrated disability and workers compensation or 24-hour care has not taken off. Therefore, add-ing productivity to the value equation has met with little success.

Even though medical inflation exceeded general inflation, it was still low enough from 1988 through 1998 for most employers to feel comfortable that they were getting value. The only exception to this came when there was significant customer service deterioration as a result of several large national health plan mergers and system conversions. When employees start complaining to employer benefit staff, value is questioned.

LOOKING FOR VALUE: 2000 AND BEYOND

As we enter the new millennium, the pressures of the late 1980s (high cost increase, customer service deterioration, increased government intervention) have returned. Many of the interventions mentioned previously no longer have the dramatic impact that they had in the early 1990s. For example,

- We cannot introduce managed care (HMO, POS, PPO) again.
- We cannot induce employees to move to efficient plans again.
- We should not expect a 5-year abatement of health care cost increases again.

Employers are now looking to a series of interventions working in concert to impact value rather than a single intervention solution. They are evaluating these interventions in broader terms than just medical cost reduction or simple quality measures as a proxy for value. They are now considering a new definition of value that

---

Table 42–3 Advantages and Disadvantages of Market Driven Interventions

Advantages	Disadvantages
Greater efficiency in use of resources, less inpatient and more outpatient	Excessive micro-management of providers
Greater integration of preventive services with active treatment	Reduced provider/patient ratios
	Avoidance of sick patients and denial of care
	Wide variation in practice patterns
	Anti-managed care sentiment

Courtesy of Towers Perrin, New York, New York.

includes the impact of health care delivery on people and business drivers within their business. They are also looking at the overall alignment of health care delivery with their business strategy.

This new employer value equation is just emerging and is driven by a greater understanding of the impact of employee reward systems (pay, benefits, learning and development, and work environment) on business results.[6] The two main drivers of business performance are business drivers and people drivers. Using these new concepts, the value equation for the 1988–1998 interventions is now illustrated in Table 42–4.

Quality of health care has been subsumed into productivity and employee satisfaction.

If we continue to use the single interventions of 1988–1998, in 2000 and beyond, the value equation worsens for all components, as illustrated in Table 42–5.

Therefore, in 2000, employers need to deploy multiple managed care interventions designed to impact the business and people drivers back to the 1988–1998 levels and better.

A list of managed care interventions, classified into three key areas, is provided in Table 42–6.

For example, an employer could elect to use a variety of interventions with the health plan, namely, rate negotiations, use of a smaller network, and disease management at the plan level. The employer may not choose to intervene with providers but use some interventions with employees. These might be additional choices of

Table 42–4 Drivers of Business Performance 1

Driver	Area	Value
Business driver	Cost	+++
Business and/or people driver	Productivity and/or retention	+
People driver	Employee perception/ satisfaction	+

Courtesy of Towers Perrin, New York, New York.

Table 42–5 Drivers of Business Performance 2

Driver	Area	Value
Business driver	Cost	—
Business and/or people driver	Productivity and/or retention	0
People driver	Employee perception/ satisfaction	—

Courtesy of Towers Perrin, New York, New York.

delivery systems supported by a new contribution strategy and greater focus on demand management.

The key to obtaining value from these multiple interventions is to make sure that they are aligned properly and are continuously measurable for their effect on the business and people drivers. Large employers by their visibility and influence and small to medium employers by collective action such as coalitions will have to work in partnership with the health plans and provider community to make these multiple interventions work. Partnership has been tried before but has remained a difficult concept to implement. A 1998 survey jointly conducted by the Washington Business Group on Health and Watson Wyatt Worldwide showed that 33 percent of employers viewed their health care providers as partners, 45 percent viewed them as suppliers, and 18 percent viewed their relationship as an adversarial/uneasy truce.[7]

In the short term, we can characterize what employers can do as a new era of experimentation. This era represents the end of the good old days. Experimentation will involve multiple interventions that require benefit reductions, plan consolidations, and continued managed care emphasis with a few new twists such as risk-adjusted contributions and performance incentives for quality and service.

In the long-term, employers will need to react to faster and more dramatic trends, such as E-health and individual health consumerism. The aligned, multiple intervention strategy may give

Table 42–6 Interventions with Health Plans, Interventions with Providers, and Interventions with Employees

Health Plans	Provider Community	Employees
Rate negotiations	Direct contracting	Choice of cost sharing options
Network development/ expansion	Employer-owned clinics	Choice of delivery systems
Report cards—plan level	Clinical pathways/protocols— local	Choice of competing options
Data management	Pressure to properly allocate spending	Plan design/cost sharing
Provider profiling		Communications reflecting quality
Clinical pathways/protocols— universal	Community-based initiatives	Demand management/ preventive focus
Use of specialty vendors	Report cards—provider level	Health risk assessments
Coalition purchasing	Telemedicine	Consumer-based web applications
Care model redesign	Inclusion of alternative care providers	Contribution strategies
Provider reimbursement models	Reconfigured models for accessing care	Information sharing (report cards)
Financial arrangements	Encouragement for physician extenders	Total health management
User groups	Centers of excellence	24-hour care
Performance guarantees	External physician review	
Disease management—plan level	Disease management—plan level	

Courtesy of Towers Perrin, New York, New York.

way to more defined partnerships between employees and the health care delivery system.

FUTURE TRENDS

Consumerism and technology are the dominant themes for the next several years. Health care consumerism is being driven by technology, aging demographics, and increased employee cost sharing. Either by design or by default, this will cause individual employees to take more responsibility for their own health. This will lead to more accountability for both service and quality from individual employees and employers.

Competition for the hearts, minds, and wallets of consumers will increase. There will continue to be the large national HMOs, but there will also be substantial competition in local market-

places from smaller regional players, including many plans controlled by provider groups.

Medicare + Choice (see Chapters 55 and 56) for seniors has already started this process. The complexities of a segmented, mass customization approach have been formidable. Until the recent reimbursement cutbacks with the Balanced Budget Act of 1997, individual Medicare HMO enrollment was growing at 10 percent per year, covering more than 6 million beneficiaries in 1998. The enrollment in Medicare by employer retiree groups was just getting started. Local HMOs and a few national HMOs started to compete for Medicare members with the early advantage going to the local HMO. With the decreased reimbursement and other effects of the Balanced Budget Act of 1997, the advantage has moved to the national HMOs with the resources to withstand the decreased profitability for a longer time period. However, the individual consumer remains the primary buyer and has been quite vocal about health plan exits from geographical markets and decreases in benefits, mostly drugs.

Health care consumerism is now inextricably linked to technology and the Internet. Internet penetration will exceed 50 percent at both the workplace and home in the next 4 years. Health care is a growing electronic commerce (e-commerce) market with growing numbers of consumers conducting health care transactions and seeking information from e-health businesses. Approximately 15,000 to 20,000 health-related sites are currently on the Internet; many of them have been around for several years. Approximately 33 million adults will use the Internet to research health issues in 1999, and these numbers are increasing rapidly. Passive patients will become motivated, empowered, and informed with greater focus on self-care. Report cards on all aspects of health plan and physician performance will become a commodity. The topic of e-commerce is also discussed in Chapters 35 to 37.

Medical practice also has the potential to become systematized and evidence based through the use of tools and technology for reducing the wide variation in medical practice. A dramatic increase in the use of medical protocols and guidelines has occurred in the last few years. Disease management also has the potential to continue the drive toward using protocols to eliminate unnecessary variation in practice. These areas are covered in Part III of this book.

These two future trends in health care and managed care have significant implications for employers. The major implication is the role of the employer in providing health benefits for its employees. As the employers look at people and business drivers and the impact of health benefits on the value of their employees, some employers may consider getting out of providing health care benefits directly. They may prefer to contribute a defined amount and let the employee decide. They are questioning whether there is adequate business value in continuing to act as the buffer between unhappy health care consumers and unhappy providers. At the mo-

ment there appears to be a spectrum of views on the employer role in providing health care benefits. It can be represented as active versus passive management as shown in Figure 42–2.

Some of this passive activity will be supported by federal tax law changes in Congress. Some in Congress are advocating a system of parallel credits for those who do not have access to employer coverage or who decline such coverage in favor of an individual market. Others are more explicit in their objectives of removing employers from the health care financing system by repealing the employers' tax deduction for providing health care benefits. These changes will not come about overnight and could be influenced in the near term by the outcome of the 2000 election. However, such changes consistent with these objectives can occur through incremental legislation, such as proposals to authorize medical spending accounts (MSAs) for all employees or to permit unused flexible spending account (FSA) balances to be carried forward from year to year.

CONCLUSION

Employer health care cost increases are back with a vengeance, and the broad brush interventions like adding POS or HMOs previously used by employers are going to be less effective than before. The sustained managed care backlash in the media is also a major concern. Employer leverage with the large national health plans has diminished for both large and small employers. The value equation for health care is also changing.

A clear understanding of the dynamics of health care and the impact of the newer trends such as the Internet and the rise in consumerism is critical to managing health care for value in this millennium. Managing multiple interventions is going to consume greater resources from the employer or the outsourced network manager.

The tantalizing prospect of some larger employers using a defined contribution approach in which individuals pick and manage their own health care is moving slowly ahead. At the same time, the government is considering adding to its role as architect and financier of health care with the prospect of adding drug coverage to Medi-

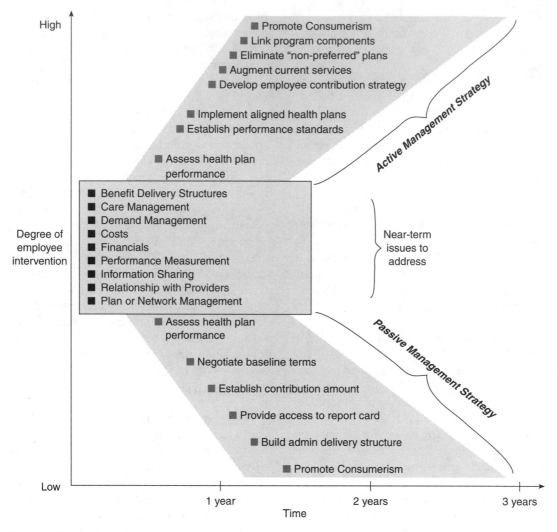

Figure 42–2 Active versus Passive Health Care Strategy. Courtesy of Towers Perrin, New York, New York.

care and regulating the managed care industry around patient rights and certain medical care treatment.

Although indemnity coverage is still alive, it has reached a stable state of 10 percent penetration in the employed population. Managed care is here to stay and employer-managed care is evolving into a value-driven exercise that will require significant attention in the years after the dawn of this millennium.

As Bette Davis said in *All About Eve*: "Fasten your seat belts, it is going to be a bumpy night"—for managed care and for employers' quest for value.

REFERENCES AND NOTES

1. J. Gabel, P. Ginsberg, and K. Hunt, Small Employers and Their Health Benefits, 1988-1996: An Awkward Adolescence, *Health Affairs* 16 (1997): 5, 103–110.

2. P. Ginsberg, J. Gabel, and K. Hunt, Tracking Small Firm Coverage, 1988-1996, *Health Affairs* 17 (1998): 1, 103–110.

3. Towers Perrin, *1995 Medicare HMO Initiative Bulletin* (New York: Towers Perrin, 1995).

4. Gabel, Ginsberg, and Hunt, Small Employers and Their Health Benefits, 1988-1996.

5. Towers Perrin, *1999 Health Care Cost Survey* (New York: Towers Perrin, 1999).

6. Towers Perrin, *The Changing Role of Employee Benefits in Today's Evolving Business Environment* (New York: Towers Perrin, 1998).

7. Washington Business Group on Health and Watson Wyatt Worldwide, Partnership or One Time Purchase? *Third Annual Survey on Purchasing Value in Health Care* (Washington, DC: WGBH, 1998).

SUGGESTED READING

Christianson, J. 1998. The Role of Employers in Community Health Care Systems. *Health Affairs* 17, no. 4: 158–164.

Briscoe, M.F., Davidson, S., Eisen, L., Robbins, M., Temin, P., and Young, C. 1998. Managed Competition in Practice: Value Purchasing by Fourteen Employers. *Health Affairs* 17, no. 3: 216–226.

CHAPTER 43

The Impact of Consumerism on Managed Health Care

Jacqueline A. Lutz and Hindy J. Shaman

Consumerism is rapidly becoming a well-established movement in American business. For health care, the trend is in its formative stage, making it difficult to fully predict how consumer-driven health care products and services will evolve. But as other industries change their products, services, and distribution to meet the increasing demands of the marketplace, consumers will bring expectations of choice, responsiveness, and convenience to the health care industry. In order to effectively meet the needs of consumers and succeed in the marketplace, organizations across all sectors of the industry must develop strategies that incorporate the rapidly evolving needs of this population.

Managed care companies are making investments—information technology and electronic commerce (e-commerce) capabilities, customer service programs, product development—in response to consumerism at a time when they are under increasing cost pressure. Complicating the situation is the ongoing integration and consolidation of the industry, which blurs business relationships among constituency and customer groups. In this environment, making appropriate investments in response to consumer needs and desires is becoming integral to an organization's long-term success.

This chapter defines the significant drivers of health care consumerism and explores how managed care organizations (MCOs) can understand and address this trend. In addition, it identifies the major implications and offers examples of consumer-oriented practices across the major business functions of the typical managed care organization.

WHY IS CONSUMERISM A SIGNIFICANT TREND?

In a May 1999 *Marketing News* article, Don E. Schultz, a professor at Northwestern University's Medill School of Journalism, notes that until recently marketing organizations were in control because they had information about customers, products, and the distribution system.[1] Today's marketplace, according to Schultz, involves a totally different interactive system in which the customer or consumer has control because he or she has access to information and technology.

Access to information and technology are only two factors influencing today's marketplace. Additional factors at the root of the

Jacqueline A. Lutz, MBA, is an Associate Director in Ernst & Young's health consulting practice. She focuses on developing strategy and planning techniques for use by clients across the health industry, including provider systems, managed care organizations, and life sciences companies.

Hindy J. Shaman, MBA, is an Associate Director in Ernst & Young's health consulting practice. She directs the firm's research and development initiatives in the managed health care industry, including examinations of health plans' efforts to transform their operations and enhance customer service through streamlined business processes, electronic commerce, and performance management systems.

growth of consumerism in society are some basic demographic trends, noted as follows.

- *Education:* The number of individuals who attended college increased from 20 percent in 1965 to more than 50 percent in 1995. Because Americans are more educated, they do more research, ask more questions, and are generally more discerning in their purchases.
- *Income:* The number of families making more than $50,000 per year has nearly doubled over the last three decades. Affluence drives an increase in demand for higher quality goods and services.
- *Time spent working:* Americans work nearly an extra month per year than they did 30 years ago, which is creating demand for goods and services that simplify or eliminate household chores and increase time spent with family and friends.
- *Aging of the work force:* With the "Baby Boom" generation reaching their 50s, and one of the smallest generations ("Generation X") following behind, an increasing percentage of the work force will be in the later, and typically lucrative, stages of their careers. This means markets will be flooded with consumers empowered with the experience, knowledge, and resources to demand performance and quality from the goods and services they buy.

These demographic changes mean consumers have less time and a greater need for fast, efficient, and convenient services. Given the proliferation of customer choices in all arenas, consumers are quick to grow impatient with organizations that are unable, or unwilling, to meet their increasing demands. As businesses find ways to respond to these demands, customers are more likely to seek an alternate source than voice their discontent—leaving organizations to ponder the root causes of decreasing market share and revenue.

In the health care industry specifically, there are many drivers of consumerism. The first of these is the growth of consumerism in society. In general, consumerism forces businesses to be customer focused, requiring them to identify consumer needs and preferences and to develop products and services that meet these needs. As companies demonstrate an ability to meet customer needs, consumers establish an expectation of higher levels of service and quality from a broad range of organizations that provide goods and services.

Other drivers of health care consumerism are:

- employers
- government purchasers
- private accreditation and advocacy groups
- media and public perception
- information technology
- societal trends

Each of these drivers is discussed below.

Employers

Employers are the single largest purchaser of health care coverage for nonelderly Americans. As health care costs skyrocketed in the 1970s and 1980s, employers pressured payers to reduce costs. In response, payers offered managed care plans that met the purchasers' price requirements. But employer purchasing requirements, which typically focus on the structure and cost of health plans, do not necessarily overlap with the decision criteria used by their employees in evaluating and selecting a health plan, as shown in Table 43–1. In the managed health care industry, the customer has been both the employer (the "wholesale" aspect) and the individual employees and their families (the "retail" aspect). As consumerism grows in this industry, the requirement to meet the needs of employers hasn't diminished, but the need to meet consumer expectations has steadily increased.

Under pressure from their employees to improve the overall quality of their health plan choices, companies began looking for ways to address patient concerns without significantly increasing costs. As a result, employers became a major driver of consumerism by demanding greater value from payers while forcing employees to become more involved—both financially and intellectually—in the purchase, use, and

Table 43–1 Top Five Criteria in Selecting a Health Plan: Percentage Citing a Factor As Extremely Important

Employers' Answers		Patients' Answers	
Access and geographic coverage	72%	Seeing the same physician all the time	61%
Annual cost and premium	67%	Being able to get an appointment quickly	48%
Clinical quality of care	60%	Going to physician who spends	
Financial strength and stability	48%	enough time	44%
Member satisfaction	44%	Affordable office visit	42%
		Free choice of physicians	40%

Courtesy of VHA, Inc., 1997, Irving, Texas and Deloitte & Touche, 1997, Wilton, Connecticut.

payment of health care services. Particularly in large or fragmented managed care markets with a number of players, many employers are now willing to do "comparison shopping" and change health plans in order to get the desired benefits at an attractive price.

In most industries, improvements in quality are accompanied by decreases in cost. Employers followed the example set in their own industries to compel health care organizations to create performance measures that could be used to evaluate the quality of health plans. In response to these demands, the National Committee for Quality Assurance (NCQA; see also Chapter 44) developed the Health Plan Employer Data and Information Set (HEDIS; see Chapters 35 and 44). While there is disagreement regarding the impact of HEDIS on cost and quality, the data set has successfully established baseline performance measures and initiated discussion and research into the subject.

Many employers participate in purchasing coalitions that provide members with comparative performance information on local health plans and frequently enable members to negotiate collectively with payers. For example, the Pacific Business Group on Health, representing 33 public and private sector employers covering more than two million employees, uses a website and other media to distribute a decision tool, report cards of providers and plans, and different health care topics of interest to their members. The New York Business Group on Health

developed a small business pool to address the significant cost differential between health plan costs for a small business—about $250 per enrollee per month—compared with larger firms; according to Milliman & Robertson data, the average citywide 1999 cost per enrollee per month for an HMO is $175.70.[2] The Greater Milwaukee Business Group on Health chose a St. Louis company to rank area HMOs, provide comparative information to members, and negotiate on behalf of the group for the best possible rates. General Motors varies its contributions to an employee's health coverage based on the cost and quality ratings of the health plan the employee chooses.[3]

The growth of defined contribution plans is also affecting health care consumerism. Viewed as an effective cost-shifting alternative, the number of these plans nearly doubled between 1985 and 1993,[4] with more than 75 percent of today's employees paying part of their health care premiums.[5] The trend for defined contribution plans is particularly strong in the small employer market, presumably because these companies are less able to absorb cost increases or to afford high cost health insurance in the first place. In other words, the growth in defined contribution does not necessarily mean that employers with defined benefits are changing; it could just as easily mean that defined contribution is the alternative to no health insurance coverage at all, especially in the small group market.

To illustrate this, a study by William M. Mercer, Inc. concluded that despite the growth in defined contribution plans, employers still absorbed most of the cost of health coverage inflation (estimated at 7.5 percent in 2000 and 7.3 percent in 1999) and actually added new benefits such as dental and vision coverage.[6] The study's authors speculate that the tight labor market in 1999 required employers to compete for qualified employees. How the dynamic will play out between defined benefit and defined contribution plans in the various commercial market sectors (Medicare+Choice is a totally retail market) remains difficult to predict at this time.

Even in defined benefit plans, employees are also paying deductibles, copayments, and higher costs for services that fall partially or completely outside the benefits and services included in many managed care plans (for example, branded pharmaceuticals, new treatment modalities, or alternative therapies), as well as higher cost sharing for out-of-network care in point-of-service (POS) plans and preferred provider organizations (PPOs).

The net effect of using defined-contribution plans and greater cost sharing as a way of controlling health care costs is that as employees take a larger role in paying for health care services, they are more motivated to seek out and use consumer-focused information in their decision making. The use of cost-shifting mechanisms was a hallmark of the response to health care inflation before the widespread adoption of managed care. The return of cost shifting may be seen as a response to the conflicting consumer demands for wide network access with less restrictions, and the need to keep costs under control. The difference between now and the early 1980s is that consumers have far more information and ability to use that information, as is discussed throughout this chapter.

Employers are also fueling health care consumerism by providing greater choice in the number and type of health plans available to their employees. Eighty percent of covered employees in 1998 were working for firms that offered more than one health plan, up from 78 percent in 1997. Larger employers are more likely to offer a greater number of plans, and the percentage of employers (31 percent) offering a selection of three or more HMO plans is much higher than other plan types. Only 6 percent offer three or more indemnity plans, 7 percent offer PPO plans, and 14 percent offer POS plans.

Regulators and analysts who study defined contribution plans and their impact on plan choice note that when employers contribute a fixed dollar amount to health care premiums, employees must absorb any cost differential resulting from their selection of higher priced plans. This may lead to selection and viability problems of certain plans. In general, a higher fraction of employees choose a high-cost, high-benefit plan if employers contribute a proportional share of the premium or adjust their contribution for risk selection. Proponents of managed competition have argued that employers should contribute equally to all health plan premiums, a practice that would force employees to bear the real cost differences across health plans. However, a 1997 study by Hunt et al. suggests that 88 percent of large employers that offer multiple health plan options continue to subsidize more expensive health plans.[7]

Clearly, many employers are reluctant to implement health benefits strategies that encourage employees to choose plans that offer better overall value in order to reduce costs for the employer as well as the employee. Some believe this reluctance stems from a company's traditional commitment to cover all health care costs and is encouraged by pressure from labor organizations that work to maintain health benefits. And as noted earlier by other analysts, another explanation may be tight labor markets in which employers risk losing employees due to benefits packages that are not competitive in the market.[8]

Government Purchasers

State and federal regulators and purchasers view consumerism as the rationale for addressing public concerns over managed care as well as outstanding problems with health care coverage and costs in the United States. A number of public policy initiatives are being proposed and hotly debated that address consumer protection and empowerment in the health care market.

Federal Initiatives

The Clinton Health Security Act (1993), despite its failure, brought attention to the deficiencies of the American health care system, as well as the growing public concern over the growth of managed care. Since then, a series of federal initiatives focused on establishing a national health care policy regarding consumer protection and health care quality. The Health Insurance Portability and Accountability Act of 1996 (see Chapter 67) addressed the issue of portability of commercial insurance. In 1997 the Balanced Budget Act (BBA) included a Medicare Information Campaign and increased enforcement of Medicare fraud and abuse rules. The current debate over the Health Care Consumer Bill of Rights focuses on nonfederal health care programs because it already applies to Medicare, Medicaid, and all federal employees. Table 43–2 provides an overview of major federal initiatives.

In anticipation of Congress passing some form of the bill, the managed care industry in 1999 began implementing new consumer-focused initiatives based on ensuring consumer protection and increasing consumer choice. For example, many MCOs assign a personal representative for each member. The representative not only welcomes and introduces new members to the health plan, but also functions as the primary liaison between the individual and the organization.

In another attempt to respond to consumer demands and legislative pressures, some MCOs have remodeled their appeal process to allow members to appeal denials of coverage to independent physicians. One company's chief medical officer believes that the policy will "reach out to protect the interests of [individual] mem-

Table 43–2 Overview of Federal Initiatives

Health Care Policy Issues	Health Security Act (1993)	HIPAA (1996)	BBA (1997)	FY 1999 Federal Budget
Primary Market	Commercial	Commercial	Medicare and Medicaid	All segments
Consumer Information	Information brokers		Medicare Information Campaign	Consumer Bill of Rights
Uninsured	Subsidies and employer mandate	Guaranteed issue and portability	KidsCare	Medicare expansion and small group purchasing
Access to Providers				Consumer Bill of Rights
Fraud and Abuse		Increased Medicare enforcement	Increased Medicare enforcement	
Risk Selection	Risk pooling		Risk-adjusted payment	

bers . . . [and] will help [the organization] gain greater understanding about how managed care can work best for the consumer."[9] It should be noted that appeal to external reviewers has been mandated by many states (see Chapter 69), and it is a generally noncontroversial aspect of possible federal legislation.

Additionally, consumer protection legislation is likely to have significant impact on the daily operations of health plans. The National Association of Insurance Commissioners (NAIC), a group that seeks to develop uniform insurance policy for the United States and its territories, believes that implicit in the legislation is the requirement for MCOs to reengineer their processes and make major management information systems changes in order to administer some of the new requirements.[10] Examples of potential new requirements by operational area include:

- *Medical management:* Specific timeframes for eligibility verification and utilization review, retrospective external review process
- *Member services*: Standards for an internal appeal process, specific information available to members
- *Network management*: Access standards, definition of type of doctor that can be assigned as PCP members

The NAIC supports the operational changes but appears to be concerned over the potential cost impact of a broad reengineering effort and the growing intrusion of the federal government in the area of insurance regulation.

State Initiatives

California is a leader in using state agencies to drive consumerism in the health care market. CalPERS, a state agency that administers state employee retirement benefits (and may also be considered a purchaser), produces and distributes health plan report cards that enable residents to make appropriate comparisons of health plans. The state is also debating the creation of a new regulatory agency responsible for ensuring that health plans follow state mandated consumer protections.

Other states have also been promoting health care consumerism through legislation. For example, New York passed a Managed Care Bill of Rights that allows consumers to take a dispute with a health plan to an outside arbiter. Connecticut, along with many other states, passed legislation to require coverage of certain benefits, including 48-hour hospital stays for mastectomy patients, alcoholism treatment, home health, some alternative drug therapies, and well-baby visits. Texas passed an "enterprise liability" bill that holds health plans accountable for the effects of their policies.

Greater discussion of state legislation and regulation in this arena is found in Chapter 69.

Private Accreditation and Advocacy Groups

In managed care, one of the most active private groups is the NCQA. A not-for-profit organization, NCQA's mission is to provide information that enables purchasers and consumers of managed health care to distinguish among plans based on quality, thereby allowing them to make more informed health care purchasing decisions. Founded in 1990 with the support of the Robert Wood Johnson Foundation, the large employer community and managed care trade organizations, NCQA's activities involve both accreditation and performance measurement. Their first accreditation survey was conducted in 1991, and participation in NCQA's accreditation program has quickly become a virtual requirement for HMOs. As of 1999, 75 percent of Americans enrolled in an HMO were members of plans participating in the NCQA accreditation program.[11]

NCQA regularly publishes and distributes the results of their surveys and research in both print and electronic media. In 1998 traffic on their website, which now has a "consumer page," reached 40,000 visits per month. The organization's most recent effort to guide health plan purchasing decisions was the announcement of an elite group of health plans meeting their new "excellent" accreditation status. The report, which listed 40 plans meeting this designation, clearly attempts to differentiate health plans based on clinical excellence, customer service, and continuous improvement. The report was released in October 1999, just in time for the open enrollment period for a large percentage of employers.

Media and Public Perception

For the media, bad news is good news. Between 1992 and 1997 the number of critical stories regarding the managed care industry doubled, while the number of positive stories went down.

Most major news magazines have run a cover story critical of the managed care industry. Typical cover stories read, "How HMOs Decide Your Fate," "What Your Health Plan Won't Cover," and even "HMO Hell."

Advertisements by attorneys, once focused on medical malpractice, now include "HMO abuse" in their list of specialties, while groups of attorneys attack the managed care industry on any possible front, looking for a huge settlement or award. In all cases, the attorneys claim that they are pursuing such cases to punish the managed care industry and protect the consumer from the alleged dangerous business practices of managed health care.

As negative media mentions increase, and public perception forms, HMOs are routinely accused of a variety of acts of wrongdoing. Examples include approving "drive-by" deliveries and mastectomies, dumping mentally ill and other at-risk groups, restricting expensive lifesaving therapies, prohibiting physicians from disclosing expensive treatment options, denying "reasonably needed" emergency care, and paying physicians to practice poor medicine. The lack of credible studies (as opposed to "horror stories" and anecdotal reports*) to support such allegations has not served as a barrier to negative media reports. The repetition of negative stories

---

*As one reporter for a national newspaper remarked to the editor of this book when asked why his newspaper did not report a more balanced set of stories on managed care: "We don't report on safe airplane landings at LaGuardia either."

has also been useful for politicians and has led to highly negative rhetoric in political debate.

Media exposure of the managed care industry has led to a flood of individual and group efforts to systematically increase awareness and protect patients from potential abuse. In August 1999 the American Medical Association (AMA) issued a news release about a new patients' rights advertising campaign. The corresponding ads, which ran in 37 newspapers across the United States, asked, "What Are HMOs So Afraid of?" and alerted readers to the money spent by health plans in an effort to defeat patients' rights legislation being debated by Congress. The ads were part of a focused effort by the AMA to discredit what they termed an "irresponsible propaganda campaign" and build support for a patients' bill of rights.[12]

Information Technology

The Internet now offers at least 15,000 health care sites. In 1999 almost 25 million Americans used the Internet to search for health information. Cyber Dialogue, a market research firm focused on interactive customer relationships, expects health-related Internet traffic to grow to 30 million in the year 2000.[13] While the growth of the Internet is unstoppable, its use within health care is still being explored and defined. Certainly the proliferation of health care sites demonstrates its potential, but skeptics of e-health wonder about the long-term potential of the Internet in health care due to the strong dependence in the industry on personal interaction and relationships. E-commerce is a rapidly evolving aspect of this industry, though, and is discussed in greater measure in Chapter 37 as well as many other chapters in this book.

While the Internet is unlikely to replace provider-patient relationships, the Institute for the Future cites four driving forces that ensure the integration of the Internet into health care[14]:

1. *Twenty-first century health care consumers*: In the future, health care consumers will be actively involved in making health care decisions and will expect high levels of choice, control, customer service, and access to information.

2. ***Experiences with other industries:*** As growth of e-commerce and e-mail explode, consumers will learn to expect the responsiveness, choice, and interactivity they get using these Internet-based media.

3. ***Characteristics of the Internet:*** The Internet is an inexpensive, user-friendly, globally accessible provider of expansive health care information, enabling the creation of a global network of users with common interests.

4. ***Market forces in health care:*** Managed care increases the diversity and urgency of information flow, and web technologies serve as a platform for disseminating information across vertically and horizontally integrated health care organizations.

Societal Trends

There are subtler, yet still significant trends that drive consumerism. Some of these were identified by DYG SCAN, a social and consumer trend identification program that uses various focus groups to track shifts in social values. DYG identified additional elements that will shape the consumer agenda during the next decade. Two of these have significant implications for health care. The first, the spread of anti-institutional sentiment that leads consumers to question authority, means patients are more likely to question not only the advice of doctors and care givers, but also the policies and procedures of the organizations involved in the decision process, namely health plans. The second, value placed on self-reliance, means patients expect to take responsibility for their own health and health care. The prerequisites of the self-reliant consumer are (a) choice, which is provided by the marketplace, and (b) control, which is fueled by the growing sophistication and power of information technology and the Internet.

WHO IS THE NEW HEALTH CARE CONSUMER?

In general, today's health care consumer is educated, demanding, informed, time-con-

strained, and choice hungry. The new consumer is also responsive—willing to get involved in health care decisions by asking questions, seeking and investigating alternatives, and demanding answers and action. Above all, the health care consumer of the millennium is clear about his or her demands:

- I am in charge.
- Treat me with respect.
- Minimize my risk.
- Give me the best.
- Help me improve my quality of life.[15]

At the root of these demands is an evolving set of values and attitudes about health and health care. Identified by DYG through a study sponsored by the Center for the Advancement of Health,[16] changing views about both personal and community health affect how individuals relate to the health care industry and impact the types of policies and reforms sought by government and regulatory agencies. Perhaps the most significant finding from the study is that Americans possess an expanded view of what contributes to both personal and community health. Health in the 1990s has a positive spin. As opposed to being "not ill" or simply a matter of luck or fate, "health" today implies an ongoing state of well-being. This state goes beyond one's physical or medical state to include: being fit and in shape, having energy, psychological and spiritual well-being, absence of stress, a positive outlook and good mood, a safe and clean environment, being in control of one's life, and having a sense of achievement and value. At the community level, in addition to the local providers, things like a strong economic base and a good, safe environment for children all contribute to the overall health of the community.

In their study, DYG also uncovered attitudes about improving and maintaining health that fit well into the description of today's health care consumer:

- More self-reliance and less subservience to the medical establishment is leading to significant behavioral changes by patients.

—More self-diagnosis
—More self-monitoring
—More self-care

- Empowerment via information is central to the patient's ability to become more self-reliant.
- Embracing technology—because we believe technology solves problems.
- Opening avenues to alternative medicine and approaches for creating and preserving health are necessary.

It is particularly interesting that these last two trends are happening simultaneously. DYG asserts that the blending of the technical and the nontechnical is prevalent in modern American society. In the context of health care, perhaps it suggests that technology best supports the diagnosis and solving of illness but that nontechnological approaches are better for maintaining health.[17]

WHAT ARE THE IMPLICATIONS OF CONSUMERISM?

Clearly, consumer demands are both varied and unlikely to wane. To succeed in an increasingly competitive and consumer-oriented marketplace, MCOs must:

- disseminate meaningful, understandable information on clinical care and quality
- develop innovative products and services that satisfy consumers' specific preferences for choice, convenience, and access
- encourage and support consumer and patient empowerment in treatment decisions
- streamline administrative functions to keep costs in line and prices competitive.

These new strategic demands of the marketplace necessitate changes to virtually all aspects of a managed care organization's operations, including general management and governance, sales and marketing, medical and network management, back-office operations and customer service, and the supporting infrastructure. The types of operational changes that may be adopted by MCOs in addressing these various consumer demands are discussed below. The purpose of this discussion is not to advocate or promote any specific practices (many of which may likely change subsequent to this writing). Rather, the intent is to highlight examples that may foretell future operational changes in the managed care industry. To date, relatively few MCOs have fully implemented these changes, although many have strategic plans or development under way in selected areas.

Consumer Demand for Meaningful Information

Consumers' almost insatiable thirst for information requires the managed care organization to be a major avenue and filter for information. Many payers have already developed personal, print, and electronic channels to support communications with members. The issue of quality is of major concern to consumers, as seen in the proliferation of guidelines on how to choose a health plan or provider (see Exhibit 43–1).

The demand for health information is growing so quickly that health websites are now hosted by a broad range of organizations, such as government organizations (e.g., HCFA), accrediting organizations (e.g., NCQA), business coalitions, industry associations, private companies, and the media. These sites offer a variety of health-related information and services, including:

- ratings of hospital, physician, health plan quality and performance
- provider directories
- guidelines for choosing hospitals, physicians, and health plan
- glossary of health terms
- health-related news and articles
- links to health search engines
- physician malpractice/sanctions
- hospital accreditation, volume, level of emergency services, and malpractice actions
- general information about conditions and procedures
- questions for patients to ask about their medical conditions

Exhibit 43–1 Sample Guidelines for How To Choose a Health Plan

1. Check the plan's Health Plan Report Cards and HMO Report Cards ratings. Read health plans carefully. Do not rely on summaries.
2. Check the Physician Report Cards ratings of physicians in the plan. Check the Hospital Report Cards ratings of hospitals in the plan.
3. Are the plan's physician(s) and hospital(s) close to your home/work?
4. Are physicians in the plan board-certified?
5. What is the plan's NCQA accreditation status?
6. Are you required to select a primary care physician?
7. Is your current physician a member of the network?
8. Are you allowed to receive care from providers outside the network? At what cost?
9. How restrictive is the physician list? What restrictions apply to your choice of hospital?
10. What physicians provide specialty care?
11. How easy is it to be referred to a specialist?
12. Does the plan have patient surveys? Can you see the results?
13. Call the plan's customer service number. How long are you on hold? Is the customer service staff helpful?
14. Ask friends and coworkers about their experience with the plan.
15. How many people leave the plan? How many consumer complaints has the plan received?
16. What is the plan's process for appeals? Is it prompt?
17. What does your current physician think of the plan?
18. What is the process for receiving emergency care in the plan?
19. Can you easily get a second opinion in the plan?
20. What services important to you are not covered in the plan?
21. If applicable, find out the plan's policies on preexisting conditions.
22. What are the plan's pharmacy benefits?
23. What costs to you are associated with the plan (premiums, deductible, co-payments, out-of-network costs, out-of-town costs, emergency care costs, etc.)?
24. What limits exist in the plan (lifetime, treatment, cost, etc.)?
25. How are physicians compensated and incentivized by the plan?

Source: Reprinted with permission from Sample Guidelines for How to Choose a Health Plan, from www.healthgrades.com/Healthtools/How to Choose/hg choose plan.cfm?

- policy monitoring
- shopping for health care products.

Despite this wealth of data, consumers are confused. The majority of seniors enrolled in Medicare HMOs report knowing "none or little of what they need to know" about the Medicare program on which they depend.[18] In response, the 1997 BBA requires HCFA to provide Medicare recipients with specific consumer information, as listed in Exhibit 43–2. Even for health-savvy consumers, sorting through the volumes of sites is time consuming and potentially risky.

A study by the University of Michigan Health System found that much of the information on websites may be inappropriate, inaccurate, misleading, or not reviewed by doctors.[19] The health plan quality ratings are based on a variety of indicators, ranging from consumer satisfaction surveys, self-reported patient comments, physician preferences, accreditation reports, covered benefits, percent of members receiving preventive care, disenrollment rates, and so on. While most are based in part on HEDIS information, the methodologies for applying and reporting HEDIS data vary widely. Consequently, results are often contradictory; the same organization can receive a different score, depending on the rating system used.

Clearly, there is a growing need for MCOs to provide information to ensure members have what they need to enhance their own health status and support any health-related decisions. They need to consider the impact of consumerism on the physician-patient relationship and look for opportunities to drive, support, and

Exhibit 43–2 Consumer Information Required by the Balanced Budget Act

---

- *Product comparison charts*—consumer-focused charts comparing health plan benefit, premium, and member cost-sharing information
- *Medicare+Choice membership rules*—membership policies and procedures, including how to enroll or disenroll, how to file a claim or an appeal, and how to access care in a managed care organization
- *Quality measures*—dissemination of the Medicare HEDIS measures that are most comprehensible and usable for consumers
- *Member satisfaction*—distribution of the CAHPS survey to measure beneficiaries' perceptions of and experiences with membership rules, customer service, and access to care
- *Quality of life indicators*—measurement of self-reported quality of life status over time of a sampling of Medicare+Choice members
- *Disenrollment rates*—comparative tables on the rates of disenrollment in competing Medicare+Choice plans

Source: Reprinted from Health Care Financing Administration, Department of Health and Human Services.

---

integrate these efforts. Says one physician quoted in an October 1999 *Wall Street Journal* report on the future of health care: "The public is crying out for access to the best information, and doctors must learn that the decisions have to be made with a patient who is correctly informed."[20]

In addition to information about treatment decisions, today's consumer wants to make intelligent decisions about which health insurance plan to purchase and which providers to use. To respond effectively, MCOs must develop and communicate data about their operations and performance in a meaningful, understandable manner. But to date few standard performance measures exist and management reporting is generally lacking in the managed care industry. There are significant inconsistencies in data definitions across and even within MCOs.[21]

Performance measurement and reporting have implications for MCOs' back office operations. Some MCOs have begun to benchmark themselves against other health plans and major banks with large customer service centers. Key performance measures include claims turnaround time, payment and coding accuracy, and average phone answering times. In large employer contracts, they incorporate financial incentives geared to meeting measurable quality objectives. To help attain these objectives, they use sophisticated telephone switches and other equipment to track historical data and trends, so they can predict call volume for every hour of the day and assign work shifts accordingly. Reported results include shorter hold times and higher call volume per agent because the number of staff on duty at any time is matched precisely to expected needs.[22]

Performance measurement has implications for provider networks and medical groups as well. Some MCOs have started to release clinical and service quality data for the medical groups in their provider networks. They distribute reports of medical group quality to businesses and employees during open enrollment. Ratings are based on clinical quality measures (for example, physician qualifications and credentialing processes, utilization management performance, and preventive service use rates) and service measures (for example, satisfaction with physician group and primary care physician, primary care access complaints, ease of scheduling, ability to handle appeals and grievances, and member disenrollment due to dissatisfaction). One MCO found that high-scoring groups attract significantly more new enrollees than lower-scoring groups.[23]

Consumer demand for information will require significant investments in information systems and technology. But it affords an opportunity to better understand, and ultimately change, member behaviors that affect health status and costs. For example, information systems can be used to profile member needs and usage and to assist consumers in finding, researching, and selecting desired services and providers of services. Health plans can provide medical information and decision-making tools for members who have an injury or illness. They can match members to preventive care and exercise programs based on their interests, health status, and lifestyles. Providers can develop clinical computing systems that function as information filters and decision support tools for doctors and patients.

Consumer Demand for Innovative Products and Services

Managed care organizations have traditionally employed a mass-market, retail-oriented market strategy. During the sales cycle, the primary focus is typically on the broker and employer as customer, rather than the employee (or member). Market segments are usually defined in terms of employer characteristics (employer size and location are common criteria). As a result, insurance products have been developed to meet employer criteria, with most plans in a given market offering benefits and network designs that are similar or identical in nature.

Few plans currently segment their markets based on consumer attributes such as age, gender, lifestyle, or other indicators that reflect their health care decision-making and purchasing behavior (these tend to be used solely for actuarial and underwriting purposes). As consumers become more empowered, they will select products and services that directly align with their particular health care needs. Consumer-oriented sales and marketing approaches will target specific market segments and increase variety of product features and options to enable consumers to choose what they want. Distribution strategies will emphasize retail sales techniques and direct selling to targeted consumer segments via multiple channels.

Regardless of how an MCO chooses to segment its customers, it is clear that consumerism requires health plans to understand the defining characteristics of each group, along with its preferences in terms of choice, service, and information. As an example, many industries and companies use basic demographic cohorts as an initial segmentation strategy. The characteristics

and preferences relate to broad national trends for each group but are likely to carry over to the local and regional level (see Exhibit 43–3).

Health plans can use comprehensive knowledge about their local markets and customer segments to develop innovative products and services. Some examples are described below.

Consumer Products

Some MCOs are expanding beyond their medical insurance offerings to market health-related products and services directly to consumers via the Internet. Aetna U.S. Healthcare and Johns Hopkins University have marketed health information and personal care devices through their InteliHealth joint venture for a number of years. Some MCOs market health-related services at a discount, in exchange for an annual membership fee. Typical offerings include prescriptions, dental care, alternative health treatments, nutritional supplements, eyeglasses, and vision exams.

Alternative Care and Other Lifestyle Benefits

Market research has found that young adults (so-called "Gen Y'ers") and other market segments desire coverage for health products and services to which they have had personal exposure, including alternative medicine (including chiropractic care, homeopathy, massage therapy, acupuncture, and so on), oral contraceptives, and vision and dental benefits. Many MCOs have offered coverage for these services for the past several years. Additionally, a few are offering limited coverage for services that are lifestyle- rather than health-related, such as health club dues and employee transportation.

Amenities

Research has shown that wealthy consumers prefer to purchase products from specialty stores or boutiques, demand high-quality products and services, and desire customized, individual attention. Many health care providers have begun to respond with renovations to improve the ambiance of their facility, after-hours care, longer visits, shorter waiting times, and house calls.[24,25]

Exhibit 43–3 Demographic Cohorts and Their Health Care Preferences

Cohort	Characteristics	Health Care Preferences	Implications for Payers
Generation Y[1]	• Large generation (60 million) born after 1979 • Racially and ethnically diverse • First generation to grow up with direct-to-consumer advertising • Little product loyalty (switch easily) • Internet generation—nearly four times more likely than their elders to use Internet to access health care information • Less likely to be offered health insurance (between 1987–96, the number of workers < age 25 who were offered insurance through jobs decreased by 8 percent) • Only 34 percent of 18- to 24-year-olds have a regular place where they receive health care	• Less likely to elect health insurance (take-up rates for young workers decreased by 13 percent from 1987–96) • Price is biggest factor in saying "no" to health insurance • Need maintenance health care: flu shots, pap smears, physicals • Have high expectations for information and use it comparatively • Want flexibility to choose alternative medical care (35 percent of people age 18–24 used alternative medicine in last 12 months)	• Little attention has been paid thus far to this cohort, and general good health of the young adult population makes them a good risk for insurers • Implement tracking mechanism to follow young adults after they roll off their parents' insurance policies • Design packages around "frills" of health care: alternative medicine, vision and dental, contraceptives, health club discounts, lifestyle enhancements • Internet capabilities are essential • Price competitive
Generation X[2–5]	• Generation born between 1965 and 1979 • Seem to be marketing-resistant; like to be self-reliant and independent • Soon to be core earners in economy (now 34 percent of workforce) • Spent $30 billion on eating out during past year • Skeptical about future; poll found that young people are more likely to believe in UFOs than in the availability of social security when they retire • Not politically active and generally distrustful of large institutions • In past few years, GenXers have started their own businesses at more than twice the rate of other Americans	• Prefer job advancement at the expense of job (and benefits) security; 51 percent of GenXers put "success" before "integrity" • Study products and contemplate spending decisions more carefully than any generation before them, but willing to spend money on what they want and need • Need to be involved with decisions, and are typically more aggressive investors than Boomers • See physicians and health care providers as the means to an end (good health) rather than as a caretaker	• Provide information to generate trust in organization • Offer choice and involvement in health plan selection • Develop "personalized" marketing that supports need to study product and service offerings carefully • Build networks and benefits that allow members to access services needed to meet their individual health goals • Define value of products and services in terms that go beyond cost • Internet capabilities are essential
Baby Boomers[6–8]	• Largest generation (76 million) born between 1946 and 1964	• Boomers don't want choice—they want what they want, when they want it	• Create and deliver augmented products to meet needs

continues

Exhibit 43–3 continued

Cohort	Characteristics	Health Care Preferences	Implications for Payers
	• Well-educated, more demanding, more individualistic, more sophisticated, more self-indulgent than any 50+ generation before them • Bulk of health consumer population for the coming decades • Value brand names • Spend freely; largest spenders in economy; $203 billion out of pocket on health care in 1995 or 18 percent of overall U.S. health care spending • "Sandwich" generation—raising children and caring for aging parents • Determined to maintain their vigor and quality of life; new consciousness about health	• "Dealing direct" is perceived to be the ultimate bargain and Boomers like bargains • High-quality health coverage upon retirement • Expect a dialogue with physicians, not a hearing • Willing to fight for their best interest and make their concerns public	• Offer more out-of-pocket services that Boomers are willing to pay for • Incorporate alternative and complementary therapies to plan offerings • Provide information via Internet and other accessible venues • Offer supplemental "luxury" packages • Convey "value" • Offer retirement planning assistance
Seniors[9–11]	• Over-65 population will grow from about 34 million in 1998 to 70 million by 2030 ("graying of America") • Politically active (voting rate of elderly is twice that of nonelderly) • Life expectancy is longer than ever before • Not as "health care literate" as younger generations and ability to care for medical problems is limited • Typically hold doctors and medical establishment in high regard; less likely to confront provider regarding treatment or care	• Personal relationship with physician and insurer; stay with same physicians • Stability and security in their health care coverage (particularly Medicare HMOs) • Low-cost care; particularly for pharmaceuticals • Comprehensive coverage (drug benefits, nursing home, and so on) • Like a sense of community • User-friendly, convenient (close to home) services	• Senior-specific services are needed (welcoming groups, personal assistants, and so on) • Create something "human" and "personal" about organization that seniors can identify • Promote organizational stability and commitment to seniors • Geographic coverage is needed to facilitate senior access • Communicate information in ways seniors can understand and access

[1] Neuborne, E. "Generation Y" *Business Week.* February 15, 1999, 79–88.

[2] Maurer, R. Don't Resist Generation X, http://www.reinforce.com/spotlight/generation_x/

[3] The Pages of Generation X, http://www.vex.net

[4] "The Misplaced Generation?" *New York Post.* September 7, 1999, page 28.

[5] Miller, M. "Smashing the Gen-X Stereotype," *Los Angeles Times.* September 3, 1999, A1.

[6] Bartlett, D. "The New Health Care Consumer," *Journal of Health Care Finance.* Spring 1999, volume 25, 44–51.

[7] "Health Care Organizations are Listening to the Newly-found Voice of the Consumer," *Health Care Strategic Management.* March 1, 1998.

[8] "The New Rules: For Marketing to the 25 Million Baby Boomers Over Fifty," *Drug Store News.* April 7, 1997, page 1.

[9] Howgill, M. "Health Care Consumerism, the Information Explosion, and Branding," *Managed Care Quarterly.* Autumn 1998, 33–43.

[10] Gazmariarian, J. "Health Literacy Among Medicare Enrollees in a Managed Care Organization," *Journal of the American Medical Association.* February 1999, 545–551.

[11] Zimmermann, S. "Old Folks, New Options," *Chicago Sun-Times.* October 5, 1998, J1.

Source: Data from references 1–11 above.

Some medical groups rely exclusively on physicians rather than physician assistants or nurse practitioners, and guarantee "personal doctors dedicated to a one-on-one relationship." Some providers are targeting executives by providing a lounge complete with phones, fax machines, and jacks for laptops. Although one such program charges $1,600 for a 2-day physical and has never advertised, it maintains a 6-month waiting list and experiences 2,500 visits annually.[26] Patients usually pay directly for these high-end services.

Personal Attention

Many MCOs have assigned personal representatives to greet new members and handle most of their subsequent interactions with the health plan. The personal representatives are cross-trained to deal with most issues and know where to refer the rest. More complicated and overflow calls are shifted to a claims unit dedicated to deal with more complex issues. The personal representatives often provide an outreach phone call to all new members, ensure members have received a legible ID card, explain the toll-free nurse-advice line, and verify that the member has the correct number. One MCO has reported a drop in its Medicare HMO disenrollment rate from slightly more than 20 percent to less than 10 percent as a result of the program.[27]

Some plans also offer a personal service specialist to deal with issues that may arise for the enrollee's employer. If an employee complains that a claim has not been paid and asks the employer for help, the employer can call the same personal service representative.[28] One national MCO has set up what it calls "customer clusters" to serve the special needs of large national accounts and deal with their specific questions and service needs. It holds day-long "customer-supplier workshops" once or twice a year, during which sales personnel and operations staff meet with employer representatives to clearly understand each employer's strategies and needs.[29]

Services To Address Special Needs

Some MCOs provide value-added services for members, such as telephone access to counselors who can deal with issues of stress, family relationships, and substance abuse; as well as phone access to financial advisors and attorneys who can deal with such issues as divorce, child support, wills, estate planning, and taxes. Phone consults are available for employers dealing with difficult management issues; onsite services are available to help deal with traumatic workplace events.[30]

Some MCOs ensure customer service representatives are sensitive to members with special needs. In their call centers, translators can help Spanish-speaking members. In addition, customer service representatives working with Medicare HMO enrollees are trained to spend extra time if necessary, speak clearly, and ask questions to ensure that the member understands what has been said. Representatives go through a special three-day sensitivity training program in which they wear fogged-up glasses, plug up their ears, and are shown materials in tiny type so they develop an awareness of the special challenges Medicare patients may face.[31]

Branding Strategies

Consumer demand for innovative products and services also requires MCOs to integrate branding strategies into their overall market approach. Consumer-oriented companies in other industries have long recognized the need to clearly define an organization's relationship to its consumers through a branding strategy. Effective branding allows companies to fully understand and serve the needs of its customers and concentrate its performance in those areas. For example, Sears identified its brand as higher echelon consumer goods and services and sold its periphery insurance and financial units. Companies can adopt a general branding strategy across all their customers, with targeted branding for specific market segments. The brand needs to address issues of interest or concern to consumers.

In the health industry, branding efforts have been fairly limited to name changes, corporate logos, and sporadic advertising. A few plans have attempted mass promotion and advertising to the general consumer population. Some groups and coalitions have been formed to explore the potential to use mass advertising to counter negative public sentiment regarding managed care. (Coordinate Care Coalition was formed in 1997 by Aetna U.S. Healthcare, Humana, United Health Care, PacifiCare, and other HMOs to enhance public relations.) But to date, the majority of health plans do not have an articulated brand and offer identical or similar products.

Consumer Demand for Empowerment in Treatment Decisions

For more than a decade, MCOs have modified their network and medical management policies in response to consumer demand for increased access. Enrollment in restrictive staff and group model HMOs has leveled off in favor of more open IPA models and PPO plans. Gatekeeping restrictions have been relaxed. Most health plans allow women direct access to OB/GYNs and many allow members with certain chronic conditions (for example, cancer or AIDS) to select a specialist as their primary provider. Some allow members to self-refer to certain specialties to speed their access to desired services.[32] In response to consumer demands for alternative care, some health plans include nontraditional providers such as chiropractors and acupuncturists in their networks.

Health plans' network design and medical management policies can drive member satisfaction and influence retention. Research has shown that members who are allowed to choose their personal physician are more likely to rate their satisfaction as "excellent" or "very good" than those who are assigned a physician.[33] While consumers generally believe that MCOs have improved access to preventive care and prescription drugs and have helped to control costs, they also believe that managed care has negatively affected the doctor-patient relationship. Surveys show that consumers believe managed care has reduced the time patients spend with their doctors, access to specialists, and physician control of treatment decisions.[34]

As consumers become more selective, they will seek health insurance options that offer advantages in addition to cost control. Consumer-oriented medical and network management approaches will address the dissatisfiers—access to care, time with physicians, and so on—by increasing physician involvement and member empowerment in medical decision making. Some examples of recent efforts to address these issues are described below.

Delegation of Treatment Decisions

Vocal consumers, patient protection legislation, and the negative public perceptions of managed care create incentives for health plans to cede control of care authorization and treatment decisions. Many MCOs are delegating more responsibility for these decisions to providers, third-party organizations, and case managers. A number of MCOs have remodeled their appeals processes to allow members to appeal denials in insurance coverage to independent physicians. Some have reevaluated the cost versus benefit of their medical management efforts, and a few have considered dropping use of precertification review and other specific techniques and relying instead on physician decisions regarding necessity of covered services.[35]

Disease and Demand Management

Managed care organizations have long encouraged employers and members to take charge of their health and manage their own medical care by providing prevention, wellness, and education services. Many offer disease management programs that encourage members to proactively manage chronic conditions such as diabetes, high risk pregnancy, congestive heart failure, asthma, HIV/AIDS, and cancer. Nurse lines allow members to obtain personalized health information, guidance on prescription drug use, choices on treatment options, or physician referrals directly via a phone call to registered nurses, registered pharmacists, or health benefit specialists.

Online Self Care

The Internet has opened another channel for MCOs to reach consumers and encourage them to manage their own medical care. Many MCOs offer members online health risk assessments through either their own websites or links to a vendor.[36] Some provide members with online health care information tailored to their personal lifestyle. This not only provides added value to the member, but it also creates a profile that can be used in preventive care and disease management programs and as an entry for the health plan or an associated business line to market-related services. Other MCOs allow members to use the Internet to make doctor's appointments, seek advice about prescriptions, and find information on diseases and symptoms. Members also can complete an online health assessment or e-mail questions to a pharmacist about medications and possible side effects.[37]

*   *   *

Consumer demand for empowerment in treatment decisions will require that health plans reexamine their approaches to medical management and how they involve members and providers. While MCOs can greatly impact those areas that they wholly control (such as claims handling, member services, plan design, public relations), they have a smaller impact on areas that are more directly related to health service delivery (such as quality of care, thoroughness of treatment, access to care, provider availability, and meeting consumer care needs). To meet consumers' needs in these areas, MCOs must work with their provider groups to effect changes in the care provided and the provider-patient relationship. Recognizing the need to collaborate with providers, some organizations have reconsidered delegating more medical management responsibilities to provider organizations (although many of these relationships faltered in the mid-1990s). They are examining providers' attitudes toward managed care and investing in education efforts to reach consumers through informed, supportive providers.

Consumer Demand for Efficient and Streamlined Administrative Functions

Research indicates that consumers have a generally poor opinion of administrative performance and customer service in the managed care industry. In one study, only 45 percent of re-

spondents rated managed care as having "good" customer service, exceeding only the tobacco industry with 32 percent (hospitals, telephones, and the airlines each had "good" ratings exceeding 70 percent).[38]

The Internet offers the opportunity for health plans to replace traditional administrative processes and reach customers through a new avenue to improve performance, reduce costs, and improve satisfaction. A variety of Internet-based enrollment, member service, and claims functions are feasible through current technology (see Exhibit 43–4). Although research has shown that administrative best practices can be leveraged across plans,[39] most of these functions have thus far been confined to a few pilot programs. A recent study found that, while most health plans distribute information and some communicate through their websites, few are offering financial or two-way transactions through them.[40]

A few health plans have begun to offer interactive, self-service capabilities for members through their websites. Some of the more advanced sites provide members with direct, live access to their individual medical claims and benefit and eligibility data, in addition to information on providers. Members and customer service representatives have concurrent access to identical information. Members can send e-mail messages to customer service representatives, which are automatically routed to specifically designated customer service areas. MCOs designed this capability to save members time and money by reducing telephone inquiries typically made to customer service departments or human resources departments.[41]

In response to employee benefits managers' requests for less paperwork, some MCOs provide online connectivity between employers and the health plan. Workers can fill in their information sitting at a computer screen; the health plan administrator only needs to press a button to transmit the form. One plan reports a resulting reduction in the time to receive a membership card from two weeks to one.[42]

Some health plans have begun to automate many of their sales and enrollment functions through the Internet. These applications are pri-

Exhibit 43–4 Potential Internet-Based Administrative Functions

Function	Information	Transactions	Personalization
Enrollment	• Marketing collateral • Enrollment materials delivered online	• Online price quotes • Choice of Internet, IVR, or paper enrollment • Automatic, electronic life status and other eligibility changes	• Customized answers to questions on benefits • Integration between sales and enrollment to automatically track new members and trigger instantaneous ID card generation
Member service	• Provider directories, maps, and driving instructions • Online customer service • Glossary of health insurance-related terms • Links to health sites and community services	• Automatic pharmacy ordering with printable versions of member and prescription drug claim forms • Details on performance of primary medical group and/ or primary care physicians	• Specialist referrals • Proactive care management • Information on handling specific diseases (e.g., child's asthma) • Develop a community of interest around a disease or special set of health needs
Claims	• Easy-to-read explanation of benefits, including co-payments, deductibles, and benefit maximums	• Online coordination of benefits • Prompt and accurate claims submission and payment	• Claims/Medical management one process vs. separate processes • Claims tracking • Online claims correction

Courtesy of Ernst & Young LLP, 2000, Washington, DC.

marily focused on employer accounts and brokers, but some have features for seniors and other individuals who purchase their health insurance directly. Additionally, a number of Internet companies offer self-service quotes and enrollment for self-insured employers and individuals (e.g., healthaxis.com, ehealthinsurance.com, and insweb.com).

Such direct-to-consumer administrative functions offer MCOs the potential to reduce overhead costs. While most MCOs are offering self-enrollment functions as an adjunct to their traditional sales and marketing efforts, others are focusing on electronic self-enrollment as a way to bypass independent insurance brokers altogether. One MCO has projected being able to reduce broker commissions by 20 to 50 percent by enrolling most of its members directly over the Internet.[43] Yet research indicates that most MCOs have not yet achieved savings (and some have even experienced increased costs) as a re-

sult of electronic commerce; for the present, these functions are supplementing rather than replacing traditional administrative processes.[44]

HOW CAN ORGANIZATIONS DEVELOP A CONSUMER STRATEGY?

Consumer demands affect every aspect of a managed care organization's operations. The investments required to develop and execute a comprehensive consumer strategy are likely to be significant. Given the current financial pressures in the industry, and the lack of a clear direction for the health care consumer trend, it is obvious that health plans must invest wisely. Some considerations for developing an organization's consumer strategy include:

• At the local market level, the drivers and characteristics of consumerism may differ from the general trends at play on a national level. It is important to understand how consumerism is developing in the local market. The MCO can research the relevant investments made by different players in the market, and understand the impact of those investments.

- When generating ideas for consumer-oriented initiatives, MCOs can look at industries outside of health care that have a track record for redefining their business operations around the customer (for example, banking and financial services). Programs developed in these industries can be adapted, in whole or in part, to the health care industry.
- Initiatives that support the consumer strategy have to be effective in the local market but also must leverage the organization's current capabilities, resources, and infrastructure.
- The initiatives supporting the strategy should reflect a broad range of investments in terms of scale and scope of resources and time frame for development and implementation. The planning process could incorporate a process for reevaluating investments over time, to ensure projects reflect latest knowledge and direction regarding consumerism.

WHAT CONSUMERISM MEANS FOR THE MANAGED CARE INDUSTRY

HealthCast 2010, a report compiled from interviews and surveys of four hundred experts in the field and health care executives, concluded that dynamic forces, including consumerism, "will threaten the status quo . . . but also will create exciting new opportunities for improved quality of care, greater efficiencies, and e-business." [45] The report also noted that only 14 percent of the survey participants thought insurers were prepared to deal with empowered consumers. Interestingly, 25 percent of the participants thought providers were prepared.

Clearly, the implications and opportunities for individual organizations are profound, but will the consumer movement cause a restructuring of

the managed health care industry? Consumerism is redefining customer relationships and the overall structure in some industries, such as banking and financial services. Yet in managed health care, other counterbalancing forces may prevail. The industry is heavily dependent on personal interaction and trust between patients and physicians; Internet technologies and other innovative approaches are unlikely to completely replace those relationships. Patients rely on health practitioners for medical treatment and advice; self-care and education may supplement their expertise but not supplant it.

Health insurance is feasible because payers can aggregate and distribute medical risk across a population. Thus, individuals are able to pool their risk to obtain affordable health insurance. If consumers were allowed to obtain the "ultimate" in tailored services and obtain coverage for only those medical services they will use, more healthy individuals would most certainly save money. But those with chronic or catastrophic acute conditions would just as certainly be unable to afford any coverage. Thus, the concept of viable (particularly universal) health insurance—what consumers need—depends on them *not* being able to get everything they want. While pressured to defend the rights of individuals, the government is also bound to protect the collective interests of all its citizens. Thus the greater interests of society may prevail over at least some of the demands of individual consumers.

CONCLUSION

As illustrated in this chapter, MCOs, on aggregate, have implemented a broad range of service, information, and operational programs aimed at addressing certain aspects of consumerism. These same companies, however, will be challenged by the market to develop more comprehensive strategies that are supported by focused tactical initiatives and broader cultural and operational changes.

Health care consumerism, as noted in the beginning of this chapter, is in its formative stage, but clearly is a major driver of change for

MCOs. They will need to redefine their strategies and operations in order to meet increasing consumer demands for information, service, access, and quality. At present there is no correct strategy, but there are myriad examples from health care and other industries that can help the managed care organization define a consumer strategy that will address consumer demands and help payers better manage the health care decisions, and ultimately the costs, of their customers.

REFERENCES AND NOTES

1. Don Schultz, Perhaps the 4Ps Really Should Be the 4Rs, *Marketing News*, May 24, 1999, 7.

2. Ron Shinkman, Making Room in the Pool: New York Business Group on Health Creating Buying Organization for Small Business, *Modern Healthcare*, March 29, 1999, 66.

3. Howard Larkin, Doctors Starting To Feel Report Cards' Impact, *American Medical News,* July 26, 1999.

4. Employee Benefits Research Institute, Aggregate Trends in Defined Benefit and Defined Contribution Plan Sponsorship, Participation, and Vesting, *EBRI Databook on Employee Benefits*, 4th ed.,1994.

5. U.S. Department of Labor, 1995.

6. Phil Galewitz, "Employers Paying More for Health Insurance, But Not Their Workers," Associated Press Newswires, December 14, 1999.

7. Hunt as cited in M. Susan Marquis and Joan L. Buchanan, Simulating the Effects of Employer Contributions on Adverse Selection and Health Plan Choice, *Health Services Research*, October 10, 1999.

8. Marquis and Buchanan, Simulating the Effects of Employer Contributions.

9. P. Galewitz, HMO Giant to Give Consumers Right to Appeal to Outside Experts, Associated Press Political Service, January 12, 1999.

10. Notes from Fall 1999 NAIC meeting.

11. *www.ncqa.org/pages/main/timeline.htm.*

12. Press release from AMA dated August 24, 1999, *www.ama-assn.org/ad-com/releases/1999.*

13. Madeleine Bickert, The Impact of Ecommerce on Legacy Health-Care Companies. Report prepared for Cyber Dialogue, July 1999.

14. Center for the Advancement of Health Report, Results of a Literature Search and Analysis of the Public's Health Care Values and Attitudes. DYG, Inc. (*www.cfah.org*).

15. Center for the Advancement of Health Report, Results of a Literature Search.

16. Center for the Advancement of Health Report, Results of a Literature Search.

17. Center for the Advancement of Health Report, Results of a Literature Search.

18. California HealthCare Foundation Announces: New Poll Shows California Seniors Overwhelmed by Changing Medicare Program; Foundation Launches New Education Effort To Help, *BW HealthWire*, September 8, 1999.

19. Study Finds Much of the Consumer Health Advice on Internet Is Wrong, *Modern Healthcare*, August 9, 1999.

20. The Evolution of a Partnership, *Wall Street Journal,* October 18, 1999.

21. Ernst & Young, Critical Calibration: Metrics and Benchmarking in Managed Care, February, 1999.

22. What Plans Are Doing to Improve Customer Service, *Managed Care Week*, March 8, 1999.

23. H. Larkin, Doctors Starting To Feel Report Cards' Impact, *American Medical News*, July 26, 1999.

24. M. Pulaski, Marketing Medical Services to the Affluent, *Medical Group Management Journal* 44 (September–October 1997): 26–39.

25. HMNo: Denver Doctors J.Sheldon & H. Sowell, 1997. *www.hmno.com.*

26. L. Armour, Me and the Mayo, *Fortune*, July 21, 1997, 86.

27. What Plans Are Doing to Improve Customer Service, *Managed Care Week*, March 8, 1999.

28. What Plans Are Doing, *Managed Care Week*.

29. What Plans Are Doing, *Managed Care Week*.

30. What Plans Are Doing, *Managed Care Week*.

31. What Plans Are Doing, *Managed Care Week*.

32. E.B. Severoni, A Checklist for Consumer-Centered Health Plans, *Healthplan*, September–October 1999, 67–70.

33. J. Schmittdiel, J.V. Selby, K. Grumbach, and C.P. Quesenberry, Choice of a Personal Physician and Patient Satisfaction in a Health Maintenance Organization, *JAMA* 278 (November 19, 1997): 19.

34. P.D. Hart and T. Tiehle, *Wall Street Journal*/NBC News Poll, *American Opinion*, 1998.

35. Big H.M.O. To Give Decisions on Care Back to Doctors, *Dow Vision,* November 9, 1999 (Press release).

36. Ernst & Young, How Payors Are Using the Internet to Reach Customers, March 2000.

37. Site of the Week, *Los Angeles Daily News*, September 19, 1999.

38. Harvard University and Kaiser Family Foundation, Kaiser/Harvard Survey of Americans' Views on Consumer Protection of Managed Care, January 1998.

39. Ernst & Young, Critical Calibration: Metrics and Benchmarking in Managed Care, February 1999.

40. Ernst & Young, How Payors Are Using the Internet.

41. Blue Cross Introduces New Interactive Internet Service for Members; New Technological Advances Demonstrate Commitment to Meeting Members' Changing Health Care Needs, *Business Wire*, November 19, 1998.

42. What Plans Are Doing to Improve Customer Service, *Managed Care Week*, March 8, 1999.

43. Aetna Cuts Brokers' Commissions, May Mean Focus on Internet Enrollment, *World Reporter*, Knight Ridder Business News, November 7, 1999 (Press release).

44. Ernst & Young, How Payors Are Using the Internet.

45. Consumerism, E-Commerce, and Biotechnology Advances To Cause Disruptive Changes in Health System over Next Decade, Worldside PricewaterhouseCoopers Study Reports, *PR Newswire,* October 28, 1999 (Press release).

Accreditation and Performance Measurement Programs for Managed Care Organizations

Margaret E. O'Kane

INTRODUCTION

Since 1996, accreditation and performance measurement have become dominant features in the managed care landscape. Practice patterns, information systems, and key administrative and management functions have all been refined or even built from the ground up to promote quality and satisfy the demands of external oversight. Driven by employer mandates and a growing need to demonstrate quality objectively as a condition of market success, about half the nation's health maintenance organizations (HMOs) and point-of-service (POS) health plans now participate in some form of accreditation, and the vast majority measure their performance—although far fewer publicly report their results.

Over the same period, the oversight process has evolved from its initial exclusive focus on HMOs; accreditation, certification, and performance measurement programs now, or soon will, cover the full spectrum of affiliated organizations—man-

aged behavioral health care organizations, credentials verification organizations (CVOs), preferred provider organizations (PPOs), and provider groups. Growing legislative and market forces will likely advance this trend further until accountability in health care applies not just to health plans but also to facilities, provider groups, and even to individual providers. Consumers, employers, and others need and want to know about the quality of their health care.

Despite the trend, it is notable that accreditation and performance measurement in managed care remain largely voluntary. No federal legislation exists compelling health plans to report on their performance or to achieve any form of external accreditation. At the state level, selected states require health plans to do either or both, sometimes as a condition of licensure and in other instances in order to gain entry into the state employee market. In place of legislative mandates, however, the market has developed its own mandate. Dozens of the nation's leading corporations will not do business with a health plan that has not earned some form of external accreditation—in particular by the National Committee for Quality Assurance (NCQA), whose seal of approval is now required by several states and more than 30 percent of the nation's largest firms. An even larger number of employers require their health plan partners to report on their performance, a prerequisite to assessing value.

Three organizations, each of which approaches its oversight role from a different per-

---

Margaret E. O'Kane is President of the National Committee for Quality Assurance, an independent, nonprofit organization whose mission is to evaluate and improve the quality of health care in the United States.

The sections of this chapter related to the activities of the Joint Commission on Accreditation of Healthcare Organizations and Utilization Review Accreditation Committee were authored by representatives of those organizations. Both submissions were subsequently edited for style, length, and clarity to facilitate their inclusion in this chapter.

spective and each of which specializes in a different sector of the market, have developed managed care oversight programs of note. The NCQA, the Utilization Review Accreditation Commission (URAC), and the Joint Commission on Accreditation of Healthcare Organizations (Joint Commission) all now accredit managed care organizations (MCOs) and each offers related accreditation or certification programs. These organizations and the various oversight programs they offer are described in this chapter. In addition, NCQA defines the predominant form of performance measurement as it relates to managed care plans through its Health Plan Employer Data and Information Set (HEDIS), the measurement tool used by about 90 percent of all health plans.

It is important to note that there are differences among the accreditation programs offered by each organization. These differences reflect the accreditors' varied histories and perspectives for which their programs were designed. For NCQA, the major emphasis is on providing the market—consumers and employers—with compelling information that will help to distinguish between the organizations on the basis of quality. Hence, NCQA's focus is on the quality of the systems, process, care, and service that an organization delivers to its enrollees. NCQA also puts special emphasis on those mechanisms that the organization has established for continuous improvement in quality. Historically, NCQA focused on evaluating HMO and POS plans, but its agenda has expanded considerably in recent years and now includes behavioral health care organizations and PPOs. NCQA believes that by providing the market with this information, it rewards those health plans that are providing excellent care and service, thus giving all health plans a strong incentive to focus on quality.

URAC was formed in 1990 with the backing of a broad range of consumers, employers, regulators, providers, and industry representatives to provide an efficient and effective method for evaluating utilization review (UR) processes. The organization has since branched out beyond UR oversight and into the evaluation of PPOs by ac-

quiring an existing PPO accreditation program. URAC is infrequently referred to as the American Accreditation HealthCare Commission.

An independent, nonprofit organization, the Joint Commission is the nation's oldest and largest standards-setting and accrediting body in health care, evaluating and accrediting nearly 20,000 hospitals and other health care organizations throughout the United States. In 1965 Congress passed the Medicare Act, which "deemed" hospitals with Joint Commission accreditation to be in compliance with the Medicare program's Conditions for Participation. The Joint Commission's stated mission is to "improve the quality of care provided to the public by setting standards and evaluating the performance of organizations against those standards." The organization is largely provider-governed, although its board of directors includes representatives from many other constituencies, such as employers, consumers, and labor representatives.

OVERSIGHT BY TYPE OF ORGANIZATION

Managed care is a loosely defined term that might be applied to any number of different types of organizations, including HMOs, POS plans, PPOs, independent practice associations (IPAs), UR firms, and a host of other derivative organizational models. Accreditation has not weighed equally on the various systems of care. On the contrary, only the most tightly managed delivery systems, HMO and POS plans, have typically been prompted to seek external accreditation. No doubt the reason for the focus on HMO and POS plans is partly in response to extensive media coverage of HMO "horror stories" and the public's general reluctance to accept change in the health care system, or the introduction of a third party into the physician-patient relationship.

HMOs' participation in accreditation and performance measurement programs over the years has paid an important dividend: improved quality. Since 1992, the percent of HMOs earning the highest levels of accreditation, Excellent or

Commendable, from the nation's leading HMO accreditor, NCQA, has risen from about 20 percent to nearly 70 percent, evidence that an increasing number of HMOs are endeavoring to ensure quality and to improve over time. Similarly, data collected since 1996 show that most HMOs that publicly report on their performance in such areas as immunization and mammography rates have steadily, and in some cases dramatically, improved their performance. For example, participating HMO and POS plans have gone from treating just 62 percent of heart attack patients with beta blockers to treating 80 percent, an improvement that annually saves thousands of lives.

By contrast, there have historically been few regulatory or accreditation mechanisms for PPOs and little information available either about what proportion of PPOs have quality-assurance programs or about the efficacy of those programs. The vast majority of PPOs do not pursue external accreditation by *any* oversight organization in large part because appropriate oversight programs have not existed. This is likely to change in the future, however, as all three major oversight organizations are now working with their various constituencies to build pressure for PPO accreditation and performance measurement.

The simplest type of MCO is the UR firm, which does not typically include a defined delivery system. As more tightly managed systems of care such as HMO, POS, and PPO plans continue to grab an increasing portion of the health care market, the UR firm that contracts with a health care purchaser to help manage medical costs for its employees is becoming increasingly rare. While UR is a key part of any cost management effort, there are real limitations to effective quality management with *only* a UR system. For example, in a UR-only system, no central body has control over who provides medical services, providers cannot be credentialed, and it is impossible to monitor for underutilization, misdiagnosis, or incompetent use of the right treatment. Although a number of states have enacted regulations for UR firms, few address the need for quality assurance mechanisms.

As indicated previously, the accreditation programs offered by the three MCOs discussed in this chapter are unique, as are the organizations behind each program. These differences are reflected in the focus of their review process, in the governance of the organizations, and in the actual accreditation process.

NATIONAL COMMITTEE FOR QUALITY ASSURANCE

The NCQA accredits HMOs, including traditional staff and group model HMOs, network and IPA model HMOs, mixed models, and open-ended HMOs or POS products. These various types of plans are sometimes referred to as MCOs. Eligible organizations must provide comprehensive health care services to enrolled members through a defined benefit package in both ambulatory and inpatient settings, have been in operation and actively caring for members for at least 18 months, have an active quality management system, and have the capacity to report on their performance according to the specifications laid out in NCQA's HEDIS. Copies of NCQA's accreditation standards, HEDIS specifications, and application materials can be obtained by contacting NCQA's Publications Department, 2000 L Street N.W., Suite 500, Washington, D.C. 20036; (800) 839-6487; fax: (202) 955-3599; or on the Internet: *www.ncqa.org*.

History

NCQA was established in 1979 by the Group Health Association of America and the American Association of Foundations for Medical Care (both organizations have since joined to become the American Association of Health Plans), the trade associations at that time for HMOs. Original NCQA governance was by the HMO industry. In 1987 HMO industry leaders, believing that NCQA provided a good base for external quality review, studied a broader role for NCQA and began a process to separate it from the trade associations and make it independent, a recognized prerequisite for its credibility. As part of that process, the board was restructured to empower purchasers and other users.

In 1988 the Robert Wood Johnson Foundation funded a series of meetings to explore interest in the purchaser community in NCQA's potential as an independent external review organization. The group of purchaser representatives, benefits managers from Fortune 500 companies who were at the leading edge of external quality assessment, gave a resounding mandate for NCQA to go forward. In late 1989 the foundation awarded NCQA a grant to support its development as an independent entity. As evidence of industry support, the grant required that matching monies be raised from the managed care industry. Industry contributions demonstrated support, and NCQA was officially launched in March 1990.

To date, NCQA has reviewed about half the nation's HMOs, which collectively enroll about 75 percent of all Americans covered by HMOs.

Reviewers

NCQA review teams typically consist of one or two administrative reviewers and two or three physician reviewers. Administrative reviewers are nonphysician clinicians or quality assurance experts with extensive experience in quality assurance in managed care. Physician reviewers are medical directors, associate medical directors, or directors of quality management from noncompeting MCOs.

Areas of Review

Quality Management and Improvement

The first and most intensive area of NCQA review is an organization's own internal quality control systems. To meet NCQA standards, an organization must have a well-organized, comprehensive quality assurance program accountable to its highest organizational levels. The program's scope and content must be broad, covering the full spectrum of services included in its delivery system; the program should focus on important aspects of care and service and address clinical issues with major impact on the health status of the enrolled population.

To ensure physician participation in quality improvement activities, contracts with physicians and other health care providers must be explicit about the need to cooperate with the plan's quality activities or about the contractor's delegation of quality assurance responsibilities. NCQA also calls on organizations to actively monitor any delegated quality assurance activity.

Most important, an organization must be able to demonstrate program effectiveness in improving its quality of care and service. Typically this is achieved by comparing successive years' HEDIS results in the areas in which the health plan has chosen to focus (e.g., immunization rates, eye exams for diabetics, and so on). NCQA establishes compliance with its standards by thorough on-site review of an organization's quality assurance program description and related policies and procedures, quality assurance studies, projects and monitoring activities, quality assurance and governing body minutes, interviews with key staff, tracking of issues uncovered by the quality assurance system to ensure resolution, and documented evidence of quality improvement.

Another consumer issue addressed by NCQA's accreditation standards deals with the related issues of provider turnover and continuity of care. To help ensure continuity of care when a provider leaves or is removed from a health plan's network, NCQA requires that members who are undergoing an active course of treatment be allowed to receive care from that provider for up to an additional 90 days in the event that that provider is removed from the network. This will allow patients to complete ongoing treatment or stabilize their condition before initiating care with a new practitioner. The standard also applies to obstetrical care being delivered to pregnant women in the second or third trimester and to new mothers.

Utilization Management

Utilization management (UM), a keystone of effective managed care, is an important determinant of both the cost and the quality of an MCO. To earn NCQA accreditation, an organization must meet rigorous utilization management standards designed to ensure that this key health plan function promotes good medicine rather than acting as an arbitrary barrier to care. For instance, NCQA requires that review decisions be made by qualified medical professionals and that the organization has written UM protocols based on reasonable scientific evidence.

NCQA recently added a standard specifying that in any instance where a UM decision results in a denial, a similarly trained specialist must make the determination during at least one level of the internal review process. The standard ensures that if, for example, a neurologist appeals a decision to deny a requested treatment, another neurologist or similarly trained practitioner will rule on the appeal. This issue is an especially critical consideration for appeals dealing with complex medical questions where simply referring to preexisting medical guidelines may not adequately account for a specific patient's situation.

To ensure that UM decisions and appeals are processed in a timely manner, NCQA sets specific "turnaround time" requirements that specify the maximum allowable time between appeal and determination by the plan. While consumers and others are typically most concerned about overaggressive UM, insufficient UM can be problematic as well, leading to unnecessary care and expense. Thus, NCQA requires that a health plan's UM system monitor for under- as well as overutilization.

Compliance with UM standards is determined by pulling UR files and interviewing relevant staff.

Credentialing

NCQA's accreditation process includes a thorough review of an organization's credentialing system. NCQA requires that the MCO conduct primary verification of such credentialing information as licensure, malpractice history, good standing of hospital privileges, Drug Enforcement Agency certification, and so forth. Additionally, for IPA model organizations, NCQA requires the MCO to conduct a structured review of primary care physician offices.

An important part of ensuring delivery system integrity is periodic recertification or reappointment of providers. Aside from reverifying the paper credentials, NCQA requires a periodic performance appraisal to include information from quality assurance activity, risk management and UM, member complaints, and member satisfaction surveys. Organizations delegating credentialing responsibility retain responsibility for ensuring that they meet NCQA standards. Compliance with credentialing standards is ascertained by reviewing an organization's credentialing policies and procedures, sampling individual provider files, conducting interviews with relevant staff, and tracking issues identified through the complaint system or quality assurance findings.

In 1995 the NCQA released standards and began pilot testing a program to certify CVOs, thus eliminating the need for MCOs to conduct an annual review of those organizations. This program is described in more detail later in this chapter.

Member Rights and Responsibilities

To meet NCQA standards, an organization must have written policies that recognize such member rights as voicing grievances and receiving information regarding the organization, its services, and its practitioners. These written policies must also address such member responsibilities as providing information needed by the professional staff and following practitioners' instructions and guidelines. The NCQA requires an organization to have a system for resolving members' complaints and grievances, to aggregate and analyze complaint and grievance data, and to use the information for quality improvement.

NCQA standards require communication to members of certain types of information about how the health plan works, including the organization's policies on referrals for specialty care; provisions for after-hours and emergency coverage; covered benefits; charges to patients; procedures for notifying patients about terminations or changes in benefits, services, or delivery sites; procedures for appealing decisions regarding coverage, benefits, or relationship to the organization; disenrollment procedures; and complaint and grievance procedures. The standards require that member information be written in readable prose and be available in the languages of the major population groups served. Organizations must also have mechanisms ensuring confidentiality of specified patient information and records.

As noted earlier, a notable recent addition to NCQA's requirements includes a standard that requires plans to give members an opportunity to appeal UM decisions to an external body. The requirement means that if members exhaust a health plan's internal appeals process, they can then take the matter to an independent third party for final resolution. The independent appeal standard addresses widespread consumer concern that appeal decisions are sometimes based on financial considerations or poor medical judgment, rather than what is truly best for the patient.

Consistent with NCQA's emphasis on consumer protection, NCQA requires that organizations have mechanisms to protect and enhance member satisfaction with its services, including member satisfaction surveys and studies of disenrollment. NCQA further requires organizations to use this information to improve its quality of service.

Preventive Health Services

HMOs have traditionally prided themselves on their commitment to preventive health services. Moreover, because they serve defined populations, HMOs are in a better position than the fee-for-service system to ensure that preventive services are used appropriately. NCQA preventive services standards require adoption of specifications (clinical policies or practice guidelines) for the use of preventive services, communication of this information to providers and patients, and yearly measurement of performance in the delivery of two such services chosen from a list developed by NCQA. These results are audited by NCQA.

Medical Records

NCQA supplements management systems review with a sample of ambulatory records to assess both the quality of documentation and the quality of care. NCQA physician reviewers, guided by a 21-item medical record review form, assess the adequacy of diagnosis, the appropriateness and continuity of care, and the use of preventive services. NCQA surveyors also look closely for documentation of adequate coordination of care between medical and behavioral health providers, a critical determinant of quality.

HEDIS Performance

NCQA added a powerful new dimension to its accreditation program in 1999 by incorporating selected performance measures into the process. The measures are drawn from specifications in NCQA's HEDIS, the performance measurement tool used by about 90 percent of the nation's health plans.

HEDIS is a set of standardized performance measures designed to ensure that purchasers and consumers have the information they need to reliably compare the performance of managed health care plans. The measures in HEDIS are related to many significant public health issues, such as cancer, heart disease, smoking, asthma, and diabetes. HEDIS also includes a standardized member satisfaction survey. To earn NCQA accreditation, health plans must report on their performance on the following HEDIS measures.

Effectiveness of Care

- childhood immunizations
- adolescent immunizations
- breast cancer screening
- cervical cancer screening
- prenatal care in the first trimester
- advising smokers to quit
- beta-blocker treatment after a heart attack
- eye exams for people with diabetes
- check-ups after delivery
- follow-up after hospitalization for mental illness
- flu shots for the elderly

Consumer Survey Results

- getting care quickly
- getting needed care
- claims processing
- customer service
- rating of experience with health plan

HEDIS results will initially count for 25 percent of a plan's accreditation score. The remaining 75 percent will be based on a plan's degree of compliance with NCQA's standards. In the future, NCQA anticipates increasing the proportion of the accreditation score based on a health plan's performance. HEDIS results will initially be evaluated relative to national and regional averages, and national benchmarks.

To ensure that quality and performance are maintained between on-site surveys (which occur at least every three years), plans will be required to submit independently audited HEDIS results to NCQA annually. Should these results, or other factors such as regulatory action, suggest a lapse in quality, NCQA may elect to resurvey the health plan sooner. NCQA will also resurvey a plan sooner if its initial compliance with NCQA standards is low. HEDIS is discussed further later in this chapter, as well as in Chapter 35.

NCQA Accreditation Review Process

At the time of application, the applicant organization fills out a preliminary information form, which contains detailed descriptions of the plan's delivery system, including information about delegated quality assurance, UM, and credentialing activity. NCQA uses this information to determine the size and composition of the review team and the duration of the on-site review, both of which are used to determine the price of the review. Before the review, the applicant organization fills out a detailed preassessment information form that contains information regarding the plan's compliance with each of the accreditation standards.

The on-site review typically lasts three days and includes extensive review of documentation, such as minutes of quality assurance committee and board meetings; policies and procedures relating to various areas of the standards; provider contracts; quality assurance studies, reports, and case files; UM review criteria, reports, and files; credentialing files; complaint and grievance files; and member satisfaction and disenrollment surveys.

Interviews are conducted with the chief executive officer; the medical director; the directors of quality assurance, UM, provider relations, and member services; members of the quality assurance committee; a member of the board of directors; and participating physicians. The review team inspects for evidence of compliance with each of the NCQA standards and presents a summary of its findings at the end of the site visit. A member of the review team prepares a report that is submitted to NCQA.

The report is reviewed by NCQA staff and the NCQA Review Oversight Committee, an independent group of medical directors and others. This committee makes compliance determinations for each of the NCQA standards as well as for the overall accreditation decision.

Accreditation Decisions and Information

Following an on-site survey, NCQA will issue one of several possible accreditation decisions:

- *Excellent:* NCQA's highest accreditation status is granted only to those plans that demonstrate levels of service and clinical quality that meet or exceed NCQA's rigorous requirements for consumer protection and quality improvement. Plans earning this accreditation level must also achieve HEDIS results that are in the highest range of national or regional performance.
- *Commendable:* This accreditation level is awarded to plans that demonstrate levels of service and clinical quality that meet or exceed NCQA's rigorous requirements for consumer protection and quality improvement. This designation is equivalent to the NCQA's former "Full Accreditation" designation.
- *Accredited:* Health plans that earn this designation must meet most of NCQA's require-

ments for consumer protection and quality improvement. "Accredited" is equivalent to the former "One-Year" designation.

- *Provisional:* This accreditation indicates that a health plan's service and clinical quality meet some but not all of NCQA's requirements for consumer protection and quality improvement.
- *Denied:* This designation is an indication that a health plan did not meet NCQA's requirements during its review.

The NCQA since 1994 has made the results of all its accreditation surveys available to the public through its Health Plan Report Card. This list is now available on-line at NCQA's website, and it is searched or downloaded nearly 20,000 times each month.

To help consumers and others better understand each health plan's strengths and weaknesses, reports based on NCQA surveys will indicate plan performance in five categories. Each reporting category reflects a plan's performance on several related measures and standards. For example, the "staying healthy" category reflects plans' scores on the mammography, cervical cancer screening, and immunization measures and on several preventive health and quality improvement standards.

The categories are:

- access and service
- qualified providers
- staying healthy
- getting better
- living with illness

Other NCQA Accreditation and Certification Programs

The current managed care era has given rise to a diverse array of managed systems of care beyond HMOs and POS plans—PPOs, physician-hospital organizations, IPAs, managed behavioral health organizations, and many others—about which quality information has historically been scarce. To help address the need for information about these organizations and to facilitate NCQA's core MCO accreditation program by reducing the oversight burden for health plans, NCQA sponsors a number of other accreditation and certification programs. Taken together, these programs point to one of the trends for the future of quality oversight—targeted accreditation and certification programs suited to particular types of managed care systems.

Managed Behavioral Healthcare Organization Accreditation

About 100 million Americans currently are covered by a Managed Behavioral Healthcare Organization (MBHO)—more than are covered by HMOs by a wide margin (see also Chapter 25 for discussion of managed behavioral health programs). Nevertheless, little standardized information about the quality of these organizations has been available. That is problematic both for consumers and for MCOs seeking to delegate behavioral health services to such organizations. NCQA's MBHO accreditation program helps fill that void. The program is as rigorous as the MCO accreditation program and involves a similarly comprehensive survey. It provides health plans, consumers, and employers with the information they need to help select the best MBHO for their needs.

Initially, the Behavioral Health Accreditation Standards differ from the MCO standards in several significant ways in order to address issues of special concern with respect to managed behavioral health care. For example, a new category of standards covering access and triage addresses was included in the MBHO standards. These unique standards were designed to ensure that patients can see appropriate clinicians in a timely manner. The standards also covered such areas as network adequacy—whether the MBHO contracts with a sufficient number of providers in a particular area—and introduced stricter confidentiality requirements, since confidentiality concerns are traditionally greater in the mental health and substance abuse arenas than with regular medical care.

The standards also required that an MBHO demonstrate well-established lines of communication between members' primary care physicians and their behavioral health practitioners.

Effective coordination of care is closely related to treatment efficacy. The coordination of care encouraged by these standards marks a turning point in efforts to manage an individual's overall health across systems of care.

To help ensure high quality behavioral health care regardless of the system in which it is provided, NCQA is in the process of applying these same requirements to MCOs. To ensure that health plans have sufficient time to prepare to meet the additional behavioral health standards, they are or are being phased in according to the following schedule:

- *In 1999* health plans were required to meet the new coordination and continuity of care standards requiring plans to facilitate open and ongoing communication and coordination between behavioral health and medical providers.
- *In 2000* core behavioral health standards relating to access, confidentiality, credentialing, and timeliness of review decisions apply to MCOs.
- *In 2001* other behavioral health standards such as those relating to member input into treatment goals, clinical practice guidelines, rights and responsibilities policies, and preventive health guidelines will apply to MCOs.

As with the MCO survey process, survey teams (which may include psychologists, psychiatrists, and/or clinical social workers) and other quality experts conduct an in-depth, on-site review of an MBHO's clinical and administrative systems to gauge how well the organization complies with NCQA MBHO standards. The standards cover the same broad areas as the MCO standards but also include an additional (aforementioned) section on accessibility, availability, and triage of services.

PPO Accreditation

PPOs outnumber HMOs 1,035 to 650 and cover millions more Americans, but they have rarely been asked to report performance data or undergo any sort of accreditation process. Even URAC, to date the nation's leading accreditor of PPOs, has evaluated only a handful of such organizations (for details, see "The Utilization Review Accreditation Commission," below). The absence of data about PPOs has proven frustrating to employers and consumers. To fill this void, in 1999 NCQA announced plans to expand the scope of its current oversight programs to include PPOs. In late 1999 the NCQA introduced a survey tool to assess PPO members' experience with their plans. A more comprehensive PPO evaluation program will follow in mid-2000. This survey will be adapted from the existing Consumer Assessment of Health Plans Study (CAHPS) 2.0H instrument (see "The CAHPS 2.0H Survey," below). The survey will include questions designed to rate the members' experiences with the PPO and will address specific issues, such as how well appeals procedures work, whether there are any obstacles to getting needed care, claims processing, and customer service.

The full-fledged PPO accreditation program slated for release in mid-2000 will be modeled on NCQA's existing HMO accreditation program. This program will feature on-site reviews of the core systems and processes that define a PPO—appeal procedures, provider evaluation processes, medical review systems, and quality improvement efforts. NCQA's review of these systems, combined with the PPO's results on the member experiences survey, will determine its overall accreditation decision.

NCQA's CVO Certification Program

A CVO is any independent organization that verifies the credentials of physicians for MCOs or other health delivery organizations. Reliance on CVOs to conduct credentialing is becoming increasingly commonplace among health plans, hospitals, and medical groups.

NCQA's certification program for CVOs is designed to reduce the burden of oversight efforts for MCOs, CVOs, and physicians alike. It does so by, in effect, replacing many surveys with a single survey; a health plan contracting with a certified CVO is excused from NCQA requirements that it audit that CVO. For CVOs with multiple health plan clients, the savings in terms of time, effort, and financial resources are substantial.

Current NCQA accreditation standards for MCOs require health plans to review annually any delegated credentialing services. MCOs contracting with certified CVOs, however, are excused from this oversight responsibility for the elements in which their CVO has been certified. Quality is instead verified during the NCQA CVO certification survey. This represents a greater level of efficiency for both CVOs and MCOs.

NCQA's CVO standards are essentially a subset of the requirements specified in NCQA's MCO accreditation standards. The survey process is equally rigorous and includes a review of the organization's policies and procedures, internal quality assurance processes, mechanisms for maintaining credentials integrity and confidentiality, physician application components, and capabilities for ongoing data collection and reporting of physician disciplinary actions.

CVO certification is not meant as a blanket endorsement of all services offered by a CVO. Instead, CVOs are certified to verify 10 specific credentials:

- licensure
- hospital privileges
- drug enforcement agency registration
- medical education and/or board certification
- malpractice insurance
- liability claims history
- National Practitioner Data Bank queries
- medical board sanctions
- Medicare/Medicaid sanctions
- provider application

A CVO may be certified to verify any number of the above credentials from one to all 10. NCQA CVO certification decisions are valid for two years, representing another efficiency of the program as compared to the annual health plan audits that would otherwise be required.

Accreditation of New Health Plans

NCQA maintains an accreditation program designed for MCOs that otherwise would not be eli-gible to participate in NCQA accreditation. The program, designed especially for organizations less than two years old, is fundamentally similar to our regular MCO accreditation program, except for two key differences: the program contains no requirement that a plan demonstrate improvement over time (an unrealistic expectation given the short history of the plan), and results are on a pass-or-fail basis (to distinguish it from NCQA's main MCO accreditation program). Plans may apply for new health plan accreditation only once, and the accreditation period for plans that receive a "pass" designation is two years.

Physician Organization Certification

Another program with a rationale similar to that of NCQA's CVO certification program is NCQA's Physician Organization Certification (POC) program. This program allows physician organizations, IPAs, medical groups, and other such organizations to substitute one NCQA survey for the many overlapping annual surveys they may currently face from their MCO partners.

Physician organizations have recently emerged to play an important role as delegated providers of a wide range of administrative and clinical services for HMOs and other MCOs. Historically, the more MCO contracts these organizations held, the more annual audits they faced from plans seeking to satisfy NCQA accreditation requirements.

The POC standards are comprised largely of a subset of NCQA's MCO accreditation standards. Although a few new program-specific standards were added—requiring open, ongoing communication between the physician organization and the MCO—no significant changes were made to the existing MCO standards in order to apply them to physician organizations. The survey process for physician organizations is fundamentally similar to that of MCOs.

Performance Measurement: NCQA's HEDIS

The discussion of NCQA's MCO accreditation program looked briefly at how the incorporation of performance measures from HEDIS has transformed the way health plans demonstrate accountability. HEDIS will now be discussed in more detail, examining its role in the health care system, its content, and the process by which it evolves.

First, a definition: HEDIS is a set of standardized measures that look at plan performance across a variety of important dimensions, such as delivery of preventive health services, member satisfaction, and treatment efficacy for various illnesses. By specifying not only what to measure, but also how to measure it, HEDIS allows true "apples-to-apples" comparisons between health plans in these and other areas. HEDIS allows health plans to manage and improve quality and it allows purchasers of health care to make informed choices. Every year, dozens of national news magazines, local newspapers, employers, and others use HEDIS data to generate health plan "report cards" during open enrollment.

HEDIS consists of approximately 60 measures (not including the CAHPS 2.0H survey, which includes dozens of individual questions) that fall into eight broad categories or domains. The broad areas covered by HEDIS are:

- *Effectiveness of Care:* Measures in this category underlie such oft-reported statistics as childhood immunization rates and mammography rates. These and other measures seek to establish whether or not the health plan is responding to the needs of those who are ill ("Does the health plan make me better when I am sick?") and also to the needs of those who are well ("Does the health plan keep me healthy when I am well?").
- *Access/Availability of Care:* Measures in this category assess whether care is available to members when they need it in a timely manner. Accessibility is a precondition of high-quality care.
- *Member Satisfaction:* These measures provide important information about whether a health plan is able to satisfy the diverse needs of its members. Two different sur-

veys—one for adults, the other related to parents' impressions of the care their children receive—include numerous questions related to many key consumer issues, including average office wait times, satisfaction with choice of provider, difficulty receiving care, and overall satisfaction.
- *Use of Services:* How a health plan uses its resources is a signal of how efficiently care is managed. Measures in this category permit users to understand patterns of service use across different health plans. Measures look at such key areas as Caesarean section rates, maternity length of stay, well-child visits, mental health utilization, and the frequency of selected procedures.
- *Cost of Care:* Used in conjunction with other measures, these measures (rate trends, frequency of high-cost procedures) permit comparison between plans based on the "value" of the services they deliver.
- *Informed Health Care Choices:* This new section of HEDIS—for which measures are currently being developed—was included to encourage health plans to help members become active partners in their health care decisions by providing them with enough information about treatment options to allow them to make informed choices.
- *Health Plan Descriptive Information:* While not technically "measures," HEDIS includes several general questions about aspects of a health plan that employers and consumers have found useful when selecting among plans.

All these measures can be used not only to help consumers and employers select among health plans but also to help manage care and service as well. That explains why about 90 percent of the nation's health plans collect HEDIS data, whether for internal purposes or for release to employers and the public.

Significantly, HEDIS is applicable to both the public and private sectors. The same measurement standards are applied to care provided to Medicaid beneficiaries, commercial enrollees, and Medicare risk populations. This not only increases the efficiency of measurement but also allows for performance comparisons across populations and health plan types.

The standards for including a measure in HEDIS are high. The evolution of HEDIS is managed by NCQA's Committee on Performance Measurement (CPM), a broad-based committee whose members reflect the diverse constituencies affected by performance measurement. Measures included in HEDIS typically undergo exhaustive testing and review prior to inclusion and must possess three key attributes:

- *Relevance:* Measures must address health issues of significant concern, and performance on measures should be controllable (at least to some extent) by the health plan. Also, information produced by a given measure should be useful to consumers and employers.
- *Scientific soundness:* Measures must generate reproducible, valid, and accurate results. Measures also must be sensitive enough to detect meaningful differences in performance between health plans.
- *Feasibility:* It should be possible to collect the data required for a measure at a reasonable cost and without threatening the confidentiality of patient medical information.

To ensure that it has a rich pool of measures to draw from in the future, the CPM also manages a "testing set" of performance measures comprised of likely candidates for inclusion in future iterations of HEDIS. As the name implies, measures in the testing set are actively tested and periodically reviewed by the CPM for possible inclusion in HEDIS.

The CAHPS 2.0H Survey

The member satisfaction survey has long been a popular means of assessing plan performance, and such a survey has been featured in HEDIS since the release of version 3.0 in 1996. Previously, information about member satisfaction was gathered using a variety of surveys and instruments developed by the health plans for use with their enrolled population. Because no standardized survey was in broad use, what little member satisfaction data were available could not be used to compare plans since the survey instruments and survey methodology varied from plan to plan.

At the insistence of various constituencies—including health plans, which were often required by their clients to field dozens of different satisfaction surveys annually—satisfaction survey data are now collected in a more rational, efficient manner using a standard tool. Today, the satisfaction survey instrument of choice among health plans is the CAHPS 2.0H survey, which was jointly developed by NCQA and the federal Agency for Health Research and Quality (AHRQ). CAHPS 2.0H is part of HEDIS and, like HEDIS, is designed to be applicable to all health plans regardless of the population they serve: Medicare, Medicaid, or commercial. CAHPS 2.0H actually consists of several different surveys: one for the adult population, another designed to assess parents' impressions of their children's health care, and a third for use specifically with the Medicare and Medicaid populations. To ensure that CAHPS 2.0H data are collected using only the approved, standardized methodology, health plans are required to contract with an NCQA-certified third-party vendor to administer the survey.

While each CAHPS 2.0H survey consists of dozens of questions, the questions are grouped in "composites" to make comparisons between plans easier. The composites provide information on plan performance in the following areas:

- getting needed care
- getting care quickly
- how well doctors communicate
- courteous and helpful office staff
- customer service
- claims processing
- overall rating of health plan

The HEDIS Compliance Audit™

There has been strong interest, from employers and others, in developing a means by which to validate HEDIS data that are collected and reported by health plans. It is recognized that, despite the clear specifications defined in HEDIS, data collection and calculation methods employed by health plans may vary, and other errors may taint the results, diminishing the usefulness of HEDIS data for MCO comparison.

In order for HEDIS to reach its full potential, NCQA and others concluded that an independent audit of HEDIS collection and reporting processes, as well as an audit of the data that are manipulated by those processes, would be necessary in order to ensure that HEDIS specifications are met. In response, NCQA developed the HEDIS Compliance Audit Program, a precise, standardized methodology for verifying the integrity of HEDIS collection and calculation processes. It is a two-part program consisting of an overall information systems capabilities assessment (IS standards) followed by an evaluation of the MCO's ability to comply with HEDIS specifications. NCQA-certified auditors using standard audit methodologies help enable purchasers to make more reliable "apples-to-apples" comparisons between health plans.

NCQA licenses organizations and certifies selected employees of licensed organizations to conduct audits using NCQA's standardized audit methodology. Auditors use the first half of the audit—the overall IS review— to identify data areas to focus on during the second half of the review (HEDIS compliance standards). This allows for customization of each audit depending on the individual health plan's strengths and weaknesses. The audit adds a higher degree of integrity to HEDIS data and enables MCOs to provide consumers and purchasers with consistent and comparable HEDIS reports.

The audit is principally designed to verify the compliance of HEDIS production processes with specifications. To this end, auditors verify a sample of HEDIS measures to confirm that HEDIS results are based on accurate source information. The focus of the audit is on data management processes and on the translation of captured data into HEDIS statistics, according to the specifications defined by NCQA.

A list of the licensed organizations and certified auditors can be found on NCQA's website.

NCQA's Quality Compass™

For performance measurement to be of value, the results must reach consumers and employers. NCQA's Quality Compass, a national database of comparative information on the quality of the nation's managed care plans, makes HEDIS data accessible to employers and the media. In the past, HEDIS data were used almost exclusively by large employers due to cost issues. Quality Compass corrects that situation, making data broadly available at a reasonable cost.

Quality Compass integrates summary NCQA accreditation information and data from NCQA's HEDIS from hundreds of the nation's health plans, making comparisons between plans easier, and allowing for identification of important national and regional benchmarks. The benchmarks can help guide employers seeking to establish reasonable performance goals for their health plan partners.

The data gathered for Quality Compass also support the generation of NCQA's *State of Managed Care Quality* report, an annual assessment of the overall performance of the industry.

THE UTILIZATION REVIEW ACCREDITATION COMMISSION

History and Governance

URAC was established in December 1990 from an initiative led by the American Managed Care and Review Association (AMCRA), a trade association for UR firms, PPOs, and HMOs. AMCRA's goal was to address providers' concerns and frustration with the diversity of UR procedures and with the growing impact of UR on physicians and hospitals. As a result of this provider frustration, legislative initiatives were underway in a number of states to pass legislation that, according to managed care advocates, would severely limit the impact of UR in some instances and make it impossible to conduct UR in others. The URAC Health Utilization Management standards were in large part a response and alternative to these legislative initiatives. In late 1994 URAC announced its intention to develop standards and an accreditation program for health care networks ineligible for NCQA accreditation. In 1999 URAC introduced revised health network standards for the accreditation of less integrated health care systems, such as PPOs. Also in 1999 URAC introduced health plan standards for the accreditation of more highly integrated health care systems, such as HMOs.

URAC Accreditation Process

The URAC accreditation process begins with a desktop review of a detailed application. At the conclusion of the desktop review, the URAC reviewer sends a letter to the applicant requesting any further information or documentation that may be necessary. At this time, the applicant has 30 days to respond to the request for information.

Upon receipt of a satisfactory response to the request for information, an on-site visit is scheduled. During that visit, the reviewer conducts interviews of members of the applicant's staff and reviews documents to ensure compliance with URAC standards. At the conclusion of the on-site review, the reviewer writes an executive summary of the findings of the desktop and on-site review. This summary serves as the basis for the reviewer's report to the accreditation committee, which consists of representatives from URAC member organizations and industry experts.

The accreditation committee then reviews the "blinded" executive summary, discusses the application with the assigned reviewer, and makes a determination as to whether in its view the applicant has met the minimum standards for accreditation. The accreditation committee then sends the executive summary and its recommendation to the executive committee, which makes the formal determination as to whether to grant accreditation. The executive committee may request an organization to take corrective action if the accreditation committee or the executive committee has reason to believe that the organization is not in compliance with URAC standards. URAC accreditation is for two years, starting the first day of the month following URAC's executive committee approval. Accredited companies remain on their current cycle, even if executive commit-

tee approval should occur after the accreditation expiration date.

Accredited organizations must continue to remain in compliance with the applicable standards throughout the accreditation cycle. URAC may rescind accreditation status if an accredited company is unable to comply with URAC standards.

Following are summaries of URAC's health UM, health network, and health plan standards. Copies of the URAC standards and application materials can be obtained by writing to URAC, 1275 K Street NW, Suite 1100, Washington, D.C. 20005, or calling (202) 216-9010. Summaries of all URAC accreditation standards are at their website, *www.urac.org.* The summaries provide an overview of the standards. Should there be a conflict between the summaries and the full standards, the wording of the full standards always governs.

URAC's Health Utilization Management Standards

URAC's UM standards may be applied to "stand-alone" UM organizations or to the UM functions that are integrated into health benefits programs, such as indemnity insurance, HMOs, or PPOs. The standards cover the following categories.

Confidentiality

Under the confidentiality section, an organization must comply with two standards. The first standard states that the UM organization must have written policies and procedures in place that ensure information obtained during the UM process will be kept confidential in accordance with the law. That information must be limited to only what is necessary for UM of the services under review and must be used solely for the purpose of UM, quality management, discharge planning, and case management.

The second standard states that if provider-specific data are to be released to the public, the UM organization must have policies and procedures for exercising due care in compiling and releasing such data. The policies and procedures must address things such as how data are obtained and verified, how subjects of such disclosures are informed of the disclosures, how potential users of the information are informed about the uses of the data, and so on.

Staff Qualifications

Under the seven staff qualifications standards, a UM organization must maintain a UM staff that is qualified, trained, and supervised, as well as supported by written clinical review criteria. It must limit the types of data collection, intake screening, and scripted clinical screening that a nonclinical administrative staff may perform. It also must establish the proper procedure for who may perform initial clinical review. The standards in this section also include procedures for conducting peer clinical review for cases where clinical determination to certify cannot be made by initial clinical review and procedure for the availability of health professionals who conduct peer review. The UM organization is also strongly encouraged to require clinical peers who render review determinations to be in active practice.

Program Qualifications

The 10 standards of the program qualifications section include a requirement that the organization have a medical director in place who has professional postresidency experience in direct patient care. The organization must maintain written policies and procedures that govern all aspects of the UM process and exercise oversight to make sure that all delegated or subcontracted functions of the UM program are in compliance with URAC UM standards. The standards require the utilization of explicit clinical review criteria for scripted clinical screening and also require the implementation and documentation of a staff management program to orient and train all clinical reviewers. The program qualifications standards also specify that the UM organization conduct a periodic formal program for training and maintain and document a quality management program that includes a written plan addressing the ongoing monitoring of compliance with URAC UM standards.

Accessibility

The accessibility and on-site review procedures standards require that the UM organization must provide a telephone service that provides access to review staff during normal business hours. This service must also provide a mechanism for timely callbacks from providers. A UM organization also must require on-site reviewers to follow reasonable and standard hospital or faculty procedures.

UM Information

When conducting prospective, concurrent, or retrospective review, a UM organization is required to follow the guidelines outlined in the UM standards. It is also recommended, but not required, that the UM organization limit its requirements for data to the categories listed in this section of the standards.

Review Determination

Under the standards covering procedures for review determination, the UM organization must have written procedures that ensure reviews and second opinions are conducted in a timely manner. The standards also require written procedures for providing notification of its review determinations and for addressing the failure or inability of a provider, patient, or representative to provide the information needed for review. A UM organization is also required to provide an opportunity for discussion when an initial determination is made not to certify an admission.

Appeals

The standards addressing appeals of determinations not to certify require a UM organization to provide a mechanism to appeal such decisions. The UM organization also must inform the provider of the right to initiate appeals when there is a difference of opinion regarding the determination not to certify. Under an additional expedited appeal standard, a UM organization is required to provide a documented process, under procedures listed in the standards, for expedited appeals by telephone when review is required of a current service.

PPO Accreditation

Since 1995 URAC has also offered a PPO accreditation program that it acquired when it purchased the American Accreditation Program Inc. The program has accredited about 20 PPOs and until recently was the only accreditation program available tailored specifically to the PPO community. NCQA and the Joint Commission have both, however, recently released or announced their own PPO accreditation programs. URAC's PPO accreditation program features standards in the following areas.

Network Management Standards

To be eligible for URAC accreditation, URAC requires that PPOs define, in writing, the scope of the services they offer, including type of service, region serviced, and populations served. A network must also establish goals for access to care, availability of providers, and provider selection criteria related to the services most commonly used by eligible persons. A health network must measure its performance against the established goals. A network must also implement written policies for covered services not available through participating providers and emergency care both in and out of the network.

The organization management category requires health networks to designate a medical director with expertise appropriate in the type of services provided. Health networks must implement policies to integrate administrative and clinical operations and to establish and maintain data collection and retention methods. URAC recommends that data systems capture demographic, cost, and diagnostic data and provide reports to assist the operations of the health network.

URAC's PPO accreditation standards are designed to encourage incorporating providers' perspectives in all relevant clinical or administrative areas. Thus, URAC requires plans to maintain good communications between the network and the provider and specify in its provider contracts the terms between the network and the provider. URAC also bars "gag clauses" that would restrict providers from discussing available treatment options with eligible persons.

Provider Credentialing

URAC's credentialing standards fall into three distinct areas: credentialing plan, credentialing delegation, and credentialing implementation. Under the credentialing plan section, the network must develop and implement a written plan for credentialing that is approved by the executive staff of the network. The plan must specify which types of providers must be credentialed and should define the structure of the program, including naming the medical director as the overseer of the clinical aspects. The plan must provide the selection criteria for participating providers (including facilities) and a list a credentialing information to be gathered, as well as the method of collection. The program must include the biennial recredentialing of providers.

URAC requires a network to complete its provider credentialing plan within a required period. Specifically, the network must complete program infrastructure design, implementation, and credentialing of at least 15 percent of providers by the end of the first year after URAC awards initial accreditation. The network must credential 50 percent of the providers by the end of the second year and 100 percent by the end of the third year. The network must submit progress reports to URAC every six months until it completes 100 percent credentialing.

Member Protection

URAC's member protection standards focus on confidentiality and marketing. Under the confidentiality section, the health network must implement a policy of confidentiality for maintaining protected information. All staff with access to protected information must be annually oriented on their responsibilities in preserving confidentiality and be required to sign a confidentiality statement.

The marketing section requires the health network to implement a mechanism to communicate information effectively and accurately about network services to eligible persons. The network must also maintain a responsive complaint and grievance policy.

Quality Management

URAC's standards also prescribe certain features of a health plan's quality management structure and organization and the quality management process. URAC's quality management standards specify that networks must designate a senior-level staff member to oversee the quality management program and establish a quality management committee to provide guidance for the health network on related issues. The quality management process standards also require the network to implement a program designed to improve clinical and nonclinical services. The committee must identify priorities by reviewing data about network performance and must choose at least two performance improvement projects, of which one should be clinical. Before each project, the committee must assess current levels of performance, establish goals for improvement, establish time frames for improvement, and periodically measure their progress.

HMO Accreditation

URAC also accredits HMOs with standards that focus on the same areas as its PPO accreditation program. HMOs seeking URAC accreditation must comply with URAC's UM standards and establish a mechanism giving members access to an external appeals process. URAC's HMO accreditation program was introduced in 1999 and to date has accredited only a handful of organizations. For a complete list of URAC-accredited HMOs, visit the organization's website, *www.urac.org.*

JOINT COMMISSION ON ACCREDITATION OF HEALTHCARE ORGANIZATIONS

Best known for its pioneering work in accrediting the nation's hospitals and other medical facilities, the Joint Commission on Accreditation of Healthcare Organizations is an independent, nonprofit organization that is the nation's oldest standards-setting and accrediting body in health care. The Joint Commission evaluates and ac-

credits nearly 20,000 hospitals and other health care organizations across the country each year.

Mission

The mission of the Joint Commission is to improve the quality of care provided to the public through the provision of health care accreditation and related services that support performance improvement in health care organizations.

History

The Joint Commission's roots can be traced back to 1951 when the American College of Surgeons transferred its Hospital Standardization Program to the Joint Commission on Accreditation of Hospitals, which was formed with the purpose of providing voluntary accreditation. In 1987 the Joint Commission changed its name to the Joint Commission on Accreditation of Healthcare Organizations to reflect this expanded scope of activities. Today, the Joint Commission offers accreditation programs in seven health care areas: ambulatory care organizations, behavioral health care organizations, clinical laboratories, health care networks, home care and hospice organizations, hospitals, and long-term care organizations.

The Joint Commission's governing board of commissioners consists of 28 individuals having diverse experience in health care, business, and public policy. The board includes physicians, consumers, medical directors, health care administrators, a nurse, a business representative, a labor representative, quality experts, ethicists, a health insurance administrator, and educators.

Health Care Network Accreditation Program

Since 1994, the Joint Commission has accredited MCOs under its network accreditation program. This program provides comprehensive, yet flexible accreditation services to managed care plans, integrated delivery networks, provider-sponsored organizations, and PPOs. Related accreditation services for managed behavioral health care organizations are provided through the behavioral health care accreditation program. The Joint Commission is the only accrediting body that evaluates the actual health care delivery sites where patients receive care—hospitals, home care agencies, ambulatory care centers, nursing homes, and behavioral clinics—in addition to the network's central operations. The standards used to evaluate the health care network's overall performance address issues related to systemwide integration, coordination, and accountability. These standards were developed in collaboration with a national advisory group of more than 100 health care executives, managed care experts, policy makers, business leaders, and consumers. The standards cover the following areas:

- *Rights, responsibilities and ethics:* Standards in this area address ethical issues that arise in the provision of care and services to network members at the network, component, and practitioner-site levels.
- *Continuum of care:* Standards in this area focus on how services and service-delivery settings should be linked into a network, providing a seamless continuum of care that is accessible, communicates with members and practitioners, plans and develops effective member-centered services, and considers the impact of financial performance on the network providers' ability to provide health care services.
- *Education and communication:* Standards in this area emphasize the need to educate members so that they can be knowledgeable participants in their health care.
- *Health promotion and disease prevention:* Standards in this area address maintenance of health, prevention of acute diseases and injuries, avoidance or delay of morbidity and disability, and health care resource use associated with chronic and degenerative diseases.
- *Network leadership:* Standards in this area provide a framework for planning, directing, coordinating, providing, and improving health care services that are cost effective and responsive to member and community needs, while improving member outcomes.
- *Management of human resources:* Standards in this area help ensure that the right number of qualified, competent, and motivated staff are available to fulfill the network's mission and meet members' needs. Credentialing of physicians and other licensed independent practitioners practicing in the networks is addressed.
- *Management of information:* Standards in this area encourage networks to manage and use information to improve member outcomes as well as individual and network performance of member care, governance, management, and support processes.
- *Improving network performance:* Standards in this area encourage the network to continuously evaluate and improve the performance of the network, including its use of resources. This covers the most up-to-date ideas about performance improvement, including continuous quality improvement, total quality management, and how to apply those principles to the network's own performance-management efforts.

Scope of Surveys

During the survey, the Joint Commission evaluates all functions performed by the network and renders an accreditation decision appropriate to the evaluation. A network must be prepared to provide evidence of its compliance with each standard and its intent statement that applies to its operations. To be accredited, a network must demonstrate that it is in overall compliance with the standards.

The Survey Process in Brief

During an accreditation survey, the Joint Commission evaluates a network's performance of functions and processes aimed at continuously improving member outcomes. The survey process focuses on assessing performance of important member-centered and organization functions that support quality care. Surveys are designed to be individualized to each network, to be consistent, and to support the network's efforts to improve performance. Depending on the scope of the survey, networks receive a two-, three-, four-, or five-day survey of the network central office and a sample of individual practitioner sites. The surveys are conducted on a triennial basis.

Survey Team Composition

Accreditation surveys are conducted by a team of Joint Commission surveyors. The composition of a network's survey team is based on the information provided in its application for survey. The Joint Commission will structure the survey team to the network's specific characteristics. For example, when a network component (e.g., a nursing home) is not already accredited or certified, the component is subject to survey under selected standards during the network's survey. The composition of the survey team will reflect this requirement. Furthermore, when certain services are provided in high volume, the survey team may also include surveyors who have special expertise in that service. All surveyors assess and provide consultation regarding all functions addressed by the standards.

Opening Conference

After the network has completed the pre-survey steps, the first actual survey activity involves an opening conference. This conference lays the groundwork for the survey.

Document Review

After completing the opening conference and the performance improvement review, the surveyors begin the assessment process by reviewing key documents that focus on the network's performance. Documents include committee minutes, reports of performance-improvement activities, measurement data, and reports to network committees and the governing body. Certain bylaws, planning documents, and other evidence of performance also will be included.

Interviews with Network Leaders

Interviews with the network's leaders occur both early and at later stages in the survey process. The purpose of these interviews is to provide an opportunity for surveyors to assess the level of communication among the network leaders, the role that each plays in its management, and the extent to which the standards' requirements for communication and cooperation are being met by the network. Interviews address the collaboration of senior leaders in the performance-improvement process and the roles each leader plays. Participants should be able to provide information that illustrates how the network's leaders work together to develop, review, and revise the network's mission, strategic plans, budgets, bases for resource allocation, operational plans, and policies.

Function Interviews

These interviews gather a multidisciplinary group of the network's staff who have important responsibilities related to a given function (e.g., education and communication). They follow up on issues identified in the document review and investigate any observations made by surveyors in visits to care settings.

Scoring Compliance against Track Record Requirements

Accredited organizations are expected to remain in continuous compliance with the standards and their intent statements throughout the interval between surveys. However, for practical purposes in conducting the survey, surveyors will ordinarily limit their evaluation of the organization's track record of compliance. In addition to the performance expectations of each standard, and subject to exercise of appropriate discretion, networks ordinarily will be expected to show a track record of compliance for one year before a triennial survey. Surveyors may evaluate over a shorter or longer time frame depending on circumstances encountered during the survey.

Feedback Sessions

Final scores about compliance are not reached until all selected care settings have been visited and all other assessment interviews and activities have been conducted. However, surveyors will communicate their observations at daily briefings.

Final On-Site Survey Activities

At the leadership exit conference, the survey team will present complete survey findings and a potential accreditation decision.

Accreditation Decisions

Organizations that are surveyed by the Joint Commission are placed in one of six accreditation categories, as follows:

- *Accreditation with Commendation:* This is the highest accreditation level awarded to a health care organization; it is given to those that demonstrate exemplary overall performance.
- *Accreditation:* This category indicates that a health care organization meets Joint Commission standards in all performance areas.
- *Accreditation with Recommendations for Improvement:* This accreditation level is given to a health care organization that generally meets the standards but does not meet important standards in at least one performance area. In order to remain accredited, the health care organization must demonstrate that it meets all standards within a specified period of time.
- *Conditional Accreditation:* This designation is awarded when an organization is not in substantial compliance with Joint Commission standards but is believed to be capable of achieving acceptable standards compliance within a stipulated time period. Evidence of correction must be found through a timely follow-up survey in order for the organization to be considered for full accreditation status.
- *Preliminary Nonaccreditation:* This designation applies when an organization is initially denied accreditation because of significant noncompliance with Joint Commission standards or when its accreditation is withdrawn by the Joint Commission for other reasons. An organization remains in this status until a final decision is made.
- *Not Accredited:* This designation means that an organization has been denied accreditation or has had accreditation withdrawn because it does not meet Joint Commission standards.

Public Access to Information

The Joint Commission is committed to making relevant information about surveyed health care organizations available to interested persons. Information on Joint Commission-accredited health care organizations, such as the organization's name, address, phone number, accreditation decision, and effective date, can be obtained on-line through Quality Check™, which is accessible through the Joint Commission website at *www.jcaho.org*. Performance reports, based on the accreditation evaluation, that provide more detailed, useful, and understandable information about each accredited institution are also available through Quality Check™.

Major Initiatives

The Joint Commission shares with health care providers a commitment to the continual improvement of the quality of health care. Standards utilized in on-site surveys are patient-centered and focused on systems and processes rather than structures. They are used to evaluate actual performance, rather than only capability. In recent years this standards-based accreditation process has been expanded through several new initiatives.

Reduction in Duplication: Cooperative Accreditation Agreements

Cooperative agreements permit the Joint Commission to substantially rely on the process, findings, and decisions of other accrediting bodies in circumstances where the Joint Commission would otherwise conduct potentially duplicative surveys of organizations seeking accreditation.

Under these cooperative agreements, the Joint Commission will accept the accreditation decision of the other accrediting body or government agency for specific components of health care organizations undergoing Joint Commission review. For those Joint Commission standards areas not covered by the other accrediting body, the Joint Commission may conduct a limited survey.

The cooperative accreditation initiative is part of the Joint Commission's national duplication reduction effort that is focused on improving the efficiency and reducing the cost of quality oversight activities by enhancing the communication and coordination among various public- and private-sector organizations that have responsibility for these activities.

Currently, the Joint Commission has finalized cooperative accreditation agreements with the following organizations:

- Accreditation Association for Ambulatory Health Care
- American Association of Blood Banks
- American College of Radiology
- American College of Surgeons, Commission on Cancer
- American Society for Histocompatibility and Immunogenetics
- College of American Pathologists
- CARF—The Rehabilitation Accreditation Commission
- Commission on Office Laboratory Accreditation
- Community Health Accreditation Program.

ORYX Initiative

The ORYX initiative, introduced in 1997, assists in measuring performance and supports quality improvement efforts within the health care organization by integrating outcomes and other performance measurement data into the accreditation process.

When fully implemented, each accredited organization will collect standard—"core"—performance measures that are relevant to the type of organization and its services, and these data will be regularly transmitted to the Joint Commission to be used in the accreditation process.

Over the next five years, a three-phase strategy for ORYX activities in health care networks will be implemented. This strategy is designed to transition organizations from the current performance measurement requirements to a comprehensive, integrated performance measurement framework that encompasses the organization and its provider organization components.

Phase I will allow organizations to replace any of the previously selected measures from five consensus-based measure sets with measures that more effectively meet their unique measurement needs by December 31, 1999. The organizations may select measures from the universe of existing performance measures.

Phase II will include pilot testing of the proposed model for data collection and transmission and the ability to evaluate data trends for quality management. Core measures specific to these organizations also will be identified and tested.

Phase III will involve the progressive introduction of a comprehensive, integrated performance measurement framework for the organizations. Core measures for organizations, as well as for all types of provider organizations, will be incorporated into the framework, which is targeted to be fully operational by 2005.

Other Joint Commission Accreditation Programs

In addition to network accreditation, the Joint Commission operates accreditation programs serving organizations in the following areas:

- hospital accreditation services
- home care accreditation services
- ambulatory care accreditation services
- laboratory accreditation services
- long-term care accreditation services
- behavioral care accreditation services

CONCLUSION

This chapter has presented a summary of the three primary organizations that currently accredit MCOs, as well as a detailed look at the oversight programs they offer. Like the organizations they review, the three organizations vary in their goals and in their approach to external review. Although they vary considerably in their approach, all of these organizations hold the potential for rationalizing and consolidating current external review processes for state, federal, and individual purchasers. These processes are sometimes duplicative or contradictory in their requirements and, in some cases, this can have a detrimental impact on managed care programs. Ultimately, however, their effectiveness must be judged in terms of their ability to improve the quality of care and service that health care organizations provide to their customers.

CHAPTER 45

Risk Management in Managed Care

Barbara J. Youngberg

INTRODUCTION

Risk management has been in a period of evolution since it first became a process utilized in the health care setting. In the mid 1970s, the health care risk management profession emerged in response to the malpractice crisis surrounding the availability of liability insurance.[1] Although the basic concepts for health care risk management were adopted from the insurance industry, over the past two decades the discipline of health care risk management has taken on many important characteristics and unique functions. Risk management takes on many functions of a managed care organization (MCO) as discussed in various chapters throughout this book, especially those in the section on legal and regulatory issues and those that discuss managing quality and utilization. Although clear risks are associated with benefits administration, contracting, and other activities, the bulk of risks

in managed care is associated with the provision of health care services and coverage decisions surrounding that care. In addition, providers face risks associated with managed care beyond those faced by health plans. Therefore, this chapter focuses particularly on those issues.

With the federal "Patient's Rights" legislation (the outcome of which is undetermined at the time of publication) and many similar types of bills currently pending or already passed in state legislatures (see Chapter 69), including expanded rights for patients to sue their MCOs, it is clear that the risks inherent in operating an MCO have never been greater. So too is the need for comprehensive, proactive risk management. In California, sweeping legislation was signed into law by Governor Gray Davis on September 27, 1999; additional provisions also allow for a number of other MCO reforms that will benefit patients but increase MCO cost and risk including:

- a bill to establish an independent medical review system by January 1, 2001, that will handle patients' disputes over claims when treatment has been delayed, denied, or modified by the plan
- a bill that requires health service plans to provide all enrollees with written responses to grievances, which expands the right to external review for experimental treatments
- the establishment of a new state agency referred to as the Department of Managed Care devoted exclusively to the licensing and regulation of health care service plans

Barbara J. Youngberg, BSN, MSW, JD, is Vice President of Insurance, Risk and Quality, and Legal Services Management for the University HealthSystem Consortium (UHC). In this capacity she has responsibility for the design and management of group professional liability and provider excess insurance programs and for supporting risk and quality management for 86 academic medical centers in the United States, Switzerland, Australia, and Finland. Ms. Youngberg is also on the faculty of the Loyola University College of Law, Health Law Institute, and the Chicago Medical School, Finch University College of Health Sciences.

and an Office of the Patient Advocate, which will assist health plan enrollees with complaints and education about their MCOs

- a bill requiring health service plans to provide a second opinion at the patient's request
- a bill requiring that all telephone advice be provided by persons with a medical license
- a bill that limits and, in some cases, prohibits the release of medical information regarding a patient's participation in outpatient treatment with a psychotherapist
- bills that prohibit the unauthorized selling, sharing, or use of medical information for any purpose not necessary to provide health care services and the unauthorized marketing and selling of provider lists
- a bill that sets forth procedures and time frames for health care plans to review treatment requests made by physicians
- a bill that clarifies a prior bill dealing with a patient's referral to a specialist
- a bill requiring coverage for the screening, diagnosis, and treatment of breast cancer (Also, enrollment in a plan cannot be denied because of a personal or family history of breast cancer or breast disease.)
- a bill requiring that health care plans cover the diagnosis and medically necessary treatment of severe mental illness at any age and serious emotional disturbances of a child
- a bill adding hospice care to the basic health care services

Although these changes in California may seem beneficial for the health care consumer, the associated costs of implementing them and of managing their risks could significantly increase the MCO's administrative costs, as well as employer's costs and employee's copayments or payroll deductions. Balancing the risks and benefits provides an additional challenge.

Risk management has changed from an activity that sought solely to transfer risk through the purchase of commercial insurance or the financing of risk through the establishment of a self-insured trust or investment fund to a profession where education, proactive risk control and risk modification, and risk financing and risk transfer are merged into a partnership. The overall goals of the partnership enable the organization to be responsive to the needs and demands of the health care industry and to provide safe and effective care to patients. The organizational goals of ensuring financial stability in the event of an adverse outcome are still consistent with the goals of the health care risk manager, but risk managers also find that their work takes them out of the finance department and into those clinical and operational areas where the risks are created. In addition, the many changes occurring in the law mandating change in the ways MCOs historically conducted their business come with significant associated costs and risks.

Specific objectives in risk management programs relate to the organization's desire to ensure survival, maximize efficiency, and sustain growth and effectiveness. This is accomplished through the identification, control, management, elimination, transfer, or financing of risk. Achievement of these objectives is accomplished by interacting with internal and external customers of the organization that demand low-risk, high-quality, cost-effective service. Management may have different priorities in seeking efficiency and growth, while achieving high levels of consumer satisfaction, particularly as managed care continues to dominate the marketplace.

The primary targets or strategies of management could relate to gaining market share, increasing the overall number of relationships and contracts with payers, increasing sales or service volume, ensuring continuity of performance, maintaining the quantity of controlled resources, or other items expected to produce desired long-term financial results. These targets may be sought without appropriate consideration of the inherent risks that may also be assumed by adopting those strategies.

The goals identified to achieve market success may not be the most efficient or effective strategies from a risk management perspective. To achieve favorable results from both a risk management and an organizational perspective, the risk manager must recognize how the internal and external changes in health care created by managed care and the legal system influence or enhance risk. The risk manager should begin to plan a strategy by first identifying how the organization is influenced from a risk perspective caused by managed care (Exhibits 45–1 and 45–2). After this assessment, the risk manager should work with administration to determine critical success factors that will define risk management success for the organization (Exhibit 45–3).

Once the key measures of success have been agreed on, the risk manager can develop a plan to protect the organization and help it progress. The risk manager's role and the challenges posed by that role will not differ significantly if the risk manager is employed by an MCO, a hospital that seeks to be the hub of an integrated delivery system (IDS), or a network that forms to be able to compete under managed care. Thus, this chapter has been written to focus on the key risk management issues created by managed care as opposed to a specific job that a risk manager might assume given potentially differing structures. Many of the legal and risk management challenges created by managed care will exist regardless of the employer. The customers of the risk manager will include not only those in administration and finance but also physicians, nurses, and patients and other consumers. As the scrutiny on MCOs and the providers of care working for those organizations increases, risk managers must develop new knowledge and use existing and new skills and techniques to identify the new risks created, design creative strategies for managing those new risks, and provide education and information to an ever-increasing and divergent customer base.

CHANGES IN THE HEALTH CARE ORGANIZATION RELATED TO MANAGED CARE

Managed care initially started out as "discount medicine," but it has now evolved to actual management of medical care by providing the patient with the appropriate level of care in the appropriate setting. In his book *Making*

Exhibit 45–1 Internal Environment Assessment

From	To
Focus on acute care hospital	→ Part of an integrated delivery system or network
Focus on clinical risk	→ Increasingly complicated with diverse risks
Focus on patients as customers	→ Many customers identified
Risks contained within single like entities	→ Risks extremely varied and increasingly complex
Reactive approach	→ Proactive approach
Multiple managers with autonomy	→ Streamlined individual management with shared responsibility
Focus on individual incidents	→ Focus on "big picture," requiring ability to track, trend, and benchmark
Data generated for internal use	→ Risk management data provided to payers and consumers
Risk management activities centralized and well defined	→ Risk management activities shared or delegated
Monopolistic	→ Focus on free market
Volume-driven staffing	→ Organization streamlined by function
Internal stability	→ Chaotic environment with multiple changes
Physician driven	→ Market driven
Professional roles clearly defined	→ Roles of health care professionals blurred by multidisciplinary and crossfunctional training

Source: Reprinted from B. Youngberg, Risk Management Strategic Planning for a Changed Health Care Delivery System, *Managing the Risks of Managed Care*, p. 25, © 1996, Aspen Publishers, Inc.

Exhibit 45–2 External Environment Assessment

From		To
Managing episodes of care	→	Managing covered lives
Managing illness	→	Managing health
Primary risk of clinical exposure	→	Organizations at significant financial risk due to changes in payment and access
Appropriate care determined and quality defined by providers	→	Reimbursable care and definition of quality determined by payers and legislators
Ethical decisions regarding health care made by hospitals and providers	→	Ethical standards set by consumer and various legislators
"Hospital-contained" risks	→	Risks prevalent in many settings, varied, and unique
Risk management reliant on conceptual and philosophical skills	→	Risk management requiring enhanced technical and theoretical skills while retaining interpersonal and communication skills
Privileged data not shared	→	Data widely shared

Source: Reprinted from B. Youngberg, Risk Management Strategic Planning for a Changed Health Care Delivery System, *Managing the Risks of Managed Care*, p. 26, © 1996, Aspen Publishers, Inc.

Exhibit 45–3 Organizational/Risk Management Critical Success Factors

- Develop a systematic process for proactively identifying the nature and severity of risks created or acquired through the expansion into diverse health care services that might include for-profit activities.
- Collaborate on a methodology for quantifying the financial risk inherent in managing the care of populations through capitated arrangements or other payer-driven financing strategies.
- Determine the risk tolerance of the organization, and design the most advantageous risk transfer and risk sharing program.
- Develop a strategy for managing and controlling the clinical, administrative, and contractual liabilities arising out of delivering care in the changing health care environment.
- Develop and provide innovative strategies and tools that will contribute to improvement of patient care and service.

Managed Health Care Work: A Practical Guide to Strategies and Solutions, Peter Boland states the following: "Managed care alters the decision making of providers of health care services by interjecting a complex system of financial incentives, penalties, and administrative procedures into the doctor-patient relationship. Managed care often attempts to redefine what is best for the patient and how to achieve it most economically."[2(p.3)] This economic focus, however, has been challenged recently by numerous state legislatures and state courts and has shifted dramatically in the direction of the patient-consumer, often without consideration of the cost.

Managed care administrators, insurance providers, and risk managers are becoming increasingly aware of the development of new case law associated with managed care, particularly how quality or access is limited by strict use or financial restrictions and how that limitation can pose a significant financial and legal risk to the organization. Learning how to identify proactively these and other potential new exposures associated with managed care and how to control or eliminate them will be a challenge and will be at the core of the risk manager's responsibility.

Historically, MCOs have faced minimal professional liability exposure, especially compared with other health care organizations. In large part, this is the result of the broad and well-publicized protection provided by the Employee Retirement Income Security Act of 1974 (ERISA; see Chapter 66).[3] That protection includes barring jury trials and punitive damage awards, limiting compensation to medical expenses, and preempting actions against an MCO for the administration of an ERISA-qualified employee benefit plan.[4] The Federal Employee Health Benefits Act (see Chapter 54) can also afford some protection for federal employee benefit plans.[5] These statutory protections have their limits, however, and as has already been described, in some states (California and Texas by legislative action and Illinois by their state Supreme Court), have already been eroded. Risk managers must develop a clear understanding of the new risks that may be created under managed care that are not afforded statutory protection and must develop strategies to manage them. Fundamental to these strategies will be the development of policies, procedures, protocols, marketing information, and patient contractual and benefits information that specifically limits the exposure of the organization and that also limits the corporate entity from directly (and negatively) interfering with the patient-provider relationship and plan of care.

The changes in the organization relative to managed care create new operational and clinical risks and opportunities for risk management. No longer are the risks contained within the walls of a provider organization; rather, the risks now follow the patients to whom the MCO has agreed to provide services. This may result in making the environment more difficult to control for the risk manager. In addition, with the movement away from high-technology specialties, many organizations may find the need to identify and engage providers with a focus on primary care and prevention. This group of professionals may include physicians but may also include nurse practitioners, physician assistants or extenders, social workers, and other health care professionals. Credentialing, reappointment, privilege delineation, and definition of the scope of service for an enhanced range of caregivers will be essential components of the risk manager's job.

OPERATIONAL RISKS UNDER MANAGED CARE

Operational risks are enhanced under managed care. For example, a provider organization becomes more complex as it attempts to compete by becoming part of an IDS (see Chapter 4). New business risks can create corporate liability, both direct and indirect (vicarious). A risk manager whose responsibility is to manage the risks of the MCO must be mindful of the business and clinical risks created. *Managed care plans can pose the following risk concerns that will be new challenges for the organization's risk manager:*

- coordinating the appropriate amount and level of care, by appropriate providers, through utilization management activities, being certain that needed care is not denied because of the organization's desire to cut costs and educating patients and providers about the appeals process available to argue against decisions that are made
- negotiating arrangements with selective providers with proven skills and competence to provide comprehensive services identified in the contracts and clearly spelling out the relationship between the provider and the MCO in the contracts with providers and patients
- ensuring that the operational protocols developed by management are sufficient to sustain the organization and that the potential for catastrophic financial risk is understood and appropriately funded for or transferred
- relative to physician compensation, the risk manager should also be cognizant of the government's current position relative to gainsharing programs that use financial incentives to financially reward providers who manage (or in the mind of the consumer, limit) care for Medicare patients. For physicians that an MCO contracts with directly, there are limitations on the amount of financial risk that the physician can be given (see Chapters 8 and 55). Given recent Office of the Inspector General (OIG) and

Health and Human Services (DHHS) opinions, the use of gainsharing by IDSs as a method of provider compensation should be avoided; see Chapters 9 and 65 for further discussion of this issue

- understanding the nature of the new clinical risks created and proactively designing systems or structures to eliminate or control them (This would include gaining an understanding as to consumer expectations regarding use of all treatment options.)

Figure 45–1 illustrates the relative risk for managed care structures on the basis of the degree of influence and relationships that the MCO maintains with its providers.[6] It is only through an analysis of the MCO's business and an understanding of the relative risk associated with that business that one can develop a comprehensive risk management plan to ensure that all risks created are eliminated, managed, controlled, or transferred.

MANAGING CORPORATE NEGLIGENCE

Direct Liability

Corporate negligence claims arising from managed care pose new risks for the risk manager. Corporate liability claims are based on the premise that the health care entity or MCO has a legal duty to protect the patient from harm. This responsibility can be deemed to be abrogated when negligent providers are employed by the MCO or IDS and render care to patients that is determined to be negligent. The need to develop rigorous screening procedures for potential staff members and to follow those procedures is an important risk management function in this new environment and should be carefully monitored to verify adherence.

Under the doctrine of corporate negligence, an MCO and its physician administrators may be held directly liable to patients or providers for failing to investigate adequately the competence of health care providers it employs or with whom it contracts, particularly when the MCO actually provides health care services or restricts the patient's/enrollee's choice of physician. MCOs and their physician administrators may be held liable for bodily injury to patients/enrollees resulting from improper credentialing of physicians or for economic or compensatory damages to providers as a result of credentialing activities (e.g., unlawful exclusion from provider networks or staff decertification). The doctrine of corporate negligence may also apply to other managed care activities besides credentialing, such as performance of utilization review. As already stated under recently enacted legislature and various state court opinions, an MCO can now also be found directly liable for administrative decisions that have a negative impact on patient outcomes or that prevent or limit certain types of services.

Under the theory of negligent or improper design or administration of cost-control systems, an MCO and its physician administrators may be held liable when they design or administer cost control systems in a manner that interferes with the rendering of quality medical care or corrupts medical judgment. To date, most litigation involving allegations of negligent administration of a cost-control system have involved utilization review activities of MCOs.

Figure 45–1 Relative Risk for Managed Care Structures. PPO, preferred provider organization; IPA, independent practice association; HMO, health maintenance organization.

MCOs and their physician administrators are also susceptible to antitrust liability for violations of federal and state antitrust laws, which generally prohibit the unlawful restraint of trade, monopolies, price fixing and discrimination, group boycotts, illegal tying arrangements, exclusive dealing, and other arrangements that are anticompetitive. Antitrust problems may arise when entities engage in collective actions that reduce competition in a given market. Antitrust problems can arise early in a market when managed care encourages the combining of the services of former competitors to facilitate service delivery. A balancing test must be performed to ensure that the benefits gained by combining outweigh the danger posed by limiting competition of those entities outside the agreement. Managed care networks are also likely to face an increased number of antitrust lawsuits from providers and competitors as they gain increased market share. The larger an MCO becomes in a particular area, the fewer opportunities are available to the provider who is not part of the network. This issue is discussed extensively in Chapter 63.

In addition, MCOs and their physician administrators face corporate exposure and direct liability for various forms of discrimination, for example discrimination in benefit design, underwriting, claims adjudication, credentialing, treatment, employment, and contracting. The following pieces of legislation may give rise to allegations of discrimination in specific managed care plans:

- the Family and Medical Leave Act of 1993
- the Americans with Disabilities Act of 1992
- the Civil Rights Act of 1991
- the Age Discrimination in Employment Act of 1967, including the Older Workers Benefit Protection Act of 1990
- Title VI of the Civil Rights Laws of 1964, as amended (1983), including the Pregnancy Discrimination Act of 1978
- the Civil Rights Act of 1966, Section 1981
- the Fifth and Fourteenth Amendments of the U.S. Constitution

MCOs and their physician administrators may also face corporate liability for invasion of the privacy of providers for improper dissemination of information regarding credentials or competence to the National Practitioner Data Bank or other third parties or of patients/enrollees for improper dissemination of their records or information pertaining to their health. They may also be sued by providers, patients, or employees for defamation, particularly in connection with their peer review activities. In such an event, however, they may be entitled to qualified immunity under the Health Care Quality Improvement Act of 1986 (HCQIA).

Vicarious Liability

Under the theory of vicarious liability or ostensible agency, hospitals and provider entities, including MCOs, have been held vicariously liable for the acts, errors, and omissions of their independent contractors. Until recently, a provider of an MCO was deemed to be an independent contractor in independent practice associations and direct contract models. Therefore, the MCO was not held responsible for negligent acts unless it had given the impression that these providers were acting as agents of the MCO. The decisions of the courts to uphold claims based on ostensible agency depend on many factors, applicable state statutes, the ability of the plaintiff's attorney to demonstrate the apparent agency relationship, and other aspects of the provider-MCO relationship as viewed by the courts. As has already been stated, court decisions and state legislatures are rapidly changing this area of liability.

Because appearance or perception seems to be the major issue driving the ostensible agency argument, it might be wise for the risk manager to consider some of the circumstances that might lead the public to assume that an agency relationship exists and to make the necessary arrangements to control these potential exposures. ***Factors that may give rise to the presumption of the existence of an agency relationship include:***

- supplying the provider with office space
- keeping the provider's medical records

- employing other health care professionals, such as nurses, laboratory technicians, and therapists, to support the physician provider
- developing promotional or marketing materials that allow a relationship to be inferred

The risk manager may wish to review documents provided to patients to ensure that the physician is described as an independent practitioner and that there is a clear distinction between those services provided by the MCO and those provided by the physician.

Clinical Risks

Managing clinical risks has been an activity of pivotal importance for the health care risk manager. This activity continues to be important, but there have been changes in its complexity under managed care. Specific risks that require control and relate to the provision of clinical care include risks associated with credentialing, risks associated with clinical decision making (e.g., rationing of care), risks associated with utilization review, and risks associated with adhering to externally imposed standards of care.

Credentialing

Credentialing is a risk management function that considers who the health care provider is in the MCO and what the provider can do.[7] In an effort to facilitate the credentialing process and reduce administrative burdens and costs, some entities may choose to participate in a joint credentialing process. This process might include a consolidation of credentialing procedures and a sharing of the information requested as part of the process. It will be important to have appropriate releases signed by the professional being credentialed so that there can be no subsequent claims for breach of confidentiality.

In general, a credentialing process must be developed that allows for the successful selection and retention of high-quality providers who understand and support the mission and vision of the organization or network with which they

work. See Chapters 7, 44, and 64 for further discussion of credentialing.

Measures that might be instituted to prevent or limit liability associated with credentialing include establishing realistic criteria, ensuring that the data being measured and evaluated are accurate, conveying and evaluating the criteria on a consistent basis, and creating a paper trail clearly tying quality to the economic credentialing process.[8] *The following is a checklist for risk managers to keep in mind when setting up a credentialing process:*[9]

- Review credentialing criteria for compliance with state statutes, standards for MCOs, Joint Commission on Accreditation of Healthcare Organizations standards, Medicare conditions of participation, National Committee for Quality Assurance, and court decisions.
- Review policies, procedures, bylaws, and contracts to ensure that all credentialing criteria are clearly stated and consistently applied.
- Review application forms for compliance with standards and local, state, and federal regulations.
- Review credentialing policies and procedures of other hospitals, facilities, and credentialing services whose credentialing decisions are used instead of an internal process.
- Review protocols for investigating and verifying an applicant's credentials. Do these protocols minimize the risk of inadequately screening and verifying the credentials of practitioners?
- Observe the methods by which these protocols are applied in reviewing individual applicants. Are protocols applied equally to all applicants whether they are well known or not?
- Evaluate the organizational structure of the credentialing process. Are checks in place to minimize the involvement of direct economic competitors in the credentialing process? Does the structure minimize the risk of creating antitrust liability?

- Review due process provisions to ensure that practitioners who are denied medical staff membership or have had privileges restricted are afforded a fair hearing in accordance with federal and state laws and standards.
- Require all practitioners to report claims, disciplinary proceedings, or adverse actions taken against them at other facilities or hospitals. Ensure risk management access to these records.
- Ensure that HCQIA regulations are complied with and that information from the National Practitioner Data Bank is used appropriately in credentialing and privileging determinations.
- Establish rapport with practitioners to facilitate open communication, education, and resourcefulness regarding risk management issues.

CLINICAL DECISION MAKING

One of the most frequently verbalized fears relative to managed care is that it will create a system whereby care is predicated on a person's ability to pay or on an externally imposed system of values that dictates which medical conditions are appropriate for specific types of intervention. In general, when these issues and concerns are voiced, they relate to the denial of interventions deemed to be extraordinary or experimental to patients with terminal conditions or conditions for which the treatment may not result in a cure but may only serve to delay inevitable furtherance of the disease. Although much of the discussion thus far seems to be fueled more by fear than fact, making care decisions based on reasons other than best medical judgment is risky and thus should be avoided. Risk managers can assist in limiting these types of risks by determining that policies are in place that clearly indicate that care decisions are not predicated on the ability of the patient to pay or the willingness of the payer to reimburse but rather on sound medical judgment that is rendered consistent with appropriate professional standards of care. Many of these decisions also are linked to an area of well-developed case law

in managed care, that law related to utilization review activities.

UTILIZATION MANAGEMENT ISSUES

Controlling the parameters of care through a well-detailed utilization review process is an important component of cost controls associated with managed care. Court cases have demonstrated that a plan's utilization review process is an operational exposure with the potential for considerable financial risk. A well-structured utilization review program is designed to limit the potential risks associated with attempts to structure care around predetermined criteria. The program should allow for retrospective, concurrent, and prospective review of care provided under the managed care plan and should provide for an appeal process that can be used by a provider and a patient. It should be remembered that underutilization presents potential threats to quality and risk just as overutilization presents threats to cost control.

EMERGING CASE LAW

The seminal case describing the liability that can attach to an organization with inappropriate utilization criteria is *Wickline v. State of California*.[10] This case addressed the legal implications of preadmission certification of treatment and length-of-stay authorization. In this case, suit was brought against the state of California alleging that its agency for administering the medical assistance program was negligent when it approved only a 4-day extension of the plaintiff's hospitalization when an 8-day extension was requested by the physician. Plaintiff's attorney alleged that the discharge was premature, resulting in the ultimate amputation of the plaintiff's leg. The physician requesting the 8-day extension did not appeal the decision of the state agency. Neither the hospital nor the physician was the defendant in this action.

A jury returned a verdict in the plaintiff's favor on the grounds that the plaintiff had suffered harm as a result of the negligent administration of the state's cost-control system. The trial court's decision was reversed by the appellate court, which found that the state had not been negligent and therefore was not liable. The court held that the state was not responsible for the physician's discharge decision and that a physician who complies without protest with limitations imposed by third-party payers when the physician's medical judgment dictates otherwise cannot avoid ultimate responsibility for the patient's care. The court did acknowledge, however, that an entity could be found liable for injuries resulting from arbitrary or unreasonable decisions that disapprove requests for medical care. The court emphasized that a patient who requires treatment and is harmed when care that should have been provided is not provided should recover for the injuries suffered from all those responsible for the deprivation of such care, including, when appropriate, health care payers. The court went on to say that third-party payers can be held legally accountable when medically inappropriate decisions result from defects in the design or implementation of cost-containment mechanisms. The court concluded from the facts at issue in this case that the California cost-containment program did not corrupt medical judgment and therefore could not be found liable for the resulting harm to the plaintiff.

In another case, *Wilson v. Blue Cross of California*, plaintiffs alleged that their son's suicide was directly caused by the utilization review firm's refusal to authorize additional days of inpatient treatment.[11] The patient had been admitted for inpatient psychiatric care for depression, drug dependency, and anorexia. His physician recommended 3 to 4 weeks of inpatient care, but the utilization review firm only approved 10 days. The patient was discharged and committed suicide less than 3 weeks later by taking a drug overdose. The trial court granted summary judgment in favor of the defendants. The appellate court reversed this decision, concluding that the insurer could be held liable for the patient's wrongful death if any negligent conduct was a substantial factor in bringing about harm. Testimony of the treating physician indicated that, had the decedent completed his planned hospitalization, there was a reasonable medical prob-

ability that he would not have committed suicide. The court concluded that whether the conduct of the utilization review contractor's employee was a substantial factor in the patient's suicide was a question of fact precluding summary judgment and remanded the case for further review. On retrial, the jury entered a verdict in favor of the defendants.

Litigation for utilization review decisions may also be brought under theories of bad faith and breach of contract on the basis of the contractual nature of the relationship between the MCO and its patient members.

REDUCING UTILIZATION MANAGEMENT EXPOSURE

The risk manager attempting to work with providers in the organization can provide the following advice to assist physicians in the reduction or elimination of exposures related to utilization review:

- *Devise a comprehensive utilization management program that integrates with quality and risk management.* Individuals performing utilization management functions should use patient outcome indicators as a means of identifying quality of care or risk problems.
- *Physicians must exercise independent medical judgment that meets with the standard of care.* Utilization management decisions should not influence the physician's clinical decisions in any way that the physician would consider truly harmful to the patient.
- *Providers must advise the MCO of their medical judgment.* The physician needs to be aware of each plan's utilization review process and to advise the plan of his or her medical judgment in clear terms. If a disagreement arises, the physician may need to support the validity of the clinical recommendations with documentation as to the medical necessity. Including diagnostic test results and providing an opinion as to the possible adverse outcomes should the request be denied will also be helpful.

- *Develop a "fast-track" second opinion program.* Providers need to support the development of a system that can quickly render a second opinion in case of disagreement surrounding clinical judgment. Ideally, the second opinion should be rendered by a health care professional whose skill and training are commensurate with those of the provider whose judgment is being questioned.
- *The patient should be informed of any issues that are being disputed relative to the physician's recommended treatment plan and the MCO's coverage decision.* Alternative approaches and the potential cost and outcome of those approaches should be discussed with the patient. Also, the patient should be informed that, if the plan continues to deny coverage, the patient may be responsible for payment. The patient should continue to be informed throughout the appeal process.
- *Exhaust the appeals process.* In the event that the treating physician firmly believes that the MCO has made an incorrect decision, the best defense in cases of treatment denials is staunch patient advocacy. The physician should request to speak to the medical director in charge of the utilization decision and explain the rationale behind the intended treatment. If a plan continues to deny coverage for a service that the physician believes is necessary, the process that allows for a second opinion fails to support treatment, and the physician continues to believe that the denial of coverage is in error, then the decision should be appealed aggressively. All avenues of appeal should be exhausted. If unsuccessful, the physician should inform the patient of treatment opinions without regard to coverage. The patient must ultimately decide whether to continue treatment at his or her cost. If the patient should wish to proceed at his or her own expense, the physician should have the patient sign an informed consent signifying awareness that such expenses may not be covered by the health plan.

- *Ascertain that insuring agreements include coverage for utilization review activities.*

EXTERNALLY IMPOSED PRACTICE GUIDELINES OR STANDARDS OF CARE

Many clinicians are particularly concerned about the development of practice guidelines that seek to define appropriate services that should be provided to a patient given a specific condition. In some instances, these guidelines are used to support utilization management decisions; in others, they may be developed in attempts to define best practice. Although developers often argue that best practice determinations are predicated on an evaluation of effectiveness, some providers believe that under managed care best practice really means lowest cost. To avoid the risks that are likely to be associated with the use of guidelines, clinicians should be assured that the existence of a guideline does not in and of itself create a standard of care and that guidelines, although they may be instructive, do not set standards of care (although well-developed guidelines should articulate agreed-upon standards of care; see Chapter 29). Risk managers should advise clinicians that, despite the existence of a guideline, their skill and judgment based on a careful assessment of the patient's condition can and should preempt the recommendations of a guideline. Case law, at least to date, supports this position.

MULTI-SITE CHALLENGES

The sheer number of sites where clinical care may be provided or that have affiliation or network agreements makes it essential that the risk manager create tools that can empower staff at these sites to understand and manage their own risks. Risk management will increasingly become a responsibility of all staff who will rely on the risk manager for support and advice but will ultimately be responsible for on-site control of risks inherent in the operation of their business. Tools that are developed should focus on those proactive strategies that enable all health care professionals working in a particular area to identify issues unique to their area that may give rise to risk and to modifying those risks in a manner that will allow for a safer environment with staff increasingly aware of the risks inherent in providing care in a specific area or setting. Tools that contain specific questions about an area can be developed and are useful for assisting managers and clinicians in recognizing and managing their own risks.

THE CONVERGENCE OF FINANCIAL AND RISK MANAGEMENT

Capitation

Managed care contracts create both opportunity and risk for health care organizations. Under many contracts the reimbursement from payers is capitated, with the health care organization receiving a fixed sum per member per month regardless of the intensity of services that the member receives. Understanding the financial risks assumed under these contracts and either funding for those risks or transferring them to a third party require many of the same skills that the risk manager uses to manage the clinical risks that are part of all health care organizations. Once the total risk being assumed is quantified, the risk manager, working with the chief financial officer or managed care plan administrator, can evaluate the best ways either to fund for or to transfer this risk.

Financial Incentives and Cost Control Programs

Incentive payment systems link provider compensation to the provision of cost-effective health care. An incentive system is meant to encourage providers to render only care that is necessary and appropriate (see Chapters 8, 9, 10, and 11). Financial incentives can take a variety of forms, and depending on the outcome of care, patients may view the incentive programs as having influenced their providers' medical decision making.

Cases are beginning to emerge that allege that physicians whose salaries are based in part on an incentive structure that predicates payment for services based on utilization of services make treatment decisions based more on their financial reward than on the well-being of the patient. It is imperative that financial incentives be structured in such a way that they do not have the appearance of encouraging this type of behavior.

Whether the cost control program of the MCO creates a financial incentive for physicians to provide inadequate treatment was raised in a recent legal opinion.[12] The case involved a delay in the diagnosis of cervical cancer because of the failure of the primary care physician to order a Pap smear. In this case, an MCO participant brought suit against the MCO alleging that the contractual agreements between the MCO and its providers encouraged physicians not to refer patients to specialists. The court found that the plaintiff had offered evidence establishing that the cost-control system contributed to the delay in diagnosis and treatment. A formal opinion on this issue was never rendered, however, because the case was settled during trial for an undisclosed amount.

In another well-publicized case, *Fox v. HealthNet*, a California jury awarded nearly $90 million to the estate of a breast cancer patient arising from the refusal of the MCO to pay for a bone marrow transplant; $77 million was awarded as punitive damages.[13] The MCO considered this procedure experimental and would not pay for any experimental treatment until it was proven effective. According to reports in the press, testimony at the trial included that of two women for whom the MCO had approved identical treatments as proof that the treatment might have worked.[14] Furthermore, it was shown that the physician executive who denied payment for the bone marrow transplant received bonuses on the basis of denial of costly medical procedures. The jury concluded that the MCO acted in bad faith, breached its contract of care with its subscriber, and intentionally inflicted emotional distress.

This case represents a good example of how denial of access to treatment can expose an

MCO to liability. It also demonstrates how the emotional impact and negative publicity associated with the denial of treatment, even if the treatment has not been proven effective, can influence the ultimate decision and the damage award. In a managed care environment, the primary care physician, in conjunction with the MCO, acts as a gatekeeper in determining what hospital or specialty physician services should be provided. The failure to meet the applicable standard of care in making these decisions can expose the primary care physician and the MCO to liability. In the Fox case, the treating physician recommended the treatment with the support of the two other MCO physicians who had used it for the two witnesses in the case, and the MCO, as gatekeeper, refused to pay for it.

These cases reveal that courts are willing to impose liability on MCOs when inappropriate medical decisions result from defects in the design or implementation of the cost-containment programs, breach of contract, or bad faith in the denial of payment. The impact of an MCO's financial incentives to contain costs has also been tested. If financial incentives result in inadequate treatment being rendered, the MCO could be held liable. These cases indicate that members will seek redress if harmed as a result of the administration of cost control programs that deny them access to care, that delay care, or that deny payment for necessary care.

The OIG and the DHHS have recently issued clear proclamations disfavoring gainsharing as a form of compensation, which is predicated on the control of cost and service. Risk managers and financial officers should be wary of using any type of compensation structure that could be viewed as a gainsharing arrangement.

Avoiding Liability Associated with Cost-Control Programs

The design and administration of cost-control programs should promote efficient care but must not corrupt the medical judgment of the physician. If an MCO overrides the medical judgment of the physician, it could be held liable for the consequences of the treatment or discharge deci-

sion. ***To avoid liability in this regard, an MCO needs to ensure that its financial incentive and cost-control programs include procedures that accomplish the following:***

- use medical necessity criteria that meet acceptable standards of medical practice
- review all pertinent records in determining the necessity of treatment
- contact the treating physician before certification is denied
- allow sufficient time to review the claim before denial
- ensure that medical personnel approving payment denials are appropriately trained, have met established minimum qualifications, and have the requisite knowledge to assess the appropriateness of care
- maintain policies and procedures that ensure that operations do not interfere with the physician-patient relationship regarding the duration and level of medical care
- carefully document procedures used to deny certification of care (coverage restrictions need to be adequately described in materials given to MCO members, especially with respect to experimental or investigational treatments)
- devise a mechanism for communicating programs to members

Risk Financing

The professional liability and business risks that are associated with managed care have fairly consistently been insurable under standard insurance contracts. Many creative products and concepts are being developed for the control or minimization of the financial risks that are inherent in capitated contracts or for the balance sheet fluctuations that are possible during a period of time when there is considerable volatility in the financing of health care services. The concepts underlying the financing of all these risks are the same and are consistent with the risk-financing skills that were practiced by many risk managers before the emergence of managed care.

USING THE RISK MANAGEMENT PROCESS TO CONTROL THE RISKS OF MANAGED CARE

The risk management process is generally structured around loss reduction techniques (which include the identification of risk, the elimination of risk whenever possible, and the control or management of risk when it cannot be entirely eliminated) and loss transfer (techniques that include determining the economic risk associated with various types of loss and selection of the best methods either to finance risk internally or to transfer those risks to a third party, generally through the purchase of insurance). These processes can be successful in managing the emerging risks that are created by a managed health care system. Obviously, the techniques will need to be tailored to the specific needs of each organization, particularly as managed care becomes increasingly dominant.

Because it is essential that the risk manager understand the scope of potential risk in the hospital, health network, or IDS, the first step will be to develop effective communication links with those parts of the organization that are responsible for the strategic growth of the hospital into a managed care partner or into the hub of a managed care network. Anticipating risk and being able to plan for it will greatly enhance the likelihood that risks created by the new delivery model will be capable of being controlled. Educating all staff, including administration and health care providers, about the emerging risks that are associated either with the delivery system created by managed care or with the clinical delivery system that is more decentralized because of managed care will be an important function for the risk manager. The risk manager may achieve the greatest success by developing tools that can be used by others to assess and manage their own risk. Making each member of the health care team responsible for managing the risks created by this complicated new health care delivery model will be the only way to ensure success.

CONCLUSION

Risk managers must continually monitor emerging risks and design comprehensive strategies for managing them. Unlike the traditional role of the risk manager in a hospital, where a single person or a designated risk management staff is central to the risk management effort, in an MCO or IDS everyone will have to become engaged in the process of proactively identifying and managing risks. *A brief checklist follows that will assist the risk manager in managing the process of providing health care in a managed care environment:*

- Design department-, unit-, or function-specific assessment tools that can be used easily by managers and clinicians to assess risks associated with specific environments or activities. Make risk management everyone's responsibility!
- Continually monitor case law and legislative actions that have an impact on managed care and design a system to provide information about new developments to all staff working in the MCO or network and to proactively manage the new risks created.
- Never underestimate the importance of a rigorous credentialing process that allows for the careful screening of all health care providers, physicians, and advanced practitioners. Make certain that this process is in compliance with state and federal law and that it measures both credentials and competence.
- Verify that a comprehensive process exists for utilization management activities. Ascertain that decisions about patient care are based on the best interest of the patient, not primarily the financial interest of the provider or the MCO.
- Develop a system that allows risk managers to be involved in the assessment of potential new business opportunities or entities before they become part of the organization

or network. This will allow for a clear understanding of the risks to be assumed and for the development of a plan to control, eliminate, or transfer those risks.

- Develop the risk management role as one of a consultant whose advice and expertise are

sought whenever issues of potential liability arise.

- Limit the degree of risk that an individual physician bears for medical costs.
- Avoid the use of gainsharing in an IDS as a method for physician compensation.

REFERENCES AND NOTES

1. B. Youngberg, *Essentials of Hospital Risk Management* (Gaithersburg, MD: Aspen Publishers, 1990).

2. P. Boland, *Making Managed Health Care Work: A Practical Guide to Strategies and Solutions* (Gaithersburg, MD: Aspen Publishers, 1993).

3. Employee Retirement Income Security Act of 1994, 29 U.S.C. Section 1001 et seq.

4. *Corcoran v. United Healthcare, Inc.*, 965 F.2d 1321 (5th Cir. 1992), *cert. denied*, 113 S.Ct. 812 (1992).

5. Federal Employees Health Benefits Act, 56 U.S.C.A., Section 8901 et seq.

6. R.J. Hester, *Managed Care Liability Concerns*, in 1992 Health Care Law Update (Florida Bar Lecture Program, 1992).

7. B. Youngberg, *Managing the Risks of Managed Care* (Gaithersburg, MD: Aspen Publishers, 1996).

8. C.S. Doyle, Managing the Risks of Managed Care, *Journal of Healthcare Risk Management* 14 (1995): 3–7.

9. S. Hagg-Rickert, Medical Staff Credentialing and Privileging Determinations: The Emerging Role of the Risk Manager, *Perspectives in Healthcare Risk Management* 11 (1991): 2–4.

10. *Wickline v. State of California*, 192 Cal.App.3d 1630, 239 Cal. Rptr. 810 (Ct. App.); *cert. granted*, 727 P.2d 753, 231 Cal. Rptr. 560 (1986); *review dismissed, case remanded*, 741 P.2d 613, 239 Cal. Rptr. 805 (1987).

11. *Wilson v. Blue Cross of California*, 271 Cal. Rptr. 876 (Cal. Ct. App. 1990), *review denied*, No. S017315, 1990 Cal. LEXIS 4574 (Cal. 1990).

12. *Bush v. Dake*, File No. 86-25767 No-2 (Mich. Cir. Ct. 1987).

13. *Fox v. HealthNet*, No. 219692 (Cal. Super. Ct. 1992).

14. *Los Angeles Times* (7 April 1994): D-1.

SUGGESTED READING

American Society of Healthcare Risk Management. *Journal of Healthcare Risk Management*. Chicago, IL: American Hospital Association. A quarterly journal devoted to relevant risk management issues.

Benda, C.G., and Rozovsky, F.A. 1996. *Managed Care and the Law*. Boston: Little, Brown & Co.

Berkowitz, S. 1991. *Managing Risks and Quality in Hospital Related Managed Care: A Guide to Hospitals*. Chicago, IL: The Institute on Quality Care and Patterns of Practice, The Hospital Research and Education Trust, American Hospital Association.

Creed, B.B., Corcoran, M.E., and Leitner, M. 1993. Managing the Legal Risks of Managed Care Programs, 390–

395. *Driving Down Health Care Costs: Strategies and Solutions*. New York: Panel Publishers.

Harding, J. 1994. Risk Management in an IPA Setting. Part I. *Physician Executive* 20 (5): 32–37.

Harding, J. 1994. Risk Management in an IPA Setting. Part II. *Physician Executive* 20 (6): 21–24.

Thomasson, G.O. 1994. Participatory Risk Management: Promoting Physician Compliance with Practice Guidelines. *The Joint Commission Journal on Quality Improvement* 20 (6): 317–329.

Youngberg, B.J. 1996. *Managing the Risks of Managed Care*. Gaithersburg, MD: Aspen Publishers.

Youngberg, B.J. 1994. *The Risk Manager's Desk Reference*. Gaithersburg, MD: Aspen Publishers.

CHAPTER 46

Common Operational Problems in Managed Health Care Plans

Peter R. Kongstvedt

INTRODUCTION AND BACKGROUND

Before the rise of managed health care, the health insurance industry, which was largely not-for-profit, would experience a predictable three-year cycle often referred to as the "underwriting cycle." The health insurer or Blue Cross Blue Shield plan would experience three years of positive margins (considered contributions to reserves in the not-for-profit plans) followed by three years of negative margins (or reductions in reserves). There is still debate about why this regular cycle occurred. Some believe it was due to state regulators requiring health plans with large reserves to lower their rates to take those reserves down and then raise rates when reserves became low. Others believe that it was market forces creating competitive pressures to lower rates when the plan could afford it to gain market share. Still others believe that it was basically inertia that caused the plan's underwriters to continually be writing premium rates based on data that were 18 months old at best and two years old in most cases. Whatever the reasons, this cyclic phenomenon was part of the business cycle in health insurance and was considered a routine event. The appearance of stability was deceptive.

By the 1980s, premium rates began to climb at an intolerable rate, and managed health care became an increasingly sought option for the provision of health benefits. Managed health care introduced not only new ways of managing medical care and controlling costs but also an increasing element of competition; the growing for-profit health insurance industry (and for-profit hospital) did likewise. The downward swings of the cycle began to exceed the positive ones, primarily in the old-line health insurers. Losses exceeded gains over the course of the cycle, and many older health plans found themselves in serious financial difficulties, failing to adapt to the new environment.

By the early 1990s, the predictable three-year cycle disappeared as managed care became the dominant form of health benefit.* What took its place was a more volatile period, with managed care organizations (MCOs) and insurance companies making large margins in some years and suffering substantial losses in others. Although these losses and gains were experienced by the managed care industry as a whole, there was no longer a predictable cycle. A drift toward a lower amplitude of swings in positive margins or losses began toward the late 1990s, and there has been some relative stabilization of this volatility as we have moved into the twenty-first century. Continual downward market pressure on premiums in the face of upward pressure on medical costs prevents a return to high profits: the days of MCOs making large profits because of their ability to control costs compared with unmanaged indemnity insurance have diminished as managed care has become predominant in the market.

---

*Whether the three-year cycle (or some other type of predictable cycle) will return is unknown, but there is no reason to believe that it will.

During this shift in the environment (i.e., the two last decades of the twentieth century), many new MCOs, primarily health maintenance organizations (HMOs) but also preferred provider organizations (PPOs) and other forms of financial risk-bearing MCOs, appeared and grew. And many of them failed. Acquisitions of financially weak plans by stronger rivals became common, but some of the newly merged health plans found themselves facing financial difficulties not long thereafter.

Consolidation continued, as did the continual appearance of new start-ups. Most mergers and acquisitions occurred because it made good business sense to the MCOs involved, not because of MCO failure or weakness. But failures did continue as well, especially among the smaller health plans. Failure was not rampant, however. The percentage of MCOs that have failed or were acquired to prevent failure has always been low: between 2 percent and 5 percent, with the notable exception of 1988, when roughly 14 percent of existing HMOs either failed or were acquired as a consequence of poor financial performance.

By the end of the 1990s, consolidation had reached the point where the number of operating Blue Cross Blue Shield plans had dropped dramatically because of regional mergers of smaller independent plans. The number of commercial managed care and health insurance companies likewise fell as a small group of large and successful companies acquired their smaller rivals, and several multiline commercial insurance companies decided to exit the health insurance business entirely and focus on nonhealth products and financial services. These events were less a consequence of financial failure than of business strategy.

Health plan failures still occurred, however. Although most health plan failures occurred in smaller plans as was always the case, some large and allegedly successful health plans experienced catastrophic financial losses. In all cases, the causes of the poor performance did not occur abruptly but took years. In some cases of failure, the financial hemorrhaging was drawn out over many years; in other cases the financial catastrophe appeared to be abrupt, but this was a result of poor financial management and reporting within the plan, not a sudden event. Some of these large, failed MCOs were acquired by healthier MCOs (often at the urging of the state insurance commissioner), a few obtained recapitalization and struggled to regain solvency (not always making it), and others were simply seized by the state and liquidated, and the members moved to the remaining health plans.

A similar set of events occurred in many integrated delivery systems (IDSs), large provider groups (e.g., large physician groups or independent practice associations [IPAs]), and physician practice management companies (PPMCs). As described in more detail in Chapter 4, some of these IDSs, IPAs, and PPMCs took on global capitation for all medical expenses but were utterly unable to manage it. Several massive failures, especially in PPMCs, occurred in the late 1990s, causing significant disruption to members, physicians, and MCOs. Although these provider organizations only carried out certain functions, primarily medical and reimbursement functions, the problems they encountered are still common to the industry and are part of the set of problems discussed in this chapter.

COMMON VERSUS UNIQUE PROBLEMS OR EVENTS

It is certainly possible that a failure or severe financial condition may occur as a result of an atypical condition or event. One common such event is a lawsuit in which an adverse judgment against the plan results in a financial penalty so severe and punitive, and so unexpected from the point of view of the merits of the case, that the plan is unprepared to absorb the blow. Post-award settlements may reduce the severity, and insurance may likewise offset the impact, so that a single lawsuit is an uncommon reason for outright failure.

In a far different vein, a state or even the federal government may pass legislation that has profound unintended consequences, causing all operating MCOs to suffer severe financial losses. This is something that is becoming increasingly a part of operating in this industry, but it does affect all MCOs in that state, or in the case of federal legislation, the nation. The exception to the concept that all plans are affected equally is when the legislation or regulation applies only to one market segment such as Medicare or Medicaid, in which case MCOs with higher enrollment in those segments are disproportionately affected. In the latter situation, financial catastrophe may well occur caused primarily by this effect if the MCO is highly concentrated in an entitlement market that suddenly becomes untenable (e.g., a state may lower Medicaid payments to a point where no MCO can sustain operations).

Outside these two situations, some still may argue that all failures or severely negative operational results are unique to each situation. That may be true for certain specifics (e.g., the personalities of the senior executives), but it is not true on the whole. All industries have in common sets of reasons for failure or operational difficulties. The managed health care industry is no different from any other type of business in that regard. It is possible to define that set of reasons, and that is the purpose of this chapter: to briefly define the most common causes of operational problems and mistakes in MCOs so as to help make a manager aware of them. Early detection could prevent severe damage to the plan.

Whether a problem occurs and how serious that problem is will depend on a variety of factors. None of the problems and common mistakes that are discussed in this chapter occur in isolation. Certain problems will be exacerbated by the presence of other, concurrent problems. It is rare for an MCO to proceed to a seriously adverse financial condition or even failure without several of the problems described in this chapter occurring simultaneously.

Not *all* of these problems would be found in the same plan at the same time, and as noted above, rarely will only one problem exist at a time. In general, troubled health plans will have problems in logical combinations. For example, if significant problems are occurring with expenses that are incurred but not reported (IBNRs), it is likely that the plan will also be having problems with claims processing and in-

accurate utilization reports. In some types of plans the relative dangers will be far less than in others. For example, plans that do not take risk for medical expenses (e.g., a MCO that serves primarily the self-insured market) may have less exposure to problems associated with utilization and cost but will be more vulnerable to problems associated with general administration.

COMMON PROBLEMS IN MANAGED CARE ORGANIZATIONS

This section provides brief descriptions of the most common problems and conditions that can occur in managed health care plans. Because it is an overview, it is necessarily high level rather than detailed. A problem described here will always have a root cause or causes, but there are too many such possible causes to enumerate. By recognizing the existence of one or more of these common problems, a manager may then know where to focus her or his attention and analyze the root causes. It is unlikely that a single root cause will be found, however, because there is such interrelationship between all activities of an MCO. Through the identification and resolution of one major cause of a problem, other related problems will be uncovered. The other chapters of this book provide the detail to understand the operational issues involved.

Undercapitalization

A classic problem in business, particularly for start-ups but also applicable to acquisitions and geographical expansions, undercapitalization is just as troublesome for health plans as for any other business. Losses can mount more quickly than anticipated, and if the pricing strategy was too low, losses can continue for quite some time. It is not uncommon for new plans to spend between $5,000,000 to $10,000,00 before getting to break-even status. Prevention is the best approach to this problem (that can be said for all the problems described in this chapter, but especially so here). The use of experienced actuaries to develop premium and cost models is always necessary, and a thorough analysis of market conditions should lead to the development of several different scenarios (best case, worst case, and expected case) that the actuary can use. Contingency plans must also be developed if enrollment expectations are not met (discussed later) but operational costs continue to be significant. The ability to leverage operational functionality on the basis of low capital commitment can also be a preventive option; for example, leasing or outsourcing basic enrollment and claims service to a competent third party for the first few years.

Undercapitalization can also occur as the result of sustained operating losses in a plan that has been operating for quite some time. Another cause for undercapitalization is an acquisition or acquisitions that result in a large decrease in capital caused by the acquisition cost and operating losses in the acquired entity. There are plenty of other ways for an MCO to lose serious money, but the point has been made. Although the use of the term "undercapitalization" is traditionally applied to start-up companies, a dangerous lack of capital for any reason will have some elements in common. The need to obtain capital will apply in any case, even though the causes for that need and the corrective actions will differ.

Unless an undercapitalized plan is amenable to fast repairs (e.g., sharp reductions in administrative cost or medical cost, or rapid increases in premium revenue), there are a limited number of responses available to management. One response is to lower cost outlays to the providers to assume the expenses, perhaps through mandatory fee reductions, or to use a reimbursement method that shifts significant financial risk for medical expenses to provider systems (which is a complicated strategy; see Chapters 4 and 8).

If the plan is large enough and has considerable assets that are nonadmitted, or not allowable, as part of the calculation of reserve requirements of the state (i.e., are not considered a liquid asset under the state's statutory accounting principles—see Chapter 47), then it may be able to arrange a sale/lease-back of the asset to convert it into cash. For example, the plan sells the nonadmitted assets such as furniture, the computer system, or even the building if it owns that, to a financing company. The financing company provides cash to the plan, and the plan leases back the furniture, etc. on a long-term basis. Although the total long-term cost of a sale/lease-back will be higher than owning the assets, the need for liquid capital far outweighs that cost.

Other routes for obtaining money from outside sources are issuing debt or selling equity. In either of these cases, the troubled plan is obviously dealing from a position of weakness and will usually pay the price of failing to obtain adequate capital earlier. If the plan has adequate reserves such that it is not in danger of state insurance department intervention, it may be able to obtain capital on terms that are acceptable, if costly. If the plan is in danger of not meeting minimum state reserve requirements, then obtaining capital will be quite difficult. In the case of bond issuance, the bonds may be rated as "junk bonds" and be required to pay a large return. A for-profit plan may be required to dilute current shareholders and sell any retained equity (assuming that there is any value in that) but will surely have to sell a high amount of equity at a very low price, with accompanying terms that allow the new investors to seize control and assets of the plan if conditions do not improve. Obtaining a bank loan or letter of credit may be difficult in a plan that is in danger of not meeting reserve requirements because the infused capital must be subordinated to the reserve requirement (i.e., the capital may only be used to meet reserve requirements and not reclaimed by the debt issuer as long as it is needed for reserves). Also, a loan or letter of credit cannot be secured by any asset that is also being used for purposes of calculating the reserves.

Expansion or start-up plans that are part of a large corporate parent may also turn to that parent corporation for capital, which may stave off insolvency but does not address the reasons that the plan was undercapitalized in the first place. Types of capital infusion would include the actual transfer of subordinated capital to the plan or more commonly a subordinated surplus note (i.e., promises to provide such capital, again subordinated to the troubled plan for purposes of meeting reserve requirements). In some states, the reserves of the parent company are considered in the aggregate for all subsidiaries if the parent corporation has clear responsibility for financial adequacy. However, some companies have crafted local incorporation terms such that the parent company cannot be held directly liable for reserve requirements or capital infusions; in those cases, the state insurance department will treat the subsidiary as though it were a free-standing plan.

In addition to the severe negative impact on operations and payment to providers, failing to have adequate capital may mean failing to meet state solvency requirements. When a plan reaches that stage, it may wind up in a forced merger with a healthy plan, in receivership to creditors, or seized by the state insurance department, which then controls its fate. Once the state has seized control, options include the state allowing the plan to work its way out, declaring bankruptcy to stave off creditors so that financial obligations to members and providers are always met first, forced sale of the plan, or the declaration of permanent insolvency, which results in the plan being shut down. If the plan is shut down, the members are usually allowed to enroll in the other health plans in the same service area, or the state may determine that only certain alternative health plans are strong enough to handle the forced increase in membership.

Unrealistic Projections

Any and all categories of revenue and expense are subject to unrealistic projections and expectations, but two stand out: overprojecting enrollment and underprojecting medical expenses.

In new plans, it is common to overestimate enrollment. The reasons are probably a combination of high optimism, inexperience of the marketing director, failure to correctly forecast and reforecast enrollment on an account-specific basis, and an unrealistic start date. Unless the marketing director is a seasoned veteran, the forecast may include accounts considered sold that were only being polite, a factor may be added for new business even when the source and probability of that business are in doubt, or a standard penetration factor may be used that fails to address competitiveness in the account. If the plan does not go operational when antici-

pated or if the delivery system is weaker than the anticipated delivery system used to forecast enrollment, significant negative variations in projected growth can occur.

In the case of existing or mature plans, the common types of unrealistic projections are predicting a percentage growth consistent with past growth without knowing how that growth rate will be sustained. If the market has become saturated, customer service has eroded, premiums are too high, or competitors' products are more attractive, the impact on growth will be negative.

Certainly unanticipated events can blindside even the most experienced marketing director. Competing or invading plans may spark a price war, or a regulator may delay certification for unexpected reasons. For all these reasons, the best marketing projections are conservative ones. Some executive directors believe that enrollment projections should always be high to motivate the director of marketing through his or her bonus. Other executive directors may simply dictate to the marketing director what the growth rate will be, on the basis of desired performance, not market reality. Unfortunately, enrollment projections drive financial projections, so care must be taken, especially in new plans. It is one thing to create financial incentives to sales and marketing personnel on the basis of aggressive growth; it is another to base financial projections on unrealistic growth, no matter how fervently that growth rate is desired.

Underprojecting medical expenses, or overestimating ability to manage utilization, is equally common in new plans. As has been mentioned earlier, naïve managers sometimes assume that if they call themselves an HMO or a PPO and put some rudimentary controls in place, they will have the same results as an experienced and successful plan. If the medical director is inexperienced, or if the physicians on the panel are not used to effective medical management, it is unlikely that good utilization results will occur, unless by good luck.

Luck can also be bad. During the early stages of a plan's life, enrollment will be small enough so that a few bad cases can have an excessive impact on expenses. A common and critical mistake for new plan managers to make is to project utilization as though there will be few serious cases. When the cases occur, management keeps factoring out the cost of caring for those sick patients and measures utilization on the basis of the remaining members. Clearly, if one factors out sick patients, utilization will always look reasonable. This mistake can be partially offset by purchasing adequate reinsurance, but that comes at a cost.

Unrealistic projections of medical costs are especially likely to occur in IDSs or large provider groups taking on a high level of risk for medical expenses. This is usually due to the dual factors of adverse selection (discussed later) and a naïve grasp of medical management (i.e., a belief that utilization may be effectively managed without the need to perform the functions of medical management).

Predatory Pricing or Low-Balling

This refers to premium rates that are intentionally well below the actual cost of delivering care. This is usually found in start-up plans, although a mature plan may low-ball to preserve or rapidly gain market share in response to a competitor's rates. Price undercutting is a venerable tradition in a capitalistic system and has great usefulness in enhancing one's competitive stance. Buying market share is not necessarily a mistake under all circumstances, but it is a risky strategy that must be undertaken with great care.

There is an old cliché in business that goes: "If you sell dimes for a nickel, you can't make it up on volume." This is even more true in managed health care than in manufacturing. The manufacturer may hope to sell a service contract with the widget and recoup the loss or raise the price of widgets after a few months. The only thing a health plan sells is service; there are no benefits riders that will make up for a grossly underbid base premium. Further, once the plan signs up a group for a set premium rate, it usually has to live with that rate for at least a year, or longer if the plan "wins" a multiyear contract due to low rate guarantees. Even in accounts in which the plan is not bearing financial risk for medical ex-

penses (such as an administrative services only or self-funded account), the plan may suffer a financial penalty if it has guaranteed medical expense trends, and it will doubtless suffer a tarnished reputation for effective management, veracity, or both.

The purpose of low-balling is to drive enrollment up and buy market share. If a low-ball rate loses $10 per member per month (PMPM), and if the MCO succeeds in increasing enrollment by 5,000 members, it has succeeded in increasing losses by 5,000 x $10 PMPM, or $50,000 per month, or $600,000 per year. You cannot make it up on volume.

Occasionally, managers may low-ball primarily to cover high overhead costs (in other words, to get some cash flowing in) rather than as an attempt to get market dominance. In those cases, the losses from the fixed overhead are in fact attenuated by the premium revenue brought in, at least initially, even though the medical loss ratio is unacceptably high. Low-balling may provide a short-term fix for highly leveraged plans such as closed panels, but the long-term result is the same: As enrollment increases, the overhead required to provide service increases as well, leading to a continuing loss situation that may become more severe than anticipated.

In addition to sustained losses, low-balling is a market strategy that appeals to the most price-sensitive customers. That can be a set-up for a raid by a competitor that low-balls the rates even further. Unless another strategy is available, the plan could then end up in a price war and never recoup its losses.

None of this is to say that a plan may not have to hold rates down or even lower them for competitive reasons. This is to say that low-balling should never be the only competitive strategy. It should really be used only as an adjunct to a longer range strategy, and even then only with caution. Far too many plans have found that their pockets were not as deep as they thought or that they underestimated how deep those pockets would need to be.

A common and critical mistake by plan managers facing price competition is to lower the rates to unrealistic levels and simply budget expenses lower, usually medical expenses. Unless there is a clear and believable strategy for lowering those expenses, the savings will not materialize. It is not enough to order the medical director to harass the physicians and get costs down; there needs to be a more cogent plan for reducing expenses. Sadly, a manager under pressure frequently indulges in a combination of magical thinking and rule by decree. In other words, by decreeing that expenses must be reduced, the other managers will magically figure out how to do that despite not having succeeded the previous year. The lesson here is that if the rates are intentionally lowered, managers had better figure out specifically how they are going to reduce expenses in each category. If they cannot come up with a clear plan for each category, they should budget the loss.

Assuming that the decision has been made to try to recover some of the losses, the main question is whether to raise the rates in one breathtaking rate hike or to phase it in over a number of years. That decision must be made by analyzing the plan's financial resources, the market conditions, the customer's willingness to put up with a rate hike, the danger of losing significant enrollment in that group (which may or may not be a bad thing, depending on the degree of losses the plan is sustaining in the group; in turn this may lead to adverse selection, which is discussed later), and the plan's ability to control expenses. Of course, if the situation is bad enough, the state insurance commissioner may wind up making the decision unilaterally.

Overpricing

The antithesis of low-balling, overpricing simply refers to rates that are unacceptably high in the marketplace (i.e., overpriced for the market). This is usually found in mature plans, but occasionally it occurs in new plans that anticipate high costs or that have incurred unusually high preoperational expenses. Overpricing is becoming more rare in the current, highly competitive marketplace because purchasers simply will not overpay when good, less expensive alternatives exist. Nevertheless, overpricing is not extinct and remains an identifiable and even predictable problem for health plans.

There are four primary reasons for overpricing:

- A panic response to previous low-balling
- Excessive overhead
- Failure to control utilization properly
- Adverse selection

A panic response to previous low-balling is not unusual. As losses mount, plan management feels unable to weather the losses and tries to make up the revenue quickly. This is particularly true when a plan is being pressured by investors or regulators or when the plan's financial reserves are projected to be dangerously low. If the low-balling strategy has driven out competition (not a likely event), exorbitant rate hikes may occur simply as a natural course.

Excessive overhead may also lead to overpricing. If plan management is unable to improve efficiency, the price must be paid. Excessive overhead may occur in any plan. It occurs in new starts when required administrative support has been estimated on the basis of enrollment projections that fail to materialize. In mature plans, excessive overhead usually is traced to a combination of internal politics, or turf battles, and management's unwillingness or inability to explore new methods of managing the plan. If a mature plan is operating with grossly outmoded systems and/or multiple legacy systems, then the administrative cost to maintain those systems and perform the manual workarounds will add greatly to overhead.

High medical cost is a common reason for overpricing. If rising medical costs are due to endemic reasons, it is likely to affect all plans in the area. For example, rapid increases in drug benefit costs are usually not confined to a single plan. In that case, it is also likely that all plans will raise prices and less likely that one single plan will do so. The occurrence of cost inflation is not the same as overpricing.

If a plan's utilization is high compared with competitors, it may be easier to raise prices than to deal with the causes of overutilization. The usual rationalization goes something like this: "The reason we have the highest rates is that we have the best physicians, and so we have the sickest patients. It's all adverse selection!" In these cases, the plan has often marketed benefits comparable to or better than those of competing plans and has assumed utilization rates similar to those of experienced HMOs (after all, if you call yourself an HMO, you should perform like one, right?) but has imposed fewer controls on physicians and hospitals. Rather than impose restrictions on the network and tighten management, managers (especially medical managers) indulge in the common fantasy that they are doing the best they can and it is all the fault of external events.

Bear in mind, however, that excessively high rates do indeed lead to adverse selection. This is especially true in two situations. The first situation is when an account allows more than one health plan to market to employees, in contrast to a total replacement account, where no competing health plans are allowed to market (an increasingly uncommon situation). In a multiple-choice environment, if the plan becomes too expensive for most people, only those facing high medical costs will choose to enroll because the plan's premiums are still less than the coinsurance and deductibles they would face with the competition. A related phenomenon has been a classic problem with indemnity insurance when multiple HMOs are offered: Despite high premium rates in the indemnity plan, individuals with high medical costs and an affinity with a provider not in the managed care plan will enroll at almost any premium cost. This is often referred to as the "insurance death spiral."

The second common situation is in a free-choice environment, such as is found in a purchasing cooperative or in the public sector market (i.e., Medicare and Medicaid). In this situation, analogous to what was just described, each individual can choose between several alternatives. A high-priced plan with a large provider panel will remain attractive to sick individuals, whereas healthy individuals may choose a less-expensive plan despite a smaller network because they feel healthy and have other bills to pay (and can thus use the savings for other needs). This situation is especially dangerous for provider-sponsored health plans that may easily enroll existing patients but not attract nonpatient members with few health problems.

Uncontrolled Growth

Rapid growth is usually greeted with applause. In fact, many readers of this book may be saying to themselves, "I wish we had such problems," but rapid growth is not always a good thing (dandelions and kudzu come to mind). Certainly growth is a necessary ingredient to long-term success, but if growth is too rapid, it can lead to problems that are long in resolving. There are several reasons for rapid growth. The market may be hot, the products and prices highly competitive (but if prices are low-balled, then problems are magnified as discussed previously), the sales and marketing department may be extremely well run, the competition left town, or other reasons.

Rapid growth may also be a result of an acquisition of a competing health plan or even multiple acquisitions over a short time. Mergers and acquisitions create their own host of management and operational issues surrounding the need to integrate the combined companies. Some of those issues are the same as discussed in this chapter, whereas others are unique to mergers (e.g., rationalization of services and the number and location of employees required to operate the plan). Those unique issues are not within the scope of this chapter.

Although it is uncommon, a plan may also experience rapid growth because of the failure of a competitor. If the competing health plan is known to be financially unstable, it is common for that plan's customers and members to seek out an alternative health plan that will provide stability. If the weak plan actually fails, then the state's insurance commissioner may dissolve the plan and apportion the failed plan's enrollment to the remaining plans.

Closely related to the problem of overextended management (see later), the problems of uncontrolled growth have a generalized impact: rapid growth not only may quickly outstrip the ability of the plan's managers to keep up, but may outstrip the system's capabilities as well. Dysfunctional patterns can set in, such as referral patterns or utilization behaviors that are more difficult to change after the fact than if they were addressed early on. Because the systems and management capabilities in the plan may now be inadequate, the developing problems will not be picked up until they are serious.

Rapid growth also means rapid expansions in the delivery system. The same attention paid to recruiting and credentialing in the development stages may not be present, and there may be little or no time spent properly orienting new providers to the plan's policies and procedures. That ultimately leads not only to inefficient practice patterns but to frustration on the part of those new providers.

Conversely, rapid growth can lead to saturation of the delivery system before there is adequate recruiting to take up the volume. This becomes especially problematic when practices begin to close to new patients more quickly than directory printing can accommodate, and new groups are enrolled with inaccurate directories of providers (or directories are distributed with addendums falling out onto the floor). Although a plan may be able to update directories on their Internet websites, a large number of members and physicians still rely on printed directories. In many cases, the physician practices will decide to close before they even notify the plan, and new members are signed up for those practices only to be turned away when calling for an appointment.

Service erosion is common when growth has been too rapid. Identification cards are not produced on time (and produced inaccurately), claims are not paid properly, telephone calls to the plan are not answered in a timely or quality manner, evidence of coverage statements are not sent out on time, inadequate information is given to new members, and so forth. Poor service leads to a vicious circle of ever-escalating problems resulting in a poor reputation that takes a long time to recover from.

Rapid growth may also result in insufficient claims reserves. In periods of rapid growth, the usual methods of calculating claims reserves and

IBNR become less reliable. This issue is discussed later in this chapter.

Last, rapid growth may lead to inadequate reserves. If reserves were adequate for a small plan, utilization in a plan suddenly grown large may take those reserves down to a dangerously low level, and the reserve requirements rise in proportion to the enrollment of insured members (usually on the basis of the risk-based capital formula discussed in Chapter 49).

One approach to the problem of rapid growth is to limit increases in enrollment through decreased offerings and marketing. This has been done by a few plans in the past and is a viable approach. The risk to this is that the competition will pick up the members, and the plan will never catch up. For that reason, most plan managers are reluctant to turn off the tap unless it is a critical situation.

If rapid growth is possible or even certain, strategies and tactics for dealing with rapid growth can be ready for implementation before the MCO's back is against the wall. Plan for expansion of the plan's information and computer systems. Groom potential candidates for managerial promotion; consider delegating certain responsibilities before such delegation is required. Some amount of physician recruiting activity should always be occurring, especially in areas without a great deal of capacity, although the rate of actual contracting needs to be coordinated with projected enrollment increases. Careful attention to staffing levels and training lead times in service areas such as claims and member services will help a great deal, although if projected enrollment does not occur, the overhead to the plan can become crushing. For this reason, having the strategies and tactics planned out is valuable, but overstaffing in anticipation of growth that may not occur may be harmful.

Failure To Manage a Reduction in Growth

There are two major components to this topic: failure to grow and failure to manage the consequences of a flattened or even negative growth rate. The first subject, failure to grow, is a fundamental issue of marketing that is addressed in

Chapter 41 and will not be addressed here. The second subject, failure to manage the consequences of flattened or negative growth is addressed here. In other words, the focus of this discussion is not on what should be done in sales and marketing to stimulate growth but rather the effects on other aspects of the health plan.

Periods of rapid growth commonly cause the claims liabilities and IBNR to be understated. When growth flattens, the claims lag catches up and the medical loss ratio begins to rise rapidly. In other words, the numerator (medical costs) goes up as costs come in, while the denominator (revenue) remains flat because of flattened growth. This important topic is discussed separately later in this chapter.

As a health plan grows, the administrative and operational requirements must grow along with the enrollment. Growth can outstrip operational capabilities as noted earlier. Sooner or later, though, operations expands to meet the need. This expansion will be a mix of automated support and human resources, although the more complex the operations (e.g., unusual benefits plans being sold, or reimbursement methods that cannot be supported by the plan's information systems), the more the need for personnel to manually provide the service.

Theoretically, this expansion in operations should provide economies of scale because lesser-paid clerical personnel are added more rapidly than higher-paid management personnel. This theoretical advantage is almost always negated by the creation of new departments and functions that require staffing of their own, and the surreptitious creation of management activities that seem to function solely to serve other management activities that serve solely to support other management activities, and so forth until the circle is complete. As MCOs grow larger, more management and reporting activities take place that are more distant to the actual operating needs of the company.

As long as growth is robust, this is tolerable. But if growth flattens or diminishes, the ability to support the cost of administration becomes strained. If this flattening takes place early in the plan's life, adjustments in the cost structure may

be relatively easy because management is less complex. Furthermore, if a small plan fails to successfully address lack of growth for long, managing overhead will be a function of being acquired or liquidated and so need not be further addressed here.

Mature plans experiencing flattened or negative growth face more complex issues. The diminished ability to afford the current level of overhead does not mean that costs can be easily cut, although it is common for an organization in this situation to simply demand a 10 percent cost reduction in all departments as a first measure. This meat-ax approach will provide some temporary relief, and if the plan has never undergone cost reductions before it can sustain an across-the-board cut without a great deal of disruption in operations.

More insidious are the costs associated with having become a more complex MCO. There are several aspects to this, but the most important is an inadequate management information system (MIS), which is discussed later in this chapter; the diminished ability to produce meaningful reports in an adequate time frame, which is also discussed later in this chapter; and the need for manual interventions caused by complex or irregular benefits plans and provider reimbursement mechanisms, which are discussed in various chapters in this book (e.g., Chapters 8, 11, 12, 38, 39, and 40). Meeting new regulatory requirements such as are found in the Health Insurance Portability and Accountability Act (HIPAA; see Chapter 67) and Medicare+Choice (see Chapter 55) compound the problem.

With the specifics of each of these major aspects of high operational overhead addressed elsewhere, the point of this section is that management cannot wait until flattened or negative growth becomes acute before action is taken. If the market signals that growth may be sluggish or negative, planning and actions should be initiated early, although not precipitously. Growth projections should be supportable by environmental and competitive information, as well as product analysis, and not by simple declarations or sovereign decrees. If growth projections do not appear to have a sound basis, management must be ready to deal with poor results, not hope that enrollment will pick up again in the near future unless there is a concrete reason for such a hope.

Reacting to diminished growth by reducing costs is required of most plans, but it is far better to have addressed those costs earlier. Increasing automation, reducing the number of needlessly complex business arrangements, increasing the self-service capabilities for members and providers, improving efficiency in processes, and increasing the use of electronic interchange and electronic commerce are all required. More difficult but equally important is the routine identification and elimination of activities that do not add value. This last task will usually be resisted by those whose jobs are involved in those activities or who are unable to comprehend that the activity has low importance. Once an activity or business process is in place, there is strong momentum to keep it in place.

The last issue to mention here in regard to flattened or negative growth is medical costs. The management of medical cost and quality is the subject of Part III (Chapters 16 to 34) of this book, so the only issue to be raised here is the increase in focus on medical cost management that occurs when growth is not present. This will result in a greater level of discomfort in some medical directors and in some providers in the network. But failure to become more proactive in managing medical costs will result in even greater financial pressure, which will undoubtedly have an even more negative effect on the providers.

Failure To Use Underwriting

As discussed in Chapters 49 to 52, state and federal laws and regulations have limited the degree to which MCOs and insurance companies may medically underwrite accounts (i.e., choose whether to offer coverage and under what terms). Except for some requirements under HIPAA, the specifics of these limitations vary from state to state. But an MCO that fails to adapt its underwriting functions to meet current market conditions will experience lower premium yields, lower growth, and adverse selection.

Even in the face of market reform, underwriting has a place, and in the desire to grow, proper underwriting guidelines may be neglected. This is most likely to occur in a new plan trying to grow, but it can occur in any plan where marketing representatives and managers are inadequately supervised at the same time that they are being pressured to produce growth. Proper information must be obtained and acted on both to determine what product to offer (or even whether the group qualifies for coverage under any circumstances) and to determine proper premium rates. New automated tools that span underwriting and sales go far to offset this problem, but the judgment of the salesperson and the underwriter remain critical. If those two functional areas fail to communicate and have a common purpose, suboptimal results will occur.

The plan's approach to rate setting must also occur in the context of the market, or problems will arise. If a plan uses standard book rates or basic community rating while the competition uses more advanced rating methods, it is likely that the risk selection will be skewed. Conversely, if advanced approaches to rating are used simply to lower the price, the plan will not obtain the required premium revenue yield in the budget.

Last, operational underwriting should be used to identify areas of high cost or high risk. This will provide important information during the product development cycle so that a new product will not result in a large but costly enrollment. Retrospective review of underwriting activities may also reveal that guidelines are either not being followed or are no longer appropriate and useful and require updating.

Adverse Selection

As has been noted several times in this chapter, adverse selection refers to an MCO enrolling a population of members that have higher medical needs than those enrolling in other health plans (i.e., the members are sicker than average). Adverse selection can occur either though the addition of new members or the loss of existing members. A disproportionately high loss of members who use fewer medical services means that the remaining members of the MCO are by definition higher utilizers on average. If this results in higher premiums, the exodus of healthier members accelerates and medical costs for the remaining pool of members rise even more rapidly. As noted earlier in this chapter, this can continue until the plan enters an "insurance death spiral" in which it is not possible to collect adequate premiums to cover the costs of a small, sick but loyal group of members. Failure to reverse this trend early increases the odds of entering the death spiral. The first obvious warning sign that this is occurring is when an MCO's premium rates are significantly higher than the competitor's for similar products. One year of such a disparity of rates will usually not cause a substantial loss of existing members, although it will certainly diminish new enrollment. If the premium rate disparities persist over several years, the loss of positive risk members and retention of adverse risk members will surely occur.

On the sales and marketing side, when the MCO is offered in an account with multiple other carriers or plans competing to enroll employees, the MCO is essentially retail selling. It is much harder to accurately assess the actuarial risk in a multiple choice environment because it is possible to enroll only those members who have high medical needs or vice versa. In other words, the possibility of adverse selection occurring within a group is very real. This is a particular problem in a highly competitive market, where the pressure on the marketing department is high. If the sales representative is on a pure commission basis, the pressure may be overwhelming. If emphasis is placed on the ease of access to high-cost specialists and hospitals and if any restrictions to that access are downplayed, it can lead to adverse selection within an otherwise normal risk group.

The problem of adverse selection is especially important to provider-owned or sponsored health plans. Provider-sponsored plans often look at members as patients and fail to truly understand that a health plan needs more members than patients. In other words, all patients may be members, but not all members may be patients.

There will always be a pool of relatively young and healthy people who will choose price over provider selection because they have needs in their lives greater than health-related needs (e.g., they need to pay their mortgage or car loan). Young and healthy individuals may also believe that they are simply not going to need much in the way of medical care and therefore look more to price than to any other attribute. A provider-sponsored health plan appeals primarily to the patients of the owner-providers, not the general population. If the provider-sponsored health plan has a smaller network than the competition and is at price parity (or even more expensive, which often is the case after several years of operation), it will have no appeal to individuals who have no deep affiliation with a particular provider. This means that the provider-sponsored health plan is less appealing to new enrollment of relatively young and healthy individuals compared with plans that are less expensive and have broader networks, and thus the provider-sponsored plan will have adverse selection.

Improper Incurred But Not Reported Calculations and Accrual Methods

As discussed in Chapter 47, the calculation and booking of liabilities in managed care plans is different from that found in most other industries, including the health care provider sector. There have been quite a few health plans where accruals were based on the bills that came in the mail that month or on historical data only. A health plan that is standing risk for medical services must estimate accurately the cost of those services and accrue for them. If the costs are simply booked as they come in, disaster is certain.

The usual culprit here is failure to accrue properly for expenses that are IBNR With data from lag studies and the plan's MIS (i.e., the authorization and encounter data systems) and prior experience, sufficient accruals must be made each month for all expenses, regardless of whether the bills came in or not. Calculation of proper accruals and IBNRs becomes especially difficult in plans that are experiencing rapid growth. A new member's premium payment contributes to revenue on day one, but generally does not incur medical costs until some later date. Also, new members are not familiar with the plan and may not comply with policies and procedures, incurring medical costs that the plan will ultimately have to pay, but are not well controlled. If the plan fails to perform good lag studies, the problem will be compounded because a trend of higher claims in past periods may not be picked up. For all the reasons discussed earlier, a rapidly growing plan will have a diminished capacity to capture data accurately and will have lessened efficacy of medical utilization management. Rapid growth should always lead management to boost IBNR reserves unless there is a concrete reason why that is unnecessary. Boosting the IBNRs is safer than the opposite. Taking down excess reserves is always more pleasant than posting an unexpected negative adjustment, the latter action often being considered a career-limiting move.

In plans that have failed to accrue properly for expenses, actual expenses may exceed accruals as early as the first six months. The malignant feature of this problem is that it can continue inexorably for another six months or even more, especially if the plan is experiencing a claims-processing problem, as most plans undergoing rapid growth do. Each month's accruals have to be adjusted for expenses related to past months, and financial performance suffers not only for performance to date but for past periods as well. The plan cannot stop the financial hemorrhage quickly because the expenses were already incurred and will keep rolling in. Monthly performance gets muddied up with adjustments for prior performance, and managers find themselves chasing their tails. This problem becomes intensified if the plan is generating inadequate premium revenue either through intentional low-balling or through faulty rate calculations or poor underwriting. If adverse selection is also present, the plan is in for a really rough ride, with a possible crash landing at the end.

This problem has accounted for a disproportionate number of health plan failures. Lack of experienced or strong financial management is a common root cause. An experienced outside ac-

tuary may be able to detect the problem, but unless plan management suspects this problem, the outside actuary may only come in during the annual audit. If the other senior managers, particularly the executive director, are also inexperienced, the environmental pressures that increase the risk of inadequate IBNRs may not be recognized (e.g., rapid growth, a rapidly expanding network or service area, a new product with lesser medical management). Inadequate accruals for IBNR liabilities do not occur as isolated problems and are usually accompanied by serious operational problems such as poor claims processing, poor MIS reporting capabilities, and inadequate management of utilization. Failure to accrue properly is preventable with experience, vigilance, an understanding of market dynamics, and early detection.

Failure To Reconcile Accounts Receivable and Membership

Typical managed care plans have considerable changes occurring in membership each month. When the plan is standing risk for medical expenses, capitates providers, capitates administration fees, books some accruals based on PMPM historical cost, and so forth, it is vital to have as accurate a reconciliation of membership as possible. Most importantly, accounts receivable are directly tied to membership and billing.

It is common for plans to have difficulty with this activity. In some accounts (e.g., the federal employee health benefit program; see Chapter 54), the account is chronically late in providing accurate enrollment information. In other cases, the plan receives information from an account but never properly reconciles it every month because it is such a labor-intensive process. In any case, if the plan pays medical expenses for members who are no longer eligible or fails to collect premiums for members who are newly enrolled, losses are likely to follow. More devastating is the need to make a huge downward adjustment on the balance sheet to write off uncollectable premium receivables.

The early warning sign of this problem is a progressively aging premium accounts receivable. Regular reconciliation of enrollment and premiums for accounts is necessary, and the larger the account, the more often it requires reconciliation. As electronic commerce capabilities increase (see Chapter 37), the ability to automate this activity increases as well, although this requires MIS capabilities that may not exist in older systems.

Overextended Management

What may have been appropriate or even generous staffing at the start-up stage can become understaffing after significant growth, especially if that growth has been rapid. The problem is more complex than the number of management bodies available; it is really one of span of control and experience of managers.

It is not uncommon in any industry for management requirements to change over time. Frequently, the methods used by the pioneers become dysfunctional as plans reach significant size. Tight control concentrated in a few managers, overreliance on central decision making, heavy hands-on involvement by senior managers, and so forth all can lead to paralysis and calcification as a plan becomes large and complex. The few managers with the control are unable to keep up with all the necessary details and demands of running operations, and failure to delegate properly prevents the plan from recruiting and retaining talented second-level managers.

Conversely, an MCO may be started up by individuals who excel at sales and marketing but have less skill in general management. If the leadership of the new and rapidly growing MCO is focused heavily on growth and less on other operational needs (i.e., the value placed on executive talent is in sales, not operations), there will be fewer and possibly less-experienced managers in the operational functions. In some highly entrepreneurial MCOs that were heavily focused on growth, not only were there relatively fewer operations managers than would be expected, but the executive leadership in operations often came from sales and marketing.

As a plan grows, its ability to change and adapt to the competitive environment becomes diminished. All the details necessary for proper operations become overwhelming. If senior managers are personally responsible for all these details, they may be unable to keep up, and things will get missed. Change becomes even less likely when overloaded managers cannot handle the prospect of having to learn yet another set of management skills while still having to use the old ones. This becomes demoralizing to subordinates and providers when plan management is seen as unresponsive, inattentive, or both.

A full discussion of appropriate delegation of authority and responsibility is beyond the scope of this chapter. Here it is sufficient to point out the dangers inherent in failing to create proper tiers of management as a plan grows. This is not to imply that senior managers should insulate themselves from the operations of the plan, overdelegate, create unnecessary new layers of management hierarchy, or drive up administrative costs for no good reason. Rather, this is to emphasize that health plans are complex organizations, and nobody can do it all.

Failure of Management To Produce or Understand Reports

Difficult as it may be to believe, managers may not always understand how reports are developed and written. A report may be labeled as one thing, but the data that are put into the report are really something else. For example, there may be a report that gives the rate of disenrollment from the plan. Depending on how the MIS department inputs the data or how the computer was programmed, the disenrollment rate may include any member who changes status (e.g., goes from single to family) or coverage (e.g., changes jobs but continues with the plan under the new group). If that is the case, the disenrollment rate will be spuriously high. Failure to understand the meaning behind the disenrollment rate can lead to inaccurate forecasting and budgeting. Failure to understand the data elements in medical management and utilization reports is obviously far more serious.

To prevent this, senior management should be involved in developing the formats of reports and deciding what data will be used. The decisions about how to collect data and how to input them should not be made solely by the MIS department. In the event that the plan has experienced changeover in managers, it is important for the new manager not to assume anything and to ask explicitly what data go into each report. This last may seem embarrassing to a manager, but that type of compulsive behavior could prevent a serious mistake in the future.

The evil doppelgänger of an inability to produce and understand reports is the crushing production of so many reports that management is overwhelmed with trivial or conflicting information. The more senior the executive in the management of the MCO, the more the reports need to be summary reports that will allow the senior executive to focus on the overall state of the plan and to identify the broad areas that require more attention. When serious issues are identified, the senior executive may want more detailed reports during the time the problem is being addressed. As one moves down through the organization, the information and reports required for managers become narrower but more detailed.

Failure To Track Correctly Medical Costs and Utilization

This is a special subset of the problem just discussed, that of failure of management to understand reports. The problem of tracking medical expenses and utilization is so important that it merits brief discussion by itself.

As growing plans develop problems with operations (the authorization system, claims, or data gathering in general), medical expense and utilization reports frequently suffer. If the plan is accruing for IBNRs on the basis of historical data because current data are inaccurate, expenses may be allocated to categories primarily because that is where the expenses have been found before. For example, if a plan historically has had high costs in orthopedics and if the data system is unable reliably to provide current utilization data, finance may accrue expenses to orthopedics even if the medical director has been

able to reduce costs in that area. It may take six months for the data to come through the system that show a reduction in orthopedics expenses, but by that time the medical director has resigned in frustration.

Another example would be a plan that has an authorization system for referrals but that system allows for subauthorizations, automatic authorization of return visits, and self-referral. Because of the loose nature of the system, the finance department cannot rely on it when calculating accruals. If there is a concomitant problem with claims processing, there will be no timely and accurate data about utilization. In that case, finance will calculate accruals by using lag studies and best guess numbers and will assign the expenses where they fell as the claims were processed. In this way, high expenses may really be reflective of a combination of two things: what was happening in utilization some time back, and what type of claims were processed that month.

If the calculation of these numbers is sufficiently removed from senior management and if the medical director does not know how the numbers are derived, tremendous efforts may be expended in dealing with problems that are neither timely nor high priority. As mentioned in Chapter 30 on quality management, a plan's ability to implement continuous quality improvement in its business operations will be hampered if efforts are wasted trying to solve problems that are not indicative of the true problems facing management.

Closely related is the problem of not properly tracking utilization. For example, if a plan has an authorization system for referrals that tracks initial referrals from the primary care physician but fails to track adequately subauthorizations, self-referrals, and repeat visits, the referral rate may be grossly inaccurate. Another example would be a plan that is able to report high rates of utilization but is unable to provide the details about why those rates are high.

In a perverse twist, in those cases in which data are presented in an inaccurate or inadequate form but the medical director understands why that is so, a false sense of complacency can develop. For example, if a hospital utilization report consistently and inaccurately reports high utilization for a certain physician (perhaps because that physician performs all inpatient admissions for a three-physician group), the medical director may continually make adjustments when reviewing the report and fail to recognize a genuine increase in utilization.

Recent advances in software support systems for medical management help address this problem. These newer systems are able to produce useful reports in addition to supporting the operational aspects of medical management. Some of the newer full-capability systems (i.e., the systems that support all the operations, for example enrollment, claims, finance) also have medical management reporting capabilities, but these are generally less sophisticated than dedicated medical management systems. There are also systems that are dedicated solely to the production of medical management reports and practice profiles (Chapter 32), but those systems are dependent on data from other MIS in the MCO. If a MCO does not have any of these more advanced capabilities, it will be at a disadvantage to a competitor that does.

Systems Inability To Manage the Business

As a health plan grows in the marketplace, it must continue to evolve to meet ever-changing needs. When the plan does so, it is not uncommon that the MIS is unable to change at the same pace without a prohibitively high cost in programming and time. Manual workarounds are put into place, custom programming is undertaken, and soon the MIS is a cat's cradle of code, and the administrative costs have escalated. Multiple systems are used to manage different parts of the business, and they do not tie or even match up. This problem is quickly compounded when innovative managers invent new ways of doing business (e.g., invent a new reimbursement system) that appears to make sense but cannot be supported by the MIS.

MCOs that have acquired other MCOs face the added problem of using the legacy systems from the acquired plan. Although converting the acquired plan to the MCO's MIS would seem

logical, it has so many complications that such a conversion is often undertaken only after several years. The ability of one system to support the acquired MCO's benefits plans, reimbursement methods, enrollment data, and the need to convert history to the new system create high barriers to conversion. What usually ends up happening is that the MCO that has acquired other MCOs continues to run all of the legacy systems that came along with the acquisition. In the case of some large commercial carriers and Blue Cross Blue Shield plans, the company may be running different systems for different products, with little ability to tie information together.

Unfortunately, the most obvious way to prevent this problem is also the least useful answer: never change anything. But a health plan that fails to change and innovate soon becomes stale in the market and begins losing to the competition. At the other end of the spectrum, a viable solution is to migrate to an entirely new system, with the attendant headaches that accompany any conversion. This is a long, expensive, and exhausting process but, if accomplished successfully, has large advantages. Solutions in between the two extremes involve the addition of systems designed to bridge the gaps between legacy systems and to provide a common interface for users so as to reduce confusion and training requirements.

The rise of e-commerce, as discussed in Chapter 37, adds new dimensions to the need for MIS capabilities. Enabling internal and external users to communicate and conduct business electronically by way of the Internet or other electronic channels is a functionality that is only just appearing in most MCOs' MIS. Plans that fail to keep pace with this rapidly rising form of business and consumer interaction will soon be at a serious disadvantage.

Complicating all of this are the new data security and privacy requirements and transaction requirements under HIPAA. Although this is not a common problem at the time of publication, that is solely because these new requirements are not yet in force. They will be some time in 2002 to 2003 and will become a common problem for MCOs. The need for changing policies and procedures to accommodate privacy and security needs and to remediate or surround MIS to accommodate the transaction requirements will represent serious challenges to MCOs.

On a managerial basis, what is most important is for information systems managers to be involved in management policies and procedures so that alternative approaches are explored and the entire team understands the systems implications of policy changes. Even more important, the information systems managers need to be able to engage in strategic planning to stay in front of the demands of the industry. As discussed in Chapter 35, the MIS must be flexible and designed such that change is accommodated at an acceptable cost.

Failure To Educate and Reeducate Providers

An all too common sin of omission is the failure to properly educate providers. As discussed in Chapter 7, proper orientation of new providers and office staff is an important success factor. All too often the providers are simply given a procedure manual and a metaphorical kiss on the cheek. Even in those situations where proper orientation has taken place, it is unlikely that the information will stick unless there are already a large number of patients coming in through the plan. This is even more of a problem when there are a number of competing health plans, each with its own unique way of doing things.

Just as important as the initial orientation is a program of continuing education in the procedures and policies of the plan, especially as the plan undergoes operational changes (e.g., due to e-commerce or HIPAA compliance). Regular maintenance of the knowledge base of the providers and their office staff will help prevent problems caused solely by lack of communication.

Examples of this problem abound in most open panels. Physicians may fail to use properly the authorization system, may provide or promise benefits that the plan does not cover, may allow open-ended authorizations to specialists, and so forth. Although none of these occurrences is dangerous in itself, they all can be addi-

tive. In a large plan, failure to communicate properly with providers can lead rapidly to a loss of control. Far more energy is spent trying to repair damage than would have been spent in maintenance.

Failure To Deal with Difficult or Noncompliant Providers

Perhaps the most difficult of all the tasks of a medical director is dealing with difficult and noncompliant physicians. The same task applies to nonphysician providers, but that is generally easier for most medical directors. Because dealing with difficult physicians is so onerous to physician managers, they tend to avoid it or at least procrastinate. Assuming that the plan is reasonably well run and not subject to a justified physician mutiny, difficult physicians, like difficult patients, make up only a tiny minority of the total panel but consume an inordinate amount of managerial energy. Failure to deal with such physicians has both direct and indirect ramifications.

The direct result of failing to deal with an uncooperative physician is the expense associated with that physician's utilization of resources. This problem is obvious, although easy to rationalize away ("Well, maybe they have sicker patients"). The indirect results are less obvious. The most important is the effect on members. If the physician has a truly bad attitude, that will be transmitted to members. A little bit of this "blame the bogeyman" behavior can be tolerated and understood, but if it becomes chronic, the plan can find itself fighting off unwarranted attacks by members and employee benefits managers. Other indirect effects include promoting a poor attitude among the other physicians and lowering the morale of the plan staff who have to deal with that particular physician.

The most frequent objection to dealing with difficult physicians is that the plan needs them because they are so prestigious or popular. In many cases, that physician also has a large number of members, and there are fears that if the physician leaves or is recorded, the plan will lose membership. It is up to plan management to determine whether the plan is worse off with or without the physician. Regarding the issue of prestige, it is far worse to have that physician bad mouthing the plan directly to the members than it is to have him or her deriding the plan in the hospital lounge (where he or she is probably doing it anyway). It is also probable that a sizeable number of members stick with the plan and agree to change physicians.

If education and personal appeals fail to effect the needed change, the medical director must take action. Failure to take action is the mark of weak and ineffectual management.

Hubris

The final category of common problems is hubris. This is especially dangerous when MCO senior executives are publicly lauded for their superior acumen and results. An MCO may be achieving rapid growth and apparent financial success (although see previously for reasons why such financial success may not be real) and be praised by investors and the media. At some point, the managers begin believing their own press, which is always dangerous. In other cases, an MCO is indeed large and successful, and senior management has come to believe that they are truly superior to their competition and have

little to learn about the industry (but the industry could learn a lot from them). Pride of accomplishment is justifiable, but not if that pride prevents management from seeing things as they really are.

Senior executives flush with hubris are also more likely to believe that they will succeed in any venture and that they possess skills and vision so superior that whatever they undertake will be successful. Self-confidence is a good attribute for an effective executive, but arrogance is not. It becomes too easy to commit the company to a course that is ill fated and to refuse to heed the danger signs as they appear.

CONCLUSION

This chapter presents some of the common problems that can occur in managed care plans. There are few plans in existence today that have not experienced at least a few of these difficulties at some point. The list is not exhaustive, and there are certainly many other difficulties that a plan can experience. The important point is to recognize that managed care plans do indeed develop predictable problems and to be ever vigilant for their emergence.

PART V

Finance and Underwriting

"Being good in business is the most fascinating kind of art....
Making money is art and working is art and good business is the best art."

Andy Warhol
(1928—1987)
From A to B and Back Again, ch. 6 [1975]

CHAPTER 47

Operational Finance and Budgeting

Dale F. Harding

To manage successfully a managed care organization (MCO), the challenge lies in the financial manager's ability to interact with operational and medical managers, manage changes in the regulatory environment, gather timely information to facilitate communication of financial results to the organization and its constituencies, and react appropriately to sustain or exceed financial goals. Accuracy of the reported financial results is impacted by significant accounting estimates that are based on historical trends and results and appropriately adjusted for recent changes affecting such estimates. The interaction between operational managers and financial managers is key to developing timely, accurate financial results.

Overall financial management of an MCO begins with the MCO's product pricing strategies. Strategic pricing is based on an assessment of the competition, targeted profitability, the MCO's estimate of costs incurred for the provision of health care, and its ability to control costs, in particular, medical costs. Detailed operating budgets are then developed under the same assumptions used in the pricing strategy. Financial managers rely significantly on information captured and monitored by operational departments to develop the detailed budgets.

Information provided by operational departments is also used as the basis for certain accounting estimates recorded in financial statements. The financial manager's ability to report on actual results, analyze budget variances, and assess the reasonableness of pricing strategies in a timely manner is dependent on the support of operating functions.

In this chapter, through a review of the components of the financial statements of a health maintenance organization (HMO), key information and operational procedures that the financial manager will need and rely on are discussed. The discussion addresses typical problems that occur in gathering information and provides insight into challenging the integrity of information.

Dale F. Harding, from Aetna US Healthcare, is the project manager to the Core Integration Team assigned to the Prudential HealthCare acquisition. Just before her current position, Dale was the Chief Financial Officer of NYLCare Health Plans of New York, formerly a subsidiary of New York Life Insurance Company. Before that, Dale was a senior manager in the East/Great Lakes Healthcare Practice of Ernst & Young LLP, where during her 12-year career, she focused on the insurance and health care fields, specializing in managed care organizations.

BACKGROUND

Accounting policy for MCOs is set by many regulatory entities. MCOs are primarily regulated at the state level, although certain federal regulations may be imposed if an MCO offers federally regulated products such as Medicare risk contracts. State regulation may be imposed by both the Department of Insurance and the Department of Health. In addition, there are many publicly held MCOs that are subject to the rules and regulations of the Securities and Exchange Commission (SEC).

The state's Department of Insurance is generally concerned with the fiscal solvency of the MCO to ensure that the health benefits of enrollees will be provided. The state's Department of Health is generally concerned with quality of care issues and access to care issues, including the location of providers within specific geographical boundaries and the mix of primary care physicians and specialists to serve the population within these boundaries.

Financial management of MCOs must consider the interests of each of the users of financial information, whether they are senior management, insurance regulators, the SEC, tax authorities, or investors. Balancing the concerns of each interested party represents a challenge for the financial manager. Senior management is concerned with the profitability of products and market segment performance. Management will require internal reporting that focuses on line of business management and also meets regulatory reporting requirements. Regulators are concerned with protecting the insured members and focus on liquidity of the MCO. The SEC is concerned with the protection of investor interests. Balancing conservatism and positive performance with the best return on investment is a difficult task.

The requirements imposed by the state's Department of Insurance and Department of Health can be found in the state laws and regulations. The National Association of Insurance Commissioners (NAIC) is an organization comprising the state commissioners of insurance, who set guidelines at a national level. The NAIC has no governing authority over the individual states, however. Generally, states will introduce legislation modeling NAIC guidelines. The NAIC has adopted an annual statement report format that has been adopted by most states. The financial information is prepared in accordance with statutory accounting practices (SAP). Other financial statement users (lenders, the SEC, and investors) require that financial statements be prepared in accordance with generally accepted accounting principles (GAAP). The American

Institute of Certified Public Accountants issued an audit and accounting guide for health care providers that provides additional guidance on audit, accounting, and reporting matters for prepaid health plans.

The financial manager should also be aware of the continuous changes taking place in the regulatory arena. For many states, managed care market penetration has historically been minimal, and legislation has not kept pace with recent growth in managed care. Many varieties of MCOs or managed care strategies are emerging, such as physician-hospital organizations (PHOs), integrated delivery systems, management services organizations, direct contracting arrangements among employers and providers, and so forth (see Chapters 3 and 4), and regulators acknowledge that there is little or no legislation governing these emerging areas (see Chapters 51 and 69). For example, many regulators have imposed policy (absent legislative authority) to exercise financial restrictions on PHOs or other provider organizations that contract directly with self-insured plans. Other developments include the NAIC's development of risk-based capital requirements for health insurers, including HMOs, which impose stricter minimum capital requirements. Also in the past few years, expanded financial disclosure requirements regarding changes in claims reserves have been imposed on health insurers.

FINANCIAL STATEMENT COMPONENTS

Operating Statement

A typical high-level profit-and-loss statement for an HMO is depicted in Exhibit 47–1. For internal management reporting purposes, the ability to develop profit and loss reports by product line/market segment is critical to the financial management process. Assumptions and financial benchmarks may vary widely by product or market segment. For example, medical cost estimates are based on utilization patterns and provider reimbursement strategies that will differ by product and market segment. Likewise, ad-

Exhibit 47–1 Sample Profit-and-Loss Statement for an MCO—Percentage of Total Revenue

Percentage revenue
  Premiums earned: 95
  Other income: 5
  Total revenue: 100
Percentage expenses
  Health care expenses: 84
  General and administrative expenses: 11
  Total expenses: 95
Percentage income or loss before income
  taxes: 5

ministration of lines of business may be different. For example, the costs associated with supporting a Medicare or Medicaid product will differ from those associated with the commercial population because the customers have unique service needs and because dedicated staff with specific skill sets will be needed to service Medicare and Medicaid enrollees. Pricing is based on the medical cost and administrative cost components; therefore, premium pricing by product will vary consistent with the variations in these cost components. In the following discussion of the components of the financial statement, keep in mind the importance of segregating the reporting by product line or market segment. Analyzing financial results by line of business not only will enhance management's ability to understand the fluctuations from budgeted results but will provide information needed to redirect strategies to preserve the overall success of the operation.

Premium Revenue

Premium revenue is the primary revenue source for HMOs. Premiums are generally received in advance of the coverage period, which is usually monthly. Premium rates are generally effective for a 12-month period. Rates or rating methods are usually filed with and must be approved by the state's Department of Insurance. MCOs may file revisions to the rates or method, which will also be subject to approval by the Department of Insurance. New rates will not be effective for existing groups until the renewal of the annual contract.

Premiums are determined using actuarial and underwriting techniques, as discussed in Chapters 49 through 51. Premiums are intended to cover all medical and administrative expenses and to provide a profit margin. Premium rates are therefore directly related to medical expense and administrative expense projections. If the premium rates are not adequate to cover the actual medical expenses and administrative costs, expected profit margins will diminish. If losses for a line of business are anticipated, a premium deficiency exists. Under GAAP accounting, because premium rates are fixed until the end of the coverage period, the aggregate anticipated net loss for the line of business may need to be recorded immediately, not ratably over the remaining coverage period.

Certain premium rates may not be controlled by the MCO, such as those for Medicare risk contracts or Medicaid. These rates are set by the government. For example, Medicare premium rates are based on the rates set by the federal government. The sufficiency of these rates therefore is dependent, in part, on the federal government's ability to capture and analyze data when determining the rates and also on the ultimate product benefit design and the ability of the MCO to manage benefits and expenses to the rates. It is then the responsibility of the MCO to be able to perform medical management and administrative expense management so that the premium is sufficient to cover costs and yield a profit.

Rating methods derive rates on the basis of an evaluation of demographic data (e.g., the age and sex mix or geographical location) of the population to insure. Rates may be determined using a community rating method or an experience rating method. Community rating is often used for small groups (less than 50 subscribers) or individuals, and experience rating is used for large groups. In many states community rating is mandatory for small groups and individuals. States may also mandate community rating for all groups regardless of size.

Basic community rating entails the application of a standard rate to all groups within the community being underwritten. The standard rate is applied to groups on the basis of the number of rate tiers quoted, the average family size, and the contract mix assumed for the group. Rate tiers are developed on the basis of the age and sex of members and the classification of individual versus family. Community rating by class considers an adjustment to the basic rate for specific demographics and/or industry classification of the group. Adjusted community rating allows for adjustments to the base rate for group-specific information other than demographics and industry classification.

The experience rating method develops a group rate on the basis of a group's actual experience. After determining actual past experience, expenses are trended forward. Experience-rated contracts can be retrospectively rated or prospectively rated. Retrospective rate adjustments allow for an adjustment to the current period premium on the basis of actual experience. The premium adjustment should be accrued in the current financial statement period and may need to be estimated if the settlement date is subsequent to the end of the accounting period. Prospectively rated premiums provide for increases in rates in the next contract period on the basis of the actual experience of the previous period. When premium adjustments are prospectively rated, there are no accounting entries required in the current reporting period.

Revenues are recorded in the financial statements as a function of the underlying billing process. The effectiveness of the billing process further depends on the membership or enrollment process. Membership data must be gathered in sufficient detail from the enrollment forms to allow for the proper classification of the enrollee to ensure that the appropriate rates are charged. Timely updating of enrollment records for changes in membership status not only ensures the accuracy of rates charged but also ensures that medical services are provided only to active enrollees. Furthermore, compliance with billing and enrollment procedures may affect whether the MCO will incur costs for health care services provided to inactive enrollees. Subscribers, providers, and the MCO each have contractual obligations related to updating and verification of the enrollee's status. Failure to meet contractual obligations to maintain enrollment records properly and accurately could result in additional costs to the MCO. Therefore, the financial manager should have the information needed to ensure that revenue is being billed for all active enrollees and that business processes are functioning in a manner to prevent loss because of noncompliance with contract terms.

Premium billing may occur under two methods: self-billing or retroactive billing. The self-billing method permits the subscriber (or the group) to adjust the invoice for changes in enrollment. In this situation, the amount billed and recorded as premium revenue receivable will differ from the actual amounts paid by the group. Differences in the amount billed and received require adjustment to revenue and accounts receivable records. A secondary process should include communication of changes to ensure timely updating of enrollment records and notification of enrollment changes to providers. If processes are not in place to ensure that such differences are reconciled and resolved on a timely basis, revenue and accounts receivable may not be recorded properly in the financial statements, and health care benefits may be provided to individuals who are no longer insured.

The retroactive billing method results in adjustments to be recorded in the next month's billing cycle. Under this method, payments made by the group should equal amounts billed. Any changes in enrollment will be adjusted on the next billing. Any changes in enrollment noted should also be forwarded to the appropriate department to ensure updating of enrollment records.

For either billing method, the financial manager must develop a method of estimating adjustments affecting the current accounting period. Because the actual adjustments are not known until payment is received or reported in the next billing cycle, an estimate of expected adjustments should be accrued in the current reporting cycle.

Certain large commercial or government clients remit payment without detailed hard copy explanation of the adjustment. These customers often request electronic data transfer for billing purposes. Financial managers should be aware that significant resources may be needed to service these customers. Information systems personnel will be needed to deal with technical aspects of the electronic data transfer process. Support personnel with specific training will be needed to handle the unique challenges associated with large accounts. The process of reconciling the MCO's records with the customer's records can be time consuming but is absolutely necessary. The financial manager should monitor the status (timeliness and completeness) of the reconciliations of these accounts to ensure that any potential problems with the reconciliations do not also affect other financial statement components, such as medical expense accruals.

Other Revenue Sources

Because many HMOs offer preferred provider organization (PPO) products, a growing revenue source is fee revenue derived from PPO members. Subscribers selecting a PPO product generally pay an access fee for use of the provider network established by the MCO. For example, PPO product fees are generally based on a specified per member per month charge. Fees for PPO products vary depending on the level of service. There is a base fee for accessing the provider network, but enhanced services such as utilization management or providing a gatekeeper mechanism to manage utilization would increase the PPO access fee charged. Pricing of access fees should consider costs of performing administrative functions related to maintaining the provider network, such as credentialing, contract negotiations, and monitoring physician practice patterns.

Coordination of benefits (COB) recoverable is another source of revenue for the HMO. MCOs must have sufficient procedures in place to identify recoveries of costs under COB. COB usually exists when there is a two-wage-earner family and individuals will have insurance coverage under two policies with a different insurer or health plan.

Policies and procedures are established by insurance organizations to determine which insurer or health plan will serve as the primary or secondary payer. Procedures need to be in place to ensure that costs that are the responsibility of the other carrier are recovered. The data necessary to perform this procedure are usually gathered during the enrollment and billing process. Again, accuracy and completeness during the enrollment process are key to securing the data necessary to determine the amounts recoverable.

There are two primary methods of recovering COB: pay and pursue, and pursue and pay. Under the pay and pursue method, claims are paid, and COB recovery is sought later from the other carrier. Under pursue and pay, the claim net of any COB is paid. To ensure that medical expenses are not recorded net, it is important that gross claim costs and COB recoverable are identifiable by the financial manager. See Chapter 39 for a detailed discussion of this issue.

Reinsurance recoverable is another source of income to the MCO. Reinsurance against catastrophic claims or claims in excess of specified dollar limits is often obtained to reduce the risk of individual large losses for the MCO. MCOs may forgo obtaining reinsurance on the basis of the cost versus benefit of the coverage. The financial manager needs to perform a risk assessment to determine whether stop-loss insurance is appropriate. Procedures need to exist to ensure that costs recoverable under reinsurance are identifiable, so that the MCO receives the full benefit to which it is entitled under the reinsurance arrangement. Reinsurance premiums should be recorded as health care costs, and reinsurance recoverable should be shown net of health care costs. See Chapter 53 for a discussion of stop-loss insurance for IDSs, a related topic.

Another source of income for HMOs is interest income. Excess cash is generally invested in short-term instruments to ensure cash availability for the payment of claims.

Medical Expenses

Table 47–1, imported from Chapter 49 (Table 49–2 in *Underwriting and Rating Functions*

Table 47–1 Sample Actuarial Cost Model

	Medical Service	(1) Annual Utilization per 1,000 Members	(2) Allowed Average Charge Per Service	(3) Per Member Per Month Medical Cost	(4) Copay Frequency	(5) Copay	(6) Cost Sharing Per Member Per Month	(7) Per Member Per Month Net Claim Costs
Hospital inpatient	Medical-surgical	247 days	$1,276.76	$26.28				$26.28
	Psychiatric/substance abuse	67 days	$657.31	$3.67				$3.67
	Extended care	5 days	$250.00	$0.10				$0.10
	Subtotal	**319 days**	**$2,184.07**	**$30.05**				**$30.05**
Hospital outpatient	Emergency room	261 visits	$159.99	$3.48	196	$25.00	$0.41	$3.07
	Surgery	85 visits	$1,172.46	$8.30				$8.30
	Other	512 services	$149.53	$6.38				$6.38
	Subtotal			**$18.16**			**$0.41**	**$17.75**
Primary care capitation	Office and inpatient visits	2,152 visits	$42.77	$7.67	2,035	$10.00	$1.70	$5.97
	Immunizations and injections	154 procedures	$17.14	$0.22				$0.22
	Subtotal			**$7.89**			**$1.70**	**$6.19**
Fee-for-service physician	Surgery	374 procedures	$266.63	$8.31				$8.31
	Anesthesia	78 procedures	$575.38	$3.74				$3.74
	Office and inpatient visits	1,025 visits	$45.78	$3.91	944	$10.00	$0.79	$3.12
	Other	3,277 services	$75.00	$20.48				$20.48
	Subtotal			**$36.44**			**$0.79**	**$35.65**
Other	Prescription drugs	5,209 scripts	$36.00	$15.63	5,209	$5.00	$2.17	$13.46
	Home health care	29 visits	$228.21	$0.55				$0.55
	Ambulance	15 runs	$322.43	$0.40				$0.40
	Durable medical equipment	32 units	$269.54	$0.72				$0.72
	Subtotal			**$17.30**			**$2.17**	**$15.13**
Total medical costs PMPM				$109.84			$5.07	$104.77
Retention load PMPM (12.69% of the required rate)								$15.23
Required rate PMPM								$120.00

Source: Courtesy of Milliman and Robertson, 2000, Brookfield, Wisconsin

Common to Most Markets, by Cigich and Sturm) summarizes the breakdown of medical costs among hospital, physician, and ancillary services. Medical expenses may be incurred on a capitated basis, fee schedule, or per diem arrangement. Another form of reimbursement that is similar to capitation is percentage of premium. Capitation and percentage of premium represent risk transfer arrangements. Risk transfer arrangements place the providers at risk if utilization exceeds expected results. Reimbursement strategies are discussed in more detail in Chapters 8 through 12.

Medical expenses reported in the financial statements should represent paid claims plus accruals for claims reported but unpaid and claims incurred but not reported (IBNR). The development of the accruals for both reported and unreported claims is an accounting estimate whereby the accuracy of the estimate depends on the data captured by operations personnel and communicated to the financial managers. For reported claims, the incidence of claims is known (e.g., estimated length of stay for inpatient service, number of referred visits for outpatient services), and the type of claim is known (e.g., inpatient procedure codes, type of outpatient service). The costs related to the claim incident must be estimated. For reported claims there is less unknown, and there can be more accuracy when ultimate costs are projected, although the ultimate disposition of the claims must still be estimated.

For IBNR claims, both the incidence of claims and the type of claims are unknown and must be estimated. IBNR estimates are often developed with the assistance of actuaries. A preferred method for estimating IBNR is the development of loss triangles (Table 47–2). These triangles graphically depict the lag between either the date of service and the payment date or the date of service and the date the claim is reported. From the lag analysis, completion factors are developed to estimate the remaining claims to be reported or paid at each duration. Claim severity, or the estimated average claim costs, is then used to calculate the total projected costs yet to be incurred. The total projected costs

are the basis for accruals to be recorded in the financial statements for the IBNR claims.

Loss triangles are often developed separately for hospital and physician claims. Physician claims can also be further analyzed by type of specialty claim where appropriate. Also the IBNR claims analysis should be segregated by line of business. Although a greater level of details can assist in a more refined estimate, caution should be used when one is developing estimates from small population sizes. The smaller the base population, the less precise the estimates. It is prudent to limit the level of detail used in the analysis.

As discussed previously, the adequacy of the estimates for reported claims developed by financial managers depends on the availability of data from the operating areas within the MCO. These data are usually developed from the utilization management program. Inpatient care, excluding nonemergency care, typically requires preauthorization; therefore, if the utilization managers are keeping accurate records of admissions and length-of-stay statistics, the data needed by the financial managers to estimate admissions and cost of services should be readily available. For outpatient services and specialist services, referrals are usually required for more services. Again, if the utilization management program is properly monitoring outpatient and specialist utilization and is maintaining accurate records of referrals, the data needed to estimate outpatient and specialist visits should be readily available to the financial manager. To be usable, the authorization information must be carefully controlled so that authorizations unlikely to be used are eliminated before ultimate utilization is estimated. It is extremely important that the utilization managers understand the significance of their responsibilities in that utilization managers not only are vital to controlling overall utilization but also provide necessary information to predict medical costs accurately, prepare reports on financial results, and develop budgets and financial forecasts. See Chapter 19 for a detailed discussion of authorization systems and types of authorizations.

Because the tools used by the financial managers to estimate medical costs also rely heavily

Table 47–2 Loss Triangles

Inpatient services
Claims paid by month of receipt

Service Month	Jan	Feb	Mar	Apr	May	Jun	Jul	Aug	Sep	Oct	Nov	Dec
Jan	10	100	150	50	35	2	1		1		4	1
Feb		7	126	164	44	22	1	1		6		
Mar			24	89	201	33	46	53			5	1
Apr				12	109	177	3	25	2	2	1	
May					1	188	156	45	59	3	4	2
Jun						3	255	189	67	55	4	1
July							9	163	198	84	54	8
Aug								33	127	199	87	62
Sep									27	244	149	88
Oct										17	155	205
Nov											5	104
Dec												12
Total	10	107	300	315	390	425	471	509	481	610	468	484

Inpatient services
Completion factors by month of receipt

Service Month	Cur	+1	+2	+3	+4	+5	+6	+7	+8	+9	+10	+11	Total
Jan	0.03	0.31	0.73	0.88	0.97	0.98	0.98	0.98	0.99	0.99	1.00	1.00	
Feb	0.02	0.36	0.80	0.92	0.98	0.98	0.98	0.98	1.00	1.00	1.00		
Mar	0.05	0.25	0.69	0.77	0.87	0.99	0.99	0.99	1.00	1.00			
Apr	0.04	0.37	0.90	0.91	0.98	0.99	1.00	1.00	1.00				
May	0.00	0.41	0.75	0.85	0.98	0.99	1.00	1.00					
Jun	0.01	0.45	0.78	0.90	0.99	1.00	1.00						
Jul	0.02	0.33	0.72	0.88	0.98	1.00							
Aug	0.06	0.31	0.71	0.88	1.00								
Sep	0.05	0.53	0.83	1.00									
Oct	0.05	0.46	1.00										
Nov	0.05	1.00											
Dec	1.00												
Jan–Jun	0.02	0.36	0.78	0.87	0.96	0.99	0.99	0.99	1.00	1.00	1.00	1.00	

on the accuracy of paid claims data, the claims processing department also plays an important role in financial management. The accuracy of claims data and the timely processing of claims will affect the reliability of the data used to develop the loss triangles. The extent of any backlogs in claim processing must be communicated in timely fashion to the financial manager. See Chapter 38 for a detailed discussion of claims.

Loss triangles represent the most frequently used method to estimate claim costs. Other analyses can also be performed to substantiate further the reasonableness of the estimates for IBNR claims. Analyzing the monthly trends in claims costs or loss ratios by service type (inpatient, outpatient, physician services by specialty, etc.) within product lines and on a per member per month basis provides a basis for determining whether the overall trends in claim costs are consistent with expected results and, where appropriate, industry benchmarks. ***Factors that may affect the trends include:***

- significant changes in enrollment
- unusual or large claims (isolated occurrences versus changes in utilization/cost patterns)
- changes in pricing or product design
- seasonal utilization or reporting patterns
- claim processing backlogs
- major changes to the provider network or reimbursement methods

Each of these factors provides a basis for explaining fluctuations when one is preparing trend analyses. It is important to note, however, that significant changes in enrollment also affect the financial manager's ability to determine reasonable estimates used in financial statements. For example, during periods of enrollment growth, it is difficult to estimate medical cost trends because there is little history associated with the current enrollment base and revenue begins on the first day of enrollment but medical costs generally do not; this may lull an inexperienced financial manager into believing that the medical costs ratio is low. In times of significant disenrollment, there is a risk of adverse selection. Adverse selection exists when the characteristics of the remaining population of insureds are weighted toward a high-risk group. Significant disenrollment often occurs when it is generally not an optimal condition for the enrollee to maintain the current coverage. Usually, those insureds with less choice (e.g., those who are unable to opt for other coverage because of current health status) remain enrolled. Medical cost estimates must be adjusted under these circumstances.

Administrative Expenses

Administrative expenses include salaries, as well as sales, marketing, and other operating expenses. Administrative expenses also vary by product and market segment. Administrative expenses can be measured using percentage of premium and per member per month benchmarks.

Administrative expenses may also be tracked by functional area (e.g., finance, sales, underwriting, member services). Administrative expenses will vary with volume as a result of economies of scale. In growth periods, administrative expenses tend to be high as a percentage of premium.

Tracking of administrative expenses by product and market segment allows management to identify whether the appropriate resources are being allocated to product lines. In addition, if the HMO experience rates certain groups, management needs to track adequately costs associated with a particular group's business to ensure that costs are appropriately allocated to the group and are recovered. The financial manager should also be aware that certain products or market segments, such as government groups and Medicare or Medicaid, place limits on administrative expense allocations to these product lines.

BALANCE SHEET

Cash and Investments

Cash and investments represent a significant balance sheet account for an HMO. The major source of cash is premium revenue. An HMO's investment portfolio usually consists of short-term investments because cash outlays for claims are frequent. As a result, the financial manager is not significantly affected by investment strategies, and typically there is limited investment risk associated with an HMO's investment portfolio. Because cash does churn quickly through the HMO, management may benefit from implementing strong cash management practices, such as using lock-box arrangements for premiums.

Premium Receivable

Another significant balance sheet account is premium receivable. Premiums are generally collected monthly; therefore, problems with the aging of accounts will probably arise from many old items that are not reconciled often. Unreconciled differences may occur when billing problems exist or as a result of discrepancies in the enrollment records of the MCO in comparison with customer records.

Timely update of membership records ensures the accuracy of premium billings and further ensures that claims are paid appropriately. Policies and procedures to ensure timely updating of membership records protect the MCO from paying claims for terminated members or ensures the recoverability of amounts paid incorrectly. In general, if membership records are not up to date and the MCO bills incorrectly for terminated or inactive members, on remittance a group will adjust the payment accordingly. If the MCO does not have procedures in place to reconcile remittances to billed amounts, premium receivable records will show amounts outstanding and past due. Because of the large number of individual members within a group and the potentially large number of billings, management must monitor closely the status of premium reconciliation procedures.

The reconciliation process related to premium receivable for government accounts is usually a more complex problem. For example, federal and state employers often remit premium on a cycle that differs from the normal billing cycle of the MCO. The remittances by these institutions are consistent with the institution's payroll cycles. Premium is remitted only for those employees noted as active on the payroll. There are many events that affect the active status of federal and state employees (e.g., leave of absence, summer recess for educators), but these employees may still be eligible for health benefits. For this reason, the MCO will bill and accrue for premium that will not be paid until the employee's status on the institution's records is reinstated to active status. Often, MCOs that provide coverage to federal and state groups will have dedicated resources to support the reconciliation process.

The reconciliation process for certain large groups may also be complex. The high enrollment volume or the need to accept enrollment data in compatible electronic format may present a challenge for the MCO.

Other Assets

The significance of other assets of an MCO will vary. Another typical large asset may be fixed assets, particularly if the HMO is organized as a staff model HMO and owns and operates physician offices.

Unearned Premiums

Unearned premiums are premiums received by the MCO that at the close of the financial reporting period have not been earned, principally because the premiums are for the ensuing month and are in actuality premiums received in advance. Because most MCOs bill on a monthly basis, unearned premium is generally not a major accounting issue. If premiums are billed and collected other than monthly (e.g., quarterly), an unearned premium reserve would be required.

Claims Payable and IBNR

As discussed earlier, the basis for the recording of claim reserves, including IBNR, depends on information provided by other operating areas of the MCO. Claim liabilities are separated between hospital claims and physician claims. In addition to the matters discussed for medical expenses, the financial manager should prepare further analyses of claim reserves and IBNR estimates.

The financial manager should compare the actual claim payments since the close of the accounting period with the original estimates. Significant differences in the actual results compared with estimated results should be investigated. Information obtained from the investigation should be considered when the sufficiency of current estimates is evaluated.

Risk Pool Liabilities

As discussed in Chapters 8 through 12, reimbursement strategies may provide for risk pools, which will require the MCO to maintain accurate records of payment withholds from hospitals and physicians. Amounts payable to the providers from the withhold should be maintained in separate accounts. In addition, shortfalls in the risk pool that must be recovered from the providers need to be evaluated to ensure that the amounts are recoverable, and where necessary the financial manager should consider the need for a provision for unrecoverable amounts. In addition, any contributions to be made by the MCO for its participation in a risk pool should be appropriately accrued in the financial statements.

Equity

The MCO will need to track its SAP and GAAP basis equity. SAP equity generally differs from GAAP equity as a result of certain assets being nonadmitted and also, where permitted, certain liabilities being recognized as equity. For example, the statutory balance sheet may permit certain surplus notes to be classified as equity for purposes of determining statutory net worth (issues regarding statutory net worth are discussed later). Surplus notes are obligations to investors that meet certain requirements of the state insurance laws, which are generally subordinated to all obligations of the MCOs. Repayment of surplus notes is subject to the approval of the state's commissioners of insurance. Other transactions affecting equity that are generally subject to the approval of the state's commissioners of insurance include restrictions on the payout of dividends.

REGULATORY REPORTING CONSIDERATIONS

Generally, HMOs are required to file quarterly financial statements with the state Department of Insurance, which are due 45 days after the close of the quarter. An annual statement filing is also required. The annual filing is due March 1. Effective with the reporting for calendar year 1998, changes were made to the NAIC annual statement format. The changes to investment reporting (Schedule D to the NAIC annual statement) resulted in MCOs' reporting of investment activity, which is identical to that reported by other types of insurance organizations (e.g., life and health insurers and property/casualty insurers). Previously, MCOs were not required to submit such detailed information of their investment activity and holdings at the end of the reporting period. Another important change included the addition of Schedule L to the NAIC annual statement, which reports information and activities with intermediaries including the concentration of business with intermediaries and whether the intermediaries are subject to regulatory oversight, including risk-based capital requirements, and provides an indication as to whether the requirements have been met. Schedule L provides the regulators with more up-to-date information on the extent of risk transfer arrangements between the MCO and an intermediary organization that may not in turn be subject to regulatory oversight. This is particularly important to the regulators because when risk is transferred to unregulated entities, there is an increased risk that the assuming entity may not have adequate capital to sustain adverse underwriting risk. In these situations, the funds for the provision of care have already been disbursed by the MCO. If the intermediary is in financial distress, the funds may no longer be available, further increasing the financial risk to the MCO.

The information provided on both Schedules D and L also facilitated the development of the data to be reported in the MCO's risk-based capital filing. There is a direct feed of information from both Schedule D and Schedule L to the risk-based capital filing.

Many states also require the filing of a certification on claims reserves prepared by a licensed actuary. Audited financial statements are also required; the filing deadline may vary by state but is generally June 1. Any differences in the amounts reported in the audited financial statements and the annual filing due on March 1 must be disclosed in the footnotes to the audited financial statements. Depending on the applicable state's requirements, the audited financial statements may be prepared on either an SAP basis or a GAAP basis.

GAAP focuses more on the matching of revenue and expenses in a given reporting period to measure the earnings of an entity. The state insurance departments that have jurisdiction over the MCO are concerned with the MCO's ability to pay claims in the future. For example, certain expenditures (e.g., capital assets) may benefit future earnings ability and therefore are likely to be capitalized and expensed ratably over future periods for GAAP. However, such costs are expensed immediately in accordance with SAP because moneys expended are no longer available to pay future liabilities.

The many differences between SAP and GAAP accounting are generally based on the premise of the state insurance department's ability to determine liquidity of the MCO. *Some of the major differences include the following:*

- treatment of certain assets and investments as nonadmitted under SAP (e.g., fixed assets other than electronic data processing equipment, past due premium receivables, certain loans and other receivables, and investments not authorized by statute or in excess of statutory limitations)
- deferred tax accounts
- carrying value of investments in subsidiaries (which is primarily affected by limitations in the carrying amount and the amortization period of goodwill)

The state Department of Insurance imposes minimum statutory capital requirements for HMOs. The NAIC adopted a model act for HMOs that specified that minimum capital for HMOs should be determined as follows:

- the greater of $1,000,000, or
- 2 percent of annual premium as reported on the most recent annual financial statement filed with the commissioners of insurance on the first $150 million of premium and 1 percent of annual premium on premium greater than $150 million, or
- an amount equal to the sum of three months' uncovered health care expenditures as reported on the most recent financial statement filed with the commissioners, or

- an amount equal to the sum of:
  — 8 percent of annual health care expenditures except those paid on a capitated basis or a managed hospital payment basis as reported on the most recent financial statement filed with the commissioner, and
  — 4 percent of annual health care expenditures paid on a managed hospital payment basis as reported on the most recent financial statement filed with the commissioner

Managed hospital basis means agreements wherein the financial risk is primarily related to the degree of utilization rather than to the cost of services. Uncovered expenditures means the costs to the HMO for health care services that are the obligation of the HMO, for which an enrollee may also be liable in the event of HMO insolvency and for which no alternative arrangements have been made that are acceptable to the commissioner.

Many states are in the process of adopting the NAIC model act. Other states maintain separate minimum surplus requirements. The requirements of each of the states generally call for plans of action when an entity's capital falls within a close range of the minimum requirement.

Although the states' minimum requirements have provided a means to measure the financial viability of an insurance entity, the states' requirements were often a flat minimum and disregarded the size of an entity or the differing degrees of risk to which different entities are exposed. Insurance entities' exposure to risk has become more diverse, and although some are conservative in investment and underwriting practices, others have been more aggressive.

The NAIC began examining existing capital requirements and concluded that consumers should be further protected by having companies that assume a more aggressive, risk-taking approach be subject to higher capital requirements. Risk-based capital (RBC) requirements were first required for life and health insurers and property/casualty insurers. A working group was formed in 1993 to develop a separate RBC formula for health organizations, including traditional health insurers, HMOs, Blue Cross/Blue Shield plans, and health service plans. The working group completed its assignment, and now RBC for Insurers Model Law published by the NAIC (the Law) covers the RBC requirements for such health organizations. In the final stages of development of the Law, MCOs were required to complete model filings using financial information reported in prior reporting periods; for the calendar year ended 1998, MCOs were required to file electronic and paper filings with the NAIC and to respective state regulators. Beginning with the calendar year ended 1999, MCOs need to complete the "RBC Plan" to be submitted as required by the Law in the event the reporting MCO's RBC requirements are not met. Consistent with the deadline for filing the MCO's NAIC annual statement, the RBC filing is due on March first.

RBC is a method of measuring the minimum amount of capital appropriate for an MCO to support its overall business operations on the basis of its size and degree of risk taken in each of the five major categories of risk: asset risk-affiliates, asset risk-other, underwriting risk, credit risk, and business risk. An MCO's RBC is calculated by applying factors to various asset, premium, and reserve items that result in a charge to the MCO's actual capital and arrives at "adjusted capital." The MCO's actual capital is compared with varying levels of the adjusted capital to determine levels of actions, if any, to be taken to improve actual capital. For example if the MCO's actual capital is greater than 200 percent of the adjusted capital, no action is required. At 200 percent of adjusted capital, the MCO is required to develop and submit a plan of action. If actual capital is below 150 percent, regulatory action is required; if the actual capital falls to 70 percent or less, then mandatory control of the MCO is required.

Of the five categories of risk, underwriting risk results in the largest charge to adjusted capital. The development of this charge was to protect against the risk of fluctuation in underwriting experience. The net charge for underwriting risk is offset by credits that are based to a great extent on the positive effect that management care arrangements may have on underwriting risk. There is a presumed benefit from certain managed care arrangements that may reduce the uncertainty about future claims payments. For example, capitated fee arrangements with no risk-sharing features are generally fixed costs per member per month and therefore reduce the MCO's risk associated with adverse fluctuations in utilization or intensity, thus providing for a more defined estimate of the cost of the capitated fee arrangement. The impact on an MCO's RBC for the other categories of risk includes protection against investments in assets of affiliates, including subsidiary entities with their own RBC requirements, investments in other assets whose value may be subject to fluctuation in market value, credit risk associated with the recoverability of amounts owed to the MCO (i.e., premium receivables, recoverables from providers), and business risk including the effect of excessive business growth on the MCO's capital.

The regulatory environment under which MCOs operate is continuously changing to meet market changes, and entities need to prepare themselves in particular to meet the challenges imposed by new or expected legislation.

BUDGETING AND FINANCIAL FORECASTING

The importance of maintaining detailed budgets has been discussed throughout this chapter. Financial forecasts, which project activity and results beyond the current period, are also important management tools. Financial forecasts are often developed several months in advance of the actual reporting period. In developing the forecasts, a balance between complexity and simplicity is sought by the financial manager. Although it is essential to capture much detail to develop the overall forecast, the detail information must roll up to a summary level that will facilitate presentation to senior decision makers within the organization and to provide ease for monitoring variances in actual results. At the early stages of development, if the financial forecast evolves from the appropriate level of detail, the overall summaries discussed by senior management teams will be more meaningful.

At the highest level, membership data priced at blended premium rates must be presented. The development of both the aggregate membership growth and the blended premium rates is based on input from personnel within sales and marketing, underwriting, and actuarial functions and should have considered specific assumptions for the different array of products offered by the MCO. It is important to verify assumptions with the sales function's expectations and the organization's underwriting policies and pricing strategies.

Because both new and renewal membership and premium rate changes are affected by seasonal patterns, the assumptions should trend from quarterly, if not monthly, baseline data. Developing the overall financial forecasts from this level of detail will assist the financial manager in providing the most accurate report of actual versus budgeted results. Understanding variances in planned to actual premium revenue will support whether or not expected rate changes or net membership growth assumptions were achieved. Sometimes the rate increase by product and the net membership growth may meet expected targets; however, changes in the membership by product type could still result in the aggregate premium levels not being achieved. The ability of the financial manager to identify the root cause of variances between forecast and actual results is essential to achieving an organization's overall financial goals.

The baseline for the medical expense component of the financial forecast is generally developed from a historical "look back" of the results. At the time that financial forecasts are being developed, there is still some level of estimation in the historical results that further complicates the development of the baseline estimate of medical expenses. This baseline must then be adjusted for expected changes, including but not limited to medical inflation trends, expected changes in regulations (e.g., new benefit mandates), changes in provider contracting arrangements, and enhancements to patient management programs. The effects of changes in provider contracts may depend on whether the changes have an impact on a significant portion of the overall membership. In addition, the effects of patient management programs often require a period of time before the financial impact of the benefit is achieved and/or measurable.

It may also be beneficial, to the extent it is practicable, to segregate average medical costs by types of provider contract arrangements. For example, identifying expected per member per month costs for global contract arrangements, fee for service arrangements, specialty capitation, and other ancillary arrangements could provide critical information for monitoring the success of the various types of provider arrangements. If it is difficult to identify expected or actual costs for these arrangements, one may question the appropriateness of the arrangement and the viability of the rate that was negotiated with the provider.

Other key components of forecasting medical expenses include the impact of risk-sharing arrangements with providers and the cost and/or benefit of the historical settlement in addition to regulatory imposed costs, such as interest assessed on late payment of claims or surcharges assessed as subsidies to finance the cost of individual and small employer insurance and care for the uninsured.

Administrative costs need to be forecast. Consideration of the cost to invest in planned growth and to sustain existing membership volumes is necessary. The most significant component of the administrative costs is typically salary and related expenses.

Whether the financial manager is developing premium revenue, medical expense, or administrative costs, the development of the financial forecast is an iterative process, and the financial model must be flexible to facilitate this process while being responsive and not unreasonably complex.

The financial forecasting process must also include the development of a projected balance sheet. This is particularly important to evaluate the impact of the projected growth in operations on minimum capital requirements. In addition, the forecasting process should require variations from the baseline projections to determine the risks and exposures if the actual results fall short of the baseline and also to project the impact if actual results are better than expected. Cash flow analyses are also important to ensure that cash will be generated from operations or to determine the extent to which cash reserves will be needed, particularly as new lines of business are pursued.

CONCLUSION

Whether the financial manager is developing budgets or financial forecasts or preparing financial statements, he or she must depend on the information prepared and maintained by the operating departments. This information is an integral part of the financial manager's decision-making process. Communication among the various functional areas in the MCO will be key to the successful operation of the entity. Timely financial reporting enhances management's ability to determine performance against anticipated results and redirect its strategies to minimize exposure to loss and preserve a favorable financial performance.

CHAPTER 48

Tax Issues Relating to Health Risk-Bearing Entities

Phillip G. Royalty and Terry A. Jacobs

This chapter discusses the federal income tax treatment of taxable and tax-exempt health maintenance organizations (HMOs) and certain other types of health risk-bearing entities.

TAXABLE HEALTH RISK-BEARING ENTITIES

Status As an Insurance Company

Regulation Section 1.801-3(a) defines an insurance company as a company whose primary and predominant activity is the business of issuing insurance contracts. This is a subjective test, one that is generally met if a company can demonstrate that more than 50 percent of its business relates to the issuance of insurance contracts.

Phillip G. Royalty, JD, CPA, is a partner and director of the National Tax Department Health Industry Group of Ernst & Young LLP in Washington, D. C. Before joining Ernst & Young, Mr. Royalty was a tax lawyer with the Internal Revenue Service Exempt Organizations Division in Washington, D.C.

Terry A. Jacobs, JD, CPA, is the National Director of Insurance Tax Services for Ernst & Young LLP, based in Washington, D.C. He oversees the firm's technical tax services and helps clients identify and strategically respond to issues and opportunities arising from a changing business environment and legislative, regulatory, and tax policy changes. Mr. Jacobs previously served as Attorney Advisor to the Assistant Secretary of the Treasury for Tax Policy and has worked with the Internal Revenue Service on tax matters relating to insurance companies and products.

Generally, an insurance contract exists if the contract shifts and distributes risk. These concepts were first applied by the Supreme Court in *LeGierse* and have further developed over the years.[1,2] Generally, the courts have held that an insurable risk of economic loss must be shifted from an insured to an insurer for an insurance relationship to exist. That risk must also be distributed among several unrelated insureds. Applied to an HMO, risk is shifted from the member to the HMO when the HMO contractually assumes an obligation to provide a service for the member on illness or injury for a premium payment representing a fraction of the possible loss. The risk is distributed among the number of members.

The application of the LeGierse risk shifting and distributing concepts to an HMO is complicated by the fact that many HMOs assume an obligation to satisfy a member's loss by providing physician services rather than providing financial indemnification to the member. The Internal Revenue Service (IRS) has focused on services provided by physicians rather than the HMO's payment for these services. In Revenue Ruling 68-27, the IRS determined that an organization that provided medical service contracts was not an insurance company because its primary business was not issuing insurance contracts.[3] The IRS concluded that there was no hazard or peril inured with respect to the preventive care portion of the medical service contracts. Although there was a risk with respect to the sick or disabled phase of the medical service contracts, it was a business risk of an organization furnishing medical services on a fixed-price basis, not an insurance risk. Because the essential element of an insurance contract, the transfer of an insurance risk, was lacking, the medical service contracts were not insurance contracts.

Similarly, in *Group Life & Health Insurance Co. v. Royal Drug*, the Supreme Court examined an arrangement between an HMO and a provider of health care services.[4] The court stated that if an insurance company were to acquire a chain of drugstores to control the cost of satisfying its obligations, the acquisition would not be the business of insurance. The court reasoned that insurance is a relationship between the insurer and the insured, not between the insurer and a third party.

The IRS distinguished the principles of Revenue Ruling 68-27 in Technical Advice Memorandum (TAM) 9412002 and concluded that two IPA model HMOs were insurance companies for federal income tax purposes. The HMOs were not licensed to provide medical services and contracted with physicians to provide care on a fee-for-service basis. The HMOs were not liable for any malpractice claims against affiliated physicians. Other than deductibles, copayments, and coinsurance, the HMOs had full responsibility for payments to the affiliated physicians. The HMOs were subject to the control of the state Department of Insurance in their state of domestication. The department maintained control and approval of premiums and required the filing of an annual statement and state income taxes under the rules applicable to domestic accident and health insurance companies. The HMOs were subject to examination by the insurance department, including a review of the unearned premiums and incurred claims reserves; were required to furnish solvency deposits; and were subject to assessments to subsidize health insurance for high-risk subscribers. More than 90 percent of the HMOs' revenues were from actuarially determined member premiums.

The IRS analyzed whether the predominant business activity of the HMOs was the issuance of insurance contracts. It found that the contracts issued by the HMOs provided for risk shifting

and risk distribution and were therefore insurance contracts. Because the premiums from the insurance contracts constituted more than 90 percent of the revenues, the IRS concluded that the primary and predominant business activity of the HMOs was the issuance of insurance contracts and that they should be treated as insurance companies for tax purposes. The IRS distinguished the facts from the organization in Revenue Ruling 68-27, in which the taxpayer had hired physicians, nurses, and technicians to provide care to its members.

The IRS reached a similar conclusion in TAM 9416001. Although the taxpayer in TAM 9416001 was not an HMO, the analysis of the federal income tax treatment of the company was quite similar to that of a health care plan. The taxpayer was a provider of home warranty contracts, under which it agreed to repair or replace certain systems and appliances that broke down during the contract period. The IRS held that, unlike the taxpayer in Revenue Ruling 68-27, the taxpayer in question did not provide any services through salaried staff but rather contracted with independent contractors and technicians to provide services. Thus, the home warranty contracts were insurance contracts, and, because the predominant activity of the taxpayer was issuing such contracts, it was an insurance company.

In TAM 9601001, the IRS held that a corporation that sells motor vehicle service agreements to the general public is an insurance company even though it reinsures 100 percent of the risk of loss it assumes under the motor vehicle service agreements. The IRS concluded that the indemnification under the reinsurance agreement is immaterial to the determination of the corporation's status as an insurance company for federal income tax purposes. Based on this position, the IRS may classify taxable HMOs as insurance companies even though they capitate all or most of their providers.

If an HMO is considered an insurance company for federal tax purposes, it is taxed as a corporation. Its taxable income is determined under rules applicable to insurance companies, including the unique treatment provided for unearned premiums, discounting of unpaid losses, proration adjustments, and salvage and subrogation.

An HMO that is considered an insurance company is faced with a unique issue. The U.S. Code and regulations presume that an insurance company annually files a uniform annual statement, the National Association of Insurance Commissioners' (NAIC's) yellow book, with the applicable state insurance department. Many accounting methods and tax calculations are based on the NAIC statement. HMOs do not file a yellow book, however, and may not file any statement with a regulatory authority. These companies will, therefore, experience a problem in that their information or financial statements are not in conformity with the yellow book. In some instances, this may be a mere mechanical problem, but in other instances the issue may be more troublesome.

Accrued Claim Liability

At year end, many HMOs accrue liabilities for outstanding claims. If the HMO is an insurance company, it is allowed to include in its unpaid losses a reasonable estimate of its incurred losses. If the HMO is not an insurance company, however, the liability must meet the all-events test and the economic performance requirements of Section 461(h). The all-events test requires that all of the events have occurred that determine the fact of the liability and the amount of the liability must be determined with reasonable accuracy.[5] In addition, the all-events test generally cannot be satisfied sooner than when economic performance occurs. If the liability of the taxpayer arises out of the providing of services to the taxpayer by another person, economic performance occurs as the person performs the services.[6]

In interpreting the all-events test, the Supreme Court in General Dynamics held that the last event necessary to fix the taxpayer's liability was not the receipt of medical care by members but rather the filing of medical reimbursement claims.[7] Furthermore, the court continued, if the all-events test permitted the deduction of incurred but not reported claims, there would have been no need for Congress to enact Sections

832(b)(5) and 832(c)(4), which explicitly allow insurance companies to deduct these reserves.

General Dynamics, however, involved self-insurance of the company's employees. The court recognized that the employees had certain motivations relating to job security to prevent or dissuade them from actually making a claim even though the medical expense was incurred. This fact is not present in a prepaid health plan such as an HMO. The physicians are motivated to file claims. Furthermore, an HMO contractually assumes an obligation to cover a member's medical loss and contracts separately with physicians. This may factually distinguish an HMO from General Dynamics.

In a technical advice memorandum, the IRS allowed the deduction for accrued claims in the year the services were provided to the member for a firm operating much like a staff model HMO.[8] The firm offered mental health and substance abuse counseling services through its own clinics. It entered into contracts with certain third-party vendors to provide special services beyond the skills of the firm's clinic staff. Under the contracts, after the firm preauthorized the patient care to be provided by the outside vendor, the vendor was required to offer the service, and the firm was required to pay for it.

Under the firm's accrual method of accounting, the firm recorded a liability at the time of preauthorization on the basis of the number of authorized days or visits and the specific contract or average historical rate. The firm also recorded a liability for preauthorized services to be performed in the next taxable year, relying on the recurring item exception to the economic performance rules. The firm adjusted the recorded liability if actual invoice amounts differed from the accrual, which occurred when the treatment varied from that originally authorized.

The IRS held that preauthorization of services does not constitute economic performance because all events that determine the fact of the liability will not occur until the preauthorized services are performed. In addition, the IRS stated that, because the company had failed properly to adopt the recurring item exception method of accounting, the company could not accrue amounts for services to be performed in the next taxable year. The firm had to accrue the expenses in the year the services were performed.

The recurring item exception to the economic performance rules is provided in Section 461(h)(3)(A). Under this exception, a deduction is permitted if:

- The all-events test, without regard to economic performance, is satisfied during such taxable year
- Economic performance occurs within the shorter of 8.5 months or a reasonable time after the close of such taxable year
- The item is recurring in nature, and the taxpayer consistently treats similar items as incurred in the taxable year in which the all-events test is met
- The item is not material, or the accrual of the item in the year that the all-events test is met results in a better matching of income and expense

The all-events test, discussed above, is the threshold requirement for claiming a deduction. The second and third requirements are not usually troublesome because HMOs normally pay claims within 8.5 months, and the claims are recurring in nature. Accrued claims may not be an immaterial item, however, so that an HMO must prove that the accrual of such liability in the taxable year results in more proper matching of income and deductions to satisfy the last requirement. Because a taxpayer's financial treatment of an item is considered evidence of the proper period for matching of income and deductions, HMOs that deduct accrued claims should expense these liabilities in the same period on their financial statements. Such a financial statement presentation normally is permissible under generally accepted accounting principles.

Revenue Ruling 98-39 held that accrued cooperative advertising costs were deductible before receiving the claims.[9] The IRS distinguished General Dynamics because filing the claims for the advertising costs was merely a "ministerial act." If the rationale in Revenue Ruling 98-39 is applied to HMOs, then HMOs should be able to deduct their incurred but not reported (IBNR) costs. The ratio-

nale of Revenue Ruling 98-39 should apply to HMOs because health care providers are unlikely to fail to submit claims.

Withhold Arrangements

Some plans provide an incentive to providers to meet certain objectives through a withhold mechanism. Under these arrangements, a portion of the fee paid to the provider is withheld and not paid to the provider unless the provider meets certain economic criteria. Typically, the withhold is not paid until after the year end of the plan.

In TAM 9723005, the IRS applied Section 404 to deny a loss reserve deduction to an HMO. The HMO, an individual practice association taxed as an insurance company, had provider contracts with individual physicians, hospitals, and other health care providers. These provider contracts included a specified reimbursement formula with a risk-sharing plan under which participating providers would share financial risks and rewards with the HMO, depending on the ultimate health care costs compared with the HMO's health care budget.

Under the risk-sharing plan, the providers could be compensated in three ways. Initially, the providers would be paid 85 percent of the standard fee schedule amount, and the remaining 15 percent of the fee schedule amount would be allocated to a "risk withhold" account. If anticipated medical efficiencies are achieved, the funds in that account would be paid to the provider. Otherwise the amounts would be applied to cover the HMO's health care costs. If there is an overall health care budget surplus, the provider could receive a surplus distribution. Although the amounts to be paid to a specific provider are unknown at the end of the year, the total payments to be paid to all providers can be estimated by use of actuarial methods.

The HMO estimated its liability for payment of risk withholds and surplus distributions to the providers on the basis of the claims incurred (reported and unreported). In computing its taxable income, the HMO included that liability in unpaid losses. The IRS disallowed the deduction, holding that the liability was deferred compensation subject to the timing rules of Section 404. Therefore, if the providers are on the cash basis method of accounting, Section 404 essentially requires the deductibility of the liability for the risk withhold amounts and surplus distributions with respect to the HMO to be limited to a cash basis (unless paid within two and a half months).

The HMO argued that because it is an insurance company, the estimated liabilities are for amounts to satisfy the insureds' claims, and those estimated amounts are included in loss reserves and not subject to Section 404. The IRS agreed that the HMO spread its risk of loss over a large number of insureds; however, the IRS found the managed care aspect of the HMO's business to be a distinguishing factor. Under the risk-sharing system, the HMO provided financial incentives to providers to control use of health care services by linking the providers' compensation to use. The IRS equated this risk-sharing agreement to a performance-based deferred compensation arrangement used in other industries. Citing legislative history, the IRS stated that Section 404(a) has broad application to deferred compensation arrangements, and even if the liability was correctly included in losses incurred, the timing rules of Section 404(a) would take precedence.

The HMO also argued that Section 404 cannot apply to losses incurred. The IRS, on the basis of Section 832(c)(4) and several cases that it cited, rejected the argument that losses incurred are actually an exclusion from insurance company gross income and not a deduction.

State Premium Tax

Generally, states subject premiums received by regulated insurance companies to a premium tax. Depending on the state (and type of business), premium tax rates can range from 0.5 percent to 3 percent. Many states exempt an insurance company that is subject to a premium tax from the state's corporate income tax. Several states subject insurance companies to both an income tax and the premium tax. Also, several states subject regulated HMOs to the state's corporate income tax and exclude them from the state's premium tax.

Many state tax statutes and regulations do not specifically provide for the taxation of other types of health risk-bearing entities. A position that is likely to be adopted by many states, however, is that an entity regulated by a state as an insurance company will be subject to taxation by that state as an insurance company. Thus the regulation of a health risk-bearing entity as an insurance company will probably subject the entity in many states to a premium tax.[10]

Other Types of Taxable Health Risk-Bearing Entities

The rules previously discussed with respect to taxable HMOs apply generally to other types of health risk-bearing entities. If a health risk-bearing entity is determined to be an insurance company for federal income tax purposes, it is taxed as a corporation regardless of its legal form and is subject to special accounting rules. Generally, these special rules result in favorable tax treatment for an insurance company relative to a noninsurance company. In certain situations, however, these rules may result in the acceleration of income tax for many health risk-bearing entities.

For federal income tax purposes, an insurance company is a company whose primary and predominant business activity during the taxable year is the issuing or reinsuring of contracts that have the elements of risk shifting and risk distribution. Although its name, charter powers, and subjection to state insurance laws are significant in determining the business that a company is authorized to conduct, it is the character of the business actually conducted in the taxable year that determines whether a company is taxable as an insurance company under the Internal Revenue Code.

Generally, health risk-bearing entities will meet the risk distribution test because, to gain efficiencies and provide cost-effective services, the entity must provide services to a significant number of lives. Thus, the essential issue is whether the contract contains risk shifting or the provision of health services. Factors that may affect the determination of whether a contract involves risk shifting or the provision of health services include the state regulatory treatment of the contract and the issuing entity, the malpractice liability retained by the entity, and the payment mechanism to the entity and to the entity's providers (i.e., salaried employees, contracted providers on a capitation basis, or contracted providers on a fee-for-service basis). Each of these, on its own, may not determine insurance company status. Taken together, however, these factors are relevant in determining whether a contract involves risk shifting or the provision of health services.

TAX-EXEMPT HEALTH RISK-BEARING ENTITIES

Before the Enactment of Section 501(m)

Before the enactment of Section 501(m) in the 1986 Tax Reform Act, in determining whether an HMO qualified for exempt status under Section 501(c)(3) of the Internal Revenue Code, the IRS generally followed the tax court's decision in *Sound Health Association v. Commissioner*.[11] Sound Health held that a staff model HMO that provided health care services to its members on a prepaid basis and to nonmembers on a fee-for-service basis, and which also provided free emergency care to indigents, qualified for exempt status under Section 501(c)(3). In holding that Sound Health qualified for Section 501(c)(3) status, the court made an analogy between the HMO and the tax-exempt hospital described in Revenue Ruling 69-545.[12]

General Counsel Memorandum (GCM) 39057 stated, however, that an HMO affiliated with an IPA did not qualify under Section 501(c)(3) because it was organized and operated primarily for the benefit of the IPA physician members.

Also, *Geisinger Health Plan v. Commissioner* held that arrangements for the provision of health care to members through contracts with other entities does not qualify an HMO for exempt status under Section 501(c)(3).[13] The court applied a flexible community benefit standard, and concluded that the HMO did not demonstrate that it benefitted anyone other than its subscribers.

HMOs not resembling Sound Health may be able to qualify for exemption under Section 501(c)(4) as a social welfare organization even though there are no published revenue rulings concerning this issue. Although Revenue Ruling 86-98 held that IPAs do not qualify for tax-exempt status under Section 501(c)(4) or (6), the IRS did not adopt a blanket prohibition against exempt status for IPA model HMOs.[14] Over the years, several IPA model HMOs have received favorable determination letters under Section 501(c)(4).

After the Enactment of Section 501(m)

Effective for taxable years beginning after December 31, 1986, Section 501(m) provides that an organization described in Section 501(c)(3) or (4) may be exempt only if no substantial part of its activities consists of providing commercial type insurance.[15] A Section 501(c)(3) or (4) organization with insubstantial commercial insurance activities is exempt from tax, but the activity of providing commercial-type insurance is an unrelated business activity. The organization is treated as an insurance company for purposes of Subchapter L with respect to this commercial insurance activity in lieu of the tax on unrelated business income of tax-exempt organizations imposed by Section 511.

Commercial-type insurance does not include insurance provided at substantially below cost to a class of charitable recipients (Section 501(m)(3)(A)), or incidental health insurance provided by an HMO of a kind customarily provided by such organizations (Section 501(m)(3)(B)).

Although the statutory language of Section 501(m) relating to HMOs may be ambiguous, the committee reports are not. The conference report to the 1986 Tax Act states that Section 501(m) is not intended to affect the exemption of any HMOs:

> The conference agreement does not alter the tax-exempt status of [HMOs]. HMOs provide physician services in a variety of practice settings, primarily through physicians who are either employees or partners of the HMO or through contracts with individual phy-

sicians or one or more groups of physicians (organized on a group practice
basis or individual practice basis).[16]

Congress again explained the application of
Section 501(m) to HMOs in the Technical and
Miscellaneous Revenue Act of 1988 (TAMRA)[17]:

Under the 1986 Act, the provision relating to organizations engaged in commercial-type insurance activities did not
alter the tax-exempt status of [HMOs].
HMOs provide physician services in a
variety of practice settings, primarily
through physicians who are either employees or partners of the HMO or
through contracts with individual physicians or one or more groups of physicians (organized on a group practice or
individual practice basis). The conference agreement clarifies that, in addition to the general exemption for
[HMOs], organizations that provide
supplemental [HMO]-type services
(such as dental or vision services) are
not treated as providing commercial-
type insurance if they operate in the
same manner as [an HMO].[18]

Despite the express congressional language in
the 1986 Tax Act and TAMRA, the IRS concluded in two general counsel memoranda that the
intended meaning of the HMO exception to Section 501(m) is unclear. In GCMs 39828 (August
30, 1990) and 39829 (August 30, 1990), the IRS
stated that it does not read the legislative history to
Section 501(m) as indicating that HMOs should
be recognized as not providing commercial-type
insurance within the meaning of the section. Instead, whether an HMO is providing Section
501(m) commercial-type insurance is based on the
particular facts and circumstances involved, not
solely on whether an HMO operates as a staff,
group, or IPA model.

The IRS position as stated in these GCMs is
that Section 501(m) will not affect the tax-exempt status of any of the common, existing
HMOs that compensate primary care physicians
exclusively on a salary, capitation, or other

fixed-fee basis, even though the HMO may pay
other providers on a fee-for-service basis.[19] The
term "common, existing HMOs" refers to
HMOs as they were commonly structured at the
time of the 1986 Tax Act. The IRS maintains
that, although called HMOs, many of the hybrid
organizations, such as point-of-service plans or
open-ended HMOs, closely resemble indemnity
insurers in operation and that these hybrid
HMOs are precluded from exempt status if a
substantial part of their activities consists of providing out-of-plan benefits on a fee-for-service
basis. Furthermore, if the activities are not substantial, the income from those activities is
treated as unrelated business income.

In addition to meeting the requirements of
Section 501(m), an HMO must satisfy the requirements for exempt status under Section
501(c). In GCM 39828, the IRS listed several
factors that are relevant in determining whether
an HMO qualifies as a tax-exempt charitable organization under Section 501(c)(3). These factors are not all inclusive, nor is any one factor
determinative. They include the following:

- Actually providing health care services and
  maintaining facilities and staff
- Offering services to nonmembers on a fee-
  for-service basis
- Providing care and extending reduced rates
  to indigent persons
- Caring for persons covered by Medicare,
  Medicaid, and similar programs
- Making emergency department facilities
  available to the community regardless of an
  ability to pay (and informing the community about the services)
- Operating a meaningful subsidized membership program
- Forming a board of directors that is broadly
  representative of the community
- Offering health education programs that
  are open to the community
- Conducting health research programs
- Having health care providers who are paid
  on a fixed-fee basis
- Using surplus funds to improve facilities,
  equipment, patient care, or any of the programs described in the list

GCM 39828 lists other factors to determine whether an HMO meets the Section 501(c)(3) requirement that no meaningful restrictions be placed on membership that would preclude the HMO from serving the community as a whole. An HMO meets these requirements if:

- Individuals compose a substantial portion of membership
- An active program exists to attract individual members
- Uniform rates for prepaid care are provided by a community rating system
- Individual and group members have similar rates
- No substantive age or health barriers exist for determining eligibility for individuals or groups

Both HMOs considered in GCM 39828 failed to qualify, in the IRS's view, for exempt status under Section 501(c)(3). The IRS ruled that the HMOs lacked sufficient community benefit and that their membership was not open to the community. The IRS also concluded that both HMOs were providing commercial-type insurance under 501(m).

GCM 39830 (August 30, 1990) held that a separately incorporated nonstaff model HMO that is controlled by a tax-exempt parent organization of a nonprofit health care system, and that does not qualify for exemption under Section 501(c)(3) on its own merits, cannot qualify for exemption as an "integral part" of its exempt parent. The IRS has subsequently stated that an HMO may qualify for exempt status under the integral part doctrine if it serves only the patients of the health system that controls the HMO. See Chapter 27, *IRS Exempt Organizations Examination Guidelines Handbook* (Appendix 48–A), sections 27.8.2.2 and 27.9.2.

In GCM 39829, the IRS considered whether a particular HMO qualified as a tax-exempt social welfare organization under Section 501(c)(4), taking Section 501(m) into consideration. The HMO had received a letter in 1978 from the IRS determining that it was exempt under Section 501(c)(4). Exemption standards under Section 501(c)(4) are similar to those outlined for Section 501(c)(3) organizations, only less restric-

tive. Standards under Section 501(c)(4) focus on whether membership is open to individuals and groups; whether the HMO serves low-income, high-risk, medically underserved, or elderly persons; and whether premiums are established on a community-rated basis. Provided that the HMO had not materially changed its operations from the previous determination letter, the IRS stated that the HMO could rely on its 1978 letter granting exempt status under Section 501(c)(4), at least until Section 501(m) became effective.

In determining whether commercial-type insurance under Section 501(m) is being provided, GCM 39829 lists the following factors that must be analyzed:

- Whether an insurance risk is being transferred and distributed
- Whether, and to what extent, the entity is operated in a manner similar to that of for-profit insurers or Blue Cross/Blue Shield organizations
- Whether, and to what extent, the entity is marketing a product similar to that of for-profit insurers or Blue Cross/Blue Shield organizations
- Whether, and to what extent, the entity provides health care services directly
- Whether, and to what extent, the entity has shifted any risk of loss to the service providers through salary or fixed-fee compensation arrangements

The IRS concluded that the IPA model HMO retained its exempt status under Section 501(c)(4) even after Section 501(m) became effective. The HMO capitated its contracted physicians, and the capitation represented about 50 percent of the HMO's total payments for medical benefits.

In GCM 39829, the IRS made the following observations about the applicability of Section 501(m) to HMOs:

- The term "insurance company" in Treasury Regulation 1.801-3(a) is not the same as commercial-type insurance under Section 501(m). This suggests that the IRS may not agree that an HMO that is barred from tax-exempt status under Section 501(m) necessarily qualifies as an insurance company for federal tax purposes.

- The only practical way to distinguish an HMO from commercial insurers or Blue Cross/Blue Shield organizations is the fact that an HMO employs its own staff, operates its own facilities, or otherwise fixes its costs by shifting a substantial portion of the risk to providers.
- Nonstaff, nongroup HMOs that pay providers on a fee-for-service basis, even when the providers are subject to a percentage withhold or reduction for overutilization, are much harder to distinguish from commercial insurance companies and Blue Cross/Blue Shield organizations. No opinion was expressed as to whether these types of HMOs primarily provide services or an insurance-type benefit, or whether they fit within Section 501(m)(3)(B).
- In determining whether an HMO's insurance aspects are incidental, salary, or capitation agreements with primary care physicians ordinarily should be accorded greater weight than agreements with specialists or hospitals.[20]

IRS Revokes HMO's Section 501(c)(3) Status

In an unreleased technical advice memorandum that was published in *Tax Notes* in December, 1998,[21] the IRS concluded that a Section 501(c)(3) HMO's exempt status should be revoked. The IRS also concluded that the HMO is providing substantial commercial-type insurance within the meaning of Section 501(m)(1), preventing it from qualifying for exempt status under Section 501(c)(3) or 501(c)(4).

The HMO is a member of a nonprofit, multicorporate health care system and was recognized as exempt in 1985. The system's parent (M) is the sole member of the HMO and is also the parent of N, which owned or operated 25 acute care hospitals in three western states. The HMO was recognized as exempt under Section 501(c)(3) on June 5, 1985; 6 months later, it was licensed as a qualified HMO.

The HMO does not operate an emergency room, does not treat nonmember patients, and does not have a Medicare risk-sharing contract. The HMO arranges inpatient and outpatient hospital services to its enrollees primarily through M hospitals and provides primary and specialty care physician services through contracts with physicians. The HMO provides coverage only through accepted employer groups with 25 or more employees. Employer groups with fewer than 25 employees were subject to medical underwriting and could be accepted on a case-by-case basis. Some employees or conditions were excluded from coverage. The HMO's trustees were appointed, and subject to removal, by M. The bylaws provide that at all times a majority of the board will consist of individuals who are community representatives and do not have a financial interest in the operations of the HMO.

The physicians, who are either employed by M or maintain independent practices in their local communities, are paid the greater of a capitated fee or 85 percent of the physician's customary charges. The HMO does not withhold any portion of fees paid to physicians. In the event of budget surpluses, the physicians may be eligible to receive additional payments. However, in the event of a budget deficit, the physicians have no financial obligations. The HMO uses an adjusted community rating method to determine its premiums.

Approximately 90 percent of the inpatient and outpatient hospital services provided to HMO enrollees were provided by M hospitals. During a period covered by the examination, the HMO paid 70.4 percent of the total amount paid for physician services to physicians who were not employed by M, comprising 52.4 percent of the total amount paid by the HMO for all medical services (i.e., professional and hospital services) during the same period.

The IRS ruled that because the HMO does not provide medical services at its own facilities, does not operate an emergency room, and does not provide services regardless of an individual's ability to pay, it does not satisfy the community benefit standard under Rev. Rul. 69-545 and Sound Health. In addition, the IRS ruled, because the HMO provides services almost exclusively to its enrollees, it does not satisfy the flexible community benefit standard in *Geisinger*, which requires a benefit to the community as a whole and not just a benefit to the HMO subscribers and a limited number of nonsubscribers. The IRS noted that the HMO does not subsidize premiums for, or retain as members, persons who become unable to pay. Further, although the HMO does not terminate a person's enrollment on the basis of health conditions or experience, offers a variety of free programs to enrollees, provides health care prevention and education services at cost, and establishes premiums using an adjusted community rating method, these benefits are almost exclusively available to the HMO's enrollees.

The IRS also concluded that the HMO does not qualify for exempt status under the integral part doctrine because a substantial portion (52.4 percent) of the amount paid by the HMO for medical services was paid to physicians not employed by M (i.e., for services for individuals who were not patients of M under Revenue Ruling 68-376, 1968-2 C.B. 246).

Analyzing the arrangement under Section 501(m)(1), the IRS concluded that the HMO's fee-for-service arrangement shifts only an incidental portion of the HMO's total economic risk of loss to the physicians. The IRS did note that physician compensation based on capitated payments, or a discounted fee-for-service arrangement (minimum 15 percent discount), coupled with a significant withhold provision (minimum 15 percent of the discounted fee), would constitute shifting the economic risk to the providers. If it shifts the risk, the HMO will not be considered to be engaged in a commercial-type insurance activity under Section 501(m). In this case, although fees paid to physicians were discounted, they were not subject to a withhold. Because the amount of fees paid to nonemployee physicians was substantial (52.4 percent of the total amount paid by the HMO for all medical services), the IRS concluded that a substantial part of the HMO's activities consists of providing commercial-type insurance under Section 501(m)(1).

The IRS did not consider limiting the retroactive effect of the exemption revocation because the taxpayer expressly requested the IRS not to exercise its discretionary authority to do so under Section 7805(b).

HMO Challenges IRS's Revocation of Exempt Status

IHC Health Plans has challenged the revocation of its Section 501(c)(3) status, filing a petition for declaratory judgment in the Tax Court.[22] The Utah-based HMO claims that its activities are an integral part of an exempt health care system and that no substantial part of its activities constitutes "commercial-type insurance" within the meaning of Section 501(m).

In its Tax Court petition, IHC argues that it continues to be operated exclusively for the charitable purpose of promoting health for the benefit of the community under the Sound Health decision. Further, IHC argues that its activities are an integral part of the activities of Intermountain Health Care Inc. and IHC Health Services Inc., both of which are Section 501(c)(3) organizations. IHC's mission, according to the petition, is "the development of alternative health care delivery systems" for the benefit of the integrated system. IHC points out that it offers a selection of six health plan alternatives through its own resources and those of its two subsidiaries. "By balancing pricing options with choices of physicians in a variety of ways, the health plans offered to the community can be tailored to meet the differing needs" of its enrollees, IHC argues.

IHC further argues that its activities enable the integrated system to reach more people and to deliver health care more efficiently to the communities it serves. In addition, because it arranges for the provision of health care through numerous hospitals and other facilities, it enables the integrated system to provide services that "transcend the typical services offered by health systems."

With regard to physician compensation, IHC notes that its methods include capitation, discounted fee for service, and discounted fee for service with withholds or bonuses. The compensation is set by contract in a reasonable manner and does not result in inurement, IHC maintains. It argues that no substantial part of its activities constitutes the provision of "commercial-type insurance" within the meaning of Section 501(m)(1).

IRS Guidelines on Examinations of Tax-Exempt HMOs

In May 1999 the Internal Revenue Service issued a chapter in the Internal Revenue Manual (IRM) Exempt Organizations Examinations Guidelines Handbook that provides guidance for IRS examinations of tax-exempt HMOs.[23] The chapter covers the following four areas:

- Definitions and a general description of the different types of HMOs, physician and hospital compensation methods, and methods of determining enrollment and setting premiums
- Factors the IRS will take into account in determining whether an HMO qualifies for exempt status under Section 501(c)(3) and the examination guidelines for Section 501(c)(3) HMOs
- IRS exemption criteria and examination guidelines for Section 501(c)(4) HMOs
- Guidelines for determining whether an HMO is precluded, under Section 501(m), from exempt status under Section 501(c)(3) or 501(c)(4) because of substantial commercial-type insurance activities

The Section 501(m) guidelines include guidance for determining whether the exceptions to the definition of commercial-type insurance set forth in Section 501(m)(3)(A) (relating to insurance provided substantially below cost to a class of charitable recipients) and Section 501(m)(3)(B) (relating to incidental health insurance provided by an HMO of a kind customarily provided by such organizations) may apply, as well as guidance for determining unrelated business income from insubstantial commercial-type insurance activities under Section 501(m)(2).

In general, the chapter incorporates the IRS positions discussed previously on tax-exemption issues relating to HMOs. A copy of Chapter 27, *Exempt Organizations Examination Guidelines Handbook* on Health Maintenance Organizations is attached as Appendix 48–A.

Other Types of Tax-Exempt Health Risk-Bearing Entities

Integrated Delivery Systems (IDSs)

The IRS has issued several rulings recognizing the tax-exempt status under Section 501(c)(3) of IDSs.[24] To obtain recognition of exemption, an IDS generally must demonstrate that it is benefiting the community through some combination of charity care, treatment of Medicare and Medicaid patients, research and education activities, and the like. Also, the IRS generally requires that a majority of its board be comprised of individuals who are independent of the organization, and that the organization adopt a conflict of interest policy.[25] In addition, in situations in which an IDS is buying a physician practice, the IRS closely reviews the method used in valuing the practice to ensure that no more than fair market value is paid for the practice.[26] Finally, the IRS reviews incentive compensation arrangements between the IDS and physicians to guard against the possibility of private benefit or private inurement.[27]

Physician-Hospital Organizations (PHOs)

The IRS's position is that PHOs generally will not qualify for tax-exempt status on the basis that their activities further the private interests of the physician members of the PHO.[28] A PHO affiliated with the University of Kansas Hospital, however, received an IRS determination letter recognizing its tax-exempt status under Section 501(c)(3) on the basis of a rather narrow fact pattern.[29] Participants in the PHO were limited to the University of Kansas Hospital; 14 faculty group clinical practices associated with the hospital, all of which were tax exempt under Section 501(c)(3); and physicians who are employees of the faculty practices and on the faculty at the University of Kansas Medical Center. The hospital had veto power over any activities of the PHO. Furthermore, the PHO's contracts for medical services were with the affiliated hospital and the faculty practices.

Management Service Organizations (MSOs)

As with PHOs, the IRS's position generally is that MSOs do not qualify for tax-exempt status because they are not engaged in charitable activities.[30] Conceivably, an MSO formed along the lines of the PHO affiliated with the University of Kansas Hospital discussed previously could qualify for tax-exempt status, but so far the IRS has not published any rulings to that effect.

Unrelated Business Income

A tax-exempt health risk-bearing entity may jeopardize its exempt status if it engages in substantial insurance activities. Insubstantial insurance activities will not threaten the entity's exemption but may be taxed as unrelated trade or business under Section 501(m).

Participation of Tax-Exempt Hospitals in Taxable Health Risk-Bearing Entities

Tax-exempt hospitals participating (for example, as an investor) in a taxable health risk-bearing entity arrangement with physicians should structure the arrangement so as not to jeopardize their exempt status. A hospital may make commercially reasonable loans or reasonable nonvoting stock investments in the entity. However, private benefit or inurement may result if the physicians are being paid more than reasonable compensation for their services or if the hospital receives less than a fair portion of the entity's income. In addition, penalty excise taxes in the form of intermediate sanctions under Section 4958 may be imposed on certain physicians who receive excessive compensation or other excess benefits directly or indirectly from the hospital.

Under Section 501(o), participation by a Section 501(c)(3) hospital in a provider-sponsored organization (PSO) is treated as an activity in furtherance of the hospital's tax-exempt purposes. However, any persons with a material financial interest in the PSO may be subject to the intermediate sanctions excise taxes if such persons receive an excess benefit from participating in the PSO. Also, such persons are treated as private shareholders or individuals with respect to the hospital for purposes of the prohibition against private inurement of the net earnings of the hospital.

REFERENCES AND NOTES

1. 312 U.S. 531 (1941).
2. The courts have recognized the similarities between HMOs and insurance companies and have held that HMOs are insurance companies. See for example, *United States Fidelity & Guaranty Co. v. Group Health Plan of Southeast Michigan, 131 Mich. App. 268, 345 N.W. 2d 683 (1983),* and *West Michigan Health Care Network v. Transamerica Insurance Corp. of America, 167 Mich. App. 218, 421 N.W. 2d 638, 642 (1988).*
3. 1968-1 C.B. 315.
4. 440 U.S. 205 (1978).
5. Reg. Section 1.461-1(a)(2).
6. I.R.C. Section 461(h)(2)(A)(i).
7. 107 S. Ct. 1732, 87-1 U.S.T.C. 9280 (April 27, 1987).
8. Ltr. Ruls. 9203002 and 9203003.
9. 1998-2 C.B. 56.
10. National Association of Insurance Commissioners (NAIC), Suggested Bulletin Regarding Certain Types of Compensation and Reimbursement Arrangements between Health Care Providers and Individuals, Employ-

ers, and Other Groups (Kansas City, Mo.: NAIC, 1995). In this bulletin, the NAIC clarified its position that any organization assuming all or part of the risk for health care expenses is in the business of insurance.
11. 71 T.C. 158 (1978), acq., 1981-2 C.B. 2.
12. 1969-2 C.B. 117, amplified by Revenue Ruling 83-157, 1983-2 C.B. 94. To qualify for tax exemption under Section 501(c)(3), a not-for-profit hospital must be organized and operated exclusively in furtherance of some purpose that is considered charitable (e.g., the promotion of health), and the hospital may not be operated, directly or indirectly, for the benefit of private interests. A hospital will be considered tax exempt if it is operated to serve a public rather than a private interest even though the class of beneficiaries eligible to receive a direct benefit from its activities does not include all members of the community. In determining whether a hospital is providing services to the community as a whole, key factors include a provision of services to Medicare and Medicaid recipients, and, except for certain specialty hospitals, the provision of emergency services to anyone without regard to their ability to pay.

13. *Geisinger Health Plan v. Commissioner, 93-1 U.S.T.C. Paragraph 50,123 (3d Cir. 1993).* In a subsequent decision, the court held that the HMO did not qualify for Section 501(c)(3) status on the basis that it was an integral part of the Geisinger system (*Geisinger Health Plan v. Commissioner, 94-2 U.S.T.C. Paragraph 50,398 [3d Cir. 1994]*).

14. 1986-2 C.B. 74.

15. The General Explanation to the Tax Reform Act of 1986 at 585 refers to *Haswell v. United States, 74-2 U.S.T.C. 9591 (Ct. Cl. 1974), Seasongood v. Commissioner, 56-1 U.S.T.C. 9135 (6th Cir. 1955),* and Section 501(h) for a definition of substantial.

16. H.R. Rep. 841, 99th Cong., 2d Sess., Vol. II at 346 (1986).

17. P.L. 100-647, 102 Stat. 3342.

18. H.R. Rep. 1104, 100th Cong., 2d Sess., Vol. II at 9 (1988).

19. G.C.M. 39829.

20. *See generally* Philip S. Neal, *IRS Perpetuates Confusion over the Status of Health Maintenance Organizations,* Taxes (February 1991), at 90, which concludes that the IRS analysis in GCM 39829 of Section 501(m) is erroneous.

21. 98 TNT 243-15.

22. *IHC Health Plans, Inc. v. Comm'r., No. 14600-99X* (September 3, 1999).

23. IRS Manual Handbook, EO Examination Guidelines Handbook, Chapter 27, Health Maintenance Organizations (May 25, 1999).

24. See, for example, I.R.C. Section 501(c)(3) ruling letters (unnumbered) issued to Harriman Jones Medical Foundation (letter dated 3 February 1994), 9 Tax Analysts Exempt Organization Tax Review 719 (March 1994), and to Friendly Hills Healthcare Network (letter dated 29 January 1993), 7 Tax Analysts Exempt Organization Tax Review 490 (March 1993). Also see IRS Exempt Organizations Continuing Professional Education Technical Instruction Program for FY 1996, at page 384.

25. IRS Exempt Organizations Continuing Professional Education Technical Instruction Program for FY 1997, at page 17, and for FY 2000, at page 45.

26. IRS Exempt Organizations Continuing Professional Education Technical Instruction Program for FY 1996, at page 404.

27. G.C.M. 38283, 38905, and 39674.

28. IRS Exempt Organizations Continuing Professional Education Technical Instruction Program for FY 1996, at page 401.

29. University Affiliated Health Care, Inc., TNT 95-2398 (February 17, 1995).

30. IRS Exempt Organizations Continuing Professional Education Technical Instruction Program for FY 1996, at page 157.

Internal Revenue Service Manual Exempt Organizations Examination Guidelines Handbook—Chapter 27: Health Maintenance Organizations

27.1 (05-25-1999)
OVERVIEW

1. This chapter provides descriptions and guidelines for examiners of health maintenance organizations (HMOs).
2. The examination of HMOs has the following objectives:
   a. to determine whether the organization qualifies for exemption under either IRC 501(c)(3) or IRC 501(c)(4);
   b. to determine whether the organization is precluded from qualifying for exemption by IRC 501(m)(1); and
   c. to determine whether any part of the organization's activities is subject to tax under IRC 501(m)(2).

27.2 (05-25-1999)
EXAMINATION GUIDELINES—
IN GENERAL

1. Due to the varied character of HMOs and the rapidly changing nature of the health care industry, examiners should be flexible in applying these guidelines.

Source: Reprinted from Health Maintenance Organizations, EO Examination Guidelines Handbook, *IRS Manual Handbook,* Ch. 27, May 25, 1999, Internal Revenue Service.

27.3 (05-25-1999)
ACTIVITIES

1. HMOs directly provide, or arrange for the provision of, health care services to members on a prepaid basis typically through a managed care arrangement.
   a. Direct Provider. A direct provider HMO provides health care services to its members principally by its employed health care providers at facilities that the HMO either owns or leases. (This arrangement is sometimes referred to as a "staff model" HMO.) An HMO's services may consist of only primary care or may also include specialist care, inpatient and outpatient hospital care, mental health care, vision care and dental care.
   b. Arranger. An arranger HMO arranges for the provision of health care services to its members principally through a network of contracted health care providers at the providers' own facilities. An arranger HMO's services may consist of arranging for only primary care or may also include arranging for specialist care, inpatient and outpatient hospital care, mental health care, vision care and dental care.
   c. Managed Care Arrangement. A managed care arrangement describes an HMO that uses its employed and/or contracted primary care providers as "gatekeepers." Members choose or are assigned a primary care provider and must obtain a re-

ferral from the primary care provider to utilize inpatient or outpatient hospital services, specialist physician services, and ancillary health care services.

2. Point-of-service. An HMO may permit members to obtain health care services from providers who are not employed or contracted by the HMO. These benefits, referred to as "point-of-service benefits," may be available to members within the HMO's service area or may be limited to emergency situations where the member is out of the HMO's service area.

3. An HMO may also engage in other activities, such as:
   a. Providing whole or partial subsidies of premiums for persons who cannot afford to pay the established premiums;
   b. Health care education programs; or
   c. Health research programs.

4. Stop-loss insurance. To reduce its risk of loss associated with providing, or arranging for the provision of, health care services to its members, an HMO may purchase insurance from an insurance company, a state or local government agency or from another organization in the HMO's health care system.

27.4 (05-25-1999)
PROVIDERS

1. An HMO employs or contracts with physicians and other health care professionals. An HMO may also contract with hospitals or clinics. Under these contracts, the providers agree to provide health care services to the HMO's members.

27.4.1 (05-25-1999)
PHYSICIANS

1. An HMO's physicians may be employed by the HMO, or may be independent physicians in private practice who contract with the HMO, or both.
   a. Contracts with physicians in private practice are typically on a non-exclusive basis.
   b. Contracted physicians may practice individually, in a group of several physicians,

or as an individual practice association (IPA).
   c. An HMO may employ or contract with primary care physicians, specialists, or both.
   d. An HMO may employ or contract with other health care professionals, such as osteopaths, registered nurses, nurse practitioners, physician assistants, psychologists or social workers.

27.4.1.1 (05-25-1999)
PHYSICIAN COMPENSATION METHODS

1. An HMO usually compensates its employed physicians on a salaried basis. Some HMOs may also pay bonuses.

2. An HMO compensates its contracted physicians using various compensation methods:
   a. Capitated Fee. An HMO pays the physician a fixed monthly fee for each HMO member for whom the physician serves as the member's primary care provider. This compensation method usually applies only to primary care physicians.
   b. Fee-For-Service. An HMO pays the physician a predetermined fee for services the physician actually provides to a member. The fee schedule may reflect a discount below the usual and customary fees charged by similarly situated providers for comparable services. The fee schedule may be based on the Medicare fee schedule (Resource Based Relative Value Scale or RBRVS) or the state Medicaid fee schedule. This method may be used to compensate primary care providers, specialists, or both.
   c. Withholding. An HMO may withhold a percentage of the fees paid to its contracted physicians and place the amount withheld in a reserve. Withholding arrangements generally are found only in fee-for-service arrangements with primary care physicians. (Withholding rates generally range from 10 percent to 20 percent). The physician may be eligible to recover all or a portion of the amount

withheld based on a variety of factors, for example, if the physician achieves certain predetermined budget goals and certain patient satisfaction standards, quality care standards or efficiency standards.

    d. Bonuses. An HMO may agree to pay its contracted physicians a bonus. If the HMO withholds from the physicians' fees, the bonus may be limited to the amount withheld or it may also include additional amounts.

    e. Point-of-service. If an HMO offers point-of-service benefits, the HMO either directly compensates the provider or reimburses the member based on a predetermined fee schedule.

27.4.2 (05-25-1999)
HOSPITALS

1. An HMO may contract with hospitals and clinics to provide members with inpatient and/or outpatient health care services. The contracted hospitals and clinics may be related to the HMO or may be independent organizations.

27.4.2.1 (05-25-1999)
HOSPITAL COMPENSATION METHODS

1. For inpatient hospital services, an HMO usually pays hospitals on a per diem basis. For outpatient hospital services, an HMO usually pays hospitals based on a predetermined fee schedule.

2. For clinic services, an HMO usually pays clinics based on a predetermined fee schedule.

27.5 (05-25-1999)
ENROLLMENT

1. An HMO may offer enrollment to certain groups, such as commercial employer groups, state or local government employer groups, insurance companies, other HMOs, Medicaid beneficiaries, Medicare beneficiaries, or individuals unaffiliated with any group.

2. Generally, individuals are not rejected for enrollment based on pre-existing conditions or excessive utilization of the HMO's services. HMOs commonly impose a reasonable waiting period, such as six months to one year, before a member is eligible to receive treatment of pre-existing condition.

27.6 (05-25-1999)
PREMIUMS

1. An HMO determines its premiums using various methods, such as a community rating method or an experience rating method. In the case of HMOs that enroll Medicaid and Medicare beneficiaries, the government program generally sets the premiums.

    a. Community Rating. Premiums are determined without regard to the member's utilization of services. All members pay the same premium regardless of the extent of health care services they require. An HMO may use an adjusted community rating method under which the premiums are the same for all members in a particular class.

    b. Experience Rating. Premiums vary based on utilization of services. Members who require more health care services pay higher premiums.

    c. Medicaid and Medicare. State Medicaid agencies generally establish the premiums for enrolled Medicaid beneficiaries. The Health Care Financing Administration (HCFA) determines the premiums it pays for enrolled Medicare beneficiaries.

27.7 (05-25-1999)
CONTROL

1. An HMO's governing body, such as its board of directors, may consist of independent members of the community. In addition, an HMO may be controlled by:

    a. One or more IRC 501(c)(3) organizations, such as hospitals, which may be related to each other or may be unrelated;

b. One or more HMOs, which may be exempt under IRC 501(c)(3) or IRC 501(c)(4), or may be non-exempt;

c. Physicians, either individually or as part of a group or IPA; or

d. Enrollees in the HMO.

27.8 (05-25-1999)
IRC 501(c)(3)

1. To qualify for exemption as an organization described in IRC 501(c)(3), an HMO must be organized and operated exclusively for one or more exempt purposes.

2. An HMO is organized exclusively for one or more exempt purposes if it satisfies the organizational test in Reg. 1.501(c)(3)-1(b).

3. An HMO is operated exclusively for one or more exempt purposes if it satisfies the operational test in Reg. 1.501(c)(3)-1(c).

4. The promotion of health is considered an exempt purpose. See IRM 3.11.1 (Exempt Organizations Handbook). However, not every activity that promotes health supports tax exemption. See, for example, *Federation Pharmacy Services, Inc. v. Commissioner,* 72 T.C. 687 (1979), *aff'd,* 625 F.2d 804 (8th Cir. 1980).

5. No part of net earnings may inure to the benefit of private shareholders or individuals. Reg. 1.501(c)(3)-1(c)(2). See IRM 3.11.1 (Exempt Organizations Handbook.)

27.8.1 (05-25-1999)
DIRECT PROVIDER

1. The promotion of health in a charitable manner may be accomplished by the direct provision of health care services.

2. An HMO that operates exclusively as a direct provider of health care services accomplishes the charitable promotion of health if it operates in a manner comparable to the hospital described in Situation 1 in Rev. Rul. 69-545, 1969-2 C.B. 117, or to the HMO described in *Sound Health Association v. Commissioner,* 71 T.C. 158 (1978), *acq.* 1981-2 C.B. 2.

27.8.2 (05-25-1999)
ARRANGER

1. Under certain circumstances, the promotion of health in a charitable manner may be accomplished by arranging for the provision of health care services.

2. In determining whether an arranger HMO qualifies for tax-exempt status under IRC 501(c)(3), the totality of the circumstances must be examined, with an eye toward discerning whether the HMO benefits the community as a whole in addition to its subscribers. *Geisinger Health Plan v. Commissioner,* 985 F.2d 1210 (3rd Cir. 1993), *rev'g* 62 T.C.M. (CCH) 1656 (1991).

3. Under this community benefit standard, the HMO's activities must be directed toward achieving a charitable purpose, such as benefiting the community as a whole in addition to its members, rather than merely arranging for the provision of health care services to its members for a fee.

27.8.2.1 (05-25-1999)
MEDICAID HMO

1. An HMO that arranges for the provision of health care services to its members, consisting exclusively of persons eligible under Medicaid, a comparable state program, or persons having special health care needs, promotes the health of the community if it also actively engages in the following programs that provide related health care services to its members:

a. Educational programs regarding the benefits available.

b. Counseling and assistance in making the transition to managed care.

c. Preventive health care programs.

d. Coordinating health care services among providers.

e. Facilitates access to the plan's providers.

27.8.2.2 (05-25-1999)
INTEGRAL PART

1. An HMO that arranges for the provision of health care services and is part of an IRC

501(c)(3) health care system may qualify for exemption under IRC 501(c)(3) as an integral part of the health care system. See Reg. 1.502-1(b); Rev. Rul. 78-41, 1978-1 C.B. 148.

2. To be considered as an integral part, an HMO must be financially and structurally controlled by either:

   a. One organization in the health care system that is exempt under IRC 501(c)(3), or

   b. Two or more organizations in the health care system that are exempt under IRC 501(c)(3) and related to each other through common control.

3. An HMO must perform an essential function of one or more related IRC 501(c)(3) organizations in the health care system of which it is a part. For related organizations that are hospitals, the HMO must serve only the patients of these hospitals. Thus, the HMO's members must also be patients of the related exempt hospitals. *Geisinger Health Plan v. Commissioner,* 100 T.C. 394 (1993), *aff'd on other grounds,* 30 F.3d 494 (3rd Cir. 1994); Rev. Rul. 68-374, 1968-2 C.B. 242; Rev. Rul. 68-375, 1968-2 C.B. 245; Rev. Rul. 68-376, 1968-2 C.B. 246.

27.8.3 (05-25-1999)
EXAMINATION GUIDELINES FOR IRC 501(c)(3)

1. The following guidelines should be used for examining an HMO that otherwise satisfies the organizational and operational tests to determine whether it qualifies for exemption under IRC 501(c)(3) on the basis that it promotes health or relieves the poor and distressed.

27.8.3.1 (05-25-1999)
OPEN ENROLLMENT

1. Determine whether the HMO enrolls more than an insubstantial number of persons who generally are unable to obtain affordable health care services or health care insurance, or who have special health care needs, such as:

   a. Individuals;

   b. Employer groups consisting of employers having 50 or fewer employees;

   Note: The Health Insurance Portability and Accountability Act of 1996, P.L. 104-191, § 102; 42 USC § 300gg- 91(e)(4), defines the term "small employer" as an employer who employed an average of at least 2 but not more than 50 employees.

   c. Elderly persons, such as persons qualifying for benefits under Medicare;

   d. Low income persons, such as persons qualifying for benefits under Medicaid, a comparable state program, or who cannot obtain affordable health insurance; and

   e. Other individuals having special health care needs, such as persons who are disabled or who suffer from substance abuse.

27.8.3.2 (05-25-1999)
PREMIUM METHODOLOGY

1. Determine whether the method the HMO uses to determine the premiums it charges to the members described in IRM 27.8.3.1(1) results in premiums that are generally affordable. A community rating methodology is one method that generally results in premiums that are generally affordable.

2. This guideline does not apply to enrollees who are beneficiaries under Medicaid, a comparable state program, beneficiaries under Medicare, or other persons having special health care needs, where a government agency determines the premiums.

27.8.3.3 (05-25-1999)
COMMUNITY CONTROL

1. Determine whether the HMO is controlled by community interests rather than by health care providers or others who can benefit personally from the HMO's operations. See *Sound Health Association v. Commissioner,* 71 T.C. 158 (1978); *Geisinger Health Plan v. Commissioner,* 985 F.2d 1210 (3rd Cir. 1993).

   a. An HMO that satisfies the "community benefit standard" discussed above and in

Rev. Rul. 69-545 is controlled by community interests.

b. One factor demonstrating control of an HMO by community interests is an HMO that is controlled by one or more organizations exempt under IRC 501(c)(3), all of which satisfy the "community benefit standard" discussed above.

c. One factor demonstrating that the HMO has taken sufficient steps to prevent any private inurement or impermissible private benefit is that the HMO has adopted a substantial conflicts of interest policy or is controlled by an IRC 501(c)(3) organization that has adopted a substantial conflicts of interest policy that applies to the HMO.

d. An HMO that is controlled by one or more organizations exempt under IRC 501(c)(4) is not alone sufficient to demonstrate that the HMO is controlled by community interests.

27.8.3.4 (05-25-1999)
PROMOTION OF HEALTH

1. Determine whether as its primary purpose, the HMO operates programs that accomplish the charitable promotion of health as:
   a. A direct provider, consistent with IRM 27.8.1;
   b. An arranger, consistent with IRM 27.8.2; or
   c. As an integral part, consistent with IRM 27.8.2.2.

27.8.3.5 (05-25-1999)
RELIEF OF THE POOR AND DISTRESSED

1. If the HMO does not primarily operate programs that accomplish the charitable promotion of health, determine whether the HMO operates, as its primary purpose, programs that otherwise accomplish charitable purposes, such as the relief of the poor and distressed or of the underprivileged. Reg. 1.501(c)(3)-1(d)(2).

27.8.3.5.1 (05-25-1999)
MEDICAID HMO

1. An HMO that enrolls only Medicaid beneficiaries, or beneficiaries of a comparable state program, and arranges for the provision of health care services to these individuals by a group of health care providers, should be considered as providing relief of the poor and distressed because it facilitates the provision of health care services to low-income individuals (a group having special health care needs) if it also actively engages in programs that provide related health care services to its members.

2. Determine whether the Medicaid HMO:
   a. Provides educational programs relating to the benefits available.
   b. Provides counseling and assistance in making the transition to managed care.
   c. Provides preventive health care programs.
   d. Coordinates health care services among providers.
   e. Facilitates access to the plan's providers.

27.9 (05-25-1999)
IRC 501(c)(4)

1. To qualify for exemption as an organization described in IRC 501(c)(4), an HMO must be not organized for profit and must be operated exclusively for the promotion of social welfare.

2. An HMO is operated exclusively for the promotion of social welfare if it is primarily engaged in promoting in some way the common good and general welfare of the people of the community. Reg. 1.501(c)(4)-1(a)(2).

3. If an HMO does not qualify for exemption under IRC 501(c)(3), it may qualify for exemption under IRC 501(c)(4). For examination guidelines for IRC 501(c)(4), see IRM 27.9.3.

27.9.1 (05-25-1999)
MEDICAID HMO

1. An HMO that arranges for the provision of health care services to its members, consisting exclusively of persons eligible under Medicaid, a comparable state program, or persons having special health care needs, and provides its members with related health care education, counseling and preventive health care services, qualifies for exemption under IRC 501(c)(4) if it satisfies the examination guidelines in IRM 27.9.3.

27.9.2 (05-25-1999)
INTEGRAL PART

1. An HMO that arranges for the provision of health care services to its members and is part of a health care system may qualify for exemption under IRC 501(c)(4) as an integral part of the health care system. See Reg. 1.502-1(b); Rev. Rul. 78-41, 1978-1 C.B. 148.
2. To be considered an integral part, an HMO must be financially and structurally controlled by either:
   a. One organization in the health care system that is exempt under IRC 501(c)(3) or IRC 501(c)(4), or
   b. Two or more organizations in the health care system that are exempt under IRC 501(c)(3) or IRC 501(c)(4) and are related to each other through common control.
3. An HMO must perform an essential function of one or more related IRC 501(c)(3) or IRC 501(c)(4) organizations in the health care system of which it is a part. For related organizations that are hospitals, the HMO must serve only the patients of these hospitals. Thus, the HMO's members must also be patients of the related exempt hospitals. *Geisinger Health Plan v. Commissioner,* 100 T.C. 394 (1993), *aff'd on other grounds,* 30 F.3d 494 (3rd Cir. 1994); Rev. Rul. 68-374, 1968-2 C.B. 242; Rev. Rul. 68-375, 1968-2 C.B. 245; Rev. Rul. 68-376, 1968-2 C.B. 246.

27.9.3 (05-25-1999)
EXAMINATION GUIDELINES FOR IRC 501(c)(4)

1. The following guidelines should be used for examining an HMO to determine whether it qualifies for exemption under IRC 501(c)(4).

27.9.3.1 (05-25-1999)
ORGANIZATION AND OPERATIONS

1. Determine whether the HMO is:
   a. Not organized for profit;
   b. Operated exclusively for the promotion of social welfare by primarily engaging in activities that promote the common good and general welfare of the people of the community (Reg. 1.501(c)(4)-1(a)(2)); and
   c. No part of its net earnings inures to the benefit of any private shareholder or individual.

27.9.3.2 (05-25-1999)
OPEN ENROLLMENT

1. Determine whether the HMO enrolls more than an insubstantial number of persons who generally are unable to obtain affordable health care services or health care insurance, or who have special health care needs, for example:
   a. Individuals;
   b. Employer groups consisting of employers having 50 or fewer employees;
   Note: The Health Insurance Portability and Accountability Act of 1996, P.L. 104-191, § 102; 42 USC § 300gg-91(e)(4), defines the term "small employer" as an employer who employed an average of at least 2 but not more than 50 employees.
   c. Elderly persons, such as persons who qualify for benefits under Medicare;
   d. Low income persons, such as persons who qualify for benefits under Medicaid or a comparable state program; or

e. Other individuals who have special health care needs, such as persons who are disabled or who suffer from substance abuse.

27.9.3.3 (05-25-1999)
PREMIUM METHODOLOGY

1. Determine whether the method the HMO uses to determine the premiums it charges to the members described in IRM 27.9.3.2(1) results in premiums that are generally affordable. A community rating methodology is one method that generally results in premiums that are generally affordable.
2. This guideline does not apply to enrollees who are beneficiaries under Medicaid, a comparable state program, beneficiaries under Medicare, or other persons having special health care needs, where a government agency determines the premiums.

27.9.3.4 (05-25-1999)
COMMUNITY CONTROL

1. Determine whether the HMO is controlled by community interests rather than by health care providers or others who can benefit personally from the HMO's operations. See *Sound Health Association v. Commissioner,* 71 T.C. 158 (1978); *Geisinger Health Plan,* 985 F.2d 1210 (3rd Cir. 1993).
   a. An HMO that satisfies the "community benefit standard" discussed above and in Rev. Rul. 69-545 is controlled by community interests.
   b. One factor demonstrating control of an HMO by community interests is an HMO that is controlled by one or more organizations exempt under IRC 501(c)(3), all of which satisfy the "community benefit standard" discussed above.
   c. One factor demonstrating that the HMO has taken sufficient steps to prevent any private inurement or impermissible private benefit is that the HMO has adopted a substantial conflicts of interest policy or is con-

trolled by an IRC 501(c)(3) organization that has adopted a substantial conflicts of interest policy that applies to the HMO.
   d. An HMO that is controlled by one or more organizations exempt under IRC 501(c)(4) is not alone sufficient to demonstrate that the HMO is controlled by community interests.

27.10 (05-25-1999)
EXEMPTION PRECLUDED BY IRC 501(m)

1. An HMO that satisfies the requirements for exemption under IRC 501(c)(3) or IRC 501(c)(4) is precluded from qualifying for exemption if a substantial part of its activities consists of providing commercial-type insurance. IRC 501(m)(1).

27.10.1 (05-25-1999)
EXAMINATION GUIDELINES FOR IRC 501(m)

1. In determining whether a substantial part of an HMO's activities consists of providing commercial-type insurance, all the surrounding facts and circumstances should be taken into account.
   a. The law does not define the concept of "substantial," which is dependent on all the facts and circumstances. However, as a safe harbor guideline, if less than 15% of an HMO's activities consists of providing commercial-type insurance, it should be considered that no substantial part of the HMO's activities consists of providing commercial-type insurance.
   b. See, for example, *Haswell v. U.S.,* 500 F.2d 1133 (Ct. Cl. 1974), *cert. den.,* 419 U.S. 1107 (1975) (16.6% to 20.5% was "substantial"); *Seasongood v. Commissioner,* 227 F.2d 907 (6th Cir. 1955) (5% was not "substantial"); Rev. Rul. 71-529, 1971-2 C.B. 234 (less than 15% was not "substantial").

c. However, if more than 15% of an HMO's activities consists of providing commercial-type insurance, whether a substantial part of the HMO's activities consists of providing commercial-type insurance depends on all the facts and circumstances.

2. In measuring an HMO's activities for a particular year, the following factors should be considered:

   a. That year's activities; or

   b. An average of the activities of that year plus the immediately preceding three years.

3. One factor demonstrating that an HMO's activities do not consist of providing commercial-type insurance is an HMO that has shifted a significant portion of its risk of loss to its primary care providers. See Rev. Rul. 68-27, 1968-1 C.B. 315.

4. An example of an HMO that has shifted a significant portion of its risk of loss to its primary care providers is an HMO that uses one or more of the following methods for compensating its primary care providers:

   a. Salary (and bonus);

   b. Capitated fees; or

   c. Fees-for-service.

   Note: The fee schedule consists of fees that are substantially discounted; and the fees paid are subject to a substantial withhold.

5. Substantially Discounted Fee Schedule. An example of a substantially discounted fee schedule is a fee schedule that is at least 15% less than the usual and customary fees charged by similarly situated primary care providers for comparable services.

   a. An example of a fee schedule that is not a substantially discounted fee schedule is one that permits the provider to recover the discount. See IRM 27.10.1 for a discussion of the term "substantial."

6. Substantial Withhold. An example of a substantial withhold is a withholding arrangement where the HMO withholds from the primary care provider at least 15% of the discounted fees paid. The provider may recover all or a portion of the amounts withheld based on a variety of factors, for example, if the physician achieves certain predetermined budget goals and certain patient satisfaction standards, quality care standards or efficiency standards.

   a. An example of a withholding arrangement that does not involve a substantial withhold is a compensation system that permits the provider to recover automatically the amount withheld. See IRM 27.10.1 for a discussion of the term "substantial."

7. Whether a fee schedule that is equal to the Medicare fee schedule (Resource Based Relative Value Scale or RBRVS) or the state Medicaid fee schedule shifts a significant portion of the HMO's risk of loss depends on all the facts and circumstances.

27.10.2 (05-25-1999)
RISKS ASSUMED BY HMO

1. Stop-Loss Insurance. An HMO that compensates providers using a fee-for-service arrangement may obtain stop-loss insurance from an unrelated party to protect itself from a portion of the financial risk associated with operating the HMO. Whether a stop-loss insurance arrangement obtained by an HMO shifts a significant portion of the HMO's risk of loss depends on all the facts and circumstances.

2. Deficit Sharing. An HMO that compensates providers using a fee-for-service arrangement may enter into an arrangement with the providers for the providers to share a portion of the HMO's operating losses. Whether a deficit sharing arrangement that an HMO has with its providers shifts a significant portion of the HMO's risk of loss depends on all the facts and circumstances.

   a. An HMO that has a deficit sharing arrangement with a related organization does not shift a significant portion of its risk of loss because the related organization is part of the HMO's "economic family." See Rev. Rul. 77-316, 1977-2 C.B. 53; Rev. Rul. 78-338, 1978-2 C.B. 107.

27.10.3 (05-25-1999)
STATUTORY EXCEPTIONS TO COMMERCIAL-TYPE INSURANCE

1. Certain activities of an HMO should not be considered as providing commercial-type insurance:
   a. An HMO that provides insurance at substantially below cost to a class of charitable recipients. IRC 501(m)(3)(A).
   b. An HMO that provides incidental health insurance of a kind that is customarily provided by HMOs. IRC 501(m)(3)(B).

27.10.3.1 (05-25-1999)
EXAMINATION GUIDELINES FOR IRC 501(m)(3)(A)

1. The following guidelines should be used for examining an HMO to determine whether insurance that it provides is substantially below cost to a class of charitable recipients.
2. An HMO that contracts with a government agency to directly provide or arrange for the provision of health care services to persons who have special health care needs, such as persons who are Medicaid beneficiaries, indigent, disabled or substance abusers, should not be considered as providing commercial-type insurance at substantially below cost.
   a. See Rev. Rul. 71-529, 1971-2 C.B. 234; H.R. Rept. No. 99-426, 99th Cong., 2d Sess. 662 (1986), 1986-3 C.B. Vol. 2 664; *Nonprofits' Insurance Alliance of California v. U.S.,* 94-2 USTC (CCH) ¶ 50,593 (Fed. Cl. 1994); and *Paratransit Insurance Corporation,* 102 T.C. 745 (1994).

27.10.3.2 (05-25-1999)
EXAMPLES UNDER IRC 501(m)(3)(B)

1. Examples of incidental health insurance of a kind that is customarily provided by HMOs are:
   a. Dental care, vision care and mental health care services. See H.R. Conf. Rep. No. 100-1104, 100th Cong. 2d Sess II-9 (1988).

   b. Inpatient and outpatient hospital services, specialist physician services and ancillary health care services that are provided by an HMO as a result of referral by a member's primary care provider under a managed care arrangement.
   c. Point-of-service benefits relating to emergency health care services provided to the HMO's members out of the HMO's service area.

27.11 (05-25-1999)
UNRELATED TRADE OR BUSINESS

1. If an HMO that satisfies the requirements for exemption under IRC 501(c)(3) or IRC 501(c)(4) is not precluded by IRC 501(m) from qualifying for exemption, any commercial-type insurance activities of the HMO should be considered as an unrelated trade or business and the HMO should be considered as an insurance company for applying Subchapter L to such activity. IRC 501(m)(2).

27.11.1 (05-25-1999)
EXAMINATION GUIDELINES FOR IRC 501(m)(2)

1. For guidelines to determine whether any activities of an HMO constitute the provision of commercial-type insurance, see IRM 27.10.1 and IRM 27.10.2.
2. Premiums that are not directly related to commercial-type insurance activities should be allocated. Allocations should be based on all the facts and circumstances. In making allocations, direct expenses paid to providers for commercial-type insurance activities and total numbers of patient encounters should be taken into account.
3. Expenses that are not directly related to commercial-type insurance activities should be allocated. Allocations should be based on all the facts and circumstances. In making allocations, premiums paid directly for commercial-type insurance should be taken into account.

CHAPTER 49

Underwriting and Rating Functions Common to Most Markets

Stephen M. Cigich and Michael G. Sturm

Underwriting and rating are two important functions within a health plan. Successful underwriting and rating create a balance among adequacy, competitiveness, and equity of rates. It can be a difficult and delicate balance to achieve. Moving too far in any direction can lead to financial disaster for a health plan.

Adequate rates are high enough to generate sufficient revenue to cover all plan expenses and yield an acceptable return on equity. Competitive rates are low enough to sell enough cases and enroll enough members to meet health plan growth targets. Equitable rates will approximate any given group's costs with a reasonable amount of cross-subsidization among groups. Equitable rates are achieved by applying various

Stephen M. Cigich, FSA, MAAA, is a Consulting Actuary with the Brookfield, Wisconsin office of Milliman & Robertson, Inc. Having managed accounting and actuarial functions in both large and mid-sized MCOs, his area of expertise is in managed health care programs. His specialty is in the areas of medical delivery systems design and evaluation, product and rate manual development, experience analysis, benchmarking, and actuarial projections.

Michael G. Sturm, FSA, MAAA, is an Actuary with the Brookfield, Wisconsin office of Milliman & Robertson, Inc. He consults with HMO and insurance company staff, physicians, and self-funded plan sponsors about group, individual, and international health consulting matters. He assists these clients with various projects, including experience analysis, underwriting strategy, product and rate manual development, and actuarial projections.

rating factors and result in higher persistency if groups realize they are being charged a fair amount for their insurance.

A health plan should continually assess its success in each of these areas. This is particularly true for a newly established plan or product offering. For example, a plan cannot be sure whether a high volume of sales or successful renewals is good or bad until adequacy is assessed because competitive (and perhaps equitable) rates are not necessarily adequate.

This chapter discusses underwriting and rating functions common to most major health insurance markets. Major markets include individual nongovernment, commercial group (both small and large), and government (Medicare and Medicaid). Each major market segment has several components with unique risk characteristics that require different approaches to underwriting and rating. Unique underwriting and rating characteristics for these markets are discussed in Chapter 50, "Underwriting and Rating Functions by Market."

UNDERWRITING

Most of the underwriting discussion is contained in Chapters 50 and 52 because underwriting varies significantly among the major health insurance markets. However, the following discusses highlights common to all markets.

Underwriting involves gathering information about applicants or groups of applicants to determine an adequate, competitive, and equitable rate to insure them. The type of underwriting and level of scrutiny depends on many factors, including the time at which it is done (i.e., at issue, during the plan year, or at renewal).

At Issue

Effective underwriting at issue determines individual and/or group applicants':

- health status
- ability to pay the premium
- other coverage (if any)
- historical persistency (applies mainly to groups with high start-up costs)

Health Status

Information gathered to determine health status varies from requesting:

- physical examinations and/or attending physician statements (individual) to
- individual medical questionnaires (small group) to
- an employer disclosure listing major health conditions (large group) to
- medical cost experience (large group) to
- no health status information (e.g., Medicare and Medicaid risk contracts)

Some carriers use health status information in certain markets (where allowed by law) to apply a pre-existing condition limitation or exclusion (i.e., a temporary limit on medical payments for existing health conditions). Pre-existing condition limitations are often used in conjunction with underwriting to provide incentive to prospective enrollees to apply for coverage before becoming sick.

Various underwriting policies are also used with groups that screen for health status at both issue and renewal. These policies prevent groups with higher than average morbidity from being issued coverage at average rates (thereby avoiding adverse selection). The chance of adverse selection increases as the group size decreases because individual applicants and small groups are likely to buy insurance only if they need it. This occurs for various reasons, including cost concerns, the need to offer health ben-

efits to attract employees, and whether health insurance premiums are tax deductible. Therefore, underwriting with medical questions to determine health status is common for individuals and small groups and less common for large groups. Medical underwriting for the purpose of setting rates is not allowed in Medicaid and Medicare risk contracts.

Ability To Pay

Information gathered to determine an applicant's premium-paying ability might include income and credit history. Income can be verified through tax returns. Credit history can be verified through independent credit agencies (such as Dun & Bradstreet). Insurers do not necessarily have to decline coverage to applicants with poor credit histories. Insurers customarily require groups with a poor credit rating to produce some form of collateral or a letter of credit (for up to two months of premium) instead of declining coverage. Insurers nearly always require individual policyholders to pay their premium before the coverage period, thus ensuring their ability to pay the premium.

Other Coverage

Insureds are often asked on the application (or surveyed during the plan year) whether they have other health insurance coverage. The presence of other coverage should be noted so the claim adjudicator can determine which insurer is responsible for payment of claims on the basis of coordination of benefit rules. Coordinating payment for benefits allows insurers to keep premiums lower.

Persistency

Insurers should be cautious when writing groups that frequently change carriers because a significant amount of fixed costs (e.g., advertising and commissions) are involved when writing a new group. Small groups that frequently change carriers can be placed in the highest rating tier. Large groups with more than two carriers in the past five years might not be offered coverage.

Carriers' actions (based on underwriting information) include issuing coverage at the standard rate, issuing coverage at a higher rate, or declining coverage (when allowed by law).

During the Plan Year and At Renewal

Underwriting during the plan year and at renewal varies enough by major market segment that they are discussed under each market segment in Chapter 50. However, in general, underwriting during the plan year involves checking for adverse selection. At renewal, the underwriter has more information on the specific risks and implements rate changes on the basis of experience and projected changes to the experience.

RATING

Rating involves calculating the premium to be charged for a specific individual or group on the basis of information gathered through underwriting. The premium calculation is usually done using a rate formula. The result of the rate formula is sometimes called the book or manual rate. The book rate represents the experience (i.e., historical medical costs) of all individuals or groups in a specific block (or pool).

The final rate might be solely a result of the book rate or a combination of the book rate and rate projections using other information, such as a specific group's experience. Adjusting an individual's rate (whether he or she has individual or group coverage) on the basis of the individual's experience is not allowed by law.

Group-specific experience rating can be thought of as varying the book rate (i.e., the combination of all the groups' experience) on the basis of a specific group's experience. Experience rating can be thought of as the converse of pooling experience because recognizing a group's experience in their rate calculation reduces the extent to which groups subsidize each other.

The rate formula should recognize all health plan costs, be easy to apply in most situations, and result in a premium rate. Health plan costs include medical services, sales and marketing expenses, administrative expenses, applicable rate changes, and profit. The rate formula typically expresses rates on a per member per month (PMPM) basis that must be transformed into rates for each individual or employee on the basis of the number of covered members in the individual's/employee's family.

The rate formula is updated through various reports that measure experience. These reports can also be helpful in establishing budgets by medical service category or department; establishing funding for provider-based risk pools; and identifying, quantifying, and prioritizing medical management opportunities within the health plan. Timely analysis of the reports will allow the health plan to establish the proper provider-based education and incentives necessary to realize opportunities within the health plan.

Rate Formula

Base Rate Development

Most rate formulas start with a base rate. That is, a PMPM incurred medical cost (a.k.a., starting cost). The base rate reflects a specific:

- population (e.g., commercial, Medicare, Medicaid, or other population)
- covered services (including limits)
- cost-sharing provisions
- provider reimbursement arrangements
- demographics (i.e., age and gender)
- geographical area
- occupation/industry
- health status
- degree of health care management
- coverage effective date
- out-of-network usage (if applicable)
- presence or absence of worker's compensation insurance
- use of pre-existing condition clauses
- underwriting practices
- claim administration practices
- distribution method (i.e., agents, brokers, direct)
- other variables impacting medical costs

The projection period base rate is developed by analyzing historical incurred medical costs for a given time period (a.k.a., the base period) and projecting (i.e., trending) it forward to the projection period recognizing actual and anticipated changes in the block of business. Historical medical costs are often summarized in 12-month segments of paid medical costs to provide a credible base and avoid any seasonal fluctuations.

Paid claim data are usually converted to an incurred basis by use of various estimation techniques (e.g., claim lag analyses and/or loss ratio techniques). Incurred claims (which should include any capitation payments to providers) are then matched with health plan exposure measured in member months to develop a base period PMPM medical cost.

Incurred claim estimation techniques should account for a health plan's unique payment arrangements. The actuary should know whether the paid claim triangles include capitations, withhold payments, stop-loss recoveries, and/or coordination of benefit savings and make any necessary adjustments. In addition, the actuary may need to modify incurred claims for any accrued medical incentives (i.e., provider bonuses).

Projection adjustments should recognize changes in health plan operations between the base period and projection period. Exhibit 49–1 presents elements to consider that may change between the base period and projection period. The elements listed in Exhibit 49–1 may be offsetting. For example, the underlying demand to use more health care services may be offset by anticipated medical management improvements.

The projection period base rate can be summarized in an actuarial cost model. Exhibit 49–2 displays a sample actuarial cost model. The model contains: annual utilization per 1,000 members (column 1), the allowed average charge per service (column 2), PMPM medical costs not reflecting cost-sharing provisions (column 3), cost-sharing adjustments composited across the underlying benefit plans (columns 4, 5, and 6), and PMPM medical costs net of cost sharing (column 7) by medical service category.

Each medical service category is defined by a unique set of procedure codes. For example, hospital inpatient services can be grouped by diagnosis-related group (DRG). Physician services are usually grouped using current proce-

Exhibit 49–1 Adjustments to Convert the Historical Base Rate to the Projection Period Base Rate

Actual or anticipated changes in incurred claims caused by changes in:
- The underlying demand for medical services
- Medical management
- Provider reimbursement
- Contractual benefit levels or member cost sharing
- The insured population (i.e., age, gender, Medicare/Medicaid eligibility)
- The geographical area of the insured population
- Claim administration
- Underwriting requirements
- Distribution method (i.e., the method used to sell the policy)
- Intensity (i.e., amount of services per day or visit)
- Other variables affecting health care costs

dural terminology (CPT). The medical service categories can be further grouped into risk allocation pools. For example, Exhibit 49–2 presents the cost for primary care physician services (as defined by specific CPT codes) in a separate section to support a primary care capitation payment for those services.

A key component of the cost model is the rate at which the population is assumed to use medical services (i.e., utilization). Utilization can vary substantially depending on the efficiency of network providers. Two or more utilization scenarios are often developed to estimate medical costs under current levels of health care management and well-managed levels.

Average charge per service is based on provider reimbursement negotiated in the contracts. The average charge per service can be in the form of discounts from billed charges, per diems, case rates, fee schedules, capitation payments, or other forms of reimbursement. The impact of copays depends on the benefit plan design and the plan's policy for their collection. The PMPM medical cost equals the annual utilization per 1,000 members, multiplied by the average charge per service, divided by 12,000 less

Exhibit 49–2 Sample Actuarial Cost Model

Medical Service		(1)	(2)	(3)	(4)	(5)	(6)	(7)
		Annual Utilization per 1,000 Members	Allowed Average Charge Per Service	Per Member Per Month Medical Cost	Copay Frequency	Copay	Cost Sharing Per Member Per Month	Per Member Per Month Net Claim Costs
Hospital inpatient	Medical-Surgical	247 days	$1,276.76	$26.28				$26.28
	Psychiatric/substance abuse	67 days	657.31	3.67				3.67
	Extended care	5 days	250.00	0.10				0.10
	Subtotal	**319 days**	**$2,184.07**	**$30.05**				**$30.05**
Hospital outpatient	Emergency room	261 visits	$159.99	$3.48	196	$25.00	$0.41	$3.07
	Surgery	85 visits	1,172.46	8.30				8.30
	Other	512 services	149.53	6.38				6.38
	Subtotal			**$18.16**			**$0.41**	**$17.75**
Primary care capitation	Office and inpatient visits	2,152 visits	$42.77	$7.67	2,035	$10.00	$1.70	$5.97
	Immunizations and injections	154 procedures	17.14	0.22				0.22
	Subtotal			**$7.89**			**$1.70**	**$6.19**
Fee-for-service physician	Surgery	374 procedures	$266.63	$8.31				$8.31
	Anesthesia	78 procedures	575.38	3.74				3.74
	Office and inpatient visits	1,025 visits	45.78	3.91	944	$10.00	$0.79	3.12
	Other	3,277 services	75.00	20.48				20.48
	Subtotal			**$36.44**			**$0.79**	**$35.65**
Other	Prescription drugs	5,209 scripts	$36.00	$15.63	5,209	$5.00	$2.17	$13.46
	Home health care	29 visits	228.21	0.55				0.55
	Ambulance	15 runs	322.43	0.40				0.40
	Durable medical equipment	32 units	269.54	0.72				0.72
	Subtotal			**$17.30**			**$2.17**	**$15.13**
Total medical costs PMPM				$109.84			$5.07	$104.77
Retention Load PMPM (12.69% of the Required Rate)								$15.23
Required Rate PMPM								$120.00

the value of cost sharing (i.e., the copay frequency multiplied by the copay, divided by 12,000). The values in the actuarial cost model will differ for each group, depending on the group's characteristics as discussed previously.

Rate Formula

Exhibit 49–3 contains a sample rate formula (i.e., case-specific adjustments to the projection period base rate). Step 2 and subsequent steps in

Exhibit 49–3 Sample Rate Formula

Step 1: Incurred medical costs PMPM (i.e., the projection period base rate)
Step 2: Add or subtract:
—Covered services (not) reflected in the base rate
—Net pooling charges (if applicable)
Step 3: Multiply by:
—Benefit plan factor
—Geographical area factor
—Care management
—Provider reimbursement differences
—Trend
—Other factors
Step 4: Retention load (multiply or add)
—Administrative expenses
—Contingency reserves
—Coordination of benefits savings
—Profit
Step 5: Convert the member rate to a contract rate

the formula adjust the projection period base rate to reflect the specific plan's characteristics. This is because the projection period base rate assumes that all characteristics of a particular insured individual/group have the same characteristics as the average historical medical costs of the block of policies the base rate represents.

The rate formula adjustments should consider important factors that predict medical cost differences among individuals/groups, yet be easy to measure and apply. The adjustments might be additive or multiplicative, depending on the type of adjustment and user's preference. For example, the base rate may need to add costs to reflect additional covered services for mandated benefits in certain states. In addition, the base rate may need to be lowered to reflect lower utilization of services resulting from an efficient health care provider network (i.e., degree of health care management).

Retention

Retention items are usually built into the rate formula once medical costs are calculated. Re-

tention can include administrative expenses, a buildup of contingency reserves, coordination of benefit savings, and profit. Retention can be combined with medical costs to arrive at the PMPM premium by dividing the medical costs by a target loss ratio (possibly different by group size) or adding specific PMPM retention costs.

Retention must be sufficient to cover all functions performed by the carrier. This might include only a subset of normal carrier functions if the targets are developed for a physician-hospital organization or other provider-based group that is responsible for only a portion of the administrative duties.

Conversion of Rates from Member to Employee

The PMPM rate target must be converted into rates by family status. Individual and some small group contracts generally build a family rate by adding together the appropriate rates for each member of the family on the basis of their age and gender (a.k.a., list bill rating). Large groups (and some small groups) often charge employees rates according to specific family groupings or tiers, such as employee only, couple, and so forth, without varying rates by age or gender (a.k.a., composite rates). Composite rates need to be set such that the total premium generated for the groups reflects the average number of members per contract type in the groups. Medicare and Medicaid rates are nearly always stated on a per member (i.e., individual) basis.

Data Sources

The best data source for any health plan is experience because it implicitly recognizes all the plan-specific characteristics. However, carriers often have trouble collecting their experience in the necessary format, might be expanding into a new market, or have recently been established. As a result, many health plans look to published sources or actuarial consulting firms to provide initial medical cost targets based on data relevant to their situation. The carrier can substitute experience for the estimates with data from their own health plan as it becomes available.

Managing the Business

The rate formula should be routinely updated (at least once per year, some carriers do it quarterly). Updates are done with data from various management reports. *The management reports might include:*

- **financial gain/loss summaries by:**
  - total block of business
  - large group vs. small group business
  - calendar year
  - commercial vs. Medicare and/or other business
  - each group
- **incurred claim costs by:**
  - total block of business
  - geographical area
  - large group vs. small group business
  - commercial vs. Medicare or Medicaid business
  - policy year duration of the individual/ group (not usually applicable to large groups)
- **group-specific reports (applies mostly to large groups) including:**
  - paid premium
  - paid claims
  - medical loss ratio
  - large claim information
  - subscriber and membership counts by contract type
- **A development of incurred but not reported (IBNR) claims.** This report should contain paid claim triangles; a lag development of incurred claims; a projection development of incurred claims; paid claim lags (to monitor the speed of claim processing); medical cost trends; and monthly, quarterly, and annual incurred claim estimates. Carriers might produce IBNR reports by:

  - type of population (i.e., commercial or Medicare)
  - HMO vs. point-of-service
  - type of medical service (i.e., hospital inpatient, hospital outpatient, physician, prescription drugs, and other)
- **membership by:**
  - group size
  - contract tier
  - product
  - age
  - gender.

These reports will allow for analyzing experience and updating the rate formula.

The financial area of most carriers will also produce traditional accounting reports such as the income statement, balance sheet, and cash flow reports. These reports help a business measure its financial goals. One measure might be return-on-equity, a popular and universal measure of the value of a business. Return-on-equity is universal because it allows a business to compare its value with other types of investments, such as investing the carrier's surplus in a money market account, bonds, or the stock market. Carriers that target a percent of premium might find it difficult measuring the value of the business versus non-insurance–oriented businesses. Accounting reports are discussed in more detail in Chapter 47.

CONCLUSION

Underwriting and rating goals should produce adequate, competitive, and equitable rates. Underwriting involves gathering information to analyze applicants' risk characteristics. Rating includes using the information gathered through underwriting and management reports to develop a final rate.

SUGGESTED READING

Bluhm, W.F. 1992. *Group Insurance*. Winsted, CT: Actex Publications.

O'Grady, F.T. 1988. *Individual Health Insurance*. Schaumberg, IL: Society of Actuaries.

Pyenson, B.S. 1998. *Managing Risk*. Chicago, IL: AHA Press.

Sutton, H.L., and Sorbo, A.J. 1993. *Actuarial Issues in the Fee-For-Service/Prepaid Medical Group*. 2d ed. Englewood, CO: Center for Research in Ambulatory Health Care Administration/MGMA.

CHAPTER 50

Underwriting and Rating Functions by Market

Michael G. Sturm

This chapter discusses underwriting and rating functions specific to the various major health insurance markets. Please refer to Chapter 49 for a general discussion of underwriting and rating functions common to most markets. The major markets discussed in this chapter include:

- individual nongovernment
- commercial group
  — small (2 to 50 eligible employees)
  — large (51 or more eligible employees)
- government
  — Medicare supplements
  — Medicare risk contracts
  — Medicaid risk contracts

In general, underwriting and rating differs among markets on the basis of the probability of adverse selection (i.e., insuring risks with significantly higher morbidity than anticipated by the rate formula) in a given market and whether underwriting is even allowed. The chance of adverse selection increases as the group size decreases because individual applicants and small groups are likely to buy insurance only if they need it. This occurs for various reasons, including cost con-

Michael G. Sturm, FSA, is an Actuary with the Brookfield, Wisconsin office of Milliman & Robertson, Inc. He consults with HMO and insurance company staff, physicians, and self-funded plan sponsors regarding group, individual, and international health consulting matters. He assists these clients with various projects, including experience analysis, underwriting strategy, product and rate manual development, and actuarial projections.

cerns, the need to attract employees with health benefits, and whether health insurance premiums are tax deductible. Medicaid and Medicare risk contracts do not allow any underwriting. Rate setting also differs among the markets on the basis of whether the insurer sets the rates (as in most markets) or the government sets the rates (as in the Medicare and Medicaid risk markets).

INDIVIDUAL NONGOVERNMENT MARKET

The individual nongovernment market includes self-employed individuals (such as insurance agents and/or farmers) and employees (usually of small employers) not offered group health insurance.

The comments in this chapter apply mainly to individual major medical policies that reimburse insureds on the basis of actual expenses after any provider discounts and/or insured cost-sharing provisions are applied. The comments do not necessarily apply to hospital income, per diem, fixed indemnity, disability, credit insurance, long-term care, Medicare supplement, or accident-only policies. Medicare supplement policies are discussed in a separate section of this chapter.

Underwriting

Issue

Underwriting at issue varies depending on state regulations. However, underwriting at issue is usually quite strict in states that do not prohibit its use. This is because individual health insurance applicants usually exhibit higher morbidity costs, on average, than group applicants because of the high degree of adverse selection (i.e., those applying for coverage are usually those that need it most). Underwriting encourages individuals to obtain insurance before needing it.

Most carriers use long form underwriting. In addition, many carriers require a paramedical or medical examination. Examinations range from a simple physical to specific tests that check for certain conditions (e.g., an electrocardiogram, urinalysis, and/or blood test). The underwriter might also request an attending physician statement (APS) or follow-up with a telephone call to verify the information on the application. An APS is a record prepared by the applicant's personal physician that discusses a specific condition, examination, or operation. APSs provide more detail than the application and can be more useful than a medical examination.

Maternity coverage is a highly selective benefit. Applicants expecting a child or contemplating childbirth are more likely to request maternity coverage than single adults or elderly couples. The underwriter should consider this when issuing coverage and determining an appropriate rate.

Many insurers assess relative morbidity using a debit point system. Each applicant is assigned debits on the basis of historical and current medical conditions. A lower debit point assignment is associated with a healthier applicant. Each debit point is usually related to a percent of average claim costs (e.g., 1 percent). The percent of extra medical costs per debit point can then be translated into a dollar amount.

Debit point systems are only estimates of a person's medical costs. For example, two people with the same condition can have significantly different costs, depending on their age, physician, medical delivery patterns by geographical area, and available treatments. Therefore, most insurers employ a medical director to assist the underwriter in estimating future costs on the basis of available information.

Any existing health conditions might cause the insurer to decline the applicant (if allowed by law), exclude the specific conditions from reimbursement for a specified number of months (commonly 12, although possibly for the life of the policy), or charge an extra premium for the condition. These actions may seem quite punitive. However, their purpose is to encourage individuals to purchase insurance before becoming ill.

Exclusion riders (a.k.a., pre-existing condition exclusions) have the disadvantage of removing coverage for the medical services needed most. However, the advantage of exclusion riders is that they allow coverage to be issued to applicants who would normally be declined or offered a significantly more expensive policy (a.k.a., "rated-up"). Extra premium can be assessed on a temporary or permanent basis and be a flat dollar amount or a percent of the base policy premium.

The degree of underwriting must be weighed against the time and cost of the various tests. Spending too much time underwriting can result in less new business if applicants enroll with another company. Spending too little time underwriting can result in higher than expected morbidity experience.

The Health Insurance Portability and Accountability Act (HIPAA) requires insurers to offer coverage to *eligible individuals*. *Eligible individuals* are defined as individuals who have at least 18 months of creditable coverage as of the date on which they apply for individual coverage. In addition, the most recent prior creditable coverage must be through a group health plan, government plan, or church plan. Also, *eligible individuals* cannot be eligible for coverage under a group health plan, Medicare, or Medicaid. Finally, *eligible individuals* must have applied for and exhausted all available COBRA and state health insurance pool coverage.

Renewal

Certain states prohibit insurers from varying rates at renewal on the basis of health status. Other states restrict health status variation from the average rate to a specific percent.

Insureds often seek out new policies at renewal. Those who pass underwriting are offered rates reflecting a healthy applicant through a new block of policies. Insureds who do not pass underwriting usually remain in the old block and receive a higher rate increase than would a mixture of less healthy and healthy insureds. This "re-entry" effect results in less healthy insureds from the original block funding a larger portion of their own medical costs because there are fewer healthy insureds subsidizing them.

Many states require that individual policies have a clause to automatically renew unless the insurer cancels the whole block of policies. If insurers choose to cancel the whole block, they are usually prohibited from marketing a similar form of insurance for a specified time period (e.g., five years) from the date of cancellation.

Rating

Rates for new blocks can be priced using existing blocks of business adjusted for benefit, underwriting, claim administration, marketing, and other differences. Carriers' rates in many states are public information that can be found on file with the state department of insurance (where required by law). Insurers can also find consultants who have experience in pricing individual health insurance.

Individual health insurance rates and medical cost experience vary directly with the strictness of underwriting (i.e., how underwriters decline applications, rate-up applications, and how claim administrators enforce pre-existing condition limitations and exclusions). Medical cost experience, on average, increases significantly from the time since underwriting on blocks with very strict underwriting at issue. This is due to healthy groups "regressing to the mean" health status of the population (a.k.a., underwriting "wear-off") as the duration since issue increases. However, premium might increase at a slower rate than medical costs if the premium at issue is set higher than the medical costs to reflect the durational increase in medical costs.

State Laws

Rating restrictions vary significantly depending on the state. Some states have passed laws that limit rate differences for noncase characteristics within and among classes (a.k.a., blocks) of business (i.e., modified community rating). Case characteristics are defined differently among the various states. Case characteristics generally include family status (i.e., the type and number of dependents within a family unit) and benefit plan. States vary as to whether they allow carriers to rate for age, gender, geographical area, and occupation. Some states require individual insurance to be sold on a guarantee issue, pure community-rated basis (i.e., allowing rate differences for only the benefit plan and number of family members). Experience has shown declines in the number of individually insured people in states that have implemented guarantee issue coupled with pure community rating by age.

Guarantee issue type of legislation effectively forces healthier insureds to subsidize less healthy insureds. It prompts the debate of whether health insurance is a right or a privilege. Some healthy insureds will terminate or reduce coverage if they are required to subsidize too much of the less healthy insureds' costs in a voluntary insurance system. Each insured's risk profile varies substantially. Therefore, it is difficult to determine the level of cross-subsidization in a given situation that will cause healthy insureds to terminate or reduce coverage.

State insurance departments often regulate individual policies through rate filings. States often require a rate filing for new products that demonstrate minimum loss ratios (i.e., incurred claims divided by earned premium) will be achieved. They also often require filings that demonstrate the need for any planned rate increases. The insurer must demonstrate that the future loss ratio and cumulative lifetime loss ratio are projected to be higher than the state minimum loss ratio (e.g., 60 percent).

COMMERCIAL GROUP MARKET

The commercial group market can be subdivided into small groups (defined as two to 50 eligible employees for purposes of this chapter) and large groups (51 or more eligible employees). These two markets share many underwriting and rating characteristics as discussed in the following. This section also discusses underwriting and rating functions specific to each of the markets.

Small groups possess different risk characteristics than large groups. The underwriting and rating process must recognize that small groups often choose not to provide coverage for their employees. This voluntary nature of coverage presents an opportunity for the small group to adversely select against a health plan that does not underwrite and rate this risk prudently.

Adverse selection is not unique to the small group market. Carriers can experience adverse selection on large groups if employees are allowed to choose among competing health plans through an open enrollment process. Adverse selection may also occur, for example, within a poorly designed open network plan. The design, rating, and underwriting process used by the health plan must recognize the potential for adverse selection and ensure that rates will be adequate, competitive, and equitable.

Underwriting Common to Small and Large Groups

Issue

Group underwriting requirements are enforced at issue to ensure that groups applying for coverage have an average health status in relation to the insurer's current block. Rates would not be equitable if an insurer required responsible groups that obtain insurance before becoming less healthy to fund groups that apply at the time they need insurance. *Group underwriting ensures:*

- the group has a valid employer/employee relationship (i.e., it is not formed for the sole purpose of obtaining insurance)
- a minimum percent of employees and dependents enroll, excluding employees with other coverage (usually 50 percent to 100 percent on the basis of employer contribution)
- the employer contributes a minimum portion of the costs (e.g., 50 percent of the single employee costs)

- the group is currently insured
- the group submits current claim experience (large groups only)
- the group is permanent in nature, financially stable, and has a regular influx of healthy lives (e.g., no seasonal groups)
- only full-time, active employees are covered
- groups sold are on a "total replacement" basis only (this requirement may be relaxed for large groups)

Information required from the employer might include a group's:

- legal name
- address
- phone number
- date of application submission
- requested date the quote is due back to the broker
- broker (along with name, address, and telephone number)
- commission paid to the broker
- number of years in business
- credit history
- recent layoffs (if any)
- worker's compensation policy (if any)
- Standard Industrial Classification (SIC) code
- definition of employee eligibility for the health plan
- medical history (e.g., employer disclosure form for large groups)
- renewal date
- employer contribution
- expected percent of employees electing coverage
- waiting periods
- demographics (i.e., employees' age, gender, income, and family status)
- number of employees in the service area
- wage and tax data
- proposed rate increase (if available)
- historical benefit plans and rates (for at least two years)
- funding arrangement (i.e., fully insured, self-funded)
- historical claim experience (usually applies to large groups only)

Information required from the employee might include:

- legal name
- address
- phone number
- social security number
- title
- hours worked per week
- earnings (if disability coverage is offered)
- height and weight
- medical history (i.e., individual medical questionnaires for small groups)
- other health insurance coverage (if any)
- other employment (if any)
- information on dependents (e.g., name, relationship, date of birth, gender, and any other coverage)
- signed refusal statements indicating the reason for refusal (e.g., coverage through a spouse) for employees declining coverage

HIPAA has limited some historical group underwriting requirements. For example, HIPAA has limited HMO affiliation periods (i.e., a "waiting" period after the application for which there is no coverage) and pre-existing condition limitations. Affiliation periods are limited to 2 months (3 months for late enrollees).

Pre-existing condition limitations can only exclude/deny payments for 12 months (18 months for late enrollees) on future claims because of health conditions *treated* within 6 months (i.e., the "look-back" period) before applying for coverage. Historically, carriers have applied the "prudent person" rule with respect to the "look-back" period. The prudent person rule denies coverage on conditions for which a prudent person would have sought treatment. HIPAA prohibits use of the prudent person rule. In addition, carriers can no longer exclude medical costs because of pregnancy as a pre-existing condition.

Finally, the insurer must decrease the exclusion period (on a month-for-month basis) if the applicant has prior insurance coverage. For example, the maximum exclusion period for any health conditions treated within 6 months of applying for coverage is 4 months if the insured has had

8 months of continuous prior coverage with any coverage lapses during the prior coverage period not exceeding 62 days per lapse period. A lapse in coverage longer than 62 days is considered a significant break in coverage. Any coverage before a significant break in coverage does not have to be considered "creditable coverage" for the purpose of decreasing the exclusion period.

A late enrollee is defined as an insured who initially declines coverage without a valid reason, then applies for coverage after the group enrolls. The maximum exclusion period for late enrollees is 18 months. Insurers do not have to accept late enrollees at all; however, they cannot accept them on an ad-hoc basis. Stated differently, insurers must accept all late enrollees if they accept any late enrollees.

Coverage generally becomes effective on the first day of the month after receipt of an enrollment form and completion of any waiting period. Late entrants may have to wait longer (assuming they are offered coverage at all).

During the Plan Year

New employees are occasionally required to wait before being enrolled in the plan (a.k.a., waiting period). Waiting until the first day of the next month or 30 days is common; however, many carriers use longer waiting periods for businesses with high turnover (e.g., beauty salons, retail stores, and restaurants). HIPAA requires that time elapsed during the waiting period does not count as a break in coverage. Also, waiting periods must run concurrently with any exclusion periods.

HIPAA requires "special enrollment" periods for employees and their dependents lasting at least 30 days from a qualifying event. Qualifying events include marriage, birth, adoption, or a loss of other coverage an employee had when he or she originally refused to enroll in the plan. Qualifying events are viewed as circumstances not controllable by the employee and therefore virtually preclude adverse selection. Carriers are not allowed to increase the rates on a group because of enrollees qualifying for coverage through special enrollment periods until renewal.

Note, carriers can apply a pre-existing condition limitation or affiliation period on employees with a significant break in coverage who qualify through a special enrollment period. However, pre-existing condition exclusions *cannot* be applied to pregnancy costs, newborns, adopted children, or children placed for adoption who qualify for coverage through a special enrollment period and enroll within 30 days, unless the insured subsequently incurs a significant break in coverage as defined previously.

Renewal

As stated in Chapter 49, the underwriter has more information on the specific risks at renewal and usually implements rate changes on the basis of experience and projected changes to the experience. Renewal rates for a given group can be calculated on the basis of historical experience of the total block, historical experience of the specific group, and/or projected changes to historical experience.

Projected changes in historical experience might include increased medical management, changes in provider reimbursement, medical cost and expense trend, stricter application of underwriting requirements, claim administration changes, distribution method changes, and/or any other changes that will have an impact on future medical costs. Please refer to Exhibit 49–1 for a more detailed list of projection factors.

Most group underwriting requirements applied at issue should also be applied at renewal. For example, the underwriter should make sure the group still meets minimum participation requirements, minimum employer contribution requirements, and there is still a valid employer/employee relationship at renewal. Medical costs for groups that do not pass these (and other) group underwriting requirements will increase much faster than groups that do pass underwriting requirements.

HIPAA requires carriers to renew groups except for stated reasons, which include:

- nonpayment of premium
- fraud
- not meeting minimum contribution or participation requirements

- the employee moving out of the carrier's service area
- termination of the block (the carrier must offer other coverage)
- termination of all health business (the carrier is then prevented from offering any health products for five years)

In any case, a carrier cannot discontinue or not renew any coverage on the basis of claim experience or health status. This requirement is not too significant for small group carriers because many states have already passed small group laws guaranteeing renewability. Similarly, it is not too significant for large group carriers because they have less restrictions on setting renewal rates.

Eligible Enrollees

Insurers only offer coverage to eligible employees. The definition of eligible employees varies among insurers. ***Common definitions for eligible employees include:***

- actively at work
- full-time (i.e., a minimum of 30 hours per week)
- those receiving 100 percent of their income from the employer
- COBRA eligibles
- retirees

Common definitions for eligible dependents include:

- spouses
- unmarried children dependents, including:
  — adopted children,
  — stepchildren through a legal marriage
  — other children dependent on the employee

Eligible children might be subject to other requirements. For example, insurers might only cover them if they are age 19 or less unless they are a full-time student, totally disabled, or mentally retarded and still dependent on the parent for most of their financial support.

The insurer usually coordinates with Medicare for retirees and Medicare-eligible active employees (a.k.a., the working aged) when possible. Medicare is always the primary payer for Medicare-eligible retirees. However, the primary payer for the working aged can vary, depending on the employer's total employees (including those not enrolled in the health plan). Employers with 20 or more total employees are primary payers. Employers with less than 20 employees can elect Medicare as the primary payer if they notify Medicare.

Rating Common to Small and Large Groups

Carriers use various approaches to calculate group-specific rates. Group-specific rates vary with respect to the rate structure and degree of community rating.

Rate Structure

Group rate structures vary depending on the number of dependents per employee and whether they recognize age and/or gender within a group. List billing recognizes each employee's age, number of dependents, and possibly gender. Composite billing recognizes the number of de-

pendents per employee but does not recognize each employee's age or gender. Generally, only small groups use list billing (where allowed by law) because the substitution of one member (e.g., a 20-year-old man) for another member (e.g., a 65-year-old woman) has the potential to significantly change the total group's premium. However, some small groups and most large groups use composite billing.

Table 50–1 presents common family tier categories used when composite billing.

Degree of Community Rating

The phrase community rating can have various meanings. The degree of community rating refers to the extent a specific group's rates reflect the group's characteristics or the total block's characteristics (i.e., the extent to which the many possible rating formula adjustments are recognized among groups). The most common approaches used to establish group-specific rates are pure community rating, community rating by class (CRC), and adjusted community rating (ACR).

Pure community rates are the same for every group with the same benefit plan and located in

---

Table 50–1 Common Employer Billing Bases

Number of Family Tiers*	Family Tier Categories
One	Employee
Two	Employee
	Employee with family
Three	Employee
	Employee with one dependent
	Employee with two or more dependents
Four	Employee
	Employee with spouse
	Employee with child(ren)
	Employee with spouse and child(ren)
Five	Employee
	Employee with spouse
	Employee with child
	Employee with children
	Employee with spouse and child(ren)

*These family tiers may also be list billed in the small group market, with premium rates being calculated by employee age and/or gender.

the same geographical area. Pure community rating recognizes only benefit plan differences among and within groups, family status differences within groups, and sometimes geographical area differences among groups. Other group-specific rate formula adjustments are not used; they are based on the total block experience.

CRC rating uses benefit plan, family status, and more rate formula adjustments to create unique rates for each group. The purpose of CRC is to recognize additional group characteristics without using the group's medical cost experience. CRC rating, at a minimum, adjusts a group's rates on the basis of their demographic factors (i.e., age, gender, and number of members per contract). Some CRC rate formulas adjust for additional group characteristics (e.g., geographical area or occupation).

Illustrative age and gender factors by type of contract are shown in Table 50–2. These factors reflect the expected rate requirements for an employee of a particular age, gender, and contract status compared with the carrier's average per member per month (PMPM) rate target.

For example, the expected revenue for a single male employee younger than 30 years is 50 percent (i.e., 0.50 from Table 50–2) of the carrier's average PMPM rate target. Note that the composite of all factors from Table 50–2 is equal to 2.32, the average number of members per employee contract. This ensures that the overall PMPM revenue is obtained when these factors are applied to the number of employee contracts.

ACR is similar to CRC, except it also recognizes the group's historical medical costs. ACR is normally only used with large groups.

Despite the rating method used, premium rates depend on the PMPM rate requirements, demographics underlying the development of the required rate, and targeted premium relationships. As noted previously, the demographic assumptions may be expected block demographics (pure community rating) or employer demographics (CRC).

Table 50–3 shows the development of four-tier composite bill rates. This example assumes 2.32 members per employee. Column 1 contains the percent of employees by contract type. Column 2 contains the average number of members for each contract type and illustrates that the weighted average of members per contract equals the total average members per contract of 2.32. Column 3 contains the factor necessary to convert (i.e., the conversion factor) the average PMPM rate across all contracts to a specific rate for each contract and illustrates that the weighted average conversion factor equals the average members per contract. Column 4 displays the PMPM rate required. Column 5 contains the required rate by contract (equal to the conversion factor in column 3 multiplied by the average PMPM rate contained in column 4).

The conversion factor in column 3 relates to a member cost relativity of 1.00 and is based on medical claims for each family tier. The single conversion factor in Table 50–3, the ratio of the single premium to the PMPM revenue, is esti-

Table 50–2 Illustrative Age/Gender Factors for a Two-Tier Rate Structure*

| | Employee | | Employee with Family | |
Employee Age	Male	Female	Male	Female
< 30	0.50	1.20	2.90	2.80
30–39	0.70	1.30	2.80	2.60
40–49	1.00	1.40	2.70	2.50
50–59	1.40	1.50	2.90	3.10
>60	1.90	1.80	3.40	3.50

*Overall composite of factors = 2.32 using a standard labor force population.

Table 50–3 Four-Tier Premium Rate Development

Contract Type	(1) Contract Distribution (%)	(2) Members Per Contract	(3) Conversion Factor	(4) PMPM Rate Requirement	(5) Target Premium Rate ($)
Employee	41	1.0	1.19	120.00	$142.80
Employee and spouse	15	2.0	3.08	120.00	369.60
Employee and child(ren)	10	2.5	2.04	120.00	244.80
Employee with spouse and child(ren)	34	4.0	3.42	120.00	410.40
Composite	100	2.32	2.32	120.00	278.40

mated to be 1.19. The single premium is an adult (or employee) only rate, whereas the PMPM revenue reflects average member costs when adults and children are combined. The employee-only premium is higher than the PMPM rate because child costs are, on average, lower than adult costs.

A carrier's rates for a specific group can be set to reflect the same rate relativities among family tiers as the competition. For example, a carrier wishing to bid on a large group may modify the conversion factor to reflect the group's current rate relativity. The employer may insist that family rates equal 3.0 times the single rate (i.e., $142.80 × 3.0 = $428.40).

Table 50–4 illustrates how the carrier can accomplish this, yet still collect the PMPM rate requirement of $120.00. Note the relative change in the conversion factors from Table 50–3. This is necessary to maintain the required PMPM $120 ($278.40 ÷ 2.32) rate.

A CRC rate development that recognizes a specific group's demographics is provided in Table 50–5. The calculation uses the age/gender factors from Table 50–2. The example at the bottom of the table contains the calculation of an employee-only rate; however, the process is similar to that for other family tiers. The resulting employee-only rate is 15 percent greater than the PMPM rate target (i.e., the employee-only conversion factor equals 1.15) and 3 percent less than the average PMPM rate for all contract types (1.15 divided by 1.19). CRC results in more rate variability among groups than community rating because each group's demographics are recognized in the rate development.

Table 50–4 Competitively Adjusted Four-Tier Premium Rate Development

Contract Type	(1) Contract Distribution (%)	(2) Standard Conversion Factor	(3) Competitive Conversion Factor	(4) Resulting Competitive Premium Rate ($)
Employee	41	1.19	1.19	$142.80
Employee and spouse	15	3.08	2.86	343.20
Employee and child(ren)	10	2.04	1.89	226.80
Employee with spouse and child(ren)	34	3.42	3.57	428.40
Composite	100	2.32	2.32	278.40

Employee with spouse and child(ren) is set equal to 3.0 (3.57 divided by 1.19) times the employee rate.

Table 50–5 Community Rating by Class Example Assuming a $120.00 Health Plan PMPM Target Rate

Employee Age (Years)	Employee	
	Male	Female
< 30	5	6
30–39	4	5
40–49	3	4
50–59	2	3
>60	1	2
Total	15	20

Employee only premium = $120.00 × [(5)(0.5)+(4)(0.7)+ (3)(1.0)+(2)(1.4)+(1)(1.9)+(6)(1.2)+ (5)(1.3)+(4)(1.4)+(3)(1.5)+(2)(1.8)] ÷ (15+20)

= $120.00 × (40.4 ÷ 35)

= $138.51

Table 50–5 could be modified to illustrate list billing for small employer groups. For example, the rate for male employees younger than 30 years old would equal $60 (0.50 × $120, from Tables 50–2 and 50–3).

Rates are generally guaranteed for 12 months. However, some carriers allow large employers to negotiate multiyear rate guarantees. Multiyear rate guarantees increase the probability of significant losses caused by unexpected medical cost increases.

Small Group Underwriting

This section differentiates small group underwriting from large group underwriting. One should consider the previous section, "Underwriting and Rating Common to Small and Large Groups," in addition to this section when determining all small group underwriting requirements.

The percent of small employers offering health insurance to their employees is much less than large groups for various reasons, including cost concerns. Similar to individual coverage, small groups, on average, tend to purchase insurance when they anticipate or contract illnesses (i.e., adverse selection). Insurers underwrite small groups to charge them equitable rates.

Issue

Effective underwriting at issue maintains equitable rates on a group-by-group basis. This leads to higher persistency and an average pool rate that, after applicable state rate restrictions are applied, will still be competitive enough to attract new, healthy groups. Adverse selection, potentially leading to a rapid escalation in required premium rates, can occur if carriers do not assign equitable rates among groups. This occurs as healthy groups enroll with carriers that recognize their experience. Subsequently, the total pool rates will increase, leading to rapid rate escalation.

Unlike the individual market, insurers are *not* allowed to decline less healthy small group applicants. HIPAA requires all carriers doing business in the small group market to issue coverage in their open policy forms to all small group applicants. Historically, medical costs for groups passing underwriting would start at something less than the ultimate rate for all groups (i.e., new and renewal) in year 1 and, on average, increase to the ultimate rate. Guarantee issue requires carriers to insure groups greater than, at, and less than the ultimate rate. It therefore has created multiple medical cost durational curves (to the extent groups greater than and at the ultimate rate accept coverage) that, on average, should regress to the ultimate rate.

Medical underwriting in the small group market is almost always done at issue and sometimes at renewal to maintain equitable rates among groups. Carriers might collect forms from the employer disclosing current health conditions (at a minimum) and/or individual medical questionnaires (IMQs). IMQs can be short form (e.g., 1 to 10 questions) or long form. The general rule is to use forms capturing more detail as group size decreases.

Underwriting at issue results in a group being assigned a health status adjustment (where allowed by law). Some carriers still require IMQs at issue in states not allowing a health status adjustment to identify individuals that could benefit from increased medical attention.

IMQs are required for groups from 2 to 10 employees by virtually all carriers in states that allow a health status adjustment. Carriers vary regarding the minimum number of employees at which they will waive individual medical questionnaires. Many carriers require long form IMQs up to 25 employees and short form above that to 50 employees. However, carriers may have to use the same application forms for all groups with 2 to 50 eligible employees if state small group insurance laws do not allow for different rating adjustments by case size. The number of employees at which carriers stop requesting IMQs varies by carrier, geographical market, and competitors' practices.

Typical "short form" questions include:

- Are you or any of your dependents currently under medical care, treatment, or consultation by a medical practitioner (including medication)?
- Have you or any of your dependents been prevented from performing your usual duties or activities in the past 12 months?
- Have you or any of your dependents ever been treated or told that you had heart trouble, high blood pressure, sugar in urine, diabetes, tuberculosis, cancer, tumor, ulcer, arthritis, asthma, epilepsy, lung or respiratory disorder, or mental disorder?
- Have you or any of your dependents been hospitalized or had a surgical operation in the past five years?
- Are you or any of your dependents currently pregnant?
- Have you or any of your dependents had more than $5,000 in medical charges during the past 12 months?
- Have you or any of your dependents had any physical examinations within the past five years that resulted in any adverse findings?
- Have you or any of your dependents used drugs other than prescribed by your physician, been advised to have treatment, or been treated for alcohol or drug abuse?
- Do you or any of your dependents currently smoke?

    If any of the preceding questions have been answered "yes," please give details

(name of patient, dates of treatment, names of prescriptions, names of hospital and/or attending physician, etc.) below. Make reference to the question you are answering.

In addition, IMQs should be signed by the employee and be less than 30 days old to prevent the carrier from assigning rates based on outdated medical information.

Similar to individual medical underwriting, many insurers assess relative morbidity with a debit point system. Each applicant in a group is assigned debits on the basis of historical and current medical conditions. Each debit point is usually related to a percent of average claim costs. The percent of extra medical costs per debit point can then be translated into a dollar amount, depending on the average medical costs per member for the block of policies being medically underwritten.

The carrier usually calculates an average debit point per group calculated as the sum of debits for the group divided by the group's exposure. The average debit points per group are then translated into a relative rate (which might differ from the relative medical cost) through a table mapping debit points to tiers. Table 50–6 displays a mapping of average debit points to relative rates.

The numbers in Table 50–6 are for illustration purposes only. The tier groupings have been randomly selected. Carriers could assign a separate relative rate for each average debit point if desired. Alternatively, carriers could further pool the groups by combining tiers one and two (or any combination of consecutive tiers). Combining tiers one and two effectively requires expected healthier groups (i.e., average debits per exposure unit less than five) to subsidize groups expected to be less healthy that are assigned average debit points between five and eight. The mapping of debit points to relative rates depends on the specific state's regulations, the carrier's administrative flexibility, and the carrier's strategy to pool groups with varying health statuses.

Note, the relative rate column in Table 50–6 has been set such that it complies with state regulations that require a plus or minus 25 per-

Table 50–6 Sample Mapping of Average Debit Points Per Exposure Unit Per Group to a Rate Relativity

Tier	Range of Average Debit Points per Exposure Unit per Group	Expected Percent of Groups (%)	Relative Medical Cost	Relative Rate
1	0–4.99	27.5	0.63	0.80
2	5–7.99	13.6	0.75	0.86
3	8–10.99	11.3	0.84	0.92
4	11–13.99	9.9	0.93	0.98
5	14–16.99	6.7	1.02	1.05
6	17–19.99	6.3	1.12	1.12
7	20–22.99	4.7	1.21	1.20
8	23–25.99	3.6	1.30	1.28
9	26+	16.4	1.80	1.33
Total/average	14.18	100.0	1.00	1.00

cent health status rate adjustment from the index rate (i.e., 1.33/0.80 is approximately equal to 1.25/0.75). In addition, a group can be moved up two tiers and still comply with most state requirements that groups cannot receive more than a 15 percent annual increase for health status.

In addition, the average debit points assigned by a given underwriter (14.18 in Table 50–6) will vary on the basis of many factors, including, but not necessarily limited to:

- the underwriter's level of conservatism when assigning points
- the amount of information requested (i.e., employer disclosure form, individual short form, and/or individual long form)
- the group's demographics (older groups should, on average, be assigned more debit points)
- statistical fluctuation

The underwriter should track the average debit points assigned per group to ensure the average rate target is met (i.e., the average tier factors for all groups composite to 1.00). In addition, tracking assigned debit points allows the underwriter to develop an aggregate debit point distribution. Multiple underwriters may need to assign points to a sample set of groups to equate their level of conservatism, ensuring consistent

ratings among underwriters for the same group. If not, brokers will sense which underwriter assigns the most favorable rate tiers and submit their business to that underwriter.

As stated in the individual underwriting section, debit point systems are only estimates of a person's claim costs. For example, two people with the same condition can have significantly different medical costs, depending on their age, doctor, provider practice patterns by geographical area, available treatments, and many other factors. Therefore, most insurers employ a medical director to assist the underwriter in estimating future costs on the basis of available information.

Underwriters must be aware of companies that enroll an abnormally high portion of extended family members. Extra measures should be taken to validate the employer/employee relationship in groups with a high number of insured family members because some small employers place family members that require immediate medical care on their payroll to obtain health insurance for them. These people rarely fund their own costs before needing insurance. Therefore, other members of the insurance pool must subsidize their health costs.

Quoting groups that request multiple options (i.e., closed panel plans alongside point-of-service plans) is generally not a problem if the carrier insures the total group (a.k.a., full replacement). However, most carriers in the small group market avoid quoting groups with multiple carriers because of the potential for adverse selection and higher administrative costs as a percent of premium.

During the Plan Year

Groups will occasionally request benefit changes during the plan year. Most carriers do not allow small groups to increase benefits during the year because of the selective nature (i.e., groups that need more coverage will be primarily the ones that request it).

Renewal

As discussed in the Commercial Group section, "Underwriting Common to Small and Large Groups," most group underwriting requirements applied at issue should also be applied at renewal. For example, the underwriter should make sure the group still meets minimum participation requirements, minimum employer contribution requirements, and there is still a valid employer/employee relationship at renewal. Medical costs for groups that do not pass these (and other) group underwriting requirements will increase much faster than groups that do pass underwriting requirements.

Small Group Rating

Rates for a given group in the small group market are usually based on the employee's age, gender, and the number of dependents (a.k.a., "list bill"). A given group's list bill rates might also vary by geographical area, benefit plan, industry, health status, contract effective date, case size, and other variables as permitted by law. Carriers use list bill rates for small groups because each insured's age and gender can have a significant impact on the group's required premium.

NAIC Model Laws and State Regulations

Before small group regulations, most carriers historically charged each group a rate that largely reflected their historical or projected ex-

perience. This resulted in small groups with less healthy employees not being able to afford insurance and/or experiencing significant renewal rate increases as the favorable morbidity experience in the first few years achieved through strict underwriting dissipated.

Rates quoted at issue and renewal varied significantly and led to instability in the small group market. The public protested to legislators and the insurance industry about perceived unfair treatment by insurers because of the fluctuations in the rates.

The industry, led by the National Association of Insurance Commissioners (NAIC), responded by drafting model insurance laws that states could choose to adopt. Many states have adopted the NAIC's small group model laws.

The NAIC model laws provide for various restrictions, including a maximum amount rates can vary for any given group within a block of policies. For example, the NAIC model law limits rate differentials for noncase characteristics (which include health status or claim experience). Case characteristics are defined differently among the various states. They include, but are not necessarily limited to, family status, benefit plan, age, gender, industry, case size, and geographical area.

Rate increases for noncase characteristics are limited to 15 percent plus the increase in the overall block of policies (i.e., the change in the new business rate). Some states require pure community rating (i.e., rates can only vary by family size and benefit plan). Other states vary as to whether they allow carriers to rate for age, gender, geographical area, and industry on a group-specific basis.

In states allowing a health status variation, carriers might assign each group's health status rate adjustment (a.k.a., rate tier and/or underwriting adjustment) based on, but not necessarily limited to, the:

- medical underwriting results of the group
- number of insureds that are expecting children
- frequency with which the group changes carriers

- presence of worker's compensation insurance
- employee turnover, and/or
- the group's proposed rate increase from their current carrier

Reducing the rate variation for health status requires healthy groups to subsidize less healthy groups. Some legislators favor no health status adjustment. This can be interpreted as the view that health care is a right and healthy individuals should be required to subsidize less healthy individuals.

However, other state legislators favor an unlimited health status adjustment (i.e., charging groups entirely on the basis of their own experience). One view supporting this position is that forcing subsidization in a voluntary market can lead to healthy groups declining or reducing coverage if they realize that they are not paying a fair price. This leaves less healthy groups funding their own health costs (i.e., a rate spiral, also known as cumulative adverse selection theory*). This can lead to an erosion of the number of insureds and an increase in health insurance premiums as healthy individuals refuse to subsidize less healthy insureds.

State regulations (based on NAIC model laws) usually allow separate rate bands for significantly different blocks of business. Their level of underwriting, type of distribution, and whether they purchased the block from another carrier often define blocks. However, states still apply maximum index rate differences among blocks (e.g., 20 percent). Last, states that have passed these laws often require an actuarial certification that carriers are complying with the law. The certification is usually due in March or April and certifies that a carrier's rates in the previous year are in compliance with the state's small group laws.

Renewal

Carriers usually recalculate the group's rate for the upcoming year based on the rate formula.

---

*For a detailed discussion and modeling of cumulative adverse selection theory, you may want to refer to Bill Bluhm's paper, "Cumulative Antiselection Theory."

This might include age, gender, industry, health status, and more rate factors, depending on the state. Carriers evaluate historical experience (e.g., loss ratio) and projected future experience (e.g., current diagnoses) when assigning health status. Some carriers assign groups a higher health status tier if both historical and projected experience are poor, lower the health status tier if both are good, and maintain the same health status tier if one is poor and the other is good.

Large Group Underwriting

For purposes of this chapter, I have defined large groups as having 51 or more eligible employees. This section does not necessarily apply to association groups. Associations are different from large groups in that there is a greater opportunity for adverse selection, especially if underwriting requirements are lax.

The large group market operates differently than the individual and small group markets. Selection problems are less significant because a randomly selected group will experience average medical costs as the size of the group increases (a.k.a., the law of large numbers). In addition, participation of all eligible employees (those healthy and less healthy) is encouraged with group insurance because health insurance premiums are not taxed as part of compensation.

Large group underwriting seldom involves IMQs because most carriers require medical cost experience before quoting a fully insured rate or setting equivalent claim estimates on a self-insured group. Underwriters also request an employer disclosure form that lists employees' serious health conditions. However, the employer disclosure form has shortcomings to the extent large employers are not aware of the serious conditions or underreport them to obtain a lower rate.

Underwriting at issue also involves determining a group's ability to administer the plan (e.g., submitting enrollment data and contributions to the insurer, assisting with collecting claim submissions, and identification of COBRA eligibles). A carrier might want to charge groups more for administrative expenses to the extent groups cannot perform these functions.

HIPAA's pre-existing condition requirements are of less importance in the large group market because pre-existing conditions are often handled under a "no gain/no loss" arrangement. In this situation, the new carrier pays for existing health conditions covered under the group's prior benefit plan. However, the pre-existing condition limitations might apply to new benefits.

Certain large groups invite multiple carriers to offer products to their employees. Employees then sign up for desired health plans during an open enrollment process. These situations must be treated with caution from an underwriting and rating perspective because much opportunity exists for adverse selection (especially for carriers offering products with broader networks). The number of rate tiers (e.g., single, family) in these situations should either equal or exceed the number of tiers used by the other carriers. Fewer rate tiers than competing plans will also likely result in adverse selection.

A risk of adverse selection also exists in multiple carrier situations when a specific carrier's rate is substantially higher than the competitor's rate or certain high-profile benefits are reimbursed higher in the carrier's plan. For example, some carriers do not allow employee contributions for their plan to be more than $10 to $15 per month for single employees ($25 to $40 per month for families) than competing carriers because the people willing to pay more for health insurance are likely going to use more health insurance. High-profile benefits include prescription drug coverage, infertility treatment, mental health, and substance abuse.

The adverse selection caused by the premium differential and benefit selection can be mitigated by reducing benefits (and hence premium). Another option to mitigate adverse selection caused by the premium differential is to increase the employer subsidy on the more expensive plan, thereby reducing the employee's contribution differential on the plans.

Large Group Rating

Rates *among* groups in the large group market will vary on the basis of most (and possibly all) of the rating factors mentioned in the Rate Formula section in Chapter 49. However, rates for employees *within* a specific group do not usually vary by age or gender of the employee but still vary by the number of dependents (a.k.a., tier or composite rated).

For example, five-tier composite rates might be defined as: employee, employee and spouse, employee and child, employee and child[ren], and family (employee, spouse, and child[ren]). Actual demographics (especially members per contract) should be used at issue or compared with expected demographics at renewal (if a group does not have actual demographics at issue) or if a group is composite rated, and appropriate adjustments should be made if necessary.

Carriers will also allow large groups to customize their benefit plans. For example, they will often accommodate special cost sharing, covered services, and/or benefit limitations. In addition, large groups are often allowed to change benefit plans throughout the year, especially when they are self-funded.

Rates for a given large group will often recognize the group's historical medical costs, utilization statistics, or other measures of historical medical costs (a.k.a., experience). This differs from individual and small group rating, in which medical costs among groups are largely pooled for rating purposes. Large group rates for groups with 51 to 500 or 1,000 employees are often a weighted average of the book (a.k.a., manual or pooled) rate and the rate suggested by the group's experience. The general formula to blend the book rate with the manual rate is:

$$\text{Experience rate} \times \text{Credibility factor} + \text{Book rate} \times (1 - \text{Credibility factor})$$

The Rate Formula section in Chapter 49 discusses book rate development. The experience rate is often developed starting with paid claims and making adjustments for:

- pooled claims (i.e., claims above the individual or aggregate stop-loss levels)
- incurred but not reported medical costs
- other trend factors that convert historical costs to projected costs (as listed in Exhibit 49–1)

Rates for groups with more than 1,000 employees are often based purely on experience. However, these groups will usually have individual and/or aggregate stop-loss insurance as well.

Careful judgment must be used when group-specific experience is used to set future rates. The experience must be scrutinized carefully for inconsistencies. The underwriter must determine whether the experience data are credible (i.e., whether the experience represents the group's long-term average medical costs or whether it is highly volatile and potentially under/overstated). The underwriter should determine whether the data are paid or incurred (or a mixture), current, stable over time, and whether any reserves being held are reasonable.

Many methods are available to rate an employer group on the basis of prior experience. The method chosen can be based on the quality and type of information available. A simplified example of claims-based experience rating is shown in Table 50–7. Two years of claims information is used in this example to illustrate the blending of multiple years of data. Multiple years are often used to reduce the impact of fluctuation that may occur in a group's year-to-year medical cost experience.

Steps 1 and 2 calculate incurred claims on the basis of paid claim data. As discussed previously, large claims are pooled in steps 3 and 4.

This reduces the impact of experience fluctuation caused by an unexpected number of large claims. The pooling adjustment replaces actual claims above the pooling point with the health plan's expected claim amount.

Step 7 calculates the actual-to-expected ratios for two years. No explicit adjustments are made between the time periods for trend, benefit design, or demographics in this example because both steps 6 and 7 reflect the group's characteristics for the time period shown. More credibility (60%) is assigned to the most current year's data.

Step 8 contains the 2000 projected PMPM book rate calculated from the rate formula that also reflects the group's characteristics. Step 10 combines the employer's experience ratio for each year with the expected cost calculated from the projected book rate using credibility assignments listed in step 9. In this example, 60 percent, 20 percent, and 20 percent weight is given to the employer's most recent, second most recent, and the projected book rate, respectively.

MEDICARE SUPPLEMENT

Medicare supplement policies pay for medical services that are not reimbursed through Medicare, including both cost-sharing provisions for covered services and services not covered (e.g., prescription drugs). More than half of

Table 50–7 Experience Rating Example Using Historical Medical Costs

Experience Rate Formula Steps	Projected Book Rate	Group-Specific Medical Costs	
		1998	1999
1. Paid claims	NA	$50	$68
2. Incurred claims		65	82
3. Pooling charge		7	8
4. Pooled claims		(2)	(10)
5. Experience claims (2 + 3 + 4)		$70	$80
6. Book rate for experience period		$60	$75
7. Actual-to-expected ratio (5 ÷ 6)		1.17	1.07
8. 2000 PMPM projected book rate	$120	NA	NA
9. Credibility assignment	20%	20%	60%
10. Final rate = $129.12 = $120 × [(1.00 x 20%)+(1.17 × 20%)+(1.07 × 60%)]			

all Medicare enrollees have a Medicare supplement policy. Supplements can be purchased in the open market on an individual basis or provided through an employer as part of the employee's retirement package on a group basis.

The Federal government has defined ten standard Medicare supplement benefit plans (labeled A through J, in order of increasing benefits). Carriers' Medicare supplement policies must conform to these plans (with the exception of carriers operating in states with federal waivers and plans offering innovative benefits).

Underwriting

Medicare supplement policies vary whether they are offered on an underwritten or guarantee-issue basis. Medicare supplement carriers must guarantee issue applicants older than 65 who apply for coverage within six months of becoming eligible for Medicare Part B (i.e., the open enrollment period). In addition, carriers cannot charge these individuals higher premiums related to health status during the open enrollment period. However, the carrier is allowed to exclude services that result from pre-existing conditions for a maximum of six months during the open enrollment period. Medicare supplement carriers can underwrite applicants after the open enrollment period.

Rating

There are generally four rate structures used by Medicare supplement carriers. They include:

- community rated (CR)
- issue age (IA)
- attained age (AA)
- age-banded rates (a blend of IA and AA rating)

Rates within and among any of these four structures might vary because of benefit plan, geographical area, and health status. In addition, the rates will generally change with medical cost trend and the duration because of issue (to reflect the "wearing-off" of underwriting [if applicable]).

The rates among the four structures differ by whether age and/or gender is used as a rate adjustment and whether the rate reflects increases in medical costs because of age (i.e., pre-funds for age). Pre-funds simply means to change more premium than necessary in the early years of the policy to fund costs higher than the premium in later policy years. A CR policy establishes the same rate for individuals of different ages and genders (assuming all other rate adjustments are constant). A CR may need to be lowered if new enrollees cause the average age to decrease or raised if new business declines, causing the average age of the policies to increase.

The rate for an IA (a.k.a., entry age) policy varies by age and pre-funds the increase in medical costs because of age. The rate for an AA policy varies by age but does not pre-fund the increase in medical costs because of age. A rate that varies by age bands (i.e., 65 to 69, 70 to 74), by definition, varies by age and partially pre-funds for medical cost increases because of age within each band.

Medicare supplement pricing information can be obtained through various sources, including medical costs for similar policies sold by the company, consultants, and/or rate filings required by state insurance departments. Carriers sometimes review existing rates in the marketplace and shadow price. However, this can be dangerous, especially if the competition is not charging an adequate rate.

MEDICARE RISK

A Medicare risk contract is an agreement between the Health Care Financing Administration (HCFA) and an HMO or competitive medical plan (CMP) for the HMO/CMP to provide Medicare's benefits (and usually more benefits at the plan's option) to Medicare enrollees for a fixed payment per member per month to the HMO. Risk contracts are authorized through Section 1876 of the Social Security Act.

HCFA has promoted risk contracts for different reasons. First, risk contracts often coordinate and manage health care better than the traditional fee-for-service (FFS) system, thereby increasing quality of care. Second, Medicare is one of the fastest growing components of the national budget and reducing the deficit is at the top of the government's agenda. Risk contracts are a way the government can gain more control over Medicare's expenditures. Last, risk contracts theoretically have saved the government money by historically paying HMOs 95 percent of the average FFS enrollee's cost. However, recent studies have been performed to determine whether HCFA has been losing money on risk contracts because some assert that the average medical cost of a risk contract enrollee may be less than 95 percent of average FFS costs.

A consumer might choose a Medicare risk contract to receive additional benefits (beyond Medicare's benefits) for little or no cost. In addition, the premium for risk contracts has historically been less than the cost of Medicare supplement policies, and risk contract enrollees do not have to be involved in the claim payment process.

Alternatively, a consumer might avoid Medicare risk contracts because he or she is locked into using a certain set of providers. However, HCFA has established point-of-service (POS) rules allowing enrollees to have the choice of using a plan's providers for less cost sharing or paying more cost sharing and have their choice of providers. Last, consumers might avoid risk contracts because their premiums at the time this material was written were rising because of HCFA's recent revisions to the payment rates.

Underwriting

Underwriting for the purpose of declining coverage or charging a higher rate to enrollees is not allowed. However, the risk contractor might still ask medical questions of the enrollees to determine their medical needs so they can effectively manage their care (which might include implementing early prevention measures).

Rating

Carriers determine premium rates charged to the consumer on the basis of their revenue from the government and anticipated expenses. Revenue is projected by multiplying the average adjusted per capita cost (AAPCC, as published by HCFA) by a demographic factor. The demographic factor varies based on the following characteristics:

- age
- gender
- institutional status
- insured status

There are five age categories: 65–69, 70–74, 75–79, 80–84, and 85+. Institutional status has four categories: non-institutionalized–non-Medicaid, institutionalized, Medicaid, and working aged. Insured status has three categories: aged, disabled, and enrollees with end-stage renal disease.

Expenses consist of medical costs, administrative costs, risk charges, and profit. An actuarial cost model (as in Table 50–2) can facilitate in the estimation of these expenses. A key component of the cost model is the rate at which the population is assumed to use medical services (i.e., utilization). Utilization can vary substantially, depending on the efficiency of network providers. Two or more utilization scenarios are often developed to estimate profitability of the risk contract under current levels of health care management and well-managed levels.

The plan must also give HCFA an adjusted community rate (ACR) filing, which proves to HCFA that the plan is providing benefits that are greater than or equal to the average payment rate (APR) received from HCFA (on an actuarially equivalent basis). The ACR is developed by starting with a plan's commercial utilization experience (for benefits covered by Medicare) and adjusting it to the Medicare population using volume and complexity factors published by HCFA that reflect the difference of the number of services and their complexity between the commercial and Medicare population.

If the APR is greater than the ACR, the plan must provide extra benefits or refund a portion of the AAPCC to HCFA. When calculating the actuarial equivalence of the extra benefits, the plan must use published sources.

MEDICAID RISK

Historically, providers were paid on a fee-for-service basis to provide medical services to the Medicaid population. There were few controls on the utilization of services. Subsequently, costs for the Medicaid program grew substantially. Medicaid health care costs currently consume approximately 20 percent of states' budgets and slightly less than 10 percent of the federal government's budget.

To gain budgetary control, many state governments have applied for a special waiver from the federal government allowing the states to shift their medical cost risk by contracting with managed care plans for Medicaid services. Some states receiving a waiver mandate that all Medicaid enrollees join a Medicaid risk plan. Other states allow Medicaid enrollees to join risk plans on a voluntary basis.

Underwriting

Similar to Medicare risk contracts, underwriting for the purpose of declining or charging a higher rate to enrollees is not allowed because the government requires guarantee issue to Medicaid eligibles and generally determines the payment rates (to a lesser extent in bid situations). Similar to Medicare risk contracts, risk contractors might still ask medical questions of the enrollees to determine their medical needs so they can effectively manage their care (which might include implementing early prevention measures).

Rating

States have shifted risk to plans by paying them a fixed monthly payment per enrollee to provide health care to the Medicaid population. States that offer fixed payment rates set them at 90 percent to 100 percent of historical fee-for-service program costs, anticipating plans will lower medical costs through care management. The payment cells are also defined by the states. They usually vary by Medicaid eligibility category, age, and gender. Carriers are not allowed to charge Medicaid enrollees a premium for coverage.

States vary as to how the payment is determined. They determine payments through either a "take-it-or-leave-it" or "bid" method. States explicitly offer the same payment amounts by rate cell to all plans in a "take-it-or-leave-it" system. States may implicitly set rates under a "bid method" by setting a predefined range of payments under the "bid" method. The predefined payment range prevents plans from underbidding (which could lead to underutilization) or overbidding (resulting in excessive profits).

Under both methods, plans can receive preferential treatment from the state based on various factors, including their network size, quality of care, provider agreements, office hours, clinic locations, and bid (if applicable).

CONCLUSION

Underwriting and rating vary significantly by type of market. Underwriting is generally more intense for individuals and small groups because applicants in these markets do not always buy insurance before its need. This is due to a variety of reasons, including the high cost of insurance, the need to attract employees with health benefits, and whether health insurance premiums are tax deductible. Some markets, such as the Medicare and Medicaid risk markets, do not allow underwriting.

Rating practices in the individual and small group market are regulated in many states. Rates for Medicare and Medicaid risk contracts are generally set by the government.

SUGGESTED READING

Bluhm, W.F. 1996. *Group Insurance*. 2d ed. Winsted, CT:Actex Publications.

O'Grady, F.T. 1988. *Individual Health Insurance*. Schaumburg, IL: Society of Actuaries.

Pyenson, B.S. 1998. *Managing Risk*. Chicago, IL: AHA Press.

Sutton, H.L., and Sorbo, A.J. 1993. *Actuarial Issues in the Fee-For-Service/Prepaid Medical Group*. 2d ed. Englewood, CO: Center for Research in Ambulatory Health Care Administration/MGMA.

CHAPTER 51

Actuarial Services in an Integrated Delivery System

Stephen M. Cigich

The integrated delivery system (IDS; see Chapters 4 and 65), whether it is a global system of providers accepting the risk to provide all health care services under a health maintenance organization (HMO) contract or a subset of providers accepting the risk for a limited scope of services, creates uses for the services of actuarial science. These services can help the IDS achieve success in many areas critical to the design and operation of the IDS.

Beyond survival, the major goal of an IDS is to make its providers attractive to the customers of its services; customers are the members whom the providers treat and the payers who provide these members. This goal is achieved by the IDS providing value by focusing on improving efficiency and demonstrating quality in the delivery of medical services.

Improved efficiency will benefit customers by keeping IDS costs low. Done properly, improved efficiency will improve the quality of the care outcome by removing the variation in care caused by inefficiencies. Demonstrating quality will provide customer satisfaction.

Stephen M. Cigich, FSA, is a Consulting Actuary with the Brookfield, Wisconsin office of Milliman & Robertson, Inc. Having managed accounting and actuarial functions in both large and mid-sized MCOs, he is an expert in managed health care programs. His specialty is in the areas of medical delivery systems design and evaluation, product and rate manual development, experience analysis, benchmarking, and actuarial projections.

SUMMARY OF ACTUARIAL SERVICES

Actuarial services can help provide financial focus to identify and realize opportunities, create incentive structures, and measure results. In particular:

- actuarial cost modeling to:
  - establish total budgetary targets
  - allocate revenue among providers
  - establish risk pool funding levels
  - identify and prioritize provider contracting opportunities
  - design and determine the value of various provider capitation arrangements
  - establish financial benchmarks for future measurement
  - quantify medical management policy
- fee structure analysis to:
  - determine equitable payment structures among similar providers
  - negotiate provider fee schedules
  - determine supportable payment levels by provider risk pools
- clinical efficiency benchmarking analysis to:
  - examine particular providers to identify and prioritize clinical processing efficiency opportunities within their practice
  - aid HMOs or other payers to select providers to include or exclude from contracting
  - determine equitable payment levels
- claim distribution analysis to assess specific or aggregate stop-loss reinsurance risks

- risk pool disbursement design to determine operational (i.e., at the time of service or monthly) payments for medical services during the year and allow for incentive distributions at year end
- incentive structure designs to make regular, budgeted payments or periodic bonus payments to providers from IDS gains
- develop reporting structures for and monitoring medical cost and administrative expenses

The use of these services, together with accepted clinical practice guidelines, education forums, feedback reporting, and incentives for efficiency and quality improvement, can create an IDS with both perceived and real value to its owners, its providers, and the customers it serves.

IDENTIFYING AND REALIZING OPPORTUNITIES

Actuarial Cost Modeling

Actuarial cost models reflect the interaction of an IDS's important expense-generating variables. The models can be designed to focus on logical groupings of medical services to quantify utilization and cost levels. Dependent cost-generating variables include service utilization and service cost. Independent cost-generating variables commonly include member age, gender, and benefit plan.

Combining actuarial modeling with clinical analysis is a powerful process to help an IDS achieve its goals. Clinical analysis techniques are beyond the scope of this chapter but may include operational assessments, resource use assessments, and assessments against best clinical practice guidelines.

Traditionally, opportunities for IDS efficiencies have been quantified using the clinical service–based actuarial cost model described in Chapter 49. Recent developments in claim coding structures and claim systems information capturing have expanded the scope of actuarial modeling.

In addition to modeling the costs of each medical service, actuarial cost modeling may include place of service, diagnosis, and service provider (e.g., physician specialty).

Claim coding systems (and thereby actuarial modeling) continue to evolve. For example, the Health Care Financing Administration is in the process of standardizing Medicare's hospital outpatient coding. This standardization is scheduled for 2000 implementation and will allow uniformity in hospital outpatient service coding. Such evolution not only expands modeling capability but will also drive negotiated payment standardization for all hospital outpatient populations.

Fee Schedule Analysis

Fee schedule analysis allows comparison of compensation levels among similar providers by evaluating provider fee schedules using consistent assumptions. Fee schedule analysis transforms each provider fee schedule (which may contain fees for hundreds of services) to a per member per month (PMPM) compensation level. The PMPM compensation levels are determined by combining each provider's fee schedule with service utilization targets. Consequently, equity can be created among providers by ensuring that different fee schedules produce the same compensation.

Fee schedule analysis requires a uniform service coding structure and expected service utilization targets on a similar basis. As previously mentioned, coding structures are evolving and claim systems are accepting additional coding information to allow fee level analyses. At the time of publication, the current coding structure standards are emerging:

Commonly Accepted Financial Coding Standards

Provider Services	*Coding Standards*
Hospital inpatient	Diagnosis-related groups (DRG)
Hospital outpatient	Ambulatory payment classification (APC)
Physician	Resource-based relative value scale (RBRVS) using CPT-4 coding
Skilled nursing care	Resource utilization groups (RUG)

Payers may use fee schedule analysis to select and negotiate payment contracts with certain providers within an IDS. For example, fees charged by various community hospitals may be evaluated by use of actual hospital contracts and estimated diagnosis-related group (DRG) utilization. Fees charged by various cardiac surgeons may be evaluated using each surgeon's fee schedule and estimated current procedural terminology-4 (CPT-4) utilization.

A provider risk pool within an IDS may be funded by a health plan on a PMPM capitated basis for all services, but payments to individual providers may be on a fee-for-service basis. These structures typically require a fee-for-service payment schedule that is the same for each service provided, regardless of the type of provider performing the service. Risk pool funding should be consistent with expected service utilization and fee schedules, otherwise unintended risk pool gains or losses could occur.

Utilization models used in fee schedule analysis may be developed from IDS data, but IDS data are often not well developed or credible. Consequently, IDSs look to consulting firms to provide standard utilization measures for use in fee schedule evaluation.

Clinical Efficiency Benchmarking

Clinical efficiency benchmarking compares the results of a provider's clinical processes with his or her peers. Peers could include other physicians within the same practice group, local competitors, or nationwide observed "best-practice" benchmarks. Such comparisons help identify,

prioritize, and catalyze action for clinical process improvement. The topic of profiling is addressed in detail in Chapter 32.

The following example centers on hospital inpatient services, but a similar process may be applied to other IDS providers.

Good Care Hospital is a tertiary facility that is experiencing longer than average lengths of stay than other hospitals in its service area. But are the longer lengths of stay caused by Good Care Hospital's more complex cases or by process inefficiencies?

Actuarial consulting firms have created statistically determined "best-practices" length of stays benchmarks by DRG and case severity coding to determine the answer to such a question. In such a comparison, Good Care Hospital's DRG and case severity mix are used as weightings in comparison to "best-practices" length of stay benchmarks. This type of comparison not only provides an answer to the preceding question but will also pinpoint areas where Good Care Hospital's processes are less efficient compared with both other areas within Good Care Hospital and also to Good Care Hospital's competition.

Payers, using the results of these studies, can negotiate payment levels and better design provider networks. Less efficient hospitals would be contracted on a case rate or DRG basis, whereas more efficient hospitals would be contracted on a per diem basis.

Claim Probability Distributions

Actuarial cost models, by their design, represent the average, or expected, utilization and cost levels within an IDS. These models do not reflect the randomness of medical cost for an individual or the probable variation in expected medical costs for a grouping of individuals.

The risks associated with large claims for an individual or unusually large fluctuation for a grouping of individuals are analyzed by use of claim probability distributions (CPDs). IDSs, using the analysis from CPDs, can establish reserve pools within their structure to immunize their operational payments from large, random claims.

For example, global capitation payments may be made to a hospital from an IDS risk pool to provide all medical services to a certain population up to $50,000 in yearly medical expenses for any one individual. To fund individual claims greater than $50,000, the IDS can withhold a percentage of total expected medical costs and disburse amounts for these expenses when they occur. Thus individual hospitals within the IDS take the risk for all expenses up to $50,000 on individuals assigned to them, but the risk on claims greater than this amount is held at the IDS level. The IDS may then retain this risk or seek reinsurance protection from an outside source.

Individual CPDs may be aggregated to model the variation in total claims expected for a population of individuals. The actuarial cost model produces a point estimate for expected costs under a certain set of assumptions. This point estimate is expected to exceed actual costs approximately 50 percent of the time and to be less than actual costs about 50 percent of the time. The variation about the point estimate becomes smaller as the number of members covered by an IDS increases. This expected variation in costs by membership size can be measured by mathematically combining several individual CPDs. This is useful in assessing and quantifying the need for aggregate reinsurance protection.

Other actuarial services that assess additional opportunities within an IDS, such as provider staffing, resource models, and compensation planning models, are beyond the scope of this chapter.

CREATING INCENTIVE STRUCTURES

Quality-based reimbursement has the potential to reshape the health care industry by providing incentives to deliver what is ultimately most important to patients and their families—quality care and outcomes. Linking financial rewards with demonstrated quality will reward the best physicians and encourage others to improve. Information on quality in the hands of providers, health plans, and purchasers will empower all parties to transform the evaluation of health care from a question of cost to a question of quality and value.

Incentive structures provide either financial or other reinforcement to focus providers within the IDS on attaining commonly determined goals. With proper design and monitoring, incentive structures can help achieve operating efficiency and quality.

Incentive structures are created by identifying logical groupings (or pools) of providers to share the risk/reward of managing a clinical segment of the IDS. Equally important in identifying these groupings is the operational disbursement, the method of distributing gains/losses periodically, and the monitoring of each pool to ensure solvency. Actuarial tools and analyses can aid this process at each step.

For example, assume an IDS establishes a risk pool for specialty care physicians. An actuarial cost model can determine the PMPM amount available for their services on the basis of expected utilization and fee payment. Risk pool disbursements are designed to pay providers on an operational basis (i.e., ongoing, on the basis of service performance at a reduced amount from the fee schedule) and an incentive basis (i.e., annually, on the basis of the quality and quantity of services performed). Monthly or quarterly risk pool financial reports can determine whether sufficient funds exist to continue to discharge payments at the given fee schedule level.

Although most risk pools and incentive structures use provider-based definitions, other designs may be used. For example:

- event-based to fund certain medical events, such as pregnancies and urgent care
- disease-based to fund cost of specifically identified diagnoses such as hemophilia and diabetes

Risk pools and incentive structures based on managing events provide incentives to handle the event in the most efficient fashion and require coordination among different providers. Events that focus solely on high-cost items handled by mainly one type of physician specialty (e.g., pregnancies handled by obstetricians) typically include the facility charges as well. This provides incentives to plan care in a fashion to minimize unnecessary steps in care delivery.

Events handled by multiple specialties (e.g., laminectomies, which may be handled by neurosurgeons or orthopaedic surgeons) will typically pay all specialties at the same fee level from a self-supporting risk pool. Fee schedules will be reduced if providers are unable to manage costs consistent with pool funding.

Latitude exists in defining the responsibilities of each of these event pools. For example, provider payments may be limited to specific physician procedure costs or may include the handling of all costs (including facility and prescription drugs) associated with treatment. Again, actuarial analysis can be used with clinical input to determine fair cost allocations into these risk pools.

Risk pools based on managing diseases typically will adjust payments on the basis of patient classification. For example, the costs associated with hemophiliacs may be gathered and classified into disease severity categories to assess the cost for treatment of various severity categories. Cost and clinical processes may be further studied to determine areas where cost efficiency can be achieved without sacrificing quality of care.

The funding of risk pools and incentive structures will typically be done as a fixed percentage of the medical cost component of premiums for each different office copay plan level. Although the allocation of premium revenue will vary on the basis of the many factors identified in Chapters 49

and 50, it is assumed these factors are addressed in the level of premium charged by the payer.

The reader needs to be mindful, however, that the entire area of incentives in managed care is under continuous scrutiny and change. This is particularly so in IDSs and medical groups, and doubly so in programs involving Medicare and Medicaid. The reader is referred to Chapters 9 and 65 for further discussion and is also cautioned to keep current as to laws and regulations that may affect incentive plans.

MEASURING RESULTS

The actuarial cost models and other models described in this chapter provide insight into identifying the important cost-generating variables in the delivery of IDS services. These models are constructed with historical data and assumptions developed from many sources. They allow the IDS to identify, prioritize, and act on opportunities.

Report monitoring systems designed to capture IDS data in a format similar to these models can be used to perform actual-to-expected analyses. Such analyses allow the IDS to substitute historical data and assumptions based on outside sources with its own experience. These analyses are useful in setting future pricing levels and refining risk pool allocations and medical management policy. Actual-to-expected analyses are also used to identify, quantify, and prioritize a new set of IDS opportunities.

CONCLUSION

An IDS has many financial and clinical needs in its formation and operation. The tools of actuarial science allow focused analyses to help identify, quantify, and prioritize risk and opportunities within the IDS. Careful implementation and consideration of these tools in conjunction with accepted clinical practice guidelines, education forums, feedback reporting, and incentives for efficiency and quality improvement can help the IDS achieve long-term success.

SUGGESTED READING

Cigich, S.M., and Mischler, N.E. 1996. *Success in Managed Care: A Disciplined Approach to Achieving Clinical Quality and Efficiency Improvement*. Milliman & Robertson, Inc. Research Report.

Girod, C.S. 1999. *APCs: A Prospective Payment System for Outpatient Hospital Services*. Milliman & Robertson, Inc. Research Report.

Melek, S.P. 1996. Behavioral Healthcare Risk-Sharing and Medical Cost Offsets. Milliman & Robertson, Inc. Research Report.

Pyenson, B.S. 1998. *Managing Risk*. Chicago, IL: AHA Press.

Sutton, H.L., and Sorbo, A.J. 1993. *Actuarial Issues in the Fee-For-Service/Prepaid Medical Group*. 2nd ed. Englewood, CO: Center for Research in Ambulatory Health Care Administration/MGMA.

CHAPTER 52

Operational Underwriting in Managed Care Organizations

Gregory J. Lippe

Reviewing critical success factors in a managed care organization (MCO) usually prompts discussion of medical management, marketing, provider relations, and finance.* The chapters immediately preceding this one (Chapters 49–51) focused primarily on actuarial services, though with considerable attention paid to underwriting issues. But even experienced managed care personnel often underestimate the importance of underwriting in a voluntary market. This chapter reviews underwriting from an operations perspective to supplement the actuarial perspective provided earlier. Knowledge of risk factors and underwriting principles can benefit the MCO, its customers, and those organizations contracting with the MCO on a risk basis.

---

*This discussion defines an MCO as any payer organization that usually assumes some level of financial risk in the coordination and delivery of health care services to covered persons.

Gregory J. Lippe, MBA, is Principal, Ernst & Young LLP, Milwaukee, Wisconsin. He assists payers and providers with managed care strategy, operational assessments, mergers, acquisitions, and business development. Previously, Lippe was employed by United HealthCare Corporation, EQUICOR, and Time Insurance in a variety of executive positions.

The author wishes to thank Cory Lynn, manager of client services and senior technical analyst at the Chicago office of Seabury & Smith, for his research and review contributions.

HISTORICAL OVERVIEW

Underwriting within an MCO can be defined as processes to attract, maintain, and manage the cross section of risk anticipated in the actuarial and financial assumptions of the organization's business plan. Successful underwriting yields the membership, the revenue per member per month (PMPM), and utilization levels incorporated in the MCO business plan.

Many MCOs did not historically develop strong underwriting processes. Federally qualified health maintenance organizations (HMOs) were limited in their underwriting practices by federal regulation and related interpretations. Where not constrained by federal or state regulation, underwriting was an infrequent MCO priority. This often reflected the competencies of existing MCO management and their limited knowledge of and appreciation for underwriting. Some managed care personnel still continue to view sales and underwriting activities as a roll of the dice rather than as integrated processes that should be managed to maintain the competitive position of the MCO.

Despite limited appreciation for and use of underwriting techniques, many MCOs were successful in the 1980s with their pricing and risk selection approaches. Previously, the dominant indemnity carrier or Blue Cross/Blue Shield (BCBS) plan serving a large employer group generally ignored the upstart MCO. The dominant carrier's arrangement with the employer often limited or eliminated health insurance risk.

In many instances, the dominant carrier functioned as a third-party administrator (TPA) of the employer benefit program. As a TPA, the carrier may have been paid based on the number or level of claim payments processed by the carrier. The higher the utilization of services, the greater the administrative fee paid by the employer group to the TPA.

Focus on larger cases tended to mitigate the MCO risk of ignoring or applying limited underwriting practices. Many large employers, particularly in the 1980s, offered multiple benefit plans of several different MCOs and insurance companies. In this dual or multiple choice environment, MCOs with relatively closed delivery systems often attracted a favorable risk selection. The closed panel delivery system (see Chapter 3) of many MCOs was a concern to potential members with an established physician relationship and whose physician did not participate in the MCO. MCO benefit program emphasis on preventive or routine services tended to appeal to younger and healthier individuals. These and other factors such as a mandated minimum employer contribution at that time helped to protect MCOs despite their limited use of underwriting techniques.

Most MCOs possessed the ability to increase premium to levels to fund the projected risk or claim costs during most of the last 30 years. These periods were marked by the willingness of employers and their employees to accept significant premium increases, especially when indemnity insurance premium levels were even higher. When an MCO suffered adverse claim experience, it could increase its premium to offset the higher than anticipated utilization or cost experience. This ability to raise premiums when necessary or desired dampened MCO interest in underwriting. In some MCOs, underwriting was often viewed as merely an improved pricing methodology, secondary to achieving enrollment targets.

During the 1990s most MCOs were confronted by many market factors, including increasing buyer price sensitivity. Even where premium increases could be justified by higher than anticipated utilization and cost, these increases were difficult to sell in the competitive market. Ultimately, premium compression helped to send MCOs back into what many in the industry refer to as the underwriting cycle. At the same time, managed health care became the dominant form of health insurance, thus enrolling a more normalized member risk profile rather than attracting members who were somewhat healthier than average.

All insurers strive to consistently earn a sufficient financial return. Pricing and underwriting processes are driven by multiple assumptions. Some of those key assumptions include average contract size, age and gender demographics, and the ability of the MCO to control medical utilization and cost. Adjusting those assumptions even slightly can greatly impact enrollment and financial results. By being too aggressive the insurer may be risking financial performance to protect or build market share. Being too conservative subjects the insurer to potential loss of market share.

The health insurance industry has experienced a recurring financial cycle over the years, usually referred to as the underwriting cycle. This phenomenon reflects the cyclical industry results produced when comparing premium received with corresponding health and administrative costs. A simplistic view is that when financial conservatism is the controlling influence, bottom line results are strong, albeit sometimes at the cost of MCO market share. Conversely, when member growth or sales gains control of price and risk decision making, MCO market share increases but usually with deteriorating MCO financial results. While the underwriting cycle impacts the entire industry, not every carrier is at the same point in the underwriting cycle. As the decade of the 1990s came to a close, many insurers were beginning a financial recovery after previously waging an intense battle over market share that undermined their short-term financial results.

While an insurer cannot escape the forces of the health underwriting cycle, it can more effectively manage through the cycle than its competitors. *Some of the actions to manage through the cycle include:*

- Developing a superior management information system. Timely reporting of accurate data is fundamental to optimizing long-term pricing and enrollment strategies.
- Maintaining an ongoing competitive database to identify trends in pricing and products. Tracking competitor products, their approach to pricing, and their financial results will help the MCO make optimal decisions over the long term.
- Striving for a partnership between actuarial, underwriting, and marketing personnel to maximize the MCO's market position and attempt to achieve the elusive goal of profitable growth, regardless of the stage of the underwriting cycle.
- Sustaining competitive agreements with providers for the delivery of health care services.

SALES AND UNDERWRITING COLLABORATION

To encourage effective underwriting and ongoing sales results, personnel from underwriting and marketing/sales should share responsibilities. Collaboration by sales and underwriting personnel within MCOs:

- encourages rational risk taking and innovative customer solutions
- improves management of factors influencing sales and underwriting results
- includes an underwriting perspective in overall MCO decision making
- influences the marketing approach and sales plan of the MCO
- balances membership growth and financial results
- utilizes underwriting information to manage new member risk

To support ongoing collaboration between marketing/sales and underwriting personnel, several MCOs have aligned compensation and bonus arrangements to balance sales growth and MCO profits. Proper alignment encourages the underwriter to build market share at a profitable premium level. Similarly, sales personnel are encouraged and rewarded for profitable business and improved member/group retention, not just new membership growth.

MANAGEMENT INFORMATION SYSTEM

To operate an effective underwriting function, the MCO must possess an effective management information system (MIS). Underwriting is dependent on access to, analysis of, and interpretation of administrative, claim, and encounter data. These data must reflect all MCO health services.

Many MCOs contract out or capitate certain health services or risks, such as mental health/substance abuse (see Chapter 25), laboratory (see Chapter 20), and prescription services (see Chapter 24). Regardless of short-term contract arrangements, the MCO must capture, analyze, and routinely track services and risks managed by outside vendors. Access to and analysis of all health care data are essential for effective underwriting as well as for MCO initiatives involving outcomes research and disease management.

The MCO MIS must also track and monitor selected administrative services. Managing risk and improving product design can benefit from routine feedback from member services and provider relations. Consistent questions or complaints related to a benefit may suggest that in the next product design cycle new wording should be added or substituted. Benefit redesign may also be considered given the frequency and risk associated with the questions or complaints. Similarly, feedback from provider relations should help identify concerns that may be causing administrative problems for the provider. Some of these concerns may affect the utilization and cost of the benefits provided. Consequently, even if the MCO relies on an outside vendor or affiliated entity to provide member services or a 24-hour nurse advice line, the MCO's MIS should still capture and be able to analyze the activities of these services.

Fundamentally, data must be available at the group level to assist in new case and renewal underwriting decisions. The MCO must be able to roll up data by industry, product type, market segment, and age and gender. Properly managed data can also contribute to measuring the effectiveness of a sales representative, independent agent, and an MCO distribution channel. It is essential to measure both the level of activity and the actuarial and financial results of all MCO distribution channels, products, and market segments. The need for all these data elements and their analysis emphasizes the importance of an effective MIS to an MCO and its management challenges, including underwriting.

REGULATION

The underwriting function must understand and comply with regulations from several sources. If the MCO is a state-licensed HMO or a BCBS plan, it could be subject to special enabling legislation and state regulation (see Chapter 69). When enacted, insurance reform at the state level has produced regulations affecting MCO product design, pricing, and in some instances MCO compensation paid to independent agents or the sales force. Serving the Federal Employees Health Benefits Program (see Chapter 54), Medicaid (see Chapter 57), and Medicare (see Chapters 55 and 56) under risk contracts lends additional underwriting requirements. Although this discussion encourages a proactive approach to underwriting, it views regulatory compliance as an absolute necessity and ultimately the most effective approach.

The Health Insurance Portability and Accountability Act (HIPAA; see Chapter 67), passed in 1996, established federal minimum standards for the availability of small group policies. The act required each state to adopt these minimum standards (or more stringent standards) by July 1, 1997.

Under HIPAA, a small employer group is defined as having at least 2 but not more than 50 employees on business days during the proceeding calendar year and who employs at least 2 employees on the first day of the plan year. *Carriers and MCOs that serve the small employer market as defined above are subject to the following rules:*

- Each carrier or MCO must offer to a small employer in the state all approved products for sale that it is then actively marketing to the small group market.
- The insurance issuer must accept for enrollment every individual who applies (with certain differences depending on whether or not the individual has been "continuously enrolled," by the definition under HIPAA, with another carrier).
- Insurance carriers can limit plan availability based on service area.
- Insurers are required to renew in-force coverage at the option of the plan sponsor.
- Exceptions to guaranteed coverage renewal include nonpayment of premiums, fraud, violation of minimum participation or contribution rules, insurer exits the market, all participating insured under the plan leave the network service area, and the termination of an employer's membership in a bona fide association.
- Carriers are not required to issue coverage to late enrollees.
- Additional rating restrictions for the small group market are reserved for each state.

HIPAA does not require carriers to issue coverage to late enrollees. The act allows each state to define additional rating restrictions for the small group market. The act does limit the circumstances under which a preexisting medical condition exclusion may be imposed on an employee applying for group health coverage with an employer. HIPAA places a cap of 12 months on the preexisting medical condition exclusion and requires that the 12-month cap be reduced by periods of prior coverage. Therefore, HIPAA requires employers to issue certificates of coverage to all employees who terminate their employment and had insurance through their employment.

Given the act's requirements, MCOs have been subject to increased risk primarily through the guarantee of coverage and renewal requirement, subject to any rate limitations imposed by the state. Given this increased risk, MCOs have explored the following actions:

- Evaluate options to tighten guidelines for group participation, collection of waivers, increasing the employer contribution percentage and minimum service area requirements.

- Review current benefit programs for small groups to determine whether some of the "rich" benefit designs should still be offered.
- Establish small group multiple rate tiers, subject to state limitations, so that small groups can still be rated up depending on the medical costs of the type of group.
- Consider whether the investigation of pre-existing conditions is cost effective.

Even with these potential underwriting changes, risk of small group coverage has increased. Similarly, HIPAA has added administrative complexity for both the employer group and the insurance entity. New reporting standards under HIPAA are expected to drive significant efforts at MCOs in the first years of the new millennium.

To comply with all this regulation, the MCO must possess an MIS that is capable of tracking and modeling certain activities and outcomes. As an example, state regulation may require MCO pricing to return a minimum specified percentage of premiums to members or covered persons in the form of health care benefits provided. In other cases, the MCO may be required to subsidize a high-risk pool established by the state. Similarly, the MIS needs to monitor key benefit and premium relationships when products are offered to the Medicare and Medicaid markets. Finally, the MCO MIS must be able to meet the regulatory and reporting challenges defined under HIPAA.

MAJOR RISK FACTORS

Although some suggest that underwriting is more an art than a science, experienced underwriters generally emphasize the importance of first understanding the science. Much of the science is described from an actuarial perspective in the preceding chapters. This chapter supplements the actuarial material by identifying and discussing the key elements of risk to an MCO that underwriters must bear in mind. These same risk factors are indirectly assumed and should be understood by vendors that contract with the MCO under a fixed-price, percentage of premium, or capitated arrangement. The major risk factors include the following:

- ***Demographic factors***—The age and gender of members of the group to be covered are key predictors of future utilization. Predicting utilization, even when all health care costs are fixed under capitation arrangements, is necessary to ensure that adequate resources remain available to deliver high-quality and effective services. Even when the demographic factor is not specifically adjusted on a group basis, it should be tracked by the MCO. Similarly, vendors contracting with the MCO are encouraged to analyze and track demographic factors to understand their utilization experience and assist with subsequent contract negotiations with the MCO. While age and gender factors have their limitations as to predictors of future utilization, absent prior claim experience or detailed medical histories, these factors can help the MCO assess its level of risk for health services.
- ***Economic factors***—The actual costs of services and applicable rates of inflation influence reimbursement paid to providers regardless of the payment methodology because long-term, even capitated contracts get renewed. Incorporating these economic factors into the pricing methodology is essential for employer group renewals at premium levels projecting the expected future cost for the MCO.
- ***Enrollment factors***—Apart from potential administrative efficiencies, the larger the group of covered persons, the more likely a consistent claim pattern, level of health care cost, or utilization of services will emerge and be planned for accordingly. Larger groups of 1,000 or more employees and dependents are generally viewed as credible; that is, the group's previous claim experience or utilization of services should be a good predictor of future health care

service requirements, assuming that no major changes occur in the group's composition.

- *Industry factors*—Populations employed within a specific industry have historical claim patterns or health service requirements defined by claim experience over many years. Certain industries have been shown by actuarial studies consistently to use less than average, average, or above average levels of health care services. Even when the industry factor is not priced for on a group-specific level, it should be tracked by the MCO and considered in various analyses. Vendors contracting with the MCO under a risk arrangement would be prudent to assess and track the composite industry factor of the MCO's block of business.

- *Probability*—Variations from expected or typical utilization rates even for large groups occur over time. For the claim patterns of groups smaller than 100 covered lives, there is increased likelihood of variance and a greater range of variance from the average or MCO norm compared with a group of 1,000 covered lives. Even with several years of experience, groups with less than 100 covered lives are not fully credible and therefore difficult to predict as to claim experience or utilization of required services.

- *Provider practices*—The practice orientation of providers in both owned health centers and contracted physician networks significantly influences the use and location of health services. These practices can vary even within an MCO's service area. Understanding the impact of provider practices contributes to more effective pricing and improved projection of health services. Provider practices are critical to the MCO and to health care vendors contracting with the MCO on a risk basis.

- *Selection factors*—As discussed more fully in Chapter 43 regarding consumerism, individuals joining an MCO act in their own best interests. In a multichoice environment where the employee has two or more benefit options to choose from, the type of enrollment appeal, including product design or delivery system, can influence member selection of a health plan and hence MCO risk selection. When the MCO is the only or dominant health care option, selection factors reflect the group's composite characteristics.

The more an MCO identifies, analyzes, and reacts to these variables in its operations, the greater the likelihood of improved financial performance. Underwriting should be a responsibility shared by personnel throughout the MCO. Similarly, if a vendor contracting with an MCO understands these variables, there is a greater likelihood that the vendor will sustain a long-term financially sound relationship with the MCO.

UNDERWRITING AS AN INTERNAL CONTROL

Understanding the variables of risk enables MCO leadership to select prudent and realistic approaches to managing risk. These approaches reflect the art of underwriting. One fundamental process involves routinely evaluating and tracking changes and trends in the entire block of business. The MCO should also monitor performance and trends at the industry, product line, and market segment levels. Variations and potential concerns should be identified, explained, and corrected. Effective group-specific underwriting is fundamental to consistent MCO enrollment and financial success.

An effective underwriting function acts as an important internal control for the MCO. The underwriting function, through analysis of claim data, can help identify emerging trends and abuses at the employer, employee, and provider level. Examples of trends or issues that have been previously identified or clarified by experienced underwriting personnel using standard analyses include the following:

- the need for benefit plan changes (for example, increase the office visit copayment, amend the approach to prescription drug benefits and mental health/substance abuse services, address utilization concerns involving the use of rehabilitation services or coverage of nondurable medical equipment)

- the need for updated review of the pricing basis as the competitive position of the MCO significantly deteriorates (or improves) as noted by the level of underwriting and sales activity and the ratio of closed or successful new business sales to completed quotations
- opportunities for cost reductions for health services (for example, channeling certain services, such as mental health, laboratory, or specified radiology procedures, to an alternative or single vendor)
- the need for review of sales procedures and enrollment appeals based on monitoring of risk selection of new members joining the MCO for the first six months after joining the MCO (a common MCO procedure is to review the level of hospital inpatient usage of new members during their first six months of coverage; these analyses should be done on an ongoing new member basis as well as for new groups).

The underwriting function should contribute to the enrollment and revenue PMPM assumptions included in the annual MCO business plan. Underwriting should also help determine the demographic and industry factors of the MCO's enrollment to project future resource or health service requirements. Demographic and industry factors are explained later in the overview of MCO pricing methodologies.

EMPLOYER GROUP UNDERWRITING

Some MCOs confuse a simple pricing approach with the concepts of underwriting. These MCOs merely reply to employer group requests for quotations on specific benefit packages. Although a simple pricing approach quickly fills the request for rate quotes, it is not as productive, innovative, or proactive as group-specific or market segment underwriting.

Underwriting should be much more than filling orders and finalizing price. As previously defined, underwriting is a set of integrated processes that attract, maintain, and manage the cross section of risk anticipated in the MCO's business plan. Effective MCO underwriting is most easily demonstrated at the employer group level.

The sales and underwriting process to identify and close a new employer group includes the integrated steps shown in Exhibit 52–1. While reviewing these steps, note the desirability of strong collaboration between sales and underwriting. The new employer sales efforts are directed and include the input and influence of underwriting. Similarly, the final proposal developed by underwriting reflects the input of the sales team.

Renewal of an existing account should follow a pattern similar to that shown in Exhibit 52–1 to ensure that the MCO understands the current employer group environment. Making an assumption that nothing has changed at the employer group can lead to significant and unplanned variances in enrollment, risk selection, and ultimately financial performance.

Group level analysis and decisions contribute to the overall formation and management of the MCO business block. Underwriting success at a group level should be measured in several ways. Increased enrollment, improvement or maintenance of risk profiles, and improvements in premium adequacy are three key indicators. The old adage among hospitals, "No margin, no mission," also applies to MCOs today, regardless of their tax status.

Group underwriting is dependent upon employer group information. Most data on new potential employer groups are supplied to underwriting by the marketing/sales force. Many long-time and established MCOs still quote premiums and benefit plans lacking fundamental employer group information. MCO management often concludes that it has no apparent choice but to quote without all or any of the desired information. This conclusion ignores at least three alternatives. First, the MCO may not be required to quote on a particular case (depending on the specifics of the group requesting

Exhibit 52–1 Steps in the Sales and Underwriting Process

Step 1: Sales and underwriting personnel collaborate on identifying and targeting key employers, industries, and/or employer characteristics for use by the sales force.
Step 2: Sales personnel contact targeted groups and collect data, prequalifying the employer group using checklist or criteria supplied by underwriting.
Step 3: Sales personnel prepare and submit a request for a quotation to underwriting.
Step 4: Underwriting reviews the request, qualifies the employer group, and identifies any additional questions that sales is requested to pursue.
Step 5: A clerk prepares an analysis of basic group characteristics and runs the initial pricing of the requested benefit plan(s) and contract effective date(s).
Step 6: An underwriter reviews the case materials, including updated data from sales, and determines whether the case should be declined or quoted.
Step 7: Through an iterative process, the underwriter develops the benefit plans, pricing, conditions, and/or options that the MCO will tentatively offer to the employer group.
Step 8: Sales reviews the underwriting proposal, and any questions or differences between sales and underwriting are resolved.
Step 9: Sales presents the MCO proposal to the targeted group, closes the sale, and assists the employer group throughout the enrollment process.
Step 10: Underwriting reviews the actual group enrollment and identifies any major variations from the assumptions made during the sales/underwriting process.

coverage and applicable state and federal laws). Second, the quotation prepared with limited information could reflect conservative assumptions that will encourage enhanced information gathering efforts by sales personnel in the future.

Third, a quotation could be prepared with some contingencies or requirements that serve to protect the MCO when quoting a case without basic information.

One such contingency might be a minimum level of enrollment to avoid attracting a very limited enrollment at an employer group that causes administrative difficulties for both the employer and the MCO. This contingency also indirectly considers the potential adverse risk selection that could occur in a limited employer enrollment. Other contingencies could relate to changes in carriers offered, the employer's contribution strategy, or the benefit design by the self-funded employer group base benefit plan. Admittedly, selling proposals with contingencies is more difficult. Such contingencies will often encourage the marketing/sales personnel to eliminate the need for the contingency through securing and supplying more information to underwriting.

Collection and interpretation of employer group information produce understandable tension between underwriting and sales/marketing personnel. In difficult situations with emotions running high, all MCO personnel should recall three concepts. First, even the best medical management system cannot completely offset poor or deteriorating risk selection. Second, the MCO needs more members than patients. Third, employer group decisions affect the group under review and contribute to the results for the entire block of business. These three concepts are particularly important for the MCO with a limited enrollment and capital base.

KEY EMPLOYER GROUP DATA

Employer group-specific data usually required by a proactive underwriting department include the following:

- address of business and number of years in operation
- industry of the proposed employer group and activities performed in the service area
- number and location of employees by 5-digit ZIP code within the MCO's service area

- number of contract tiers or required premiums (for example, single, couple, family, and so on)
- mix of contracts and average number of persons covered per contract
- age and gender characteristics of at least the employee work force
- prior year premiums of at least the dominant carrier in the group
- benefit plan options available to employees and the number of employees choosing each option
- employer contribution policy
- employee out-of-pocket cost for health care options
- requested benefit plan and tier structure of the employer or its consultant.

Marketing and sales representatives who have not previously collected employer group-specific information will have understandable concerns about its availability and the ease and value of collecting it. The proactive underwriting function addresses these concerns by ensuring that the sales representative understands the need for collection and use of group-specific information. As automation becomes an increasingly common factor in sales and underwriting, it becomes easier for the sales personnel to collect much of that information. Underwriting and rate setting need not be a "black box" to marketing and sales personnel.

By utilizing group-specific and market segment information, the MCO substantially increases its chances to attract a cross section of risk and reasonably project the size, characteristics, and health care needs of new MCO membership. The availability and use of group-specific information helps the MCO maintain and better serve employer groups during its annual renewal period. Increasingly, much of the information tracked and analyzed by the underwriting function is being requested by the employer group to improve its assessment of MCO performance and that of its benefits program. The MCO underwriting function can play an important role in responding to the data requests of employer groups. Underwriting personnel can

assist sales and marketing in responding to employer requests for data. Through sales and underwriting collaboration, the MCO can offer the employer group-specific data and, more important, analysis that turns the data into information of use to the employer group.

MARKET FACTORS AND TRENDS

The marketplace evolution in the last several years has underscored the need for proactive underwriting competencies in MCOs. ***Trends or factors present and projected in most markets that encourage MCO interest in underwriting include the following:***

- continual downward pressure on premiums
- deteriorating or poor MCO financial results
- competitors apparently buying market share
- stagnation or even loss of market share by the MCO
- complexity in renewing large employer groups
- groups requiring more data, more options, and lower health care costs
- MCO risk as the dominant carrier or insurance option at the employer group
- increased focus on midsize (100 to 500) and medium-size (25 to 99) groups
- MCO initiatives to serve small groups of less than 25 employees
- consolidation of carriers and health options within larger groups
- complexity of point-of-service and triple-option programs
- entry into the Medicaid market on a risk basis
- entry into the Medicare market on a risk basis
- responding to state reform initiatives and federal regulation, such as HIPAA.

These trends or factors have prompted MCOs to review their underwriting and marketing/sales processes. Through review and analysis, many MCOs have significantly evolved their pricing and underwriting methodologies.

COMMUNITY RATING METHODOLOGIES

The pricing methodology chosen by the MCO affects and is affected by ongoing marketing, sales, and underwriting processes; further, rating methodologies may be affected by state or federal laws for certain types of groups of individuals. In past years HMOs were required to use community rating, and even now many MCOs have adopted some derivation of community rating. Under community rating, the MCO charges a similar premium to employer groups and individuals with like benefits and the same contract renewal date.

There are three related but distinct standard community rating methodologies: simplified community rating, adjusted community rating (ACR), and community rating by class (CRC). Each of these pricing methodologies is explained and demonstrated below. This section uses rates generated for Dream Group, Inc., a hypothetical employer. After discussing common MCO pricing methodologies, the section focuses on underwriting concepts.

Summarized in Exhibit 52–2 is the assumed group-specific information provided primarily

---

Exhibit 52–2 Key Assumptions and Factors for Dream Group, Inc.

The group includes 500 employees all located in the same MCO service area.

The chosen benefit plan and effective date require $150 revenue PMPM.

The group has a three-tier premium scheme with single, couple, and family contracts.

The couple rate is 1.95 times the single rate; the family is 2.85 times the single rate.

The percentage mix of contracts within the group is 30/20/50 for single/couple/family.

The company reports that its average family size is 3.8 just for family contracts.

The age and gender factors of the group equal a 0.98 demographic factor.

The industry factor of the group according to an actuarial table is 0.95.

---

by the sales force to the underwriting function. The importance and use of the factors are examined through review of the three rating methodologies. Note that some of the employer information is not directly used by the less sophisticated rating methodologies. Also, an MCO might use a hybrid of the rating methodologies discussed. Additionally, some MCOs use multiple pricing methodologies, selecting a pricing methodology that responds effectively to a particular market segment. MCOs started during the 1980s and 1990s probably began with a more sophisticated approach to pricing and underwriting than many HMOs started earlier. Regardless of the commencement date for operations, the evolution of pricing methodologies within an MCO varies significantly among organizations.

Simplified Community Rating

Simplified community rating uses planwide assumptions as to levels of utilization, cost per unit, administrative costs, membership composition (that is, age and gender), contract mix, and charging ratio or ratio of the rates. The charging ratio refers to the desired relationship of various premium tiers to the single premium quoted. For example, a charging ratio of 1.95 for the couple premium tier means that the MCO or employer group desires the couple premium to be 1.95 times the single premium quoted by the MCO. Most MCOs using simplified community rating will not make group-specific adjustments for the charging ratios. Instead, the MCO will use a standard set of charging ratios in preparing premium quotations. By using so many standard rating assumptions, an MCO needs only to know the contract effective date, the plan of benefits, and the desired tier structure of the group to quote premiums using a simplified community rating methodology.

Simplified community rating does not use the actual group-specific contract mix, in this case the 30/20/50 percentage mix for single/couple/family contracts. A standard mix assumption would probably be applied based on actuarial recommendation. This pricing methodology also does not adjust for the group-specific average family size. Average family size refers to the average number of covered persons included in a family tier contract. The demographic factor and the industry factor are adjustments typically utilized only by the CRC methodology. These factors are discussed later.

In all three pricing methodologies, the underwriter calculates a conversion factor. The conversion factor is a statistic that, when multiplied by the required revenue PMPM produces the MCO's desired single premium. The conversion factor is dependent upon assumptions as to contract mix, contract size for each tier, and charging ratios or the ratio of the rates. Exhibit 52–3 summarizes the three steps to calculate the conversion factor, the subsequent steps to calculate premiums using simplified community rating, and the pricing methodology and mathematical result and calculated premium related to each of the steps.

To verify that these premiums will yield the required revenue of $150.00 PMPM, as stated in the Dream Group assumptions, review the check of the computations shown in Table 52–1, which calculates the projected average premium per contract and divides this revenue per contract into the average contract size or number of covered persons per contract. This calculation yields the average projected revenue PMPM.

As shown in Table 52–1, the projected weighted average premium is $345.08. Dividing this average premium by the projected average contract size (2.30 as determined in Exhibit 52–3) yields the projected average revenue PMPM. If the rating is performed correctly, it yields the required premium PMPM, in this case $150.00 PMPM, except for a potential (and immaterial) rounding error. Dividing $345.08 (the average contract revenue PMPM) by the average contract size of 2.30 members per contract yields a projected revenue of $150.03 PMPM, reflecting rounding error and verifying the mathematical accuracy of the proposed premium rates prepared using simplified community rating.

Exhibit 52–3 Calculation To Develop Simplified Community Rates for Dream Group, Inc.

Step 1: $(0.40 \times 1.00) + (0.20 \times 2.00) + (0.40 \times 3.75) = 2.30$
Average weighted contract size = Mix (column A) times contract size (column B)

Step 2: $(0.40 \times 1.00) + (0.20 \times 1.95) + (0.40 \times 2.85) = 1.93$
Average weighted charging ratio (CR) = Mix (column A) times CR (column C)

Step 3: $2.30 / 1.93 = 1.192$
Single conversion factor = Step 1 result divided by step 2 result

Step 4: $150.00 \text{ PMPM} \times 1.192 = \$178.80$
Single conversion factor times required premium PMPM equals single premium

Step 5: $\$178.80 \times 1.95 = \$348.66$
Single premium times couple CR equals couple premium

Step 6: $\$178.80 \times 2.85 = \$509.58$
Single premium times family CR equals family premium

Contract Type	(A) Contract Mix (%)	(B) Contract Size	(C) Charging Ratios	Computed Conversion Factor	Required or Estimated Premiums ($)
Single	40	1.00	1.00	1.192 (3)	178.80 (4)
Couple	20	2.00	1.95		348.66 (5)
Family	40	3.75	2.85		509.58 (6)
TOTAL	100	2.30 (1)	1.93 (2)		

Table 52–1 Premium Proof of PMPM

(A) Contract Tier Mix	(B) Calculated Premium ($)	(A × B) Weighted Average Premium ($)
Single, 40%	178.80	71.52
Couple, 20%	348.66	69.73
Family, 40%	509.58	203.83
Total weighted premium		345.08
Projected weighted premium per contract*		150.03

*Total weighted premium divided by average contract size (2.30).

If the group-specific characteristics varied from the standard MCO assumptions, the MCO would recognize a revenue excess or shortfall PMPM. For example, if a group with more than the assumed number or mix of large families was quoted, the MCO would experience a premium deficiency PMPM when dividing actual premiums collected by the higher than anticipated actual number of covered persons per contract.

Adjusted Community Rating

The financial risks assumed by the MCO in using so many standard assumptions caused many management teams to seek improvement in the pricing methodology. Competitive pressures also encouraged many MCOs to differentiate their premiums further on a group-specific basis while still retaining a community rating methodology. The limitations of simplified community rating and increasing competitive pressures helped encourage the development and use of ACR by many MCOs.

The use of ACR often reflects an MCO's recognition of the need for a pricing methodology that will allow it to be more price competitive while reducing the risk inherent in applying so many standard assumptions. Many MCOs found that premiums developed using simplified community rating were most price competitive in the highest-risk groups. Furthermore, groups that had significant variations from MCO standard assumptions as to contract mix, size, and charg-

ing ratios were often quoted rates that yielded unfavorable financial results.

In some MCOs the marketing program encourages the sales force to sell the standard community rate to any interested group. This approach reflects the belief that in the long run the underlying actuarial assumptions will be achieved. In some cases the underlying actuarial assumptions were not understood or even considered by the MCO. Therefore, although the MCO added new membership, it often attracted risk that required above average use of health services, or it experienced a degree of adverse risk selection.

Increasingly, many MCOs saw the need to make at least some group-specific adjustments to their pricing methodology. The changes were intended to improve competitive position, avoid adverse risk selection, and appropriately charge an ACR to groups with unique contract mixes, average contract sizes, or charging ratios. In making these adjustments, MCOs were also responding to increasing employer group requests for data and rationale behind the rates charged to a particular group.

ACR provides the MCO a better opportunity to attract a cross section of risk and to quote premiums that are more likely to fund the membership risk. These improvements allow the MCO to be more proactive rather than merely hope that the actuarial assumptions will be right in the long run.

One way to understand the ACR pricing methodology is to compare it to simplified community rating. The ACR methodology uses group-specific assumptions rather than standard planwide assumptions for contract mix, contract size, and charging ratios. Like simplified community rating, this pricing methodology does not consider the demographic factor or the industry factor.

Using Dream Group, Inc. as a basis for quotation, Exhibit 52–4 calculates premiums determined by the ACR methodology using the same revenue requirement of $150.00 PMPM. Note that ACR uses the same steps as simplified community rating shown in Exhibit 52–3. Instead of planwide assumptions, ACR uses group-specific assumptions to calculate the conversion factor and proposed premiums.

Notice how different the community rates are for the same group using the ACR methodology versus the simplified approach. Compare, for example, the single rate of $178.80 under simplified community rating to $184.35 as determined by ACR. There is a family rate difference

of approximately $16.00 per month. In fact, if the group-specific assumptions in Dream Group, Inc., are accurate and the membership achieved by the MCO during enrollment reflects those characteristics, the simplified approach would leave the MCO with an estimated monthly premium deficiency of $4.55 PMPM. The actual group premium, reflecting the simplified community rates but divided by the actual group contract size of 2.6 produces a premium yield of $145.45 PMPM instead of the targeted revenue of $150.00 PMPM. If the MCO enrolled 1,000 members (employees and dependents) in the group, the monthly shortfall to the MCO for this single group would be $4,550. This shortfall would need to be made up, assuming that the MCO targeted or required premium PMPM is accurate.

Clearly, ACR allows the MCO to quote group-specific community rates more accurately that yield the same revenue PMPM targeted by simplified community rating. The adjustments improve the matching of revenue and expense. ACR also

---

Exhibit 52–4 Calculation To Develop ACR for Dream Group, Inc.

Step 1: $(0.30 \times 1.00) + (0.20 \times 2.00) + (0.50 \times 3.80) = 2.60$
Average weighted contract size = Mix (column A) times contract size (column B)

Step 2: $(0.30 \times 1.00) + (0.20 \times 1.95) + (0.50 \times 2.85) = 2.115$
Average weighted charging ratio (CR) = Mix (column A) times CR (column C)

Step 3: $2.60 \div 2.115 = 1.229$
Single conversion factor = Step 1 result divided by step 2 result

Step 4: 150.00 PMPM $\times 1.229 = \$184.35$
Single conversion factor times required premium PMPM equals single premium

Step 5: $184.35 \times 1.95 = \$359.48$
Single premium times couple CR equals couple premium

Step 6: $184.35 \times 2.85 = \$525.40$
Single premium times family CR equals family premium

Contract Type	(A) Contract Mix (%)	(B) Contract Size	(C) Charging Ratios	Computed Conversion Factor	Required or Estimated Premiums ($)
Single	30	1.00	1.00	1.229 (3)	184.35 (4)
Couple	20	2.00	1.95		359.48 (5)
Family	50	3.80	2.85		525.40 (6)
TOTAL	100	2.60 (1)	2.115 (2)		

helps the MCO to manage its block of business and to price both new and renewing groups.

Using ACR creates questions. Members under the same benefit plan and contract effective date, but in separate employer groups with different characteristics, pay different monthly premiums. The increase in rate variation through use of ACR places greater demands on the sales force to respond to employer group questions concerning pricing. In many MCOs the evolution from simplified community rating to ACR is where confusion arose as to pricing methodology. The arithmetic of ACR is straightforward. Inadequate communication by those in charge of pricing or overestimation of the complexity of determining premiums by marketing and sales personnel helps create and perpetuate the "black box" of premium determination. If an individual can multiply and divide, he or she can develop premiums that reflect the ACR methodology. Given the simplicity of the arithmetic, MCOs developed computer spreadsheets to ensure that the routine calculations were properly and consistently completed. With spreadsheet software, a clerk could quickly develop premiums that reflected the group-specific assumptions.

Although ACR represented a significant advancement in pricing compared with simplified community rating, it did not address all the issues that many MCOs identified and verified as pricing difficulties. Management of MCOs recognized that the age and gender of members affect usage of health services. Moreover, MCO claim experience and encounter data often showed a correlation between the utilization of health services and the industry of the employer group. These observations were consistent with the advice and studies of consulting actuaries serving the health insurance industry. Recognition of the importance of age, gender, and industry factor in a competitive marketplace contributed to the development of a more sophisticated pricing methodology.

Community Rating by Class

Conditions in the marketplace, specifically the use of experience rating by insurance companies, encouraged more sophistication in the MCO community rating methodology. MCOs were competing in groups whose premiums for alternative health options to the MCO reflected prior claim experience. Without additional adjustments, MCOs found themselves being competitive on groups with above average risk and higher than average claim experience. Conversely, MCOs found it more difficult to price competitively in groups with favorable claim experience. Accordingly, the CRC pricing methodology arose and was applied by MCOs.

Just as the ACR methodology builds on simplified community rating, the CRC approach builds upon the ACR approach. The CRC methodology merely adds to the ACR methodology adjustments for classes that have an actuarial basis for predicting future levels of utilization.

There are two common classes defined and used by MCOs in their pricing methodology. The first class reflects the composite age and gender characteristics of the employer group. The second class considers the industry factor associated with the employer group. These two classes are independent of each other. The class factors can offset one another or be either favorable or unfavorable. In groups with favorable demographic and industry factors, the MCO charges a lesser premium for the selected benefit plan. In groups with unfavorable factors, the MCO charges a higher premium for the selected benefit plan.

The CRC methodology adjusts the ACR premiums for class adjustments tied to the demographic and industry factors. These adjustments are made to the underlying revenue requirement PMPM for the specific benefit plan under review. For example, if a group had a relatively older membership, it would possess a group-specific demographic factor over 1.00, with 1.00 representing the MCO average age and gender profile. Groups with a demographic factor over 1.00 are projected to use more than average health services over the long term. To adjust for this class, the MCO would increase the revenue requirement PMPM and apply the standard ACR methodology.

Demographic Factors

Hypothetical utilization factors by age and sex are listed in Table 52–2; these factors are

Table 52–2 Hypothetical Utilization Factors by Age and Gender

Age Range (Years)	Male	Female
0–10	0.50	0.50
11–25	0.80	1.15
26–45	1.00	1.25
46–65	1.25	1.25

supplied only for demonstration purposes. A mature MCO with a significant claim history can develop its own utilization factors that, when multiplied by group membership, derive the group-specific weighted demographic factor. Utilization factors also can be obtained from consulting actuarial firms for a nominal fee. Normally, the factors are summarized in quinquennial tables (five-year ranges) broken down by gender.

Note that males and females of the same age generally have the same utilization factor except for the impact of maternity during the childbearing years of women. Multiplying the stated utilization factors by the number of members in each age and gender cell produces the weighted average demographic factor for the group. For example, a group with 10 potential enrollees in the 26- to 45-year-old male cell and 10 potential enrollees in the 46- to 65-year-old female cell would have a demographic factor of 1.125. Adjustment for the group-specific demographic factor and industry factor of Dream Group, Inc. is shown in Exhibit 52–5. Most MCOs determine the demographic factor for a new employer group based on the overall employee and (if available) dependent pool. For renewing groups, the starting point for estimating the demographic factor is the previous enrollment into the MCO program.

While this discussion focuses on group underwriting, some comment is appropriate about underwriting and pricing of individual health care contracts and very small groups, such as groups

Exhibit 52–5 Calculation To Derive CRC Rates for Dream Group, Inc.

Step 1: $(0.30 \times 1.00) + (0.20 \times 2.00) + (0.50 \times 3.80) = 2.60$
Average weighted contract size = Mix (column A) times contract size (column B)

Step 2: $(0.30 \times 1.00) + (0.20 \times 1.95) + (0.50 \times 2.85) = 2.115$
Average weighted charging ratio (CR) = Mix (column A) times CR (column C)

Step 3: $2.60 \div 2.115 = 1.229$
Single conversion factor = Step 1 result divided by step 2 result

Step 4: $\$139.50 \text{ PMPM} \times 1.229 = \$171.45$
Single conversion factor times required premium PMPM equals single premium

Step 5: $\$171.45 \times 1.95 = \$334.33$
Single premium times couple CR equals couple premium

Step 6: $\$171.45 \times 2.85 = \$488.63$
Single premium times family CR equals family premium

Contract Type	(A) Contract Mix (%)	(B) Contract Size	(C) Charging Ratios	Computed Conversion Factor	Required or Estimated Premiums ($)
Single	30	1.00	1.00	1.229 (3)	171.45 (4)
Couple	20	2.00	1.95		334.33 (5)
Family	50	3.80	2.85		488.63 (6)
TOTAL	100	2.60 (1)	2.115 (2)		

under 15 employees. Individual and small group pricing often reflects consideration of the same age and gender factors used to generate a group-specific demographic factor. Age and gender pricing ties health insurance cost to the projected actuarial need of those proposed for coverage. That generally means that older individuals pay more for the same benefits than younger adults, independent of the adjustment for the cost of maternity. While age and gender factors often impact pricing for individual and small group coverage, the underwriting decision itself is usually based on a review of responses to a medical history form. For individual contract applicants and very small groups, each employee applicant usually completes a medical history form that summarizes the health status of the employee and any dependents. After review of these forms, the underwriter, subject to state and federal regulation, decides to offer or decline coverage, in compliance, of course, with HIPAA and state regulations.

When coverage is extended, pricing often reflects the applicant's age and gender factors, subject to heavy state regulation as to product design, initial and renewal pricing, and other requirements. For very small groups, the MCO will often list each covered employee and their own particular premium rate. When a group's size exceeds, say, 15 or 20 employees, an average premium by enrollment category (single, two-party, family) is calculated reflecting in part the overall age and gender factors for the small group.

Industry Factors

Industry factors primarily reflect the actuarial study of years of indemnity claim experience. The historical utilization patterns of particular industries are accepted as an actuarially sound class for use in CRC. MCOs should not arbitrarily adopt a list of industry factors without understanding the context of how the factors were developed. Like the age and gender demographic factors, industry factor lists are available from actuarial firms serving the health care sector.

A standard industry factor list is a necessary resource for CRC methodology to adjust premiums on a group-specific and actuarially sound basis for the class defined as industry. A typical list would include a description of the industry, a definition of the standard industry classification range, and an industry or medical factor that can be used to predict future utilization of services. Hypothetical examples of industry factors are illustrated in Table 52–3.

An employer group assigned an industry factor greater than 1.00 would be expected to use more than an average level of health services over the term of the contract. Therefore, the MCO would adjust the revenue requirement to price the product so that the group would yield revenue PMPM that reflected its actuarially sound industry factor. Those industries assigned a factor less than 1.00 would receive a reduction or discount from standard or average MCO premium requirements. Those industries with a 1.00 factor would receive the standard MCO amount; that is, no adjustment to the revenue requirement would be made.

Other Aspects of CRC

Adjusting the revenue requirement for actuarially sound classes such as industry and demographic factors causes the range of community rates to expand significantly. It is common for small groups to have appropriately assigned industry factors or demographic factors that increase or decrease the standard revenue requirement PMPM by 10 percent or more from the

Table 52–3 Hypothetical Industry Factors

Industry Type	Industry Factor
Agriculture	1.05
Mining and quarrying (excluding metals and fuels)	1.15
Air transportation	1.00
Banking	0.95
Hospitals	1.20
Insurance companies	1.00
Public administration	1.10
Services for engineering, accounting, research	0.95
Retail (apparel, furniture)	1.00

standard MCO norm. This increasing flexibility in pricing requires strong oversight of the pricing activities. Left unattended, MCO pricing functions have fallen into common pitfalls, such as pricing to the market or assuming unrealistic demographic factors to justify a lower price, especially for a first-time offering.

If the MCO uses the CRC methodology to reduce rates but fails to sell groups with net industry and demographic factors above 1.00 the required higher rate, the pricing approach is merely a discounting technique. Such an approach does not comply with the spirit of community rating. In some cases, inappropriate discounting from the standard community rating requirements fails to comply with the direction of regulatory agencies and requirements of such groups as the Federal Employees Health Benefits Program (see Chapter 54).

Using CRC to calculate premiums for Dream Group, Inc., reflects the ACR methodology with a simple adjustment of required revenue PMPM. In the case of this group, both the demographic factor (0.98) and the industry factor (0.95) were less than 1.00. Accordingly, Dream Group would receive a discounted rate based on the actuarially sound class adjustments. A simple discount of 7 percent could be used by the MCO to reflect the net favorable demographic (2 percent) and industry (5 percent) factors. Instead of a revenue requirement of $150.00 PMPM, the premiums quoted Dream Group will yield a revenue of $139.50 PMPM, or 7 percent less than $150.00.

In Exhibit 52–5, note that steps 1 through 3 to derive the conversion factor of 1.229 are identical between ACR and CRC. Both methodologies use group-specific assumptions. Steps 4 through 6 are also identical to those in ACR, the only change being a discounted revenue requirement PMPM of $139.50 instead of $150.00.

Summary of Community Rating Methodologies

Table 52–4 offers an actuarially sound community rate for Dream Group, Inc., as prepared by each of the three community rating methodologies reviewed. Without full understanding of the CRC pricing methodology, managed care competitors, employers, and even the MCO sales force were prone to question how community rates could vary so much, particularly when they were above the norm. Given the adjustments for mix, contract size, charging ratio, and demographic and industry factors, significant rate variation among groups with the same benefit plan and contract effective date is probable.

Given the transition to more sophisticated pricing methodologies, many employers and regulators increasingly view MCO pricing practices as similar to those used by insurance companies. Instead of charging everyone the same community rate, the MCO has adapted its community rating approach to the competitive and experience-rated marketplace. Considering the marketplace and the limited capitalization of many MCOs, these pricing adaptations were desirable and in some cases necessary for survival.

When demographic and industry factors directly affect product pricing, their impact is often limited or moderated. The MCO could consider both demographic and industry factors in

Table 52–4 Community Rating Summary for Dream Group, Inc.

| Contract Tier | *Premiums Reflecting Community Rating* | | |
	Simplified Community Rating	*ACR*	*CRC*
Single	178.80	184.35	171.45
Couple	348.66	359.48	334.33
Family	509.58	525.40	488.63

choosing to cover (or decline) the group but could establish a limit for price adjustments. The MCO might limit the impact of favorable group-specific demographics to a revenue PMPM reduction of no more than 10 percent. Unfavorable demographic characteristics could be capped at 20 percent above standard.

Similar moderation could be applied to the industry factor. With proper actuarial support, all industries could be condensed within a limited range of industry factors. The majority of industries would probably be assigned a neutral factor of 1.00. The industries with significant outlier claim histories could be assigned reasonable factors while still maintaining a fairly tight range.

In these manners, the rate variation caused by demographic and industry factor impact is limited to a tighter range. This approach produces rates that reflect more closely the historic community rating philosophy. At the same time, the moderation of these factors complies with increasing regulation of pricing at the state level.

Even MCOs that choose not to adjust rates for such classes as age, gender, and industry often apply these concepts in developing their operational plan. MCOs utilize demographic and industry information to focus new business sales and plan renewal activities at existing clients. Analysis of demographic and industry factors is also useful in predicting the utilization levels of a particular large group or the entire MCO membership. Similarly, in assessing merger candidates or blocks of business, demographic and industry factors are components of a comprehensive analysis.

UNDERWRITING PRINCIPLES

Given this lengthy discussion of the rating methodology for a community-rated MCO, one might mistakenly conclude, "So that's how managed care underwriting is done." That conclusion would fail to understand the relationship between a pricing methodology and underwriting. The pricing methodology is an important element of underwriting, but underwriting is much more than understanding and operating a pricing methodology.

In MCOs that operate "pricing mills," rate quotes are often prepared by clerks using a spreadsheet program on a personal computer. In these environments, underwriting is sometimes confused with the mere preparation of a rate quote. The rate quote reflects, where possible, exactly what the potential customer or sales representative requested. No additional analysis is performed. Other, more creative options are not generally identified or presented to the customer.

Today, many MCOs view the pricing process as an integral part of a successful underwriting function. Increasingly, MCOs recognize the importance of attracting a cross section of risk and properly managing millions of premium dollars. Accordingly, the compensation paid has moved the underwriting position from a clerk to an experienced person with important skills and broad operational understanding of the MCO and the marketplace. Clerks still work within the pricing and underwriting function, but their output is often the starting point for underwriting rather than the end point of a client proposal.

Regardless of the pricing methodology applied, there are several underwriting principles that most MCOs consider and apply. The most common underwriting principles or criteria that an employer group must satisfy include the following.

Employer Stability

Companies lacking 1 year of operations experience and those that have not previously offered an employee health insurance program generally are considered high risks. Some MCOs choose to decline to offer coverage in this situation. Similarly, if a company consistently changes carriers or MCOs, it suggests that a long-term relationship with the employer may be difficult to achieve. Without employer stability and a chance for a long-term relationship, it is more difficult for the MCO to fund the insurance risk of the group. Industries subject to large-scale layoffs pose an additional risk: mass individual conversions and extension of health benefits to former employees on a voluntary basis. Conversely, stable employer groups with rapidly expanding work forces are usually attractive groups for the MCO.

Employee-Employer Relationship

Entities assuming insurance risk want to attract a cross section of risk. When the normal employee-employer relationship does not exist, the ability to attract a cross section of risk comes into question. Historically, part-time or seasonal workers have generally demonstrated much higher risk or have required much higher levels of health services.

Employee Participation

Commonly, at least 75 percent of employees who are eligible for coverage should select some form of health care coverage. In a group with lower than 75 percent participation, employees who participate are generally those who intend to utilize their coverage. Those who believe that they need not participate are assumed to be the better risk.

Employee Eligibility

An eligible employee is often defined in terms of a minimum number of hours worked per week (say, 30 hours per week). Under this definition, ineligible employees could include seasonal workers, part-time employees, and officers and directors of the company who are not full-time employees. By covering otherwise ineligible employees, the MCO increases its chance of adverse selection. Normally, all MCOs and insurance options accept the same eligibility definition in large employer groups. In small employer groups of fewer than 50 people, the definition of an employee is critical. Employers that have a defined waiting period (subject to limitations for certain individuals or groups under applicable state regulations and HIPAA) help to reduce some of the underwriting risk, particularly for groups with high rates of employee turnover. When possible, the MCO may also include an "actively at work" clause in its contract with the small employer group. When allowed and prop-

erly constructed, this clause requires an employee to be discharged from a hospital and to return to work and be capable of carrying on normal tasks associated with employment before coverage commences under the MCO contract. In some cases, the "actively at work" clause also applies to dependents of the eligible employee. Once the employee returns to work and is eligible for coverage, the actively at work clause no longer applies. Hospitalization and disability of a covered person subsequent to his or her initial eligibility would be covered by the MCO. The actively at work clause provides some protection to the MCO against enrolling, without its knowledge or approval, disabled individuals or individuals confined to a hospital or home who are unable to return to work on the date of their otherwise initial eligibility date for the MCO program.

High-Risk Groups

Certain types of businesses have historically been avoided because of their perceived high risk (for example, bars, massage parlors, and escort services). Many MCOs have lists of groups that would at least not be aggressively pursued. In some cases, some MCOs will choose not to quote a business that they believe is properly described as high risk. High-risk groups often violate several of the underwriting principles being discussed, such as low employee participation and the prevalence of part-time employees or personnel under contract who lack the typical employer-employee relationship.

Premium Differential

To attract a cross section of risk, the MCO's premium generally must be competitive. If too expensive, the MCO would attract only a small enrollment of employees and dependents who choose to pay more to gain coverage afforded by the MCO. If substantially cheaper than other options, the MCO may have misunderstood the risk and underpriced the coverage. The MCO could be efficient and therefore much cheaper, but most underwriters are somewhat skeptical rather than perpetual optimists. The concept of premium differential must also be reviewed from an employee perspective.

Employee Out-of-Pocket Cost

Most employees pay less than 50 percent of the total cost of their health care benefits. Cost to the employee is what he or she is required to pay for a particular health care option, typically expressed on a monthly basis. Although most employers generally treat all health care options similarly, the employee out-of-pocket cost for each health care option should be considered. Historically, it was thought that an employee would pay an additional monthly amount up front in lieu of a deductible. Still, in some groups that historically did not require the employee to pay for his or her health insurance, even a small added monthly out-of-pocket cost could significantly curtail chances for a reasonable enrollment in terms of numbers and cross section of risk.

Minimum Contract Size

Some MCOs establish administrative requirements as to the minimum size of the group. In some cases, the group minimum reflects in part the added cost of billing and premium collection in a small group. From a risk perspective, the minimum group size also serves to protect the MCO from coverage of groups that would substantially increase the risk to the MCO. Thus by stating a minimum group size, the MCO is trying to prevent potential abuse, decrease risk, and encourage the sales force to focus on groups offering a better chance of sizable enrollment in the MCO.

Employer Contribution

An eligible employer must contribute at least 50 percent, and preferably more, to the single cost of the MCO premium. The employer contribution encourages a wider number of employees to participate, making it easier to spread out and manage the risk of health insurance. A low employer contribution will affect the overall level of employee and dependent participation and reflect in part the strength and stability of the employer group.

Demographic Factor Norms

The community rating approach presumes that all groups will use generally the same level of services. Groups with significantly different characteristics are often carefully reviewed before a proposal is prepared. Some MCOs will choose not to quote a business group on a risk basis whose demographic factor is substantially above the norm—say, 1.25—regardless of the ability to charge a loaded premium.

Benefit Plan Compatibility

The level of benefits offered to a group is often determined solely by the group; the employer group states what coverages it desires the MCO to offer. Blindly filling this request is not proactive underwriting as envisioned in this discussion. The MCO should ensure that the benefit plan and related premium will be compatible and competitive with the other options offered. No MCO would routinely want to be the richest benefit plan offered with a comparatively high employee out-of-pocket cost because of the probability of adverse selection. Similarly, the MCO may not wish to offer its most economical benefit plan with high copayments if other options have low deductibles and/or small copayments. Product design and compatibility are often difficult and controversial issues, particularly in a multiple choice environment. This refers to where the aggregate employer risk pool is split among competing carriers, each of which assumes risk for its enrollees. Where possible, the MCO should maintain control over the benefit plan offered. This is a more critical issue in the MCO with open provider access and fee-for-service reimbursement.

Summary of Community Rating and Underwriting

These principles and criteria offer a good foundation for understanding the underwriting mindset. Do not conclude that that's all there is. Moreover, do not assume that underwriting is essentially the same for each employer group or product line. While methodologies must be consistently applied and actuarially sound, underwriting challenges vary substantially from group to group.

The approach to underwrite a group of 7 employees is different from that for a group of 47 employees. The underwriting process is different for a group of 470 or 4,700 employees. As many inexperienced MCOs began to serve associations of employer groups, or participate in programs that target small businesses and the uninsured, the complexities of underwriting were promptly recognized. In many instances the risk assumed by these inexperienced MCOs was poorly understood in terms of both composition and amount. Similarly, experienced MCOs entering new markets are encouraged to critically assess the underwriting requirements of the market, necessary products, and use of alternative distribution channels.

Many groups of more than 100 employees want to share risk or attempt to self-fund their employee health insurance program. These variable funding arrangements further complicate the underwriting challenges.

ADMINISTRATIVE SERVICE ONLY UNDERWRITING

Some employer groups, typically more than 500 employees but sometimes less (for example, 100 employees), attempt to minimize the cost of their health benefits by assuming the underlying risk of claim cost. Under an administrative service only (ASO) contract, the employer group pays an MCO, conventional payer, or TPA to process its claims. In most cases, the ASO vendor also provides the covered persons access to a managed care network. Before offering an ASO arrangement, the MCO must gain necessary regulatory approvals and develop underlying operational capabilities tied to ASO contracts.

Under an ASO arrangement, the insurer functions as an administrator. The employer group funds the payment of eligible claims from a special bank set up by the insurer. Underwriting an ASO contract requires the payer to determine its administrative break-even levels by product and employer group size. After determining the break-even price, the insurer then adjusts for the targeted profit level for its ASO business. This profit is commonly expressed on a PMPM basis. Final ASO quotes generally take four forms: (1) a combination of the PMPM price, (2) a per employee per month charge, (3) a charge per claim, and (4) a percentage of defined network savings.

Insurers offering ASO contracts can usually provide coverage to help mitigate the employer's risk in the form of individual stop loss (ISL) and aggregate stop loss (ASL). ISL is an insurance policy that caps the maximum employer group liability on any covered member in any given calendar year. For example, an ISL level of $50,000 would mean the employer group would be at risk for the first $50,000 of claims incurred during the policy year for any member. Thereafter, the insurer would be liable for any claims over the $50,000 level in the given year.

Under ASL, the employer group is protected in the event that total claims experience reaches a specified threshold in any given year. Once the threshold is reached, the insurer becomes responsible for any claims (or a percentage of claims) over the agreed upon threshold. The ASL threshold is usually expressed as some percentage of the total annual predicted claim cost, such as 125 percent of the ASL. The underwriter predicts the total claim experience for any given group, and the ASL coverage becomes liable only after the total claims experience comes in higher than the stated prediction. For example, if the underwriter determines that the total claims experience for a given group in a given year will be $1,000,000, then coverage provided after reaching 125 percent of the ASL will take place when the group's claims experience crosses the $1,250,000 threshold in this example. Many employer groups acquire both ISL and ASL coverage to help manage the risk associated with a self-funded program.

EFFECTIVE UNDERWRITING: LESSONS LEARNED

MCOs with consistently successful underwriting have adapted their processes to the changing environment. These organizations have responded to the emerging regulation of underwriting, particularly in the small employer group market. Rather than viewing underwriting as merely a pricing methodology, these MCOs have recognized the importance of underwriting and have treated it accordingly in terms of staff, salaries, scope of responsibilities, and range of influence. *It is appropriate at this point to reflect upon several of the basic lessons learned by MCOs with successful underwriting activities:*

- The underwriting function requires a mix of personnel with defined career paths. Mathematical, spreadsheet, and database skills are core competencies of an underwriting function.
- Underwriting assistants can efficiently prepare various analyses, determine the demographic characteristics of the group, and run the initial pricing model.
- Underwriters are key MCO personnel who share management of a revenue stream in the millions of dollars. The compensation and performance requirements for underwriters should reflect this scope of responsibilities.
- Good underwriters have broad operations knowledge and can help develop realistic planning assumptions for the MCO.
- Underwriting must identify the impact of catastrophic or shock claims in the preparation of various analyses. Failure properly to consider shock claims (claims greater than $75,000 per member per year) could lead to faulty decision making.
- Underwriting analyses should help focus the efforts of the sales force and support renewal activities. Some MCOs have used the list of industry factors to direct sales activities to certain industries or businesses. Internal MCO analysis of loss ratio by industry type is also beneficial to direct future sales efforts in terms of new groups and product designs for a particular industry or market segment.
- The actual pricing/underwriting activity is usually an iterative process. The underwriter uses the initial output of the pricing

spreadsheet model to ultimately tailor the most effective approach for the client. During the process, the proposed premiums and benefit design are evaluated for the specific employer group environment. Several factors, such as projected employee out-of-pocket cost, benefit differences, and network issues, are reviewed for each of the projected health care options to be offered by the MCO and its competitors.

- For large, complex groups, the entire underwriting process generally takes several days of work after all the necessary data are collected. Various scenarios should be modeled with corresponding estimates as to the impact on enrollment, risk selection, revenue PMPM, and other factors. Given the slim historical margins within the health care industry, the MCO always needs to have a realistic rate for large groups.
- The MCO will be prudent if it aligns incentives for marketing/sales and underwriting personnel. Ideally, underwriters should share marketing and sales goals, and sales personnel should share accountability for financial results along with underwriting.
- Generally, the MCO should be leery about competing on the basis of offering the richest benefits or the most choice relative to certain services, such as mental health, substance abuse, prescription services, and transplants. This approach to competition is a particular concern when the MCO is at risk for the financial results.
- Increasingly, underwriters need to understand funding arrangements in which the employer group shares at least a portion of the risk with the MCO. The MCO should be cautious in approaching these arrangements because much of the MCO's profitability is tied to the assumption and management of risk. If the MCO transfers both risk and profitability to employer groups that are producing sound financial results, it will increase the challenge of funding the less attractive groups with more variable outcomes.
- Experienced underwriting personnel can contribute to a myriad of MCO decisions

that influence sales and risk selection. What are the themes of the upcoming advertising campaign? Will all contracted specialist physicians be listed in the provider directory, and, if so, how will they be listed? Should the MCO contract with the academic medical center, be listed, and under what terms? Should the MCO change its copayment for office visits or prescriptions? All these questions (and many more) can benefit from an experienced underwriting perspective.

- As the MCO expands its product portfolio and means of distribution, it is necessary to reassess the underwriting function to support these changes.
- The data gathered by underwriting, often at the individual employee or dependent level, should be used by the MCO to meet member needs and/or manage health care services more effectively. Underwriting identification of members with special needs should be routinely provided to the MCO medical management function.
- For market opportunities such as Medicaid and Medicare risk contracting, the underwriting department should assist in the assessment of the opportunity and creation of a comprehensive implementation program.
- As the MCO MIS provides increasing access to and analysis of data, the MCO must be cautious to preserve patient and member confidentiality while providing meaningful information to employer groups and other interested parties.

These lessons can be used to implement or enhance an effective underwriting function. An existing MCO may use these lessons to assess its current underwriting structure, incentives, and processes.

CONCLUSION

This chapter has provided a historical overview of MCO pricing and underwriting. It identified and discussed marketplace trends, risk factors, adaptations of pricing methodologies, and underwriting principles. Collaboration between marketing/sales and the underwriting function within the MCO was strongly encouraged.

This discussion underscores the importance of underwriting to an MCO's success even as insurance reform and government regulation increasingly limit individual and group-specific underwriting. Organizations providing health services and contracting on a risk basis with an MCO are encouraged to understand basic underwriting principles and techniques used by many MCOs.

During the next decade, sound underwriting will continue to help the MCO attract and manage a cross section of health care risk amid trends of consumerism, the continuing public opinion backlash toward managed care, rising employee cost for health insurance, and direct sales to the consumer. Underwriting processes will need to be adapted for interactive sales using the Internet. Previous benchmarks as to underwriting performance, measured in days or weeks, will be replaced with decisions made in seconds or minutes. Emerging technology will allow underwriting function to help lead the MCO toward greater success in the new millennium.

CHAPTER 53

Provider Excess Loss Coverage

Scott A. Walker

INTRODUCTION

When discussing financial risk for medical expenses, costs and utilization are often considered on a population basis. For example, a per member per month (PMPM) cost for a type of service may be given as $2.00 PMPM. This cost represents what an actuary predicts (see Chapter 51 for a discussion of actuarial services in integrated delivery systems [IDSs]) or operational finance reports (see Chapter 47) as the cost of all

---

Scott A. Walker is the Senior Manager of Managed Care Services for AIG Consultants' Healthcare Management Division. In this role, Mr. Walker assists clients in addressing a wide variety of managed care business needs, including analysis and guidance of managed care contracting, development of responsibility matrices, valuation of services, determination of provider excess insurance needs, integration of utilization management with excess claims reporting, and implementation of the provider excess loss reporting processes.

Mr. Walker joined AIG Consultants in his present role after more than 14 years of success as an underwriter, assistant vice president, and regional underwriting manager. His underwriting experience includes employee benefits, employer stop loss, and provider excess liability. While working in the provider excess liability arena, he was responsible for managed care contract review, development of coverage for inpatient diagnosis-related group risk contracting, analysis of utilization benchmark data relative to provider excess liability, development of provider excess programs and coverage, and provision of education on provider excess liability.

services spread across all members. In reality, those average costs represent the collection of individual patient costs, which may be exceedingly high or may be nonexistent for that type of service. The larger the population considered, the less overall variance from the prediction; conversely, the smaller the population considered, the more likelihood that considerable fluctuations will occur.

Large payer organizations account for this through their budgeting and reserving processes and, depending on the size of the health plan, may also purchase reinsurance to cover large, catastrophic, or "shock" claims. The plan may also provide levels of stop-loss protection for individual physicians to prevent financial catastrophes, as discussed in Chapters 8 and 11.

A detailed discussion of capitation is found in Chapters 4 and 8 through 12. As noted in those chapters, capitation exists in many forms. Readers are urged to read those chapters if they are not familiar with the various forms of capitation because the content of this chapter is predicated on that knowledge. The remainder of the chapter will therefore not provide cross-references to those chapters.

The problem of high medical costs and the financial tools to manage those costs is often better understood by health plans than by those providers who accept risk for medical expenses under capitation. The broader the level of capitation (i.e., the more types of services covered under the capitation contract), the greater the risk of fluctuating costs. The focus of this chapter, then, is on provider excess loss insurance or reinsurance. Although the chapter focuses on provider organizations, it should be noted that reinsurance for health plans is not substantially different except for matters of degree.

CAPITATION—THE NEED FOR PROTECTION

Capitation reimbursement, defined as a fixed amount of funds a provider receives irrespective of the number of services provided, gained increasing popularity in the 1990s. The fixed amount is typically expressed on a PMPM basis, with "member" corresponding to a covered member assigned to the provider panel under an agreement between the provider-contracting entity and managed care organization (MCO) or health maintenance organization (HMO). Indeed, capitation has become the predominant method of reimbursement for the primary care physician under contract with HMOs as indicated in Table 53–1. Capitation reimbursement to specialists and hospitals, although not the leading method of payment, has made signifi-

cant gains in recent years. It appears, however, that at the time of publication, the amount of global risk capitation contracting has declined caused in part by the failures of some large practice management companies. Whether that trend continues, flattens, or reverses is not clear. Nevertheless, capitation remains an important feature of the managed care landscape, as does the financial management of risk for medical expenses.

By accepting a defined fixed payment to provide contractual services, providers assume the financial risk expressed as the medical loss ratio, defined as the cost of contracted services divided by revenue from capitation and member copayments. For capitation contracting to be efficient, it must apply over a sufficient number of covered members. This spread of risk enables providers to minimize volatility and absorb losses associated with a fixed payment reimbursement method. Although MCOs often contract with individual providers and pay capitation for the physician's own services, it is not efficient, practical, or reasonable to contract with individual physicians for capitation on a larger scale (i.e., for medical costs that are well

---

Table 53–1 Percentage of HMOs Using Each Provider Reimbursement Method, Showing the Percent of HMOs Using Reimbursement Methods for Any Portion of Provider Payments

	July 1993	*July 1995*	*July 1997*	*July 1998*
Primary Care Physicians				
Capitation	64.3%	66.9%	56.6%	78.7%
Fee for Service	21.7%	17.9%	32.7%	69.7%
Relative Value Scale	5.2%	4.7%	7.1%	27.2%
Salary	8.8%	10.5%	3.6%	9.8%
Specialty Care Physicians				
Capitation	47.4%	49.1%	32.8%	56.4%
Fee for Service	39.0%	35.6%	48.6%	75.5%
Relative Value Scale	9.7%	9.2%	17.6%	32.2%
Salary	3.9%	0.1%	1.1%	3.3%
Hospitals				
Fee for Service	NA	16.9%	15.8%	71.7%
Per Diem Rates	NA	42.9%	53.2%	86.2%
Diagnosis Related Groups (DRGs)	NA	14.1%	12.0%	49.5%
Capitation	NA	26.1%	19.0%	32.5%

Source: Reprinted with permission from InterStudy Publications, The Interstudy Competitive Edge Part II: HMO Industry Report 9.1, p. 54, © 1999, InterStudy Publications.

outside the individual physician's ability to manage or influence and that represent considerable financial risk).

For purposes of contracting with providers for the broader forms of capitation, the MCO generally contracts with a physician-hospital organization, independent practice association (IPA), management services organization, or in some cases with a corporate entity that employs the providers. Hospitals often assume risk by directly contracting with HMOs for institutional and ancillary services. Professional services may be covered under a separate contract with the IPA or medical group. Networks of providers who contract with HMOs are loosely referred to as provider organizations (POs) or more commonly as IDSs. These types of organizations provide managed care contract and capitation reimbursement management for participating providers, thus leaving the health care professional to the practice of medicine. IDS structures are discussed in more depth in Chapter 4, and legal issues important to IDSs are discussed in Chapter 6. The term IDS will be used generically, with the understanding that it does not refer to any single type of PO, and the issues discussed in this chapter will be more or less applicable to any given type of IDS.

Risk contracting under capitation has four major advantages for providers:

- fixed revenue stream
- advanced revenue payment
- allocated profits from risk pools
- increased control over utilization management (UM) functions

Fixed Revenue

The fixed revenue stream afforded by capitation is much easier to budget and should increase over time, given an increase in covered members. Fee-for-service (FFS) revenue, on the other hand, can fluctuate with the volume of services provided. Traditional FFS income is vulnerable to reduction from both private and public payers.

Advanced Revenue

The timing of payments under capitation is usually in advance each month, thereby eliminating the problem of receiving payment after the service is provided.

Risk Pool Profit Allocation

Capitation accounts known as risk pools are typically reconciled on a quarterly and annual basis. Risk pools are generally segregated by type of service: hospital, professional, and ancillary. The capitated revenue of each pool is offset by the actual cost of services provided and allowance for services incurred but not reported. The assumption of risk enables the IDS and participating providers to share in risk pool surpluses if such surpluses exist.

Increased UM Control

Capitation and the inherent risk assumption provide for the opportunity of increased control over UM functions. UM protocols, which the IDS participates in developing, implementing, and monitoring, encourage common goals on all levels of the organization.

Capitation risk contracting brings with it the following disadvantages:

- allocated deficits from risk pools
- increased investment in systems
- exposure to catastrophic losses

Risk Pool Deficit Allocation

The cost of actual services on the basis of utilization can exceed revenue, thus creating a loss, for which the IDS must bear some or all responsibility. Depending on the contract language, prior deficits may be paid by reducing future capitation payments. The need to manage utilization becomes a critical element to the success of provider risk through capitation. There are two basic components to the derivation of capitated revenue: utilization and cost of service. Because the cost of service is negotiated up front between the HMO and IDS on the basis of a number of factors, such as location, size of covered members, type of service, and type of population (e.g., commercial, Medicare, Medicaid), its influence is largely predetermined. Utilization, or the level of service consumption, is less certain and is factored into the capitation revenue on the basis of HMO prior experience and estimated levels from a set of assumptions. The actual capitation PMPM formula is shown in Exhibit 53–1. The IDS receives the PMPM amount derived from an estimated level of utilization; therefore, it stands to reason that the IDS can profit should it manage to lower utilization below levels inputed in the PMPM. Providers are confronted with cuts in prevailing fees due to increased managed care penetration and reduction in rates from Medicare and Medicaid. In some markets, fees have been refined to the point that they no longer cover operating expenses. Utilization becomes the area in which providers can benefit by eliminating inefficiency and directing care to less costly settings.

Increased Investment in Systems

Accepting capitation risk requires initial and periodic capital expenditures for information and administrative systems essential to monitoring and evaluating performance. Proper due diligence in this area will turn what initially is a disadvantage into an advantage as revenue from capitation increases.

Exhibit 53–1 PMPM ($) Formula for a Given Service Area

$$\frac{\dfrac{\text{Utilization of Service}}{\text{Unit per Thousand}} \times \dfrac{\text{Cost per}}{\text{Service Unit}}}{12,000} = \text{PMPM}$$

For example, assume:

The service is hospital inpatient medical/surgical bed days
Medical/surgical bed days are 250/1,000
The average cost per medical/surgical bed day is $1,200
The PMPM value for medical/surgical bed days is $25.00 [(250 × $1,200)/12,000]

Large Claims

Catastrophic losses can have an adverse impact on profitability, especially for IDSs with a relatively small member base over which to spread such losses. The most effective means to minimize the impact of large claims is through the use of provider excess loss (PEL) or stop-loss coverage. Using stop-loss coverage is nothing new to employers who self-insure their medical benefits, as well as insurance companies, including HMOs, who provide fully insured benefits to individual and group members. The incidence and severity of large claims occurring from organ transplants and neonatal events are difficult to predict. It is logical for IDSs to transfer some of the risk resulting from low-frequency, high-severity items. The insurance coverage available to accept the transfer of risk of catastrophic losses is referred to as specific or individual excess. The remainder of this chapter will focus exclusively on the discussion of PEL coverage, including aggregate excess, which protects the IDS against overutilization. Less time will be spent on aggregate excess because of its limited availability in the marketplace and its refined applicability for single specialty risk contracting.

PEL UNDER PROVIDER RISK CONTRACTING

In the early days of provider risk contracting, the IDS purchased PEL coverage from the MCO or HMO. This is known as buying coverage "inside the contract." The primary advantage of purchasing stop-loss coverage from the HMO is the reduced administrative burden associated with reporting losses. Typically, the HMO retains the claims adjudication responsibility, and transactions to account for stop-loss recoveries are internal to the HMO. Premium payments are deducted from the capitation payment each month. The IDS rarely has to comply with the burden of producing lengthy claim documentation for proof of loss. Purchasing PEL coverage from the HMO carries one major disadvantage—price. PEL coverage may be more expensive if arranged through the HMO. Depending on the health plan, additional loads for profit, excess rates based on a broad service area, and broader excess coverage account for much of the difference.

As the PEL premium became a significant expense, IDSs turned to insurance carriers providing PEL coverage, known as purchasing "outside the contract." The two primary advantages of buying the stop-loss coverage outside the contract relate to price and flexibility. The coverage may be less expensive as indicated earlier from the additional loads used by the HMO. PEL carriers have the flexibility to combine multiple contracts under one PEL policy.

TYPES OF PEL COVERAGE

There are two types of PEL coverage: specific and aggregate. Specific coverage, the most common coverage purchased, provides for reimbursement of eligible expenses above a given attachment or deductible level per member, per policy period. Separate attachment levels quite often apply to hospital and professional expenses. The average deductible for hospital expenses ranges from $50,000 to $75,000, but can be as low as $25,000. For physician services, deductibles tend to average $10,000 to $15,000, with a low of $5,000 to $7,500. Reimbursement above the specific attachment is typically 90 percent up to $1 million. The purpose of partial reimbursement is to give the insured a financial incentive to manage large claims. Specific attachments vary according to the number of members covered and the type of

risk (i.e., commercial less than age 65, Medicare, Medicaid) as shown in Table 53–2.

Aggregate stop-loss, which is limited in its availability, provides for reimbursement above a predetermined attachment point expressed as a dollar amount PMPM. The purpose of aggregate stop-loss is to afford the IDS some protection should actual medical expenses exceed capitated revenue. The aggregate attachment ranges from 105 to 125 percent of medical capitated revenue PMPM. Actual medical expenses can be quite volatile, especially for smaller groups. From the PEL carrier perspective, aggregate coverage is either not available or restricted to certain at-risk contracts covering specific areas such as mental health, prescription drugs, or single specialty professional services. Exhibit 53–2 shows how specific and aggregate stop-loss coverage works.

SPECIFIC EXCESS RATE DEVELOPMENT

Variables Affecting Manual Specific PEL Rating

With this basic understanding of what PEL coverage is, let us look at the variables that interact to determine the specific manual stop-loss premium. The term "manual" refers to a premium rate derived from a data set of homogenous observations (excluding the IDS's own experience) large enough to yield predictive results given a set of variable values. Homogenous refers to a similar risk group such as commer-

Table 53–2 Suggested Specific Attachments per Member per Policy Year (PMPPY)

Covered Members	Commercial		Medicare and Medicaid	
	Hospital	Physician	Hospital	Physician
< 1,000	$25,000–$35,000	$5,000–$7,500	$25,000–$50,000	$5,000–$10,000
1,000–5,000	$40,000–$50,000	$7,500–$10,000	$50,000–$75,000	$10,000–$15,000
5,000–10,000	$50,000–$100,000	$10,000–$15,000	$75,000–$125,000	$15,000–$25,000
10,000–25,000	$100,000–$125,000	$15,000–$25,000	$125,000–$175,000	$25,000–$35,000
> 25,000	$125,000 +	$25,000 +	$175,000 +	$35,000 +

Source: Reprinted with permission from PEL Underwriting Manual, p. 11, © 1998, Lexington Insurance Company.

Exhibit 53–2 Examples of How Specific and Aggregate PEL Coverage Works

Specific PEL coverage example	
Variables assumed (apply over 12-month policy period)	
Hospital specific attachment	$ 75,000
Hospital claims paid for member for eligible services incurred	$ 150,000
Reimbursement factor	90%
Specific reimbursement due insured (PO)	$ 67,500
Eligible claims paid	$ 150,000
Less specific attachment	$ 75,000
Times reimbursement factor	90%
Equals reimbursement	$ 67,500
Aggregate PEL coverage example	
Variables assumed (apply over 12-month policy period)	
Expected claims PMPM use for attachment purposes	$ 35.00
Attachment percentage above expected claims PMPM	115%
Aggregate attachment point PMPM	$ 40.25
Actual claims PMPM for eligible services covered under aggregate	$ 42.00
Reimbursement factor	90%
Aggregate reimbursement PMPM due insured (PO)	$ 1.58
Actual claims PMPM	$ 42.00
Less aggregate attachment point PMPM	$ 40.25
Times reimbursement factor	90%
Equals reimbursement PMPM	$ 1.58

Multiply reimbursement PMPM by total member months for actual dollar value of reimbursement.

cial. Observations are defined as a collection of individual dates of service.

The variables that follow combine to determine an IDS's expected hospital claim costs above a given specific attachment. Some variables affect pricing more than others. The phrase "all other things being equal" will be used when referring to the impact of a single variable.

Manual Hospital-Specific PEL Rating

Specific Attachment Per Member, Per Policy Period of 12 Months

The threshold at which covered services qualify as excess greatly affects the frequency of members exceeding the specific attachment, and subsequently the total amount of specific excess expenses for the IDS. Lower specific attachments will result in greater frequency and cost, thus requiring a higher premium, all other things being equal.

Reimbursement Factor

Sometimes referred to as the coinsurance factor, the reimbursement factor is the percentage of excess expenses that the IDS will collect as reimbursement. Varying the reimbursement factor will cause an equal reaction on PEL premium rates. For example, changing the reimbursement percentage from 90 to 80 percent results in an 11.1 percent premium rate reduction [1 − (.80 /

.90)]. This is true because the reimbursement factor applies only to excess expenses.

The Method of Reimbursement for In-Network Hospital Expenses

HMOs and IDSs use several methods to reimburse hospitals (and may combine them as well): per diem (or amount per day), fixed rates for defined procedures (e.g., maternity admissions or cardiac surgery), diagnosis-related groups (DRGs), and percent of charges; capitation of hospitals also exists, although it is less prevalent than the other methods listed. The method of hospital service reimbursement determines how services will accumulate toward the specific attachment. Excess hospital expenses are lower under per diem reimbursement because the average cost per inpatient day is equal to the per diem amount, regardless of whether the admission is for 3 days or 30. This applies to manual rating models. In the real world, hospitals are reimbursed using a variety of per diem amounts that vary by bed type (i.e., medical, surgical, intensive care) and intensity (i.e., higher per diems for the first few hospital days or the use of an outlier payment triggered at a given threshold). In contrast to the per diem method, the discount off billed charges generates significant variation around the average cost per inpatient day. Admissions with expensive services incurred over a disproportionate number of days can generate extremely high average cost per day values compared with the overall average cost per day for all admissions. Because of the variation and extreme costs observed with the discount off billed charges method, the expected cost of hospital expenses penetrating the specific attachment is higher. Although discount charges may be viewed favorably by some hospitals, PEL carriers oppose writing coverage under this reimbursement method without a limit, known as a "per diem limit" or "average daily maximum." Another factor to consider is that billed charges vary widely by location, so premium rates in Los Angeles would be higher than Columbia, South Carolina, because of the billed charge differential between the two locations. The inherent flaw in using a discount off billed charges as the accumulation method is that a facility's billed charge master bears little correlation to actual cost.

Per Diem Limit or Average Daily Maximum

It is not uncommon for PEL coverage to contain limits on the accumulation of eligible expenses under the specific attachment. Such limits known as per diem or average daily maximums generally apply to inpatient expenses provided by out-of-network (OON) or out-of-area (OOA) providers. OON providers are those facilities with whom there is no contracted reimbursement but that reside in the service area. OOA expenses are those expenses provided by facilities outside the service area as defined in the managed care contract with the HMO. Without any contract to govern reimbursement, OON/OOA providers will usually bill using charges (retail), particularly for commercial members. Expenses will accumulate much faster without limits on billed charges in addition to the volatility factor caused by the dispersion around the average charge per day. PEL carriers will place a limit on the amount allowed per inpatient day, typically $2,500 to $3,500, to reduce the volatility and cost. IDSs should assess the impact of per diem limits using their own experience, provided the experience is credible. In-network expenses, including expenses incurred at the IDS's own facility, may be limited as well should inpatient expenses accumulate on the basis of a percent of billed charges. Per diem by definition applies to inpatient expenses, whereas average daily maximum could encompass outpatient and subacute expenses. Exhibit 53–3 illustrates how member claims are revalued using per diem limits and average daily maximums. The PEL policy should clearly state how the limits apply; for example, does the per diem limit apply to total member days or on a per confinement basis?

Type of Population Covered

The type of members (commercial, Medicare, or Medicaid) can have a significant impact on hospital PEL pricing. Because utilization among Medicare beneficiaries aged 65 and older is

Exhibit 53–3 Hospital Claim Re-priced Based on Per Diem Limit

Example:	
Total member's inpatient hospital billed charges	$250,000
Valuation basis that inpatient hospital expenses accumulate toward specific attachment	60% of billed charges
Total inpatient days associated with member's inpatient claims	60
Inpatient per diem (per day) limit for eligible inpatient expenses	$2,000
Eligible expenses based on 60% of billed	$150,000 (A)
Maximum expenses allowed based on per diem limit	$120,000 (B)
Lesser of (A) or (B)	$120,000

In this example, $120,000 would apply toward the specific attachment before the reimbursement factor is applied.

higher than commercial, expected excess claim costs are higher as well. The degree of difference depends on the specific attachment; the greater the attachment, the smaller the ratio of Medicare excess costs to commercial excess costs. Because the specific retention exceeds $250,000 or more, expected excess claims begin to equalize for both commercial and Medicare. The reason for this is attributed to acuity. Excess claims observed in a Medicare population reflect chronic conditions and co-morbidity, resulting in multiple admissions and expensive medication therapy. Such services, when applied to a relatively low stop-loss threshold, will result in more frequent claims above the threshold, thus resulting in greater excess claim costs. In contrast, excess claims observed from a commercial population exhibit a higher incidence of severe claims resulting from organ transplants, trauma, and neonatal care. Although less frequent, enough observations can be seen to reduce the difference in excess claims between the two risk groups at the higher attachments.

Two demographic groups categorize Medicaid risk: Aid to Families with Dependent Children (AFDC; the term has recently been changed to Temporary Assistance to Needy Families, or TANF) and Disability or Aged. The expected excess claim costs associated with AFDC/

TANF risk are similar to commercial. Although utilization of hospital services, particularly emergency department services, is higher for a Medicaid population, the cost basis at which claims accumulate toward the specific attachment is much lower, thereby producing a counterbalance effect. Excess claims observed among the Medicaid disabled exhibit excess costs similar, but to a lesser degree, to Medicare.

In-Network Average Cost per Inpatient Day

The average cost per inpatient bed day is critical to manual PEL price development. The average cost is the valuation basis that inpatient expenses are assumed to accumulate toward the specific attachment. The greater the average cost, the greater the expected excess claim costs, all other things being equal. To determine the cost per day for manual rating, a blended cost per day is derived from the contracted (in-network) hospital reimbursement rates. MCOs typically reimburse hospital inpatient expenses using per diem rates. Exhibit 53–4 illustrates how a blended cost per day is developed using separate rates for medical, surgical, and intensive care. For manual rate development, the weighted cost is inputted as the average cost per day. Calculating a blended cost on the basis of a

Exhibit 53–4 Example of Weighted In-Network per Diem Rate Using Separate Rates for Medical, Surgical, and Intensive Care

	Weight	Per Diem/Day	Weighted
Medical	20%	$800	$160
Surgical	50%	$950	$475
ICU/CCU/NICU	30%	$1,400	$420
Weighted per diem in-network			$1,055

Source: Weight data from *1999 Provider Stop-Loss Rate Manual: Hospital Excess,* p. II.2, © 1998, Towers Perrin, Minneapolis, Minnesota.

percent of billed charge reimbursement is more subjective than the method using per diem rates. PEL rating manuals often include a list of average billed charge amounts per day by ZIP code. The results reflect a survey average for several hospitals in a given ZIP code, which may not accurately reflect the individual hospital system rated. In addition, the charge data may be two years old, failing to reflect increases in charges. Adjusting the charge amounts by a trend factor would help offset the effect of data that are considered out-of-date. A more accurate method is to calculate an average charge per day from the hospital's own admission experience reflecting the discount off charge reimbursement basis utilized in the risk contract.

OON Cost per Day

PEL pricing must take into consideration the effect of services delivered by OON providers. These are providers that reside in the service area but are free to charge what they are able to get. Without a written contract formalizing any negotiated discount, costs for OON services are more expensive and generally reflect billed charges. As previously mentioned, PEL carriers will quite often place a cap on OON costs through the use of per diem limits. The overall impact of OON costs on manual rate development depends on the estimated percentage of services provided OON and how those services are valued. Manual rating models will calculate both in-network and OON expected excess claim costs and blend the two using the percent-

age distribution of in-network versus OON.[1] For example, if 90 percent of the hospital services are delivered from in-network contracted providers, the OON expected excess claim costs will be weighted 10 percent. The distribution may vary by type of plan (i.e., point-of-service [POS] plans will tend to experience greater use of OON utilization compared with traditional HMO plans). The cost basis in which eligible hospital services will accumulate toward the specific attachment for OON providers is significant in determining the OON rate. Manual rating typically uses the average charges based on the location of the hospital for OON expenses, notwithstanding any discounts or limits applied by the PEL coverage.

OOA Cost per Day

Expenses submitted from OOA providers are those hospital services provided to covered members while the member is beyond the service area boundaries, usually defined in the contract as a list of counties or within a maximum radius of the insured's location. OOA utilization is random and virtually impossible to predict. Consequently, few IDSs accept risk for OOA services. If covered, however, the impact on manual rating is minimal because of the low frequency of OOA utilization.

Outpatient Hospital Services Included?

Outpatient hospital services can account for approximately one fifth (or sometimes more) of the total manual premium rate PMPM.[2] Outpatient services represent technical or facility charges associated with procedures performed in an outpatient setting and include:[3]

- surgical
- emergency department
- radiology
- pathology
- other (i.e., supplies, durable medical equipment)

If the contract simply states that "outpatient services" are covered, all the above would be included in the rate development. Over the past few years, more contracts have shifted the responsibility of technical services associated with outpatient radiology and pathology to the physician risk pool. There may be an instance in which a separate physician group contractually provides and bills for those services separately. A more likely scenario is one in which a medical group performs certain laboratory and imaging services using stand-alone centers distinct from the hospital. Manual rating models are unlikely to allow the user to differentiate technical expenses associated with free-standing facilities from an outpatient hospital environment.

Mental Health/Substance Abuse Covered?

Like OOA services, mental health and substance abuse hospital services are generally excluded from the IDS's risk pool, but for a different reason. Psychiatric services within a managed care contract are often subcontracted to a provider entity specializing in behavioral health. The impact to PEL rates is minimal though because of low severity, low provider costs, and plan limits; however, recent legislation providing for expanded benefits may ultimately have some impact on the cost.

Deductible Carryover

PEL coverage commonly includes what is known as a "deductible carryover" or "thirty-one-day carryover provision." Its impact on expected excess claims development manifests itself in the subsequent years of a PEL policy. The purpose of 31-day carryover coverage is to allow the insured to submit hospital expenses incurred in the month before renewal effective date against the renewal deductible, provided the member has not yet reached the specific attachment in the current period (i.e., the period preceding the renewal date). Exhibit 53–5 shows how the provision works using expenses from a hospital admission less than 31 days before the PEL coverage renewal date.

Claim Eligibility Basis

Claim eligibility basis refers to determining the eligibility of covered expenses for reimbursement under the PEL policy on the basis of the time period the service was delivered (incurred) and paid. For noncapitated services, payment denotes the date the check is issued for payment of service. Capitated services are prepaid services based on covered members, irre-

---

Exhibit 53–5 Application of 31-Day Deductible Carryover Provision within PEL Coverage

Hospital expenses incurred in last month of policy period (calendar year) 1	$24,000
Member admitted 12/6/98	12/6/98
Member discharged 12/26/98	12/26/98
Specific attachment is $50,000 policy period 1	$50,000
Specific attachment is $50,000 policy period 2	$50,000
Amount eligible for carry forward to policy period 2 attachment	$24,000

Explanation: the member failed to reach the specific attachment in policy period 1; thus, eligible expenses incurred within the prior 31 days of policy period 2 are carried forward to apply toward the specific attachment in policy period 2.

spective of the individual services delivered. PEL carriers will normally use the date that the service was presented as an offset against capitated revenue in the risk pool. A timeline diagram illustrating the various common eligibility parameters is shown in Figure 53–1. PEL carriers may choose to discount PEL rates in the first year based on the claims eligibility basis. The discount may vary by the type of eligibility basis as shown in Figure 53–1 and by specific deductible. PEL carriers are moving away from discounting their rate development based on claims eligibility basis, which is removed for rate development in the renewal years. Much of the PEL book of business includes IDSs that have had both risk contracts and stop-loss for several years, and the credibility of the discount is questionable.

Duration of Policy Period

The length of the PEL coverage period over which eligible claims accumulate toward the specific attachment can reduce or increase the expected excess claim costs. Reducing the period of accumulation while leaving the specific attachment unchanged will lower excess claims. Incurred expenses have a shorter period of time to penetrate the threshold, thereby reducing excess frequency and cost. In contrast, a longer accumulation period will result in a greater number of claims and increased excess cost given those members have more time to incur claims. Stan-

dard PEL rate development assumes a 12-month accumulation period.

PEL Carrier Expense Ratio or Target Loss Ratio

Until now, we have frequently referred to hospital manual PEL rate development as expected excess claim costs. Providers of PEL coverage load expected costs to factor in company expenses and profit objectives, which include:

- general and administrative expenses (i.e., salaries, rent)
- acquisition expenses (i.e., brokerage commission)
- underwriting profit objective

Although the expense load varies by carrier, a general rule of thumb is 35 percent. In other words, if the manual expected excess claim expense is $1.00 PMPM, the premium rate charged would be $1.54 ($1.00 divided by .65).

Manual Physician-Specific PEL Rating

Because of separate risk pools and cost basis, it is necessary to develop stop-loss rates unique to professional or physician services covered under an MCO risk contract. Like hospital rate development, several variables contribute to determining excess professional claims. Several of the variables are the same as their counterparts in hospital rating and warrant little discussion

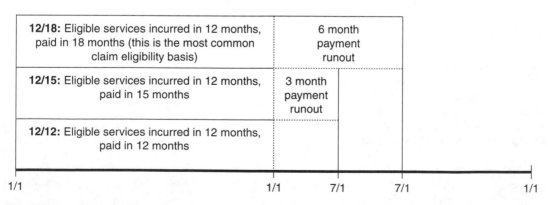

Figure 53–1 The Three Forms of Claim Eligibility Basis Typically Allowed by PEL Carriers

other than what was previously stated. Those variables unique to physician services will be discussed with greater detail.

Specific Attachment Per Member, Per Policy Period of 12 Months

The specific attachment or threshold for professional expense functions the same way as it does for hospital services. The one difference worth noting is specific attachment levels are much lower given the low severity and high frequency of services.

Reimbursement Factor

The percentage of excess physician claims reimbursable under the PEL policy is usually the same percentage for excess facility reimbursement (i.e., 90 percent). The method and degree of impact on pricing are the same as well.

Distribution of Services: In-Network versus OON

The percentage of professional services provided by in-network professionals greatly affects expected excess claim costs because of the vast cost differences between contracted (in-network) fee schedules and noncontracted reasonable and customary rates. Although the percentage of OON services is relatively low, their cost is much higher compared with contract fee schedules. Traditional HMO plans exhibit approximately 98 percent in-network use.[4] POS plans show a tendency for greater OON utilization where members can self-refer to a specialist of their choice.

In-Network Fee Schedules

Medicare resource-based relative value scale (RBRVS) is the most common fee schedule used in risk contracts because of its simple application and availability (published in the Federal Register).[5] In 1992, the Health Care Financing Administration (HCFA) began using RBRVS, a form of reimbursement based on the concept of developing quantitative values or relative value units (RVUs) for the resources used by a physician for any given procedure.[6] RVUs are derived separately for resources associated with:

- work (the physician's time used while providing the service)
- practice expense
- malpractice expense

Since its implementation, RBRVS has been continually updated, assigning RVUs to an increasing number of codes listed in the American Medical Association's Common Procedural Terminology (CPT). RBRVS uses a conversion factor to convert RVUs to dollar fee amounts. It is impractical for a manual rating model to encompass more than 10,000 CPT codes. Fortunately, only a small number of codes are needed to develop a relative conversion factor for any fee schedule. Conversion factors provide the basis to adjust the level of reimbursement using RVUs. Given the same level of utilization and location, a higher conversion factor will result in greater valuation of physician services, which in turn will accumulate more rapidly toward the specific attachment. The result is a higher expected excess claim expense.

RVUs within the Medicare payment system are adjusted on the basis of geographical location using geographic practice cost indices (GPCIs). Separate GPCIs apply to work, practice, and malpractice RVUs. The GPCIs' relative value is actually the sum of the three individual GPCI products (see Exhibit 53–6). Critics of the GPCIs argue that their use is limited given the lack of specific data.[7] HMO plans covering commercial and Medicaid risk may choose not to adjust RVUs on the basis of GPCIs. Because a wide variety of risk contracts use stop-loss, manual rate development must have the ability to both adjust for and neutralize the impact of GPCIs.

Rating models may use different approaches to determine the impact on excess claims from a given fee schedule; however, for purposes of this discussion the focus will be on medical excess expenses observed at various specific attachments and conversion factors. Because the conversion factor allows us to adjust the professional fee amount for any set of RVUs (i.e., Medicare RBRVS), reimbursement amounts can be manipulated in a database containing a credible number of CPT services utilized by a study

Exhibit 53–6 GPCI Relative Value

Work value units	× Work GPCI	= Adjusted work value units (**A**)
Practice expense value units	× Practice GPCI	= Adjusted practice expense value units (**B**)
Malpractice expense value units	× Malpractice GPCI	= Adjusted malpractice expense value units (**C**)
		GPCI Relative Value Units = (**A**) + (**B**) + (**C**)

Source: Data from *St. Anthony 1999 Complete RBRVS,* 1999, St. Anthony Publishing, Reston, VA.

population. The mix of actual CPT codes is the key. RVUs and varying conversion factors are incorporated into the CPT code mix, and then fee amounts are generated. Once the professional fees (cost) are calculated, they are accumulated on a per member basis to determine excess expense factors at any given attachment. The result is a table of excess expense factors matrixed by conversion factor and specific attachment.

When developing a manual PEL physician rate, the top 40 to 50 contributing codes are used to develop a relative conversion factor that can be matched with values from the table of excess expense factors described previously. The top revenue-producing codes include surgical procedures and specialty and primary care. Before 1998, HCFA published separate conversion factors for surgical, nonsurgical/nonprimary care, and primary care. Since then, a single conversion factor has been used. Commercial and Medicaid fee schedules often use multiple conversion factors, creating incentives for primary care physicians who perform evaluation and management services. Manual rate models will typically segregate the top contributing codes by the following groupings: surgical, radiology, pathology, and medicine.[8] The conversion factor is multiplied by the RVU (GPCI RVU if location specific) for each of the codes within each grouping. The resulting fee amounts are weighted by their relative utilization. A relative conversion factor is then derived for each of the four groupings by dividing the weighted total fee amount by total RVUs. Each relative conversion factor from each grouping is weighted to calculate an overall relative conversion factor. The weighted conversion factor represents the weighted average conversion factor, which is then matched up with its corresponding excess expense factor. Exhibit 53–7 illustrates the step-by-step derivation of the weighted average conversion factor.

Risk contracts make use of other fee schedules aside from Medicare RBRVS. Manual PEL models should be able to evaluate the impact on excess claims from any fee schedule. Commercial risk contracts often use an FFS schedule that is unique to that particular contract. To determine its impact on PEL pricing, individual fee amounts corresponding to the top volume codes in the rating model are input. From there, the weighted-average conversion factor is calculated in the same manner as described in Exhibit 53–7.

OON Fee Schedule

Medical excess expense factors are derived separately for both in-network and OON expenses. OON expenses are associated with those services delivered by physicians with whom there is no contract. Authorized referrals to certain specialists outside the panel should be addressed in the contract (i.e., pediatric subspecialties). OON expenses are typically valued at the reasonable and customary (R&C) charge. Because of the inherent inflationary element and the lack of association with true cost, PEL carriers may place limits on the valuation of OON professional services such as a maximum percent of billed amount. R&C may be further defined in the PEL contract as an amount not to

Exhibit 53–7 Excess Physician Expense: Conversion Factor Estimate—RBRVS Fee Schedule

Locality	DC & MD/VA Suburbs
Zip code	20036
Percent of RBRVS	100%
1998 Medicare conversion factor	36.6873
Medicare work RVU adjuster included?	Yes
Work GPCI	1.051
PE GPCI	1.177
Malpractice GPCI	1.006

CPT Code		RBRVS Units	×	Conversion Factor	=	Fee	×	Weighting Factor	=	Product
Surgical services										
19318	Reduction mammaplasty	34.99328	×	36.6873	=	1283.809	×	0.030591	=	39.27277
22554	Arthrodesis, anterior interbody technique	44.80283	×	36.6873	=	1643.695	×	0.026592	=	43.70917
27447	Total knee replacement	53.49393	×	36.6873	=	1962.548	×	0.024893	=	48.85278
29881	Knee arthroscopy with meniscectomy	19.36133	×	36.6873	=	710.315	×	0.038289	=	27.19691
29888	Arthroscopically aided anterior cruciate ligament repair	34.59177	×	36.6873	=	1269.079	×	0.029391	=	37.29972
30520	Septoplasty	13.83902	×	36.6873	=	507.7163	×	0.019994	=	10.15128
33533	Coronary artery bypass	63.72483	×	36.6873	=	2337.892	×	0.037989	=	88.81325
43239	Upper GI endoscopy, biopsy	6.973393	×	36.6873	=	255.835	×	0.023993	=	6.138198
45378	Diagnostic colonoscopy, w/o biopsy	8.819288	×	36.6873	=	323.5559	×	0.022293	=	7.213132
45380	Diagnostic colonoscopy, biopsy	9.904936	×	36.6873	=	363.3853	×	0.019994	=	7.265527
49505	Repair inguinal hernia, age 5+	12.50876	×	36.6873	=	458.9126	×	0.020894	=	9.588396
50590	Lithotripsy, extracorporeal shock wave	21.50646	×	36.6873	=	789.014	×	0.022893	=	18.063
56308	Laparoscopy, with vaginal hysterectomy	26.8103	×	36.6873	=	983.5977	×	0.028791	=	28.31912
56340	Cholecystectomy	21.84285	×	36.6873	=	801.355	×	0.050585	=	40.5364
56341	Cholecystectomy w/cholangiography	23.28053	×	36.6873	=	854.0997	×	0.029991	=	25.61531
58150	Total abdominal hysterectomy	28.04418	×	36.6873	=	1028.865	×	0.049985	=	51.42783
59400	Routine obstetrical care, vaginal delivery, and postpartum	43.35852	×	36.6873	=	1590.707	×	0.327502	=	520.9593
59510	Routine obstetrical care, Caesarean delivery, and postpartum	49.10479	×	36.6873	=	1801.522	×	0.103069	=	185.6812
63030	Laminectomy, one interspace, lumbar	29.92846	×	36.6873	=	1097.995	×	0.044587	=	48.95587
66984	Cataract removal	24.16503	×	36.6873	=	886.5499	×	0.047686	=	42.27575
	RBRVS Average									1287.335
	1998 St. Anthony's complete RBRVS average units									33.34213
	1998 St. Anthony's complete RBRVS surgical CF (1287.335/33.34213)									38.60985
Radiology										
70553	Magnetic resonance, without contrast material	33.11222	×	36.6873	=	1214.798	×	0.1	=	121.4798
71020	Front and lateral chest X-ray	1.074459	×	36.6873	=	39.41899	×	0.3341	=	13.16988

continues

Exhibit 53–7 continued

CPT Code		RBRVS Units	×	Conversion Factor	=	Fee	×	Weighting Factor	=	Product
76091	Bilateral mammography	2.446999	×	36.6873	=	89.77379	×	0.1564	=	14.04062
76805	Lymphangiography, pelvic/abdominal, bilateral	4.038979	×	36.6873	=	148.1792	×	0.2177	=	32.25862
76856	Echo exam, pelvic (nonobstetric)	2.899189	×	36.6873	=	106.3634	×	0.1918	=	20.4005
	RBRVS Average									201.3494
	1998 St. Anthony's complete RBRVS average units									4.84097
	1998 St. Anthony's complete RBRVS radiology CF (201.3494/4.84097)									41.59279
Pathology										
80054	Clinical chemistry tests				=		×		=	
81000	Urinalysis				=		×		=	
85023	Hemogram and platelet count, automated				=		×		=	
88305	Surgical pathology (Level IV)	2.015615	×	36.6873	=	73.94748	×	0.682691	=	50.48326
88307	Surgical pathology (Level V)	3.44215	×	36.6873	=	126.2832	×	0.317309	=	40.07081
	RBRVS Average									90.55408
	1998 St. Anthony's complete RBRVS average units									2.294714
	1998 St. Anthony's complete RBRVS pathology CF (90.55408/39.46204)									39.46204
Medical Services										
90807	Individual psychotherapy, approx 45 to 50 minutes	2.643594	×	36.6873	=	96.98633	×	0.09529	=	9.241873
99203	Office visit, new patient, detailed	1.963848	×	36.6873	=	72.04827	×	0.045795	=	3.29481
99204	Office visit, new patient, comprehensive	2.926074	×	36.6873	=	107.3498	×	0.040896	=	4.390166
99212	Office visit, established patient, detailed	0.783375	×	36.6873	=	28.73992	×	0.056594	=	1.626517
99213	Office visit, established patient, detailed	1.123164	×	36.6873	=	41.20585	×	0.39816	=	16.40653
99214	Office visit, established patient, detailed	1.688884	×	36.6873	=	61.96058	×	0.161984	=	10.03661
99215	Office visit, established patient, comprehensive	2.670808	×	36.6873	=	97.98472	×	0.050495	=	4.947734
99232	Subsequent hospital care	1.591483	×	36.6873	=	58.38721	×	0.045795	=	2.673867
99283	Emergency department visit	1.812041	×	36.6873	=	66.47889	×	0.058094	=	3.862038
99284	Emergency department visit, detailed	2.763606	×	36.6873	=	101.3892	×	0.046895	=	4.754679
	RBRVS Average									61.23949
	1998 St. Anthony's complete RBRVS average units									1.624846
	1998 St. Anthony's complete RBRVS medical CF (61.23949/1.624846)									37.68943
	Weighted average 1998 St. Anthony's complete RBRVS conversion factor (56% surgical + 12% radiology + 5% pathology + 27% medical)									38.7619

Source: Data from *1999 Provider Stop-Loss Rate Manual: Physician Excess*, worksheet 2D, © 1999, Towers Perrin.

exceed a percentile of providers within the same geographic area. For example, R&C expenses may be limited to the 80th percentile of HIAA (Health Insurance Association of America) or some other national database. What this means is that for any given procedure the physician's charge is limited to the amount that 80 percent of the physicians in the same area would have charged for the same procedure.

Type of Population Covered

The particular type of population (i.e., commercial, Medicare, or Medicaid) has a similar impact on physician PEL rates as it does for hospitals. Medicare patients aged 65 and older can generate physician excess rates over five times compared with a commercial risk group, all other things being equal.[9] The elderly suffer from chronic conditions related to aging such as diabetes, cerebrovascular disease, and end-stage renal disease. The treatment of these conditions requires the services of specialists over a long period of time. Surgical fees associated with procedures such as hip replacements occur more frequently. The degree of difference in PEL rates caused by higher utilization of a Medicare-aged population begins to taper off as the physician attachment increases; a similar trend is experienced with hospital excess rating. Utilization of physician services observed from a Medicaid population is higher compared with a commercial population. The degree of difference over the same fee schedule (i.e., the same level of RBRVS) ranges from 25 to 50 percent for AFDC/TANF, and 300 to 350 percent for Disabled or Aged.[10] This difference, however, can be offset by the low fee schedules attributed to Medicaid risk. Fee schedules used within Medicaid risk contracts when converted to an RBRVS equivalency average anywhere from 50 to 80 percent of Medicare payments. Thus, stop-loss rates for AFDC/TANF can be lower than commercial at a given specific attachment because of the lower cost of accumulated services. The impact from utilization observed from a Medicaid Disabled or Aged population is greater than the counter impact resulting from lower fees, thus contributing to excess claims greater than commercial risk. Manual PEL rating models optimally should provide the user with the capability to compute separate rates for AFDC/TANF and Disabled or Aged.

Outpatient Technical Services

Today, more IDSs are accepting risk for technical or facility expenses under the physician pool. Inclusion of technical services associated with outpatient procedures increases physician stop-loss rates because of the greater number of services accumulating toward the specific attachment. The areas where the technical or facility component is sometimes transferred to the physician risk pool include:[11]

- surgical procedures
- emergency department procedures
- imaging
- laboratory
- chemotherapy agents

The most common technical risk areas assumed within physician pools are chemotherapy agents, imaging, and laboratory. More medical groups today have the capability to perform certain imaging and laboratory tests within their practice. The trend of medical groups accepting risk for chemotherapy agents presents a substantial risk for consideration under PEL rate development. Quantifying the impact of chemotherapeutic injectables on PEL rates remains somewhat subjective. The definition of covered hospital outpatient services traditionally includes all nonprofessional facility charges associated with chemotherapy. Although rating models possess the ability to identify how outpatient services are distributed among major categories such as radiology, pathology, emergency department, and surgical, they are unable to identify separately the impact of injected substances administered in an outpatient setting. The developers of manual PEL models tend to conform to the needs of their customers, PEL carriers. Because carriers have a need to quantify more accurately the impact of injected substances such as chemotherapeutic agents, one would expect models to include the enhancement in future releases.

Much less common under physician responsibility is the acceptance of outpatient facility charges related to surgical and emergency department procedures. Physicians have virtually no control over these expenses, and accepting responsibility is contrary to risk contracting; that is, you tend to accept risk for what you can control. Specialty practices such as orthopaedics are increasingly developing stand-alone same-day surgical facilities completely separate from hospitals. Surgical group facilities afford the opportunity for the medical group to control facility expenses against revenue from managed care contracts.

PEL Coverage Effective Date

The effective date of coverage provides the parameter for trend adjustment relative to R&C (OON fee schedule) costs. Trend factors are applied from the midpoint of the experience period used to develop the base R&C conversion factors to the midpoint of the coverage period. A monthly trend component is derived by dividing the annual trend factor by 12. The monthly component is then multiplied by the number of months between the two midpoints.

Claims Eligibility Basis

This variable definition is the same as for hospital rating, although the discount available is generally less and may be nonspecific to the attachment. The impact on rate development is minimal, and as previously mentioned, many carriers are removing the discount altogether because of the question of efficacy.

Duration of Policy Period

The variable definition and its applicability are the same as previously described for hospital excess rating.

PEL Carrier Expense Ratio or Target Loss Ratio

PEL physician rates are increased in the same manner and by the same factor as described in hospital excess rating.

Exhibits 53–8 and 53–9 list the covered services included in hospital and physician PEL coverage on the basis of the standard risk contract. This concludes the discussion on manual PEL rate development for specific excess coverage. Attention is now directed to experience rating, which is blended with manual rates on the basis of credibility factors.

EXPERIENCE-SPECIFIC PEL RATING

Experience rating is the process of determining excess claims at any given specific attachment from actual claims experience obtained from the insured. Rate development using actual experience should encompass a minimum of two to three years of loss data. Excess claims can be converted to a PMPM basis using covered member data corresponding to the loss period. Experience rating is performed by PEL carriers and can vary by carrier; however, the conceptual methodology is similar. The experience rating process can be broken down into sequential steps, which are summarized in Exhibit 53–10.

Step 1: Identifying the Loss Data Elements Required for Experience Rating

Data elements must include information pertaining to all factors affecting the cost of excess claims. Hospital services may be limited by a per diem amount applicable to inpatient services. Given that case, loss data for each member should include inpatient services separated from outpatient services and the number of inpatient days. PEL carriers can rely somewhat on their internal claims system for complementary data such as inpatient days associated with each member; however, these data are not as current as data obtained from the insured, and obtaining the data internally may be a painstaking exercise in futility. If excess claims are affected by valuation parameters such as per diem limits or daily maximum amounts, it is best for the PEL carrier to establish the data reporting capabilities of the insured before binding coverage.

Step 2: Obtain Loss Data from Insured

PEL carriers will send out a request for loss data before their initial evaluation of the risk and annually as part of the renewal information required for annual rate development. Much of the

Exhibit 53–8 Definition of Hospital Services

Listed below is a summary of the services that we have assumed are included in the definition of inpatient hospital and outpatient hospital services for purposes of developing the premium rates. These services are representative of those typically included in a capitation arrangement with the exception of mental health services, which have been excluded.

Hospital inpatient (including all related nonprofessional ancillary facility charges)
  Medical
  Surgical
  Boarder baby
  ICU/CCU/NICU
  Maternity
  Skilled nursing facility

The inpatient hospital service category generally includes all nonprofessional facility charges associated with an inpatient hospital stay. Thus, any ancillary services (i.e., laboratory, radiology, anesthesia) associated with an inpatient hospital stay will be included. Professional services are typically billed separately and are not included as inpatient hospital services. Charges for hospital-based physicians who are employed by the hospital and paid a salary may be built into the hospital's daily rates and, therefore, included in the inpatient hospital category. Hospital-based physicians who are not employed by the hospital will submit a separate bill, and have not been included in the inpatient category.

Hospital outpatient (including all related nonprofessional ancillary facility charges)
  Same-day surgery
  Emergency room
  Radiology and radiation oncology
  Laboratory
  Ambulance
  Durable medical equipment
  Therapies (physical, occupational, speech, IV)
  Anesthesia
  Home health
  Hospice
  Dialysis
  Chemotherapy
  Miscellaneous

The outpatient hospital service category generally includes all nonprofessional facility charges that are not associated with an inpatient hospital stay. Any ancillary services (i.e., laboratory, radiology, anesthesia) associated with an inpatient hospital stay have not been included. Professional services are typically billed separately and are not included as outpatient hospital services. Charges for hospital-based physicians who are employed by the hospital and paid a salary may be built into the outpatient facility rates and, therefore, may be included in the outpatient hospital category. Hospital-based physicians who are not employed by the hospital will submit a separate bill, and have not been included in the outpatient category.

Source: Data from *1999 Provider Stop-Loss Rate Manual: Hospital Excess,* VI-1, © 1999, Towers Perrin.

---

loss data required, if not all, are usually reported on a regular basis by the insured to satisfy both internal management and the reporting requirements in the PEL policy. Regular reporting allows the insured to avoid the trouble of creating special ad-hoc reports specifically for the purpose of experience rating.

Step 3: Structure the Loss Data in a Spreadsheet or Database Application

Constructing experience models on a spreadsheet or database application enables the user to manipulate, query, and tabulate results more efficiently. Quite often, the user will develop rates on the basis of several options by changing variables such as specific attachment, inpatient per diem, or percent of billed allowed. Carriers should encourage insureds to transmit data electronically in the same format for both loss reporting and annual rating. The final experience model should consist of records of data, with each record containing the required data elements for a member who has exceeded the stop-loss threshold for each experience period.

Exhibit 53–9 Definition of Capitated Physician Services

Listed below is a summary of the services that we have assumed are included in the definition of capitated physician services for purposes of developing the premium rates. These services are representative of those typically included in a risk or capitation arrangement that transfers financial risk for medical services to either a group practice or an IPA. The definition was developed based on a review of a number of these contracts from Towers Perrin files. Please note that mental health and substance abuse professional benefits have been excluded from standard coverage.

Capitated physician services
- Office visits and services routinely provided in the physician's office
- Consultations, inpatient, outpatient, or at office
- Hospital visits
- SNF visits, when medically necessary
- Home and nursing home visits, when medically necessary
- Authorized referrals to outside physicians
- Emergency room visits/physician fees
- Radiology services (inpatient and outpatient)
- Laboratory and pathology services (inpatient and outpatient)
- Other diagnostic tests, including ECGs and EEGs (inpatient professional and outpatient professional)
- Injectable medications
- Allergy testing
- Therapeutic radiology, professional component
- Preventive services
- Elective physical
- Well-baby care
- Pediatric and adult immunizations
- Pap tests
- Surgery, including assistant surgeon (professional charges only)
- Anesthesiology
- Family planning benefits
  —Vasectomy and tubal ligation
  —Infertility studies and treatment
- Vision and hearing examinations for members under 18
- Health education
- Obstetrical services including delivery and pre- and postnatal care
- Newborn care, including initial exam in hospital
- Short-term physical, speech and occupational therapy (outpatient)
- Outpatient detox (professional services only)
- Emergency care in area—physician services
- Nonoral drugs

Source: Data from *1999 Provider Stop-Loss Rate Manual: Physician Excess,* V-1, © 1999, Towers Perrin.

Step 4: Calculate Excess Claims above the Specific Attachment

Total the excess claims for all members for each experience period. At this point the excess claims column should represent the valuation of covered services applicable for each individual loss year. Covered services or valuation in historical experience years may not coincide with the current covered services or valuation basis.

Exhibit 53–10 Steps for Developing Provider Stop-Loss Rates from Experience

Step 1 Identify loss data elements for experience rate development (i.e., total inpatient days are needed for each excess member if a per diem limit is utilized).

Step 2 Obtain loss data from insured (PO).

Step 3 Input or transfer the data into a spreadsheet or database application. Construct the experience loss model for preparation of experience rate development.

Step 4 Calculate the excess claims above each specific attachment option.

Step 5 Multiply the total excess claims above the specific attachment by the loss development factor.

Step 6 Multiply the developed total excess claims by the reimbursement or coinsurance factor.

Step 7 Convert the total developed excess claims net of coinsurance to a per member, per month (PMPM) basis by dividing by total member months (lagged if necessary).

Step 8 Divide the developed excess claims net of coinsurance PMPM by the administrative load factor to arrive at the experience rated premium PMPM.

Step 9 Blend the manual premium rate PMPM with the experience premium rate PMPM using the credibility factor as the basis for weighting.

Variables can be easily changed to reflect those changes directly related to PEL coverage such as specific attachment or per diem limit. However, accounting for a change in covered services is much more difficult to quantify objectively given the type of experience data available to the user. Adjusting the manual rates to reflect previous covered services or valuation is preferred to attempting to adjust the experience in prior years. The manual rates are matched up with their corresponding experience rates to ensure a more "apples to apples" comparison. When confronted with eligible excess claims based on a discount off billed charges, trending the charge data to reflect current billed charges must be considered. Thus, the excess claims developed from the adjusted charges will be accurate.

Step 5: Adjust the Excess Claims by the Loss Development Factor

Of all the areas integral to PEL rate development, loss development is the one area that has been misjudged by PEL carriers, thus being the primary reason for rate inadequacy and industry losses. Determining accurate loss development for PEL claims has been difficult to calculate for several reasons including:

- The MCO or HMO adjudicates many of the covered services, particularly hospital. The insured may have limited access to loss information, and the timing of data transfer lags behind the normal claims lag that occurs between the date of service and claim processing date.
- Many insureds lack the necessary information systems to capture and report loss data efficiently as a means to minimize lag associated with data warehousing and transmission.
- Although PEL contracts require the insured to report loss data, they often do so at the very latest point of time allowed, which can be three to six months after the renewal is effective.
- Risk pools are typically finalized 120 days after the end of the annual contract period.

Risk pool reconciliation within the risk contract places an explicit value on annual settlement after the effective date. Conversely, PEL rate development for the subsequent policy year is completed 30 to 60 days before the effective date.

- Little has been done in the way of developing PEL loss development factors from statistical models.

The most complete year of experience may not be the most recent one. For example, of experience loss data obtained as of 4/1/99 for both 1998 and 1997, 1997 would likely be considered complete or fully developed. A fully developed loss year has a loss development factor of 1.00, thus requiring no further adjustment. In our example, 1998 may require a loss development factor greater than 1.00. One way to determine whether the loss data are incomplete is to compare dates of service with paid claim dates among the members in the excess pool. If there is little incurred claim activity in the last few months, there may be additional claims outstanding that have yet to be reported. This method is effective if the loss data reflect a credible volume of excess claims. When dealing with a few large claims, identifying which claims are ongoing versus those cases that are considered to be closed can be an effective way to determine the extent of additional claims expected. For example, a member diagnosed with hemophilia could very well be incurring monthly charges for blocker medication that will continue in future months.

In lieu of loss development factors applicable for the development of excess claims within PEL coverage, loss development assessed from the total claim activity covering all covered members provides a starting benchmark for completing immature loss data. The information required for the assessment is usually derived from what is known as a *claims lag report*. It is next to impossible for PEL carriers to obtain claims lag information from the insured. IDSs and MCOs consider such information proprietary and confidential and rarely release the data. Carriers are becoming more conservative in their approach toward loss development when confronted with limited data. An example would be assigning little weight to current or incomplete loss years.

Step 6: Multiply the Total Developed Excess Claims by the Reimbursement Factor or Coinsurance

For example, IDS ABC had $200,000 in excess facility claims in 1998 at a $75,000 specific attachment level. The excess claims net of coinsurance of 10 percent is $180,000, or $200,000 × .90.

Step 7: Convert the Excess Claims Derived in Step 6 to a PMPM Value Using Total Covered Member Months Corresponding to the Developed Loss Period

Member months are the cumulative value of monthly covered members. Because insureds typically remit stop-loss premium on a monthly basis, covered member data for each month is information that can be quickly accessed by the PEL carrier. Member months may be adjusted or "lagged" to accurately determine the member months correlating with the loss experience. PEL carriers will use member month lags when confronted with member growth over the loss period. Table 53–3 illustrates an example of lagging covered members three months. Lagging covered members by three months produced a member months' total of 79,591, 12,546 less than the nonlagged total.

To convert excess claims to a PMPM value, divide the excess claims by the lagged member months.

Step 8: Convert the Excess Claims PMPM to a Premium Value PMPM

Divide the excess claims PMPM by the administrative load factor to gross up the claims PMPM. The administrative load factor is equal to 1 minus the underwriting expense ratio. For example, if the PEL carrier uses an expense ratio of 35 percent, the administrative load factor is .65.

Table 53–3 Illustration of Three-Month Lagged Member Months Compared with Zero-Month Lagged Member Months

Month	Covered Members	Covered Members April to March (0-month lag)	Covered Members April to March (3-month lag)
January	5,000		
February	5,250		
March	5,513		
April	5,789	5,789	5,000
May	6,078	6,078	5,250
June	6,382	6,382	5,513
July	6,701	6,701	5,789
August	7,036	7,036	6,078
September	7,388	7,388	6,382
October	7,757	7,757	6,701
November	8,145	8,145	7,036
December	8,552	8,552	7,388
January	8,980	8,980	7,757
February	9,429	9,429	8,145
March	9,900	9,900	8,552
Member months:		92,137	79,591

Given the lag of time that occurs from the date of service to the date the claim is processed, 79,591 member months is representative of the member months corresponding to the total claims for the same 12-month period.

Step 9: Blend the Manual Premium Rate PMPM with the Experience Premium Rate PMPM Derived from Step 8

Manual and experience are blended using a credibility factor. Credibility is the concept of assigning a numeric weight between zero and one to the premium rate PMPM. Credibility values differ for hospital and physician expenses, but the basis for derivation is the same. The most common method for establishing credibility for hospital excess claims involves member months. Credibility factors developed from a model using a large volume of claims data incorporate the expected number of excess claims per thousand as the basis of the credibility calculation. The expected number of excess claims per thousand for hospital expenses varies depending on three factors:[12]

- reimbursement basis of hospital expenses (i.e., per diem or discounted charges)
- average cost per day
- specific attachment

The general concepts of how the variables affect credibility levels are given below.

Credibility Decreases As the Specific Attachment Increases

As the specific attachment increases, members penetrate the specific threshold less frequently, and observations of frequency and severity are more volatile. The law of large numbers is observed much less at the higher deductibles. Less statistical certainty means less credibility.

Credibility Increases As the Average Cost per Day Increases

A higher average cost per day will produce greater frequency above the specific threshold, and thus greater credibility.

Credibility Is Generally Greater for Discounted Charges As Opposed to Level Per Diem

Hospital expenses reimbursed under a discounted charge method will produce a greater number of claims in excess of the specific attachment.

Cost and deductible affect credibility relative to physician expenses in the same manner. The greater the cost stated as conversion factor, the higher the credibility. The greater the specific attachment, the lower the credibility. Physician excess rating generally produces higher credibility factors compared with hospital excess for the same number of covered members. The relative higher frequency of services, less volatility of excess claim amounts observed, and a relatively greater number of excess claims given the lower specific attachment levels account for the higher credibility.

The formula to derive the credibility factor on the basis of the number of expected excess claims per thousand covered members is shown in Exhibit 53–11.

Once the experience credibility factor is derived as illustrated in Exhibit 53–10, the factor is then multiplied by the experience premium rate PMPM. The manual premium rate PMPM is then multiplied by one minus the credibility factor. The two weighted premium PMPM values are added together to derive the blended premium rate PMPM.

Credibility factors serve only as a means for developing blended rates on the basis of the manual premium rate and experience. What PEL carriers do with the results varies by each carrier. There are, however, some basic underwriting concepts that come into play:

- PEL carriers are more likely to require two or more complete years of loss data for insureds that are 50 percent or more credible.
- PEL carriers are more likely to give more weight to the most recent complete year of loss data.

Exhibit 53–11 Credibility Formula for Provider Excess Loss Rating

N = the number of expected excess claims above a given specific attachment at a given average cost basis.	Expected excess claims per 1,000 covered members are provided in lookup tables in the rating manual.
Example:	
Hospital rate development using discounted charge as the reimbursement basis, a $50,000 specific attachment, and an average cost per day of $1,500 per day. Member months are 120,000 or 10,000 average per month.	The expected excess claims per 1,000 covered members is .65 based on the variables: $50,000 attachment, $1,500 cost per day, and discounted charge reimbursement basis.

Credibility calculation: square of N divided by 11
1. N = .65 × 10 = 6.5.
2. Square root of N = 2.5495098
3. 2.5495098/11 = .2318
Credibility assigned to experience is 23.2%. The manual rating is assigned 76.8%.

Source: Data from *1999 Provider Stop-Loss Rate Manual: Hospital Excess,* V-2, © 1999, Towers Perrin.

- PEL carriers are more likely to give more weight in their final rate development to experience rates if such rates are higher than manual.

It is important to note that rate development methods serve only as guidelines for determining the final proposed rates. The final rates reflect not only sound actuarial and underwriting logic but also marketing forces as well such as creating the ability to write other lines of insurance. This concludes the discussion on specific PEL rate development. The discussion now turns to aggregate PEL rate development.

AGGREGATE EXCESS RATE DEVELOPMENT

Aggregate rate development is the process of determining the premium rate PMPM to charge for providing excess protection should total claims *less than* the specific threshold per member per period exceed a given attachment point. The attachment point is established at a given percentage above the expected claims PMPM. IDSs who purchase this type of PEL coverage do so with the objective of providing some protec-tion in the event claim expenses exceed capitated revenue. PEL carriers typically do not offer aggregate excess coverage on full medical or hospital risk contracts. Coverage is generally reserved for carved-out capitated contracts covering low-severity, high-frequency type services such as behavioral health, single specialty professional, and prescription drugs.

The objective of manual rating is to develop a PMPM medical expense value for both in-network and OON expenses.[13] Models are constructed that show the expense categories for hospital inpatient and outpatient, professional, and ancillary. PMPM values are derived for each expense category using utilization per thousand units and average cost of unit. To arrive at the net medical expense PMPM, adjustments are made for member copays and coinsurance, as well as Medicare and Medicaid utilization relative to commercial risk.[14] In-network and OON net medical expense values are weighted on the basis of the distribution of in-network and OON services.[15] At this point, further adjustments are made that will be discussed in the following section. Exhibit 53–12 shows how the net expense PMPM is derived for inpatient hospital expenses.

Exhibit 53–12 Calculation of Commercial Inpatient Hospital Expense PMPM

Inpatient Service	Days Per 1,000	Cost Per Day	Gross PMPM	Member Coinsurance/ Copay PMPM	Net PMPM
Medical/surgical	175.0	$1,300.00	$18.96	$0.00	$18.96
Maternity	32.5	$900.00	$2.44	$0.00	$2.44
Psychiatric	21.5	$500.00	$0.90	$0.00	$0.90
Substance abuse	14.8	$450.00	$0.55	$0.00	$0.55
Skilled nursing	6.3	$250.00	$0.13	$0.00	$0.13
	250.0	$1,102.80	$22.98	$0.00	$22.98

Gross PMPM = $$\frac{\text{Days per 1,000} \times \text{Cost per day}}{12,000}$$

Member coinsurance or copay PMPM = $$\frac{\text{Dollar value of coinsurance or copay per utilization unit} \times \text{units per 1,000}}{12,000}$$

Net PMPM = Gross PMPM − Member coinsurance or copay PMPM

Source: Data from *1999 Provider Aggregate Stop-Loss Manual*, II.1-II.6, © 1999, Towers Perrin.

Variables Affecting Manual Aggregate PEL Rating

The variables affecting manual rate development, some of which have already been addressed in the specific manual discussion, are listed below.

Location of Members

OON expenses are impacted by the geographical location of the service area. Providers who are not included in the contracted, in-network panel of providers will typically bill according to reasonable and customary levels. These levels vary by geographical location. The location also provides the reference point for in-network and OON utilization.

Plan of Benefits

The development of expense factors should possess the ability to handle various types of HMO and POS plans. The plan benefit has an impact on the observation of frequency or utilization. For example, a plan with an office visit copay of $15 compared with one with a copay of $5 will have fewer total office visits, all other things being equal.

Reimbursement Method

How expenses are reimbursed and the level or valuation of reimbursement has an impact on the cost of each unit, which is the second component of the PMPM expense calculation. For example, hospital in-network expenses may be reimbursed using a per diem schedule that includes one rate for medical/surgical bed days and another rate for intensive care bed days.

Type of Population Covered

The type of risk (i.e., commercial, Medicare, or Medicaid) has an impact on the net expense PMPM factor. Adjustments are made on the basis of observed utilization differences between Medicare or Medicaid and commercial risk.

Age/Sex Adjustment

The net medical expense PMPM is adjusted by the composite age/sex factor, which applies to commercial and Medicaid risk, if Medicaid demographics are available.[16] Medicare aged 65 and older may not require any demographic input (i.e., a default factor is used).

Group Size

The observed medical expenses exceeding the attachment point (aggregate claims) under simulation analysis decrease as the covered member population increases.[17] This is explained by the presence of increased dispersion observed around the average aggregate claims exceeding a given attachment point. The volatility lends weight to the argument that aggregate coverage is volatile and too risky for PEL carriers to offer, given that most potential clients are IDSs with relatively small member bases.

Specific Attachment

Aggregate coverage is generally written, and sometimes required, with specific excess coverage. The two coverages must be coordinated to remove the impact of specific excess claims PMPM from the expected total claims PMPM. The higher the specific attachment point, the greater the expected aggregate excess claims because of a larger value of each member's total claims accumulating under the aggregate coverage.

Attachment Point above the Expected Medical Expense PMPM

Aggregate coverage seldom attaches at the expected claim level. Attachment points, the level where excess claims must exceed for coverage to respond, range from 105 to 125 percent of expected claims PMPM. As the attachment point increases, the claims expected to exceed the attachment decrease.

Reimbursement Factor or Coinsurance

Aggregate PEL coverage promises to reimburse the insured for eligible claims that exceed the attachment point. The reimbursement may be 100 percent of the excess amount, or less (i.e., 50 to 90 percent). There appears to be no rule established for aggregate coverage other than 90 percent might be selected more often simply because it is the standard for specific coverage.

PEL Carrier Expense Ratio or Target Loss Ratio

The aggregate claims PMPM is adjusted in the same manner as described for specific rating.

Aggregate PEL coverage is ideally suited for single service specialty contracts because of the high frequency and low severity of individual claims. Self-insured employers who have been carving out their mental health and prescription drug benefits recognize the financial savings realized through specialty vendors capable of delivering improved performance from large economies of scale measured in member purchasing power. Vendors who specialized in single-service risk bring innovative systems and provider network management. Single-service professional risk remains relatively immature among the various types of risk contracting. The number of members required to reduce volatility to achieve significant confident levels can range from 5,000 to 75,000, depending on the specialty. Nephrology, for example, requires a minimum of 75,000 members to obtain acceptable actuarial credibility on a single-service capitated basis.[18] PEL carriers are more likely to entertain aggregate coverage for carve-out contracts; however, the HMO often provides built-in contract protection in the case of utilization fluctuation over a specified percentage of the capitated rate.

Aggregate coverage has its purpose, but PEL carriers will remain reluctant to offer this type of protection over a full-service or hospital risk contract. Carriers normally require either two complete years of actual experience or the actuarial development of the capitated rate. Both are difficult to come by. Single-service capitated rates are often derived from the experience pool of the HMO, subject to adjustments through the negotiation process. HMOs seldom release experience to the PEL carrier at the request of the potential insured. Actuarial capitated rate development from an objective third party is always suggested, even if the HMO provides the IDS with its methodology of rate development. For aggregate PEL coverage to become more prevalent, risk pool results measured as actual claims against capitated revenue must improve overall and exhibit less volatility.

PEL POLICY COVERAGE FORM

Once the carrier determines the premium rates it will propose and if successful coverage is bound, a policy is then issued that stipulates the terms and conditions of the coverage. The insured does not have to wait until coverage is bound to view the policy. Insurers customarily send out specimen policy forms to insurance brokers and potential insureds. The provider excess policy issued to the insured contains several provisions that are similar to other excess insurance contracts covering morbidity risk. PEL coverage does, however, contain some unique definitions and provisions that are discussed in the following, beginning with definitions.

Definitions

Types of Care Facilities Defined

Covered members receive care at a variety of facilities, all within the network. The various types of facilities defined in the PEL policy are considered to be standard for medical insurance and are similar to the MCO's set of facility definitions. The major facilities, providers, or care programs defined include:

- chemical dependency treatment facility
- extended care facility
- home health care agency
- hospice
- hospital
- intensive care unit
- physician
- primary care physician
- rehabilitation facility
- specialty care physician

Eligible Service

This definition restricts an eligible service as one that is not only medically necessary but is defined as a covered service for which the insured is financially responsible. The insured's financial responsibility of covered services is often depicted in what is referred to as a "responsibility matrix" (see Exhibit 53–13).

In-Network

The in-network definition according to the standard PEL policy associates in-network providers as those who have entered into a written contract with the insured to provide contracted services at predetermined rates. Many IDSs, such as IPAs, accept risk for hospital services, yet the IPA is not a party to the hospital contract between the facility and the HMO. The empha-

Exhibit 53–13 Responsibility Matrix

		Hospital	IPA	Health Plan	MH Provider	Not Covered
				Responsibility		
Inpatient hospital	Medical	X				
	Surgical	X				
	ICU	X				
	CCU	X				
	NICU	X				
	PICU	X				
	Boarder baby	X				
	Maternity—normal delivery	X				
	Maternity—C section	X				
	SNF/ECF	X				
	OOA admissions			X		
	Chemotherapy drugs—inpatient	X				
	Hemodialysis—inpatient facility	X				
	Organ & tissue transplants	X				
	Rehabilitation—inpatient facility	X				
	Transitional care—inpatient	X				
	Psychiatric				X	
	Substance abuse				X	
	Detox—facility				X	
Outpatient hospital	Outpatient surgery—facility	X				
	Emergency department in area—facility	X				
	Emergency department OOA—facility			X		
	Radiology—outpatient technical[a]	X				
	Radiation therapy—facility	X				
	Chemotherapy drugs—outpatient	X				
	Nuclear medicine—facility	X				
	Hemodialysis—outpatient facility	X				
	Pathology—outpatient technical[a]	X				
	Anesthesia—facility	X				
	Physical therapy, OT, ST—facility	X				
	Rehabilitation—outpatient facility	X				
	Other outpatient facility	X				
Physician	Allergy testing		X			
	Anesthesia—professional		X			
	Authorized referrals		X			
	Chemotherapy—drugs (office)		X			
	Chemotherapy—professional		X			

continues

Exhibit 53–13 continued

		Responsibility				
		Hospital	IPA	Health Plan	MH Provider	Not Covered
	Chiropractic		X			
	Consultations		X			
	Detox—professional				X	
	Family planning		X			
	Hearing screening		X			
	Hemodialysis—professional		X			
	Home care visits		X			
	Hospital visits		X			
	Immunizations		X			
	Injections—admin. by medical professional		X			
	Laboratory—professional		X			
	Mammograms		X			
	Mental health—professional				X	
	Nuclear medicine—professional		X			
	OB/GYN—C section		X			
	OB/GYN—normal delivery		X			
	Office visit medical supplies		X			
	Office visits		X			
	Organ transplants—professional		X			
	Outpatient diagnostic services		X			
	Physical exams		X			
	Physical therapy, OT, ST—professional		X			
	Radiation therapy—professional		X			
	Radiology—professional		X			
	Rehabilitation—professional		X			
	SNF visits		X			
	Surgery fees		X			
	Vision screening		X			
	Well adult		X			
	Well baby/child		X			
	Unlisted codes		X			
Other (Ancillary)	Injections—self-administered			X		
	Insulin & syringes			X		
	Medications—O/P self-administered			X		
	Outpatient prescription drugs			X		
	Home health total care	X				
	Home health infusion	X				
	Hospice	X				
	Contacts/glasses					X
	TMJ					X
	Infertility treatment					X
	DME	X				
	Prosthetics/orthotics	X				
	Ambulance	X				

[a]Services for hospital-based physicians who bill separately are not included.

sis for satisfying the definition is placed on the words "written contract." HMO agreements that are established in writing with facilities for the purpose of a global risk contract would be considered in-network as defined by the provider agreement with the HMO. The fact that the IPA reciprocates to the HMO hospital contract does not nullify the in-network status.

OOA Emergency

The purpose of this definition is to clearly define what is considered OOA treatment. Emergency services can be delivered in-network, OON, or OOA. By definition, OOA emergency refers to emergency services delivered by providers outside the area. MCOs tend to insert the word "service" in front of "area" so that the reference is to emergency services outside the service area, which is defined in the provider agreement between the MCO and IDS.

OON

In contrast to in-network services, OON services are those services that are delivered by providers with whom the HMO or IDS does not have a written agreement—that is to say, those providers who do not meet the definition of in-network.

Paid

The definition of "paid" is unique to stop-loss insurance. It carries a similar definition to its counterpart in employer stop-loss contracts but has been modified for capitated services. For noncapitated services, paid is defined as the date a check or draft is issued for payment of service. Capitated services are treated differently because a check or payment directly related to the specific service is never generated. Providers who accept capitated payments are prepaid on the basis of the assigned members regardless of the number of services performed. PEL carriers generally define a paid capitated service by the date the service is debited to the individual provider's risk pool or capitated account.

Referral Services

Referral services are defined in the provider agreement and the PEL policy. Referral services

qualify as eligible services provided such services are authorized by the IDS or HMO and are listed as covered services in the provider agreement.

Reported

The definition of "reported" is critical to the reporting of potential excess claims under the PEL policy and is expanded on further in the policy section covering the administration of claims. Reported refers to the date that the PEL carrier receives written notice of claim.

Totally Confined

The definition of "totally confined" refers to a covered member confined to a hospital or any other institution. The purpose of the definition relates to the totally confined limitation, which will be discussed in the next section.

Limitations

PEL coverage is designed to cover the exact services the insured is financially responsible for as outlined in the provider agreement with the HMO. Any limitations stated in the provider agreement apply to the PEL coverage as well. One limitation found in PEL coverage is unique—the totally confined provision. The provision has its history with employer stop-loss. In the late 1970s and continuing through today, self-funded medical plans have become increasingly popular among employers. Insurance companies offering stop-loss coverage to employers self-funding for the first time were able to limit their exposure in the first year of coverage by excluding claims incurred by employees and dependents who were considered totally disabled on the effective date of coverage. The provision was generally removed in the subsequent coverage years provided the insured disclosed potential large claim activity to the carrier.

The provision made its way to PEL policies in much the same manner with a different definition of totally disabled. The intent of the provision is to exclude claims incurred by covered members who are confined in a hospital or other such institution. Eventually, carriers began using the phrase "totally confined." The limitation is applied as follows:

- A covered member must be considered totally confined by satisfying the definition of totally confined.
- If the member is totally confined, any charges incurred before the date the member ceases to be totally confined are excluded from accumulation toward the attachment.

This provision can have serious implications for insureds. Its applicability in risk contracting and provider stop-loss is challenged for two reasons:

- The limitation focuses on institutional claims, which are adjudicated in many instances by the HMO. The insured seldom receives timely information to quantify the risk or provide disclosure to the carrier with any confidence and accuracy.
- Risk contracting is dynamic in that insureds are constantly expanding their penetration in at-risk contracts. Additional contracts are added and large volumes of members are transferred to an existing contract. The possible risk resulting from the totally confined provision is considered to be impossible to assess by most insureds, therefore making it nearly impossible to absorb the potential risk. In recent years, carriers have begun to waive the provision, but contingencies for binding coverage have become more stringent through the use of disclosure of known claims and even the right to change the renewal rates retroactively because of developed excess losses exceeding those expected.

Policy Provisions

Changes to Provider Agreement

PEL carriers reserve the right to review any changes relating to policyholder, provider agreement or HMO subscriber agreement by requesting advance notice of such changes. After completion of its review, the carrier can either alter the terms of the existing policy or terminate coverage subject to proper written notice. The provision may be further expanded in contract language to include right of review should the insured add new contracts.

Premium Change

The premium change provision allows the carrier to change the premium under specific circumstances:

- change in the PEL coverage provided
- policyholder change
- provider agreement change
- HMO subscriber agreement change
- on any renewal date

Most PEL policies stipulate a 31-day notice for the premium change.

Termination and Cancellation

The essential message to comprehend from this provision is that the obligations of the stop-loss carrier cease on termination or cancellation. If termination occurs before the end of the coverage period, the incurred period coinciding with the original coverage period ends at the termination date. The extended payment period allowed for eligible claims to be paid, typically six months from the end of the coverage period, becomes six months from the end of the termination date.

Administration of Claims or Reporting Eligibility of Claims

This provision addresses the insured's responsibility to report claims and the conditions in which reported claims are eligible for reimbursement. Although likely to vary depending on the PEL carrier, certain items are common among all carriers such as:

- the requirement for the insured to notify the stop-loss carrier when a covered member's claims exceed 50 percent or are likely to exceed 50 percent of the specific attachment
- a time limit for the insured to submit claims to the stop-loss carrier for which it has no record of receiving prior notification

- a time limit for the insured to submit claims to the stop-loss carrier for which it has received prior notification

Some carriers will use the provision to list the detailed information acceptable for excess claim adjudication. This is difficult to do for documentation relating to excess reimbursement requests because of the variance observed among the type of information and systems maintained by insureds. Instead, any specific data elements listed in the policy provision typically correspond to 50 percent notification.

Time limits available for the insured to report potential or known excess claims may vary by PEL carrier but typically range from 6 to 12 months for claims with no prior written notification, and 12 to 24 months for claims with prior notification.

Do carriers strictly enforce the claim administration rules all the time? In the world of procedural manuals, yes. In the real world, however, clients that carry substantial premiums occasionally push the envelope when it comes to loss reporting. Furthermore, the information carriers require to adjudicate excess claims is just now beginning to become standardized. Carriers are encouraging insureds to invest in the technology to capture the data elements for excess loss submission. This will ultimately benefit the insured by reducing the time stop-loss claim examiners spend to review each claim, thus improving reimbursement turnaround time. The loss reporting guidelines used by PEL carriers will be explained in detail after the conclusion of PEL policy coverage form.

Subrogation

Subrogation is the process of the PEL carrier establishing its right to pursue any possible recovery of an equal portion of the benefits it has paid from third parties should the covered member become ill or injured through the act or omission of a third party and if the expenses incurred under the risk contract relate to that illness or injury. What that really means is that the PEL policy stipulates that the insured must exercise its subrogation rights whenever possible and in-

vestigate, collect, and pay the PEL carrier its portion of the recovery. Types of claims that are potential candidates for subrogation are those that involve accidents (i.e., motor vehicle accidents). The provision further states that the PEL carrier will subrogate and coordinate benefits for all excess payments when potential subrogation and coordination of benefits is evident.

Appendix 53–A includes sample contract language for the definitions, limitations, and provisions described previously. This is not intended to be a complete PEL coverage form document but rather a description of the language somewhat unique to the provider stop-loss contract.

Loss Reporting Guidelines Relative to PEL

Although the actual PEL policy often contains no reference to specific data or forms, stop-loss carriers must receive timely notification and complete documentation of eligible excess claims. The insurance company distributes claim submission guidelines to the insured once coverage is bound or to potential insureds as part of the proposal. The guidelines outline the specific information sufficient for a complete claim submission. The information is separated into three areas:

- notification of members who have exceeded 50 percent of the specific attachment, as well as notification of members who have the potential to exceed the specific attachment on the basis of primary diagnosis
- verification of member eligibility
- proof of loss documentation

Each area has a required set of data elements relative to the individual claimant. These data elements are shown in Exhibit 53–14.

Notification

Notifying the carrier of potential excess claims serves two purposes: (1) it satisfies the notification requirement in the policy, and (2) it enables the carrier to establish a file and reserve amount for the claimant. PEL carriers supply their own forms but will accept other forms pro-

Exhibit 53–14 Required Data Elements for Provider Excess Loss Reporting

Data elements required for 50% or early notification
- Patient name
- Date of birth
- Sex
- Social security number or member identification number
- Plan name
- Type of member—commercial, Medicare, or Medicaid
- Member effective date
- Member termination date
- Patient relationship—self, spouse, child, or other
- Primary diagnosis code
- Primary diagnosis narrative description
- Secondary diagnosis, if known
- Expenses incurred to notification date, if known
- Projected expenses for policy period, if known
- Preparer information—name, address, telephone, fax, and e-mail address

Data elements required for verification of member eligibility (submitted to insurer when member exceeds the specific retention; member now becomes claimant)
- Plan name
- Claimant effective date
- Claimant date of birth
- Type of member—commercial, Medicare, or Medicaid
- Claimant relationship—self, spouse, child, or other

- Employer subscriber effective and termination date with the HMO
- COBRA effective and termination date, if applicable
- COB information, if applicable
- Basis of Medicare enrollee under the age of 65, if applicable
- Verification of other coverage for Medicaid claimants, if applicable (i.e., dual eligibles)

Data elements required for individual claimant request for reimbursement (detail by date of service)
- Provider name
- Beginning date of service
- Ending date of service
- Place of service (i.e., inpatient, outpatient, emergency)
- ICD-9 classification code
- Procedure code (i.e., CPT code for professional service)
- Procedure code narrative description
- Unit value (i.e., number of inpatient days)
- Billed amount
- Eligible/allowed amount—amount allowed based on valuation of covered services net of member copays
- Paid amount
- Paid date—capitation services for which individual paid dates do not exist use date credited to risk pool
- Check number—applicable to noncapitated providers
- In network, OON, OOA designation (i.e., was the service performed in-network, OON, or OOA)

Source: Data from *Provider Excess Loss Submission Guidelines II-IV,* 1999, Lexington Insurance Company, Boston, Massachusetts.

vided the information required is reported. Member threshold reports showing a list of members who have exceeded 50 percent of the attachment are generally created monthly to ensure timely notification. Developing queries to list members containing certain diagnoses such as premature birth and organ transplants can identify claimants with the potential to exceed the specific attachment.

Member Eligibility

Member eligibility data are obtained from the insured typically in the form of screen prints from the eligibility file maintained by the insured or the health plan (HMO). Insureds will sometimes include member eligibility information as part of the computerized documentation submitted for proof of loss. The purpose of eligibility data, aside from verifying that the member is covered, is to identify the existence of other coverage, a process known as coordination of benefits. The primary concern resides with commercial members, but insureds with Medicaid risk are exposed to members qualifying for Medicare coverage as a dual eligible.

Proof of Loss

Once a member exceeds the specific attachment, a minimum amount of documentation is required to adjudicate reimbursement to the insured. The information, which is shown in Exhibit 53–14, is provided in a variety of formats, ranging from manual to electronic submission. Requests for reimbursement should be sent to the PEL carrier on a quarterly basis for insureds who experience a high volume of excess claims. Regular claim submissions will provide for timely reimbursement. Insureds are beginning to improve their capabilities in the loss reporting area through software vendors offering managed care claim processing inclusive of a PEL reporting module.

COVERAGE AVAILABILITY

The sources of PEL coverage are expanding despite poor results for the 1996 and 1997 underwriting years. New entrants are able to secure reinsurance, although the conditions for reinsurance approval are becoming tighter. Reinsurance is utilized quite heavily among PEL writers. The most common form of reinsurance obtained is known as "treaty." Under treaty reinsurance, the PEL writer will cede a portion of the risk to a number of reinsurers participating on the provider excess loss treaty. In return for the proportional premium and claim risk it receives, the reinsurers remit a fee known as a ceding commission to the ceding company. The treaties are renewed each year, with the recent 1999 renewal year indicating much tougher terms for ceding companies such as large premium cases reviewed by the lead treaty underwriter.

PEL writers can be classified in one of the following categories:

- for-profit insurance companies
- managing general underwriters (MGUs)
- licensed state HMOs
- reinsurers writing on a direct basis (i.e., competing with ceding companies)
- insurance captives
- state agencies providing stop-loss protection over Medicaid contracts

Insurance companies are more stable and accept a greater percentage of the risk compared with MGUs, which appear to be at the complete mercy of the treaty reinsurers.

Although HMOs are generally more expensive, the gap is expected to shrink as carriers increase rates as a result of losses. Direct reinsurers are increasing their market presence, often at the dismay of the competition they reinsure. As long as large insurers can benefit from PEL recoveries in a marketplace characterized by increased capacity, capitalizing an insurance captive for the purpose of provider excess loss risk will remain less prominent. State agencies offering stop-loss protection for Medicaid-risk contracts to prepaid health plans is viewed as a temporary market. As states increase Medicaid managed care enrollment through the use of HCFA 1115 waivers mandating enrollment, states expect to attract private writers of PEL coverage.

CONCLUSION

The provider excess loss market thus far has been characterized by extreme volatility in pricing. The bulk of our discussion has focused on the principles of rate development. Although these principles apply industrywide, they do not guarantee that written stop-loss rates will be close to one another or reflect with any accuracy the manual rates. The use of comprehensive manual rates is less than five years old. Credible experience rating using account-specific PEL data is just recently beginning to earn widespread application. Initially, several insureds utilized PEL coverage as a profit center. PEL carriers were inexperienced in dealing with provider reimbursements. Hospitals who were accepting capitation were placing stop-loss coverage on a discounted-billed charge basis. Many of these hospitals resided in very high charge areas such as Southern California. The percent of charge generated excess claims reimbursement at a rate greater than the premium, thus supplementing the insured's risk pool balances.

In the near term, provider excess coverage will be going through its first industrywide price increase. HMO rates have bottomed out in many areas of the country and are experiencing price increases as well. Losses among PEL carriers are expected to improve for the 1998 and 1999 underwriting years but will need to improve further to meet the profit objectives of reinsurers. In response to unprofitable loss development, PEL carriers are undertaking several steps to improve profitability:

- increasing premium rates
- increasing specific attachments
- restricting coverage terms (i.e., mandating per diem limits for discounted charge innetwork and OON services)
- requiring experience for loss rating
- enforcing the claim submission guidelines to ensure quality of documentation
- reviewing the financial viability of insureds as part of the underwriting process
- implementing value-added consulting services

PEL coverage remains a viable risk-transfer option for IDSs who accept risk from MCOs. Its rate of expansion, however, is vulnerable to industry losses. The principles relative to how the coverage works, the variables affecting rate development, and basic policy form will remain constant.

REFERENCES AND NOTES

1. *1999 Provider Stop-Loss Rate Manual: Hospital Excess* (Minneapolis, MN: Towers Perrin, 1998), II-1.
2. *1999 Provider Stop-Loss Rate Manual: Hospital Excess,* IV-Table 5.
3. *1999 Provider Stop-Loss Rate Manual: Hospital Excess,* III-2.
4. *1999 Provider Stop-Loss Rate Manual: Physician Excess* (Minneapolis, MN: Towers Perrin, 1998), II-2.
5. *1999 St. Anthony's Complete RBRVS* (Reston, VA: St. Anthony Publishing, Inc., 1999), Preface.
6. R.A. Bereson and R.N. Lieberman, *Special Report: Using Medicare's RBRVS to Evaluate Capitation and Fee Schedules* (Reston, VA: St. Anthony Publishing, Inc., 1995), 5.
7. *1999 St. Anthony's Complete RBRVS,* 14.
8. *1999 Provider Stop-Loss Rate Manual: Physician Excess,* III-Worksheet 2A-2E.
9. *1999 Provider Stop-Loss Rate Manual: Physician Excess,* IV-Table 5.
10. *1999 Provider Stop-Loss Rate Manual: Physician Excess,* IV-Table 2.
11. *1999 Provider Stop-Loss Rate Manual: Physician Excess,* II-2.
12. *1999 Provider Stop-Loss Rate Manual: Hospital Excess,* V-Exhibit 1.
13. *1999 Provider Aggregate Stop-Loss Manual* (Minneapolis, MN: Towers Perrin, 1998), II-1-II-6.
14. *1999 Provider Aggregate Stop-Loss Rate Manual,* II-1-II-6.
15. *1999 Provider Aggregate Stop-Loss Rate Manual,* II-1-II-6.
16. *1999 Provider Aggregate Stop-Loss Rate Manual,* II-1-II-6.
17. *1999 Provider Aggregate Stop-Loss Rate Manual,* II-1-II-6.
18. *Membership Enrollment Guidelines for Single Specialty Risk Contracting* (Atlanta, GA: Milliman and Robertson, 1996).

SUGGESTED READING

1999 Provider Stop-Loss Rate Manuals: Hospital, Physician and Aggregate. 1998. Minneapolis, MN: Towers Perrin.

1999 St. Anthony's Complete RBRVS. 1999. Reston, VA: St. Anthony Publishing, Inc.

Bereson, R.A., and Lieberman, R.N. 1995. *Special Report: Using Medicare's RBRVS to Evaluate Capitation and Fee Schedules.* Reston, VA: St. Anthony Publishing, Inc.

Appendix 53–A

Sample PEL Policy Language

I. DEFINITIONS

Types of Care Facilities:

Chemical dependency treatment facility means an institution licensed by the laws of the state where it is located as a Chemical Dependency Treatment Facility, and which:

(1) operates within the scope of its license;
(2) provides 24-hour-a-day nursing care furnished or supervised by registered graduate nurses;
(3) maintains daily clinical records on each patient;
(4) has the services of a physician available at all times under an established agreement;
(5) has treatment policies developed with the advice of, and reviewed by, a group of professionals who are specialists in the care and treatment of chemical dependency;
(6) has a utilization review plan in effect;
(7) has transfer arrangements with at least one hospital; and
(8) uses appropriate methods to dispense and administer drugs and medicines.

Source: Reprinted with permission from *Provider Excess Loss Indemnity Policy,* pp. 7–22, © 1999, Lexington Insurance Company, Boston, Massachusetts.

Extended care facility means:

(1) an institution owned, operated by or affiliated with a hospital (by written agreement); or
(2) a separate and distinct part of a hospital; or
(3) any other institution or part of an institution meeting the requirements established for approved operation under Medicare.

Such institution must be operated and licensed in accordance with the laws of the state and locality where located. It must maintain daily medical records for each patient and be primarily engaged in providing, under the supervision of a physician or staff physicians whose services are available at all times:

(1) room and board; and
(2) 24-hour-a-day inpatient skilled nursing services by, or under the supervision of, a full-time registered nurse (RN); and
(3) other necessary medical services.

Home health care agency means an agency or organization which:

(1) is primarily engaged in and is federally qualified or state certified as a home health agency and duly licensed, if such licensing is required, by the appropriate licensing authority, to provide nursing and other therapeutic services;

(2) has policies which are established by a professional group associated with such agency or organization, including at least one physician and at least one registered nurse (RN);

(3) provides for full-time supervision of such services by a physician or by a registered nurse (RN);

(4) maintains a complete medical record on each patient; and

(5) has its own administrator.

Hospice means a facility or program engaged in providing palliative and supportive care of the terminally ill, which is licensed, certified or otherwise authorized pursuant to the law and jurisdiction in which the services are performed and received.

Hospital means an institution which:

(1) is licensed and operated as a hospital under the laws of the jurisdiction where it is located; and

(2) provides, as its primary function, for pay on an inpatient basis:
   (a) facilities for medical and surgical diagnosis and therapy; and
   (b) treatment and care of the sick and injured; and

(3) is under the direction of a staff of physicians; and

(4) provides 24-hour-a-day nursing services by registered nurses (RN); and

(5) has facilities on the premises for major surgery.

An institution which lacks surgical facilities may still be considered a hospital if it has a written contractual arrangement with an accredited hospital for the performance of major surgery.

Hospital will *not* include an institution used as a facility for:

(1) rest; or

(2) custodial care; or

(3) nursing; or

(4) care for the aged; or

(5) care for alcoholics or drug addicts.

Intensive care unit means a type of hospital accommodation to provide the level of services necessary for:

(1) the care of critically ill patients who require constant audio-visual observation under the supervision of a registered graduate nurse that is prescribed by a physician; and

(2) the provision of all necessary life saving equipment, drugs, and supplies for immediate use.

Physician means a person duly licensed or certified to treat the type of injury or illness for which a claim is made, and one who is practicing within the scope of his/her license.

Primary care physician means a physician under contract with the policyholder that is selected by a covered member to be responsible for providing or arranging for the covered member's eligible services, and for maintaining the covered member's medical records.

Rehabilitation facility means an institution licensed as a rehabilitation hospital by the laws of the state where it is located, and which:

(1) is operated within the scope of its license;

(2) provides 24-hour-a-day nursing care furnished or supervised by registered graduate nurses;

(3) maintains daily clinical records on each patient;

(4) has the services of a physician available at all times under an established agreement;

(5) uses appropriate methods to dispense and administer drugs and medicines;

(6) has transfer arrangement with at least one hospital;

(7) has a utilization review plan in effect; and

(8) has treatment policies developed with the advice of, and reviewed by, a group of professionals who are specialists in the care and treatment provided by the institution.

Specialty care physician means a physician that is under contract with the policyholder to provide physician services of a specialized nature to a covered member upon referral of that covered member's primary care physician.

Eligible Service:

Eligible service means a medically necessary service, treatment or supply which is:

(1) included as a covered service in the subscriber agreement;
(2) specified in the capitated provider agreement as being the responsibility solely of the policyholder to provide to a covered member; and
(3) shown in the schedule of insurance as an eligible service.

In-Network:

In network means any hospital, physician or other health care or medical service provider, who has entered into a written agreement with the policyholder to provide health care services and/or treatment to covered members in exchange for pre-determined pricing. It also means any provider in which or in whom the policyholder has an ownership interest.

Out-of-Area Emergency:

Out-of-area emergency means those hospital services, physicians services and all other medical services provided to a covered member and which, due to an emergency, are provided outside the network of the named insured. An emergency exists when there is a sudden onset of illness or accidental injury that occurs outside the network of the named insured and requires such immediate treatment that the life of the covered member might be jeopardized if taken to a hospital, physician, or surgeon within the network of the named insured.

Out-of-Network:

Out-of-network means those providers of health care services who do not meet the definition of in-network provider.

Paid:

Paid means the date on which the policyholder tenders a draft or check in payment, the date on which an itemized bill is generated by a provider or the date the provider otherwise settles any such amount due for eligible expenses incurred by a covered member. If no date is indicated on an itemized bill, it will be treated as if billed on the 7th day before receipt by the company.

Referral Services:

Referral services means those eligible expenses which, due to the specialized nature of the service or facility required, are not available and cannot be provided in network. These services must be specifically authorized by the policyholder and/or the managed care organization, and such services, treatments or supplies must be covered services under the subscriber's agreement.

Reported:

Reported means the date that written notice of claim is received by the company.

Totally Confined:

Totally confined means that due to illness or injury, a covered member is confined in a hospital, extended care facility or other such institution.

II. LIMITATIONS

Totally Confined:

If a covered member is totally confined on the effective date of this policy, any charges incurred prior to the date such covered member ceases to be totally confined will be excluded from the definition of eligible services and will not be used to satisfy the specific retention amount, nor will such charge serve as the basis of any benefit payable under this policy.

III. POLICY PROVISIONS

Changes to Provider Agreement:

The policyholder shall give the company written notice at least 45 days in advance of any policyholder change, capitated provider agreement change or subscriber agreement change, as defined herein.

Upon receipt of the written notice of a policyholder change, capitated provider agreement change, or subscriber agreement change, the company shall have the right to review each change on an individual basis and either accept or reject the change. If the change is rejected, the company shall have the right to terminate this policy by giving written notice by registered mail, which shall set forth the date of such termination which shall not be sooner than thirty-one (31) days after the date of delivery of such notice.

If the company elects to accept the policyholder change, capitated provider agreement change, or subscriber agreement change, it shall have the right to change the premium or provisions of the policy. Such change will become effective, either concurrent with the effective date of such policyholder change, capitated provider agreement change, subscriber agreement change, or on some other date mutually agreed upon by the company and the policyholder.

Premium Change:

Premium change: The company has the right to change the premium as a result of:

(1) change in the insurance provided herein;
(2) a policyholder change;
(3) a capitated provider agreement change;
(4) a subscriber agreement change;
(5) or at any renewal date as specified in Section IX, Renewal.

The company will provide the policyholder with at least 31 days written notice of such premium change.

Termination and Cancellation:

Termination: This policy and all insurance provided hereunder will terminate upon the earliest of:

(1) the due date of any premium not paid, subject to the grace period;
(2) the premium due date next following the company's receipt of written notice from the policyholder that this policy is to be terminated;
(3) the end of the policy period shown in the schedule of insurance, unless the company and the policyholder agree upon renewal terms;
(4) the date of termination of the subscriber agreement; capitated provider agreement or the covered plan(s);
(5) the date the policyholder suspends or ceases active business operation or is placed in bankruptcy or receivership;
(6) the date the policyholder's business is dissolved; or
(7) the cancellation date as explained under the terms of the cancellation provision of this policy.

Cancellation: This policy may be canceled by the policyholder by mailing to the company written notice which states when thereafter such cancellation shall be effective. This policy may be canceled by the company by mailing to the policyholder at the address shown in the schedule of insurance, written notice which states when, not less than 30 days thereafter, such cancellation shall be effective for any of the following reasons:

(1) fraud, misrepresentation or failure to comply with the terms and conditions of this policy by the policyholder;
(2) policyholder change, capitated provider agreement change or subscriber agreement change as defined in this policy;
(3) failure of the policyholder to act in accordance with the subrogation provision.

Termination or cancellation of this policy shall not terminate the rights or liabilities of either the policyholder or the company which arise during any period this policy was in force, provided that nothing herein shall be construed to extend the company's liability for payments under this policy for any losses incurred by the policyholder on or after the date of termination or cancellation of this policy. If the policyholder's insurance under this policy terminates prior to the end of the policy period, then the claims basis period shall also end on that date. However, claims basis payment will continue to be considered for any charge incurred for eligible services prior to the termination date for a period not to exceed 6 months from said termination date.

Administration of Claims:

The policyholder shall be responsible, at its own cost and expense, for the investigation, settlement, or defense of any claim made, or suit brought, or proceedings instated against the policyholder. The company, at its own election and expense, shall have the right to participate with the policyholder in the defense or appeal of any action, suit or proceedings in which they may, in their sole judgment, become involved.

The policyholder shall:

(1) Supervise the administration and adjustment of all claims and verify the validity, accuracy, and computation;
(2) Maintain accurate records of all charges for eligible services;
(3) Submit monthly reports to the company giving details of eligible services for all covered members where the total sum of eligible services at the close of each month exceeds fifty percent (50%), or can reasonably be expected to exceed fifty percent (50%) of the specific retention amount shown in the schedule of insurance. Details to include name of the covered member, date enrolled under the covered plan, date injury or illness first manifested itself, nature of injury or illness, date of admissions as an inpatient, date of commencement of hospital inpa-

tient services and estimated likely total costs during the policy period.

The company shall not be liable for claims for which written notification was not provided to the company within seven (7) months after the expiration date of the policy period shown in the schedule of insurance.

Claims that have been put on notice to the company may not be filed under the policy any later than twelve (12) months after the expiration date of the policy period as shown in the schedule of insurance.

The company shall not be liable for the fulfillment of any obligation prior to the receipt of information in reasonable form satisfactory to the company. Incorrect information furnished may be corrected, if the company has not acted to its prejudice by relying on it.

Subrogation:

Subrogation: If a covered member is injured or becomes ill through the act or omission of a third party, and if expenses are incurred under the covered plan due to that injury or illness, then to the extent the policyholder recovers any amount for expenses incurred for that same injury or illness from the covered member due to reimbursement from a third party, or its insurer, the company shall be entitled to a refund of an equal portion of the benefits it has paid as a result of the policyholder's expenses incurred for that same injury or illness. The policyholder shall prosecute any and all valid claims against third parties arising out of a loss which results in incurring expenses under the covered plan. Any amount of payment recovered by the policyholder from a third party or insurer shall be accounted for.

The policyholder shall fully exercise its rights under any coordination of benefits provision incorporated in the covered plan. Should the policyholder fail to fully exercise its coordination of benefits rights under the covered plan, or prosecute any valid claims against third parties or insurers, and the company thereupon becomes liable to make payment to the policyholder under terms and conditions of this policy, the company shall then be subrogated to all of the policyholder's coordination of benefits rights under the covered plan, and rights against such third parties or insurers. Any amount of payment the company recovered due to the exercising of the coordination of benefits provision, or from a subrogated third party or insurer for any amount that it may have paid or becomes liable to pay to the policyholder under the terms of this policy, shall be used to pay for expenses incurred for collection and reimbursement from such coordination of benefits, or subrogated third party or insurer. All remaining amounts shall be paid to the policyholder.

PART VI

Special Market Segments

"We're One
But we're not the same"

Bono [1991]

CHAPTER 54

The Federal Employees Health Benefits Program and Managed Care

Christine C. Rinn

The Federal Employees Health Benefits Program (FEHBP), with its coverage of approximately 10 million federal employees and annuitants and their dependents, represents the largest employer-sponsored health benefits program in the United States today. The Federal Employees Health Benefits Act, 5 U.S. Code 8901 et seq. (FEHBA) established the FEHBP. The federal Office of Personnel Management (OPM) administers the FEHBP. The FEHBA authorizes OPM to offer certain choices of health benefits plans to federal employees. These choices include government-wide plans and employee organization plans, as well as comprehensive health plans. Most of the comprehensive health plans are health maintenance organizations (HMOs) and represent a significant presence by OPM as a purchaser of managed care services. Government-wide and employee organization plans are experience rated, and HMOs are predominantly community rated.

The focus of this chapter is the FEHBP's relationship to HMOs, with particular emphasis on continuing controversies over HMO rating practices under the FEHBP. Also discussed are issues related to benefit design, federal employee–HMO relationships, and federal preemption of state laws.

One of the key reasons why rating issues are particularly significant is that FEHBP contracting is not a competitive bidding process. More-

over, historically, OPM did not exercise its purchasing power (at least on the front end of the rate proposal process) to achieve a better rate. More recently, however, OPM has adopted rating requirements for the FEHBP that, in effect, achieve the financial benefits of competitive bidding for the FEHBP with respect to the health plan's two employer groups that are most similar in size to the FEHBP.

OPM contracts with approximately 350 comprehensive medical plans, almost all of which are community-rated plans. Comprehensive medical plans may be group practice, individual practice, or mixed model plans, depending on the configuration of the HMO's provider delivery system. Community rating, in its most simplistic terms, means that the rates charged to an employer group represent costs spread across the community and not just the experience of a particular account. HMOs that are federally qualified under the federal HMO law are required to be community rated by that statute, and OPM, under the FEHBA, has an affirmative obligation to offer federally qualified HMOs that meet the requirements of the FEHBP.[1]

Amendments to the federal HMO law changed community rating over the years, thereby adding to the complexity of determining whether the HMO is truly offering a community rate to the FEHBP. In light of this complexity, OPM is concerned whether certain HMO contractors are engaged in a pattern of discounting of certain nonfederal employer groups. In an effort to curb these abuses and simplify program

Christine C. Rinn is a principal in the law firm of Michaels & Bonner, P.C., in Washington, DC.

administration, OPM has moved away from community rating requirements to a "market price" concept in which the focus is on how the rates charged to the FEHBP compare with those charged to the contractor's two subscriber groups that are most similar to the FEHBP. How similarity is defined varies with the contract year and is discussed later.

THE APPLICATION PROCESS

Plans interested in participating in the FEHBP must submit an application letter to OPM by January 31 of the year preceding the year in which their contract will be effective.[2] To be approved for the FEHBP, a carrier must demonstrate substantial compliance with standards adopted by OPM, including stable management with experience pertinent to the prepaid health care provider industry and sufficient operating experience to enable OPM to evaluate realistically the plan's past and expected future performance, a rate of enrollment that ensures equalization of income and expenses within projected time frames and sufficient subscriber income to operate within budget thereafter, a health care delivery system providing reasonable access to and choice of quality primary care and specialty care throughout the service area, and establishment of firm budget projections and demonstrated success in meeting or exceeding those projections on a regular basis.[3] Once a contract is entered into, the carrier has an ongoing obligation to notify OPM of the occurrence of certain "significant events" that could affect the carrier's ability to satisfy the foregoing standards on an ongoing basis or could impair the carrier's ability to perform its contractual obligations.[4]

Participation in the FEHBP is open to any carrier that satisfies OPM's requirements. In addition, as noted earlier, OPM is statutorily obligated to contract with federally qualified HMOs,[5] so an abbreviated application process is available to federally qualified HMOs.[6] OPM has sought to restrict applications from community-rated plans. In 1994, OPM indicated its intention to stabilize the FEHBP by not permitting any new plans for contract year 1996 and limiting the entry of new plans thereafter. The

agency's intention was formally communicated in interim regulations published in the *Federal Register* in December 1994.[7] The interim regulations provided that "The Director of OPM shall consider applications to participate in the [FEHBP] from comprehensive medical plans (CMPs) at his or her discretion. If the Director of OPM determines that it is beneficial to enrollees and the [FEHBP] to invite new plans to join the program, OPM will publish a notice in the *Federal Register*."[8]

In response to industry objection and threatened legal action, OPM modified the language of the final rule. Under the final rule, CMPs are "automatically" invited to submit applications annually unless otherwise notified by OPM.[9] If the Director of OPM determines that it is not "beneficial" to enrollees and the FEHBP to consider applications for a specific year, the Director is required to publish a notice with a 60-day comment period in the *Federal Register* no less than seven months before the due date for applications for that year.[10]

PREMIUM CONTRIBUTION AND BENEFIT DESIGN

Under 5 U.S. Code Section 8906, OPM pays a portion of the premium, and the employee or annuitant is responsible for the remainder. OPM uses a formula to develop the contribution. OPM determines the weighted average of the premium charges for the upcoming contract year for self-enrollments and for self and family enrollments. In general, the government's contribution for health benefits for an employee or annuitant is adjusted to equal 72 percent of the weighted average premium charge for applicable tier of coverage (i.e., self only or self and family). For example, in the 2000 contract year, the government will pay up to $2,049.60 for self-only enrollment and $4,575.24 for self and family enrollment. These amounts are subject to the overall limitation that the government contribution shall not exceed 75 percent of the total premium of any plan. Therefore, if OPM's contribution would be more than 75 percent of an HMO's premium, the HMO receives a contribution from OPM equal to 75 percent of its premium.

As for benefit design, OPM is authorized to establish reasonable minimum standards. These minimum benefits include hospital benefits, surgical benefits, in-hospital surgical benefits, ambulatory patient benefits, supplemental benefits, and obstetrical benefits.[11] OPM requires HMOs to offer the basic benefits mandated for federally qualified HMOs.[12] *These required benefits include:*

- nonexperimental bone marrow, cornea, kidney, and liver transplants
- short-term rehabilitative therapy
- family planning services including artificial insemination
- home health services
- in-hospital administration of blood and blood products, including blood processing
- surgical treatment of morbid obesity when medically necessary

OPM's expectations and requirements regarding benefit design for the FEHBP are described in annual "call letters" that the agency sends to carriers. In recent years, OPM has attempted to standardize benefits among FEHBP contractors. In the call letter for contract year 2000, all plan-initiated benefit change proposals must be cost-neutral.[13] Despite this requirement, OPM has indicated that it does not limit HMOs to zero cost benefit tradeoffs. However, HMOs are generally not allowed to change a benefit unless the change is part of the HMO's community benefits package and is offered to all groups and not just the federal account. OPM's benefit instructions to HMOs specifically state that it is OPM's intention to purchase the benefit package purchased by most of the carrier's nonfederal subscribers. If OPM subsequently determines that a carrier failed to disclose its most prevalent benefit package to OPM and OPM purchased a benefits package that is not the community benefits package purchased on behalf of the majority, then OPM will adjust the carrier's premium rates.

PATIENTS' BILL OF RIGHTS AND RESPONSIBILITIES

Pursuant to an Executive Memorandum signed on February 20, 1998, OPM is directed to bring the FEHBP into contractual compliance with the Patients' Bills of Rights and Responsibilities requirements by the end of 1999 (see also Chapter 2).[14] Since then, OPM and FEHBP carriers have implemented several of the requirements relating to information disclosure, access to emergency care, access to obstetricians and gynecologists, access to specialists for enrollees with special health care needs, and access to appropriate providers including out-of-network providers.

Certain requirements of the Patients' Bill of Rights may necessitate changes to participating provider contracts. OPM gave carriers until contract year 2000 to address these requirements either through provider contract changes or the adoption of compliance strategies. One of these requirements is to permit certain members to continue to see their specialty providers for up to 90 days after the member "involuntarily changes health plans" or the provider is terminated from the carrier's network other than for cause. Members affected by this new requirement are those with chronic or disabling conditions or in the second or third trimester of pregnancy at the time of the change or termination.

Another requirement relates to access to medical records. Members must be allowed to review and obtain copies of their medical records on request and promptly. In addition, a patient may request that a physician amend a record that is not accurate, relevant, or complete. If the physician does not make the requested change, then the member patient may add a brief statement to the record. This provision is similar to one found in the Health Insurance Portability and Accountability Act of 1996 (HIPAA; see Chapter 67).

PREMIUM RATING UNDER THE FEHBP

There are two rating options under the FEHBP. One option, as mentioned earlier, is community rating. The other option is experience rating.[15] Both are discussed later. In addition, the reader is referred to Chapters 49 to 52 for detailed discussions of rating and underwriting.

Experience Rating

Under the experience rating option, carriers charge the FEHBP a rate that is based on the utilization of health care services by the federal account. This rate is retrospectively determined and should not be confused with adjusted community rating (ACR), in which the experience of an account is prospectively factored into the rate charged the group. The FEHBP Acquisition Regulations (FEHBAR),[16] which govern the FEHBP, define an experience rate as follows:

> [a] rate for a given group that is the result of that group's actual paid claims, administrative expenses, retentions, and estimated claims incurred but not reported, adjusted for benefit modification, utilization trends, and economic trends. Actual paid claims include any actual or negotiated benefits payments made to providers of medical services for the provision of health care such as capitation not adjusted for specific groups, per diems, and [diagnosis-related group] (DRG) payments.[17]

Before 1990, the definition of experience rate did not specifically recognize provider capitation payments as paid claims. This gap in the regulation was a barrier to HMOs to contract with OPM on an experience-rated basis because capitation payments are a typical provider compensation payment arrangement used by HMOs.[18] Since the regulatory amendment was promulgated, experience rating has become a contracting option for HMOs that no longer wish to contract on a community-rated basis but want to remain in the program. However, the financial reporting and other requirements imposed on experience-rated FEHBP contractors, as well as the limitation on contractors' profit,[19] make experience rating an unattractive option for many HMOs. These requirements include:

- The experience analysis must include coordination of benefits and subrogation recoveries and exclude marketing costs and interest expense.

- The HMO's administrative load cannot exceed a specific percentage of premium, which tends to range from 5 percent to 10 percent.
- Administrative expenses that cannot be allocated to the FEHBP on a direct basis must be allocated on an indirect basis, typically by number of claims or member months.

Community Rating

OPM has adopted the methods of community rating established by the federal Department of Health and Human Services (DHHS) Health Care Financing Administration (HCFA) for federally qualified HMOs. These are traditional community rating (TCR), community rating by class (CRC), and ACR. Although OPM has adopted DHHS' methods of community rating, the agency has not limited its requirements for and interpretation of the three methods to those adopted by DHHS. OPM's community rating requirements are contained in the agency's annual instructions to plans.

Before the 1991 contract year, the premium rate development of community-rated carriers participating in the FEHBP was severely restricted by OPM's rating requirements. These requirements included the following definition of a community rate: a "rate of payment that is equivalent to that charged on the effective date to all subscriber groups of the carrier for the same contract period for the same level of benefits."[20] Under this definition, any rating discrepancies between the rate charged the FEHBP and that charged any other group by the carrier that were discovered on audit were subject to challenge as improper discounts.

OPM amended the FEHBAR definition of a community rate to "a rate of payment based on a per member per month capitation rate or its equivalent that applies to a combination of the subscriber groups for a comprehensive medical plan...."[21] Under this definition, OPM no longer requires that a single community rate be applicable to all of a carrier's groups, including the FEHBP. The revised definition substantially relaxes the rating restrictions imposed by OPM on its community-rated carriers. In fact, one of the stated purposes of the revised definition was to "recognize the increasing diversity in community rating in the insurance industry and, specifically, within the [FEHBP]."[22]

Traditional Community Rating

Under TRC, OPM expects carriers to develop rates from a community-based revenue requirement (typically a capitation rate) that is documented and verifiable. Acceptable documentation includes a state rate filing or actuarial memorandum. The capitation rate is then adjusted by demographic factors to convert the capitation rate into single and family rates. Contractors must include supporting documentation for the conversion process. OPM also accepts as an acceptable form of TCR a standard set of two-tiered rates for all of the contractor's groups.

Community Rating by Class

CRC permits the introduction of classes, such as age and gender, in determining the HMO's revenue requirement for its enrolled population. Again, the starting point should be a capitation rate. The amount charged an employer is then based on the composition of the employer's work force and dependents.

Carriers using CRC for the FEHBP must provide OPM with a standard presentation of their method. OPM provides carriers with a standard CRC format in the annual rate instructions. If a carrier cannot comply with OPM's standard format, then it must submit its rate manual and/or "official documents" that demonstrate the actuarial soundness of the carrier's CRC method.

OPM accepts age and gender as legitimate CRC factors. If a carrier proposes to use another factor, it must provide documentation showing that the factor predicts utilization. One factor that was used by many HMOs was an industry adjustment factor (IAF). OPM does not accept IAFs as legitimate predictors of health care utilization but views them as a potential means to provide discounts relative to the FEHBP. As a result, OPM adopted a policy that if an FEHBP contractor uses an IAF of less than 1.00 (thereby reducing the rate ultimately charged) for a simi-

larly sized subscriber group (SSSG), then the contractor must give the same IAF to the FEHBP. If both SSSGs receive IAFs of less than 1.00, then the FEHBP must receive the lower of the two IAFs. In no event, however, may the FEHBP be charged an IAF greater than 1.00.

Adjusted Community Rating

OPM also recognizes ACR as an acceptable method for FEHBP carriers. An adjusted community rate is a "community rate which has been adjusted for expected use of medical resources of the FEHBP group. An ACR is a prospective rate and cannot be retroactively revised to reflect actual experience, utilization, or costs of the FEHBP group."[23] OPM currently accepts two methods of ACR: a method based on utilization data and a prospective method based on actual FEHBP claims data. Under both methods of ACR, the contractor must keep on file all data necessary to justify the ACR rate, including backup tapes of the contractor's claims database.

OPM's rules for a claims-based ACR are:

- The experience period may not change in the reconciliation from that used in the federal rate proposal.
- If completion factors are used to convert paid claims to incurred claims, the completion factors must be the same for all groups for which the contractor used a claims-based ACR.
- Any method used to convert paid claims to incurred claims should be consistent for all groups that are rated using a claims-based ACR method.
- If claims include special benefit claims, the contractor may not charge the FEHBP special benefit loadings.
- If claims include annuitants age 65 or over, claims must be reduced by the amount received from Medicare or the FEHBP must receive a credit to reflect the income received from Medicare.
- Loadings for administrative expenses must be either (a) a flat community rate per member per month amount or (b) a standard percentage of claims.

- If a trend factor is used for the FEHBP, then it must be the same as that used for other groups.

Similarly Sized Subscriber Groups

The concept of SSSGs is one of the most significant changes for the FEHBP in the area of rating requirements. Under the FEHBAR provisions that were in effect before 1991, a contractor had to certify that the rate charged the FEHBP was charged to all its subscriber groups that had the same contract period and benefit package as the FEHBP. Since then, contractors have been required to certify that the FEHBP rates were developed in a manner consistent with the rating method used to rate the carrier's SSSGs and approved by OPM.[24,25]

At the time of their adoption, the SSSG regulations were viewed as potentially reducing the substantial audit adjustments/controversies that were common under OPM's prior community-rating regulations. Focusing on the rating of two groups rather than the entire community would enhance contractor compliance with OPM's rating requirements for the FEHBP. However, regulatory ambiguity, conflicts between OPM's regulations and instructions on the criteria for identifying SSSGs, conflicts within OPM on the SSSG criteria, and other factors caused the SSSG requirements to be viewed as potentially more onerous than OPM's prior requirements. As a result, the SSSG requirements have been modified several times since their promulgation on July 2, 1990.

Identifying the SSSGs

Although the criteria for identifying the SSSGs are substantially different now compared with what they were when OPM first adopted them, it is nevertheless important to review the criteria as they have changed over time because audits of these earlier years may still be unresolved for some contractors.

Contract years 1990–1992. On July 2, 1990, OPM promulgated final regulations that introduced the SSSG concept to the FEHBP.[26] Under those regulations, the SSSGs were defined as the contractor's

[T]wo employer groups which best meet all of the following conditions:

(a) Have total number of contracts at the time of the rate proposal arithmetically closest in size to the previous September's FEHBP subscriber enrollment, as determined by OPM;
(b) Purchase substantially the same basic benefit package proposed for the Federal group; and
(c) Are renewed during the plan's fiscal year. Contracts with a governmental authority or program or any health benefits program for employees of states, political subdivisions of states and other public entities may be used if they are community rated.[27]

Starting with the 1991 contract year, OPM required contractors to identify their two SSSGs at the time of the rate proposal *and* at the time of the rate reconciliation. Instructions included in the 1991 and 1992 rate proposal forms provided the following guidance to contractors in identifying the SSSGs:

OPM will purchase the community benefits package that is purchased by the greatest number of the plan's other subscribers. There may be riders or other additions to the basic package, but the basis for determining the similarly sized subscriber groups will be the core package covering the largest number of the plan's subscribers. Once the groups that purchase this package have been determined, the two groups from this set that are closest in size to the Federal group will be the two similarly sized subscriber groups.

Included among the same 1991 and 1992 instructions to the contractors, from which those quoted above are taken, was a directive that contractors select the SSSGs from among those groups that purchase the contractor's "core" community benefits package that is purchased by the greatest number of non-FEHBP subscribers.

In addition to identifying the SSSGs, contractors were required to submit an executed "Certificate of Accurate Pricing" to OPM certifying to the appropriateness of the rates charged the FEHBP. OPM required contractors to make these certifications at the time of the rate reconciliation and to refer to the SSSG rates that were in effect at the time of the rate reconciliation. OPM's requirement for making the certification at the time of the rate reconciliation with the use of current information, and not at the rate proposal, was arguably contrary to OPM's regulations then in effect. Specifically, those regulations stated that:

> When a carrier proposes a community rate…the Contracting Officer shall require the carrier to execute the Certificate of Accurate Pricing for Community Rated Plans contained in this section unless the carrier has been exempt from filing certified cost or pricing data. *The Certificate shall be executed each time a proposal is made* (emphasis added).[28]

The text of the certificate is repeated below:

> This is to certify that, to the best of my knowledge and belief, the cost or pricing data submitted, either actually or by specific identification in writing, to the Contracting Officer or the Contracting Officer's designee in support of the __* FEHBP rates were developed in accordance with the requirements of 48 C.F.R. chapter 16 and the FEHBP contract and are accurate, complete, and current as of the date this certificate is executed. The FEHBP rates were developed in a manner consistent with the rating

methodology used to rate the Carrier's similarly sized subscriber groups… and approved by OPM….

Based on the language of OPM's regulations, OPM apparently should have required contractors to submit the Certificate of Accurate Pricing at the time of the rate proposal and not at the time of the rate reconciliation. Moreover, contractors should have certified to the consistency with rate methods that were in effect for SSSGs identified at the time of the rate proposal and not as of the rate reconciliation.

Despite the language of the regulations, audit findings of defective pricing have been made on the basis of the Office of the Inspector General's (OIG) identification of SSSGs as of the rate reconciliation for these years either by using subscriber counts or rates charged the SSSGs (or both) at the time of the reconciliation. Contractors' identification of the SSSGs for these years has been further complicated by the fact that the OIG has, in general, ignored benefit differences between the potential SSSGs and the FEHBP in making SSSG selections. This is the case despite OPM's regulations and instructions that the SSSGs purchase substantially the same basic benefits package as the FEHBP and that the SSSGs be selected from groups that purchase the most popular community benefits package.

Confusion also exists for these years on the issue of whether governmental accounts are eligible as potential SSSGs. Under OPM's proposed SSSG regulations, which were published in 1989, governmental accounts could not be used as SSSGs. The final rule published in 1990 stated that governmental accounts "may" be used if they are community rated. Staff of OPM's Office of the Actuary indicated that plans had the discretion to use or not use governmental accounts as their SSSGs, provided that only a community-rated governmental account could be an SSSG. In conducting audits, the OIG has taken the position that once a contractor identifies a governmental account as an SSSG, other governmental accounts are also eligible.

With respect to the benefit similarity requirement referenced in (b) previously, OPM never

---

*Identify the time period to which the rates apply. The rate must be either the actual rate in effect for the current contract term or a quoted rate for the next contract term.

published guidelines or other instructions about the meaning of "substantially the same basic benefit package." As a result, contractors were left to select groups on the basis of their own interpretation of the regulation. The lack of OPM guidance on this issue has resulted in adverse audit findings against community-rated contractors that selected their SSSGs on the basis of benefit package similarities when, in practice, OPM focused principally on the size of the group in determining whether it was or was not an SSSG. With respect to (c) above, the contract renewal date, plans interpreted this criterion to mean that groups that had a multiyear term were ineligible for SSSG purposes if these groups did not renew during the plan's fiscal year that included the FEHBP contract year. Again, contractors have learned on audit that the renewal date requirement can be problematic.

Contract Years 1993 and 1994. For contract years 1993 and 1994, OPM revised its instructions to contractors on how to identify the SSSGs although the agency did not amend the regulatory criteria for the SSSGs. Specifically, OPM instructed contractors as follows:

> [B]eginning with the 1993 rate year, the following rules will apply:
> 1) The definition of SSSGs will be changed so that it depends only on the enrollment for the rate year under consideration. For example, for the 1993 rate year, 1993 group enrollment will be used. Note that under the previous definition, September, 1991 enrollment would have been used.
> 2) We will not request information concerning the names and the rate development for the SSSGs at the time of the FEHBP proposal. Rather, we will ask the plan to furnish all such information at the time it submits its reconciliation. For the 1993 rate year, this will be around March, 1993.

Starting with the 1993 contract year, OPM instructed contractors to identify SSSGs only at the time of the rate reconciliation using the most current enrollment statistics. The community benefits package requirement no longer appeared to be a specific requirement based on OPM's rating instructions for those years, although contractors were still required to propose to OPM the community benefits package in their benefit proposals. In addition, OPM continued its practice of requiring contractors to submit the Certificate of Accurate Pricing at the time of the rate reconciliation. The governmental account issue was not addressed by OPM.

Contract Years 1995 and After. On March 24, 1994, OPM promulgated new regulations that amended the definition of the SSSGs.[29] These regulatory changes became effective for the 1995 contract year. The apparent intent of the regulations was to clarify the many uncertainties and ambiguities that existed in OPM's SSSG requirements and to restrict a plan's ability to provide preferential rates to other accounts of comparable size to the FEHBP without passing those rating preferences on to the FEHBP.

Under the 1994 regulations the SSSGs were defined as a contractor's

> [T]wo employer groups that:
> (a) As of the date specified by OPM in the rate instructions, have a subscriber enrollment closest to the FEHBP subscriber enrollment; and
> (b) Use any rating method other than retrospective rating; and
> (c) Meet the criteria specified in the rate instructions issued by OPM.[30]

The new regulations eliminated much of the ambiguity that existed before 1995 with respect to identifying the SSSGs. Specifically, the regulations eliminated benefits package differences as a consideration in identifying the SSSGs. In addition, the exception that existed for governmental accounts was eliminated. The new regulations also make clear that the FEHBP is entitled to the lowest rates using the method used for the SSSGs.

In 1997, OPM further amended the definition of SSSGs to add that any group with which an FEHBP carrier enters into an agreement to provide health care services is a potential SSSG (including separate lines of business, government entities, groups that have multiyear contracts, and groups having point of service products). However, certain groups must be excluded from SSSG consideration:

- groups that are rated using a retrospective experience rating method
- groups consisting of the carrier's own employees
- Medicaid groups, Medicare groups, and groups that have a stand-alone benefit (such as dental only)
- a purchasing alliance whose rate-setting is mandated by a state or local government[31]

Other SSSG Issues

Multiyear Contracts. OPM has clarified its position on multiyear contracts and whether and how groups with a multiyear contract term can be the basis for a premium rate adjustment for the FEHBP. OPM's position is:

> If an SSSG's rate is extended beyond twelve months (i.e., the carrier allows an SSSG to change its renewal date), a premium adjustment must be made for the SSSG in the following year, or the OPM audit staff may interpret the rate extension as a discount.[32]

Multiple Rating Regions. Identifying the SSSGs can be complicated by the fact that some contractors may have distinct rating regions within a particular state and have established different community rates for those regions. In these cases, it has been unclear how contractors should select their SSSGs. For plans with multiple rating regions, OPM's policy as reflected in the 1996 rate instructions was that groups in different rating areas than the FEHBP are also eligible for SSSG purposes. Any group that is enrolled in the same legal entity that contracts with OPM is potentially an SSSG even if it is in a different rating region.

OPM announced a change in its policy effective for the 1999 contract year. OPM now requires that both SSSGs be chosen only from groups that have enrollees in the federal group's region. OPM's

policy also addressed the significance of a carrier's rate code in the selection of SSSGs:

> Our SSSG policy with regard to federal groups in different regions under the same rate code is as follows:
> a) those federal groups in the same state or in the same metropolitan area must be combined and the carrier must choose two SSSGs for the combined federal groups.
> b) those federal groups in different states (but not in the same metropolitan area) must be combined in each state, and the carrier must choose two SSSGs for the combined federal groups in each state.

OPM's rate instructions for the 2000 contract year include examples of SSSG selection in multiple rating regions.

OPM AUDITS AND APPEALS

As government contractors, HMOs participating in the FEHBP are subject to periodic audit by OPM. For community-rated carriers, this means that auditors from OPM's OIG will seek to verify that the rate charged the FEHBP was a community rate or "market price" as defined by the FEHBAR and that any benefit and other loadings to the FEHBP rate were reasonable and appropriate.

Record Retention and Audits

To assist OPM in the conduct of audits, contractors are required to maintain their records relating to a contract year for 5 years after the expiration of that contract year.[33] Plans must retain and make available all records that support the annual statement of operations and the rate submission for that contract term for a period of 5 years after the end of the contract term to which the records relate. Although there is no limitations period within which OPM's OIG must conduct an audit, the OIG uses the five-year record retention requirement described previously as a self-imposed time limit.

As noted previously, the specific documents that must be retained are not clear. *However, as a general rule, contractors should retain the following documents for five years after the end of the contract year:*

- FEHBP rate proposals and reconciliations.
- Enrollment data used in selecting the SSSGs (as of March 31 or earlier in the year) for the top 20 accounts including the FEHBP. Relevant data include subscriber/member counts by rating tier, contract mix, average family size, and age/sex statistics by rating tier.
- If enrollment data other than in-force statistics are used, supporting documentation for the enrollment data that were used in the development of each group's (top 20 including the FEHBP) rates. For example, if group-wide demographics are used, the enrollment data furnished by the employer should be retained. If assumed demographics are used, data regarding (a) the reason(s) why assumed demographics were used and (b) supporting documentation for the demographics actually used, should be retained.
- If a plan uses regional rates, group-specific documentation of enrollment in each rating region for the top 20 groups including the FEHBP.
- Rating sheets used in the development of the premium rates charged the top 20 accounts including the FEHBP.
- Group contracts including benefit schedules for the top 20 accounts including the FEHBP.
- Premium billing invoices for the top 20 accounts.
- Plan rating manual or rating policies and procedures.
- Group-specific experience data for the top 20 accounts including FEHBP if the plan uses adjusted community rating. Plans should save backup tapes of their claims, utilization, etc.
- Community rates including trend factors. Documentation could be state rate filings, book rates, actuarial memorandum, etc.

The Audit Process

Five-Year Audits

The typical audit conducted by the OIG covers a period of five years. The audit process begins with a notice of audit letter to the carrier from the OIG. The letter notifies the plan what contract years will be audited and when the audit will commence. The notice includes a standard information request. Contractors are required to assemble the requested material and forward it to the OIG before the on-site portion of the audit. *The requested information typically includes:*

- the plan's community rates for all standard benefit packages and riders for the years under audit
- the plan's written procedures for rating groups, including a detailed model for each rating method used by the plan for the audited years
- any audit report or review made by a state regulatory agency within the last two years
- a corporate organizational chart
- sample hold harmless clause used in provider contracts
- the plan's commercial (non-FEHBP) benefit brochure for each audited year that corresponds to the benefit package sold to the FEHBP
- the plan's audited financial statements for the last accounting year
- the plan's interim financial statements for the most recent period
- a listing of the plan's top 20 groups (including the FEHBP) for each year to be audited; the list of groups should include the following information for each year:
  — number of contracts and members and the renewal dates for each of the groups
  — benefit package and riders that were purchased by each of the groups
  — total number of plan contracts and members
  — identify all groups that were rated using retrospective experience rating techniques

— identify the two SSSGs that were used in the plan's rate submissions for each year under audit and provide a written narrative describing the criteria used to select these groups

— if the FEHBP rates were based on a rating method that is different from the SSSGs, explain the reason(s) for rating the FEHBP differently and submit a recalculation of the FEHBP rates using the same method as was used for the SSSGs

Once the auditors are on site at the plan, they will require ready access to rate folders, marketing folders, group billings, demographic statistics used in rate development, rating manuals, and all documentation supporting calculations for the groups described previously.

The on-site portion of the audit begins with an entrance interview between the OIG auditors and plan staff. During the entrance interview, the auditors explain the purpose of the audit and the information they will review for audit purposes. The auditors conduct an exit interview at the conclusion of the audit to review their initial findings with plan staff.

The OIG issues a draft audit report to the plan that summarizes the auditors' preliminary findings and recommendations. The issuance of the draft audit report can take from three months to a year or longer after the on-site audit. The plan is allowed to submit comments to the draft audit report, which are taken into consideration and incorporated into the final audit report. The OIG submits the final audit report to OPM's Office of Insurance Programs, which is charged with responsibility for resolving the audit's findings and recommendations. The plan is permitted another opportunity to respond to the audit's findings in response to the final audit report. The Office of Insurance Programs resolves audit findings either by settlement negotiations with the contractor or by accepting the OIG's findings and issuing a final decision, from which the contractor can pursue an administrative appeal or seek judicial review if it disagrees with the audit's findings and recommendations.[34]

Special Audits

In the 1997 rate instructions, OPM notified contractors that the OIG would perform audits of the 1996 rate reconciliations on a selected basis. OPM's Office of the Actuary used the results of these audits in setting the final rates for the audited groups. OPM informed contractors that although these "special audits" focused on the 1996 rate reconciliation, OIG auditors may need to analyze rate information for the FEHBP and other groups for previous years. Documentation must be kept readily available in the event of a special audit.

OPM has continued the special audits to the present. In its 1999 Reconciliation Guidelines, OPM notified contractors that the OIG will not conduct a subsequent audit of any contract year that has been reviewed by special audit. In addition, once the rates are finalized, OPM will not permit any change to the rates or accept additional information that is intended to change the audit results or final rates. The only condition under which rates finalized in conjunction with a special audit will be changed is when the rates are affected by a subsequent audit performed on previous contract years.

Defending and Settling Adverse Audit Findings

FEHBP contractors that are charged with defective pricing typically have two formal opportunities to defend themselves at the agency level. The first opportunity is in response to the findings contained in the draft audit report. The second opportunity is after receipt of the final audit report, which is issued after OPM has received the contractor's comments to the draft audit report. It is critical that both responses be comprehensive submissions that defend the contractor's rating practices, where possible, and put forth alternative analyses for the calculation of the FEHBP's damages. In this regard, there are many analyses available to a contractor. Alternative analyses serve two purposes: The first is to show the unreasonableness of the amount recommended by the auditors by showing that the government's actual damages as a result of the contractor's rating practices are much lower. The second is to serve as the basis of settlement negotiations between OPM and the contractor.

If OPM and the contractor are unable to settle their dispute, the contracting officer will issue a final decision. Although settlement negotiations may continue after a final decision has been issued, once the final decision is issued the time period for appealing the government's decision starts to run. In addition, interest on the claimed amount begins to accrue 30 days after the decision is issued.

Contract appeals are subject to the Contract Disputes Act of 1978, 41 U.S. Code Section 601 et seq. In appealing the contracting officer's decision, the contractor can appeal to the Armed Services Board of Contract Appeals. Alternatively, the contractor can make an appeal to the U.S. Court of Federal Claims. Although several contractors have appealed agency final decisions, with the exception of lost investment income claims, most contractor claims have been settled at the agency level.

Lost Investment Income or Interest Claims

In 1994, OPM began to include with audit findings a claim for lost investment income or interest on the overpayments made by the government as a result of the contractor's defective rating practices. Because the government would calculate interest from the date the overpayment was made as opposed to when the audit findings were finalized by a final decision, these interest claims often represented substantial sums.

Several contractors challenged OPM's authority to collect interest from the date the overpayment was made. The legal grounds for these challenges differed for contract years 1988 to 1989 and 1991 forward.[35] In June of 1998, the Armed Services Board of Contract Appeals (ASBCA) upheld OPM's right to claim lost investment income from the date of the overpayment for contract years 1988, 1989, and 1991.[36] The United States Court of Appeals for the Federal Circuit affirmed the ASBCA's decision on the record in that case.[37]

In making its decision, the Federal Circuit affirmed the ASBCA's factual findings with respect to contract year 1991 and did not consider whether there is a legal difference between a violation of the FEHBP contract by engaging in "defective community rating and defective pricing" and a violation of the contract by submitting "defective cost or pricing data."

QualMed Plans for Health of New Mexico ("QualMed") also appealed OPM's lost investment income claim, but it pursued its appeal in the U.S. Court of Federal Claims rather than before the ASBCA. When the Federal Circuit rendered its decision in *PCA,* QualMed argued that the Court of Federal Claims was not bound by the factual finding in *PCA.* The Court of Federal Claims agreed and granted QualMed's motion for summary judgment.[38] The Court held, as a matter of law, that the contract and incorporated regulations treat defective community rating and defective pricing differently from defective cost and pricing data. The terms "defective community rating and defective pricing" concern errors relating to the SSSGs, e.g., selecting the wrong SSSGs or affording the SSSG(s) a discount that is not given to the FEHBP. "Defective cost or pricing data," on the other hand, relates to errors in the development of FEHBP specific-loadings, such as special benefit loadings, and demographic adjustments made to a contractor's community rate to derive FEHBP-specific single and family rates.

The contract years at issue in the *QualMed* decision are 1991 and 1992. To date, the Government has not appealed the decision in *QualMed.*

FEHBP AND FALSE CLAIMS LIABILITY

One of the more serious developments in the FEHBP contracting area is the potential for a community-rated plan to be held liable for filing a false certification with OPM. Before the adoption of the SSSG rules, plans were required at the time of the rate proposal and at the time of the reconciliation to certify that the rate charged the FEHBP was a community rate. Given the vagaries as to how a community rate is defined and the variety of ways in which community-rating principles can be applied to different employer groups, however, questions may arise as to whether the rate certifications provided to OPM at the time of rate reconciliation were true and accurate.

The application of SSSG principles to the FEHBP rates further narrows the scope of the analysis of whether certifications provided to OPM by the plan were true and accurate. One of the certifications that the plan is required to make at the time of the rate reconciliation is that the method used to determine the FEHBP rates is consistent with the method used to determine the rates for the plan's SSSGs. With the 1994 and 1997 amendments to the FEHBAR that made the universe of comparable groups more precise and defined cost and pricing data for certification purposes, the exposure for false claims liability may be even greater for plans.

In the process of auditing certain HMOs, OIG has referred certain matters to the U.S. Attorney for the District of Columbia to evaluate whether a certification filed by a plan resulted in the filing of a false claim with the federal government as prohibited by 31 U.S. Code Section 3729 et seq. Section 3729(a) provides in part that any person who knowingly presents, or causes to be presented, to an officer or employee of the U.S. government a false or fraudulent claim for payment or approval is liable to the government for a civil penalty of not less than $5,000 and not more than $10,000, plus three times the amount of damages that the government sustains because of the act of that person. Knowingly, as defined under Section 3729(b), means that a person with respect to information has actual knowledge of the information, acts in deliberate ignorance of the truth or falsity of the information, or acts in reckless disregard of the truth or falsity of the information. No proof of specific intent to defraud is required under the statute.

The issue of whether a contractor engaged in filing a false certification either as to its community rate or as to the methodology used in rating its SSSGs has yet to be litigated. This is due to plan exposure to treble damage liability, as well as the adverse publicity associated with the filing of a false claim. OIG has been able to recover substantial amounts of money as part of the settlements of these investigations between the plans and the U.S. Attorney, the results of which are reported to Congress semiannually by the OIG. Careful review of the plan's rates and files before the execution of these certifications can diminish the potential for false claim liability. The issue of false claims and audit liability exposure, however, is particularly problematic in cases involving the acquisition of one health plan by another. The scope and extent of FEHBP audit and false claim liability is often not known at the time of the acquisition, yet the successor to the government contract is fully liable for all prior acts of the selling party under the contract. Indemnification commitments that are received by the purchaser from the selling party need to be sufficiently well defined and secured to deal with an exposure that often is not identified for many years after the acquisition occurs.

OPM'S POLICY ON ERROR REPORTING

In the 1999 Reconciliation Guidelines, OPM notified HMOs that if they discover that a previous rate proposal and/or rate reconciliation submitted to OPM is incorrect, the carrier must: (1) notify OPM, and (2) prepare and submit to OPM an amended proposal and/or reconciliation (including a newly executed Certificate of Accurate Pricing). The policy does not apply to proposals and/or reconciliations that have already been audited by OPM's audit staff and resolved by OPM's insurance programs.

The legal significance of OPM's new policy in reporting errors is unclear. However, at a minimum, the policy appears to create a contractual obligation for contractors to disclose and correct any rating errors of which they have knowledge.

MISCELLANEOUS CONTRACTING ISSUES

Enrollment Reconciliations with Local Payroll Offices

A common problem faced by FEHBP contractors is the inability to obtain timely enrollment and disenrollment information from OPM and the local payroll offices. As a result, many contractors find that they are carrying FEHBP enrollees on their membership lists and may be paying capitation payments to providers for federal enrollees long after these individuals have been terminated from the FEHBP.

Before the 1997 contract year, OPM was contractually obligated to maintain or cause to be maintained adequate enrollment information to allow contractors to maintain an accurate record of their FEHBP enrollees. Moreover, contractors were entitled to rely on this information. Despite these contractual obligations, however, OPM's position was that it is the responsibility of the contractors and the individual payroll offices to reconcile enrollment records to ensure that the contractor's records are accurate. Unfortunately, most payroll offices were unwilling or unable to work with the contractors to reconcile their enrollment records. The problem continues today. Thus the contractors are left without any definitive source in seeking to maintain accurate records.

The inability to obtain accurate and timely enrollment information has been the subject of several contractor lawsuits against OPM.[39] In at least one case, the government conceded liability, but the amount of money due the contractors was left to be determined through an audit of the contractors' databases. As a result of these lawsuits, OPM has paid millions of dollars to contractors.

Apparently in light of these lawsuits and the fact that other contractors may pursue similar lawsuits, OPM amended its standard contract with community-rated plans to limit its exposure for failing to maintain accurate enrollment information and providing it to plans in a timely manner.[40]

Starting with the 1997 contract year, OPM included in its Standard Contract for Community-Rated Comprehensive Medical Plans a 1 percent loading for community-rated CMPs "in full resolution" of all discrepancies between enrollment and actual payments to carriers.[41] In consideration for the 1 percent adjustment, contractors agree to waive any rights they may have under other sections of the contract relating to OPM's obligation to provide or ensure the accuracy of enrollment information. The enrollment

reconciliation process and 1 percent adjustment are to be reviewed by OPM and contractors for the 2001 contract year.

In a Benefits Administration Letter issued in September 1999, OPM indicated that it is still receiving reports from FEHBP carriers that they are not receiving quarterly enrollment reconciliation reports from federal agency employing offices.[42]

Department of Defense Demonstration Project

OPM will conduct a demonstration project with the Department of Defense (DoD) to make FEHBP coverage available to up to 66,000 Medicare-eligible military retirees and related beneficiaries. The demonstration project will commence with the 2000 contract year and run through the 2002 contract year.

The demonstration project was mandated by the 1999 National Defense Authorization Act.[43] OPM identified HMOs with service areas in the demonstration site areas that are required to participate in the project in the areas that have been identified by OPM.[44] The demonstration sites are Dover Air Force Base, Delaware; Puerto Rico; Fort Knox, Kentucky; Greensboro/Winston-Salem/High Point, North Carolina; Dallas, Texas; Humbolt County, California; Naval Hospital, Camp Pendleton, California; and New Orleans, Louisiana.

For carriers participating in the demonstration project, the SSSG requirements are not applicable to determine the reasonableness of the carrier's demonstration project premium rates. Rather, carriers are required to "benchmark" demonstration projection premiums against ACRs if available, Medigap offerings, or other similar products.[45]

Health programs in the DoD are discussed in Chapter 58.

Federal Preemption of State Laws

Terms of the FEHBP Contract

FEHBP contractors can sometimes face conflicting requirements as federal government contractors and as state-licensed HMOs (see Chapter 69 for a discussion of state requirements). These conflicts can relate to benefits, rates, and terms of the federal subscriber documents. FEHBA contains a preemption provision that can eliminate the need of contractors to comply with some state laws that affect the contractors' FEHBP operations. The FEHBA states: "The terms of any contract under this chapter [5 U.S.C.A. § 8901 et seq.] which relate to the nature or extent of coverage or benefits (including payments with respect to benefits) shall supersede and preempt any State or local law, or any regulation issued thereunder, which relates to health insurance or plans."[46]

Section 8902(m)(1) can preempt state-mandated benefit requirements to the extent that the state benefits are inconsistent with those offered by the contractor to the FEHBP. In addition, it is possible that the preemption clause may be used to preempt state laws that may not appear, on their face, to affect the nature of coverage or extent of benefits. For example, Section 8902(m)(1) could be used to preempt state prohibitions on such practices as subrogation.

The FEHBP is also outside the scope of the Employee Retirement Income Security Act (ERISA; see Chapter 66).[47] As a result, ERISA preemption of state law claims does not extend to claims against FEHBP contractors.[48] The FEHBP brochure given to enrollees, however, limits recoveries to the benefits under the contract. This has been construed to limit the ability of a claimant to recover punitive damages for bad faith denials.[49] FEHBP procedures and remedies are the sole procedures and remedies for claim denials in the FEHBP, and state actions for claims may therefore be preempted by Section 8902(m)(1).[50] Although the true scope of federal preemption of state laws under Section 8902(m)(1) has not been definitively established, the case law seems to suggest that the scope of federal preemption is broad, similar to that under ERISA.[51]

State Premium Taxes and Similar Laws

FEHBA also preempts state premium tax and similar assessment laws.[52] The statute provides that

> No tax, fee, or other monetary payment may be imposed, directly or in-

directly, on a carrier...by any State, the District of Columbia...or other governmental authority thereof, with respect to any payment from the [Employees Health Benefits] Fund.

Contractors that operate in states that impose a premium tax must ensure that their FEHBP subscription rates do not include an allocation for the tax. This is accomplished by charging the FEHBP a "negative loading" to back out the applicable amount.

The preemption is not limited to state premium taxes. Other state fees have also been preempted.[53] Preemption does not apply, however, to state assessments of general applicability.[54]

QUALITY ASSURANCE

FEHBP carriers are required to develop and maintain a quality assurance program.[55] The quality assurance program must include procedures for (1) accuracy of payments; (2) timeliness of payments to members or providers; (3) quality of services and responsiveness to members; (4) responsiveness to FEHBP members' requests for reconsideration; (5) quality assurance plan; (6) physician credentialing; and (7) appointment scheduling. OPM's Standard Contract sets forth the required standards for aspects of the contractor's quality assurance program. Carriers are required to collect data on measures endorsed by the Foundation for Accountability (FACCT) in assessing the quality of health care. Carriers are also required to participate in either the National Committee for Quality Assurance (NCQA) Health Plan Employer Data and Information Set (HEDIS) consumer survey or any FEHBP-specific consumer survey to provide feedback to enrollees on enrollee experience with the health plan. Accreditation and HEDIS are discussed in Chapter 44.

CONCLUSION

The FEHBP will continue to be the largest employer-sponsored health benefits program. OPM's ability to administer successfully this ever-growing program and to retain desirable contractors will depend on its ability to demand accountability from its contractors while maintaining consistency in the application of its rules on rates and benefits. In this regard, one of the most important developments to date has been the move away from traditional community-rating requirements toward a focus on the

FEHBP's comparability to other SSSGs. This approach appears to be preferred from the perspective of both OPM and the contractors because the latest SSSG rules define with more precision the standards by which FEHBP contractors' rates will be evaluated.

REFERENCES AND NOTES

1. *See* 5 U.S.C. Section 8902(1). The federal HMO law is at 42 U.S.C. Sections 300e *et seq.*

2. 5 C.F.R. Section 890.203(a)(1) (1999).

3. 5 C.F.R. Section 890.203(a)(3) (1999).

4. 48 C.F.R. Section 1652.222-70 (1999).

5. 5 U.S.C. Section 8902(1).

6. 5 C.F.R. Section 890.203(a)(5) (1999).

7. 59 Fed. Reg. 62,283 (December 5, 1994).

8. 59 Fed. Reg. 62,284.

9. *See* 60 Fed. Reg. 15,074 (March 22, 1995) (codified at 5 C.F.R. Section 890.203).

10. 5 C.F.R. Section 890.203(a)(1) (1999).

11. *See* 5 U.S.C. Section 8904.

12. Carrier Letter 1999-016 (April 9, 1999).

13. Carrier Letter, see note 12.

14. *See* Consumer Bill of Rights and Responsibilities, Report to the President of the United States, President's Advisory Commission on Consumer Protection and Quality in the Health Care Industry, November 1997.

15. Pursuant to 42 U.S.C. 300e-1, with limited exceptions, the premium rates charged by federally qualified HMOs must be based on a community rating system. *See also* 42 C.F.R. Section 417.104. Subject to state HMO law restrictions, entities operating federally qualified HMOs may offer a non-federally-qualified product that is experience rated.

16. 48 C.F.R. Sections 1601.100-1653.000 (1999).

17. 48 C.F.R. Section 1602.170-6 (1999).

18. *See* 55 Fed. Reg. 27406-27419 (July 2, 1990).

19. *See* 48 C.F.R. Section 1615.905(b).

20. 48 C.F.R. Section 1602.170-2 (1989).

21. 48 C.F.R. Section 1602.170-2(a) (1993).

22. 54 Fed. Reg. 43,089 (October 20, 1989).

23. 48 C.F.R. Section 1602.170-2(b) (1993).

24. 48 C.F.R. Section 1615.804-70 (1993).

25. OPM promulgated final regulations in 1997 that also require CMPs to certify cost and pricing data. *See* 62 Fed. Reg. 47,569 (September 10, 1997). Cost or pricing data for community rated carriers is "the specialized rating data used by carriers in computing a rate that is appropriate for the Federal group and the [SSSGs]. Such data include, but are not limited to, capitation rates; prescription drug, hospital, and office visit benefits utilization data; trend data; actuarial data; rating methodologies for other groups; standardized presentation of the carrier's rating method (age, sex, etc.) showing that the factor predicts utilization; tiered rates information; 'step-up' factors information; demographics such as family size; special benefit loading capitations and adjustment factors for capitation." 48 C.F.R. Section 1602.170-5 (1997).

26. Even though the SSSG regulations were not finalized until well after the 1990 contract year had commenced, OPM announced that, for the 1990 contract year, the agency would assess a contractor's compliance with applicable rating requirements on the basis of the rates charged the SSSGs.

27. 48 C.F.R. § 1602.170-11 (1990).

28. 48 C.F.R. Section 1615.804-70 (1990).

29. 59 Fed. Reg. 14,761 (March 30, 1994).

30. 48 C.F.R. Section 1602.170-11 (1994).

31. 62 Fed. Reg. 47,574 (September 10, 1997) (codified at 48 C.F.R. Section 1602.170-13).

32. OPM Reconciliation Guidelines—1999.

33. *See* 48 C.F.R. Section 1652.204-70 (1999).

34. Contractor appeals of adverse audit findings that are reflected in an agency final decision are governed by the Contract Disputes Act, 41 U.S.C. Sections 601 *et seq.*

35. OPM acknowledges that it lacks authority to claim interest from the date of the overpayment for contract year 1990.

36. *PCA Health Plans of Texas, Inc.*, ASBCA No. 48711, 1998 ASBCA LEXIS 108 (June 24, 1998).

37. *PCA Health Plans of Texas, Inc. v. United States*, 191 F.3d 1353 (Fed. Cir. 1999).

38. *QualMed Plans for Health of New Mexico, Inc. v. United States,* No. 98-145 C (January 11, 2000).

39. *See, e.g., MD-Individual Practice Association, Inc. v. United States of America*, No. 93-460C (Ct. Fed. Cl. filed 23 July 1993) and *Kaiser Foundation Health Plan of the Mid-Atlantic States, Inc. v. United States of America*, No. 92-855C (Ct. Fed. Cl. filed 18 December 1992).

40. *See* FEHBP Letter No. 95-27c (August 10, 1995).

41. *See* Section 3.6, "Discrepancies between Enrollment and Payments to Carrier," Federal Employees Health Benefits Program Standard Contract for Community-Rated Comprehensive Medical Plans 1997.

42. OPM Retirement and Insurance Service Benefits Administration Letter Number 99-410 (September 17, 1999).

43. 10 U.S. Code Section 1108 (1999).

44. 5 C.F.R. Section 890.1308 (1999).

45. Section 3.2(c), "Accounting and Price Adjustment, Federal Employees Health Benefits Program Standard Contract for Community-Rated Comprehensive Medical Plans 2000. *See also* 64 Fed. Reg. 36,237 (July 6, 1999).

46. 5 U.S. Code Section 8901(m)(1).

47. 29 U.S. Code Section 1003(b).

48. *See Pilot Life Insurance Company v. Dedeaux*, 481 U.S. 41 (1987), wherein the U.S. Supreme Court held that the civil enforcement provisions of ERISA are preemptive and provide a federal remedy for state law claims such as tortuous breach of contract or bad faith conduct. Suits by enrollees challenging the denial of benefits under an employee health benefit plan may therefore be removed to federal court, where only ERISA remedies are available.

49. *See Hartenstine v. Superior Court of San Bernardino County*, 196 Cal. App. 3d 206 (1987), *cert. denied*, 488 U.S. 899 (1988).

50. *See Hanson v. Blue Cross Blue Shield of Iowa*, 953 F. Supp. 270 (N.D. Iowa 1996).

51. *See Negron v. Patel*, 6 F. Supp. 2d 366 (E.D. Pa. 1998) (FEHBA did not preempt federal enrollee's claim to impose various liability on HMO for medical malpractice, but did preempt enrollee's corporate negligence claim). Other cases addressing the scope of FEHBA preemption include: *State of Connecticut v. U.S.*, 1 F. Supp. 2d 147 (D. Conn. 1998); *Arnold v. Blue Cross and Blue Shield of Texas*, 973 F. Supp. 726 (S.D. Tex. 1997); *Sarkis v. Heimburger*, 933 F. Supp. 828 (E.D. Mo. 1996); and *Santitoro v. Evans*, 935 F. Supp. 733 (E.D.N.C. 1996).

52. 5 U.S. Code Section 8909(f).

53. *Health Maintenance Organization of New Jersey v. Whitman,* 72 F.3d 1123 (3rd Cir. 1995).

54. 5 U.S. Code Section 8909(f)(2).

55. *See* Section 1.9, Standard Contract for Community-Rated Comprehensive Medical Plans.

CHAPTER 55

Medicare and Managed Care

Carlos Zarabozo and Jean D. LeMasurier

INTRODUCTION

Observing the current debate on the future of the Medicare program and the role of private health plans in that future calls to mind certain metaphors of family life in America. The Medicare program, which seems to have been around forever, only dates from 1965 and is now in its younger middle-aged epoch, whereas the Medicare risk program dates from 1985—not "old," but not a toddler either. Medicare managed care is a teenager, but nearly half the age of its parent. Like many teenagers, it is still growing, and it is still finding its way in the world. Meanwhile, its parent is having a midlife crisis, trying to keep up with a fast-changing world and wondering what to do with its teenage offspring. Will the Medicare program act on its life crisis by buying a sports car and riding off into the sunset—with the teenager at the wheel? Or will the old family car, the this-*is*-your-father's Oldsmobile, get only a little body work and a paint job, with a morose teenager relegated to the back seat for those Sunday drives?

However that domestic scene resolves itself, the teenager has had an interesting adolescence. It was one of the stars of the Balanced Budget Act of 1997 (BBA), which gave new prominence to the role of private health plans in Medicare; expanded the types of options available to Medicare beneficiaries; and introduced a number of changes in payment, enrollment rules, contracting standards, and other requirements. Not that the program necessarily needed an extra boost. By some measures, the program did quite well in its adolescence without the BBA. The percent of beneficiaries enrolled in what is now known as Medicare + Choice (M+C) has increased, as of 1999, to about 16 percent of the nationwide Medicare population. In terms of managed care "penetration," among beneficiaries with access to M+C plans (about 70 percent of the population), 23 percent are M+C enrollees. In some counties penetration rates exceed 50 percent of the population—the teenager has surpassed the parent in certain counties in Oregon and California.

The largest increases in Medicare risk enrollment occurred before the BBA, at about the

Carlos Zarabozo is a social science research analyst in the Office of Strategic Planning of the Health Care Financing Administration (HCFA). He previously held a number of positions in HCFA's managed care office, including Director of the Operational Analysis Staff and Special Assistant to the Director.

Jean D. LeMasurier is Deputy Director of HCFA's Health Plan Purchasing Administration, Center For Health Plans and Providers. The office is responsible for implementing the newly enacted Medicare + Choice program. She previously was Deputy Director of the Plan and Provider Purchasing Policy Group, the office that developed the Medicare + Choice regulation.

Note: The views expressed in this chapter are the authors and not those of HCFA. All addresses and telephone numbers listed were accurate at the time of publication; however, such numbers and addresses occasionally change, and the authors make no warranty as to their currency.

same time as the surge in managed care enrollment in the private sector and in Medicaid. One-half million beneficiaries were added to the Medicare managed care rolls in 1994; 800,000 in 1995; and more than one million were added in both 1996 and 1997. The latter two years were also the years in which overall HMO enrollment had its greatest rate of increase in this decade (InterStudy).

The BBA did a number of things to attempt to continue the expansion of Medicare managed care and other private options while changing almost all aspects of the Medicare managed care program. Hence much of this chapter discusses new or revised standards introduced by the BBA. It contains what might appear to be endless references to the BBA and its implementing regulations and how the BBA differs from earlier statutory and regulatory provisions governing what was known in its earlier incarnation as the TEFRA risk program (after the enabling legislation, the Tax Equity and Fiscal Responsibility Act of 1982) or the Medicare risk HMO program. The chapter includes the modifications to the BBA made by the Balanced Budget Refinement Act of 1999 (BBRA), which made changes to BBA provisions affecting the M+C program.

ORGANIZATION OF THE CHAPTER

This chapter discusses the M+C program from a primarily "operational" viewpoint. The sections of the chapter are ordered in a way that roughly matches the decision process of a person or organization deciding whether to enter into a Medicare contract. The chapter explains what kind of organization may enter into a risk contract, how the contractor is paid and what limits there are on the sources and uses of revenue under the contract, what the contractor is required to do (a very large part of the chapter), how marketing and information dissemination occurs, how enrollment occurs, what rights beneficiaries and providers have, and what changes might be in store for the program in the future. Entire sections may be skipped by particular readers, for example, readers who believe they know inti-

mately how payment works may skip the entire section on payment.

WHO IS ELIGIBLE FOR A MEDICARE RISK CONTRACT?

State Licensure

One of the major changes in the BBA involves greater reliance on state standards than on federal standards in certain areas. Before the BBA, eligibility for a Medicare managed care contract depended on a federal determination of whether the organization could meet the definition of an "eligible organization." The determination was made by the Health Care Financing Administration (HCFA), the federal agency that administers the Medicare program. An eligible organization could be one of two types of entities, federally qualified HMOs, as defined by the federal HMO Act, or competitive medical plans, defined by Medicare law as organizations essentially meeting most of the same standards as federally qualified plans in their structure and benefit offering in the non-Medicare sector. With the BBA, the kind of organization that can "come in the door" includes any health care organization licensed by a state as a risk-bearing entity. A 100-year-old licensed insurance company offering health care coverage that had no HMO experience (admittedly a rare breed in today's world) would meet this initial qualification requirement under the BBA, but it would not have been a pre-BBA "eligible organization."

For all organizations, HCFA requires that the state provide a certification that the nature of the licensure or authority to offer risk products is, in the opinion of the state, consistent with the requirements for assumption of risk as an M+C organization. Under HCFA's regulatory interpretation of the statute, an entity need not be formally licensed by the State regulatory body overseeing HMOs and health insurers, as long as that regulatory body finds the legal status and financial status of the organization to be sufficient to manage the risk entailed by a Medicare risk contract. For example, an organization operating in a state as a "state-defined" Medicaid HMO that was not licensed by the insurance department (as the state regulatory body licensing HMOs in the particular state), but was instead authorized to operate as a Medicaid plan by the state health department, could have an M+C contract as long as the insurance department consented—agreeing, for example, that the state health department's standards for Medicaid contracts were sufficient for the purposes of M+C contracting.

Repeal of 50/50

The same Medicaid-only HMO that the state has blessed would have had another insurmountable hurdle in pre-BBA days because of its inability to comply with the "50/50 rule," the rule requiring that at least 50 percent of an organization's enrollment be non-Medicare, non-Medicaid enrollment. This requirement not only prevented "Medicaid-only" HMOs from participating in Medicare, but it also prevented the expansion of organizations to new Medicare markets because the 50/50 rule was applied to the membership within a particular service area. An organization seeking to expand its Medicare business to a new geographical area not contiguous to its current area would have to establish a commercial presence in the new area before being able to enter into a Medicare contract in the new area. Or an organization could approach the goal in a different way by adding contiguous counties to its existing service area and offering Medicare in the new counties one by one, until the desired county could be added on as the last contiguous county (a somewhat difficult feat if, for instance, a Los Angeles HMO wanted to enter the Medicare market in New York).

Minimum Enrollment: Waiver of Requirement

The BBA also modified the minimum enrollment requirement so as to encourage new contracts. Under the BBA policy, there is a requirement that to have an M+C contract an organization must have at least 5,000 members, or 1,500 members if operating in a rural area. Members are defined by the BBA differently from pre-BBA days,

when the members had to be prepaid, capitated members, not members of an indemnity plan, for example. To further encourage new organizations, the BBA gives HCFA authority to waive this minimum enrollment requirement for up to three years under certain conditions (generally if the organization and its providers show the ability to manage a risk contract).

THE EXCEPTION IN STATE LICENSURE: PROVIDER-SPONSORED ORGANIZATIONS

Because Medicare law requires that Medicare coordinated care contractors be state-licensed entities and because state laws governing entities that assume risk for comprehensive services are geared toward the more traditional HMO model, the BBA allows provider-sponsored organizations (PSOs) meeting certain standards to have a waiver of the state licensure requirements that would otherwise apply to all M+C organizations. Although other M+C organizations must meet state solvency standards for risk-bearing organizations, the BBA directed HCFA to establish federal solvency standards for PSOs that avail themselves of the waiver of state licensure provision. The solvency standards were established through a negotiated rule-making process, with the standards published in the *Federal Register*, preceded by an earlier notice providing a definition of a PSO. The state licensure waiver is available to PSOs until November 1, 2002. A waiver is limited to three years' duration and can be granted only under certain conditions, including, for example, when a State requires a PSO to meet solvency standards for coordinated care plans that are more stringent than the federally established PSO solvency standards.

PSOs must meet all other standards applicable to M+C coordinated care plans, except for the minimum enrollment requirement, as explained in the following. Although the state licensure requirement may be waived, there is no waiver of other state standards that apply to M+C organizations (e.g., quality and consumer protection standards in a state).

For purposes of the BBA exceptions, a PSO is defined as an organization that delivers a substantial proportion of services directly through the sponsoring provider(s) or through affiliated providers. In an urban area 70 percent of health care services (as measured by expenditures) must be provided directly or through affiliated providers (but only 60 percent in a rural area). Providers are considered affiliates if they have direct or indirect financial risk for the overall organization. Providers must have majority ownership of the organization. For organizations meeting the BBA definition of a PSO, the minimum precontract enrollment requirement is reduced to 1,000 members (500 in a rural area), a requirement that may also be waived.

OTHER NEW OPTIONS

Medical Savings Account Plans

The BBA includes authority for a demonstration of a medical savings account (MSA) option for up to 390,000 Medicare beneficiaries. The MSA is combined with an M+C "high-deductible" plan (which may be a network plan such as an HMO) that is responsible for paying 100 percent of the cost of covered care after the deductible is met. A portion of the capitation that would otherwise be paid to the M+C organization is deposited in an account that the beneficiary can use to finance the cost of medical care, including medical care that is not covered by Medicare. The Medicare payment to the account is made at the beginning of the year for use during the year or in subsequent years. The Medicare contribution may also be used to finance the cost of items or services that the Internal Revenue Services does not define as qualified medical expenses, but in such a case the withdrawal would be taxable.

The rationale for MSA plans is that they eliminate "first dollar" coverage by a third party and thereby make individuals more prudent purchasers of health care. That is, until the deductible is met, a Medicare beneficiary uses his or her own money—including any money available from the MSA account—to pay for the cost of care. The actual expenses a person must incur out-of-pocket will vary with his or her health care needs, by the size of the deductible (no

minimum has been established, but the maximum is $6,000 per year), and by the level of contribution available from Medicare. In some cases, it may take several years to accumulate a Medicare contribution equal to the deductible.

Under the law, MSA options would first be available beginning in January 1999, although as of the end of 1999 there were no operating MSA plans. On choosing this option, a Medicare beneficiary must remain enrolled in the M+C MSA plan for at least one year (or until the next M+C annual coordinated election period if coverage began during a person's initial period of Medicare eligibility during the calendar year). Certain beneficiaries are not eligible to enroll in the MSA option: those on Medicaid, individuals obtaining health care coverage through certain federal programs, and others who have primary coverage other than Medicare or coverage that covers all or part of the annual deductible. A person must also reside in the United States at least half the year to be eligible to enroll.

Preferred Provider Organizations

As noted previously, the BBA makes changes to some definitions and standards in hopes of expanding available options. The BBA defines coordinated care plans as including HMOs (a category that would encompass what are defined as competitive medical plans in prior law), preferred provider organizations (PPOs), and PSOs. Before the BBA, a PPO offered by an indemnity insurer might not have been able to enter into a Medicare risk contract as a competitive medical plan (CMP) because it would not have met the definition of a CMP—that is, the organization may not have assumed full risk on an exclusively prepaid capitated basis for its *non-Medicare* enrollees, as required by the prior Medicare statute. The new law and regulations require that any M+C plan, including a PPO, assume prepaid capitated risk for its *Medicare* enrollees and that it be able to provide the full range of covered services through network providers. The statute as changed by the BBA no longer specifies the nature of the risk arrangement for *non-Medicare* members and no longer specifies any limitation on the extent of non-network use by non-Medicare enrollees (who under prior law had to obtain service "primarily" through CMP providers). The BBA only requires that a PPO—or any entity wishing to have an M+C contract—be licensed as a risk-bearing entity by the state, and that its members be individuals "who are receiving health benefits through the organization," regardless of the exact nature of the risk arrangement (insurance risk versus prepaid capitated risk). As noted previously, the state determines whether the type of license held by a PPO, a PPO sponsor, or any other risk-bearing entity would enable the organization to enter into a contract with HCFA to assume risk for the comprehensive range of Medicare services.

A significant change made in the BBRA was to classify PPOs as non-network plans for the purposes of the quality standards that apply to M+C plans. That is, PPOs follow the quality standards applicable to private fee-for-service (PFFS) plans and non-network MSA plans. The BBRA also clarified the definition of M+C PPOs. A PPO is a plan offered by an organization not licensed by the state as an HMO, which has a network of providers that agree to a specific rate of reimbursement for covered services, and which reimburses members for services received through non-network providers.

Private Fee-for-Service Plans

An organization may choose to enter into a contract with HCFA to offer a private insurance plan that reimburses providers on a fee-for-service basis and does not limit enrollees to the use of network providers. As an enrollee of an M+C PFFS plan, a Medicare beneficiary may use any Medicare-participating provider who agrees to provide services to the beneficiary, and the organization sponsoring the PFFS plan (e.g., a private insurer) will make payment for covered services in a manner similar to a traditional indemnity plan operating in the private marketplace. A PFFS plan may not pay its providers on other than a fee-for-service basis, and it may not place providers at financial risk for the utilization of services.

The PFFS plan may have a network of providers who agree to the terms of the plan, but the law also provides for "deemed" participating providers. A provider is deemed to be a participating provider if he or she (or the entity) is aware of the beneficiary's enrollment in the PFFS plan and the provider is aware of, or has been given a reasonable opportunity to be made aware of, the terms and conditions of payment under the plan "in a manner reasonably designed to effect informed agreement" to participate, as stated in the regulations. A noncontracting provider may only receive, in total payments (from the PFFS plan and from enrollee cost sharing), an amount equal to what would have been paid in total under original Medicare. Contracting and deemed providers may also receive additional payments from the enrollee ("balance billing") up to 15 percent of the PFFS plan payment amount. The PFFS organization is charged with ensuring that providers adhere to the limits on permissible balance billed amounts; failure to monitor adherence to the requirement can result in HCFA's decision not to renew the organization's contract. Enrollees may incur additional liability if the PFFS retrospectively denies coverage (as not Medicare-covered or for non-Medicare-covered benefits not covered under the plan).

As noted in the Conference Report accompanying the BBA legislation, the PFFS option is the first Medicare option that has the structure of a defined contribution. That is, the government contribution toward the cost of the option is limited to the M+C payment amount, but there are no limits on what the organization may charge as a member premium for the benefit package. (For Medicare-covered services, other M+C plans are limited to charges (premiums and other cost-sharing) that do not exceed the actuarial equivalent of cost-sharing under original Medicare, as explained in the following.)

Point of Service: Old Wine in New Bottles

Among the "new" options "introduced" by the BBA were Medicare point-of-service (POS) plans to be offered by M+C organizations. This was actually a reintroduction of an option available under the risk program since 1995. Perhaps it was reintroduced with greater fanfare because it had not enjoyed great popularity among risk contractors (for a number of reasons, some having to do with state regulatory standards). HMOs may offer a POS benefit (coverage of care obtained out of network) to their Medicare enrollees. The regulations provide great latitude in the design of the benefit, how it is financed (including as an additional benefit funded by Medicare capitation payments), charges to beneficiaries, and the extent to which it must be made available (e.g., it can be a benefit solely available to employer group retirees). However, organizations offering a POS option are subject to additional monitoring by HCFA to ensure continued compliance with standards pertaining to financial solvency, availability and accessibility of care, quality assurance, member appeals, and marketing standards.

Repeal of the Cost Plan Option

Since the beginning of the Medicare program, HMOs have been allowed to participate in the program under a cost reimbursement arrangement. As of August 5, 1997, the Secretary is prohibited from entering into any new cost-based contracts. The cost-based payment authority is repealed and all cost contracts are terminated as of December 31, 2004. Until that time, cost contractors adhere to the rules applicable before enactment of the BBA.[1]

MUDDYING THE WATERS: PLANS VERSUS ORGANIZATIONS

A terminological excursus is necessary before we can proceed. There are many good reasons why bureaucrats are considered great enemies of the English language. Among our crimes against the English language are mere misdemeanors, such as the use of *timely* as an adverb ("your appeal was denied because you didn't file timely"), and more serious offenses such as HCFA's hi-

jacking of the term *provider* to mean only institutional providers and home health agencies. Although the "plain English" meaning of the term *health plan* is known throughout the land, the BBA has forced HCFA into another linguistic miasma by requiring a distinction between an organization holding an M+C contract and the "plans" that organization offers. One organization may offer multiple "plans" in a given service area or multiple areas (including noncontiguous areas, as alluded to in the previous discussion of the 50/50 rule), as long as each plan meets applicable M+C standards. The plans may differ slightly (e.g., POS benefits are or are not included) or they may be significantly different: the same organization offers a PFFS plan and a traditional HMO option. Where one organization has multiple plans, HCFA will treat plans as "severable" if, for example, the need arises to impose a corrective action on a given plan or if a termination or nonrenewal of a particular plan of the organization is deemed appropriate.

Service Area: "Flexible Benefits"

In olden times (the mid-1980s), an organization's Medicare service area was required to match its commercial service area, although one would be hard put to find specific statutory language expressing such a requirement. Because olden times were simpler times, the statute contemplated (as the lawyers say) a situation in which an organization merely added Medicare business to its products, with much of the remaining structure untouched (service area, provider network).

As time passed, HCFA changed its policy and permitted organizations to operate in a smaller area for Medicare, as long as "county integrity" was maintained. That is, an organization could choose which counties within its authorized service area it wanted to include in the Medicare contract, but a geographical unit smaller than a county could not be designated as the Medicare service area for a given county unless the organization served only that portion of the county in its other lines of business. HCFA approved

Medicare service area designations requested by applicants on the basis of network adequacy (the ability to provide the full range of services under the contract in the service area), using standards to prevent discrimination or other "gaming" through service area configurations. This is essentially the policy under the BBA, but with the county integrity rule (subject to limited exceptions) particularly emphasized. The BBA introduces a wrinkle in the service area issue because the BBA also requires that within the service area of a plan, the benefits and premiums must be uniform. The uniform premium and benefits requirement leads to certain decisions on the part of organizations with regard to the "plans" they offer and the areas in which those plans are offered.

The uniform benefits policy of the BBA was both a departure from and a return to pre-BBA policy. To clarify this seemingly oxymoronic statement, before the BBA, HCFA permitted organizations to vary benefits by county under what was known as the "flexible benefits" policy. The legal basis for the flexible benefits policy was not well understood, or at least not widely understood, with the result that the BBA policy became fixed based on an erroneous assumption regarding the legal underpinnings of the flexible benefits policy. A new policy was developed that allowed organizations to continue the flexible benefits approach within the parameters of the BBA.

Under pre-BBA law there was in fact a uniform benefits policy that applied to all enrollees under one contract (and hence to an entire service area): all beneficiaries residing in the service area had to be charged the same premium for Medicare enrollment and had to receive all extra benefits that the organization was obligated to provide. That is to say, any surplus Medicare revenues, after normal profit, had to be returned equally to all beneficiaries in the service area (as part of the adjusted community rate proposal computation described in detail later). However, on the basis of a legal opinion declaring that the requirement only applied to the disposition of *Medicare* dollars (i.e., the Medicare capitation), HCFA permitted organizations to use *non-Medicare* money to enhance benefits for some

Medicare beneficiaries and not for others. But there were limits placed on who could or could not benefit from an organization's generosity. Although HCFA initially allowed differing benefits to be provided on the basis of an individual's choice of provider network within an organization, HCFA eventually determined that "flexible benefits" could vary only at the county level—all Medicare beneficiaries in a county had to enjoy the same level of nongovernmental largesse.

The BBA's uniform premium and benefits policy nearly put an end to flexible benefits, until the concept of segmented service areas was developed. This policy allows organizations to subdivide a service area under a single contract and provide varying benefits within the subareas. The segmented service area approach is described as a transitional policy that essentially allows the continuation of flexible benefits in the same pre-BBA geographical configuration, although the regulations do suggest that there should be some standards calling for a segmented area to have characteristics that are usually associated with the concept of an independent service area or a regional component (e.g., a provider network for the subarea, different rating for the subarea). The BBRA modified the statutory language so that now what was developed as a transitional policy has become the statutorily determined approach to segmented service areas. The BBRA requires uniformity of premiums and benefits at the level of the "segment" of a service area, defined as one or more M+C payment areas (with the BBA defining M+C payment areas as counties).

One byproduct of the segmented service area policy is that the computation of surplus Medicare revenues to be "returned" to beneficiaries as extra benefits occurs at the level of the segmented area, not at the level of the contract area. Hence, where Medicare capitation rates vary significantly among counties, an organization can, through segmenting of service areas, vary the generosity of benefit packages solely as a function of the level of Medicare capitation. The organization no longer has to have recourse to a policy that required a "lowest common denominator" benefit package across all counties and only allowed *non-Medi-*

care revenue to be parceled out differently among neighboring counties (although it is quite likely that the revenue used for "flexible benefits" was in fact Medicare revenue despite the legal underpinning of the policy). Thus, the BBA and BBRA policy continues the flexible benefits approach but it has now sanctioned, or institutionalized, variation in the use of *Medicare* dollars at the subcontract level.

Continuation Areas: Service beyond the Service Area

A new provision allows M+C plans to have enrollment "continuation areas," areas that are not part of the service area but in which an enrollee moving to the area can retain enrollment in the M+C plan, with the organization arranging for coverage of services in the new area. Generally, the same requirements apply in the continuation area as apply in the original service area for both the organization and the enrollee. However, the law as it is currently written does not require the provision of additional benefits (i.e., non-Medicare benefits financed by surplus Medicare revenue) in the continuation area.

The BBRA introduced a change that permits an organization to offer continued M+C enrollment to residents of an area affected by a "service area reduction" (i.e., the organization chooses to drop a county or counties from its M+C service area, but retains the M+C contract in a reduced service area). The M+C organization, at its option, may offer continued enrollment to residents of all, or some, of the discontinued areas, as long as the Medicare enrollee agrees to receive all (non-emergent) services in the surviving service area, and as long as no other M+C options are available in the discontinued area.

Payment, or the Art of Phasing In and Phasing Out

It is an immutable law of human nature, it seems, that payment is an important issue, just as it appears to be an immutable law that the payment method the government uses cannot be ex-

plained in a sentence or two, as illustrated by the next sentence. The capitation payments for M+C plans after 1997 are based on a formula for updating the 1997 rates combined with certain provisions that increase or decrease payments in certain areas, under certain conditions, for certain items or for certain people—in some cases, and sometimes on a gradual basis.

Perhaps recourse to a foreign language will help. *"L'avenir de la France dépend de son futur,"* was the seemingly profound campaign statement of a French politician. This gem can be translated loosely as "What will become of France depends on its future." The relevance of this to payment under a Medicare risk contract is that your statutorily determined Medicare payment rate determines how much you will get paid for each enrollee. That is, Medicare uses an "administered" pricing mechanism to set rates for M+C plans. The rates for each calendar year for each county (or for each state, in the case of payments for enrollees with end-stage renal disease [ESRD]) are published early in the preceding year.[2] Rates for individuals vary by fixed demographic factors applicable across the entire population, and, as of the year 2000, payments are risk adjusted at the level of the individual enrollee. You may not want to know about the details of how the rates are determined (you will not be tested on your knowledge of the rate-setting mechanism, except perhaps in the sense of being "sorely tested"), but at a minimum you would want to know what to expect in the way of payment changes from one year to the next. (Recourse to tables also helps. See Table 55–1.)

Until 1997, Medicare's capitation payments were based on historical fee-for-service costs in the geographical area (the county, except for beneficiaries with ESRD, who have a statewide payment rate). County-level capitation rates were set at 95 percent of the expected level of costs in the traditional Medicare fee-for-service program for a calendar year. Actuarial projections were made on the basis of the historical relationship between local fee-for-service expenditures and national expenditures, and adjustments were made at the county level to reflect any differences in the demographic makeup

Table 55–1 Variables Affecting M+C Payments

Year	Medical Education Removed	Local/National Blend, if Budget Neutral	Risk Adjustment Applies to . . .	Reduction in Update
1998	20%	90% local/10% national	0	.8 (point reduction in projected growth %)
1999	40%	82/18	0	.5
2000	60%	74/26 (first year of actual blend payments)	10% of payment (inpatient data only)	.5
2001	80%	66/34	10%	.5
2002	100%	58/52	no more than 20%	.3
2003		50% local/ 50% national	not yet determined	0
2004			not yet determined	0

Source: Reprinted from the Balanced Budget Act of 1997, the Balanced Budget Refinement Act of 1999, and the *Federal Register* of June 16, 1998.

of the county compared with the nation as a whole. This was the much-reviled adjusted average per capita cost methodology.

The pre-BBA methodology resulted in wide variation across counties. In 1997, for example, the base payment rate for the lowest-paid county in the 50 states, Arthur, Nebraska, with its 79 Medicare beneficiaries, was $221 per month, whereas in Miami-Dade the rate was nearly $750 per month or more than three times the rate of Arthur. In the year 2000, the Miami-Dade rate will be only twice as high as the rate that Arthur receives (the national minimum rate). The new payment method made a number of changes that, among other things, even out these regional differences and may serve to increase the availability of M+C options in rural areas, for example. Whereas in 1997, there would have been one (long) answer to the question, why are we paid X dollars in this county and only Y dollars in this neighboring county?, in 2000 there would be a different (long) answer to the question.

Minimum Payments and Increases

Under the BBA the payment is no longer based on local fee-for-service costs but is instead subject to a variety of provisions that determine the change in payment levels from one year to

the next. Beginning with payments for 1998, each county's rates are the highest of three possible rates:

- a minimum payment level or "floor," set initially at $367 for 1998 and $402 in 2000 (for the 50 states and the District of Columbia)
- a minimum increase in payment from year to year of at least two percent
- a blended rate of local-level rates and input-price–adjusted national rates (i.e., average national costs by category of service adjusted by the ratio of local input prices to national average input prices)

The 1997 rates are the payment rates that form the basis of subsequent updates and changes. Updates to payment rates from year to year will be made on the basis of a projection of the growth in Medicare's per capita expenditures. Under BBA provisions, the projected update amounts are required to be reduced by a fraction of a percent through the year 2002, as shown in Table 55–1.

Blended Rate

The blended rate is phased in so that beginning in 2003, there is a 50/50 blend of local and national rates. The law also provides state governors the opportunity to request a reconfiguration of geographical payment areas to use an alternative other than the county as the geographical unit (e.g., metropolitan areas). However, the blend is adjusted for budget neutrality to ensure that aggregate Medicare payments to M+C plans throughout the country do not exceed the amount that would otherwise have been paid in the absence of the blend (i.e., had all counties received a payment based entirely on local rates rather than a local/national blend). Thus, blended rates were not paid until the year 2000.

Removal of Medical Education

Medical education costs paid by the Medicare program (direct and indirect medical education payments) are removed from M+C rates and are to be paid by the Medicare program directly to providers and organizations incurring medical education costs for M+C enrollees. This reduction and shift in payment began in 1998 on a phased-in basis and will be fully implemented in 2002.

Risk Adjustment

An important change in payment policy addresses the issue of selection bias among Medicare risk plans. Beginning in the year 2000, on a phased-in basis, payments to M+C plans will be adjusted for the health status of individual enrollees. To make appropriate adjustments, HCFA has required M+C plans to submit patient data on their inpatient admissions dating from July 1, 1997, with full encounter data required for services on or after July 1, 1998 (consistent with the BBA statutory authority). Payment on the basis of risk-adjusted amounts for the year 2000 are based only on inpatient hospital data, with comprehensive risk adjustment, including inpatient and outpatient data, set to begin in 2004, the year in which risk adjustment is fully phased in.

HCFA exercised its discretion and chose to phase in risk-adjusted payments. For 2000 and 2001, the actual payment to the plan is 90 percent demographically adjusted and 10 percent risk adjusted. The risk-adjusted payments are computed for each beneficiary using three fac-

tors—demographics (age, sex), health status, and "other" factors (previously disabled, Medicaid, and working aged status). The only demographic factor not used for the new risk-adjusted payments is the separate set of factors used for beneficiaries who reside in an institution, a factor found to be no longer necessary because of the new risk adjustment method.

The risk adjustment is at the individual level (it "follows" the individual if the person changes plans), and, under the current method, is based on recent, but "lagged," information on hospital admissions for the individual and the diagnosis for the hospital admission. The method is the principal inpatient diagnostic cost group (PIP/DCG) method, which uses inpatient stays as a predictor of *total* Medicare expenditures for an individual. Individuals who have no history of hospitalization during the relevant prior period, or individuals for whom HCFA has no hospitalization records (e.g., new Medicare beneficiaries at age 65), have their payments risk-adjusted (as opposed to health-status-adjusted) only by the demographic factors for the individual. One-day hospital stays do not qualify for a health status adjustment.[3]

New Entrant Bonus

The BBRA added a provision to the law that calls for bonus payments to M+C organizations entering new markets in 2000 or 2001. For the first 12 months of the M+C contract, there is a five percent increase in payments for an organization entering a new market, and a three percent bonus in the second 12 months. The bonus is available only if the area has not had a Medicare plan since 1997, or if all organizations previously serving the area notified HCFA, by October 13, 1999, of their departure from the area as of January 1, 2000. The bonus is available only to the first new entrant, unless there are multiple new entrants entering the market on the same date.

User Fees

One more factor affects payments, which is a reduction in payments on the basis of a pro-rata user fee collected from all M+C organizations for the cost of M+C information activities described in the following, and for counseling and assistance programs.[4]

Announcement of Rates: Computation of Rates

The announcement of rates for each calendar year occurs early in the year to allow time for development of the informational material necessary for the coordinated open enrollment period introduced by the BBA. On January 15 each year, HCFA's actuaries announce, for purposes of public comment, any changes in the method. On March 1, the rates for the subsequent year are published.

Because payments are based on a blend of the old purely demographic rates and the new risk-adjusted rates, there are two "rate books" that HCFA publishes that need to be consulted to determine how much a particular organization will be paid. One is an update of the purely demographic rate book for 1997. This rate book lists rates for all U.S. counties, Medicare part A and part B base rates for the aged and the disabled (beneficiaries younger than 65 years entitled to Medicare because of their disability), together with a table of nationally used demographic factors, by which the county rates are multiplied to determine payment for an individual falling within a given "rate cell." State-level rates are given for individuals with ESRD. The updated rate book reflects the minimum payments, blends, and floor called for in the BBA.

The rate book for risk adjustment provides separate aged and disabled part A and part B rates showing:

- a base rate for each county
- a "rescaling" factor that is necessary to convert the base rate because the risk adjustment factors are not the same as those used in the 1997 methodology (e.g., institutionalization is no longer a factor)[5]
- demographic factors for the categories used with the PIP/DCG method

Data are also available on the average risk "scores" in each county, indicating the relative health status of Medicare beneficiaries in the county as a whole. (Individuals with ESRD continue to have their capitation payments computed on a statewide basis outside of the PIP/DCG method.)

PIP/DCG factors are person-specific factors that HCFA provides to organizations for enrolled individuals. Only the highest PIP/DCG risk factor is applied to an individual. Demographic factors that apply to the individual are "additive," which means that the PIP/DCG risk factor is combined with all other applicable risk factors to come up with a total expected level of expenditures (and, therefore, capitation payment level) for a given individual.

For years in which there is a blend of purely demographic and PIP/DCG rates, the relevant percentages shown in Table 55–1 apply to the determination of the combined payment from each of the two methods.

Benefits and Charges: Adjusted Community Rate Proposal Requirements

As noted previously, HCFA uses an administered pricing mechanism to pay M+C plans (oops!, we mean organizations). There is no negotiation over rates, and, given that all plans must include at least the Medicare benefit package, there would be no negotiation over the minimum benefit package required, nor is there negotiation over any supplemental or "additional" benefits. But just as the law specifies payment rates, the law also specifies charges that are possible, certain aspects of benefit offerings, and requirements that apply to the disposition of Medicare revenues.

An administrative process determines what premiums and other charges an organization may impose and determines whether Medicare's payments exceed the revenue needs of the organization for the provision of the Medicare benefit package. That process—submission of the adjusted community rate (ACR) proposal—is an accounting exercise to determine what it would cost a buyer other than HCFA to buy the Medicare benefit package for a group similar to the group HCFA is "insuring" (adjusted for the health care needs of the particular population and including administrative costs and the normal profit of a for-profit organization).[6] An element of the process is the comparison of the revenue needs to the revenue projected to be received from HCFA—i.e., the computation of an average payment rate (APR) using the process described in the Payment section.[7] Revenues in excess of those needed for providing the basic benefit must be "returned," dollar-for-dollar, to Medicare enrollees in the form of "additional benefits," which the law defines as reduced premium or cost-sharing for covered services, or the provision of extra, non-Medicare-covered benefits, or any combination of the two.[8]

ACR proposals are due July 1 of each year for the following calendar year, or they form a part of an initial application for an M+C contract. ACRs are filed electronically using an HCFA-prepared format. Each *plan* that an organization intends to offer must have a separate ACR.[9] Although the actuaries and the research community have been busy adding bells and whistles to the payment process, other elements within HCFA have made some modifications to the ACR process, as it is commonly known. Through regulations, HCFA changed the manner in which these proposals are to be computed beginning in the year 2000. Categories of commercial premium costs were modified to allow for more accurate accounting of the types of costs incurred and to provide a better measure of costs incurred for Medicare enrollees. In addition, the BBA requires HCFA to audit one third of all ACR proposals each year.

Limits on Charges for Medicare Services

As part of the rate determination and publication process, each year HCFA's actuaries determine the national actuarial equivalent of Medicare beneficiary liability amounts, expressed as a monthly average amount that Medicare beneficiaries have to pay for out-of-pocket expenses in fee-for-service Medicare for covered services (such as the coinsurance for physician services or the deductible a person pays on entering a hospital). When a Medicare beneficiary joins an

M+C plan, the beneficiary deductible and coinsurance requirements are usually satisfied by having the beneficiary pay a monthly premium to the HMO and/or copayments or other charges for services. The actuarial equivalent is the maximum total of premiums, copayments, and other charges that an organization may charge its Medicare members for Medicare-covered services (other than under a POS option, or in a PFFS plan). Plans for which the ACR proposal requires that "additional benefits" be provided use this limit as the starting point for reduction of cost sharing. For plans in which the ACR exceeds the APR, the published actuarial value of coinsurance and deductibles is the limit on total charges for Medicare-covered services; that is, no additional revenue may be obtained from the beneficiary (other than in a PFFS plan), such as through balance billing on the part of providers.

Supplemental Benefits: Waiving of Charges

In addition to required "additional benefits," M+C plans may include other benefits as either optional or mandatory supplemental offerings. Optional supplemental benefits are those offered to M+C enrollees through payment of an additional premium. Beneficiaries are free to choose or decline the offering. Plans may also include mandatory supplemental benefits, which are benefits a Medicare beneficiary must purchase as a condition of enrollment (e.g., because Medicare does not cover many types of preventive care, a health plan may choose to add a benefit that all enrollees must have). Charges for each type of supplemental benefit are subject to HCFA review and are limited to the adjusted community rate for the items and services. For optional supplemental benefits, any Medicare beneficiary may choose the benefit (without health screening, for example), although the periods during which the benefits are available can be limited. HCFA will also review proposed mandatory supplemental benefits to ensure that the level of premium is not likely to limit enrollment to only higher income individuals.

An organization may also add "free benefits" not otherwise required, or the organization may elect to waive collection of premiums or other charges that could otherwise be collected under M+C rules, as long as the "free benefits" or reduced charges are available to all Medicare enrollees of a plan.

Benefit Information Form and Its Successors

A component of the electronic submission of the ACR proposal is submission of the Benefit Information Form (BIF), which forms the basis of the description of each plan used for the Medicare Compare information discussed later (see Information Dissemination). HCFA is working on further consolidation of the various premium and benefit reports and other reporting requirements to streamline reporting and simplify the process of conveying information to enrollees and prospective enrollees. What was known as the BIF will have a new name but will serve the same purpose of providing plan benefit information.

Mid-Year Benefit Changes

Organizations are obligated to provide the ACR-approved benefits throughout the contract year. However, benefit packages can be enhanced (but not reduced) during the course of the contract year by decreasing premiums or other charges or by adding extra benefits. This practice is subject to HCFA approval and is permitted to take effect no earlier than February 1 of each year (in part because of the desire to provide accurate information to Medicare beneficiaries making decisions during the open enrollment period).

Special Treatment of Employer Group Retirees

Medicare beneficiaries who wish to enroll in an M+C plan available to them as the retiree benefit offering of an employer or union may pay a higher or lower premium than individual Medicare enrollees. Often, employers or unions include, in their retiree benefit packages, additional services not covered by Medicare, and the union or employer contributes toward the cost of such benefits (wholly or partly). However, because all such enrollees (other than the working aged) continue to be primarily Medicare enrollees of an M+C plan, most M+C rules apply to the coverage for retirees. Hence, the employer group must be offered the same benefit plans available to individual enrollees (i.e., the same choices must be available to employer-group connected retirees as are available to individual Medicare beneficiaries, even though the employer-sponsored option or options may not match any of the individually available options).

The employer or union may include supplemental benefits beyond those available to individual M+C enrollees, and any possible higher charges would be outside the M+C contract (i.e., negotiated between the employer/union and the health plan). The employer or union may also "buy out" the cost of premium or other charges for its enrollees. If an employer or union wishes to offer a less generous package (in terms of charges to individuals, given that the benefits cannot be less generous than M+C benefits available to individuals), this can be done only if such a package is available to individual Medicare beneficiaries. For example, if an employer wishes to offer a plan that has physician copayments of $10 while all other Medicare enrollees pay only $5, the M+C organization may provide such a package to the employer only if the level of copayments is also a feature of a plan available to individual Medicare beneficiaries and there is an approved ACR establishing appropriate charges for such a package in what might be called the "individual Medicare" market.

FEDERAL PREEMPTION

Premium Tax Prohibition and Other Preemption of State Laws

The law giveth and the law taketh away. Before talking about what a contract with the federal government under the M+C program requires, we can have a brief change of pace by discussing what is no longer required. Because the states were given the principal role in determining the kinds of organizations eligible for

M+C contracts, the BBA, true to its name of being a balanced act, balanced the new role of the states with new restrictions on the extent to which states could regulate or tax M+C plans.

In addition to a provision prohibiting states from imposing premium taxes on HCFA payments to M+C organizations, the BBA included provisions preempting state law in the M+C program. Federal law supersedes state law with regard to the operation of the M+C program when state law is inconsistent with M+C provisions, as was the case before the BBA. The BBA added specific preemptions ("preempting the field") for three areas in which state laws do not apply at all: benefits (no mandated benefits), provider participation rules (no mandatory inclusion of specific providers), and coverage determinations under M+C contracts (Medicare law applies exclusively in coverage decisions for services covered under the M+C contract).

HCFA has applied a narrow interpretation of the preemption provisions, allowing, for example, beneficiary recourse to state appeals, grievance, and judicial review for matters *related to* a Medicare coverage decision but not for the coverage decision itself. That is, the question of whether an item or service is covered under the contract and the issue of how much the person has to pay for a covered item or service falls solely within Medicare rules, but claims that denial of the service that is being disputed resulted in damage to a person's health or other adverse consequences can be addressed under state law.

Employer Group Benefits and Preemption

In the preceding discussion of differing benefits for employer group retirees, it was mentioned that the arrangements fall outside the M+C contracting rules. One consequence of this is that federal preemption does not apply to the employer group arrangement, meaning, for example, that if an M+C organization includes particular benefits only in employer group plans, state laws regarding those benefits, including any state mandates, would apply (to the extent that there is no other basis for federal preemption, such as under the Employee Retirement In-

come Security Act of 1974 (ERISA); see also Chapter 66).

WHAT THE CONTRACT REQUIRES (FINALLY!)

Are we there yet?, the youngster in the Oldsmobile would be asking by now. If there are readers still left after the payment section or for the readers who skipped payment, it is time to talk about the contract requirements. All M+C organizations sign a standard contract; there is no negotiation over the terms of the contract. The contractor must comply with the terms of the contract, federal regulations and statute governing the contract, and certain other federal laws, as outlined in the standard contract (e.g., the Civil Rights Act of 1964, the Americans with Disabilities Act, among others). However, federal acquisition regulations do not apply to M+C contracts.

In contrast to prior regulations, the M+C regulations are much more explicit in listing the contracting requirements that an M+C organization must comply with and their responsibilities with respect to subcontractors. The standard for "administrative and management capability" is carried over from prior regulations but now includes a compliance plan to ensure that the M+C organization has dedicated and accountable resources to ensure compliance with M+C contract requirements.

HCFA has also exercised regulatory discretion in certain areas, for example, in departing from the practice of making renewals of contracts "automatic" in the absence of notice by either party of an intent not to renew. Instead, HCFA will make a determination each year as to whether a contract should be renewed. HCFA may choose not to renew a contract if the organization has failed to implement quality improvement, has an insufficient level of enrollment, or has committed an action that would subject the organization to a civil money penalty under M+C rules.

Due process provisions for contract nonrenewals and terminations are clarified in the regulations implementing the BBA. There is also a provision allowing HCFA to immediately terminate a contract before the outcome of any appeal of the decision if a situation arises in which the health of enrollees is put at risk because services are not made available.

Some Basic Requirements

It goes without saying (even though we are saying it) that an organization must have sufficient administrative ability to carry out the terms of a Medicare contract. As one might guess, even post-BBA, organizations are still required to be able to provide at least the Medicare benefit package to their Medicare enrollees, following Medicare coverage rules. A contractor must make available all the Medicare services available in fee-for-service Medicare to beneficiaries residing in the service area and must use Medicare-certified "providers"—hospitals, skilled nursing facilities, and home health agencies. The plan's physicians and suppliers must not be barred from participation in either Medicare or Medicaid because of program abuse or fraud. For network plans, services must be available through staff providers or providers that are under contract with the organization.

Organizations are required to provide the benefits in a manner that ensures quality, availability, and accessibility of services. However, some of the requirements vary between network plans (HMOs, PSOs, MSAs offered by such organizations) and non-network plans (PFFS plans, PPOs, and indemnity-based MSA plans). For example, PFFS plans need only *pay* for services covered by any Medicare-eligible provider and may also cover supplemental services. Such plans are not required to have networks and are not required to have contracts with Medicare peer review organizations (PROs) for external quality review.

Under a network plan, an organization must be able to provide 24-hour emergency services and must have provisions for the payment of claims for emergency services within the service area and for out-of-area emergent or urgently needed services. All services that an organization is required to render (including any non-Medicare services in the benefit packages) must be accessible with reasonable promptness, and there must be a recordkeeping system that ensures continuity of care. The organization is required to maintain the confidentiality of the medical and nonmedical records of its Medicare members.

Quality Standards

Whereas the pre-BBA law contained a grand total of one sentence that referred to quality standards, the BBA dwells a little more on what is expected in the way of quality standards. The regulations on quality standards are extensive and detailed. All plans must collect and analyze health information, ensure that it is accurate, and make the information available to HCFA. Non-network plans are required to measure and report performance and meet specific requirements regarding utilization review procedures to the extent that the plan has written procedures. The findings on quality are disseminated to Medicare beneficiaries, as discussed in the following.

Among the requirements related to quality of care, the law and regulations require that organizations:

- have an ongoing quality assessment and performance improvement program that focuses on health outcomes and measurable change
- conduct quality improvement projects in clinical and nonclinical focus areas and demonstrate measurable improvement
- provide for peer review within the quality assurance system
- report on standardized measures, currently HEDIS® (the Health Plan Employer Data Information Set; see also Chapters 35 and 44), and conduct or participate in satisfaction surveys
- collect and interpret data systematically to make necessary changes in the provision of health services
- include written procedures for remedial action to correct problems.

For the required quality improvement projects, in some cases the focus areas for quality improvement projects will be selected by HCFA. In 1999, for example, all plans conducted an improvement project in the area of diabetes. In other cases, plans may select their own projects that focus on the needs of their enrolled populations. When HCFA establishes a minimum performance level, plans will have a year to come into compliance or be terminated from the program.

Reporting and Surveying

In addition to the reporting and auditing of HEDIS® data, which is the responsibility of M+C organizations, Medicare enrollees of health plans participate in satisfaction surveys, the Consumer Assessment of Health Plans Survey (CAHPS), and the Health Outcomes Survey (HOS). HCFA arranges for and pays for administration of the CAHPS survey, whereas M+C organizations are responsible for administering the HOS survey.[10]

External Review

Coordinated care plans are subject to external review of the quality of care they render. The PROs that are under contract to HCFA to review the quality of care of hospitals in fee-for-service Medicare also review the quality of care among M+C enrollees. The current approach to the role of the PROs moves away from review of individual cases and toward a collaborative approach focusing on patterns of care. PROs are also authorized to provide technical assistance to plans when they design their quality improvement projects and to evaluate the results of these projects. PROs also review complaints by M+C enrollees about the quality of care in an M+C plan. As in fee-for-service Medicare, PROs process beneficiary requests for review of hospital discharge decisions.

Evolving Quality Standards

The "state of the art" in evaluating health plan quality has advanced significantly in the last decade, and this area has become increasingly important for all purchasers, both private and public. HCFA has often led the way, or been a significant participant, in developing quality standards for plans and in promoting public/private partnerships to improve health plan stan-

dards and the reporting of information on quality. However, much remains to be done in measuring the performance of plans and determining what information is appropriate for consumers to use in evaluating competing plans. HCFA continues to refine the development of the Quality Improvement System for Managed Care (QISMC), a set of standards to be used for both Medicare and Medicaid health plans.

QISMC adopts a very broad definition of "quality" to include the "measurement of health outcomes, consumer satisfaction, the accountability of managed care organizations for achieving ongoing quality improvement, the need for intervention to achieve this improvement, and the importance of data collection, analysis, and reporting." HCFA continues to develop health plan performance measures that are to be disseminated to beneficiaries by using a public process that will include health plans, other purchasers, experts on quality measurement, beneficiaries and their advocates, and other interested parties. HCFA will publish a notice describing data elements to be collected and summarizing the process used for making the determination of what is to be reported.

Deemed Compliance with Quality Requirements

The BBA and BBRA allow M+C organizations to meet a number of quality standards through accreditation by a private accrediting body. The accrediting organization must be approved by HCFA, with approval subject to notice and comment in the *Federal Register*. Approval of the accrediting body may be withdrawn under certain conditions.

LIMITATIONS ON PHYSICIAN INCENTIVE PLANS

The M+C statute contains a specific prohibition on certain types of financial incentives and provides that certain requirements must be met in the event that physicians or physician groups are placed at "substantial" financial risk. To quote the statute on the outright prohibition, "No specific payment is made directly or indirectly under the plan to a physician or physician group as an inducement to reduce or limit medically necessary services provided with respect to a specific individual enrolled with the organization."

If physicians or physician groups are placed at "substantial" financial risk for services they do not directly render, the organization must provide stop-loss protection for the providers, and the organization must conduct periodic satisfaction surveys of current and former enrollees (a requirement that can be met through the CAHPS survey otherwise required of many organizations). The regulations specify the requirements for stop-loss insurance and also define what is considered "substantial" financial risk. To oversimplify the standard, physicians or groups are considered to be at substantial risk if more than 25 percent of their potential payments are at risk.

Each year, M+C organizations must provide descriptive information about their physician incentive plan in sufficient detail to enable HCFA to determine whether that plan complies with these requirements. Organizations must also disclose to Medicare beneficiaries, on request, whether the M+C organization uses a physician incentive plan, the type of incentives used, whether stop-loss protection is provided, and, if the M+C organization was required to conduct a survey, a summary of the survey results.

CONSUMER PROTECTIONS

Access Standards

One of the areas in which HCFA may be said to have exercised the greatest level of regulatory discretion in establishing M+C standards is in the area of requirements relating to what may generally be termed access to care. Prior law contained a general requirement regarding the guarantee of access to covered care. *As a result of the BBA and an executive order relating to the Consumer Bill of Rights and Responsibilities, the regulations contain new requirements, including:*

- requiring unrestricted communication between patients and health care profession-

als through the prohibition of "gag" clauses (a codification of existing HCFA policy)
- using the "prudent lay person" definition of what constitutes an emergency, clarification of the liability of the M+C organization for the cost of such care, and a requirement to cover appropriate maintenance and poststabilization care after an emergency
- covering out-of-area dialysis during an enrollee's temporary absence from the service area
- limiting copayments for emergency services to no more than $50
- specifying that the decision of the examining physician treating the individual enrollee prevails regarding when the enrollee may be considered stabilized for discharge or transfer (codification of existing policy)
- requiring plans to permit women enrollees to choose direct access to a women's health specialist within the network for women's routine and preventive health
- requiring plans to have procedures approved by HCFA for identification of individuals with complex or serious medical conditions, assessment of such individuals, and development of an appropriate treatment plan, including the right to direct access to specialists under the treatment plan
- requiring that services be provided in a "culturally competent" manner (i.e., with sensitivity toward cultural, ethnic, and language differences)

Information on Advance Directives

M+C organizations must meet the same requirements applicable to hospitals under Medicare with regard to maintaining written policies and procedures for advance directives.

Member Appeals and Grievances

M+C enrollees have the right to an administrative and judicial appeals process and a grievance process for matters in which the Medicare appeals process does not apply. The rules for Medicare appeals (referred to in regulations as "organization determinations," another anti-English locution) pertain to decisions regarding coverage or cost of an item or service included in the Medicare contract (Medicare-covered items and services and additional and supplemental benefits), including payment for out-of-network services received in an emergency.

The steps of the appeals process include:

- the determination by the organization (or a subcontracted entity)
- reconsideration by the organization, or, if the organization proposes a reconsideration decision adverse to the beneficiary, review of that decision by an external review entity under contract to HCFA
- review by an Administrative Law Judge (for claims valued at $100 or more) of the external review entity's decision if adverse to the beneficiary (The M+C organization is not entitled to appeal a decision by the external review entity when the decision is in favor of the beneficiary.)
- review of the Administrative Law Judge decision by the Departmental Appeals Board of the U.S. Department of Health and Human Services (a right available to members and to the M+C organization)
- judicial review in federal court for claims valued at $1,000 or more

The M+C regulations established new timeliness standards for appeal rights of Medicare beneficiaries enrolled in private plans and incorporated certain clarifications of HCFA policy on appeals. Although not required until the BBA, HCFA has used an independent contractor for the processing of health plan coverage denials for the past 10 years. HCFA, through regulations, had also already begun to implement expedited appeals procedures in cases in which a delay could endanger a beneficiary's health and had implemented time frame standards for health plan decisions where none were specified in statute.

Under the M+C regulations, for both M+C organizations and for the independent reviewer, time frames are shortened, or newly added, such that the first-level determination is to be made by the M+C organization within 14 days (or "as expeditiously as the enrollee's health condition requires" but no later than 14 days), and a reconsideration decision (by the organization or the review entity) is to be made within 30 days (with the same requirement for expeditious processing). For expedited appeals, the standard is that a decision must be rendered within 72 hours.

PROs also review beneficiary complaints, including beneficiary appeals about the appropriateness of a hospital discharge. Expedited time frames similar to those of fee-for-service Medicare apply in such a case.

Grievances

Grievances against a plan, as opposed to Medicare appeals, are subject to different standards. Beneficiaries must currently be afforded a "meaningful" grievance right when the matter in dispute is an issue other than coverage or cost of an item or service the M+C organization is obligated to provide. HCFA is considering imposing timeliness standards for the processing of grievances against M+C organizations. The BBA requires organizations to provide data on the number of grievances and their disposition in the aggregate on an enrollee's request.

Avoiding Speed Traps

You should be warned that one of the favorite findings or "gotchas" of reviewers who go on site visits to M+C contractors is to cite organizations for their failure to distinguish between a complaint or claim that is subject to the Medicare appeals process and complaints that are classified as grievances under Medicare rules.

PROVIDER PROTECTIONS AND RIGHTS: CONSCIENCE PROTECTION

The M+C statute contains provider protections, including:

- a provision prohibiting discrimination against particular providers, in selection of providers or payment or indemnification provisions, solely on the basis of the provider's licensure status

- appeal rights afforded to providers in the event of exclusion from a network
- a requirement that M+C organizations consult with plan physicians regarding medical policy, quality, and medical management procedures

The M+C statute also permits a health care professional to refuse to provide advice, counseling, or referral for a service that the provider objects to on moral and religious grounds, as long as the M+C organization provides notification to enrollees of the applicability of this provision.

Prompt Payment to Noncontracted Providers

M+C plans and their subcontractors are required to meet the same prompt payment standards that apply to Medicare carriers and intermediaries in fee-for-service Medicare with respect to the timeliness of payments made to noncontracted physicians and other providers. The standards apply to "clean" claims; that is, claims having no "defect or impropriety" as the law says and not lacking "substantiating documentation" or "requiring special treatment." The standard is that 95 percent of clean claims must be paid within 30 days.

INFORMATION DISSEMINATION

Coordinated Open Enrollment

Until the BBA, marketing and information dissemination regarding private health plan options were primarily functions undertaken by the contracting organizations themselves. The BBA sought to increase HCFA's role in the dissemination of information and also took a number or steps to facilitate M+C enrollment in certain cases, such as when a person first becomes eligible for Medicare. Beginning with an information campaign in 1998 and a coordinated open enrollment in 1999, the BBA directed HCFA to provide comparative information containing comprehensive, detailed information about health plan choices. This activity is funded by user fees imposed on participating M+C plans.

HCFA is also required to maintain a toll-free number accessible to beneficiaries residing in areas with M+C plans.

The national Medicare education program includes a Medicare handbook with prominent mention of private health plan options and the Internet site at www.medicare.gov (known as Medicare Compare), which provides comparative information on all plan choices. The outreach and education program also includes an 800 toll-free number (1-800-Medicare or 1-800-633-4227), local health fairs before the November coordinated election period, and other outreach efforts with various partners, such as the American Association of Retired Persons (AARP).

Information on Plan Performance

As part of the information to be provided to beneficiaries, the BBA requires the inclusion of information on health plan quality and performance: disenrollment rates, satisfaction levels, health outcomes information, and compliance information, to the extent any of this information is available.

ENROLLMENT

Who May Enroll?

During an open enrollment period, any Medicare beneficiary residing in the service area of an M+C plan is entitled to enroll in the plan, as long as the person has both part A (hospital insurance) and part B (supplementary medical insurance) of Medicare.[11] Medicare beneficiaries who are Medicaid recipients may also enroll. The only Medicare beneficiaries not entitled to enroll (and to whom a plan must refuse enrollment under the law) are beneficiaries who have ESRD (whether aged, disabled, or entitled to Medicare solely because of their disease). However, enrollees who acquire ESRD after enrollment in the plan may not be disenrolled because they have ESRD, including in the case of individuals enrolled in the plan as non-Medicare members immediately before Medicare eligibility.

Open Enrollment: Coordinated Open Enrollment

Under the BBA, there are important changes in the periods when M+C plans must permit enrollment and the times that beneficiaries may select a health plan option. As often occurs in the private sector, there is now a single time when all M+C organizations must be open—the month of November. During this "annual election period" beneficiaries will receive comparative information on all of their health care options, including fee-for-service Medicare and its Medigap (supplemental coverage) options. They may elect new coverage and switch back and forth between M+C and traditional fee-for-service Medicare, effective the following January. Newly eligible enrollees who do not choose an M+C plan are deemed to have chosen the original Medicare fee-for-service option, except that the HCFA may establish procedures under which "age-ins" enrolled in a contracting plan may be deemed to have elected the entity's M+C plan.

M+C plans are also required to be open during special election periods, for example plans must accept beneficiaries when they turn 65 and become newly entitled to Medicare, and they must be open when another organization in the service area terminates a Medicare contract. Organizations that have M+C contracts are required to offer the option of continued enrollment as Medicare members to current non-Medicare enrollees when they become eligible for Medicare and meet M+C eligibility criteria (e.g., having both part A and part B).

Before the BBA, there was no "lock-in" period or minimum enrollment period beyond one month for Medicare health plan enrollees. The BBA introduced a lock-in, which, when fully phased in, in 2003, can last up to nine months. (See Table 55–2 for the phase-in schedule and the requirements for when a beneficiary may enroll or disenroll.)[12]

Capacity Waivers

Health plans that demonstrate that they are no longer able to handle new enrollees because of limits in provider capacity may request a waiver of the annual election period and special election periods as long as they meet certain criteria. For example, they must demonstrate that they have made an effort to find new providers and are not discriminating against certain types of beneficiaries. In the case of a plan with limited capacity, enrollment is to be accepted on a first-come, first-served basis. In determining capacity for Medicare enrollees, the organization may set aside vacancies for expected commercial enrollees during each Medicare contract period.

Disenrollment

Beneficiaries who are enrolled in an M+C coordinated care plan will be able to disenroll from their elected plan option once during the first 6 months of 2002. Beneficiaries who enroll in an M+C plan at the time they become eligible for Medicare will be permitted to disenroll at any time during the first year of enrollment.

Beginning January 1, 2003, beneficiaries may only disenroll from an M+C coordinated care plan and choose another plan, leave Medicare fee-for-service to enroll in an M+C plan, or return to Medicare fee-for-service, one time during the first 3 months of the calendar year. Beneficiaries will be effectively locked in to their M+C plan election for the remaining nine months after this window. Exceptions to the lock-in period are available for enrollees under the following circumstances: the M+C plan contract is terminated, the beneficiary leaves the plan service area, the M+C plan fails to provide covered benefits or is found to be improperly marketing the Medicare product, or under other conditions specified by the HCFA.

Involuntary Disenrollment

An M+C organization may involuntarily disenroll a Medicare beneficiary if the person leaves the service area permanently (defined by regulations as an absence lasting more than 12 months); if the person has committed fraud in enrolling in a plan or permits others to use his or her enrollment card to obtain care; for failure to pay premiums in a timely manner (including optional supplemental premiums); or because of disruptive or abusive behavior, subject to HCFA approval.

Table 55–2 Enrollment and Disenrollment in M+C Plans

	1999–2001	2002	2003 and after
Availability of Enrollment in an M+C Plan			
Open enrollment month to month	Yes, if plan open for enrollment	No	No
Modified open enrollment		Beneficiary may change election once during first 6 months of year	Beneficiary may change election once during first 3 months of year
In the 3 months before first eligibility for A and B of Medicare	Yes	Yes	Yes
Annual election period	Yes	Yes	Yes
Immediately after first becoming eligible for Medicare A and B	Only if plan open for enrollment	Yes, within 6 months of first entitlement (or Dec. 31, if earlier)	Yes, within 3 months of first entitlement (or Dec. 31, if earlier)
Current M+C plan terminated or no longer offered	Yes	Yes	Yes
Move to a new geographical area	Yes	Yes	Yes
Special circumstances (M+C failure to provide care, misrepresentation)	Yes	Yes	Yes
Disenrollment from M+C Plan			
Disenrollment possible month to month	Yes	No	No
Modified open disenrollment		Only once during first 6 months of year	Only once during first 3 months of year
Newly eligible individual		Yes, during first 6 months of entitlement to Medicare A and B (or Dec. 31, if earlier)	Yes, during first 3 months of entitlement (or Dec. 31, if earlier)
65-year-old who elected M+C in 3 months before or 3 months after entitlement to Medicare at age 65		Yes, if within 12 months of effective date of enrollment in M+C plan	Same as 2002
Move to a new geographical area	Yes	Yes	Yes
Special circumstances (M+C failure to provide care, misrepresentation)	Yes	Yes	Yes

Source: Reprinted from the Balanced Budget Act of 1997, the Balanced Budget Refinement Act of 1999, and the *Federal Register* of June 16, 1998.

MARKETING RULES

The marketing rules have been left for the end of the section on requirements in keeping with the general structure of the chapter, with our goal being to give you all the facts about what you will be asked to do and how you will be paid so that you can determine whether you will get as far as having to figure out how to market a product to Medicare beneficiaries.

Basic Requirement

The basic marketing requirement is that an organization must market its M+C plan or plans throughout the entire service area in a nondiscriminatory manner. All marketing materials, including membership and enrollment materials, must be approved by HCFA before use. Prospective enrollees must be given descriptive material sufficient for them to make an informed choice. One of the required marketing documents is a standardized summary of benefits form that uses standard benefit definitions and a standardized format to allow beneficiaries to make "apples to apples" comparisons among M+C offerings and between M+C and fee-for-service.

Prohibited Marketing

Prohibited marketing activities include door-to-door solicitation, discriminatory marketing (avoiding low-income areas, for example), and misleading marketing or misrepresentation. These activities are subject to sanctions, including suspension of enrollment, suspension of payment for new enrollees, or civil monetary penalties (the government's euphemism for fines).

M+C plans are prohibited from giving monetary incentives as an inducement to enroll and from completing any portion of the enrollment application for a prospective enrollee.

Prior Approval

All marketing and enrollment material (including enrollment forms) an organization proposes to use must have HCFA prior approval.

HCFA has 45 days to review marketing materials. If 45 days pass without HCFA comments on the material, it is deemed approved. If an M+C plan's marketing materials were approved for one service area, they will be deemed to be approved in all of the plan's service areas, except with regard to area-specific information.

Description of Plan (Evidence of Coverage)

The BBA specifies the kind of information an M+C member must receive on enrollment and annually thereafter. This includes information on benefits and exclusions; the number, mix, and distribution of plan providers; out-of-network and out-of-area coverage; emergency coverage—how it is defined and how to gain access to emergency care (including use of 911 services); prior authorization or other review requirements; grievances and appeals; and a description of the plan's quality assurance program. On request, the organization must provide information on utilization control practices, the number and disposition of appeals and grievances, and a summary description of physician compensation.

Notifications to Enrollees

Medicare enrollees must be notified at least 30 days in advance of changes in plan membership rules (which must be approved by HCFA). However, for the change in benefits occurring from one year to the next, the notice must be sent by October 15 before the applicable coordinated open enrollment period.

INTERACTIONS WITH YOUR GOVERNMENT

Contractor Monitoring

Once an organization signs a Medicare contract, HCFA maintains ongoing monitoring of the plan. One aspect of the monitoring is accomplished through self-reporting of financial and other information by the organization on a quarterly basis. If certain criteria are met, the information may be reported on a yearly basis.

Specific to Medicare is a monitoring process that is performed by The Health Plan Purchasing Administration of HCFA's central office and, principally, by the 10 regional offices of the HCFA. By the end of the first year of contracting, each plan will have a monitoring visit, during which the reviewers will determine whether the health plan is complying with regulatory requirements in such areas as financial arrangements, legal and financial requirements for the entity as a whole, quality of care issues, marketing practices, enrollment/disenrollment, claims payment, and grievance and appeals procedures. The reviewers follow a specific written protocol in conducting the review.[13] After such a monitoring visit, a report is prepared, and if necessary the organization is required to submit a corrective action plan to correct any deficiencies. Close monitoring of the plan continues until HCFA is satisfied that the problems have been resolved. If the initial review goes well, there may not necessarily be a review of the same plan for another two years.

A new requirement under the BBA is that HCFA must conduct a financial audit of one third of the plans each year. This means that HCFA and its contractors will visit each plan every three years to review financial records, including documentation used to develop ACRs, establish administrative costs, and pay providers.

Also new under the BBA is the requirement that an organization provide a certification of the accuracy of its claims for payment from the government in ACR submittals and in each of the monthly enrollment and encounter data reports that are the basis for HCFA's monthly electronic funds transfer to the plan. Subcontractors or delegated entities producing the data would also be obligated to make such a certification. If there is cause to believe that the certifications are fraudulent, the Department of Justice may seek damages under the False Claims Act.

The Right to Inspect and Evaluate Records

Not surprisingly, the statute gives the government the right to audit and inspect financial records, including among related parties, records relating to services provided, and enrollment and disenrollment records. The BBA extended the period of record retention to six years and clarified that records of subcontractors and related entities are also subject to these requirements.

THE CONTRACTING PROCESS

Anyone who has read this far in the chapter deserves to have a contract. To obtain a contract, you must submit an application to HCFA so that HCFA can determine whether you meet all the requirements for the granting of a contract, as listed previously, and whether you have a sufficient understanding of how the requirements are to be implemented.

There are various types of applications, matching the types of entities eligible for contracts: coordinated care plans, federally waived PSO plans, and PFFS plans. These are available at the HCFA web site, www.hcfa.gov/medicare/mgd-apps.htm.

The following are some of the issues addressed in the application:

- legal and financial structure of the organization
- types, numbers, and location of providers the plan will use
- listing of benefits
- description of the Medicare marketing strategy
- copies of marketing material to be used
- evidence of coverage or subscriber agreement listing membership rules, enrollee rights, and plan benefits
- quality assurance plan
- enrollment and disenrollment procedures
- grievance and Medicare appeals procedures

The application review is done jointly by HCFA's central and regional offices and will involve a site visit.

Getting Out of the Contract

It is possible to modify or terminate an M+C contract. Officers of an organization taking such action will not be stripped of their citizenship and deported. For either a termination of a contract or a reduction in the service area of a contract, the organization must advise HCFA by July 1 of its intentions for the following calendar year. If HCFA does not receive an ACR submission and a signed contract, this lack of interest is treated as a notification of the organization's intention not to renew the contract. Enrollees of the organization must be informed of the decision not to renew or a decision to exclude a county from a service area by October 15.

A statutory provision modified by the BBRA prevents an organization that has terminated an M+C contract from re-entering the program within 2 years of the deed. However, this is a discretionary rule that permits the Secretary of the Department of Health and Human Services (often in the guise of HCFA) to decide not to limit re-entry if "special circumstances" are involved. The BBRA provided for a specific exemption if, within 6 months of an organization's notifying HCFA of a withdrawal, a legislative or regulatory change in policy increased payments in the affected area. HCFA also permits exceptions if the area of re-entry has two or fewer M+C plans.

WEB RESOURCES AND OTHER CONTACTS

Through the miracle of the World Wide Web it is now possible for an organization to do everything electronically, except maybe for having some living individual sign the M+C contract. This is a slight exaggeration, although HCFA is moving to a paperless process for distributing documents and for receiving submissions from M+C contractors and prospective contractors. In fact, HCFA prefers that you use the Web site, taking as its official position the following: "you are encouraged to use the appropriate Web site and to contact HCFA only if you cannot locate the documents or need further information."

The M+C areas of the HCFA Web site are relatively easy to navigate and are easy to get to starting from home plate, hcfa.gov. The following are specific site locations:

- M+C applications and the state certification form are located at *www.hcfa.gov/medicare/apps.htm*

- point-of-service guidelines: *www:hcfa.gov/medicare/benefit.htm*
- Health Plan Management System information and to obtain an identification number for use of the system: *www.fu.com/hpms*
- ACRP information and electronic submission: *www.gravity.lmi/org/lmihcfa/acrseminar.htm*
- encounter data and risk adjustment: *http://www.hcfa.gov/medicare/encntqr.htm*
- QISMC: *www:hcfa.gov/quality/3a.htm*
- operational policy letters (so frequently alluded to in the chapter) and National Marketing Guidelines: *www:hcfa.gov/medicare/mgdcar1.htm*

Although we cannot call it "snail mail" because they are our brethren in public service (or semipublic service), HCFA does have an address and phone number for M+C issues related to applications, ACR filings, and monitoring:

HCFA
Health Plan Purchasing
  Administration Group
Center for Health Plans and Providers
Room C4-22-27
7500 Security Boulevard
Baltimore, MD 21244-1850
(410) 786-4297

FUTURE DIRECTION OF THE PROGRAM

Returning to the Oldsmobile versus the sports car, in the last few years Medicare reform has been a matter of concern to the entities and deliberative bodies that make and execute America's laws, mainly because of the looming demographic tsunami, as one policy expert put it, of the aging of the baby boom generation. Faced with the prospect of an insolvent Medicare trust fund and increasing shares of the federal budget dedicated to Medicare, Congress, the White House, and others began to examine the options for reform of the program.

The BBA authorized the formation of a bipartisan commission to examine the issues and make recommendations for reform of the Medicare program. The National Bipartisan Commission on the

Future of Medicare consisted of senators and congressmen, industry representatives, and policy experts.[14] Someone will eventually write the story of how the commission, referred to as the Breaux-Thomas commission (after its co-leaders, Senator John Breaux and Representative Bill Thomas), went about its task, just as many people have written about the (do you remember?) Health Security Act and its history. The commission was unable to develop recommendations supported by a "super majority" of members as required by the law authorizing the commission. Although no commission recommendation could be presented to the Congress, a majority of commissioners did endorse a set of recommendations that Senator Breaux and Mr. Thomas would attempt to fashion into legislation.

Always a difficult issue to grapple with (Medicare is one of those "third-rail" issues guaranteeing instant political death at a mere touch), over time the sense of urgency over Medicare reform waned a bit, thanks to the effects of the BBA in cutting expenditures (particularly among certain provider categories such as skilled nursing facilities and home health agencies) and because of successful efforts to combat fraud and abuse in Medicare program payments. The combined effect extended the life of the Medicare part A trust fund.

Both the Breaux-Thomas commission and the proposal put forth by the President for Medicare reform call for the introduction of competitive pricing for private health plans.[15] The variables in each of the proposals include how the government contribution is to be set, what can or cannot be included in the benefit package, and who will oversee the program (a newly created board rather than HCFA, as proposed by Breaux-Thomas). A major issue of contention is how the traditional fee-for-service Medicare program fits in with the private health plan options—will it be a direct, unsubsidized competitor (meaning that beneficiaries would be likely to have to pay more than they currently do for fee-for-service Medicare in some areas) or will it, as the President's plan has it, be some sort of benchmark, or a component of the benchmark for competition among private plans.

The question of the status of fee-for-service Medicare in relation to private health plan options is influenced by what FFS Medicare will be. Both the commission and the President's plan call for inclusion of a drug benefit as part of the basic Medicare package—in the former plan solely for low-income individuals and in the latter for all beneficiaries. The Breaux-Thomas proposal required private plans (including Medigap) to offer drug coverage, whereas in the President's plan the inclusion of drugs as a benefit for all (as an option with a premium and with annual dollar caps on coverage) would mean that all plans would include the benefit in their package and would be "bidding" on drug coverage as an element of the required basic package.

For the purpose of making fee-for-service Medicare more "competitive" in relation to private plans, to reduce expenditures in the program, and to "rationalize" the benefit package, reform proposals call for changes in the traditional program. Among the possible changes are more reliance on cost-control mechanisms used in the private sector, such as the development of preferred provider options, selective contracting along the lines of Medicare's "centers of excellence" providers, primary care case management, and disease management. There are also proposals to reform Medigap coverage to offer a plan that does not include the kind of first-dollar coverage that is believed to lead to higher utilization.

Some of the elements of the President's plan are proposals that have been tried out as HCFA demonstrations, some of which have been successful (centers of excellence) and some of which have yet to see the light of day. A perennially postponed demonstration project is the competitive pricing demonstration for M+C plans. The demonstration seeks to find an alternative to the administered pricing mechanism for paying health plans by using a competitive approach to establishing the government payment. To that extent, it is similar *in concept* to the President's proposal and to the Breaux-Thomas proposal, although it is quite different from either in its details.[16]

What role M+C organizations are to play in Medicare's future is unclear. The issue has been clouded of late because of the relatively high number of organizations leaving the program in the recent past (reminding the historically minded of a similar retreat in the late 1980s). Our editor has forbidden us from opining and speculating on this issue, so that we, too, must close by using the tack of the French politician and saying that "the future of M+C depends on what will become of the program."

REFERENCES AND NOTES

1. The BBA also permits religious fraternal benefit organizations to have M+C contracts. Specific rules apply regarding the structure of such organizations, including offering health care coverage to affiliated non-Medicare individuals. Payment to such organizations would be on an experience-rated basis, and they are not required to comply with the open enrollment requirements discussed later in the chapter.

2. The rates are available on the HCFA Web site at www.hcfa.gov/stats/hmorates/aapccpg.htm.

3. Additional information on the risk adjustment method can be found in HCFA's report to Congress, *Proposed Method of Incorporating Health Status Risk Adjusters into Medicare + Choice Payments,* March 1, 1999. Available at the HCFA Web site, http:/www.hcfa.gov/ord/rpt2Cong.pdf.

4. In the interest of full disclosure, there is also a reduction in payment for enrollees with end-stage renal disease. The BBA requires a reduction of 50 cents per dialysis session, with the amount payable to dialysis network administrators.

5. For the working aged (Medicare beneficiaries whose employer coverage is primary and coordinated with Medicare), the PIP/DCG risk adjustment method assumes that 21 percent of the capitation that would otherwise be payable is payable for a working aged person.

6. Hospice services, although covered by Medicare, are not covered by M+C organizations. M+C enrollees have the right to elect Medicare hospice coverage (which also requires an "election" in fee-for-service Medicare because of special coverage rules), and although the individual may remain enrolled in the M+C plan, items and services related to the terminal condition are provided or arranged by the hospice, which receives a capitation for the services. M+C plans only receive, as an HCFA payment, the amount corresponding to the dollar value of the "additional" benefits that are required to be provided under the plan (which the hospice enrollee continues to be entitled to receive) and may receive payment, on a fee-for-service basis, for services provided to the individual for the treatment of conditions unrelated to the terminal condition.

7. Such a computation is admittedly difficult for a newly contracting entity in a risk-adjusted world. Relevant information is the average risk "score" for the population of county or counties in which the organization will do business. Otherwise, it is a matter of projecting the composition of Medicare enrollment in the organization. HCFA can also assist organizations in the development of ACRs, and the law specifically states that new organizations that have insufficient enrollment experience can have their expected average payment rate and ACR determined by HCFA "using data in the general commercial marketplace" and data from other contractors.

8. Organizations may "return" the additional benefits in the contract year to which the ACR applies or they may reserve all or a portion of the excess revenue in a benefit stabilization fund administered by HCFA for use in a later contract period.

9. The premiums and other amounts, such as the deductible of MSA plans, and the premiums of private fee-for-service plans, are not subject to HCFA approval.

10. For additional information on the survey and data requirements, see HCFA Operation Policy Letter (OPL) 99.078, available at the HCFA Web site (http:/www.hcfa.gov).

11. Requiring people to have part A of Medicare is a new requirement. Some organizations may continue to cover people with only part B that are carried as "grandfathered" members of plans. Previously there was a prohibition on enrollment of Medicare beneficiaries who had elected Medicare hospice coverage. That prohibition is not found in the BBA, but for individuals who have elected Medicare hospice coverage and are newly enrolling in an M+C plan, the payment provisions explained previously apply from the first date of enrollment.

12. As mentioned previously, religious fraternal benefit societies would not enroll unaffiliated individuals. Special enrollment rules also apply to MSA plans, both with regard to who may enroll and the length of enrollment, as noted previously. See the regulations published in the *Federal Register* on June 26, 1998, pp. 34967–35116, available through the Government Printing Office Web site, www.gpo.gov.

13. The monitoring guide is available at the HCFA Web site, www.hcfa.gov/medicare/monitor.htm.

14. The proposal of the Commission and various other documents related to its work can be found at the Commission's Web site, http://thomas.loc.gov/medicare.

15. The President's plan can be found at the White House Web site, depending on who is occupying that house (www.whitehouse.gov).

16. An advisory group, the Competitive Pricing Advisory Committee, oversees the implementation of the demonstration. It has public meetings and its proceedings and additional documentation on the demonstration are available at the HCFA Web site.

CHAPTER 56

Medicare + Choice: The Health Plan's View

Craig S. Schub and Nick Franklin

INTRODUCTION

This chapter briefly explains the history and growth of Medicare health maintenance organizations (HMOs) and discusses the potential for Medicare HMOs in the senior market, a market that is expected to double in size within the next 30 years. It takes a look at what plans need to do to be successful Medicare contractors, particularly in light of the Balanced Budget Act of 1997 (BBA), and at some of the marketing, administrative, clinical, and customer service challenges posed by this unique population. Because this chapter represents the view of Medicare risk from a health plan's perspective, the authors' opinions will also be given regarding certain as-

pects of the current program. The chapter also deals with ways to prepare the delivery system for the special needs of the elderly and discusses the relationship with the government as both a payer for and a partner in the delivery of care. The reader is also strongly urged to review Chapter 55 for additional discussion of Medicare managed care.

TODAY'S ELDERLY

Today's seniors expect to enjoy good health during their second adulthood, a term that author Gail Sheehy coined to describe postretirement years that are richer in challenge and variety than ever before in our history. Indeed, only 10 percent of Americans older than 65 experience any significant limitations on their physical activities because of illness or disease. On the contrary, many are taking up new interests and hobbies. Approximately 12 percent are eschewing retirement, preferring instead to continue to work at least on a part-time basis.[1]

Seniors want to stay healthy as long as possible, but they are also realists. They have begun to feel the aches and pains of aging but want to maintain their independence and dignity by staving off the inevitable for as long as possible. Still, the issue of how they will pay for the health care they know they will need over the years remains a key concern. As a result of government budget limitations and a growing population of seniors, predictions of Medicare insolvency or restructuring are of great concern to most seniors.[2]

Craig S. Schub is President of Secure Horizons USA, a subsidiary of PacifiCare Health Systems, Inc. Since 1985, he has been involved in the development of the Secure Horizons Medicare + Choice program, the largest of its kind in the United States, with more than one million members in 12 states. He serves as a trustee for the Alliance for Aging Research in Washington, DC.

Nick Franklin is Senior Vice President of Public Affairs for PacifiCare Health Systems, Inc., where he leads public policy and external communications activities. He represents the company in a number of industry groups, including the American Association of Health Plans (AAHP) and the Council for Affordable Quality Health Care. He is Chair-Elect of the Public Affairs Council. He joined PacifiCare in 1997, after serving as senior vice president of public affairs for FHP International.

Medicare was designed 35 years ago to cover acute episodes of illness. Today, we recognize the value of preventive care and of providing coordinated care for chronic or debilitating conditions that often plague today's longer-living seniors. But despite the addition of some preventive measures, such as flu shots and mammograms, the traditional Medicare program still does not cover such basic services as regular physicals, outpatient prescription drugs, vision, or dental services, although proposals afloat would address some of these items. Other valuable adjuncts to healthy aging, such as general fitness and nutrition classes or group sessions on coping with aging, are not linked closely enough with an acute illness to be considered part of coverage. Meanwhile, the percentage of seniors' total health care costs that Medicare pays is decreasing.

Health Care Options for Seniors

Most seniors have availed themselves of an additional benefit option to help bridge the gap between what Medicare will cover and what they perceive they may need. More than 66 percent have some form of Medigap insurance policy to supplement Medicare coverage, paid for either by seniors themselves or by previous employers.[3]

Others choose to belong to managed care plans. In August 1997, Congress passed the BBA, which among other things created the Medicare + Choice program, designed to offer more managed care choices to seniors. As of May 1999, approximately 6.2 million or more than 16 percent of the nearly 40 million Medicare beneficiaries were enrolled in 301 Medicare + Choice plans, according to the Health Care Financing Administration (HCFA), the federal agency that administers Medicare.

Before the BBA, a growing number of seniors had opted to join HMOs with Medicare risk contracts. In these Medicare risk HMOs, they enjoyed an increased level of benefits, usually including preventive care and some prescription drug coverage. This additional level of coverage was generally provided with no deductible or coinsurance and low copayments for small or no additional monthly premiums.

For each senior who joined the Medicare risk plan, the government paid the HMO 95 percent of the average adjusted per capita cost (AAPCC), a statistic that represented the estimated cost of providing medical care through traditional fee-for-service (FFS) methods (adjusted for age, sex, county of residence, and other factors).

However, there were some concerns about the Medicare risk program that Congress addressed in the BBA, the result of which is likely to be debated for some time. Historically, some in government have believed that Medicare paid too much for basic benefits delivered through managed care. The BBA sought to address the payment issue and other perceived inequities and to provide more choices in health plans for Medicare beneficiaries. Indeed, the BBA produced more changes in Medicare than had occurred in its previous 35-year history.

The result was the creation of the Medicare + Choice program, which allows new types of health plans for seniors. These health care options include HMOs; preferred-provider organizations, in which physicians and hospitals organize into a restricted network; provider-sponsored organizations, in which physicians and hospitals can organize their own managed care plan; medical savings accounts; and private FFS plans, which can pay physicians more than the Medicare fee schedule and charge seniors an extra premium for the standard Medicare package of benefits.

The BBA also created a new way to pay managed care organizations. One of the changes is called the risk-adjustment payment method. Beginning in 2000, payments will be phased in and will attempt to reflect the relative health status of managed care enrollees, with plans getting more money for their sickest beneficiaries. BBA provisions also will reallocate HMO payments in rural and urban areas. Before BBA, HMO rates were based entirely on FFS costs in their local area as noted earlier. This meant that HMOs in lower-cost rural areas received lower payments than those in higher-cost urban areas. Under the BBA, plan rates are based on a combination or "blend" of local and national rates. This blend is designed to help encourage the development of managed care plans by increasing rates in lower cost or rural areas, where many Medicare enrollees have limited managed care choices.[4] But regardless of how the payments are allocated, managed care plans are more concerned about the future reduction in the growth of payments to them under the BBA that will not keep pace with FFS growth in payments.

Overall, the changes in plan requirements were designed to attract more managed care plans to the program. These changes may result in new plans in some areas, but the payment reforms in the BBA, coupled with new regulatory requirements, have already had the unintended effect of discouraging health plans from participating, resulting in fewer choices at the time of publication.[5]

THE DEMOGRAPHIC IMPERATIVE: AGING POPULATION AND UNPREDICTABLE HEALTH CARE COSTS

Seniors currently represent just 13 percent of the U.S. population, yet they account for more than 36 percent of total health care expenditures. By 2030, seniors, defined as those 65 years of age and older, will represent more than 20 percent of Americans, posing a significant threat to future federal budgets and the generation that will have to help pay for their care.

The growth of this age group will result partly from the aging of the large number of Baby Boomers. People are also living longer as a result of better nutrition, preventive care (especially early cancer detection), and advances in medical technology. The other side of the coin is that the birth rate has dropped, meaning fewer working-age people (as a percentage of the total) to support a growing retired population. At the turn of the last century, life expectancy was 47 years. In 1935, the average life expectancy was 62 years. Today, Americans can expect to live until at least 75 years, with women who are free of heart disease and cancer at age 50 predicted to reach an average age of 92 years. Ten million Baby Boomers will reach the age of 90. One million will become centenarians.

These demographic changes are putting unprecedented pressures on our nation's financial resources. Medicare spending, for example, rose from $146 billion in 1993 to $214.6 billion in 1997. Seniors already account for more than one third of the pharmaceutical industry's budget and the same proportion of our health care dollars. If the trends of the past decade or two continue until 2020, the elderly's health care consumption will be approximately $25,000 per person (in 1995 dollars) compared with $9,200 in 1995.[6]

Both Medicare and Medicaid programs are feeling the strain, and the BBA attempted to address a number of issues with a variety of policy changes. More are being considered, and in some cases implemented, to address this crisis. Yet, the private sector in the United States is already providing at least part of the answer in the form of HMOs. In various important ways they have had an undisputed impact in lowering the cost of health care for Americans older than 65 while offering comprehensive care and benefits that better meet the needs of an aging population. The benefits and nature of our entire health care system, which is designed to meet acute health care needs, however, are out of sync with the chronic care needs of older adults.

In short, Medicare HMOs, which emphasize continuity of care, health maintenance, and total patient management, are a much-appreciated option for today's longer-living, more active, and more value-conscious seniors. Medicare HMOs can provide equal or better care, frequently better service, fewer claims hassles, and certainly more benefits than FFS Medicare and at lower cost.

PUBLIC POLICY INITIATIVES: FROM 1965 TO THE BALANCED BUDGET ACT

Brief History of Medicare

Medicare was introduced in 1965 to provide a baseline of acute health care services to the elderly. Authorized under Title XVIII of the Social Security Act in 1965, the government insurance program is divided into two parts: hospital insurance (part A) and supplementary medical insurance (part B). Individuals entitled to Social Security are automatically entitled to benefits when they reach age 65, as are persons with end-stage renal disease (ESRD) and individuals younger than 65 who are eligible for Social Security disability and have been disabled for at least 2 years. Part A covers some inpatient, skilled nursing facility, home health, and hospice care. Medicare part B is voluntary, and enrollment is open to those 65 and older or those entitled to part A benefits. Part B covers physician and other outpatient medical services.

Medicare benefits, however, were designed to cover episodes of illness and injury rather than to preserve the long-term health of beneficiaries. In the 1960s, that approach made plenty of sense in a fragmented FFS environment, and Medicare was an instant success in the eyes of beneficiaries. Even today, as seniors battle with Medicare's increased cost sharing, claim form procedures, and the extra cost of Medigap insurance, most remain firmly supportive of Medicare and are quick to come to the program's defense.

The strain that Medicare is placing on the federal government's budget, however, has not gone unnoticed. Since 1980 at the direction of Congress and various administrations, HCFA has made major changes in the way the program pays hospitals, physicians, and other health care providers in an effort to control medical cost inflation. Medicare introduced the prospective payment system for inpatient hospital care in 1983 to limit Medicare's liability for costs per hospitalization. (There is no volume limit, just a dollar limit on hospitalization. Without volume limits, overall liability is not limited.) In 1992, Medicare implemented the Medicare fee schedule for physician payment, which combined aggregate volume controls with price constraints in an effort to control expenses for physician services. The BBA contains similar initiatives for outpatient, skilled nursing facilities, and home health payments.

To reduce Medicare expenses and to provide Medicare beneficiaries with an option similar to managed care products available in the private market, Medicare managed care was authorized by the Tax Equity and Fiscal Responsibility Act of 1982. Medicare HMOs began operation in 1985. In 1997, the program was revised significantly as a result of the BBA and the Balanced Budget Revisions Act (BBRA) which was enacted in late 1999.

Participation and Growth in Response to Public Policy

In 1985, 87 Medicare risk plans were on the market. By 1987, this figure had climbed to 161. During the next few years, those plans that were not successful either went under or left the market, and by 1990 the number of HMOs with risk contracts sank to 96. Since then, however, the industry has learned from the experience of successful plans that the senior market differs from the commercial market in significant ways. Senior HMOs began adjusting their delivery systems, benefits, and marketing approaches to take these differences into account. They also adjusted to dealing with administrative pricing and increased regulatory actions of a government program as opposed to market pricing and limited regulatory oversight of the commercial market. In 1998 the number of Medicare risk plans reached 350. And in 1999, once again the number of plans declined in response to changes in public policy under the BBA. Indeed, an estimated 450,000 seniors were affected in 1999 as 54 health plans announced their intent to reduce the size of the markets they serve and 45 did not renew their contracts. Another 327,000 will either have to move to other managed care plans or use FFS in 2000 because Medicare + Choice plans had to notify HCFA of their intent to stay in markets by July 1, 1999. Of that group, an estimated 70,000 will have no choice but to use traditional Medicare FFS.

Enrollment had grown steadily from 441,000 in 1987 to 6.2 million in 1999. Since the implementation of the BBA, growth has slowed to an average of 5,000 new members per month from levels nearly twice that during much of the 1990s. It is unknown at the time of publication how enrollment trends will look over the next several years because so much change is taking place within the program.

As of 1999, Medicare + Choice enrollment has been concentrated in a few states, although the percent of beneficiaries in Medicare managed care plans exceeds the national percentage of 16 percent in 15 states. California leads the way in numbers with nearly 1.5 million enrollees or 39 percent of the state's senior population as of this writing. Others with high numbers include Florida (nearly 800,000), Pennsylvania (nearly 540,000), Arizona (more than 250,000 or 40 percent of eligibles), Massachusetts (nearly 210,000), Colorado (more than 140,000), and Oregon (more than 135,000). These clusters of membership tell their own story: If seniors are satisfied with their care, they will tell friends and peers about their experiences. Word of mouth is still the most effective marketing tool among this generation. Seniors are quick to challenge poor performance, so that a reputation for quality care and service is proving to be an invaluable asset for some HMOs.

Balanced Budget Act Curtails Growth and Reduces Choice

With the advent of the BBA, Medicare + Choice plans must cope with new rules for participation and added administrative costs because the makeup of traditional Medicare risk plans has changed to such a degree. New reporting requirements and a new payment method are among the key changes. Medicare + Choice plans, for example, must now submit hospital encounter data, which will be used to help determine payments beginning in the year 2000.

The new payment methodology established under the BBA sets each county's rates (before risk adjustment) at a greater of: (1) a blend of a local and national rate; (2) a minimum floor rate; or (3) a rate reflecting a 2 percent minimum increase from the previous year's rate. (Before the BBA, it was common to give annual increases similar to FFS to reflect health care cost increases. The increase to managed care, now reduced to about 2 percent, will widen the gap of what is paid for FFS and managed care and is viewed by some as a threat to already low operating margins, which hover around 3 percent for successful plans in 1999.)

The controversial new health-status–based risk adjustment mechanism will be phased in between 2000 and 2004. The risk adjustment will be based on inpatient hospital utilization, raising sincere concerns among managed care plans regarding inappropriate incentives. Other factors include certain geographical and demographic characteristics (e.g., age, sex, Medicaid eligibility, working aged status, and under 65 disability status). The risk-adjustment payment transition, as was recently changed by the BBRA, will ease out the previously used demographically adjusted payment, is scheduled to be 10 percent in 2000, 10 percent in 2001, 20 percent in 2002, and 80 percent in 2003 with 100 percent comprehensive health-status–based risk adjustment in place by 2004. The second stage, beginning in 2004, is planned to include full encounter data, including physician visits, not just inpatient data.[7]

Risk adjustment is a means of modifying/redistributing payments received by risk-bearing entities within a health insurance system to more accurately reflect the level of services that the entity will provide. For example, an individual with a history of cardiovascular disease will require a higher payment than an individual without any such acute health care risk. The higher premium anticipates hospitalization and medication costs. The goal of risk adjustment is to more equitably compensate entities on the basis of the amount of risk they bear by making accurate estimations of an individual's future health care costs and adjusting the payment to the health plan accordingly.

Although the concept makes sense on some level, HCFA's chosen approach already is having a negative effect on the Medicare + Choice program. Rather than merely reallocating funds to plans with sicker enrollees and away from plans with healthier enrollees, it reduces program payments by more than $8 billion on top of the $22.5 billion reduction already planned by the BBA. First, it will reduce total Medicare + Choice payments, widening the gap with FFS Medicare. Second, built-in flaws, both conceptual and operational, will likely underpay plans.

Medicare originally paid Medicare HMOs 95 percent of FFS reimbursement in part to account for risk adjustment. The BBA reduces these payments to well below 95 percent to as low as 82 percent by some estimates in 2004. Indeed, it is estimated in 2004 that FFS will be paid an average of $1,500 more per Medicare patient than managed care plans.

The widening gap between health care costs and payments over the next few years will likely see fewer providers willing to contract with plans, leaving beneficiaries with fewer, more expensive options. Providers continue to view the threat of reduced Medicare + Choice payments and the relatively more generous payments under the FFS Medicare as a "lose/win" proposition.

The current risk adjuster penalizes effective care management in outpatient settings and undermines the real value of HMOs to manage beneficiaries' health. For example, one-day hospitalizations do not qualify for risk-adjusted payment. Yet if a health plan is effectively managing care, it will have a greater percentage of these hospitalizations than those who are not. The risk adjuster also fails to take into account medical advances that reduce the need for hospitalization, does not fully account for costs in the last year of life, and preventive care efforts that reduce hospitalization would not be reimbursed.

This much is certain: The expansion of senior HMOs to all markets will not occur unless the payment method from HCFA is viewed as both fair and viable in the market.

Public Policy Challenges

Although managed care programs have grown rapidly, membership is mostly concentrated in a few states where these programs are highly successful. Medicare from a national perspective, unlike the private market, which has experienced a significant shift toward managed care, remains overwhelmingly a discounted FFS system.

There is enough room in the system for FFS and Medicare + Choice plans. Historically, providers have called for protectionist legislation, largely on the commercial side of HMOs. These more traditional health care interests represent a powerful group. As a result, legislative initiatives arise from time to time designed to slow the growth of HMOs or to regulate the freedom of HMOs to manage covered services.

On the Medicare side, the pressures for changes are largely financial and are coming from the government and policy makers as they search for ways to control health care costs. Traditionally, providers have focused their lobbying efforts on increasing their own Medicare payments, not on regulating Medicare HMOs.

Despite these challenges, the success of HMOs in offering a variety of benefit plan options to seniors and delivering satisfactory, affordable care underscores the importance of allowing free market principles to drive down costs among this population. Still, there is a deep distrust of the private sector among many legislators, government officials, and policy makers.

The Government As a Regulator and Competitor

Medicare FFS reimbursement is a cost-based and production-based program. Over time, this structure has grown to become extremely costly for both Medicare enrollees and the federal government, which pays for more than a third of medical costs in the country. Medicare HMOs have demonstrated the ability to assume risk for the government, making costs more predictable, reducing unnecessary utilization, and at the same time increasing benefits to Medicare eligibles with equal or greater quality and satisfaction.

Historically, HCFA has been a supportive and responsive partner in introducing managed care to the Medicare market. First set up as a regulatory body to oversee the Medicare program, however, HCFA has developed an identity crisis of sorts in its role as both a purchaser of health services and regulator of its competition. Indeed, HCFA has arguably become the largest self-insured health organization in the world. It is hardly surprising, therefore, that HCFA is reluctant to preside over its own demise. Instead, the organization from time to time attempts to bring in new regulations to improve the financing and delivery of health care in the FFS model. Unfortunately, many of these activities simply perpetuate the problems inherent in old-style FFS. Until it is clear that HCFA, supported by Congress, sees the long-term viability of the managed care industry as an important policy goal, it will limit the industry's willingness to capitalize fully on the development of efficient, accountable delivery systems across America.

Competitive Bidding and a Level Playing Field

Competitive bidding among health plan options is one avenue being discussed as a means of achieving savings for the government. Indeed, the BBA mandated that a competitive pricing demonstration project be conducted to test this method of paying for Medicare + Choice organizations; however, as of the publication date, the project has been delayed. Competitive bidding could significantly reduce the incentives for health plans to offer Medicare managed care plans, however, especially if the traditional Medicare FFS program is not required to compete under the same terms as health plans.

The debate is not so much on the concept but how it is structured and whether FFS also is required to participate. With more than 80 percent of beneficiaries still in traditional Medicare and with an expected 10 percent annual increase in health care expenditures, it would seem logical to encourage the growth of Medicare + Choice programs rather than have them compete with each other for their current market share. Competition is already intense in markets where numerous Medicare + Choice contractors provide service, which is reflected in increased benefits and lower premiums for seniors.

EVOLVING CHALLENGES AND OPPORTUNITIES OF MEDICARE + CHOICE (RISK) CONTRACTORS

HCFA's Center for Health Plans and Providers has lead responsibility for approving applications to operate Medicare plans. HCFA's dual responsibility for stimulating innovation and competition in managed health care for the elderly, while also operating a huge FFS insurance system, creates unique conflicts and pressures for the agency, the administration, and Congress. HCFA's regional offices are responsible for monitoring plan quality, access, provider networks, marketing and member materials, continuous improvement programs, and outcomes data.

Medicare + Choice programs must meet federal regulatory requirements in four major areas:

- *Organizational and contractual:* Does the plan have state authority to operate? Are provider contracts adequate? Do they contain the National Association of Insurance Commissioner's hold-harmless clause (see Chapters 62 and 69) and indicate provider willingness to serve Medicare recipients? Are provider compensation and incentives adequately detailed?
- *Financial:* What is the plan's fiscal soundness, net operating surplus, and member protection against insolvency?
- *Medicare:* Are all Medicare regulations adhered to in all regards?
- *Health care delivery:* Is there adequate availability, access, and quality monitoring?

Once applications are received, it takes approximately 24 weeks or more to gain approval if all the facts in the application are complete and accurate. Site visits are performed at HCFA's discretion. If the application is for a start-up plan, an expansion into a new region, or a large multicounty expansion, HCFA will usually conduct a site visit. If the application is a one-county expansion in an area where the HMO is already doing business or is immediately adjacent to a county that HCFA has recently reviewed, a site visit may not be conducted. The purpose of the site visit is to conduct interviews with HMO staff and contracting providers to evaluate their knowledge and skills required for the successful implementation of a Medicare + Choice contract. During the site review, HCFA regulators verify information included in the application and obtain additional details and understanding of the HMO's operations. The site visit is also an opportunity for HCFA staff to validate information relating to trends in the HMO industry by obtaining feedback from multiple health plans.

The single most common problem preventing speedy approval is the failure of the plan to have a provider network in place or contracts with appropriate language signed with providers before implementation. Other frequent mistakes include the failure to develop adequate informational material or provide sufficient financial support and quality assurance processes. In developing marketing materials, HMOs must consider HCFA's extreme sensitivity to language that is at all exaggerated and should review materials that HCFA has previously approved.

Once plans are approved, sales and marketing techniques and materials are likely to come under continuing close scrutiny by HCFA to make sure that they are not misleading to the public. Plans would be wise to err on the side of caution in explaining their benefit packages.

Once a Medicare + Choice contract has been implemented, HCFA performs monitoring site reviews once every two years, usually lasting five days. Plans should be prepared to establish long-term relationships with HCFA and be sensitive to the demands, both time and resource related, made on this government organization. Respect and perseverance will pay off in the long run.

The Market

Seniors present an interesting marketing challenge. They are not, as some believe, a homogenous group; rather, they are individuals with different needs and ideas about the way health care should be delivered. Their health care options today are much broader than ever before, and as discriminating buyers, they are likely to take their time in making decisions. Furthermore, the senior health care market is extremely competitive.

Medicare HMOs compete for customers with Medigap insurance policies, employer-sponsored coverage, and those with only Medicare FFS coverage. Many people cannot afford Medigap premiums and find Medicare + Choice plans an affordable alternative for comprehensive coverage. Retirees age 65 and older whose previous employers provide Medigap policies may have no price incentive to choose HMO coverage. Employers paying Medicare supplemental premiums, however, have significant incentives to reduce their direct costs and future liabilities, especially because the Federal Accounting Standards Board requires employers, as of 1993, to account for their total liability based on projected future costs of paying for retiree care.

Before a plan offers a Medicare + Choice product, it is important to evaluate the market and determine opportunities for growth within that market. Market research should be done to find out the number of Medicare eligibles and multiyear payment trends. Most important is to assess the community's provider mix and familiarity with managed care and the penetration and performance of Medicare and commercial HMOs in the area. Sufficient provider interest is required to build an adequate network. Seniors living in areas with low HMO penetration may be less familiar with managed care and require more information about managed care concepts.

In 1998, 72 percent of eligibles had access to at least one Medicare + Choice HMO, and 62 percent had access to two or more plans. Yet, despite significant growth over the past decade, only 16 percent of beneficiaries belonged to Medicare + Choice plans because of a lack of awareness about the benefits that managed care can offer seniors, lack of incentives to leave FFS, and reluctance to change providers. Plans entering new markets must therefore be prepared to invest in education and public relations programs to improve understanding of HMOs as a category while building and maintaining quality provider networks. In addition, they need to invest in advertising that clearly communicates the real advantages of their particular products.

In addition, to manage risk and to maintain an adequate return on investment, Medicare HMOs must constantly grow and replenish their base of members. As the market becomes more competitive and the gap widens between health care costs and reimbursement, HMOs must reinvest in the product by finding creative ways to offer benefits and to become more efficient managers of medical costs.

Geographical Distribution

As noted earlier, Medicare membership is disproportionately high in a few states. This distribution has resulted from several factors. First, the presence of organized medical groups that could effectively manage care for the senior population created a platform for early success and growth. Second, word of mouth has proved a powerful marketing tool, resulting in exponential growth where plans have most members. Third, several of these areas enjoyed reasonably high AAPCC rates, the method of payment before the BBA. The areas with higher AAPCCs were usually the most attractive to plans seeking a reasonable return on investment. Fourth, managed care is familiar to individuals younger than 65 in these states, leading to greater acceptance of Medicare HMOs and the existence of a provider network already familiar with capitated arrangements. Finally, some of these states, particularly Florida, have a disproportionate number of the elderly living within their borders.

These factors are all important in assessing the relative value of beginning operations in a given market, particularly the presence of providers educated in the delivery of care in a capitated environment and who want to work in a managed care environment.

Special Groups within the Market

Retirees

Employer-sponsored retiree health benefits cover approximately 30 percent of Medicare eligibles, representing a significant market segment with unique needs, particularly as companies recognize the impact of their generous retiree plans on their bottom line. Seniors also share their previous employers' concerns about the rising costs of health care, especially as they see other companies cut back on commitments that retirees thought were a lifetime entitlement.

Medicare managed care plans are making more and more sense, especially as corporations all over America have become accustomed to the savings that commercial HMOs have

brought to their health care expenditures. The retiree market has the potential for growth as companies seek to escape the high costs of postretirement medical coverage, especially because this liability is often unfunded and creates a negative drain on net worth.

At the time of publication, however, Medicare plans still have difficulty penetrating the retiree market. The mobility of recent retirees and the instability as a result of the BBA, coupled with incompatibility of locally driven HMO benefit structures with nationally standardized retiree benefits, creates special problems. As employers convert to a defined contribution approach to retiree benefits, however, the beneficiary begins to have more flexibility in the choice of plans available within each community. Likewise, many HMOs have become more flexible in providing customized plans to match the defined benefit plans of larger employers. Finally, a few plans have begun to arrange for member reciprocity with plans in other states, helping solve the service problems that go with member mobility.

Medicare-Medicaid Eligibles

A small percentage of the population is eligible for both Medicare and Medicaid benefits (often referred to as "dual eligibles" or more prosaically as "Medi-Medi's"), and HCFA estimates that about half of all Medicaid beneficiaries are now enrolled in managed care. The Medicaid program, through both federal and state funding, covers primarily long-term care and a number of other costs for the impoverished elderly.

The Medicaid eligibility status of these beneficiaries may change quickly, however, which can create problems for health plans. The unilateral ability of the government to set payment policy retroactively and regulate its subcontractors suggests that plans should use caution in this area. Further, state Medicaid program requirements and oversight can add significantly to a plan's overhead and political exposure.

Despite these difficulties, however, there is a real opportunity to improve patient care and increase efficiency in this population. By combining state and federal funding into one capitation payment to an HMO, the government can be assured that there is an accountable delivery system bringing discipline to the market and access to the patient. An accountable delivery system also brings cost control and quality health care, including preventive care, to this needy and often neglected population. Success with this group often requires additional outreach efforts, transportation support, and active coordination with community resources and support groups.

Medicaid is discussed in detail in Chapter 57.

Pricing and Benefit Design

Plans will be challenged to devise products that continue to include the added benefits that traditionally were their hallmark before the BBA. New products will likely include more cost sharing in the form of increased copayments and premiums and reduced benefits.

Indeed, a 1999 survey of large health plans covering 4 million Medicare + Choice beneficiaries showed nearly 1.5 million will see an increase in their premiums and nearly 60 percent will see reduced drug benefits in 2000. The survey was conducted among the 23 largest members of the American Association of Health Plans by Peter D. Hart Research.

Added benefits typically include 100 percent hospitalization coverage, low office visit copayments, preventive care, wellness programs, limited prescription drug coverage, vision care, worldwide emergency care, hearing examinations, and in some cases even hearing aids and additional chiropractic and podiatry services. If most plans in a market offer comprehensive benefits for little or no extra monthly premiums, seniors must rely more on the perception of added value than on pricing differences in making decisions regarding which Medicare + Choice plan to buy.

Less obvious but often attractive features of managed care plans include the lack of claims forms and related paperwork and free nutrition and fitness classes, which serve the dual purpose of keeping members healthy and satisfied with what they perceive as extra perks. Health plans can use their imagination in adding features that increase the value of the plan to seniors, from memberships in local health clubs to free coun-

seling sessions addressing aging, bereavement, and loss. Under BBA, the gap between health care costs and payments, however, will give HMOs less room to maneuver.

Marketing and Sales

Before enrolling members, plans must prepare their staff for handling the particular needs and sensitivities of the senior market. Bear in mind that seniors' good health holds the key to their happiness, personal security, and quality of life. Changing health plans is not a decision that should or can be made lightly. In making the sale, your plan is beginning a long-term relationship with the senior. Nurturing this relationship should be the primary goal of plan providers and customer service representatives, and all plan exclusions and limitations should be disclosed fully from the start. Because of the high degree of education required, Medicare HMOs have predominantly been marketed through a direct sales organization as opposed to using brokers or any other third-party arrangement.

High-pressure sales techniques are a guarantee of failure. If the market does not turn on you, HCFA will. ***There are several key ways to generate interest in the program:***

- direct mail
- print, television, and radio advertising
- media or public relations programs
- educational seminars
- special events, such as sponsorships of Senior Olympics or wellness fairs

These methods all help raise awareness of and generate interest in the plan. Sales can be gained through group and one-on-one meetings or over the telephone.

It is of great importance to make sure, after the sale, that the senior has fully understood the implications of joining your health plan. Some plans have member service representatives call new enrollees several days after the sale; others hold follow-up educational meetings to explain in greater detail how members access care and can best use their benefits. Some do both.

Customer Service

Member service representatives are particularly important links to senior members, especially because member retention and reputation are both keys to profitability. Some estimates put the cost of acquiring a new member at between $500 to well over $1,000. A minimally sized plan (usually estimated at 10,000 members) with even a 5 percent annual voluntary disenrollment could experience a significant shortfall in premium revenues. Customer service representatives should be well trained and polite and regard it as a requirement of their job to treat senior customers with the utmost respect. Plans that encourage member services staff to spend time on the phone with members, solve their problems promptly, and always call back with either a solution or a promise to look further into the problem at hand will find themselves winners in a competitive marketplace. Quality of care complaints should trigger quality audits, so that consistently good care is delivered. After all, the ideal scenario is for members to stay with the plan for the balance of their lifetimes, so that risk can be managed and health care resources allocated appropriately. Keeping members happy is, therefore, of great importance. This requires all staff, from claims processors to contracted providers, to be honest, straightforward, respectful, and patient in all their dealings with members.

Education

Educational and informational needs of seniors are often served by sending regular newsletters and magazines that emphasize the importance of staying healthy and may include feature articles about seniors pursuing active and healthy lifestyles. Newsletters also serve an important role in educating seniors about the philosophy of HMOs, the role of the primary care physician, and the value of the nurse case manager or triage nurse. Stories about members' experiences can reinforce the educational message. HMOs can also use these communications to remind members of services such as toll-free member service phone numbers and health care information lines. For all printed materials, use a 10-point or larger typeface and contrasting colors rather than shades or pastels and avoid glossy paper, which can contribute to glare.

CHANGING DYNAMICS OF THE DELIVERY SYSTEM

Having a health plan and provider groups that share aligned incentives to manage both quality of care and costs is the key to success. Physicians who are already accustomed to working in a capitated environment are ideal recruits for Medicare HMO contracts. Unfortunately, they are in short supply so health plans need to play an active role in their development. This development includes helping physicians understand the need to approach health care in a much more inclusive manner, managing the overall care of the member and establishing an ongoing relationship rather than providing episodic treatment for disparate illnesses or injuries followed by piecemeal referrals to specialists. The successful provider group understands that managed care saves money and improves quality by rewarding teamwork, efficiency, and the delivery of the appropriate acuity of care in a clinically appropriate setting.

More often, they understand the value of preventive care and the creative use of resources to achieve the desired result. Effective providers follow up complex consultations with regular phone calls to encourage compliance in taking prescription drugs, such as blood pressure medication. Many others conduct health risk assessments followed, where indicated, by consultation or inspection of the senior's home environment in an effort to prevent the kinds of injuries or complications that result in extended hospital stays. Another example is providing frail patients with a free shower chair, immediately cutting down on the number of falls that are likely to result in expensive hospital stays and hip replacements. These and other creative approaches, stimulated by capitated arrangements, have a significant impact on the life of senior members, keeping them healthy, improving the quality of their lives, and at the same time ensuring a return on the investment made by the provider group in this new approach to care.

If organized well, providers with existing contracts with Medicare-managed care companies appreciate the consistent cash flow and upfront capital that accompanies capitated arrangements. They have in many cases adjusted their practices accordingly, reengineering their administrative infrastructure to focus on prevention, service, and outcomes data rather than simply the payment of physicians' claims.

Challenges of the Elderly and Disabled

The elderly usually require longer appointments than patients younger than 65 for several reasons: They may have more questions to ask or more health problems to discuss, and they are often less rushed for time than their Baby Boomer children. That must be taken into account in scheduling time with the physician. Consulting rooms may need to be a little larger to accommodate spouses or family who accompany the elderly patient to a consultation. Bathrooms should be fitted with handrails, and more handicapped parking should be available. Even more than these alterations to the physical space, providers of care to the elderly must be patient, respectful, and willing to listen.

This does not mean that physicians need to throw their productivity standards out the window. Most successful medical groups in Medicare HMO contracts have learned to use teams of professionals and paraprofessionals to address their HMO members' needs, resulting in both better care and increased overall efficiency.

Impact on Network Design and Staffing

More than any other factor, the design and management of the delivery system determine the success or failure of a senior HMO, and the control of hospitalization is the single most likely contributor to financial success. ***There are generally four***

main formats of provider groups that, when properly designed and managed, currently seem best suited to managing health care for seniors within a capitated environment:

- integrated multispecialty groups with good primary care capacity
- primary care medical groups with a limited network of contracted specialists
- independent practice associations (IPAs) with a selective network of providers and with policy driven by primary care providers
- integrated delivery systems, which are challenged by size and complexity (This category includes such models as physician-hospital organizations [PHOs], management service organizations [MSOs], or medical foundations. However, assuming that they are well run, selective in network participation, market driven, and have redistributed the dollars and incentives to support growth and service, they can be effective [see also Chapter 4].)

Each medical delivery system model has different advantages and disadvantages, but all will experience significant patient care demand from senior members. Medicare members use more services, including office visits, than commercial members. As noted in Chapters 7 and 18, commercial enrollees younger than 65 have an average of 3.6 to 3.8 physician encounters per year, of which 2.5 are primary care visits. Medicare members average 7.0 encounters per year for Medicare risk enrollees, and 6.4 encounters per year for Medicare cost enrollees[8]; these data refer to total physician encounters, not necessarily those for primary care only, and do not include encounters with nonphysicians. Nevertheless, the implications for staffing are clear: Staffing needs are greatly increased when a substantial Medicare population is served. As pointed out in Chapter 7, most closed-panel HMOs increased their staffing ratios for Medicare members to a mean of 1.6 per 1,000 Medicare enrollees.[9]

Although components of any of these accountable delivery systems may be paid by means of some form of per diem, case rate, or other FFS basis, the value of capitation is emphasized because of its power in aligning the delivery system's incentives with those of the patient and plan. With capitation, the delivery system is motivated to prevent health problems, treat them well and efficiently when they occur, and keep members happy, all of which are critical variables to properly serve older adult members.

Administrative and leadership requirements are also significant and include:

- the ability to add physician capacity when membership grows
- the ability to influence practice patterns and change physician behavior to avoid unnecessary hospitalizations or referrals
- the ability to process coverage authorizations and medical claims payments within the bounds of government policy, which is generally stricter than that of the average commercial population
- the ability to manage complex cases involving a number of different specialists, hospitalizations, and prescription drugs within a variety of clinical settings
- the ability to interface with and use the many community agencies and support services that add value to the total care of this population

These demands have different implications for different medical group models (these model types are discussed in Chapter 4; reimbursement to different types of medical groups, including specific financial incentive regulations applicable to physicians in Medicare + Choice plans, is discussed in Chapter 8). IPAs can generally be more flexible because they can extend their physician capacity quickly by contracting with physicians in the community at large. IPAs also often have well-established links with the community. The IPA's weaker commitment to a centralized administrative management and governance, however, may diminish the consistency and therefore the effectiveness of the group's referral and authorization policies. In addition, the lack of any centralized governance

over IPA's provider system resources prevents them from driving efficiencies through office consolidation or capitalizing either expansion sites or alternative treatment centers.

The primary medical group (PMG) can provide a closer level of coordination between the clinical and business sides of the operation and simplify the implementation of coordinated patient care management through a tighter governance structure concentrated among primary group owners. A PMG without distributed medical offices, however, may be less marketable than a contracted primary care physician network. In addition, PMGs must be particularly sensitive, as must primary care–driven IPAs, to the more complicated medical conditions found in their senior population. For example, as noted in Chapters 7 and 18, an internist or medical subspecialist may be a more effective care manager than a general practitioner in some cases.

Integrated multispecialty groups have the greatest potential to control inpatient and outpatient specialist costs and the ability to implement effective and efficient disease management programs for chronic conditions such as diabetes or cardiopulmonary disease. These groups, however, may also be more departmentally structured and traditional in their approach to the delivery of care, less likely to work as a team, and more resistant to accepting the central role of primary care as it relates to policy and income redistribution. Foundations vary; they may exhibit some of the strengths and weaknesses of multiple models.

PHOs and MSOs are the newest of the preceding models and, depending on their organizational structure, could exhibit all the best or all the worst of the aforementioned traits. In general, most PHOs are limiting their potential for success by failing to support the necessary redistribution of policy and income away from hospital and specialty care toward primary care. They have also typically failed to build the experienced management infrastructure and have resisted the need to push strong financial incentives down to the individual physician level. Nevertheless, if they could overcome this understandable resistance, PHOs and MSOs have better potential access to capital and organizational support than many IPAs, primary group structures, or not-for-profit foundations. Strong leadership and a willingness to accept new ways of approaching health care for seniors will go a long way toward improving the likelihood of success with every delivery model.

No matter how a plan's provider relationships are structured, there are some critical areas to examine to assess how compatible the groups are with the philosophy of capitation and its financial impact on their practices:

- governance
- commonality of purpose
- sharing of financial risk
- control of primary care physician activities, training, and reporting
- control over hospital admissions and lengths of stay
- control of specialist and ancillary expenses
- ability to finance growth
- ability and willingness to recruit new primary care physicians
- marketability
- sensitivity to the special needs of the senior population
- willingness to work as a partner with the health plan in total patient care management

Role of Care Coordinators, Ancillary Providers, and Guidelines

Managed care has been defined as the delivery of the appropriate care at the appropriate time in the appropriate setting by the appropriate provider. The provider may be a primary care physician or specialist, but in many cases an ancillary provider, such as a nurse practitioner, physician assistant, or home health nurse, may be more appropriate and effective.

Older members of the population, in particular, may benefit from extended conversations with nurse practitioners, who can help allay fears and discuss symptoms in some detail before giving a summary to the physician. It is important, however, to let the elderly patient know that the nurse is an added value and not a substi-

tute for physician care. Neither should the nurse or physician assistant treat the senior in a patronizing manner; instead, all caregivers should provide an opportunity for the patient to provide full details of his or her physical problems. This level of detail can be extremely helpful in arriving at accurate diagnoses and ultimately can save time for the busy practitioner.

It is not unusual for successful medical groups to have developed extensive clinical care guidelines and active patient care committees to help their physicians decide how to provide quality care in the most cost-efficient way. Such guidelines, coupled with aggressive development of alternative care sites, have allowed medical groups to decrease significantly their number of hospital days. This reduction in expensive hospital days is achieved through using more appropriate and less expensive settings such as surgicenters, diagnostic clinics, skilled nursing or subacute care facilities, and home-based therapies. Plans and medical groups should also contract with home health agencies (see Chapter 26) and hospice care (see Chapter 28) to provide clinical services as appropriate.

Most large and successful capitated groups have gone beyond simple clinical care guidelines and have developed whole multidisciplinary programs to manage chronic diseases or problematic conditions. For example, one medical group serving more than 25,000 capitated senior lives has developed a program called Options to help manage the last few months of life for terminal patients. The purpose is twofold: to prevent unnecessary hospital readmissions and, more important, to improve the quality of life for the dying patient. A multifunctional team, including specialists, the primary care physician, pharmacy representatives, medical technologists, home health nurses, and family members, all take part in the decision-making process. Twenty-four-hour emergency care is made available, as well as a 24-hour help line and respite or home health care to support family members and the patient during difficult times. As a result of this approach, hospital admissions have fallen dramatically, and family members report greater satisfaction with the care and quality of life of their loved ones during their final days. Not incidentally, the medical group in question also reduced expenses per member per month.

A customer service and quality focus, combined with creativity and resourcefulness, is the best indicator that a medical group is likely to be successful in a capitated, risk-sharing arrangement caring for seniors.

Working with Special Populations

In addition to the wide range of health care needs found within the senior population, there are a number of segments that present particular opportunities and challenges, particularly because as the population ages, more Americans are living longer with chronic or disabling conditions. These special populations include the disabled, the frail elderly, those with ESRD, and the hospice population. Plans should consider carefully whether their organizational structure, physician mix, and incentive systems are set up to provide adequate care to these groups while maintaining plan viability as a business.

Each special population has different financing sources, payment methods, and levels. Because legislation has designated funding for programs that address specific needs, older persons with complex needs for both acute and chronic services must often rely on a number of funding sources and programs. Funding can include federal, state, and private sources.

With some populations, the integration of state programs with the federal Medicare program through contracts or other methods will be necessary to resolve issues in fragmentation and to merge the acute and long-term care funding streams. HCFA has initiated a number of demonstration projects to finance the care of special populations through capitation and to test various payment rates, benefit designs, risk adjustment methods, and combined funding sources. Some plans use disease management programs (see Chapter 23) to monitor proactively the situations of at-risk enrollees. Case managers (see Chapter 22) assess need, develop care plans, make arrangements for care with appropriate providers, and provide follow-up and monitoring to ensure that the care selected continues to be appropriate. And home care (Chapter 26), subacute care (Chapter 27), and hospice and end-of-life care (Chapter 28) are likewise important adjuncts to clinical care for this population.

The Disabled

According to HCFA's 1998 Medicare Chart Book, the disabled represented an estimated 10 percent of its Medicare beneficiaries. This population is expected to grow to 16 percent in 2017. In providing services for this group, it is important for plans to develop strategic and contractual arrangements with ancillary providers such as physiatrists, physical therapists, podiatrists, chiropractors, and other specialized therapists who serve this population, as well as with rehabilitation facilities, skilled nursing facilities, and long-term care facilities.

Strategies that are used to manage chronic medical conditions in the general Medicare population must be applied even more vigorously to the disabled, including close coordination with community resources and programs. Upfront risk assessment and health status profiling are key. Resources must be allocated efficiently, and strategies must be applied that enhance the best possible health status for these individuals by preventing the exacerbation of existing problems. Consistent outreach is important; so is education of members and their families regarding nutrition and how best to handle their physical challenges and maintain relative health.

The Frail Elderly

Nursing home expenditures are consuming increasing levels of our nation's resources; predictions are that the cost to Medicaid alone will rise to $9 billion by 2010. Overall, about 70 percent of all public and private long-term health care dollars are currently spent for institutional care. Also, the number of those older than 65 who are severely impaired was expected to increase by 30 percent between 1990 and 2000. An estimated 1.6 million are now living in 16,800 nursing homes. Given these statistics and demographic trends suggesting that the over-85 population is likely to increase substantially in the next 10 years, the frail elderly population (those who have a physical, cognitive, or medical condition that affects their ability to perform the activities of daily living) presents Medicare + Choice plans with significant opportunities and challenges.

Plans that develop programs specifically designed to manage the particular problems associated with the frail elderly are likely to be the most successful. The successful plans will also be those that combine home care services and community-based resources in the most efficient manner, usually through a dedicated care manager. In addition, advocacy on the part of the member should become an overriding responsibility of the care manager, particularly when he or she is working with impaired members who cannot negotiate the system for themselves.

End-Stage Renal Disease

The number of Medicare beneficiaries with ESRD grew at an average annual rate of about 10 percent from 1982 to 1992. This population, which is also likely to grow substantially in the coming years, has been the subject of much research and is part of HCFA demonstration projects in California, Tennessee, and Florida. There are more than 230,000 ESRD patients nationwide, and more than 6,000 of these are currently enrolled in Medicare managed care organizations. Medicare HMO plans cannot actively recruit members with ESRD, although this group may provide an opportunity to apply managed care principles to the benefit of both the patient and the plan.

If enrollees develop ESRD after they are already enrolled, Medicare + Choice contractors cannot automatically disenroll them. Plans must monitor the chronic care needs of ESRD enrollees and take proactive measures to improve their functioning and avoid acute care crises. For several years, there has been an interest in refining or adjusting the capitation rate for ESRD enrollees, particularly to cover the large cost outlays

for transplant surgery and to reflect cost differences related to whether the enrollee is receiving maintenance dialysis or has successfully received a transplant.

Of note, members with ESRD who are enrolled in the plan as commercial members, not Medicare + Choice members, become eligible for Medicare and the plan may apply coordination of benefits rules to coverage of those members after a 30-month period. The reader is referred to Chapter 39 for a discussion of the complex policies and procedure of this issue, as well as a discussion of coordination of benefits for commercial members who are also Medicare eligible.

Hospice Care

In 1995, Medicare fiscal year expenditures on hospice care were estimated at close to $1.4 billion compared with $90 million in 1988.[10] Part of the reason for this dramatic shift was the decrease in the use of hospitals to take care of the elderly in the last month of life, when most expenditures occur. The net effect of this market shift is financially positive; Medicare beneficiaries with cancer who were enrolled in a hospice cost Medicare on average $2,737 less than nonusers in the last year of life.[11]

Hospice care helps terminally ill patients spend their last months of life in the most comfortable setting possible, providing palliative care rather than making unwanted and unnecessary heroic efforts that will provide little benefit. Most managed care payers provide coverage similar to Medicare coverage for hospice services. HMOs offer these benefits in the belief that it is more cost-effective to provide a person with less expensive (though prolonged) hospice care than to encourage fruitless attempts to halt the progress of a terminal disease. Expanded use of hospice benefits could represent significant potential savings to the country, given that Medicare beneficiaries in their last year of life account for approximately 27 percent of Medicare expenditures.

Managed care plans offering hospice benefits may find this feature an attractive added value to potential members and a cost-saving technique for the plan in the long term. This niche market, however, is also fraught with the danger of possible litigation. The attempt to persuade a patient to enter hospice care may be regarded as a sign of the plan's attempt to lower cost rather than an action taken in the interest of the patient. This is, understandably, a difficult and emotional time for the family. In fact, the most successful medical groups and risk contractors often educate their members about wills, advance directives, and powers of attorney, preparing both the family and the patient to deal better with these tough issues before the need for difficult decisions arises.

Quality Issues

As previously discussed in this chapter and in Chapter 30, the power of managed care to improve coordination and appropriateness of care is proving an added bonus for seniors, some of whom have been overmedicated in the past or undergone surgeries of doubtful value in a system in which incentives were skewed toward an oversupply of services and procedures.

Competition among senior HMOs, unheard of among the general Medicare population, has resulted in plans offering an unparalleled level of benefits. A 1997 report from the Prospective Payment Advisory Commission estimated that, on average, health plans offer benefits worth about $95 more per month than the traditional FFS Medicare program. A 1998 HCFA survey of managed care plans showed 97 percent covered routine physicals, 83 percent covered eye examinations, 72 percent covered ear examinations, 66 percent covered outpatient drugs, and 37 percent covered dental costs. In addition, many plans offered fitness and nutrition classes and educational newsletters with information about health maintenance. These are benefits that Medicare generally does not cover.

In addition to improvement in the quality of care through added benefits, plans set up quality assurance programs that monitor the amount and kind of care delivered by providers and flag inappropriate care. Members also have access to grievance procedures should they have any concerns about their benefits or care (see Chapter 40). Because of the competitive nature of the market in the most highly penetrated areas, a reputation for quality becomes a valuable marketing asset and a moral imperative. Further, the reality that managed care plans are providing quality care is shown through a number of studies conducted over the past few years.

According to an HCFA study, elderly HMO members with cancer were more likely to be diagnosed at an early stage than elderly people in old-style FFS plans. In that study, breast, cervical, and colon cancer, along with melanomas, were diagnosed significantly earlier in HMOs than FFS plans.[12] Another study comparing treatments and outcomes in myocardial infarction found that HMO patients received hospital care that was generally better in terms of process than that reviewed by patients in a national FFS sample.[13] In addition, a study comparing treatment decisions among 140,000 Californians with clogged coronary arteries found that HMOs offered the best way to avoid unnecessary treatment without sacrificing needed care. HMO patients underwent less surgery, yet there was no difference in death rates for HMO and FFS patients.[14] A study published in the November 17, 1997, issue of the *Journal of the National Cancer Institute* found that women enrolled in two HMOs participating in Medicare had survival outcomes at least equal to or possibly better than women in traditional Medicare. Researchers attributed more regular and widespread screening examinations that led to detection at earlier stages, which meant smaller tumor sizes as partial reasons for the lower overall mortality rate for HMO enrollees. These are just a few of an expanding list of studies that suggest that innovation and quality are increasingly the accepted hallmarks of successful Medicare HMO plans.

Moreover, studies show that seniors have high levels of satisfaction with their Medicare health plans. A recent survey by Sachs Group of 16,000 seniors in 33 markets assessed satisfaction in seven categories: plan benefits, cost, network access, physician access, perceived medical quality, medical management, and member services.

The study showed Medicare HMO members are just as satisfied as Medicare supplemental and Medicare-only members. In fact, in six of the seven survey categories, HMO members are as satisfied or more satisfied than seniors with only Medicare coverage. And chronically ill HMO members are as satisfied or more satisfied than seniors with Medicare supplemental coverage in five areas studied: member services, physician access, medical quality, cost, and plan benefits.

The study challenges industry perceptions that managed care might not be appropriate for seniors with chronic conditions and that managed care better serves the healthy. In fact, the research showed that in highly competitive, mature HMO markets such as Denver, Los Angeles, Phoenix, San Francisco, and Seattle, plans enroll an equal share of chronically ill members and healthy seniors. And more than half of the chronically ill seniors had been enrolled in their plans for more than five years.[15]

HCFA's 1998 beneficiary satisfaction survey, collected through the Consumer Assessment of Health Plans (CAHPS) survey, included approximately 136,000 Medicare beneficiaries, who were asked to assess their health plans on a scale of 1 to 10. With 10 being the highest score, 84% of Medicare HMO enrollees rated their health plan an "8" or higher with one-half of all enrollees rating their health plan at a "10."

Quality Initiatives

While independent organizations have conducted numerous surveys on quality issues, HCFA has established its own reporting mechanisms during the past few years.

The Quality Improvement System for Managed Care (QISMC) is an HCFA initiative to strengthen managed care organizations' efforts to protect and improve the health and satisfaction of Medicare and Medicaid beneficiaries. For Medicare + Choice organizations, QISMC standards took effect on January 1, 1999. During the first year organizations are required to report on Health Plan Employer Data and Information Set and CAHPS measures, but they do not have

to meet any minimum performance levels. They are required to initiate two performance projects. Neither project has to achieve any demonstrable improvement until the end of the third contract year.[16] For the year 2000, HCFA has decided that the agency-sponsored project will focus on pneumonia.

The quality initiatives, according to HCFA, are designed to ensure Medicare + Choice organizations have a common goal of ensuring a consistently high-quality and cost-effective standard of care by measuring improved outcomes of health care and services. It is hoped that this type of quality initiative will be introduced for the FFS program to improve the care of all Medicare beneficiaries.

Corporate Compliance

Medicare + Choice contains many requirements that have been referenced in this chapter. Requirements include quality reporting, consumer protections and service, data reporting, and many others. The reader is referred to Chapter 68 for a full discussion of the corporate compliance requirements that must be met on an ongoing basis.

FUTURE TRENDS

Congressional interest in the power of managed care to reduce Medicare costs is spurring new demonstration projects and heated debate over future reimbursement issues and the impact of the BBA on Medicare + Choice plans, which so far seems to have lessened the choices of seniors rather than increased them. As the discussion broadens to long-term Medicare restructuring, there are also likely to be many new challenges and opportunities for managed care companies. During this period of transition, it will be important to keep a dialog going among seniors, providers, plans, and legislators to prevent the passage of well-meaning but misguided laws that could have an adverse effect on the senior market.

Indeed, these are fascinating times. The senior market presents some interesting and exciting opportunities for health plans and providers to find resourceful new ways to improve quality and efficiency. The longer-living, more active, healthier seniors of the future will be able to select plans that are best suited to their physical needs, financial situation, and delivery system preferences, all of which will become important as the discriminating Baby Boomers reach their mid-60s with higher expectations of the health system than ever before. The managed care industry will need to continue to evolve to keep up with this highly dynamic market.

REFERENCES AND NOTES

1. 1995 Retirement Guide, *U.S. News & World Report* (June 12, 1995), 62–69. *Excerpt from New Passages: Mapping Your Life Across Time* (New York: Random House, 1995).

2. If You Build It, They Will Come, *IBC's Capitation Alert!* 1, no. 6.

3. *Profile of Medicare Chart Book*, U.S. Department of Health and Human Services, 1998.

4. *Medicare and Managed Care Fact Sheet*, Health Care Financing Administration, February 1999.

5. P. Newman et al., Medicare Choice Explosion? Implications for Beneficiaries, *Health Affairs* (January–February 1999): 152.

6. V. Fuchs, Health Care for the Elderly: How Much? Who Will Pay for It? *Health Affairs* (January–February 1999): 11.

7. *Medicare + Choice Risk Adjustment Methodology Policy Brief*, American Association of Health Plans (February 1999).

8. Group Health Association of America, *HMO Industry Profile* (Washington, DC.: Group Health Association of America, 1994).

9. T.H. Dial et al., Clinical Staffing in Staff- and Group-Model HMOs, *Health Affairs* (Summer 1995): 168–80.

10. S. Becker and R.J. Pristave, Managed Care and the Provision of Hospital Care, *Managed Care Quarterly* 3 (1995): 1, 39-43.

11. *An Analysis of the Cost-Savings of the Medicare Hospice Benefit: Lewin-VHI Inc.,* Study prepared for the National Hospital Association, May 21, 1995.

12. G. Riley et al., Stage of Cancer at Diagnosis for Medicare HMO and Fee-For-Service Enrollees, *American Journal of Public Health* 84 (1994): 10, 1598–1604.

13. D. Faze et al., HMO Bests Fee-For-Service Care of Older Persons with Acute Myocardial Infarction, *American Journal of Public Health* 82 (1992): 12, 1626–30.

14. Group Health Association of America, *HMO Fact Sheet* (Washington, DC: GHAA, 1995).

15. L. Garvy, Debunking the Myths of Medicare HMOs, *Managed Healthcare* (December 1998).

16. *Quality of Care Information Project Activities*, Health Care Financing Administration (September 1998).

CHAPTER 57

Medicaid Managed Care

Robert E. Hurley and Stephen A. Somers

INTRODUCTION

Medicaid agency officials, like their private employer counterparts, have turned to managed care strategies to pursue more value for the money they are spending to buy health services for their beneficiaries. After a modest start, they have moved expeditiously with more than 17 million beneficiaries—more than half of the eligible population—enrolled in managed care arrangements by 1999. Embracing managed care has been especially challenging for Medicaid agencies because it represents a major philosophical change from being relatively passive claims processors and bill payers to becoming proactive, prudent purchasers. As in the private sector, it has taken time for Medicaid agencies to develop the commitment, skills, and experience to become proficient in these new responsibilities. Because Medicaid fee-for-service programs have long been characterized by low payment rates and limited provider participation, translat-

ing private sector managed care techniques such as price discounting and tight networks has not been easy. Moreover, in many instances, worries about access and quality have overshadowed cost concerns in Medicaid.

Much of the interest in and concern about Medicaid managed care has centered on how well Medicaid agencies are assuming the role of sponsor or prudent buyer, particularly in light of their ambivalent attitudes toward managed care organizations and their conflicting purchaser and regulator roles. Medicaid agencies, whose beneficiaries are among the most vulnerable populations, may be especially susceptible to this ambivalence as they attempt to do business with the same organizations that are being criticized and sometimes vilified by other public officials and consumer advocacy groups.

In this chapter, we examine some of the history and background of Medicaid and Medicaid managed care that has contributed to, in many instances, Medicaid managed care still being more Medicaid than managed care. However, many purchaser functions, including program design, planning, implementation, and management, actually reflect more similarities than differences with those of aggressive employee benefits managers, and these areas are described and detailed. We detail the successes and failures that have characterized the past 15 years of Medicaid's foray into managed care and then turn to several issues that are looming over what has become a turbulent period for many states with Medicaid managed care initiatives. Finally,

Robert E. Hurley, PhD, is a faculty member at the Medical College of Virginia at Virginia Commonwealth University. He has been conducting managed care research, primarily in the public sector, for more than a decade.

Stephen A. Somers, PhD, is President of the Center for Health Care Strategies, Inc. and a Senior Visiting Researcher and Lecturer at the Woodrow Wilson School of Public and International Affairs at Princeton University. He has served as the Program Director for the Robert Wood Johnson Foundation's Medicaid Managed Care Program since 1995.

the chapter concludes with a series of as yet unanswered questions that linger over the future of Medicaid managed care.

MEDICAID—ORIGINS AND EVOLUTION

Medicaid, the principal public program for low-income persons, was developed largely as an afterthought to the passage of Medicare legislation in 1965.[1] Cost estimates about this jointly financed federal and state program were quickly discovered to be far off the mark. Over the next 30 years there was inexorable growth in the expenditures as Medicaid encountered the dual consequences of expanding enrollment and rampant medical care cost inflation. By 1998, the cost of this program covering approximately 35 million Medicaid beneficiaries reached $170 billion.[2]

At the outset, there was an expressed aim for Medicaid to be patterned after private insurance coverage to gain access to the same providers of care serving commercially insured persons.[3] In addition, like Medicare, Medicaid was intended to be a claims payer for those covered services determined to be appropriate by providers, with minimal intrusion into provider discretion, further conforming the new public sector programs with private health insurance of that era. However, escalating costs soon eroded commitment to maintaining full program parity; payment rates to providers began to lag private sector rates, which, in turn, led to declining provider participation and many other problems discussed in the following.[4]

Beneficiary Growth

Medicaid is three distinct programs reflecting different constituencies. The largest covered group, generally healthy women and children who qualify on the basis of their low incomes, represents 70 percent of the persons enrolled in Medicaid. The second largest group includes both aged and younger persons with chronic illness and disability who qualify on the basis of their disabled status, which may keep them out of the workforce or, in some instances, prevent them from obtaining private insurance. The third group, a subset of the second group, is an institutionalized population including persons in nursing homes or specialized facilities for the developmentally disabled or mentally retarded. It is because of this group that Medicaid is the principal financier of nursing homes in the nation.[5]

Taken as a whole, the latter two groups are so much more costly on average that, although they represent only 30 percent of the population with Medicaid coverage, they consume about 70 percent of expenditures. The combination of persons eligible for Medicaid has important implications for Medicaid's forays into managed care. Most managed care enrollment has been among low-income women and children, whose medical needs are generally similar to persons found among private managed care enrollment. Thus, despite dramatic increases in Medicaid managed care enrollment, the ability of states to extract large aggregate savings is constrained by the fact that most Medicaid expenditures are still not exposed to managed care. And there are major obstacles to be overcome to convert high-need/high-cost beneficiaries from Medicaid fee-for-service to managed care arrangements.

The Medicaid Environment

Medicaid is a complex program. Len Kirschner, one time director of the Arizona Medicaid program likes to say "Medicaid is not rocket science: it's actually more complicated and costly than that." It is the prototypical *federal* program, with administrative and financing responsibilities shared between national and state (and in some cases county) agencies. In many states, the Medicaid program represents 20 percent or more of all expenditures despite the fact that the growth rate has tapered off in the last two years.[6] Policies, rules, and regulations pertaining to eligibility, coverage, payment, and services are voluminous and often arcane. There are more than fifty variations on all of these elements because of variability among the states and territories. And, in recent years, major pieces of national legislation, including the

Americans with Disabilities Act, welfare reform legislation, the Balanced Budget Act of 1997, and the State Children's Health Insurance Program (S/CHIP), have had sweeping consequences for Medicaid, even though it was not the direct target of much of this legislation.

The complexity is intensified by the political context of Medicaid. General debates and disputes about public spending on human service programs often focus on Medicaid because of the size and growth of the program and the populations who have benefited from it. The program has also been a battleground for the "devolution" struggle between states and the federal government. States have contended that the federal government has burdened them with unfunded mandates. Moreover, they assert federal heavy-handedness denies states the flexibility to be innovative and creative in program developments and enhancements—requiring them to petition for waivers to deviate from federal policies for such initiatives, including most of those undertaken in the expansion of managed care. On the other hand, some critics raise concerns that the federal government is relinquishing too much control to states. They contend this is contributing to even greater disparities among the states in terms of who is covered, what benefits are being covered, and how much providers are being paid.[7]

MEDICAID MANAGED CARE— BACKGROUND AND MODELS

Initial efforts to make managed care available to Medicaid beneficiaries involved promoting enrollment in HMOs on a voluntary basis.[8] Only a small number of plans tried this and by the early 1980s less than 1 percent of beneficiaries were in HMOs, at a time when commercial HMO penetration was running between 5 and 10 percent. But several states began to look to managed care models to address some of the problems endemic to Medicaid with its low payment rates and low-income constituency. The problems included declining provider participation, limited access to primary and preventive care, dependence on inappropriate sites of care such as emergency departments, and a general concern about the quality of services that many beneficiaries were able to receive.[9] Notably, concerns about costs were not paramount at this time, although this would change at the end of the 1980s, when major eligibility expansions led to rising program expenditures.

State Approaches to Buying Managed Care

Two major models emerged to address these challenges. Several states, led by Michigan and Utah,[10] began in the early 1980s to devise primary care case management (PCCM) or gatekeeper programs. The PCCM arrangement guaranteed Medicaid beneficiaries a medical home, and it required primary care physicians to authorize and manage services for patients who were now formally enrolled in their practices. PCCM programs paid physicians fee-for-service and a modest case management fee for their round-the-clock availability and care management responsibilities and left most other features of Medicaid unchanged.

These programs grew quite rapidly across a number of states. Their ability to add value lay in the guarantee of access and modest savings caused by care coordination and reduced emergency department use. PCCM was also a model that was well accepted in the medical community, in part because it was *not an HMO*, and it was suitable in both urban and rural markets. The growth in utilization management and gatekeeping in the private sector contributed to acceptances of this relatively benign intrusion into physician practice prerogatives. The PCCM model, although limited by contemporary managed care standards, has proven robust with more than four million beneficiaries enrolled in these arrangements in 1998. Enrollments may be poised to grow faster given other developments in the Medicaid managed care arena discussed in the following.[11]

The other model adopted by Medicaid managers was HMO enrollment of beneficiaries. In most instances, this involved offering HMOs as an alternative to traditional fee-for-service Medicaid, just as a private purchaser might offer an HMO choice alongside the standard indemnity plan. Established HMOs were initially less than enthusiastic about entering this line of business.[12] They were concerned about rate adequacy and their capacity to serve this population, whose intermittent eligibility could undermine the ability of plans to promote preventive service use. There were also concerns about the ability of beneficiaries to navigate managed care processes like plan choice, restrictive networks, and preservice authorization. A few plans were created to serve this population, but their growth was constrained by requirements that their membership eventually had to be at least 25 percent non-Medicaid (the so-called 75/25 rule was removed by the Balanced Budget Act of 1997). Despite these problems, voluntary enrollment in HMOs gave states their first experiences in contracting with health systems for the total benefit package, in establishing prepaid rates, and in developing capacity to monitor care being bought in a very different fashion from fee-for-service.

A few states took the bolder approach of making HMO enrollment mandatory. Arizona finally implemented its Medicaid program in 1982 by building it entirely around prepaid health plans. Under a major federal policy waiver, Arizona Health Care Cost Containment System (AHCCCS) became, in many respects, the first of the new generation of Medicaid programs.[13] Prepayment prevailed throughout the state as health plans that won a competitive bidding process and signed long-term contracts (currently for five years) became responsible for virtually the entire Medicaid benefit package. Although there were some severe implementation problems, by the late 1980s AHCCCS had stabilized and attracted growing acclaim. Other states adopted similar mandatory HMO enrollment approaches in selected cities including Milwaukee, Kansas City (MO), and Minneapolis.[14]

Armed with broad waivers issued by the Health Care Financing Administration, the list of states with mandatory HMO enrollment programs lengthened in the early 1990s (Tennessee, Rhode Island, Delaware, Hawaii) at least for low-income women and children or within selected urban areas in their states (California,

Pennsylvania, Ohio). Many states also offered combinations of HMO and PCCM programs sometimes operating them side-by-side (Oregon, Florida, Texas) and sometimes making HMO enrollment mandatory in metropolitan areas and requiring PCCM enrollment in the remainder of the state (Virginia, North Carolina). By 1999, 20 states had only HMO programs, 4 had exclusively PCCM programs, and 25 had some combination.[15] About 75 percent of the 17 million beneficiaries in managed care (Figure 57–1) are in HMO or fully capitated programs.

Some of the programs are mandatory for all noninstitutionalized populations, whereas others exempt certain special need beneficiary groups. A number of others states operate specialized managed care programs for benefits that are carved out of the medical benefits package, most commonly mental/behavioral health or pharmacy services. In this regard, Medicaid agencies have mimicked the experience of private purchasers but probably have moved even more cautiously because of interagency and intergovernmental complications. Some carveouts are undertaken not only because of clinical desirability but also because they are used by public purchasers to protect existing providers and delivery systems. Carveouts may also be designed to give additional time to certain vulnerable providers, such as public hospitals or community mental health centers, to adjust managed care demands. This is one example of how public sector purchasers of managed care cannot simply import commercial managed care approaches without customizing them to their special needs and responsibilities.[16]

OPERATIONAL FEATURES

The origins and distinctiveness of Medicaid managed care help explain why Medicaid purchasers have had to translate cautiously the experience gained in private sector managed care.[17] Several other factors influence the operations of Medicaid managed care programs. Health and human service needs of beneficiaries may be more complex than those commonly found in commercially insured populations.

Enrollees in 000s

Figure 57–1 Medicaid Managed Care Enrollment 1985–98. *Source:* Reprinted from Health Care Financing Administration, Department of Health and Human Services.

Beneficiaries typically have little or no cost participation to shape and constrain their use of services. Many traditional Medicaid providers may not be well represented in managed care plan networks. In a mandatory enrollment program, techniques are needed to facilitate choice among plans for beneficiaries and to arrange for persons who do not make a choice to find a medical home. Taken together these obstacles constitute daunting challenges for those trying to make managed care work in Medicaid and illustrate how Medicaid operational features are both similar to and different from those in the private sector.

Design, Planning, and Implementation

The traditional Medicaid program is similar to a *rich* indemnity product offered by a private employer that has limited features of managed care: extensive benefit package; few restrictions on provider choice; and no premium contribution, deductibles, or copayments. In moving toward managed care, states must consider what the implications will be for the covered population, existing providers, new contractors, and the buyer itself. Such decisions require evaluation of alternatives, assessment of acceptability of the modifications to both beneficiaries and providers, and a well-planned implementation schedule with realistic timetables. The more extensive the changes, the more preparation and transition time required, if disruption and confusion are to be avoided.

Medicaid programs have a mixed record on these transitions. Some states like Virginia have been quite successful in preparing beneficiaries for forthcoming changes and encouraging providers to timely affiliations with managed care organizations. Others like Missouri have modulated the implementation of major initiatives until a managed care market is more fully developed or deferred the extension of the program to more challenging populations (e.g., the disabled) or more difficult locations (e.g., rural areas) because of lack of readiness. Some states, however, have taken the tack of moving expeditiously, if not precipitously, to preempt resistance. The most notable example of this was in 1994, when the TennCare program enrolled more than 700,000 beneficiaries in prepaid organizations in less than two months. Critics suggest that TennCare managers spent much of the next several years dealing with remedial problems resulting from lack of advance planning and preparation. As an apparent response to the notoriety of the Tennessee experience, state implementation plans and schedules seem to have become more cautious and well considered.

Program Models

One of a state's first steps is to identify the potential models appropriate to its strategic purposes and the structure and maturity of their managed care market. Typically, states study the experience of their peers, then convene a planning group that may include interagency staff and perhaps outsiders like medical association representatives and beneficiaries/consumers. PCCM program design can be seen as analogous to a private employer developing a PPO network for a self-insured product. To date most states have chosen to administer their PCCM programs directly, but there is some growth in the use of outside contractors for various functions including network development and management.

States committing to a prepaid health plan strategy may be more likely to buy "off-the-shelf" managed care products, meaning those that are already being offered by an established HMO. In these instances, states develop contractor qualifications and issue a request for proposal that details expectations and requirements. Plans may be selected on a competitive basis in which only a limited number of awards will be made on the basis of a predetermined scoring scheme. In other cases, all plans meeting specified qualifications may enter the market and compete to enroll beneficiaries. The requests for proposals and the proposals themselves have to be explicitly customized to reflect the Medicaid benefit packages, its specific regulations and requirements, the role of traditional Medicaid providers in health plan networks, and appropriate sensitivity to serving the populations covered by the program.

It is during this phase that state Medicaid officials must decide if they will consider contract-

ing with organizations that are not licensed as HMOs. If so, they may have to coordinate with other state agencies like health and insurance departments to determine what requirements will be in areas like risk reserves, market conduct, and network adequacy. Along these lines, some states have explored the option of contracting with provider-sponsored managed care entities as a means to protect traditional Medicaid and safety net providers. It also is used in states where there is concern that established HMOs may not enter or may not remain in the Medicaid market. The downside risk for this option lies in the potential for increasing enrollment of Medicaid beneficiaries in plans serving only Medicaid beneficiaries. This development signals one of the practical and philosophical crossroads that Medicaid is currently approaching: does it give up on the elusive goal of "mainstreaming" beneficiaries in commercial plans to ensure that some measure of capitated managed care will continue to be available.

Eligibility, Enrollment, and Choice

Irrespective of the model(s) developed, other major design questions have to be addressed: which populations will be covered; which services will be included or carved out; will enrollment be voluntary or mandatory or some combination of both; and which markets/regions of the state will be included or excluded. Most states have made substantial progress toward enrolling most low-income women and children in managed care arrangements. But only a few states have attempted to reach the institutionalized population. Relatively few states enroll persons with disabilities and chronic illnesses in HMOs on a mandatory basis. Resistance to managed care arrangements remains strong among these beneficiaries, their advocates, and their traditional providers, and most states have exercised considerable caution with these populations. There are also important technical problems to be overcome including developing purchasing specifications for the special needs that many of these individuals have, risk adjustment methods for rates, and performance indicators that can be used to evaluate how well these persons are being served. Once again, it is worth noting that most private sector buyers have not had to tackle these issues. Medicaid purchasers have had to be pioneers in these areas and are breaking new ground that will ultimately benefit both private and other public purchasers, including Medicare, when they attempt to design and implement managed care approaches for persons with disabilities and chronic illnesses.

Another realm where Medicaid agencies have developed expertise is in the use of independent enrollment brokers or benefits counselors to engineer the selection of plans by beneficiaries and to execute auto-assignment for persons who fail to exercise choice. This development reflects the convergence of several trends. Medicaid agencies have at times had negative experiences with some health plans engaging in dishonest or overly aggressive direct marketing practices, often aimed at trying to promote favorable selection of less costly beneficiaries.[18] In addition, rapid expansion of enrollment in managed care taxes the resources of Medicaid agencies to provide sufficient information to support informed choice. Finally, there has been long-standing concern about how well HMOs can communicate with beneficiaries who have little exposure to managed care and who may have additional educational, linguistic, and/or cultural barriers to overcome.

At present, more than half the states contract with an outside organization to provide information to beneficiaries about their managed care options, respond to their questions and concerns about choice making, and complete the enrollment process with a plan.[19] States have limited direct marketing by plans and have funneled most plan information sharing through the enrollment broker. Marketing abuses have been dramatically reduced by this strategy, although questions remain about how well brokers may be educating beneficiaries about their options and how to negotiate the complex world of managed care. Brokers may also play a major role in assigning to a plan those persons who fail to make a choice of a managed care plan or PCCM. This auto-assignment process is carried out in various ways across the country,[20] ranging from matching with providers and plans on the basis of prior service use to pure random assignment among participating plans. Some states even use allocation of auto-assignees as a means to reward plans that have received high scores in the bidding process or that are sponsored by or include safety net providers as a way to increase membership for these particular plans.

Buying Value—It's All in the Contract

The complexity of the Medicaid program and its operating environment means that state purchasers are not able to buy the same generic managed care products that employer benefit managers may be purchasing. When enrollment was voluntary and beneficiaries could opt into HMOs or revert to traditional fee-for-service Medicaid on demand, the customization of managed care carried less import. But in recent years, the role of the contract has grown and become a major focus for Medicaid managers and health plans. Rosenbaum contends that managed care is in fact a cascade of contracts through which an entire delivery system is crafted and thus attention to the contract is essential.[21] Moreover, because the relationship of beneficiaries to the Medicaid program is a more dependent one than in the private sector, purchasing for them carries added responsibilities that must be expressed explicitly in contract terms.

A number of examples can illustrate the significance of contractual terms. Although a private purchaser may rely on HMO licensure and perhaps accreditation as indications of network adequacy, Medicaid programs commonly go much further. They may specify types of providers who must be incorporated (e.g., federally qualified health centers), the capacity of providers who are in the network (e.g., ratio of members to primary care physicians), and access standards like travel time (primary care physicians must be within 30 minutes of all members). For special need groups, additional requirements may be included to ensure that an HMO has a more comprehensive network than what would normally be the case; or that members may be able to nominate current providers of care to be incorporated in the network; or that disease specialists may qualify to be primary care case managers for persons with chronic conditions. In a relatively new trend responsive to the diversity of the Medicaid population, health plans are also being required to demonstrate cultural and linguistic competency to gain or retain contracts.[22]

The expansiveness and specificity of these contracts is not without its critics—especially among commercial HMOs—who note that these demands widen the gap between what they do for their commercial accounts and what Medicaid is requiring. The failure to conform Medicaid requirements to private sector requirements means added systems and costs for plans. For some, this is one reason why they either avoid Medicaid or have chosen to exit from the Medicaid market. Many plans simply believe Medicaid is not prepared to pay for all that it demands in terms of services and administrative requirements. Some beneficiary advocates also worry that this forced customization for Medicaid may further contribute to crystallizing a two-tiered system of managed care. As discussed in the section on future challenges, alignment of expectations and payments is an elusive goal that will have to be reached to achieve a viable Medicaid managed care market.

Compensation and Rates

Medicaid's tradition of being a meager fee-for-service payer for most services has affected its managed care experience in a number of ways. For states with PCCM programs, the case management fee paid to providers has been seen as an overdue fee increase and has assisted in promoting provider participation. For states with HMO programs, the setting of capitation rates has often been contentious. Rates may be set in a variety of ways in the pursuit of actuarial soundness, which is federally required but difficult to define. However, rates cannot exceed the fee-for-service equivalent payments that would have been made for the enrolled beneficiaries. This program requirement is called the "upper payment limit" (UPL) and essentially ensures that HMOs will be paid something less than the UPL for states to both meet the administrative costs of

a managed care program and garner some level of savings. How much less normally depends on how aggressively states wish to pursue savings by means of rate setting.

The adequacy of rates has been one of the major battlegrounds around Medicaid managed care and perhaps the most visible reason why some plans refuse to participate or have discontinued participation. Some simply believe they cannot deliver the kind of product that purchasers are requesting for the rates Medicaid is paying. These plans contend that they are unable to offer adequate compensation to attract desired providers and to promote effective incentives. They argue that Medicaid has been able to achieve below-market fee-for-service rates because of its public program status and its largely captive high-volume Medicaid provider base. Consequently, health plans cannot obtain savings in negotiations with providers but may in fact have to pay them *more* than what Medicaid was paying to get them to participate in a network. Rate adequacy and rate adjustments for high-cost, special-need beneficiaries have proven to be a complex problem. This concern rarely surfaced with private group accounts because of their small numbers of seriously ill and extraordinarily costly beneficiaries. But Medicaid managed care may bring major clusters of these individuals to a health plan. There may be great heterogeneity in costs among these individuals, and rates that are simply adjusted by age, gender, and eligibility category fail to reflect their actual cost of care. Faced with lack of risk adjustment in rates, plans may resort to avoiding enrolling persons with above average costs such as shunning providers who may have disproportionate numbers of such patients. Various administrative remedies may be needed to compensate for imprecision in rates. Fortunately, new techniques of risk adjustment are emerging in Medicaid managed care, and several states such as Colorado, Maryland, and Oregon are working to apply and refine them.[23]

Quality Monitoring and Oversight

The test of buying value is whether a purchaser can establish that outcomes have improved, or at least not declined, while costs are being controlled or reduced. The need to know about outcomes in a managed care environment has focused attention on performance monitoring and has launched a whole industry of organizations that measure outcomes and the capacity of organizations to improve outcomes. Private purchasers have promoted accreditation agencies, most notably the National Commission on Quality Assurance (NCQA), and detailed sets of performance indicators, in particular the Health Plan Employer Data Information Set (HEDIS), to contribute to these efforts. Medicaid agencies were late comers to some of these efforts but have now become integral participants in HEDIS indicator development, advancing the adoption of a number of Medicaid-pertinent indicators in HEDIS. A number of states now require reporting of HEDIS indicators on a regular basis by their MCO contractors.[24]

Medicaid has also been a participant in efforts to develop standardized measures of consumer satisfaction in the Consumer Assessment of Health Plan Surveys (CAHPS) initiative that has been mounted by the federal government.[25] The aim of CAHPS is to develop a set of satisfaction surveys built off a core of standardized items and supplemented by additional targeted elements that make the surveys both adaptable to different subpopulations and suitable for making cross-group comparisons. Special Medicaid modules have been developed that accommodate educational, linguistic, and cultural differences in this population. CAHPS is a good example of efforts to conform Medicaid requirements with those of the Medicare and commercial sectors, and it provides an opportunity to contrast the experience of Medicaid beneficiaries with private sector enrollees in managed care plans.

There is a more mixed picture of Medicaid agency support for private accreditation. In part, states have moved ahead with their own initiatives to promote quality assurance and development of quality assurance infrastructures. This has been most notable in the PCCM programs with the Quality Assurance Reform Initiative (QARI). In the case of HMOs, some states have developed detailed requirements that parallel private accreditation standards, and a new set of quality improvement standards and requirements is being proposed by the Health Care Financing Administration for health plans serving both Medicare and Medicaid members. Some critics have challenged the development and enforcement of separate quality standards for public sector beneficiaries. They argue that Medicaid should consider treating private accreditation as a surrogate for meeting public sector requirements (called "deemed status"), as is done when states accept Joint Commission on Accreditation of Health Care Organizations accreditation in lieu of state licensing inspections. Many Medicaid officials and advocates counter that the special needs of Medicaid beneficiaries demand customization of standards and performance monitoring.

SUCCESSES OF MEDICAID MANAGED CARE

With more than 15 years of experience with Medicaid managed care, it is becoming easier to assess its positive and negative impacts. The picture is a mixed one, both owing to extraordinary state variation and also to continuing program evolution. Successes are described in six areas that reflect aims for these initiatives: access, cost, quality/outcomes, consumer responsiveness, accountability, and devolution or changes in state-federal relations.

Access

Medicaid managed care has clearly succeeded in securing a medical home for its beneficiaries. Even the most modest PCCM programs provide a contractually obligated source of continuing care that is to be available 24 hours per day and 7 days a week. Most states audit this availability, and evaluations have generally found that improved use of primary care is a direct consequence of such arrangements.[26] This access reduces reliance on sites of episodic care like emergency departments. It has also contributed to continuity of care for managed care enrollees, although this pattern is more difficult to measure. There have been gains in access to prenatal care in some states because of managed care enrollment, and some other states can demonstrate that immunization levels and child health screening rates have improved through managed care.[27, 28]

Medicaid managed care has not only increased access to services, it has also broadened access to coverage itself. A number of states that obtained waivers in the early 1990s used the argument that savings gained through managed care could be used to offset, in part, expansions in eligibility. This seems to have been the case in states like Tennessee, Oregon, Hawaii, and others that expanded coverage and used managed care models to deliver services to newly covered persons.

Demonstrating that use of services has been increased has been hampered by data collection and reporting problems. Many states have not been able to collect reliable data or to develop good indicators of use of services for members enrolling in HMOs. The growing use of HEDIS measures should address these concerns. Adapting indicators like HEDIS that are in widespread use in the private sector will also enable states to address questions of how access to specific services for Medicaid members compares with persons with commercial coverage.

Cost

Although early managed care programs in Medicaid were more likely to stress improved predictability in costs than actual cost savings, evidence over time suggested that modest savings over fee-for-service Medicaid were possible for persons enrolled in managed care arrangements. A review of 25 programs conducted in 1991 indicated savings of 5 to 15 percent for the AFDC population, with some states claiming even more substantial savings.[29] These higher claims may have induced other states to set higher expectations for savings when they began to convert existing beneficiaries to managed care models. Several states attempted to guarantee savings by paying capitation rates that were substantially below fee-for-service equivalents. These states shifted the risk to HMOs, which in turn sought to obtain reduced provider payment and utilization rates that fit within the discounted capitation rates. This has set some states on a collision course with their health plan contractors, which is now being manifested in loss of plans and threats to the fundamental viability of prepaid programs.

The improved predictability of payments did provide some relief to states who saw Medicaid expenditures soar after mandated expansions in eligibility started in 1989. States like Arizona that had mandatory enrollment of all beneficiaries in HMOs could modulate expenditure increases by controlling the rate of increases in capitation payments, an opportunity not available to states with PCCM or voluntary HMO enrollment. However, because most enrollment has been centered on the AFDC (later called Temporary Assistance to Needy Families or TANF) population, the potential for overall savings is limited. The beneficiaries who represent nearly 70 percent of the Medicaid budget remain largely unaffected by managed care.[30] It is still unclear what the impact of formal managed care programs will be on these special need populations because there have been very few studies—other than in Arizona—that have demonstrated that substantial savings can be achieved. In fact, proponents argue that the real value of managed care for these population is not so much in potential savings but rather that capitation can liberate providers to deliver a different mix of services to achieve better outcomes at no additional costs.

Quality/Outcomes

One of the most appealing aspects of managed care for Medicaid beneficiaries, as it is for private managed care plan members, is that it becomes possible to organize the care and measure the experience of persons who are *enrolled* in a way not possible in fee-for-service medicine. In the latter system, care is, at best, benignly distributed among a variety of providers or, at worst, rendered in a fragmented or duplicative manner. For many years Medicaid managed care initiatives have been promoted on this basis. States that have made the investment in data collection, analysis, and reporting can now generate performance measures to support this contention. But evidence of the impact of Medicaid managed care on quality has progressed more slowly than in the private sector or the Medicare program. When programs cannot produce this kind of evidence, they cannot support claims that value is being improved, and the promise of improved performance measurement wears thin on both skeptics and supporters alike. Such evidence is especially critical to address concerns among higher need beneficiaries with chronic illnesses and disabilities, who need proof of potential gains to counteract the lurking suspicion about the incentives to skimp or stint on services in prepaid health care.

The previously described enhancements to HEDIS represent a renewed promise that measures will emerge that are reliable, timely, and actionable. Certainly, such measures will far exceed anything done in the fee-for-service Medicaid world. In addition, some states, such as Massachusetts, have taken on a more interactive role with their health plan contractors to develop plan-specific quality improvement targets and reflect improvements in performance in rate negotiations. This pay-for-performance corresponds to what is arising among some of the more sophisticated and aggressive private employers and business coalitions, although they too are plagued with measurement and data collection problems and often seem more focused on administrative performance in areas like timeliness of provider payment and customer service. There may be a more compelling reason why performance measurement must continue to improve in Medicaid managed care: to persuade state agencies to pay plans adequately. As the ability to rely on historical fee-for-service data to benchmark payment rates fades away, states will have to find new means to ascertain whether they are, in fact, getting what they pay for. Meaningful plan performance indicators will be critical to make these assessments.

Consumer Satisfaction and Responsiveness

Medicaid agencies have rarely been noted for their consumer responsiveness. Converting to a managed care mode of thinking and operating has forced many agencies to examine the Medicaid experience more through the eyes of their beneficiaries than they have in the past. They have had to do this to prepare these populations for a new experience and to assess which features of managed care will be the most unfamiliar and challenging for them to negotiate and what will be most attractive to them. This may seem paternalistic but, unlike in the private sector where employees typically have options and financial resources to allow them to exercise choice or to go "out-of-network" when they wish to, the impact of mandatory enrollment programs in Medicaid is far more momentous. There have been instances of exploitation of beneficiaries in managed care situations dating back to the California scandals of the early 1970s and continuing through to the mid-1990s in states like Florida.[30]

Satisfaction with managed care has tended to be high in the many states that have been monitoring it, although such high levels are typically observed in most medical care satisfaction surveys. Acquiring a bona fide medical home has been a valued experience and for some the opportunity to go *where they want to go* rather *where they have to go* has been welcomed. When states have implemented programs precipitously, confusion has ensued and beneficiaries may have experienced disruptions in continuity and resultant anxiety. Some features of managed care like gatekeeper authorizations of specialty referrals or emergency department visits have grated on beneficiaries, just as they have on private sector managed care enrollees. Restricted panels of providers seem to have been less of a problem because most Medicaid beneficiaries have already experienced restricted access. They are more likely to be troubled by reconfiguration of networks that again may be confusing or disruptive. Plan departures from the Medicaid market represent an extreme case of this dislocation.

Use of enrollment brokers to support plan selection has succeeded in addressing concerns about exploitation and offering balanced, useful information. States are focusing now on both auto-assignment rates and disenrollment rates to appraise how well these brokers are performing and how well beneficiaries are navigating the choice process.[31] Advocates and providers complain that they must provide a substantial amount of remedial assistance to explain to beneficiaries their rights and responsibilities in managed care arrangements. All these experiences resonate with those of private benefits managers who struggle to ensure that employees have the necessary information and guidance to make informed choices.

Accountability

The view of many Medicaid agency executives toward managed care is captured well by the observation of Bruce Bullen, former Massachusetts Medicaid Director and past Chair of the National Association of State Medicaid Directors. From his vantage point, the greatest contribution of managed care is that the contract with the plan gives Medicaid directors an entity that can be held accountable for the well-being of beneficiaries. This was never possible in the fee-for-service world, in which responsibility for care was diluted and diffuse and payers had little or no leverage to extract preferred performance. This view also underscores why the contract and the detailed language of the contract has moved to center stage in Medicaid managed care—it represents the clearest specification of what the agency is buying and how it is to be delivered.

This perspective also illustrates how contracting with prepaid health plans offers advantages over operating PCCM programs, where the delivery system remains largely unbundled, and the role of PCCM as care coordinator is not sufficient to assign full responsibility. However, the single point of accountability argument also represents one of the reasons that some plans are reluctant to participate in Medicaid. They fear that they will be held responsible for things beyond their control such as behaviors or life circumstances of their members, performance of providers they are required to include because of state mandates, or unreasonable performance targets that were never even approached in the fee-for-service environment. They view this

"laying it on the plans" philosophy as misguided or disingenuous or both.

Devolution

Assessing the achievements of Medicaid managed care would not be complete without acknowledging that for many states their forays into managed care reflect notable efforts to innovate and to improve health care delivery to low-income citizens. Although states have portrayed obtaining federal permission through waivers as irksome and frustrating, Medicaid managed care has been one arena in which the sought-after devolution of authority from federal to state governments is being achieved.[32] Many states have availed themselves of Section 1115 waivers to completely transform their Medicaid programs and to adopt managed care models that previously only one state, Arizona, had achieved in the first 25 years of the program. How successful and desirable the shifting of control to states has been depends on one's point of view. State legislators and policy makers tend to rate their success highly, expressing frustration that devolution is still too slow and too reluctantly accepted by federal officials. Critics, including advocates representing many of the other constituencies of Medicaid, point out that the decentralization of Medicaid may undermine beneficiary protections, program uniformity, and its overall equity.

SHORTFALLS OF MEDICAID MANAGED CARE

A balanced scorecard requires attention to areas where Medicaid managed care has failed to deliver or stumbled in its efforts to improve value. As with its successes, conclusions must be qualified by recognizing that there are more than 50 Medicaid agencies in the states and territories, and that their experiences have been varied. Problems in initial development may give way to solid performance after a program matures. Well-established programs may be destabilized by changes in the Medicaid or broader managed care environment that can lead to the loss of key contractors.

Lack of Data/Evidence of Impact

The relatively modest savings and the scarcity of data on outcomes contrasts with the enthusiasm shown for Medicaid managed care as measured by its sevenfold to eightfold growth in the past decade. Clearly, many state policy makers have embraced Medicaid managed care as an act of faith in lieu of more convincing evidence. This is not entirely different from what private employee benefits managers have done—although it can be argued that the latter have, in fact, been better able to document real reductions in rates of premium increases. Medicaid executives generally have not had such persuasive evidence. Savings may not be carefully calculated, data may not be reliable, or voluntary enrollment programs may experience selection bias.

Evidence on outcomes is even more difficult to come by because of data collection, reporting, and measurement problems. Few states have invested the resources needed for rigorous program evaluations to be completed, so findings tend to be fragmentary or anecdotal. In addition, the episodic eligibility for Medicaid creates problems in calculating rates of service use, as well as frustrating the ability of managed care organizations to have a significant impact on the well-being of members. Virtually no state has succeeded in getting reliable encounter level data from plans necessary to gain a full picture of program effects. Nor are federal requirements on data submission by states detailed enough to force states to produce information comparable to that in fee-for-service programs. So despite the fact that managed care carries with it the promise of improved measurement, monitoring, and accountability, most state agencies are still not able to use data from the managed care experience to fully compare it with fee-for-service experience. Consequently, even if they are achieving cost savings, they are simply unable to prove that they are buying a product that is as good as or superior to fee-for-service Medicaid.

Administrative Capacity and Performance

It has taken time for state Medicaid officials to grow into the new role of prudent, "value-based" purchaser. The role requires new attitudes, personnel, skill sets, and infrastructure to achieve success. Marshaling these resources has not been easy in a period of retrenchment in state government. When many managed care programs were started, they were directed by small compartmentalized units scrambling to build a PCCM network or crafting the state's initial managed care contracts and capitation rates. In time, however, managed care has emerged from its experimental, alternative status to be the mainstream delivery system in state Medicaid programs. Few states have retooled to accommodate these changes and most have struggled to recruit, retain, or replace key staff members, many of whom found attractive opportunities in the booming managed care industry.

Even if the technical challenges of program design and development can be met with internal or external resources, the effort to mount massive planning and implementation initiatives, often on compressed timetables in a politically charged environment, has required near heroic efforts. Few, if any, private employee benefits managers have attempted projects of this scale within these time frames. The fact that confusion has characterized many of these efforts, or that they almost always take much longer to achieve than projected, is often more a testament to the frenzied context within which they are implemented than to the skills or commitment of the staff engineering them.

Adversarial Contracting Environment

New problems have arisen in the recent years in terms of increasing tensions between state Medicaid purchasers and plans. This has contributed to increasing numbers of plan withdrawals from the Medicaid market, reversing the trend of rapid growth in new entrants.[35] As shown in Table 57–1, the number of plans with predominantly commercial membership (as opposed to predominantly Medicaid membership) has declined sharply over the past two years and the percentage of enrollees in commercial plans is declining. Some of these tensions may be attributable to the downturn in the overall finan-

Table 57–1 Commercial Plans in Medicaid Managed Care, 1994–1998

	1994	1995	1996	1997	1998
Participating plans					
Number of commercial plans	101	124	153	145	126
Pct of participating plans exiting	8	8	7	18	15
Pct change in net participating plans	31	23	23	−5	−13
Enrollees					
Enrollees served by commercial plan (000s)	2,293	3,201	3,982	4,742	4,648
Pct of Medicaid enrollees served by commercial plans	62	62	66	64	60

States: AZ, CA, CT, FL, IL, MI, MO, NJ, NY, OH, OR, PA, TN, WA, WI.

Source: This publication was reprinted with permission of the Henry J. Kaiser Family Foundation of Menlo Park, California. The Kaiser Family Foundation is an independent health care philanthropy and is not associated with Kaiser Permanente or Kaiser Industries.

cial performance of the managed care industry, leading some to question whether they want to continue to participate in a low or no-margin line of business like Medicaid. But some of the tension is attributed by plans to the attitudes and activities of state agencies that seem to be becoming more demanding and arbitrary in their relations with plans. In the minds of some plans, state officials simply do not understand how to develop and foster long-term business relationships. They do not recognize the plans as their partners, but simply as vendors selected by means of a procurement process.

Some states have sharply reduced capitation rates or set them without attention to their actuarial soundness. Others have instituted selection processes that have not been seen as fair because they include unqualified plans or are stretched to satisfy other agendas such as preservation of safety net providers. Some plans worry that competitive bidding or selection criteria may not weight the appropriate factors properly and may encourage new plans with limited market commitment to enter, take short-term gains, then depart. Other states have set limits on plan profitability or justified low rates on the basis of the unreasonable expectation that plans can and will cross-subsidize Medicaid losses with profits from other lines of business. All these concerns have found their way into the rationales for some plans choosing to exit the Medicaid market and raising longer term worries about what plans

will remain interested in sustained relationships with state Medicaid agencies.[34]

Serving Special Need Groups

The slow progress made in serving special need groups may be seen as both a shortfall or a success, depending on whether one believes these persons would or would not benefit from managed care. Generally speaking, slow implementation probably reflects lack of readiness on the parts of purchasers, plans, providers, and beneficiaries. It also indicates that in the absence of evidence as to how managed care can improve the care and well-being of persons with serious chronic illnesses or disabilities, it is difficult to build momentum toward implementation and enrollment. The evidence that coordinated care has real benefits or that capitation can liberate caregivers to provide services more flexibly and effectively is available for only relatively small samples of persons or narrowly defined populations.[35] Promising new disease management programs that may be especially well suited for beneficiaries with chronic conditions have only had limited use in Medicaid managed care to date.

The emergence of more robust models of care with more convincing indications of superior performance will take more time and innovation and a more hospitable climate in which such models could flourish. An adversarial relationship between state agencies and plans is a major impediment. Absence of well-proven risk adjustment schemes is another. Ambivalence about whether generic or special need plans are preferable and whether a competitive bid or limited franchise award approach is sensible are additional areas that will have to be resolved to make progress. Because a substantial number of these persons have dual eligibility for Medicaid and Medicare, the nearly insurmountable problems of coordinating these two programs will have to be tackled forthrightly.

THE CHALLENGING CONTEMPORARY CONTEXT

Medicaid managed care is reaching a crossroads because it has now become the dominant delivery model for low-income beneficiaries of the program. This is consistent with the status of the managed care marketplace as a whole. Managed care models have become the mainstream delivery systems and purchasers, providers, and consumers seem reconciled to the fact that there will not be a return to the days of unmanaged care. Both public and private sectors have experienced substantial relief from rampant health care inflation, and there is little generalizable evidence of reduced quality of services. Nonetheless, a number of concerns with the managed care experience cannot be ignored. Premiums are beginning to rise more quickly. Provider and, perhaps to a lesser extent, consumer disgruntlement has become more vocal and policy makers have responded by layering on new mandates and strictures. The health plan industry has experienced a reversal of fortune and reports of consolidation, market withdrawals, and failures are becoming more commonplace.

Medicaid managed care, especially its prepaid models, has been more fragile and less firmly entrenched than commercial managed care and seems to be experiencing some of the current market turbulence more intensely. Many states have seen plans withdraw from participation in the past two years for the reasons described earlier. In some instances, withdrawals have stymied state plans to further expand managed care, and in other cases they have threatened the

sustainability of mandatory HMO enrollment programs because of the requirement of a minimum of two competing plans in an area. In other states, plans have struggled with a hostile contracting environment or engaged in acrimonious public disputes with policy makers over rate adequacy. The fact that plans may ultimately prevail to some degree in these disputes, such as they have in New York and Pennsylvania, does not alter the impression that the pain of being in the Medicaid line of business may not exceed the possible gain for health plans.

It is far from clear whether some states will be able to sustain markets with several competing plans or whether they will have to move, by default or by design, to more orchestrated arrangements with a limited number of awards to selected plans. Recent research underscores the enormous variability in rates, with some states paying twice as much as others for a similar benefit package to similar beneficiary groups.[36] Rates alone are not the sole determinant of the viability of a market. Other facets of the contracting environment play roles in making participation attractive and sustainable for plans, and states may find that they will have to devote more attention to these other mechanisms. Setting suitable rates is likely to become more challenging as the fee-for-service base disappears and states continue to struggle with getting good information on what they are buying in terms of outputs and outcomes.

Two responses by states to these market developments are notable. Some states are revising plans to phase out PCCM programs and others are bolstering these programs. This strategy can be a hedge against the loss of plans or the possibility that the number of plans would shrink to a point where Medicaid programs are disadvantaged in their negotiations with the plans. The PCCM program also retains appeal for rural areas where prepaid managed care simply has not flourished, and few states see Medicaid as strong enough to overcome resistance in such areas. The flexibility of a fee-for-service PCCM program allows it to be adapted to serve special need populations with some modest improvements in care coordination while avoiding the operational and financial difficulties associated with enrolling these beneficiaries in prepaid health plans.

Another response of state agencies has been to broaden the range of entities that qualify for contracts or to provide transitional time for provider organizations to develop managed care capacity. Both of these developments are consonant with changes occurring in the Medicare markets with provider-sponsored organizations and in the private market with some employers or groups of employers contracting directly with provider groups. Adopting these models in Medicaid programs may have an additional benefit: a means to offer traditional providers of care for Medicaid and the uninsured an opportunity to sustain revenue flows and market share. Safety net providers have warned that aggressive, self-interested buying by managed care runs the risk of having an adverse impact on those organizations that have relied on cost-shifting to finance some of their commitment to the uninsured. They suggest that because of their "open door" status, their patients continue to seek care from them whether the patient retains Medicaid eligibility or not. Critics of this strategy express concern that these entities will likely remain Medicaid-only plans and that their reliance on this single (and low paying) revenue stream will make them vulnerable managed care enterprises.[37]

In addition to turbulence in the managed care world, Medicaid purchasers face uncertainty in the policy realm as well. Both state and national initiatives in welfare reform are changing the size, composition, and possibly the average per person cost of the population enrolled in Medicaid. Despite the fact that Medicaid eligibility and public assistance eligibility are no longer linked, many persons who could continue to qualify for Medicaid are allowing their coverage to lapse when their welfare benefits are terminated. It is possible that those leaving the Medicaid rolls for employment may be in better health than those remaining. If this residual population is more costly, capitation rates will have to be adjusted accordingly.

States are also in the midst of implementing diverse Children's Health Insurance Programs. Although many approaches are extensions of Medicaid, determining how to integrate these programs with existing Medicaid managed care arrangements is a challenge to states across the country. Finally, the Balanced Budget Act of 1997 introduced some of the most sweeping changes in Medicaid policies in more than a decade, many of which target managed care. Some reduce waiver requirements for states, but others raise the bar in terms of oversight for both states and health plans. It will be a number of years before the consequences of these changes can be fully appreciated.

LONGER TERM QUESTIONS AND CONCERNS

We close this overview of Medicaid managed care by posing five questions that are not only rhetorical but also essential to one's consideration of the future of Medicaid managed care.

1. How can public policy makers reconcile their ambiguous roles and ambivalent attitudes as both buyers and regulators of managed care organizations?

Walking the talk of prudent, value-based purchasing is more difficult in the public sector than it is for private employee benefits managers because of the multiple, and sometimes conflicting, roles of public agencies. In some respects, this is even more apparent for the Medicare program than Medicaid. On the one hand, Congress criticizes, castigates, and regulates managed care organizations for their shortfalls, while attempting to promote expanded managed care for beneficiaries through Medicare + Choice. Medicaid agencies are in a similar situation given the fact that many program managers express ambivalence about the motives and methods used by managed care organizations and the impact that managed care–related cost savings may have on certain hard-pressed providers. Medicaid purchasers are also subjected to pressures from state legislators, sister state agencies, local governments, provider associations, and consumer advocates, as well as various federal oversight agencies—all expressing varying preferences and concerns about managed care. There is little relief in sight to this conundrum, but it is possible that more and better information on program impacts could assist state policy makers to feel more convinced that their managed care strategies are worth the investment.

2. Can Medicaid agencies align their expectations for real management of care with their ability to pay plans accordingly?

The short answer to this question may simply be that they will have to. The propensity to see managed care as a panacea or a kind of Christmas tree on which to load many ornaments is disconcerting to health plans. They and other observers believe this reflects a misguided belief that plans have the capacity and responsibility to solve many problems that have been endemic to Medicaid for many years—some that public officials may be unwilling to resolve themselves for fear of the political consequences. Some even think that burdening plans with unreasonable expectations is a sinister effort by managed care critics to undermine plan credibility and demonstrate that managed care is a misbegotten strategy. But the fact remains that if plans do not believe they are paid adequately to perform what they can reasonably be expected to accomplish, then those that can leave Medicaid will do so. States will be left in the dangerous position of contracting only with plans that cannot afford to leave: plans that are completely Medicaid-dependent or built around providers who rely heavily on Medicaid patients and revenues. There are serious doubts about whether these types of plans have the infrastructure necessary for the authentic management of care that Medicaid purchasers are seeking.

3. Will Medicaid agencies succeed in developing sustainable relationships with high-quality managed care plans?

Several states like Arizona, California, Massachusetts, Missouri, Pennsylvania, Wisconsin, and others have longstanding HMO contracting relationships with health plans in some or all parts of the state. These include plans that are serving predominantly commercial members and some with predominantly or exclusively Medicaid memberships. They have weathered marketplace changes, contract renewals, rate adjustments, and changes in the types of beneficiaries being enrolled. Some of these states do as well or better than private employers in terms of supporting plan choice for beneficiaries and extracting performance data and improvement

strategies from their health plan contractors. But the picture is an uneven one across the country, as evidenced by the fact that some large multimarket HMO companies are entering some states for the first time while exiting others that have proven to be poor or unpromising opportunities. More work is needed to understand the full range of factors that contribute to state success so that these positive experiences can be converted into clear prescriptions for improvement that can be shared across the country.

4. How will Medicaid managed care mesh the competing aims of mainstreaming beneficiaries while maintaining safety net providers?

This question will continue to bedevil Medicaid managed care as long as Medicaid programs carry responsibilities beyond simply getting the best value for the persons they are currently covering. No issue sets Medicaid managed care managers further apart from their private sector counterparts who have license to single-mindedly do the best they can for their own people. And this concern certainly works at cross-purposes with the mainstreaming goal that Medicaid has pursued for more than three decades because, in many instances, Medicaid beneficiaries are the conduits through which dollars are being funneled to safety net providers to allow them to serve the uninsured. The new wave of Children's Health Insurance Programs takes states a step closer to paying for care for all low-income persons by means of an insurance model. Unless safety net–based health plans become stronger, more diversified entities, many Medicaid agencies will continue to shape and, at times, distort their Medicaid managed care initiatives to preserve and protect those providers most jeopardized by managed care.

5. Will state Medicaid agencies reach a point at which they can evaluate whether they are getting value for the rates they are paying for their beneficiaries?

Evidence of savings alone is not proof that value has been increased. Only a few states have already reached the point in their appraisals of their managed care strategies where they know how managed care has affected both costs and outcomes. The fact that some states are paying more than twice as much as other states for comparable services for similar beneficiaries[38] suggests much more must be done to try to understand what Medicaid agencies are buying. Consider the response of a Medicaid director who was asked how he explained to his legislature the fact that his state's rates to HMO were among the highest in the country. He replied by saying that when he looked at the HEDIS indicators provided to him by his contracting plans and compared them with commercial member experience, he believed he was getting what he was paying for. It is likely that not all states are getting what they are paying for, but until they have the information necessary to make this appraisal, they will be engaged in an elusive pursuit of value.

CONCLUSION

Like the broader Medicaid program in which Medicaid managed care initiatives are nested, the current picture is one of successes and failures; high hopes and undelivered promises; genuine progress and real disappointments in terms of inequities and the pace of improvement. The fact that some states have registered notable accomplishments in terms of cost containment and improved outcomes bolsters hopes that managed care can succeed in remaking Medicaid into a more clearly successful program. But there are several current uncertainties in the managed care realm and in the policy environment that cast shadows over some of the enthusiasm. The jury is still out on how to surmount serious threats like rate adequacy, performance measurement, and extension of managed care to special need populations. The one fact that most observers seem to agree on is that irrespective of the future shape of managed care in Medicaid, there will be no return to the not-so-felicitous days of fee-for-service.

REFERENCES

1. R. Stevens and R. Stevens, *Welfare Medicine in America* (New York: Free Press, 1974).

2. J. Iglehart, The American Health Care System—Medicaid, *New England Journal of Medicine* 340 (1999): 5, 403–408.

3. Stevens and Stevens, *Welfare Medicine in America.*

4. Stevens and Stevens, *Welfare Medicine in America.*

5. Iglehart, The American Health Care System—Medicaid.

6. Iglehart, The American Health Care System—Medicaid.

7. J. Holahan, T. Coughlin, L. Ku, D. Lipson, and S. Rajan, Insuring the Poor Through Section 1115 Waivers, *Health Affairs* 14 (1995): 1, 199–216.

8. R. Hurley, D. Freund, and J. Paul, *Managed Care in Medicaid* (Ann Arbor, MI: Health Administration Press, 1993).

9. Hurley, Freund, Paul, *Managed Care in Medicaid.*

10. D. Freund, *Medicaid Reform: Four Studies of Case Management* (Washington, DC: American Enterprise Institute, 1984).

11. National Academy for State Health Policy, *Medicaid Managed Care: A Guide for States,* 4th ed. (Portland, ME: NASHP, 1999).

12. Hurley, Freund, Paul, *Managed Care in Medicaid.*

13. N. McCall, Lesson From Arizona's Medicaid Managed Care Program, *Health Affairs* 16 (1997): 4, 194–199.

14. Hurley, Freund, Paul, *Managed Care in Medicaid.*

15. National Academy for State Health Policy, *Medicaid Managed Care: A Guide for States,* 4th ed. (Portland, ME, 1999).

16. R. Hurley and S. Wallin, Adopting and Adapting Managed Care for Medicaid Beneficiaries: An Imperfect Translation, *New Federalism: Issues and Options for States, Series A, no. A-7* (Washington, DC: Urban Institute, 1998).

17. Hurley and Wallin, Adopting and Adapting Managed Care for Medicaid Beneficiaries: An Imperfect Translation.

18. Hurley and Wallin, Adopting and Adapting Managed Care for Medicaid Beneficiaries: An Imperfect Translation.

19. M. Kenesson, *Medicaid Managed Care Enrollment Study Report of Findings from the Survey of State Medicaid Managed Care Programs* (Princeton, NJ: Center for Health Care Strategies, Inc., 1997).

20. K. Maloy, S. Rosenbaum, C. DeGraw, C. Sonosky, and J. Teitelbaum, *The Role of Auto-Enrollment in Mandatory Medicaid Managed Care* (Princeton, NJ: Center for Health Care Strategies, Inc., 1999).

21. S. Rosenbaum, et al., *Negotiating the New Health Care System: An Analysis of Contracts Between State Medicaid Agencies and Managed Care Organizations* (Washington, DC: The George Washington University Medical Center—Center for Health Policy Research, 1997).

22. National Academy for State Health Policy, *Medicaid Managed Care: A Guide for States*, 4th ed.

23. R. Kronick and T. Dreyfus, *The Challenge of Risk Adjustment for People with Disabilities: Health-Based Payment for Medicaid Programs, A Guide for State Medicaid Programs, Providers, and Consumers* (Princeton, NJ: Center for Health Care Strategies, Inc., 1997).

24. National Academy for State Health Policy, *Medicaid Managed Care: A Guide for States,* 4th ed.

25. A. Epstein, Performance Reports on Quality—Prototypes, Problems, and Prospects, *New England Journal of Medicine,* 329 (1995): 57–61.

26. Hurley, Freund, Paul, *Managed Care in Medicaid.*

27. J. Griffin, J. Hogan, J. Buechner, and T. Leddy, The Effect of a Medicaid Managed Care Program on the Adequacy of Prenatal Care Utilization in Rhode Island, *American Journal of Public Health*, 89 (1999): 4, 497–501.

28. K. Piper and P. Bartels, Medicaid Primary Care: HMOs or Fee-for-Service, *Public Welfare*, Spring (1995): 18–21.

29. Iglehart, The American Health Care System—Medicaid.

30. Hurley and Wallin, Adopting and Adapting Managed Care for Medicaid Beneficiaries: An Imperfect Translation.

31. Maloy, Rosenbaum, DeGraw, Sonosky, and Teitelbaum, *The Role of Auto-Enrollment in Mandatory Medicaid Managed Care.*

32. J. Holahan, S. Zuckerman, A. Evans, and S. Rangarajan, Medicaid Managed Care in Thirteen States, *Health Affairs* 17 (1998): 1, 43–63.

33. S. Felt-Lisk, *The Changing Medicaid Managed Care Market: Trends in Commercial Plans' Participation* (Washington: Kaiser Commission on Medicaid and the Uninsured, 1999).

34. M. McCue, R. Hurley, D. Draper, and M. Jurgensen, Reversal of Fortune: Commercial HMOs in the Medicaid Market, *Health Affairs* 18 (1999): 1, 223–230.

35. R. Hurley and D. Draper, "Special Plans for Special Persons: The Elusive Pursuit of Customized Managed Care," in *Remaking Medicaid: Managed Care and the Public Good*, eds. S. Davidson and S. Somers (San Francisco: Jossey-Bass Publishers, 1998).

36. J. Holahan, S. Rangarajan, and M. Schirmer, Medicaid Managed Care Rates in 1998, *Health Affairs* 18 (1999): 3, 217–227.

37. McCue, Hurley, Draper, and Jurgensen, Reversal of Fortune: Commercial HMOs in the Medicaid Market, 223–230.

38. Holahan, Rangarajan, and Schirmer, Medicaid Managed Care Rates in 1998, 217–227.

CHAPTER 58

CHAMPUS and the Department of Defense Managed Care Programs

Steve Lillie and Larry Sobel

The Military Health System (MHS) is a large and complex health care system designed to provide, and to maintain readiness to provide, medical services and support to the armed forces during military operations and to provide medical services and support to members of the armed forces, their dependents, and others entitled to Department of Defense (DOD) medical care. To accomplish these missions, the Army, Navy, and Air Force operate more than 500 medical and dental treatment facilities, including nearly 100 hospitals, located throughout the world. This "direct care system" is augmented by care purchased from civilian sources under the Civilian Health and Medical Program of the Uniformed Services (CHAMPUS). This chapter focuses on

Steve Lillie is Associate Director, Program Design and Innovation in the TRICARE Management Activity, Department of Defense. He has more than 20 years of experience in policy development and evaluation of federal health care programs in the Department of Health and Human Services and the Department of Defense.

Larry Sobel is Director, Special Programs and Demonstrations, TRICARE Management Activity, Department of Defense. He has more than 20 years of experience in managed health care in the Department of Health and Human Services and the Department of Defense. He holds a bachelor's degree from Harvard College and a doctoral degree in jurisprudence from Harvard Law School.

The views expressed within the chapter are those of the authors and not necessarily those of the Department of Defense.

the development of TRICARE, DOD's worldwide managed health care program. TRICARE was initiated in 1995, integrating health care services provided in the direct care system of military hospitals and clinics with services purchased under CHAMPUS.

The impetus for the transition to TRICARE came from several factors. As a result of Base Realignment and Closure actions, 35 percent of the DOD medical treatment facilities (MTFs) providing services in 1987 had been closed by the end of 1997. The beneficiary population shrank by less than 10 percent during this time. In addition, retirees and their family members made up an increasing proportion of the beneficiary population—growing from approximately 8 percent of beneficiaries in the 1950s to approximately 50 percent in the 1990s. The combination of general medical inflation and higher health care demand from this older population produced rising health care costs for DOD. The closure of military bases and their medical facilities required the department to initiate an intensive reengineering effort to design new ways to provide the military health care benefits.

The TRICARE managed health care system uses the existing military infrastructure as the basis for a managed care program modeled after civilian managed care standards and managed by the military in partnership with civilian contractors. This system provides comprehensive, cost-effective care to active-duty members, their families, and other eligible beneficiaries in all the uniformed services. The TRICARE system offers expanded access to care, a choice of health care options, consistent high-quality health care benefits, and reduced health care costs for beneficiaries and taxpayers alike. For each of 11 designated health service regions in the United States, as well as in Europe, the Pacific, and Latin America, a senior military health care officer, called the lead agent, is responsible for coordinating the delivery of all health care to eligible beneficiaries who live in that region. Day-to-day health care decision making is done by primary care managers, with oversight by local military medical treatment facility commanders.

LEGAL AUTHORITY AND RESPONSIBILITIES

Title 10, Chapter 55 of the U.S. Code authorizes the operation of the military health system and defines eligibility for care, covered services, cost sharing, and other program details. The Secretary of Defense, the Secretary of Health and Human Services, and the Secretary of Transportation jointly prescribe regulations (at 32 Code of Federal Regulations, Part 199) for the administration of TRICARE and CHAMPUS, the predecessor program. Title 10, Chapter 55 also authorizes the Secretary of Defense to administer TRICARE/CHAMPUS for the Army, Navy, Air Force, and Marine Corps under DOD jurisdiction; the Secretary of Transportation to administer TRICARE/CHAMPUS for the Coast Guard (when the Coast Guard is not operating as a service in the Navy); and the Secretary of Health and Human Services to administer TRICARE/CHAMPUS for the Commissioned Corps of the U.S. Public Health Service and the National Oceanic and Atmospheric Administration.

The Secretary of Defense has delegated authority to the Assistant Secretary of Defense (Health Affairs) to provide policy guidance, management control, and coordination for TRICARE and CHAMPUS. The Secretary of Health and Human Services has delegated authority to the Assistant Secretary for Health, Department of Health and Human Services to consult with the Secretary of Defense or a designee

and to approve and issue joint regulations implementing title 10, Chapter 55. The Secretary of Transportation has delegated authority to the Commandant of the U.S. Coast Guard to consult with the Secretary of Defense or a designee and to approve and issue joint regulations implementing title 10 U.S. Code, Chapter 55.

In 1998, the Secretary of Defense established the TRICARE Management Activity (TMA) as a DOD field activity. TMA works with the components of the military health system—military hospitals and clinics, health care managers in the Army, Navy, and Air Force, regional TRICARE lead agents, and regional at-risk TRICARE managed care support contractors—to operate the TRICARE program day to day. The Office of the Assistant Secretary of Defense (Health Affairs) provides policy guidance and direction for the operation of TRICARE.

THE MILITARY MEDICAL BENEFITS PROGRAM

Historically, military beneficiaries obtained health care services from military facilities, as space and capabilities were available, and from civilian sources, with government cost sharing of civilian care under CHAMPUS. CHAMPUS is a program of medical benefits provided by the U.S. government under provisions of title 10 U.S.C. sections 1079 and 1086. Specified categories of individuals qualify for these benefits by virtue of their relationship to one of the seven uniformed services (Army, Navy, Air Force, Marine Corps, Coast Guard, Commissioned Corps of the U.S. Public Health Service, and Commissioned Corps of the National Oceanic and Atmospheric Administration). In general, persons eligible for CHAMPUS benefits include families of active-duty service members; retired service members, their spouses, and their unmarried children; survivors of active duty or retired service members; and certain former spouses of members of the military. Active-duty members of the services are not covered by CHAMPUS, nor, in general, are retirees, survivors, or family members of a retiree if they are eligible for Medicare on the basis of age. Active-duty members are entitled to receive all care from military facilities; Medicare-eligible beneficiaries retain eligibility for space-available care in military facilities in addition to their Medicare benefits.

Although similar in structure to an insurance program in many respects, TRICARE/CHAMPUS is not an insurance program. That is, it does not involve a contract guaranteeing the indemnification of an insured party against a specified loss in return for a paid premium. Furthermore, TRICARE/CHAMPUS is not subject to state regulatory bodies or agencies that control the insurance industry generally. Instead, it is a program whereby the federal government provides or pays for certain medically or psychologically necessary services provided by an authorized health care professional to eligible beneficiaries. Specifics about program eligibility, basic program benefits, provider authorization, claims processing, and other program features are detailed in federal regulations at 32 CFR Part 199.

When the TRICARE program was initiated in 1995, a major revision to the regulations was published, detailing both the operational features of TRICARE (32 CFR 199.17) and the benefit changes (32 CFR 199.18). Those regulatory changes appeared in the *Federal Register* October 5, 1995 (60 *Federal Register* 52078).

ELIGIBILITY FOR TRICARE

In general, three categories of beneficiaries are eligible for services covered under TRICARE: active-duty members of the uniformed services; spouses and children of active-duty members; and retirees from the uniformed services, and their spouses and children. Importantly, beneficiaries who become eligible for Medicare on the basis of age lose their CHAMPUS entitlement and thus are not eligible for TRICARE. A demonstration program begun in 1998, called TRICARE Senior Prime, tests TRICARE enrollment of Medicare-eligible beneficiaries, with capitated payments from the Medicare Trust Funds to six military sites that have been qualified as Medicare + Choice plans.

TRICARE OPTIONS

A major feature of the TRICARE program is its triple option benefit. *Beneficiaries are offered three options; they may:*

- enroll to receive health care in an HMO-type program called "TRICARE Prime"
- use the civilian TRICARE provider network on a case-by-case basis, under "TRICARE Extra"
- choose to receive care from non-network providers and have the services reimbursed under "TRICARE Standard" (TRICARE Standard is the same as historical CHAMPUS.)

Enrollees in TRICARE Prime obtain most of their care within the network and pay substantially reduced cost shares when they receive care from civilian network providers. Enrollees in TRICARE Prime retain freedom to use non-network civilian providers, but they have to pay cost sharing considerably higher than under TRICARE Standard if they do so. Beneficiaries who choose not to enroll in TRICARE Prime will preserve their freedom of choice of provider for the most part by remaining in TRICARE Standard. These beneficiaries face standard CHAMPUS cost-sharing requirements, except that their coinsurance percentage is lower when they opt to use the TRICARE provider network under TRICARE Extra. All beneficiaries continue to be eligible to receive care in military facilities, but TRICARE Prime enrollees have priority over other beneficiaries.

TRICARE BENEFITS

Benefits covered under TRICARE roughly parallel those of high-option programs available under other public and major private health care plans. TRICARE coverage includes most inpatient and outpatient health services, prescription drugs, a substantial portion of physician and hospital charges, medical supplies and equipment, and mental health services.

TRICARE COST SHARING

Aside from the TRICARE Prime "enrollment fee" of $230 or $460 annually for retiree families, TRICARE beneficiaries do not pay premiums for their health care coverage. Military facility care continues to be free under TRICARE (aside from nominal daily subsistence charges for inpatient care), but TRICARE does include cost sharing for civilian sector care. As a rule, retirees and their family members pay more than families of active-duty members. TRICARE Standard outpatient cost sharing is 20 percent for active duty families and 25 percent for retiree families after a deductible of $300 per family ($100 for junior enlisted families).

Under TRICARE Prime these cost sharing requirements are replaced by a standard charge for most civilian provider network outpatient visits of $12 per visit or $6 per visit for family members of junior enlisted sponsors. For retiree families, the deductible of $300 per family and 25 percent cost sharing for outpatient services are also replaced by a standard charge of $12 for most outpatient visits. Retiree families also are charged a $230/$460 annual individual/family enrollment fee.

TRICARE BENEFICIARY ASSISTANCE

The TRICARE system has several unique features especially designed to help beneficiaries manage their own health care and gain quick and easy access to the system at their appropriate level of need. TRICARE service centers are located in each health service region, normally one at every military facility or located nearby. Qualified health professionals answer questions, make appointments, and help beneficiaries decide which health care option is best for them. Health benefits advisors assist them with claims paperwork and answer questions about any of the TRICARE programs. Health care finders make beneficiaries' referral appointments to physicians and specialists participating in the TRICARE network. For Medicare-eligible retirees, they locate physicians who accept Medicare payments for treatment when space is not available in a military hospital or clinic. Another feature available in most regions is the nurse advisor, who is accessible by telephone to provide health care advice and assistance 24 hours a day, 7 days a week.

ORIGINS OF TRICARE—MANAGED CARE DEMONSTRATIONS

In the 1980s and early 1990s, DOD implemented a number of demonstration programs to test the feasibility of using certain managed care mechanisms and to explore their impact on the delivery of health care services in military facilities and the purchase of civilian health care services. The demonstrations, which varied in design and scope, tested cost and utilization management controls in a variety of health care settings. The projects ranged in size from small-scale demonstrations at a single site for a given population to systemwide implementation of managed care mechanisms. Among the principal demonstration programs were the following:

- the CHAMPUS reform initiative (CRI)
- the New Orleans managed care demonstration
- several catchment area management (CAM) projects
- the Southeast region preferred provider organization (PPO) demonstration
- the contracted provider arrangement (CPA) in Norfolk

The CHAMPUS Reform Initiative

The CRI was a demonstration program designed to improve CHAMPUS through competitive selection of a financially at-risk contractor to underwrite delivery of CHAMPUS health care services. The primary goal of the CRI was to improve the program's quality and cost-effectiveness through the application of proven managed health care techniques. In February 1988, in accordance with requirements of the Federal Acquisition Regulation, the DOD awarded a contract to Foundation Health Corporation to conduct the demonstration in California and Hawaii. At the beginning of the demonstration, approximately 800,000 CHAMPUS-eligible beneficiaries lived within the demonstration area, or about 14 percent of the total number of program eligibles. Foundation Health began delivery of health care services in August 1988, subcontracting with three health plans and offering two alternatives to the standard CHAMPUS program: CHAMPUS Prime and CHAMPUS Extra.

In CHAMPUS Prime, which was similar to a health maintenance organization (HMO), beneficiaries enrolled, selected a primary care provider, and were required to obtain all their care through that provider. The designated provider was on staff in one of the MTFs located in the demonstration area or was a participating civilian provider. Enrollees were also referred to participating specialists as needed. Beneficiaries paid only a small cost for each office visit or hospital day, and little paperwork was involved. CHAMPUS Extra was essentially a PPO plan. Beneficiaries sought care from either a network provider or a non-network provider; if they used the former, however, their portion of the allowable fee for the service was reduced by 5 percent on an already discounted provider fee. The beneficiaries' out-of-pocket costs, therefore, were reduced, although they paid somewhat more than CHAMPUS Prime enrollees.

From numerous surveys conducted by independent, objective investigators, satisfaction with CRI in general, as well as with the medical care received therein, was high among all beneficiary categories. The most popular features of CHAMPUS Prime among beneficiaries included the small copayments, reduced paperwork, and reasonable visit fees. From the providers' perspective, the patient referral system and the professionalism shown in the program's utilization and quality management functions were most commonly cited. In addition to features common to many managed care plans, the CRI also included several innovative features that contributed to its successes. CHAMPUS service centers, established in all military hospitals and clinics in the demonstration area, employed registered nurses as "health care finders" to coordinate all patient referrals.

These personnel managed more than 10,000 referrals per month.

Another successful feature of CRI was called resource sharing, which involved the establishment of agreements between the CRI contractor and MTFs. Under these agreements, the contractor provided personnel, supplies, or equipment to an MTF to enhance patient care capability. By 1992, more than 200 resource-sharing agreements had been executed. Enhancing the capacity of MTFs by selectively increasing staff and material resources, resource sharing enabled facilities to operate more productively and therefore proved to be a valuable component of the CRI demonstration.

The CRI demonstration ended in February 1994, when a follow-on managed care contract for California and Hawaii began operations. Many of the design features of CRI were carried forward into TRICARE.

New Orleans Managed Care Demonstration

Congressionally directed, the New Orleans demonstration project was designed to test the application of managed care techniques in an area without an inpatient MTF. After a competitive procurement, a contract was awarded in June 1991 to Foundation Health Federal Services, a wholly owned subsidiary of Foundation Health Corporation. Health services delivery under the demonstration began on December 1, 1991. The design features of the project were similar to those of the CRI: a risk-based contract with a triple option (i.e., HMO, PPO, and standard CHAMPUS), provider networks, and comprehensive utilization management and quality assurance programs. In 1996, managed care services in New Orleans came under TRICARE.

Catchment Area Management (CAM) Demonstration Projects

CAM projects were initiated to pursue alternative management techniques within CHAMPUS in an effort to contain costs at the local level. Under CAM, a military hospital commander had responsibility for managing the delivery and financing of health care services for the entire beneficiary population residing in the hospital's catchment area (an area surrounding the facility, specified by ZIP codes, with a radius of roughly 40 miles). In these projects, CHAMPUS funds were allocated to the hospital commander, who was then responsible for distributing the combined CHAMPUS and direct care system funds appropriately for all services within the catchment area. Although funding was limited to that which would have been spent in the absence of a demonstration, commanders were given authority to pursue alternative health care delivery methods that were not generally possible outside the demonstration area.

Within the guidelines of demonstration authority and the overall design approach established by the DOD, the Army, Navy, and Air Force implemented separate demonstration projects. The first CAM site became operational in June 1989, and ultimately the program became operational at five demonstration sites. At each site, attempts were made to maximize the opportunities for innovation available through CAM to take advantage of local geographical and health care environments. Therefore, although there was a central CAM design, significant operational differences, both interservice and intraservice, existed among CAM sites.

Among the design features common to all CAM projects were a health care finder service, enhanced claims management, enrollment, and modifications to the standard CHAMPUS benefit package. All demonstrations required enrollment for a minimum of 1 year as a condition of CAM participation. Enrollment was limited to CHAMPUS-eligible beneficiaries within the catchment area, with the family being the unit of enrollment. All CAM demonstrations entailed reduced or eliminated deductibles and/or copayments, and some inpatient and outpatient services charges were discounted.

All the CAM designs also included both utilization management and quality assurance features. Preadmission review of inpatient care and retrospective case review were the common mechanisms applied. Some sites also conducted case management of either all patients or those with selected high-cost diagnoses. All contracted civilian providers were subject to the same utilization and quality management procedures as military providers.

Claims-processing functions under CAM were simplified to relieve beneficiaries of the paperwork of claims preparation and submission. Although all the claims-processing functions were similar in concept, implementation of simplified claims-processing functions was site specific, depending on demonstration design and Fiscal Intermediary (FI) requirements and capabilities.

The CAM projects provided key information on how best to integrate military facility health care management into TRICARE.

The Southeast Region Preferred Provider Organization (PPO) Project

The Southeast region demonstration was undertaken as a response to Congressional direction to modify a regional CHAMPUS FI contract to implement managed care techniques. The primary goals were to reduce CHAMPUS cost growth and to improve beneficiary satisfaction by organizing an accessible, cost-efficient network of health care providers.

In July 1990, an FI contract was awarded to Wisconsin Physicians Service. Under the contract, a PPO was established in a five-state Southeast region of the United States to offer beneficiaries a low-cost alternative to standard CHAMPUS. To develop PPO networks and to perform utilization management, Wisconsin Physicians Services subcontracted with a national firm having expertise in those areas. In the design of the demonstration, participants retained freedom of choice and did not enroll, but they had several incentives to use preferred providers. In particular, there were fee discounts, a 5 percent reduction in coinsurance rates, and direct claims filing by providers. The program, which covered nearly 900,000 beneficiaries in 20 military hospital catchment areas, was viewed as a support contract for individual hospital commanders in establishing relationships with civilian providers.

Additional features of the demonstration included a quality assessment program and contractor personnel on site in the military hospitals. A key component, as in the CRI and CAM demonstration projects, was that the military hospital was considered the most preferred provider. Furthermore, civilian networks were seen as complementing, rather than competing with, the MTFs.

Throughout the demonstration, where PPOs were operational, management reports were provided to military hospital commanders on all aspects of the networks, including percentage of network use by beneficiaries, type and cost of services delivered, utilization review activity, savings from provider discounts, and estimates of savings from utilization review.

The Southeast Region PPO Demonstration Project provided important information about the ability of DOD to extend managed care into locations where commercial managed care experience was limited. This was significant for national implementation of TRICARE because many military facilities are located away from metropolitan areas.

Contracted Provider Arrangement-Norfolk

One of the first managed care demonstration programs initiated by DOD was limited to mental health services. During the 1980s, CHAMPUS costs for mental health care represented a substantial portion of the CHAMPUS budget. Before 1986, the Tidewater area of Virginia presented a particular concern because per capita costs for mental health care were found to be twice the national average. As a result of this finding, the CPA-Norfolk demonstration project was initiated to test the effects of cost and utilization controls on the delivery of mental health services in this area. The design of the demonstration included an at-risk, fixed-price contract for all necessary mental health services; case management as a prerequisite for payment; a contracted provider network with negotiated rates; claims processing and administrative

functions performed by the contractor; a partial hospitalization benefit; and independent quality monitoring.

After a competitive procurement process, the DOD contracted with Sentara First Step for delivery of services, and operations commenced on October 1, 1986. Sentara First Step implemented all features of the design, including intake and case management processes, a network of preferred providers with significantly reduced rates, and an internal quality assurance program. For government monitoring purposes, an external quality monitoring effort was undertaken through a separate contract with SysteMetrics/McGraw-Hill. Delivery of services by Sentara First Step under the demonstration ceased on March 31, 1989, and after another procurement effort a follow-on contract was awarded to First Hospital Corporation-Options (FHC-Options). In the follow-on contract, FHC-Options was responsible for all mental health care provided to CHAMPUS beneficiaries in the geographical region of the demonstration. Utilization management of all inpatient care and all outpatient care beyond the twenty-third visit was required. The contractor was allowed to reduce or eliminate cost-sharing requirements as an inducement for beneficiaries to use those providers who joined the preferred provider network. All contracted providers were required to accept assignment on all claims and were not allowed to bill CHAMPUS beneficiaries for charges above the allowable amount. In addition, all noncontracted providers were required to comply with utilization management activities at least 95 percent of the time or risk losing certification as CHAMPUS-authorized providers for a period of 1 year.

THE TRICARE PROGRAM

In general, the demonstrations discussed previously were successful in providing evidence that innovations in the delivery and financing of health care services can help in containing the rising costs of health care, at least in the short term. The demonstrations also showed that such approaches can have a positive effect on provider and beneficiary behavior and on maintaining or improving the quality of care delivered. Therefore, many features of the DOD demonstration projects have been incorporated into TRICARE, the DOD's recently implemented, systemwide managed care initiative.

As noted earlier, the goal of TRICARE is to bring together the health care delivery systems of each of the military departments and CHAMPUS to use most efficiently the resources available to military medicine and to best serve its beneficiaries. Under TRICARE, the military service medical departments and MTF commanders have the tools, authority, and flexibility needed to perform the health care/medical mission more effectively, and the DOD, in general, is better able to accomplish its mission by improving beneficiary access to health care services, controlling health care costs, and ensuring quality care to all MHS beneficiaries.

To implement TRICARE, the DOD has established 11 health service regions and a new administrative structure to oversee the delivery of health care. The regions are designated on a geographical basis, and each encompasses medical facilities from all three of the military services. Within each region, the commanding officer of a component tertiary medical center is designated as the regional lead agent. Lead agents are responsible for planning, coordinating, and monitoring all health care delivered throughout their region.

The linchpin of the delivery system is a primary care manager: a specific primary care clinic, site, provider, or group of providers where each enrolled beneficiary will establish and maintain a medical affiliation. Some differences in the delivery of care occur geographically because of differences in the relative capacity of MTFs. That is, in some areas MTFs have the ability to deliver extensive primary and specialty care. In other locations, MTF commanders must rely on civilian providers to deliver care not available within the facility. In still other areas, beneficiaries rely completely on civilian providers.

MANAGED CARE SUPPORT CONTRACTS

In addition to providing new options for health care and a new regional structure, TRICARE expands on the DOD's experience in using contracted providers in demonstration programs to the entire MHS. Under TRICARE, seven managed care support contracts have been procured competitively for 11 TRICARE regions (that is, every region is supported by a contract, but some contracts cover more than one region). Each contract augments the care available within the direct care system in the region and provides administrative support to the lead agent.

The TRICARE managed care support contracts are procured centrally by the Office of the Assistant Secretary of Defense (Health Affairs). A standard request for proposals is used in the procurements, augmented by any unique or region-specific requirements identified by the lead agent that go beyond the standard specifications. The contracts are bid on a competitive basis and are considered fixed-price, at-risk contracts. Only the administrative portion of the contract has a fixed price; however, the health care price is subject to adjustments on the basis of risk-sharing provisions in which the contractor and the government share losses or gains beyond certain levels. Adjustments can be based on factors such as inflation, MTF workload shifts, and beneficiary population changes. The risk-sharing and bid price adjustment features are intended to protect both the contractor and the government from large risks associated with these complex contracts.

COMPARING TRICARE AND MEDICARE MANAGED CARE

It may be useful to compare the development of managed care under the Medicare and CHAMPUS programs. A significant difference in this development is that, after a brief demonstration period, the Medicare HMO risk program was implemented through permanent statutory and regulatory authorities (see Chapters 55 and

56 for a detailed discussion of Medicare managed care). In contrast, TRICARE was implemented after nearly 10 years of demonstration projects. The managed care demonstrations that gave rise to TRICARE were quite varied, including a multibillion dollar, triple-option, risk-based program; a much smaller triple-option, risk-based program in an area without a military hospital; a five-state, dual-option, cost plus incentives reimbursement project; and five similar service-designed managed care projects managed by MTF commanders at the local level.

A second significant difference between the Medicare HMO risk program and the major DOD risk-based contracts is the reimbursement mechanism. Whereas Medicare HMOs are totally at risk for cost overruns in the enrolled program, there are adjustments in TRICARE in the fixed price paid to the managed care support contractor for circumstances outside contractor control (e.g., the workload in the MTF). Also, there is risk sharing (and sharing in savings) between the contractor and the DOD for cost overruns (and underruns) in the contract price. In addition, each DOD managed care support contractor is at risk for all nonenrolled beneficiaries in the relevant health service region, not just those beneficiaries in the enrolled option. As a result, there are no issues of adverse selection or skimming with which to contend. In fact, it is in the contractor's best financial interest to have the individuals with the more severe health problems enroll in the more closely managed TRICARE Prime option.

CONCLUSION: NEXT STEPS FOR THE TRICARE PROGRAM

In addition to the usual and important functions of a primary care manager coordinating different types and levels of care, TRICARE must support military medical readiness and include the essential function of coordination between the military direct care system and the civilian health care system. Along with quality, cost, and access, integrating the civilian and direct care systems of the MHS has been a focal point of TRICARE and will continue to be a major challenge as TRICARE evolves.

TRICARE represents a major reengineering of the way health care is managed in the MHS. Significant components include an enrollment system, cost-sharing incentives, a system of primary care managers and health care networks, and comprehensive utilization management and quality assurance programs. A key factor that was not anticipated when TRICARE was designed was the rapid pace of change in the health care system overall, in managed care, and in the military health system. It will be important to improve the ability of the system to respond to external and internal changes to maintain a viable, cost-effective health care delivery program for military beneficiaries.

CHAPTER 59

Managed Care Organizations in Rural Areas

Keith J. Mueller

The evolution of managed care in rural areas will differ from experiences in urban areas. Although the roots of managed care can be traced to application in a rural setting,[1] the rapid spread of managed care in recent years has been concentrated in urban (metropolitan) areas. Some of the building blocks of successful managed care organizations are difficult to assemble in rural areas, such as:

Keith Mueller, PhD, is a Professor and the Director of the Nebraska Center for Rural Health Research, University of Nebraska. He was the 1996–1997 President of the National Rural Health Association and the recipient of the Association's Distinguished Rural Health Researcher Award in 1998. Dr. Mueller's doctorate in Political Science is from the University of Arizona. He is the author of a University of Nebraska Press book, *Health Care Policy in the United States*, and has published more than 30 articles on health planning, access to care for vulnerable populations, rural health, and access to care among the uninsured. He is the Chair of the Health Panel, Rural Policy Research Institute, and primary author of a number of its publications dealing with rural implications of health reform legislation, analysis of legislation focused on rural health, analysis of the Balanced Budget Act of 1997, and analysis of changes in Medicare policy. Dr. Mueller has directed major health services studies funded by the U.S. Agency for Health Care Policy and Research, the Federal Office of Rural Health Policy, and the Robert Wood Johnson Foundation. He has testified on numerous occasions before committees of Congress and in other forums, including the Bipartisan Commission on the Future of Medicare.

- enrolling sufficient numbers of individuals to accept risk for the costs of care (overcoming adverse risk selection)
- securing discounted pricing from competing physicians and hospitals
- establishing cost-effective alternatives to acute care in clinical practices

Combining managed care with desires for competing health plans, an argument can be made that managed competition cannot work in rural areas.[2] However, the unique characteristics of the rural environment are reasons to think about different ways of applying the practices of managed care, not reasons to abandon the concept.

One rural difference is the lack of development of managed care in rural areas in the past 20 years. As a result, rural providers are less prepared (lacking knowledge and experience) to participate in risk-sharing plans, and health plans are not experienced in adapting management strategies on the basis of high-volume business to sparsely populated areas. Since the Medicare and Medicaid programs have expanded use of managed care for their enrollees, interest among providers and health plans in rural areas has grown. Especially in the case of Medicare, public programs represent significant sources of revenue for providers and opportunities for health plans. In Medicare, there has been very little use of managed care in rural areas as of the year 2000, but changes in Medicare payment may create incentives for rural providers to participate in managed care plans (see also

Chapter 55). The Medicaid experience is especially instructive. Typically, conversions to managed care in Medicaid programs begin in urban counties, and application in rural areas may be different. In rural areas, Medicaid managed care plans are more likely to be characterized as primary care case management (PCCM) programs (physicians receive a monthly fee for managing the care of the patients, but no change in basic fee for service reimbursement) than as risk contracts (see Chapter 57 for a discussion of Medicaid and managed health care). In sum, historical differences between urban and rural areas in use of managed care are being overcome by new strategic approaches in health care finance and financial pressures to escape the limitations of fee-for-service payment.

Before proceeding with the substance of this chapter, some definitions are needed. In this chapter rural will include all counties not part of metropolitan statistical areas, the definition used by the U.S. Office of Management and Budget and most federal programs. Managed care organizations include any insurance plans that fall within the continuum of managed care, from managed indemnity plans to closed-panel HMOs. This chapter will pay special attention to plans that share financial risk with providers and those that accept per-member per-month payments as the total revenues for the plan and manage within those revenue constraints.

STATUS OF MANAGED CARE IN RURAL AREAS

There has been very little enrollment in managed care plans in rural areas. Although more than 80 percent of all rural counties were in the service areas of HMOs in 1995, enrollment in commercial plans in states where such data were available was quite low, ranging from 0.6 percent in Wyoming to 17.0 percent in Wisconsin. Only one other of 8 states, Pennsylvania with 12.0 percent, had rural enrollment greater than 10 percent (the other states were Florida, Minnesota, Missouri, North Carolina, and South Carolina).[3] InterStudy estimated that approximately 9 percent of all HMO enrollees were in rural areas

in 1996.[4] More than 50 percent of rural counties were included in Medicare managed care areas in May 1997, although fully capitated programs were operating in only 10 percent of rural counties.[5] As of the end of 1998 all but two states (Alaska and Wyoming) enrolled at least some rural Medicaid recipients in managed care plans, but only Tennessee, Washington, Montana, Utah, and Colorado enrolled more than 90 percent of rural recipients in managed care plans.[6] There was also substantial rural enrollment in Medicaid managed care plans in Arizona and Oregon.

Experiences in attempting to establish managed care plans in rural areas have been mixed. Decisions by health plans to discontinue offering Medicare managed care plans in certain counties have affected rural beneficiaries disproportionately.[7] In 1999, only 27 percent of rural Medicare beneficiaries lived in counties served by HMOs.[8] States are experiencing similar problems in the Medicaid program and in expansions building from Medicaid to offer insurance to the previously uninsured. For example, Oregon's Health Plan, originally implemented exclusively through HMOs, is now open to groups of primary care physicians unaffiliated with an HMO because HMOs are withdrawing from sparsely populated areas.[9]

In contrast with the examples of HMO withdrawals that receive a great deal of publicity, there are illustrations of successful (as of the time of publication) rural managed care plans. Urban-based managed care plans have expanded into rural areas in North Carolina (base is Greensboro), Iowa and Wisconsin (base is Dubuque, Iowa), Oregon (base is Portland), and Montana (base is Billings). In North Carolina, 17 percent of the plan's 160,000 commercial members reside in nonmetropolitan areas, served by a network of primary care providers.[10] In the Dubuque, Iowa, area a plan that started in 1982 has grown to include rural satellite practices in Iowa, Wisconsin, and Illinois, but the plan remains modest in size—28,000 members.[11] A very large HMO in Oregon, Regence HMO Oregon, based in Portland, included 53,000 commercial enrollees in rural counties,

55,000 rural Oregon Plan (publicly supported) enrollees, and 6,700 rural Medicare enrollees as of 1996.[12] However, since that time that same HMO has pulled out of 16 counties and in late 1999 left 7 more.[13] Other managed care plans have developed from a rural base. One very large example is the Rocky Mountain HMO in Colorado. This plan, based in Mesa County, began in western Colorado, in the mid-1970s. At that time, Mesa County was considered nonmetropolitan (it has grown into a metropolitan area since then). At the end of 1996 the plan included 96,000 members, 64,200 of whom were commercially insured.[14] NorthMed HMO in Michigan serves a 13-county region from its base in a rural community and remains modest in size, 16,000 members.[15] A small rural HMO, Missouri Advantage, was started in southern Missouri in 1996 and as of early 1997 enrolled 5,800 commercial members.[16] The Yellowstone Community Health Plan in Billings, Montana, serves that small metropolitan area and surrounding rural counties. As of May 1999 the plan had 11,500 commercial enrollees, 600 Medicaid recipients, and 2,600 Medicare beneficiaries.[17]

A common approach to managed care in state Medicaid programs has been to use the PCCM model, in which primary care physicians are paid a monthly stipend (usually between $2 and $5 per enrollee, inclusive) to coordinate all care for the Medicaid recipients enrolling through their practices. For example, in Louisiana the Medicaid program pays physicians $5 per enrollee for a management fee and reimburses on the basis of charges to 106 primary care physicians in 19 rural parishes. An assessment of that program, based on interviewing participating physicians, found high understanding of how the system works and appreciation of financial stability but concerns about limits on medical decision making, added paperwork burden, and insufficient communication.[18]

APPRECIATING THE RURAL CONTEXT FOR MANAGED CARE

Any effort to establish managed care in rural areas will require investment in information systems and development of care management plans. Doing so in a manner that ensures return on investment requires a sufficient base of patients. The reality for much of rural America is that rural managed care plan service areas will need to span large geographical areas and encompass multiple hospitals, physicians, and other health care providers. An alternative is to assume that managed care plans based in urban areas will encompass adjacent rural areas. The most likely scenario for developing a rural population base sufficient to support managed care is for rural providers to form service delivery networks that can either develop their own managed care plans or participate in managed care plans offered through large insurance organizations.

For rural health care delivery service networks to be effective, they must be formally organized and supported by their members. The relationships among members must be governed by specific bylaws, with binding legal commitments to live by those bylaws (which could be in the format of memoranda of understanding, contracts, or articles of incorporation). A variety of members would compose the network, which would be capable of providing a continuum of care (primary care in ambulatory settings, hospital-based care, postacute care). Members of the networks contribute resources toward achieving a common, specified purpose.

Rural health networks may encompass single counties, as is the case in Itasca County, Minnesota (Itasca Medical Care), and in Tioga County, Pennsylvania (Laurel Health System), or multiple counties as is true for the Marshfield Clinic in Wisconsin (14 counties), and for Av-Med Santa Fe in Florida (5 counties). Rural health networks may cross state lines to encompass large geographical areas such as West River Health Services in North Dakota, South Dakota, and Montana.[19] The service areas in these examples vary significantly in size, both in numbers of persons in the service area and in the size of the area. The two single-county service areas have populations of approximately 40,000 each. The service area for the West River network is quite large, with 18,000 square miles, but encompasses only 25,000 to 30,000 persons. The larger systems include many more persons, 292,000 in Florida and 511,000 in Wisconsin.[20] Those larger systems offer health plans for which network members accept financial risk.

Networks can obtain the critical mass necessary to support information systems and other critical management tools to move toward establishing managed care plans, even if such plans are not created by the networks. Recognizing the value of rural networks, the federal government created a grant program in 1997 to encourage the establishment of more networks. As of late 1999, there were more than 34 recipients of these grant awards. Network development is an ambitious, time-consuming, and long-term task. After completing case studies of the networks identified in the previous paragraph, the authors offered these lessons[21]:

- The formation and operation of rural networks is an incremental process involving political and economic decisions that require a substantial amount of time.
- Integrated networks need product lines that provide revenue.
- There is no single approach to organizing rural networks.
- External catalysts can stimulate or retard growth of integrated rural networks.

These conclusions about the difficulties in developing and nurturing rural health networks also apply to developing managed care plans in rural areas because for much of rural America, one development (networks) is a predecessor to the other (rural-based managed care plans).

Public policies designed to encourage development of managed care in rural areas recognize the importance of forming service delivery networks. For example, the Minnesota health reform legislation of 1994 authorized community integrated service networks (CISNs) in rural areas. Four networks that developed under the authorization included 10, 16, 20, and 47 counties. Even with those aggregations of counties, the CISNs are unable to garner sufficient populations in rural areas to guarantee the enrollment of the 20,000 to 30,000 persons considered necessary for HMOs to be cost-effective.[22]

In a notable effort to encourage development of managed care in rural areas, in 1994 the federal Agency for Health Care Policy and Research (AHCPR) awarded to university-based centers five grants whose intent was to foster the development of rural-based managed care plans. In 1997 and 1998, an evaluation of those grants revealed that forming rural networks and moving them toward development of managed care plans is a lengthy and often unpredictable process.[23] *Three of the conclusions from the evaluation are particularly important:*

- The motivation of providers to form networks increases with the presence of immediate external threats to their patient base and/or revenue (e.g., incursion of urban based plans into the rural service area).
- Local provider leadership is important to successful network development.
- Technical assistance, as provided by the five centers, has little power to independently influence the pace of network development and movement toward creating or participating in managed care plans.[24]

The principal investigators of the five projects reached similar conclusions, identifying the following prerequisites for success in increasing the use of managed care in rural areas:[25]

- provider leadership from both hospitals and physicians
- organized medical communities (typically in the form of independent physician associations and horizontal hospital networks)
- persistence among those engaged in network and managed care development (A long time frame is needed to overcome the initial lack of experience with different strategies of health care financing and organization of services.)
- external funds (Rural providers and communities are unlikely to have the resources needed to learn about and develop organized systems and the capital required to offer locally based health plans.)
- information systems to manage medical care and network administration

- ability to overcome local biases against managed care
- nurturing managed care experience among the local leadership

REASONS TO EXPECT MANAGED CARE DEVELOPMENT IN RURAL AREAS

As the AHCPR centers have learned, a major motivator for action by rural providers to develop independent health plans is the threat of losing financial and clinical autonomy to large urban-based plans. Large HMOs experienced slow growth in the late 1990s, including, for some, reduced service areas. As that occurred, rural providers and communities were secure in thinking that preemptive development of managed care plans was unnecessary. However, although there have been well-publicized financial woes for large HMOs, the use of managed care continues to grow. For example, in Nebraska enrollment in HMOs grew from 149,631 in 1994 to 236,818 in 1998.[26] Health plans based in urban areas may include rural enrollees, such as state employees, federal employees, and workers in large national firms. As a result, rural physicians find themselves working with managed care contracts. A survey of rural physicians in nine states found that nearly 70 percent participated in contracts that had them sharing financial risk through capitation, withholds, or bonuses. The share of physician practice revenue through managed care contracts, though, remained modest—18 percent of all revenue for those who participated in contracts using capitation.[27] In short, the seeds of managed care have been planted in many rural areas already. Further, managed care firms are recovering from the economic dip of the late 1990s, and another effort to increase enrollment can be expected. Therefore, the motivation of preempting an external threat remains.

A second motivation is the new program created in Medicare by the Balanced Budget Act (BBA) of 1997, Medicare + Choice, which includes more attractive payment for managed care plans enrolling rural beneficiaries. The same legislation includes changes in traditional fee-for-service Medicare payments that make continuing to rely on those payments unattractive to rural providers. These changes include conversion to prospective payment to generate savings in payment for skilled nursing care, home health care, and hospital outpatient care. In addition, payments have been reduced for durable medical equipment, disproportionate share payments, graduate medical education, and hospice care. Subsequent analyses predict significant shortfalls for rural hospitals, home health agencies, and skilled nursing facilities. Conversely, changes in the payment formula for risk contracts will result in higher payments in rural counties than had been true.[28] The impetus created by the BBA may be enhanced by other structural changes in the Medicare program. Proposals being debated in 1999 and 2000 would have Medicare rely more on contracts with private health plans, for the purpose of offering more choices to beneficiaries, including choices with more comprehensive benefits than the traditional Medicare program. Given this policy preference, the opportunities for managed care plans in the Medicare program will grow. Because Medicare is a major source of patient revenue for rural providers, the result will be an increased incentive to contract directly with Medicare or intermediaries to capture the risk contract dollars. There will be an opportunity for rural providers to use the full Medicare capitated payment for all enrollees rather than to rely on the reduced payment for services rendered to those who need care.

BUILDING SUCCESSFUL MANAGED CARE IN RURAL AREAS

The first step toward a successful managed care plan supported by rural health care providers is to develop specific reasons to create a plan. Without a commitment to succeeding in the development of managed care, providers and health plans in rural areas are unlikely to sustain the effort required to succeed. Initial reasons can include a desire to ward off urban plans who are seen as predators and enhancing local provider income. These reasons may not be sufficient, though, to argue for an expensive investment in a local system versus contracting with an urban-based system, particularly if the pace of expansion of managed care plans is slow. An additional reason, to provide better service in local communities, may help sustain the effort, especially if this reason is linked with a desire to control the decisions related to providing care (rather than following the utilization precepts set forth by external plans).

Health care providers are more likely to support a new scheme such as managed care because they believe they can provide care in a more cost-effective manner by making decisions themselves. They also are likely to link a new system with improvements in the quality of care. This can be done by engaging in projects with their peers in rural communities and by improving their control over the continuum of care needed by their patients. Primary care providers are well positioned to do this in rural communities, particularly through the PCCM model. The model can be carried out under the auspices of rural independent practice associations (IPAs), who offer access to their members as the preferred provider organizations (PPOs) in a managed care arrangement. The PPO model for managed care has gained favor as HMOs lost favor in recent years—between 1997 and 1998 the share of workers in employer-sponsored plans accounted for by HMOs decreased, whereas the PPO share increased.[29]

Once the commitment exists to develop a health plan, an organization has to be created (unless it already exists) that can span rural communities and providers such that a critical mass of potential enrollees is present. An early planning document needs to develop an estimate of the number of enrollees from an assessment of the ability of the providers to control utilization and total costs of services; the tighter the control, the lower the population base needed. There also are tradeoffs between the number of persons enrolled and the level of reinsurance needed to protect against high-cost cases. Some HMOs have succeeded with very few enrollees, such as the Heart of America HMO in Rugby, North Da-

kota, which as of 1995 had 15 years of operation and only 3,000 enrollees.[30]

The next logical step for an aspiring rural HMO is a thorough market assessment, which includes an analysis of the ability to garner patients from three principal (excluding self-pay) sources of payment: commercial insurance, Medicare, and Medicaid. *The commercial market can be assessed by answering these questions:*

- How many persons are insured through commercial vendors?
- What are the sizes of groups of insured lives (e.g., how many in groups of more than 50 employees)?
- Are insurance brokers and employers willing to consider a locally based managed care plan (some employers may be regional or local managers of national corporations)?
- What are the demographic characteristics of the insured population that might predict health care utilization?

For the Medicare population the relevant questions include:

- How many Medicare beneficiaries reside in the service area?
- What percentage of them are willing to consider enrolling in a managed care plan?
- What is the age distribution of the Medicare population?
- What strategies might succeed in enrolling Medicare beneficiaries least likely to use services?
- What is the current pattern of using Medigap policies among the beneficiaries and can a managed care plan compete effectively, given the federal payment for Medicare + Choice plans in the service area?

The following questions are important to ask about the local Medicaid eligible population:

- What is the state plan for Medicaid and is payment sufficient to warrant aggressive pursuit of Medicaid managed care enrollment?
- What has been the pattern of health care utilization among Medicaid beneficiaries and can it be affected to lower expenditures?

- Are the providers in the rural network willing to treat all Medicaid patients?

Assuming the preliminary market analysis indicates at least some likelihood of success, the next step is to develop a strategic plan designed to have a managed care plan in place by a certain date. The plan would cover these elements: financing, plan design, organizational design, quality assurance, marketing, and negotiations.

Financing

Initial financial analysis is focused on creating capital to absorb the startup costs for any managed care plan. If organizers are starting from ground zero to create a plan, the following costs will need to be covered: reserves, working capital, consulting and actuarial fees, attorney fees, information systems, office setup, preoperational staff, marketing, and first year operational loss. These costs are variable, depending on the size of the market, potential for partnering with existing health plans (lowering reserve and setup requirements), and willingness of member organizations to contribute existing resources. Most rural organizations are unlikely to have the several millions of dollars on hand to cover capital requirements, so these options will need to be considered: securing financial partners, such as an insurance carrier; "taxing" the members of the rural network interested in creating a managed care plan; soliciting local contributions to the new plan from those in the community anxious to see locally based options for health insurance; and/or selling shares in the venture, generally to providers and the community, with the expectation of return on that investment.

The second level of financial planning is the creation of an appropriate balance of expected revenues and expenses, both of which are subject to strategic decisions of the network. Revenues are affected by the premiums charged and copayments built into any plan. Expenses are related to administrative costs and utilization of medical services. The decisions about financial stability can be illustrated using the decision to initiate a Medicare managed care plan. The premium paid by the federal government is based on the total expenditures by Medicare for the

beneficiaries in each county in the service area, trended forward from 1997. Any offering in managed care is likely to include more benefits than were not paid for by Medicare (such as prescription drugs), so there is a need to add a premium to be paid by the enrollee, given the added value of the plan over what Medicare offers. The market analysis, completed earlier, will include the prices for Medigap policies that cover the additional benefits, which provide a boundary for what the new managed care plan should charge. That same market analysis will provide parameters for what can be assessed as deductibles and copayments when Medicare beneficiaries receive services. The revenue side of a Medicare managed care plan, then, equals the adjusted Medicare premium (initial amount adjusted for demographics of enrollees) plus a premium charged to beneficiaries, plus deductibles and copayments. The cost side of the equation will include the health care expenditures (commonly referred to as the medical loss ratio) plus administrative expenses (sales/marketing, product development, financing, information system, eligibility verification and claims processing, member services, and provider relations), plus a special assessment by the Health Care Financing Administration to cover costs of beneficiary education. Actuarial analysis can determine the possible range of monthly costs to the plan by using previous experience in the service area, using Medicare claims information and estimates for benefits not covered by Medicare. These estimates can be presented as per member per month costs, and then the costs can be compared with the revenues. One outcome of such analysis will be a clear illustration of the importance of managing care: if use of expensive services such as inpatient hospital care and emergency department visits can be reduced, the managed care plan will be more attractive to potential enrollees because the additional monthly premium will be lower.

Plan Design

The results of financial analysis will influence the design of the plan to be offered. For example, any prescription drug benefit will be costly, but the cost to the plan can be lowered by designing a benefit with appropriate deductible and copayments. This is an aspect of developing a rural managed care plan that is influenced by the decisions made within the rural context. Although other plans might develop formularies for medications and encourage use of a single supplier (often by mail), the rural plan may not want to impose a formulary on participating physicians who may want to support local pharmacists. Rural plans offering prescription benefits will need to balance local availability with the effects on premiums and copayments. Another critical element in plan design will be the benefits associated with preventive services and management of chronic illness. Designing a plan requires use of the market analysis as well, which may differ between rural and urban areas as a function of the preferences of local residents.

The plan must be designed to be competitive in the local market while being fiscally prudent. Major service categories should be considered separately: hospitalization, optical services, physician services, dental care, prescription medication, emergency services, and postacute care (including home health). Plan design also includes specifying member rights and responsibilities, a grievance procedure, and rules governing enrollment and disenrollment.

Organization Design

Organizing to deliver care in a managed care model may require more detailed considerations than are necessary when forming the initial network. The organization that markets a health plan to the service area will need to meet a host of legal requirements, including those related to securities, taxes, and liability, as described in other chapters of the *Handbook*. Integrating all the providers who will participate in the health plan into a single organization may involve vertical integration that was not part of network development because previous relationships may have been within categories of network members, such as physicians or hospitals. In developing a cost-effective health plan, those groups will need to create a board of directors and by-laws. The board will create separate committees to review contracts, consider financing issues, establish and implement quality assurance processes, and review member complaints. In rural areas where large health care delivery systems have not been developed previously, sharing decision power that influences both incomes for providers and the clinical protocols used to treat patients will be a major challenge. Some level of trust will have to precede agreements between various providers, and decision rules will need to anticipate areas of disagreement and establish methods for achieving consensus. Principles of majority rule do not apply when each participant's cooperation is required to make the venture a success, as is true when managing patient care.

Another part of organizational design is working to maintain the interest and commitment of providers participating in the health plan. Initially, there should be some criteria for membership in the health plan, so that the providers meet expectations related to providing cost-effective medical services. For example, the organization will need to determine whether board certification, or board eligibility, is to be a requirement for participation by physicians. Organizations can retain the providers' continued interest and commitment by using continuing education sessions for health care professionals; career development for administrators of the network and of member institutional providers; committee activities related to governance of the health plans; and services to practices and institutions, such as purchasing agreements, discounts on necessary products and services, and organizational development.

Quality Assurance

This is an especially important area of activity for any rural-based managed care plan. Rural health care providers fight a perception that they are not capable of performing all services at the same level of quality as their urban counterparts. The perception is related to the "bigger is better" myth and to the proximity of subspecialty providers and institutions that have more high-tech equipment available. Rural health plans have to be able to promote the high quality of care they deliver because it is their strongest asset. Rural systems begin with a comparative advantage over many urban systems. The entry point to care for rural residents is the local primary care physician, who can manage the entire episode of care because there is a greater likelihood for contact with the patient because of advantages of proximity. In the context of quality assurance systems for health plans, this rural advantage is improved by using specific techniques and tools that make tracking a patient's care easier and more efficient. Rural health care organizations can engage in quality improvement efforts by establishing and following set protocols that are developed and reviewed by their own physician members.

Quality assurance programs should be patient focused. This can begin with assessing health risks of each new enrollee into the plan, so that conditions are detected at appropriate times, when treatment is less intrusive (and happily for the plan, often less expensive). For rural enrollees this includes assessing occupational risks associated with farming, ranching, and mining. After the risk assessment, quality assurance includes providing counseling and self-education for persons to lower their own risks. In rural practices this may require providing counseling in ways that protect confidentiality of the individuals. Well-functioning health plans will include disease management programs for the chronically afflicted, through either formal disease-specific programs or less formal general "good practices" efforts.

Marketing

Rural health plan managers must develop and execute a plan for marketing themselves and the health plan they establish. It is appropriate to consider marketing immediately after a discussion of quality because the product to be marketed is high-quality health care delivered in the local community. General principles of effective marketing can be followed. The first principle is that the managers must know the product and

providers being marketed. This means they must know the coverage provided by the plan and how their plan compares with other health plans on the market. The providers are of course the local rural providers, as well as the specialists and institutions used from outside the local community. This is one of the special rural differences—the combination of the "home town" provider of high quality, with choices of whom to see when other services are required. The second principle is to communicate effectively with the target customers. This may entail parallel but distinct marketing activities to reach subgroups in the rural community. The approaches to human resource managers of local firms and to the elderly will be parallel rather than separate because the volume of enrollment needed for a successful plan will be an aggregation of several groups. The third principle is to engage in marketing activities constantly and consistently. A major marketing advantage for rural plans is the ability to establish and enhance a local reputation for customer service (quality health care delivered with a focus on the customer, who is also a neighbor) that will spread quickly in small communities.

The following are a few of the variety of specific strategies, as applied to Medicare beneficiaries, that can be used in marketing a local health plan. Marketing guides can be developed that are simple and easy to understand. They should be honest representations of the product and may include comparisons with other products. In the case of Medicare, the comparisons are to other managed care plans and to the combination of Medicare and supplemental coverage. Guides are useful during open enrollment periods, when mass distribution to persons choosing among options is the most effective means of enrolling new clients. Much of marketing, though, may involve more personal contacts. In the Medicare context, methods that reach individuals and couples have to be developed because they make their own decisions (compared with employees and dependents in the commercial market). In rural areas, for example, word of mouth communications through local senior centers, civic organizations, and community events (such as community dances) is perhaps the most effective marketing tool. All these strategies for marketing should be assessed against two criteria. First, the strategy should be cost effective. Second, the resulting mix of enrollees creates an appropriate risk pool (sick and healthy persons) for the plan.

Negotiations

Health plan administrators will find themselves negotiating both internally and externally. Internally, the integrated network supporting the health plan is held together through relationships among different providers, including hospitals and physicians. In rural areas, with some exceptions, not all providers will be under contract as employees of the same system. The implication is that different provider groups, and in some instances individual providers, will need to agree to the ingredients of the health plan, including pricing, quality assurance programs, and accepting eligible patients. Health plan administrators will need to negotiate with external organizations. Rural networks may not have sufficient capital to assume risk for insurance plans, so the negotiations may be with insurance company partners. In all of the negotiations rural providers, who form the network and provide the services to the insured population, need to carefully monitor the following plan components: fees and charges specified by contract, timeliness of payment, any gag clauses, and confidentiality of patient records.

THE FUTURE

Given the current landscape in health care finance in rural areas and the prospects for more activities in managed care in rural areas, what will the landscape look like in 2010? Recent swings in enrollment into HMOs, both commercial and public, make any prediction rather tenuous. However, two realities temper the publicity generated by health plans withdrawing Medicare managed care plans and the "consumer rebellion" related to HMOs. First, in the case of Medicare, aggregate enrollment in managed care plans continues to increase. Even in rural counties the total enrollment was more as of June 1999 than it was before the market pullouts began. Second, in the commercial market enrollment is changing very little, and the shift in market share is to other types of health plans that also restrict choice of providers, such as preferred provider organizations and point-of-service plans. Elements of a consumer backlash apply to any health plan that restricts payment for services deemed unnecessary, a practice not limited to HMOs, and not common to all HMOs. Consumer satisfaction with HMOs remains high overall, an indication there are specific issues to address, but not general unhappiness with plan design. In sum, there is no compelling evidence that HMOs will become dinosaurs, and there are reasons to believe that managed care will grow as a share of the insured market in rural areas.

A reasonable approach to predicting the future is to examine the present as a foundation. In the case of managed care in rural areas, a review of experiences of some rural plans and how they are evolving is instructive. Different models have been able to show success in rural areas. At one extreme is the very small plan, Heart of America HMO, in Rugby, North Dakota. This plan's success is based on having a significant share of a small market, appropriate purchase of reinsurance, and use of medical management. At another end of the spectrum, the Marshfield Clinic in central Wisconsin enrolled 90,000 members in its Security Health Plan as of 1997. The network supporting this plan includes 450 physicians, 23 additional group practice branches, 12 affiliated hospitals including the large tertiary hospital in Marshfield, and 12 regional centers. The Marshfield example is the one more worthy of emulation, with its ability to integrate the spectrum of care and grow in size by building a large regional network. Most rural areas, though, do not have tertiary facilities or the capital available to build large integrated systems anchored by a single institution (exceptions would be the Mayo Clinic in Minnesota and the Penn State–Giesinger Health System in Pennsylvania). Neither of these two extreme examples of size and scope is likely to characterize rural plans of the future; they are the boundaries within which to characterize expectations. Importantly, they do illustrate that extremes are possible. A network with size and scope falling between the first two examples is First Health West, in Comanche County, Oklahoma. A tertiary care hospital in Lawton, Oklahoma, anchors this network that encompasses 11 counties, 34 clinics, and 93 physicians. The First Health West network has partnered with insurance companies to offer an HMO product in that region.[31]

There are three models that rural-based managed care plans could follow. One possibility is for health care providers and local businesses to form Physician-Hospital-Community-Organizations (PHCOs). PHCOs provide investment opportunities for rural community organizations and provide a stake in the development and sponsorship of the health plan. The PHCO model is very difficult to implement because it magnifies the difficulties inherent in forming successful rural integrated health delivery systems by adding another set of organizations to the mix. If successful, it holds a great deal of promise for local communities because the employers in a community share a direct financial interest in keeping the local health care delivery system financially sound. Conversely, this model also requires that the health care providers cede some of the decision making about their business activities to organizations outside of health care delivery. Popular during the early 1990s when national health care reform seemed possible,[32] this model has not proven to be a sustainable option.

The second model, provider-sponsored managed care (HMO) plans, is a more likely scenario. This option at times has been equally popular in urban and rural areas. In recent years it has fallen out of favor, particularly in urban areas. Nationally, the percentage of HMOs owned by hospitals fell from 8 percent in 1997 to 7.6 percent in 1998. Provider-based plans in large urban markets seemed most vulnerable, suffering large losses and being forced out by large competing plans. One conclusion drawn from a survey of HMOs and offered by proponents of the provider-sponsored plan model is that such plans are most likely to succeed in small or regional markets.[33] However, doing this in a rural market requires the capitalization described earlier in this chapter, which precludes many providers in many small markets because they are unable to raise the requisite cash investment to start a plan and sustain the early losses that are likely to occur. However, rural networks with a sufficient number of investors will continue to consider this approach, and rural networks anchored by a large institution, such as the Marshfield Clinic, will continue as provider-owned plans.

A variation of the second model, and a transition to the third (contracting with other health plans), is to establish a partnership between local providers and a commercial insurance entity. This is the organizational structure, for example, used by the Yellowstone Community Health Plan in Montana. This plan grew from enrolling 3,100 lives in a commercial insurance product in December 1995 to enrolling 11,500 people with commercial insurance, 600 Medicaid beneficiaries, and 2,600 Medicare clients in May 1999 (the plan withdrew from Medicare in January 2000 because of inadequate payment from Medicare). The plan is a partnership of a large hospital and health center in Billings, Montana, with Blue Cross & Blue Shield of Montana.[34]

The third model is a rural provider network that contracts on behalf of its members with managed care plans. Rural providers may resist forming their own plans because of inherent opposition to managed care. When faced with increased enrollment into managed care plans by the insured persons in their communities, these providers may be more willing to join forces in negotiations with plans than to form their own plan. Such was the case in Porterville, California, an eastern county that was not part of the initial movement in the cities of California to managed care but by 1992 became an area that plans from Bakersfield began to find attractive. As a result, local physicians, who had resisted any efforts to organize for the purposes of participating in managed care, formed an IPA. By 1995 the IPA included 190 physicians with an annual operating budget of $5 million. The physicians then joined with the hospital in the county to form a physician-hospital organization (PHO), the Sierra Health Network. The goal of the PHO was to enter into favorable contracts with managed care organizations by using capitation as the method of provider payment, so that provider income would remain secure. As of the end of 1995 the network had enrolled 15,000 persons and had created a successful risk pool that yielded $400,000 annually. Sierra Health Network was successful because it followed the practices described earlier in this chapter to help market the managed care plan locally and followed practices of medical management (quality assurance) that lowered utilization of services and yielded higher returns from the risk pool.[35] This third model is not one, then, of simply signing agreements with insurance plans for the purposes of seeing patients enrolled in those plans. Instead, it is one of choosing plans and negotiating terms that enhance local provision of health care services. The most effective negotiation strategies are to learn as much as possible about what will make the plan successful and to participate in those elements of the plan that affect the practice of care. For example, successful managed care relies on medical management of episodes of illness, and local rural providers

should negotiate a role in that effort. Local rural providers should have a role in marketing the plan and in determining what is the best design of the plan for their unique rural environment.[36]

CONCLUSION

Managed care plans involving networks of rural health care providers can be designed by and for rural communities. Doing so, though, requires at least as much effort as is needed in competitive urban environments. Providers scattered over greater geographical areas, and working independently or for different organizations, need to be knit together as providers of choice in a managed care plan. In many rural areas this alone will require a great deal of time and effort on the part of plan administrators. Additional time is required to allow rural providers to develop the management skills and systems needed to make a managed care plan work in their unique environment. This time can be shortened through partnerships of rural organizations with urban-based health plans that have more mature systems of financing, marketing, and pricing health benefits.

REFERENCES AND NOTES

1. A. Birenbaum, *Managed Care: Made in America* (Westport, CT: Praeger, 1997).

2. R. Kronick et al., Special Report—The Market Place in Health Care Reform: The Demographic Limitations of Managed Competition, *The New England Journal of Medicine* 328 (1993): 148–52.

3. I. Moscovice et al., *Rural Managed Care: Patterns and Prospects* (Minneapolis, MN: Rural Health Research Center, University of Minnesota, 1997).

4. S. Krein and M. Casey, Research on Managed Care Organizations in Rural Communities, *The Journal of Rural Health*, 14 (1998): 3, 180–99.

5. R.T. Slifkin et al., Medicaid Managed Care Programs in Rural Areas: A Fifty-State Overview, *Health Affairs* 17, (1998): 6, 217–27.

6. From the Health Care Financing Administration web site: www.hcfa.gov/medicaid.omcpr98.htm

7. Rural Policy Research Institute Rural Health Panel, *Implementation of the Provisions of the Balanced Bud-*

get Act of 1997: Critical Issues for Rural Health Care Delivery (Columbia, MO: Rural Policy Research Institute, July 29, 1999).

8. K. Haddadd and L. Slass, *Rural Neglect: Medicare HMOs Ignore Rural Communities* (Washington, DC: Families USA, 1999).

9. S.D. Jones, Oregon Prepares To Revise Its Struggling Health Plan, *Wall Street Journal*, April 28, 1999.

10. M. Casey and A. Wellever, United Health Care of North Carolina, *The Journal of Rural Health* 14 (1998): 3, 200–10.

11. A. Wellever and J. Christianson, Medical Associates HMO, *The Journal of Rural Health* 14 (1998): 3, 224–32.

12. M. Casey and I. Moscovice, Regence HMO Oregon, *The Journal of Rural Health* 14 (1998): 3, 244–56.

13. Jones, Oregon Prepares To Revise Its Struggling Health Plan.

14. A. Wellever and I. Moscovice, Rocky Mountain HMO, *The Journal of Rural Health* 14 (1998): 3, 211–23.

15. J. Christianson and S. Krein, NorthMed HMO, *The Journal of Rural Health* 14 (1998): 3, 233–43.

16. M. Casey and B. Yawn, Missouri Advantage, *The Journal of Rural Health* 14 (1998): 3, 257–67.

17. C. Beam, Is Medicare Managed Care a Viable Option for Your Organization? Paper presented at the annual meeting of the National Rural Health Association; May 1999; San Diego, CA.

18. A.H. Butcher and J.C. Szekely, Report from the Front Lines: Rural Medicaid Primary Care Providers as Gatekeepers of Rural Health Service Networks, *Journal of the Louisiana Medical Society* 150 (1998): 372–83.

19. I. Moscovice et al., Rural Health Networks: Concepts, Cases and Public Policy, *Report of the Rural Health Research Center* (Minneapolis, MN: University of Minnesota, 1996).

20. Moscovice, Rural Health Networks: Concepts, Cases and Public Policy.

21. Moscovice, Rural Health Networks: Concepts, Cases and Public Policy.

22. M. Casey, Integrated Networks and Health Care Provider Cooperatives: New Models for Rural Health Care Delivery and Financing, *Health Care Management Review* 22 (1997): 2, 41–58.

23. N.J. Fasciano et al., Preparing Rural Communities for Managed Care: Lessons Learned, *The Journal of Rural Health* 15 (1999): 1, 78–86.

24. Fasciano, Preparing Rural Communities for Managed Care: Lessons Learned.

25. D. Hartley et al., AHCPR-Funded Rural Managed Care Centers: Report from the Field, *The Journal of Rural Health* 15 (1999): 1, 87 93.

26. S. Jordon, HMOs Say Higher Premiums Await, *Omaha World-Herald*, August 21, 1999: 1-M.

27. Rural Health Research Center, Rural Physician Risk-Sharing: Insights and Issues, Minneapolis, MN: Division of Health Services Research and Policy, School of Public Health, University of Minnesota. April, 1998.

28. K. Mueller, Rural Implications of the Balanced Budget Act of 1997: A Rural Analysis of the Health Policy Provisions. RUPRI Rural Health Panel P97-10 (Columbia, MO: The Rural Policy Research Institute, 1997). Available: www.rupri.org

29. M.D. Dalzell, PPOs: A Better Brand of Managed Care? *Managed Care Magazine.* July 13, 1999 www.managedcaremag.com/archiveMC/9906/9906.ppos.html

30. B.Z. Harness, Innovative Approaches to Integrated Rural Health Delivery. Paper presented at the 20th annual conference, National Rural Health Association; May 1997.

31. The illustrations used thus far were taken from: B.Z. Harness, Innovative Approaches to Integrated Rural Health Delivery. Paper presented at the 20th annual conference, National Rural Health Association; May 1997.

32. A.J. DeFail (interviewed), Three's Company: Hospital, Physicians, and Community Make a Strong Alliance, *Hospitals & Health Networks,* October 20, 1993: 10.

33. C. Rauber, Market Deflates for Provider-Owned HMOs: Survey Shows Many Plans Are Losing Ground to Growing National and Regional Players, *Modern HealthCare,* June 14, 1999: 34.

34. C.A. Beam, Is Medicare Managed Care a Viable Option for Your Organization? Paper presented at the annual meeting of the National Rural Health Association; May 1999; San Diego, CA.

35. C.F. Haberkern, Developing Managed Strategies: A Case Study in Progress. Paper presented to the Rural Health Care Leadership Conference; February 1996; Scottsdale, AZ.

36. M. Martell, *Coordinated Managed Care: A Handbook for Rural Providers* (Portland, OR: Oregon Health Sciences University Office of Rural Health, 1992).

CHAPTER 60

Managed Care Dental Benefits

Fred L. Horowitz, Bruce H. Safran, Wayne A. Paul, and Evelyn F. Ireland

Before we discuss this topic, we must first define the term, "managed care" as it relates to the field of payment for dental care. In the dental benefits marketplace, this term represents any program that provides dental benefits and is designed to affect the cost of the benefits and quality of the care through changes to either the system of delivery or the provider reimbursement. Managed dental care benefit plans fall into three broad categories:

- dental health maintenance organizations (DHMOs)

This chapter was originally drafted by Fred L. Horowitz, DMD, who is currently President of Affiliated Network Services, an administrative and consulting firm specializing in the dental care benefits industry. He has been involved with the dental managed care industry for the past 18 years as both provider and administrator. Formerly, Dr. Horowitz served as Vice-President of Dental Products for Employers Health Insurance Co., a wholly owned subsidiary of Humana, Inc., and President of TDC/The Dental Concern, Ltd., a Midwestern dental HMO that was purchased by Humana. He has served on the Board of Directors of the National Association of Dental Plans and now chairs the Board of its nonprofit foundation for research in the dental benefits industry.

In 1999, the original chapter was updated by NADP's Executive Director, Evelyn F. Ireland, CAE, and two members of the NADP Board of Directors, Dr. Bruce H. Safran, Vice-President of National Marketing for Healthplex (New York) and Wayne A. Paul, Executive Vice-President of United Concordia Companies Inc. (Maryland).

- dental preferred provider organizations (DPPOs)
- dental referral plans often referred to as discount, or access, plans

In most states companies offering DHMO products must obtain a separate license. Until the mid-90s most DHMOs were stand-alone companies. In the late 1990s the phenomenal growth of DHMO enrollment resulted in more public trading of stand-alone DHMOs and acquisitions by traditional insurers. Thus, the structure of the dental managed care industry, which was initially largely focused on the DHMO product, has changed. Today, many companies hold licenses both as DHMOs and as insurers authorized to write both indemnity and PPO products.

DPPOs are a product line that can be offered by conventional indemnity or insurance companies. These companies may also offer other dental products with certain features of managed care such as preauthorization of services or utilization review. Dental referral products are offered by companies that offer only this product line, as well as DHMOs and traditional insurance companies that offer other dental product lines.

DENTAL HMOs

A dental HMO, also referred to as a prepaid or capitation plan, is an organization that provides dental services to enrollees (members) for some form of prepayment. Those services are provided through a group practice or network of dentists, and payment for dental services rendered is usually through a combination of per member per month (PMPM) capitation payments to the practitioners paid by the dental HMO and copayments for services paid by the enrollee. Co-payments can be made on a schedule of dollar amounts or percentages. A schedule of dollar amounts is most common.

Differing significantly from the indemnity world, claims are a minor or nonexistent part of dental HMOs. A gatekeeper approach to specialty care and some form of quality improvement program are hallmarks of these programs. As marketed today, they are really the most extensive form of truly "managed" dental care on the market because they have some quality of care oversight components in addition to a payment system that "incentivizes" cost-conscious care.

Dental HMOs currently operate in all of the states and at least three countries outside the United States (Canada, Mexico, and Great Britain). Most dental HMOs in the United States were formed in the mid-to-late 80s. Since 1990, the growth of dental HMOs has been phenomenal, from approximately 7.8 million members in 1990 to 26.5 million in 1997 in the United States alone (Table 60–1). According to the National Association of Dental Plans (NADP), in 1998 the industry was projected to grow an additional 17.5 percent. About 10 percent of this growth is in Medicaid programs.

As would be expected, participation in dental HMOs is concentrated in the most populous states and regions. California has the most enrollment, with approximately 8 million residents participating in dental HMOs. California, Florida, Texas, Illinois, and Pennsylvania combined account for about 60 percent of the total enrollment. The top 10 states account for more than 75 percent of the total enrollment in the United States.[1]

Concomitantly, the location and numbers of participating practitioners follow a similar pattern. More than 21,000 general dentists and 10,600 specialists report participating in one or more dental HMOs.[2] This represents more than 21.6 percent of all dentists in private practice.

Most dental HMO benefit plans are sold to employer groups. Of those, approximately 55 percent are paid for in whole or in part by the employer.[3] Another 21.5 percent are sold on a voluntary basis through employers with no employer contribution. Of the remaining 23.5 percent, individual plans represent 2.6 percent; those plans serving the public sector, Medicare and Medicaid, have grown to 7 percent and 11.6 percent, respectively.

DENTAL PPOs

Dental PPOs are generally not companies but a benefit design that is sold by indemnity insurance companies. Dental PPOs take various forms in terms of structure and design. The PPO models can, and most often do, provide many of the managed care components of the dental HMO model such as credentialing, gatekeeper provisions for specialty care, quality assurance, and utilization review (UR). PPOs, in their least managed form, can simply be a contracted network of dental providers giving discounts.

There are two principal benefit models delivered through dental PPOs. The first is known as a "passive PPO." In this model, the member may seek care from any dentist; however, the employer benefits from payer discounts when the employee uses a contracted network provider. The more common "patient direction" model is one in which patients are directed to network providers to receive the maximum benefit. Care provided by non-network dentists is paid at a reduced benefit. This patient direction model can provide the same managed care features as the dental HMO; however, PPO services are typically reimbursed on a discounted fee-for-service basis or a fee schedule.

Dental PPOs offer employers several advantages, which can include:

- larger, more accessible networks
- minimal geographical restrictions
- patient direction and managed care provisions
- effectiveness at managing cost

The dental PPO model has experienced significant growth, growing at almost four times

Table 60–1 The Dental Benefits Industry at a Glance

Line of Business	1994	1995	1996	1997	1997 Growth Rate	1997 % of Total Market
Dental HMO	18,301,250	20,697,452	24,359,434	26,457,650	8.61%	18.0%
Dental PPO fully insured	9,708,907	11,479,177	9,936,816	12,927,842		
Dental PPO self-insured	1,989,335	2,606,004	8,505,400	11,532,220		
Dental PPO subtotal	11,698,242	14,085,181	18,442,216	24,460,062	32.63%	16.6%
Dental referral networks	2,248,399	1,920,330	5,033,866	5,453,264	8.33%	3.7%
Dental managed care subtotal	32,247,891	36,702,963	47,835,516	56,370,976	17.84%	38.3%
Dental indemnity fully insured	18,944,655	20,600,903	29,841,309	32,657,379		
Dental indemnity self-insured	5,135,613	10,367,339	20,688,556	20,189,509		
Estimated additional indemnity		49,287,104	37,793,938	37,793,938		
Indemnity subtotal	24,080,268	80,255,346	88,323,803	90,640,826	2.62%	61.7%
Estimate: Total dental benefits market	56,328,159	116,958,309	136,159,319	147,011,802	7.97%	100.0%

Source: Reprinted with permission from NADP/InterStudy 1998 Dental HMO/PPO Industry Profile and InterStudy reports, *1999 NADP Foundation Dental Plan Accreditation Standards v.1 (DPAS v.1),* September 12, 1999, p. 5, National Association of Dental Plans Foundation and the National Association of Dental Plans.

the rate of growth of dental HMOs in 1997. At the end of 1997 more than 24 million individuals were covered through dental PPOs.

REFERRAL PLANS

Access or referral plans are neither a form of dental insurance nor dental managed care. Rather, they are a form of marketing large networks of providers to the public for a small fee. The benefit offered is access to a provider network that has agreed to reduce fees. However, the individual must pay the entire fee, albeit discounted, of the provider for the services received. The referral plan pays no part of the provider's fees but simply negotiates the discounts. At the end of 1997, 5.4 million individuals were receiving dental benefits through dental referral plans.

For the remainder of this chapter, the discussion of "managed care" will be focused on dental HMOs (prepaid plans) and dental PPOs as the primary forms of dental managed care in the market today.

Like medical HMOs and insurance carriers, dental HMOs are regulated at the state level under one of the following enabling statutes:

- limited health service organization (8 states)
- single-service HMOs (9 states)
- prepaid dental plans (18 states)
- dental service corporation or plan (29 states)
- dental-only health corporation (1 state)
- no regulation (states and the District of Columbia)

Note: Some states have multiple licensing statutes allowing both for profit and not-for-profit dental plans. Dental PPOs are currently regulated in 24 states.

In addition some states allow life and health indemnity carriers to offer prepaid products and dental PPOs. Unlike medical HMOs, dental HMOs cannot be licensed at the federal level. Thus, homogeneity of operating structure is sometimes absent in dental HMOs.

The NADP, the trade association of network-based dental plans, was founded to respond to the development of a standard licensing statute for dental HMOs. The Prepaid Limited Health Service Organization (PLHSO) model was promulgated by the National Association of Insurance Commissioners with input from the NADP in 1989. To date, this enabling act has been adopted in eight states with minor variances. As the industry matures and more national companies become involved, state statutes and regulations should become more constant from state to state.

THE DENTAL DELIVERY SYSTEM

Dental HMOs and dental PPOs offer benefits through a network of practicing dentists. These networks take several forms. Many dental HMOs are now using a combination of these models to offer their members more variety and stable rates from year to year. Dental PPOs generally follow the independent practice association (IPA) model.

The staff practice model is similar to the earliest forms of medical HMOs. In this model, the carrier or plan owns the facilities and uses employee dentists and ancillary personnel to provide care. This is usually the most restrictive network in that choice is limited to those sites that the plan operates. Although no conclusive research has been done, anecdotal surveys indicate that this is the most profitable type of arrangement for the plans and has the most predictable costs.

The IPA model is a network made up of independently practicing dentists, usually at many sites, who contract individually with the plan to provide care at a predetermined rate. The benefit to the member is usually a larger selection of practitioners from which to choose. The payment mechanism to those dentists may be more complex and usually is not as predictable as in the staff model because a degree of control is relinquished to the practicing dentist. At the same time, the risk is more often shared by those dentists to a larger degree. This is the most common form of dental HMO and dental PPO available today.

The group model is similar to the IPA model except that the dentists are organized into one or more groups, which in turn contract with the carrier or plan. This may give the groups a better negotiating edge with the carrier, but the needs of the individual dentists may be lost to the homogeneity of the group contract.

RECRUITING

The first step in organizing a dental HMO or dental PPO, after licensure and plan design, is recruiting the providers to participate in the program. Here a major difference occurs between medical prepaid plans and dental programs. In medical plans, one or more hospitals are the focus of the program, and the networks of practicing physicians are recruited to complement those care centers. In contrast, the dental delivery system is focused on the individual dental office, so that there is no central organization around which to recruit. Most dental HMOs start by recruiting a core group of dentists and then extending the network, by referral, from that core group. The recruitment process can be tedious and slow because there are no central bodies, such as hospitals, to endorse one plan or another or to aid in recruitment through its membership and the methods of payment are unique. This difference becomes a bit less apparent if the network is a staff or group model. Recruitment for dental PPOs is somewhat less difficult because the method of payment is based on fee-for-service albeit reduced.

CREDENTIALING

Because of the patchwork of state regulation, the credentialing process varies greatly from state to state and from company to company. Some states, such as California, prescribe specific quality assessment standards that affect the credentialing process for dental HMOs. Others have no requirements or standards for credentialing.

A survey by NADP in 1998 found that all dental HMOs and virtually all dental PPOs credential providers before admitting them to the network. However, there is a wide variety in the information collected. Plans that contract with medical HMOs to provide a dental benefit often use the credentialing guidelines established by the National Committee for Quality Assurance (NCQA; see Chapter 44) for consistency with the medical plan's requirements. This organization has standardized the credentialing process into 10 elements and certifies companies that can demonstrate their ability to follow the guidelines within certain time frames. The process includes, but is not limited to, verification of the following items: dental school graduation, a license to practice dentistry, DEA registration, malpractice insurance/claims history, and a query of the National Practitioner Databank.

Most dental HMOs also conduct site visits of participating dental offices. This is done to verify that the dentists are complying with Occupational Safety and Health Administration regulations, are properly sterilizing their equipment, maintain an emergency medical kit, and are following plan guidelines for treating and referring members. Credentialing and site visits are extremely important functions for managed care plans because they lend credibility to a health care delivery system that is frequently challenged in the media. The NADP Foundation published the Dental Plan Accreditation Standards (DPAS) in the fall of 1999. The intent of DPAS is to identify credentialing elements for dental plans to create consistency across state lines and regions.

COMPENSATION

Because dental plans are less complex than their medical counterparts, so too are their compensation mechanisms. Because there are no hospitals involved in the delivery system, dental HMOs contract directly with their participating providers or a group representing those providers (an IPA). Most dental HMOs compensate their participating general dentists on a capitated basis (PMPM or per subscriber per month[4]). Most dental PPOs use a schedule of fees or reduced fees for services.

There are two commonly used methods for determining the amount of capitation and any member copayment. The first involves calculating the anticipated number and type of procedures that will be performed in a specified time period for a specific population and assigning a fee-for-service equivalent to those procedures. After member copayments are determined (for the most part a market-driven event), the PMPM amount can be derived from the anticipated fee-for-service equivalent. The amount is usually discounted on the basis of factors such as reduced billing costs, marketing and collection activities, and increased volume. The second, and probably more accurate, method is to assign relative time units to each anticipated procedure. These time units can then be assigned a dollar value, depending on geographical, population, and practice style factors. From this a PMPM amount can be determined.

Specialty practitioners can also be compensated on the basis of a similar capitation process. To be successful, however, a large volume of prospective patients is required. Many dental HMOs do not have adequate membership to make this a viable alternative, so that compensation is usually made on a negotiated fee-for-service basis, similar to a PPO. As the industry matures, more plans will turn to capitating their participating specialists. In parts of the country where dental HMOs have not reached a level of sophistication comparable with that of their medical counterparts, specialty services may be offered on a discounted fee-for-service basis to the member with no compensation (no risk) from the dental HMO.

UTILIZATION REVIEW

UR is a statistically based system that examines the distribution of treatment procedures on the basis of claims or encounter information. By identifying variation and aberrance from normative patterns established in claims and/or encounter data, opportunities for improvement can be identified. In dental HMOs or PPOs, UR helps to determine whether the organization or benefit plan is meeting its goals to its members, clients, and providers.

In dental PPOs, UR is based on extensive claims data whereas, in dental HMOs, sampling techniques are often used.

In addition to broad analysis, UR examines individual practice profiles to verify that the population assumptions as well as the specific compensation compared with that of the group are correct. For the client, this UR determines whether the premiums being paid are in line with the amount and type of services being performed.

QUALITY IMPROVEMENT

Dentistry has relatively few valid performance measures. Historically, performance in dentistry has been evaluated on the basis of "technical proficiency" in the dental "art" or "craft."[5] During the 80s the dental profession broadened its evaluation of quality using a "structure, process, and outcome" model.[6] This limits quality improvement activities in any form of dental managed care benefits program.

Interest has increased in the development and application of quality and performance measures to network-based dental plans. A number of corporations and organizations have created a variety of tools and techniques designed to measure performance in dentistry and, specifically, in network-based dental plans like dental HMOs and PPOs.

At present, the predominant type of company with functional, formalized quality assessment and improvement programs in place is the dental HMO. The programs range from "performance report cards,"[7] oral health status indices, and site and dental record audits.[8] Seven dental professional organizations have developed or are developing dental practice guidelines or "parameters," although none are universally accepted and most are not measurable.[9]

Development of true quality assessment measures is critical to the long-term success of dental HMOs and dental PPOs. A key element of measurement is the development of diagnostic codes. The American Dental Association released the first set of diagnostic codes in the summer of 1999. It is expected to take several years for the codes to be put into wide enough use for them to be used as a basis for measurement purposes.

SPECIALTY CARE

Provision for specialty care providers is key to obtaining and maintaining the dental health of an insured population. In addition to recruiting networks of primary care providers, maturing dental HMOs and PPOs must recruit, credential, and maintain networks of specialty care dentists, including oral and maxillofacial surgeons, endodontists, orthodontists, periodontists, pedodontists, and prosthodontists. Access to these specialists is usually provided through some form of gatekeeper approach. The primary care provider and the dental HMO or PPO, working in combination, control the referral process. When the need for a specialist to provide care is determined by the general dentist, a referral is made to a previously credentialed member of the specialty network following the procedures and protocols of the specific carrier or plan. For a routine procedure, this usually involves the general dentist submitting a written request to the carrier, along with a narrative and supporting radiographic documentation, requesting that certain benefits be approved at the specialist's office. After review, the carrier then notifies the referring dentist, the patient, or (in the best of circumstances) both of the approved procedures and benefit levels. The member is then able to make an appropriate appointment with the specialist. In some programs, the carrier or the primary provider actually makes the appointment for the member. In the event of a dental emergency, plans will generally allow the primary care dentist to refer directly to a participating specialist without prior approval. They also will usually allow a fixed dollar amount toward emergency care if such treatment is needed when the member is out of the plan's service area or if the patient's primary care dentist cannot be reached. Also, many programs allow the primary dentist and the patient a choice of specialists, so that a referral can be made taking into account convenience of location, hours of service, and specific skill sets required.

With the evolution of electronic data interchange, some carriers are streamlining this process for routine referrals, allowing online, real-time approval of specialty care referrals. As the technology improves and becomes more widespread, it is anticipated that this will become the standard for referrals.

ACCREDITATION

Unlike the case for medical managed care organizations, there is not an accreditation program for dental managed care organizations. The NCQA currently has credentialing protocols for medical HMOs that contract with dentists for delivery of certain medical services. These protocols are based on the medical practice model and are not applicable to a stand-alone dental network organized to deliver dental benefits.

NCQA, the Joint Commission on Accreditation of Healthcare Organizations, and URAC accreditation guidelines for medical managed care organizations were reviewed by a cross section of the dental industry in a 1998 Summit meeting sponsored by the NADP Foundation and found not to be appropriate for application to dental managed care organizations. Although multiple reasons were cited for this, a key reason cited was available funds to conduct administrative activity (see Figure 60–1).

On the basis of the discussions at that 1998 Summit meeting, the NADP Foundation developed DPAS. Version 1 of these standards was published in September 1999. NADP and the NADP Foundation are negotiating with several vendors to implement DPAS V.1 for network-based dental plans. The first accreditations are expected in 2001. Until that time, the industry is using DPAVV.1 as a voluntary standard.

CONCLUSION

By far the largest growing segment in the dental benefits industry, as in the medical benefits industry, is comprised of various forms of managed care delivery. In fact, recent market data show that indemnity dental plan enrollment is relatively flat. Statistics from various sources indicate the strong growth of the dental HMO and

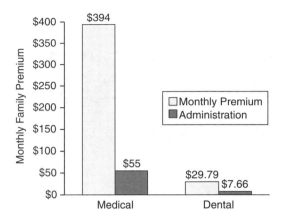

Figure 60–1 1997 Portion of Family HMO Premium Available for Administrative Expense. *Source:* Reprinted with permission from NADP/InterStudy 1998 Dental HMO/PPO Industry Profile and InterStudy reports, *1999 NADP Foundation Dental Plan Accreditation Standards v.1 (DPAS v.1),* September 12, 1999, p. 5, National Association of Dental Plans Foundation and the National Association of Dental Plans.

PPO markets at the expense of the traditional indemnity plan. The specific plan type varies from geographical area to geographical area, with dental HMOs being strongest in large metropoli-

tan centers and dental PPOs being strongest in smaller cities and more rural environs.

As these plans mature, their success will depend on the cooperative working relationship of dentists, carriers, and employers to ensure that proper plan designs, access, delivery of care, and compensation are provided. As in the medical managed care industry, this maturation process seems to occur in large population centers first and then migrates to smaller communities over time. If successful, these types of plans will become the dominant form of dental insurance as we cross into the new millennium because they provide cost predictability, comprehensive coverage, and access to care for the largest population at the most appropriate cost.

Most dental benefit companies—managed care organizations and traditional dental insurers—are represented by the NADP, located in Dallas, Texas. This trade organization was established in 1989 to act as a forum and voice for the industry. Further information about this growing industry may be obtained by contacting the NADP at 5001 LBJ Freeway, Suite 375, Dallas, Texas 75244-6160, calling (972) 458-6998, or visiting NADP Direct, their website at www.nadp.org.

REFERENCES AND NOTES

1. InterStudy, *1998 Dental HMO/PPO Industry Profile* (Dallas, TX: InterStudy Publications and National Association of Dental Plans, 1998), 25.

2. InterStudy, *1998 Dental HMO/PPO Industry Profile*, 30.

3. InterStudy, *1998 Dental HMO/PPO Industry Profile*, 15, 17.

4. A subscriber is the "paying unit"; members are subscribers and their dependents.

5. J. Bader and D. Shugars, Variation, Treatment Outcomes, and Practice Guidelines in Dental Practice. *Journal of Dental Education* 59 (1995): 61–62.

6. Bader and Shugars, Variation, Treatment Outcomes, and Practice Guidelines in Dental Practice, 83.

7. *The Prudential Develops Industry's First Managed Dental Report Card.* Press Release. The Prudential Insurance Company of America, April 6, 1995.

8. D.S. Mayes, *Managed Dental Care: A Guide to Dental HMOs* (Brookfield, WI: International Foundation of Employee Benefit Plans, 1993), 122–128.

9. Bader and Shugars, Variation, Treatment Outcomes, and Practice Guidelines in Dental Practice, 82–83.

CHAPTER 61

Workers' Compensation Managed Care: The Search for Integration

Alex L. Swedlow and Gregory L. Johnson

INTRODUCTION

Recent spikes in medical costs, coupled with the intense competitive pressures faced by employers, have fueled an increased focus on controlling medical costs while not reducing the quality and outcome of services. Although the use of health maintenance organizations (HMOs), preferred provider organizations (PPOs), and point-of-service plans was successful in slowing the rate of health care inflation in group plans, it is only in recent years that employers and insurance carriers have taken additional steps to control inflation in workers' compensation medical costs.

This chapter identifies the key trends, successes, and promises in workers' compensation managed care. The most important long-term trend is the integration of the health care, workers' compensation, and group disability industries. Al-

---

Alex L. Swedlow, MHSA, is a principal at Applied Outcomes Research in Sacramento, California. He has over 13 years of senior level experience in applied research to the fields of health services research, medical and disability program design and management, workers' compensation, and data and analytics development.

Gregory L. Johnson, PhD, is a partner in the strategic change practice at Pricewaterhouse Coopers in San Francisco. He has directed organizational transformations and merger integration efforts at managed care organizations, property casualty insurance companies, and major computer manufacturers.

though complete integration may elude the market for some time to come, the impact of changes in the larger health care industry is already having a dramatic effect on workers' compensation.

WORKERS' COMPENSATION: THE ORIGIN OF THE SOCIAL CONTRACT

Workers' compensation was the United States' first widely developed form of no-fault insurance—a system in which employees do not have to prove an injury was the result of worksite conditions in order to receive medical and replacement wage (disability) benefits for an on-the-job injury. Workers' compensation operates as a social contract between the employee and employer, in which the employee receives prompt benefits and medical treatment, if necessary, and the employer provides the "exclusive remedy" for the injured employee. The no-fault system was designed to eliminate litigation over employer negligence or "fault." Litigation contributes to other issues, such as whether injuries occurred on the job or what amount of benefits an injured worker is entitled to receive. *The array of benefits injured employees are eligible to receive includes:*

- medical care designed to "cure and relieve" the effects of an injury or illness
- temporary disability benefits intended to provide coverage until the employee is able to return to work

- permanent disability benefits, if the injury or illness causes some degree of permanent impairment
- vocational rehabilitation services, designed to rehabilitate the injured or ill employee back into the work force
- death benefits provided to the family

Since workers' compensation is a mandatory benefit paid to relieve the effects of a work-related injury or illness, no copayment is required from the individual receiving care. This leaves the major mechanisms for controlling medical expenditures—risk-sharing with the medical providers of care, access to specialists, and referral to specialists—more difficult to manage within the workers' compensation system.

Workers' compensation is essentially a state system with variations in benefit levels, medical reimbursement schedules, and the degree to which an employer can control the medical choices made by the employee. The existence of state regulations governing workers' compensation, however, does not prohibit the employer from exercising a degree of control over medical costs. In fact, most states allow employers to direct how employees are cared for after a work-related injury, although the degree of control allowed varies greatly. These state variations must be understood before appropriate managed care products can be designed for employers across the country. Although state regulations differ, the trend is clearly toward integrating workers' compensation into a managed, single-source health care delivery system. As one of the last fee-for-service systems, workers' compensation has often been the victim of cost shifting from more managed payment systems or upcoding of conditions by physicians, who know that workers' compensation often allows greater levels of utilization and reimbursement. These differences in medical practice patterns were documented in recent studies by researchers at the California Workers Compensation Institute and the Minnesota Department of Labor and Industry, which indicated that workers' compensation charges for injuries were 30 to 250 percent more expensive when handled as a workers' compensa-

tion claim compared with the average group health indemnity plans for a similar mix of injuries.[1,2]

EARLY CONTROLS ON MEDICAL COSTS

The trend toward integrating workers' compensation with traditional health care delivery systems has been driven in part by the changing role that insurers have played in the market. Nearly 70 percent of all American employers are currently covered for their workers' compensation costs through property and casualty insurance on a guaranteed-cost, fully insured basis. This trend is the converse of traditional group health, where 60 percent of companies are self-insured and only 40 percent are in fully insured plans. Insurance carriers generally have viewed workers' compensation medical and indemnity costs as a pass through to the insured employers, to be recouped the following year in higher premiums.

What was the impetus for cost containment efforts in the workers' compensation system? As shown in Figures 61–1 and 61–2, a 44 percent relative spike in medical losses and a 108 percent increase in indemnity losses (replaced wages due to time loss from work) over a 10-year period, coupled with cut-throat insurance price competition during the 1990s, led many workers' compensation carriers to seek solutions to control their costs more effectively, especially medical costs. This cost crisis led to the first generation of medical cost containment: hospital and medical bill audits and PPO discounts. Bill audits—a fee adjustment of billed charges against state-regulated fee schedules or usual and customary charges, further reduced by provider and hospital PPO discounts—produced varying results, depending on the effectiveness of their execution. The highest-yield programs audit all hospital and medical bills and drive more than 30 percent of all provider billings into PPO networks, with discounts averaging 25 percent. Most payers continue to rely on these first-generation controls. Despite the unit price cost controls of fee schedules and PPO discounts, utilization quickly eroded the early success of this strategy.

Figure 61–1 Average Medical Payment per Indemnity Claim. *Source:* Data from the Workers' Compensation Insurance Rating Board.

The second generation of cost control rests on a cardinal principle of managed care: To be effective, both unit price and volume of services must be controlled. Second-generation techniques apply utilization controls, including hospital, surgical, and diagnostic test preauthorization, as well as focused management of high-volume, specialized providers (such as chiropractors and physical therapists). To be optimally effective, utilization management must be closely integrated with the claims function, as well as with first-generation techniques.[3,4] For

Figure 61–2 Average Indemnity Payment per Indemnity Claim. *Source:* Data from the Workers' Compensation Insurance Rating Board.

example, the claims adjuster must be aware of the utilization review findings because the adjuster can override any decision. Claims adjusters control millions of dollars in medical reserves and are key members of the carrier's team. Although many do not have any clinical training, they can be roadblocks to effective managed care. In addition, the utilization review decision must be part of the bill audit process because some unauthorized services may be paid without timely input from utilization review.

Employers and carriers recently have begun to address the indemnity portion of workers' compensation. Disability costs represent almost half of all workers' compensation expenditures. No payer would approve a plan that drives up disability costs while controlling medical costs. Like hospital utilization review, disability management uses injury-specific templates of expected lengths of disability. The most effective disability management programs adjust these templates for variations in sex, age, and occupation. In addition to disability duration guidelines, advanced disability management programs utilize clinical personnel to verify impairment, establish disability, determine functional capacity, and promote early return to work.

KEY SUCCESS FACTORS

HMOs have demonstrated the ability to manage and control group health costs and slow the growth rate of medical inflation. Employers and policymakers have encouraged HMOs to deliver workers' compensation services, and now more than 100 HMOs have workers' compensation departments. HMO products range from enhanced delivery of workers' compensation medical care to complete equity ownership of a workers' compensation carrier.

In identifying physicians, organized health plans must be attentive to the difference between primary and occupational care. Many primary care physicians do not understand occupational medicine beyond the most rudimentary treatment. These primary physicians must understand when the appropriate time is to refer a patient to an occupational medicine specialist.

Such specialists understand the difference between functional capacity and disability. Rather than simply labeling the worker disabled, it is essential to understand whether the person can actually carry out the specific job at which he or she is working. Technology now exists to identify selectively and profile physicians on a case-matched basis based upon their degree of efficiency in delivering occupational medical care.

TWENTY-FOUR HOUR COVERAGE: A SOLUTION IN SEARCH OF CUSTOMERS

Perhaps no phrase has stimulated as much product innovation and customer confusion in the insurance world over the past five years as "24-hour coverage." Since 1992, carriers and health plans have introduced more than 40 different products integrating portions of group health, group disability, and workers' compensation coverage. While the demand for new products has slowed over the past three years because of the availability of lower rates for workers' compensation, the interest in integrated products remains. The existence of three separate benefits systems leads to administrative waste and uneven medical and disability outcomes.

Recent studies have shown that an episode of care rendered under a workers' compensation program is three times as expensive to administer, on average, as a similar medical problem addressed through a group health plan. On the other hand, the duration of disability for the *identical* diagnosis is twice as long in group disability as it is in workers' compensation. Additionally, an uncoordinated approach leads to the development of loss prevention and return-to-work programs that can ignore the overlap between occupational and nonoccupational illnesses. For example, more than half of group disability claims are attributed to factors in the workplace, according to claimants.

Unfortunately, bundling health, disability, and workers' compensation benefits into one "coverage" (one risk, one financial policy) has not been possible because the underlying underwriting assumptions for each type of coverage differ dramatically. For example, an occurrence-based workers' compensation policy may require an insurer to pay for a single injury for 20 or more years. In the group health arena, the same 20-year medical problem may be covered by multiple carriers as the insurer is changed over time.

Product integration also presents licensing and regulatory complexities. This reflects the fact that employers purchase the three products from separate companies—a workers' compensation policy from a property and casualty insurer; group health and group disability from a property and casualty or life company; and group health from a life or health insurer or HMO. In many states the bureaucracy regulating workers' compensation may be different from that for life insurers and health plans. Under such circumstances, achieving consolidated operations or a joint venture can be challenging.

Because of the difficulty of attaining unified financing, efforts to date have focused on administrative integration, including unified policy forms, customized distribution through specially trained brokers, and coordinated underwriting and billing. In an integrated product sale, a single organization collects underwriting information, assists in comparing coverage and financing options, and helps the employer with enrollment. Members are given a single identification card, a unified benefits brochure, and a single 800-number to call for claims, along with a multibenefit provider directory. Some products also have attempted, with varying success, to designate a specialized cadre of workers' compensation health care providers who should be used for occupational illnesses and injuries.

Case Study: Kaiser Permanente/State Compensation Insurance Fund of California Alliance Project

In what might be judged as the most successful integration of insurance operations and HMO service delivery, the Kaiser Permanente/State Compensation Insurance Fund of California Alliance Project serves as a model for how to leverage core competencies of managed care with coordinated case management. The "Alliance" between the State Compensation Insurance Fund and Kaiser Permanente was structured as a partnership between the state's largest workers' compensation carrier and the state's largest HMO.

Employers enrolled in the Alliance received a discount in premium for enrolling workers in the project. Injured workers were directed into one of Kaiser's occupational health clinics and triaged for care throughout the system. The injured workers were treated by a physician skilled in the knowledge of workers' compensation health care, the importance of return to work, and early referral to a specialist, if appropriate. The results of the four-year pilot completed in June 1999 are significant and represent dramatic decreases in both medical and disability (indemnity) costs for all claims in the study. In the controlled study of more than 10,000 Alliance and non-Alliance employees, the Alliance program showed:

- 20 percent and 24 percent relative decrease in average medical costs for claims *without* temporary disability and claims *with* temporary disability
- 16 percent difference in average total costs for all claims
- 11 percent reduction in average length of temporary disability on claims with temporary disability
- 32 percent reduction in litigation rate for claims with *and* without temporary disability

As found in the Alliance program profiled above, successful HMOs must retool their group health provider networks to provide comprehensive workers' compensation services. Less than 10 percent of group health medical providers understand workers' compensation medical treatment and reporting protocols. Knowledgeable providers must be identified, and specialists should be linked to primary care providers through specific referral procedures.

ADDRESSING WORKER EXPECTATIONS

When treating and counseling injured workers, the managed care professional must understand the concepts of entitlement and secondary gain. The injured worker, protected by law from copayments and deductibles, often feels entitled to benefits. This perspective can inflate workers' compensation medical costs when workers demand excessive medical services and delay their return to work as long as possible. Although most workers (85 percent) do not respond to an injury this way, the 15 percent who do account for a disproportionate share of cost to the employer.

Moreover, the majority of workers' compensation costs (55 percent) are not for medical benefits, but for disability benefits, primarily wage replacement. These benefits create, especially for low-wage workers, a secondary gain from the injury, whereby the worker benefits from a more exaggerated injury and higher medical expenses, which create a greater disability award.

These two simple concepts help us understand the opportunities and limitations in applying the precepts of managed care to workers' compensation. The most effective techniques to control workers' expectations involve clarity of clinical directions, treatment, and return to work date.

DEVELOPING PROTOCOLS FOR CASE MANAGEMENT

The most effective managed care plans will carefully incorporate medical and disability protocols into utilization management. Disability protocols will be based not simply on duration guidelines (specific target disability days by diagnosis) but rather on a complex understanding of the injury, the age and occupation of the injured worker, and the match of the functional capacity of the worker with specific job skills.

Medical protocols will be attentive to the requirement of some workers' compensation claims for intensive medical treatment early in the claim, including physical therapy and diagnostic testing. This type of treatment, which sometimes facilitates return to work, differs significantly from group health managed care protocols. Moreover, the most successful plans will incorporate methods for educating, monitoring, and reeducating providers regarding adherence to both types of protocols.

THE EMPLOYER PERSPECTIVE: CHANGING THE CORPORATE CULTURE

Managed workers' compensation has been a vendor-driven phenomenon. Employers are starting to realize its importance as a way of integrating benefits. Savvy employers now recognize that employee health benefits, workers' compensation, group disability, wellness, and employee assistance programs must be administered in a more unified fashion. The risk management department, on the finance side of the organization, traditionally administers workers' compensation as part of its property and casualty responsibilities. Human resources and employee benefits, a separate corporate silo, take responsibility for health benefits.

Long-term disability may not be on anyone's radar screen because it is often insured rather than offered as a benefit by a self-funded plan under the Employee Retirement Income Security Act (ERISA; see also Chapter 66). Thus the transition operation will probably include the removal of organizational silos and the fusion of a time-loss management program. In addition to these internal barriers, purchasers have been faced with a proliferation of specialty vendors that promise to manage certain elements of the employer's exposure more effectively. On the health benefits side, these carve-outs include behavioral health, various drug programs, wellness, and, more recently, disease-specific management. In workers' compensation, employers can choose third-party administrators, medical and hospital bill review organizations, case management, specialty providers for back or repetitive motion injuries, and a host of others. The cost of administering a multitude of carve-out vendors has led some employers to conclude that they are giving back the medical management savings in administrative friction and expense. For these employers, the prospect of carving in, or consolidating the management of all benefits, is attractive.

THE NEXT STEP: COMPREHENSIVE MEDICAL EVENTS MANAGEMENT

The goal of comprehensive medical event management is to minimize administrative expenses by creating centralized management of the entire range of health care services provided to employees, both occupational and nonoccupational. Although the concept may appear simple and straightforward, major changes in corporate culture and organizational structure must occur, and territorial issues between human resource departments and risk managers must be settled. Not to be underestimated, demands and expectations of workers must be addressed.

After a vision is developed of how medical events and overall employee down-time will be managed in the future, the challenge is how to get there from the current state of normal operations. Designers of a corporate benefits network must look at all the benefit components that impact employee productivity, whether it be a workers' compensation injury, other illness, or even a family crisis, with an eye on integration of those benefits so that workers do not migrate from a restricted managed care medical benefit into an unlimited workers' compensation and disability program. For many employers seeking to control both occupational (workers' compensation) and nonoccupational medical and disability costs and to maximize productivity, comprehensive medical event management will be the foundation of future health care savings. The core function in such a management system will be a single point of entry for notification and tracking of all medical events. This front end will be a robust triage system for tracking calls from employees and supervisors. There are three key benefits to establishing a single point of entry: early capture of lost-time events so that they can be managed optimally, construction of a data file for tracking multiple calls concerning a single event, and creation of a foundation for developing an enterprise-wide database on lost time.

An essential capability of the single-point-of-entry function will be integrated partnerships with managed care organizations. These organizations will have the ability to manage occupational or nonoccupational acute medical events efficiently and appropriately. In addition, future delivery models will have a mechanism for placing individual providers at partial risk for return to work.

The totally managed model will incorporate process maps for the optimal claims administration of each of the benefit systems that flow from the single entry point. For disability and workers' compensation, these claims-processing maps will include claims notification, case man-

agement, reserve setting, diagnosis-specific treatment protocols, return-to-work protocols, medical direction systems, and payment systems. For medical benefits, the administrative flow will be directed toward utilizing credentialed and contracted medical providers proficient in disability management. Finally, future savings strategies will include various programs such as comprehensive demand management, including self-care and lifestyle management, health promotion and disease prevention, safety, and ergonomics.

Case Study: Nationwide Puts It All Together

Further successes toward integration were found in a recent pilot project administered in 1997 by the Nationwide Insurance Company. This program featured an end-to-end tracking system, triggered by a centralized and integrated toll-free call center that recorded all employee time-loss events. Employees would contact the call center to report any time-loss event—whether workers' compensation, sick leave, family medical event, and so on. The call center and underlying databases would alert appropriate support structures including case management, Human Resources, or medical oversight. The key was in the creation of a centralized comprehensive disability management system that was able to measure direct and indirect costs and savings through effective participation of all parties involved (treating physician, employer, supervisor, and case managers). The program integrated on-line, reporting, monitoring, and disability management with a strong emphasis on return to work. A recent evaluation of program findings by Ernst & Young LLP showed a significant 20 percent reduction in lost-time days when compared to a comparable control group.[5]

CONCLUSION

Given the fact that more than $40 billion was paid to workers' compensation beneficiaries in 1998, it seems inevitable that managed health care techniques will be applied increasingly to the workers' compensation market. Farsighted managed care organizations and carriers will continue to emphasize high-quality, efficient medical event management.

Furthermore, employer interest in reducing employee downtime and the focus on return to work offer opportunities for organizations to integrate the management of both workers' compensation and group short- and long-term disability. The positive results achieved through the State Compensation/Kaiser Alliance, Nationwide Insurance, and other models leave significant optimism for employers, as costs are likely to increase in the near term. *The successful programs will likely include common elements:*

- An emphasis on return to work and productivity needs to be an essential component in all managed care programs involving employee disability.
- Physicians trained to handle the many clinical and medical-legal complexities of the workers' compensation system and skilled in return-to-work principles should be the primary caregivers for injured workers.
- Physicians should be rewarded for their success in returning employees to work and productivity.
- Payers and managed care organizations should actively cooperate in the medical and disability management of all workers' compensation claims.

Twenty-four-hour integration of two disparate benefits systems (one voluntary and one state mandated) continues to be slow in development due to the myriad complexities and infrastructures within both systems. Well-planned coordination and integration of medical management across these programs can create significant gains in total employee benefit plan value and productivity.

REFERENCES

1. B. Zaidman, Industrial Strength Medicine: A Comparison of Workers' Compensation and Blue Cross Health Care in Minnesota (Minneapolis: Minnesota Department of Labor and Industry, 1990), 83.

2. California Workers Compensation Institute (Oakland, CA, September 1994).

3. Final Florida Pilot Shows Big Gains from HMO, PPO, Workers' Compensation Managed Care (September 1994): 7.

4. J.R. Douglas, *Managing Workers' Compensation* (New York: Wiley Law Publications, 1994), 11.

5. Ernst & Young LLP, An Evaluation of the Nationwide Comprehensive Disability Management Program (January 1999).

PART VII

Regulatory and Legal Issues

"A wise government knows how to enforce with temper or to conciliate with dignity."

George Grenville
(1712–1770)
Speech against expulsion of John Wilkes, in Parliament [1769]

CHAPTER 62

Legal Issues in Provider Contracting

Mark S. Joffe

The business of a managed health care plan is to provide or arrange for the provision of health care services. Most managed health care plans such as health maintenance organizations (HMOs) or preferred provider organizations (PPOs) provide their services through arrangements with individual physicians, individual practice associations (IPAs), medical groups, hospitals, and other types of health care professionals and facilities. The provider contract formalizes the managed health care plan-provider relationship. A carefully drafted contract accomplishes more than mere memorializing of the arrangement between the parties. A well-written contract can foster a positive relationship between the provider and the managed health care plan. Moreover, a good contract can provide important and needed protections to both parties if the relationship sours.

This chapter offers the managed health care plan and the provider a practical guide to reviewing and drafting a provider contract. In the appendixes that follow the chapter are an HMO-primary care physician agreement and an HMO-hospital agreement. These contracts, which have been provided solely for illustrative purposes, have been annotated by the author. Although these agreements are used by an HMO, most provisions have equal applicability to other managed care plans.

Contracts need not be complex or lengthy to be legally binding and enforceable. A single-sentence letter agreement between a hospital and a managed health care plan that says that the hospital agrees to provide access to its facility to enrollees of the managed health care plan in exchange for payment of billed charges is a valid contract. If a single-paragraph agreement is legally binding, why is it necessary for managed health care plan-provider contracts to be so lengthy? The answer is twofold. First, many terms of the contract, although not required, perform useful functions by articulating the rights and responsibilities of the parties. As managed care has become an increasingly important revenue source to providers, a clear understanding of these rights and responsibilities correspondingly becomes increasingly important. Second, a growing number of contractual provisions are required by state licensure regulations (for example, a hold harmless clause) or by government payer programs, such as Medicare and Medicaid.

An ideal contract or contract form does not exist. Appropriate contract terms vary depending on the issues of concern and objectives of the parties, each party's relative negotiating strength, and the desired degree of formality. Although the focus of this chapter is explaining key substantive provisions in a contract, the importance of clarity cannot be overstated. A poorly written contract confuses and misleads the parties. Lack of clarity increases substantially the likelihood of disagreements over the

Mark S. Joffe is an attorney in private practice in Washington, DC, and specializes in legal and business issues affecting managed health care organizations.

meaning of contract language. A contract should not only be written in simple, commonly understood language but should be well organized so that either party is able to find and review provisions as quickly and easily as possible.

The need for clarity has become more important as contracts have become increasingly complex. Many managed health care plans may act as an HMO, PPO, and a third-party administrator. Those health care plans will frequently enter into a single contract with a provider to supply services in all three capacities. In addition, this single contract may obligate the provider to furnish services not only to the managed health care plan enrollees but to enrollees of a number of affiliates or nonaffiliates of the managed health care plan.

The following discussion is designed to provide a workable guide for managed health care plans and providers to draft, amend, or review contracts. Much of the discussion is cast from the perspective of the managed health care plan, but the points are equally valid from the provider's perspective. Most of the discussion relates to contracts directly between the managed health care plan and the provider of services. When the contract is between the managed health care plan and an IPA or medical group, the managed health care plan needs to ensure that the areas discussed below are appropriately addressed in both the managed health care plan's contract and the contract between the IPA or medical group and the provider.

GENERAL ISSUES IN CONTRACTING

Key Objectives

The managed health care plan should divide key objectives into two categories: those that are essential—the "musts"—and those that, although not essential, are highly desirable. Throughout the negotiations process a managed health care plan needs to keep in mind both the musts and the highly desirable objectives. Not infrequently, a managed health care plan or a provider will suddenly realize at the end of the negotiation process that it has not achieved all its basic goals. The managed health care plan's key objectives will vary. If the managed health care plan is in a community with a single provider of a particular specialty service, merely entering into a contract on any terms with the provider may be its objective. On the other hand, the managed health care plan's objectives might be quite complex, and it may demand carefully planned negotiations to achieve them.

Most objectives may derive from state and federal regulations, which may require or prohibit particular clauses in contracts. Managed health care plans need to be aware of these requirements and make sure that their contracting providers understand that these provisions are required by law.

Beyond the essential objectives are the highly desirable ones. Before commencing the drafting or the negotiation of the contract, the managed health care plan should list these objectives and have a good understanding of their relative importance. This preliminary thought process assists the managed health care plan in developing its negotiating strategy.

Annual Calendar

Key provider contracts may take months to negotiate. If the contemplated arrangement with the provider is important to the managed health care plan's delivery system, the managed health care plan will want to avoid the diminution of its bargaining strength as the desired effective date approaches.

The managed health care plan should have a master schedule identifying the contracts that need to be entered into and renewed. This schedule should include timelines that identify dates by which progress on key contract negotiations should take place. Although such an orderly system may be difficult to maintain, it may protect the managed health care plan from potential problems that may arise if it is forced to operate without a contract or to negotiate from a weakened position.

Letter of Intent Compared to Contract

The purpose of a letter of intent is to define the basic elements of a contemplated arrangement or transaction between two parties. A letter of intent is used most often when the negotiation process between two parties is expected to be lengthy and expensive. A letter of intent is a preliminary, nonbinding understanding that allows the parties to ascertain whether they are able to agree on key terms. If the parties agree on a letter of intent, the terms of that letter serve as the blueprint for the contract. Some people confuse a letter of intent with a letter of agreement. Because a letter of intent is not a legally binding agreement, regulators will not consider it in evaluating whether a managed care organization has made available and accessible the full range of services. Therefore, the use of a letter of intent should be limited to identifying the general parameters of a future contract.

Negotiating Strategy

Negotiating strategy is determined by objectives and relative negotiating strength. Depending on the locale or market dynamics, either the managed health care plan or the provider may have greater negotiating strength. Except in circumstances in which the relative negotiating strength is so one-sided that one party can dictate the terms to the other party, each party should identify for itself, before beginning negotiations, the negotiable issues, the party's initial position on each issue, and the extent to which it will compromise. Because a managed health care plan may use the same contract form as the contract for many providers, the managed health care plan needs to keep in mind the implications of amending one contract for the other contracts that use the same form.

A recurring theme presented at conference sessions discussing provider contracting and provider relations is the need to foster a win-win relationship, where both parties perceive that they gain from the relationship. The managed health care plan's objective should be fostering long-term, mutually satisfactory relationships with providers. When managed health care plans have enough negotiating strength to dictate the contract terms, they should exercise that strength cautiously to ensure that their short-term actions do not jeopardize their long-term goals.

CONTRACT STRUCTURE

As mentioned above, clarity is an important objective in drafting a provider contract. A key factor affecting the degree of clarity of a contract is the manner in which the agreement is organized. In fact, many managed health care plan contracts follow fairly similar formats. The contract begins with a title describing the instrument (for example, "Primary Care Physician Agreement"). After this is the caption, which identifies the names of the parties and the legal action taken, along with the transition, which contains words signifying that the parties have entered into an agreement. Then, the contract includes the recitals, which are best explained as the "whereas" clauses. These clauses are not intended to have legal significance but may become relevant to resolve inconsistencies in the body of the contract or if the drafter inappropriately includes substantive provisions in them. The use of the word *whereas* is merely tradition and has no legal significance.

The next section of the contract is the definitions section, which includes definitions of all key contract terms. The definitions section precedes the operative language, including the substantive health-related provisions that define the responsibilities and obligations of each of the parties, representations and warranties, and declarations. The last section of the contract, the closing or testimonium, reflects the assent of the parties through their signatures. Sometimes the drafters of a provider contract decide to have the signature page on the first page for administrative simplicity.

Contracts frequently incorporate by reference other documents, some of which will be appended to the agreement as attachments or exhibits. As discussed further below, managed health care plans frequently reserve the right to amend some of these referenced documents unilaterally.

The contract's form or structure is intended to accomplish three purposes: to simplify a reader's use and understanding of the agreement, to facilitate amendment or revision of the contract where the contract form has been used for many providers, and to streamline the administrative process necessary to submit and obtain regulatory approvals.

Clarity and efficiency can be attained by using commonly understood terms, avoiding legal or technical jargon, using definitions to explain key and frequently used terms, and using well-organized headings and a numbering system. The ultimate objective is that any representative of the managed health care plan or the provider who has an interest in an issue be able to find easily the pertinent contract provision and understand its meaning.

Exhibits and appendixes are frequently used by managed health care plans to promote efficiency in administering many provider contracts. The managed health care plan, to the extent possible, could design many of its provider contracts or groups of provider contracts around a core set of common requirements. Exhibits may be used to identify the terms that may vary, such as payment rates and provider responsibilities. This approach has several advantages. First, it eases the administrative burden in drafting and revising contracts. Second, if an appendix or exhibit is the only part of the contract that is being amended and it has a separate state insurance department provider number, the managed health care plan need only submit the amendment for state review. Third, when a contract is under consideration for renewal and the key issue is the payment rate, having the payment rate listed separately in the appendix lessens the likelihood that the provider will review and suggest amending other provisions of the contract.

COMMON CLAUSES, PROVISIONS, AND KEY FACTORS

Names

The initial paragraph of the contract will identify the names of the parties entering into the agreement. It is always a good idea to ensure that the parties named in the opening paragraph are the parties who are signing the agreement. If one organization is signing the agreement on behalf of affiliates, you may want to have the signing

party represent and warrant that it is authorized to sign on behalf of the nonsigning party. This is also the case where a physician group or intermediate entity is signing on behalf of its member physicians. If the nonsigning party is much stronger financially than the signing party, it would be worthwhile to have a representation directly from the nonsigning party that the signing party may enter into the agreement on its behalf. In reviewing a contract, providers should be particularly sensitive to the responsibilities of nonparties to the agreement. If a managed care organization is offering services to self-insured employers, is the self-insured employer a party to the agreement? If not, what assurances does the provider have that the self-insured employer will fulfill its responsibilities?

Recitals

A contract will typically contain in rather legalistic prose a series of statements describing who the parties are and what they are trying to accomplish. These statements, called recitals, are relatively unimportant because they should not contain substantive contractual obligations. However, managed health care organizations and providers should review these statements to confirm their accuracy and that each party is not assuming any unintended responsibilities.

Table of Contents

Although a table of contents has no legal significance, the reader will be greatly assisted in finding pertinent sections in a long contract. One common failing in contract renegotiations is neglecting to update the table of contents after the contract has been amended.

Definitions

The definitions section of a contract plays an essential role in simplifying the structure and the reader's understanding of a contract. The body of the contract often contains complicated terms that merit amplification and explanation. The use of a definition, although requiring the reader to refer back to an earlier section for a meaning, simplifies greatly the discussion in the body of the agreement. A poorly drafted contract will define unnecessary terms or define terms in a manner that is inconsistent with their use in the body of the agreement.

Defined terms are frequently capitalized in a contract to alert the reader that the word is defined. Definitions are almost essential in many contracts, but their use may complicate the understanding of the agreement. Someone who reads a contract will first read a definition without knowing its significance. Later, when he or she reads the body of the contract, he or she may no longer recall a term's meaning. For this reason, someone reviewing a contract for the first time should read the definitions twice: initially and then in the context of each term's use. Definitions sections tend to err on the side of containing too many definitions. A term that is used only once in a contract need not be defined. On the other hand, a critical reader of a contract will identify instances in which the contract could be improved by the use of additional definitions.

In reviewing a contract, managed health care organizations and providers should not underestimate the importance of the definitions section. A provider's right to payment may depend on how such terms as emergency, covered services, or medical necessity are defined. It is important to review the definitions section of a contract initially as well as in the context of the terms usage in the body of the contract.

An occasional defect in some contracts is that the drafter includes substantive contract provisions in definitions. A definition is merely an explanation of a meaning of a term and should not contain substantive provisions. This does not mean that a definition that imposes a substantive obligation on a party is invalid. In reviewing a contract, if a party identifies a substantive provision in a definition, the party should ensure that its usage is consistent with the corresponding provision in the body of the contract.

Terms that are commonly defined in a managed care context are *member, subscriber, medical director, provider, payer, physician, member, primary care physician, emergency,* *medically necessary,* and *utilization review program.* Some of these terms, such as *medically necessary,* are crucial to readers' understanding of the parties' responsibilities and should be considered carefully in the review of a contract. In many managed care agreements, payers other than the managed health care organization are responsible for payment under the contract. In this case, who is a payer and how they are selected and removed become very important to the provider. The definition of *member* or *enrollee* is also important. The contract should convey clearly who is covered under the agreement and who the managed health care organization can add in the future. The managed health care plan and provider should ensure that these terms are consistent, if appropriate, with those in other contracts (for example, the group enrollment agreement).

It is important to note that a number of the definitions in the contract may be controlled by state or federal law. For example, Medicare and Medicaid law and a number of state laws set forth a definition of *emergency services.* In addition, Medicare law and an increasing number of states set forth standards for *medical necessity.* The contracting parties should be aware of the law and should, at a minimum, ensure that the definitions in the contract are consistent with such law.

Provider Obligations

Provider Qualifications and Credentialing

Provider contracts should include the provider's representations and warranties that the provider meets the managed care plan's applicable requirements for network participation. These representations and warranties should include, at a minimum, that the provider has a valid license, has not been excluded from participation in any federal health care program and, in the case of an institutional provider, meets any relevant accreditation standards and Medicare conditions for participation. As discussed later in this chapter, it is important that the provider be obligated to notify the managed care plan if any of this information changes.

In addition, the contract should include a provision requiring the provider to comply with any of the managed care plan's policies and procedures for credentialing and recredentialing of providers.

Provider Services

Because the purpose of the agreement is to contract for the provision of health services, the description of those services in the contract is important. As mentioned above, the recitation of services to be furnished by the provider could be either set out in the contract or set out in an exhibit or attachment. An exhibit format frequently allows the party more flexibility and administrative simplicity when it amends the exhibited portion of the agreement, particularly when the change requires regulatory approval.

Contracts may use the term *provider services* to denote the range of services that are to be provided under the contract. Managed health care organizations frequently adapt physician contracts to apply to ancillary providers. In so doing, the managed health care organization may not revise language that applies only to physicians.

The contract needs to specify to whom the provider is obligated to furnish services. Although the answer is that the provider furnishes services to covered enrollees, the contract needs to define what is meant by *covered enrollee,* explain how the provider will learn who is covered, and assign the responsibility for payment if services are furnished to a noncovered person. Managed care organizations and providers frequently disagree on this issue. The providers' view is frequently that if the managed care organization represented that the individual was covered, the managed care organization should be responsible for payment. In contrast, the managed care organization frequently asserts that they should not be responsible for the costs of services provided to noncovered enrollees and that the provider should seek payment directly from the individual. This issue is particularly important when the enrollee population includes Medicaid beneficiaries who are unlikely to be able to pay the provider for services. Oftentimes the issue is resolved based on relative negotiating strength.

Provider contracts should also cover adequately a number of other provider responsibilities, including their responsibilities to refer or to accept referrals of enrollees, the days and times of days the provider agrees to be available to provide services, and substitute on-call arrangements, if appropriate. Provider contracts may also specify the qualifications necessary for the provider of backup services when the provider is not available. Some of these requirements may be posed as conditions of participation in public programs, such as the Medicare program.

If the provider is a hospital, the contract will include language identifying the circumstances in which the managed health care plan agrees to be responsible or not responsible for services provided to nonemergency patients. A fairly common provision in hospital contracts states that the hospital, except in emergencies, must as a prerequisite to admit have the order of the participating physician or other preadmission authorization. The hospital contract also should have an explicit provision requiring that the managed health care plan be notified within a specified period after an emergency admission. A particularly sensitive issue is whether the managed health care plan's coverage of emergency medical services meets state and federal requirements for such coverage. Medicare, Medicaid, and a number of state laws require managed care plans to pay for screening and stabilization services in situations in which a prudent layperson reasonably believed that an emergency medical condition existed. A related policy and contracting issue is whether such a law automatically entitles a hospital to reimbursement for performing the initial screen that is required when a patient goes to the emergency room.

A good provider contract must be supplemented by a competent provider relations program to ensure that problems that arise are resolved and that the providers have a means to answer questions about their contract responsibilities. Providers will be frequently given the opportunity to appeal internally claim denials and decisions of nonmedical necessity by the managed care organization. Moreover, Medicare+Choice organizations are required to provide physicians the right to appeal the organization's decision to terminate or suspend the physician's plan participation and to note these appeal rights in their physician contracts.

Nondiscriminatory Requirements

Provider agreements frequently contain clauses obligating the provider to furnish services in the same manner as the provider furnishes services to nonmanaged health care patients (that is, not to discriminate on the basis of payment source). In addition, a clause is used to prohibit other types of discrimination on the basis of race, color, sex, age, disability, religion, and national origin. Government contracts may require the use of specific contract language, including a reference to compliance with the Americans with Disabilities Act and the Rehabilitation Act of 1973. As an alternative, the managed care organization and provider may want to add a second contract clause that requires compliance with all nondiscrimination requirements under federal, state, and local law. These obligations may also apply to subcontractors of the provider.

Compliance with Utilization and Quality Management Programs

The success of the managed care organization is dependent on its providers being able and willing to control unnecessary utilization. To do so, the providers need to follow the utilization review guidelines of the managed health care plan. The contract needs to set out the provider's responsibilities in carrying out the managed health care plan's utilization review program. The managed health care plan's dilemma is how to articulate this obligation in the contract when the utilization review program may be quite detailed and frequently is updated over time. One option used by some managed care organizations is to append the utilization review program to the contract as an exhibit. A second option is merely to incorporate the program by reference. In either case, it is important for the managed health care plan to ensure that the contract al-

lows it to amend the utilization review standards in the future without the consent of the provider. If the managed health care plan does not append a cross-referenced standard, the managed health care plan should give each provider a copy of the guidelines and any amendments. Without this documentation, the provider might argue that he or she did not agree to the guidelines or subsequent amendments.

The contract needs to inform providers of their responsibilities to cooperate in efforts by the managed health care plan to ensure compliance and the implications of the provider not meeting the plan's requirements. Contracts differ on whether the managed health care plan is seeking the providers' "cooperation" or "compliance." The current Health Care Financing Administration (HCFA) guidelines for provider contracts require that the provider "cooperate with and participate in" the managed health care plan's quality assurance, member grievance system, and utilization review programs. Providers generally favor an obligation to cooperate rather than to comply with these programs because a requirement to comply with the programs' decisions seems to preclude the right to disagree.

The same basic concepts and principles apply to the provider's acceptance of the managed health care plan's quality assurance program. Some managed health care plans tend to equate their utilization review and their quality assurance programs. This attitude not only reflects a misunderstanding of the objectives of the two programs but is likely to engender the concern or criticism of government regulators who view the two programs as being separate. In the last several years, as managed health care plans have placed greater emphasis on their quality assurance and quality improvement programs, provider compliance responsibilities have correspondingly increased. To provide some guidance on the nature of these responsibilities, some managed health care organizations have appended summaries of these quality programs to the contracts in order to give providers a better idea of their responsibilities.

The contract should include a provision requiring the provider to cooperate both in furnishing information to the managed health care plan and in taking corrective actions, if appropriate.

Acceptance of Enrollee Patients

A provider contract, particularly with a physician or physician group, will need a clause to ensure that the provider will accept enrollees regardless of health status. This provision is more important when the risk-sharing responsibilities with the providers are such that the physician has an incentive to dissuade high utilizers from becoming part of his or her panel. Most provider contracts with primary care physicians also include a minimum number of members that the physician will accept into his or her panel (for example, 250 members). The contract should also include fair and reasonable procedures for allowing the provider to limit or stop new members to his or her panel (at a point after the provider has accepted at least the minimum number of members) and a mechanism to notify the managed health care plan when these changes take place. The managed health care plan needs to have data regarding which providers are limiting panel size in order to comply with regulatory requirements.

The contract should also specify the circumstances in which the provider, principally a primary care physician, can cease being an enrollee's physician. Examples may be abusive behavior or refusal to follow the recommended course of treatment. This contract language would need to be consistent with language in the member's or subscriber's agreement and in compliance with licensure requirements and federal health care program requirements, which frequently identify the grounds in which a physician may end the physician-enrollee relationship.

Enrollee Complaints

The contract should require the provider to cooperate in resolving enrollee complaints and to notify the managed health care plan within a specified period of time when any complaints are conveyed to the provider. The provider should also be obligated to advise the managed health care plan of any coverage denials so that the managed health care plan might anticipate future enrollee complaints. To the extent governmental payer programs require special enrollee grievance procedures, the language in the contract should be written sufficiently broadly to ensure provider cooperation with those procedures.

Maintenance and Retention of Records and Confidentiality

Provider contracts should require the provider to maintain both medical and business records for specified periods of time. For example, these agreements could provide that the records must be maintained in accordance with federal and state laws and consistent with generally accepted business and professional standards as well as whatever other standards are established by the managed health care plan. If the managed health care plan participates in any public or private payer program that establishes certain specific records retention requirements, those requirements should be conveyed to the providers. The contract should state that these obligations survive the termination of the contract.

The managed health care plan also needs a legal right to have access to books and records. The contract will want to state that the managed health care plan, its representatives, and government agencies have the right to inspect, review, and make or obtain copies of medical, financial, and administrative records. The provider would want the availability of this information to be limited to services rendered to enrollees, after reasonable notice, and during normal business hours. The cost of performing these services is often an issue of controversy. If there are no fees for copying these records, the contract should so state. When the managed health care organization is acting on behalf of other payers, it is desirable to have language acknowledging that the other payers have agreed to comply with applicable confidentiality laws.

In addition to the availability of books or records, the managed health care plan might also want the right to require the provider to prepare reports identifying statistical and descriptive medical and patient data and other identifying information as specified by the managed health care plan. If such a provision is included in the contract, the managed health care plan should inform the provider of the types of reports it might request to minimize any future problems. Finally, the provider should be obligated to provide information that is necessary for compliance with state or federal law.

An often neglected legal issue is how the managed health care plan obtains the authority to have access to medical records. Provider agreements periodically contain an acknowledgment by the provider that the managed health care plan is authorized to receive medical records. The problem with this approach is that the managed health care plan might not have the right to have access to this information and, if it does not, an acknowledgment of that right in the contract has no legal effect. Some state laws give insurers and HMOs, as payers, a limited right of access to medical records. This right may arise if the managed health care organization is performing utilization review on behalf of an enrollee. Managed health care plans should review their state law provisions, and any applicable federal law provisions, on this issue and their plan's procedures for obtaining the appropriate consents of their members to have access to this information. Many managed health care plans obtain this information through signatures that are part of the initial enrollment materials. These consents could also be obtained at the time health services are rendered.

Managed health care organizations frequently include provisions in contracts in which the provider acknowledges that the managed health care organization has the right of access to enrollee records. The provider should be reluctant to agree to this provision without consulting state law. Although the clause acknowledging the right of access may make it easier to persuade a reluctant provider to release an enrollee's medical records, the managed health care plan needs to remember that that statement, or for that matter similar statements in the group enrollment agreement, does not confer that right. Finally, the contract should explicitly state that the provisions concerning access to records should survive the termination of the agreement.

A related provision almost always included in provider contracts is a requirement that the provider maintain the confidentiality of medical records. A common clause is a provision that will only release the records in accordance with the terms of the contract, in accordance with applicable law, or upon appropriate consent. State law will frequently allow disclosure of information without patient identifiers for purposes of research or education. Managed health care plans and providers need to be sensitive to confidentiality concerns with regard to minors, incompetents, and persons with communicable diseases for which there are specific state confidentiality statutes governing disclosure of information.

A medical records issue may arise when a managed health care plan wants the right to perform certain medical tests outside the hospital before an enrollee's admission. The contract between the managed health care plan and the hospital may allow for such tests and the inclusion of the test results into the hospital's medical records. The hospital may insist that the results of the tests be in a format acceptable to the hospital's medical records committee, that the laboratory results be properly certified, and that the duties performed shall be consistent with the proper practice of medicine.

Payment

The payment terms of the agreement often represent the most important provision for both the provider and the managed health care plan. As mentioned earlier, the payment terms are frequently set forth in an exhibit appended to the contract and are cross-referenced in the body of the agreement. A number of payment issues should be covered in the contract. For example, who will collect the copayments? Another issue concerns the managed health care plan's payment responsibilities for uncovered services. A provision needs to state that unauthorized or uncovered services are not the responsibility of the managed health care plan. To avoid members receiving unexpected bills from providers for noncovered services, contracts may say that the provider must first inform the member that a service will not be covered by the health plan prior to providing the service. In addition, the contract may preclude the provider from ever billing an enrollee when the managed health care organization has determined that the service is not medically necessary.

From the provider's perspective, he or she needs a clear understanding of what is necessary for a service to be authorized. If the provider submits claims to the managed health care plan, the contract should set out the manner in which the claim is to be made and either identify the information to be provided in the claim or give the managed health care plan the right to designate or revise that information in the future. If the contract specifies the information to be included in a claim, the managed health care plan should also have the unilateral right to make changes in the future.

The agreement should also obligate the provider to submit claims within a specified period and the managed health care plan to pay claims within a certain number of days. The latter requirement should not apply to contested claims. The parties should ensure that the number of days for claims payment set forth in the contract is consistent with any state or federal laws regulating such payment. While Medicare+Choice law does not set forth a specific time frame in which contracting providers must be paid, it does require that Medicare+Choice organizations set forth in their provider contracts a "prompt payment" provision as negotiated by the contracting parties. Special provisions regarding timing of payment will apply to claims for which another carrier may be the primary payer. A common way to address the coordination of benefits issue in a balanced manner is to allow a two-month period for collection from the purported primary carrier. If unsuccessful, the managed health care plan would pay while awaiting resolution of the dispute.

At issue is the time in which the managed health care organization is required to pay on claims. Contracts frequently identify a specific time period (for example, 30–60 days) during which payment on clean claims is to be made. Provider contracts rarely impose an interest penalty for late payment, reflecting the greater bargaining strength of the managed health care or-

ganization. Some contracts require the managed health care organization to make a good faith effort to pay within a specified period. From the provider's perspective, the weakness of this provision is that "good faith" is probably too ambiguous to be enforceable. Some states have laws requiring insurers and HMOs to pay interest on late claims.

The contract needs also to address reconciliations to account for overpayments or underpayments. To avoid these issues from lingering an inordinately long period of time, some managed health care plans limit the adjustment period to a specified time period (for example, 6 months). Also, some managed health care plans use contract provisions that do not allow for a reconciliation if the amount in controversy falls below a specified amount.

Risk-Sharing Arrangements

The most complex aspects of provider contracts are often the risk-sharing arrangements. Risk can be shared with providers in significantly varying degrees depending on the initial amount of risk transferred, the services for which the provider is at risk, and whether the managed care organization offers stop-loss protection. Risk pools with complicated formulas determining distributions are frequently used both when services are capitated or payments are based on a fee schedule. Although the primary objective of these arrangements is to create incentives to discourage unnecessary utilization, the complexity of many of these arrangements has confused providers and engendered their distrust when their distribution falls below expectations. Some managed health care plans that had complex risk-sharing arrangements are now realizing that simpler, more understandable arrangements are preferable. If the arrangement designed by the managed health care plan is somewhat complex, the provider's understanding will be greatly enhanced by the use of examples that illustrate for providers the total payments they will receive in different factual scenarios.

Managed care plans should be aware of and comply with any state and federal laws that regulate risk-sharing arrangements. For example, under the Medicare and Medicaid managed care programs, managed care plans must comply with the requirements for physician incentive plans (PIPs). The PIP requirements impose stop-loss and enrollee survey obligations on managed care plans when payment arrangements for the provision of services to Medicare or Medicaid beneficiaries put a physician or physician group at risk for more than 25 percent of total potential payments for services the physician or group does not directly provide. Moreover, managed care plans providing services to commercial enrollees with Medicare as a secondary payer may also need to comply with the PIP obligations in order to qualify for an exception from the compensation prohibitions under the personal services exception to the federal physician self-referral law (also known as Stark II).

Payment and Physician-Hospital Organizations

The most significant trend in provider payment arrangements has been the growth of arrangements where physician-hospital organizations are willing to accept a percentage of the managed care organization's payment from a payer in return for agreeing to provide all or a substantial portion of the organization's health care services. This arrangement has become prevalent in the Medicare risk contract program. In developing these relationships, the parties need to identify carefully the obligations of the provider organization. The agreement needs to clearly identify the services that will and will not be covered under the agreement. Will the managed care organization have the right to have the services performed by other providers if it is not satisfied with the contracted provider's performance? What assumptions have been made regarding the demographics and health needs of the covered population? When a provider is financially responsible for services furnished by a different provider, will the first provider or the health plan be paying the second provider for services furnished?

Other-Party Liability: Subrogation and Coordination of Benefits

Provider contracts should contain provisions to address situations in which a party other than the enrollee or managed health care plan is financially responsible for all or part of the services provided to an enrollee.

Such provisions should set forth the provider's obligation to assist the managed health care plan in identifying other parties that are responsible for paying for, or providing, services to an enrollee. In addition, the provision should identify the party with the responsibility for billing another payer and indicate the party to which the payment belongs. Some managed health care plans allow their providers to collect and keep third-party recoveries, whereas others will require that the information be reported and deducted. Often, the specific procedure depends on how the provider is paid, for example, on a fee-for-service basis, a capitation basis, or by some other mechanism.

A sensitive issue is the potential liability of a managed health care plan if a provider collects from Medicare inappropriately when the managed health care plan had primary responsibility under the Medicare secondary payer rules. Under the regulations of HCFA, the managed health care plan is legally responsible and may be forced to pay back HCFA even if the payment was received by the provider without the knowledge of the managed health care plan. Managed health care plans should include a contract provision transferring the ultimate financial liability to the provider in this circumstance.

Another issue that should be addressed in the contract is the responsibility of the managed health care plan as a secondary carrier if the provider bills the primary carrier an amount greater than the amount the provider would have received from the managed health care plan. From the managed health care plan's perspective, it will want a contract provision relieving the managed health care plan of any payment responsibility if the provider has received at least the amount he or she would have been entitled to under the managed health care plan-provider contract. However, there is an important exception to this general rule where Medicare is primary payer. If the amount the provider bills Medicare is greater than the amount the provider would have received from the managed care plan, either the managed care plan or the beneficiary must pay the Medicare cost-sharing amounts. Otherwise, the provider will potentially be violating three laws. The first is the Medicare law that requires that the Medicare cost sharing be paid. Second, the anti-kickback law may be violated because the waiver of cost sharing is being done in return for the referral of a patient. Third, the False Claims Act may be violated because the provider has submitted a bill to HCFA for an amount greater than the provider's "actual charge."

Other Payment-Related Issues

In recent years, as providers gain more experience with managed health care plans, they are becoming more sophisticated in analyzing and evaluating payment arrangements and are more aware of the ability or inability of managed health care plans to produce the volume promised. A growing number of contracts are being renegotiated in light of the actual volume of patients a managed health care plan is able to deliver to the provider. Contracts are also now beginning to allow volume as a factor affecting payment amount.

A few other payment-related issues that should be addressed in a contract are: What if services are provided to a person who is no longer eligible for enrollment? What if services are provided to a nonenrollee who obtained services by using an enrollee's membership card?

Hold-Harmless and No-Balance-Billing Clauses

Virtually all provider contracts contain a hold-harmless clause under which the provider agrees not to sue or assert any claims against the enrollee for services covered under the contract, even if the managed health care plan becomes insolvent or fails to meet its obligations. A no-balance-billing clause is similar (and may be used synonymously) and states that a provider may not balance bill a member for any payment owed by the plan, regardless of the reason for nonpayment; the provider may bill the member for any amount that the member is required to pay, such as copayment or coinsurance, or for services not covered under the schedule of benefits (for example, cosmetic surgery). Many state insurance departments (or other agencies having regulatory oversight in this area) will not approve the provider forms without inclusion of a hold-harmless clause with specific language. HCFA also has adopted recommended model hold-harmless language applicable to federally qualified HMOs and Medicare+Choice organizations that was approved by the National Association of Insurance Commissioners.

Relationship of the Parties

Provider contracts usually contain a provision stating that the managed health care plan and the provider have an independent contractual arrangement. The purpose for this provision is to refute an assertion that the provider serves as an employee of the managed health care plan. The reason is that under the legal theory of respondeat superior the managed health care plan would automatically be liable for the negligent acts of its employees. Although managed health care plans frequently include a provision such as this in their provider contracts, it has limited value. In a lawsuit against the managed health care plan by an enrollee alleging malpractice, the court is likely to disregard such language and to focus on the relationship between the managed health care plan and the provider and the manner in which the managed health care plan represented the provider in evaluating whether the managed health care plan should be vicariously liable.

A related clause frequently used in provider contracts states that nothing contained in the agreement shall be construed to require physicians to recommend any procedure or course of treatment that physicians deem professionally inappropriate. This clause is intended, in part, to affirm that the managed health care plan is not engaged in the practice of medicine, an activity that the managed health care plan may not be permitted to perform. Another reason for this clause is to protect the managed health care plan from liability arising from a provider's negligence.

Use of Name

Many provider contracts limit the ability of either party to use the name of the other. This is done by identifying the circumstances in which the party's name may or may not be used. Contract clauses may allow the managed health care plan the right to use the name of the provider for the health benefits accounts, the enrollees, and the patients of the participating providers. Otherwise the party needs the written approval of the other party. The use applies not only to the name but to any symbol, trademark, and service mark of the entity. The managed health care plan and the provider will want to ensure that proprietary information is protected. The contract should require that the provider keep all information about the managed health care plan confidential and prohibit the use of the information for any competitive purpose after the contract is terminated. With medical groups frequently switching managed care affiliations, this protection is important to the managed health care plan.

Notification

The managed health care plan needs to ensure that it is advised of a number of important changes that affect the ability of the provider to meet his or her contractual obligations. The contract should identify the information that needs to be conveyed to the managed health care plan and the time frames for providing that information. For example, a physician might be required to notify a managed health care plan within 5 days (or less) upon loss or suspension of his or her license or certification, loss or restriction of full active admitting privileges at any hospital, issuance of any formal charges brought by a government agency, change in or loss of liability insurance coverage, or the initiation of a civil action by an enrollee. Although specific events should be identified in the contract, a broad catchall category should also be included, such as an event that if sustained would materially impair the provider's ability to perform the duties under the contract. The contract should require immediate notification if the provider is sanctioned under a federal health care program. If the managed care organization is contracting with

a provider who has been sanctioned, the organization may no longer be eligible to receive federal funds.

In a hospital contract, the corresponding provisions would be when the hospital suffers from a change that materially impairs its ability to provide services or if action is taken against it regarding certifications or licenses by federal agencies or private accrediting bodies.

Insurance and Indemnification

Insurance provisions in contracts are fairly straightforward. The obligations in the contract may be for both professional liability coverage and general liability coverage. The managed health care plan wants to ensure that the provider has resources to pay for any eventuality. The contract will state particular insurance limits, provide that the limits will be set forth in a separate attachment, or leave it up to the managed health care plan to specify. A hospital agreement may require only that the limits be commensurate with limits contained in policies of similar hospitals in the state. From the managed health care organization's perspective, it will probably want a specific requirement in order to ensure adequate levels of insurance. A provision should also be included requiring the provider to notify the managed health care plan of any notification of cancellations of the policy. Another needed notification in a physician context is notification of any malpractice claims.

Cross-indemnification provisions in which each party indemnifies the other for damages caused by the other party are common in contracts. One weakness of the clause is that some professional liability carriers will not pay for claims arising from these clauses because of general exclusions in their policies for contractual claims. Although these clauses are frequently used, this limitation and the fact that a provider should still be liable for his or her negligent acts suggest that these indemnification clauses are not essential.

Term, Suspension, and Termination

One section of most contracts identifies the term of the contract and the term of any subsequent contract renewals. Many contracts have automatic renewal provisions if no party exercises its right to terminate. Both managed health care plans and providers should give careful thought to the length of the contract and the renewal periods.

Some contracts give a right of suspension to the managed health care plan. In suspension, the contract continues, but the provider loses specific rights. For example, if a provider fails to follow utilization review protocols a specified number of times, the provider will not be assigned new HMO members or perhaps will receive a reduction in the amount of payment. The advantage of a suspension provision is that total termination of a contract might be counterproductive for the managed health care plan, but a suspension might be sufficiently punitive to persuade the provider to improve.

Termination provisions fall into two categories: termination without cause and termination with cause. The value of having a provision that allows the managed health care plan to terminate without cause is that the managed health care plan need not defend a challenge by the provider on the substantive issue of whether the grounds were met. A 90-day period is fairly common. However, managed care plans should be aware that state or federal law may affect a managed care plan's ability or procedures for terminating without cause. For example, the Medicare+ Choice regulations require 60 days' prior notice before terminating without cause. If the managed health care plan has the right to terminate without cause, frequently the provider will also be given that right. Another regulatory issue to be aware of is that some state laws require providers to continue to provide services for a specified period of time after their contract has terminated. Such provisions are likely to become even more common because, as a federal advisory body on patient's rights* advocated, such an approach is intended to ensure continuity of care for persons being treated by a provider at the time of the provider's termination. These requirements may also relate to the state's requirements for the managed health care plan to have protections against insolvency and have to be re-

flected in the contract. If a managed care plan includes a requirement to continue care in the contract, it should ensure that the provider will continue meeting the contractual requirements with regard to the services for which the plan continues to cover after the termination. Specifically, the provider should continue to meet the managed care plan's hold-harmless requirements, reporting requirements, and quality assurance requirements.

Terminations with cause may allow the health plan to terminate faster and should be used in situations where the managed health care plan needs to act quickly. The contract might establish two different categories: immediate termination and termination within a 30-day period. Many contracts give either party a period of time to cure any contract violations. This time period, although useful to the managed health care plan if it has allegedly violated the agreement, extends the period of time in which it can terminate the contract. Grounds for termination for cause may be suspension or revocation of license, loss of hospital privileges, breach of the contract, failure to meet accreditation and credentialing requirements, failure to provide services to enrollees in a professionally acceptable manner, bankruptcy, and refusal to accept an amendment to the contract agreement.

A provision allowing for termination if the provider takes any actions or makes any communications that undermine or could undermine the confidence of enrollees in the quality of care provided by the managed health care plan may be included in a provider contract. However, a managed care plan should be aware that such provisions are sensitive and may be interpreted as a "gag clause." So called gag clauses, which prohibit physicians from fully discussing a patient's treatment options and medical condi-

---

*This obligation is included in the Consumer Bill of Rights and Responsibilities, which was developed by the President's Advisory Commission on Consumer Protection and Quality in the Health Care Industry (November 20, 1997). The president has directed federal agencies to implement these protections to the extent possible through regulatory action.

tions, are prohibited under federal health care programs and a number of state laws. If the managed care plan elects to use such a provision, the clause should make clear that the intent is to prohibit disparagement of the managed care plan and that a physician remains free to advise his or her patients regarding all medically indicated treatment options, regardless of whether such treatments are covered under the managed care plan, to discuss the patient's medical condition and to make medical recommendations within the scope of the provider's licensure.

The contract should give the managed care plan the right to immediately terminate the contract upon the occurrence of certain events, including the provider's loss of licensure or accreditation or exclusion from a federal health care program. A good contracting practice is to include a general provision that allows for immediate termination of the contract if, in the opinion of the managed care organization, continuation of the contract would endanger the health or well-being of the managed care plan's members. Such a clause would allow the managed care organization the flexibility to terminate the contract immediately in the case of an unforeseen contingency of sufficient gravity to endanger the managed care plan's enrollees.

The contract should be clear that a provider, upon termination, is required to cooperate in the orderly transfer of enrollee care, including records, to other providers. The provider also should agree to cooperate in resolving any disputes. Finally, the provider should continue to furnish services under the terms of the contract until the services being rendered to enrollees are complete or the managed health care plan has made appropriate provisions for another provider to assume the responsibility. The contract should also be clear that the provider is entitled to compensation for performing these services. In general, too little consideration has been given to preparing for contract terminations. When the provider and the managed health care plan enter into a contract, little thought is given to what will occur when the contract ends. Often, relationships end acrimoniously, and it is in both parties' best interest to consider how their interests will be protected in the event the contract is terminated.

"Flow Down" Clauses and Provider Subcontracts

A managed care plan may be obligated to "flow down" certain clauses that are included in the contract between the managed care plan and the payer. For example, if a managed care organization has a contract with the federal government or a state Medicaid agency, the managed care plan is obligated to include in its provider contracts a clause recognizing that the payments the provider receives from the managed care plan to provide services to enrollees under the applicable federal health care program are, in whole or part, from federal funds and that the provider and any of its subcontractors are therefore subject to certain laws that are applicable to individuals and entities receiving federal funds, including, but not limited to, Title VI of the Civil Rights Act of 1964, the Age Discrimination Act of 1975, the Rehabilitation Act of 1973, and the Americans with Disabilities Act. The managed care plan should be aware of any contract provisions that must be "flowed down" to its contractors. Moreover, the managed care plan should carefully note whether those provisions must be included in the contracts of all downstream providers, that is, subcontractors entering into agreements to provide services to the managed care organization's members.

In addition to clauses that must be "flowed down" from the plan-payer contract, if a provider will be a subcontractor to another provider that contracts directly with the managed care plan, the contract between the managed care plan and the first-tier provider should include a provision that sets forth the requirements that must be included in the downstream subcontracts. This provision may set forth the terms of the provider's contract that must be included in any of the provider's subcontracts. Medicare+ Choice policy specifically identifies a number of contract provisions that must be included in downstream contracts to provide services to members of Medicare+Choice organizations.

Managed care plans should make sure that they comply with similar requirements under other federal or state law.

In addition, if the provider will be subcontracting, the contract should specify whether the managed care plan or the provider will credential any subcontracting providers. If the managed care plan delegates its credentialing function, it should generally state the standards under which the provider will be credentialing its subcontractors. The managed care plan may want to reserve the right to approve, suspend, or deny the participation of any of the provider's subcontractors.

Declarations

In declarations, the parties provide answers to a number of "what if" questions. These clauses are common to all contracts.

A *force majeure* clause relieves a party of responsibility if an event occurs beyond its control. In a provider contract this instance is more likely to arise if the provider is no longer able to provide services. In considering *force majeure* clauses, the parties need to distinguish between events that are beyond a party's control and those that disadvantage a party but for which the party should still be obligated to perform the contract's responsibilities.

A choice of law provision identifies the law that will apply in the event of a dispute. Absent a violation of public policy in the state in question, a court will apply the agreed-upon law. Frequently, lawyers draft contracts using the state in which their client is located without consideration of the advantages and disadvantages of the underlying law. In provider contracts where the managed health care plan and the provider are located in the same state, this clause has little relevance.

A merger clause specifies that only the language in the agreement shall constitute the contract. Such a clause prevents a party from arguing that oral conversations or other documents not included in the contract modify the contract's terms.

A provision allowing or not allowing parties to assign their rights is frequently included in contracts. Provider contracts usually prohibit a provider from assigning its rights under a contract. Some contracts are silent on the right of the managed health care plan to assign the contract. Silence would generally allow the managed health care plan to assign the contract. An option is to allow the managed health care plan to assign the contract only to an affiliate or a successor without the written consent of the provider.

A clause identifying how the contract will be amended is almost always included in a provider contract. A contract will frequently give the managed health care plan the unilateral right to amend the contract absent an objection by the provider. This procedure is necessary when the managed health care plan has a large provider panel and it is administratively difficult to obtain the signatures of all the providers.

A severability clause allows the contract to continue if a court invalidates a portion of the contract. This is a common provision in a contract, but it is unlikely that the problem will arise.

Contracts also set forth a notice requirement identifying how notices are provided to parties and to whom. The manner in which notice is provided is important. If a notice requires that the communication be conveyed by certified mail with return receipt requested, an alternative form of delivery is not valid. Parties should consider what is administratively feasible before agreeing on how notice will be given.

Closing

Both parties need to confirm that the parties identified at the beginning of the contract are the parties that sign the contract. Also, if a corporation is one of the parties, the signatory needs to be authorized on behalf of the corporation to sign the agreement.

CONCLUSION

The provider contract establishes the foundation for the working relationship between the managed health care plan and the provider. A good contract is well organized and clearly written and accurately reflects the full intentions of the parties. In drafting and reviewing provider contracts, the managed health care plan and the provider need to keep in mind their objectives in entering the relationship, the relationship of this contract to other provider contracts and agreements, and applicable regulatory requirements.

The appendixes to this chapter contain two sample provider contracts. The author has annotated each contract to point out strengths and weaknesses of the provisions. These two contracts are provided for illustrative purposes and are not represented as ideal agreements.

Sample Physician Agreement

AGREEMENT BETWEEN

_____

AND

PRIMARY CARE PHYSICIAN

THIS AGREEMENT, made and entered into the date set forth on the signature page hereto, by and between _____, Inc, a _____ corporation (hereinafter referred to as "HMO"), which is organized and operated as a health maintenance organization under the laws of the State of _____ and the individual physician or group practice identified on the signature page hereto (hereinafter referred to as "Primary Care Physician").

WHEREAS, HMO desires to operate a health maintenance organization pursuant to the laws of the State of _____;

WHEREAS, Primary Care Physician is a duly licensed physician (or if Primary Care Physician is a legal entity, the members of such entity are duly licensed physicians) in the State of _____, whose license(s) is (are) without limitation or restriction;[1] and

WHEREAS, HMO has as an objective the development and expansion of cost-effective means of delivering quality health services to Members, as defined herein, particularly through prepaid health care plans, and Primary Care Physician concurs in, actively supports, and will contribute to the achievement of this objective; and

WHEREAS, HMO and Primary Care Physician mutually desire to enter into an Agreement whereby the Primary Care Physician shall provide and coordinate the health care services to Members of HMO.

NOW, THEREFORE, in consideration of the premises and mutual covenants herein contained and other good and valuable consideration, it is mutually covenanted and agreed by and between the parties hereto as follows:

---

[1]Although there is nothing wrong with having a statement here that the primary care physician's license is not restricted, the body of the contract, as is the case in this contract in Section IV. H, needs to contain this requirement and provide that the failure to maintain the license is grounds for termination.

PART I. DEFINITIONS

A. *Covered Services* means those health services and benefits to which Members are entitled under the terms of an applicable Health Maintenance Certificate which may be amended by HMO from time to time.[2]

B. *Emergency Services* means those Medically Necessary services provided in connection with an "Emergency," defined as a sudden or unexpected onset of a condition requiring medical or surgical care which the Member secures after the onset of such condition (or as soon thereafter as care can be made available but which in any case not later than twenty-four (24) hours after onset) and in the absence of such care the Member could reasonably be expected to suffer serious physical impairment or death. Heart attacks, severe chest pain, cardiovascular accidents, hemorrhaging, poisonings, major burns, loss of consciousness, serious breathing difficulties, spinal injuries, shock, and other acute conditions as HMO shall determine are Emergencies.[3]

C. *Encounter Form* means a record of services provided by Physician to Members in a format acceptable to the HMO.[4]

D. *Health Maintenance Certificate* means a contract issued by HMO to a Member or an employer of Members specifying the services and benefits available under the HMO's prepaid health benefits program.

E. *Health Professionals* means doctors of medicine, doctors of osteopathy, dentists, nurses, chiropractors, podiatrists, optometrists, physician assistants, clinical psychologists, social workers, pharmacists, occupational therapists, physical therapists, and other professionals engaged in the delivery of health services who are licensed, practice under an institutional license, and are certified or practice under other authority consistent with the laws of the State of _____.

F. *Medical Director* means a Physician designated by HMO to monitor and review the provision of Covered Services to Members.

G. *Medically Necessary* services and/or supplies means the use of services or supplies as provided by a hospital, skilled nursing facility, Physician or other provider required to identify or treat a Member's illness or injury and which, as determined by HMO's Medical Director or its utilization review committee, are: (1) consistent with the symptoms or diagnosis and treatment of the Member's condition, disease, ailment or injury; (2) appropriate with regard to standards of good medical practice; (3) not solely for the convenience of the Member, his or her physician, hospital, or other health care provider; and (4) the most appropriate supply or level of service which can be safely provided to the Member.[5] When specifically applied to an inpatient Member, it further

---

[2]This definition notes the HMO's right to revise the covered services that the primary care physician is required to provide. If the physicians were capitated for those services, a mechanism would need to be available to revise the capitation rate accordingly. If the services were not limited to HMO enrollees (for example, covered persons under an administrative services only arrangement with a self-insured employer), this definition would have to be written more broadly.

[3]The definition for emergency services would be coordinated with the definition used in the HMO's group enrollment agreement. The examples are a useful method of illustrating the types of conditions that are considered emergencies. Some contracts will exclude deliveries during the last month of pregnancy while the mother is traveling outside the service area.

[4]By stating that the encounter form must be acceptable to the HMO, the contract allows the HMO to change its requirements in the future.

[5]This clause gives the HMO the authority to deny coverage for a medically appropriate procedure where another procedure is also appropriate. Although this clause does not explicitly address the subject, it is intended to give the HMO the right to cover the most cost-effective, medically appropriate procedure. An alternative way of addressing the issue is to state explicitly as one of the criteria that the procedure performed is the least costly setting or manner appropriate to treat the enrollee's medical condition.

means that the Member's medical symptoms or condition requires that the diagnosis or treatment cannot be safely provided to the Member as an outpatient.[6]

H. *Member* means both a Subscriber and his or her eligible family members for whom premium payment has been made.[7]

I. *Participating Physician* means a Physician who, at the time of providing or authorizing services to a Member, has contracted with or on whose behalf a contract has been entered into with HMO to provide professional services to Members.

J. *Participating Provider* means a Physician, hospital, skilled nursing facility, home health agency or any other duly licensed institution or Health Professional under contract with HMO to provide professional and hospital services to Members.

K. *Physician* means a duly licensed doctor of medicine or osteopathy.

L. *Primary Care Physician* means a Participating Physician who provides primary care services to Members (e.g., general or family practitioner, internist, pediatrician or such other physician specialty as may be designated by HMO) and is responsible for referrals of Members to Referral Physicians, other Participating Providers and if necessary non-Participating Providers. Each Member shall select or have selected on his or her behalf a Primary Care Physician.

M. *Referral Physician* means a Participating Physician who is responsible for providing certain medical referral physician services upon referral by a Primary Care Physician.

N. *Service Area* means those counties in _____ set forth in Attachment A and such other areas as may be designated by HMO from time to time.

O. *Subscriber* means an individual who has contracted, or on whose behalf a contract has been entered into, with HMO for health care services.

PART II. OBLIGATIONS OF HMO

A. *Administrative Procedures.* HMO shall make available to Primary Care Physician a manual of administrative procedures (including any changes thereto) in the areas of record keeping, reporting, and other administrative duties of the Primary Care Physician under this Agreement. Primary Care Physician agrees to abide by such administrative procedures including, but not limited to, the submission of HMO Encounter Forms documenting all Covered Services provided to Members by Primary Care Physician.[8]

B. *Compensation.* For all Medically Necessary Covered Services provided to Members by Primary Care Physician, HMO shall pay to Primary Care Physician the compensation set forth in Attachment B.[9] Itemized statements on HMO Encounter Forms, or approved equivalent, for all Covered Services rendered by Primary Care Physician must be submitted to HMO within ninety (90) days of the date the service was rendered in order to be compensated by HMO. The purpose of the risk sharing/incentive compensation arrangement set forth in Attachment B is to monitor utilization, control costs of health services, including hospitalization, and to achieve utilization goals while maintaining quality of care.

---

[6]This last sentence is a good addition to the definition. It makes clear the preference of outpatient care over inpatient care.

[7]Member is usually regarded as synonymous with enrollee. The definition of member should be consistent with the definition used in the group enrollment agreement.

[8]This paragraph allows the HMO to designate and amend the information, including the claims form, that the primary care physician provides the HMO without obtaining the prior approval of the primary care physician.

[9]This contract reimburses primary care physicians on a fee-for-service basis. Attachment B also sets forth alternative language if an HMO pays its primary care physicians on a capitated basis.

C. ***Processing of Claims.*** HMO agrees to process Primary Care Physician claims for Covered Services rendered to Members. HMO will make payment within thirty (30) days from the date the claim is received with sufficient documentation. Where a claim requires additional documentation, HMO will make payment within thirty (30) days from date of receipt of sufficient documentation to approve the claim.[10]

D. ***Eligibility Report.*** HMO shall provide Primary Care Physician with a monthly listing of eligible Members who have selected or have been assigned to Primary Care Physician.

E. ***Reports.*** HMO will provide Primary Care Physician with periodic statements with respect to the compensation set forth in Attachment B and with utilization reports in accordance with HMO's administrative procedures. Primary Care Physician agrees to maintain the confidentiality of the information presented in such reports.

PART III. OBLIGATIONS OF PRIMARY CARE PHYSICIAN

A. ***Health Services.*** Primary Care Physician shall have the primary responsibility for arranging and coordinating the overall health care of Members, including appropriate referral to Participating Physicians and Participating Providers, and for managing and coordinating the performance of administrative functions relating to the delivery of health services to Members in accordance with this Agreement. In the event that Primary Care Physician shall provide Member non-Covered Services, Primary Care Physician shall, prior to the provision of such non-Covered Services, inform the Member:

1. of the service(s) to be provided,
2. that HMO will not pay for or be liable for said services, and
3. that Member will be financially liable for such services.[11]

For any health care services rendered to or authorized for Members by Primary Care Physician for which HMO's prior approval is required and such prior approval was not obtained, Primary Care Physician agrees that in no event will HMO assume financial responsibility for charges arising from such services, and payments made by HMO for such services may be deducted by HMO from payments otherwise due Primary Care Physician.[12]

B. ***Referrals.*** Except in Emergencies or when authorized by HMO, Primary Care Physician agrees to make referrals of Members only to Participating Providers, and only in accordance with HMO policies. Primary Care Physician will furnish such Physicians and providers complete information on treatment procedures and diagnostic tests performed prior to such referral. Upon referral, Primary Care Physician agrees to notify HMO of referral. In the event that services required by a Member are not available from Participating Providers, non-Participating Physicians or Providers may be utilized with the prior approval of HMO. HMO will periodically furnish Primary Care Physician with a current listing of HMO's Participating Referral Physicians and Participating Providers.

C. ***Hospital Admissions.*** In cases where a Member requires a non-Emergency hospital admission, Primary Care Physician agrees to secure authorization for such admission in accordance with HMO's procedures prior to the admission. In addition, the Primary Care Physician agrees to abide by HMO hospital discharge policies and procedures for Members.[13]

---

[10]This paragraph allows the HMO to delay payment to the physician while waiting for sufficient documentation.

[11]This prior notification requirement is an important requirement and often required by state law.

[12]It is important for the HMO to make sure that the physicians know the circumstances or conditions for which prior HMO approval is required.

[13]Here, again, it is important for the HMO to ensure that the primary care physicians have full notice of all the requirements for prior authorization and discharges.

D. *Primary Care Physician's Members.* The Primary Care Physician shall not refuse to accept a Member as a patient on the basis of health status or medical condition of such Member, except with the approval of the Medical Director. Primary Care Physician may request that he/she does not wish to accept additional Members (excluding persons already in Primary Care Physician's practice that enroll in HMO as Members) by giving HMO written notice of such intent thirty (30) days in advance of the effective date of such closure. Primary Care Physician agrees to accept any HMO Members seeking his/her services during the thirty (30) day notice period. Primary Care Physician agrees to initiate closure of his/her practice to additional Members only if his/her practice, as a whole, is to be closed to additional patients or if authorized by HMO. A request for such authorization shall not be unreasonably denied. HMO may suspend, upon thirty (30) days prior written notice to Primary Care Physician, any further selection of Primary Care Physician by Members who have not already sought Primary Care Physician's services at the time of such suspension.

   In addition, a physician who is a Participating Provider may request, in writing to HMO, that coverage for a Member be transferred to another Participating Physician. Participating Physician shall not seek without authorization by HMO to have a Member transferred because of the amount of services required by the Member or because of the health status of the Member.

E. *Charges to Members.* Primary Care Physician shall accept as payment in full, for services which he/she provides, the compensation specified in Attachment B. Primary Care Physician agrees that in no event, including, but not limited to, non-payment, HMO insolvency or breach of this Agreement, shall Physician bill, charge, collect a deposit from, seek compensation, remuneration or reimbursement from, or have any recourse against Subscriber, Member, or persons other than the HMO acting on a Member's behalf for services provided pursuant to this Agreement. This provision shall not prohibit collection of copayments on HMO's behalf made in accordance with the terms of the Health Maintenance Certificate between HMO and Subscriber/Member.

   Primary Care Physician agrees that in the event of HMO's insolvency or other cessation of operations, services to Members will continue through the period for which the premium has been paid and services to members confined in an inpatient hospital on the date of insolvency or other cessation of operations will continue until their discharge.

   Primary Care Physician further agrees that:
   1. this provision shall survive the termination of this Agreement regardless of the cause giving rise to termination and shall be construed to be for the benefit of the HMO Member, and that
   2. this provision supersedes any oral or written contrary agreement now existing or hereafter entered into between Primary Care Physician and Member, or persons acting on their behalf.[14]

   Any modifications, addition or deletion to these provisions shall become effective on a date no earlier than 15 days after the _____ Department of Insurance has received written notice of such proposed changes.

F. *Records and Reports.*
   1. Primary Care Physician shall submit to HMO for each Member encounter an HMO Encounter Form which shall contain such statistical and descriptive medical and patient data as specified by HMO. Primary Care Physician shall maintain such records and provide such medical, financial and administrative information to HMO as the HMO determines may be necessary for compliance by HMO with state and federal law, as well as for program management purposes. Primary Care Physician will further provide to HMO and, if required, to authorized state and federal agencies, such access to medical records of HMO Members as is

---

[14]State regulatory agencies often dictate the precise language of this clause.

needed to assure the quality of care rendered to such Members. HMO shall have access at reasonable times, upon request, to the billing and medical records of the Primary Care Physician relating to the health care services provided Members, and to information on the cost of such services, and on copayments received by the Primary Care Physician from Members for Covered Services. Utilization and cost data relating to a Participating Physician may be distributed by HMO to other Participating Physicians for HMO program management purposes.

2. HMO shall also have the right to inspect, at reasonable times, Primary Care Physician's facilities pursuant to HMO's credentialing, peer review and quality assurance program.

3. Primary Care Physician shall maintain a complete medical record for each Member in accordance with the requirements established by HMO. Medical records of Members will include the recording of services provided by the Primary Care Physician, specialists, hospitals, and other reports from referral providers, discharge summaries, records of Emergency care received by the Member, and such other information as HMO requires.[15] Medical records of Members shall be treated as confidential so as to comply with all federal and state laws and regulations regarding the confidentiality of patient records.[16]

G. *Provision of Services and Professional Requirements.*

1. Primary Care Physician shall make necessary and appropriate arrangements to assure the availability of physician services to his/her Member patients on a twenty-four (24) hours per day, seven (7) days per week basis, including arrangements to assure coverage of his/her Member patients after-hours or when Primary Care Physician is otherwise absent, consistent with HMO's administrative requirements. Primary Care Physician agrees that scheduling of appointments for Members shall be done in a timely manner. The Primary Care Physician will maintain weekly appointment hours which are sufficient and convenient to serve Members and will maintain at all times Emergency and on-call services. Covering arrangements shall be with another Physician who is also a Participating Provider or who has otherwise been approved in advance by HMO. For services rendered by any covering Physician on behalf of Primary Care Physician, including Emergency Services, it shall be Primary Care Physician's sole responsibility to make suitable arrangements with the covering Physician regarding the manner in which said Physician will be reimbursed or otherwise compensated, provided, however, that Primary Care Physician shall assure that the covering Physician will not, under any circumstances, bill HMO or bill Member for Covered Services (except copayments), and Primary Care Physician hereby agrees to indemnify and hold harmless Members and HMO against charges for Covered Services rendered by physicians who are covering on behalf of Primary Care Physician.

2. Primary Care Physician agrees:

   (a) not to discriminate in the treatment of his/her patients or in the quality of services delivered to HMO's Members on the basis of race, sex, age, religion, place of residence, health status, disability, or source of payment, and

---

[15]This paragraph contains an important requirement. The primary care physician serves as a gatekeeper and the coordinator of care for this HMO. To serve this function, the primary care physician needs information from referral providers. There, of course, needs to be a requirement in the contracts with referral physicians that this information be provided to the applicable primary care physician.

[16]For this sentence to be effective, the HMO needs to ensure that its staff and the primary care physician understand state and federal confidentiality laws. Special requirements often arise in some areas, such as for acquired immunodeficiency syndrome and mental health and substance abuse services.

(b) to observe, protect and promote the rights of Members as patients. Primary Care Physician shall not seek to transfer a Member from his/her practice based on the Member's health status, without authorization by HMO.

3. Primary Care Physician agrees that all duties performed hereunder shall be consistent with the proper practice of medicine, and that such duties shall be performed in accordance with the customary rules of ethics and conduct of the applicable state and professional licensure boards and agencies.

4. Primary Care Physician agrees that to the extent he/she utilizes allied Health Professionals and other personnel for delivery of health care, he/she will inform HMO of the functions performed by such personnel.

5. Primary Care Physician shall be duly licensed to practice medicine in _____ and shall maintain good professional standing at all times. Evidence of such licensing shall be submitted to HMO upon request. In addition, Primary Care Physician must meet all qualifications and standards for membership on the medical staff of at least one of the hospitals which have contracted with HMO and shall be required to maintain staff membership and full admission privileges in accordance with the rules and regulations of such hospital and be otherwise acceptable to such hospital. Physician agrees to give immediate notice to HMO in the case of suspension or revocation, or initiation of any proceeding that could result in suspension or revocation, of his/her licensure, hospital privileges, or participation under a Federal health care program or the filing of a malpractice action against the Primary Care Physician.

H. *Insurance.* Primary Care Physician, including individual Physicians providing services to Members under this Agreement if Primary Care Physician is a legal entity, shall provide and maintain such policies of general and professional liability (malpractice) insurance as shall be necessary to insure the Primary Care Physician and his/her employees against any claim or claims for damages arising by reason of personal injuries or death occasioned, directly or indirectly, in connection with the performance of any service by Primary Care Physician. The amounts and extent of such insurance coverage shall be subject to the approval of HMO. Primary Care Physician shall provide memorandum copies of such insurance coverage to HMO upon request.[17] Primary Care Physician agrees to notify HMO within five (5) days of any reduction to or cancellation of such insurance coverage.

I. *Administration.*

1. Primary Care Physician agrees to cooperate and participate in such review and service programs as may be established by HMO, including utilization and quality assurance programs, credentialing, sanctioning, external audit systems, administrative procedures, and Member and Physician grievance procedures. Primary Care Physician shall comply with all determinations rendered through the above programs.

2. Primary Care Physician agrees that HMO may use his/her name, address, phone number, picture, type of practice, applicable practice restrictions, and an indication of Primary Care Physician's willingness to accept additional Members, in HMO's roster of physician participants and other HMO materials. Primary Care Physician shall not reference HMO in any publicity, advertisements, notices, or promotional material or in any announcement to the Members without prior review and written approval of HMO.

3. Primary Care Physician agrees to provide to HMO information for the collection and coordination of benefits when a Member holds other coverage that is deemed primary for the pro-

---

[17]The HMO should have this insurance information on file. Thus the HMO, as a matter of course, should request this information and require notification of changes in the insurance coverage.

vision of services to said Member and to abide by HMO coordination of benefits and duplicate coverage policies. This shall include, but not be limited to, permitting HMO to bill and
process forms for any third party payer on the Primary Care Physician's behalf for Covered
Services and to retain any sums received. In addition, Primary Care Physician shall cooperate in and abide by HMO subrogation policies and procedures.

4. Primary Care Physician agrees to maintain the confidentiality of all information related to
   fees, charges, expenses, and utilization derived from, through, or provided by HMO.

5. In the event of:
   (a) termination of this Agreement,
   (b) the selection by a Member of another Primary Care Physician in accordance with HMO
       procedures, or
   (c) the approval by HMO of Primary Care Physician's request to transfer a Member from
       his/her practice,
   Primary Care Physician agrees to transfer copies of the Member's medical records, X-rays,
   or other data to HMO when requested to do so in writing by HMO, at the reasonable, customary and usual fee for such copies.

6. Upon termination of the Agreement, the Primary Care Physician shall not use any information
   obtained during the course of the Agreement in furtherance of any competitors of the HMO.

7. Primary Care Physician warrants and represents that all information and statements given to
   HMO in applying for or maintaining his/her HMO Primary Care Physician Agreement are
   true, accurate and complete. The HMO Physician application shall be incorporated by reference into this Agreement. Any inaccurate or incomplete information or misrepresentation of
   information provided by Primary Care Physician may result in the immediate termination of
   the Agreement by HMO. Primary Care Physician shall notify HMO as soon as possible, but
   no more than five (5) days after, of any changes to the information provided in the HMO
   Physician application.

8. Primary Care Physician shall cooperate with HMO in complying with applicable laws relating to HMO.

PART IV. MISCELLANEOUS

A. ***Modification of this Agreement.*** This Agreement may be amended or modified in writing as
   mutually agreed upon by the parties. In addition, HMO may modify any provision of this Agreement upon thirty (30) days prior written notice to Primary Care Physician. Primary Care Physician
   shall be deemed to have accepted HMO's modification if Primary Care Physician fails to object to
   such modification, in writing, within the thirty (30) day notice period.[18]

B. ***Interpretation.*** This Agreement shall be governed in all respects by the laws of the State of
   _____. The invalidity or unenforceability of any terms or conditions hereof shall in no way
   affect the validity or enforceability of any other terms or provisions. The waiver by either party of
   a breach or violation of any provision of this Agreement shall not operate as or be construed to be
   a waiver of any subsequent breach thereof.

C. ***Assignment.*** This Agreement, being intended to secure the services of and be personal to the
   Primary Care Physician, shall not be assigned, sublet, delegated or transferred by Primary Care
   Physician without the prior written consent of HMO.

---

[18]This is a common provision and useful in simplifying the administrative work associated with amending the
agreement. Needless to say, it is important for the HMO to explain clearly the nature of the amendment to the
primary care physician.

D. ***Notice.*** Any notice required to be given pursuant to the terms and provisions hereof shall be sent by certified mail, return receipt requested, postage prepaid, to HMO or to the Primary Care Physician at the respective addresses indicated herein. Notice shall be deemed to be effective when mailed, but notice of change of address shall be effective upon receipt.[19]

E. ***Relationship of Parties.*** None of the provisions of this Agreement is intended to create nor shall be deemed or construed to create any relationship between the parties hereto other than that of independent entities contracting with each other hereunder solely for the purpose of effecting the provisions of this Agreement. Neither of the parties hereto, nor any of their respective employees, shall be construed to be the agent, employer, employee or representative of the other, nor will either party have an express or implied right of authority to assume or create any obligation or responsibility on behalf of or in the name of the other party. Neither Primary Care Physician nor HMO shall be liable to any other party for any act, or any failure to act, of the other party to this Agreement.

F. ***Gender.*** The use of any gender herein shall be deemed to include the other gender where applicable.

G. ***Legal Entity.*** If Primary Care Physician is a legal entity, an application for each Physician who is a member of such entity must be submitted to and accepted by HMO before such Physician may serve as a Primary Care Physician under this Agreement.

H. ***Term and Termination.*** The term of this Agreement shall be for three (3) years from the "effective date" set forth on the signature page. This Agreement may be terminated by either party at any time without cause by prior written notice given at least sixty (60) days in advance of the effective date of such termination. This Agreement may also be terminated by HMO effective immediately upon written notice if Primary Care Physician's (or if a legal entity, any of the entity's physicians') medical license, participation under a Federal health care program or hospital privileges are suspended, limited, restricted or revoked, or if Primary Care Physician violates Part III(E), (G)(3), (G)(5), (H), (I)(1) or (I)(4) herein. Upon termination, the rights of each party hereunder shall terminate, provided, however, that such action shall not release the Primary Care Physician or HMO from their obligations with respect to:

1. payments accrued to the Primary Care Physician prior to termination;
2. the Primary Care Physician's agreement not to seek compensation from Members for Covered Services provided prior to termination; and
3. completion of treatment of Members then receiving care until continuation of the Member's care can be arranged by HMO.

In the event of termination, no distribution of any money accruing to Primary Care Physician under the provisions of Attachment B shall be made until the regularly scheduled date for such distributions. Upon termination, HMO is empowered and authorized to notify Members and prospective Members, other Primary Care Physicians, and other persons or entities whom it deems to have an interest herein of such termination, through such means as it may choose.

In the event of notice of termination, HMO may notify Members of such fact and assign Members or require Members to select another Primary Care Physician prior to the effective date of termination. In any event, HMO shall continue to compensate Primary Care Physician until the effective date of termination as provided herein for those Members who, because of health reasons, cannot be assigned or make such selection during the notice of termination period and as provided by HMO's Medical Director.

---

[19]Before adopting this paragraph, an HMO should consider whether it is necessary to require that all notifications be sent by certified mail, return receipt requested. If the HMO has a large provider panel, it might prefer the right to send information by regular mail.

IN WITNESS WHEREOF, the foregoing Agreement between _____ and Primary Care Physician, is entered into by and between the undersigned parties, to be effective this _____ day of _____, 20___.

PRIMARY CARE PHYSICIAN

_____   By: _____
(Name of Individual Physician or of
Group Practice—Please Print)

_____   _____
(Mailing Address)   (Date)

_____
(City, State, ZIP)

_____
(Telephone Number)

_____
(Taxpayer Identification Number)

_____
(DEA#)

_____
(Signature)

_____
(Name and Title if signing as authorized
representative of Group Practice)

_____
(Date)

ATTACHMENT B
COMPENSATION SCHEDULE

PRIMARY CARE PHYSICIAN AGREEMENT

I. Services Rendered by Physicians

For Covered Services provided by Primary Care Physician in accordance with the terms of this Agreement, HMO shall pay Primary Care Physician his/her Reimbursement Allowance, less any applicable copayment for which the Member is responsible under the applicable Health Maintenance Certificate, and less the Withhold Amount, as described below. "Reimbursement Allowance" shall mean the lower of (i) the usual and customary fee charged by Primary Care Physician for the Covered Service, or (ii) the maximum amount allowed under the fee limits established by HMO.

II. Withholds from Reimbursement Allowance

HMO shall withhold from each payment to Primary Care Physician a percentage of the Reimbursement Allowance ("Withhold Amount") and shall allocate an amount equal to such withhold to an HMO Risk Fund. HMO shall have the right, at its sole discretion, to modify the percentage withheld from Primary Care Physician if, in its judgment, the financial condition, operations or commitments of the HMO or its expenses for particular health services or for services by any particular Participating Providers warrant such modification.

III. Withhold Amount Distributions

HMO may, at its sole discretion, from time to time distribute to Primary Care Physician Withhold Amounts retained by HMO from payments to Primary Care Physician, plus such additional amounts, if any, that HMO may deem appropriate as a financial incentive to the provision of cost-effective health care services. HMO may, from time to time, commit or expend Withhold Amounts, in whole or in part, to assure the financial stability of or commitments of the HMO or health care plans or payers with or for which the HMO has an agreement to arrange for the provision of health care services, or to satisfy budgetary or financial objectives established by HMO.

Subject to HMO's peer review procedures and policies, a Primary Care Physician may be excluded from any distribution if he/she does not qualify for such distribution, for example, if he/she has exceeded HMO utilization standards or criteria. No Primary Care Physician shall have any entitlement to any funds in the HMO Risk Fund.

IV. Accounting

Primary Care Physician shall be entitled to an accounting of Withhold Amounts from payments to him/her upon written request to HMO.

ATTACHMENT B (ALTERNATE)
CAPITATION PAYMENT

PRIMARY CARE PHYSICIAN AGREEMENT

Compensation

I. Capitation Allocation

The total monthly amounts paid to Primary Care Physician will be determined as follows:

For each Member selecting Primary Care Physician ("selecting" also includes Members assigned to a Primary Care Physician), 90 percent of the monthly Primary Care Service capitation set forth below for Primary Care Services shall be paid by HMO to Primary Care Physician by the 5th day of the following month. The capitation shall be set according to the particular benefit plan in which each Member is enrolled. Where the capitation is not currently adjusted for age and/or sex, HMO reserves the right to make such age and/or sex adjustment to the capitation rates upon thirty (30) days notice. In consideration of such payments, Primary Care Physician agrees to provide to Members the Primary Care Services set forth in the Agreement.

Health Plan shall allocate the remaining 10 percent of the monthly capitation payments to a Risk Reserve Fund which fund is subject to the further provisions of this Attachment. The capitation payments to Primary Care Physician for Primary Care Services, subject to the above withhold, are as follows:

Coverage Plans

Age/Sex	Commercial Plan__ Capitation Payment	Commercial Plan__ Capitation Payment	Commercial Plan__ Capitation Payment
0–24 Months/M/F	$ _____	$ _____	$ _____
2–4 Years/M/F	$ _____	$ _____	$ _____
5–19 Years/M/F	$ _____	$ _____	$ _____
20–39 Years/F	$ _____	$ _____	$ _____
20–39 Years/M	$ _____	$ _____	$ _____
40–49 Years/F	$ _____	$ _____	$ _____
40–49 Years/M	$ _____	$ _____	$ _____
50–59 Years/F	$ _____	$ _____	$ _____
50–59 Years/M	$ _____	$ _____	$ _____
>60 Years/F	$ _____	$ _____	$ _____
>60 Years/M	$ _____	$ _____	$ _____

Primary Care Physician is financially liable for all Primary Care Services rendered to Members under the above capitation. If Primary Care Physician fails to do so, HMO may pay for such services on behalf of Primary Care Physician and deduct such payments from any sums otherwise due Primary Care Physician by HMO.

Sample Hospital Agreement

_____.

HEALTH MAINTENANCE ORGANIZATION

PARTICIPATING HOSPITAL AGREEMENT[1]

THIS AGREEMENT, made and entered into the date set forth on the signature page hereto, by and between _____ (the "Hospital"), a facility duly licensed under the laws of the State of _____ and located at _____, and _____ ("HMO"), a corporation organized under the _____ law, and located at _____.

WHEREAS, HMO provides a plan of health care benefits (the "Plan") to individuals and their eligible family members and dependents who contract with HMO or who are the beneficiaries of a contract with HMO for such benefits ("Members"), and in connection with such Plan, arranges for the provision of health care services, including Hospital Services, to such Members; and

WHEREAS, the Hospital desires to provide Hospital Services to Members in accordance with the terms and conditions of this Agreement as hereinafter set forth; and

WHEREAS, HMO desires to arrange for the services of the Hospital for the benefit of the Members of the Plan.

NOW, THEREFORE, in consideration of the foregoing recitals and the mutual covenants and promises herein contained and other good and valuable consideration, receipt and sufficiency of which are hereby acknowledged, the parties hereto agree and covenant as follows:

PART I. DEFINITIONS

A. *Covered Services* means those health services and benefits to which Members are entitled under the terms of the applicable Health Maintenance Certificate, which may be amended by HMO from time to time.

B. *Emergency Services* means those Medically Necessary services provided in connection with an "Emergency," defined as a sudden or unexpected onset of a condition requiring medical or surgi-

---

[1]For consistency, the HMO has used the same definitions for this agreement and the preceding primary care physician agreement. This agreement also uses some of the same provisions as in the primary care physician agreement. Comments made to those provisions in the primary care physician agreement will not be repeated here.

cal care which the Member receives after the onset of such condition (or as soon thereafter as care can be made available but not more than twenty-four (24) hours after onset) and in the absence of such care the Member could reasonably be expected to suffer serious physical impairment or death. Heart attacks, severe chest pain, cardiovascular accidents, hemorrhaging, poisonings, major burns, loss of consciousness, serious breathing difficulties, spinal injuries, shock, and other acute conditions as HMO shall determine are Emergencies.

C. *Health Maintenance Certificate* means a contract issued by HMO to a Member or an employer of Members specifying the services and benefits available under the HMO's prepaid health benefits program.

D. *Hospital Services* means all inpatient services, emergency room, and outpatient hospital services that are Covered Services.

E. *Medical Director* means a Physician designated by HMO to monitor and review the provision of Covered Services to Members.

F. *Medically Necessary services and/or supplies* means the use of services or supplies as provided by a hospital, skilled nursing facility, Physician or other provider required to identify or treat a Member's illness or injury and which, as determined by HMO's Medical Director or its utilization management committee, are: (1) consistent with the symptoms or diagnosis and treatment of the Member's condition, disease, ailment or injury; (2) appropriate with regard to standards of good medical practice; (3) not solely for the convenience of the Member, his/her Physician, hospital, or other health care provider; and (4) the most appropriate supply or level of service which can be safely provided to the Member. When specifically applied to an inpatient Member, it further means that the Member's medical symptoms or condition requires that the diagnosis or treatment cannot be safely provided to the Member as an outpatient.

G. *Member* means both an HMO subscriber and his/her enrolled family members for whom premium payment has been made.

H. *Participating Physician* means a Physician who, at the time of providing or authorizing services to a Member, has contracted with or on whose behalf a contract has been entered into with HMO to provide professional services to Members.

I. *Participating Provider* means a Physician, hospital, skilled nursing facility, home health agency or any other duly licensed institution or health professional under contract with HMO to provide health care services to Members. A list of Participating Providers and their locations is available to each Member upon enrollment. Such list shall be revised from time to time as HMO deems necessary.

J. *Physician* means a duly licensed doctor of medicine or osteopathy.

K. *Primary Care Physician* means a Participating Physician who provides primary care services to Members (e.g., general or family practitioner, internist, pediatrician, or such other physician specialty as may be designated by HMO) and is responsible for referrals of Members to referral Physicians, other Participating Providers, and if necessary, non-Participating Providers.

PART II. HOSPITAL OBLIGATIONS

A. Hospital shall provide to Members those Hospital Services which Hospital has the capacity to provide. Such services shall be provided by Hospital in accordance with the provisions of its Articles of Incorporation and bylaws and medical staff bylaws and the appropriate terms of this Agreement.

B. Hospital shall render Hospital Services to Members in an economical and efficient manner consistent with professional standards of medical care generally accepted in the medical community. Hospital shall not discriminate in the treatment of members and, except as otherwise required by this Agreement, shall make its services available to Members in the same manner as to its other patients.[2] In the event that an admission of a Member cannot be accommodated by Hospital, Hospital shall make the same efforts to arrange for the provision of services at another facility approved by HMO that it would make for other patients in similar circumstances. In the event that Hospital shall provide Member non-Covered Services, Hospital shall, prior to the provision of such non-Covered Services, inform the Member:

1. of the service(s) to be provided,
2. that HMO will not pay for or be liable for said services, and
3. that Member will be financially liable for such services.

C. Except in an Emergency, Hospital shall provide Hospital Inpatient Services to a Member only when Hospital has received certification from HMO in advance of admission of such Member. Services which have not been so approved or authorized shall be the sole financial responsibility of Hospital.[3]

D. If, and to the extent that, the Hospital is not authorized to perform preadmission testing, the Hospital agrees to accept the results of qualified and timely laboratory, radiological and other tests and procedures which may be performed on a Member prior to admission. The Hospital will not require that duplicate tests or procedures be performed after the Enrollee is admitted, unless such tests and procedures are Medically Necessary.

E. In an Emergency, Hospital shall immediately proceed to render Medically Necessary services to the Member. Hospital shall also contact HMO within twenty-four (24) hours of the treatment of the emergency treatment visit or emergency admission. HMO has twenty-four (24) hour on-call nurse coverage for notification of Emergency Services or admits.

   If Hospital fails to notify HMO within the required time period, neither HMO nor the Member shall be liable for charges for Hospital Services rendered subsequent to the required notification period that are deemed by HMO not to be Medically Necessary.[4]

F. Hospital shall cooperate with and abide by HMO's programs that monitor and evaluate whether Hospital Services provided to Members in accordance with this Agreement are Medically Necessary and consistent with professional standards of medical care generally accepted in the medical community. Such programs include, but are not limited to, utilization management, quality assurance review, and grievance procedures. In connection with HMO's programs, Hospital shall permit HMO's utilization management personnel to visit Members in the Hospital and, to the extent permitted by applicable laws, to inspect and copy health records (including medical records) of Members maintained by Hospital for the purposes of concurrent and retrospective utilization management, discharge planning, and other program management purposes.

G. Hospital shall cooperate with HMO in complying with applicable laws relating to HMO.

---

[2]This requirement serves the same purpose as its counterpart in the primary care physician agreement of requiring the hospital to treat HMO members in the same manner as fee-for-service patients.

[3]A growing issue, not addressed in this provision, is the HMO's responsibility for hospital charges incurred to provide a medical screening examination, as required by Section 1867 of the Social Security Act, to enrollees seeking care from the hospital's emergency department. The hospital may want to seek an explicit statement requiring the HMO to cover the cost of that examination.

[4]To avoid disputes, the hospital and HMO need a common understanding of the meaning of the term Medically Necessary. The definition of that term used in this contract favors the HMO by allowing for its interpretation.

PART III. LICENSURE AND ACCREDITATION

Hospital represents that it is duly licensed by the Department of Health of the State of _____ to operate a hospital, is a qualified provider under the Medicare program, and is accredited by the Joint Commission on the Accreditation of Healthcare Organizations ("Joint Commission"). Hospital shall maintain in good standing such license and accreditation and shall notify HMO immediately should any action of any kind be initiated against Hospital which could result in:

1. the suspension or loss of such license;
2. the suspension or loss of such accreditation; or
3. the imposition of any sanctions against Hospital under a Federal health care program.

Hospital shall furnish to HMO such evidence of licensure, Medicare qualification and accreditation as HMO may request.

PART IV. RECORDS

A. Hospital shall maintain with respect to each Member receiving Hospital Services pursuant to this Agreement a standard hospital medical record in such form, containing such information, and preserved for such time period(s) as are required by the rules and regulations of the _____ Department of Health, the Medicare program, and the Joint Commission. The original hospital medical records shall be and remain the property of Hospital and shall not be removed or transferred from Hospital except in accordance with applicable laws and general Hospital policies, rules, and regulations relating thereto; provided, however, that HMO shall have the right, in accordance with paragraph (B) below, to inspect, review, and make copies of such records upon request.

B. Upon consent of the Member and a request for such records or information, Hospital shall provide copies of information contained in the medical records of Members to other authorized providers of health care services and to HMO for the purpose of facilitating the delivery of appropriate health care services to Members and carrying out the purposes and provisions of this Agreement, and shall facilitate the sharing of such records among health care providers involved in a Member's care. HMO, and if required, authorized state and federal agencies, shall have the right upon request to inspect at reasonable times and to obtain copies of all records that are maintained by Hospital relating to the care of Members pursuant to this Agreement.

PART V. INSURANCE AND INDEMNIFICATION

A. Hospital shall secure and maintain at its expense throughout the term of this Agreement such policy or policies of general liability and professional liability insurance as shall be necessary to insure Hospital, its agents and employees against any claim or claims for damages arising by reason of injury or death, occasioned directly or indirectly by the performance or nonperformance of any service by Hospital, its agents or employees. Upon request, Hospital shall provide HMO with a copy of the policy (or policies) or certificate(s) of insurance which evidence compliance with the foregoing insurance requirements. It is specifically agreed that coverage amounts in general conformity with other similar type and size hospitals within the State of _____ shall be acceptable to HMO and be considered satisfactory and in compliance with this requirement.[5]

---

[5]This paragraph reflects the difference in relative bargaining strength that the HMO has with hospitals and physicians. Although the HMO–primary care physician agreement gives the HMO the right to approve malpractice coverage, no such right is contained in the HMO–participating hospital agreement. Another factor may be that the concern of inadequate coverage may be greater for a physician than a hospital.

B. Hospital and HMO each shall indemnify and hold the other harmless from any and all liability, loss, damage, claim or expense of any kind, including costs and attorney's fees, arising out of the performance of this Agreement and for which the other is solely responsible.

PART VI. MEDICAL STAFF MEMBERSHIP

Notwithstanding any other provision of this Agreement, a Participating Physician may not admit or treat a Member in the Hospital unless he/she is a member in good standing of Hospital's organized medical staff with appropriate clinical privileges to admit and treat such Member.[6]

PART VII. HMO OBLIGATIONS

A. HMO shall provide to or for the benefit of each Member an identification card which shall be presented for purposes of assisting Hospital in verifying Member eligibility. In addition, HMO shall maintain other verification procedures by which Hospital may confirm the eligibility of any Member.
B. HMO shall provide thirty (30) days' advance notice to Hospital of any changes in Covered Services or in the copayments or conditions of coverage applicable thereto.
C. HMO will, whenever an individual, admitted or referred, is not a Member, advise Hospital within thirty (30) days from the date of receipt of an invoice from Hospital for services to such an individual. In such cases, Hospital shall directly bill the individual or another third party payer for services rendered to such individual.
D. In the event continued stay or services are denied after a patient has been admitted, HMO or its representative shall inform the patient that services have been denied.

PART VIII. USE OF NAME

Except as provided in this paragraph, neither HMO nor Hospital shall use the other's name, symbols, trademarks or service marks in advertising or promotional material or otherwise. HMO shall have the right to use the name of Hospital for purposes of marketing, informing Members of the identity of Hospital and otherwise to carry out the terms of this Agreement. Hospital shall have the right to use HMO's name in its informational or promotional materials with HMO's prior approval, which approval shall not be unreasonably withheld.

PART IX. COMPENSATION

Hospital will be compensated by HMO for all Medically Necessary Covered Services provided to Members in accordance with the provisions of Attachment A annexed hereto and incorporated herein.[7]

---

[6]Requiring the HMO's physicians to comply with the hospital's medical staff requirements is important and reasonable.

[7]Attachment A provides for payment as a percentage of charges. By structuring the agreement in this manner, the HMO is able to negotiate different payment arrangements with hospitals without revising the body of the agreement.

PART X. PAYMENT TO HOSPITAL BY HMO

For Hospital Services rendered to Members, Hospital shall invoice HMO at Hospital's current charges. [Alternative: For Hospital Services rendered to Members, Hospital shall invoice HMO.[8]] Except for Hospital Services which HMO determines require further review under HMO's utilization management procedures, or when there are circumstances which are beyond the control of HMO, including submission of incomplete claims, HMO shall make payment of invoices for Hospital Services within thirty (30) calendar days after the HMO's receipt thereof. HMO authorized copayments shall be collected by the Hospital from the Member and the Member shall be solely responsible for the payment of such copayments. All billings by Hospital shall be considered final unless adjustments are requested in writing by Hospital within sixty (60) days after receipt of original billing by HMO, except for circumstances which are beyond the control of Hospital.[9] No payment shall be made unless the invoice for services is received within sixty (60) days after the date of discharge of the Member or date of service, whichever occurs later. Hospital shall interim bill HMO every thirty (30) days for patients whose length of stay is greater than thirty (30) days.

PART XI. PROHIBITIONS ON MEMBER BILLING

Hospital hereby agrees that in no event, including, but not limited to, nonpayment by HMO, HMO's insolvency or breach of this Agreement, shall Hospital bill, charge, collect a deposit from, seek compensation, remuneration or reimbursement from, or have any recourse against a Member or persons other than HMO acting on a Member's behalf for services provided pursuant to this Agreement. This provision shall not prohibit collection of copayment on HMO's behalf in accordance with the terms of the Health Maintenance Certificate between HMO and Member.

Hospital agrees that in the event of HMO's insolvency or other cessation of operations, services to Members will continue through the period for which the premium has been paid and services to members confined in an inpatient hospital on the date of insolvency or other cessation of operations will continue until their discharge.

Hospital further agrees that:
1. this provision shall survive the termination of this Agreement regardless of the cause giving rise to termination and shall be construed to be for the benefit of the Member; and
2. this provision supersedes any oral or written contrary agreement now existing or hereafter entered into between Hospital and Member, or persons acting on their behalf.

Any modifications, addition or deletion to these provisions shall become effective on a date no earlier than 15 days after the _____ Department of Insurance has received written notice of such proposed changes.

PART XII. INSPECTION OF RECORDS

Upon request, and at reasonable times, HMO and Hospital shall make available to the other for review such books, records, utilization information and other documents or information relating directly to any determination required by this Agreement. All such information shall be held by the

---

[8]This broader alternative language along with the cross-reference to Attachment A in the preceding paragraph allows the body of the contract to be used for any type of payment arrangement. An alternative Attachment A is offered that establishes per diem rates for inpatient stays and a percentage of charges for outpatient services.

[9]To avoid potential disputes, the hospital and the HMO should have some general understanding of the meaning of the term beyond the control of Hospital.

receiving party in confidence and shall only be used in connection with the administration of this Agreement.

PART XIII. COORDINATION OF BENEFITS

Hospital agrees to cooperate with HMO toward effective implementation of any provisions of HMO's Health Maintenance Certificates relating to coordination of benefits and claims by third parties. Hospital shall forward to HMO any payments received from a third party payer for authorized Hospital Services where HMO has made payment to Hospital covering such Hospital Services and such third party payer is determined to be primarily obligated for such Hospital Services under applicable Coordination of Benefits rules. Such payment shall not exceed the amount paid to Hospital by HMO. Except as otherwise required by law, Hospital agrees to permit HMO to bill and process forms for any third party payer on Hospital's behalf, or to bill such third party directly, as determined by HMO. Hospital further agrees to waive, when requested, any claims against third party payers for its provision of Hospital Services to Members and to execute any further documents that reasonably may be required or appropriate for this purpose. Any such waiver shall be contingent upon HMO's payment to Hospital of its (HMO's) obligations for charges incurred by Member. This paragraph shall not be interpreted as a waiver of Medicare beneficiary cost sharing obligations to the extent that such waiver is in violation of Federal law.

PART XIV. TERM AND TERMINATION

A. This Agreement shall take effect on the "effective date" set forth on the signature page and shall continue for a period of one year or until terminated as provided herein.
   1. Either party may terminate this Agreement without cause upon at least ninety (90) days written notice prior to the term of this Agreement.
   2. Either party may terminate this Agreement with cause upon at least thirty (30) days prior written notice.
B. HMO shall have the right to terminate this Agreement immediately by notice to Hospital upon the occurrence of any of the following events:
   1. the suspension or revocation of Hospital's license;
   2. the suspension, revocation or loss of the Hospital's Joint Commission accreditation or Medicare qualification; or
   3. breach of Part II(E) or Part XI of this Agreement.
C. HMO shall continue to pay Hospital in accordance with the provisions of Attachment A for Hospital Services provided by Hospital to Members hospitalized at the time of termination of this Agreement, pending clinically appropriate discharge or transfer to an HMO designated hospital when medically appropriate as determined by HMO. In continuing to provide such Hospital Services, Hospital shall abide by the applicable terms and conditions of this Agreement.

PART XV. ADMINISTRATION

Hospital agrees to abide by and cooperate with HMO administrative policies including, but not limited to, claims procedures, copayment collections, and duplicate coverage/subrogation recoveries. Nothing in this Agreement shall be construed to require Hospital to violate, breach, or modify its written policies and procedures unless specifically agreed to herein.

PART XVI. MEMBER GRIEVANCES

Hospital agrees to cooperate in and abide by HMO grievance procedures in resolving Member's grievances related to the provision of Hospital Services. In this regard, HMO shall bring to the attention of appropriate Hospital officials all Member complaints involving Hospital, and Hospital shall, in accordance with its regular procedure, investigate such complaints and use its best efforts to resolve them in a fair and equitable manner. Hospital agrees to notify HMO promptly of any action taken or proposed with respect to the resolution of such complaints and the avoidance of similar complaints in the future. The Hospital shall notify the HMO after it has received a complaint from an HMO Member.

PART XVII. MISCELLANEOUS

A. If any term, provision, covenant or condition of this Agreement is invalid, void or unenforceable, the rest of the Agreement shall remain in full force and effect. The invalidity or unenforceability of any term or provision hereof shall in no way affect the validity or enforceability of any other term or provision.
B. This Agreement contains the complete understanding and agreement between Hospital and HMO and supersedes all representations, understandings or agreements prior to the execution hereof.
C. HMO and Hospital agree that, to the extent compatible with the separate and independent management of each, they shall at all times maintain an effective liaison and close cooperation with each other to provide maximum benefits to Members at the most reasonable cost consistent with quality standards of hospital care.
D. No waiver, alteration, amendment or modification of this Agreement shall be valid unless in each instance a written memorandum specifically expressing such waiver, alteration, amendment, or modification is made and subscribed by a duly authorized officer of Hospital and a duly authorized officer of HMO.
E. Hospital shall not assign its rights, duties, or obligations under this Agreement without the express, written permission of HMO.
F. None of the provisions of this Agreement are intended to create nor shall be deemed to create any relationship between HMO and Hospital other than that of independent entities contracting with each other hereunder solely for the purpose of effecting the provisions of this Agreement. Neither of the parties hereto, nor any of their respective employees shall be construed to be the agent, employer, employee or representative of the other.
G. This Agreement shall be construed in accordance with the laws of the State of _____.
H. The headings and numbers of sections and paragraphs contained in this Agreement are for reference purposes only and shall not affect in any way the meaning or interpretation of this Agreement.
I. Any notice required or permitted to be given pursuant to the terms and provisions of this Agreement shall be sent by registered mail or certified mail, return receipt requested, postage prepaid, to:

_____

_____

_____

_____

and to Hospital at:

_____

_____

_____

_____

IN WITNESS WHEREOF, the foregoing Agreement between _____
and Hospital is entered into by and between the undersigned parties, to be effective the _____ day of
_____, 20___.

HOSPITAL

By: _____   By: _____

Title: _____   Title: _____

Date: _____   Date: _____

ATTACHMENT A
PARTICIPATING HOSPITAL COMPENSATION

Subject to the terms and conditions set forth in this Agreement, HMO shall pay Hospital
_____ (_____%) of Hospital's schedule of charges effective _____
as submitted and approved by HMO, for Medically Necessary Covered Services provided to Members.

ATTACHMENT A (ALTERNATE)
PARTICIPATING HOSPITAL COMPENSATION

Subject to the terms and conditions set forth in this Agreement, HMO shall pay Hospital, as follows:

Service	Type of Reimbursement	Total Reimbursement
Inpatient care		
Nonmaternity—Secondary	Per Diem	$_____
Nonmaternity—Tertiary	Per Diem	$_____
Maternity	Per Diem	$_____
Psychiatric	Per Diem	$_____
Well newborn children	Per Diem	$_____
Outpatient care		
Other than outpatient surgery	Percentage Discount	_____%
Outpatient surgery	Hospital will be reimbursed (1) the percentage discount stated above, (2) any guaranteed maximum "global" rate program adopted by the Hospital for ambulatory surgical procedures,[10] or (3) 125 percent[11] of the per diem payment amount had the Enrollee been admitted to the Hospital, whichever is least.	

---

[10]If Medicare adopts a global fee for reimbursement of outpatient hospital costs, an increasing number of HMO-hospital contracts are likely to adopt a similar approach.

[11]This percentage commonly varies from 100% to 125%.

CHAPTER 63

Antitrust Remedies for Managed Care: Attacking Barriers to Free Markets

William G. Kopit and Robert Hudock

INTRODUCTION

As competition intensifies and combines with other factors to squeeze the bottom line, health maintenance organizations (HMOs) and other managed care organizations (MCOs) have demonstrated an increased willingness to use the antitrust laws to challenge the behavior of competitors and suppliers. A variety of arrangements, including alleged price fixing, boycotts, most favored nations (MFNs) clauses in provider contracts, exclusive provider arrangements, and provider unions have all come under heightened scrutiny. Where competitors or suppliers wield sufficient economic power to force increased prices or to force participation or nonparticipation in provider networks, some sort of antitrust challenge reasonably can be expected. This chapter explores the recent trend in antitrust enforcement undertaken by HMOs and MCOs, acting either for themselves or through complaints to antitrust enforcement agencies.

The antitrust laws are designed to protect consumers. The basic premise behind these laws is that if competition is preserved, consumers will get the lowest prices possible (at any given level of quality) and the greatest number of choices possible. On the other hand, the antitrust laws are not designed to protect competitors. Thus, an action that merely benefits one competitor at the expense of another, but does not have the potential to harm consumers, is generally not actionable under the antitrust laws, at least if the action is undertaken by a private party. This simple but important concept is central to the analysis of almost every antitrust question involving a challenge, or potential challenge, to conduct brought by an HMO or MCO. In fact, although a number of seemingly complex doctrines have developed under the antitrust laws, in virtually every antitrust case it helps to focus the inquiry by asking, "How does the conduct upon which the complaint is based harm consumers?"[1]

ENFORCEMENT OF THE ANTITRUST AND UNFAIR COMPETITION LAWS

The United States has what has been described as a three-level antitrust enforcement system because the federal antitrust laws can be enforced by two agencies at the federal level, as well as by the states, usually acting through state attorney generals ("AGs"), and by private parties like complaining HMOs and MCOs themselves. The federal antitrust agencies—the Federal Trade Commission (FTC or Commission) and the Antitrust Division of the United States Department of Justice (Antitrust Division) (collectively, the Agencies)—administer and en-

William G. Kopit is a senior member of the health law section of Epstein Becker & Green, P.C., located in Washington, DC. He specializes in antitrust, managed care, and policy litigation.

Robert Hudock is a senior at Cornell Law School and was a summer associate at Epstein Becker & Green, P.C. in the summer of 1999. He will become a permanent associate at the law firm in September 2000.

force the federal antitrust laws. State AGs and other state agencies can enforce state-enacted antitrust laws, which are usually modeled after the federal Sherman Act, as well as the federal statutes. However, state enforcers are most often concerned with activity within the borders of their respective states. Still, health care typically has local consequences, and, as a result, many state AGs have expressed considerable interest in the issues.[2] Finally, both the federal and the state antitrust laws permit private parties injured by anticompetitive conduct to bring actions and seek, among other remedies, treble damages. Because both the federal government and the state enforcers have limited resources, HMOs and MCOs faced with serious economic injury, or the threat of serious economic injury, have begun to seriously consider self-help through private antitrust actions.

THE ANTITRUST LAWS

Standing

To have standing under Section 4 of the Clayton Act, a private plaintiff must prove that he was injured, that the injury was to business or property, that the injury was caused by an antitrust violation, that the injury was an antitrust injury, and that he has antitrust standing. See *Amerinet, Inc. v. Standard Oil Co.,* 405 U.S. 251 (1972). As one court has explained:

> Even an act of pure malice by one business competitor against another does not, without more, state a claim under the federal antitrust laws; those laws do not create a federal law of unfair competition or "purport to afford remedies for all torts committed by or against persons engaged in interstate commerce."

Brook Group Ltd. v. Brown & Williamson Tobacco Corp., 113 S. Ct. 2578, 2589 (1993) (quoting *Hunt v. Crumboch,* 65 S. Ct. 1545, 1548 (1945)).

In some situations a potential plaintiff who is a competitor is not injured by a defendant's

wrongful conduct; for example, in a conspiracy to raise prices or reduce output, if higher prices are charged by a competitor, the plaintiff in actuality is benefited by the higher prices for his goods or services. See *Matsushita Electric Industrial Co., LTD. v. Zenith Radio Corporation,* 475 U.S. at 582-583. However, plaintiffs have been able to establish standing for unreasonably exclusionary conduct by competitors. See *Key Enterprises,* 919 F.2d at 1559 (recognizing antitrust laws where designed to prevent unreasonably exclusionary practices); see also *U.S. Healthcare, Inc. v. Healthsource, Inc.,* 986 F.2d 589 (1st Cir. 1993) (presupposing that plaintiff MCO had standing to sue defendant MCO for exclusionary practices).

In addition, a plaintiff must establish that injury was direct. The Supreme Court has recognized that the antitrust laws will be more "effectively enforced" by those who have been directly injured and thus has declined to allow everyone who may have been potentially affected by the illegal conduct to recover. See *Illinois Brick Company v. Illinois,* 431 U.S. 720, 733-735 (1977). Establishing a direct injury of the MCO should not be a problem, provided the MCO directly pays the provider's fees. See *Todorov v. DCH Healthcare Authority,* 921 F.2d 1438, 1455 (11th Cir. 1991) (recognizing that both the insurer and the patient have standing to sue physicians for overcharges resulting from activity that violates the antitrust laws); see also *Blue Cross & Blue Shield United of Wisconsin v. Marshfield Clinic,* 65 F.3d 1406 (7th Cir. 1995) (recognizing that if the patient paid clinic fees and was reimbursed, then the insurer was not directly injured).

A potential private plaintiff must establish that its injury was to business or property. Thus, personal injury is excluded. See *Reiter v. Sonotone Corporation,* 442 U.S. 330, 340-342 (1979). The plaintiff's injury must "flow from that which makes the defendants' acts unlawful." See *Brunswick Corp. v. Pueblo Bowl-O-Mat, Inc.,* 429 U.S. 477, 489 (1977) (plaintiff lacked standing to sue where it alleged that competitor's acquisition of bowling alleys would harm plaintiff because absent the acquisition the bowling alleys would fail, resulting in less competition and greater market power for the plaintiff). Not only must the plaintiff's injury have resulted directly from defendant's wrongful conduct, there must be sufficient "physical and economic nexus between the alleged violation and the harm to the plaintiff." See *Blue Shield of Virginia v. McCready*, 457 U.S. 465, 478 (1982). More importantly, the injury must be of a type that Congress intended to protect the plaintiff against making the defendant's conduct unlawful under the Sherman Act. *Id.*

Section 1 of the Sherman Act

Section 1 of the Sherman Act condemns "every contract, combination…or conspiracy in restraint of trade." 15 U.S.C. § 1 (1998). Section 1 condemns both horizontal agreements between competitors and vertical agreements between market participants at various levels of production and distribution. On its face, Section 1 requires that a potential plaintiff establish an agreement and that the alleged agreement be anticompetitive. However, courts have applied Section 1 differently, depending on whether the agreement is viewed as "per se" illegal.

The standard for establishing liability under § 1 of the Sherman Act is far less forgiving than the standard for establishing liability under § 2. Section 2 of the Sherman Act, which covers unilateral, as well as concerted activity, typically imposes liability only when a firm "actually monopolizes or dangerously threatens to do so." *Spectrum Sports, Inc. v. McQuillan*, 506 U.S. 447, 459 (1993) (citing, *Copperweld Corp. v. Independence Tube Corp.*, 467 U.S. 752, 767 (1984)).

Concerted Conduct

To prevail on a § 1 claim of the Sherman Act, which only applies to concerted, not unilateral, conduct, a plaintiff need not establish that the defendants are monopolists or are likely to become monopolists as a result of the challenged conduct. Instead, the plaintiff must prove only "that the defendants' concerted action established an unreasonable restraint of trade." *Advanced Health-Care Services, Inc. v. Radford*

Community Hosp., 910 F.2d 139, 144 (4th Cir. 1990). As the Supreme Court has explained, the difference in the standards of liability has been imposed precisely because concerted activity is inherently "fraught with anticompetitive risk." *Spectrum Sports*, 506 U.S. at 459 (citing *Copperweld Corp. v. Independence Tube Corp.*, 467 U.S. 752, 767-69 (1984)). As the Court explained in *Copperweld*:

> The reason Congress treated concerted behavior more strictly than unilateral behavior is readily appreciated. Concerted activity inherently is fraught with anticompetitive risk. It deprives the marketplace of the independent centers of decision making that competition assumes and demands....Of course, such merging of resources may well lead to efficiencies that benefit consumers, but their anticompetitive potential is sufficient to warrant scrutiny even in the absence of incipient monopoly.

Copperweld, 467 U.S. at 768-69 (1984).

Per Se Illegality

Since the advent of the Sherman Act in 1890, the Supreme Court has certain limited business arrangements that are per se illegal under § 1. Because these arrangements have historically been considered to lack any redeeming virtue, they "are conclusively presumed to be unreasonable and therefore illegal without elaborate inquiry as to the precise harm they have caused or the business excuse for their use." *United States v. Topco Associates, Inc.*, 405 U.S. 596, 607 (1972). "Today, the only serious candidates for this label are price (or output) fixing agreements and certain group boycotts or concerted refusals to deal." *U.S. Healthcare, Inc., v. Healthsource, Inc.*, 986 F.2d 589, 593 (1st Cir. 1993). All other agreements and other concerted arrangements are treated under the so-called rule of reason, which was first enunciated in 1918 by Mr. Justice Brandeis. *Topco*, 405 U.S. at 606-7 (citing *Chicago Board of Trade v. U.S.*, 246 U.S. 231, 238 (1918)). "An analysis of the reasonableness of a particular restraint includes consideration of the facts peculiar to the business in which the restraint is applied, the nature of the restraint and its affects, and the history of the restraint and the reasons for its adoption." *Topco*, 405 U.S. at 607 (1972) (citing *Chicago Board of Trade v. U.S.*, 246 U.S. at 238 (1918)).

Vertical and Horizontal Restraints

The risk of anticompetitive harm is substantially reduced in the context of a vertical arrangement between market participants at various levels of production and distribution than in the context of a horizontal arrangement between competitors. Compare *Maricopa County Medical Society*, 457 U.S. at 332 (holding that maximum fee schedule among competing physicians is per se illegal), with *State Oil Co. v. Kahn*, 522 U.S. 3 (1997) (holding that vertical maximum price fixing is not per se illegal). Further, unlike horizontal restrictions, all nonprice vertical restrictions, including customer, territorial, or product limitations, are evaluated under the rule of reason. See *Continental T.V., Inc. v. GTE Sylvania Inc.*, 433 U.S. 36 (1977). Virtually the only type of vertical agreements evaluated under the per se rule are agreements between suppliers and distributors about the specific prices to be charged on the resale of products (vertical price fixing agreements). See *Monsanto Co. v. Spray-Rite Service Corp*, 465 U.S. 752 (1984). Consequently, courts will usually end up applying the rule of reason to vertical restraints.

The "Rule of Reason"

Under the "rule of reason," the plaintiff must make an initial showing that the defendant's conduct has caused harm to competition in general (in the form of causing consumers to suffer higher prices or lower quality or output). *NCAA v. Board of Regents*, 104 S. Ct. 2948, 2962-63 (1984); *Jefferson Parish Hosp. v. Hyde*, 104 S. Ct. 1551, 1568 & n.52 (1984); *Capital Imaging Assocs. v. Mohawk Valley Medical Assocs.*, 725 F. Supp. 669, 676 (N.D.N.Y. 1989) ("Capital I"); *Capital Imaging Assocs. v. Mohawk Valley Medical Assocs.*, 791 F. Supp 956 (N.D.N.Y.

1992), *afford*, 996 F.2d 537 (2d Cir.), *cert. denied*, 114 S. Ct. 388 (1993).

To prevail on a "rule of reason" claim analysis, the plaintiff can make a showing of damage to competition in one of two ways. One way is for the plaintiff to actually demonstrate detrimental effects on competition (such as a reduction in output). *Capital III*, 996 F.2d at 546 (citing *F.T.C. v. Indiana Fed'n of Dentists*, 106 S. Ct. 2009, 2019 (1986)). If the plaintiff can do this, he has met the initial burden under the "rule of reason" test and need not offer a detailed market analysis or proof of the defendant's market power. *Id.*[3] As the Eleventh Circuit has stated, "rule or reason" analysis requires the Plaintiff to establish "(1) an anticompetitive effect to the defendant's conduct on the relevant market, and (2) that the conduct has no procompetitive benefit or justification." *Levine v. Cent. Florida Med. Affiliates*, 72 F.3d 1538, 1551 (11th Cir. 1996). "In order to prove an anticompetitive effect on the market, the Plaintiff may either prove that the defendants behavior had an 'actual detrimental effect' on competition, or that the behavior had 'the potential for genuine adverse effects on competition.' In order to prove the latter, the Plaintiff must define the relevant market and establish that the defendants possess power in that market." *Id.* (citing *Indiana Fed. of Dentists*, 476 U.S. at 460-61).

Inferring Concerted Conduct

Sometimes, the challenge for a potential plaintiff is establishing the existence of an agreement between or among competitors. An agreement may be inferred when the parties undertake parallel actions that are truly interdependent, where the benefits accrue to the parties only if all participate, and where there is no other rational business reason for the parties taking such actions independently. See *Interstate Circuit, Inc. v. United States*, 306 U.S. 208 (1939); see also *Theater Enterprises v. Paramount Film Distributing Corp.*, 346 U.S. 537 (1954). Although agreements may be inferred from parallel interdependent conduct between competitors, courts do not consider parent corporations and wholly owned subsidiaries competitors. Thus, a wholly owned subsidiary cannot conspire, for purposes of Section 1. See *Copperweld Corp. v. Independence Tube Corp.*, 467 U.S. 752, 771 (1984) (recognizing that unity of purpose between parent and subsidiary makes conspiracy for Section 1 purposes impossible).

PROVIDER NETWORKS

In an attempt to reduce costs and increase efficiencies, providers (e.g., physicians) have begun to form provider networks to market their services to MCOs. Of course, providers are interested in collective bargaining to gain leverage in dealing with MCOs. Thus, a provider network may also conceal attempts to increase the bargaining power of the members when dealing with MCOs. If a network has sufficient market power, the MCO will have to pay the members of the network higher rates and consequently charge enrollees higher fees and/or reduce services.

Under certain circumstances, collective bargaining by independent providers is illegal under Section 1 of the Sherman Act. Nevertheless, independent providers may collectively bargain where they are clinically or financially integrated. The Department of Justice and the FTC have articulated antitrust safety zones that allow collaborations that increase efficiency through integration, while at the same time discourage collaborations that may hurt competition. See *Department of Justice and Federal Trade Commission Statements of Antitrust Enforcement Policy in Health Care*, 4 Trade Reg. Rep. (CCH) ¶ 13,153, at 20,815 (August 28, 1996). The Joint FTC and Justice Department guidelines present two safety zones for conduct that is "highly unlikely to raise substantial competitive concerns." *Id.*

The Safety Zones

Under Statement 8, physician network joint ventures are divided into exclusive and nonexclusive joint ventures. An exclusive arrangement is one in which the agreement between the network and the providers prohibits or discour-

ages the providers from contracting outside of the network, either with other networks or directly with payers. Exclusive arrangements are more likely than nonexclusive ones to harm competition because, particularly when combined with a large share of the physicians in the relevant market, they may prevent or hinder the formation of competing networks.

In determining whether a network is exclusive, the Agencies will look beyond the language of the agreements to determine whether an arrangement is, in fact, exclusive. The following factors are considered indicia of nonexclusivity:

- That viable competing networks or plans with adequate provider participation currently exist in the market
- That providers in the network actually participate in other networks or contract individually with health benefits plans, or there is other evidence of their willingness and incentive to do so
- That providers in the network earn substantial revenue outside the network
- The absence of any indications of significant departicipation from other networks in the market
- The absence of any indications of coordination among the providers in the network regarding price or other competitively significant terms of participation in other networks or plans

Enforcement Statements at 69-70.

Where an exclusive physician network consists of no more than 20 percent of the physicians in a specialty and the member physicians share substantial financial risk, then "absent extraordinary circumstances" such collaborations do *not* raise substantial competitive concerns. *Id.* Further, a nonexclusive physician network consisting of 30 percent of the physicians in specialties in which the member physicians share a substantial financial risk also falls within the antitrust safety zone. *Id.*

The Guidelines emphasize the importance of looking beyond the terms of the contractual arrangement to determine whether an arrangement is exclusive. *Id.* The Agencies will consider five indicia of nonexclusivity in determining whether a physician network is nonexclusive: The *Enforcement* Statements and the safety zones that they establish do not have the effect of law and are not binding on courts. Thus, although the Agencies would be highly unlikely to challenge conduct falling within a safety zone, it would be possible for state attorneys general—who have authority to enforce federal, as well as state, antitrust laws—or private plaintiffs to challenge conduct falling within an antitrust safety zone. However, because the safety zones basically immunize only conduct that the courts had already deemed legitimate under traditional antitrust analysis, any challenge of conduct falling within a safety zone would be highly unlikely to succeed.

Nonexclusive Physician Networks

Statement 8 provides that a nonexclusive physician network joint venture will fall within an antitrust safety zone—meaning that it will not be challenged by the Agencies absent extraordinary circumstances—if it includes "30 percent or less of the physicians in each physician specialty with active hospital staff privileges who practice in the relevant geographic market and share substantial financial risk." *Id.* at 69. However, if the relevant market contains fewer than four physicians in a particular specialty, a venture otherwise qualifying for the safety zone may include one physician from that specialty, even though the venture will then have more than 30 percent of the physicians in that specialty.

Exclusive Physician Networks

Similarly, Statement 8 provides that an exclusive physician network joint venture will fall within an antitrust safety zone if it includes "20 percent or less of the physicians in each physician specialty with active hospital staff privileges who practice in the relevant geographic market and share substantial financial risk." *Id.* at 68. Again, if the relevant market contains fewer than five physicians in a particular specialty, a venture otherwise qualifying for the

safety zone may include one physician from that specialty, on a nonexclusive basis, even though the venture will then have more than 20 percent of the physicians in that specialty.

Risk Sharing

To qualify for either safety zone, the physicians in the network must share substantial financial risk. The agencies have recognized two types of risk sharing that may satisfy this requirement: capitation and withholds. Under a system of capitation, the venture agrees to provide services to a health benefits plan in return for a fixed, predetermined payment per covered life.[4] A "withhold" is an amount of money retained by the joint venture from all members out of the amount of compensation due to them, with distribution of that amount to the members only if the cost-containment goals are met. Capitation automatically satisfies the "substantial financial risk" requirement. However, whether a withhold is sufficient will depend on the particular facts of each case. The inquiry is whether, given the surrounding circumstances, the withhold is large enough to create significant financial incentives for the members of the network to achieve specified cost-containment goals. The Agencies have expressed a willingness to consider other types of risk-sharing arrangements but have recognized no others to date.

Networks Falling Outside of the Safety Zones

The antitrust safety zones for exclusive and nonexclusive networks apply only to physician network joint ventures. There is no safety zone for multiprovider networks. However, networks—whether physician networks or multiprovider networks—that fall outside of the safety zones will not necessarily violate the antitrust laws. Rather, they must be evaluated under general antitrust principles to determine whether they are permissible. Arrangements that fall outside the antitrust safety zones may still be considered to have significant efficiencies and not raise substantial antitrust concerns. Even when a network does not have shared financial risk, but there exists significant clinical integration, then the network may be considered a legitimate joint venture reasonably necessary to accomplish procompetitive efficiencies. *Id.* at 20,820. The Guidelines list three examples of clinical integration: (1) ventures that establish "mechanisms to monitor and control utilization of health care services that are designed to control costs and assure quality of care"; (2) ventures that selectively admit physicians that "are likely to further efficiency objectives"; and (3) ventures that invest significant resources in an infrastructure to "realize claimed efficiencies" *Id.* Generally, credentialing, basic utilization review, and quality assurance programs do not constitute substantial clinical integration.

Per Se and the Rule of Reason

Agreements among competitors to fix prices are generally deemed per se illegal. Thus, a provider network that is merely a "naked" agreement to fix prices will violate Section 1 of the antitrust laws. In contrast, when a network is a "true" or "legitimate" joint venture—that is, one in which the physicians have integrated their practices and share substantial financial risk—the arrangement is likely to have procompetitive effects that could outweigh its anticompetitive effects and, thus, is evaluated under the rule of reason. Capitation will generally be sufficient to qualify a network as "integrated," whereas a withhold may suffice to make the network integrated, depending on the surrounding circumstances. Whether a withhold is sufficient to bring a network within the rule of reason analysis depends on whether it is likely to create a sufficient incentive for physicians to limit utilization and thus generate efficiencies that could outweigh the potential anticompetitive effects of the agreements on price or fees.

Anticompetitive Effects

Anticompetitive effects are likely in a provider network where the network includes a large percentage of the providers in each product market within the relevant geographical market and where the venture is exclusive—that is, where providers' ability to contract outside of the network is restricted. When a network is nonexclusive (both according to the agreement and in practice), it is unlikely that it will have any anticompetitive effect.

When an agreement between a network and providers is exclusive—that is, when the providers are prohibited from or restricted in their ability to contract outside of the network, either with payers directly or with other managed care entities—the risks of antitrust liability are greater. However, although such exclusive agreements often harm competitors, they do not violate the antitrust laws unless they also harm competition. Thus, the mere insistence of an exclusive dealing clause in a contract with a provider-controlled organization does not establish an antitrust violation. *Bob Maxfield, Inc. v. American Motors Corp.*, 637 F.2d 1033, 1036 (5th cir.), *cert. denied*, 454 U.S. 860 (1981).

Indeed, exclusive agreements of this sort can create a number of efficiencies, including enhanced price or quality competition between networks or plans, lower administrative costs, improved quality control, and a stable supply of services to plan subscribers. Because they may be procompetitive, exclusive agreements between health plans and providers are almost always evaluated under the rule of reason rather than the per se rule.

The primary antitrust risk of exclusive arrangements with provider-controlled organizations is the possibility of "foreclosure." As the court explained in *U.S. Healthcare v. Healthsource*,

> [T]here is one common danger for competition; an exclusive arrangement may "foreclose" so much of the available supply or outlet capacity that existing competitors or new entrants may be limited or excluded and, under certain circumstances, this may reinforce market power and raise prices for consumers.

986 F.2d at 595.

In *Tampa Electric*, the Supreme Court explained that, in evaluating exclusive arrangements, a court should weigh the probable effect of the contract on the relevant area of effective competition, taking into account the relative strength of the parties, the proportionate volume of commerce involved in relation to the total volume of commerce in the relevant market area, and the probable immediate and future effects which pre-emption of that share of the market might have on effective competition therein.

365 U.S. at 328-29.

Foreclosure. When a network or similar entity has contracts with a large percentage of the providers in a given area and those contracts restrict or eliminate the ability of those providers to contract outside of the plan or network, it may not be possible for competing ventures or networks to develop because they may not be able to obtain the necessary providers. In contrast, if a network or managed care plan has a very small market share, the fact that it requires providers that contract with it to enter into exclusive contracts is probably not, in and of itself, problematic from an antitrust perspective. In such a case, absent other indications of anticompetitive effect, a finding of an antitrust violation is unlikely.

In *Ryko Mfg. Co. v. Eden Servs.*, 823 F.2d 1215, 1233 (8th Cir. 1987), *cert. denied*, 484 U.S. 1026 (1988), the court explained:

Where the degree of foreclosure caused by the exclusivity provisions is so great that it invariably indicates that the supplier imposing the provisions has substantial market power, we may rely on the foreclosure rate alone to establish the violation. However, where, as here, the foreclosure rate is neither substantial nor even apparent, the plaintiff must demonstrate that other factors in the market exacerbate the detrimental effect of the challenged restraints.

The other factors that must be considered when market foreclosure is not substantial include: "the willingness of consumers to comparison shop and their loyalty to existing distributors, the existence of barriers to entry by new distributors, the availability of alternative methods of distribution, and any trend toward growth or decline in the level of competition at the supplier level." *Id.* at 1234.

In determining the degree of foreclosure caused in a market for physician services by an exclusive arrangement, it is necessary to determine the number of physicians within the relevant geographical market who would be available to entities seeking to contract with physicians outside of the exclusive network or plan. Certain physicians within the geographical area would not be included in this number because of retirement or unwillingness to participate in certain types of health plans. *Healthsource*, 986 F.2d at 596.

The number of participants. Because an MCO must offer a variety of types of physicians, it is necessary to determine whether a sufficient number of each type of physician required by networks remains outside of the exclusive arrangement. For purposes of this inquiry, the percent of the area's primary care physicians that are in the network and the percent of the physicians in each necessary specialty, such as obstetrics, must be considered. Other factors that may be considered include the fact that new physicians are constantly finishing school and entering the market and that competing plans may be able to encourage physicians to move into the market from other geographical areas. See *id.* In *Healthsource*, the First Circuit, affirming the decision of the district court, held that the defendant's foreclosure of at least 25 percent of all of the primary care physicians in the relevant geographical market was not sufficient to establish an antitrust violation. 986 F.2d at 596-97.

The duration of the agreement. Also significant is the duration of the exclusive arrangement and its termination penalties. An exclusive for a year, with termination at will without substantial penalty, is unlikely to have anticompetitive effects. See Letter from Jeffrey Zuckerman, Director, FTC Bureau of Competition, Consumer Protection, and Economics, to David Gates, Insurance Commissioner, State of Nevada (Nov. 5, 1986) at 3.

Efficiencies

If it appears that the network may have anticompetitive effects, the next step is to consider the procompetitive efficiencies that it will create. *Capital III*, 996 F.2d at 543. Because the evil to be prevented by the antitrust laws is a decrease in competition, procompetitive effects, or efficiencies, are viewed as redeeming virtues that can justify the defendant's conduct if they outweigh the anticompetitive effects of that conduct.

Recent Cases

Networks that are exclusive and have neither clinical nor financial integration and have the purpose and effect of fixing prices by preventing or impeding competition will be considered per se illegal by the federal antitrust enforcement agencies. *Id.* at 20,821. Two recent complaints filed by the Department of Justice illustrate how physician networks can use joint negotiation to fix prices, and thus extract supracompetitive salaries from managed organizations.

On January 25, 1999, the Department of Justice filed suit against the Federation of Certified Surgeons and Specialists for a Section 1 violation of the Sherman Act. See *United States v. Federation of Certified Surgeons and Specialists, et al.,* No. 99-167-CIV-T-17F, 2 (M.D. Fla. January 25, 1999). The Defendants, 29 general and vascular surgeons, formed a corporation that hired an independent consulting firm to negotiate with managed care plans. *Id.* The new corporation informed health plans that their participating surgeons would not participate in the plan's networks unless the plans contracted with all participating surgeons at higher rates. *Id.* at 3. Further, in one instance, the physicians terminated their existing contracts with a health plan before the plan capitulated. *Id.* at 4. The complaint alleged that the average annual salary of each participating physician was increased by $14,097. *Id.* at 5. The parties have agreed to a consent decree that enjoins the physicians from joint negotiations with MCOs.

In August of 1998 the Department of Justice filed a suit against the Federations of Physicians and Dentists, Inc., which comprised almost all of the independent orthopaedic surgeons in Delaware. See *United States v. Federation of Physicians and Dentists, Inc.,* No. 98-475, 1-3 (D. Del. August 8, 1998). Members of the Federation allegedly agreed to negotiate through the plan, so as to prevent Blue Cross and Blue Shield of Delaware from reducing the fees paid to orthopaedic surgeons to a level equal to what other medical specialists in Delaware were paid. *Id.* Consequently, most members ended up terminating their agreement with Blue Cross and Blue Shield of Delaware. *Id.* The federation allegedly justified its efforts as an attempt to implement the messenger model arrangement. *Id.* at 4. Trial has been set for April of 2000. Both the *Federation of Certified Surgeons and Specialists* and the *Federation of Physicians and Dentists, Inc.* illustrate attempts to use the "messenger model" to circumvent the antitrust prohibition on collective bargaining.

PHYSICIAN UNIONS

Faced with an imbalance of bargaining power, independent physicians are organizing into unions. In addition, the American Medical Association voted on June 23, 1999, to create a physician labor union. Amy Goldstein, *AMA Votes to Form Labor Union Reaction to HMOs Reflects Radical Change for Doctors*, Washington Post, June 24, 1999 at A01. Texas has signed into law legislation that will allow physicians to unionize. At present, there is legislation before congress that will allow health care workers to unionize. A physician union exemption to the antitrust laws would create a major obstacle to MCOs being able to negotiate the most economically efficient rates with their physician provider (and, in the case of Texas, all health care providers).

There is currently a labor exemption for certain "bona fide" trade unions; however, the contours of this exemption are strictly limited. Specifically, the labor exemption requires that conduct arise out of a labor dispute, acting in its own self-interest, and must involve unilateral conduct of a labor organization. Independently employed individuals typically are not exempted from the antitrust laws, with certain limited exceptions—e.g., owner-driver truckers, musicians, and screen directors. See *Local 24, International Brotherhood of Teamsters v. Oliver*, 358 U.S. 283 (1959) (exempting owner-driver truckers); see also *American Federation of Musicians v. Carroll*, 391 U.S. 99 (1968) (exempting Musicians); see also *Home Box Office Inc. v. Directors' Guild of America, Inc.*, 531 F. Supp. 578 (S.D.N.Y. 1982), *aff'd*, 708 F.2d 95 (2nd Cir. 1983) (exempting screen directors). In general, the courts allow independent contractors to join unions where there is job or wage competition between employed personnel and independent contractors. Under those circumstances the legitimate interests of the unions would be severely undermined if independent contractors were prohibited from joining. *Home Box Office Inc.*, 531 F. Supp at 588. However, that rationale does not appear to apply to most situations involving independent physicians.

As a result, under current law, independently employed physicians do not appear to fall within the statutory or common law exemption. Consequently, they will be judged under the same standards as other provider networks. Without economic or clinical integration their conduct can be "per se" illegal.

In a recent effort to avoid the constraints of Section 1 of the Sherman Act, Local 56 of the United Food and Commercial Workers sought certification from the National Labor Relations Board (NLRB) to act as the collective bargaining representative for 652 independent physicians in southern New Jersey that had contracted with AmeriHealth, an HMO subsidiary of Independence Blue Cross, a Blue Cross plan headquartered in Philadelphia. The physicians did not argue that the interests of the union would be jeopardized if they were not permitted to join, notwithstanding their status as independent contractors. Instead, they argued they were "de facto" employees of AmeriHealth because of the amount of actual control the HMO exercised over them. As a result, the physicians argued that they were entitled to have the union certified as their bargaining agent under the National Labor Relations Act so that they could bargain collectively with AmeriHealth.

Had the NLRB agreed with the physicians and certified the union as a legitimate bargaining agent, then collective bargaining by the union on behalf of the physicians would have been exempt from the antitrust laws as a result of the labor exemption. However, the NLRB refused to certify the union, finding that the physicians were not employees under applicable legal principles. The NLRB concluded that the relevant issue was not whether collective bargaining by the physicians would benefit their patients or redress an inequality in bargaining power or whether the physicians had become "agents of the HMO in its efforts to control healthcare costs." According to the NLRB, the issue was whether the physicians were "so integrated with and controlled by AmeriHealth that they meet the statutory definition of employees, which, in turn, is based on the common law definition of 'servants'" AmeriHealth Inc./AmeriHealth HMO, Case-4RC (Reg'l Dir. Decision (May 24, 1999)). In determining that the physicians were not employees, the NLRB noted that the physicians contract with other insurance companies, supply their own equipment and places of work, do business and advertise in their own names, and have discretion in staffing their offices, managing their practices, and expanding their offices. *Id*. Unless the decision is overturned on appeal, which appears unlikely, independent physicians contracting with MCOs will remain subject to the antitrust laws, at least in the near term. That means that, in appropriate situations, there may be legal action taken against collective negotiations.

The FTC, in fact, already has challenged a number of physicians' unions and similar arrangements where the Agency believed there was evidence of boycotts and/or price fixing. For example, in *College of Physicians-Surgeons of Puerto Rico*, FTC File No. 971-0011, Civil No. 97-2466-HL (District of Puerto Rico) (Oct. 2, 1997), eight thousand independently employed physicians ceased providing nonemergency services to patients in an attempt to get the government of Puerto Rico to recognize the College of Physicians-Surgeons of Puerto Rico as the exclusive agent of all physicians in Puerto

Rico. The FTC obtained a consent decree prohibiting the defendants from boycotting or refusing to deal with third-party payers.

In *North Lake Tahoe Medical Group Inc.,* FTC File No. 981-0261, 64 Fed. Reg. 14730 (Mar. 26, 1999), 91 physicians comprising 70 percent of the physicians practicing in the Lake Tahoe area collectively refused to deal with various third-party payers when they refused to acquiesce to their plans. The proposed consent order prohibits the independent practice association (IPA) from engaging in collective negotiations, boycotting, or refusing to deal. Further, the IPA must terminate the membership of any physician who refuses to deal.

In *Mesa County Physicians Independent Practice Association, Inc.,* Dkt. No. 9283 (May 4, 1999) (consent order), 85 percent of physicians in Mesa County, Colorado, belonging to the Mesa County IPA collectively negotiated through the IPA's Contract Review Committee using IPA-approved guidelines and fee schedules. The consent order prohibits collective negotiation but allows qualified clinical integration and allows any conduct that is reasonably necessary to operate a qualified risk-sharing joint arrangement. The consent order permits the FTC to determine whether "a risk-sharing joint venture" is "qualified."

Of course, in the future, the FTC, the Justice Department, and private plaintiffs will be unable to challenge the aforementioned conduct if physician unions become exempted specifically from the antitrust laws. In that regard, there is currently pending legislation at both the state and federal level that would allow independent physicians to unionize. See, e.g., HR 1304, 106th Cong. (1999). At the federal level the "Quality Health-Care Coalition Act of 1999" (H.R. 1304) would exempt physicians from antitrust laws as they apply to collective negotiations between physicians and health care plans or health insurers. The exemption would be similar in function to collective bargaining that is currently permissible when undertaken by labor organizations under the National Labor Relations Act.*

Significantly, Texas already has passed a similar statute under state action immunity exemption to the antitrust laws that will take effect on September 1, 1999.* S.B. No. 1468, 76th Leg., available at <http://www.capital.state.tx.us>.** (Other states are discussing similar legislation.)

VIRTUAL MERGERS

Like an actual merger, a virtual merger results in the combination of two competitors and often a substantial increase in market concentration. As a consequence, MCOs may be unable to negotiate successfully if, for example, there are only two principal hospitals in a given market. When virtual mergers involve a change in control and/or substantial efficiencies, they are judged under the rule of reason. However, when they do not, they may be challenged as per se illegal.

In February of 1998, the Attorney General of New York filed suit against Saint Francis Hospital, Vassar Brothers Hospital, and their joint operating company, Mid-Hudson Health. *New York v. Saint Francis Hospital*, No. 98-0939 (S.D.N.Y. February 10, 1998) for the hospitals' price fixing and illegal market allocation. Through their joint operating company, the hospitals jointly negotiated with payers and allocated particular services between the two hospitals. *Id.*

The Department of Justice, in evaluating the legality of a joint venture between hospitals forming a new company for the purpose of joint negotiations with managed care plans, has highlighted the importance of the "alignment of the

---

*As noted, collective negotiation by independently employed physicians is per se illegal under the antitrust laws. However, H.R. 1304, the "Quality Health-Care Coalition Act of 1999" would allow independent physicians to collectively negotiate. It has been estimated that the proposed legislation would result in an increase of between $35 and $80 billion in health care expenditures. Charles River Associates, *Antitrust Waivers for Physicians: Costs and Consequences* (visited July 10, 1999) <http://www.hiaa.org/news/news-state/antitrustreport.htm>.

**Unlike the federal statute, the Texas statute exempts all health care workers.

corporations' economic interests and the ability of the parent company to ensure the aligned interests are pursued." Mark J. Botti, *Comments on the Antitrust Aspects of Hospital Virtual Mergers: When might the antitrust laws condemn joint negotiation with managed care plans as per se illegal?,* at the American Health Lawyers Association Annual Meeting in San Diego, CA (July 1, 1998).

EXCLUSIVE DEALING ARRANGEMENTS BY COMPETITORS

Exclusive dealing arrangements imposed by competing MCOs or hospitals also can violate the Sherman Act. Although these exclusive contracts often may be benign, "there is one common danger for competition: an exclusive arrangement may 'foreclose' so much of the available supply or outlet capacity that existing competitors or new entrants may be eliminated or excluded and, under certain circumstances, this may reinforce market power and raise prices for consumers." *U.S. Healthcare*, 986 F.2d at 595. See also, *Jefferson* Parish Hosp. Dist. No.2 v. Hyde, 466 U.S. 2, 45 (1984) (concurring opinion of Justice O'Connor) ("[e]xclusive dealing arrangements may, in some circumstances, create or extend market power of a supplier . . . party to the exclusive dealing arrangement. . . . Exclusive dealing can have adverse economic consequences by allowing one supplier of goods or services unreasonably to deprive other of a market for their goods. . . .").

On August 10, 1999, a hospital located in Brevard County, Florida ("Wuesthoff"), filed an antitrust case against a competing hospital in state court. (Case No. 99-27250-CA-F, Eighteenth Circuit of Florida). Specifically, since its formation in 1995, the plaintiff alleged that a competing Health First tied or bundled its two hospital facilities—Cape Canaveral with Holmes Regional—for purposes of contracting with managed care plans. That is, neither Health First hospital would contract with a third-party payer unless the payer also agreed to contract with the other Health First hospital. According to the plaintiff, Health First offered no credible competitive or legitimate business justification for its conduct other than to divert managed care plans and other third-party payers from Wuesthoff to Cape Canaveral. In addition, the plaintiff claimed that Health First would not offer an MCO a substantial discount unless the MCO excluded the plaintiff from its hospital network.

The defendant, Health First, operates the only acute care hospital facilities in the Southern portion of Brevard County (which includes the city of Melbourne), the most densely populated portion of the county. According to the plaintiff, Melbourne is the largest community in Florida without any hospital competition. Health First was formed in August 1995 as a partnership between Holmes Regional Medical Center, Inc. and Cocoa Beach Area Health Services, Inc. The plaintiff alleged that after the creation of Health First, the defendants initiated conduct designed to foreclose plaintiff's access to, what they assert is, a significant and growing population—enrollees of MCOs. Specifically, plaintiff alleged that the Health First hospitals excluded Wuesthoff from the Health First HMO, which is owned by the hospitals. According to the plaintiff, the defendants also undertook exclusionary managed care contracting arrangements to the detriment of Wuesthoff and competition.

By bundling Holmes with Cape Canaveral, the plaintiff asserted that payers that would prefer to contract with the plaintiff were required instead to contract with Cape Canaveral Hospital. Plaintiff claims that as a result of the policy Wuesthoff was excluded from several managed care hospital networks, including Allmerica Financial, AmeriPlus, American Medical Securities, Blue Cross and Blue Shield (preferred provider organization) (PPO), Blue Cross and Blue Shield (health options), CIGNA, Foundation Health, Health Choice (PPO), Health First Health Plan, Marco Underwriters, McRae Industries (Kanawha HC Solutions), Med-Care Advantage, PruCare, SunHealth, and WellCare (HMO). Plaintiff claimed a substantial economic loss as a result.

MOST FAVORED NATION CLAUSES

The Justice Department has gone to great lengths to establish the illegality of certain favored nations clauses, which are generally used by dominant health insurers to the disadvantage of their competitors. MFNs generally provide that the provider will give the contracting plan the best of all its prices. In *United States v. Delta Dental of Rhode Island*, 943 F. Supp. 172, 174 (D.R.I. 1996), the district court found Delta Dental's "Prudent Buyer Policy" anticompetitive. The "Prudent Buyer" clause specifically provided that "Delta Dental reserves the right to limit reimbursements to dentists to such levels as such dentists have agreed to accept as reimbursement from other non-government dental benefit reimbursement programs." See Complaint at 4-5, *Delta Dental of Rhode Island* (No. 96-113). Delta Dental subsequently agreed to discontinue use of its Prudent Buyer Policy. See Consent Decree at 3, *Delta Dental of Rhode Island* (No. 96-113). The District Court in *Delta Dental* recognized that MFNs have the effect of "excluding potential rivals, retarding expansion by existing competitors, and substantially increasing the costs to Rhode Island consumers of dental insurance and dental services." *Id.* at 177 (internal citation omitted); but see *Ocean State Physicians Health Plan v. Blue Cross and Blue Shield Island*, 883 F.2d 1101 (1st Cir. 1989) (upholding MFN as reasonable).

A similar MFN was involved in another case; the MFN clause provided that contracting ophthalmologists would not charge fees to Vision Service Plan that were any higher than those charged to the doctor's non-VSP patients. See *U.S. v. Vision Service Plan*, 1996-1 Trade Cas. (CCH) ¶ 71,404 (D.D.C. 1996). The Vision Services Plan signed a consent decree with the Department of Justice enjoining the use of the MFN contract clause. *Id.*

The Arizona Attorney General's Office in conjunction with the Antitrust Division filed suit to stop defendant from violating Section 1 of the Sherman Act and a parallel provision of Arizona state law.[5] The defendant, Delta Dental Plan of Arizona, Inc. (Delta Dental)—a not-for-profit corporation whose participating providers comprise dentists licensed to practice in Arizona—enforced an MFN in its contracts with its member dentists, who composed about 85 percent of the dentists in Arizona. The State AG and Antitrust Division al-

leged that the MFNs in Delta Dental's agreements limited discounts to other plans.

As a result of the joint legal action, the parties entered into a settlement agreement whereby Delta Dental was enjoined from continuing to enforce the MFNs it had in its contracts with all its member dentists and from engaging in various other anticompetitive activities. The Antitrust Division and Arizona AG retained jurisdiction over Delta Dental and retained access to any Delta Dental corporate documents and information. Also, Delta Dental may be required to submit written reports at the request of the Antitrust Division or Arizona AG.

The Justice Department also obtained a consent decree enjoining Medical Mutual of Ohio from using a "Most Favorable Rate" clause that required hospitals to charge Medical Mutual's competitors 15 to 30 percent more than they charged Medical Mutual. See Complaint at 1, *Medical Mutual of Ohio* (No. 1:98-CV-2172); see also Consent Decree at 1-3, *Medical Mutual of Ohio* (No. 1:98-CV-2172). Thus, an MCO that finds itself receiving less than competitive rates from health care providers because of MFN clauses found in contracts between its providers, and a competitor may be able to obtain relief under the antitrust laws.

SECTION 2 OF THE SHERMAN ACT

Section 2 of the Sherman Act makes it illegal "to monopolize, or attempt to monopolize, or combine or conspire with any person or persons, to monopolize any part of the trade or commerce among the several States, or with foreign nations." 15 U.S.C. § 2 (1998). Despite the breadth of Section 2, it does not forbid the mere possession of monopoly power nor does it proscribe monopolies resulting from a "superior product, business acumen, or historic accident." See *United States v. Grinnel Corp.*, 384 U.S. 563, 570 (1966). Rather, Section 2 makes it illegal to monopolize or attempt to monopolize.

Monopolization

To establish a Section 2 violation of monopolization a plaintiff must prove that a firm possesses monopoly power in a relevant market and the firm has taken some predatory or exclusionary conduct to acquire or maintain that power. *Id.*

Monopoly Power

Monopoly power is the ability to control prices or exclude competition. See *United States v. E.I. Du Pont De Nemours and Co.*, 351 U.S. 377, 392 (1956). Monopoly power and market power are similar concepts. Market power "is inferred from the seller's possession of a predominate share of the [product and corresponding geographic] market." See *Eastman Kodak v. Image Technical Services*, 504 U.S. 451, 464 (1992) (citing *Jefferson Parish*, 466 U.S. at 17). Market power is defined by the cross-elasticity of demand between a product and its substitutes. *Id.* at 394. Monopoly power is found where a firm possesses a market share far in excess of what would be necessary to establish market power. *Compare Id.* at 481 (80 percent market share sufficient to establish monopoly power), *with Standard Fashion Co. v. Margrane-Houston Co.,* 258 U.S. 346 (1922) (40 percent market share sufficient to establish market power).

Determining the relevant product market and corresponding geographic market can sometimes be difficult. See *United States v. Mercy Health Services*, 902 F. Supp. 968, 976 (N.D. Iowa 1995) (highlighting the importance of looking at future conditions such as expansion by other hospitals and willingness of managed care enrollees to make changes for financial reasons); see also *FTC v. Tenet Healthcare Corporation*, 17 F. Supp. 2d 937 (E.D. M.O. 1998) (recognizing that geographical market definition includes an "examination of practical alternatives from a consumer's perspective" including "managed care coalitions and third party payers"). Generally, courts begin with the "Elzinga-Hogarty" test, which looks at patient flow "to determine (1) the area from which the hospitals draw their patients and (2) where the residents in that area go for hospital care." *Mercy*, 902 F. Supp. at 977. Where hospitals draw 90 percent of their patients from within the proposed geographical area and 90 percent of the residents in that geographical area go to hos-

pitals within that geographical area, the market definition is said to be strong, whereas numbers less than 75 percent indicate a weak geographical market definition. *Id.* However, courts must also consider the effect of entry barriers, possible expansion, and financial incentives on consumers to travel in the future. *Id.* at 976.

Even within the health care industry there is a diverse array of potential product markets including primary care services, general acute care hospitals, and anchor hospitals. See generally *United States v. Long Island Jewish Med. Ctr.,* 983 F. Supp. 121, 140 (E.D.N.Y. 1997). Generally, "the outer boundaries of a product market are determined by the reasonable interchangeability of use or the cross-elasticity of demand between the product itself and substitutes for it." *Brown Shoe Co. v. United States*, 370 U.S. 294, 325 (1962). The Supreme Court in *Brown Shoe* highlighted practical indicia in determining the boundaries of a product submarket: recognition of a submarket as a separate economic entity by consumers, the product's peculiar characteristics and uses (fungible versus differentiated), unique production facilities, customers, price, price sensitivity, specialized vendors, and barriers to entry. *Id.*

The Requirement of Wrongful Conduct

Monopoly power by itself is not enough to establish a violation of Section 2 of the Sherman Act; a potential plaintiff must establish that the defendant has engaged in some type of wrongful or predatory conduct. See *United States v. Grinnel Corp.,* 384 U.S. at 570. Examples of predatory conduct include predatory pricing, refusal to deal, or other exclusionary acts.

To establish predatory pricing a potential plaintiff must prove that the defendant has sold its product below cost (either average variable or average fixed cost) and that the defendant has a dangerous probability of success (recovering the monies spent in below-cost pricing with monopoly prices after the competitor has gone out of business). See *Brooke Group, Ltd. v. Brown & Williamson Tobacco Co.,* 509 U.S. 209 (1993); see also *Matsushita Electric Industrial Co., LTD. v. Zenith Radio Corporation,* 475 U.S. 574, 582-583

(1986). Predatory pricing is extremely difficult to prove; courts are unwilling to discourage what appears to be competitive conduct. *Id.*

Another type of wrongful conduct is the refusal to deal in certain situations. Generally, even a monopolist can deal with whomever it wants. However, the Supreme Court has articulated two exceptions. See *Colgate*, 250 U.S. at 307. The first exception is the essential facility doctrine. To establish an essential facility claim one must prove that: (1) the competitor controls an essential facility, (2) the plaintiff is unable to reasonably duplicate the facility, (3) the plaintiff has been denied use of the facility by his competitor, (4) it is feasible for the competitor to provide access to the facility, and (5) the competitor lacks a legitimate business reason for denying access. See *MCI Communs. Corp. v. AT&T*, 708 F.2d 1081, 1132-33 (7th Cir. 1983); see also *Pontius v. Children's Hosp.*, 452 F. Supp. 1352, 1370 (W.D. Pa. 1982) (denying essential operating room to surgeons judged unqualified by hospital did not raise an essential facility claim).

However, at least one Supreme Court case has held that where the monopolist's cooperation is necessary for a competitor to effectively compete the conduct can be viewed as predatory. See *Aspen Skiing Co. v. Aspen Highlands Skiing Corp.*, 472 U.S. 585 (1985) (recognizing that cutting plaintiff ski area out of the multi-ski-area package plan created no efficiencies and needlessly hurt plaintiff).

Another example of predatory conduct occurs when a monopolist needlessly modifies a product so that a competitor cannot compete. See, e.g., *C.R. Bard, Inc. v. M3 Systems, Inc.*, 157 F.3d 1340, 1382-1383 (Fed. Cir. 1998) (affirming jury's finding that C.R. Bard had needlessly modified its biopsy gun, thereby hampering M3 System's ability to produce replacement needles for its biopsy gun). That case also reaffirmed that under some circumstances the relevant market can be limited to a single brand. *Id.*

Attempts To Monopolize

Section 2 of the Sherman Act also prohibits attempts to monopolize. 15 U.S.C. § 2. A firm can be found guilty of attempted monopolization where the firm's relevant market power falls far short of monopoly power. See *supra* (discussion of monopoly power). To prevail on a claim of attempted monopolization a potential plaintiff must prove: (1) that the defendant has engaged in predatory or anticompetitive conduct, (2) with a specific intent to monopolize, (3) and the defendant had a dangerous probability of achieving monopoly power. See *Lorain Journal v. United States*, 342 U.S. 143 (1951); see *supra* (for discussion of predatory conduct). Specific intent may be inferred from predatory conduct. See *M&M Medical Supplies & Serv., Inc. v. Pleasant Valley Hosp.*, 981 F.2d 568, 574 (6th Cir. 1992). Further, the defendant's dangerous probability of success depends on proof of the defendant's market power. See, e.g., *Pennsylvania Dental Association v. Medical Service Association of Pennsylvania*, 574 F. Supp. 457, 472, *aff'd*, 745 F.2d 248 (3d Cir. 1984), cert. denied, 471 U.S. 1016 (1985) (recognizing that 40 percent is not a sufficiently large market share to create a dangerous probability of success); see also *C.A.T. Indus. Disposal, Inc. v. Browning-Ferris Indus.*, 884 F.2d 209 (5th Cir. 1989) (50 percent market share requires consideration of other factors including barriers to entry, consumer demand, strength of competition, and market concentration); see also *Total Benefit Servs. v. Group Ins. Admin.*, 875 F. Supp. 1228 (E.D. La. 1995) (market share of 50 percent or more sufficient).

Leveraging can also constitute predatory conduct. Leveraging occurs where a defendant uses its monopoly or market power in one market to gain a competitive advantage in another market. See *Berkey Photo, Inc. v. Eastman Kodak Co.*, 603 F.2d 263, 275 (2d Cir. 1979), *cert. denied*, 444 U.S. 1093 (1980); see also *Kerasotes Michigan Theaters, Inc. v. National Amusement, Inc.*, 854 F.2d 135 (6th Cir. 1998). The Ninth and Third Circuits have explicitly rejected the theory, requiring that the firm have monopoly power in or attempt to monopolize the second market. See *Alaska Airlines, Inc. v. United Airlines, Inc.*, 948 F.2d 536, 547 (9th Cir. 1991), see also *Fineman v. Armstrong World Indus., Inc.*,

980 F.2d 171 (3d Cir. 1992), *cert. denied*, 507 U.S. 921 (1993). Leveraging does not require coercion of a customer to buy a second product, only that customer's reason for buying the product results from the defendant's market power. See *Key Enterprises of Delaware, Inc. v. Venice Hosp.*, 919 F.2d 1550 (11th Cir. 1990), *vacated as mute,* 919 F.2d 1550 (11th Cir.1992) (recognizing that defendant hospital improperly used its market power to gain a competitive advantage in the home health care equipment market).

There is some case law supporting the proposition that monopoly leveraging does not necessarily require the use of monopoly power in one market to achieve a monopoly, or come close to achieving a monopoly, in a second market. There is considerable question, however, whether a monopolist violates section 2 when it uses its monopoly power solely to achieve an advantage in a second market without threatening to monopolize that market. Drawing from prior Supreme Court jurisprudence, in *Berkey Photo, Inc. v. Eastman Kodak Co.*, 603 F.2d 263, 275 (2d Cir. 1979), *cert. denied*, 444 U.S. 1093 (1980), the Second Circuit adopted an expansive view of "monopoly leveraging" and stated that "a firm violates § 2 by using its monopoly power in one market to gain a competitive advantage in another, albeit without an attempt to monopolize the second market." The court emphasized, however, that the offense requires the abuse of "monopoly power" as opposed to a defendant's merely taking advantage of its size. *Id.* at 276.

Still, the federal courts of appeal clearly are split between those that hold that a monopoly-leveraging claim can succeed if the defendant merely gains a "competitive advantage" in the second market and those that require a plaintiff to demonstrate that the defendant has achieved monopoly power (or at least that there is a dangerous probability that it will do so) in the second market. In the decade after *Berkey*, several courts of appeals reserved judgment on whether they would follow *Berkey* and hold that leveraging violates § 2, even when there is no threat of monopolizing the second market.[6]

More recently, two courts of appeals have flatly rejected *Berkey*. In *Alaska Airlines, Inc. v.*

United Airlines, Inc., supra. fn. 26, the Ninth Circuit became the first court of appeals explicitly to reject *Berkey*. After noting that the antitrust laws tolerate natural monopolies and those that arise from efficiency, the Ninth Circuit explained that "[u]nless the monopolist uses its power in the first market to acquire and maintain a monopoly in the second market, or to attempt to do so, there is no Section 2 violation." *Id.* at 548. Similarly, in *Fineman v. Armstrong World Indus., Inc.*, 980 F.2d 171 (3d Cir. 1992), *cert. denied*, 507 U.S. 921 (1993), the Third Circuit held that *Berkey* erroneously permits actions for unilateral restraints of trade, in disregard of the statutory scheme under which concerted restraints are judged under the relatively strict standards of the Sherman Act § 1, whereas unilateral restraints are judged under the more lenient standards of § 2.

The Supreme Court's opinion in *Spectrum Sports, Inc. v. McQuillan*, 506 U.S. 447 (1993), which notes that "§ 2 makes the conduct of a single firm unlawful only when it actually monopolizes or dangerously threatens to do so," casts further doubt on the *Berkey* doctrine. *Id.* at 459. Indeed, at least one lower court has held that *Spectrum Sports* precludes the imposition of liability under § 2 unless there is a likelihood of achieving monopoly power in the second market.[7]

The Health First Litigation

The "Health First" Case described previously also contains allegations of monopolization and attempted monopolization. The plaintiff has asserted that in Central Brevard County, managed care plans historically have been able to contract selectively by choosing between, or threatening to choose between, Wuesthoff Hospital and Cape Canaveral Hospital for inpatient hospital services. As a result of this competition, the plaintiff claims that net hospital prices (and particularly prices charged to managed care plans) have been lower in Central Brevard County than in South Brevard County.

In 1995 Holmes Regional affiliated with Cape Canaveral to create Health First. Since the affiliation, the plaintiff claims that the combined entity has exercised its economic power by increasing prices and engaging in exclusionary conduct in both South and Central Brevard County, with the result of substantially lessening inpatient hospital competition in those markets and throughout Brevard County.

According to the plaintiff, the Health First hospitals (defendants Holmes Regional and Palm Bay, both located in South Brevard County, and defendant Cape Canaveral located in Central Brevard County) exercised their economic power to maintain monopoly power in South Brevard County and to obtain monopoly power in Central Brevard County. The allegedly unlawful behavior included:

- the refusal by Health First to make Holmes Regional available for managed care contracts unless the plan agreed to contract with Cape Canaveral as well
- the negotiation of meaningful discounts only if the managed care plan agreed to exclude Wuesthoff from its hospital network in favor of the Health First hospitals
- the use of sham arguments in regulatory proceedings to prevent and delay Wuesthoff from building a new hospital to compete with Holmes Regional in South Brevard County
- the improper exclusion of Wuesthoff from contracting with Health First Health Plans, one of the largest HMOs operating in Brevard County

CONCLUSION

Faced with a variety of economic threats, suppliers and competitors of MCOs sometimes resort to conduct that is questionable under the antitrust laws. As this chapter has demonstrated, those laws can be used to ensure the continuation of competition through free and open markets.

REFERENCES AND NOTES

1. Of course, an antitrust plaintiff must itself face economic injury as well. Section 4 of the Clayton Act provides that "any person who shall be injured in his business or property by reason of anything forbidden in the antitrust laws may sue…and shall recover threefold the damages by him sustained and the cost of suit, including a reasonable attorney fee." 15 U.S.C. § 15 (1998). In *Key Enterprises of Delaware, Inc. v. Venice Hospital,* 919 F.2d 1550, 1568 (11th Cir. 1990), *vacated as mute* 919 F.2d 1550 (11th Cir.1992) the eleventh circuit reinstated a jury award of more than \$2 million in a private antitrust action brought by a durable medical equipment supplier against a competitor partially owned by the defendant hospital. The defendant hospital conditioned continued access to patients by home health care nurses on the recommendation of the defendant hospital's affiliated DME company. *Id.* at 1557. Like the plaintiff in *Key Enterprises*, MCOs are currently and will be in the future facing antitrust injury by new forms of collaborations by health care providers.

2. Federal and state antitrust officials often work together to investigate antitrust issues of mutual concern. Through the Executive Working Group for Antitrust (EWG), the Antitrust Division, FTC and state AGs share complaints and information to encourage joint investigations. Moreover, both the FTC and the Antitrust Division of the Department of Justice often tend to involve state AGs in their investigations when those investigations involve local markets or activities.

3. Several cases have noted that, without market power, there can be no harm to consumers and thus no liability under the antitrust laws. *See NCAA,* 468 U.S. at 110; *Capital III,* 996 F.2d at 546. Although it is certainly true that to have harm to consumers, and thus to have antitrust liability, market power must *exist,* this does not mean that a plaintiff who has proved actual harm to competition must also *prove* that market power exists. On the contrary, market power is simply used as a surrogate for actual harm to competition when actual harm cannot be proven directly, *Capital III,* 996 F.2d at 546.

4. In Statement 9, the Agencies explain that, as long as the network is paid by the payer on a capitation basis, the individual providers can be reimbursed either through capitation or fee-for-service—either way, the arrangement will be considered "capitation" and will satisfy the requirement that the physicians share substantial financial risk. *Enforcement Statements* at 93 n.34.

5. *United States and State of Arizona v. Delta Dental Plan of Arizona, Inc.,* 1995-1 Trade Cas. ¶ 71,048 (1995).

6. *See, e.g., Willman v. Heartland Hosp. East,* 34 F.3d 605, 613 (8th Cir. 1994) (even if monopoly leveraging theory

is valid, evidence was insufficient here), *cert. denied*, 514 U.S. 1018 (1995); *M & M Med. Supplies & Serv. Inc. v. Pleasant Valley Hosp. Inc.*, 981 F.2d 160, 169 (4th Cir. 1992) (en banc) (reserving judgment on *Berkey* doctrine), *cert. denied*, 508 U.S. 972 (1993); *Key Enters. of Delaware, Inc. v. Venice Hosp.*, 919 F.2d 1550, 1566-68 (11th Cir. 1990) (expressing reservation about *Berkey*'s conclusion that leveraging is illegal even without an attempt to monopolize the second market, but affirming judgment for plaintiff because such an attempt was proven), *vacated*, 979 F.2d 806 (11th Cir. 1992), *app. dismissed as moot*, 9 F.3d 893 (11th Cir. 1993), *cert. denied*, 511 U.S. 1126 (1994); *Advanced Health-Care Servs. Inc. v. Radford Community Hosp.*, 910 F.2d 139, 149 n.17 (4th Cir. 1990) (reserving judgment on *Berkey* doctrine); *Association for Intercollegiate Athletics for Women v. NCAA*, 735 F.2d 577, 586 n.14 (D.C. Cir. 1984) (while noting "the substantial academic criticism cast upon the leveraging concept," the court reserved judgment on whether the leveraging offense described in *Berkey* constitutes "an independent Section 2 offense separate from monopolization and attempted monopolization").

7. *See, e.g., Spruce Oil Corp. v. Archer-Daniels-Midland Co.*, 870 F. Supp. 1005, 1007 (D. Colo. 1994).

CHAPTER 64

Legal Liability Related to Medical Management Activities

James L. Touse

Managed care organizations (plans) are subject to a variety of legal and regulatory obligations related to the development and operation of their medical management programs. This chapter briefly discusses those obligations and plans' legal liability exposure if they fail to satisfy those obligations. The reader is urged to review the other chapters in Part V for additional discussion of related issues.

The terms *medical management program* and *medical management activities* are used to refer to the types of activities that plans utilize to control the cost and quality of health care services provided to their members. Those activities can be broadly categorized as utilization management, quality assurance, and dispute resolution programs. Utilization management activities may include referral management programs; preadmission, concurrent, and retrospective review programs; utilization reporting and evaluation programs; case management programs; and

James L. Touse is the Vice President and General Counsel of BlueCross BlueShield of Tennessee (BCBST). He has previously served as legal counsel to other insurance companies, health maintenance organizations, and the Ohio Department of Insurance.

The views presented in this chapter are intended to stimulate consideration and discussion concerning an evolving area of the law and should not be interpreted to constitute legal advice or to describe standards applicable to BCBST or any other managed care organization related to the conduct of its medical management activities.

provider incentive arrangements. Quality assurance activities may include provider selection, credentialing, or privileging programs; quality assurance and assessment programs; peer review activities; and the implementation of medical policies, protocols, and practice guidelines. All these subjects are discussed in various chapters in Parts II and III. Although member and provider grievance programs have not traditionally been considered to be medical management activities, they are also discussed in this chapter. Those programs may permit plan management to identify and resolve disputes related to other medical management activities before they escalate into costly and time-consuming legal or regulatory actions against the plan. Member grievance programs and consumer affairs are discussed in Chapter 40.

The statutory and common (that is, case) law related to plans' medical management obligations has dramatically changed during the past 20 years, as managed care has evolved from the health maintenance organization (HMO) movement to the predominant form of health benefits coverage in the United States. That evolution will presumably continue and even escalate as state and federal legislatures, regulators, and courts enact, clarify, and enforce laws and regulations governing plans' medical management activities. At the time this chapter was written, Congress was considering sweeping patient protection legislation, and several states have already enacted laws permitting plans to be held liable for their medical management determinations. Those laws, which will be discussed in greater detail in Chapter 69, will certainly affect plans' future medical management obligations, liability exposure, and programs.

Plans must conduct effective medical management programs in order to be successful in an increasingly competitive market. The question confronting plan management and counsel is how to structure and operate effective medical management programs, while avoiding foreseeable liability exposures related to those activities.

If there is any generally accepted rule concerning what plans should do to avoid liability, it is that they must understand their obligations and act in a reasonable manner when making medical management determinations. If an organization acts reasonably, it should minimize its legal liability exposure while still conducting effective medical management activities.

OBLIGATIONS TO CONDUCT MEDICAL MANAGEMENT ACTIVITIES

Plans must implement and operate medical management programs pursuant to applicable laws, accreditation standards, and agreements with customers. Failure to comply with those obligations may, at best, expose a plan to increased regulatory oversight, legal liability, or loss of business. At worst, the plan might be ordered to cease doing business by regulatory agencies or be forced out of business by a loss of customers or a catastrophic liability judgment.

This section discusses state and federal statutes, regulations, and administrative requirements (laws) requiring plans to implement medical management programs. It is clearly beyond the scope of this chapter to evaluate all the laws that are applicable to plans' medical management activities.

Most plans can fairly easily comply with such medical management laws because they establish minimum requirements to obtain and maintain a license or certificate of authority in a state. The term *plan* is used throughout this chapter, but there are many different types of managed care organizations. Those distinctions are most

relevant when determining what laws are applicable to a plan's medical management activities.

HMOs are generally required to establish medical management programs pursuant to state HMO licensure laws. As an example, the National Association of Insurance Commissioners (NAIC) Model HMO Act (see Chapter 69), which served as a model for most states' HMO statutes, requires HMOs to conduct medical management activities as a condition of licensure. That model act requires licensed plans to ensure that the health care services provided to enrollees are rendered in accordance with reasonable standards of quality that are consistent with prevailing professionally recognized standards of medical practice.[1] HMOs are also required to establish grievance procedures to address and attempt to resolve member grievances, including grievances related to such organizations' medical management activities,[2] as discussed in greater detail in Chapter 40.

If an HMO is federally qualified, it will also have to comply with the requirements of the federal HMO statute. That statute requires HMOs to have an ongoing quality assurance program that stresses health outcomes and provides for peer review of the services provided to members. It also requires qualified HMOs to have an effective procedure for collecting, evaluating, and then reporting information concerning the utilization of services to the secretary of the Department of Health and Human Services (DHHS).[3] The Health Care Financing Administration also requires Medicare + Choice plans (see also Chapters 55 and 56) to implement quality assessment and performance improvement programs, contract with an approved independent quality review and improvement organization to provide external review of the plan's medical management activities, and implement specified grievance procedures,[4] as conditions of contracting with such plans to serve Medicare beneficiaries.

Regulatory oversight of an HMO's medical management activities varies, depending on the jurisdiction where the HMO is licensed and whether it is federally qualified. The Model HMO Act empowers the state regulatory agency to fine, suspend, or revoke an HMO's license if it fails to comply with its statutory obligations.[5] The secretary of DHHS may also revoke the federal qualification of any HMO that fails to comply with the assurances given to DHHS concerning its medical management activities.[6]

There are generally fewer regulatory requirements applicable to the medical management activities of other types of managed care organizations, such as preferred provider organizations (PPOs). The NAIC Model PPO Act requires plans to include mechanisms to control utilization and determine if services are medically necessary. It does not require plans to implement other medical management programs, such as quality assurance or grievance procedures.[7]

An increasing number of customer groups contractually require plans to be accredited as a condition of being offered to the groups' employees. One possible explanation for such accreditation requirements is the concern that those groups will be held liable for breaching their fiduciary duties pursuant to the Employee Retirement Income Security Act (ERISA) of 1974, as amended (see Chapter 66 for a full discussion of ERISA),[8] or for negligence if they fail to exercise reasonable care when selecting and supervising the activities of contracting plans.[9]

There are a number of private accreditation organizations, but the most widely accepted HMO accreditation agency is the National Committee for Quality Assurance (NCQA; see Chapter 44). The NCQA accreditation process evaluates an applicant's compliance with specific quality management and improvement, utilization management, credentialing, member rights and responsibilities, preventive health service, and medical records' standards.

Other groups do not require accreditation, but require contracting plans to satisfy specified medical management standards as a condition of being offered to the groups' members. As an example, the Federal Employees Health Benefit Program (FEHBP; see Chapter 54) requires contracting plans to develop and implement a quality assurance program that assesses the utilization of services, credentialing of providers, risk arrangements with providers, and member satisfaction with the plan.

COMMON LAW MEDICAL MANAGEMENT LIABILITY ACTIONS

Creative plaintiffs' attorneys are constantly dreaming up new and novel liability theories in actions against plans. The most recent actions have alleged violations of the Federal Racketeer Influenced and Corrupt Organizations Act ("RICO") on behalf of a class of the defendant plan's members.[10] The Supreme Court of the United States has held that RICO actions are not preempted by state insurance laws, in *Humana, Inc. v. Forsyth*,[11] but, as of the end of 1999, no case had held a plan liable for violating RICO. In fact, in September 1999, the U.S. District Court for the Eastern District of Pennsylvania dismissed a class action civil RICO action against a plan in *Maio v. Aetna, Inc.*[12] The plaintiffs alleged that Aetna had engaged in a fraudulent scheme to induce members to enroll based upon its commitment to provide quality care, when it was really motivated by cost and administrative considerations. The Court concluded the plaintiffs had failed to prove any actual injuries; an actionable fraud claim; or that Aetna could conspire with its subsidiary, as required to establish an actionable RICO claim. While plan counsel and management must be concerned about potential RICO actions, which permit treble damage awards, this chapter will focus on current trends in contract and negligence liability actions against plans. Such actions currently represent the most significant medical management liability exposure for plans.

Most reported liability actions against plans have either alleged that the plan violated its contractual obligations to members or was directly or indirectly negligent when conducting medical management activities. The fundamental difference between a contract and a negligence action is the basis of the alleged duty to the other party and the type of damages arising from the failure to comply with such duties.

A contract action is based upon the duties specified in the agreement between the parties.

Contractual damages are limited to the economic losses caused by the failure to perform those agreed-upon duties.

A negligence action is based upon an alleged failure to exercise the degree of care required by law, which directly or proximately causes injuries to a member. If a plan fails to exercise reasonable care, the injured party may be awarded compensatory damages for past and future expenses arising from or related to that injury.

Damages are generally limited to the amount necessary to compensate the other party for contractual losses or personal injuries. Punitive damages may be awarded in certain circumstances, however, to punish a defendant and create an example for others, if the defendant acted in an intentional, malicious, wanton, willful, reckless, or outrageous manner.

CONTRACT ACTIONS RELATED TO MEDICAL MANAGEMENT ACTIVITIES

Most medical management issues, to date, have involved the denial of claims for services or failure to authorize providers to render services to members (referred to as adverse determinations) when such services allegedly should have been covered pursuant to a plan's certificate of coverage. Those cases have generally considered whether an adverse determination was reasonable based upon the terms of the certificate and factual circumstances of that case. One of the most significant issues in such cases has been the question of whether the member's benefit plan is governed by ERISA.

The media and elected officials have convinced the public that ERISA prevents members from suing their plan if it fails to authorize or pay for covered benefits. In fact, as demonstrated by the number of cases against plans cited in this chapter, ERISA imposes no such limitation on suing a plan. It does, however, limit the damages that can be assessed against a plan to amounts that should have been paid pursuant to the member's certificate of coverage.

Such damages are appropriate in a breach of contract action, but plaintiffs' attorneys and the media argue that such damages are inadequate when a denial of authorization effectively precludes members from receiving desired services. Those arguments ignore the fact that not all treatments are covered by health insurance. They also fail to differentiate between benefit or payment determinations, which are made by plans, and treatment decisions, which are made by providers in consultation with their patients. Providers can always render treatment and then dispute the plan's denial of authorization or refusal to pay claims, if they believe that such services are medically necessary and covered by the member's certificate. Unfortunately, the perception that the remedies available under ERISA are inadequate has caused certain courts and legislators to expand plans' liability for their medical management determinations beyond that specified in the ERISA statute.

ERISA provides that it preempts "any and all State laws insofar as they now or hereafter relate to any employee benefit plan."[13] The Supreme Court has stated that the preemption provision should be liberally construed as follows: "a law 'relates to' an employee benefit plan, in the normal sense of the phrase, if it has a connection with or reference to such a plan."[14] ERISA also includes what is referred to as the savings clause, which states that "nothing in this subchapter shall be construed to exempt or relieve any person from any law of any State which regulates insurance, banking, or securities."[15]

The apparent conflict between the broad preemption of any law related to an ERISA plan and the savings clause was addressed in *Pilot Life Insurance Co. v. Dedeaux*.[16] In that case, the Supreme Court decided that ERISA preempted a bad faith judgment against an insurance company because Mississippi's bad faith law was not specifically directed at regulating the insurer's activities. *Pilot Life* held that ERISA only permits a plan participant or beneficiary "to recover benefits due to him under the terms of his plan, to enforce his rights under the terms of the plan, or to clarify his rights to future benefits under the terms of the plan."[17]

Although *Pilot Life* held that ERISA preempts bad faith actions, plans must not ignore their potential bad faith liability exposure when conducting medical management activities. ERISA is not applicable to government, church, or nongroup benefit plans.[18] FEHBP imposes limitations similar to those of ERISA, but actions by state or local government employees will probably not be preempted by ERISA. Not all states have adopted a cause of action for bad faith benefit determinations, but as of 1996, that theory of liability had been accepted by 43 states, with 14 of those states imposing some type of cap on punitive damage awards.[19]

Bad Faith Actions

The basis for a bad faith action is an allegation that a plan breached its implied duty of good faith and fair dealing when conducting medical management activities. The consequences of violating that implied duty can be catastrophic.

The two most notable bad faith cases have both been decided by juries in California, *Goodrich v. Aetna,* ("*Goodrich*") and *Fox v. HealthNet* ("*Fox*").[20] As trial court decisions, they have limited precedental value (that is, the requirement that the decision be followed by lower courts in the same jurisdiction). They also have limited precedental value because there was no written decision in either case explaining the legal and factual bases for either jury's decision. Finally, the *Goodrich* case is being appealed and the *Fox* case was settled upon undisclosed terms after the jury issued its decision, so we do not yet know if higher courts will affirm, reverse, or modify those trial court decisions.

It is important to examine those cases, however, to determine what incited the juries to award such extraordinary punitive damages against the defendant plans. Published reports concerning the *Goodrich* case and the pleadings filed in the *Fox* case provide valuable information about the factual circumstances of each case.

In *Goodrich*, a jury in San Bernardino, California, awarded a total of $120,564,363.40 against Aetna U.S. Healthcare of California in January 1999. Of that amount, $747,655.88 was awarded for unpaid medical bills, $3,790,603.52 for wrongful death, and $116,026,104 in puni-

tive damages. The plaintiff's attorney, Michael Bidart, wrote a commentary summarizing the facts of that case from the plaintiff's perspective.[21] Mr. Bidart reported that Mr. Goodrich, a deputy district attorney for San Bernardino County, was diagnosed with a rare form of stomach cancer after collapsing in court on June 5, 1992. Goodrich's primary care physician authorized a referral to the City of Hope Hospital for consultation and assessment to determine if he was an appropriate candidate for high dose chemotherapy and a bone marrow transplant (the "transplant"). Aetna's consulting oncologist agreed that Goodrich should be referred to that hospital on July 21, 1992. The authorization request was then referred from the contracting provider group, Redlands Medical Group, to Aetna's local medical director, who forwarded it to Aetna's home office in Hartford, Connecticut. Aetna ultimately denied authorization on November 18, 1992, because it deemed the procedure to be experimental. Bidart claims that Goodrich's evidence of coverage did not exclude coverage for experimental and investigational procedures. Unfortunately, by the time Aetna issued its decision, the cancer had metastasized, which disqualified Goodrich as a candidate for the proposed transplant.

Goodrich's primary care physician then requested authorization to refer him for potential cryosurgery at St. John's Medical Center on August 26, 1993. That request was again referred from the local medical group, to the local Aetna medical director and to the company's home office. Aetna denied coverage on November 3, 1993, because the medical center was not a participating provider. According to Bidart, the treating oncologist testified that performing the surgery would have extended Goodrich's life by 15 to 20 months and improved the quality of his life during that period.

Finally, on January 11, 1995, Goodrich's primary care physician requested authorization to hospitalize him at St. John's for surgery and chemotherapy. This time, Goodrich's providers did not wait for authorization from Aetna and performed the surgery on January 17. According to Bidart, Aetna denied authorization on January

18 in a letter from a registered nurse that was delivered to Goodrich's wife while he was in the intensive care unit. Goodrich remained hospitalized until his death on March 15, 1995. He died believing that he had left his family owing $750,000 in medical bills, although his wife had secondary coverage that ultimately paid those bills.

Aetna disputes many of the facts cited by Bidart. It has also publicly stated that it will vigorously appeal the jury's verdict. Aetna specifically claims that the trial court excluded critical evidence from the jury's consideration. That evidence included the facts that: (1) Ms. Goodrich's health plan had precertified the out-of-network treatment; (2) there was an addendum to the evidence of coverage that listed covered benefits and the experimental exclusion; (3) Goodrich was not an appropriate candidate for high dose chemotherapy because his cancer had metastasized by the time he was referred for treatment; (4) the services performed by out-of-network providers had been approved if they were performed by participating providers; (5) Goodrich did not take advantage of the case management services available to him; (6) he did not utilize Aetna's internal grievance and appeals procedures; and (7) Aetna's conduct in the case did not contribute to shortening Goodrich's life.[22]

The jury's decision might have been different had they been given the opportunity to consider those facts. It appears, however, that the most significant factor in their decision was Aetna's failure to respond to Goodrich's treating physicians' authorization requests in a timely manner. The jury apparently believed that Goodrich's life could have been saved or the quality of his remaining life improved if Aetna had promptly authorized the proposed treatments. It is unclear from the published reports why the authorization requests were not given expedited consideration. Aetna may ultimately have made the same benefit determinations, but the jury might have concluded that the plan acted in good faith and not awarded punitive damages if Aetna had permitted expedited reconsideration of the initial adverse determination. An expedited reconsideration process would have permitted the treating

physicians to attempt to justify their proposed treatments to an objective qualified medical reviewer on an expedited basis, as recommended at the conclusion of this chapter.

In the *Fox* case, a jury in Riverside, California, awarded the family of a schoolteacher, Nelene Fox, $89.3 million based upon the plan's failure to authorize coverage for a bone marrow transplant to treat her metastatic breast cancer.[23] That award included $212,000 plus interest to pay for the cost of the transplant, $12.1 million for breach of the duty of good faith and infliction of emotional distress, and the remainder as punitive damages.

Fox was diagnosed with breast cancer in June 1991. The tumor had metastasized to her bone marrow by December. Her treating oncologist requested that HealthNet's contracting medical group approve a referral to the University of Southern California (USC) for further evaluation, which was denied by the medical group. Fox was evaluated, despite that decision, and USC agreed to perform the bone marrow transplant. HealthNet subsequently received a request to authorize the transplant on June 5, 1992, received requested medical records on June 10, and denied the transplant as investigational on June 12. The Foxes conducted extensive fundraising activities and paid for the transplant after the plan's denial of coverage. The transplant was performed at USC in late August, but Fox died in April 1993.

At trial, the plaintiff's attorney, who was Fox's brother, alleged that HealthNet had breached the covenant of good faith and fair dealing by refusing to cover the transplant procedure. His trial brief alleged that Fox's certificate specifically provided coverage for bone marrow transplants under the following provision: "The member must satisfy the medical criteria developed by HealthNet Participating Medical Group and by the referral facility performing the transplant."[24] The attorney argued that Fox had satisfied those conditions because her treating oncologist had recommended the bone marrow transplant and referred her to USC, which agreed to perform that procedure. The oncologist allegedly changed his mind about the need for the transplant only after a discussion with the plan's associate medical director, during which "financial issues" were discussed. The trial brief further alleged that the experimental and investigative procedure exclusion of the certificate was ambiguous as evidenced by the facts that: the plan subsequently expanded that exclusion from one sentence to an entire page, the plan's 1990 independent technology assessment concluded that the procedure had gained widespread acceptance, and the plan had paid for bone marrow transplants for two other members in similar circumstances. Finally, the brief alleged that the bonus of the medical director, who made the decision to deny coverage, was based on the plan's medical loss ratio, which provided an incentive for him to deny the transplant.

The lesson of the *Fox* case is that a plan must consider how a jury will view its conduct when it decides to deny coverage for a procedure recommended by a participating provider. In that case, the plaintiff was able to persuade the jury that the plan had acted in bad faith based upon: its interpretation of the coverage and exclusion provisions of an ambiguous provision of the certificate (as evidenced by the revision of the exclusion language), its efforts to get the oncologist to change his mind (as evidenced by the discussion of financial issues after he had written letters supporting the transplant), differentiating in the treatment of members with similar conditions, and paying a reported $5.5 million in bonuses to key executives of the plan at the same time that it was denying coverage for Fox's transplant.

A critical issue in both the *Goodrich* and *Fox* cases was the question of whether the member's certificate clearly excluded coverage of the proposed transplants. Other cases have upheld denials of coverage in similar circumstances when the plan specifically excluded autologous bone marrow transplants for breast cancer; excluded coverage for transplants that were not specifically listed as being covered; or referenced objective sources of information, such as the Medicare coverage manual, to determine whether a procedure was experimental. [25–27]

Even if a plan has a clear exclusion in its certificate, the *Warne v. Lincoln National Adminis-* *trative Services Corp.* case illustrates the importance of making certain that the plan's promotional materials are consistent with the terms of that certificate.[28] In that case, a jury awarded the plaintiff, who was also covered by a school district plan, $26.8 million for the plan's failure to cover Warne's liver transplant, despite the fact that transplant was clearly excluded by Warne's certificate. Unfortunately, the plan's benefit brochure stated that the cost of organ transplants was a covered benefit. The jury found that the denial of coverage in such circumstances constituted bad faith and awarded the plaintiffs $320,000 for breach of contract, $1.5 million for pain and suffering, and $25 million in punitive damages.

The decision in another bad faith case, *Hughes v. Blue Cross of Northern California*, provides a good example of what a plan should not do when making a medical management decision.[29] In that case, the California Court of Appeals upheld an award of $150,000 in compensatory damages and $700,000 in punitive damages against Blue Cross based upon its denial of claims totaling $17,000 for psychiatric inpatient services. The court stated:

> There was evidence that the denial of respondent's claim was not simply the unfortunate result of poor judgment but the product of the fragmentary medical records, a cursory review of the records, the consultant's disclaimer of any obligation to investigate, the use of a standard of medical necessity at variance with community standards, and the uninformative follow-up letters sent to the treating physician. The jury could reasonably infer that these practices, particularly the reliance on a restrictive standard of medical necessity and the unhelpful letter to the treating physician, were all rooted in established company practice. The evidence hence was sufficient to support a finding that the review process operated *in conscious disregard of the insured's rights.* (emphasis added) [30]

In short, the plan acted in bad faith because it did not conduct a reasonable evaluation, give the treating physician the opportunity to provide additional information, or, most important, balance the member's interests in having services covered against the plan's interests in containing costs when making medical management decisions. Other bad faith cases have held plans liable for failing to contact the member's attending physician concerning the member's condition before denying coverage on the basis of a preexisting condition, failing to obtain pertinent sections of a patient's medical record, not requiring medical review of a claim before determining that services were not medically necessary, or failing to inform members of their right to appeal an adverse determination.[31–33]

Contract Actions Governed by ERISA

The *Hughes* case also illustrates the scope of ERISA's preemption. It was subsequently overturned by the Supreme Court of California, which concluded that California's bad faith common law was preempted by ERISA based on the *Pilot Life* decision.[34] If state law claims are preempted by ERISA, members cannot recover damages for pain and suffering, emotional distress, or punitive damages, in contrast to the plaintiffs in the *Goodrich, Fox*, and *Warne* cases. They may only recover benefits due them under the terms of the plan, enforce their rights under the terms of the plan, or clarify their rights to future benefits under the terms of the plan.

While ERISA may limit the damages that may be awarded, it does not relieve a plan of its responsibility to act in a reasonable manner when making medical management determinations. Plan administrators are prohibited from acting in an arbitrary and capricious manner when making such determinations.

If the plan has been granted discretionary authority to make benefit determinations by the ERISA plan sponsor, the courts generally defer to the administrator's determination unless it is clearly unreasonable. In *Jett v. Blue Cross and Blue Shield of Alabama*, the court stated: "The function of the court is to determine whether there was a reasonable basis for the decision based on the facts known to the administrator at the time that the decision was made."[35]

A decision may be found to be arbitrary and capricious, however, if a plan fails to act in a reasonable manner when making medical management determinations. The following has been held to be arbitrary and capricious conduct: relying on undisclosed medical criteria that are more restrictive than the policies utilized by other insurers, basing an adverse determination on an ambiguous provision of the member's benefit agreement, and failing to comply with the notification and reconsideration procedures mandated by ERISA, which precluded the member from requesting reconsideration of an adverse determination.[36–38]

In *Brown v. Blue Cross and Blue Shield of Alabama*, the Eleventh Circuit Court adopted a higher standard when a plan has an inherent conflict of interest.[39] In that case, the plan offered insured coverage to the plaintiff's employer, so any benefits were paid from the plan's funds. The court stated: "When a plan beneficiary demonstrates a substantial conflict of interest . . . the burden shifts to the fiduciary to prove that its interpretation of plan provisions committed to its discretion was not tainted by self-interest. That is, a wrong but apparently reasonable interpretation is arbitrary and capricious if it advances the conflicting interest of the fiduciary at the expense of the affected beneficiary."[40] Not all courts have accepted that higher standard when a plan underwrites coverage for an ERISA group. The Second Circuit Court of Appeals expressly rejected the *Brown* decision, in *Whitney v. Empire Blue Cross & Blue Shield.*[41] That court concluded that an administrator's benefit determination should not be held to be arbitrary and capricious as long as the interpretation is reasonable, in light of competing interpretations, and the evidence does not show that the administrator was, in fact, influenced by its potential conflict of interest.

The question of whether a plan acts in an arbitrary and capricious manner is important because, if a plan acts in an arbitrary and capricious manner, ERISA permits courts to require the plan to pay the member's attorney's fees and legal costs, which can be a significant penalty. As an example, in *Egert v. Connecticut General Life Insurance Co.*, the insurer utilized inconsistent and undisclosed medical coverage policies to deny coverage for Ms. Egert's infertility treatments.[42] The court ordered the insurer to pay for treatments that had already been rendered and to cover Egert's future infertility treatments. It also awarded her $160,000 in legal fees and costs to "deter plan administrators from developing unreasonable interpretations of ERISA plans as a means of wrongly denying coverage to plan participants."[43]

NEGLIGENCE ACTIONS RELATED TO MEDICAL MANAGEMENT ACTIVITIES

An increasing number of actions have alleged that plans have acted in a negligent manner when performing medical management activities. Negligent conduct is defined as "conduct which falls below the standard established by law for the protection of others against unreasonable risk of harm."[44] In other words, plans are required to exercise the level of care that would be exercised by a reasonably prudent managed care organization in similar circumstances to avoid causing foreseeable injuries to their members.

The enactment of plan liability statutes and the trend to consider vicarious liability actions against plans represent the most significant developments affecting plans' liability for their medical management activities during the past several years. Although there have been relatively few cases alleging direct or corporate negligence related to plans' medical management activities, that may change if Congress and/or additional states adopt "patient protection laws" permitting plans to be held liable for their medical management activities. There have also been an increasing number of cases alleging that plans should be held liable for the acts of employed or contracting providers, which is referred to as vicarious liability.

Negligent Design of Medical Management Programs

Wickline v. State of California was the first widely reported case that suggested that a plan might be held liable for the negligent design of its utilization review program.[45] The court stated, in dicta (a statement of opinion that did not support the ultimate decision in that case), that the failure to offer a physician the right to appeal a nonauthorization decision might be negligent. The court ultimately decided, however, that the failure to offer such an appeal procedure did not cause Wickline's injuries, despite the plan's refusal to authorize continued hospitalization, because her attending physician had discharged her without any effort to appeal that decision. The court concluded that the attending physician was solely responsible for the consequences of his decision to discharge Wickline. That is consistent with the generally accepted rule that an attending physician is ultimately responsible for making treatment decisions concerning the care of his or her patients.[46]

In *Wilson v. Blue Cross of Southern California*, however, the court stated that Blue Cross might be held liable for negligence even though the attending physician had not appealed the denial of authorization to continue Wilson's hospitalization.[47] The court noted that the plan only had an informal reconsideration process and concluded that the plan would not have reversed its initial decision even if the attending physician had attempted to appeal that decision. It returned the case to the trial court, which ultimately decided that Blue Cross's failure to authorize continued hospitalization did not directly contribute to Wilson's death.

Despite the trial court's decision, the *Wilson* case has been interpreted to erode the traditional distinction between a physician's obligation to make treatment decisions and a plan's obligation to make benefit determinations. In the future, courts may decide that plans have a duty to exercise reasonable care, even if the attending physician does not appeal an adverse determination, if it is reasonably foreseeable that a denial of authorization will preclude members from receiving necessary covered services.

If members are covered by ERISA plans, the courts have generally held that actions alleging that plans have acted negligently when conducting medical management activities are preempted by ERISA. The Supreme Court has refused to review lower court decisions holding that ERISA preempts negligence actions against plans for failing to authorize the hospitalization of a mother during a high-risk pregnancy, allegedly resulting in the death of her unborn child, in *Corcoran v. United Healthcare, Inc.,* or for failing to authorize heart surgery for a member in *Kuhl vs. Lincoln National Health Plan of Kansas City,* because such determinations relate to the administration of the ERISA plan.[48,49]

Negligence Actions Related to the Selection and Supervision of Participating Providers

There have been a number of cases in which hospitals have been held to be liable for failing to exercise reasonable care when selecting or supervising their staff physicians (see also Chapter 7 for additional discussion about physician credentialing). The landmark case holding hospitals liable in such circumstances is *Darling v. Charleston Community Memorial Hospital.*[50] In that case, the court concluded that the hospital had an independent duty to oversee the care provided to patients in accordance with applicable licensing regulations, accreditation standards, and the hospital's own bylaws. The court rejected the hospital's argument that it should not be held liable for a physician's negligence, noting "the state licensing regulations and the defendant's bylaws demonstrate that the medical profession and other responsible authorities regard it as both desirable and feasible that a hospital assume certain responsibilities for the care of the patient."[51]

Similar issues can be raised concerning a plan's obligation to exercise reasonable care in selecting and supervising its participating providers. The most widely reported case addressing a plan's potential liability for such negligence is *Harrell v. Total Health Care.*[52] In that case, the member's negligence action against the HMO was dismissed based upon a unique Missouri statute that immunized nonprofit HMOs against liability in such circumstances. The Missouri Court of Appeals stated, however, that the HMO might have been held liable, absent such immunity, because it failed to exercise reasonable care when credentialing the participating special-

ist who caused Harrell's injuries. The court noted that the HMO had solicited applications from specialists by mail and had limited its evaluation of such applications to determining whether the applicant was licensed, could dispense narcotics, and had hospital admitting privileges. It had not conducted personal interviews, checked references, or otherwise investigated the applicant's credentials before accepting that physician as a participant. The court concluded that the failure to conduct a reasonable investigation created a foreseeable risk of harm to members who were required to utilize that specialist.

There is a question of whether ERISA preempts a negligent credentialing action against a plan. In *Altieri v. Cigna Dental Health, Inc.*, the court dismissed a member's claim that the plan was negligent when evaluating a participating dentist's competence during its credentialing process. The court concluded that such claims have a substantial enough effect on a benefit plan to trigger preemption because "plaintiff's negligence, misrepresentation . . . and breach of contract claims have one central feature: the circumstances of [the plaintiff's] medical treatment under his employer's [dental] services plan."[53]

Other cases and the liability statutes discussed below differentiate between a plan's administrative duties under ERISA and its duty of care to members, which is not preempted by ERISA. Plans should, therefore, exercise reasonable care when selecting and supervising participating providers because of the increasing possibility that a state law negligence action will not be preempted by ERISA.

Negligence Actions Related to the Compensation of Participating Providers

An evolving theory of liability contends that implementing provider compensation arrangements that provide incentives to limit the utilization of covered services is either negligent or a breach of a plan's fiduciary obligations pursuant to ERISA. In *Bush v. Dake*, the court decided that a plan might be liable for negligence if it implements an incentive compensation arrangement that encourages participating providers to withhold necessary treatment from members.[54] That case conflicts with the decision in *Pulvers v. Kaiser Foundation Health Plan*, however, which held that "the use of such incentive plans is not only recommended by professional organizations, but that they are specifically required by section 1301 of the Health Maintenance Act."[55]

The most recent development concerning provider incentive programs is the decision that such programs may constitute a breach of the plan's fiduciary duties pursuant to ERISA. In *Shea v. Esensten,* the plaintiff, Mr. Shea, visited his long-time family physician after experiencing severe chest pains on a business trip.[56] The physician advised that Mr. Shea did not need to see a cardiologist, despite his offer to pay the cardiologist's fee. Several months later, Mr. Shea died of heart failure and his widow brought an action in state court against the physician and the plan. Ms. Shea alleged that the plan's non-disclosure and misrepresentation about its physician incentive arrangement, which created incentives to limit referrals to specialists, had limited Shea's ability to make an informed decision about consulting a cardiologist. The plan removed the case to federal court because Shea was covered by an ERISA benefit plan. Ms. Shea then amended her complaint to allege that the plan's failure to disclose its incentive arrangements breached its fiduciary duties under ERISA. The 8th Circuit Court of Appeals concluded that ERISA preempted Ms. Shea's state law claims, because those claims related to the administration of the ERISA benefit plan, but found that she had stated a potential breach of fiduciary duty claim against the plan. The Court concluded that a fiduciary of an ERISA plan has a duty of loyalty requiring the disclosure of any material facts that might adversely affect a member's interests. The court reasoned that Mr. Shea had a right to know that his physician would be penalized for making too many referrals and could earn a bonus for "skimping on specialized care," which might affect his judgment about the need for a referral to a cardiologist.

The 5th Circuit Court of Appeals reached a different conclusion in *Ehlmann v. Kaiser Health Plan of Texas et al.*[57] That Court concluded that the ERISA statute and regulations do not require plans to disclose provider incentive arrangements, despite numerous other provisions detailing an HMO's disclosure duties, demonstrating that Congress and the Department of Labor did not intend to require such disclosure. The Court distinguished the *Shea* decision, noting that the Court in that case had not addressed the statutory interpretation issue. It also noted that the ERISA plan members, who were the plaintiffs in the *Ehlmann* case, had not specifically inquired about the plan's provider compensation arrangements nor established any special circumstances requiring the disclosure of material information about such arrangements. That distinguished the *Ehlmann* case from the *Shea* case, where Mr. Shea, who had asked to be referred to a cardiologist, was not informed of the plan's incentive arrangement that discouraged such referrals.

The question of whether a plan has a fiduciary duty to disclose its financial arrangements with participating providers to members should be resolved during the 1999–2000 term of the U.S. Supreme Court. The Court has granted *certiorari*, or agreed to review, the *Herdrich vs. Pegram* decision, which held that a plan could be found to have breached its fiduciary duties to members by providing incentives to physicians to limit treatment of their member patients.[58]

In that case, the plaintiff, Ms. Herdrich, was covered by an ERISA plan. Her physician, Dr. Pegram, who was employed by the plan, discovered that Herdrich's appendix was inflamed but required her to wait eight days before having a diagnostic ultrasound at a plan facility located approximately 50 miles from her home. Her appendix ruptured before she received that test, resulting in peritonitis. Herdrich filed suit in state court against Dr. Pegram, her employer, the plan, and the plan's affiliated entities, alleging both medical malpractice and fraud. She subsequently amended her complaint to allege a breach of the defendants' fiduciary duty after the case was removed to federal district court. The district court dismissed the breach of fiduciary duty claim, and she appealed that dismissal to the Seventh Circuit Court of Appeals.

A divided Court of Appeals reversed the district court decision on August 18, 1998. The majority first concluded that the defendants were fiduciaries under ERISA because they retained discretionary authority to decide disputed claims. As fiduciaries, the defendants were required to act solely in the interests of participants and beneficiaries pursuant to ERISA. The court then noted that clinic physicians, who owned and administered the plan, made all medical management decisions and received bonuses based upon cost savings achieved during the year, which created an incentive to limit treatments to increase their bonuses. The majority of the Court then devoted most of the remainder of their decision to excoriating the "bottom line" orientation of managed care organizations, including their opinion that physicians, "not insurance bureaucrats dictating policies from the boardroom," should make care-related decisions.[59] They concluded that Herdrich's allegation that the defendant's incentive system depleted plan assets to benefit physician-owners was sufficient to submit the issue of whether the defendants breached their fiduciary duty to a trial court.

Irrespective of the ultimate decision in the *Herdrich* case, the lower court's decision and the decisions in the *Bush* and *Shea* cases should concern plan management and counsel. They illustrate that courts believe that physician incentive arrangements create such an inherent conflict of interest that failing to disclose such arrangements is either negligent or breaches a plan's fiduciary obligation to its members. The concern that incentive arrangements might inappropriately influence provider treatment decisions has resulted in 16 states enacting legislation requiring plans to disclose such arrangements in certain circumstances and the requirement that Medicare + Choice plans disclose incentive arrangements that place providers at substantial financial risk.[60]

Liability for the Negligence of Participating Providers

Perhaps the most significant development affecting plans' medical management liability exposure during the past several years has been the trend to hold plans liable for the negligence of their participating providers. A plan, as an employer, may be held liable for the conduct of its employees. The basis for such liability, referred to as respondeat superior, is that the employer is able to control its employees' conduct. It should, therefore, be held responsible if they injure someone when acting within the scope of their duties.

Another legal theory, referred to as the ostensible agent theory, permits a plan also to be held liable for negligence of an independent contractor if a member reasonably believes that the contractor is acting as an employee or agent of the plan. Such actions are referred to as vicarious liability actions because, unlike cases seeking to hold a plan liable for its own negligence, vicarious liability actions seek to hold the plan liable solely because of its relationship with the negligent provider.

The courts have consistently held that actions against plans based upon their administration of an ERISA benefits plan are preempted by ERISA. The question is whether an action based upon the quality of care rendered to a member by an employed or contracting provider involves the administration of an ERISA plan? In *Nealy v. U.S. Healthcare*, the plaintiffs alleged that the plan should be held liable for the failure of a contracting primary care physician to refer Nealy to a cardiologist before he died from a heart attack.[61] The court concluded that the negligence action was preempted by ERISA, because the ERISA plan created the relationship between the plan and Nealy. The court, therefore, decided that the malpractice action, in which the plaintiffs claimed that the plan failed to provide timely and adequate treatment, related to the administration of Nealey's ERISA benefit plan. In response to an allegation that the plaintiffs would be left without an adequate remedy, the court noted that the preemption of the action against the plan did not affect the plaintiff's state law malpractice action against the involved providers.

The Nealy decision appropriately differentiates between administrative medical management determinations and treatment decisions by participating providers. Unfortunately, other courts have not made that distinction and have decided that such quality of care actions are either not preempted by ERISA or that the ERISA preemption defense is properly addressed in state courts (that is, the case is not removable to the federal courts).

The leading case distinguishing between administrative and quality of care related actions is *Dukes v. U.S. Healthcare, Inc.*[62] In that case, the plaintiffs claimed that the plan should be held vicariously liable for the negligence of its contracting providers, who allegedly failed to order blood tests that would have prevented Duke's death. The court held that the malpractice action should not be removed to the federal courts because it was not a claim for benefits or to clarify the member's right to benefits under the ERISA plan. The court returned the case to the state court to determine whether the plan should be held vicariously liable for the malpractice of its contracting providers. The Supreme Court refused to consider an appeal of that decision.

The issue of whether the federal or state courts are the proper forum to consider allegations concerning the quality of care provided to a member of an ERISA plan was addressed more recently in *Giles v. NYLCare Health Plans, Inc.*[63] In that case, Giles sued the plan for negligence, vicarious liability, breach of contract, misrepresentation, and breach of warranty following her son's death while being treated by the plan's participating providers. When the plan attempted to remove the case to the federal district court, Giles dropped the breach of contract, misrepresentation, and breach of warranty claims and moved to remand, or return, the case to state court. The federal court granted that motion based upon the *Dukes* decision. The Fifth Circuit Court of Appeals affirmed that decision, explaining that there are two types of ERISA preemption: complete and conflict preemption. Completely preempted claims, such as those seeking to enforce the ERISA remedies, may not be remanded to state courts because they involve exclusively federal issues. The court explained that ERISA simply provides a defense to other state law actions that fall outside of ERISA's civil enforcement remedies, such as vicarious liability claims. Such actions must be remanded to

the state court for resolution of that preemption defense.

Another federal circuit court has gone even further, in *Pacificare of Oklahoma, Inc. v Burrage*, holding that a vicarious liability claim against a plan based upon the alleged malpractice of its contracting primary care physician was not preempted by ERISA.[64] The court reasoned that the claim did not involve the administration of the benefit plan and was, therefore, "too tenuous, remote or peripheral . . . to warrant a finding that the law 'relates to' the plan."

Even if vicarious liability actions are not preempted by ERISA, the generally accepted common law rule holds that plans should not be held vicariously liable for the negligence of an independent contractor.[65] In *Williams v. Good Health Plus, Inc.,* the court not only refused to hold the plan liable for the actions of its contracting provider but also emphasized that an HMO could not practice medicine pursuant to the Texas Medical Practice Act.[66] It stated that the plan could not, therefore, be held liable for negligence related to the provision of medical services to members.

Other courts are beginning to challenge that rule, however, particularly when members are required to be treated by a designated participating provider. As an example, in *Schleier v. Kaiser Foundation Health Plan,* the court held the plan liable for the malpractice of a contracting cardiologist.[67] It based that decision on the facts that the plan restricted members' access to a limited number of physicians, paid those physicians to provide services that it was obligated to provide pursuant to its member certificate, and had some right to control the contracting physician's behavior. The court concluded that those were all attributes of an employer-employee relationship, so that the plan could be held vicariously liable for the contracting specialist's negligence.

In *Boyd v. Albert Einstein Medical Center*, the court reversed a summary judgment against the plaintiffs because it concluded that there was a question of fact concerning whether the contracting provider was acting as the plan's ostensible agent when he negligently treated Boyd.[68] The court noted that the plan advertised that its participating providers were competent, required members to utilize network physicians, required primary care physicians to refer members to participating specialists, made capitation payments to primary care physicians, and exercised some control over the physicians' conduct pursuant to the terms of its participation agreement. On that basis, the court concluded that Boyd could reasonably have believed that her primary care physician was acting as an agent of the plan when he instructed her to have diagnostic tests performed at his office instead of at the hospital emergency department. Unfortunately, Boyd died of a heart attack after leaving the emergency department. The court concluded that summary judgement was not appropriate because the trial court might find that the physician was acting as the plan's ostensible agent when he failed to authorize the diagnostic tests that would have disclosed Boyd's heart condition.

Those cases illustrate the danger that courts will increasingly hold plans vicariously liable for the conduct of contracting providers in the future. In fact, that liability exposure may increase as plans implement medical management programs that include practice guidelines, financial incentives to practice cost effectively, and tightly restrict which providers can treat their members. Unfortunately, the very actions that plans take to control the cost and improve the quality of services provided to members may lead to the conclusion that they either control such providers' conduct or are permitting them to act as representatives of the plan.

State and Federal Liability Laws

As of 1999, Texas, California, and Georgia have adopted laws holding plans accountable if they are negligent when conducting medical management activities. On October 7, 1999, the U.S. House of Representatives adopted the Bipartisan Consensus Managed Care Improvement Act of 1999, commonly referred to as the "Patient Protection Act," which also creates a cause of action if a plan is negligent when performing medical management activities. It does not appear likely that version of the Patient Protection

Act will be enacted, because of significant disagreements among the House of Representatives, the Senate, and the President. That act and the referenced state liability statutes clearly reflect a trend to hold plans liable for certain medical management activities. Advocates of such legislation, including plaintiffs' attorneys, claim that such laws will prevent "insurance bureaucrats" from becoming involved in treatment decisions. Ironically, such laws may simply increase premium costs, while requiring plans to restrict network participation, require indemnification from participating providers, and require greater oversight of their practices; plans may be held directly liable if they disagree with a provider's treatment recommendations.

It is beyond the scope of this chapter to examine each of those liability statutes in detail, so this section will briefly examine the Texas liability statute. It is appropriate to consider that statute because Texas was the first state to adopt such a statute, which has served as a model for the other states that have either enacted or considered such liability statutes. It is also appropriate to consider that statute because a federal district court has addressed the question of whether the statute is preempted by ERISA.

The Texas Health Care Liability Act (the "Act") was adopted in 1997. It provides that a health insurance carrier, HMO, or other managed care entity has a duty to exercise reasonable care when making health care treatment decisions. The Act further provides that a plan is liable for damages proximately caused by treatment decisions made by its employees, agents, ostensible agents, or representatives acting on its behalf over whom it exercises or has a right to exercise influence or control. The Act provides a defense to a liability action if the plan does not control, influence, or participate in a treatment decision; or deny or delay payment for any treatment prescribed or recommended by a provider. The Act prohibits plans from removing participating providers because the provider advocates for coverage of medically necessary services on behalf of an enrollee. It further prohibits plans from requiring providers to indemnify or hold the plan harmless for their acts or conduct. Finally, the Act requires members to exhaust the plan's internal appeals process and submit their claim for review by an independent review organization as a precondition to initiating a legal action against the plan in most circumstances.

In *Corporate Health Insurance, Inc. v. The Texas Department of Insurance,* Corporate Health and several Aetna affiliates initiated an action against the Texas Department of Insurance, its commissioner, and the Texas attorney general seeking a declaration that the Act was preempted by ERISA and the FEHBP.[69] On September 18, 1998, the Federal District Court for the Southern District of Texas issued a decision finding that the liability provisions of the Act were not preempted. The court did find that: the provisions prohibiting plans from removing providers for advocating on behalf of their patients, the indemnification prohibition, and the independent review requirement of the Act were preempted by ERISA. The reason that the court held that the liability provisions of the Act were not preempted was because the Act created a standard of care for regulated health insurers and HMOs when making treatment decisions, while specifically excluding ERISA plans from the definition of a managed care entity. The administrative provisions were preempted, however, because they placed restrictions on how managed care entities structure their programs (e.g., prohibiting provider indemnification or hold harmless clauses), which affects ERISA plans that purchase such programs. The Court decided that such interference with the structure and administration of the plans conflicts with Congress's intent to permit uniformity in the administration of ERISA plans.

The court distinguished the *Corcoran* and *Rodriguez v. Pacificare of Texas, Inc.* decisions, in which the 5th Circuit Court of Appeals decided that ERISA preempted claims seeking to hold plans liable for adverse determinations.[70] The district court noted that the *Dukes* decision had subsequently distinguished between an action based on a denial of benefits from one based upon the quality of benefits actually received by a member. The court, therefore, concluded that the Act permitted plaintiffs to seek

to hold a plan liable for failing to exercise reasonable care in its capacity as an arranger of health care services, as distinguished from denial of coverage allegations, which would be preempted by ERISA.

The *Complete Health* decision is currently on appeal to the Fifth Circuit Court of Appeals. If the Appeals Court upholds that decision, it is likely that other states will promptly enact MCO liability laws patterned after the Texas Act. Even if reversed, it is apparent that legislators and the courts, under pressure from consumer advocates, plaintiffs' attorneys, and providers, will continue to search for ways to hold plans liable for their medical management decisions.

It also appears likely that Congress will enact some type of "patient protection" legislation within the next several years. President Clinton and all of the candidates running for president in the 2000 election have endorsed holding MCOs liable for their medical management activities in certain circumstances, so it is likely such legislation will be signed into law if enacted by Congress.

RECOMMENDATIONS

The prospect of state and/or federal liability laws being enacted, together with the continuing trend by courts to hold plans liable for their medical management activities, should encourage plan counsel and management to carefully evaluate and oversee the operation of their plans' medical management programs. The objective of such evaluation and oversight should be to ensure that those programs achieve their objectives of providing high quality covered services to members in a timely and cost-effective manner without creating unnecessary liability exposures for the plan. As stated at the beginning of this chapter, the key to achieving those objectives is to act reasonably and in good faith when selecting participating providers; establishing medical management policies, procedures and criteria; drafting contracts and membership materials; making medical management determinations; and resolving disputes with members and providers. More specifically, this recommends plans should take the following actions to comply with their medical management obligations and to minimize their liability exposure related to their medical management activities:

- Monitor significant court decisions and proposed legislation through trade publications, seminars, and discussions with legal counsel to understand how those developments may affect the plan's medical management obligations.
- State that the plan has discretionary authority to make eligibility and coverage determinations in agreements with insured groups. Reserving such discretionary authority should encourage the courts to defer to the plan's determinations in ERISA cases. If the plan contracts with self-funded or ASO groups, clearly specify who will make and assume liability for such determinations.
- Comply with ERISA's notice and reconsideration requirements. Failure to provide the specific information required by ERISA might be deemed to be arbitrary and capricious, bad faith, or negligent conduct if it deprives members of their right to request reconsideration of an adverse determination.
- Periodically update the plan's certificates to ensure that they clearly express the intended contractual obligations to members. As examples, plans should incorporate specific definitions (for example, of medical necessity, emergency services, experimental or investigational procedures, and custodial care) and specifically explain any exclusions or limitations (for example, of dental, cosmetic, rehabilitation, mental health, and other services) to avoid any ambiguity concerning what services are covered by their certificates. Although there is no generally accepted source of model contract provisions, plans should attempt to use provisions that have been tested and found to be enforceable instead of developing novel contract provisions that courts may find to be ambiguous in future benefit disputes.
- Ensure that marketing brochures accurately describe the benefits, exclusions, and limi-

tations of the certificate to avoid conflicts between those documents.
- If the plan makes exceptions to the exclusions or limitations of the certificate, those extra-contractual benefits should be described in a separate written agreement with the member. That agreement should explain the reason for that exception, state that it is not intended to create a precedent in future cases, and prohibit the member from disclosing any information about that agreement, including its existence, to third parties.
- Make a reasonable effort to ensure that any medical management issues are thoroughly investigated before the plan makes an adverse benefit determination. As an example, it may be advisable to develop a checklist of the type of information that should be obtained before making an adverse determination. That checklist will document that the plan has fully and fairly evaluated the circumstances of each case before making an adverse determination. It might require reviewers to affirm that they review applicable provisions of a member's certificate, review relevant medical policies, contact the member's attending physician(s), obtain pertinent medical information, refer issues requiring specialized knowledge or training to a qualified physician specialist, and generally follow established policies or procedures before making an adverse determination. Many plans further require that a medical director approve any adverse determination that may affect members' access to services (e.g., nonauthorization of services). That procedure helps ensure that relevant medical issues have been appropriately evaluated and identifies whom the attending physician should be directed to contact if he or she disagrees with that determination.
- Ensure that bonuses payable to those plan employees who are responsible for making medical management decisions are not based primarily upon the plan's utilization experience.

- Establish medical policies that are consistent with generally accepted standards of medical practice. As an example, it may be advisable to submit proposed policies and review criteria to a panel of physicians to ensure that they are not overly restrictive or at variance with community standards. After those policies have been approved, they should be distributed to participating providers. Distributing those policies to providers should limit the plan's liability exposure because the plan will not need to make adverse determinations if participating providers understand those policies and do not order services that they know will not be covered by the plan.

- Implement a member complaint and grievance procedure that encourages members to contact the plan concerning anything that causes them to be dissatisfied with their coverage from the plan, including treatment received from participating providers. That procedure should establish specific deadlines for responding to inquiries, complaints, and grievances; ensure that such issues are routed to an individual who is able to evaluate and respond to member concerns; include a mechanism to identify and resolve matters causing member complaints; and provide a multi-level appeal process to disinterested persons, if members are dissatisfied with the plan's response to their concerns. If any disputes cannot be resolved to the member's satisfaction during the plan's internal review process, the plan's certificate should require that those matters be referred to an external organization, such as a specified mediation or arbitration agency. Plans should also consider requiring that the decision of such an external review organization be based upon applicable contract provisions and the information submitted by the parties and that the decision be binding upon both parties, absent a mistake of law or an abuse of discretion. Such an external review process will provide a prompt, thorough, and objective method of resolving member concerns without the delay, ex-

pense, adverse publicity, and potential liability exposure involved in litigating such matters.

- Establish a provider appeal procedure similar to that used to resolve member grievances. That procedure should permit providers to request a hearing before an impartial and appropriately qualified physician hearing officer to present and explain their arguments concerning a disputed medical management determination. The plan should also permit physicians and members to request an expedited review if an adverse determination may preclude a member from receiving urgently needed services. The ability to identify and resolve disputes quickly, or at least to demonstrate that the plan fully and fairly considered relevant information before making an adverse determination, should significantly reduce the plan's liability exposure, particularly in bad faith or negligence actions. This recommendation is also discussed in Chapter 18 on managing basic medical-surgical utilization.

- Obtain current technology assessments concerning the status of new, experimental, or investigational procedures. As an alternative the plan should consider contracting with a "centers of excellence" vendor for transplants and other high cost, but relatively low frequency procedures. Such vendors may be better able to select qualified providers, conduct assessments, and negotiate favorable reimbursement arrangements with providers because they can refer a large volume of cases to participating providers. Another advantage of such arrangements is that participating providers have an incentive to select only qualified candidates for such procedures to ensure that their outcome results satisfy the vendor's requirements for continued participation in its program.

- Base provider bonuses upon specific performance measures, such as member satisfaction, compliance with applicable administrative standards, and satisfying quality of care requirements, in addition to the provider's utilization experience (see Chapters 8–11). If applicable, plans should notify members about their provider incentive compensation arrangements and emphasize that members may appeal any denial of services that they believe may be financially motivated. If members request more detailed information concerning such incentive arrangements, plans should provide an explanation of those arrangements, although such disclosure should not include confidential information concerning amounts paid to specific providers.

- If providers are placed at substantial financial risk, the plan should provide or require those providers to obtain stop-loss coverage to limit their risk once they reach a specified risk threshold. While the Federal Medicare + Choice regulations, which require contracting plans provide such stop-loss coverage to providers, are only applicable to Medicare + Choice plans, it is advisable to extend such coverage to any incentive arrangement that places providers at substantial financial risk.[70] Such stop-loss arrangements should minimize allegations that the plan has created an incentive for providers to deny necessary care to members.

- Clearly explain the independent contractor relationship between the organization and its participating providers in certificates, brochures, and provider participation agreements. Such provisions should emphasize that providers are solely responsible for all treatment decisions and also explain how providers or members can appeal adverse determinations.

- Implement quality assurance programs to evaluate members' access to services, any underutilization of services, and patient complaints to prove that the plan has exercised reasonable care in reviewing the quality of services provided to members. Plans should structure their quality assurance programs in accordance with applicable accreditation standards, even if the plan does not seek accreditation, to demonstrate that those programs comply with generally accepted quality assurance standards.

- Adopt credentialing criteria, including verification of applicants' professional references, malpractice history, insurance coverages, hospital privileges, and licensure. Incomplete applications, unsolicited applications, or applications indicating that a provider does not meet the plan's participation requirements (for example, no staff privileges at a participating hospital) should not be accepted for further review. If applicants satisfy the plan's screening criteria, their application should be submitted to a peer review committee for evaluation of their professional reputation, qualifications, and experience.

- Thoroughly investigate any questions concerning a participating provider's conduct or competence. The plan should terminate the participation of any providers who are unable or unwilling to comply with the organization's medical management requirements. The plan's sanction procedure should also permit immediate termination if a provider's incompetence or misconduct creates a risk of harm to the organization or its members.

- Do not delegate medical management responsibilities to another entity (for example, an independent practice association) unless that entity's medical management programs are comparable with the plan's programs. The plan should retain the right to audit that entity's activities to ensure that it exercises reasonable care when performing delegated management activities. The provider entity should also be required to refer all complaints to the plan so it can promptly address any problems related to that entity's performance of its delegated duties.

- Purchase professional liability coverage to insure the plan and representatives (e.g., directors, officers, employees, and committee members) against liability and defense costs related to the plan's medical management activities. The plan should also require providers to indemnify the plan (that is, hold it harmless) if it is held vicariously liable for the provider's negligence.

- Furnish members and their attending physicians with understandable information about treatment alternatives, if any, if the plan determines that a proposed treatment is not medically necessary. If the plan denies authorization to render services, its participation agreements should require physicians to explain available treatment alternatives to patients if that physician and the plan's medical director are unable to agree upon an acceptable alternative for the denied services. Available treatment alternatives should also be mentioned in letters to members and their attending physicians to encourage discussion of the risks and advantages of the alternative treatments.

• Refer any questions related to the plan's medical management obligations or compliance with those obligations to the plan's legal counsel. Acting upon the advice of counsel may establish that plan determinations are reasonable and made in good faith. It may also provide protection against the disclosure of privileged attorney-client or attorney work product information if the plan is sued based on those determinations.

CONCLUSION

Plans have a variety of regulatory, contractual, and common law obligations related to the organization and operation of their medical management programs. Although the laws concerning plans' liability for failing to satisfy those obligations are rapidly changing and evolving, the fundamental issue in all the cases discussed in this chapter has been whether an organization acted reasonably when conducting its medical management activities. The ability to make benefit determinations to control the cost of providing covered services to members is one of the fundamental purposes of a medical management program. A plan will not be competitive if it is unable to deny claims for services that are specifically excluded by its certificate or for services that are not medically necessary or appropriately authorized by the plan. Plans should not permit their potential liability exposure to deter them from making appropriate benefit determinations, provided that they can prove that such determinations are reasonable and give the member's interest in obtaining covered services equal weight to the plan's interest in containing costs. If a plan conducts medical management activities in such a fair, reasonable, and well-documented manner, it should be able to achieve its essential medical management objectives without having to be overly concerned about the regulatory or legal liability consequences of those activities.

REFERENCES AND NOTES

1. Section 7 of the Model HMO Act.
2. Section 11 of the Model HMO Act.
3. 42 U.S.C. 300e(c)(6) and (8).
4. 42 CFR 422.
5. Section 25 of the Model HMO Act.
6. U.S.C. 300e–11.
7. Preferred Provider Arrangement Model Act, *NAIC Model Laws, Regulations, and Guidelines,* 165-1, 1987.
8. U.S.C. 1001 et seq.
9. Scogland, Fiduciary Duty: What Does It Mean? 24 *Tort & Insurance Law Journal,* p. 803 (1989).
10. 18 U.S.C. 1961–1968.
11. *Humana, Inc. v. Forsyth,* 1999 U.S. LEXIS 744 (U.S. Supreme Court, January 20, 1999).
12. *Maio v. Aetna, Inc.,* No. 99CV1969 (E.D. Pa. Files April 21).
13. 29 U.S.C. 1144(a).
14. 463 U.S. 95, 96–7, 103 S. Ct. 2890 (1983).
15. 29 U.S.C. 1144(b)(2)(A).
16. 481 U.S. 41, 107 S. Ct. 1549 (1987).
17. 29 U.S.C. 1132(a)(1)(b).
18. 29 U.S.C. 1003(b).
19. David Studdert and Troyen Brennan, "The Problems with Punitive Damages in Lawsuits against Managed Care Organizations," *The New England Journal of Medicine,* January 27, 2000, p. 280.
20. *Goodrich v. Aetna,* No. RCV 20499 (Sup. Ct. San Bernadino Co., Rancho Cucamonga District, Ca.) (1994); *Fox v. HealthNet,* No. 219692 (Superior Ct. Riverside Co., Ca.) (1994).
21. Michael J. Bidart, Esq., and Ricardo Echeverria, *Goodrich v. Aetna,* 3 *Mealey's Managed Care Liability Report* (April 28, 1999), pp. 22–24.
22. Carolyn Whetzel, California Jury Awards Record Damages against Aetna for Treatment Decision, 8 *Health Law Reporter,* p. 127 (January 28, 1999).

23. 219692 (Sup. Ct. Riverside Co., Ca.) (1994).

24. Trial Brief, *Fox v. HealthNet,* Superior Court of the State of California, Case No. 219692, November 1, 1993, p. 8, fn. 2.

25. *Roger v. Espy,* 836 F. Supp. 869 (N.D. Ga. 1993).

26. *Caudill v. Blue Cross and Blue Shield of N.C.,* 999 F.2d 74 (4th Cir. 1993).

27. *Beechtold v. Physicians Health Plan of Northern Indiana, Inc.,* 19 F.3d (7th Cir. 1994).

28. Idaho D. Ct. July 20, 1994. Reported in *Health Law Perspectives,* November 30, 1994, p. 1.

29. 245 Cal. Rptr. 273 (1988).

30. *Hughes v. Blue Cross of California,* 255 Cal. Rptr. at pp. 858–9 (1989).

31. *Linthiacum v. Nationwide Life Insurance Company,* 723 P.2d 675 (Az.) (1986).

32. *Aetna Life Insurance Company v. Lavio,* 505 So. 2d 1050 (Al. 1986).

33. *Sarchett v. Blue Cross of California,* 43 Cal. 3d 1 (1987).

34. *Hughes* at p. 813.

35. 890 F.2d 1137, 1139 (11th Cir.) (1989).

36. *Bucci v. Blue Cross and Blue Shield of Connecticut, Inc.,* 764 F. Supp. 728 (D. Ct.) (1991).

37. *Kunin v. Benefit Trust Life Insurance Company,* 910 F.2d 534 (9th Cir.), cert. denied, 111 S. Ct. 581 (1991).

38. *DePina v. General Dynamics Corp.,* 674 F. Supp. 46 (E.D. Mass.) (1987).

39. 898 F.2d 1556 (11th Cir.) (1990).

40. *Brown* at pp. 1566–67.

41. *Whitney v. Empire Blue Cross and Blue Shield,* U.S. Ct. App. (2d Circuit), No. 96-7635 (February 10, 1997).

42. 768 F. Supp. 216 (N.D. 111) (1991).

43. *Egert* at p. 218.

44. Restatement (Second) of Torts, Section 282.

45. 183 Cal. App. 3d 1064, 228 Cal. Rptr. 661 (1986).

46. See Boyd, Cost Containment and the Physician's Fiduciary Duty to the Patient, 39 *DePaul L Rev.*

47. 271 Cal. Rptr. 876, 222 Cal. App. 3d 660 (1990).

48. 965 F.2d 1321 (5th Cir.), *cert. denied,* 113 S.Ct. 812 (1992).

49. 999 F.2d 298 (8th Cir. 1993), *cert. denied,* 114 S.Ct. 694 (1994).

50. 211 N.E. 2d 253 (1965), *cert. denied,* 383 U.S. 946 (1966).

51. *Darling* at p. 257.

52. 1989 W.L. 153066 (Mo. Ct. App.) (1989), *aff'd on other grounds,* 782 S.W.2d 58 (Mo. 1989).

53. 753 F. Supp. 61, 64 (D. Comm. 1990), citing *Rollo v. Maxicare of Louisiana, Inc.,* 695 F. Supp. 245, 248 (E.D. La.) (1988).

54. No. 86–25767-NM (Mich. Cir. Ct., Saginaw City, April 27, 1989).

55. 99 Cal. App. 3d 560, 565 (1980).

56. 107 F.3d 625 (8th Cir. 1997).

57. 198 F.3d 552 (5th Cir. 2000).

58. 154 F.3d 362 (7th Cir. 1998).

59. 154 F.3d 362 (7th Cir. 1998).

60. Joel L. Michaels and Robert S. Canterman, "Disclosure of Physician Incentive Arrangements to Members of Managed Care Plans," member briefing of the HMOs and Health Plans Substantive Law Committee of the American Health Lawyers Association, www. healthlawyers.org, March 8, 2000.

61. 844 F. Supp. 966 (S.D.N.Y. 1994).

62. 57 F.3d 350 (3rd Cir. 1995) U.S. Sup. Ct., No. 95–442, *review denied* 12/4/95.

63. *Giles v. Nylcare Health Plans,* 1999 U.S. App. LEXIS 6370 (5th Cir., Apr. 9, 1999).

64. 59 F.3d 151 (10th Cir. 1995).

65. 478 N.Y.S. 2d 911 (App. Div. 1984).

66. 743 S.W. 2d 373 (Tex. App. 1987).

67. 876 F.2d 174 (1989).

68. 547 A.2d 1229 (Pa. Super. 1988).

69. 12 F. Supp. 2d 597; 1998 U.S. Dist. LEXIS 14831; 22 E.B.C. 1973.

70. 980 F.2d 1014 (5th Cir. 1993).

SUGGESTED READING

BNA's Health Law Reporter and *Managed Care Reporter.* Washington, DC: Bureau of National Affairs.

Health Law Digest, Health Lawyers News, and other publications from the American Health Lawyers' Association. Washington, DC. www.healthlawyers.org.

Government Affairs Bulletin, In the States, and other publications from the American Association of Health Plans, Washington, DC. www.aahp.org.

Legal Affairs Bulletin. Chicago, IL: Blue Cross and Blue Shield Association.

Managed Care Law Manual. 1995. Gaithersburg, MD: Aspen Publishers, Inc.

Health Law Week. Atlanta, GA: Strafford Publications.

CHAPTER 65

Legal Issues in Integrated Delivery Systems

Jerry R. Peters

DEFINITIONS

An integrated delivery system (IDS; see also Chapter 4) is an organization or group of legally affiliated organizations in which hospitals and physicians combine their assets, activities, risks, and rewards to deliver comprehensive health care services. This classic definition of an IDS is often confused in two ways.

First, there are numerous terms that are used in place of IDS, including *integrated health care organization, integrated health care system, integrated health care network, integrated service network,* and *organized delivery system.* The particular label one gives to the IDS is unimportant; the fundamental question is whether there is a legally affiliated system that controls the delivery of hospital and physician services.

The second area of confusion arises from the use of the term *IDS* to describe arrangements that are actually physician-hospital organizations (PHOs) or management service organizations (MSOs). From a legal perspective, the

PHO and MSO are both arrangements in which a hospital is not legally affiliated with the physician practice, but enters into a joint venture (the PHO) or contractual arrangement (the MSO) with the legally separate physician organization. In fact, this much looser use of the term IDS is found frequently throughout this book, including Chapter 4 (which is focused solely on IDSs), since the much looser terminology is in widespread use.

To better understand the differences among an IDS (representing an actual legal entity as noted above), PHO, and MSO, one must first identify the two types of integration: structural integration and operational integration. Structural integration occurs when previously separate businesses combine into either a single organization or a group of affiliated organizations that are under common ownership and control. This may occur when a hospital and a physician practice merge into a single organization or when a hospital or physician practice places itself under the common control of a single parent holding company.

Operational integration is the merger and consolidation of previously separate business operations into a single business operation. Typically, it is evidenced by factors such as the common

Jerry R. Peters, Esq., is a partner practicing in the San Francisco office of Latham & Watkins and national chair of their health care practice group. He has spoken extensively and published several books and numerous articles on physician-hospital business arrangements, including integrated delivery systems. He was an adjunct professor in health care law at the University of San Francisco Law School. He received his degree in economics at the University of California, Berkeley, and received his law degree from Hastings College of the Law.

*An analogue to this is the use of the term *independent practice association* (IPA) to describe a type of physician organization that contracts with an HMO, or negotiates with the HMO so that the health plan may contract directly with the physicians.

development of operational systems, the consolidation of management into a single management team, the joint planning and implementation of services by the hospital and physician practice, and the general consolidation of staff and other functions. There is no clear standard to determine when an operational integration has occurred. Instead, there are degrees or levels of operational integration. A hospital and physician practice achieve more operational integration when they operate under a consolidated budget, consolidated management and governance, a consolidated strategic plan, a unified marketing program, a single payer contracting process, and a coordinated operating system.

Structural integration is often the first focus of developing an IDS. As difficult as the merger of a hospital business into a physician practice may be, such structural integration is often more simple than operational integration. In fact, many IDS efforts have foundered in the waters of operational integration, and there is a backlash against IDSs because of the costs, time, and lost opportunities associated with operational integration.

Given this distinction between operational integration and structural integration, the difference among an IDS, PHO, and MSO is that the IDS includes both structural and operational integration between a hospital and a physician practice. Both the PHO and the MSO do not undergo structural integration; instead, the hospital and the physician practice maintain separate businesses from each other. This lack of structural integration in a PHO and MSO means that such arrangements have additional legal risks (compared with an IDS), and there might be less economic incentive to implement operational integration between the parties (that is, a hospital may not be willing to invest significant capital in a medical practice that is free to leave the hospital's sphere of influence or otherwise use the capital to the detriment of the hospital).

Because the terms *IDS, PHO,* and *MSO* are often used interchangeably, it is important to determine whether the parties intend to integrate structurally (that is, merge their businesses into a single economic enterprise—IDS) or whether each party will remain a separate business (that

is, each retains the right to its own revenue stream and controls its own means of production—PHO and MSO). In addition, one should determine what level of operational integration the parties intend to implement, recognizing that it is possible (even if not always economically preferable) to implement a significant degree of operational integration regardless of the level of structural integration between the parties.

IDS MODELS

There are several variables that combine to create numerous IDS models (for example, nonprofit model, for-profit model, foundation model, integrated health care organization model, and so on). Important variables include the number of organizations in the IDS, whether the organizations are nonprofit or for profit, whether the organizations are taxable or tax exempt, the degree to which the organizations are operationally integrated, the relationship between the IDS and the physicians (that is, employees or independent contractors), who controls the IDS (physicians, shareholder-investors, or nonprofit community directors), and how physicians are compensated. In developing an IDS, an advisor should examine each of these issues with his or her clients to determine what structure best meets the clients' goals. A few examples are illustrative of how one might structure an IDS.

The California foundation model typically involves a parent holding company, which is a nonprofit corporation that obtains tax exempt status. This parent holding company has two subsidiaries: one that operates the hospital and another that operates a medical practice (the medical practice corporation is typically called the foundation). The California foundation model is inherently a nonprofit, tax-exempt model because California's corporate practice of medicine doctrine and licensure laws require that the physician practice organization (that is, the foundation) be tax exempt. The Internal Revenue Service (IRS) will impose restrictions on the number of physicians who may serve on the board of directors of the foundation. California's corporate practice of medicine doctrine requires that the physicians be independent contractors to the foundation (thus the physicians are not employees of the foundation but instead organize their own professional corporation, which enters into a professional services agreement with the foundation under an independent contractor arrangement). Under this model, the IDS is ultimately controlled by nonprofit community directors (who typically control the parent holding company and the subsidiaries). Although this model has been copied in other states, there is no legal requirement that the structure be adopted in states that either do not have a corporate practice of medicine doctrine or have a more lenient doctrine than California.

In some states (other than California), the parties might establish a single for-profit IDS organization that is exclusively or predominantly owned by physicians (often called an integrated health care organization). This organization may acquire a hospital and then enter into contracts with payers to provide comprehensive hospital and physician services. This model is a for-profit organization whereby physicians own and are employed by the organization.

Another alternative is for physicians to own their medical practice and to establish a separate organization that owns the means of production (that is, space, equipment, staff, and so on) for the physicians to operate their practice. This separate organization is often referred to as an MSO. The MSO may acquire a hospital and its assets. The MSO might also have investors (in addition to the physician owners, who typically control a majority of the MSO). The MSO leases its assets to the physician practice, and the physician practice pays a fee to the MSO that must, at a minimum, equal the cost of operating the MSO.

This alternative illustrates the blurry distinction between an IDS and an MSO. In this example, the physician practice effectively functions as an IDS (it controls the revenues of both the physician and hospital practice and controls the operations of the hospital through the MSO lease arrangement), even though the hospital is technically owned by a separate organization. The common control by the physicians over both organizations, however, combined with the unification of economic incentives between the hospital and physicians, arguably makes this arrangement an IDS.

Given the various options for structuring an IDS, there are numerous models that can be developed. It is important for the parties to begin their integration process by identifying their goals and structuring the IDS to meet those goals. If the parties encounter significant differences in their goals or are unable to agree on the fundamental structural issues (nonprofit or for profit, physician controlled or community director controlled, and so on), the parties should not be afraid to postpone or discontinue their integration discussions. It is most often better to use these warnings signs to avoid a bad marriage than to embark upon integration efforts with an incompatible partner.

PROVIDER-SPONSORED ORGANIZATIONS

Complicating the taxonomy of IDSs is the provider-sponsored organization (PSO), as defined by the Health Care Financing Administration (HCFA). PSOs were specifically enabled in the Balanced Budget Act of 1997 (BBA) as part of the Medicare + Choice program, for purposes of contracting directly between HCFA and providers for Medicare risk plans. As such, the PSO is actually a form of a licensed health plan. The BBA provides for PSOs to be state licensed, but if state licensure is not forthcoming, then the BBA allows for HCFA to license the PSO directly and to allow the PSO to conform to somewhat lesser solvency requirements than those applied to a state-licensed managed care plan such as an HMO.

PSOs are mentioned here because they are organizations in which providers must have majority ownership and deliver a substantial proportion of services to enrolled Medicare beneficiaries directly through the sponsoring provider(s) or through affiliated providers. In an urban area 70 percent of health care services (as measured by expenditures) must be provided directly or through affiliated providers. Providers are considered affiliates if they have direct or indirect financial risk for the overall organization. For this reason, a PSO may be considered a form of IDS. But since PSOs contract directly with HCFA and operate as licensed health plans, they are not the focus of this chapter. PSOs are discussed further in Chapters 55 and 68, and the reader is referred to those chapters for additional discussion.

GOVERNANCE

If the IDS is organized as a professional corporation (or some other type of professional organization under state law), the state's corporate practice of medicine doctrine or other licensing laws may restrict who may serve on the board of directors of the organization (typically, only physicians or other licensed persons may serve on the board). If the IDS is formed as a nonprofit corporation under state law, state corporate law may again restrict the number or types of persons who may serve on the board (for example, some laws require that no more than 49 percent of the board members be interested directors, as that term is defined in the state corporate law). Finally, if the IDS applies for federal tax exempt status under Internal Revenue Code Section 501(c)(3), it will most likely need to address the safe harbor requirements regarding governance that are imposed by the IRS. The IRS has set forth its safe harbors in its 1994, 1995, and 1996 Continuing Professional Education Exempt Organizations Technical Instruction Program (CPE guidelines), copies of which may be obtained from the IRS.

To meet IRS requirements, no more than 49 percent of an IDS board should consist of persons (including management and physicians) who are financially related, directly or indirectly, to the IDS. The requirement includes physicians who have retired from a medical group. In the IRS's view, any physician who sells assets to, is employed by, or receives significant referrals from an IDS is "tainted" and can never serve as a disinterested physician on the board of directors.

COMMITTEES

Any committee or subcommittee created to consider the business or charitable operations of

the IDS must be independent and broadly representative of the community. Although the meaning of the phrase *independent and broadly representative of the community* was previously unclear, the IRS now requests that IDS committees, with a few exceptions, comply with the 49 percent safe harbor.

The IRS and legal counsel should carefully consider the strength of the IRS's position before enforcing it against an IDS. This is particularly true when the committees are advisory to the board (but see below). Nonetheless, the IRS's rationale for limiting committee participation should be reviewed and understood by the client before the client decides to assume the risk of noncompliance (IRS rationale is addressed in the 1996 CPE guidelines).

The IRS has made particular statements about two committees: the compensation committee and the fee committee. The IRS insists that physicians who have (or have had) a financial relationship with the IDS (or the predecessor physician group) may not serve on any committee that recommends or determines physician compensation. The problem with this limitation is that it prevents the IDS from utilizing physician expertise regarding compensation and physician incentives. As long as the compensation committee is advisory to the board and the board has the full power to accept, reject, and modify the committee's recommendations, some physician representation on this committee might be beneficial. In general, the physicians are likely to know more about physician compensation than the average person. This expertise should not be lost to the IDS.

At the same time, the IDS board should not simply accept the committee's recommendation without scrutiny. The board should have outside expertise to verify the committee's report. The board should also examine regional or national compensation surveys. If the committee's report is unreasonable, the board must appoint nonphysicians to negotiate physician compensation with the physicians and reject the committee's recommendation.

This issue may be a red herring in that physicians might not serve on the committee directly but will participate via their negotiations with the committee. Practically speaking, physicians will participate in compensation deliberations however the organization is structured.

The IRS also requires that physician participation on the committee that determines IDS fees be limited to a minority of the total committee members. Physician participation on the committee may not be equal to nonphysician participation. Because the IRS is allowing significant physician participation on the fee committee, its position is more palatable to physicians and most likely would be defensible in court. Therefore, IDS participants should consider compliance with this particular requirement.

Finally, the 1996 CPE guidelines specifically differentiate between the board-delegated authority committees and advisory committees:

> Most IDS organizations have provisions in their bylaws for the creation and operation of various committees. Normally, an IDS organization will have an executive committee, finance and planning committee, and provisions for various other committees or subcommittees. Often these committees have substantial authority to study, create, implement, and review charitable and business activities as well as the clinical aspects of the organization's operations. Generally, a committee has either advisory authority or specific powers delegated to it by the board of directors.[1]

DELEGATED BOARD AUTHORITY

In situations where an organization's bylaws grant board of directors powers to a committee or subcommittee, the IRS requests that the organization's bylaws state that no more than 20 percent of its committee members may be physicians who are financially interested or related, directly or indirectly, to any owner, partner, shareholder, or employee of the medical group or other physicians providing services in conjunction with the IDS organization. It should be

noted that the IRS's position allows unlimited physician representation on any committees or subcommittees that have authority over the clinical aspects of the organization's activities.[2]

ADVISORY COMMITTEES

Committees that do not have board of directors powers but are merely advisory in nature may also create concerns for the IRS. To elucidate these issues, some background information may be useful. The tax exempt status of the IDS presents several difficult issues. Generally speaking, IDS organizations are created through the purchase of one or more existing private medical practices, and the individual physicians become employees or contractors of the IDS organization. These are factually intensive cases with important issues that the IRS must address. The benefit to the community from the formation of the IDS must be carefully weighed against the benefit to the physicians from the sale of their practices and subsequent professional services agreements. Unless there is a significant community benefit, these transactions may benefit the physicians more than unsubstantially.

Integration also raises serious concerns for physicians. After integration, physicians face a totally different employment or service environment; they may be hesitant to relinquish control of their former medical practice. The IRS, on the other hand, is concerned that the community receive a substantial benefit because of the large amount of charitable assets involved in the purchase of physicians' medical practice assets. In contrast, the physicians may believe that, as the former owners of a valuable business, they should continue to exert considerable control. The IRS acknowledges this expertise but seeks to ensure that there is a significant community benefit, which in certain situations may conflict directly with the interests of the physicians.

Because of the perceived loss of control, physicians often seek to become designated members of committees having substantial day-to-day operational powers as well as considerable influence over business and charitable programs. In many cases, these committees are the important bodies that weigh all the facts and circumstances in a complicated proposed action. These committees often make recommendations based upon complex fact patterns to the board of directors. Typically, the full board of directors meets infrequently. Because of workload demands, the limited expertise of board members, and the complexity of issues, the board often is unable to give detailed attention to every item that comes before it for a vote. Under certain circumstances, the IRS is concerned that the board will routinely accept the recommendations of committees that have significant control by financially interested parties.

CONFLICT OF INTEREST POLICY

The IDS should be careful to comply with state law regarding the development of a conflict of interest policy and its operations. This is particularly important if the IDS is a nonprofit organization because most states regulate conflicts of interest with respect to nonprofit directors and officers. In addition, if the IDS seeks tax exempt status, the IRS has set forth guidelines as to how it prefers to see the conflict of interest policy developed for the IDS. In the 1996 CPE Guidelines, the IRS states:

> The Service has expressed concerns about interested party control of IDS organizations through its 80 percent community board safe harbor. The Service is also concerned about private benefit and inurement issues that may arise because of the relationship between an exempt organization providing IDS services and its physician employees/contractors, officers, directors and key employees. In most situations, the best protection for a charitable trust is well-defined, written policy governing conflicts of interest. This serves to educate affected individuals and limit their activities under appropriate circumstances. Because most IDS organizations include some financially interested individuals on their governing boards, they

may wish to adopt a clear conflicts of interest policy.[3]

Although not required, the IRS favorably views organizations having policy statements in their bylaws that clearly identify situations where a conflict might arise. The IRS believes that directors of tax exempt IDS organizations must exercise their powers in good faith and in a manner that they believe to be in the organization's best interests. Furthermore, organizations that educate their new directors, employees, and officers regarding conflicts of interest and concerns about private benefit and inurement help eliminate problems arising from lack of knowledge.

An example of a conflict of interest policy that is viewed favorably by the IRS is one that requires that, in the event that the board of directors considers entering into any transaction or arrangement with a corporation, entity, or individual in which a director has an interest:

- the interested director must disclose the potential conflict of interest to the board
- the board may ask the interested director to leave the meeting during the discussion of the matter that gives rise to the potential conflict
- the interested director will not vote on the matter that gives rise to the potential conflict
- the board must approve the transaction or arrangement by a majority vote of the directors present at a meeting that has a quorum, not including the vote of the interested director
- the board meeting minutes must state which directors were present for the discussion and vote, the content of the discussion, and any roll call of the vote

In addition, if a director has any interest in a transaction or arrangement that might involve personal financial gain or loss for the director, the policy should contain the following provisions:

- If appropriate, the board may appoint a noninterested person or committee to investigate alternatives to the proposed transaction or arrangement.

- To approve the transaction, the board must first find, by a majority vote of the directors then in office without counting the vote of the interested director, that the proposed transaction or arrangement is in the IDS organization's best interest and for its own benefit, that the proposed transaction is fair and reasonable to the IDS organization, and, after reasonable investigation, that the board had determined that the IDS organization cannot obtain a more advantageous transaction or arrangement with reasonable efforts under the circumstances.
- The interested director will not be present for the discussion or vote regarding the transaction or arrangement.
- The transaction or arrangement must be approved by a majority vote of the directors, not including interested directors.

The IRS has released a model conflicts of interest policy, which it modified and re-released. Practitioners should review that policy with their clients.

TAX EXEMPTION AND CHARITABLE BENEFIT

In addition to the restrictions mentioned above, the IRS will impose additional requirements on an IDS that seeks federal tax exempt status under Internal Revenue Code Section 501 (c)(3). For this reason, many parties should consider carefully whether tax exemption is in their best interest. Some of the advantages of tax exemption are that net income is not subject to federal income taxes (except unrelated business income tax); that the organization may qualify for exemption from state, sales, and property tax; that the organization may qualify for tax exempt bond financing (this is limited to only a few situations); and that contributions to the organization are tax deductible (thereby increasing the probability of the organization receiving grants). The disadvantages include the restrictions placed by the IRS on the organization, the requirement to disclose the tax exemption application and Form 990 to the public (thereby disclos-

ing the salaries of key employees and officers), limitations on the organization's ability to dissolve, and limitations on the use of facilities that were financed by tax exempt bond proceeds.

If the IDS decides to seek exemption from federal taxation under Internal Revenue Code Section 501(c)(3), it must demonstrate that it serves a charitable purpose more than incidentally. This is a facts and circumstances test in which the IRS (or the court) considers all the activities of the IDS to determine whether its primary function is charitable.

The IRS has set forth several requirements, based on Revenue Ruling 69–545, which sets forth guidelines for a hospital to qualify for Section 501(c)(3), for an IDS to qualify for tax exempt status under Section 501(c)(3). *Although no single factor is determinative, certain factors are more important (and the probability of obtaining tax exempt status is low if such factors are not present):*

- *Open medical staff*—Any hospital operated by an IDS must have an open medical staff. Although clinic facilities (in which physicians practice medicine) are not required to have an open medical staff, this policy has created some controversy because of the need for an IDS to control hospital utilization (which is best done by the IDS physicians, not independent physicians who have no economic incentive to control hospital utilization).
- *Medicare/Medicaid patients*—The IDS must be receptive to providing services to all Medicare and Medicaid patients in a nondiscriminatory manner at IDS sites. This has been generally interpreted to mean that the IDS may not open specific Medicaid clinical facilities and refer all Medicaid patients to those facilities. If the IDS is in a state that has a Medicaid contracting program, the IDS must negotiate in good faith to enter into such a contract with the government. Although this is a financially difficult requirement for an IDS to meet, it is a significant factor that the IRS is likely to treat as mandatory.

- *Emergency services*—All IDS facilities must treat emergency or urgent care patients regardless of their ability to pay. This applies to both the hospital facilities and the physician clinical facilities. Exceptions might be available where emergency services are not offered, but this requirement is relatively important to the IRS.
- *Charity care*—Although the IRS does not always require that an IDS provide a specific amount of charity care, in those situations where the IRS determines that the organization is unlikely to provide charity care, the IRS may require the IDS to budget a specific amount of charity care to be provided each year. If the IDS can show that it benefits the community in significant other ways (see the other requirements), there is a chance that the IRS will not require charity care by the IDS.
- *Miscellaneous*—The 1995 CPE guidelines listed the following factors as indicators of community benefit:
  — All medical functions and records are integrated for each individual patient.
  — Anyone in need of care is treated at any clinic location without regard to ability to pay.
  — The IDS treats patients seeking urgent care at its urgent care centers without regard to ability to pay.
  — The clinic participates in, or has made good faith efforts to participate in, the Medicaid program in a nondiscriminatory manner.
  — Contract physicians do not discriminate against patients based on ability to pay and will see Medicaid patients on a nondiscriminatory basis.
  — A specified minimum amount is spent each year for charity care.
  — The IDS conducts health education programs.
  — A substantial number of the physicians provide coverage in the hospital emergency department and render care in those emergency departments without regard to the patients' ability to pay.

PHYSICIAN COMPENSATION

An IDS must be careful that it distributes its income to physicians in a manner that complies with the Ethics and Patient Referrals Act of 1989 (the Stark law) as amended. In addition, any state antireferral laws should be examined before a physician compensation arrangement is finalized.

Generally, the IRS is concerned that a tax exempt IDS does not share its net profits with physicians or otherwise use the IDS organization as a joint venture with physicians. This leaves significant leeway for a tax exempt organization to develop a physician compensation plan based on production, quality of care delivered to patients, and other quantifiable measures (other than the net profits of the organization).

The IRS has made clear that it will closely scrutinize situations where an IDS pays significant amounts for the intangible value of the acquired practice and, at the same time, pays significant annual compensation to the physicians. In the 1996 CPE guidelines, the IRS discusses its concerns regarding compensation and sets forth a list of the data that it will examine to determine whether compensation paid to the physicians is reasonable under all of the circumstances. The 1996 CPE guidelines state: "Compensation issues often arise in IDS organizations, faculty group practice plans, clinics, hospitals converting from for-profit to nonprofit status, and joint ventures and partnerships involving exempt organizations, as well as ruling requests regarding these entities. Compensation arrangements often provide for base salaries, fringe benefits, deferred payments, income guarantees, contingencies to compensation, and incentive bonuses."[4]

In most situations, the IRS wants to review certain basic information involving compensation arrangements. Although the compensation arrangements and the accompanying professional services agreement may be included in the file, they are complex, and often it is difficult ultimately to determine actual compensation. Thus the IRS often requests more specific information, adding additional time to the rulings process. The following is a reproduction of the typical compensation information that the IRS requests (it expedites matters if this information is included in the original submission to the IRS):

- How many physicians do you employ, and how many do you contract with for professional services?
- Please submit a compensation contract for each physician employee. You may black out the physician's name and assign a letter or number to each contract if you are concerned about privacy issues.
- For each compensation arrangement, please provide the following:
    1. A realistic estimate of *total* projected physician's compensation (including base, bonus, benefits, and managed care risk pool withholds or other risk pool participation) for a *3-year period* (the estimate could be for 1 year of actual operation and 2 years of projections, depending upon how long you have been operational). The estimate must be based on the terms contained in the compensation agreement.
    2. A realistic estimate of 3 years' projected gross receipts (the estimate could be for 1 year of actual operation and 2 years of projections, depending upon how long you have been operational). The estimate must be supported by data used in preparing actual or future financial reports or projections.
    3. A statement establishing that the physician's total compensation is reasonable based on the geographic locale and the physician's specialty. You can establish reasonableness by the use of compensation data for the physician specialty based upon compensation studies produced by local, regional, or national medical associations; the American Hospital Association, the Medical Group Management Association, the Hay Group, or other knowledgeable consultants.
    4. Are there any caps (ceilings) on total compensation?
    5. Before total compensation of all physicians (base and benefits minus bonus and risk pool withholds) is determined, how much surplus remains for the exempt organization? After total compensation is determined, how much surplus remains? What percentage of surplus do the physicians receive? What percentage does your organization receive?

Physician compensation in IDSs and medical groups is also discussed in Chapter 9, and restrictions on the amount of risk individual physicians may accept under Medicare are discussed in Chapter 8.

PRACTICE ACQUISITIONS/ VALUATION

If the IDS will acquire assets from an existing physician practice, a tax specialist should be consulted as to the tax consequences of the transaction to any for-profit organization (either the IDS or the physicians). Tax issues for managed care organizations and IDSs are discussed in Chapter 48.

If the IDS is a tax exempt organization, the parties should consult the guidelines set forth in the 1996 CPE guidelines with respect to physician practice acquisitions. These guidelines include a discussion of how the IRS would prefer to see valuations performed, and they indicate a variety of methods recognized by the IRS as to how valuations may be performed. Instead of insisting on the discounted cash flow valuation method, the IRS recognizes that various valuation methods are appropriate in different situations.

One particularly difficult situation occurs when an IDS acquires a small or solo practice (especially in a rural area, where the intangible value of the practice is low). In these situations, the IDS does not wish to pay for a valuation fee (often, the valuation fee is higher than the intangible value to be paid to the physician). In these situations, the IDS should obtain an independent valuation for this first practice acquisition. Thereafter, someone employed by the IDS should use the same procedures used by the independent valuation association (and should pay careful attention to the 1996 CPE guidelines) and document the value of the practice. As long as the IDS has carefully demonstrated the reason why it has paid fair market value to the physician, the IRS is unlikely to challenge the arrangement in court.

MEDICARE/MEDICAID PROVIDER NUMBERS

Medicare/Medicaid part B payment rules only allow for payment to the patient or to the patient's physician. In addition, the physician is not allowed to assign his or her right to such income to another party. There are two relevant exceptions to this assignment prohibition: Payment may be made to the employer of the provider of services if the employee is required, as a condition of employment, to pay over such amounts to the employer; and if the services are provided in a hospital, rural primary care hospital, or other facility, payment may be made to the facility in which the service was provided if the facility has a contractual agreement with the provider of services and that agreement requires the facility to submit the bill for such service.

If an IDS acquires a physician practice (including accounts receivable), the assignment of Medicare and Medicaid accounts receivable by the physician to the IDS might constitute a violation of the assignment prohibition. In addition, if physicians are contractually established as independent contractors of the IDS, the IDS may have difficulty receiving the Medicare or Medicaid receivables for the performance of services. Practically speaking, most physicians are employed by the IDS, and this problem does not arise. If the problem exists, however, the IDS may contract with the physician for everything except Medicaid services, and the physician's Medicaid provider number might be used to bill and collect all revenues for Medicaid patients. The total amount paid by the IDS to the physician would be net of any Medicaid receipts received by the physician.

The reader should note that under the Health Insurance Portability and Accountability Act of 1996 (HIPAA; see Chapters 35, 36, and 67), the provider identification numbers are scheduled to be replaced with the National Provider Identification Number (NPID) beginning in 2002 or 2003. The reader is referred to those other chapters for a brief discussion of this issue, and the reader is also urged to keep up to date with recent regulations and implementation issues by checking the HCFA website at *www.hcfa.gov*.

ANTITRUST LAW

There are two types of risks that potentially arise from the development of an IDS: the risk from developing the IDS (that is, monopoly and other risks associated with consolidating a hospital and a physician practice), and the risk arising from the ongoing operations of the IDS (that is, tying arrangements and other illegal activities conducted by the IDS).

With respect to the development of an IDS, the parties should carefully examine Section 7 of the Clayton Act, which prohibits mergers and acquisitions that have the potential to restrain competition in the market unreasonably. If the development of an IDS creates a monopoly power or even market dominance with respect to any particular service (for example, outpatient surgery or other services), the IDS arrangement might be challenged. Nonetheless, the parties should review the Marshfield Clinic case and assess whether the facts of that case are applicable to their own particular IDS.[5] In addition, the parties should review the enforcement policy statements issued by the Department of Justice and the Federal Trade Commission on September 27, 1994, to assess the risk of government action against the proposed IDS.[6]

In assessing whether the development of an IDS presents risk, the parties should first determine whether the formation creates too much market power for the IDS and its participants. Critical to this analysis is the definition of the market, which can be summarized as the area in which consumers will freely move to receive similar services. This is a highly factual determination. If physicians who join the IDS previously competed with each other and, through the merger of their practices into the IDS, effectively eliminated competition among themselves, the risk of an antitrust challenge increases as the percentage of physicians who otherwise would have competed with each other (absent the IDS) increases.

If the IDS has an exclusive relationship with a significant number of physicians so that no other hospital can contract with a sufficient number of physicians to develop a competing IDS product, the monopolist IDS may be subject to a successful challenge. Presently, exclusive dealing arrangements can tie up to 35 percent of total physicians in a particular specialty in the market without raising significant antitrust concerns.

Another issue is that the IDS may not participate in an agreement among competitors by which it refuses to deal with other competitors (or causes others not to deal with those competitors). Such group boycotts generally are illegal if they exclude competitors from something that those competitors need to compete effectively in the market. A fourth issue is that the IDS, which has market power (as defined under antitrust law), should not condition its sale of a service (such as hospital services) upon the payer's agreeing to purchase another service offered by the IDS (such as physician services). Finally, the parties should be careful not to engage in any price-fixing activities before they form the IDS and should not engage in any price-fixing activities with independent physicians after they form the IDS.

Although it is not common in the IDS setting, the parties should determine whether they need to file a Hart-Scott-Rodino notification. *This premerger notification must be filed if the parties merge, if one party acquires the assets or stock of other parties, or if new legal entities are established to operate the IDS and if all three of the following conditions are met:*

1. The IDS or at least one participant is engaged in or affects commerce.
2. The transaction (merger of the parties or acquisition) involves the acquisition of assets or voting securities, the acquired firm has total assets of $10 million or more, and

the acquiring firm has annual net sales or total assets of $100 million or more; or the acquired firm has total assets or annual net sales of $100 million or more; and the acquiring firm has total assets or annual net sales of $10 million or more.

3. If the transaction results in the acquiring party obtaining 15 percent or more of the voting securities or assets of the acquired party, or the acquiring party obtains voting securities or assets of the acquired party that in aggregate exceed $15 million, the third condition is met.

The reader should also read Chapter 63 for additional, specific discussion of antitrust issues.

INDEPENDENT CONTRACTOR STATUS

The IDS must decide whether it will employ its physicians or contract with them as independent contractors. This decision will have several ramifications, including the IDS's liability for the actions of the physicians and the inclusion of physicians in the employee benefits plans of the IDS. In addition, this decision will determine whether the IDS issues a W-2 or 1099 form to the physicians.

Most often, this issue is resolved by law, not by the business decision of the parties. Even if the IDS enters into a contract with a physician as an independent contractor, the law may reclassify the physician as an employee of the IDS (and assess back taxes and penalties against the IDS). Thus it is important for a tax specialist to determine whether the physician should be treated as an employee or independent contractor for the purposes of tax reporting and for an employee benefits specialist to determine whether the physician must be offered employee benefits.

An employer must withhold payroll taxes from the wages that the employer pays to its employees.[7] These payroll taxes include federal income tax withholding, Federal Insurance Contribution Act (FICA) taxes, and Federal Unemployment Tax Act taxes. If a physician is not an employee (but is an independent contractor) of the employer, the employer is not fully responsible for these taxes. Thus employers prefer to classify workers as independent contractors, but the IRS prefers that workers be classified as employees (thereby ensuring collection of the taxes).

The IRS recently has given increased attention to the classification of individual service providers as independent contractors. The Comprehensive Audit Program conducted by the IRS has specifically targeted this issue as an area of focus (because the IRS might be able to collect revenues from the exempt organization if it finds that a worker has been misclassified as an independent contractor). Typically, the structure and documentation of the worker's arrangement will determine proper classification.

An employer–employee relationship generally exists if the employer has common law control over the worker. The IRS has established a list of 20 factors that are used to determine whether sufficient control exists to constitute an employer–employee relationship (see Exhibit 65–1).[8] The 20 factors are weighed as part of a

---

Exhibit 65–1 IRS's 20 Factors Used in Determining Employer–Employee Relationship

1. *Instructions.* An employer may require an employee to follow instructions. An independent contractor may only be required to follow overall project specifications.
2. *Training.* An employer generally trains an employee as to its methodologies and practices. An independent contractor generally has his or her own style and does not require training.
3. *Integration.* When a person is so integrated into a business that the success or failure of the business depends a good deal on such person's performance, the worker is under the employer's control. An independent contractor is generally not necessary for the longevity of the employer.
4. *Services rendered personally.* Employees provide services personally. An independent contractor can generally assign a task; qualified people are fungible.
5. *Hiring, supervising, and paying assistants.* An employee generally works with other people who are also employees of the employer; an employee does not hire, fire, supervise, or pay assistants. Independent contractors, however, hire, supervise, and pay their own assistants.
6. *Continuing relationship.* The longer a relationship continues between an employer and a worker, the more likely it is that relationship is an employer–employee relationship. This may include services that recur frequently, even if at irregular intervals (e.g., either on

call by the employer or whenever the work is available).
7. *Set hours of work.* The more formal and rigid a worker's hours, the more control the employer has over the worker. An independent contractor generally works on his or her own schedule and only has specified overall project or task deadlines.
8. *Full time required.* When a worker works substantially full time for an employer and does not work for any other employers, the employer has control over the worker's time. An independent contractor usually works for several employers at the same time. An employee may also have more than one employer, however.
9. *Doing work on employer's premises.* Evidence of control over an employee exists when an employer can designate the place where work is to be done and has control over that environment.
10. *Order or sequence set.* If an employer retains the right to control the order or sequence of the work that is to be performed and the type of work does not naturally dictate the order or sequence, evidence of control over the worker exists.
11. *Oral or written reports.* The more often a worker reports to an employer, the more likely it is that the employer controls the worker. It is acceptable for an independent contractor to issue progress reports as phases of a project are completed, however.

continues

Exhibit 65–1 continued

12. *Payment by hour, week, or month.* An employee generally receives a set wage based upon a time period. On the other hand, an independent contractor receives payment based upon a project or straight commission. A contract may specify when payments are due. The independent contractor should invoice the employer for amounts due, however. The payments should not be made automatically.

13. *Payment of business and/or traveling expenses.* When an employer controls expenses, the employer also controls the worker's activities. Generally, independent contractors take care of their own incidental expenses.

14. *Furnishing of tools and materials.* The more tools and materials supplied by the employer, the more likely it is that the worker is an employee. The weight of this factor will depend on the occupation of the worker and the type of tools and materials supplied.

15. *Significant investment.* If a worker makes an investment in facilities or tools that are not normally invested in by employees, this factor will show a lack of control by the employer. Use of an employer's facilities generally indicates control by the employer. Facilities include premises and equipment, such as office furniture and machinery.

16. *Realization of profit or loss.* Employees have no opportunity to realize a gain or loss. Independent contractors, however, are business people who take risks expecting either to enhance their return or to suffer a loss.

17. *Working for more than one firm at a time.* When an individual works for more than one firm and performs de minimis services for each, it is likely that none of the firms will have control over the individual. Even if a person works for more than one employer, however, if enough control exists, the person could be considered to be an employee of more than one employer.

18. *Making services available to the general public.* The more a person offers services to the general public, the less likely it is that control will be found to exist. Indicia of making services available to the general public are advertising, business cards, stationery, telephone listings, holding a license, and the like.

19. *Right to discharge.* If a person can be discharged at will, then the person is an employee. The person who possesses the right to discharge is an employer. Independent contractors cannot be fired so long as they are in compliance with the contract.

20. *Right to terminate.* Independent contractors cannot quit; employees can terminate at will. Therefore, to be an independent contractor there must be a legal obligation to complete the contract.

subjective balancing test. The *Internal Revenue Manual* states: "Any single fact or small group of facts is not conclusive evidence of the presence or absence of control."[9] Taken together, the 20 factors are balanced on a case-by-case basis to determine whether a worker (or a class of workers) is an employee. When the 20 factors determine that an employer–employee relationship exists, it is immaterial to the IRS which label the parties attach to the relationship.[10]

The IRS has established audit guidelines that focus on specific factors for assessing whether physicians should be classified as independent contractors, including the following[11]*:*

- whether the physician has a private practice
- whether the hospital pays wages to the physician
- whether the hospital provides supplies and support staff to the physician
- whether the hospital bills and collects revenues for the physician
- whether the physician and hospital divide the physician's professional fees on a percentage basis
- whether the hospital regulates or otherwise has the right to control the physician
- whether the physician has specific hours to be on duty at the hospital

- whether the physician's uniform has the hospital's logo or name
- whether the hospital pays the physician's malpractice insurance premiums

The audit guidelines instruct IRS agents to pay particular attention to hospital-based specialists, such as radiologists, pathologists, and anesthesiologists. The IRS particularly believes that such physicians should be employees of the hospital for purposes of federal employment taxes (regardless of the state's corporate medicine doctrine).

The IRS has instituted a health care industry specialization program, pursuant to which it conducts coordinated audits of tax exempt health organizations. As part of this program, the IRS has developed a physician issue paper that sets forth the IRS's proposed position regarding the independent contractor/employee classification of hospital-based physicians. This paper still relies on the 20-factor test identified in Exhibit 65–1 but attempts to assign emphasis to certain of the 20 common law factors for the analysis of relationships with physicians. Its approach is to give less emphasis to factors that are common to all hospital–physician relationships, thereby making it easier to isolate the factors that are strong indicators of employee versus independent contractor status. The paper identifies several factors as important in classifying a physician as an employee of a hospital, including whether the hospital reserves the right to specify the physician's hours, whether the hospital is entitled to the physician's professional fees, and whether the hospital bears the risk and expenses associated with the physician's delivery of services (for example, operating costs).

The paper also provides examples of when a hospital-based physician would be classified as an independent contractor, when a physician should be characterized as an employee of his or her own professional corporation, and when the physician must be recognized as having dual status (that is, the physician is both an employee and an independent contractor of the same organization when he or she is acting in more than one capacity for that organization). It also states

categorically that residents and interns are almost always common law employees of the hospital at which they are being trained.

Internal Revenue Code Section 530 precludes the IRS from challenging an employer for failure to withhold federal employment taxes with respect to certain independent contractor arrangements. *An employer can avoid retroactive assessments of federal employment taxes caused by reclassification of workers from independent contractors to employees if each of the following three requirements is met:*

1. The employer must have a reasonable basis for treating the worker as an independent contractor (it is not clear whether this reasonable basis must have existed before December 31, 1978). There are four safe harbors for meeting this requirement: reliance on a published IRS ruling or judicial precedent; reliance on the outcome of a prior audit by the IRS if the IRS reviewed workers who held similar positions as the position that is at issue; reliance on the long-standing recognized practice of a significant segment of the industry, even if the practice of treating the worker as an independent contractor is not uniform throughout the entire industry; or any other reasonable basis for not classifying a worker as an employee.[12]
2. The employer must not have treated the worker as an employee anytime after 1977. In particular, the employer should not have withheld federal income tax or FICA taxes from the worker's wages, must not have filed certain employment tax returns for the worker, and must not have treated any worker holding a similar position as an employee for any period after December 31, 1977.
3. The employer must have filed all appropriate federal tax returns in a manner that is timely and consistent with the worker not being treated as an employee (for example, 1099 forms must have been filed properly).

The IRS has published form SS-8, which may be used by a taxpayer to request that the IRS determine whether a person is an employee or an independent contractor. This form may be submitted either by an employer or an employee. It may not always be advisable to submit this form, however, because once an answer is received, the employer has no basis for treating a worker contrary to the IRS's determination.

If a worker is misclassified as an independent contractor and is later determined to be an employee, the employer is then liable for the employment taxes not previously paid plus interest and any penalties that may be imposed by the IRS. If an independent contractor is reclassified as an employee, the employer must review the tax-qualified pension and employee benefit plans for the years at issue. In situations where qualification was marginal, the reclassification of independent contractors may disqualify pension or benefit plans.

Failure to classify a worker properly as an employee and then having a nonfavorable redetermination can cause severe financial hardship to an enterprise and to the enterprise participants. Past payroll taxes and the associated penalties and interest can bankrupt many small enterprises. If the enterprise cannot pay the IRS's payroll tax assessment, the participants in the enterprise may be personally liable for the assessment, depending on the enterprise participant's role in the enterprise or the type of entity chosen for the enterprise. Last, if payroll taxes are assessed personally against an enterprise participant, the taxes may not be discharged in bankruptcy proceedings.

COVENANTS NOT TO COMPETE

In its first determination letters (for example, the Friendly Hills determination letter), the IRS put certain restrictions on the covenants not to compete that an IDS may enforce against physicians. This created a controversy because it restricted the IDS from realizing the full benefit of its covenant not to compete and thereby prevented the IDS from realizing the full benefits of the amounts paid to physicians in exchange for the covenants not to compete (the IRS would counter that the IDS should have simply paid

less for the covenant not to compete). In the 1996 guidelines and in more recent determination letters, the IRS appears to have dropped this issue. It is not clear presently whether the IRS has any restrictions upon covenants not to compete. Parties should negotiate a significant covenant not to compete between themselves and should wait for the IRS to make any modifications (and then argue with the IRS regarding those modifications before conceding the point).

CONCLUSION

The development of an IDS involves an examination of numerous business issues. Most important, the parties should be careful that their cultural differences (for example, physicians are independent and hospital administrators are committee oriented) are identified and addressed. Numerous miscellaneous legal issues (for example, employee benefits law, labor law, tax identification numbers, certificate of need law, corporate/partnership law, financing law, state licensuring and corporate practice of medicine law, malpractice liability law, rate and review law, real property laws, recordkeeping laws, state antireferral laws, securities law, tax law and tax exemption law, insurance issues, intellectual property law, medical staff issues, and possibly environmental law) must be considered.

One should not expect an IDS to be developed overnight, but one also should not languish into the 18- to 24-month backwater of merger negotiations. Most important, the parties must recognize that, after the merger is done, the real work begins. They must work well together, and they should not try to integrate themselves operationally more than they are culturally capable of tolerating. Often, an IDS will simply allow the physician organization to operate separately from the hospital organization and will look for common areas where capital allocations improve the overall delivery of health care services to the community. The parties must commit themselves to some level of operational integration (including capital planning, strategic planning, payer contracting, and so on), or else they should question why they developed the IDS in the first place. Nonetheless, they should be careful not to integrate their operations excessively if such integration will cause undue burden or strains upon the parties.

Finally, the parties should be careful to address any political issues that arise from the formation of the IDS. Most important, reaction of independent physicians who are not part of the IDS can be a fatal factor if IDS leadership does not properly address those physicians' concerns. An IDS is not for everyone, and the parties should be careful before expending the time and money in developing an IDS to determine that the effort will generate appropriate benefits for themselves and their constituents.

REFERENCES AND NOTES

1. 1996 CPE at p. 388.
2. See 1994 CPE at p. 227 for more information about the 20 percent safe harbor.
3. 1996 CPE at pp. 386–87.
4. 1996 CPE at p. 391.
5. *Blue Cross and Blue Shield United of Wisc. and Compcure Health Services Insurance Corp. v. The Marshfield Clinic and Security Health Plan of Wisc., Inc.,* 881 F. Supp. 1309 (W.D. Wisc. 1994).
6. *Statements of Enforcement Policy and Analytical Principles Relating to Health Care and Antitrust,* U.S. Department of Justice and Federal Trade Commission (September 27, 1994).
7. I.R.C. Section 3402.
8. Rev. Rul. 87-41, 1987-1 C.B. 296.
9. 2 *Internal Revenue Manual* (CCH) 8465 (1988).
10. Treas. Reg. Sections 31.3306(i)–1(d), 31.3121(d)–1(a)(3), and 31.3401(b)–1(e).
11. *IRS Audit Guidelines for Hospitals,* Manual Transmittal 7 (10) 69–38; *Exempt Organizations Guidelines Handbook* Section 331(1) (27 March 1992).
12. See Priv. Ltr. Rul. 8733004.

SUGGESTED READING

Peters, G.R. 1995. *Healthcare Integration: A Legal Manual for Constructing Integrated Organizations.* Washington, D.C.: National Health Lawyers Association.

National Health Lawyers Association. 1994. *Health Law Practice Guide.*

Health Law Center. 1995. *Managed Care Law Manual.* Gaithersburg, MD: Aspen.

CHAPTER 66

ERISA and Managed Care

Jacqueline M. Saue and Gregg H. Dooge

Few federal laws have a greater impact on the operations of managed care organizations (MCOs) than the Employee Retirement Income Security Act (ERISA) of 1974, as amended.[1] Although ERISA does not directly regulate MCOs, it does regulate most employer-sponsored employee benefit plans to which MCOs market their products. ERISA will affect the nature, design, and administration of such products by MCOs. Moreover, ERISA will determine what state laws can be applied to such products, as well as what legal challenges can be made to the administration of such products.

This chapter is designed to provide MCOs with a working knowledge of the provisions of

ERISA that are likely to affect their operations. Topics addressed include ERISA's documentation, reporting, and disclosure requirements; benefit plan design considerations; the amendment of benefit plans; the duties of ERISA fiduciaries, which may include MCOs; challenges to benefit denials; ERISA's civil enforcement scheme and remedies; and the effect of ERISA preemption of state laws and causes of actions on MCOs' operations.

DOCUMENTATION, REPORTING, AND DISCLOSURE REQUIREMENTS

A plan maintained by a nongovernment employer that provides health care or health care benefits to employees (including plans providing coverage or benefits through a managed care arrangement) generally constitutes an employee benefit plan subject to ERISA.[2] Such plans must meet the documentation, reporting, and disclosure requirements set forth in ERISA.

Plan Document

Every employee benefit plan governed by ERISA is required to be set forth in a written plan document (or documents) that details the operative provisions governing benefits under the plan.[3] In the case of health care benefits that are provided through an insurance contract or a contract with an MCO, the sponsoring employer might maintain a simple plan document that describes certain of the plan's rules, such as a de-

Jacqueline M. Saue is a partner with the firm of Foley & Lardner in Washington, DC. She received her law degree from Georgetown University Law Center in 1975 and her bachelor's degree magna cum laude from Mount Holyoke College in 1972. She is a member of the District of Columbia Bar and the State Bar Association of Maryland. Ms. Saue concentrates her practice in the area of health law and has written and spoken frequently on health law issues, including managed care, ERISA, and health antitrust.

Gregg H. Dooge is a partner in the Milwaukee, Wisconsin, office of Foley & Lardner, practicing in the area of employee benefits. He is a 1981 graduate of the University of Wisconsin-Madison and a 1984 graduate of Stanford University Law School. In addition to his private practice, he is an Adjunct Professor at Marquette University School of Law and is a member of Wisconsin Retirement Plan Professionals, Ltd. and the Greater Milwaukee Employee Benefits Council.

scription of the plan's eligibility and amendment provisions, but that otherwise refers to the insurance or managed care contract for the description of plan benefits.

Summary Plan Description

A summary plan description is a booklet that describes the operative provisions of a plan in lay language. The Department of Labor has prescribed the types of information that are required to be included in the summary plan description.[4] For insured or managed care plans, employers often use the booklet published by the insurance company or MCO as the basis for the summary plan description, although the employer generally will have to add certain administrative information to comply with the Department of Labor requirements concerning summary plan descriptions. In some cases, a health care plan contains detailed benefit schedules that are difficult to summarize. In lieu of repeating the benefit schedules, the summary plan description may provide a general description of the types of benefits provided if the summary informs participants that the complete schedules are available for their review.[5]

The summary plan description must be distributed to participants within 120 days after the date on which the plan is adopted or made effective (or, in the case of an employee who becomes a participant after the adoption or effective date of the plan, within 90 days after the date on which the employee becomes a participant).[6] In general, a new summary plan description must be issued every 5 years, although if there have been no amendments to the plan, distribution of a new summary plan description can be made every 10 years.[7]

Summary of Material Modifications

If there are changes in the plan that affect the information provided in the summary plan description at a time when the plan sponsor is not required to publish a new summary plan description, the employer must publish a summary of material modifications.[8] The summary of mate-

rial modifications explains the plan changes and acts as a supplement to the summary plan description until a revised summary plan description is distributed. The summary of material modifications must be distributed to plan participants within 210 days after the close of the plan year in which the plan amendment is adopted.[9] Alternatively, the plan sponsor may at any time publish an updated summary plan description in lieu of the summary of material modifications.

Discrepancies in Plan Documentation

Although the summary plan description and summary of material modifications are intended, as their names suggest, as summaries of the actual plan document, some courts have held that the summaries override the terms of the plan when the plan and the summaries conflict.[10] Thus, when the summary plan description provides for benefits in a situation not covered under the formal plan document, the summary plan description might govern, particularly if the participant or beneficiary is able to demonstrate reliance on the faulty summary plan description.[11]

Government Reporting Requirements

The plan administrator of an ERISA welfare benefit plan (including plans that provide benefits pursuant to a managed care contract) must file a variety of documents with either the Department of Labor or the Internal Revenue Service. Each year, the plan administrator must file an annual return unless the plan is exempt from filing.[12] Generally, an annual return (filed on Form 5500) is required for plans that have more than 100 participants as of the first day of the plan year. Plans with fewer than 100 participants as of the first day of the plan year generally are exempt from filing if benefits are provided through insurance contracts, the premiums for which are paid from the plan sponsor's general corporate assets, directly by the plan sponsor out of general corporate assets, or a combination of the two.[13] Plans in which benefits or insurance premiums are payable through a trust, and certain plans that receive employee contributions, do not qualify for the exception, and an annual return is required to be filed even though the plans might have fewer than 100 participants.[14]

Some health plans are operated in conjunction with a "flexible spending arrangement" or "cafeteria plan" under Section 125 of the Internal Revenue Code. A simple example would be a health plan in which the employer requires its employees to pay a portion of the premium. The employer then establishes a plan under Section 125 that enables a plan participant to make so-called salary reduction contributions; that is, the participant reduces his or her salary in exchange for the employer's payment of the employee premium contribution. Even if the arrangement covers fewer than 100 participants, an annual report is required with respect to the Section 125 arrangement.[15]

The annual return is due on or before the last day of the seventh month after the close of the plan year, although certain extensions are possible.[16] The return is filed with the Internal Revenue Service and is provided by the Service to the Department of Labor. The annual return is not distributed to plan participants as a general matter, although a plan participant must be allowed to review and make copies of the annual return.[17]

PLAN DESIGN CONSIDERATIONS

Substantive Regulation under ERISA

ERISA provides relatively little regulation of the content of employee welfare benefit plans (a category that includes health benefit plans), although recent ERISA amendments have begun to regulate the content of employee welfare benefit plans more extensively. In contrast to the regulation of pension plans, in which ERISA provides detailed and generally comprehensive requirements, ERISA regulation of employer-sponsored health plans has been piecemeal and is limited to the following:

- An employer-sponsored health plan is required to comply with the terms of a qualified medical child support order. A quali-

fied medical child support order is a court order or court-approved property settlement agreement that is entered pursuant to state domestic relations law or certain state Medicaid laws and that provides for health insurance coverage for a child of an employee.[18]
- A group health plan, if it otherwise provides coverage for dependent natural children, is required to provide identical coverage for children who are placed for adoption with the covered employee.[19]
- A group health plan may not reduce its coverage of pediatric vaccines below the level of coverage that it provided as of May 1, 1993.[20]
- A plan of an employer with 20 or more employees is required to provide employees and their covered dependents whose coverage under the plan would otherwise cease as a result of termination of employment or certain other "qualifying events" the opportunity to purchase continued coverage under the plan for a limited period of time.[21] (State law insurance continuation rules may also apply.)
- A group health plan generally may exclude coverage for preexisting conditions only for those conditions that were diagnosed or for which the participant received treatment within 6 months before enrollment, and the exclusion generally cannot extend for more than 12 months after enrollment. Further, a group health plan generally must credit periods of prior coverage toward the 12-month exclusion period unless there exists a 63-day or greater gap between the prior coverage and the participant's coverage under the group health plan.[22]
- A group health plan may not establish eligibility rules that are based on an individual's health status, medical condition, claims experience, medical history, genetic information, evidence of insurability and/or disability.[23]
- A group health plan that is a multi-employer plan or a multiple employer welfare arrangement may not, with certain exceptions, deny an employer who participates in the plan and

whose employees are covered under the plan, continued access to the plan.[24]

- A group health plan may not, with certain exceptions, restrict hospitalization benefits for the delivering mother or newborn child to less than 48 hours for normal vaginal deliveries or 96 hours after a Caesarean section.[25]
- A group health plan with 50 or more employees generally may not place lower annual and/or aggregate dollar limits on mental health care benefits compared with limits placed on medical and surgical benefits.[26]
- A group health plan that provides medical and surgical benefits for mastectomies must also provide benefits for breast reconstruction, prostheses, and all physical complications related to a mastectomy.[27]

Despite the limited regulation of the content of employee welfare benefit plans, ERISA's impact is considerable.

ERISA Preemption of State Insurance Laws Affecting Plan Design

Generally

As is explained in more detail in the section of this chapter devoted to ERISA preemption, ERISA broadly preempts all state law (and state law causes of action) that relate to ERISA plans.[28] Although limited exceptions exist for state laws that regulate insurance, banking, or securities, as well as for certain generally applicable laws, ERISA's preemptive scope provides plan sponsors with great flexibility with respect to the design of their benefit programs because ERISA generally will preempt state law attempts to regulate the terms and conditions of ERISA plans.

Distinction between Insured and Self-Insured Plans

The exception for state laws that regulate the "business of insurance" creates an interesting distinction between health benefit plans that purchase insurance and those for which the plan sponsor self-insures (or self-funds) the benefits.

So-called mandated benefits laws—that is, state laws that mandate that health insurance contracts subject to the state's jurisdiction provide coverage or benefits for certain conditions or illnesses—constitute laws that regulate the business of insurance and are saved from preemption.[29] A self-insured (or self-funded) plan does not purchase insurance, however, and a provision of ERISA known as the "deemer clause" prevents a state from directly applying its insurance regulation to the employee benefit plan.[30] The result is a significant distinction between insured and self-insured plans. Although a state may not directly regulate an employee benefit plan, the state may indirectly regulate the content of an insured plan by regulating the terms and conditions of the insurance contract that the plan purchases. A state may not, however, directly or indirectly regulate the terms and conditions of a self-insured plan.

When Is a Plan Self-Insured?

Historically, most managed care programs were insured arrangements, although today a growing number of plan sponsors have adopted self-insured arrangements that incorporate a preferred provider organization (PPO), point-of-service product, or other feature generally associated within the rubric of managed care. Because of the significance of the distinction between insured and self-insured plans, courts and state regulators have been called on to determine whether certain plans are insured or self-insured.

This issue typically arises when the plan claims to be self-insured, but the plan or the plan sponsor then purchases stop-loss or excess loss insurance to protect the plan or plan sponsor from large losses. Stop-loss or excess loss insurance provides reimbursement to the plan or plan sponsor in the event that benefits paid by the plan to or on behalf of a plan participant or all plan participants as a group exceed thresholds established in the insurance policy. Stop-loss coverage is written with either or both a specific or individual attachment point and an aggregate attachment point. Above the specific or individual attachment point, the plan or plan sponsor is entitled to reimbursement for claims paid during the policy year with respect to a single plan participant. Above the aggregate attachment point, the plan or the plan sponsor is entitled to reimbursement for claims paid during the policy year with respect to all plan participants.

Plans that purchase stop-loss or excess loss insurance coverage generally have been considered self-insured for the purposes of the preemption rules described previously, so that a state is not allowed to regulate the plan indirectly through application of its mandated benefit or other health insurance laws to the terms and conditions of the insurance contract.[31] Rather, the stop-loss or excess loss contract typically is viewed as property and casualty insurance that is subject to the state's rules and regulations for such insurance. This characterization is subject to two caveats. First, the plan participant should have no rights to claim benefits directly against the stop-loss or excess loss insurer. Stop-loss or excess loss insurance is intended to provide reimbursement to the plan or the plan sponsor for losses incurred beyond certain thresholds. If the plan participant has a direct claim against the insurer, however, the stop-loss or excess loss contract arguably constitutes a direct health insurance contract that the state could regulate as such.

Second, the thresholds at which the insurance company reimburses the plan or the plan sponsor should be sufficient so that the plan or the plan sponsor bears substantial risk for the provision of benefits under the plan (other than the risk of the insurance carrier's bankruptcy). A number of courts have suggested that, if the thresholds are set so low that they constitute a disguised deductible, the insurance contract, even though treated by the parties as providing stop-loss or excess loss coverage, might be treated as direct health insurance.[32] Similarly, several states have promulgated regulations to the effect that stop-loss or excess loss policies with threshold points below certain amounts would be regulated as direct health insurance contracts, allowing the state to assert the applicability of its mandated benefit laws to the contract.[33] In 1995, the National Association of Insurance Commissioners adopted a Stop-Loss Insurance Model Act, under which a self-insured plan would be treated as

having purchased health insurance, which would be subject to all state insurance mandates, if the specific attachment point is less than $20,000. Similar rules would apply with respect to the aggregate attachment point. For groups of 50 or more, the plan will be treated as fully insured if the aggregate attachment point is less than 110 percent of expected claims. For groups of 50 or less, the aggregate attachment point must be at least equal to the greater of $4,000 times the number of employees, 120 percent of expected claims, or $20,000.[34] However, at least one court has held that ERISA preempts application of a state regulation to the effect that stock-loss insurance with an attachment point below a prescribed minimum would be treated as health insurance.[35]

Limits on ERISA Preemption

ERISA's preemptive reach is extremely broad, although not all encompassing. For example, a New York law that imposed surcharges on hospital bills was not preempted by ERISA.[36] Although the surcharges undoubtedly had an impact on a self-insured plan by increasing the cost of the benefits provided by the plan, the New York surcharge system did not relate to ERISA plans and therefore was not preempted. Although this type of indirect impact law may survive preemption, a state law that attempts to regulate the benefits provided by the plan will be preempted unless saved, in the case of an insured plan, as a law regulating the business of insurance. Thus, plan sponsors have significant flexibility with respect to the design of health benefit plans.

Other Federal Laws Affecting Plan Design

Although ERISA grants plan sponsors considerable flexibility with respect to the design of their health care plans, other federal laws may restrict a plan sponsor's discretion to some extent. For example, a plan may not discriminate on the basis of age or other protected classification.[37] Moreover, a plan may not discriminate on the basis of disability in a manner that violates the Americans with Disabilities Act (ADA).[38]

The ADA contains several rules that, apparently, were designed to protect employee benefit plans. For example, the ADA does not prohibit an insurer, health maintenance organization (HMO), hospital, or medical service company from underwriting risks, classifying risks, or administering risks in a manner that is not based on or not inconsistent with state law.[39] Similarly, the ADA does not prohibit a person or organization from establishing, sponsoring, observing, or administering the terms of a bona fide benefit plan that is not subject to state laws that regulate insurance (i.e., a self-insured plan).[40] In all cases, however, the protection provided under these provisions of the ADA is not available if the practice or plan provision is used as a subterfuge to evade the purposes of the ADA.[41]

The degree to which the ADA regulates employer-sponsored health plans is as yet uncertain. The Equal Employment Opportunity Commission has indicated that the ADA does not prohibit broad limitations on the nature and scope of services covered under the plan, such as a general exclusion on preexisting conditions or a separate annual or lifetime maximum on the amount of benefits payable for nervous and mental disorders.[42] (Although not prescribed by the ADA, a separate annual or lifetime maximum on the amount of benefits payable for nervous and mental disorders generally would violate ERISA.)[43] These broad limitations generally affect plan participants whether the plan participant is disabled or not within the meaning of the ADA. Where a plan excludes or provides limited coverage for a specific disabling condition or illness (such as human immunodeficiency virus infection), however, the Equal Employment Opportunity Commission takes the position that the provision violates the ADA.[44]

Case law on this subject overturns provisions in employer-sponsored group health plans that discriminate on the basis of disability. For example, in *Henderson v. Bodine Aluminum, Inc.*, the U.S. Court of Appeals for the Eighth Circuit issued an injunction preventing the defendant company from denying coverage for expenses incurred by a cancer patient in connection with high-dose chemotherapy treatments.[45] The health plan in question excluded coverage of high-dose chemotherapy for certain types of

cancer, an exclusion that the Eighth Circuit Court concluded might violate the ADA. Other cases, however, have determined that the ADA does not necessarily require that the benefits provided by a plan with respect to a particular disability be equivalent to the benefits provided with respect to another disability.[46]

AMENDMENT OF PLANS

Generally

ERISA requires that every employee benefit plan provide a procedure for amending the plan and for identifying the persons who have authority to amend the plan.[47] Generally, a plan sponsor reserves to itself the power and authority to amend (or even terminate) a plan. The employer's reserved amendment authority and the process by which the employer exercises that authority has been the subject of considerable debate.

Benefit Reductions

Many employers provide health plan coverage to former employees who retired after attaining a certain age and after completing a minimum period of service specified in the plan (e.g., age 55 and 10 years of service). Traditionally, the employer had few retirees relative to active employees, and health care costs were reasonable. As health care costs escalated, however, and as the employer's population shifted to include a greater number of retirees relative to active employees, employers began to modify (and in some cases terminate) the coverage provided to retirees.

Predictably, retirees whose coverage was modified or eliminated challenged many of the benefit cutbacks. Although early cases were far from uniform—some favoring the employer, some applying a refutable presumption in favor of the retiree—more recent cases, although still not entirely uniform, have become more homogenous in their approach. In particular, the cases have rejected a per se rule and have instead viewed the issue as a question of plan interpretation. Where the employer (plan sponsor) has reserved to itself the authority to amend, modify, or terminate the plan, the employer's exercise of that right has been upheld.[48] Where the employer has not reserved to itself the authority to amend, modify, or terminate the plan, however, or if the plan language is ambiguous, the courts will seek to ascertain the parties' intent when creating the plan (i.e., did the employer or, in the case of a collectively bargained arrangement, the parties to the contract intend to create vested benefit rights that cannot thereafter be modified by the employer?).[49] The starting point, however, is the plan language concerning the employer's right to amend the plan.

A developing theme in the case law is that, even where the plan documents reserve to the employer the right to amend, modify, or terminate the plan, the employer might be estopped from implementing the change as a result of prior assurances provided to plan participants. For example, in a case involving Unisys Corporation retirees, the U.S. Court of Appeals for the Third Circuit permitted a retiree challenge to proceed based on a breach of fiduciary duty theory despite the fact that the plan document had at all times reserved to the employer the right to amend, modify, or terminate benefits.[50] The retirees alleged that plan fiduciaries had violated their fiduciary duties by consistently misrepresenting to plan participants over a period of years that retiree benefits were lifetime benefits.

Amendment Procedure

Even where a plan document reserves to the employer the right to amend the plan, employees and retirees have challenged the process by which amendments have been adopted. In *Schoonejongen v. Curtiss-Wright Corp.*, the employer terminated a retiree health insurance program.[51] The plan reserved to the employer the right to amend or terminate the plan but did not specify the process by which amendments could be adopted or the persons or person with the authority to amend the plan. The U.S. Court of Appeals for the Third Circuit held that the plan amendment procedure, and thus the amendment terminating the plan, was invalid under ERISA.

The Third Circuit position was short-lived. The U.S. Supreme Court reversed, holding that the plan amendment procedure was valid even though it did not specifically identify the person or persons with the authority to amend the plan.[52] Also, the U.S. Court of Appeals for the Seventh Circuit refused to set aside an amendment terminating a retiree welfare plan even though the plan did not contain an adequate amendment procedure under ERISA.[53] It would thus appear that the courts will not easily set aside plan changes communicated by the employer to plan participants. Nevertheless, a plan sponsor would be well advised to avoid the issue altogether by specifying the amendment procedure in the plan document and, having done so, following that procedure.

FIDUCIARY DUTIES

ERISA imposes special duties on plan fiduciaries. ERISA's definition of *fiduciary* is functional, that is, a person, regardless of formal title or position, is a fiduciary to the extent that he or she exercises discretionary authority and control over the operation or administration of the plan, exercises any control over plan assets, or renders investment advice for a fee.[54]

ERISA prescribes the minimum standard of conduct applicable to fiduciaries, the so-called fiduciary duties. A fiduciary with respect to a plan must discharge his or her obligations with respect to a plan solely in the interests of the plan participants and beneficiaries and for the exclusive purpose of providing benefits to plan participants and their beneficiaries and defraying reasonable expenses of administering the plan.[55] Furthermore, the fiduciary must act in accordance with the plan documents (except to the extent that the documents are themselves inconsistent with ERISA) and with the care, skill, and diligence that a prudent person familiar with such matters would use in a similar enterprise.[56] Finally, if the plan is funded, plan investment must be diversified to minimize the risk of large losses.[57]

Often, a plan fiduciary is also an officer of the sponsoring employer, raising the question of when such a person is wearing his or her "fiduciary hat," and thus is required to act in the sole interest of plan participants and their beneficiaries, and when the fiduciary is wearing his or her "corporate hat," and thus is able to act in the best interests of the plan sponsor. Although the distinction is not always clear, the authority to amend or even terminate the plan is a "settlor function," that is, an employer is not acting in a fiduciary capacity when deciding to amend or terminate a plan.[58] Thus, an employer might prospectively amend its group health plan to eliminate certain coverages (assuming that such elimination does not violate the ADA), and this action, although detrimental to plan participants, does not implicate the fiduciary's obligations under ERISA. Similarly, the decision to terminate a plan is a "settlor" or business decision of the plan sponsor. Although certain aspects of the termination process might constitute fiduciary functions, the decision to terminate does not.

The distinction between fiduciary functions and nonfiduciary settlor functions has blurred to some extent. Although the decision to amend a plan is a settlor function, the Supreme Court has indicated that providing information about likely future plan benefits falls within ERISA's definition of a fiduciary act.[59] Moreover, a number of courts have held that plan fiduciaries have an obligation to disclose information about proposed plan amendments as soon as the proposal is under "serious consideration."[60] Generally, these courts have determined that "serious consideration" does not exist until (1) a specific proposal (2) is being discussed for the purpose of implementation (3) by management with the authority to implement the change.[61]

Other cases have viewed the "serious consideration" test as part of a broader question of whether the plan fiduciary is in receipt of material information and whether the fiduciary's duty of loyalty to plan participants and beneficiaries requires that material information relevant to a plan participant or beneficiary be disclosed.[62] Some cases have held that a plan fiduciary has an affirmative duty to disclose information,[63] whereas others have determined that the fiduciary's obligation is triggered only if the participant or beneficiary has asked.[64] Thus, certain functions that traditionally have been viewed as nonfiduciary settlor functions have been redefined, at least in part, to include a fiduciary component.

To date, cases addressing the "serious consideration" or "material information" doctrines have arisen in the context of amendments to pension programs that provide enhanced benefits to employees who retire during a prescribed window. The theory, however, is potentially applicable to proposed changes in welfare benefit plans as well.

In addition to ERISA's general fiduciary responsibility rules, ERISA also prohibits a plan fiduciary from engaging in a number of transactions known as prohibited transactions.[65] There are two sets of prohibited transactions. The first set prohibits a plan fiduciary from causing a plan to engage in certain transactions (such as sale or lease of property or extension of credit) between a plan and a party in interest. A party in interest includes a fiduciary with respect to the plan, persons who perform services for a plan, and other persons or entities related to such fiduciaries or service providers.[66] Unless advance approval is obtained from the Department of Labor, this type of related party transaction is prohibited without regard to the economic benefits of the transaction to the plan.

A second branch of the prohibited transaction rules proscribes a fiduciary from acting in certain conflict of interest situations or from receiving compensation from a third party in connection with a transaction involving the assets of the plan. For example, a fiduciary with respect to the plan may not cause the plan to retain the fiduciary (or a related party) to perform additional services for a fee. Where a fiduciary uses the authority, discretion, and control that makes him or her a fiduciary to cause the plan to pay an additional fee to the fiduciary, the fiduciary has engaged in a prohibited act of self-dealing.[67]

CHALLENGES TO BENEFIT DENIALS

Claims Procedure

Every employee benefit plan under ERISA is required to establish a procedure whereby a plan participant or beneficiary may challenge a denial of his or her claim for benefits.[68] A claims procedure will be deemed reasonable if a plan participant's or beneficiary's claim is answered in writing, with explanation of the reasons for the decision and references to pertinent plan provisions, within 90 days. If the claim is denied and the plan participant or beneficiary wishes to pursue the matter further, an appeal may be filed with the appropriate fiduciary designated by the plan. The appeal must be answered in writing, again with explanation of the reasons for the decision and references to pertinent plan provisions within 60 days after the date on which the appeal is filed. In certain cases, the 90-day and 60-day periods can be extended if the plan participant or beneficiary is notified of the need for additional time before expiration of the initial period.[69]

The Department of Labor has proposed (but not yet implemented) new requirements for benefit claims procedures that, if finalized in their present form, will dramatically alter the claim review and appeal process for group health plans.[70] The regulations will impose new notice and disclosure requirements, as well as new standards of review of benefit claims and the appeal of denied claims.

New Time Frames for Decision Making

Benefit claims involving group health plans would be governed by new, shorter time frames that in the view of the Department of Labor are more appropriate to health care decisions. In particular, initial decisions on nonurgent health care benefit claims must be made within a reasonable time period but not later than 15 days after filing. If a claim is incomplete, the plan administrator must inform the claimant of this fact within 5 days of receipt of the claim and allow the claimant 45 days to provide missing information. A decision with respect to the claimant's benefit application would be required within 15 days of the earlier to occur of the date on which the claimant provides the additional information or the end of 45-day submission period.

The period of time during which a plan must permit a claimant to appeal an adverse decision would be increased to 180 days. Decision on review on nonurgent claims is no later than 30 days after receipt of request for review (with special rules applicable for review committees or boards that meet on a quarterly basis).

Claims involving urgent care would be required to be resolved under an expedited time frame. Claims involving urgent care must be decided as soon as possible, but not later than 72 hours after receipt. The same time frame would apply to appeals of adverse determinations on urgent care claims.

New (or Clarified) Disclosure Requirements

A group health plan's claims procedure will be considered reasonable only if it is described in the summary plan description. Descriptions of all benefit claims procedures of the plan and the time limits applicable to the procedures must be disclosed.

Written notification of any adverse determination must include reference to plan provisions of which it is based, and notification must include a full description of the plan's review process, including a statement of claimants' rights to bring a civil action.

Claimants must be able to review all relevant documents, whether or not such documents or records were actually relied on in making determination, including all documents and reports created or received during the review process (e.g., expert identities and/or reports).

New Standards of Review

A claimant must be provided the opportunity for a full and fair review (appeal) of denied claims. Full and fair review must include a review of the adverse determination by an appropriate named fiduciary who was not involved in the initial determination and who is not a subordinate of someone involved in the initial determination. No deference is to be given to the initial determination as part of the review process, and the review is to take into account all comments, documents, and records. Any appeal of a claim involving urgent care must be conducted on an expedited basis. Appeals of adverse determinations on urgent care claims must be decided and communicated to the claimant as soon as possible but not later than 72 hours after receipt of request for review.

The review of any determination that is based on medical judgment must be conducted in consultation with a health care professional who is independent of the health care professional involved in the initial determination.

Standard of Review in Court Action

If the plan participant is not satisfied with the disposition of his or her claim at the plan level, he or she can file suit in state or federal court. An important threshold question involves the standard of review that the court will apply in reviewing the plan administrator's denial of the plan participant's claim.

In *Firestone Tire & Rubber Co. v. Bruch*, the U.S. Supreme Court determined that, in accordance with established principles of trust law, a plan participant's or beneficiary's challenge to a denial of benefits is to be reviewed under a de novo standard—that is, the court independently reviews and weighs the evidence and makes its decision accordingly, without deference to the decision made by the plan administrator—unless the plan document grants to the plan administrator or other appropriate fiduciary the discretionary authority and control to determine eligibility for benefits or to construe the terms of the plan.[71] Where the plan grants the administrator such discretionary authority and control, the court is to review the benefit denial under the more deferential arbitrary and capricious standard of review. Under this standard, the court reviews the evidence but overturns the plan administrator's decision only if it represents a clearly unreasonable interpretation or construction of the plan.

The Supreme Court's decision, although based on principles of trust law, is a puzzlement to many. Although the general rule is de novo review, the Supreme Court's decision creates an exception that potentially eliminates the general rule. By including appropriate language in the plan document, a plan sponsor changes the standard of review that a court will apply in the event that a plan participant challenges a benefit denial. More generally, why should a plan sponsor be allowed to select the standard of review through its decision to include or not include certain language in the plan document?

In the years after the Supreme Court's *Bruch* decision, the lower federal courts have struggled with the implications of the decision, often with potentially conflicting results. In a number of decisions, plan language was determined to be sufficient to support the more deferential arbitrary and capricious standard of review. For example, in *Kennedy v. Georgia-Pacific Corp.,* plan language to the effect that the plan administrator "shall be solely responsible for the administration and interpretation" of the plan was found to be sufficient.[72] In other cases, courts have applied the de novo standard even though the document contained evidence that the plan administrator (or other fiduciary) was intended to have considerable authority and control with respect to the plan. For example, in *Michael Reese Hospital & Medical Center v. Solo Cup Employee Health Benefit Plan*, even though the plan document gave the administrator "the authority to control and manage the operation and administration of the plan," it was held that the plan demonstrated insufficient intent to grant to the administrator discretionary authority to determine eligibility or to construe the terms of the plan.[73]

In other cases, particularly those involving self-funded arrangements for which benefits are payable from the plan sponsor's general corporate assets, courts have focused on the conflict of interest under which a plan fiduciary may operate because a denial of benefits is directly beneficial to the plan sponsor's treasury. In some conflict of interest cases, courts have applied a less deferential standard of review than the arbitrary and capricious standard that would normally be applicable.[74] In other cases, the courts have continued to apply the arbitrary and capricious standard but have indicated that the fiduciary's conflict of interest is a factor to be taken into account in determining whether the fiduciary's actions were arbitrary and capricious.[75] By whichever route, the courts are cognizant of and treat a fiduciary's conflict of interest as a relevant consideration.

Right to Jury Trial

Most courts have held that ERISA does not provide a right to a jury trial, reasoning that benefit claims under ERISA are equitable in nature.[76] The decisions are not uniform, however, and a minority of courts have found a right to jury trial on the basis that certain claims have both legal and equitable components.[77]

ERISA'S CIVIL ENFORCEMENT SCHEME AND REMEDIES

In addition to suits for benefits brought by a plan participant or beneficiary, ERISA authorizes a plan participant, beneficiary, fiduciary, or the secretary of the Department of Labor to bring a variety of civil actions. Among the more important suits are those that involve the right of a plan participant, beneficiary, fiduciary, or the secretary to bring an action for breach of fiduciary duty under Section 502(a)(2) of ERISA.[78] Also, a plan participant, beneficiary, or fiduciary may bring an action under Section 502(a)(3) of ERISA to enjoin any act or practice that violates (or to enforce the provisions of) Title I of ERISA or the terms of the plan or to obtain other appropriate equitable relief.[79]

Although ERISA authorizes a variety of civil actions, the remedies that are available to a successful plaintiff have been quite limited. An action for breach of fiduciary duty under Section 502(a)(2) of ERISA is an action brought on behalf of the plan and all recovery runs in favor of the plan. Accordingly, the U.S. Supreme Court in *Massachusetts Mutual Life Insurance Co. v. Russell* held that a plan participant or beneficiary could not recover extracontractual or punitive damages.[80] Later, the Supreme Court in *Mertens v. Hewitt Associates* held that Section 502(a)(3) authorized only traditional forms of equitable relief, not monetary damages.[81]

The Supreme Court's restrictive interpretation of Sections 502(a)(2) and 502(a)(3) takes on added significance in light of ERISA's preemption of state laws and state law causes of action that relate to ERISA-governed employee benefit plans. Because of ERISA's preemptive reach, plaintiffs may not forgo ERISA's civil enforcement scheme in favor of state law remedies, which might, if not preempted, include punitive or extracontractual damages.[82]

After the Supreme Court's holding in *Russell* and *Mertens*, the courts have struggled to attempt to provide meaningful remedies to plan participants and beneficiaries in actions brought under Section 502(a)(3) of ERISA. For example, in *Watkins v. Westinghouse Hanford Co.*, the U.S. Court of Appeals for the Ninth Circuit ruled that a plan participant could not recover under Section 502(a)(3) benefits allegedly due the plan participant as a result of a misrepresentation.[83] More recently, however, a number of decisions have embraced the possibility of monetary relief in connection with equitable claims of reinstatement or restitution. The Supreme Court, in *Varity Corp. v. Howe*, approved reinstatement of participant benefits after a fiduciary's breach of duty.[84] Further, Seventh Circuit, in a case denying the plaintiffs' claim, nevertheless determined that not all monetary relief is damages, thus suggesting that the remedies available under Section 502(a)(3) may not be as narrow as once thought. According to the Seventh Circuit, "[e]quity sometimes awards monetary damages or the equivalent and restitution is both a legal and equitable remedy that is monetary yet is distinct from damages."[85]

ERISA PREEMPTION

Arguably, no provision of ERISA has more of an effect on the operations of MCOs than ERISA's preemption clause. This section explains the general principles of preemption and discusses the impact of preemption on the following activities of MCOs: the provision of health care services, either directly or by contract; utilization review determinations; the establishment of provider networks; representations of eligibility and coverage to health care providers; and the provision of administrative and other noninsurance services to ERISA plans.

General Principles of Preemption

When Congress enacted ERISA, it intended to make the regulation of employee benefit plans an exclusively federal concern. Congress, however, also did not want to divest the states of their traditional power to regulate insurance. Pursuant to this scheme, Congress enacted three clauses relating to the preemptive effect of ERISA:

- *The preemption clause:* This clause provides that ERISA supersedes any and all state laws insofar as they may relate to any employee benefit plan subject to ERISA, except to the extent that such laws may be "saved" from preemption by the savings clause.[86]
- *The savings clause:* This clause preserves from preemption any law of any state that regulates insurance, banking, or securities except as provided in the deemer clause.[87]
- *The deemer clause:* This clause provides that an employee benefit plan shall not be deemed to be an insurance company or other insurer, bank, trust company, or investment company or to be engaged in the business of insurance or banking for the purposes of any law of any state purporting to regulate insurance companies, insurance contracts, banks, trust companies, or investment companies.[88]

The Preemption Clause

As noted previously, Section 514(a) of ERISA preempts "any and all State laws insofar as they may now or hereafter relate to any employee benefit plan." A law relates to an employee benefit plan if it has "a connection with or reference to such a plan."[89] In application, the preemption clause has been "conspicuous for its breadth," preempting not only state laws that are specifically designed to affect employee benefit plans but also those that may only indirectly affect such plans.[90,91] Those state laws that courts have found not to be preempted under Section 514(a) were generally limited to laws of general applicability that only tangentially affected ERISA plans.[92]

In recent years, however, the U.S. Supreme Court narrowed the preemptive force of Section 514(a) in a trio of cases: *New York State Conference of Blue Cross & Blue Shield Plans v. Travelers Insurance Co* ("*Travelers*"), followed by *De Buono v. NYSA-ILA Medical and Clinical Services* ("*De Buono*") and *California Division of Labor Enforcement v. Dillingham Construction N.A., Inc.* ("*Dillingham*").[93] In *Travelers*, the Supreme Court refused to preempt a New York state statute requiring surcharges on hospital bills of patients covered by commercial carriers and on HMOs on the basis of the number of Medicaid enrollees, warning against using an "uncritical literalism" when deciding the reach of ERISA preemption and stressing that preemption under ERISA was to be determined with reference to ERISA's statutory objectives.[94] The *Travelers* decision identified three categories of state laws that Congress intended to preempt: state laws that mandated employee benefit structures or their administration; state laws that provided alternative enforcement mechanisms; and state laws that bound plan administrators to a particular choice.[95] The Supreme Court in *De Buono* declined to preempt a New York state tax on the gross receipts of health care facilities operated by a trust fund established to administer an ERISA plan, emphasizing that health and safety matters were within the historic police powers of the states and that ERISA's "relate to" language was not intended to modify the starting presumption that Congress did not intend to supplant state law that fell within areas of traditional state regulation.[96] Finally, in *Dillingham,* the Supreme Court, refusing to preempt California's prevailing wage law, found that preemption would have been warranted only if the state law acted "immediately and exclusively upon ERISA plans...or where the existence of ERISA plans is essential to the law's operation."[97] Following the lead of *Travelers, De Buono,* and *Dillingham*, lower courts have begun to whittle away at the broad parameters of ERISA preemption.

The Savings Clause

A state law that relates to an ERISA plan may be saved from preemption if it falls within Section 514(b)(2)(A), which excepts from preemption those state laws that regulate the "business of insurance." In *Pilot Life Insurance Co. v. Dedeaux*, the U.S. Supreme Court used a two-part analysis to determine whether a state law regulates the business of insurance.[98,99] First, the Supreme Court took a commonsense approach, determining that, to regulate insurance, a law must be specifically directed toward the insurance industry. Second, the Supreme Court applied the three-part test for determining whether a practice constituted the business of insurance formulated for the McCarran-Ferguson Act, namely, whether the practice had the effect of transferring or spreading a policyholder's risk, whether the practice was an integral part of the policy relationship between the insured and the insurer, and whether the practice was limited to entities within the insurance industry.[100] However, in *UNUM Life Insurance Co. v. Ward,* the Supreme Court noted that a state law need not satisfy all three factors of the McCarran-Ferguson Act to be saved from preemption.[101]

The Deemer Clause

The deemer clause exempts from any direct or indirect state regulation self-funded employee benefit plans.[102] All power to regulate insurance reserved to the states under the savings clause is taken away with respect to self-insured plans under the deemer clause. The language of the deemer clause, according to the U.S. Supreme Court, is either coextensive with or broader, not narrower, than that of the savings clause.[103] Thus state laws that relate to employee benefit plans but that are saved from preemption under Section 514(b)(2)(A) are still preempted as applied to self-funded ERISA plans. Although, as discussed earlier in regard to the benefit design of ERISA plans, this interpretation establishes a disparity between the regulation of insured and uninsured plans, the Supreme Court has determined that such a dichotomy was the intent of Congress when it enacted the statute.[104]

Vicarious Liability for Medical Malpractice

Of the various tort theories used to impose liability on MCOs for the medical malpractice of health care providers to whom they refer patients, none has generated more recent litigation than that of vicarious liability for medical malpractice based on the theories of implied agency and/or apparent or ostensible agency (see also Chapter 64). Although the elements of apparent or ostensible agency vary from jurisdiction to jurisdiction, a common allegation is that the patient reasonably relied on actions or representations of the MCO, which "held out" the negligent provider as its employee or agent, the degree of reliance required of the patient being subject to judicial debate.[105] The cardinal consideration for determining the existence of implied authority is whether a party asserted sufficient control over the alleged agent so as to negate the alleged agent's status as an independent contractor.[106]

ERISA preemption has played a crucial role in determining whether an MCO will be vicariously liable for the malpractice of health care providers. In the past, however, courts have been sharply divided as to whether ERISA preempts such claims.

Courts holding that medical malpractice claims against MCOs were not preempted have found that such claims did not sufficiently relate to the employee plan to warrant preemption.[107] Such courts pointed out that such claims did not involve the administration of benefits or the level or quality of benefits provided under plan; they merely alleged negligence by a physician and an agency relationship between the physician and the MCO. Courts reaching the opposite conclusion have reasoned that a vicarious liability malpractice claim concerned the delivery of benefits under the ERISA plan and that the claim required the examination of the terms of the ERISA plan to determine the quality and quantity of services required of physicians and the relationship between the ERISA plan and the physicians.[108]

Although, historically, the lower courts were almost evenly split as to whether ERISA preempted medical malpractice claims against MCOs on the basis of vicarious liability theories, two federal Circuit Court decisions and a recent federal District Court case demonstrate the current judicial trend against preemption.

The U.S. Court of Appeals for the Tenth Circuit in the case of *Pacificare of Oklahoma, Inc. v. Burrage* identified four categories of laws that "related to" an employee benefit plan: laws that regulated the type of benefits or terms of ERISA plans; laws that created reporting, disclosure, funding, or vesting requirements for ERISA plans; laws that provided rules for the calculation of the amount of benefits to be paid under ERISA plans; and laws and common law rules that provided remedies for misconduct growing out of the administration of ERISA plans.[109] The Tenth Circuit held that a claim that an HMO was vicariously liable for the malpractice of one of its primary care physicians did not involve the administration of benefits or the level or quality of benefits promised by the plan; it merely alleged negligent care by the physician and an agency relationship between the physician and the HMO. The court pointed out that ERISA would not preempt the malpractice claim against the physician and concluded that ERISA should similarly not preempt the vicarious liability claim against the HMO if the HMO held the physician out as its agent. Reference to the ERISA plan to resolve the agency issue did not "implicate the concerns of ERISA preemption."[110] A number of courts have turned to the reasoning of *Burrage* in holding that ERISA does not preempt vicarious liability claims.[111]

In *Dukes v. U.S. Healthcare, Inc.*, the U.S. Court of Appeals for the Third Circuit addressed the issue of whether vicarious liability malpractice claims against the defendant HMO could be removed from the state court to federal court.[112] The lower federal courts had allowed such a removal and then had dismissed the claims, holding that they were preempted by ERISA. The Third Circuit reversed, noting that not all claims preempted by ERISA were subject to removal. The court held that removal was improper where plaintiffs were merely attacking the quality of the benefits received and were not claiming that the ERISA plans had erroneously withheld benefits that were due or were not seeking to enforce rights under the terms of their respective plans or to clarify rights to future benefits. The court expressly distinguished the situation where the HMO denied benefits in its utilization review role.[113,114]

It should be noted that the Third Circuit's decision in *Dukes* was limited to the issue of whether a defendant MCO could remove a medical malpractice claim from state court to federal court.[115] However, that court's discussion of the distinction between the quantity of benefits due under an ERISA plan and the quality of the benefits provided under such plan has been cited by other courts as authority for a refusal to preempt malpractice claims challenging the quality of services provided to plan participants and beneficiaries.[116]

One such court was the U.S. District Court for the Southern District of Texas. In the recent case of *Corporate Health Insurance, Inc. v. Texas Department of Insurance,* the court considered whether various provisions of the Texas Health Care Liability Act were preempted by ERISA.[117] At issue were provisions (1) making health insurers, HMOs, and other managed care entities[118] liable for failure to exercise ordinary care when making medical treatment decisions ("the managed care liability provisions"), (2) establishing an independent review process for adverse benefit determinations ("the independent review provisions"), and (3) prohibiting managed care entities from removing providers from their plans for advocating appropriate and medically necessary care on behalf of enrollees, and from including in provider contracts indemnification and hold harmless clauses for the acts or conduct of the managed care entity ("the provider contracting provisions"). The court held that the independent review and provider contracting provisions were preempted, but the managed care liability provisions were not.

After an extensive overview of the case law regarding ERISA preemption, the *Corporate Health Insurance* court held that the managed care liability provisions did not "relate to" ERISA plans, and so were not preempted because such provisions neither make "reference to" nor had "a connection with" ERISA plans. Citing the U.S. Supreme Court decisions in the *Travelers*[119] and *Dillingham*[120] cases, the court found that the managed care liability provisions did not "make reference" to ERISA plans because they did not act immediately and exclusively on ERISA plans, and the existence of ERISA plans was not essential to their operations.[121] Relying on the *Burrage* and *Dukes* decisions, the court held that the managed care liability provisions did not have "a connection with" an ERISA plan because such provisions addressed the quality of the benefit provided by the managed care entity in its role "as an arranger for the actual medical treatment for plan participants," and not its utilization review role.[122]

Finally, the *Corporate Health Insurance* court noted that in recent cases involving ERISA preemption, the U.S. Supreme Court had begun its analysis with a presumption against preemption where the statute law at issue addressed a historic police power of the state, such as a matter of health and safety.[123] Moreover, the Supreme Court had cautioned that some state laws had too tenuous or remote effect on ERISA plans to warrant a finding that the laws "related to" such plans, such as run-of-the-mill state law claims or even torts committed by ERISA plans, and had held that ERISA did not preempt state laws that had only an indirect economic effect on the relative costs of various health insurance packages available to ERISA plans, such as quality standards.[124] On the basis of these precedents, the court concluded that quality control of benefits, such as the health care benefits provided by managed care entities, was a field traditionally occupied by state regulation that Congress did not intend to preempt.[125]

Utilization Review Decisions

The consensus among courts once was that utilization review decisions by MCOs, even when they involved medical decisions, were an integral part of the administration of ERISA plans. Consequently, they related to such plans and were preempted by ERISA.

For example, in *Jass v. Prudential Health Plan, Inc.,* plaintiff sued her treating physician, the plan administrator of her husband's benefit plan ("PruCare"), and a nurse employee of PruCare.[126] Plaintiff alleged that her treating physician had been negligent when performing knee replacement surgery, and that the nurse employee of PruCare had negligently failed to authorize physical therapy to rehabilitate the plaintiff's knee, resulting in plaintiff's premature discharge from the hospital. The U.S. Court of Appeals for the Seventh Circuit held that ERISA preempted plaintiff's claim that PruCare was vicariously liable for the alleged negligence of both its nurse employee and the treating physician based on actual or ostensible agency theories.

The U.S. Court of Appeals for the Sixth Circuit reached a similar conclusion in the case of *Tolton v. American Biodyne, Inc.* The coadministrators of the estate of a mental patient who had committed suicide sued, among others, the patient's ERISA plan administrator, the plan's mental health utilization review company, and the psychologists performing utilization review on behalf of the utilization review company, alleging that the plan administrator wrongfully denied benefits for inpatient psychiatric care on the basis of the utilization review company's refusal to authorize such care.[127] Plaintiffs' state law claims based on such utilization review decision included wrongful death, improper refusal to authorize benefits, medical malpractice, and insurance bad faith. The court held that such claims clearly related to the ERISA plan and were preempted by ERISA.

In reaching its decision, the *Tolton* court relied on an earlier opinion of the U.S. Court of Appeals for the Fifth Circuit, *Corcoran v. United Healthcare, Inc.*[128] In *Corcoran*, the utilization review decision at issue was the refusal by the defendant utilization review company to pre-certify hospitalization for a high-risk pregnancy despite the recommendation of the patient's physician. Instead, the defendant authorized 10 hours per day of home nursing care. The patient, who had already been admitted to the hospital, returned home when she learned that the expenses for her hospitalization would not be covered. At a time when no nurse was on duty, her fetus went into distress and died. The patient and her husband then sued the defendant, alleging wrongful death and medical malpractice.

The Fifth Circuit Court in *Corcoran* acknowledged that utilization reviewers make medical decisions despite any disclaimers to the contrary in policy manuals or promotional materials. The court found, however, that the medical decisions made by the defendant were inseparable from its determinations regarding what benefits were available under the plan. The court found that the wrongful death claim related to a denial of benefits under the plan and so was preempted by ERISA. Other courts have followed the reasoning of the *Corcoran* case and have preempted claims arising out of utilization review decisions.[129]

Despite the preceding precedent, a couple of lower courts, relying on the *Travelers* decision and its progeny, have refused to preempt negligent utilization review decisions. For example, in *Pappas v. Asbel,* plaintiff, who was an insured of HMO-PA, an HMO operated by U.S. Healthcare, was admitted to an emergency department of a community hospital complaining of paralysis and numbness in his extremities.[130] The emergency department physician concluded that plaintiff's condition was a neurological emergency that required treatment at a university hospital. However, HMO-PA denied authorization for plaintiff's transfer to university hospital chosen by the emergency department physician and instead authorized transfer to another hospital. By the time plaintiff was admitted to the hospital authorized by HMO-PA, the compression of his spine by an abscess caused a permanent quadriplegia. Plaintiff and his wife filed suit against his primary care physician and the community hospital, claiming that they were negligent in causing an inordinate delay in transferring plaintiff to a facility equipped and immediately available to handle his neurological emergency. Whereupon, the community hospital filed a third party complaint against HMO-PA for its refusal to authorize the transfer of plaintiff to a hospital selected by the emergency department physician.

The Pennsylvania Supreme Court in *Pappas* rejected HMO-PA's argument that ERISA preempted the third-party claims against it, holding that negligence claims against an HMO did not "relate to" an ERISA plan and therefore were not preempted.[131] The court cited the *Travelers*

case for the proposition that "Congress did not intend to preempt state laws which govern the provisions of safe medical care" and found that "[c]laims that an HMO was negligent when it provided contractually-guaranteed medical benefits in such a dilatory fashion that the patient was injured indisputably are intertwined with the provision of safe medical care."[132] The court acknowledged that by allowing such negligence claims, "there will be a financial impact on HMOs" but concluded that that consideration was not enough to countermand the conclusion that such claims were not preempted."[133] At least one other lower court has followed the *Travelers* trend of limiting the breadth of the "relate to" language of ERISA preemption in the context of utilization review decisions.[134]

Credentialing Decisions

Like the analogous duty imposed on hospitals to exercise reasonable care in the selection and granting of privileges to its medical staff, an MCO has a duty to conduct a reasonable investigation of the qualifications and competence of the health care providers to whom they refer patients.[135,136] Courts have declined to describe what will constitute a reasonable investigation of a provider's credentials, stating that its scope will vary from case to case.[137] Recent cases have focused not on the nature or extent of the investigation of a provider's qualifications but on whether a claim that an MCO did not conduct the requisite investigation is preempted by ERISA. Most courts that have considered the issue have ruled in favor of ERISA preemption.

A representative case is *Kearney v. U.S. Healthcare, Inc.*[138] In *Kearney*, plaintiff filed wrongful death and survival claims against an HMO, alleging that decedent's primary care physician failed to diagnose properly decedent's condition or to refer decedent to a hospital for specialized treatment. Plaintiff claimed that the HMO breached its contract to provide needed specialized care by limiting or discouraging the use of specialists, hospitalization, and state-of-the-art diagnostic procedures; misrepresented the primary care physician's competence and was negligent in selecting and supervising the primary care physician. Plaintiff also claimed that the HMO was vicariously liable for the malpractice of the primary care physician. The court held that a "claim that an operator or administrator of a plan failed to use due care in selecting those with whom it contracted to perform services relates to the manner in which benefits are administered or provided and is preempted."[139] The court dismissed not only plaintiff's claims of negligent selection but also the claim for misrepresentation and breach of contract. However, the court held that plaintiff's claim that the HMO was vicariously liable for the malpractice of the primary care physician on ostensible agency grounds was not preempted.

Although the list of courts in agreement with the preemption of negligent selection claims is impressive,[140] there is some authority to the contrary. For example, in *Jackson v. Roseman*, plaintiff brought a medical malpractice case against his physicians and the HMO with which they contracted.[141] Plaintiff alleged that the HMO was vicariously liable for the negligence of his physicians in allowing the growth and ultimate metastasis of a malignant cancer in his mouth. The court noted that the complaint could also be read as asserting a claim of direct negligence on the part of the HMO for negligent hiring and supervision of its contracting physicians.[142] Although the court declined to address the merits of whether a negligent hiring and/or supervision claim went to the heart of the benefit plan's administration, the court indicated that it agreed with the reasoning of the U.S. Court of Appeals for the Second Circuit in a case involving claims of negligent hiring and/or supervision of a psychologist,[143] In that case, the Second Circuit rejected defendant's argument that claims of negligent hiring and supervision of health care providers so resembled a denial of benefits or a denial of some other plan-created right as to support the removal of such claims from state court to federal court.[144]

Despite the cases to the contrary, an MCO can take some comfort from the likelihood that a court will find that claims that an MCO has negligently selected or retained a participating provider who committed malpractice are preempted. The same court, however, may not preempt a claim against the MCO on the basis of vicarious liability for the malpractice of a provider, as discussed previously.

Negligent Representations by MCOs to Providers

Whether claims by a provider that an MCO misrepresented the existence or extent of coverage is preempted by ERISA may hinge on whether the provider is suing in its own capacity or as assignee of the MCO's insured or member. A majority of courts have held that state law causes of action brought by a provider suing in its own capacity are not preempted by ERISA, even though such causes of action would be preempted if the provider were suing in a derivative capacity as assignee for the insured or member.

For example, in the influential case of *Memorial Hospital System v. Northbrook Life Insurance Company*, the plaintiff hospital had treated a patient after the hospital had called the employer of the patient's husband and verified that the patient had coverage under a group insurance policy issued and administered by defendant. [145] Subsequently, the patient and her husband assigned their benefits to the hospital. On the hospital's request for payment, however, defendant informed the hospital that the patient had not been eligible for benefits on the date of her hospitalization and denied benefits. The hospital subsequently sued, alleging that the employer acted as defendant's agent in verifying coverage and asserting state law causes of deceptive and unfair trade practices under the Texas insurance code, breach of contract, negligent misrepresentation, and equitable estoppel.

The lower court in *Memorial Hospital System* dismissed the hospital's claims for breach of contract and deceptive and unfair trade practices, finding that those claims were brought by the hospital in a derivative capacity, were related to a claim for benefits under an ERISA plan, and were consequently preempted. The lower court reached the opposite conclusion with respect to the claims of misrepresentation and estoppel, however, finding that those claims were based on the hospital's independent position as a third-party health care provider, were not related to the ERISA plan, and thus "were not caught in the broad net of ERISA preemption."[146]

The hospital appealed the dismissal of the deceptive and unfair trade practices claim, alleging that the lower court had mischaracterized it as a derivative claim for benefits. The U.S. Court of Appeals for the Fifth Circuit agreed, holding that the claim was merely a Texas codification of the common law doctrine of negligent misrepresentation. Nevertheless, the Fifth Circuit felt "compelled to enter the preemption thicket" and determine whether such cause of action was sufficiently related to the employee benefit plan at issue so as to be preempted.[147] The court ultimately held that it was not sufficiently related to be preempted. It is worthwhile to examine in some detail the court's analysis of the policy issues involved in determining whether to preempt a provider's claims on the basis of an erroneous verification of a patient's eligibility and coverage because the same reasoning has been adopted by courts in subsequent cases.

Before determining the legal issue of preemption, the Fifth Circuit found it necessary to examine the "commercial realities" of the hospital's position as a health law provider:

> The scenario depicted in Memorial's appeal is one that is reenacted each day across the county. A patient in need of medical care requests admission to a hospital (or seeks treatment from a physician). The costs of medical care are high, and many providers have only limited budget allocations for indigent care and for losses from patient nonpayment. Naturally, the provider wants to know if payment reasonably can be expected. Thus one of the first steps in accepting a patient for treatment is to determine a finan-

cial source for the cost of care to be provided.[148]

The court recognized that it was customary practice for a provider to communicate with plan agents to verify eligibility and coverage and viewed the issue of a mistaken verification of eligibility and coverage by such plan agents as solely one of allocation of risks, namely, whether the risk of nonpayment of the provider's costs "should remain with the provider or be shifted to the insurance company, which through its agents misrepresented to the provider the patient's coverage under the plan."[149] The court noted that enforcing "the allocation of risks between commercial entities that conduct business in a state is a classically important state interest."[150]

The Fifth Circuit remained unconvinced that "either the commercial scenario described above, or its state law vindication, raises any issue concerning the matters that Congress intended to be regulated exclusively by ERISA."[151] Moreover, the court was unpersuaded that "insulating plan fiduciaries from the consequences of their commercial dealings with third-party providers would further any of ERISA's goals."[152] According to the court, a one-time recovery by the hospital against the insurer or its putative agent, the employer, would not affect the ongoing administration or obligations of an ERISA plan. In addition, the court found that if providers were held to have no recourse under either ERISA or state law in situations where there was no coverage under the express terms of the plan but providers had relied on assurance that there was such coverage, providers would be understandably reluctant to accept the risk of nonpayment and might require upfront payment by beneficiaries or impose other inconveniences before treatment would be rendered: "This does not serve, but rather directly defeats, the purpose of Congress in enacting ERISA."[153]

Finally, noting that a health care provider did not have independent standing to seek redress under ERISA, the Fifth Circuit in *Memorial Hospital System* found that, although employees had received protection under ERISA in exchange for certain rights to sue under previous federal and state law, the plaintiff and "the countless other health care providers were not a party to this bargain."[154] The court stated that it could not believe that "Congress intended the preemptive scope of ERISA to shield welfare plan fiduciaries from the consequences of their acts toward non-ERISA health care providers when a cause of action based on such conduct would not relate to the terms or conditions of a welfare plan, nor affect—or affect only tangentially—the ongoing administration of the plan."[155] The court concluded that ERISA's "preemption provision designed to prevent state interference with federal control of ERISA plans does not require the creation of a fully insulated legal world that excludes these plans from regulation of any purely local transaction."[156]

The Fifth Circuit had occasion to expound on its reasoning in *Memorial Hospital System* in a subsequent case, *Cypress Fairbanks Medical Center, Inc. v. Pan-American Life Ins. Co.*[157] In *Cypress*, plaintiff was admitted to the defendant hospital after the hospital received assurances from plaintiff's insurer that he was covered under an ERISA plan and he incurred charges of $178,215.44. Ultimately, the insurer refused to pay on the ground that plaintiff's "coverage was rescinded as to the effective date."[158] The Fifth Circuit held that its decision in *Memorial Hospital System* controlled, and pointed out that prior cases where it had found ERISA preemption "had two unifying characteristics: (1) the state law claims address areas of exclusive concern, such as the right to receive benefits under the terms of an ERISA plan; and (2) the claims directly affect the relationship among the traditional ERISA entities—the employer, the plan and its fiduciaries, and the participants and beneficiaries."[159] The court noted that the claims of the hospital in the *Memorial Hospital System* case fell into neither category and therefore such hospital had asserted its state law claims as an independent, third-party provider of medical services.[160] The Fifth Circuit found that the same scenario existed in the *Cypress* case and concluded that ERISA did not preempt a provider's state law claims if such claims were "premised on a finding that the beneficiary is not covered at all by an existing ERISA plan."[161]

Other courts have adopted the reasoning of the *Memorial Hospital System* line of cases and refused to insulate ERISA plans, their sponsors, or their administrators from liability when they mistakenly verify eligibility or coverage to a health care provider.[162]

Preemption of State Insurance Regulation

State insurance laws and regulations often expressly exempt ERISA employee benefit plans from their application.[163] In the absence of such express exemption, however, it has been increasingly common for state insurance authorities to attempt to apply insurance law and regulations directly to noninsurance products of MCOs, as well as to integrated delivery systems and other entities that have contracted to provide services to ERISA plans. Whether state insurance laws and regulations are preempted by ERISA depends on a combination of the nature of the state law or regulation at issue and the nature of the services being provided to the ERISA plan.

Under the traditional preemption analysis, the first issue to be addressed is whether the state law or regulation relates to the ERISA plan. If so, the law or regulation will be preempted unless it is "saved" from preemption because it regulates the "business of insurance." The nature of the services being provided to the ERISA plan and that the state is seeking to regulate, however, must constitute the "business of insurance"; it is not sufficient that the services are being provided by an insurance company or other entity subject to insurance regulation or that the state law or regulation is part of the insurance code.

The U.S. Supreme Court has held that the underwriting or spreading of risk is an "indispensable characteristic of insurance."[164] According to the Supreme Court, the spreading of risk means that the entity engaged in the business of insurance accepts a number of risks, some of which involve losses, and spreads such losses over all the risks to enable the entity to accept each risk at a slight fraction of the possible liability upon it.[165] Courts also have held, however, that an incidental element of insurance in a contract does not bring the contract within the regulatory power of the insurance laws.[166] Because some element of risk is inherent in any business transaction, the primary effect of the contract at issue must be assumption and spreading of risk.

Administrative Services Only Contracts

In the situation where the entity contracting with the ERISA plan merely provided administrative services to such plan, courts have determined that such services did not constitute the business of insurance, and therefore ERISA preempted the application of state insurance laws and regulations to such services. For example, the U.S. Court of Appeals for the Fifth Circuit held that a party administrator of an ERISA plan was not engaged in the business of insurance when it performed no risk-bearing function.[167] Consequently, ERISA preempted a Texas statute imposing regulations, fees, and taxes to the extent that the statute applied to such third party administrator.

Similarly, the U.S. Court of Appeals for the Fourth Circuit held that, where an insurer acted as a third-party administrator, providing purely claims processing functions for an ERISA plan pursuant to an administrative services agreement with the employer, the insurer was not engaged in the business of insurance.[168] According to the court, the ERISA savings clause covered the same category of state insurance regulation as the McCarran-Ferguson Act,[169] which preserves to the states the right to regulate insurance, and the McCarran-Ferguson Act did not "purport to make the States supreme in regulating all the activities of insurance *companies*;...only when they engaged in the 'business of insurance' does the statute apply."[170]

Finally, the U.S. Court of Appeals for the Third Circuit, in the often cited case *Insurance Board of Bethlehem Steel Corp. v. Muir*, found that the Pennsylvania Blue Cross and Blue Shield (BCBS) plans were not engaged in the business of insurance when they performed no underwriting function and received only an administrative fee on the basis of the number and type of plan participants, regardless of the fact that plan participants and beneficiaries used BCBS claim forms, BCBS staff processed the claims, BCBS made initial determinations regarding coverage, and BCBS paid plan participants and beneficiaries directly and was reimbursed by the employer.[171] According to the court, because "ERISA creates a scheme in which any entity engaged in the business of insurance, except an ERISA employee benefit plan, is subject to state insurance regulation," the controlling question was whether BCBS was engaging in the business of insurance when it sold administrative services to the ERISA plan.[172] The court held that it was not because it did not assume any financial risk of a valid claim, it did not provide a service that was an essential part of the insurance relationship but instead merely provided administrative services, and other entities outside the insurance industry provided the same administrative services provided by BCBS.

In summary, so long as the services being provided by contract to the ERISA plan do not constitute the assumption and spreading of risk (i.e., the "business of insurance"), any attempted state regulation of those services, including regulation under the insurance code, will be preempted by ERISA.[173] As the discussion following of the preemption of state any willing provider (AWP) laws demonstrates, however, the dividing line between the "business of insurance" and the provision of professional services is not always clear.

AWP Laws

One of the hottest legal battles in the managed care arena is the fight between states and MCOs over the applicability of AWP laws to networks that contract with ERISA plans. Although the terms of AWP statutes differ from state to state, in general, AWP statutes require that MCOs and other entities establishing provider networks not discriminate against a provider so long as the provider meets the network's general qualifications and is willing to be compensated at the network's reduced payment rate. Under some state statutes, patients also cannot be penalized through reduced benefits if they seek treatment from providers outside their designated network.

The problem with AWP laws from the managed care industry's viewpoint is that they eliminate the means by which MCOs persuade providers to accept lower rates of compensation for their services. The attraction of MCOs for health care providers, despite the reduced compensation, is the increased volume of patients that can be generated through limiting the network of participating providers. By preventing MCOs from differentiating between participating and nonparticipating providers, providers cannot be assured of a certain number of patients, thereby eliminating the leverage with which MCOs bargain for lower rate of payment.

Proponents of AWP laws argue that AWP laws protect patient choice and that the identity of the treating provider is a part of the overall package of benefits. According to such proponents, consumers should not be forced to accept providers chosen by an MCO by a threat of reduced levels of benefits.

The current judicial debate over AWP laws centers on ERISA whether MCOs that service ERISA plans are subject to state AWP laws. As explained previously, under ERISA, any state law that "relates to" an ERISA employee benefits plan may be subject to preemption. ERISA makes an exception to its broad preemption provision, however, for any state law that regulates the "business of insurance." Courts have interpreted that phrase to require a two-part analysis. First, courts look to whether common sense dictates that the state statute regulates insurance. Then they decide whether a state statute affects a practice that has the effect of transferring or spreading a policyholder's risk, is an integral part of the relationship between the insurer and the insured, and is limited to entities within the insurance industry. If it does, then the statute is not preempted by ERISA as applied to a fully insured ERISA plan. As applied to a self-funded ERISA plan, however, the statute is still preempted.

The differences of opinion regarding the scope of ERISA preemption with respect to AWP laws arise from the uncertainty as to whether regulating the identities of a network's participating provider is a regulation of the business of insurance. Defenders of AWP laws argue that AWP laws regulate the business of insurance because they define the type of policy that can be issued. HMOs and other MCOs that maintain closed provider networks increase the costs of patients who use nonparticipating providers by reducing or eliminating benefits for services received from those providers. An AWP law allows a patient to obtain care from a provider who might otherwise be excluded from a network without a reduction of benefits. The AWP law's prohibition on closed networks, it is argued, spreads the policyholders' risk insofar as it shifts from patients to MCOs the increased costs of seeking treatment from providers who otherwise would be excluded from a network.

In addition to spreading policyholder risk, defenders of AWP laws argue that such laws affect an integral part of the relationship between the insurer and the insured: treatment and cost. AWP laws help define the nature of the available services, who can provide them, and how those providers will be paid. In this respect, AWP laws have been analogized to mandated benefits laws, which require insurers to include certain types of benefits in their insurance policies. Mandated benefit laws were found to be saved from ERISA preemption because they regulate the scope of the insurance coverage and the availability of services. In the same manner, it is argued, AWP laws affect the type of benefits that an insured receives by determining who can provide covered services and how those providers are selected. Opponents of preemption assert that such regulation touches on a vital part of the insurer-insured relationship.

On the other hand, proponents of ERISA preemption contend that AWP laws do not regulate the business of insurance, although they may regulate the business of insurance companies. They argue that AWP laws do not spread policyholder risk. Instead, such laws are merely cost-saving mechanisms. According to this argument, contracts between MCOs and providers, whereby the provider receives a reduced rate of compensation in exchange for a certain volume of patients, are merely contracts for the purchase of professional services. The spreading of risk occurs when an MCO insures an ERISA plan, not when it attempts to minimize costs through its contracts with providers. The provider contracts are seen as being identical to many other arrangements whereby MCOs try to reduce costs.

Finally, proponents of preemption argue that the practice of establishing a closed network does not affect an integral part of the relationship between an insurer and the insured. The contracts at issue are between the insurer and the providers. They do not affect the amount or the type of benefit that a patient receives, only the vehicle through which such services are rendered.

Because of the runaway costs of health care and the concerted effort to find means by which to curb health care expenses, there are also strong policy reasons for finding ERISA preemption of AWP laws. As discussed previously, if MCOs are prohibited from closing their networks, they can no longer ensure a certain volume of business. In this manner, AWP laws eliminate any leverage MCOs may have had to bargain with providers for reduced rates of compensation, effectively eliminating the benefits of establishing a provider network.

Thus far, courts have reached different conclusions as to whether particular AWP laws regulate "the business of insurance." One of the first AWP laws to be challenged by the managed care industry was in Virginia.[174] Virginia's AWP statute allowed insurers to form PPOs and established terms and conditions that physicians, hospitals, or other providers had to meet to qualify as a preferred provider. The statute, however, prohibited insurers from both unreasonably discriminating against and among such providers and from excluding providers willing to meet the terms and conditions for participation in the PPO. The challenge to the Virginia statute arose after a PPO established by Aetna, which provided services exclusively to employee benefit plans, refused to allow a hospital to participate in its network. Instead, the PPO only contracted with hospitals that were already participants in

Aetna's HMO. In *Stuart Circle Hospital Corporation v. Aetna Health Management,* the hospital sued Aetna for failing to comply with the AWP statute and excluding it from the PPO network for the sole reason that it was not a member of Aetna's HMO.[175] Aetna defended on the ground that the statute was preempted by ERISA.

In the *Stuart Circle* case, the U.S. Court of Appeals for the Fourth Circuit first found that the AWP statute "related to" ERISA plans. The statute not only expressly provided that it applied to health benefit programs offered or administered by insurers but also restricted the ability of an insurer to limit the choice of providers that would otherwise confine the plan participants of an ERISA plan to those preferred by the insurer.

Next, the Fourth Circuit held that the statute was saved from preemption because it regulated the business of insurance and consequently fell within the ERISA savings clause. According to the court, the statute spread policyholder risk because insurers whose benefits otherwise would be reduced or denied if they sought treatment from nonparticipating providers would receive full benefits under the statute. In addition, the court asserted, the statute affected an integral part of the relationship between the insurer and the insured because the statute affected the provision for treatment and cost. Finally, the Virginia statute was explicitly limited to entities within the insurance industry, thus satisfying the third McCarran-Ferguson criterion. Consequently, the court held that the Virginia AWP statute was not preempted by ERISA.[176]

However, the U.S. Court of Appeals for the Fifth Circuit reached the opposite conclusion in two cases: *CIGNA Healthplan of Louisiana, Inc. v. Louisiana ex rel. Ieyoub*[177] and *Texas Pharmacy Association v. Prudential Insurance Co.*[178] The Fifth Circuit held that the AWP laws in Louisiana and Texas, respectively, were preempted because they bound employers or plan administrators to particular choices by requiring ERISA plan to purchase benefits of a particular structure (i.e., a structure that includes AWPs).[179] The U.S. Court of Appeals for the

Tenth Circuit has also preempted the Arkansas AWP law.[180]

Nevertheless, relying on the reasoning of the U.S. Supreme Court in *Travelers, Dillingham,* and *De Buono*, other lower courts have declined to follow suit. For example, in *American Drug Stores, Inc. v. Harvard Pilgrim Health Care, Inc.,* the court held that the Massachusetts AWP law, prohibiting the formation of restricted pharmacy networks, did not "relate to" ERISA.[181] The court rejected defendants' argument that the statute mandated employee benefit structures or administration.[182] Instead, the court began its analysis with the presumption that Congress did not intend to supplant the AWP law because the law fell within an area of traditional state regulation—the health care and insurance industries. The court noted that the basic thrust of the preemption clause was to avoid a multiplicity of regulation to permit the nationally uniform administration of employee benefit plans but pointed out that the establishment and operation of provider networks was not the type of activity that could become "nationally uniform" absent state interference.[183] The court concluded that the involvement of ERISA plans in the establishment and operation of provider networks should not extend the scope of ERISA preemption.[184]

Similarly, a federal court in Kentucky, after an analysis of the *American Drug* court's reasoning, found that Kentucky's AWP statute "related to" employee benefit plans in that it mandated the benefit structure of such plans.[185] Nevertheless, the court held that the AWP was "saved" from preemption under ERISA because it regulated the business of insurance.[186]

Capitated Provider Contracts

Another legal battle is brewing over the extent to which providers who have contracted to provide health care services to either MCOs or self-funded employers on a capitated basis are subject to the insurance laws. The answer depends on whether such capitated contracts are construed as insurance contracts.

In an opinion dated June 19, 1990, the Maryland Attorney General addressed whether a third-party administrator that had established a provider network and offered that network to self-funded ERISA plans was engaged in the business of insurance and, thus, needed an insurance license.[187] The Attorney General opined that it was not. The Attorney General warned, however, that the providers might need an insurance license if they agreed to be paid on a capitated basis. The rationale for the Attorney General's opinion was that, by agreeing to be paid on a capitated basis the providers had assumed risk and, therefore, were engaged in the business of insurance. The Attorney General concluded that an employer's creation of a self-funded employee benefit plan, protected from state regulation by ERISA, did not also exempt the providers of services to that plan from state insurance regulation.

On May 18, 1995, the Office of the Georgia Commissioner of Insurance notified a physician-hospital organization that offered its services on a capitated basis that the Georgia insurance statutes "do not permit a hospital or medical group or combination of both to provide health care services or benefits directly to patients for a monthly capitation fee unless fully licensed as an insurer by this department."[188] The commissioner ordered the immediate discontinuance of the physician-hospital organization's health care program unless it was being underwritten by a licensed insurer. With respect to the issue of ERISA preemption, the commissioner took the position that the health care program at issue was being offered to multiple employers but did not meet ERISA's definition of an employee benefit plan.

Similarly, the Virginia Bureau of Insurance recently notified the managed care industry that health care providers and other entities that provide health care services to self-funded employers on a capitated basis either would have to obtain insurance licenses or would have to provide such services through licensed entities, such as HMOs.[189] If the health care services were provided on a capitated basis by means of a contract with an MCO that in turn contracted with a self-funded employer for administrative services only (a so-called capitated administrative services only contract), then the capitated administrative services only contract would be considered a risk contract by the Bureau of Insurance and would be subject to the full panoply of the insurance code, including reserves requirements and assessments. The Bureau of Insurance took the position that capitated administrative services only contracts were insurance contracts and, therefore, were saved from ERISA preemption by the savings clause.

The managed care industry would disagree. It seems likely that MCOs and integrated delivery systems will seek both legislative and judicial relief from insurance commissioners' efforts to regulate capitated arrangements and that ERISA will continue to play a prominent role.

CONCLUSION

ERISA can affect many of the core functions of an MCO, from product design to administration to issues of legal liability. Accordingly, MCOs would be well advised to acquire a proficiency with respect to the requirements of this far-reaching statute and the rapidly developing body of case law interpreting it.

REFERENCES AND NOTES

1. 29 U.S.C. § 1001 *et seq.*
2. 29 U.S.C. §§ 1002(1), 1002(3), 1003.
3. 29 U.S.C. § 1102.
4. 29 U.S.C. § 1022; 29 C.F.R. § 2520.104b-2.
5. 29 C.F.R. § 2520.102-3(j).
6. 29 C.F.R. § 2520.102-3(j).
7. *Id.*
8. *Id.*
9. *Id.*
10. *See, e.g., Aiken v. Policy Management Sys. Corp.,* 13 F.3d 138 (4th Cir. 1993); *Edwards v. State Farm Mut. Auto. Ins. Co.,* 851 F.2d 134 (6th Cir. 1988).
11. *See, e.g., Marolt v. Alliant Techsystems, Inc.,* 146 F.3d 617 (8th Cir. 1998); *Fallo v. Piccadilly Cafeterias, Inc.,* 141 F.3d 580 (5th Cir. 1998).
12. 29 U.S.C. § 1024.
13. 29 C.F.R. § 2520.104-20.
14. Dep't Labor Adv. Op. 92-24A (Nov. 6, 1992).
15. 26 U.S.C. § 6039D.
16. 29 U.S.C. § 1024.
17. *Id.*
18. 29 U.S.C. § 1169.
19. *Id.*
20. *Id*
21. 29 U.S.C. §§ 1161-1168.
22. 29 U.S.C. § 1181.
23. 29 U.S.C. § 1182.
24. 29 U.S.C. § 1183.
25. 29 U.S.C. § 1185.
26. 29 U.S.C. § 1185a.
27. 29 U.S.C. § 1185b.
28. 29 U.S.C. § 1144.

29. *Metropolitan Life Ins. Co. v. Mass.,* 471 U.S. 724 (1985).
30. *FMC Corp. v. Holliday,* 498 U.S. 52 (1990).
31. *Drexelbrook Eng'g Co. v. Travelers Ins. Co.,* 891 F.2d 280 (3d Cir. 1989); *United Food & Commercial Workers & Employers Ariz. Health & Welfare Trust v. Pacyga,* 801 F.2d 1157 (9th Cir. 1986).
32. *Brown v. Granatelli,* 897 F.2d 1351 (5th Cir.), *cert. denied,* 498 U.S. 848 (1990).
33. *See, e.g.,* Mo. Code Regs. tit. 20, § 400-2.150 (1993).
34. NAIC Stop Loss Insurance Model Act (1995).
35. *American Medical Security Inc. v. Bartlett,* 111 F.3d 358 (4th Cir. 1996).
36. *De Buono v. NYSA-ILA Medical and Clinical Servs. Fund,* 520 U.S. 806 (1997); *N.Y. State Conference of Blue Cross & Blue Shield Plans v. Travelers Ins. Co.,* 514 U.S. 645 (1995).
37. *See, e.g.,* Age Discrimination in Employment Act of 1967, as amended, 29 U.S.C. § 621 *et seq.*
38. 42 U.S.C. § 12101 *et seq.*
39. 42 U.S.C. § 12202.
40. *Id.*
41. *Id.*
42. 29 C.F.R. Part 1630, EEOC Interpretative Guidance on Title I of the Americans with Disabilities Act.
43. 29 U.S.C. § 1185a.
44. *Id.*
45. 70 F.3d 958 (8th Cir. 1995).
46. *See, e.g., Ford v. Schering-Plough Corp.,* 145 F.3d 601 (3d Cir. 1998).
47. 29 U.S.C. § 1102.
48. *See, e.g., Boyer v. Douglas Components Corp.,* 986 F.2d 999 (6th Cir. 1993).

49. *Id.*

50. *In re Unisys Corp. Retiree Medical Benefit "ERISA" Litigation,* 57 F.3d 1255 (3d Cir. 1995), *cert. denied,* 517 U.S. 1103 (1996).

51. 18 F.3d 1034 (3d Cir. 1994).

52. *Curtiss-Wright Corp. v. Schoonejongen,* 514 U.S. 73 (1995).

53. *Murphy v. Keystone Steel & Wire Co.,* 61 F.3d 560 (7th Cir. 1995).

54. 29 U.S.C. § 1002(21).

55. 29 U.S.C. § 1104.

56. *Id.*

57. *Id.*

58. *Curtiss-Wright Corp. v. Schoonejongen,* 514 U.S. 73, (1995).

59. *Varity Corp. v. Howe,* 516 U.S. 489 (1996).

60. *See, e.g., Fischer v. Philadelphia Elec. Co.,* 96 F.3d 1533 (3d Cir. 1996), *cert. denied,* 520 U.S. 1116 (1997).

61. *Bins v. Exxon Company U.S.A.,* 189 F.3d 929 (9th Cir. 1999).

62. *Ballone v. Eastman Kodak Co.,* 109 F.3d 117 (2d Cir. 1997).

63. *Bins v. Exxon Company U.S.A.,* 189 F.3d 929 (9th Cir. 1999).

64. *Id.; Ballone v. Eastman Kodak Co.,* 109 F.3d 1117 (2d Cir. 1997).

65. 29 U.S.C. § 1106.

66. 29 U.S.C. § 1002(14).

67. 29 C.F.R. § 2550.408b-2.

68. 29 U.S.C. § 1133.

69. 29 C.F.R. § 2560.503-1.

70. *See* Prop. Reg. § 29 C.F.R. § 2560.503-1.

71. 489 U.S. 101 (1989).

72. 31 F.3d 606 (8th Cir. 1994).

73. 899 F.2d 639 (7th Cir. 1990).

74. *See, e.g., Peruzzi v. Summa Medical Plan,* 137 F.3d 431 (6th Cir. 1998); *Chambers v. Family Health Plan,* 1000 F.3d 818 (10th Cir. 1996).

75. *Chambers v. Family Health Plan,* 100 F. 3d 818 (10th Cir. 1996); *Peruzzi v. Summa Medical Plan,* 137 F 3d 431 (6th Cir. 1998); *Pagun v. Nynex Medical Pension Plan,* 52 F.3d 438 (2nd Cir. 1995).

76. *See, e.g., Cox v. Keystone Carbon Co.,* 894 F.2d 647 (3d Cir.), *cert. denied,* 498 U.S. 811 (1990); *Chilton v. Savannah Foods & Indus., Inc.,* 814 F.2d 620 (11th Cir. 1987).

77. *Blue Cross & Blue Shield v. Lewis,* 753 F. Supp. 345 (N.D. Ala. 1990).

78. 29 U.S.C. § 1132(a)(2).

79. 29 U.S.C. § 1132(a)(3).

80. 473 U.S. 134 (1985).

81. 58 U.S. 248 (1993).

82. *See, e.g., Pilot Life Insurance Co. v. Dedeaux,* 481 U.S. 41 (1987).

83. 12 F.3d 1517 (9th Cir. 1993).

84. 516 U.S. 489 (1996).

85. *Clair v. Harris Trust and Savings Bank,* 190 F.3d 495 (7th Cir. 1999).

86. Section 514(a) of ERISA; 28 U.S.C. § 1144(a).

87. Section 514(b)(2)(B) of ERISA; 29 U.S.C. §1144(b)(2)(A).

88. Section 514(b)(2)(B) of ERISA; 29 U.S.C. § 1144(b)(2)(B).

89. *Shaw v. Delta Air Lines, Inc.,* 463 U.S. 85, 96-97 (1983).

90. *FMC Corp. v. Holliday,* 498 U.S. 52, 58 (1990).

91. *Ingersoll-Rand Co. v. McClendon,* 498 U.S. 133 (1990); *United Wire, Metal & Mach. Health & Welfare Fund v. Morristown Memorial Hosp.,* 995 F.2d 1179 (3d Cir.), *cert. denied,* 510 U.S. 944 (1993) (a state law may be preempted even though it has no direct nexus with ERISA plans if its effect is to dictate or restrict the choices of ERISA plans with regard to their benefits, structure, reporting, and administration).

92. *See FMC Corp. Holliday,* 498 U.S. 52, 58 (1990); *Shaw v. Delta Air Lines, Inc.,* 463 U.S. 85, 100 n. 21 (1983) (some state actions may affect employee benefit plans in "too tenuous, remote, or peripheral a manner to warrant a finding that the law 'relates to' the plan"); *Mackey v. Lanier Collection Agency & Serv., Inc.,* 486 U.S. 825 (1988).

93. *New York State Conference of Blue Cross & Blue Shield Plans v. Travelers Ins. Co.,* 514 U.S. 645 (1995); *California Div. of Labor Enforcement v. Dillingham Constr. N.A., Inc.,* 519 U.S. 316 (1997); *De Buono v. NYSA-ILA Medical and Clinical Servs.,* 520 U.S. 806 (1997).

94. 514 U.S. at 656.

95. 514 U.S. at 658-660.

96. 520 U.S. at 814.

97. 519 U.S. at 325.

98. 481 U.S. 41 (1987).

99. *Id.* at 48-49 (citing *Metropolitan Life Ins. Co. v. Mass.,* 471 U.S. 724 (1985)).

100. *Id.* (quoting *Union Labor Life Ins. Co. v. Pireno,* 458 U.S. 119 (1982)).

101. 526 U.S. 358 (1999).

102. *FMC Corp. v. Holliday,* 498 U.S. 52, 64-65 (1990).

103. *Id.*

104. *Id.* ("Our interpretation of the deemer clause makes clear that if a plan is insured, a State may regulate it indirectly through regulation of its insurer and its

insurer's insurance contracts; if the plan is uninsured, the State may not regulate it").

105. *See Petrovich v. Share Health Plan*, 188 Ill. 2d 241 (1999); *Jones v. Chicago HMO Ltd.*, 301 Ill. App. 3d 103, 703 N.E.2d 502 (1998); *Raglin v. HMO Illinois, Inc.*, 230 Ill. App.3d 642, 595 N.E.2d 153 (1992); *McClellan v. Health Maintenance Org.*, 413 Pa. Super. 128, 604 A.2d 1953, *appeal denied sub nom. Health Maintenance Org. v. McClellan*, 532 Pa. 664, 616 A.2d 985 (1992); *Boyd v. Albert Einstein Medical Center*, 377 Pa. Super. 609, 547 A.2d 1229 (1988); *Decker v. Saini*, No. 88361768 N.H., 1991 WL 277590 (Mich. Cir. Ct. Sept. 17, 1991).

106. *See Petrovich v. Share Health Plan*, 188 Ill. 2d 241 (1999).

107. *See Coyne & Delany v. Selman*, 98 F.3d 1457 (4th Cir. 1996); *Jackson v. Roseman*, 878 F. Supp. 820 (D. Md. 1995); *Kearney v. U.S. Healthcare, Inc.*, 859 F. Supp. 182 (E.D. Pa. 1994); *Haas v. Group Health Plan, Inc.*, 875 F. Supp. 544 (S.D. Ill. 1994); *Dearmas v. Av-Med, Inc.*, 865 F. Supp. 816 (S.D. Fla. 1994); *Paterno v. Albuerne*, 855 F. Supp. 1263 (S.D. Fla. 1994); *Elsesser v. Hosp. of the Philadelphia College of Osteopathic Medicine*, 802 F. Supp. 1286 (E.D. Pa. 1992); *Independence HMO, Inc. v. Smith*, 733 F. Supp. 983 (E.D. Pa. 1990); *Pickett v. CIGNA Healthplan of Texas, Inc.*, 742 F. Supp. 946 (S.D. Tex. 1990); *Tufino v. N.Y. Hotel & Motel Trades Council & Hotel Ass'ns of N.Y.C. AFL-CIO Local 6*, 223 A.D.2d 245, 646 N.Y.S.2d 799 (N.Y. Sup. Ct. 1996); *McClellan v. Health Maintenance Org.*, 413 Pa. Super. 128, 604 A.2d 1053, *appeal denied sub nom. Health Maintenance Org. v. McClellan*, 532 Pa. 664, 616 A.2d 985 (1992).

108. *See Pomeroy v. John Hopkins Medical Servs., Inc.*, 868 F. Supp. 110 (D. Md. 1994); *Nealy v. U.S. Healthcare HMO*, 844 F. Supp. 966 (S.D.N.Y. 1994); *Butler v. Wu*, 853 F. Supp. 125 (D.N.J. 1994); *Ricci v. Gooberman*, 840 F. Supp. 316 (D.N.J. 1993); *Altieri v. CIGNA Dental Health, Inc.* 753 F. Supp. 61 (D. Conn. 1990).

109. 59 F.3d 151 (10th Cir. 1995).

110. *Id.* at 155.

111. *Prudential Health Care Plan, Inc. v. Lewis*, No. 95-6255, 1996 U.S. App. LEXIS 2595 (10th Cir. Feb. 21, 1996); *Lazorko v. Pennsylvania Hosp.*, No. 96-4858, 1998 U.S. Dist. LEXIS 10062 (E.D. Pa. June 30, 1998); *Negron v. Patel*, 6 F. Supp. 2d 366 (E.D. Pa. 1998).

112. 57 F.3d 350 (3d Cir. 1995), *cert. denied sub nom. U.S. Healthcare, Inc. v. Dukes*, 516 U.S. 1009 (1995).

113. The Third Circuit acknowledged that the distinction between the quantity of benefits due under an ERISA plan and the quality of those benefits would not always be clear. The court recognized that there could be cases in which the quality of care rendered was so low as to

constitute a denial of benefits or the ERISA plan had described a benefit in terms related to the quality of services and the plan participant was claiming damages resulting from a failure to provide services of the promised quality. The court also noted that an employer and an HMO could agree that a quality of care standard articulated in their contract could replace standards that would otherwise be supplied by applicable state tort law but declined to express an opinion as to whether such an agreement would be enforceable. 57 F.3d at 358-359.

114. *Id.* at 360-361.

115. The Seventh and Second Circuit Courts also have held that a vicarious liability professional malpractice claim was not removable to state court. *Rice v. Panchal*, 65 F.3d 637 (7th Cir. 1995); *Lupo v. Human Affairs Int'l, Inc.*, 28 F.3d 269 (2d Cir. 1994); *see also Muller v. Maron*, No. 94-5052, 1995 W.L. 605483 (E.D. Pa. Oct. 13, 1995).

116. *See U.S. Healthcare, Inc. v. Bauman*, Nos. 98-5222, 98-5262, 98-5263, 1999 WL 728474 (3rd Cir. 1999), *McDonald v. Damian*, 56 F. Supp. 2d 574 (E.D. Pa. 1999); *Snow v. Burden*, No. 99-1874, 1999 WL 387196 (E.D. Pa. May 6, 1999); *Miller v. Riddle Memorial Hosp.*, No. 98-392, 1998 U.S. Dist. LEXIS 7752 (E.D. Pa. May 28, 1998); *Eaccarino v. Canlas*, No. 97-CV-5497, 1998 U.S. Dist. LEXIS 4904 (E.D. Pa. Apr. 1, 1998); *Newton v. Tavani*, 962 F. Supp. 45 (D.N.J. 1997); *Hoyt v. Edge*, No. 97-3631, 1997 U.S. Dist. LEXIS 8846 (E.D. Pa. June 19, 1997); *Roessert v. Health Net*, 929 F. Supp. 343 (N.D. Cal. 1996); *Prihoda v. Shpritz*, 914 F. Supp. 113 (D. Md. 1996); *Howard v. Sasson*, No. 95-0068, 1995 U.S. Dist. LEXIS 14373 (E.D. Pa. Oct. 3, 1995).

117. 12 F. Supp. 2d 597 (1998).

118. Notably, excluded from the statutory definition of "managed care entity" was "an employer purchasing coverage or acting on behalf of its employees." 12 F. Supp. 2d at 612.

119. 514 U.S. 645 (1995).

120. 519 U.S. 316 (1997).

121. 12 F. Supp. 2d at 614.

122. *Id.* at 619.

123. *Id.* at 616-617.

124. *Id.* at 620.

125. *Id.* at 621.

126. 88 F.3d 1482 (7th Cir. 1996).

127. 48 F.3d 937 (6th Cir. 1995).

128. 965 F.2d 1321 (5th Cir.), *cert. denied*, 506 U.S. 1033 (1992).

129. *See also Danca v. Private Health Care Systems*, 185 F.3d 1 (1st Cir. 1999), *Kuhl v. Lincoln Nat'l Health Plan*, 999 F.2d 298 (8th Cir. 1993), *cert. denied*, 510 U.S. 1045 (1994) (ERISA preempted a wrongful death

claim on the basis of a delay in precertification of surgery because the precertification decision related to the administration of benefits); *Rodriguez v. Pacificare of Tex., Inc.*, 980 F.2d 1014 (5th Cir.), *cert. denied*, 508 U.S. 956 (1993); *Garrison v. Northeast Ga. Medical Ctr., Inc.*, No. *2:99-CV-8-WCO*, 1999 U.S. Dist. LEXIS 10608 (N.D. Ga. Apr. 20, 1999); *Silva v. Kaiser Permanente*, 59 F. Supp. 2d 597 (N.D. Tex. May 25, 1999); *Toledo v. Kaiser Permanente Medical Group*, 987 F. Supp. 1174 (N.D. Cal. 1997), *Bailey-Gates v. Aetna Life Ins. Co.*, 890 F. Supp. 73 (D. Conn. 1994).

130. 724 A.2d 889 (Pa. 1998).

131. *Id.* at 893.

132. *Id.*

133. *Id.* at 894.

134. *See Crum v. Health Alliance-Midwest, Inc.*, 47 F. Supp. 2d 1013 (C.D. Ill. 1999).

135. *See Johnson v. Misericordia Community Hosp.*, 99 Wis.2d 708, 301 N.W.2d 156 (1981).

136. *See Harrell v. Total Health Care, Inc.*, No. W.D. 39809, 1989 W.L. 153066 (Mo. Ct. App. Apr. 25, 1989), *aff'd on other grounds*, 781 S.W.2d 58 (Mo. 1989); *McClellan v. Health Maintenance Org.*, 413 Pa. Super. 128, 604 A.2d 1053, *appeal denied sub nom. Health Maintenance Org. v. McClellan*, 532 Pa. 664, 616 A.2d 985 (1992).

137. *See Harrell v. Total Health Care, Inc.*, No. W.D. 39809, 1989 W.L. 153066 (Mo. Ct. App. Apr. 25, 1989), *aff'd on other grounds*, 781 S.W.2d 58 (Mo. 1989).

138. 859 F. Supp. 182 (E.D. Pa. 1994).

139. *Id.* at 187.

140. *See, e.g., Butler v. Wu*, 853 F. Supp. 125 (D.N.J. 1994); *Elsesser v. Hosp. of the Philadelphia College of Osteopathic Medicine*, 802 F. Supp. 1286 (E.D. Pa. 1992); *Altieri v. CIGNA Dental Health, Inc.*, 753 F. Supp. 61 (D. Conn. 1990); *Dalton v. Peninsula Hosp. Ctr.*, 164 Misc.2d 912, 626 N.Y.S.2d 362 (N.Y. Sup. Ct. 1995).

141. 878 F. Supp. 820 (D. Md. 1995).

142. *Id.* at 824 n. 6.

143. *Lupo v. Human Affairs Int'l, Inc.*, 28 F.3d 269 (2d Cir. 1994).

144. *See also U.S. Healthcare, Inc. v. Bauman*, Nos. 98-5222, 98-5262, 98-5263, 1999 WL 728474 (3rd Cir. 1999), *Stratton v. Bryant*, No. 92-CV-3873, 1994 W.L. 837450 (E.D. Pa. Nov. 18, 1992) (ERISA did not preempt the claim against the HMO on the basis of its negligent selection, supervision, and monitoring of the treating physician who negligently delivered plaintiffs' son); *McClellan v. Health Maintenance Org.*, 413 Pa. Super. 128, 604 A.2d 1053, *appeal denied sub nom. Health Maintenance Org. v. McClellan*, 532 Pa. 664, 616 A.2d 985 (1992).

145. 904 F.2d 236 (5th Cir. 1990), *reh'g denied*, No. 89-2513, 1990 U.S. App. LEXIS 13227 (5th Cir. July 16, 1990).

146. *Id.* at 239.

147. *Id.* at 244.

148. *Id.* at 246.

149. *Id.*

150. *Id.*

151. *Id.* at 247.

152. *Id.*

153. *Id.* at 247-48.

154. *Id.* at 249.

155. *Id.* at 250.

156. *Id.*

157. 110 F.3d 280 (5th Cir.), *cert. denied sub nom. Pan-American Life Ins. Co. v. Cypress Fairbanks Medical Ctr., Inc.*, 522 U.S. 862 (1997).

158. *Id.* at 281.

159. *Id.* at 283.

160. *Id.*

161. *Id.* at 283.

162. *See Home Health, Inc. v. Prudential Ins. Co.*, 101 F.3d 600 (8th Cir. 1996); *The Meadows v. Employers Health Ins.*, 47 F.3d 1006 (9th Cir. 1995); *Lordmann Enters., Inc. v. Equicor, Inc.*, 32 F.3d 1529 (11th Cir. 1994), *cert. denied sub nom. Equicor, Inc. v. Lordmann Enters., Inc.*, 516 U.S. 930 (1995); *Hospice of Metro Denver, Inc. v. Group Health Ins. of Okla., Inc.*, 944 F.2d 752 (10th Cir. 1991); *St. Luke's Episcopal Hosp. v. Great West Life & Annuity Ins. Co.*, 38 F. Supp. 2d 497 (S.D. Tex. 1999); *Syndicated Office Sys., Inc. v. Southeast Medical Alliance*, No. 98-2355, 1999 U.S. Dist. LEXIS 12381 (E.D. La. Aug. 6, 1999); *Davis v. United Healthcare Ins. Co.*, 34 F. Supp. 2d 1044 (S.D. Miss. 1998); *Jefferson Parish Hosp. Serv. Dist. No. 2 v. Ruby Tuesday's Inc.*, No. 97-2722, 1998 U.S. Dist. LEXIS 767 (E.D. La. Jan. 23, 1998); *Variety Children's Hosp., Inc. v. Blue Cross/Blue Shield of Fla.*, 942 F. Supp. 562 (S.D. Fla. 1996); *Memorial Hosp. Sys. v. John Hancock, Mut. Life Ins. Co.*, 952 F. Supp. 449 (S.D. Tex. 1996); *Rehabilitation Inst. v. Group Adm'rs, Ltd.*, 844 F. Supp. 1275 (N.D. Ill. 1994); *Hoag Memorial Hosp. v. Managed Care Adm'rs*, 820 F. Supp. 1232 (C.D. Cal. 1993); *Gaston Memorial Hosp. Home Health Servs., Inc. v. Bridgestone/Firestone, Inc.*, 830 F. Supp. 287 (W.D.N.C. 1993); *Suburban Hosp., Inc. v. Sampson*, 807 F.Supp. 31 (D. Md. 1992).

163. *See, e.g., Md. Ann. Code §8-301(b)(2)(iv) (1998), regulating third-party administrators, which states, in relevant part, that the term *administrator* does not include a person who administers only plans that are sub-

ject to ERISA and do not provide benefits through insurance, unless any of the plans administered is a multiple employer welfare arrangement (MEWA).

164. *Group Life & Health Ins. Co. v. Royal Drug Co.*, 440 U.S. 205, 212 (1979); *Anglin v. Blue Shield*, 693 F.2d 315 (4th Cir. 1982); *GAF Corp. v. County Sch. Bd.*, 629 F.2d 981 (4th Cir. 1980) (transferring and distribution of risks are two elements of insurance).

165. *Royal Drug*, 440 U.S. at 211.

166. *See GAF Corp. v. County Sch. Bd.*, 629 F.2d 981 (4th Cir. 1980); *Jordan v. Group Health Ass'n*, 71 App. D.C. 38, 107 F.2d 239 (1939) (where the primary purpose of a corporation was to arrange for the delivery of health services to its members and not to protect against financial loss caused by unusual occurrences, the corporation was not in the business of insurance regardless of any incidental element of risk distribution or assumption that was present in its contracts).

167. *NGS American, Inc. v. Barnes*, 998 F.2d 296 (5th Cir. 1993).

168. *Powell v. Chesapeake & Potomac Tel. Co.*, 780 F.2d 419, 423 (4th Cir. 1985), *cert. denied*, 476 U.S. 1170 (1986).

169. 15 U.S.C. § 1011 *et seq.*

170. *Powell v. Chesapeake & Potomac Tel. Co.*, 780 F.2d at 423 (quoting *SEC v. Nat'l Sec.*, 393 U.S. 453, 460 (1969)).

171. 819 F.2d 408 (3d Cir. 1987).

172. *Id.* at 411.

173. *See also O'Reilly v. Ceuleers* 912 F.2d 1383, 1389 (11th Cir. 1990) (the court held that, when an HMO merely acted as a third-party administrator, it was not engaged in the business of insurance and was, consequently, not within the insurance exception savings clause); *Aetna Life Ins. Co. v. State Bd. Of Equalization*, 11 Cal. App. 4th 1207, 15 Cal. Rptr. 2d 26 (1992)

(the court held that a California premiums tax was inapplicable to fees collected by an insurance company when the company was acting in the capacity of an administrator and not an insurer); *but see Benefax Corp. v. Wright*, 757 F.Supp. 800 (W.D. Ky. 1990) (third-party administrators were subject to Kentucky administrator licensing statutes).

174. *Stuart Circle Hosp. Corp. v. Aetna Health Management*, 995 F.2d 500 (4th Cir.), *cert. denied sub nom. Aetna Life Insurance Co. v. Stuart Circle Hosp. Corp.*, 510 U.S. 1003 (1993).

175. *Id.*

176. *See also Blue Cross & Blue Shield v. Bell*, 798 F.2d 1331 (10th Cir. 1986); *Blue Cross & Blue Shield of Va. v. St. Mary's Hosp. of Richmond, Inc.*, 245 Va. 24, 426 S.E.2d 117 (1993); *Blue Cross Hosp. Serv., Inc. v. Frappier*, 698 S.W.2d 326 (Mo. 1985).

177. 82 F.3d 642 (5th Cir. 1996).

178. 105 F.3d 1035 (5th Cir. 1997).

179. 82 F.3d at 648; 105 F. 3d at 1037.

180. *Prudential Ins. Co. v. National Park Medical Center*, 154 F.3d 812 (8th Cir. 1998).

181. 973 F. Supp. 60 (D. Mass. 1997).

182. *Id.* at 69.

183. *Id.* at 66-67.

184. *Id.* at 67.

185. *Community Health Partners, Inc. v. Kentucky ex rel. Nichols*, 14 F. Supp. 2d 991 (1998).

186. *Id.*

187. 75 Op. Att'y Gen. (1990) (Opinion No. 90-030 (September 1, 1990)).

188. Letter of William C. Lorick, Deputy Insurance Commissioner, to Northwest Georgia Physician Hospital Organization dated May 18, 1995.

189. Admin. Letter 1995-10 dated September 11, 1995.

SUGGESTED READING

American Bar Association Section of Labor and Employment Law, Employee Benefits Law (1991).

The Health Insurance Portability and Accountability Act of 1996

Charles N. Kahn III, Dean A. Rosen, Marianne Miller, and Kathleen H. Fyffe

INTRODUCTION

This chapter describes the effects of the Health Insurance Portability and Accountability Act of 1996 (HIPAA; P.L. 104-191) on several constituencies in the American health care system, emphasizing regulation of the private health insurance market. First, we recount the background of the law and explain its major provisions, including its portability and access initiatives. Administrative simplification is considered next, including new provisions on confidentiality. We then discuss administration and enforcement of the new law. Finally, we examine the Act's consequences for consumers and insurers and speculate about the direction of future policy making. Although it is early yet to draw a definitive picture of HIPAA's ultimate impact, tentative conclusions suggest themselves and will be put forward.

HIPAA appears to take a long step toward greater federal regulation of health insurance. It was enacted against the background of a history that divided these responsibilities between states and the national government—not always with the greatest rationality. And that continues; for example, all recent amendments to HIPAA use different standards of preemption, which has immeasurably complicated administration and enforcement of the law and compliance with a myriad of similar state requirements. Optimal rationality that regulates fairly but not redun-

Charles N. Kahn III, president of the Health Insurance Association of America, is a nationally known health policy expert and a seasoned political player both inside the Beltway and beyond. In 1998, he served as HIAA's chief operating officer and president-designate. Mr. Kahn's career has focused principally on health care financing—one of the defining issues of the past two decades.

As senior vice president of policy and general counsel, Dean A. Rosen plays a central role in the policy formation process at the association. He directs the analysis of legislation and regulations for their potential effect on the insurance industry and health care system and oversees the association's policy research agenda. In addition, he represents the association on all legal matters. Mr. Rosen served as health policy counsel to Senate Labor Committee Chairman Nancy Landon Kassebaum during the development of the Health Insurance Portability and Accountability Act (HIPAA).

Marianne Miller, MA, a health economist specializing in health care cost and financing issues, is HIAA's director of federal regulatory affairs and policy development. In this capacity, she helps HIAA member companies understand applicable federal laws, including HIPAA, the Mental Health Parity Act, and the Newborns' and Mothers' Health Protection Act. She is also the primary staff support for member company Medicare + Choice business.

Kathleen H. Fyffe is Federal Regulatory Director at the Health Insurance Association of America (HIAA). She is responsible for a set of issues, including health insurance operations, privacy of health information, electronic data interchange, computerized patient records, provider audit guidelines, and fraud and abuse. Ms. Fyffe has 18 years' experience in the health care industry.

dantly in dividing oversight of health insurance and the delivery of care remains a distant, but still critical, goal for American health care policy.

OVERVIEW

Background of HIPAA

Most people initially think of HIPAA as a relatively modest federal initiative to ensure that Americans can maintain their health coverage if they switch jobs. It is true that the health insurance reform provisions of HIPAA were incremental relative to the Clinton Administration's sweeping Health Security Act, considered by Congress just two years earlier. And, by 1996, most states had already adopted small group insurance reform laws that met or exceeded HIPAA's minimum standards.

But HIPAA marks a dramatic departure both from the McCarran-Ferguson Act of 1945 (P.L. 79-15) and the Employee Retirement Income Security Act of 1974 (ERISA; P.L. 93-406; see also Chapter 66) in providing federal regulatory standards for private health insurance products sold in both the group and individual markets as well as for self-insured employer-sponsored plans.

Starting with the signing into law of HIPAA, states have begun to share power with the numerous federal agencies that now hold some regulatory authority over private health insurance and group health plans. Although the current division of state and federal responsibilities still flows largely from the provisions of McCarran-Ferguson and ERISA, over time HIPAA could dramatically alter the respective regulatory roles of the state and federal governments. This would contrast sharply with the previous two decades, which saw almost no change in the division of regulatory responsibilities over private health insurance and health benefit plans.

Although HIPAA represents a significant precedent, it stands as an even more momentous political paradigm. The architects of HIPAA overcame years of infighting among Congressional committees about who would have jurisdiction over private health insurance reforms.

The legislation also passed with political support (or, at least, without significant political opposition) from consumer groups, employers, unions, governors, state legislators, state insurance regulators, and many in the insurance industry. HIPAA thus stands as a ready-made regulatory framework for future federal health insurance reforms.

In fact, less than two months after HIPAA was signed into law, it was amended to add federal standards for maternity hospital stays and coverage for mental health services.[1] Since then, nearly every one of the dozens of federal legislative proposals in Congress—to mandate insurance coverage for certain health benefits or to impose broad restrictions on managed care practices—has been drafted as an amendment to HIPAA.

Moreover, HIPAA was not limited to health insurance portability and access measures. Its five titles also include tax incentives, anti-fraud and abuse initiatives, and administrative simplification requirements that set into motion still other structural changes (and further political confrontations over issues of health information confidentiality). In addition to rules relating to access to group and individual health insurance, HIPAA gradually increases the deductibility of health insurance for the self-employed, provides tax incentives for the purchase of long-term care insurance, and authorizes a demonstration program for tax-preferred medical savings accounts (MSAs).

The law also creates a framework for developing a national standard for the electronic transmission of health claims data and implements a process for adopting federal rules about the confidentiality of health information. HIPAA contemplated that Congress would enact legislation by August 1999 governing the use of identifiable personal health information. When Congress failed to do so, it then fell to the Secretary of the Department of Health and Human Services (DHHS) to promulgate regulations.

These rules, which affect claims administration, enrollment and disenrollment processes, payment and remittance advice, referrals and authorization certifications, and other matters will significantly affect the day-to-day operations of every health insurer and health plan in the

United States. These regulations—coterminous with existing state laws on patient confidentiality—show some of the pitfalls of a combined state/federal regime. The irrational regulatory structure that will flow from these rules threatens to burden insurers with additional, duplicative, and, perhaps, conflicting administrative responsibilities, unless preemption follows.

It should also be noted that HIPAA's tax code provisions relating to MSAs and long-term care insurance establish a relatively novel mechanism for federal regulation of private health insurance. Under these rules, tax preferences extend only to qualifying policies established in conformity with the requirements set forth in the Internal Revenue Code.

Federal laws such as ERISA imposed certain requirements on employer-sponsored health plans—and therefore indirectly on insurers. In addition, the Consolidated Omnibus Budget Reconciliation Act of 1986 (COBRA, P.L. 99-272) established the right of employees and their families in employer-sponsored health plans with 20 or more employees to continue their coverage under such plans for a limited period if they experienced a change in job or family status. But HIPAA marked the first, direct regulation by the federal government of the business of health insurance.

PROVISIONS: PORTABILITY AND ACCESS

HIPAA is wide-ranging legislation. Yet the public best knows HIPAA for its portability and access provisions, contained in Title I and Title IV. Congress sought to improve access to group and individual health coverage, to ensure "portability" (continuity) of coverage for employees, and to curb discrimination in the group market on the basis of health status. The following discussion links various Title I requirements to one of these broad goals.

Relationship of Federal and State Standards

HIPAA, by adding a number of new federal minimum standards, goes some way toward weighting the balance of regulation on the federal side. State law regulating health insurance is *not* preempted by HIPAA, however, unless imposing the state standard or requirement would prevent the application of a federal requirement established by the Act. The legislative history is quite specific that "the conferees intend the narrowest preemption. State laws that are broader than federal requirements would not prevent the application of federal requirements. For example, while HIPAA requires insurers in the 'small group' market to sell policies to firms with between 2 and 50 employees, states may require guaranteed availability of coverage for groups of more than 50 employees, or for groups of 1."

State laws applicable to preexisting condition exclusions, however, are subject to a different preemption rule. Congress believed that widely differing state rules in this area would be burdensome. Therefore, state laws on preexisting conditions that differ from the standards or requirements specified in the Act are superseded except in certain specified situations.

In short, HIPAA establishes *minimum* federal standards in most areas. With respect to portability and access issues, the Act generally permits states to be more generous in granting protection to consumers.

Who and What Does HIPAA Regulate?

HIPAA's portability and access requirements apply to "group health plans," to "health insurance issuers," and to the health benefits they provide. For HIPAA, a *group health plan* is an employer-sponsored or union-sponsored employee benefit plan (as defined in ERISA) that provides medical care through insurance, reimbursement, or otherwise. *Health insurance issuer* includes an insurance company, an insurance service organization, or a health maintenance organization (HMO). In this discussion, we use "insurer" to refer to health insurance issuers.

The requirements generally do *not* apply to plans providing only "excepted benefits." Examples of excepted benefits include accident or disability income insurance, limited dental or vision benefits, long-term care benefits, coverage for a specified disease or illness, Medicare supplemental insurance, and similar types of coverage. However, to be excepted, plans offering certain of these benefits must meet additional requirements.

One-life groups generally are not subject to the group market requirements. However, a state may choose to extend HIPAA's group similar requirements to insurers with respect to one-life groups. Church plans and government plans generally are subject to the requirements, except that nonfederal government plans may choose to be excluded.

Portability and Access Standards for Groups

HIPAA establishes standards for group health plans and for group health insurance coverage that are intended to enhance access to health coverage. Before HIPAA, many states had enacted similar group market reforms. However, because ERISA preempts state requirements placed on group health plans, these state provisions apply only to insurers and health insurance coverage. Passage of HIPAA was a watershed event because it is the first federal law subjecting all group health plans—including self-insured plans—to minimum standards of accessibility to health coverage.

Nondiscrimination

HIPAA's nondiscrimination provisions aim to enhance access to health coverage in the group market for people with preexisting medical conditions. The Act provides that neither group health plans nor insurers may "establish rules for eligibility (including continued eligibility) of any individual to enroll" in the plan on the basis of any health status factor. This ban applies also to rules that define the waiting periods for enrollment in a plan.

The Act clarifies that the nondiscrimination provisions are not intended to require that a plan provide benefits not otherwise provided under the terms of the contract. Nor are they meant to prevent a plan from "establishing limitations or restrictions on the amount, extent, or nature of the benefits" for similarly situated individuals

who are enrolled in the plan, apart from the specified limitations on preexisting condition exclusions. HIPAA does not dictate plan benefit design but does offer greater access to group insurance. HIPAA's legislative history explains that the intent of these provisions is to prohibit a plan or group insurer from singling out any individual on the basis of health status to deny a benefit ordinarily provided to others the plan covers.

A second nondiscrimination provision prohibits group health plans and insurers from requiring anyone, on the basis of any health status factor, to pay a premium or contribution that is larger than fees charged to a similarly situated individual. Plan sponsors and insurers may still offer premium discounts or modify deductibles and copayments "in return for adherence to programs of health promotion and disease prevention."

The Act broadly defines "health status-related factors" to include: health status, medical condition (including both physical and mental illnesses), claims experience, receipt of health care, medical history, genetic information, evidence of insurability (including conditions arising out of acts of domestic violence), and disability.

Special Enrollment Periods

HIPAA establishes special enrollment periods, when an otherwise eligible employee or dependent who did not take an initial enrollment opportunity is ensured the right to join a plan. Special enrollment periods arise from certain triggering events and generally extend 30 days beyond it. Individuals who enroll during special enrollment periods are *not* considered late enrollees. This is relevant to the length of the allowable preexisting condition exclusion period (see later).

The Act establishes a special enrollment period for employees and dependents who at first declined coverage because they had other coverage (such as through a spouse) and who have since lost eligibility for other coverage (for example, through divorce). The right to a special enrollment period also applies if the "other coverage" was COBRA (or state-mandated) continuation coverage and that coverage is now exhausted. Finally, a special enrollment period must be provided when an employee, whether currently covered or not, gains a new dependent through marriage, birth, or adoption (if the plan covers dependents). With respect to insured coverage only, states may require additional special enrollment periods.

Limits on Preexisting Condition Exclusions

Congress could have simply prohibited the use of preexisting condition exclusions in the group market. Instead, the legislators merely restricted their use. Thus, HIPAA generally preserved incentives for individuals to obtain coverage rather than waiting until illness strikes. Under the Act, preexisting condition exclusions are limited to 12 months (18 months for late enrollees) on the basis of a look-back period of six months. These periods were chosen because, at the time of HIPAA's passage, most states already met or exceeded these standards. No exclusions are allowed for pregnancy or for newborns or adoptees who are covered promptly. Genetic information may not be treated as a preexisting condition "in the absence of a diagnosis of the condition related to such information."

With respect to insured coverage only, states may require shorter exclusion or look-back periods, and they may entirely prohibit the application of preexisting condition exclusions to added situations or conditions.

Crediting Prior Coverage: "Portability"

HIPAA's group market "crediting of prior coverage" requirement ensures "portability" when someone moves into a group health plan from previous health coverage, whether that coverage was group or individual. In popular parlance, individuals are guaranteed "group-to-group portability" and "individual-to-group portability." HIPAA also guarantees "group-to-individual portability" to *certain* individuals, as explained in the section of this chapter on portability for individuals. HIPAA does *not* provide any individual-to-individual portability.

The portability provisions ensure that, regardless of health status, a person who maintains continuous coverage will not face any new preexisting condition exclusion periods—if and when he or she enrolls in a new group health plan. The term "portability" has misled some people, who wrongly believe that HIPAA guarantees that an employee who changes jobs can keep his or her *current* group health coverage. This is not the case. The protection HIPAA offers is more accurately described as health insurance "continuity"—continuous coverage without interruptions for preexisting condition exclusions. Although HIPAA protects continuously covered individuals from having to meet new preexisting condition exclusions, it does not affect an employer's ability to require a "waiting period" before any new employee, regardless of health status, becomes eligible for the group health plan.

Group insurers and group health plan sponsors must credit qualifying ("creditable") prior coverage toward any preexisting condition exclusion period under the plan, as long as coverage has not lapsed for 63 days or longer. (Drafters of the legislation tried to accommodate people who went without coverage for two back-to-back long months such as December and January, or July and August, which total 62 days.) The provision means that insurers must reduce any preexisting condition limitation period by the length of the new enrollee's aggregate period of prior creditable coverage.

Any prior coverage that preceded any 63-day (or longer) break in coverage is not "creditable" under this provision. "Waiting periods" under group health plans and "affiliation periods" for HMOs are not considered lapses in coverage. With respect to insured coverage only, states may allow longer lapses before continuous coverage is broken, setting higher standards than HIPAA if they wish.

"Creditable" prior coverage includes any group coverage (including the Federal Employees' Health Benefits Program [FEHBP; see also Chapter 54] and the Peace Corps, other governmental plans, and church plans), individual coverage, Medicaid, Medicare, military-sponsored health care programs, Indian Health Service or tribal organization coverage, state high-risk pool coverage, or a "public health plan" (as defined in the regulations). Short-term limited coverage is also included as "creditable" coverage.

An individual would establish a creditable coverage period by presenting certifications of previous coverage or through other procedures the regulations specify.

Documenting Prior Coverage

Group insurers and group health plan sponsors are required to provide documentation to individuals whose coverage is terminated. This documentation must include certification of the period of creditable coverage under the plan, the coverage under any applicable COBRA continuation provision, and the waiting period (if any) that the person fulfilled before being allowed to enroll in the plan.

This certification must be provided when the individual ceases to be covered under the plan or otherwise becomes covered under a COBRA continuation provision and after any COBRA continuation coverage ceases. If an individual asks, a second copy must be provided within 24 months after coverage ended. The Secretary of DHHS is required to establish rules to prevent an entity's failure to provide information on health benefits under previous coverage from adversely affecting any subsequent coverage under another group health plan or health insurance.

On request, Medicare, Medicaid, a program of the Indian Health Service or a tribal organization, and military-sponsored health care programs must also provide notice of previous creditable coverage to individuals who leave such coverage.

Guaranteed Renewability of Group Coverage

The Act requires all insurers who offer coverage in connection with group health plans (whether "small" or "large") to renew coverage or continue it in force at the option of the plan sponsor, subject to specified exceptions. Insurers may, however, modify a group health plan's coverage when they renew it. Any modification of a small group's coverage must be consistent with state law and be uniformly effective for all group health plans with that product.

Nonrenewal of groups is allowed for nonpayment of premiums, fraud or intentional misrepresentation, or violation of minimum contribution or participation requirements. Network plans may also not renew or discontinue a group if there is no longer any enrollee in the group who lives, resides, or works in the plan's service area (or in the area where the insurer is authorized to do business).

Nonrenewal is permitted if an insurer is discontinuing *all* coverage in either the large group market or the small group market (or both) in a state. Any such discontinuance must comply with applicable state law, and 180-day prior notice must be given to the state insurance department, plan sponsors, participants, and beneficiaries. The insurer may not reenter that market in that state for five years.

Nonrenewal of a particular *type* of coverage (in either the large group market or the small group market) is also permitted under certain circumstances. "Type of coverage" is not defined in HIPAA. The plan sponsor must receive 90 days' prior notice and "the option to purchase all (or, in the case of the large group market, any) other health insurance coverage currently being offered" by the insurer in that market. The discontinuance must be in accordance with applicable state law and be imposed uniformly— without regard to claims experience or health status. Participants and beneficiaries must also receive 90 days' prior notice.

Multiple Employer Welfare Arrangements (MEWAs) and multi-employer group health plans may not deny an employer continued access to the same or different coverage under the terms of such plans except under certain conditions. The allowable exceptions are basically the same as described previously for insurers.

Guaranteed Availability of Coverage to Small Employers

To ensure access to coverage for small employers, all insurers serving the market of employers with 2 to 50 employees must accept every small employer who applies for coverage and every eligible individual who applies when he or she first becomes eligible.[2] An "eligible individual" is determined by the terms of the group health plan, by the insurer's uniformly applicable rules, and in accordance with all applicable state laws. The federal regulations clarify that insurers must offer to any small employer any product that they make available in the small-group market.

Exceptions to the guarantee-issue requirement are allowed for inadequate network capacity, inadequate financial capacity, or if applicants are located outside the plan's service area. Use of minimum participation or employer contribution requirements is allowed according to applicable state law.

States may, at their option, choose to extend the reach of HIPAA's small group requirements by defining small group to include groups *larger* than 50 employees, and/or one-life groups. Approximately one fourth of the states have extended the definition to include one-life groups for purposes of HIPAA standards.[3]

Disclosing Information by Group Health Plans and Insurers Serving Small Employers

Disclosure requirements are intended to further widen employers' and eligible employees' access to coverage. The Act requires all group health plans to notify participants about material reductions in covered services or benefits within 60 days after such measures are adopted and to include certain other information in the summary plan description.

On request of a small employer, insurers must provide information about the insurer's right to change premium rates (and factors affecting those changes). Insurers must also communicate provisions on renewability and preexisting conditions, as well as the benefits and premiums available "under all health insurance coverage for which the employer is qualified." Further, the availability of this information must be disclosed in solicitation and sales materials directed

to small employers. Proprietary or trade-secret information need not be disclosed.

Portability and Access Standards for Individuals

Under Title I of HIPAA, all health coverage not sponsored by employers or unions is, by default, coverage in the individual market. The Act enhances access for individuals by two means: it guarantees access to coverage for certain "eligible individuals," and it guarantees the renewability of individual market health insurance policies.

HIPAA's individual market reforms do not precisely parallel the Act's reforms for the group market. Provisions pertaining to nondiscrimination, marketwide limitations on preexisting condition exclusions, requirements for crediting prior coverage toward new preexisting condition exclusions, and broad (all small group) guaranteed issue requirements apply to the group market only.

Guaranteed Availability for Certain Individuals

The Act's "group-to-individual portability" provisions proved to be the most politically controversial in the Act, and political compromises led to the establishment of a complex array of state options.

Eligibility for Guaranteed Availability of Coverage

The Act guarantees that, regardless of health status, individuals who have maintained continuous coverage and who then lose coverage under a group health plan may purchase coverage in the individual market. *To be eligible for group-to-individual portability under HIPAA, a person must:*

- have 18 or more months of aggregate creditable coverage; the most recent coverage must have come from a group health plan, governmental plan, or church plan (or health insurance coverage linked to any such plan)

- be ineligible for group health coverage, Medicare Parts A or B, Medicaid (or any successor program)
- lack other health insurance coverage
- have not been terminated from his or her most recent prior coverage for nonpayment of premiums or fraud
- have elected and exhausted COBRA or similar state-mandated continuation coverage if he or she was eligible for it

State Flexibility for Ensuring Availability of Coverage

The Act gives states a choice of alternatives for establishing this guarantee. Under the first, individual market insurers in the state must accept "eligible individuals" who apply for coverage and may impose no preexisting condition exclusions. This is commonly referred to as the "federal fallback" mechanism because a state defaults to it if the state fails to make an explicit decision about how it will provide guaranteed availability.

The second route to guaranteed individual coverage is through a "state alternative mechanism." A state submits a proposed plan to the Secretary of DHHS that, to be acceptable, must meet a number of specified standards. The "federal fallback" requirements do not apply in states that operate an acceptable alternative mechanism.

"Federal Fallback" Guaranteed Availability

The Act requires individual insurers to offer coverage to eligible individuals with no preexisting condition exclusions. An insurer must offer all forms of its currently marketed policies. Alternatively, it may elect to offer as few as two—as long as both are designed for, marketed to, and enroll a cross-section of individuals in the community, not just HIPAA "eligible individuals." The two forms offered under these provisions must be either the insurer's two leading products in the state (by premium volume) or a high option and a low-option representative of other products the insurer sells in the state.

HIPAA's product offering requirements are designed to avoid the segregation of eligible individuals into separate (high-cost) risk pools.

Although HIPAA does not limit the rates insurers may charge for their "portability" products, the legislative history shows that Congress intended that "the risk spreading mechanism and financial subsidization standards provide meaningful financial protection and assistance for eligible individuals."

Alternative State Programs

To qualify as an acceptable alternative to the federal fallback requirements, a state program must give all eligible individuals a choice of coverage without imposing any preexisting condition exclusions. Further, at least one of these choices must provide comprehensive or standard coverage.

General types of state programs that the Secretary of DHHS may find acceptable include health insurance coverage pools or programs, mandatory group conversion policies, guaranteed issue of one or more individual policies, open enrollment by one or more individual insurers, or a combination of such programs. Specifically, a state program may be found acceptable if it is consistent with specified National Association of Insurance Commissioners (NAIC) model acts.

Routes States Chose for Initial HIPAA Implementation

Most states made an explicit decision about whether to adopt the federal fallback standards or to propose an alternative mechanism.[4] Thirty-seven states proposed acceptable alternative mechanisms. Twenty-two of these states chose to provide guaranteed availability through a state high-risk pool, the mechanism several insurance industry groups favored because it provides a broad-based subsidy for this coverage. Thirteen states are operating under the federal fallback guarantee issue requirements—whether intentionally or by default. These state choices have influenced the affordability of the coverage that is available to eligible individuals, as noted later.

Guaranteed Renewability of Individual Coverage

The Act requires guaranteed renewal, or continuation in force, of all products by all individual insurers. Nonrenewal is allowed for non-payment, fraud or misrepresentation, or insurer market exit. Nonrenewal is also permissible in cases in which the individual no longer lives in the network plan's service area or in an area in which the insurer is authorized to do business, or for coverage made available to bona fide associations, if membership in the association ceases.

Documenting Prior Coverage

Individual market insurers are subject to the same requirements as group insurers to provide certificates of creditable coverage to individuals who terminate their coverage with the insurer.

NEW ACCESS INITIATIVES

Medical Savings Accounts

HIPAA established a four-year pilot project, beginning in 1997, for federally tax-favored MSAs, to be used in conjunction with high deductible health insurance coverage. The number of individuals allowed to benefit annually from a tax-favored MSA under the pilot project was capped at approximately 750,000. The pilot project ends on December 31, 2000, after which no new MSAs may be set up.

Under the pilot project, MSAs may be established only by employees covered under an employer-sponsored high-deductible plan of a small employer (50 employees or fewer) and by self-employed individuals covered under a high-deductible plan. To be eligible, such persons must not be covered under any other health plan (with limited exceptions).

The high-deductible plan must meet the following requirements. It must have an annual deductible of at least $1,500 and no more than $2,250 in the case of individual coverage and at least $3,000 and no more than $4,500 for family coverage. In addition, the maximum out-of-pocket expenses with respect to allowed costs (including the deductible) must be no more than $3,000 in the case of individual coverage and no more than $5,500 in the case of family coverage.

For 1999 and later years, these dollar amounts are indexed for inflation.

These requirements emerged from political compromises between those who wanted truly catastrophic coverage with high deductibles and those who feared that consumers would unwittingly take on more liability for medical expenses than they could afford.

Individual contributions to an MSA are deductible (within limits) in determining adjusted gross income for federal income tax purposes. In addition, employer contributions are excludable from an employee's income (within the same limits). The maximum annual contribution that can be made to an MSA is 65 percent of the deductible under the high deductible plan, in the case of individual coverage, and 75 percent of the deductible in family coverage.

Distributions from an MSA for the medical expenses of the individual and his or her spouse or dependents are generally excludable from income. "Medical expenses," although defined as they were in the tax code, did include premiums for long-term care insurance, health care continuation coverage, and health care coverage while a person is receiving unemployment compensation under federal or state law. Distributions that are not for medical expenses are includable in income. Such distributions are also subject to an additional 15 percent tax unless they are made after someone reaches age 65, becomes disabled, or dies.

Proponents of MSAs believe that individuals should, and will, manage their own health care more prudently if they pay everyday medical expenses out-of-pocket. Opponents fear that MSA/high-deductible products will create further risk segmentation of the market, assuming that relatively healthy individuals will purchase MSAs, leaving relatively less healthy people in ever-more-costly comprehensive insurance products.

During the months before and after HIPAA's enactment, MSA proponents speculated that the MSA/high-deductible product would sell extremely well and that the cap on participants would be reached in the first year. In fact, the market response has been surprisingly lackluster, despite wide availability of the product. U.S. Treasury records show that, by the end of 1997, only 41,668 MSAs had been established and that the rate of new MSA openings appeared to be slower in the first half of 1998 than in 1997.[5]

Supporters of the MSA concept believe that the HIPAA pilot project is not a good test of market demand for MSAs because the demonstration design is to blame for the low level of sales. They continue to advocate permanent federal MSA legislation that would make MSA products available to all employees and individuals; the market, not Congress, would determine the level of deductibles and out-of-pocket maximums for the high-deductible policies linked to MSAs.

Health Insurance Tax Deduction for the Self-Employed

The Act increases the percentage of health insurance premium expenses that self-employed individuals can deduct from their income for federal income tax purposes to 40 percent in 1997, 45 percent in 1998 through 2002, and ultimately to 80 percent in 2006 and following years. Two subsequent laws have expanded the favorable tax treatment of premiums paid by self-employed persons. The Balanced Budget Act of 1997 (P.L.105-33) accelerated the phase-in schedule and provided for 100 percent deductibility for 2007 and after. The Omnibus Appropriations Act for FY 1999 (P.L.105-277) again accelerated the phase-in to reach 100 percent deductibility for 2003 and after.

Expansion of COBRA Continuation Coverage

The Act enhanced the continuation of employees' coverage protections contained in COBRA (P.L. 99-272). HIPAA provides that qualified beneficiaries who, under the Social Security Act, are determined to be disabled within the first 60 days of COBRA continuation coverage may buy an additional 11 months of coverage beyond the standard 18-month coverage. Previously, a qualified beneficiary must have been determined to be disabled at the time of the qualifying event to receive 29 months of COBRA continuation coverage. This extension of continuation coverage is also available to the spouse and dependent children of the disabled beneficiary. These extensions were intended to close gaps between the time disabled individuals exhaust their COBRA rights and the time they qualify for Medicare coverage because of disability. In addition, the Act clarifies that children who are born or adopted during the continuation coverage period are to be treated as "qualified beneficiaries."

AMENDMENTS TO HIPAA PORTABILITY AND ACCESS PROVISIONS

In September 1996, a few weeks after HIPAA became law, Congress passed amendments to the new portability and access standards that established federal standards for coverage of hospital stays in connection with childbirth and for coverage of mental health services. A third amendment was enacted in October 1998 that established standards for coverage of postmastectomy reconstructive surgery. To date, all subsequent amendments to HIPAA have used different preemption standards, further complicating the division of regulatory responsibility between the states and the federal government.

Protecting Newborns' and Mothers' Health

The Newborns' and Mothers' Health Protection Act of 1996 (NMHPA) was incorporated into and enacted as part of P.L. 104-204, the Departments of Veterans' Affairs and Housing and Urban Development Appropriations Act of 1997.[6] Its provisions apply to group health plans and to health insurance coverage offered in the group and individual markets.

The NMHPA requires that a group health plan or health insurance coverage that provides maternity (including childbirth) benefits also provide coverage for associated hospital stays. It mandates coverage for at least a 48-hour (for normal vaginal delivery) and 96-hour (for Caesarean section) in-patient stay (with specified exceptions) for a mother and her newborn. The law also requires timely postdelivery care when the mother and newborn are discharged before the minimum length of stay expires. Plan sponsors and insurers are prohibited from using certain types of penalties or inducements that could motivate participants, beneficiaries, policyholders, or providers to circumvent the law's requirements.

Mental Health Parity

In a parallel fashion to the NMHPA, the Mental Health Parity Act of 1996 (MHPA) was also enacted as part of P.L. 104-204, the Departments of Veterans' Affairs and Housing and Urban Development Appropriations Act of 1997.[7] These provisions apply in the group market alone; they do not apply to individual market health insurance coverage. Specifically, the MHPA requirements apply to a group health plan or group health insurance coverage that provides both medical/surgical and mental health benefits. A sunset clause states that these requirements do not apply to benefits furnished on or after September 30, 2001.

The MHPA requires parity in the application of aggregate lifetime dollar limits and annual dollar limits between mental health benefits and medical/surgical benefits. If a group health plan offers two or more benefit packages under the plan, the requirements apply separately to each package.

Importantly, the MHPA does not require a group health plan or group health insurance coverage to provide mental health benefits. Nor does the MHPA affect the terms and conditions[8] relating to the amount, duration, or scope of mental health benefits under a plan (or coverage) except as specifically provided in regard to parity of aggregate lifetime dollar limits and annual dollar limits.

Women's Health and Cancer Rights

The Women's Health and Cancer Rights Act of 1998 (WHCRA) was enacted as part of P.L.105-277, the Omnibus Appropriations Act for Fiscal Year 1999, which became law on Oc-

tober 21, 1998.[9] The WHCRA standards apply to both the group and individual markets.

WHCRA requires that group health plans and health insurance that cover medical and surgical benefits for mastectomies also provide coverage for (1) all stages of breast reconstruction; (2) surgery and reconstruction of the other breast to produce a symmetrical appearance; and (3) prostheses and physical complications of mastectomy, including lymphedema. It requires annual written notice that these benefits are available.

The WHCRA provisions forbid (1) denying to a patient eligibility, or continued eligibility, to enroll or to renew coverage under the terms of the plan, solely for the purpose of avoiding these requirements; and (2) penalizing or otherwise reducing or limiting the reimbursement of an attending provider, or providing incentives (monetary or otherwise) to an attending provider, to induce that person to provide care to an individual participant or beneficiary in a manner inconsistent with these standards.

PROVISIONS: ADMINISTRATIVE SIMPLIFICATION

Background and Importance to Health Care Industry

Federal legislative proposals for administrative simplification (AS) were introduced in several sessions of Congress during the early 1990s. However, not until 1996 were provisions for administrative simplification enacted as part of Title II of HIPAA. These provisions aimed to reduce the costs and administrative burden of health care by enabling the standardized electronic transmission of many administrative and financial transactions formerly handled on paper.

Administrative tasks in the health care industry are manifold. They involve processes such as enrolling persons in health plans, billing or invoicing for services or products provided, and receiving and recording payments. The term "administrative simplification" refers to methods for simplifying or streamlining these processes. Until the 1980s, many processes were performed manually (i.e., on paper) by health care organizations.

Although the industry has significantly increased its automation during the past several years, it has not yet adopted a common standard for electronic communications. There are historic reasons for this. Over the past 20 years, thousands of different types of computer software have come into use among hospitals, physicians' offices, and health plans. The vast diversity of computer systems has resulted in hundreds of ways to communicate electronically, not all of which can communicate with each other.

"Electronic data interchange" (EDI; see also Chapter 35), a method of automating administrative processes, involves communication among computer systems by means of electronic transmission of data formatted into transactions (e.g., the submission of a hospital bill or invoice to an insurance company). EDI formats data in the hospital invoice into a standardized billing transaction.

AS has long been of great importance to the health care industry because of its potential for cutting costs. In 1991, Secretary of DHHS Dr. Louis Sullivan convened a forum of national health care leaders, including insurers, to discuss the challenge of reducing administrative costs in the U.S. system. At the forum, an industry-led Workgroup for Electronic Data Interchange (WEDI) was created and charged to examine the potential for uniform electronic billing.

WEDI assembled a technical advisory group of approximately 50 staff from various parts of the health care industry to analyze the use of technology to streamline health care administration. The Workgroup then issued two significant reports. A key recommendation from its 1992 report exhorted the industry to define and publish standard formats for four core administrative transactions (enrollment, eligibility, claims submission, and remittance advice) through the American National Standards Institute (ANSI) Accredited Standards Committee (ASC X12) Insurance Subcommittee.[10] The 1993 WEDI Report expanded its recommendations to include additional transactions and estimates of admin-

istrative savings. WEDI estimated that if administrative transactions were implemented through electronic data interchange, cumulative net savings would amount to $42 billion over a six-year period.[11]

Specific Administration Simplification Provisions in HIPAA

HIPAA's administrative simplification provisions include national standards for electronic transactions and standards to guarantee the security and privacy of health information. The law generally supersedes state laws pertaining to administrative simplification processes. Although HIPAA's provisions for national electronic standards mandate compliance by health insurers, health plans, and public payers, the standards are permissive with respect to providers and employers.

The law includes monetary penalties for noncompliance with national electronic standards and both monetary penalties and possible imprisonment for violating privacy standards. Although the original timetable for implementing administrative simplification was the year 2000, that deadline has slipped; the expected implementation date is 2002, according to the schedule posted on the DHHS web site:http//aspe. hhs.gov/admnsimp.

The law also includes requirements to maintain the physical security of health information. These requirements apply to any person or organization that maintains or transmits electronic health information. The law outlines standards for maintaining reasonable and appropriate administrative, technical, and physical safeguards. The safeguards aim to protect the physical security and integrity of personal health information from threats, hazards, or unauthorized uses.

The specific health care industry business transactions set forth in HIPAA include:[12]

- ***Health claims or equivalent encounter information***—a transaction used to submit health care claim billing information, encounter information, or both, from health care providers to health plans.

- *Health claims attachments*—a transaction used to transmit health care service information, such as subscriber, patient, demographic, diagnosis, or treatment data for the purpose of a request for review, certification, notification, or reporting the outcome of a health care services review.
- *Enrollment and disenrollment in a health plan*—a transaction used to establish communication between the sponsor of a health benefit and the health plan. It provides enrollment data, such as on the subscriber and dependents, as well as information on employers and health care providers. The "sponsor" is the backer of the coverage, benefit, or product. A sponsor can be an employer, union, government agency, association, or insurance company. The health plan refers to an entity that pays claims, administers the insurance product or benefit, or both.
- *Eligibility for a health plan*—a transaction used to inquire about the eligibility, coverage, or benefits associated with a benefit plan, employer, plan sponsor, subscriber, or a dependent under the subscriber's policy. It also can be used to communicate information about, or changes in, eligibility, coverage, or benefits—information from sources such as insurers, sponsors, and health plans, that is sent to recipients such as physicians, hospitals, third-party administrators, and government agencies.
- *Health care payment and remittance advice*—a transaction used by a health plan to make a payment to a health care provider, or to send an explanation of benefits or remittance advice to a health care provider, or to send both payment and data to a health care provider.
- *Health plan premium payments*—a transaction used by employers, employees, unions, associations or other entities to make and keep track of payments of health plan premiums to health insurers.
- *First report of injury*—a transaction used to report information about an injury, illness, or incident to entities interested in the information for statistical, legal, claims, and risk management purposes.
- *Health claim status*—a transaction used by health care providers and recipients of health care products or services to request from a health plan the status of a health care claim or encounter.
- *Referral certification and authorization*—a transaction used to transmit health care service referral information among health care providers, health care providers furnishing services, and health plans. It may also be used to obtain authorization for certain health care services from a health plan.

The implementing regulations for national standards for these business transactions include detailed technical specifications for both the data fields contained in a transaction and for the electronic format for transmitting a transaction.

HIPAA addresses the confidentiality of health information by prohibiting wrongful disclosures of individually identifiable health information. Unlike the other parts of the administrative simplification title, however, the confidentiality provisions do not supersede all state laws about privacy of health information.

Last, HIPAA creates two new types of identification numbers: one for providers, the other for payer organizations. The National Provider ID (NPID) will replace the current Universal Provider ID (UPID or UPIN) and will be required for all providers (using a broad definition of provider), will be unique, and will be phased in starting with providers affected by HIPAA immediately (e.g., Medicare HMO providers), and then rolled out to all providers. The NPI will use the taxonomy of the ANSI (ASC) X 12N standards. Further information may be found at www.medicarestats@hcfa.gov.

For health plans, the new PlanID is also part of HIPAA and will be rolled out over the next several years, although the timing is as yet unknown at the time of this writing. The PlanID will serve as a new form of identification for payer organizations (broadly defined) and will also serve as a directory, telephone directory, and database for all payer organizations. It will replace the current numbering and naming conventions used today for all electronic health care transactions. The PlanID assigned to an entity will be retired and never used again if the entity associated with the number ceases to exist (e.g., mergers, buy-outs). The PlanID may be used to determine an entity's processing locations and may be used to identify addresses for the routing of different types of health plans (HMO, PPO, etc.). Further information may be found at www.hlthplan@hcfa.gov.

What Administrative Simplification Means for Payers, Providers, and Other Health Care Organizations

The HIPAA administrative simplification requirements are mandatory for health insurers, health plans, and health care clearinghouses; the term "health care clearinghouse" means a public or private entity that processes or facilitates the processing of nonstandard data elements of health information into standard data elements. Such clearinghouses function as middlemen between providers and payers. For example, a provider might send nonstandard claims information to a clearinghouse, which transforms it into standard information and transmits it to a payer.

The HIPAA administrative simplification requirements are not mandatory for providers. However, if a provider wishes to transmit any health information in electronic form, the transaction must be in the named national standard electronic format.

Collectively, HIPAA's administrative simplification provisions could vastly increase administrative efficiency and reduce costs for the health care industry. Potential savings are huge, largely because the health care sector has not fully automated as quickly as some other industries. In banking, for example, administrative transactions such as consumer cash deposits, withdrawals, and transfers, are highly automated; some can even be performed on the Internet. Financial institutions routinely exchange funds and information electronically. By contrast, the health care industry's administrative transactions, such as claims submissions

and payments to providers, remain paper-intensive. Although improvements exist, many health care organizations cannot yet exchange information or conduct routine transactions electronically.

Confidentiality

There are hundreds of state laws about "confidentiality"[13] or "privacy"[14] of health information. These laws are not uniform and many overlap with one another. The laws include a variety of provisions such as corrections to erroneous medical information, disclosure of individually identifiable health information, disclosure of drug and alcohol abuse records, and disposing of medical records during acquisitions, mergers, and closings.

Federal laws address confidentiality of health information for patients in federal health programs such as Medicare,[15] but HIPAA is the only federal law that addresses the confidentiality of this information in the private sector. HIPAA took up confidentiality of certain health information in several provisions. The law required the Secretary of DHHS to submit to Congress detailed recommendations on standards of confidentiality for individually identifiable health information, and these standards have been put forth for public commentary as of late 1999. HIPAA also mandated that federal confidentiality regulations would not supersede contrary provisions of state law if states imposed more stringent requirements or standards.

Effects of Administrative Simplification

The national standards for electronic business transactions are expected to have a positive effect on the administrative tasks of the health care industry. Although many health industry organizations currently use electronic transactions to conduct business, use of national standard electronic formats is not widespread. After HIPAA's administrative simplification provisions are fully implemented, the current growth rate for use of electronic transactions is expected to accelerate so that there will be far fewer manual paper transactions than there are today. This transition from paper-bound systems to automated electronic systems is expected to reduce administrative costs.

As a public policy issue, confidentiality of health information has been politically controversial for many years. Consumer advocacy groups have expressed concerns that health care organizations do not consistently maintain adequate privacy safeguards for individually identifiable health information. Part of these concerns might exist because there is no one federal law for confidentiality of health information, instead there is a vast array of state confidentiality laws. Although federal legislative proposals for confidentiality of health information have been introduced several times in past congresses, no law has been enacted. Congress attempted to address the issue by mandating in HIPAA a certain time frame during which either Congress needed to act or the DHHS would promulgate federal regulations. Congressional enactment of a federal law did not occur according to the mandated time frame so DHHS is now responsible for promulgating federal regulations for confidentiality of health information.

The public's discomfort about the HIPAA's administrative simplification provision for a unique health identifier for individual persons is another example of the controversy surrounding confidentiality of health information. This discomfort compelled Congress to prohibit funding for the unique identifier. The Omnibus Consolidated and Emergency Supplemental Appropriations Act for Fiscal Year 1999 (P.L. 105-277) ("the Act") provided that none of the funds under the Act may be used to promulgate or adopt any final standard for a unique health identifier for an individual until legislation approving the standard is enacted.

HIPAA ADMINISTRATION AND ENFORCEMENT

Portability and Access

In many ways HIPAA is an unusual federal law, whose implementation has placed substantial demands on all parties involved. Each challenge to successful implementation that this sec-

tion describes was aggravated by the short timetable the statute mandated.

Congress directed three federal agencies (the Departments of Labor, Treasury, and DHHS) to coordinate with each other—a relatively unprecedented demand—in developing regulatory guidance for employers and insurers. But because HIPAA became the first major federal regulation of group health plans and private health insurance, the agencies lacked a large pool of federal employees knowledgeable about the private insurance market to draw on in drafting guidance.

The law contemplated state rather than federal administration and enforcement of the requirements it placed on insurers. For that to happen, however, each state had to adopt the federal standards, at minimum, in its own state law. Alternatively, states could adopt even more stringent standards. The flexibility Congress thereby gave to states in implementing HIPAA's group-to-individual portability guarantee challenged them greatly.

Complying with HIPAA's requirements has been a complicated task for insurers, particularly for multi-state insurers. Because of the statute's *narrow* preemption of state laws, the federal law establishes minimum, not uniform, federal insurance standards. As a result of this and the state flexibility regarding group-to-individual portability, insurers face a confusing patchwork of insurance standards that vary from state to state.

With few exceptions, states accepted the challenge of adopting and administering HIPAA (or more stringent) insurance standards, primarily to preserve the state's traditional role as insurance regulator. Nearly all states had already enacted HIPAA-like standards in their small group insurance markets; minor adjustments, if any, were needed to conform their state laws to HIPAA.

The individual market standards presented greater difficulty because HIPAA allowed significantly different approaches. A political impasse prevented some states from enacting necessary legislative provisions in time to meet the federal statutory deadline. Fairly early in 1997, Missouri and Rhode Island notified the DHHS that they would not be enacting conforming legislation and that, therefore, they would not be administering the federal standards. HIPAA's fallback is federal enforcement, so the Health Care Financing Administration (HCFA) in DHHS was forced to step in. Uncertainty persisted in a number of other states as to whether the state or DHHS would be responsible for HIPAA oversight. As time passed, it became clear that Michigan, California, Massachusetts, Vermont, and several U.S. territories also required federal enforcement of all, or at least some, of HIPAA's insurance standards.

Federal enforcement on this scale was not anticipated. Because of insufficient HCFA resources, full implementation and oversight have lagged, possibly causing missed opportunities for consumers and creating hardships for federal officials and insurers. Insurers have experienced delays and uncertainties, and in some cases they have been compelled to mount significant efforts to educate federal officials (central and regional office personnel) about the private insurance market.

The continuing need for education about HIPAA's requirements is a theme sounded repeatedly in the General Accounting Office (GAO) reports on implementation of the law— education not only for government officials at both state and federal levels but also for consumers, providers, and insurance agents.

Administrative Simplification

DHHS is responsible for administering and enforcing the administrative simplification provisions of HIPAA. The law includes two categories of penalties: (1) penalties for failure to comply with requirements and standards; and (2) penalties for wrongful disclosure of individually identifiable health information. In general, DHHS may impose a penalty of not more than $100 for each violation involving noncompliance with standards, except that the total amount imposed on a person during a calendar year may not exceed $25,000. The penalties for wrongful disclosure of individually identifiable health information include fines ranging from $50,000 to $250,000 and possible imprisonment for up to 10 years.

AN EARLY REPORT ON THE EFFECTS OF HIPAA PORTABILITY AND ACCESS PROVISIONS

To what extent has HIPAA fulfilled its promise to enhance access to health insurance and diminish "job lock"—the commonly cited situation in which people remain in jobs mostly because they fear losing or interrupting their health benefits? How has it affected insurers and group health plans?

It is still early to assess HIPAA's impact. The individual market provisions took effect July 1, 1997, and the group market provisions between July 1, 1997, and June 30, 1998, depending on a group health plan's fiscal year. Some evidence of HIPAA's impact is available, however, and several problems have been identified.

We should point out at the outset that there is much that HIPAA has not done—and was not intended to do, however urgent the need. Most importantly, it was not designed to make health insurance affordable for everyone—yet this is the highest barrier to coverage for many individuals and small employers. In recent years, there has been an empirical recognition (perhaps, even an emerging consensus) that expanded coverage is best achieved through financial incentives and direct subsidies rather than regulatory requirements alone.

Impact on Insurers

The first year of HIPAA implementation placed heavy demands on insurers. The federal implementation timeline was short, and the law is complex—a challenge even for lifelong insurance professionals to master. Further, each state has adopted its own approach, resulting in different HIPAA standards from state to state. Maintaining compliance over time also means that insurers— particularly those operating in many states—will incur higher regulatory compliance costs.

A Changing Market Environment

Many insurers are apprehensive because HIPAA has increased the risk of adverse selection in the small group market and in the individual market in states that adopted some variation of the "federal fallback" guarantee issue requirement. Under HIPAA, small group insurers must offer *all* their small group products on a guaranteed-issue basis. Thus, small groups are able to move in and out of the market or between less comprehensive and more comprehensive coverage according to the medical needs of their employees. The fact that HIPAA prohibits preexisting condition exclusions for maternity benefits increases these risks. Individual market insurers in states that require guaranteed issue to HIPAA "eligible individuals" are forced to make trade-offs between affordability for high-risk guaranteed issue applicants and affordability for current policyholders. Although no evidence exists that HIPAA, per se, has resulted in insurers leaving certain markets because of these increased risks, it may well have been a contributing factor.

Certificates of Coverage

Insurers have strongly objected to HIPAA's requirement that insurers (or group health plans) produce and mail millions of "certificates of creditable coverage" to individuals who leave their current coverage. Insurers argue that the requirement is unnecessary, and it is very costly. Before HIPAA, insurers administered "portability" requirements in many states without problems through simple and direct communications between the former insurer and the new one.

Moreover, few certificates issued to individuals are needed and used. Most people who switch jobs do not have preexisting medical conditions. Further, the use of preexisting condition exclusions by group health plans is increasingly rare. Already uncommon in group plans, such exclusions became even more likely candidates for extinction after HIPAA; many other group health plans have now dropped them.

Industry versus Federal Agency Regulatory Interpretations

Another troublesome aspect of HIPAA implementation has been HCFA's regulatory interpretation of certain provisions, especially the individual market guaranteed renewal requirement. HCFA has stated in regulations that, regardless of the terms of the insurance contract, insurers must renew individual policies indefinitely (e.g., beyond age 65) at the option of the policyholder.

HCFA's interpretation of "guaranteed renewability" is at odds with state insurance regulation, which generally has recognized the legitimacy of "conditions of eligibility" for insurance coverage such as attaining the age of 65. Coverage under such a policy is terminated because the policyholder is no longer eligible for the policy; it is not viewed as a nonrenewal. HCFA's interpretation also fails to harmonize with the congressional mandate that insurance coverage that supplements Medicare be limited to the 10 standardized Medigap policies. (Similarly, Congress has prohibited insurers from *selling* to seniors private insurance coverage other than an approved Medigap policy, but now HCFA requires *renewal* of non-Medigap [individual] policies.)

There is continuing uncertainty about how HIPAA affects certain other insurance operations. Two examples are the status of state discontinuance and replacement laws vis-à-vis HIPAA's "nondiscrimination in enrollment" standard and the application of IIIPAA to college plans and other specialty markets. In these areas, further clarification would help insurers and consumers alike.

Benefits to Individuals

Group-to-Individual Portability

HIPAA clearly has worked effectively in specific instances, enabling some persons with serious medical conditions to obtain individual market coverage that otherwise would have been unavailable. A March 1999 report documents

The Role of the Federal Government before HIPAA

States, not the federal government, have had responsibility for the regulation of health insurance by virtue of the McCarran-Ferguson Act of 1945 (P.L. 79-15), which exempts insurers from federal antitrust regulation to the extent that insurance is regulated by the states and indicates that no federal law should be interpreted as overriding state insurance regulation unless it does so explicitly. The Act did not prevent the federal government from regulating insurance in the future; it merely affirmed that the government had so far abstained from doing so. Three decades later the federal government began to encroach on state jurisdiction; significant legislation included the HMO Act of 1973, ERISA, the Medigap amendments of 1980 and 1990, and now HIPAA.

This chapter discusses regulation of the private health insurance market. It does not address regulation of health plans in publicly funded programs such as Medicare and Medicaid, which are discussed separately in Chapters 55 through 57. In general, the federal government regulates health plans sponsored (i.e., self-insured) by private employers. The states regulate the business of insurance, including traditional indemnity plans, health maintenance organizations (HMOs), preferred provider organizations (PPOs), and other types of managed care organizations (MCOs) that take risk for medical costs and sell health insurance coverage to individuals, employers, or other purchasers. States also oversee plans sponsored by state and local governments.

If a private-sector employer sponsors a plan that is not purchased from an insurer (i.e., the plan is self-insured under ERISA, even if it is administered by a commercial insurance company or MCO), the plan is regulated solely by the federal government. If a private-sector employer contracts with an insurer to provide managed care to that individual's workers, regulation of that plan will depend on which entity bears the risk. State regulation can have a significant, if indirect, effect on self-insured health plans. For example, to achieve administrative simplicity, insurers offering both insured products and administrative services in connection with self-insured employer-sponsored plans in a state may comply with a state's requirements for appeals procedures for both the insured product and in administering the self-insured plan.

There is no doubt that ERISA has exerted significant impact on the private health care market during the past two decades. Although the legislative debate leading to its passage emphasized pension provisions, drafters of the 1974 law also clearly intended to build a workable framework of federal rules for all private employer-sponsored welfare benefit plans (including health plans). The framework intended to balance consumer protection with incentives that encouraged employers to offer benefits voluntarily.

ERISA leaves the content and design of employer-sponsored health plans largely to employers in negotiation with workers. It does, however, establish certain regulations for health benefit plans. These relate to reporting and disclosure, fiduciary standards, claims review, and enforcement. ERISA also offers limited protection against discrimination to participants in employer-sponsored plans. (Exempt from ERISA are government plans, church plans, and plans offered by fraternal organizations, in which no employer-employee relationship exists.)

Although Congress generally permits states to enact legislation that does not conflict with federal law, ERISA more broadly preempts most state laws that "relate to" employee benefit plans. State laws regulating the business of insurance, banking, and securities are saved from preemption through ERISA's "savings clause." But states are prohibited from defining self-insured employers as insurers to bring them under state jurisdiction. As a consequence of ERISA's preemption provisions, employers that self-insure are exempt from state regulatory requirements such as taxes on insurance premiums, requirements that health plans include specific benefits or pay specific providers, solvency and funding standards, requirements to participate in the financing of state risk pools, and laws regulating various characteristics and actions of managed care plans.

Before ERISA, nearly all health benefits were provided through state-regulated insurers. But self-insurance has grown steadily over the past two decades, driven by employers' need to control cash flow more directly and their desire to avoid experience rating, state-mandated benefits, and taxes. Equally important, self-insurance gives employers greater freedom to offer innovative, cost-effective benefits and (for those with multi-state operations) greater ease of administration. About 50 percent of employees with health coverage are now estimated to be in self-insured plans.

that 527 HIPAA-eligible individuals were enrolled in Pennsylvania between January 1 and October 31, 1998; Texas issued coverage to 1,773 HIPAA-eligible individuals between January 1 and August 31, 1998; and Illinois had covered 1,699 HIPAA-eligible individuals by October 31, 1998.[16]

As the industry had predicted, states that relied on state comprehensive health insurance (high-risk) pools—where premiums were restricted to no more than 200% of standard—were relatively successful in implementing group-to-individual portability. And, as predicted, states that relied on guaranteed issue requirements on individual market insurers fared less well.[17] A risk-based premium for many HIPAA-eligible individuals necessarily would be relatively high. The federal statute placed no restrictions on rates insurers may charge for these policies, and very few states applied restrictions. The GAO reported in February 1998 that some insurers were pricing these products at 140 percent to 600 percent of the standard rate. Consequently, HIPAA portability coverage may have been financially out of reach for many people in those states. This has been a topic of some debate in the Congress, but no legislative action has resulted as of 1999.

Releasing the "Job Lock"

HIPAA's portability requirement that reduces or eliminates group health plan preexisting condition exclusions undoubtedly has paved the way for some previously "job-locked" workers to change jobs. Also, because the HIPAA portability provisions effectively cancel out preexisting condition exclusions for many new employees, group health plans are increasingly eliminating them entirely. A 1998 survey conducted by Charles D. Spencer & Associates found that the proportion of group health plans with no preexisting condition exclusions jumped from 30 percent before HIPAA to nearly 50 percent after HIPAA's enactment.[18]

Some argue that, in the big picture, HIPAA has not successfully addressed the job lock problem.[19] The high premiums for portability coverage found in some states (discussed above) may be a significant barrier for certain employees who may want to take early retirement, become self-employed, or move to employment that offers no health benefits. Prospective employers may offer health benefits but with less generous coverage than an employee currently enjoys. Also, considerable evidence suggests that many employees do not yet adequately understand the guarantees that HIPAA does provide.[20]

Greater Access for Small Groups

HIPAA established guaranteed availability of coverage for small groups of from 2 to 50 persons in all states. This seems to have expanded coverage for employees in small companies perhaps less broadly than expected. For one thing, many states had already established guaranteed availability for small groups; by 1995, 36 states had already enacted small-group guaranteed issue.[21] More open access to small employer groups, however, may have had the positive effect of bringing more Americans under the umbrella of some type of health insurance. One research study suggests that guaranteed issue in the small group market may lower rates of noninsurance.[22]

Public education about the new law has been spotty. To reach its full potential, HIPAA must be better understood by consumers, insurance agents, and employers. The Department of Labor has made a strong effort to educate its constituency of workers and employers about the law's provisions, but it is difficult to reach the millions of employers and individuals who need a better understanding of HIPAA. The GAO has recommended that the occasion of issuing certificates of coverage be used as an opportunity to educate consumers about their insurance choices.[23]

CONCLUSION

With HIPAA as a model, Congress has shown growing interest in legislation that applies federal minimum requirements to all health plans and to extending regulations to both insured and self-insured health plans. Congress is equally interested in giving states the flexibility to apply their own laws if these are consistent with—or, in some legislative proposals, more restrictive than—the federal standard. This approach is reflected in both HIPAA and the Medigap rules.

Thus, both in Congress and in the states, legislators are pushing the outer limits of their regulatory bounds to enact legislation that seems more and more redundant. Often, such legislation inadvertently imposes costly, onerous requirements on the private health insurance market. Moreover, state-born insurance regulations and mandates are rapidly making their way to the nation's capital—and being taken quite seriously for the first time. For example, federal maternity stay legislation passed Congress less than two years after the first state adopted similar legislation. The same pattern is becoming clear with other mandates, such as mastectomy length-of-stay and "anti-gag-clause" legislation.[24] Discussion of these and other state initiatives is found in Chapter 69.

Because of HIPAA and the amendments that followed it, influence flows from Washington, D.C. to the states, as well. During their most recent legislative sessions, many states reexamined their small group and individual market reform laws and reconsidered mental health parity proposals. Some states later enacted laws that surpassed the federal law's minimum standards.

In sum, HIPAA represents the federal desire to have more weight in health insurance regulation—not because of the insurance aspect so much as the public's preoccupation with improved health care. This chapter's early report on HIPAA's effects finds the legislation's possible redundancy and regulatory burden on the health care marketplace its most negative probable consequence, even though the law faithfully reflects Americans' preoccupation with access to quality health care for every citizen.

Affordability remains the greatest barrier to covering more Americans with health insurance.[25] It is the most significant obstacle to small employers in covering more workers; it is a problem for individuals that move out of group coverage. Although they are now guaranteed eligibility for some type of coverage, its affordability is not assured. HIPAA does not, and was not intended to, deal with the affordability problem, but it is difficult to imagine that Congress will not return to the issue.

REFERENCES AND NOTES

1. Another federal mandate was added in 1998 with passage of the Women's Health and Cancer Rights Act (discussed later in this chapter), included as sections 901–903 of the Omnibus Consolidated Appropriations Act for Fiscal Year 1999 (P.L. 105-277).

2. This aligned with how most states had defined "small employers"—those with up to 50 workers—in small-group reforms enacted before HIPAA. The Senate bill would have applied this provision to all employers, both small and large. As a political compromise, the Act targets this guarantee to small employers, but requires DHHS to monitor the market and report periodically on the need for large-group protections. A July 1998 study by the General Accounting Office confirmed that large employers were having no difficulty in obtaining coverage. See U.S. General Accounting Office, July 1998. *Employment-Based Health Insurance: Medium and Large Employers Can Purchase Coverage, But Some Workers Are Not Eligible.* GAO/HEHS-98-184.

3. Health Care Financing Administration, September 17, 1999. Health Insurance Standards Bulletin 99-03.

4. U.S. General Accounting Office, May 20, 1998. *Implementation of HIPAA: State-Designed Mechanisms for Group-to-Individual Portability.* GAO/HEHS-98-161R.

5. U.S. General Accounting office, December 1998. *Medical Savings Accounts: Results from Surveys of Insurers.* GAO/HEHS-99-34: 12.

6. P.L. 104-204 amended ERISA and the PHSA to add newborns; and mothers; health protection standards. Corresponding IRC amendments were contained in P.L. 105-34, the Taxpayers' Relief Act of 1997.

7. P.L. 104-204 amended ERISA and the PHSA to add mental health parity standards. Corresponding IRC amendments were contained in P.L. 105-34, the Taxpayers' Relief Act of 1997.

8. "Terms and conditions" of mental health benefit offerings include cost-sharing, limits on the number of visits or days of coverage, and requirements relating to medical necessity, prior authorization for treatment, or primary-care physicians' referrals of individuals for treatment.

9. P.L. 105-277 amended ERISA and the PHSA to add women's health and cancer rights standards. Corresponding IRC provisions had not been enacted at the time of this writing.

10. Workgroup for Electronic Data Interchange, July 1992. *Report to Secretary of U.S. Department of Health and Human Services:* 11.

11. Workgroup for Electronic Data Interchange, October 1993. *Report to Secretary of U.S. Department of Health and Human Services:* 14.

12. *Federal Register,* May 7, 1998. Health Insurance Reform: Standards for Electronic Transaction; National Standard Health Care Provider Identifier: Proposed Rules, 15178–79.

13. The term "confidential" is defined to be anything that contains information whose unauthorized disclosure could be prejudicial.

14. The term "private" is defined to be anything that is intended for, or restricted to, the use of a particular person, group, or class.

15. Federal laws such as Section 1106 of the Social Security Act, the Freedom of Information Act, the Privacy Act, and the Computer Security Act.

16. Bob Carlson, What's Happened to HIPAA in the Real World? *Business and Health.* March (1999): 52–59.

17. Health Insurance Association of America, September 15, 1997. *Statement on Implementation of the HIPAA by Bill Gradison, HIAA President, before the House Ways and Means Committee, Subcommittee on Health.*

18. Spencer study noted in Carlson 1999: 54.

19. Employee Benefit Research Institute, August 7, 1998. Job Lock: Not Diminished by New HIPAA Law, *Employee Benefit Research Institute News.*

20. U.S. General Accounting Office, May 12, 1999. *Private Health Insurance: Progress and Challenges in Implementing 1996 Federal Standards.* GAO/HEHS-99-100.

21. U.S. General Accounting Office, 1995. *Health Insurance Portability: Reform Could Ensure Continued Coverage for Up to 15 Million Americans.* GAO/HEHS-99-257.

22. L.M. Nichols and L.J. Blumberg, A Different Kind of "New Federalism"? The Health Insurance Portability and Accountability Act of 1996, *Health Affairs,* May/June (1998): 25–42.

23. U.S. General Accounting Office, May 12, 1999. *Private Health Insurance: Progress and Challenges in Implementing 1996 Federal Standards.* GAO/HEHS-99-100.

24. The "gag clause" refers to rules of some health maintenance organizations that forbid physicians to communicate to patients the full range of treatment options that may be effective.

25. *See* William S. Custer, Ph.D., *Health Insurance Coverage and the Uninsured,* prepared for the Health Insurance Association of America, 1999.

CHAPTER 68

Health Plan Corporate Compliance Programs

Mike Treash

Corporate compliance is the process of managing an organization's conformance to legal and regulatory requirements and preventing and detecting illegal behavior. Corporate compliance is a discipline in that it is transferable across industries and across legal and regulatory requirements. It is important to separate corporate compliance from legal and regulatory compliance. Corporate compliance is concerned with how management influences compliance and monitors and detects noncompliance. In contrast, legal and regulatory compliance deals with implementing and meeting specific requirements.

The value of corporate compliance is in promoting the effective management of legal and regulatory risks across the organization. The Office of Inspector General (OIG) of the U.S. Department of Health and Human Services (DHHS), in releasing its guidance, indicated it believes that requiring health care organizations to implement a compliance plan can be a "mechanism for improving the quality, productivity, and efficiency of the health care industry."[1] The government, from its perspective, benefits greatly by promoting health plan self-compliance with consumer protection requirements and public program safeguards.

By releasing its guidance on corporate compliance programs, the federal government essentially created a new senior management position,

the corporate compliance officer (CCO). The guidance, although mandatory for Medicare + Choice contracting health plans, is voluntary for all other health insurers. The fiduciary incentive for the health plan leadership to develop a corporate compliance program is to reduce the risk of legal and regulatory sanctions. The OIG and the Justice Department look for evidence of an effective corporate compliance program when they assess penalties to health plans that have violated federal law.

The most commonly cited benefits of corporate compliance are the avoidance of legal and regulatory difficulty and the reduction of penalties if in violation of the law. Those benefits are mostly avoidance of the downside risks, not benefits that will necessarily grow a business or increase profits. At a minimum, the upside of corporate compliance is an efficiently run office that keeps the organization out of legal and regulatory difficulty at the least cost. If used most effectively, corporate compliance improves communication, enhances learning, reinforces an ethical culture, aligns measures and incentives, and provides structure to legal and regulatory issues.

CORPORATE COMPLIANCE ON PAPER

Although corporate compliance may be new to many health plans, providers are familiar with corporate compliance programs. The OIG has already released similar guidance for hospitals, home health agencies, and third-party billing companies. The reason the OIG has focused

---

Kenneth M. (Mike) Treash is a Senior Manager in Ernst & Young's Health Care Advisory Services practice working primarily in the area of managed care corporate compliance.

more on providers is due to its role in protecting federal programs from fraud and abuse. The OIG, working with the Department of Justice and the DHHS has actively and successfully identified, prosecuted, and recouped large monetary recoveries from health care providers who have overbilled the Medicare and Medicaid programs. The OIG has not been focused on health plans mainly because the risk-financing arrangements in the Medicare and Medicaid programs provide clear opportunities for health plans to falsely bill the government. While the OIG planned to prepare guidance for health plans, the Health Care Financing Administration (HCFA) forced the issue by requiring Medicare + Choice contracting health plans to have a corporate compliance program in place by January 1, 2000. The OIG released its guidance on health plan corporate compliance in June 1999. The guidance was directed to Medicare + Choice contracting health plans for whom it is mandatory. The elements the OIG looks for when evaluating an effective corporate compliance program are described in Exhibit 68–1.

The OIG's guidance is based on the U.S. Sentencing Guidelines developed by the U.S. Sentencing Commission. The U.S. Sentencing Commission is an independent agency in the federal judicial system. Among its various roles, the Commission establishes sentencing policies and practices for the federal courts, including guidelines prescribing the form and severity of punishment for offenders convicted of federal crimes, for application to both individuals and organizations. The Sentencing Commission guidelines provide that the fine range for organizations in violation of federal law "should be based on the seriousness of the offense and the culpability of the organization."[2] In assessing culpability the Commission looks to "the steps taken by the organization prior to the offense to prevent and detect criminal conduct, the level and extent of involvement in or tolerance of the offense by certain personnel, and the organization's actions after an offense has been committed."[3]

CORPORATE COMPLIANCE IN OPERATION

The most important attribute a corporate compliance officer can possess is the ability to manage and execute. It is a competency more important than legal and regulatory knowledge,

---

Exhibit 68–1 OIG Corporate Compliance Guidance Office of the Inspector General, 1999

1. The development and distribution of written standards of conduct, as well as written policies and procedures, that promote the organization's commitment to compliance and that address specific areas of potential fraud
2. The designation of a chief compliance officer and other appropriate bodies, e.g., a corporate compliance committee, charged with the responsibility of operating and monitoring the compliance program and who report directly to the CEO and the governing body
3. The development and implementation of regular, effective education and training programs for all affected employees
4. The development of effective lines of communication between the compliance officer and all employees, including a process, such as a hotline, to receive complaints (and the adoption of procedures to protect the anonymity of complainants and to protect callers from retaliation)
5. The use of audits or other risk evaluation techniques to monitor compliance and assist in the reduction of identified problem areas
6. The development of disciplinary mechanisms to consistently enforce standards and the development of policies addressing dealings with sanctioned and other specified individuals
7. The development of policies to respond to detected offenses and to initiate corrective action to prevent similar offenses

Source: Reprinted from the Office of the Inspector General, Department of Health and Human Services.

industry background, or legal or audit training. The compliance officer manages the company's legal and regulatory risk. The compliance officer is a proponent for an ethical work culture. The compliance officer, when a legal or regulatory problem occurs, manages the company's investigation and response to enforcement agencies and imposes penalties and corrective actions within the organization. The components of the OIG's basic corporate compliance guidance has striking similarity to the components of organizational development models. Organizational development theory suggests that managers have at their disposal basic tools or drivers that they use to influence employee behavior. These performance drivers include structure, leadership, education and development, measures and incentives, staffing, and communication.[4] At a minimum, a compliance officer must possess some legal and regulatory knowledge and industry experience. The difference between an average corporate compliance officer and a highly effective compliance officer may be the ability of the compliance officer to recognize and use these performance drivers.

STRUCTURE

By issuing guidance on corporate compliance, the federal government essentially told health plans to put some structure to their legal and regulatory services. This maturation in the form of structure includes creating a board-level compliance committee, appointing a senior-level individual with credentials in compliance and supporting the CCO with an office and authority. The compliance committee is responsible for monitoring and guiding all compliance activities. The compliance committee approves the appointment of the compliance officer, approves the compliance program policies and procedures, and reviews the compliance program annual work plan. The OIG's guidance suggests that the compliance committee be made up of individuals with a variety of skills, including "significant professional experience in working with quality assurance, enrollment, marketing, clinical records and auditing principles."[5] In ad-

dition, the compliance committee members must be trained on the policies and procedures of the compliance program. The OIG guidance suggests that the compliance committee's responsibilities include the following:

- analyzing the organization's regulatory environment and the legal requirements with which it must comply and specific risk areas
- assessing existing policies and procedures that address these areas for possible incorporation into the compliance program
- working with appropriate departments, as well as affiliated providers, to develop standards of conduct and policies and procedures that promote allegiance to the organization's compliance program
- recommending and monitoring, in conjunction with the relevant departments, the development of internal systems and controls to carry out the organization's standards, policies, and procedures as part of its daily operations
- determining the appropriate strategy/approach to promote compliance with the program and detection of any potential violations, such as through hotlines and other fraud reporting mechanisms
- developing a system to solicit, evaluate, and respond to complaints and problems
- monitoring internal and external audits and investigations for the purpose of identifying troublesome issues and deficient areas experienced by the Medicare + Choice organization and implementing corrective and preventive action[6]

It is essential that the compliance committee establish and oversee a system of measures and incentives around the compliance program. Those incentives should cover the compliance office and be integrated into the performance measurement and incentive program for senior managers all the way down to staff line supervisors. The measures and incentives should reflect management's commitment to the compliance program. Measures can include process measures such as development of policies and procedures around regulatory issues, implementation of audits, employee compliance training, and feedback from employees, including surveys and the employee hotline. As well, measures can include performance measures such as outcomes of regulatory agency or internal compliance audits.

Corporate Compliance Officer

The OIG in its guidance allows health plans to exercise discretion on whether the compliance officer should be a new position with sole responsibility over the compliance program or if the responsibility is added to an existing position in the firm. For a health plan with any size, the depth and range of legal and regulatory issues make it essential to appoint an individual with sole responsibility as the compliance officer. Appointing legal counsel in the dual role of counsel and as the compliance officer creates conflicting issues relative to client-attorney privilege and the compliance officer's responsibility to report wrongdoing to the government. Although not unheard of, adding compliance officer to the legal counsel's title is not advisable. Possessing a law degree does not mean an individual has the operational, management, and industry experience to be a compliance officer. Because the compliance officer is a senior management level position, it is essential that the compliance officer have substantial industry and management experience. In a recent survey of hospital compliance officers, 35 percent had 21 or more years of experience in health care and 77 percent had more than 10 years of experience.[7]

In its guidance, the OIG recommends that the compliance officer have direct access to the company's governing body, the chief executive officer (CEO), and all other senior management including legal counsel. The CCO's authority extends to the following:

- the right, independent of other managers, to review documents, conduct audits, and make decisions about compliance-related issues
- advising internal audit to focus their efforts on the issues that could lead to legal and regulatory risk

- working with legal counsel to translate new requirements into policy and to manage legal and regulatory investigations
- access to department heads to identify performance issues that increase legal and regulatory risks

As evidence that the compliance officer is given the authority and support to carry out the corporate compliance program's objectives, regulators will ask the following types of questions:

- Does the compliance office have the budget and staffing to serve its mission?
- Does the CCO have comparable training and experience to fulfill a senior management position?
- Does the CCO have the authority to stop the submission of potentially inaccurate or false data?
- Does the CCO have access to and review all internal audit reports?
- Does the CCO work closely with managers to identify legal and regulatory risks?
- Does the CCO review all documents relevant to compliance activities?
- Does the CCO coordinate compliance functions with the compliance officers of contracting vendors and providers?
- What evidence is there that the compliance program is effective?

Compliance Office

The CCO requires a dedicated staff to effectively oversee and monitor the implementation and ongoing operation of the compliance program. It is essential for the compliance office staff to be trained in compliance and the OIG's guidance. Programmatic background in the legal and regulatory environment and legal or audit training are a plus. Exhibit 68–2 provides some potential measures for a compliance office.

LEADERSHIP

The leadership's commitment to an ethical work culture is imperative to the success of the compliance program. Leadership begins with se-

Exhibit 68–2 Sample Compliance Program Measures

- Completion and periodic updating of employee compliance program policies and procedures and training
- Surveys on the effectiveness of compliance program training
- Periodic employee surveys on their knowledge and experience with the compliance program

- Results of an independent review of the employee hotline and the employee exit interview programs
- Successful implementation of audits and other regulatory reviews
- Results of annual reviews by regulatory agencies

Courtesy of Ernst & Young LLP, 2000, Washington, DC.

nior management's ability to promote a clear understanding and commitment to the mission, vision, and values of the organization. A "corporate standards of conduct" provides explicit guidelines about ethical norms in the organization and what is expected of employees in supporting the mission, vision, and values of the organization. The OIG recommends that the health plan's "governing body, CEO, chief operating officer, general counsel, chief financial officer and other senior officials should be directly involved in the development of standards of conduct."[8]

The standards of conduct should not be dismissed or taken lightly. The standards of conduct are a statement of principles and will serve as the basis for acknowledging and rewarding ethical norms and behavior in daily practices and routine decision making. The standards of conduct must be dynamic, not static. In short, the

standards of conduct are the backbone of influencing an ethical organizational culture. The development and support of an ethical organizational culture is critical to corporate compliance. In the absence or breakdown of any other compliance structure or driver, the culture and norms of its employees are the last defense an organization has against unethical or illegal behavior. Organizational culture is stable and difficult to change. Ethical norms must be constantly reinforced by means such as standards of conduct, financial incentives, penalties, communications from leadership, and training.

In writing the standards of conduct there are some important content and stylistic considerations in making the document effective. Exhibit 68–3 provides a description of the content sections a health plan should consider including in its standards of conduct. In writing the Code, there should

Exhibit 68–3 Sample Provisions in the Standards of Conduct

- Compliance with laws and regulations
- Areas of legal and regulatory focus
- Quality of care issues
- Consumer privacy and confidentiality
- Proprietary interests of the organization
- Safety and health issues
- Human resources issues

- A statement on the organization's ethical principles
- The process to report violations
- Disciplinary action against violations including causes for termination
- Management's accountability to support the compliance efforts
- Letter of support from the CEO

Courtesy of Ernst & Young LLP, 2000, Washington, DC.

be parity between the sections so as not to diminish the value of some of the codes compared with others. Statements should be concise, direct, and written at the tenth grade level or below. It is important to review the codes against existing policies and procedures and training so as not to send contradictory messages to employees. The standards of conduct are an integral component of the corporate compliance program training. The standards of conduct must be updated periodically to reflect current issues and trends. As part of the compliance training, the standards of conduct are distributed to all employees. At the training session, employees should sign and date a statement that reflects their knowledge and commitment to the standards of conduct. The standards of conduct should also be part of the training for new employees, providers, and vendors.

The OIG advises that the written standards of conduct should clearly identify the procedures for handling disciplinary problems, including who is responsible for taking disciplinary action. The standards communicate that disciplinary action is to be fair and equitable for all levels of employees. The standards make managers and supervisors accountable for the consistent application of disciplinary policy.

EDUCATION AND DEVELOPMENT

Education and development may be the most important element in a compliance program. Compliance officers use education and development to socialize employees to the organization ethics and norms, help employees understand new requirements in relation to their jobs, and foster employee empowerment at all levels to make informed and ethical decisions. The OIG is descriptive in the type and frequency of policies, procedures, and training they will look for in a compliance program.

The OIG expects health plans to develop compliance-specific and programmatic-specific categories of policies, procedures, and training. The compliance-specific policies and procedures should delineate the compliance program's requirements for every employee, as well as issues specific to the compliance office. These policies cover the elements of the OIG's compliance program guidance and the organization's compliance structure. A discussion of the specific areas of concern identified by the OIG and other regulatory bodies should be a component of these policies and training.

All employees must be trained on the compliance program policies and procedures. The training is conducted for new employees and annually to update employees on changes to the compliance program and new areas of regulatory risk. The OIG feels so strongly about the compliance program training that it recommends employment be made contingent on attending the general compliance training session. An attendance log should be maintained and retained in employee records. Employees should be distributed the standards of conduct and be required to sign an attestation to their knowledge and commitment to the standards. The OIG also recommends that contractors and vendors have the opportunity to participate in the compliance training program. As a measure of effectiveness of the training, the CCO should conduct a survey of employees to evaluate their understanding of the compliance program.

Health plans, according to the OIG guidance, are required to develop focused policies and training. The focused policies and training address "all applicable statutes, rules and program instructions that apply to each function or department."[9] In its guidance, the OIG identified its area of focus for Medicare + Choice plans but indicated that the compliance program should address the concerns of other regulatory bodies. Health plans, especially Medicare + Choice plans, should incorporate the OIG's areas of focus listed in its compliance program guidance, annual work plans, and special alerts. In addition, compliance officers working with the legal and regulatory staff should regularly evaluate the areas of concern and enforcement activities of the various legal and regulatory bodies.

MEASURES AND INCENTIVES

The OIG strongly suggests that compliance is integrated into the organization's performance measurement and incentive program. This includes establishing compliance expectations in manager and staff performance measures and clearly publishing penalties for noncompliance. Department heads and line managers can be evaluated on their ability to reduce legal and regulatory risk and implement compliance requirements. Compensation can be linked to indicators such as baseline to longitudinal risk assessments, employee compliance surveys, or evidence of noncompliance discovered through the employee hotline, audits, or reporting. In the case of large national chains, compliance measures can be implemented in the measures of the local health plan executives. Software packages that can track and link risk assessments from subsidiary health plans and departments are useful in monitoring the compliance measurement and incentive system. An important caveat for a CCO is to closely control any type of risk assessment tool put on a knowledge management system such as local area network or intranet site. Individuals cannot complete risk assessments without the CCO's knowledge. In the case of an investigation by a legal or regulatory body, any reporting of noncompliance that is not acted on by the CCO is considered as blatant disregard.

Employees must have a clear understanding of the organization's disciplinary penalties and how they are applied. The CCO, through training and policies, disseminates "the range of possible disciplinary actions for improper conduct."[10] Managers in their routine training and departmental meetings review the relevant compliance policies and legal requirements and related penalties. The compliance officer verifies that managers reinforce the message with their employees that compliance with policies and legal requirements is a condition of employment. The OIG guidance instructs that managers and supervisors are to be sanctioned for failure to adequately instruct their subordinates about compliance issues. Managers and supervisors are also held responsible for the failure to detect noncompliance with policies and legal requirements, "where reasonable diligence on the part of the manager or supervisor should have led to the discovery of any problems or violations."[11]

STAFFING

An effective compliance officer recognizes and monitors the impact staffing will have on a department's performance and compliance capabilities. Staff experience is strongly associated with performance in departments such as claims and member services.[12] The compliance officer must be aware of instances in which inappropriate, poorly trained, or inexperienced staffing is having an impact on performance. The goal of the compliance program as it relates to staffing is to encourage management to:

- recruit and reward motivated employees committed to advancing the mission and vision in an ethical manner
- match skills and competencies to regulatory and process requirements
- monitor staffing and its impact on performance and compliance risk
- avoid hiring individuals barred from participation in federal programs
- promote employee respect for state and federal laws

Assessing staffing capabilities is a valuable indicator of compliance risk. Staffing capabilities can be measured by using benchmarks and by conducting employee self-assessments of their own ability, experience, and training to fulfill their job responsibilities. Compliance officers are concerned with employees who do not believe they have the training, experience, or resources to complete their job responsibilities. Employees who do not feel empowered are compliance risks that require the compliance officer's attention. The compliance officer needs to be diligent about providing training to new employees and to employees in high-risk areas. New employees in highly complex positions, such as claims processing, should be given special attention and provided regular training and oversight by managers and the compliance office.

A priority focus of the OIG is screening for individuals or entities barred from participation in federal programs. According to the OIG guidance, health plans must "prohibit the employment of or contracting with individuals or entities who have been recently convicted of a criminal offense related to health care or who are listed as debarred, excluded or otherwise ineligible for participation in Federal health care programs."[13] This requirement applies to employees, providers, and vendors. Health plans are particularly at risk for not being fully in compliance with this screening requirement. Many health plans screen employees or contractors using the National Practitioner Databank or the OIG lists of debarred and excluded individuals and entities but not the General Services Administration list, which is required under federal program participation requirements. As part of credentialing and contracting, health plans must screen "providers and suppliers that have been the subject of health care related final adverse actions in criminal, civil and administrative proceedings."[14] As well, health plans do not generally do a good job of screening providers who have had their licenses revoked by states. An unfortunate, but common, practice for providers who have their license revoked by a state is to set up shop in another state that has a licensing reciprocity agreement. The states do a poor job of sharing information about sanctioned providers. By approximately January 2000, the federal government intends to have operating the Healthcare Integrity Protection Data Bank, an online screening service to be used (for a fee) in conducting checks on employees and contractors. Other online services are available in the market.

COMMUNICATION

Communication is the most visible role of the corporate compliance officer. The ultimate goal of the compliance officer is to create a two-way exchange of information on compliance issues with employees, providers, and vendors. Effective communication can improve awareness and understanding of regulatory requirements, processes, and compliance-related issues. In return, employees must trust that they can report back potential improper behavior without fear of retribution. In addition, the compliance officer establishes processes for reporting the results of

investigations and audits to the board and, if necessary, legal authorities.

The main goals of compliance communications to employees is to reinforce an ethical organizational culture, demonstrate management's commitment to compliance, and increase awareness and understanding of legal and regulatory requirements. Procedures are put in place for employees to approach the compliance officer or the compliance committee to clarify any confusion or question over a company policy, practice, or procedure. Employee questions of this nature are documented, dated, and shared with other employees as appropriate. Posters, fliers, and monthly compliance newsletters are all effective means of reinforcing the compliance message. A company intranet site devoted to compliance issues is a powerful tool. The compliance intranet site can serve as a centralized source on statutory, regulatory, and other compliance guidance. The site can be used to answer questions and share information about compliance issues, including alerts about the activity of regulators and examples of compliance issues turned up in audits and reviews. The compliance intranet site is also valuable for increasing connectivity and oversight of health plans spread across geographical markets and for oversight of functions delegated to vendors and providers.

Detecting and investigating noncompliance and illegal behavior is what employees most associate with compliance officers. The compliance officer has many tools for monitoring and detecting compliance issues: automated reporting, regulatory reviews, compliance reviews, risk assessments, audits, employee hotlines, employee exit and postemployment interviews, and investigations.

Automated Reporting

Automated reporting for the compliance program includes monitoring organizational performance reports and reporting back to the compliance committee. Automated reporting includes routine and ad hoc automated reporting of performance and compliance issues across various intervals of time. Reports are conducted at the individual, group, department, and enterprise levels and can include the oversight of vendors and providers. Automated reporting is proactive with its priorities aligned to goals of organization. (Automated reporting in this context refers to routine or ad hoc performance reports, not special reports from investigations.)

As noted earlier, it is critical for the compliance officer to tightly control reporting of compliance issues. The compliance officer should monitor performance reports for processes that have regulated time frames. Examples include claims processing timeliness, claims backlog, days to process member appeals, Medicare + Choice disenrollment rates, and other similar process measures. Automated reporting over process performance is particularly important for functions delegated to providers or vendors. The compliance officer can access existing management reports and advocate for new reporting for high-risk regulatory issues. The proactive use of monitoring performance reports is an invaluable tool in the early identification of potential regulatory issues.

The compliance committee does not receive as much automated reporting of performance but instead receives reporting in the form of audits, reviews, and investigations. There is some automated reporting of performance appropriate for the compliance committee. Monthly employee hotline activity can be compiled in a report and monitored by the compliance officer and the compliance committee. Automated reporting of the hotline can include measures such as number of calls received, response times, resolution status, and the number of pending issues. If performance issues emerge in high-risk processes, for instance, a high claims backlog or member disenrollment rates, monitoring of management reports may be elevated to the compliance committee. Nonautomated reporting to the compliance committee includes the results of programmatic audits, audits of the compliance program, audits of the employee hotline, legal and regulatory reviews, legal and regulatory risk assessments, investigations and remedial actions, exit interviews, and similar work products of the compliance program.

Legal and Regulatory Reviews

Legal and regulatory reviews are nonsystematic reviews to determine that the organization has implemented and appears to be in compliance with applicable requirements. Legal and regulatory reviews are reactive with priorities set by environmental forces such as regulators. Medicare + Choice contracting health plans often use HCFA's Contractor Performance Monitoring Review Guide and supplement it with information from other sources such as the HCFA Operational Policy Letters. Market conduct reviews can be classified as a legal and regulatory review, but many in the industry see it as a separate and distinct type of review. Legal and regulatory reviews are nonsystematic in that they are not governed by a set of principles as is an audit. However, they are essential to the compliance program. Often the legal and regulatory review will be conducted by the government programs staff, especially in large health plans. No matter who conducts legal and regulatory reviews, the compliance officer has an active role in determining the content, timing, and corrective action or other follow-up work.

It is advisable to conduct legal and regulatory reviews annually for every product line (e.g., Medicare, Medicaid, ERISA). The goal of legal and regulatory reviews is to verify that the health plan meets legal and regulatory requirements. Often the legal and regulatory review are conducted in preparation for a formal review by a regulatory agency. The compliance officer needs to be proactive. The OIG, in its compliance guidance for Medicare + Choice plans, recommends that the compliance officer take a "snapshot" of the organization's legal and regulatory compliance as the compliance program is implemented. This review should determine whether the organization is in compliance with legal and regulatory requirements. If the compliance officer determines that the plan is not in compliance, it must investigate and correct the causes and notify legal or regulatory authorities if necessary.

Compliance Reviews

A compliance review is an assessment of the health plan's compliance program. Compliance reviews are nonsystematic evaluations of the health plan's compliance program and its ability to comply with laws and regulations and detect wrongdoing. Compliance reviews should be proactive with priorities set by the compliance committee. Results of the annual compliance review are presented to the compliance committee and are heavily factored into the compliance officer's performance appraisal. Exhibit 68–4 describes some types of compliance program reviews a health plan can conduct.

Legal and Regulatory Risk Assessment

Legal and regulatory risk assessments are a snapshot of the organization's vulnerability to legal and regulatory noncompliance. A risk assessment can be an important management tool in setting priorities for the compliance program and measuring compliance effectiveness. In identifying the organization's legal and regulatory risks, the OIG recommends that health plans not only look outwardly to the activities of regulators but also conduct an internal risk analysis. The risk "should identify and rank the various compliance and business risks the company may experience in its daily operations."[15] This analysis is an essential tool for the compliance officer in identifying risk areas for training, policy development, regulatory reviews, audits, and communications. The risk analysis establishes the compliance officer's work plan for the year and influences the activities of internal auditors and the legal and regulatory staff. A baseline risk analysis measured against subsequent risk assessments can serve as a measure of the compliance program's effectiveness and as an incentive measure for department heads and line managers.

The framework suggested here integrates into the risk assessment an external and internal risk

---

Exhibit 68–4 Compliance Program Reviews

Employee surveys—An employee survey of their perceptions and knowledge of the compliance program. The survey may be conducted with focus groups to gain qualitative information about employee perceptions.

A compliance office review—An independent verification that the compliance office has the authority to perform its duties and is, in fact, updating policies and procedures, revising the standard of conduct, performing audits and reviews, investigating and reporting fraud and abuse violations, and generally fulfilling its other responsibilities.

An exit interview and post employment program review—A review of the exit interview and post employment review program to ensure that the interviews are conducted timely, according to established procedures, and that compliance-related information is monitored and elevated for corrective action if necessary.

Company standards of conduct review—A review of the standards of conduct to determine that they are updated regularly, updates are communicated to employees, all employees have signed an attestation to the standards, the standards meet the OIG stylistic guidelines, and that the standards are not conflicting with existing policies and procedures.

Employee hotline review—A review of the hotline operations to determine that policies are written according to the OIG guidance and that procedures are in compliance. The review should verify that confidentiality is maintained, records and logs are kept, and that inappropriate behavior is investigated and resolved accordingly.

Compliance training review—A review of the training program to ensure all employees have been trained on compliance and that sign-in sheets and evaluation forms are on record. The review should ensure that the compliance training includes the elements recommended by the OIG for training and that focused training was conducted in the areas agreed upon by the compliance committee.

Courtesy of Ernst & Young LLP, 2000, Washington, DC.

assessment. By comparing internal and external risks, the compliance officer has a more complete picture of the organization's legal and regulatory risks. The external assessment of the legal and regulatory risks is made by following the activities of policy-making and regulatory bodies such as the National Association of Insurance Commissioners, state regulatory agencies, HCFA, the OIG, the Department of Justice, state and federal court decisions, the Federal Employee Health Benefits Program (FEHBP), Employee Retirement Income Security Act (ERISA) activities under the Department of Labor, and other regulatory agencies. After identifying the regulatory bodies that have an impact on the health plan, the compliance officer working with the legal and regulatory staff should

quantify external risks on the basis of the following framework:

- degree of change caused by a new rule or requirement
- clarity of the law or regulation
- level of regulatory enforcement activity
- potential penalty for noncompliance
- competitive or regulatory driven time constraints
- external reporting requirements
- risk of lawsuits over high profile issues

This analysis should be conducted for every department in the organization. Exhibit 68–5 demonstrates an external risk analysis worksheet that can be used for any department. The compliance officer completes the analysis with

Exhibit 68–5 External Risk Analysis

Department	Commercial Insurance Products	Medicare + Choice	Medicaid	FEHBP	ERISA	OIG
Degree of change caused by a new rule or requirement						
Clarity of the law or regulation						
Level of regulatory enforcement activity						
Potential penalty for noncompliance						
Competitive or regulatory driven time constraints						
External reporting requirements						
Risk of lawsuits over high profile issues						

Courtesy of Ernst & Young LLP, 2000, Washington, DC.

assistance from the legal and regulatory staff and talking with regulators. Among other sources, the compliance officer assesses recent legislation, regulations, court cases, advisory statements, and regulatory agency work plans. A score is assigned for each category, for instance a 1- to 5-point scale in which 5 is high risk. At the completion of the analysis, the compliance officer has a better understanding of the compliance risk presented to each department by the various regulatory bodies.

The second component of the risk analysis is to understand how at risk the organization is to those external legal and regulatory threats. By comparing the areas of greatest external risk to the areas of internal risk, the compliance officer is then able to set the agenda for training, auditing, and other compliance-related activities. The internal risk analysis can be completed using different approaches.

The framework suggested here evaluates internal risk on the basis of how well the organization is performing, how well management influences performance and compliance, and how well management monitors performance and compliance. In contrast to providers who most often run into legal and regulatory difficulties because of incorrect or illegal billing, the greatest risk to health plans is that poor performance will result in noncompliance. This framework has three general categories:

- performance: risks in terms of performance measured using benchmarks related to speed, productivity, and accuracy
- controls and incentives: risk in terms of management's ability to influence performance and compliance and implement specific legal and regulatory requirements
- monitoring: risk in terms of management's ability to monitor performance and compliance through the use of regulatory reviews, audits, satisfaction surveys, and oversight of delegated functions

By using standard evaluation instruments supplemented with department and regulatory specific measures, this risk assessment should be able to answer the following questions for each major functional area of the health plan:

- Have legal and regulatory requirements or standards been implemented into the appropriate processes?
- Are the requirements or standards documented in policies or procedures?
- Has training been conducted around specific requirements or standards?
- Do employee measures and incentives support compliance with the requirement or standard?
- Have the penalties for noncompliance been made aware to the employee and the organization?
- Does management use key controls and processes specific to each department to influence compliance and prevent fraud and abuse?
- How does the organization compare with performance benchmarks related to speed, productivity, accuracy, training, or staff experience that can be used as indicators of potential legal or regulatory noncompliance?
- How well does management monitor legal and regulatory risks through use of hotlines, exit interviews, audits, regulatory reviews, satisfaction surveys, and oversight of delegated functions?

Exhibit 68–6 presents a matrix for conducting the internal risk assessment analysis for each department in the health plan.

The internal risk analysis is conducted for each department. Each component is assigned a rank scoring similar to the external review. The final analysis provides the compliance officer a global snapshot of the organization's legal and regulatory risks. The analysis also provides department managers an idea of their compliance risk. On completion of the external and internal risk analysis, the compliance officer can establish the compliance program's priorities for the year using the table provided in Exhibit 68–7.

Audits

Auditing involves documentation of compliance through a formal process that may include

Exhibit 68–6 Internal Risk Assessment Framework

	Is Noncompliance Threatened by:
Performance	Speed: our ability to complete a process timely?
	Productivity: our ability to use our work force effectively?
	Accuracy: the quality and accuracy of our work?
	Customer satisfaction: customer dissatisfaction of our service?
Controls and incentives	Staffing: the experience of our employees?
	Policies and procedures: our development of policies and procedures, including legal and regulatory requirements?
	Use of technology: our use of emerging technologies to improve performance?
	Regulatory implementation: our ability to identify and implement regulatory requirements?
	Knowledge management: our ability to communicate to our employees?
	Use of leading practices: management's use of controls and processes to improve compliance and performance?
	Incentives: our performance measurements and incentives and impact on ethical behavior?
Use of indicators	Reporting: our use of reporting to monitor performance and compliance?
	Auditing: our use of audits to verify compliance?
	Satisfaction surveys: our use of internal and customer satisfaction surveys?
	Delegation oversight: our oversight of functions delegated to providers and vendors?

Courtesy of Ernst & Young LLP, 2000, Washington, DC.

the verification of controls and execution of policies and procedures. Audits are proactive, with priorities determined by management. Audits are reviews conducted according to a formal process. The OIG recommends that health plans look at the OIG's process for conducting audits. The internal audit staff or external auditors should be used in conducting compliance audits. Compliance audits are a higher level of review conducted for high-risk areas and as part of investigations when inappropriate behavior is suspected. Audits are conducted in areas in which a regulatory body, such as the OIG, has indicated great concern and in areas in which the risk as-

Exhibit 68–7 Compliance Activity Workplan

		Internal Compliance and Performance Risk	
		High	Low
External risk	High	Immediate attention and resources through training, reviews, and audits	Increased monitoring and review regularly
	Low	"Quick hits" and measured improvements to performance	Regular monitoring

Courtesy of Ernst & Young LLP, 2000, Washington, DC.

sessment has indicated high risk. The extent and frequency of audits will vary depending on the size of the company, the internal audit budget, and the relevant risk factors. The compliance officer, the internal auditors, and the department managers work together to determine the focus and content of the annual audit plan. The audit plan and the results of the audits are presented to the compliance committee for review and approval.

Employee Hotline

Employee hotlines allow employees to report inappropriate behavior in confidence without concern of management retribution. The OIG recommends that health plans create means for employees, contractors, and members to report inappropriate behavior by the organization, its employees, or agents. This requirement is fulfilled mainly by implementing an employee hotline. Employee hotlines are an important tool in combating "whistle blower" or "qui tam" lawsuits where the government rewards individuals for reporting fraudulent behavior. The health plan must communicate the availability of the hotline to all employees, contractors, and members in training, the standards of conduct, member handbooks, routine compliance announcements, and in common work areas. Medicare + Choice and Medicaid health plan should post in a prominent available area the HHS-OIG hotline telephone number.

Management of the employee hotline is complex and extremely sensitive given the high risk associated with whistle blower cases. The compliance officer needs to be concerned with the hotline structure. Hotlines operate 24 hours a day and 7 days a week. Supporting the hotline is a tightly controlled system of intake forms, logs, and standardized reporting. Explicit hotline operation policies and procedures are developed to protect confidentiality. Written confidentiality and nonretaliation policies are developed and distributed to all employees, contractors, and members. Hotline communications will indicate the investigation could reach a point where the individual's identity may become known or may have to be revealed. Finally, the hotline proce-

dures will allow for a process of categorizing hotline reports, investigating the reports, and the criteria for raising the level of investigation to a higher level if necessary. The OIG recommends that the intake forms document the date the potential problem was reported, the internal investigative methods used, the results of any investigation, any corrective action implemented, any disciplinary measures imposed, and any overpayments returned to the government.

Employee Exit and Postemployment Interviews

A valuable communication tool for the compliance officer is an exit interview and postemployment contact program. Management or the human resources department will conduct exit interviews with terminating employees. The interview includes questions about the employee's perceptions of the organization's ethics, instances of illegal behavior or other violations of the standard of conduct. Exit interview reports are analyzed and sent to the compliance committee. A postemployment interview is conducted with former employees 3 to 4 months after departure. The postemployment interview provides former employees the opportunity to reflect back on their experiences with the organization but at a time when they are removed from the experience of their actual departure.

Investigations

Investigations are formal or informal inquiries into suspected wrongdoing. It is advisable to conduct investigations with the assistance of legal counsel and professional investigators. Investigating potential violations of the law or regulations is a serious and sensitive legal issue. The compliance officer, working carefully with the compliance committee, is wise to engage outside counsel and auditors to assist in the investigation. The compliance officer is the advocate for maintaining discipline in the use of standard investigation protocols. On completion of an internal investigation, the compliance officer, the compliance committee, and counsel will develop a plan for further action including the need for additional investigation, reporting to legal authorities, and potential remediation of the situation. If disciplinary action is warranted, the OIG is concerned that the discipline is prompt and imposed according to the organization's written standards of disciplinary action. The compliance officer will review the circumstances of the violation to determine whether modifications of the compliance program are necessary.

The OIG recommends that records of the investigation include:

- documentation of the alleged violation
- a description of the investigative process
- copies of interview notes and key documents
- a log of the witnesses interviewed and the documents reviewed
- the results of the investigation

In its guidance, the OIG reminds health plans that reporting violations demonstrates good faith and a willingness to work with authorities. Reporting misconduct is considered a mitigating factor by the OIG in determining administrative sanctions. On identifying credible evidence of a violation, the OIG recommends that the health plan notify the appropriate government authority within 60 days. Failure to notify authorities of violation, including overpayments from gov-

ernment programs, within a reasonable period of time could be interpreted as an intentional attempt to conceal and trigger additional legal concerns. In its disclosure to the government, the health plan should provide all evidence relevant to the alleged violation and any potential cost impact to state or federal programs.

CONCLUSION

The popular support for consumer protection requirements increases the legal and regulatory risk for health plans. The OIG in its compliance guidance for health plans places greater accountability on health plans for legal and regulatory compliance. Regulatory agencies will increasingly look for evidence of an effective compliance program in setting penalties for noncompliance. The federal court system through the U.S. Sentencing Commission guidelines already accounts for a compliance program in its setting of penalties. Corporate compliance is a cost of doing business in health care. A highly effective compliance officer will run an efficient compliance office and will recognize upside benefits for the organization through effective management of the legal and regulatory risk. Corporate compliance officers achieve upside benefits by recognizing and using the drivers of organizational performance—leadership, education, structure, measures and incentives, staffing, and communication.

REFERENCES AND NOTES

1. The Office of the Inspector General, United States Department of Health and Human Services, Draft OIG Compliance Program Guidance for Certain Medicare + Choice Organizations, *Federal Register*, 64 (1999): 121, June 24.

2. The United States Sentencing Commission, *Federal Sentencing Guidelines Manual,* 1998.

3. The United States Sentencing Commission, *Federal Sentencing Guidelines Manual,* 1998.

4. Ernst & Young LLP, *Ernst & Young Business Change Implementation Organizational Performance Levers*, 1998.

5. The Office of the Inspector General, United States Department of Health and Human Services, Draft OIG Compliance Program Guidance for Certain Medicare +

Choice Organizations, *Federal Register*, 64 (1999): 121, June 24.

6. The Office of the Inspector General, United States Department of Health and Human Services, Draft OIG Compliance Program Guidance for Certain Medicare + Choice Organizations, *Federal Register,* 64 (1999): 121, June 24.

7. Ernst & Young LLP, *Strengthening Ethical Cultures: The Emerging Role of Compliance Programs and Officers*, 1999.

8. The Office of the Inspector General, United States Department of Health and Human Services, Draft OIG Compliance Program Guidance for Certain Medicare + Choice Organizations, *Federal Register,* 64 (1999): 121, June 24.

9. The Office of the Inspector General, United States Department of Health and Human Services, Draft OIG Compliance Program Guidance for Certain Medicare + Choice Organizations, *Federal Register,* 64 (1999): 121, June 24.

10. The Office of the Inspector General, United States Department of Health and Human Services, Draft OIG Compliance Program Guidance for Certain Medicare + Choice Organizations, *Federal Register,* 64 (1999): 121, June 24.

11. The Office of the Inspector General, United States Department of Health and Human Services, Draft OIG Compliance Program Guidance for Certain Medicare + Choice Organizations, *Federal Register*, 64 (1999): 121, June 24.

12. Ernst & Young LLP, *The 1998 Ernst & Young Managed Care Benchmarking Study*, 1998.

13. The Office of the Inspector General, United States Department of Health and Human Services, Draft OIG Compliance Program Guidance for Certain Medicare + Choice Organizations, *Federal Register,* 64 (1999): 121, June 24.

14. The Office of the Inspector General, United States Department of Health and Human Services, Draft OIG Compliance Program Guidance for Certain Medicare + Choice Organizations, *Federal Register*, 64 (1999): 121, June 24.

15. The Office of the Inspector General, United States Department of Health and Human Services, Draft OIG Compliance Program Guidance for Certain Medicare + Choice Organizations, *Federal Register*, 64 (1999): 121, June 24.

CHAPTER 69

State Regulation of Managed Care

Richard I. Smith and Kristin Stewart

INTRODUCTION

In our federal system of government, states have had the principal responsibility for the regulation of managed care organizations (MCOs). In recent years, the scope of state regulation has expanded to intervene more directly in the structure and operations of MCOs. At the same time, the federal government has begun to play a more prominent role in the managed care market, both as a regulator and as a purchaser. To date, though, federal regulation has tended to supplement rather than supplant state regulation of MCOs. Whether this pattern will remain intact is an open question, as the U.S. Congress is considering far-reaching federal standards for health plans.

This chapter highlights the role of the states in regulating MCO operations. In particular, it describes oversight of health maintenance organization (HMO) and preferred provider organization (PPO) operations, point-of-service (POS) products, and utilization review organizations (UROs). Because space limitations preclude review of every state's laws, many of the regulatory issues detailed here are based on model acts adopted by the

Richard I. Smith, JD, is Vice President, Public Policy and Research, and Kristin Stewart, MHA, is Director, Private Market Issues, at the American Association of Health Plans (AAHP).

The authors gratefully acknowledge contributions from several AAHP colleagues: Colette Desmarais, Randi Reichel, Louis Saccoccio, Marjorie Shofer, Samantha Silva, Terry Sollom, Daniel Thornton, and Liza Wexler.

National Association of Insurance Commissioners (NAIC),[1] which represents insurance departments in the 50 states and U.S. territories. One important NAIC document is the HMO Model Act, which was adopted by the NAIC in 1972 to clearly authorize the establishment of HMOs and provide for an ongoing regulatory monitoring system.[2] All 50 states have adopted either this model legislation, or substantial portions thereof, or similar laws regulating HMOs.

The NAIC has also adopted the Preferred Provider Arrangement Model Act (PPA), which permits insurers to enter into preferred provider arrangements that ensure reasonable access to covered services under the network and seek to control the cost of the health benefit plan. Thirty-one states have adopted the PPA Model Act, or similar legislation or regulation.

State regulation of PPOs is difficult to summarize primarily because PPOs are regulated in different ways depending upon the state. In addition, the regulatory authority of each state frequently is found in various statutes, rather than in a single statute. Several states require PPOs to be licensed, registered or certified. Other states require that an insurer (most often an indemnity plan) that contracts with a preferred provider network submit documentation that the network is compliant with certain state laws. PPOs also may be subject to separate laws, apart from licensure or indemnity contracts, that govern the various functions PPOs perform. For example, the majority of states have laws governing entities that perform utilization management. PPO utilization management activities typically are subject to these laws even if they may not be part of PPO licensure standards.

STATE OVERSIGHT: THE REGULATORY PROCESS

HMOs and PPOs

On the state level, HMOs usually are regulated by more than one agency, with regulatory supervision shared by the departments of insurance and health. Insurance regulators assume principal responsibility for the financial aspects of HMO operations and, in many states, for external review of adverse benefit determinations. Health regulators focus on quality of care issues, utilization patterns, and the ability of participating providers to provide adequate care. Although typical, this division of regulatory authority is not universal. For example, until recently the Department of Corporations oversaw all aspects of HMO operations in California. In 2000, its HMO oversight functions were transferred to the Department of Managed Care, and this new agency is now responsible for regulating all aspects of HMO operations. Risk-bearing PPOs are generally regulated by departments of insurance, either under the laws applicable to all insurance carriers or a special section of state insurance law.

Licensure

HMOs obtain licensure by applying for a certificate of authority (COA). An organization may be incorporated for the sole purpose of becoming licensed as an HMO, or an existing company may sponsor an HMO product line through a subsidiary or affiliated organization. Applications usually are processed by the insurance department and, among other items, include the following documents: corporate bylaws, sample provider and group contract forms, evidence of coverage forms, financial statements, financial feasibility plan, description of service area, internal grievance procedures, and the proposed quality assurance program. Payment of licensing fees is usually required.

Many states require PPOs to be licensed, registered, or certified. In those states, the standards imposed on PPOs tend to vary, depending on whether the PPO is risk bearing or not. Risk-bearing PPOs are likely to be subject to solvency and other requirements similar to those for HMOs and insurers. PPOs that do not bear risk may only have to register. Some states require the insurer with which a PPO contracts (most often an indemnity plan) to document that the PPO complies with certain state laws. The PPA Model Act, adopted by the NAIC in October 1996, reflects this approach to regulation of PPOs, providing that "if [a PPO] . . . is not engaged in activities that would require it to be licensed as a health care insurer, the entity shall file with the [state insurance] commissioner information describing its activities and a description of [its contracts with providers]."[3] Generally, the discussion of PPO regulation in this chapter focuses on risk-bearing PPOs.

Enrollee Information

The HMO Model Act sets forth requirements for communicating health plan information to HMO enrollees. Individual and group contract holders are entitled to receive a copy of their contracts. Each contract must contain basic information describing eligibility requirements, covered benefits, out-of-pocket expenses, limitations and exclusions, termination or cancellation of policies, claims processing, grievance procedures, continuation of benefits, conversion rights, subrogation rights, term of coverage, and grace period after nonpayment of premiums. Regulators require these documents to be filed with and approved by the regulatory body in charge of reviewing contracts.

In addition to individual and group contracts, the HMO Model Act requires HMOs to make other disclosures. Every enrollee is entitled to receive a document referred to as the evidence of coverage, which describes essential features and services of the HMO. Plans also must provide details about how services can be obtained through the HMO network and a telephone number at the plan for answers to additional questions. Upon enrollment or re-enrollment, members receive a list of all health plan providers, and HMOs must notify enrollees in writing if their primary care physician's (PCP's) participation terminates. Within 30 days after a material change in the plan, HMOs are to notify enrollees of the change if it has a direct impact on them.

States may require that insurers contracting with PPOs provide enrollees with a document that discloses the extent of coverage, the conditions for reimbursement, deductibles and coinsurance, and the process for addressing enrollee complaints, among other information. In addition, insurance policies offering PPO benefits must conform to the same disclosure and marketing requirements as are applicable to any other type of health insurance policy.[4] Likewise, the PPA Model Act requires plans offering a PPO option to identify clearly the differences in benefit levels for preferred and nonpreferred providers.

Access to Medical Services

Under the HMO Model Act, HMOs must ensure the availability and accessibility of medical services. HMO patients should have access to medical care during reasonable hours; emergency care should be provided 24 hours a day, seven days a week. Regulators limit an HMO's certificate of authority to designated service areas (usually established by ZIP code regions or counties) where a determination has been made that the HMO has a sufficient provider network. Regulators also establish requirements governing HMO specialty referrals to ensure appropriate accessibility.

The Managed Care Plan Network Adequacy Model Act, which was adopted by the NAIC in 1996 and applies to plans offering PPAs as well as HMOs, provides for states to choose among different ways of measuring network adequacy, including provider-enrollee ratios, geographical accessibility, waiting times, hours of operation, and the volume of technological and specialty services available in a plan's service area. It requires plans to file an access plan with the appropriate state agency to show how the plan will meet the access standard adopted by the state.[5] Fifteen states have approved legislation or regu-

lation based on, or related to, this NAIC model act (most other states have legislation or regulation based on the HMO Model Act).[6]

Likewise, the PPA Model Act requires insurers offering a PPO option to "assure reasonable access to covered services under the preferred provider arrangement and adequate number of preferred providers to render those services."[7] At least 31 states have established access standards applicable to PPOs.[8]

Provider Issues

The HMO Model Act requires organizations applying for state licensure to provide regulators with copies of provider contract forms for different classes of providers, as well as the names and addresses of all the providers with which it has contracts. It also requires each contract to include a hold-harmless clause protecting enrollees against provider claims in the event of plan insolvency. State officials review sample contracts to ensure that they do not create incentives that could compromise access to, or quality of, care.

In addition to the requirements in the HMO Model Act, the NAIC Managed Care Plan Network Adequacy Model Act includes several provisions relating to provider contracting. First, plans are required to adopt standards for selecting participating providers and to provide these standards to the appropriate state agency for review. Second, plans must give at least 60 days' notice before terminating a provider contract "without cause." Third, the act prohibits plans from offering "an inducement... to a provider to provide less than medically necessary services to a covered person" and from including in provider contracts any provision that would restrict provider-patient communications or limit a provider's ability to act as a patient advocate.

Of the states that have enacted specific PPO laws, 18 require credentialing; 12 require providers to be involved in network management activities; 23 require written provider selection criteria; and 13 states require due process for provider termination.[9] In addition, there are typically standards outside of PPO-specific laws that govern these and other areas.

Reports and Rate Filings

State regulators use a number of methods to ensure that licensed HMOs remain in compliance with the law. Generally, HMOs file an annual report with the insurance department. This report includes audited financial statements, a list of participating providers, an update and summary of enrollee grievances handled during the year, and any additional information that regulators deem necessary to make a proper review of the organization.

The HMO Model Act also specifies that HMOs file a schedule of premium rates or a method for determining premium rates with the insurance department. Regulators normally will approve the schedule or method if premiums are not excessive, inadequate, or unfairly discriminatory. Additionally, most states have enacted laws governing premium variation among small groups that health plans must adhere to. Likewise, PPOs that are offered as insured products are typically subject to state laws governing rating practices.

In addition, states require HMOs to update regulators automatically if there are changes in documents that were part of the initial certificate of authority application filing (or part of the annual filings). Regulators keep permanent records, including PCP agreements, specialist provider contracts, group and individual contracts, certificate of coverage, and other pertinent information.

Quality Assurance and Utilization Review

Most states require an HMO to file a description of its internal quality assurance (QA) program and activities before obtaining a state license. Regulators review the description and, during site reviews, interview staff and check records to ensure that the description is accurate. A few states, such as Iowa, Kansas, and Pennsylvania, also specify that HMOs obtain periodic accreditation by an independent external accrediting body.

Under the NAIC HMO Model Act, HMOs are obliged to establish procedures to ensure that services meet reasonable standards for quality of care. These procedures must include an internal program to monitor and evaluate the quality of care provided. At a minimum, this program includes a written statement of goals and objectives, a written QA plan specifying who within the HMO is responsible for implementing the plan, systems for ongoing and focused evaluations, a system for credentialing and peer review of providers, and processes to initiate corrective action when deficiencies are identified. In addition, HMOs are required to record formal QA activities; develop an adequate patient record system; make clinical records available to determine compliance with QA standards; and report QA program activities to the HMO's board, providers, and staff periodically.

Reflecting growing state interest in quality-related issues, the NAIC has also adopted three new model acts dealing in greater specificity with standards for quality assurance, utilization review (UR), and credentialing activities.

Under the NAIC Quality Assessment and Improvement Model Act, HMOs must have an internal system that identifies opportunities to improve care; measures the performance of participating providers and conducts peer review activities; collects and analyzes data on overutilization and underutilization of services; and ensures that providers have input on the quality improvement process. Twenty-six states have adopted legislation or regulation based on, or related to, the standards established in this model act.[10]

Under the Utilization Review Model Act, HMOs, PPOs, and other health carriers subject to state regulation and that provide or perform UR services are required to use documented clinical review criteria that are based on sound clinical evidence; ensure that qualified health professionals administer the UR program; and abide by strict limits on the time period for all UR decisions. The model act prohibits compensation arrangements that encourage UR staff to make inappropriate determinations and provides for a process of appealing adverse UR decisions.

The Health Care Professional Credentialing Verification Model Act requires that HMOs establish written policies and procedures for credentialing all health care professionals and apply them in a consistent manner. Among the information to be verified are licensure, status of hospital privileges, current professional liability coverage, specialty board status, and completion of educational programs. Most of this information is updated every three years. As part of the credentialing process, health plans check with the National Practitioner Data Bank, which holds information on physicians who have had malpractice or disciplinary actions taken against them (see also Chapter 7 regarding the National Practitioner Data Bank). Sixteen states have adopted legislation or regulations based on, or related to, this NAIC model act.[11]

As discussed earlier, states also regulate the QA and UR activities of PPOs. Sometimes they do so as part of laws that apply broadly to all health insurance carriers; in other cases, they have done so in PPO-specific legislation. Requirements range from filing a description of QA and UR programs to compliance with standards and certification requirements for those making UR decisions. At least 36 states have standards relating to UR activities of PPOs,[12] and at least 23 states have standards relating to their QA programs.[13]

Grievance Procedures

The NAIC Model HMO Act specifies that HMOs have written procedures, approved by the appropriate state agency, that are designed to ensure prompt and effective resolution of written grievances. A description of these procedures is to be included in the contract or evidence of coverage given to each enrollee. Such procedures must provide for the submission of written grievances on standard forms supplied by the HMO and for resolution of such grievances within 90 days of submission. A member's enrollment in the HMO generally may not be terminated while a grievance is pending. If binding arbitration is a condition of enrollment with an HMO, this fact must be disclosed in the individual's contract or evidence of coverage.

Adopted in 1996, the NAIC's Health Carrier Grievance Procedure Model Act and its Utilization Review Model Act include more detailed

requirements in this area. The former focuses primarily on the procedures for appealing grievances, which are defined as complaints about the availability and quality of services (including adverse UR determinations), claims payment, or the enrollee-plan contractual relationship. This model act applies to carriers, which are defined as insurers and HMOs that are subject to state regulation. The Utilization Review Model Act, as discussed earlier, establishes standards for UR programs and provides more detailed guidance on the procedures to be followed for appeals involving the subset of grievances based on an adverse UR determination.

In general, these initiatives require health plans to have a two-level review process for resolving grievances. The first-level review, which is based on pertinent written evidence, must be made by individuals who were not involved in the events resulting in the grievance and, if the case involves a denial, reduction, or termination of care, must involve health professionals with appropriate expertise. A written decision will be issued generally within 20 days.

The second-level review, for which an enrollee may request a face-to-face hearing, is conducted by a panel composed mostly of health professionals of appropriate expertise who were not previously involved in the grievance and, if the case involves a denial, reduction, or termination of care, must include a health professional of appropriate expertise who is not a provider in the individual's health plan (unless one is not reasonably available). If the second-level review includes a face-to-face hearing, the hearing must occur within 45 working days of the request for such review and a written decision will be issued within five working days after completing the review. If an individual has already requested and received a separate reconsideration of an adverse UR determination, he or she is permitted to skip the first level of grievance review and proceed to a face-to-face hearing.

Expedited determinations are required for cases in which the normal time frames would seriously jeopardize the enrollee's life, health, or ability to regain maximum function. A request for an expedited determination may be oral or in writing, and such determinations are to be made no later than 72 hours after the request is made. Written notice confirming an adverse expedited determination must be provided within two working days after oral notification of the determination.

Forty-two states have adopted laws or regulations based on, or related to, the UR Model Act, and 38 states have laws pertaining to the Grievance Model Act.[14]

External Appeals

A total of 31 states has adopted policies giving enrollees a right to appeal at least some cases involving a denial of coverage to an external review entity, such as a private organization approved by the state.[15] Although there is significant variation among the states in the details of these laws, external review mechanisms generally apply to coverage denials made on the basis of medical necessity criteria or a determination that the service is experimental or investigational. Other provisions may require completion of the internal appeals process before external review occurs; no conflicts of interest for external reviewer; the plan to pay the costs of the external review process; and the external reviewer's decision to be binding on the plan.

Variations in the laws include requiring that the service in question meet a minimum dollar threshold; requiring the initiator of an external review to pay a filing fee; making the external reviewer's decision binding on the enrollee; and a "pre-review" by the state regulator or external reviewer to determine that the claim meets specified requirements before it proceeds to a full external review. At least 24 states apply their external review procedures to PPOs.[16]

The NAIC's Health Carrier External Review Model Act was approved by the NAIC in October 1999. This act provides procedures for the establishment and maintenance of external review procedures to ensure that covered persons have the opportunity for an independent review of an adverse coverage determination. The model applies to all health carriers that provide UR. A unique approach has been developed to assist states in determining the extent of the insurance commissioner's role in the review pro-

cess: three options offer varying levels of administrative involvement for the state Department of Insurance (DOI)—high DOI involvement allows DOI to conduct a preliminary review to ensure that it meets the requirements to be eligible for external review, assign the independent review organization (IRO), and review the IRO decision to ensure that it is not contrary to the terms of coverage under the covered person's health plan. Low DOI involvement allows the health carrier to assign the IRO from a list of DOI-approved IROs.

Other key provisions include a definition of "adverse determination" that triggers eligibility for review that includes denials for medical necessity, appropriateness, health care setting, and level of care or effectiveness; a standard of review that requires the IRO to consider a range of information, including "appropriate practice guidelines" that are defined to include "evidence-based" guidelines as well as "generally accepted" practice guidelines; exhaustion of internal appeals for all but expedited reviews for life-threatening cases; minimum qualifications established for IROs along with criteria for approving IROs by the state DOI; reporting requirements for IROs and health carriers; binding decisions on both parties; a $25 filing fee for the health plan member that is waived under certain circumstances; and the cost of the external review is borne by the carrier.

Solvency Standards and Insolvency Protections

To prevent HMO insolvencies and protect consumers and other affected parties against the effects of insolvencies that do occur, the HMO Model Act establishes specific capital, reserve, and deposit requirements that all HMOs must meet. Before a certificate of authority is issued, an initial net worth requirement of $1.5 million must be met. After issuance, a minimum net worth must be maintained by the HMO equal to the greater of $1 million, the sum of 2 percent of annual premiums on the first $150 million of premiums and 1 percent on the excess, the sum of three months' uncovered health care costs, or the sum of 8 percent of annual health expenditures (except those paid on a capitated basis or a managed hospital payment basis) and 4 percent of annual hospital expenses paid on a managed payment basis.

Early in 1998, the NAIC adopted a new approach to determining how much capital MCOs must have. The product of a deliberative process that began in 1993, the Risk-Based Capital (RBC) for the Health Organizations Model Act responds to the diversity of organizations and arrangements that have emerged in the rapidly changing market for health benefits coverage by codifying an approach under which capital and surplus requirements will vary from one MCO to another on the basis of the specific nature and volatility of the organization's business. The RBC formula will permit state regulators to assess the specific risk profile of individual MCOs, give credit for provider contracting mechanisms that reduce the risk borne by an MCO, and determine appropriate capital requirements based on these risk profiles.

To determine the specific capital requirements for a particular MCO, the RBC formula takes into account five different kinds of risk: the risk that the financial condition of an affiliated entity will cause an adverse change in the MCO's available capital (affiliate risk); the risk of adverse fluctuations in the value of the MCO's assets (asset risk); the risk that premiums will not be sufficient to pay claims (underwriting risk); the risk of reinsurers or capitated participating providers not fulfilling contractual obligations (credit risk); and the general risk of conducting business, including the risk that expenses will exceed budgeted amounts (business risk).

RBC information will be reported to state regulators by means of annual financial statements (called blanks), which MCOs are required to file each March. On the basis of this information, an organization-specific capital requirement is computed and then compared with the MCO's total adjusted capital. If the MCO does not meet its capital requirement, it is subject to one of three levels of regulatory intervention: company action level, regulatory action level, and mandatory control level. These interventions range from requiring the submission of a corrective action plan to placing the MCO under the direct control of state regulators. As of June 1999, five states—Arkansas, Illinois, Nebraska, North Dakota, and Washington—had adopted an RBC law. As the RBC Model Act becomes more well known, other states are expected to consider this approach to determining capital requirements for a range of MCOs.

Although RBC may ultimately replace existing capital requirements in many states, it is not expected to displace other mechanisms for protecting enrollees in the event of insolvency, such as deposits and hold-harmless requirements. For example, the HMO Model Act requires a minimum deposit of $300,000 with the state insurance department. The deposit is considered an admitted asset of the HMO in the determination of its net worth, but it is used to protect the interests of HMO enrollees or to cover administrative costs if the HMO goes into receivership or liquidation. Most states also require HMOs to include hold-harmless clauses in their provider contracts. In situations where the HMO fails to pay for covered medical care, such clauses prohibit providers from seeking collection from the enrollees. California and New York have statutory hold-harmless requirements protecting enrollees even in the absence of a contractual provision.

Several states also require that HMOs enter into reinsurance arrangements to cover liabilities in the event of an insolvency. And, aside from reinsurance arrangements, six states require HMOs to participate in stand-alone guaranty fund programs.[17] These state programs provide funding to cover an HMO's potential liabilities for health care services if it becomes insolvent. Regulators may use this money to reimburse nonparticipating providers, to pay for the continuation of benefits, and to cover conversion costs.

Additional protections for consumers include continuation of benefit provisions (requiring providers to continue to treat members of insolvent HMOs who are either undergoing an ongoing course of care or are in a designated trimester of pregnancy); open enrollment (which permits the insurance commissioner to auto-assign members to other HMOs for the duration of their contract to ensure availability of care); and as noted above, increased net worth and statutory deposit requirements and hold-harmless agreements.

States often require HMOs to establish contingency plans for insolvency that allow for the continuation of benefits to enrollees during the contract period for which premiums have been paid. If necessary, insurance departments require HMOs to take further precautions to safeguard enrollee benefits. As discussed above, these additional measures might include purchasing additional insurance, entering into contracts obligating providers to continue delivering care if the HMO ceases operation, setting aside additional solvency reserves, or securing letters of credit.

Many states also require PPOs—particularly risk-bearing PPOs—to meet requirements relating to solvency and insolvency protections. Some have established PPO-specific requirements, such as posting a bond equal to 10 percent of the PPO's estimated aggregate reimbursement, whereas others require that risk-bearing PPOs abide by the solvency requirements applicable to HMOs or indemnity insurers. This latter approach should lead to increasing use of RBC solvency standards for PPOs as more states adopt the RBC model.

Financial Examinations and Site Visits

Regulators also can conduct specialized inquiries, which often examine HMO finances, marketing activities, and QA programs. In part, the objective of these regulatory reviews is to determine the HMO's financial solvency and statutory compliance and whether any trends can be identified that may cause problems in the future. For example, the HMO Model Act requires the insurance department to complete a detailed examination of the HMO's financial affairs at least once every three years. The NAIC's *HMO Examination Handbook* sets forth specific procedures for examining HMO balance sheet assets and liabilities. The goals are to verify ownership and stated asset amounts and to ensure the adequacy of the HMO's net worth to meet current and future liabilities. Examiners may review an HMO's existing cash resources; investments; premium receivables; interest receivables; prepaid expenses; restricted assets; leasehold arrangements; accounts payable; unpaid claims; unearned premiums; outstanding loans; statutory liability; building, land, equipment, and inventory lists; and other company assets and costs.

As part of the examination process, regulators may conduct a site visit to see the HMO's operations first hand, to review health plan documents, and to assess the efficiency and soundness of plan operations. The site visit may be relatively brief, or it can take place over a period of days or weeks. Occasionally, regulators contact participating providers and enrollees directly to determine how the HMO is operating. If an HMO is undercapitalized or otherwise short of funds, regulators can pursue several actions as discussed earlier. Regulators take financial shortfalls seriously, however, and will suspend or revoke an HMO's license if necessary to protect consumer interests. As has already been noted, the RBC for the Health Organizations Model Act provides for a similar, multitiered approach to regulatory interventions.

State Role in HIPAA Implementation

The federal Health Insurance Portability and Accountability Act of 1996 (HIPAA; see also Chapter 67) was designed by Congress to improve the availability and portability of health coverage by establishing federal minimum standards for access, portability, and renewability in both the group and individual coverage markets, with primary responsibility for implementation going to the states. To achieve these goals, HIPAA limits exclusions for preexisting medical conditions, provides new rights that allow certain individuals to enroll in health coverage when they lose coverage or have a new dependent, and prohibits discrimination in employer group coverage in enrollment eligibility against employees and their dependents on the basis of health status.

HIPAA established a precedent-setting model of federal-state regulation by establishing extensive standards directly applicable to insurers. HIPAA granted states primary responsibility for implementing the federal law, but it provides for federal enforcement if the state does not enforce it. Before HIPAA's enactment, most states had approved and implemented health insurance reform laws that set forth requirements similar to those under the federal law. In many cases, states' requirements exceeded the federal law. In other cases, the HIPAA standards were intended to serve as a floor, or set of minimum requirements. States were allowed to continue in effect, and are allowed to enact, laws that meet or exceed the HIPAA standards. However, states that have laws that fell short of the HIPAA standards were required to bring their standards up to the HIPAA "floor" or face federal enforcement of the relevant HIPAA requirement(s). HIPAA provided states time to take any statutory or regulatory action necessary for state enforcement. Five states have not reached compliance with the HIPAA requirements and are currently under federal enforcement.

The model also grants states some flexibility in coming into compliance with the individual market provisions. HIPAA gave states flexibility in determining how to meet the requirement that certain individuals (those with at least 18 months of coverage without a break of more than 63 days and with their most recent coverage from a group plan) losing group coverage must have guaranteed access to at least some individual market products. States may implement the individual market provisions using either a federal fallback or an alternative mechanism. Under the federal fallback approach, a carrier must guarantee access to eligible individuals by offering either all of its individual market plans, its two most popular plans, or two representative plans. States choosing the alternative mechanism under HIPAA are allowed a variety of approaches that are subject to certain requirements. Thirty-six states and the District of Columbia have elected to use an alternative mechanism.[18]

Multi-State Operations

Managed care plans operating in more than one state must comply with the regulations of each jurisdiction. Most states mandate that foreign HMOs meet the same requirements applicable to domestic HMOs. States also may require that out-of-state HMOs register to do business under the appropriate foreign corporation law and appoint an agent in the state for receipt of legal notifications.

Multi-state operations can become expensive if plans are subject to numerous financial examinations and other regulatory requirements. To alleviate this concern, some states permit regulators who are considering the application of a foreign HMO to accept financial reports and other information from the HMO's state of origin. The NAIC also has established guidelines for coordinating examinations of HMOs licensed in more than one state. The coordinated examination is called for by the lead state in which the HMO is domiciled; other states in which the HMO operates are encouraged to participate. Occasionally, regulations in one state may adversely affect or hinder the operations of an HMO licensed in another state.

Historically, group insurance policies generally have been subject to the law of the state of issuance. A policy issued in state A would be subject to that state's insurance laws and regulations, including mandated benefits. This general rule has been eroded by extraterritorial application of state insurance law. The laws of state B may require that any state B resident covered under a group health policy, even if issued in state A, receive the same coverage that would be required had the group policy been issued in State B.

STATE REGULATION OF OTHER PRODUCTS

Point-of-Service Offerings

Interest in coverage that includes a POS option continues to grow, with 11.1 million HMO enrollees participating in such plans in 1997.[19] Under a POS option, when a health plan member needs medical care, he or she chooses, at the point of service, whether to go to a provider within the plan's network or to seek medical care out of the network, in which case higher cost sharing would apply (see also Chapters 3 and 41). When an HMO offers a POS product on its own by underwriting out-of-plan benefits, this is referred to as a stand-alone product. Some state laws, however, prohibit HMOs from offering a POS product without entering into an agreement with an insurance company to cover the out-of-plan use. This is referred to as a wraparound product. In any case, the HMO option continues to be regulated as an HMO product.

In 1999, the American Association of Health Plans (AAHP) conducted a survey that examined the ability of HMOs to offer POS at the state level.[20] It revealed that as of April 1999, of the 42 jurisdictions responding, 25 states and the District of Columbia permitted HMOs to offer stand-alone POS products, whereas 14 states prohibited it. At least 37 states and the District of Columbia, however, allow HMO-sponsored POS products on a wraparound basis through statute, regulation, or rule, or after an agency review. One state—Delaware—prohibits all POS offerings.[21] A 1993 survey by the Group Health Association of America (one of AAHP's predecessor organizations) identified the following corporate relationships underpinning wraparound offerings:

- HMO-controlled offerings, in which the HMO contracts with an indemnity carrier directly (the employer signs one contract with the HMO and pays one premium)
- shared venture offerings, in which the HMO and the indemnity carrier contract separately with the employer (the employer signs two contracts and pays two premiums)
- multiple licensed parent company offerings, in which the HMO and the indemnity carrier are affiliates or subsidiaries of the same parent company, which offers both plans to the employer
- insurance company offerings, in which the HMO must be a licensed insurance company
- indemnity trust agreements, in which the indemnity carrier issues the indemnity portion to a trust, which then contracts with employer groups

In the states that allow HMOs to offer POS products under their own license, the following provisions are typical:

- a limit on the percentage (10 to 20 percent) of total health care expenditures for enrollees who obtain services outside the plan
- increased financial solvency requirements
- a tracking system to measure in-network and out-of-network utilization separately
- a mechanism for processing and paying for all out-of-plan service claims

By June 1999, 18 states had adopted laws mandating that HMOs offer POS products in certain situations.[22] In general, mandatory POS laws require HMOs to offer POS (or PPOs, or any coverage arrangement allowing enrollees to access services outside the HMO) to either purchasers of health coverage or health plan enrollees. If the mandatory offering is directed to purchasers, the purchaser decides whether to offer the POS option to employees. In addition, such laws usually include requirements that enrollees choosing the out-of-network option pay any higher premiums and cost-sharing amounts that result.

Provider-Sponsored Organizations

Provider-sponsored organizations (PSOs; see also Chapters 4 and 55) have been defined as health care delivery systems sponsored by physicians and hospitals, although many HMOs and PPOs also fit this description.[23] Before the implementation of the federal Balanced Budget Act (BBA) in 1997, proponents of PSOs argued for special regulatory treatment of PSOs, including exemptions from state health plan licensing, solvency, and QA laws to participate in the health care market. At the time, PSOs were growing rapidly in the marketplace under existing state licensure and regulatory requirements for health plans. In fact, a 1997 AAHP survey found that nearly 40 percent of HMOs licensed over the previous two years were provider-owned.[24]

The NAIC, in 1997, noted in its white paper on the regulation of health risk-bearing entities that a "great number" of states are regulating PSOs under the same licensure requirements that apply to HMOs. Also, in 1997, the Ohio legislature enacted the Managed Care Uniform Licensure Act. The law applies comparable standards to all risk-bearing managed care entities that perform the same or similar functions—regardless of their ownership or organizational structure. All risk-bearing entities must meet a set of solvency and quality standards. Solvency requirements for health insuring corporations (HICs) are based on types of services offered. Deposit requirements are the same for provider-owned and nonprovider owned corporations; net worth requirements vary by type of ownership. The law includes operational requirements for HICs, including provisions related to grievance procedures, enrollment, coverage of particular treatments or procedures, genetic testing, and provider contract terms.

The AAHP found that by June 1999, 14 states had enacted some form of PSO enabling legislation, in many instances to allow PSOs to participate in Medicare (consistent with federal law, as discussed later) but not creating separate licensure standards for participation in other segments of the market.[25] Some states have enacted laws following requirements set out by the BBA for QA, solvency, and licensure requirements for PSOs participating in Medicare, whereas other states apply such requirements to all PSOs, not just those wishing to participate in Medicare. As noted previously, however, Ohio has enacted a uniform licensure law applying the same quality performance and solvency standards for all managed care entities, not just PSOs.

Beginning in 1997, as part of the BBA, PSOs that met certain requirements were given the authority to contract directly with Medicare. In 1998, the federal Health Care Financing Administration (HCFA) issued an interim final rule that describes a PSO for the purposes of contracting under the Medicare + Choice program and specifies related requirements for meeting this definition. The interim final rule defines a PSO as a public or private entity that (1) is licensed by the state or has obtained a federal waiver of the licensure requirement; (2) is established or organized, and operated, by a health care provider or a group of affiliated health care providers; and (3) provides a substantial proportion of the health care items and services under its Medi-

care + Choice contract directly through the provider or affiliated group of providers. Despite this new opportunity to participate in Medicare, as of the end of 1999, only a few PSOs were participating in the Medicare + Choice program.

In addition, although the BBA requires that each Medicare + Choice plan be state-licensed as a risk-bearing entity, the BBA allows for a waiver of this state licensure requirement. The waiver for PSOs is available only if an organization has applied for the appropriate state license and the state has failed to act on a substantially complete application within 90 days or denied it for certain reasons such as applying solvency standards that differ from federal rules. Such waivers are good for 36 months, and federal solvency standards apply to a PSO with a waiver, but the plan would still be subject to state consumer protection and quality standards.[26]

Specialty HMOs

A specialty HMO is an entity that accepts a capitated payment to provide for (or arrange for the provision of) a limited set of medical service categories. The arrangement is a form of a carve-out. In some cases, a specialty HMO receives its capitation payment from a general HMO and in other cases (often involving dental services) directly from an employer. The latest data show that most enrollment in specialty HMOs is in three types: dental, mental health, and vision.[27]

Some states define a broad range of health services that HMOs are required to offer, making it difficult to offer a specialty HMO. Other states allow specialty HMOs, termed "prepaid limited health services organizations" by the NAIC. General regulatory requirements for specialty HMOs are similar to, but not as comprehensive as, those in the HMO Model Act. Requirements include licensure and issuance of a COA, filing requirements, review of payment methods, development of a complaint system, periodic examinations, financial and investment guidelines, insolvency protections, oversight of agents, confidentiality rules, issuance of a fidelity bond for officers and employees, and provider contracting standards.[28]

Utilization Review Organizations

The continuing demand by employers to manage utilization of health care services and to control costs has resulted in a steady proliferation over the past 10 years of independent UROs. Many states regulate independent UROs, and many also regulate HMOs' internal UR programs through state HMO acts or other statutes. This section, however, focuses only on the regulation of independent UROs. Nonetheless, it is important to note that some states apply stand-alone UR laws to independent UROs *and* HMOs, and in some states the resulting combination of stand-alone UR laws and UR requirements in separate HMO laws can create confusion and be unnecessarily duplicative for HMOs.

As of June 1998, 36 states had some form of stand-alone UR regulation.[29] As discussed earlier, there are a number of provisions that are common to state UR laws. A prevalent requirement, included in 28 laws, is that organizations that conduct UR must be licensed, registered, or certified before performing UR activities in the state. In 25 states, specific clinical review criteria must be used when making a UR determination, and in 26 states, a physician or "clinical peer" must review all adverse coverage determinations. In addition, 32 states require that UROs have appeals processes for adverse determinations. Other areas that are frequently governed by state laws include prohibitions against financial incentives that are tied to UR determinations, oversight of delegated UR, and requirements that UROs be privately accredited.

If a URO contracts on an exclusive basis with self-funded employers, its operations are regulated by the Employee Retirement Income Security Act (ERISA), and state laws do not apply. However, many state regulators argue that if a URO has even one commercial contract, in which a health plan is assuming the insurance risk of all the URO's operations, the URO is subject to state laws. ERISA itself regulates the appeals process for adverse coverage determinations.

Although UR laws share many common attributes, variations can create compliance problems for UROs that operate in multiple states. One of the major compliance concerns facing multistate UROs is same-state licensure for reviewers. Although most states require only that a reviewer be licensed in a state, but not necessarily the state in which the review takes place, at least seven states require reviewers to be licensed in the state in which the review takes place.[30] As such, URO reviewers may be required to become licensed in multiple states. Another example of a compliance issue facing multi-state UROs is access to medical records. Several states require that all UR agents who inquire about a patient's treatment be licensed in that particular state to gain access to medical records and other pertinent information.

Third-Party Administrators

A third-party administrator (TPA) is an organization that administers group benefits and claims for a self-funded company or group. A TPA normally does not assume any insurance risk. Thirty-six states require licensure of TPAs, and almost half require licensure even if there only is one plan participant residing in the state.[31] Approximately five states require licensing if a certain percentage or number of plan participants reside in the state. About one third of all states provide for an exemption from state licensure if the TPA administers only single-employer self-funded plans.

State TPA laws typically govern the following: the TPA's written agreement with insurers, including a statement of duties; payment method; maintenance and disclosure of records; insurer responsibilities, such as determination of benefit levels; fiduciary obligations when the TPA collects charges and premiums; issuance of TPA licenses and grounds for suspension or revocation; and filing of annual reports and payment of fees.

Self-Funded Plans

An employer may decide to finance its health plan through "self-funding." This is an arrangement under which an employer provides its employees with health coverage out of its general assets. Thus, the employer takes on some or all of the risk of paying for its employees' health benefits instead of shifting the risk to an insurance company or HMO. The risk of coverage can be shared with employees through deductibles and copayments. If an employer wants to limit its risk, it also may purchase insurance to cover losses beyond a certain "stop-loss" point. Most self-funded plans choose to purchase some form of stop-loss insurance to limit their risk.

Self-funded plans are regulated by the U.S. Department of Labor (DOL) through ERISA. As such, these arrangements typically are beyond the state's insurance regulatory jurisdiction. However, not all state law requirements are necessarily preempted by ERISA. In 1997, the U.S. Supreme Court held that ERISA does not preempt a New York state hospital tax that was assessed against a self-funded health plan that owned several medical centers.[32] ERISA is discussed in detail in Chapter 66.

In addition, state insurance departments have focused in the past on the point at which a self-funded plan's stop-loss insurance is triggered. Some states have contended that when the trigger point is very low, the plan is not actually self-funded, but instead is an insured health plan subject to state regulation. The NAIC has issued model legislation that sets specific and aggregate stop-loss attachment points. However, contrary to some states' positions on this issue, a federal appellate court disagreed with one state—Maryland—that a stop-loss trigger point less than $10,000 converted a stop-loss arrangement into health insurance.[33]

Employers self-funding health benefits may rely on managed care arrangements for the delivery of health benefits. MCOs that otherwise have state-licensed products usually can offer services under self-funded arrangements in at least two ways:

- *Administrative services only:* Regulated entities can offer a self-funded managed care product under an administrative services only arrangement with an employer who assumes the financial risk of the benefits plan. The MCO handles administrative functions for the employer group, which can include utilization management.

- *Use of MCO provider networks:* Under these arrangements, a self-funded employer can contract with an MCO to use its provider panel. The employer pays the MCO on a fee-for-service basis for medical services rendered to avoid transfer of insurance risk from the employer to the MCO or providers.

MANAGED CARE LEGISLATION

Overview

MCOs were designed as a response to quality and cost containment concerns experienced by traditional indemnity insurance. To address these issues, MCOs developed techniques such as QA procedures, utilization management programs, selective contracting, and capitation. In the past 10 years, as MCOs have gained a substantial foothold in the marketplace, states have moved toward redefining the regulatory framework for MCO operations.

Any Willing Provider

The creation of selective provider panels is a cornerstone of MCO operations. Many states, however, have enacted any willing provider (AWP) laws that prevent MCOs from selectively contracting with a limited group of providers.

By mid-1999, approximately 35 AWP laws affecting MCOs had been adopted in 25 states.[34] The most common type, adopted in 15 states, requires health plans to accept into the plan's network nonparticipating pharmacists willing to meet the terms and conditions of the MCO; in about half of the states, HMOs receive full or partial exemptions from such requirements. (Most AWP laws apply to specific categories of providers, rather than across the board.) Additionally, several courts have ruled that AWP laws are preempted by federal statutes.

At least 10 states have adopted AWP laws that include physicians as possible beneficiaries. Most states traditionally have exempted HMOs from such requirements. This can be explained in part because such a law would violate the federal

HMO Act, which preempts state laws designating the number or percentage of physicians who must participate in a federally qualified HMO network.

The advent of AWP proposals in the early 1990s prompted the U.S. Federal Trade Commission (FTC) to weigh in on the implications of such proposals by concurring with MCOs' position that AWP legislation would harm consumers. In many states that have considered AWP proposals, the FTC has written opinion letters indicating that AWP bills pose a serious anticompetitive threat. For instance, in 1993, the FTC wrote to the attorney general of Montana regarding the state's AWP statute that was due to expire without legislative reauthorization. In this opinion letter, FTC staff wrote: "Although the law may be intended to assure consumers greater freedom to choose where they obtain services, it appears likely to have the unintended effect of denying consumers the advantages of cost-reducing arrangements and limiting their choices in the provision of health care services."[35] The National Governors Association has repeatedly reaffirmed its opposition to AWP legislation as first articulated in a 1994 policy statement and adopted at successive annual meetings.[36]

Several studies have documented the potential costs of implementing AWP laws. A 1998 Barents Group LLC study, commissioned by the AAHP, estimated that AWP laws would increase costs for HMOs by 13 to 16 percent—and across all managed care health plans by 6.6 to 8.6 percent.[37] This cost increase is attributed to plans' reduced ability to obtain price discounts and conduct effective utilization management when state law interferes with selective contracting.

Other studies have reached similar conclusions. A study by Arthur Andersen & Company, commissioned by the Florida legislature, indicated that if the AWP proposal were implemented most savings attributable to provider discounts and reduced utilization would probably be lost.[38] As a result, the study predicted that per-member, per-month costs for private sector managed care plans would increase by approximately 15 percent.

State AWP laws are subject to legal challenge on the basis of federal preemption under the federal HMO Act, ERISA, and the Federal Employees Health Benefits Act. There have been three major legal challenges to AWP laws in the 1990s. In 1996, a federal appeals court ruled that an AWP law in Louisiana was preempted by ERISA.[39] The court held that the law affects employers' and sponsors' discretion as to the structuring of health benefits under employee benefit plans because it explicitly directs plan administrators not to structure their plans so as to exclude any willing provider. Subsequently, the U.S. Supreme Court refused to hear the state's appeal and as a result Louisiana cannot enforce the AWP law with respect to ERISA plans, both insured and self-funded.

In 1997, a federal district court ruled that ERISA preempts an AWP law in Arkansas; this ruling was upheld by a federal appeals court in 1998, and the entire AWP provision was declared invalid.[40] The basis for the lawsuit was that the AWP law is preempted by several federal statutes and would interfere with the private relationship between health plans and employers, thereby impeding health plans' ability to offer high-quality, affordable health care.

In 1997, a federal appeals court ruled that a Texas statute relating to any willing pharmacy is preempted by ERISA.[41] The court said that the statute relates to ERISA plans because it eliminates the choice of one method of structuring benefits by prohibiting plans from contracting with pharmacy networks that exclude AWP.

Access to Specialty Care

With growing frequency during the 1990s, states have considered legislation mandating specific procedures by which patients may access specialists. Like AWP laws, many specialty access laws can be costly and inconsistent with the way that some MCOs have traditionally provided access to specialty care.

One type of access to specialty care legislation is commonly called "direct access." These initiatives usually require that plans cover specialty care visits even if individuals do not first obtain a referral from a PCP. Much of the state activity in this area has focused on providing access to specific categories of providers—most commonly obstetricians/gynecologists (OBs/GYNs). By mid-1999, 36 states had enacted laws to require plans to offer women enrollees the choice of an OB/GYN as their PCP or allow self-referral for routine OB/GYN care.[42] Other providers included in some direct access laws are dermatologists, eye care providers, and chiropractors.

Another approach that states are increasingly considering allows MCO enrollees with medical conditions that need ongoing specialty care to designate specialists as PCPs—eight states have enacted such laws.[43]

A third approach adopted by 17 states provides for "standing referrals" to specialists for enrollees with ongoing medical conditions.[44]

It should be noted that over the past few years a growing number of MCOs have developed "open access" products, which offer enrollees the opportunity to self-refer to participating specialists without obtaining prior approval. Additionally, MCOs that include coordination of referrals to specialists by PCPs are increasingly streamlining the referral process. These market-based innovations are often very different from the rigid requirements that are imposed by direct access legislation.

Research shows that access to specialty care, even before the states recently began to pass laws, is a flexible process for most enrollees—more than 75 percent of HMOs surveyed by Mathematica Policy Research Inc. in 1994 allowed specialists to serve as PCPs on a case-by-case approved basis.[45]

In many instances, specialty access legislation presents a dilemma for both health plans and consumers in that many of the specialists included in these proposals do not meet health plan requirements as PCPs, and, consequently, are not able to appropriately perform PCP functions, in which case they may be required to obtain additional training.

Drug Formularies

To promote the appropriate use of prescription drugs and control costs, managed care plans have increasingly turned to prescription drug formularies. In 1997, 93 percent of HMOs used prescription drug formularies, up from 44 percent in 1990.[46] Typically, HMOs and PPOs allow for consideration of formulary exceptions on the basis of clinical considerations. By mid-1999, at least 29 states had statutes specifically governing the use of formularies by health plans.[47] Other nonformulary-specific state statutes in areas such as UR and grievances and appeals may also indirectly apply to the use of formularies.

In general, statutes regulating the use of formularies by MCOs require plans to disclose their formularies; implement procedures for health plan members to obtain nonformulary drugs in certain circumstances; and/or disclose these procedures.

As of December 1999, 31 states required managed care plans to disclose their drug formulary and 14 states required plans to disclose procedures for obtaining nonformulary drugs.[48] Of the 16 state laws pertaining to obtaining nonformulary drugs in certain circumstances, provisions vary greatly in their scope and effect on formulary use. For example, most states provide that an "exception" procedure be in place to obtain a nonformulary drug with no restrictive requirements on the procedures. A small number of states, however, require plans to provide coverage for nonformulary drugs in any circumstance in which a physician determines the nonformulary drug to be "medically necessary." The latter type of law, would, in effect, greatly diminish a plan's ability to promote quality and affordability through the use of a formulary because the plan would be compelled to cover any drug that a physician recommends.

Health Plan Liability

Beginning in the late 1990s, expanding health plan liability became a prominent issue in state legislatures. In most of the states, changes have been proposed to tort laws that would expose health plans to liability for their coverage determinations and utilization review activities. Three states—California, Georgia, and Texas—

had enacted liability laws by December 1999.

Without expanded liability, health plans may be held liable based on the principles of direct corporate liability and vicarious liability for such acts as the negligent credentialing of physicians and consumer fraud and misrepresentation. Legislation introduced in the states would effectively expand the liability exposure of health plans beyond that which already exists.

In 1997, Texas became the first state to expand health plan liability. The Texas statute holds health plans to a standard of "ordinary care" when making "health care treatment decisions." However, it is being challenged under ERISA's preemption clause; a late 1998 federal district court decision (which was being appealed as of December 1999) held that liability claims based on the quality of the benefit are not preempted, whereas claims based on a denial of benefits would be preempted. The three laws in California, Georgia, and Texas are similar in that all internal and external review processes must be exhausted before a lawsuit can be filed. External review can be bypassed if the patient alleges that harm has already occurred.

In addition, recently introduced federal legislation seeks to expand the scope of damages available under ERISA. Provisions in ERISA provide that every employee benefit plan, whether insured or self-insured, must provide an opportunity for "full and fair review" to any participant whose claims for benefits under the plan have been denied. Moreover, ERISA beneficiaries may sue in federal court for recovery of benefits due to them, to enforce or clarify their rights under their benefit plan, and to enjoin any practice that violates either ERISA or the terms of the plan. Some liability proposals seek to expand health plan liability by permitting ERISA participants to bring state law causes of action to recover damages resulting from personal injury or wrongful death. Other proposals would create new economic and noneconomic damages within a federal claim brought under ERISA. Most proposals being considered reduce the damages available if a plan follows the recommendations of an independent external review entity. At the time this chapter was written, the final outcome of these proposals was undetermined.

MCOs have raised concerns that these proposals would increase costs, thereby adding to the number of uninsured Americans, and diminish quality of care. The cost impact of expanded liability has been studied by various research groups and government agencies: The Barents Group LLC, in a study commissioned by the AAHP, projected premium increases of 2.7 to 8.6 percent, whereas the U.S. Congressional Budget Office estimated a 1.4 percent increase, the Minnesota Department of Employee Relations estimated a 5 percent increase, and a fiscal analysis prepared for the Arizona legislature estimated a 4.5 percent increase.[49]

One reason for cost increases would be the adoption of "defensive utilization review" by plans, akin to "defensive medicine" practiced by physicians. This phenomenon is characterized by the ordering of unnecessary tests that do not benefit patients, but can help avoid or mitigate costly litigation. According to researchers at Stanford University, in states with meaningful limits on malpractice liability, hospital expenditures were 5 to 9 percent lower than those in states with weak or no limits, with no effect found on health outcomes.[50]

MCOs are also concerned that quality, too, could be harmed by expanded health plan liability, as plans are compelled to tailor care management activities to jury verdicts, which have little correlation to actual negligence, rather than to medical facts. Moreover, the current liability system as applied to physicians has already been targeted by two prominent organizations. The President's Advisory Commission on Consumer Protection and Quality in the Health Care Industry has identified the liability systems as "perhaps the most significant deterrent to the identification and reduction of [medical] errors."[51] The American Medical Association has pointed out that the current system inhibits medical innovation as well as markedly increasing health care costs: "Although patients, physicians, and health care providers are most directly harmed by the present liability system, society as a whole is also harmed....The spiraling costs generated by our nation's dysfunctional liability system are borne by everyone."[52]

Physician Antitrust Exemptions

An issue of great importance to consumers, MCOs, and regulators emerged in 1999 with legislative efforts to exempt independent, competing physicians from antitrust laws and allow them to jointly negotiate with MCOs. Texas was the only state to have passed a physician antitrust exemption bill in 1999, but similar legislation will be considered in additional states in 2000 and beyond. Currently, under longstanding federal and state antitrust laws, competing physicians, like competitors in other professions, are precluded from coming together to agree on prices. However, these physicians can form legitimate joint ventures and multi-provider networks that may negotiate with MCOs. The Texas law purports to give competing physicians not part of such legitimate joint ventures the benefit of the "state action exemption" from federal antitrust law by placing physician negotiations under state supervision. Whether the Texas law establishes the supervision necessary to qualify for the state action exemption remains to be seen.

Several current and former FTC officials have spoken out against the precedent of the Texas law. In a letter to the Texas legislature, the FTC Bureau of Competition director stated his apprehensions about possible violations of antitrust statutes and the likelihood that this would cause "substantial consumer harm." In general, concerns have been raised that antitrust exemptions would undermine marketplace competition— which brings about lower costs, greater choice, higher quality, and better service for consumers—by permitting physicians to engage in anticompetitive practices such as price fixing, boycotts, and market allocation agreements.[53]

Furthermore, a statement by the assistant attorney general in charge of the Antitrust Division of the U.S. Department of Justice (DOJ), testifying before the U.S. House of Representatives Judiciary Committee in 1999, pointedly discussed the cost implications of allowing physicians to collectively bargain: "The bill's [H.R.1304] potential adverse economic impact on consumers is large. Our investigations reveal that when health care professionals jointly negotiate with health insurers, without regard to antitrust laws, they typically seek to significantly increase their fees, sometimes by as much as 20-40%."[54]

Utilization Review As the Practice of Medicine

Legislation introduced in several states would define UR as the "practice of medicine." Although a few states have considered such legislation, only one—New Mexico—has enacted such a law.

Whether UR is the "practice of medicine" has been the subject of several state attorney general opinions.[55] For instance, the attorney general of Ohio issued an opinion in August 1999 stating that "the rendering of an opinion as to the medical necessity of physician medical services for purposes of utilization review...is not considered to be the practice of medicine and does not come within the regulatory, investigatory, or enforcement authority of the Sate Medical Board." The attorney general of North Carolina said that when performing UR, an individual is not diagnosing, operating on, prescribing for, administering to, or treating any ailment, injury or deformity, but is merely deciding whether or not third party payment is available.

In 1997, a state appeals court held that the Arizona Board of Medical Examiners had authority to regulate the insurance-related decisions of health plan medical directors.[56] Essential to the court's holding was its conclusion that utilization management decision making could be characterized as the practice of medicine under state law. Specifically, the Court of Appeals of Arizona held that a decision to deny precertification for surgery was a medical decision, and that the state Board of Medical Examiners had jurisdiction over the state-licensed physician who made the decision on behalf of his employer, the health insurer.

Defining UR as the practice of medicine leaves open the possibility that MCOs could be held liable for "medical malpractice" of their medical directors as a result of the medical directors' UR determinations. The question of whether ERISA would preempt these laws is also open. In addition, this could subject medical directors to discipline by state boards over their UR determinations, as discussed earlier.

Emergency Care

Most states have considered legislation to establish rules for coverage of emergency care delivered by both participating and nonparticipating providers. For the most part, state activity has addressed prior authorization requirements, establishment of a "prudent layperson" standard, and coverage of emergency care.

For example, by June 1999, 38 states had adopted a "prudent layperson" standard for the purpose of determining whether an emergency medical condition exists.[57] Although the exact standard varies state to state, it generally defines an emergency medical condition as "a medical condition, the onset of which is sudden, that manifests itself by symptoms of sufficient severity, including severe pain, that a prudent layperson, who possesses an average knowledge of health and medicine, could reasonably expect the absence of medical attention to result in placing the person's health in jeopardy; serious impairment of bodily functions; or serious dysfunction of any bodily organ or part."[58] If a condition meets the "prudent layperson" test, the plan is then required to cover the emergency care, which typically includes screening and stabilization, as specified by the particular state law.

Clinical Mandates

In addition to laws that states have been approving to require coverage of specific benefits, many states now dictate how and for how long certain services must be provided. Specifically, legislative proposals setting minimum requirements for coverage of postpartum and postmastectomy hospital length of stay have garnered support in recent years.

This type of legislation requires that hospital inpatient length-of-stay coverage determinations

(and, in the case of mastectomy, inpatient versus outpatient setting determinations) for the specified condition be made solely by an individual physician, in consultation with the patient. Under such a clinical mandate, the involvement of health plans in length-of-stay coverage decisions is eliminated. These kinds of laws compromise affordability and quality of life.

Since 1995, mandatory postpartum hospital length-of-stay requirements have been enacted in 42 states.[59] Most of these laws specify that plans provide coverage for 48 hours of hospital care after a normal vaginal delivery and 96 hours after a Caesarean section. This is consistent with provisions in the federal Newborns' and Mothers' Health Protection Act of 1996.

Similarly, mandatory postmastectomy hospital length of stay laws have been enacted in 19 states.[60] For the most part, these laws either require insurers to provide coverage for 48 hours of hospital care after a mastectomy and 24 hours after a lumpectomy, or require insurers to cover a hospital stay for a length of time determined appropriate by the attending physician. Notably, evidence indicates that the largest number of outpatient mastectomies are performed on women in Medicare fee-for-service arrangements, not in health plans.[61]

Other research shows that a number of states have chosen not to apply such mandates to their own state employee and Medicaid populations. A 1996 report by the U.S. General Accounting Office found that of the 29 states that had maternity length-of-stay mandates, they were not made applicable to the state Medicaid program in 18 states and to state employees in 19 states.[62]

Mandated Benefits

State laws governing HMOs require that their enrollees be offered comprehensive health care services. In fact, the industry's ability to provide broad coverage has been one of its distinctive trademarks. Nevertheless, many states now require coverage of additional specified services, too. Most mandated benefits are specific to certain conditions. Such benefits include coverage for congenital defects, phenylketonuria, in vitro fertilization, temporomandibular joint syndrome, autologous bone marrow transplants, and Lyme disease, to name a few. In addition, a handful of states have mandated coverage of routine costs associated with clinical trials. In 1998 alone, approximately 94 mandated benefit laws were enacted in 33 states.[63] This trend continued into 1999—by mid-year, 44 mandated benefit laws had passed in 17 states.[64]

One mandate that has generated significant attention is a requirement that coverage of mental health illnesses be equal in some or all respects to that of medical/surgical illnesses or conditions. In 1996, Congress passed the Mental Health Parity Act, which requires group health plans that offer mental health coverage benefits to apply the same annual and aggregate lifetime dollar limits to mental health coverage as those applied to coverage of other services. The federal law applies to fully insured and self-insured plans, including state-regulated plans. However, states may enact requirements more stringent than those contained under the federal law. By June 1999, 31 states had enacted mandatory coverage for mental illness.[65]

At least 12 states have codified the federal requirements, whereas other laws contain much broader provisions. For example, although the federal law defines the term "mental illness" as that used in the health plan contract, some states clearly define a subset of illnesses to which the requirements apply, whereas others apply their coverage requirements quite broadly to any illness listed in the *Diagnostic and Statistical Manual of Mental Illnesses*. Similarly, some state laws apply coverage requirements to a defined set of benefit design features, such as day and visit limits, whereas others prohibit the establishment of any rate, term, or condition that places a greater financial burden on an insured for mental health coverage than for coverage of a physical health condition.

When state legislatures mandate coverage of specific services or mandate medical protocols that may not always be necessary, a point of diminishing returns is quickly reached. Concerns about the impact of coverage mandates resulted in an extensive analysis by a legislative committee in Florida on the status of mandates enacted in the state.[66] The committee detailed the lack of systematic review of the effects of mandates and offered numerous options for managing existing and proposed mandates, including creating a review entity to calculate the cost of mandates, limiting new mandates to the state health plan for a trial period, and requiring MCOs to comply with mandates only if Medicare and Medicaid programs provide a comparable benefit. A recent analysis by The Lewin Group LLC, a private health services research firm, found that each 1 percent real increase in health care premiums is associated with an estimated 300,000 individuals losing health coverage.[67] Mandated benefits also reduce HMOs' flexibility in structuring benefit packages to suit the needs of a particular group.

The impact of these types of mandates on access and quality is the subject of significant debate and research. Recently, researchers have concluded that, based on their review of existing research on the consequences of mandated benefit laws, workers pay for health insurance mandates in the form of lower wages and that the number of uninsured persons would have been approximately 20 to 25 percent lower except for the presence of mandates that raised premium costs.[68]

Another key concern for lawmakers should be whether the treatment that is subject to the coverage mandate has been proven to be beneficial. For instance, in late 1999, questions were raised about the value and safety of high-dose chemotherapy with autologous bone marrow transplants (HDC-ABMT) for breast cancer treatment. At that time, the National Cancer Institute released preliminary results from clinical trials showing the lack of benefit to patients of HDC-ABMT over standard therapy. Prior to the release of these clinical trial results, seven states had mandated coverage for this type of treatment.

Uncertainty about the implications of mandating health care benefits without knowing the possible impact on quality, cost, and utilization has moved several legislatures to create commissions to study mandates. Laws in at least 18 states require a fiscal impact analysis of proposed health care mandates.[69] A unique approach to studying mandate costs was approved in Kansas, where any new mandated benefit will apply only to the state employee health care benefits program for at least one year. A state employee benefits commission must submit a report to the legislature after the year's end, assessing the mandate's impact on the state employee benefit program, including data on utilization and costs of coverage.

REGULATION BY MARKET SEGMENT

Although the focus of this chapter is on state regulation, it is important to note that, because regulation is driven by market segments, a typical MCO is regulated by several entities, depending on the combination of product lines it offers. The primary regulatory bodies responsible for protecting consumers include the following entities.

State Insurance and Health Departments

State DOIs and departments of health regulate most health plans. As previously discussed, employee health benefit plans sponsored by private employers are regulated by the U.S. DOL under ERISA, although states retain regulatory jurisdiction over the insured products purchased by employee benefit plans. Accordingly, health care coverage purchased by individuals, provided to employees of a business in which the health plan retains the risk, or offered to state employees must meet state law requirements.

In most states, health plans are regulated by at least two separate departments; state insurance departments typically regulate the financial aspects of a plan, while health departments usually regulate health plan activities and policies. In a few states, a single department is primarily responsible for regulating health plan operations.

U.S. Department of Labor

If an employer elects to offer health benefits to its employees, the employer becomes subject to regulation of the DOL under ERISA, whether the employer retains the insurance risk of providing benefits, provides the benefits on an in-

sured basis, or provides benefits through a multiple employer welfare arrangement. The DOL administers Title I of ERISA, which covers all types of employee benefit plans and has been active in implementing changes to ERISA through regulatory work and participation in an *amicus curiae* program through the DOL solicitor's office.

In September 1998, the DOL issued a proposed regulation revising current requirements for benefit claims procedures of employee benefit plans governed by ERISA. The proposed regulation modifies existing regulations governing time frames for decision making, disclosure, and notice requirements; standards of review on appeal; and consequences of failure to establish and follow reasonable claims procedures. Notably, the proposed regulation failed to make any distinction between the procedures for handling requests for prior authorization of services and handling postservice claims for payment. The regulation had not been finalized by January 2000 and may be modified before being finalized.

U.S. Department of Health and Human Services

Located in the U.S. DHHS, HCFA is the primary federal agency that oversees the Medicare and Medicaid programs and the State Children's Health Insurance Program (SCHIP). Additional regulatory responsibilities include administrative simplification and portability under HIPAA.

MCOs that participate in the Medicare managed care program, known as Medicare + Choice, must comply with rules and regulations established by HCFA. These rules preempt state laws and other standards related to benefits requirements, inclusion or treatment of providers in networks, and coverage determination, including appeals and grievance processes, in cases in which state laws are inconsistent with federal Medicare + Choice requirements. The federal rules also prohibit states from imposing taxes on payments that health plans receive under the Medicare + Choice program.

HCFA's role in overseeing Medicaid managed care and SCHIP, which was established in

1997 by the BBA, differs somewhat from its responsibility for the Medicare + Choice program. For these two programs, HCFA provides general rules and frameworks under which states must administer their programs and ensure MCOs' compliance with rules and regulations.

Medicare managed care is discussed in detail in Chapters 55 and 56.

State Medicaid Departments

State social service or welfare departments and sometimes state health departments, in conjunction with HCFA, regulate Medicaid programs. Medicaid is a joint federal-state program under which states receive federal matching funds to defray part of the cost of providing medical assistance to targeted, low-income populations. HCFA reviews state plans for assurances that the state will require participating MCOs to meet standards set in the federal statute. This statute includes standards that Medicaid managed care plans must meet and requires preapproval by HCFA for every Medicaid managed care plan contract over a threshold dollar amount.

Medicaid managed care is discussed in detail in Chapter 57.

U.S. Office of Personnel Management

The Office of Personnel Management (OPM) regulates coverage offered to federal employees (i.e., FEHBP—the Federal Employees Health Benefits Program). In designing the federal employee program, Congress took steps to ensure uniformity of benefits by explicitly preempting state laws that are inconsistent with the contract between the program and the plan, as well as state premium taxes.[70] Although ERISA does not apply to FEHBP plans, the program imposes limits similar to those under ERISA on the remedies that are available to an enrollee.

OPM manages health benefits worth more than $16 billion for 10 million enrollees. Its responsibilities include determining which plans will be part of FEHBP, communicating information to plan members, requiring participating plans to perform administrative tasks, negotiating premium rates, and auditing the plans periodically. Although there is no standard benefit package under FEHBP, OPM requires the benefit packages of participating plans to include certain core benefits. Each spring, OPM sends all plan providers its "call letter," a document that specifies, among other things, the types of benefits that must be available to plan participants, as well as the cost goals and procedural changes that the plans need to adopt. In addition, FEHBP recently mandated that all participating plans cover ABMTs. In 1998, Congress also approved a measure that requires plans that cover prescription drugs to cover contraceptives, including contraceptive devices. Unlike the ABMT mandate, which is permanent, the contraceptive mandate is subject to annual congressional approval.

The FEHBP is discussed in further detail in Chapter 54.

U.S. Department of Defense

The Department of Defense (DOD) regulates coverage delivered through its military health services system (MHSS), a worldwide health care system made up of more than 500 medical and dental treatment sites called military treatment facilities that includes 115 hospitals. In addition to covering members of the armed services on active duty and their dependents, DOD also offers health care benefits to inactive armed services personnel and their dependents through its Civilian Health and Medical Program of the Uniformed Services (CHAMPUS) program. CHAMPUS has a fee-for-service option and a managed care option, known as TRICARE.

Under TRICARE, several private managed care plans provide administrative services and backup treatment facilities on an exclusive basis in the 12 regions of the MHSS.

TRICARE and CHAMPUS are discussed in Chapter 58.

Other Regulatory Agencies

MCOs also are subject to laws of general applicability and as such are regulated by various federal and state government agencies. While some of these agencies, such as the U.S. Food and Drug Administration and the Health Resources and Services Administration, primarily focus on health care issues, others do not. At the federal level, the Occupational Safety and Health Administration of the U.S. DOL has regulatory authority over MCOs, as does the National Institute for Occupational Safety and Health. MCOs are subject to tax laws enforced by the Internal Revenue Service, antitrust laws enforced by the U.S. DOJ and the FTC, civil rights and antidiscrimination laws enforced by the DOJ and the Equal Employment Opportunity Commission, and fraud and abuse laws enforced by HCFA, the Office of the Inspector General of DHHS, and the DOJ. In addition, MCOs are subject to corresponding state laws as well, which can involve enforcement by state Attorneys General, Departments of Revenue, and other agencies.

THE STATE EXPERIENCE— CONCLUSION

The regulatory structure for MCOs faces daunting challenges in the years ahead. Historically state-centered, the system increasingly is characterized by overlapping state and federal regulation. There are serious unanswered questions about whether such a regime will produce regulation that is workable for plans and offers value to consumers. In our opinion, it is more likely than not that layers of federal and state regulation will increase costs and limit access, stymie innovation, and produce conflicting signals about what managed care plans must do to comply with the law.

Furthermore, in recent years, the debate about the regulation of MCOs—at both the federal and state levels—has proceeded as if such health plans are the sole actor in the health care system. However, the policies and practices of physicians, nurses, other health care professionals, hospitals, and other institutional providers play central and independent roles in determining how well the health care system works. For instance, the serious harm that widespread underuse, overuse, and misuse of particular medical services causes to Americans will not be redressed by multiplying the volume of regulation governing managed care plans—or by weakening their ability to use the tools that already contribute to solving these problems. To make real progress in solving the American health care system's cost and quality problems, policy makers and regulators will need to redefine the issues and adopt a systemwide perspective that recognizes the role and responsibilities of each system's participants.

REFERENCES AND NOTES

1. National Association of Insurance Commissioners (NAIC), *HMO Examination Handbook*, 1990. In addition, the NAIC has adopted many model regulations for HMOs.

2. NAIC, *Model Health Maintenance Organization Act*, July 1998.

3. NAIC, *Preferred Provider Arrangements Model Act*, subsection C of section 4, 1996. A drafting note indicates that "subsection C is an optional section if a state desires to require verification of preferred provider arrangement activity of non-insurance entities."

4. American Association of Health Plans (AAHP), *The Regulation of Health Plans*, 1998, 29.

5. AAHP, see reference 4, p. 30.

6. Three states have enacted the model act and 12 states have enacted related legislation or regulation. NAIC Web site, "States That Have Enacted NAIC Health Plans Standard Model Acts," updated 1999.

7. NAIC, see reference 3, section 4 A.

8. American Accreditation Health Care Commission (AAHCC) /URAC, *The PPO Guide*, 1998; Mardan and Quigley, *Guide to State PPO Laws and Regulations*, 1995.

9. AAHCC/URAC, *The PPO Guide,* see reference 8.

10. Two states have enacted the model act and 24 states have enacted related legislation or regulation. NAIC Web site, see reference 6.

11. One state has enacted the model act and 15 states have enacted related legislation or regulation. NAIC Web site, see reference 6.

12. AAHCC/URAC, *Survey of State Health Utilization Review Laws and Regulations*, 1999.

13. AAHCC/URAC, *The PPO Guide,* see reference 8.

14. Six states have enacted the UR Model Act and 36 states have enacted related legislation or regulation; five states have enacted the Grievance Procedure Model Act, and 33 states have enacted related legislation or regulation. NAIC Web site, see reference 6.

15. AAHP, *State External Review Laws*, December 1999.

16. AAHP, see reference 15.

17. Alabama, Florida, Illinois, Vermont, West Virginia, Wisconsin. NAIC, *Compilation of State Laws on Insurance Topics*, 1999.

18. U.S. General Accounting Office, *Health Insurance Standards: New Federal Law Creates Challenges for Consumers, Insurers, Regulators*, February 25, 1998.

19. InterStudy, *Competitive Edge Part II: HMO Industry Report*, April 1999.

20. AAHP, *Survey of State Regulators Finds POS Products Often Are Associated with Restrictions That Can Increase Costs Substantially*, April 1999.

21. Of the remaining two states, Alaska does not have an HMO in the state, and Wyoming laws and rules do not address the issue of whether HMOs may offer stand-alone POS products.

22. National Conference of State Legislators (NCSL), *Major Health Care Policies: 50 State Profile*, 1998; AAHP, *Mandatory POS Requirements: Summary of 1999 State Legislative Proposals and Enacted Laws*, December 1999.

23. Medicare Payment Advisory Commission (MedPAC), *Report to Congress: Context for a Changing Medicare Program*, June 1998.

24. AAHP, *Survey Finds That Many State-Licensed Health Plans Are Provider-Owne*d, 1997.

25. AAHP, State Legislative Tracking System, 1997 & 1998.

26. MedPAC, see reference 23.

27. AAHP, *1995-1996 Managed Health Care Overview*, 1996.

28. For up-to-date information, see NAIC, Prepaid Limited Health Services Organization Model Act, I-68-1.

29. In 29 of these states, UR laws apply to HMOs' internal UR programs. AAHCC/URAC, see reference 12.

30. These laws apply only to independent UROs in Maine, Missouri, Maryland, Oklahoma, Oregon, Virginia, and Vermont. AAHCC/URAC, see reference 12, p. 14.

31. NAIC, *Society of Professional Benefit Administrators Survey and Third Party Administrator Licensure and Bond Requirements*, 1997.

32. *De Buono v. NYSA-ILA Medical and Clinical Services Fund*, 117 S.Ct. 1747 (1997).

33. *American Medical Security, Inc. v. Bartlett*, 111 F.3d 358 (4th Cir. 1997); *cert. denied*, 118 S.Ct. 2340 (1998).

34. AAHP, State Legislative Tracking Service, December 1999.

35. U.S. Federal Trade Commission, Opinion Letter to Attorney General of Montana Regarding Any Willing Provider Law [Mont. Code Ann., Title 33, Ch. 22, Part 17 (1991)], February 4, 1993.

36. National Governors Association, "Executive Committee Policy on Managed Care and Health Care Reform," effective 1998–2000, August 1998.

37. Barents Group LLC, *Impacts of Four Legislative Provisions on Managed Care Consumers: 1999–2003*, 1998.

38. Arthur Andersen & Company, *Florida Health Security Program: Actuarial Report*, 1994.

39. *Cigna v. State of Louisiana*, No. 95-30481, 82 F. 3d 642 (5th Cir. Apr. 30, 1996); *cert. denied*, No. 96-316, 519 U.S. 964 (U.S. November 4, 1996).

40. *Prudential Insurance Company v. State of Arkansas*, No. 97-2221, 154 F. 3d 812 (8th Cir. September 2, 1999).

41. *Texas Pharmacy Association v. Prudential Insurance Company*, No. 95-50807, 1997 U.S. App. LEXIS 12986 (5th Cir. February 14, 1997).

42. NCSL, Health Policy Tracking Services, December 1999.

43. NCSL, Health Policy Tracking Services, December 1999.

44. NCSL, Health Policy Tracking Services, December 1999.

45. S. Felt-Lisk, "How HMOs Structure Primary Care Delivery," *Managed Care Quarterly*, 4 (1996): 4.

46. Marion Merrill Dow, *Managed Care Digest/HMO Edition*, 1991; Hoechst Marion Roussel, *Managed Care Digest Series/HMO-PPO Digest*, 1998.

47. Hoechst Marion Roussel, *Managed Care Digest Series/ HMO-PPO Digest*, 1998.

48. Hoechst Marion Roussel, *Managed Care Digest Series/ HMO-PPO Digest*.

49. Barents Group LLC, *Impact of Legislation Affecting Managed Care Consumers*, April 1998; U.S. Congressional Budget Office, *Analysis of Cost Impact of U.S. Senate Bill 6*, 1999; Minnesota Department of Employee Relations, "Revised Fiscal Note for Senate Bill 953," April 1999; Arizona Joint Legislative Budget Committee, "Fiscal Analysis of House Bill 2600," March 16, 2000.

50. D. Kessler and M. McClellan, "Do Doctors Practice Defensive Medicine?" *Quarterly Journal of Economics*, May 1996. See also, D. Kessler and M. McClellan, "How Liability Law Affects Medical Productivity," National Bureau of Economic Research, Stanford University, February 2000.

51. President's Advisory Commission on Consumer Protection and Health Care Quality, *Final Report and Recommendations*, chapter 10, "Reducing Errors and Increasing Safety," p. 2, 1997.

Managed Health Care
at the Millennium

Peter R. Kongstvedt

INTRODUCTION—THE ROLLERCOASTER THAT NEVER STOPS

There has never been a time when the health care system in the United States has been in a prolonged state of peaceful equilibrium. Eighteenth century medicine was hampered by a lack of knowledge, and many treatments of the period caused more misery than the diseases they purported to cure. The nineteenth century can best be characterized as a free-for-all, with true advances in medicine often overwhelmed by the wide variety of individuals who were given an MD degree from all varieties of medical schools, many of which barely provided an education or promulgated strange and useless treatments. Commerce entered medicine in a big way by the nineteenth century with patent medicines, new "electrical cures," potions, and nostrums guaranteed to cure any disease, and expensive spa treatments for the well-to-do. The twentieth century brought greater discipline in medical education with the issuance of the Flexner Report, and

Thanks to Hindy Shaman, Jacqueline Lutz, and special thanks to Jean Stanford, for their invaluable contributions to the discussion around the application of chaos theory to health care markets. An earlier version of the concept of planning in chaotic managed health care markets appeared in *Equilibrium at the Edge: Planning in Chaotic Managed Care Markets* by Kongstvedt, Stanford, Shaman, and Lutz; Ernst & Young LLP, Washington, DC, 1999.

science became a central part of medicine. Advances in clinical medicine began to accelerate and have been accelerating at an increasing rate ever since.

Until the mid-twentieth century, medical care remained generally affordable and focused on fees paid to physicians. Advances in medical care, including the widespread use of hospitals, led to the increasing risk of high or unaffordable medical costs for those unfortunates who had a serious illness or injury. It was at about this same time that insurance for catastrophic health care costs appeared, as well as a few examples of early prepaid medical care systems, as is well described in Chapter 1.

To the mix of the increasing sophistication and cost of medical care, the desire of individuals to have access to that care, and the rise of third-party health insurance, Medicare and Medicaid were added in 1965. The fuse was lit and health care costs exploded off the launch pad, accelerating to higher and higher levels. By the mid-1970s, unbearable inflation in health care costs began to cause profound problems for employers who paid for health insurance for their employees and for the federal and state governments who paid for Medicare and Medicaid. Unilaterally imposed price controls, overt in the 1970s and covert thereafter in the form of prospective payments to hospitals and fee limits on physicians, were put in place by the government. Health maintenance organizations (HMOs) were given strong support by the federal government as a means of managing cost and providing af-

52. American Medical Association, testimony presented to U.S. House of Representatives, Committee on Ways and Means, Subcommittee on Health, May 20, 1993.

53. W. Baer, Director, Bureau of Competition, U.S. Federal Trade Commission, letter to Rep. Rene Oliveira concerning Texas Senate Bill 1468, May 13, 1999.

54. J. Klein, Assistant Attorney General, Antitrust Division, U.S. Department of Justice, testimony before the U.S. House of Representatives Judiciary Committee on federal bill H.R.1304, June 22, 1999.

55. Ohio AG Opinion No. 99-044 (August 31, 1999); 1989 S.C. AG LEXIS 99 (April 20, 1989); 1993 N.C. AG LEXIS 4 (April 6, 1992); 1993 Miss. AG LEXIS 280 (May 18, 1993).

56. *Murphy v. Board of Medical Examiners,* 1997 Ariz. App. LEXIS 115 (July 15, 1997).

57. NCSL, *Issue Brief: Emergency Care Services,* May 1999.

58. NCSL, see reference 57.

59. NCSL, see reference 42.

60. NCSL, see reference 42.

61. For instance, data from the New York State Department of Health found that the majority (58%) of outpatient mastectomies done in 1995 were performed on Medi-care fee-for-service beneficiaries. Of the 124 outpatient mastectomies, 72 were on women in Medicare fee-for-service and 2 in Medicare HMOs. Fifteen were performed on women in private HMOs.

62. U.S. General Accounting Office, *Maternity Care: Appropriate Follow-Up Services Critical With Short Hospital Stays,* September 1996.

63. NCSL, *Issue Brief on Mandated Benefits*, May 1999.

64. NCSL, see reference 63.

65. NCSL, *Issue Brief on Mental Health Parity*, May 1999.

66. Florida House of Representatives, Committee on Insurance, "Managing Mandated Health Benefits: Policy Options for Consideration," January 2000.

67. The Lewin Group LLC, Letter to AAHP on Estimate of Impact of Health Care Premium Increase on Insured Americans, February 4, 1999.

68. G. Jensen and M. Morrisey, "Employer-Sponsored Health Insurance and Mandated Benefit Laws," *Milbank Quarterly*, Winter 1999.

69. Florida House of Representatives, see reference 66.

70. Academy for Healthcare Management, *Managed Care Organizations: Governance and Regulation,* 1998, p. 8–15.

fordable access to care, and over time the private sector adopted managed health care as the primary vehicle for keeping costs under control without reducing benefits to useless levels.

At no time has the health care system been static for long. In the past 50 years, the pace and degree of change have become extraordinary. Some of the change has been primarily beneficial, such as improvements in the effectiveness of many treatments and the ability to diagnose diseases at an earlier stage. Other changes have not been beneficial, such as the pool of uninsured in an environment of high health care costs, creating substantial economic barriers to accessing care. By any objective view, it is not possible to refer to "the good old days" in terms that are not actually a fantasy or a highly filtered memory that does not reflect the realities of the time—Anytime.

USING THE MAGIC EIGHT BALL: THE ANSWER IS HAZY—TRY AGAIN LATER

An important feature of change in the health care system has been the inability to predict how it would evolve. This feature applies to all aspects of health care, from scientific advances to the widespread adoption of managed health care in its current form. Although highly generalized predictions have always been possible ("We will discover new drugs to treat illnesses," for example), being able to predict the course of the various components of the health care system has generally not been a successful exercise for most and has become increasingly unsuccessful over time, with a few notable exceptions.*

Cases in point of the difficulty of making predictions abound, especially in recent times. For example, in the early 1980s, many were predicting that staff or group model HMOs would provide all health care by 1995; such HMOs have been dwindling and by 2000 represent only a small percentage of total enrollment. In the mid

to late 1980s, many predicted that all health care would be paid for by capitation by the end of the century; but as of 2000, the amount of capitation has risen slowly in some areas and has actually been reduced or eliminated in some health plans. From the early to mid-1990s (and in the case of a few academics beginning in the mid-1970s), many predicted that health care would be financed and delivered by means of large, vertically integrated, mega-corporations or health delivery and financing systems (IDSs or IDFSs). These massive IDFSs would own an insurance company or HMO, physician practices, hospitals, ancillary services, and whatever else they needed to deliver and finance health care. By 2000, there are very few of these still standing,* and losses were in the mega-millions for those IDSs that attempted such hard-wired vertical integration.

Examples of correct predictions may also occur (see the 1986 Goldsmith article footnoted earlier), but most commonly, "common wisdom" is an overreaction to a trend rather than a deep understanding of complex forces at work. Changes in the health care system, especially in managed health care, occur in a nonlinear manner—a hallmark of chaotic or complexly adapting systems. It is to chaotic systems that we must now turn.

THEY WERE RIGHT ALL ALONG— MANAGED HEALTH CARE *IS* IN CHAOS

Chaotic or complexly adapting systems (CAS) theory is a branch of mathematics that was not possible until the advent of the supercomputer, which allowed for modeling of vast quantities of data. The weather is one of the best examples of a CAS; other examples include the stock market, ecosystems, evolution, and the entire universe. Because there are insufficient data over time to conduct mathematical analyses of the health care system, it is not possible to

---

*The best of which is J. Goldsmith, The U.S. Health Care System in the Year 2000, *JAMA* Dec 26, 256 (1986): 24, 3371–3375.

*Generally speaking, those that remain are struggling financially, and are frequently trying to shed themselves of their hospitals and physician practices. *Sic transit gloria mundi.*

prove that CAS theory applies, but several important attributes of CAS are seen clearly to be applicable. Five central attributes applicable to chaotic systems are briefly described as follows.

The Object Under Study Is a System That Can Be Described and Modeled

Although often described as a nonsystem, there is no denying that there is a health care system. Interrelationships exist between all aspects of it. Our ability to describe that system becomes highly complex after a certain point because there are so many variables, but to some degree we can model it. For example, actuaries can model the probabilities of certain diseases occurring in a large population, planners can anticipate need for certain medical services in a community, or pharmaceutical manufacturers can project demand for a new drug.

The System Model Contains Essential Nonlinearity

As has been noted earlier, health care systems are essentially nonlinear. Attempts have been made in the past to describe linear models of managed health care markets, but those attempts have ultimately been unsuccessful, even if widely adopted for a period of time. The most well known, although now discarded, of these is a linear model that described managed care market evolution as a series of stages progressing from a first stage of little managed care up to a fourth (then fifth) stage in which managed care was dominant. In this fourth or fifth stage, capitation was the predominant form of reimbursement, vertical integration was the primary structure of the provider systems, utilization was low, and excesses in hospital beds and specialty physicians had been removed.*

No markets have exhibited these traits in a linear fashion. For example, Minneapolis has high managed care penetration and more vertical in-

---

*No telling where those pesky physicians were supposed to have gone. Maybe they were supposed to just give up their desolate practices, move to Seattle, and open coffee shops.

tegration than most, but there is little capitation. Southern California has relatively high levels of capitation (although global capitation has recently come into disfavor), but there are still excess hospital beds and many of the organized provider groups have failed. And the number of specialty physicians has not decreased, neither in total nor as a percentage of total physicians in practice.

Vast and Numerous Complex Forces Affect the System

It is insufficient to use a small set of variables to attempt to predict the future of health care systems or markets. Simple supply and demand are confounded by third-party payment and the impact of each individual's medical condition on his or her choices or need for care. The emotional content of health care decisions is difficult to measure at best. Forces such as geographical barriers or habits, language spoken, ethnicity, transportation options, health hazards in the community, the unintended consequences of legislation or regulation, and so forth create a system in which multiple complex forces interact in ways that become extremely difficult to comprehend, even if these forces are recognized. Even more complicating, there are many forces that we do not even recognize or take into account if we do recognize them, so that we cannot ever have a completely accurate picture of the effect of those forces.

Extreme Sensitivity to Initial Conditions Exists

Small changes in initial conditions may have a large effect at a later point in time. For example, the personality of a particular executive of a health plan or hospital system would be an initial condition that produces a major effect when that executive decides to merge with another organization, creating a dominant system in a market. Or decisions in real estate purchases by a health system may affect the system's bond ratings, reducing its capital availability, leading to the acceptance of a greater discount in pricing than would have otherwise occurred. Or the lack of an experienced financial officer at a health plan may lead to the creation of a faulty accrual method, leading to a massive downward restatement of earnings that leads to sharp premium increases.

It is also necessary to understand that initial conditions do not merely exist at a single point in the past. They are actually those conditions that exist right now as well as in the past. In the example used previously, that of the personality of a particular executive, when that executive actually arrives to lead the health system, that would be the beginning of that particular initial condition. The same definition would apply to the day that the executive chooses to meet with the system's competitor to talk about merger. In other words, every event can be considered as an initial condition for *something*. The effect of changes initiated by today's initial conditions will have an impact on changes created by initial conditions in the past and will in turn be affected by initial conditions that occur in the future, making predictions of change spectacularly complex.

Feedback of Current Conditions Affects Subsequent Results, Usually with Significant (But Not Random) Variation

Feedback occurs when external events lead to change within the system.* In other words, feedback is information that comes into the health system or plan that has an effect on actions or events within the system. Often referred to as turbulence (think of a turbulent rapids in a river where the flow of water against rocks keeps the aquatic forces roiling), this refers to the ability of external forces to create change not only once but also on a continually iterative basis. A common illustration of feedback is when trade magazines in the health care industry begin to tout a particular strategy and a large number of organizations immediately attempt to emulate it. For example, physician-hospital organizations

(PHOs) were once a top trend in health care systems, and media stories supported this movement, extolling its virtues. Consultants and law firms recognized market demand when they saw it and offered services to help create PHOs. Most PHOs created during this frenzy are now quiescent if they even still exist at all, although there are a few that remain functional.

Another illustration of feedback, in this case more iterative than the preceding, is the action of a competitor. For example, if a competing managed care plan decides to drop rates in an attempt to gain market share, the other plans in the area immediately take this into consideration in trying to remain competitive, and a rate war ensues. The short-term benefit to employers of lowered rates is negated by rate increases that eventually follow, as well as the potentially catastrophic consequences of a total failure of a health plan that does not have the financial strength to subsidize rates for long.

REVERSING ENTROPY WITH A LITTLE HELP FROM PROFESSOR HEISENBERG—PREDICTING, LEADING, AND ACTING IN A CHAOTIC MANAGED HEALTH CARE ENVIRONMENT

Use of the term "chaos," or even CAS, summons feelings of helplessness, of an inability to make any predictions or forecasts, or to choose the right actions. Although predicting and acting in a chaotic environment are certainly more difficult than in a simpler, linear one, it is not impossible. An understanding of forces that currently exist will allow an improved understanding of what the future *may* hold, but not what it *will* hold. This means countering the forces of entropy (defined here as the tendency for order to proceed toward chaos unless energy is put into a system) using the energy in strategy and management, by applying an understanding of uncertainty and probability.*

---

*Feedback can occur within the system as well, when one part of the system affects another part; but this is hard enough to understand, at least for me, so why make it harder than it needs to be?

*Thus, combining the Second Law of Thermodynamics (Newtonian physics) with the Heisenberg Uncertainty Principle (quantum physics). If we force this analogy much further something might snap and someone could get hurt, so it's best we stop here.

Predicting the future of managed health care is as complex an undertaking as one can imagine and a daunting task knowing that those predictions will live on in a book rather than perishing at the bottom of the parakeet cage along with other pages from periodicals. Indeed, creating predictions that have high certainty will be limited to the obvious (e.g., premium rates will go up some amount next year). The best we can do is to understand that forces affecting managed health care create change, but exactly how those forces act remains uncertain. Starting with that understanding, each of us may proceed to creating our own models of the future of managed health care.

HANDICAPPING THE FIELD—THE STRATIFICATION OF PREDICTABILITY

Uncertainty is not uniform. Known forces or events may be stratified into categories that range from those for which the overall effect is relatively predictable to those for which the overall effect is relatively unpredictable. Examples of such forces have been discussed throughout this text, and an example of stratification of some of them is illustrated as follows.

Sources of Relative Predictability

- Increase in e-commerce by all parties.
  — Accelerating shift to the use of electronic business processes and Web-enabled products and services.
  — By 2002–2003, the Health Insurance Portability and Accountability Act's (HIPAA's) mandate of transaction and identifier standards will have turbocharged the use of the Internet as a low-cost means to automate health care's billions of transactions between health plans, providers, and consumers.
  — The use of electronic medical records will increase.
  — The attractiveness of the e-health sector to investors and new players will continue, as will consolidations in e-health businesses.

- Continued slow drift to increased consumerism.
  — Not a headlong rush, but a slow and steady movement.
  — Members/enrollees having greater demands on and expectations for a health plan, based on information from the Internet and the media.
  — Consumers wanting more and better information so they can participate in decisions about their health care.
  — Patients walking into doctors' offices with material from the Internet (not necessarily accurate or unbiased).
  — The creation of more impatient patients.
- Shifting demographics.
  — Increased life expectancy.
  — Greater health needs later in life.
  — Proportionately smaller population base to fund health care costs.
  — Declining disability in later years and higher expectations of good health.
  — Ethnic diversity.
  — Costs to society from the rising number of uninsured.
- Continued consolidation of managed care plans and provider systems but only to a point (i.e., not to the point of national mega-corporations), as larger systems absorb smaller, struggling systems.
- Power in the health care market remains at the regional and local levels.
- Continued pressures of premium-cost compression in the market, resulting in modest margins and periods of losses and modest profits.
- Increased marketplace requirements for demonstrably higher levels of administrative and medical quality but a refusal to pay significant premiums for it—i.e., high administrative and clinical quality will become a requirement just to be in the market.
- Countervailing market pressures for broad medical networks and cost control.
- Advances in medical technology, for example:
  — Telemedicine.
  — Robotics.

— Imaging.
— Surgical techniques.
— Drug therapy.
— Gene therapy.

- Increasing ability to detect and treat asymptomatic diseases (e.g., hyperlipidemia, hypertension) with ever more sophisticated and costly drugs.
- New abilities to detect and treat diseases early in their course (e.g., genetic diseases, diabetes, precancerous states) with ever more sophisticated and costly drugs and gene therapy.

Legislative Sources of Relative Predictability

- Trend toward more regulation, not less.
  — Mandatory second opinion and appeal programs and the like.
  — Consumer protections, whether actual danger exists or not.
  — Countervailing pressure from business community to not add to costs.
- The intended consequences of the HIPAA.
  — Administrative simplification.
  — Privacy and security.
  — Limited portability of insurance.
- The lack of a real alternative to the private market for health insurance in the commercial sector—i.e., insufficient support for movement from private health insurance to a governmental single payer type of health insurance beyond those already in existence: Medicare and Medicaid.*

---

*It is far more palatable for both Congress and the President to legislate without funding and to regulate the private market than it is to advocate an even greater financial drain on what is already the biggest money sink in the federal budget: health care entitlement programs. To those who think otherwise, try to find someone who was around when Walter Mondale told the public that if elected President of the United States, he would raise their taxes—an excellent object lesson when applied to the argument for a federal single payer program that would require substantial tax increases. Counter arguments about the high cost of health care to American companies and their employees ignore political reality: a hidden tax is hugely more acceptable than a direct tax.

Sources of Relative Unpredictability

- Anti-managed care sentiment.
- Ripple effects of failures of risk-bearing organizations.
- Effect of the competition's strategies on each health system and health plan (this is a microlevel form of uncertainty, but it has a major impact on any individual plan).
- Effect of lawsuits.
- Great variations and rates of evolution of provider structure and behavior in different geographical regions.
- Great variations in compensation methods to providers.
- Uncertainty about employer's actions if costs increase above general inflationary levels. For example:
  — Purchasing marts.
  — Accelerated movement toward defined contribution plans and away from defined contribution plans.
  — Movement back toward smaller, less costly networks.
  — The effect of low unemployment rates and competition for employee recruitment and retention and the countervailing pressure away from diminished benefits plans (e.g., defined contribution).
- The ability of the U.S. economy to sustain its current (circa 2000) robustness.
  — Economic growth.
  — Low unemployment.

Legislative Sources of Relative Unpredictability

- Unintended effects of federal legislation.
  — HIPAA.
    a. Cost to remediate information systems to health plans and providers.
    b. Consequences of failure to comply.
    c. Effect of standardization of transactions and identifiers on existing businesses that capitalize on the current lack of such standardization.
    d. The increased use of the Internet for health care transactions and communication that will be spurred by HIPAA.

    e. Risks from malignant morons that insist on vandalizing the servers and websites of organizations.

    f. Risks from e-criminals who will attempt to steal financial and medical information.

    g. The effect of the enormous increase in information available to consumers and physicians.

— The Balanced Budget Act of 1997.

    a. Decreased revenues to hospitals, with diminished cost shifting.

    b. Change in the attractiveness of Medicare + Choice risk plans to existing health plans.

    c. Emergence of new types of risk-based health plans.

— Erosion of the Employee Retirement Income Security Act shield and an increase in ability to file lawsuits against health plans and employers.

- Gramm-Leach-Bliley Act of 1999—see the sidebar for a discussion of this act.

- Desire of state and federal governments to be out of the health insurance business.

- State governments' increasing inability to pay their portion of Medicaid.

- Desire of state and federal governments to remain in the political business by creating unfunded mandates and compliance requirements.

- The Health Care Financing Administration's continued desire to increase Medicare managed care enrollment counterbalanced by their desire to pay less.

- Use of risk adjustors in payment of premiums by private employers and governmental agencies.

- Federal legislation under debate or consideration.

— The Patient's Bill of Rights under debate as of early 2000.

    a. Expected to pass in some form, some time on or before 2002.

    b. The ultimate resolution of provisions being hotly contested as of early 2000 (e.g., rights to sue, the role of the federal government versus state governments, mandated activities).

The Gramm-Leach-Bliley Act of 1999 (S.900/H.R. 10) has not been discussed elsewhere in this book, so a brief note is appropriate. This act repealed the Glass-Steagall Act that had been passed in 1933 in the aftermath of the crash of 1929. Glass-Stegall prohibited most U.S. commercial banks from performing investment banking activities such as helping their corporate customers bring new debt and equity issues to market or other such underwriting. More to the point of this book, Gramm-Leach-Bliley also allows affiliations between securities firms, banks, and insurance companies and allows banks and securities firms to offer a wide variety of products, including insurance products. The impact of this on the insurance industry, including the managed health care industry, has not been felt as of early 2000. That does not mean that there will be little or no impact, however, only that the degree and nature of the impact remains unknown. With the amount of money flowing through the health care economy, it is unreasonable to expect the financial services industry not to dip their cups into the revenue stream. With their expertise in customer relations and ability to manage money, it would be natural for banks and financial services firms to attempt to insert themselves between the customers and the health insurers or managed care organizations, adding perceived value and extracting profits along the way. Mergers are also possible; although the slim margins in health insurance are below those that financial institutions desire, the old strategy of bundling services and products may rise again from the rubble of the 1980s. Gramm-Leach-Bliley also contains broad privacy provisions that could apply to all markets, not just financial markets, and have unintended consequences in the managed care industry. Stay tuned.

— Change in the tax treatment of employee benefits plans.

- The effect of election politics in any even-numbered year.

— Presidential elections in 2000 and 2004.

— Congressional and (one third of) senatorial elections every two years.

— Demagoguery versus rational policy debate.

- Intended and unintended effects of state legislation and regulation.
  — State anti-managed care legislation.
  — State specific mandates.
  — State regulatory interpretations.
- Some new idea or another that it isn't even possible to conjecture on until it looks in retrospect like an obvious thing to happen.

Many forces are listed here (although not a comprehensive list because that is impossible in a chaotic environment), but not all of them are equally germane to any individual organization or to any individual situation. For example, a capital expenditure decision may not be affected by a Patient's Bill of Rights but would be affected by the rise in e-commerce. What is important to understand is that this exercise of stratifying forces along an axis of relative certainty and uncertainty should be undertaken when looking forward for purposes of predicting, planning, and acting.

DRIVING THE NITROGLYCERINE TRUCK ON A FOGGY NIGHT— LEADERSHIP, STRATEGY, AND ACTION IN THE CHAOTIC WORLD

Most people, and most organizations, seek stability. Only so much change can be absorbed before feelings of exhaustion set in, and the desire to slow down or stop change becomes paramount. Stability, though, is the one thing that is lacking in the health care system in the past, present, and foreseeable future.

A leader in health care must internalize that dynamic, not deny its existence. A leader must project a sense of stability by virtue of their actions and behaviors and the behaviors of the management team. Blaming external forces for problems may be accurate, but if used as a means of deflecting criticism rather than simply observing reality, leadership is impaired. The leader needs to be able to articulate the goals and objectives and the tactics of the organization into terms that are meaningful to the various constituencies within and without the organization. The leader must accept a changing environment, learn to use it to advantage, and learn to communicate to the organization that it is strong and agile enough to thrive.

Continuous planning and strategic adjustments should be combined with opportunism. In a chaotic environment, situations will arise that demand rapid response but will not have been considered when forecasting scenarios or future directions. The ability to recognize such opportunities is paramount to success. Failure to recognize them is to fail to take the right action at the right time to yield disproportionate results.

Strategic planning must be undertaken in a nontraditional way. The old concept of a five-year strategic plan is of far less use today than ever before. This does not mean that there is no place for vision. Vision is even more important than before because without it the organization is subject to even greater turbulence, lacking the stabilizing force of vision.

In a chaotic market, it is dangerous to observe only a few variables or market attributes and attempt to predict the future. Therefore, one cannot rely on a single strategy, and sustainable advantage comes from several complementary activities or strategies. The presence of several complementary strategies and tactics means that a competitor must match them all, not just one.

To think and plan strategically in the complexly adapting health care environment, several elements must be present. Five of the most important are briefly discussed as follows.

First, a solid, and continually refreshing fact base must be present. A survey of the environment once per year will not provide adequate knowledge of critical changes occurring that require a response or a change in strategies. For example, major events such as the failure of a health system or health plan, a new state or federal mandate, or a major shift in employment benefits would require that strategies be formally reevaluated in light of new conditions, rather than simply observed and reacted to. Other facts such as shifts in benefits trends and pricing, a new marketing campaign by a competitor, and the like must also be monitored. In short, any data or information that has an impact on strategies must be monitored on a regular basis, and the implications of changes must be evaluated.

Second, there must be a systematic removal of impeding cultural biases. Internal biases and habits exist in an organization, just as they exist in any behaviors, including physician practice behaviors as discussed in Chapter 33. Biases that impede necessary progress must be identified and managed. It is common for an organization to voice support for necessary changes, but that is often superficial because change requires moving from a zone of comfort to a zone of discomfort or instability. An example of an impeding cultural bias would be a belief that the way things are done now is the correct way and came about through a lot of hard work so cannot be abandoned for some new and untested way of doing things. A common symptom of this particular example occurs when a plan installs a new computer software system, and a great deal of extra coding is done to make the software support the processes that currently exist rather than using the power of the new software to change processes to become more efficient. Other examples include fear of change (being equated to losing one's job—a perfectly reasonable fear for some people, but one that becomes self-fulfilling if an individual is unable to adapt), a learned dislike of another organization (e.g., a hospital's dislike of a health plan), or refusal to accept the need for medical management despite clear evidence of inappropriate use of services. A note of caution is appropriate here: the vision and mission of an organization should not be confused with a cultural bias (unless that mission has changed for some reason).

Third, it is useful to pace the amount of change undertaken. This allows the organization to adapt at an acceptable rate and avoids lurching from large-scale change to large-scale change (i.e., major efforts producing change, followed by an exhausted cessation of all forward motion until the slow accretion of environmental forces requires another massive change). A culture of adaptability is required, much like the culture that exists in many new Internet companies. All organizations have cultural momentum (or inertia if one perceives the organization as immobile), and changing the course of the organization is not a trivial matter. In human and cultural terms, Force = Mass × Acceleration (F = MA) just as in Newtonian physics. Thus, the larger the organization, the greater the need for force or the more slowly it will move; and force comes at a high cost (applying once again the Second Law of Thermodynamics, but enough of physics). The best approach to this is a continually renewing strategic and tactical plan that has a measured and planned degree of significant change as an integral factor. If the leadership of the plan is well attuned to the environment, this paced level of constant change becomes a part of the internal culture and avoids the massive reorganizations and reengineering efforts so often required when a company gets into trouble.

Fourth, scenario planning that accounts for time frame, level of risk, and relationship to core mission should be undertaken when looking at strategies. Scenarios need not be fully realized, but at the least should account for potentially important changes that may or may not occur. The scenarios must then lay out the broad direction the organization would take under such conditions. This allows the organization to recover from missteps or significant changes that make current strategies suboptimal. For example, two large medical groups may be considering a merger, so the health plan needs to understand the strategic option if the groups merge or if they do not. The lack of such scenario development and planning, even if rudimentary, allows for action rather than reaction when events occur.

Fifth, the metrics and measurements used to track and manage change must be consistent with the strategies and tactics being undertaken. Once the overall strategic direction is clear, the substrategies appropriate to the processes and functions of the plan must be determined and articulated, tactics must be developed to execute on those substrategies, and critical success factors for those tactics must be determined. Once those aspects are understood, measures directly related to those critical success factors and outcomes are determined and the means for the creation and reporting of those measures are put in place. To use traditional metrics to manage new strategies will provide indirect feedback at best.

In an uncertain future, the measurement of success will change along with the environment.

A simplistic example of the concept of focused metrics and measurements related to strategies is presented here (the simple strategy, tactics, and measurements are presented for purposes of illustration only, not as a recommended course of action). In this example, if a health plan determines that its primary strategy must be significant improvements in customer service, one substrategy might focus on customer satisfaction of access to clinical services. Areas of focus in this substrategy might include fostering the member's perception that the plan provides superior added value to members and facilitates access to quality care rather than impeding it. Focusing further on the Member Services function, tactics might include increasing direct personal contacts with members by clinical staff on a proactive basis whenever nonroutine care is needed by a member (creating a crossover function between Member Services and Medical Management), and the creation of a health facilitator type of function (all tactics must be HIPAA compliant, of course). Critical success factors identified might include the ability to achieve direct contact with the member within 24 hours of first notification, the member's willingness to accept such help from the plan, and acceptance of the program by the plan's physicians. Measures might therefore focus on the time to first contact, the percentage of members who persist with the program throughout their episode of care, utilization and quality of care measures, physician satisfaction, and member satisfaction on the basis of a minimum 30 percent response rate (thus ruling out the use of postcards or direct mail to measure satisfaction). It is important to note here that the creation of measures linked to strategies means also that as strategies change, so must the measures. If procedures aren't put in place to maintain the link between measures and strategies, the measures will take on an importance of their own, eventually clogging up reporting systems and managers' brains with measures no longer relevant to existing needs.

DOOR NUMBER ONE, TWO, OR THREE—CHOOSING STRATEGIC OPTIONS

Three basic types of options are available to a leader in the chaotic health care environment. Some actions are also independent of these options, such as undertaking improvements in automation that will yield high administrative savings and need to occur in all events, so those actions are not the subject of this section. The three basic choices of options, which are not mutually exclusive, are briefly described in the following.

Option One: Shape the Future

This option refers to taking the right action at the right time. It means setting the new standards and forcing the market, and the competition, to follow. It works best when uncertainty is confined to a small number of predictable scenarios and when the competitive advantage of the organization is high. Shaping the future, sometimes referred to as leading (or bleeding) edge, requires the highest investment, has the highest risk, but also has the highest potential reward.

Option Two: Be a Fast Follower

This option refers to following behind a competitor that makes the initial investment and takes the risk. It requires speed, agility, and constant market intelligence. It works best when there are alternate strategies created for alternate but probable scenarios so that fast action is possible. This option means the organization doesn't lead the market but rather helps to push it in a direction, creating competitive advantage against all but the market leader. The advantages of this strategy are that it requires moderate investment, has lower risk, but has a moderate reward. The exception to the issue of reward is when the market leader stumbles in an avoidable way, so the fast follower can overtake the leader by avoiding the mistake the leader made.

Option Three: Hedge Your Bets

This option means making sufficient investments to cover a wide variety of alternate scenarios and carrying out only those strategies and tactics that have low risk but are necessary to remain competitive. This strategy never leads the market but is able to follow it sufficiently closely to avoid being left behind. It entails low cost, low reward, but little or no risk.

Creating the Strategic Portfolio

A mix of all three approaches is usually required, not a single option. The specific mix of the three options will depend on an accurate assessment of market attributes, the ability to create plausible scenarios, the ability to tolerate risk, and the ability to invest. Most importantly, it is the ability to execute the strategies that must determine the best approach. This means an accurate assessment of the internal abilities of the organization, as well as the internal constraints and enablers. In the best situation, this also means the ability to execute multiple strategies and actions simultaneously, creating multiple advantages in the marketplace.

CONCLUSION—SHAKE THE MAGIC EIGHT BALL AND TRY AGAIN

So what does the future of managed health care look like in the new millennium? The answer will be forthcoming in our next installment: *The Managed Health Care Handbook, Fifth Edition*, coming to you in 2004 or later.

Glossary of Terms and Acronyms*

24/7—Slang that means something is available 24 hours per day, 7 days per week. For example, the nurse advice line is available 24/7.

AAHC—American Accreditation HealthCare Commission; see *URAC*.

AAHP—American Association of Health Plans. The primary trade organization of managed care organizations. Their areas of focus include legislative and lobbying efforts, education, certification of training in managed health care operations, and representation of the managed health care industry to the public. Created in 1995 through the merger of the Group Health Association of America (GHAA) and the American Managed Care and Review Association (AMCRA), two predecessor organizations that represented slightly different types of health plan constituencies.

AAPCC—Adjusted average per capita cost. The HCFA's best estimate of the amount of money it costs to care for Medicare recipients under fee-for-service Medicare in a given area. The AAPCC is made up of 142 different rate cells; 140 of them are factored for age, sex, Medicaid eligibility, institutional status, working aged, and whether a person has both Part A and Part B of Medicare. The two remaining cells are for individuals with end-stage renal disease. The

AAPCC has been used for setting payments rates to Medicare HMOs, but is being replaced by a new risk-adjusted methodology.

Accrete—The term used by HCFA for the process of adding new Medicare enrollees to a plan. Also see *delete*.

Accrual—The amount of money that is set aside to cover expenses. The accrual is the plan's best estimate of what those expenses are and (for medical expenses) is based on a combination of data from the authorization system, the claims system, the lag studies, and the plan's prior history.

ACGs—Ambulatory care groups. ACGs are a method of categorizing outpatient episodes. There are 51 mutually exclusive ACGs, which are based on resource use over time and modified by principal diagnosis, age, and sex. Also see ADGs, APGs, and APCs.

ACH—Automated Clearing House. A company that accepts claims or other transactions from providers, reformats them into standards acceptable to each payer, and electronically transmits them to the payer. Before HIPAA, there were no functional standards in transaction definitions or data fields (there were standard definitions; it's just that the payers continued to uses their own). With the advent of HIPAA, the need for translation into multiple proprietary formats diminished considerably, but the value of a company that will convert paper forms into electronic transactions is still considerable for small provider groups.

ACR—Adjusted community rate. Used by HMOs and CMPs with Medicare risk contracts prior to risk-adjusted payments. A calculation of what premium the plan would charge for providing exactly the Medicare-covered benefits to a group account adjusted to allow for the greater intensity and frequency of utilization by Medicare recipients. The ACR includes the normal profit of a for-profit HMO or CMP. The ACR

---

*These are working definitions of common terms and acronyms in the managed health care industry and related health care sectors. In an industry this dynamic, it is not possible to list every term or acronym in use because new ones come into use faster than any publication can keep up with. Some definitions in this glossary may also be disputed by others in the industry; and the editor is open to receiving communication from any such compulsive nit-pickers. The astute reader will also note a hint of bias or opinion in some of the definitions; consider that a bonus and take it for what it is: the learned biases of the editor.

may be equal to or less than the APR (see following) but can never exceed it.

ACS contract—See *ASO*.

Actuarial assumptions—The assumptions that an actuary uses in calculating the expected costs and revenues of the plan. Examples include utilization rates, age and sex mix of enrollees, and cost for medical services.

Adverse selection—The problem of attracting members who are sicker than the general population (specifically, members who are sicker than was anticipated when the budget for medical costs was developed).

ADGs—Ambulatory diagnostic groups. ADGs are a method of categorizing outpatient episodes. There are 34 possible ADGs. Also see *ACGs* and *APGs*.

AFDC—See *TANF*.

AHCPR—The Agency for Health Care Policy and Research.

ALOS—See *LOS*.

Alternative Medicine—See *CAM*.

Amara's law—The tendency, when confronted with significant change, to overreact in the short term and underreact in the long term. The editor gratefully acknowledges Greg Lippe as the source of this highly useful aphorism.

ANSI—The American National Standards Institute. ANSI develops and maintains standards for electronic data interchange. HIPAA mandates the use of ANSI × 12N standards for electronic transactions in the health care system.

APC—Ambulatory patient classification. This is the method settled on by HCFA to use for implementing the PPS for ambulatory procedures. Like the other methods, this is a way of clustering many different ambulatory procedure codes into groups for purposes of payment.

APG—Ambulatory patient group. A reimbursement method developed by 3M Health Information Systems for HCFA. APGs are to outpatient procedures what DRGs are to inpatient days, for outpatient procedures or visits and incorporate data regarding the reason for the visit and patient data. APGs prevent unbundling of ancillary services. Also see *ACGs*, *ADGs*, and *APCs*.

APR—Average payment rate. The amount of money that HCFA could conceivably pay an HMO or CMP for services to Medicare recipients under a risk contract prior to risk-adjusted payments. The figure is derived from the AAPCC for the service area adjusted for the enrollment characteristics that the plan would expect to have. The payment to the plan, the ACR, can never be higher than the APR, but it may be less.

ASO—Administrative services only. A contract between an insurance company and a self-funded plan in which the insurance company performs administrative services only and does not assume any risk. Services usually include claims processing but may include other services such as actuarial analysis, utilization review, and so forth. Also see *ERISA*.

Assignment of benefits—The payment of medical benefits directly to a provider of care rather than to a member. Generally requires either a contract between the health plan and the provider or a written release from the subscriber to the provider allowing the provider to bill the health plan.

AWP—Average wholesale price. Commonly used in pharmacy contracting, the AWP is generally determined through reference to a common source of information.

AWP—Any willing provider. This is a form of state law that requires an MCO to accept any provider willing to meet the terms and conditions in the MCO's contract, whether the MCO wants or needs that provider or not. Considered to be an expensive form of anti-managed care legislation.

Balance billing—The practice of a provider billing a patient for all charges not paid for by the insurance plan, even if those charges are above the plan's UCR or are considered medically unnecessary. Managed care plans and service plans generally prohibit providers from balance billing except for allowed copays, coinsurance, and deductibles. Such prohibition against balance billing may even extend to the plan's failure to pay at all (e.g., because of bankruptcy).

BBA '97—Balanced Budget Act of 1997. A sweeping piece of legislation, part of BBA '97 created the Medicare+Choice program and demonstration MSAs.

Best practices—If you do not know what those are, it is suggested that you turn to page 1, begin reading, and work your way back to this point.

BIF—Benefit information form. The BIF forms the basis of the description of each plan used for the Medicare compare information under information dissemination provisions of Medicare + Choice. HCFA will replace this term with something else, but at the time of publication what it will be isn't known, although it's safe to say it will be a government-style acronym.

CAHPS—Consumer Assessment of Health Plan Survey. An initiative by the federal government for Medicare and Medicaid, the aim of which is to develop a set of satisfaction surveys built off a core of standardized items and supplemented by additional targeted elements to make the surveys both adaptable to different subpopulations and suitable for making some cross-group comparisons. Special Medicaid survey modules have been developed that accommodate educational, linguistic, and cultural differences in this population.

CAM—Complementary and alternative medicine. This is a general term that covers treatment modalities other that traditional allopathic medicine. Examples include acupuncture, chiropractic medicine, homeopathy, and various forms of "natural healing."

Capitation—A set amount of money received or paid out; it is based on membership rather than on services delivered and usually is expressed in units of PMPM. May be varied by such factors as age and sex of the enrolled member.

Carve out—Refers to a set of medical services that are "carved out" of the basic arrangement. In term of plan benefits, may refer to a set of benefits that are carved out and contracted for separately; for example, mental health/substance abuse services may be separated from basic medical/surgical. May also refer to carving out a set of services from a basic capitation rate with a provider; for example, capitating for cardiac care, but carving out cardiac surgery and paying case rates for that.

Case management—A method of managing the provision of health care to members with high-cost medical conditions. The goal is to coordinate the care so as to both improve continuity and quality of care and lower costs. This generally is a dedicated function in the utilization management department. The official definition according to the Certification of Insurance Rehabilitation Specialists Commission (CIRSC) is: "Case management is a collaborative process which assesses, plans, implements, coordinates, monitors, and evaluates the options and services required to meet an individual's health needs, using communication and available resources to promote quality, cost-effective outcomes;" and "occurs across a continuum of care, addressing ongoing individual needs" rather than being restricted to a single practice setting. When focused solely on high-cost inpatient cases, it may be referred to as large case management or catastrophic case management.

Case mix—Refers to the mix of illness and severity of cases for a provider.

CCO—Corporate compliance officer. See *Corporate compliance.*

Certificate of coverage—See *EOC.*

CHAMPUS—Civilian Health and Medical Program of the Uniformed Services. The federal program providing health care coverage to families of military personnel, military retirees, certain spouses and de-

pendents of such personnel, and certain others. Currently provided by the TRICARE program. See also *TRICARE* and *Military health system.*

Chest Pain Unit—The term used to describe a specialized unit, usually either in or associated with the emergency department. The purpose of the chest pain unit is to rapidly identify an evolving cardiac event and initiate treatment as early as possible to decrease morbidity and mortality. The other (lesser) primary value of the unit is to rapidly identify chest pain that is noncardiac in origin so as to avoid unnecessary hospitalization. Other terms that may be used include chest pain emergency room, chest pain evaluation unit, short stay ED CCU, and ED monitored observation beds.

CHIP—Children's Health Insurance Program; also referred to as SCHIP for State Children's Health Insurance Program. A program created by the federal government to provide a "safety net" and preventive-care level of health coverage for children, funded through a combination of federal and state funds, and administered by the states in conformance with federal requirements.

Churning—The practice of a provider seeing a patient more often than is medically necessary, primarily to increase revenue through an increased number of services. Churning may also apply to any performance-based reimbursement system in which there is a heavy emphasis on productivity (in other words, rewarding a provider for seeing a high volume of patients whether through fee-for-service or through an appraisal system that pays a bonus for productivity).

CLM—Career-limiting move. A boneheaded mistake by a manager. What this book is designed to try to prevent.

Closed panel—A managed care plan that contracts with physicians on an exclusive basis for services and does not allow those physicians to see patients for another managed care organization. Examples include staff and group model HMOs. Could apply to a large private medical group that contracts with an HMO.

CMP—Competitive medical plan. A pre-BBA designation of a federal designation that allowed a health plan to obtain eligibility to receive a Medicare risk contract without having to obtain qualification as an HMO. Requirements for eligibility were somewhat less restrictive than for an HMO.

COA—Certificate of authority. The state-issued operating license for an HMO.

COB—Coordination of benefits. An agreement that uses language developed by the National Association of Insurance Commissioners and prevents double payment for services when a subscriber has coverage from two or more sources. For example, a husband may have Blue Cross Blue Shield through work, and the wife may have elected an HMO through her place of employment. The agreement gives the order for what organization has primary responsibility for payment and what organization has secondary responsibility for payment. The respective primary and secondary payment obligations of the two coverages are determined by the Order of Benefits Determination (OOBD) Rules contained in the National Association of Insurance Commissioners (NAIC) Model COB Regulation, as interpreted and adopted by the various states.

COBRA—Consolidated Omnibus Reconciliation Act. A portion of this Act requires employers to offer the opportunity for terminated employees to purchase continuation of health care coverage under the group's medical plan (also see *Conversion*). Another portion eases a Medicare recipient's ability to disenroll from an HMO or CMP with a Medicare risk contract.

Coinsurance—A provision in a member's coverage that limits the amount of coverage by the plan to a certain percentage, commonly 80 percent. Any additional costs are paid by the member out of pocket.

Commission—The money paid to a sales representative, broker, or other type of sales agent for selling the health plan. May be a flat amount of money or a percentage of the premium.

Community rating—The rating method required of HMOs under the laws of many states and occasionally indemnity plans under certain circumstances used primarily in the small group (under 25 employee) market. The HMO must obtain the same amount of money per member for all members in the plan. Community rating does allow for variability by allowing the HMO to factor in differences for age, sex, mix (average contract size), and industry factors; not all factors are necessarily allowed under state laws, however. Such techniques are referred to a community rating by class and adjusted community rating. Also see *Experience rating*.

Complementary and alternative medicine—See *CAM*.

CON—Certificate of need. The requirement that a health care organization obtain permission from an oversight agency before making changes. Generally applies only to facilities or facility-based services.

Concurrent review—Refers to utilization management that takes place during the provision of services. Almost exclusively applied to inpatient hospital stays.

Contract year—The 12-month period that a contract for services is in force. Not necessarily tied to a calendar year.

Contributory plan—A group health plan in which the employees must contribute a certain amount toward the premium cost, with the employer paying the rest.

Conversion—The conversion of a member covered under a group master contract to coverage under an individual contract. This is offered to subscribers who lose their group coverage (e.g., through job loss, death of a working spouse, and so forth) and who are ineligible for coverage under another group contract (also see *COBRA*).

Cookbook medicine—A pejorative term for medical guidelines, used by physicians and others who object to such guidelines. The main complaint behind the term is that the practice of medicine requires a far greater degree of flexibility than do other activities such as making Toll House cookies for the simple reason that human bodies and human diseases are highly complex. This is a valid point, although there are clearly many conditions in which adherence to clinical guidelines improves quality and outcomes, while simultaneously lowering costs.

Copayment—That portion of a claim or medical expense that a member must pay out of pocket as a fixed amount, such as $5 in many HMOs.

Corporate compliance—The function in a health plan or provider charged with ensuring compliance with Medicare rules and regulations. These requirements for compliance have been developed by HCFA, and it is the responsibility of the MCO or provider organization (e.g., hospital) to comply. Regulations also require the existence of a corporate compliance officer (CCO).

Corporate practice of medicine acts or statutes—State laws that prohibit a physician from working for a corporation; in other words, a physician can only work for him or herself, or another physician. Put another way, a corporation cannot practice medicine. Often created through the effort on the part of certain members of the medical community to prevent physicians from working directly for managed care plans or hospitals.

Cost sharing—Any form of coverage in which the member pays some portion of the cost of providing services. Usual forms of cost sharing include deductibles, coinsurance, and copayments.

Cost shifting—When a provider cannot cover the cost of providing services under the reimbursement received, the provider raises the prices to other payers to cover that portion of the cost.

CPT-4—*Current Procedural Terminology*, 4th edition to be eventually replaced by CPT-5. A set of five-digit codes that apply to medical services delivered. Used for billing by professionals and mandated by HIPAA (also see *HCPCS*).

Credentialing—The most common use of the term refers to obtaining and reviewing the documentation of professional providers. Such documentation includes licensure, certifications, insurance, evidence of malpractice insurance, malpractice history, and so forth. Generally includes both reviewing information provided by the provider and verification that the information is correct and complete. A much less frequent use of the term applies to closed panels and medical groups and refers to obtaining hospital privileges and other privileges to practice medicine.

Critical paths—Defined pathways of clinical care that provide for the greatest efficiency of care at the greatest quality. Critical paths are also an ever-changing activity as science and medicine evolve.

Custodial care—Care provided to an individual that is primarily the basic activities of living. May be medical or nonmedical, but the care is not meant to be curative or a form of medical treatment and is often lifelong. Rarely covered by any form of group health insurance or HMO.

CVO—Credentialing verification organization. This is an independent organization that performs primary verification of a professional provider's credentials. The managed care organization may then rely on that verification rather than subjecting the provider to provide credentials independently. This lowers the cost and "hassle" for credentialing. NCQA (see *NCQA*) has issued certification standards for CVOs.

CWW—Clinic without walls. See group practice without walls.

Date of service—Refers to the date that medical services were rendered. Usually different from the date a claim is submitted.

DAW—Dispense as written. The instruction from a physician to a pharmacist to dispense a brand-name pharmaceutical rather than a generic substitution.

Days per thousand—A standard unit of measurement of utilization. Refers to an annualized use of the hospital or other institutional care. It is the number of hospital days that are used in a year for each thousand covered lives.

DCG—Diagnostic care group. A new method commissioned by HCFA to look at how to adjust prospective payments on the basis of retrospective severity. This system, which was still not quite finalized or implemented as this book was being written, looks at ICD-9 diagnoses and sorts them iteratively until the patient is classified into one of approximately 100+ DCGs that are then to be used to compensate a risk-bearing Medicare MCO or PSO.

Defined benefit—A term of insurance that refers to an employer (or governmental agency that provides benefits to employees) providing a benefit that is the same regardless of the cost (although cost-sharing with employees is not a part of the definition of defined benefit). In other words, an employee knows what type(s) of insurance or managed health care plans are offered and what the benefits are under each, and the employer's contribution to the cost of that coverage is a function of how expensive that coverage is. This is the most common form of employee health insurance benefit as of early 2000.

Defined contribution—A term of insurance that refers to an employer designating a fixed amount of money for use in purchasing health insurance but not requiring the employee to use only those health plans chosen by the employer. In other words, here's your money, now go find some health insurance.

Death spiral—An insurance term that refers to a vicious spiral of high premium rates and adverse selection, generally in a free-choice environment; typically, an insurance company or health plan in an account with multiple other plans, or a plan offering coverage to potential members who have alternative choices, such as through an association. One plan, often the indemnity plan competing with managed care plans, ends up having continually higher premium rates such that the only members who stay with the plan are those whose medical costs are so high (and who cannot change because of provider loyalty or benefits restrictions) that they far exceed any possible premium revenue. Called the death spiral because the losses from underwriting mount faster than the premiums can ever recover, and the account eventually terminates coverage, leaving the carrier in a permanent loss position.

Decimal Dust—Slang for numbers too small to matter.

Deductible—That portion of a subscriber's (or member's) health care expenses that must be paid out of pocket before any insurance coverage applies, commonly $100 to $300. Common in insurance plans and PPOs, uncommon in HMOs. May apply only to the out-of-network portion of a point-of-service plan. May also apply only to one portion of the plan coverage (e.g., there may be a deductible for pharmacy services but not for anything else).

Delete—The term used by HCFA for the process of removing Medicare enrollees from a plan. Also see *accrete*.

Dependent—A member who is covered by virtue of a family relationship with the member who has the health plan coverage. For example, one person has health insurance or an HMO through work, and that individual's spouse and children, the dependents, also have coverage under that contract.

DHHS—The Department of Health and Human Services. See *HHS*.

DHMO—Dental health maintenance organization. An HMO organized strictly to provide dental benefits.

Direct access—A term that refers to an HMO that does not use a primary care physician "gatekeeper" model for access to specialty physicians. In other words, a member may self-refer to a specialty physician rather than seeking authorization from the PCP. HMOs that use a direct access model usually have a significant copayment differential between care received from a specialty physician and care received from a PCP.

Direct contracting—A term describing a provider or integrated health care delivery system contracting directly with employers rather than through an insurance company or managed care organization. A superficially attractive option that occasionally works when the employer is large enough. Not to be confused with direct contract model (see following).

Direct contract model—A managed care health plan that contracts directly with private practice physicians in the community rather than through an intermediary such as an IPA or a medical group. A common type of model in open-panel HMOs.

Discharge planning—That part of utilization management that is concerned with arranging for care or medical needs to facilitate discharge from the hospital.

Disease management—The process of intensively managing a particular disease. This differs from large case management in that it goes well beyond a given case in the hospital or an acute exacerbation of a condition. Disease management encompasses all settings of care and places a heavy emphasis on prevention and maintenance. It is similar to case management but more focused on a defined set of diseases.

Disenrollment—The process of termination of coverage. Voluntary termination would include a member quitting because he or she simply wants out. Involuntary termination would include leaving the plan because of changing jobs. A rare and serious form of involuntary disenrollment is when the plan terminates a member's coverage against the member's will. This is usually only allowed under state and federal laws for gross offenses such as fraud, abuse, nonpayment of premium or copayments, or a demonstrated inability to comply with recommended treatment plans.

DME—Durable medical equipment. Medical equipment that is not disposable (i.e., is used repeatedly) and is only related to care for a medical condition. Examples would include wheelchairs, home hospital beds, and so forth. An area of increasing expense, particularly in conjunction with case management.

DOL—U.S. Department of Labor. Regulates coverage offered to employees when employers retain the insurance risk (i.e., self-funding pursuant to ERISA), either on a stand-alone basis or through a multiple employer welfare arrangement.

Dread disease policy—A peculiar type of health insurance that covers only a specific and frightening type of illness, such as cancer. Uncommon.

DRG—Diagnosis-related groups. A statistical system of classifying any inpatient stay into groups for purposes of payment. DRGs may be primary or secondary, and an outlier classification also exists. This is the form of reimbursement that HCFA uses to pay hospitals for Medicare recipients. Also used by a few states for all payers and by many private health plans (usually non-HMO) for contracting purposes.

DSM IV—*Diagnostic and Statistical Manual of Mental Disorders*, 4th edition. The manual used to provide a diagnostic coding system for mental and substance abuse disorders. Far different from ICD-9-CM (see following).

Dual choice—Sometimes referred to as Section 1310 or mandating. That portion of the federal HMO regulations that required any employer with 25 or more employees that resided in an HMO's service area, paid minimum wage, and offered health coverage to offer a federally qualified HMO as well. The HMO had to request it. This provision "sunseted" in 1995. Another definition, unrelated to the previous one, pertains to point of service; see POS.

Dual option—The offering of both an HMO and a traditional insurance plan by one carrier.

Duplicate claims—When the same claim is submitted more than once, usually because payment hasn't been received quickly. Can lead to duplicate payments and incorrect data in the claims file; Often referred to as "dupes."

DUR—Drug utilization review.

EAP—Employee assistance program. A program that a company puts into effect for its employees to provide them with help in dealing with personal problems such as alcohol or drug abuse, mental health, or stress issues.

E-commerce—A term that refers to the use of electronic communications to conduct business. By convention, e-commerce applies to the use of the Internet for such transactions.

ED—Emergency department. That location or department in a hospital or other institutional facility that is focused on caring for acutely ill or injured patients. In earlier times, this was often a room or set of rooms, hence the older designation of emergency room or ER. These days, at least in busy urban and suburban hospitals, volume is high, physicians are specially trained and certified in emergency care, and it has grown to be an entire department.

EDI—Electronic data interchange. A term that refers to the exchange of data through electronic means rather than by using paper or the telephone. Before the rise of the Internet, EDI was applied primarily to direct electronic communications by proprietary means. EDI may now encompass electronic data exchange by means of both proprietary channels and the Internet; but by common use, EDI is most often used for proprietary channels, whereas the term e-commerce is used most often for Internet-based electronic exchanges.

Effective date—The day that health plan coverage goes into effect, or is modified.

EFT—Electronic funds transfer. Getting paid by electronic transfer of funds directly to one's bank instead of receiving a paper check.

Eligibility—When an individual is eligible for coverage under a plan. Also used to determine when an individual is no longer eligible for coverage (e.g., a dependent child reaches a certain age and is no longer eligible for coverage under his or her parent's health plan).

EMTALA—The Emergency Medical Treatment and Active Labor Act. 1986. 42, USC 1395 dd (1986) Pub. L. No. 99-272, 9121. "Anti-dumping" legislation dictates that all patients coming to any hospital emergency department must have a medical screening examination performed by qualified personnel, usually the emergency physician. The medical screening examination cannot be delayed for insurance reasons: either to obtain insurance information or to obtain preauthorization for examination. Specific language in EMTALA states: "An emergency medical condition means a medical condition manifested by acute symptoms of sufficient severity (including severe pain) that the absence of immediate medical attention could reasonably be expected to result in: (a) placing the patient's health in serious jeopardy; (b) serious impairment to bodily functions; or (c) serious dysfunction of any bodily organ or part."

Encounter—An outpatient or ambulatory visit by a member to a provider. Applies primarily to physician office visits but may encompass other types of encounters as well. In fee-for-service plans, an encounter also generates a claim. In capitated plans, the encounter is still the visit, but no claim is generated.

Enrollee—An individual enrolled in a managed health care plan. Usually applies to the subscriber or person who has the coverage in the first place rather than to his or her dependents, but the term is not always used that precisely.

EOB—Explanation of benefits (statement). A statement mailed to a member or covered insured explaining how and why a claim was or was not paid; the Medicare version is called an EOMB (also see *ERISA*).

EOC—Evidence of coverage; also known as a certificate of benefits. The EOC is a document that describes the health care benefits covered by the health plan and provides the member with some form of documentation that they in fact do have health insurance and what that insurance covers and how it works.

EPO—Exclusive provider organization. An EPO is similar to an HMO in that it often uses primary physicians as gatekeepers, often capitates providers, has a limited provider panel, and uses an authorization system, etc. It is referred to as exclusive because the member must remain within the network to receive benefits. The main difference is that EPOs are generally regulated under insurance statutes rather than HMO regulations. Not allowed in many states that maintain that EPOs are really HMOs.

Equity model—A term applied to a form of for-profit vertically integrated health care delivery system in which the physicians are owners.

ER—Emergency room; see *ED*.

ERISA—Employee Retirement Income Security Act. One provision of this Act allows self-funded plans to avoid paying premium taxes, complying with state-mandated benefits, or otherwise complying with state laws and regulations regarding insurance, even when insurance companies and managed care plans that stand risk for medical costs must do so. Another provision requires that plans and insurance companies provide an explanation of benefits (EOB) statement to a member or covered insured in the event of a denial of a claim, explaining why the claim was denied and informing the individual of his or her rights of appeal. Numerous other provisions in ERISA are important for a managed care organization to know.

Evidence of insurability—The form that documents whether an individual is eligible for health plan coverage when the individual does not enroll through an open enrollment period. For example, if an employee wants to change health plans in the middle of a contract year, the new health plan may require evidence of insurability (often both a questionnaire and a medical examination) to ensure that it will not be accepting adverse risk. It may also be used to document eligibility to receive mandatory issue coverage under HIPAA.

Experience rating—The method of setting premium rates on the basis of the actual health care costs of a group or groups.

Extracontractual benefits—Health care benefits beyond what the member's actual policy covers. These benefits are provided by a plan to reduce utilization. For example, a plan may not provide coverage for a hospital bed at home, but it is more cost-effective for the plan to provide such a bed than to keep admitting a member to the hospital.

FAR—Federal acquisition regulations. The regulations applied to the federal government's acquisition of services, including health care services and excluding Medicare (also see *FEHBARs*).

Fast-track ED—A pathway in the ED allowing minor ailments to be managed quickly, at lower cost, often by nonphysician practitioners.

Favored nations discount—A contractual agreement between a provider and a payer stating that the provider will automatically provide the payer the best discount it provides anyone else.

Federal qualification—Applies to HMOs and CMPs. It means that the HMO/CMP meets federal standards regarding benefits, financial solvency, rating methods, marketing, member services, health care delivery systems, and other standards. An HMO/CMP must apply for federal qualification and be examined by the OMC, including an on-site review. Federal qualification does place some restrictions on how a plan operates but also allows it to enter the Medicare and FEHBP markets in an expedited way. Federal qualification is voluntary and not required to enter the market.

Fee schedule—May also be referred to as fee maximums or as a fee allowance schedule. A listing of the maximum fee that a health plan will pay for a certain service, based on CPT billing codes.

FEHBARs—Federal Employee Health Benefit Acquisition Regulations. The regulations applied to OPM's purchase of health care benefits programs for federal employees.

FEHBP—Federal Employee Health Benefits Program. The program that provides health benefits to federal employees. See *OPM*.

FFS—Fee for service. A patient sees a provider, the provider bills the health plan or patient, and gets paid based on that bill.

Flexible benefit plan—When an employer allows employees to choose a variety of options in benefits up to a certain total amount. Employees then can tailor their benefits package between health coverage, life insurance, child care, and so forth to optimize benefits for their particular needs.

Formulary—A listing of drugs that a physician may prescribe (i.e., a list of drugs approved for use within a health care setting). The physician is requested or required to use only formulary drugs unless there is a valid medical reason to use a nonformulary drug.

Foundation—A not-for-profit form of integrated health care delivery system. The foundation model is usually formed in response to tax laws that affect not-for-profit hospitals or in response to states with laws prohibiting the corporate practice of medicine (see *corporate practice acts*). The foundation purchases both the tangible and intangible assets of a physician's practice, and the physicians then form a medical group that contracts with the foundation on an exclusive basis for services to patients seen through the foundation.

FPP—Faculty practice plan. A form of group practice organized around a teaching program. It may be a single group encompassing all the physicians providing services to patients at the teaching hospital and clinics, or it may be multiple groups drawn along specialty lines (e.g., psychiatry, cardiology, or surgery).

Fraudandabuse—A term with its roots in a description applied to fraud and/or abuse by health care providers or intermediaries in the provision of services to Medicare and Medicaid beneficiaries. Since that time nobody, and I mean nobody, uses either term separately, and it has taken on a generic meaning applied to any form of perceived skullduggery on the part of a provider or health plan doing business with the government. See also *waste*, *fraud*, and *abuse*.

FTE—Full-time equivalent. The equivalent of one full-time employee. For example, two part-time employees are 0.5 FTE each, for a total of one FTE.

Full professional risk capitation—A loose term used to refer to a physician group or organization receiving capitation for all professional expenses, not just for the services they provide themselves; does not include capitation for institutional services (see *global capitation*). The group is then responsible for subcapitating or otherwise reimbursing other physicians for services to their members.

Gag clause—A clause in a provider contract that prevents a physician from telling a patient about available clinical treatment options (i.e., a "gag"). This clause is much like the Sasquatch—big, hairy, and scary, but hard to actually find. The federal government conducted a review of managed care physician contracts and was unable to find any examples. Gag clauses have been banned by many states, and federal legislation is likely as well (always politically useful to ban what doesn't exist anyway). Most or all contracts between MCOs and physicians do contain clauses that prohibit the physician from revealing business secrets such as reimbursement schedules, but this is a different matter. In some cases in the past, contracts also required a physician to contact the MCO before initiating a treatment option, which may have been interpreted or treated as such a clause, but most contracts actually require the physician to actively discuss options with the patient.

Gatekeeper—An informal, although widely used, term that refers to a primary care case management model health plan. In this model, all care from providers other than the primary care physician, except for true emergencies, must be authorized by the primary care physician before care is rendered. This is a predominant feature of almost all HMOs.

Generic drug—A drug that is equivalent to a brand name drug but usually less expensive. Most managed care organizations that provide drug benefits cover generic drugs but may require a member to pay the difference in cost between a generic drug and a brand name drug or pay a higher copay, unless there is no generic equivalent.

Glass-Steagall Act—See the *Gramm-Leach-Bliley Act of 1999*.

Global capitation—The term used when an organization receives capitation for all medical services, including institutional and professional.

Gramm-Leach-Bliley Act of 1999—The Gramm-Leach-Bliley Act (S.900/H.R. 10) repealed the Glass-Steagall Act of 1933 that had been passed in the aftermath of the crash of 1929. Glass-Steagall prohibited most U.S. commercial banks from performing investment banking activities such bringing new debt and equity issues to market, or other such underwriting, and from functioning as insurance companies. In addition to the repeal of Glass-Steagall, Gramm-Leach-Bliley also allows affiliations between securities firms, banks, and insurance companies.

Group—The members that are covered by virtue of receiving health plan coverage at a single company.

Group model HMO—An HMO that contracts with a medical group for the provision of health care services. The relationship between the HMO and the medical group is generally close, although there are wide variations in the relative independence of the group from the HMO. A form of closed panel health plan.

Group practice—The American Medical Association defines group practice as three or more physicians who deliver patient care, make joint use of equipment and personnel, and divide income by a pre-arranged formula.

Group practice without walls (GPWW)—A group practice in which the members of the group come together legally but continue to practice in private offices scattered throughout the service area. Sometimes called a clinic without walls (CWW).

HCFA—Health Care Financing Administration. The federal agency that oversees all aspects of health financing for Medicare and also oversees the Office of Managed Care (OMC). Part of HHS.

HCFA-1500—A claims form used by professionals to bill for services. Required by Medicare and generally used by private insurance companies and managed care plans.

HCPCS—HCFA common procedural coding system. A set of codes used by Medicare that describes services and procedures. HCPCS includes CPT codes but also has codes for services not included in CPT such as DME and ambulance. Although HCPCS is nationally defined, there is provision for local use of certain codes, but such local codes will be abolished under HIPAA.

Health care—You probably think you know what this means, eh? Well, maybe, maybe not. The term is generally used to refer to the services that a health care professional or institution provide you (e.g., services from a physician, at a hospital, from a physical therapist); it is this use of the term that is universally used when discussing care management. There is a broader definition, however, that encompasses services from nontraditional providers and, more importantly, the health care that individuals self-administer (which is actually most health care anyone receives). When individuals use the broad sense of the term health care, they frequently use medical care to refer to what is considered the narrow meaning just noted. Broad or narrow—it's your choice depending on the context.

Health risk appraisals—Instruments designed to elicit or compile information about the health risk of any given individual. Initially these tools were fairly uniform, but recently they have become quite specialized and targeted toward particular populations with distinctive risk profiles (e.g., Medicare, Medicaid, underserved, commercial population).

HEDIS—Health Plan Employer Data Information Set. Developed by NCQA with considerable input from the employer community and the managed care community, HEDIS is an ever-evolving set of data reporting standards. HEDIS is designed to provide some standardization in performance reporting for financial, utilization, membership, and clinical data so that employers and others can compare performance between plans.

HHS—Health and Human Services, or more correctly, the United States Department of Health and Human Services (DHHS). This is the cabinet-level federal agency that oversees many programs, including the Health Care Financing Administration (HCFA) responsible for Medicare and Medicaid (in conjunction with individual states) and oversight of HIPAA and other related federal legislation.

HIAA—Health Insurance Association of America. A trade organization that represents health insurance companies, whether those companies are managed health care organizations or not. Their primary focus has been on legislative and lobbying activities, although they have expanded their scope somewhat to include operational issues.

HIPAA—Health Insurance Portability and Accountability Act. Enacted in 1996, this act creates a set of requirements that allow for insurance portability (i.e., the ability to keep your health insurance even if you lose eligibility through certain events), guaranteed issue of all health insurance products to small groups (but only if they have met requirements for prior continuous coverage), and mental health parity (i.e., the dollar limits on mental health coverage cannot be less than that for medical coverage; it is silent, however, to the issues of differential visit limitations, differential coinsurance requirements, or restrictions on networks). HIPAA does not guarantee affordability, however HIPAA also contains significant provisions regarding "administrative simplification" and privacy standards that will have a major impact on e-commerce.

HMO—Health maintenance organization. The definition of an HMO has changed substantially. Originally, an HMO was defined as a prepaid organization that provided health care to voluntarily enrolled members in return for a preset amount of money on a PMPM basis. With the increase in self-insured business or with financial arrangements that do not rely on prepayment, that definition is no longer accurate. Now the definition needs to encompass two possibilities: a licensed health plan (licensed as an HMO that is) that places at least some of the providers at risk for medical expenses and a health plan that uses designated (usually primary care) physicians as gatekeepers (although there are some HMOs that do not). Many in the field have given up and now use the looser term "MCO" because it avoids having to make difficult definitions like this one.

HOS—Health outcomes survey—The HOS is a survey that health plans with a Medicare+Choice risk contract must conduct to look at clinical outcomes of covered Medicare beneficiaries. HCFA arranges and pays for administration of the CAHPS survey, whereas Medicare+Choice health plans are responsible for administering the HOS survey.

Hospitalist—A physician who concentrates solely on hospitalized patients. In a MCO or medical group, this physician may specialize in hospital care, or the duties may be undertaken on a rotating basis. This model allows the other physicians to concentrate on outpatient care, while the hospitalist focuses on the care of all the plan's or groups patients in the hospital.

IBNR—Incurred but not reported. The amount of money that the plan had better accrue for medical expenses that it knows nothing about yet. These are medical expenses that the authorization system has not captured and for which claims have not yet hit the door. Unexpected IBNRs have torpedoed more managed care plans than any other cause.

ICD-9-CM—*International Classification of Diseases*, 9th revision, clinical modification. The classification of disease by diagnosis codified into six-digit numbers. The ICD-10 will use alphanumeric codes and is scheduled for publication some time in the year 2000.

IDFN—See *IDS*.

IDFS—See *IDS*.

IDN—See *IDS*.

IDS—Integrated delivery system; also referred to as an integrated health care delivery system. Other acronyms that mean the same thing include IDN (integrated delivery network), IDFS (integrated delivery and financing system), and IDFN (integrated delivery and financing network). An IDS is an organized system of health care providers to span a broad range of health care services. Although there is no clear definition of an IDS, in its full flower an IDS should be able to access the market on a broad basis, optimize cost and clinical outcomes, accept and manage a full range of financial arrangements to provide a set of defined benefits to a defined population, align financial incentives of the participants (including physicians), and operate under a cohesive management structure. Also see *IHO, IPA, PHO, MSO, equity model, staff model, foundation model.*

IHO—Integrated health care organization: An IDS that is predominantly owned by physicians. Not a common term at the time this book was written and fading fast.

IPA—Independent practice association. An organization that has a contract with a managed care plan to deliver services in return for a single capitation rate. The IPA in turn contracts with individual providers to provide the services either on a capitation basis or on a fee-for-service basis. The typical IPA encompasses all specialties, but an IPA can be solely for primary care or may be single specialty. An IPA may also be the "PO" part of a PHO.

Joint Commission—Joint Commission for Accreditation of Healthcare Organizations. A not-for-profit organization that performs accreditation reviews primarily on hospitals, other institutional facilities, and outpatient facilities. Most managed care plans require any hospital under contract to be accredited by the Joint Commission.

Lag study—A report that tells managers how old the claims are that are being processed and how much is paid out each month (both for that month and for any earlier months, by month) and compares these to the amount of money that was accrued for expenses each month. A powerful tool used to determine whether the plan's reserves are adequate to meet all expenses. Plans that fail to perform lag studies properly may find themselves staring into the abyss.

Line of business—A health plan (e.g., an HMO, EPO, or PPO) that is set up as a line of business within another, larger, organization, usually an insurance company. This legally differentiates it from a free-standing company or a company set up as a subsidiary. It may also refer to a unique product type (e.g., Medicaid) within a health plan.

LOS/ELOS/ALOS—Length of stay/estimated length of stay/average length of stay.

Loss ratio—See *medical loss ratio*.

MAC—Maximum allowable charge (or cost). The maximum, although not the minimum, that a vendor may charge for something. This term is often used in pharmacy contracting; a related term, used in conjunction with professional fees, is fee maximum.

Managed health care—A regrettably nebulous term. At the very least, a system of health care delivery that tries to manage the cost of health care, the quality of that health care, and access to that care. Common denominators include a panel of contracted providers that is less than the entire universe of available providers, some type of limitations on benefits to subscribers who use noncontracted providers (unless authorized to do so), and some type of authorization system. Managed health care is actually a spectrum of systems, ranging from so-called managed indemnity through PPOs, POS, open-panel HMOs, and closed-panel HMOs. For a better definition, the reader is urged to read this book and formulate his or her own.

Mandated benefits—Benefits that a health plan is required to provide by law. This is generally used to refer to benefits above and beyond routine insurance-type benefits, and it generally applies at the state level (where there is high variability from state to state). Common examples include in-vitro fertilization, defined days of inpatient mental health or substance abuse treatment, and other special-condition treatments. Self-funded plans are exempt from mandated benefits under ERISA.

Mandatory external review—The requirement that an MCO provide a means for a physician or member who appeals a decision about medical coverage to obtain a second opinion from an unbiased external reviewer, a physician in a specialty appropriate for the clinical condition. This process has been mandated in some states and is widely undertaken on a voluntary basis in any event.

Master group contract—The actual contract between a health plan and a group that purchases coverage. The master group contract provides specific terms of coverage, rights, and responsibilities of both parties.

Maximum out of pocket cost—The most amount of money a member will ever need to pay for covered services during a contract year. The maximum out of pocket includes deductibles and coinsurance. Once this limit is reached, the health plan pays for all services up to the maximum level of coverage. Applies mostly to non-HMO plans such as indemnity plans, PPOs, and POS plans.

MCE—Medical care evaluation. A component of a quality assurance program that looks at the process of medical care.

MCO—Managed care organization. A generic term applied to a managed care plan. Some people prefer it to the term HMO because it encompasses plans that do not conform exactly to the strict definition of an HMO (although that definition has itself loosened considerably). May also apply to a PPO, EPO, IDS, or OWA.

Medical loss ratio—The ratio between the cost to deliver medical care and the amount of money that was taken in by a plan. Insurance companies often have a medical loss ratio of 92 percent or more; tightly managed HMOs may have medical loss ratios of 75 to 85 percent, although the overhead (or administrative cost ratio) is concomitantly higher. The medical loss ratio depends on the amount of money brought in and the cost of delivering care; thus, if the rates are too low, the ratio may be high, even though the actual cost of delivering care is not really out of line.

Medical policy—Refers to the policies of a health plan regarding what will be paid for as medical benefits. Routine medical policy is linked to routine claims processing and may even be automated in the claims system; for example, the plan may pay only 50 percent of the fee of a second surgeon or may not pay for two surgical procedures done during one episode of anesthesia. This also refers to how a plan approaches payment policy for experimental or investigational care and payment for noncovered services in lieu of more expensive covered services.

Medicare+Choice—The revised form of Medicare private insurance options, created under BBA '97.

Medigap insurance—A form of health insurance that covers whatever Medicare doesn't. Medigap policies are now subject to minimum standards under federal law.

Member—An individual covered under a managed care plan. May be either the subscriber or a dependent.

Member months—The total of all months that each member was covered. For example, if a plan had 10,000 members in January and 12,000 members in February, the total member months for the year to date as of March 1 would be 22,000.

Mental Health Parity Act—Passed by Congress in 1996, it requires group health plans that offer mental health coverage benefits to apply the same annual and aggregate lifetime dollar limits to mental health coverage as those applied to coverage of other services. The federal law applies to fully insured and self-insured plans, including state-regulated plans. However, states may enact requirements more stringent than those contained under the federal law.

MET—Multiple employer trust. See *MEWA*.

MEWA—Multiple employer welfare association. A group of employers who band together for purposes of purchasing group health insurance, often through a self-funded approach to avoid state mandates and insurance regulation. By virtue of ERISA, such entities are regulated little, if at all. Many MEWAs have enabled small employers to obtain cost-effective health coverage, but some MEWAs have not had the financial resources to withstand the risk of medical costs and have failed, leaving the members without insurance or recourse. In some states, MEWAs and METs are no longer legal.

MHS—See *military health system*.

Military health system (MHS)—A large and complex health care system designed to provide, and to maintain readiness to provide, medical services and support to the armed forces during military operations and to provide medical services and support to members of the armed forces, their dependents, and others entitled to Department of Defense (DOD) medical care. See also *CHAMPUS* and *TRICARE*.

MIS—Management information system. The common term for the computer hardware and software that provides the support for managing the plan.

Mixed model—A managed care plan that mixes two or more types of delivery systems. This has traditionally been used to describe an HMO that has both closed-panel and open-panel delivery systems.

MLP—Midlevel practitioner. Physician's assistants, clinical nurse practitioners, nurse midwives, and the like. Nonphysicians who deliver medical care, generally under the supervision of a physician but for less cost.

MMI—Master member index. The MMI is used in physician practice profiling to identify in a reliable manner each patient receiving care from a particular physician. Subject to the privacy and security provisions under HIPAA.

Moral hazard—An old term of insurance that remains applicable today. Loosely defined for purposes of this glossary, moral hazard refers to the concept of providing insurance to a market in which it is certain that financial losses will occur. The term is actually a bit more complex than that, but this definition will do here.

MSA—Medical savings account. Created as a demonstration under BBA '97 and under active debate in the Congress as of early 2000, MSAs are specialized savings accounts into which a consumer can put pre-tax dollars for use in paying medical expenses in lieu of purchasing a comprehensive health insurance or managed care product. MSAs require a catastrophic health insurance policy as a "safety net" to protect against very high costs. The darling of conservative policy wonks, MSAs have proven to be underwhelming in their market attractiveness. The driving theory behind MSAs is that by directly controlling the money, consumers will be incented to be wise purchasers of health care services. Unless you are either a physician or an extraordinarily well-informed consumer, it is a challenge at best to know whether a health service is really necessary or not (is that a headache you have, or is it a glioblastoma?). The real weakness of the MSA, however, is the lack of purchasing power by an individual consumer (i.e., the inability to negotiate substantial discounts from providers). The first time a consumer with an MSA is exposed to the full fury of unfettered fee-for-service charges is often also the last time ("You're going to charge me *what*??"). To make things worse, the premium cost of a catastrophic insurance policy isn't substantially less than the cost of a comprehensive policy because most costs are related to a small percentage of patients with very expensive problems, problems that would be covered under a catastrophic policy. So there.

MSO—Management service organization. A form of integrated health delivery system. Sometimes similar to a service bureau (see later), the MSO often actually purchases certain hard assets of a physician's practice and then provides services to that physician at fair market rates. MSO are usually formed as a means to contract more effectively with managed care organizations, although their simple creation does not guarantee success.

MTF—Military treatment facilities. See *military health system*.

Multispecialty group—Just what it sounds like— a medical group made up of different specialty physicians. May or may not include primary care.

NACHA—National Automated Clearing House Association. Oversees electronic transaction protocols and standards for the regional automated clearing houses. The function of ACHs will change as a result of HIPAA.

NAHMOR—National Association of HMO Regulators.

NAIC—National Association of Insurance Commissioners.

NCPDP—National Council for Prescription Drug Programs. The NCPDP developed and maintains accepted electronic data interchange standard for pharmacy claims transmission and adjudication accelerated the adoption of pharmacy e-commerce. This standard permits the submission of pharmacy claims and the adjudication of those claims in a real-time interactive mode. Recognized by ANSI and addressed under HIPAA.

NCQA—National Committee for Quality Assurance. A not-for-profit organization that performs quality-oriented accreditation reviews on HMOs and similar types of managed care plans. NCQA also accredits CVOs and develops HEDIS standards.

NDC—National drug code. The national classification system for identifying prescription drugs.

Network model HMO—A health plan that contracts with multiple physician groups to deliver health care to members. Generally limited to large single or multispecialty groups. Distinguished from group model plans that contract with a single medical group, IPAs that contract through an intermediary, and direct contract model plans that contract with individual physicians in the community.

No brainer—A term used to describe a decision so obvious that one doesn't need to engage one's brain to make the right decision. Not to be confused with a description of any figure in authority who *just doesn't get it*.

Non-par—Short for nonparticipating. Refers to a provider that does not have a contract with the health plan.

NPI—National Provider Identifier. The NPI is mandated under HIPAA and will replace all other types of provider (broadly defined) identifiers regardless of customer (i.e., commercial health plan, Medicare, Medicaid, CHAMPUS). It is expected to be implemented in a rollout manner beginning in 2002 or 2003. At the time of publication, the NPI is proposed to be a ten digit numeric identifier. The tenth position is a checksum digit that can help detect keying errors. It contains no embedded intelligence; that is, it contains no information about the health care provider such as the type of health care provider or state where the health care provider is located. For the final definition, which will be finalized after this book goes to press, refer to: http://www.hcfa.gov/stats/npi/overview.htm

OBRA—Omnibus Reconciliation Act. What Congress calls the many annual tax and budget reconciliation acts. Most of these acts contain language important to managed care, generally in the Medicare market segment.

Observation unit—A treatment room usually adjacent to the ED where rapid evaluation and stabilization of a medical problem can be managed, resulting in discharge of the patient to home (e.g., chest pain unit).

OCR—Optical character recognition. A system of hardware and software that is able to recognize written characters scanned in from a paper source and convert those characters into standard data. Used in claims-processing systems in which paper claims are routinely submitted by providers. OCR works well with typed or printer-generated documents but poorly with hand-written documents. OCR accuracy and effectiveness is enhanced when standard forms are used (e.g., the HCFA 1500-R or the UB-92) and even more when specialized forms (e.g., those that use red "dropout" ink to print the form) are used to eliminate the need for the OCR system to scan and read the characters on the form itself.

OIG—The Office of the Inspector General. This is the federal agency responsible for conducting investigations and audits of federal contractors or any system that receives funds or reimbursement from the federal government. There are actually several OIG departments in different federal programs; examples pertinent to managed health care would include CHAMPUS, Medicare, and the FEHBP.

OMC—Office of Managed Care. The latest name for the federal agency that oversees federal qualification and compliance for HMOs and eligibility for CMPs. Old names were HMOS (Health Maintenance Organization Service), OHMO (Office of Health Maintenance Organizations), OPHC (Office of Prepaid Health Care), and the Office of Prepaid Health Care Operations and Oversight (OPHCOO). Once part of the Public Health Service, the OMC and most of its predecessors are part of HCFA. This agency could be reorganized yet again as this book is being written, so heaven only knows what their new acronym will be.

OOBD—Order of Benefits Determination. See *COB*.

Open enrollment period—The period when an employee may change health plans; usually occurs once per year. A general rule is that most managed care plans will have around half their membership up for open enrollment in the fall for an effective date of January 1. A special form of open enrollment is still law in some states. This yearly open enrollment requires an HMO to accept any individual applicant (i.e., one not coming in through an employer group) for coverage, regardless of health status. Such special open enrollments usually occur for 1 month each year. Many Blue Cross Blue Shield plans have similar open enrollments for indemnity products.

Open panel HMO—A managed care plan that contracts (either directly or indirectly) with private physicians to deliver care in their own offices. Examples would include a direct contract HMO and an IPA.

OPL—Other party liability. See *COB*.

OPM—Office of Personnel Management. The federal agency that administers the FEHBP. This is the agency with which a managed care plan contracts to provide coverage for federal employees.

Outlier—Something that is well outside of an expected range. May refer to a provider who is using medical resources at a much higher rate than their peers, or to a case in a hospital that is far more expensive than anticipated, or in fact to anything at all that is significantly more or less than expected.

OWA—Other weird arrangement. A general acronym that applies to any new and bizarre managed care plan that has thought up a new twist.

Package pricing—Also referred to as bundled pricing. An MCO pays an organization a single fee for all inpatient, outpatient, and professional expenses associated with a procedure, including preadmission and postdischarge care. Common procedures that use this form of pricing include cardiac bypass surgery and transplants.

Par provider—Shorthand term for participating provider (i.e., one who has signed an agreement with a plan to provide services). May apply to professional or institutional providers.

PAS norms—The common term for professional activity study results of the Commission on Professional and Hospital Activities. Broken out by region, the Western region has the lowest average LOS, so it tends to be used most often to set an estimated LOS. Available as LOS: *Length of Stay by Diagnosis*, published by CPHA publications, Ann Arbor, MI.

Pay and pursue—Also referred to as "pay and chase." The antonym is pursue and pay or "chase" and pay. A term commonly used in OPL or COB, this refers to the order in which a health plan will deal with claims that may be the principal liability of another insurance company or managed health care plan. Pay and pursue refers to the health plan paying for the claim and then trying to recover all or some of the costs from the other insurance company. Pursue and pay refers to the plan transferring the claim to that insurance carrier that is primarily responsible for the cost and not paying the claim unless the primary carrier does not cover the cost in full, in which case the secondary plan will cover that portion of the costs that was not covered by the primary insurer. See also *COB*.

PayerID™—Payer Identifier. See PlanID.

PCCM—Primary care case manager. This acronym is used in Medicaid managed care programs and refers to the state designating PCPs as case managers to function as "gatekeepers" but reimbursing those PCPs using traditional Medicaid fee for service, as well as paying the PCP a nominal management fee such as $2 to $5 PMPM.

PCP—Primary care physician. Generally applies to internists, pediatricians, family physicians, and general practitioners and occasionally to obstetrician/gynecologists.

PEL—Provider excess loss. Refers to a stop-loss insurance policy purchased by risk-bearing provider organizations, full-risk–bearing medical groups, or IDSs to limit exposure to catastrophic claims costs.

Pended/suspended claims—Although the terms pend and suspend are often used synonymously, some MCOs differentiate between claims that examiners place on hold (pends) and those that are placed on hold automatically by one or more systems edits (suspends).

PEPM—Per employee per month. Like PMPM, but roles the unit up to the level of the employee or subscriber rather than measuring on the basis of all members (subscriber plus dependents).

Per diem reimbursement—Reimbursement of an institution, usually a hospital, on the basis of a set rate per day rather than on charges. Per diem reimbursement can be varied by service (e.g., medical/surgical, obstetrics, mental health, and intensive care) or can be uniform regardless of intensity of services.

Periodic interim payment—A method of advancing money from a payer to a provider before an exact accounting of claims is done. For example, an MCO may make a monthly PIP to a hospital and then reconcile every quarter. This used to be common between BCBS plans and hospitals but no longer is. Because of the time value of money, a PIP is usually used now only when the MCO or payer is unable to process claims quickly and correctly but needs to pay the providers in the meantime.

PHI—Protected health information. That information that reveals medical information or data about an individual. PHI is addressed specifically by HIPAA in the Privacy and Security sections.

PHO—Physician-hospital organization. These are legal (or perhaps informal) organizations that bond hospitals and the attending medical staff. Frequently developed for the purpose of contracting with managed care plans. A PHO may be open to any member of the staff who applies, or they may be closed to staff members who fail to qualify (or who are part of an already overrepresented specialty).

Physician incentive program—A generic term referring to a reimbursement method under which a physician's income from an MCO (or an IDS) is affected by the physician's performance or the overall performance of the plan (e.g., utilization, medical cost, quality measurements, member satisfaction). This term has a specific use by HCFA, which limits the degree of incentive or risk allowed under a Medicare HMO (refer to PIP regulations at 42 CFR 422.208/210 of the June 26, 1998 regulations that implement Medicare Part C). HCFA essentially bans "gainsharing" by means of a PIP altogether in an IDS receiving reimbursement under Medicare. Some states also now have laws and regulations regarding limits on PIPs and requirements for disclosure of incentives to members enrolled in MCOs. See also *SFR*.

PIP—See *periodic interim payment*, or else see *physician incentive program*.

PIP/DCG—Principal inpatient diagnostic cost group. The method in which HCFA uses inpatient stays as a predictor of total Medicare expenditures for an individual so as to apply to risk-adjusted payments to Medicare risk plans.

PlanID—Plan Identifier, mandated under HIPAA. This term replaces PayerID. These will be the identifiers used by health plans (broadly defined) when conducting all transactions, regardless of the type of customer (e.g., commercial health plan, Medicare plan) or provider. The PayerID is expected to be implemented in a rollout fashion beginning in 2002 or 2003. The definitions for this have not been released at the time of publication, so the reader is referred to: http://www.hcfa.gov/stats/npaybrf.htm

PMG—Primary medical group. A group practice made up of primary care physicians, although some may have OB/GYN as well.

PMPM—Per member per month. Specifically applies to a revenue or cost for each enrolled member each month.

PMPY—Per member per year. The same as PMPM but based on a year.

POD—Pool of doctors. See *POP*.

POP—Pool of physicians. This refers to the plan grouping physicians into units smaller than the entire panel but larger than individual practices. Typical POPs have between 10 and 30 physicians. Often used for performance measurement and compensation. The POP is often not a real legal entity but rather a grouping.

POS—Point of service. A plan in which members do not have to choose how to receive services until they need them. The most common use of the term applies to a plan that enrolls each member in both an HMO (or HMO-like) system and an indemnity plan. Occasionally referred to as an HMO swing-out plan, an out-of-plan benefits rider to an HMO, or a primary care PPO. These plans provide a difference in benefits (e.g., 100 percent coverage rather than 70 percent) depending on whether the member chooses to use the plan (including its providers and in compliance with the authorization system) or go outside the plan for services. Dual choice refers to an HMO-like plan with an indemnity plan, and triple choice refers to the addition of a PPO to the dual choice. An archaic but still valid definition applies to a simple PPO, in which members receive coverage at a greater level if they use preferred providers (albeit without a gatekeeper system) than if they choose not to do so.

PPA—Preferred provider arrangement. Same as a PPO but sometimes used to refer to a somewhat looser type of plan in which the payer (i.e., the employer)

makes the arrangement rather than the providers. A fading term.

PPM—Physician practice management company. An organization that manages physician's practices and in most cases either owns the practices outright or has rights to purchase them in the future. PPMs concentrate only on physicians, and not on hospitals, although some PPMs have also branched into joint ventures with hospitals and insurers. Many PPMs are publicly traded.

PPO—Preferred provider organization. A plan that contracts with independent providers at a discount for services. The panel is limited in size and usually has some type of utilization review system associated with it. A PPO may be risk bearing, like an insurance company or may be non–risk-bearing, like a physician-sponsored PPO that markets itself to insurance companies or self-insured companies by means of an access fee.

PPS—Prospective payment system. Medicare's terminology for determining fixed pricing for reimbursement of hospitals and facilities for care. The most well-known example of PPS is DRGs, but it also includes APCs.

Precertification—Also known as preadmission certification, preadmission review, and precert. The process of obtaining certification or authorization from the health plan for routine hospital admissions (inpatient or outpatient). Often involves appropriateness review against criteria and assignment of length of stay. Failure to obtain precertification often results in a financial penalty to either the provider or the subscriber.

Pre-existing condition—A medical condition for which a member has received treatment during a specified period of time before becoming covered under a health plan. May have an effect on whether treatments for that condition will be covered under certain types of health plans.

Preventive care—Health care that is aimed at preventing complications of existing diseases or preventing the occurrence of a disease.

Private inurement—What happens when a not-for-profit business operates in such a way as to provide more than incidental financial gain to a private individual; for example, if a not-for-profit hospital pays too much money for a physician's practice or fails to charge fair market rates for services provided to a physician. An IRS no-no.

PRO—Peer review organization. An organization charged with reviewing quality and cost for Medicare. Established under TEFRA. Generally operates at the state level.

Prospective review—Reviewing the need for medical care before the care is rendered. Also see *precertification.*

Provider—The generic term used to refer to anyone providing medical services. In fact, it may even be used to refer to any*thing* that provides medical services, such as a hospital. Most often, however, it is used to refer to physicians. How physicians migrated from being called physicians to being called providers is not very clear cut and certainly not embraced by physicians, but it is a term in general use, including in this book.

Prudent layperson—See *reasonable layperson standard.*

PSA—Professional services agreement. A contract between a physician or medical group and an IDS or MCO for the provision of medical services. Not to be confused with prostate surface antigen, a screening blood test for prostate cancer.

PSN—See *PSO.*

PSO—Provider sponsored organization. An entity allowed under the BBA '97 Medicare + Choice. A PSO is a risk-bearing managed care organization that contracts directly with HCFA for Medicare enrollees, but unlike an HMO, the PSO is made up of the providers themselves, and the providers bear substantial risk for expenses. The rules for financial solvency are somewhat looser for a PSO compared with an HMO, and if a PSO is not licensed by the state, provisions exist to seek licensure directly from the HCFA. PSOs are the result of the belief by providers and legislators that there were fat profits to be had by "cutting out the middle man" in the form of removing the HMO from the equation. A few PSOs actually got started under a demonstration program, and a few more came into being under BBA '97. Most failed utterly and are defunct as of 2000, although a few remain.

PTMPY—Per thousand members per year. A common way of reporting utilization. The most common example is hospital utilization expressed as days per thousand members per year.

Pursue and pay—See *pay and pursue.*

QA or QM—Quality assurance (older term) or quality management (newer term).

QISMC—Quality improvement system for managed care. A HCFA initiative to strengthen managed care organization efforts to protect and improve the health and satisfaction of Medicare and Medicaid beneficiaries. QISMC adopts a very broad definition of "quality" to include the "measurement of health outcomes, consumer satisfaction, the accountability of managed care organizations for achieving ongoing quality improvement, the need for intervention to achieve this improvement, and the importance of data collection, analysis, and reporting."

Qui tam sui—A provision in tort law that allows a citizen to file suit on behalf of the (federal) government and to collect one third of the proceeds of that lawsuit. Such suits are usually also subject to treble damages, making success a lucrative endeavor. The point of this is to encourage citizens with knowledge of deliberate wrongdoing to blow the whistle on the transgressor because the government cannot always know when fraud is occurring. In the context of this book, *qui tam sui* applies to health insurance programs paid with federal funds (i.e., Medicare, Medicaid, CHAMPUS or TRICARE, and the FEHBP).

Rate—The amount of money that a group or individual must pay to the health plan for coverage. Usually a monthly fee. Rating refers to the health plan developing those rates.

RBC—Risk-based capital. A formula embodied in the Risk-Based Capital for Health Organizations Model Act, created under the auspices of the NAIC. RBC takes into account the fluctuating value of plan assets, the financial condition of plan affiliates, the risk that providers may not be able to provide contracted services, the risk that amounts due may not be recovered from reinsurance carriers, and general business risks (i.e., expenses may exceed income). The RBC formula gives credit for provider payment arrangements that reduce underwriting risk, including capitation and provider withholds, bonuses, contracted fee schedules, and aggregate cost arrangements. Although only required in a handful of states and collected in approximately 40 states as of 2000, RBC is the agreed-on standard for an insurance department to determine whether a health plan meets minimum financial solvency requirements. Under the provisions of the act (adoption of which is voluntary by each state), if a plan's total capital assets fall below 200 percent of the risk-based capital requirement, state regulators may require the plan to submit its own proposal for corrective action. If total capital assets fall below 150 percent of the capital requirement, regulators may perform their own analysis and issue a corrective order defining necessary actions to correct the problem. When total capital assets fall below 100 percent of the capital requirement, the state may place the plan under "regulatory control" and when the level falls below 70 percent, they are required to do so.

RBRVS—Resource-based relative value scale. This is a relative value scale developed for HCFA for use by Medicare. The RBRVS assigns relative values to each CPT code for services on the basis of the resources related to the procedure rather than simply on the basis of historical trends. The practical effect has been to lower reimbursement for procedural services (e.g., cardiac surgery) and to raise reimbursement for cognitive services (e.g., office visits).

Reasonable layperson standard—This means that the judgment of a reasonable nonclinician should be applied in determining whether a service is warranted. This standard is almost always focused on the use of emergency or urgent care, when a layperson has good reason to believe that a medical problem must be addressed immediately, even if a trained provider may not believe that it is urgent. The specific language most often used, and addressed directly in the Balanced Budget Act of 1997 as pertaining to Medicare and Medicaid recipients, is: "*Health plans should provide payment when a consumer presents to an emergency department with acute symptoms of sufficient severity—including severe pain—such that a 'prudent layperson' could reasonably expect the absence of medical attention to result in placing health in serious jeopardy, serious impairment to bodily functions, or serious dysfunction of any bodily organ or part.*"

Rebundlers—Software programs that roll up and reprice fragmented bills and apply industry-standard claims adjudication conventions.

Reinsurance—Insurance purchased by a health plan to protect it against extremely high cost cases (also see *stop loss*).

Reserves—The amount of money that a health plan puts aside to cover health care costs. May apply to anticipated costs such as IBNRs, or may apply to money that the plan does not expect to have to use to pay for current medical claims, but keeps as a cushion against future adverse health care costs.

Retrospective review—Reviewing health care costs after the care has been rendered. There are several forms of retrospective review. One form looks at individual claims for medical necessity, billing errors, or fraud. The other form looks at patterns of costs rather than individual cases.

Risk contract—Also known as a Medicare risk contract. A contract between an HMO or CMP and HCFA to provide services to Medicare beneficiaries under which the health plan receives a fixed monthly payment for enrolled Medicare members and then must provide all services on an at-risk basis.

Risk management—Management activities aimed at lowering an organization's legal and financial exposures, especially to lawsuits.

Rule of small numbers—The notion that predictions that are based on large numbers (e.g., a population of 2 million lives) has little relevance when the numbers are small (e.g., 100 lives); chance then plays a far more important role.

RVU—Relative value unit. A number used as a multiplier to calculate the payment to a provider. The RVU is determined on the basis of the procedure, then used by a plan to multiply against a value for each RVU to determine total payment to the provider. Not consistent or uniform, the RVU is often a combination of negotiation and national standards. See also *RBRVS*.

SCHIP—See *CHIP*.

SCP—Specialty care physician. A physician who is not a PCP.

Second opinion—An opinion obtained from another physician regarding the necessity for a treatment that has been recommended by another physician. May be required by some health plans for certain high-cost cases such as cardiac surgery.

Section 1115 waiver—That section of federal law that provides for a state to opt out of the standard (as of 2000) Medicaid fee-for-service program and adopt a managed care approach to financing and providing health care services to Medicaid-eligible recipients. Usually requires that some of the savings be applied to broaden coverage of who is eligible for Medicaid.

Self-care—The series of steps "lay" individuals take to assess and treat an illness or injury, typically without the benefit of higher levels of training in the theory or science of medicine and with little or no consultation with a medical professional.

Self-insured or self-funded plan—A health plan where the risk for medical cost is assumed by the company rather than an insurance company or managed care plan. Under ERISA, self-funded plans are exempt from state laws and regulations such as premium taxes and mandatory benefits. Self-funded plans often contract with insurance companies or third-party administrators to administer the benefits (also see *ASO*).

Sentinel effect—The phenomenon that when it is known that behavior is being observed, that behavior changes, often in the direction the observer is looking for. Applies to the fact that utilization management systems and profiling systems often lead to reductions in utilization before much intervention even takes place, simply because the providers know that someone is watching.

Service area—The geographical area that an HMO provides access to primary care. The service area is usually specifically designated by the regulators (state or federal), and the HMO is prohibited from marketing outside of the service area. May be defined by county or by ZIP code. It is possible for an HMO to have more than one service area, and the service areas may either be contiguous (i.e., they actually border each other) or noncontiguous (i.e., there is a geographical gap between the service areas).

Service bureau—A weak form of integrated delivery system in which a hospital (or other organization) provides services to a physician's practice in return for a fair market price. May also try to negotiate with managed care plans but generally not considered to be an effective negotiating mechanism.

Service plan—A health insurance plan that has direct contracts with providers but is not necessarily a managed care plan. The archetypal service plans are Blue Cross and Blue Shield plans, though there are a few non-Blue service plans. The contract applies to direct billing of the plan by providers (rather than billing of the member), a provision for direct payment of the provider (rather than reimbursement of the member), a requirement that the provider accept the plan's determination of UCR and not balance bill the member in excess of that amount, and a range of other terms. May or may not address issues of utilization and quality.

SFR—Significant financial risk—A term used by HCFA that refers to the total amount of a physician's income at risk in a Medicare HMO. Such financial risk is considered "significant" when it exceeds a certain percentage of the total potential income that physician could receive under the reimbursement program. SFR most commonly is defined as any physician incentive payment program that allows for a variation of more than 25 percent between the minimum and the maximum amount of potential reimbursement.

Shadow pricing—The practice of setting premium rates at a level just below the competition's rates, whether those rates can be justified or not. In other words, the premium rates could actually be lower, but to maximize profit the rates are raised to a level that will remain attractive but result in greater revenue. This practice is generally considered unethical and, in the case of community rating, possibly illegal.

Shock claim—Also referred to as a catastrophic claim. A shock claim is an extraordinarily expensive total cost of health care for an individual patient. Shock claims are taken into account by actuaries when they determine the trends for medical costs because shock claims have a certain amount of randomness to them because they are infrequent and costly, unlike routine care that is predictable.

Shoe box effect—When an indemnity-type benefits plan has a deductible, there may be beneficiaries who save up their receipts to file for reimbursement at a later time (i.e., save them in a shoe box). Those receipts then get lost, or the beneficiary never sends them in, so the insurance company never has to pay.

SHMO—Social health maintenance organization. An HMO that goes beyond the medical care needs of its membership to include their social needs as well. A relatively rare form of HMO.

Single point of entry—A term that means that an individual uses the same system to access both group health medical benefits and benefits for work-related medical conditions. Has waned in popularity in recent years.

SMG—Specialty medical group. A medical group made up predominantly of specialty physicians. May be a single specialty group or a multispecialty group.

Specialty network manager—A term used to describe a single specialist (or perhaps a specialist organization) that accepts capitation to manage a single specialty. Specialty services are supplied by many different specialty physicians, but the network manager has the responsibility for managing access and cost and is at economic risk. A relatively uncommon model as this text is being written.

Staff model HMO—An HMO that employs providers directly, and those providers see members in the HMO's own facilities. A form of closed-panel HMO. A different use of this term is sometimes applied to vertically integrated health care delivery systems that employ physicians, but in which the system is not licensed as an HMO.

Stark regulations—Named after Fortney "Pete" Stark, congressional representative from California. The so-called Stark regulations are actually two sets of regulations: Stark I and Stark II. These regulations are not for amateurs to handle, and competent legal counsel is required for any provider system doing business with federal or state governments.

State of domicile—The state that an insurance company or MCO is licensed in as its primary location. For example, a MCO may have its state of domicile in Virginia but also be licensed and doing business in Maryland and the District of Columbia. In many states, the insurance commissioner will defer primary regulation to the insurance department in the state of domicile as long as all minimum standards of the state are met.

Stop loss—A form of reinsurance that provides protection for medical expenses above a certain limit, generally on a year-by-year basis. This may apply to an entire health plan or to any single component. For example, the health plan may have stop-loss reinsurance for cases that exceed $100,000. After a case hits $100,000, the plan receives 80 percent of expenses in excess of $100,000 back from the reinsurance company for the rest of the year. Another example would be the plan providing a stop loss to participating physicians for referral expenses greater than $2,500. When a case exceeds that amount in a single year, the plan no longer deducts those costs from the physician's referral pool for the remainder of the year. Specific coverage refers to individual cases, whereas aggregate coverage refers to the total costs rather than a specific case.

Subacute care facility—A health facility that is a step down from an acute care hospital. May be a nursing home or a facility that provides medical care but not surgical or emergency care. However, there is a step up from conventional skilled nursing facility intensity of services, adding RNs around the clock and intravenous medications.

Subrogation—The contractual right of a health plan to recover payments made to a member for health care costs after that member has received such payment for damages in a legal action.

Subscriber—The individual or member who has the health plan coverage by virtue of being eligible on his or her own behalf rather than as a dependent.

Sutton's law—"Go where the money is!" Attributed to the Depression-era bank robber Willy Sutton, who, when asked why he robbed banks, replied "That's where the money is." Sutton apparently denied ever having made that statement. In any event, it is a good law to use when determining what needs attention in a managed care plan.

TANF—Temporary Assistance to Needy Families. The new term replacing AFDC. Both terms mean essentially the same thing: Medicaid for families that meet criteria for low income and require medical assistance to mothers and children.

TAT—Turnaround time. The amount of time it takes a health plan to process and pay a claim from the time it arrives.

TEFRA—Tax Equity and Fiscal Responsibility Act. One key provision of this Act prohibits employers and health plans from requiring full-time employees between the ages of 65 and 69 to use Medicare rather than the group health plan. Another key provision codified Medicare risk contracts for HMOs and CMPs.

Termination date—The day that health plan coverage is no longer in effect.

Time loss management—The application of managed care techniques to workers' compensation treatments for injuries or illnesses to reduce the amount of time lost on the job by the affected employee.

Total capitation—See *global capitation*.

TPA—Third-party administrator. A firm that performs administrative functions (e.g., claims processing, membership) for a self-funded plan or a start-up managed care plan (also see *ASO*).

Triage—The origins of this term are grizzly: the process of sorting out wounded soldiers into those who need treatment immediately, those who can wait, and those who are too severely injured to even try and save. In health plans, this refers to the process of sorting out requests for services by members into those who need to be seen right away, those who can wait a little while, and those whose problems can be handled with advice over the phone.

TRICARE—The Department of Defense's worldwide managed health care program. TRICARE was initiated in 1995, integrating health care services provided in the direct care system of military hospitals and clinics with services purchased under CHAMPUS. See also *CHAMPUS* and *military health system*.

Triple option—The offering of an HMO, a PPO, and a traditional insurance plan by one carrier.

Twenty-four hour care—An ill-defined term that essentially means that health care is provided 24 hours per day, regardless of the financing mechanism; applies primarily to the convergence of group health, workers' compensation, and industrial health, all under managed care.

UB-92—The common claim form used by hospitals to bill for services. Some managed care plans demand greater detail than is available on the UB-92, requiring the hospitals to send additional itemized bills.

UCR—Usual, customary, or reasonable. A method of profiling prevailing fees in an area and reimbursing providers on the basis of that profile. One archaic method is to average all fees and choose the 80th or 90th percentile, although in this era a plan will usually use another method to determine what is reasonable. Sometimes this term is used synonymously with a fee allowance schedule when that schedule is set relatively high.

Unbundling—The practice of a provider billing for multiple components of service that were previously included in a single fee. For example, if dressings and instruments were included in a fee for a mi-

nor procedure, the fee for the procedure remains the same, but there are now additional charges for the dressings and instruments.

Underwriting—In one definition, this refers to bearing the risk for something (i.e., a policy is underwritten by an insurance company). In another definition, this refers to the analysis of a group that is done to determine rates and benefits or to determine whether the group should be offered coverage at all. A related definition refers to health screening of each individual applicant for insurance and refusing to provide coverage for pre-existing conditions.

Upcoding—The practice of a provider billing for a procedure that pays better than the service actually performed. For example, an office visit that would normally be reimbursed at $45 is coded as one that is reimbursed at $53.

UPIN—Universal provider identification. An identification number issued by HCFA for use in billing Medicare. The UPIN will be replaced by the NPI some time in 2002 or 2003; in fact, all provider identification numbers will be replaced by the NPI. See *NPI*.

URAC—Utilization Review Accreditation Commission. A not-for-profit organization that performs reviews on external utilization review agencies (freestanding companies, utilization management departments of insurance companies, or utilization management departments of managed care plans). Its primary focus is managed indemnity and PPOs, although they have expanded their accreditation activities. States often require certification by URAC for a utilization management organization to operate. URAC is also known as the American Accreditation HealthCare Commission (AAHC).

URO—Utilization review organization. A freestanding organization that does nothing but UR, usually on a remote basis, by telephone and paper correspondence. It may be independent, or it may be part of another company such as an insurance company that sells UR services on a stand-alone basis.

Waste, fraud, and abuse—Not the name of a law firm or a rock band, this troika is used to cast blame for greedy and sometimes illegal behavior on the part of either providers or health plans, usually by the government, but possibly by private purchasers of health care benefits as well. See also *Fraudandabuse*.

Workers' compensation—A form of social insurance provided through property-casualty insurers. Workers' compensation provides medical benefits and replacement of lost wages that result from injuries or illnesses that arise from the workplace; in turn, the employee cannot normally sue the employer unless true negligence exists. Workers' compensation has undergone dramatic increases in cost as group health has shifted into managed care, resulting in workers' compensation carriers adopting managed care approaches. Workers' compensation is often heavily regulated under state laws that are significantly different than those used for group health insurance and is often the subject of intense negotiation between man-

agement and organized labor. See *time loss management* and *twenty-four hour care*.

Wraparound plan—Commonly used to refer to insurance or health plan coverage for copays and deductibles that are not covered under a member's base plan. This is often used for Medicare.

Zero down—The practice of a medical group or provider system distributing all the capital surplus in a health plan or the group to the members of the group, rather than retaining any capital or reinvesting it in the group or plan.

Index

A

Abuse. *See* Fraud and abuse
Academic health center
  accountability, 218–219
  change
    absence of process and cost
      information, 213
    in financial support, 210–212
    in market mechanisms, 207–210
    organizational change barriers, 212–
      213
    traditional culture, 212–213
    transforming traditional culture, 218–
      220
    transition market, 213
  cost, 207
    average cost of care per admission, 207
  education, 206–225
    reinventing education and research,
      220–223
  financial challenges, 207–213
  financial risk allocation, 209–210
  importance of purchasers, 208–209
  industry-sponsored clinical research, 208
  information sharing, 219–220
  innovation, 214–215
  leadership, 214–215
  managed care organization
    defining respective roles, 223
    education and training in creating
      value, 223–225
    innovative management techniques,
      224
    long-term benefits, 224
    new role for managed care
      organization, 223–225
    price competition, 224
  network formation, 215–216
  new stakeholders, 220–223
  noncommodity identity, 209
  outcomes, 219–220
  overutilization, 209
  patient base maintenance, 215–218
  performance evaluation, 219–220
  primary care, 216–217
  report card, 219–220
  research, reinventing education and
    research, 220–223
  specialty care, 217–218
  strategies for success, 213–223
  training, 206–225
  utilization control, 209
Access, xxix, 171
  financing, 14–15
  Medicaid managed care, 1113–1114
  specialty care, 86
  Utilization Review Accreditation
    Committee, 863
Access plan, dental benefits, 1149
Accountability
  academic health center, 218–219
  Medicaid managed care, 1116
Accounting policy
  background, 907–908
  state regulation, 907–908
Accounts receivable
  aging, 898–899
  membership, 898–899
Accreditation, 849–870
  consumerism, 833–834
  dental health maintenance organization,
    1152
  dental preferred provider organization,
    1152
  health maintenance organization, 865
  Joint Commission on Accreditation of
    Healthcare Organizations, accreditation
    categories, 868
  Managed Behavioral Healthcare
    Organization, 856–857
  National Committee for Quality
    Assurance, 802
    decisions, 855–856
    new health plans, 858
    review process, 855–858
  oversight by type of organization, 850–851
  preferred provider organization, 857,
    864–865
  subacute care, 501–502
  Utilization Review Accreditation
    Committee, 864–865, 865
    member protection, 864
    network management standards, 864
    process, 862
    provider credentialing, 864
    quality management, 864
Accrete, defined, 1357
Accrual
  calculation, 897–898
  defined, 1357
Accrued claim liability, 924–925
Acquisition
  hospital, physician practices, 64–65
  integrated delivery system, physician
    practices, 64–66
Acronyms, 1357–1377
Actuarial assumption, defined, 1358
Actuarial cost modeling, integrated delivery
  system, 972
Actuarial services
  claim probability distributions, 973–974
  clinical efficiency benchmarking, 973
  integrated delivery system, 971–975
    creating incentive structures, 974–975
    measuring results, 975
  overview, 971–972
Adjusted average per capita cost, defined,
  1357
Adjusted community rate, 988–990, 1047–
  1048
  defined, 1357
  Medicare, 1070–1071
Administration. *See also* Specific type
  consumerism, 844–845
  Internet, 844, 845
  Medicaid managed care
    administrative capacity, 1117
    administrative performance, 1117
Administrative expenses, financial
  statement, 915
Administrative physician, compensation,
  158–159
Administrative services only contract
  defined, 1358

Employee Retirement Income Security
  Act, 1276
  state law, 1334
  underwriting, 997
Admissions, emergency medicine, process,
  360–361
Advance directive, Medicare+Choice, 1072
Advanced care management. *See also* Care
  management
  benchmarking, 274–275
  building, 273–276
  characteristics, 272
  components, 281–283
  context, 267–258
  current state assessment, 273–274
  defined, 268–269
  future directions, 278–280
  future state design, 274–275
  infrastructure, 282
  long-term plan, 275–277
  mission, 273–274
  model construction, 275–277
  objective, 268
  program elements of medical
    management, 281–282
  staged implementation, 277–278
  vision, 273–274
Advanced revenue, capitation, 1002
Adverse selection, 896–897
  defined, 1358
Advertising, 811–812
  direct mail, 812
  outdoor advertising, 812
  print, 812
  radio, 812
  selection of advertising media, 812
  television, 812
Advocacy group, consumerism, 833–834
After-hours call duty, 169
Agency for Health Care Policy and
  Research, 1136
Agency for Health Care Research and
  Quality, 224
Aging
  cost, 1088
  demographics, 1088
  population growth, 509
Aid to Families with Dependent Children,
  230
Alternative care, consumerism, 839
Amara's law, defined, 1358
Ambulatory care
  clinical outcome, 575–578
  cost, 403–404
  disease management, 403–404
  payment classification
    provider profile, 602–603, 604
    reimbursement, 204–205
Ambulatory patient group, 188
  provider profile, 602–603, 604
  reimbursement, 204–205
Amenities, 839–842
American Association of Health Plans,
  defined, 1357

American Institute of Certified Public
  Accountants, 908
American Medical Association, 4
Americans with Disabilities Act, plan
  design, 1261–1262
Ancillary provider, Medicare+Choice,
  1099–1100
Ancillary service, 344–349
  contracting, 347–349
  control points, 346–347
  cost, 403–404
  data capture, 346
  disease management, 403–404
  feedback, 346
  financial incentives, 346
  indications for use, 347
  limits on services authorized, 347
  physician-owned, 345–346
  reimbursement, 347–349
Antitrust law, 1203–1219. *See also* Sherman
  Act
  enforcement, 1203–1204
  exclusive dealing arrangement, 1214
  integrated delivery system, 67, 1250–
    1251
  merger, 1213–1214
  most favored nation clause, 1214–1215
  provider network, 1207–1211
    anticompetitive effects, 1209–1210
    efficiencies, 1211
    exclusive physician networks, 1208
    foreclosure, 1210
    networks falling outside of safety
      zones, 1208–1209
    nonexclusive physician networks, 1208
    per se, 1209–1211
    physician union, 1211–1213
    recent cases, 1211
    risk sharing, 1208
    rule of reason, 1209–1211
    safety zones, 1207–1208
  standing, 1204–1205
  state law, physician antitrust exemptions,
    1338
  virtual merger, 1213–1214
Any willing provider law
  any willing provider defined, 1358
  Employee Retirement Income Security
    Act, 1276–1279
  state law, 1334–1335
Appeal
  Employee Retirement Income Security
    Act, 795
  Federal Employees Health Benefits
    Program, 1051–1054
  medical necessity decision
    eligibility decision, 792
    expedited appeals process, 792–793
    information, 793
    payment, 792–793
    process, 793
    timeline, 793
  Medicare+Choice, 1072–1073
  member services, 782–783

external review of medical necessity
  decisions, 791–794
Office of Personnel Management, 1051–
  1054
Utilization Review Accreditation
  Committee, 863
Appropriateness evaluation, 548
Arbitration, grievance, 796
Arizona Health Care Cost Containment
  System, 1108
Assets, balance sheet, 915–916
Assignment of benefits, defined, 1358
Attitude, 170
Audit
  corporate compliance, 1317–1319
  Federal Employees Health Benefits
    Program, 1051–1054
    defending, 1053–1054
    interest claims, 1054
    lost investment income, 1054
    process, 1052–1053
    settling adverse audit findings, 1053–
      1054
  Office of Personnel Management, 1051–
    1054
  record retention, 1051–1052
Authorization, 305, 331–343
  categories, 335–337
  claims payment, 334
  common data elements, 338–339
    manual data elements, 338–339
    new electronic standards, 338
    nonelectronic data elements, 338–339
  concurrent, 335
  data capture and authorization issuance,
    339–341
  definition of services requiring, 331–332
  denial, 336
  drug formulary, 437–438
  electronic authorization system, 340–341
  emergency medicine, 352–354
    prudent layperson legislation, 353–354
  Health Insurance Portability and
    Accountability Act, 338–339
  non-physician-based authorization
    systems, 342–343
  open access health maintenance
    organization, 341–342
  paper-based authorization system, 339–
    340
  pended (for review), 336
  pharmacy benefit management, 437–438
  point-of-service plan, 334–335
  prohibition, 311
  prospective, 335
  report, 341
  requirements, 171
  retrospective, 336
  single visit authorizations only, 309–310
  specialty care physician, 342
  staffing, 337–338
  subauthorization, 336–337
  telephone-based authorization system, 340
  who can authorize, 332–334

Automated reporting, corporate compliance, 1313–1314
Autonomy, physician practice behavior, 621–623
Average adjusted per capita cost, 1087
Average cost, 1000
    population, 1000
    variance, 1000
Average daily maximum, provider excess loss coverage, 1006, 1007
Average payment rate, defined, 1358

B

Baby Boomer, health care preferences, 840–841
Bad faith action
    legal issues, 1225–1228
    liability, 1225–1228
    medical management activity, 1225–1228
Balance billing, defined, 1358
Balance sheet
    assets, 915–916
    cash, 915
    claims incurred but not reported, 916
    claims payable, 916
    components, 915–917
    equity, 917
    investments, 915
    premium receivable, 915–916
    risk pool liability, 916–917
    unearned premium, 916
Balanced Budget Act, 1137
    adjustments, 21
    changes to federal health care programs, 18
    consumer information required, 838
    consumerism, 837, 838
    Medicare, 1060–1085
        choice, 1090–1091
        growth, 1090–1091
    Medicare+Choice, 1086, 1087
Balanced Budget Refinement Act, 21
Bed leasing, hospital, 203
Behavioral health care, 451–479
    benefit plan design, 461–463
    carve-in, 455, 469
    carve-out, 455, 469
    case management, 465, 469–470
    channeling mechanisms, 465–466
    common problems, 456
    coverage limits, 462–463
    credentialing, 472
    crisis intervention, 458
    defined, 451
    disorder, types, 462
    dual diagnosis services, 461
    emerging issues, 477–478
    factors influencing care, 451–452
    gatekeeper, 465–467
        employee assistance program, 465–466
        mental health/substance abuse case manager, 466
        primary care physician, 466
    goals of treatment, 456
    history, 452–453
    ideal continuum of care, 458–459
    incentives, 463
    information systems, 473–476
        features required, 474–475
        integration of health care and behavioral health care systems, 475–476
    integrated delivery system
        historic structures, 467–468
        importance of planned integrated delivery systems, 467
        managed care objectives, 467–469
        move to provider networks, 468–469
        provider structures, 467–469
    levels of care, 462
    medical cost offsets, 455–456
    Mental Health Parity Act, 461
    mental health services, 460–461
    objectives of treatment, 456–457
    outcomes assessment, 472–473
    outcomes measurement, 472–473
    paradigmatic shifts in progress, 454
    provider network, 466–467
        scope, 466–467, 468–469
        selection criteria, 467, 468
        size, 466–467, 468–469
    providers, types, 463
    psychiatric hospitalization, alternatives, 458
    psychotherapy, 458
    public/private systems integration, 476–477
    quality assurance, 469–473
        external monitoring, 470–472
        inservice training, 472
        network providers, 470
        problem identification, 472
        provider credentialing, 472
        staff qualifications, 472
        utilization criteria, 471–472
    shift toward systems planning, 454–455
    strategic approaches for enhancing clinical value, 455–456
    substance abuse
        alternatives to restrictive treatment, 458
        services, 459–460
    treatment, 457–461
        principles, 456–461
        types, 463
    utilization management, 463–464, 469–470
Benchmarking, 548
Benefit design, 157
    Federal Employees Health Benefits Program, 1044–1045
    Medicare, 1095
    Medicare+Choice, 1095
Benefit information form
    defined, 1358
    Medicare, 1072
    Medicare+Choice, 1072
Benefits. See also Claims and benefits administration
Best practices, defined, 1358
Bias, 1354
Billing, claims and benefits administration, 740
Bipartisan Consensus Managed Care Improvement Act, 1234
Blue Cross, formation, 4
Blue Shield, formation, 4
Board of directors, 73–76
    composition, 74
    functions, 74–75
    liability, 75–76
Brand name
    consumerism, 842–843
    e-commerce, 685–687
    Internet, 685–687
Broker, 805–806
Budget surplus, 18
    allocating, 18–19
Budgeting, 907–922
    background, 907–908
    financial forecast, 919–921
Bundled case rate, specialty care physician, 188
Bundled charge, outpatient procedures, 204
Business cycle, health insurance, 886

C

California, risk management, 871–872
Cancer, women's health care, 86–87
Capital budgeting, information technology, 687–689
Capitation, 1000
    advanced revenue, 1002
    advantages for providers, 1002–1003
    capitated physician services, defined, 1018
    capitated provider contract, Employee Retirement Income Security Act, 1279–1280
    carve-out, 187
    defined, 1001, 1359
    fixed revenue, 1002
    hospital, 197, 201–202
    increased investment in systems, 1003
    increased utilization management control, 1002
    medical loss ratio, 1001
    Medicare, 1067–1072
    Medicare+Choice, 1067–1072
    other party liability, 766–768
        hospitals, 768
        physicians, 767–768
    point-of-service plan, non-health maintenance organization plans, 186–187
    primary care physician, 110, 111, 112–127
        age, 114–115
        benefits reductions, 127
        capitation payment calculation, 114

capitation pool, 118–121
carve-out, 116
chance, 126
copayment levels, 127
effect of benefits design on
    reimbursement, 127–129
financial risk, 116–118
full professional risk capitation, 124
gender, 114–115
inappropriate underutilization, 126
individual *vs.* pooled risk, 122–124
institutional services, 118–121
medical expenses for which primary
    care physician is not at risk, 121
pharmacy costs, 121–122
point-of-service plan, 127–129
problems with, 126–127
reasons to capitate, 125–126
referral, 118–121
reimbursement per visit, 126
reinsurance, 121–122
risk/bonus arrangement, 118
scope of covered services, 113–114
service risk, 116–118
stop-loss, 121–122
variation factors, 114–116
variation in reimbursement model by
    product, 129
withhold, 117, 118
referral, 118–121
risk, 1000–1001
risk management, 882
risk pool deficit allocation, 1002–1003
risk pool profit allocation, 1002
specialty care physician
    carve-out, 187
    common problems, 186–187
    contact capitation, 182–183
    disease management organization,
        85
    financial risk, 187
    geographic distribution, 184
    management of referral volume, 186
    organizational models, 184–186
    organized groups, 184
    potential to increase utilization, 186
    by primary care physician choice, 186
    single specialty management, 185
    specialty independent practice
        association, 184
    specialty network manager, 185
    subcapitation of specialty care
        physician by other specialty care
        physician, 183–184
    subacute care, 501
Captive group model health maintenance
    organization, 35–36
Cardiovascular Health Improvement
    Process, 649–652
Care coordinator, Medicare+Choice, 1099–
    1100
Care management, 267–280, 281–283, 799.
    See also Advanced care management
    care delivery model, 271

components
    integration, 269–272
    patient/member-population perspective,
        270
    payer-system perspective, 269
    continuum of care model, 271
    evolution, 271
    future state, 278–280
    insurance model, 271
    physician, 272–273
    value proposition, 279
Care site, 84–85
CareMap, 522
Carrier expense ratio, provider excess loss
    coverage, 1010, 1016
Carve-in, behavioral health care, 455, 469
Carve-out, 9
    behavioral health care, 455, 469
    capitation, 116, 187
    defined, 1359
Case law, risk management, 879–880
Case management, 326–327, 371–400
    assessing information, 376–377
    behavioral health care, 465, 469–470
    claims management, 397–398
    community resources, 381–382
    consent form, 379
    coordinating, 383–384
    cost benefit analysis, 398
    defined, 1359
    disease management, 399–400
        contrasted, 282
    evaluating plan, 384
    gathering information, 376–377
    independent medical exams, 380–381
    indicators, 393, 394–396
    initial needs assessment, 377
    interviewing patient, 378–379
    monitoring, 383–384
    on-site, 374–375
    payor approval, 383
    planning, 382
    process, 375–384
    report, 382–383
        concurrent review reports, 388–392
        preadmission reports, 388–392
    return on investment, 296
    second opinion exams, 380–381
    service and equipment providers, 381
    talking with family, 379–380
    talking with referral source, 377–378
    telephone-based, 374–375
    timing intervention, 393–397
    treating physician, 380
    twenty-four hour coverage program,
        399
    utilization management
        concurrent review, 384–388
        concurrent review reports, 388–392
        preadmission reports, 388–392
        preadmission review, 384–388
    wellness program, 398–399
    work format, 375–376
    flowchart, 376

workers' compensation, developing
    protocols, 1159
Case manager
    behavioral/motivational activities, 374
    credentialing, 371
    financial activities, 373
    in managed care, 375
    medical activities, 372–373
    patient profile, 372
    role, 371–374
    vocational activities, 374
Case mix
    defined, 1359
    provider profile, 600–610
Case mix measure
    home care, 608
    intensive care unit, 608
    nursing home, 608
    rehabilitation facility, 608
Case rate
    hospital, 200–201
    specialty care physician, 188
Cash, balance sheet, 915
Cash advance
    hospital, 203
    specialty care physician, 188–189
Catastrophic management, 31
Catchment Area Management
    Demonstration Project, 1128–1129
Certificate of coverage, Health Insurance
    Portability and Accountability Act, 1301
Certification of Insurance Rehabilitation
    Specialists Commission, 371
CHAMPUS, 1124–1132
    CHAMPUS Reform Initiative, 1127–1128
    contracted provider arrangement-Norfolk,
        1130
    defined, 1359
    military medical benefits program, 1125–
        1126
Change, xxix, 638. *See also* Patient behavior
    change
    academic health center
        absence process and cost information,
            213
        organizational change barriers, 212–
            213
        traditional culture, 212–213
        transforming traditional culture, 218–
            220
        transition market, 213
    effect of beliefs, 639, 640
    inability to predict, 1347
    measurements, 1354–1355
    physician practice behavior
        active involvement of managers, 627–
            628
        clinical protocol, 629–630
        discipline, 631–633
        feedback, 628–629
        formal continuing medical education,
            628
        general approaches to changing
            behavior, 626–628

practice guidelines, 629–630
programmatic approaches, 628–630
reward effectiveness, 627
sanctions, 627, 631–633
small group programs, 630
stepwise approach to changing behavior, 631
translating goals and objectives, 626–627
rate, 1354
readiness, 638–639
stages, 638–639
Charitable benefit, integrated delivery system, 1247–1248
Chest pain unit, defined, 1359
Chief executive officer, 76
Chief information officer, 77–78
CHIP, defined, 1359
Chronic subacute care, 506–507
Churning, 168
defined, 1359
Civilian Health and Medical Program of the Uniformed Services. See CHAMPUS
Claims and benefits administration, 710–754. See also Coordination of benefits
adjustments, 748–749
benefits administration, 712, 745–746
benefits configuration problems, 752
billing, 740
claims backlog, 751
claims business functions, 743–751
claims business functions reporting, 750–751
claims data, 587–588
claims incurred but not reported (IBNR), 913
balance sheet, 916
claims operations management, 718–729
claims operations management reporting, 749–750
claims payable, balance sheet, 916
claims processing flow, 743, 744
claims scanning, electronic data interchange, 663
common claims problems, 751–753
coordination with other departments, 739, 740
coordinative policies and procedures, 737–739
coverage determination, 14
data file integrity problems, 752
departmental structure, 714–716
determination of liability, 743–745
electronic claims submission, 728–729
eligibility, provider excess loss coverage, 1009–1010, 1016
enrollment, 740
financial administration, 740
inadequate front-end control, 751
informal benefits interpretation, 752–753
information and skills needs, 733
inventory control, 718–721, 722
liability protection, 712–713

management information system, 739–743
claims system information, 742
management reporting, 749–750
medical management policy administration, 712
medical-operational policy, 737–739
member services, 712, 740, 748, 781–783
claims problems compared with service problems, 790–791
opportunities, 713
organizational structure, 713–716, 717
outsourcing claims processing, 753–754
payment
authorization, 334
information system, 658–659
pended claims management, 721–724
inadequate, 751–752
plan contract administration, 711–712
policies and procedures, 737–739
positioning, 711
within managed care organization, 713–714
pricing, 746–748
productivity, 729–731
provider service, 712, 740
purpose, 711–713
quality assessment, 735–737
audit, 735–737
standards, 735
staff development, 732–734
staffing, 716–718
ratios, 718
systems support, 739–743
task allocation, 724–726
outdated, 752
training, 732–734
turnaround time, 731–732
utilization management, 740
utilization management-claims clash, 753
work distribution, 724–726
work flow, 726–728
Claims director, 714, 715
Claims examiner, 716
Claims management, case management compared, 397–398
Claims manager, 714, 715
Claims probability distributions, actuarial services, 973–974
Claims review, utilization management, 323
Claims supervisor, 714, 715
Clayton Act, 1204
Clearinghouse, electronic data interchange, 663
Clinical decision making, risk management, 879
Clinical efficiency benchmarking, actuarial services, 973
Clinical mandates, state law, 1339–1341
Clinical pathway, 521–538
activity/precedent format, 530, 531
advantages, 521
alternative formats, 529–533

application, 528–529
background, 522
development, 525–528
emergency medicine, 362
environment, 524–525
float/slack time, 533
flowchart/network format, 530, 534–535
Gantt chart, 530, 532
resource format, 531–533, 534, 536
results, 533–538
sample uses, 529–533
scopes, 522–524
terminology, 521, 522
uses, 522–524
Clinical protocol, 629–630
Clinical risk, risk management, 878
Clinical trial, managed care organization, 87
Clinton Health Security Act, 832
Closed panel, defined, 1359
Coaching, patient behavior change, 648–649
Coinsurance
defined, 1360
fee for service, 131–132
Coinsurance factor, 1005–1006
Commercial group market
rating, 954–967
underwriting, 954–967
Commission, defined, 1360
Commission for Case Manager Certification, 371
Communication
corporate compliance, 1313–1320
patient behavior change, 646, 647
Community health center, 228–243
background, 229
cost-based reimbursement, 232
delivery system integration, 242
federal funding, 231–232
formation of CHC-sponsored health plans, 237–240
alternative arrangements, 238
brand name, 239
enrollment, 238
financial strength, 238
for-profit vs. not-for-profit, 238
further collaboration among plans, 240
health maintenance organization, 238
investment return, 239
Medicaid, 239
Medicaid marketplace changes, 240
membership base, 239–240
plan characteristics, 238
plan formation, 237
rationale, 237
tensions within provider-sponsored plans, 238–239
governance, 231
history, 230–231
impact of managed care, 240–243
increasing tensions, 230
Integrated Service Network grant, 236
Integrated Services Delivery Initiative, 236

managed care
    operational responses, 234–237
    strategic responses, 234–237
managed care effects, 229–230
Medicaid managed care, 233–234
Medicaid waiver, 233
model, 231
networks, 236–237
practice management network, 236
public policy, 231–233
quality of care, 242
service model, 231
state funding, 232
structural change, 242–243
support, 231–233
technical assistance, 233
Community mental health center, 452, 453
Community outreach program, prevention, 291–292
Community rating, 910
    adjusted community rating, 988–990
    by class, 990–993
    defined, 1360
    demographic factors, 990–992
    Federal Employees Health Benefits Program, 1043, 1046–1048
        adjusted community rating, 1047–1048
        community rating by class, 1047
        traditional, 1047
    health maintenance organization Act, 6–7
    industry factors, 992
    methodologies, 986–994
    simplified community rating, 986–988
    summary, 996–997
Community rating by class, 1047
Companion, home health care, 488
Comparative risk-adjusted clinical outcome
    cost reduction, 570–572
    using control charts for dynamic view of performance, 572, 573, 574, 575
Compensation. *See also* Specific type
    administrative physician, 158–159
    dental health maintenance organization, 1150–1151
    dental preferred provider organization, 1150–1151
    faculty practice plan, 159–160
    hospital-based practitioner, 159
    integrated delivery system, 1248–1249
        physicians, 1248–1249
    medical director, 158–159
    physician, 147–165
        access, 171
        administrative policies and procedures compliance, 171
        after-hours call duty, 169
        attitude, 170
        authorization requirements, 171
        benefits, 157
        closed panel calculation example, 172
        closed panel evaluation categories, 169–170
        dependability, 169

    design alternatives, 153–156
    direct distribution pay plan, 154
    discounted fee-for-service, 178
    distribution of ancillary revenues, 152
    E-commerce, 171
    efficiency, 169
    electronic transaction, 171
    evaluation categories, 168–172
    evaluation system problems, 167–168
    factors considered, 166–167
    fraud and abuse, 152–153
    hospital-based specialist, 159
    information system, 661–662
    leadership, 170
    management of outside resources, 170
    measurement issues, 156
    medical charting, 169
    medical knowledge, 169
    multispecialty group example, 161–162
    nonutilization-based incentive compensation, 166–174
    objective criteria, 167–168
    open panel calculation example, 172–174
    open panel evaluation categories, 170–172
    panel size and status, 171
    participation, 170
    patient care management, 169–170
    patient relations, 170, 171–172
    patient satisfaction, 166, 171–172
    pay plan design issues, 150–153
    performance measure development, 162–163
    plan network use, 171
    practice profile, 167
    precertification requirements, 171
    productivity, 169
    productivity plan, 153–154
    quality, 166
    quality management, 171
    regulatory considerations, 152
    risk level, 151–152
    RVU plan example, 161
    salary plus variable pay plan, 154–156
    salary-only pay plan, 154–155
    staff relations, 170
    Stark regulations, 152
    structure contexts externally managed, 147
    by subgroup, 149
    subjective criteria, 168
    traditional concepts, 148–150
    trend in managed care organization, 620
    utilization, 170
    weighing factors, 172–174
primary care physician, 110–144, 197
    average percentage of contracts reimbursed through capitation, 112
    basic models of reimbursement, 111–113
    capitation, 111

    capitation geographic variation, 112, 113
    direct contract model health plans, 110
    fee for service, 111
    relative value scale, 111
    salary, 111
specialty care physician, 197
    ambulatory patient group, 188
    capitating specialty care physician while paying primary care physician via fee-for-service, 182
    capitation, 187
    contact capitation, 182–183
    diagnosis-related group, 188
    fee allowance schedule, 178–180
    hourly and salary arrangements, 187–188
    models, 178
    performance-based fee-for-service, 180
    relative value scale, 178–180
    resource-based relative value scale, 178–180
    risk and reward, 189
    straight fee-for-service, 178
    subcapitation of specialty care physician by other specialty care physician, 183–184
    types of reimbursement arrangements, 178–184
Competition
    choice-based, 800
    e-commerce
        differentiators, 695–696
        premium compression, 695 696
        price parity, 695–696
    employer, 817–818
    integrated delivery system, covenants not to compete, 1255
Competitive bidding
    Medicare, 1092
    Medicare+Choice, 1092
Complaint, member services, 788–789
Complementary and alternative medicine, 245–263
    consumer, 246–247
    cost, cost-offsets, 256–258
    credentialing, 252–253
        conventional providers who use complementary and alternative medicine therapies, 254–255
        special criteria, 253–254
        unregulated providers, 255
    defined, 1359
    employer, 247
    exploratory integration, 260–263
    federal funding of research, 249–250
    finding complementary and alternative medicine providers, 254
    Health Care Finance Administration, 250
    health maintenance organization, 247
    health system, 258–260
    hospital, 249, 258–260
    managed care strategies, 251

medical education, 248–249
models, 251–258
motivation for coverage, 247–248
National Institutes of Health, 249
network businesses, 252, 253
organizations, 250–251
orientation, 245–251
per member per month pricing, 255–256
physician, 248–249
professions, 250–251
scientific basis, 249–250
stakeholder, 245–251
standards development, 250
utilization, 256–258
Complexly adapting system, attributes, 1348
Comprehensive medical events
management, 1159–1160
Computer technology, 9–10
Computerized medical record, 681–682
Concurrent review
defined, 1360
utilization management, 315–323
Confidentiality, 580, 583–586
data, 684
health care information, 22–23
Health Insurance Portability and
Accountability Act, 583–586, 663–666,
684
information system, 684
provider contract, 1172–1173
Utilization Review Accreditation
Committee, 862–863
Conflict of interest policy, integrated
delivery system, 1246–1247
Congestive heart failure, disease
management, 410, 411
Consolidated medical group, integrated
delivery system, 50–52
Consolidated Omnibus Budget
Reconciliation Act
defined, 1360
Health Insurance Portability and
Accountability Act, 1290
continuation coverage, 1294
Consolidation, 887
managed care organization, 803
Consultant, 805–806
Consumer
communications, 814
complementary and alternative medicine,
246–247
consumer information, Health Care
Finance Administration, 20
Consumer affairs. See Member services
Consumer Assessment of Health Plans
Study 2.0H, National Committee for
Quality Assurance, 857, 860
Consumer Assessment of Health Plans
Survey, 785–786
defined, 1358
Consumer product, innovative, 839
Consumer protection
legislation, 21–22
Medicare+Choice, 1076–1077

Consumerism
accreditation, 833–834
advocacy group, 833–834
alternative care, 839
amenities, 839–842
Balanced Budget Act, 837, 838
branding, 842–843
consumer demand for efficient and
streamlined administrative functions,
844–845
consumer demand for innovative products
and services, 839–843
consumer demand for meaningful
information, 836–839
demographic trends, 829
drivers, 828–835
employer, 818, 824–825, 829–831
empowerment, 843–844
delegation of treatment decisions, 843
demand management, 843
disease management, 843
Internet, 843–844
online self care, 843–844
federal initiatives, 832–833
government purchaser, 831–833
impact, 828–847, 846
implications, 836–845
importance, 828–835
information technology, 834–835
Internet, 834–835
lifestyle benefits, 839
managed care organization consumer
strategy development, 845–846
media, 834
National Committee for Quality
Assurance, 833–834
new health care consumer defined, 835–
836
personal attention, 842
public perception, 834
services to address special needs, 842
societal trends, 835
state initiatives, 833
Contact capitation, 182–183
hospital, 202–203
Contact management, member services,
667–668
Continuing medical education, 628
Continuous quality improvement, 544–554
appropriateness evaluation, 548
benchmarking, 548
comparing results, 550
consumer education, 553–554
defining indicators to measure
performance, 549–550
encounter outcome measures, 546–547
establishing performance expectations,
550
feedback, 550–552
identifying processes and outcomes
meeting customer needs, 546–547
implementing improvements, 552–554
improvement agenda, 554
managing health, 547

model, 288
monitoring performance, 550
outcomes assessment, 548
peer review, 548
practice guidelines, 552–553
provider profile, 550–551
quality improvement teams, 553
quality management matrix, 549
report card, 551–52
screening, 546
service quality, 547
standards comparison, 547–548
treating disease, 546
understanding customer need, 544–546
Continuum of care, behavioral health care,
458–459
Contract, 1165, 1223–1229
clarity, 1165
Employee Retirement Income Security
Act, 1228–1229
general issues, 1166–1167
ideal contract, 1165
patient behavior change, 646
pharmacy benefit management, pharmacy
provider contract, 431–432
physician-health plan contract provisions,
88
renewal, electronic connectivity, 104–105
Contract year, defined, 1360
Contracting
ancillary service, 347–349
faculty practice plan, 99–100
independent practice association, 97–99
integrated delivery system, 98–99
medical group, 97
physician, 97
specialty care physician, 175–178
how many of each type, 175–176
types, 97–100
Contributory plan, defined, 1360
Control, 640, 641
physician practice behavior, 621–623
control of patient care, 622
control of quality, 622–623
where care is received, 622
Conversion, defined, 1360
Cookbook medicine, defined, 1360
Coordination of benefits, 755–770.
See also Claims and benefits
administration
avoidance, 757
characterized, 756
defined, 756, 1359
diversion, 757
group agreement, 758–759
National Association of Insurance
Commissioners, 756
Order of Benefits Determination, 756,
757
organizational placement, 761
procedure, 761–762
provider agreement, 759–760
recovery, 757
requirements, 758–760

staffing, 761
subscriber agreement, 758–759
Coordination of benefits recoverable, 911
Copayment
  defined, 1360
  pharmacy benefit management, 439–444
    physician response to rising
      copayments, 441–442
    relationship to formulary positioning,
      442–443
    tiers, 440, 441, 442
Coping, 640, 641
Corporate compliance, 1306–1320
  audit, 1317–1319
  automated reporting, 1313–1314
  benefits, 1306
  communication, 1313–1320
  compliance committee's responsibilities,
    1308
  compliance office, 1309
  compliance review, 1314–1315
  defined, 1306, 1360
  development, 1311
  education, 1311
  employee exit interview, 1319
  employee hotline, 1319
  employee postemployment interview,
    1319
  incentives, 1311–1312
  investigations, 1319–1320
  leadership, 1309–1311
  legal and regulatory reviews, 1314
  legal and regulatory risk assessment,
    1315–1317, 1318
  measures, 1311–1312
  Office of Inspector General, Department
    of Health and Human Services, 1306–
    1320
  in operation, 1307–1308
  on paper, 1306
  staffing, 1312–1313
  structure, 1308–1309
Corporate compliance committee, 79
Corporate compliance officer, 76, 1306,
  1309
Corporate negligence, risk management,
  876–879
  direct liability, 876–877
  vicarious liability, 877–878
Corporate practice of medicine acts or
  statutes, defined, 1360
Cost, xxix
  academic health center, 207
  aging, 1088
  ambulatory visit, 403–404
  ancillary service, 403–404
  complementary and alternative medicine,
    cost-offsets, 256–258
  employer
    cost-shifting strategies, 818
    how employers purchase value, 820–
      822
    search for value, 822–824
  graduate medical education, 210

home health care, 481–472, 483
  hospice care, 517, 518
  increasing, 803–804
  Medicaid managed care, 1114, 1121
  pharmacy, 804
  physician practice behavior, 619
  prescription drug benefit, 413–415, 416
    cost components, 415–417
  pressures, 677
  provider profile, 600
  technology, 678
  trends, 803–804
  workers' compensation, early controls,
    1155–1157
Cost benefit analysis, case management, 398
Cost control program
  avoiding liability associated with, 883
  risk management, 882–883
Cost sharing
  defined, 1360
  TRICARE, 1127
Cost shifting, defined, 1360
Cost-based reimbursement, community
  health center, 232
Credentialing
  behavioral health care, 472
  case manager, 371
  complementary and alternative medicine,
    252–253
    conventional providers using, 254–255
    special criteria, 253–254
    unregulated providers, 255
  credentialing committee, 78
  data verification, 101, 102
  defined, 1361
  dental health maintenance organization,
    1150
  dental preferred provider organization,
    1150
  direct evaluation of physician's office,
    104
  electronic connectivity, 104–105
  elements, 101, 102
  federal databases, 101–105
  Healthcare Integrity and Protection Data
    Bank, 103–105
  medical record review, 104
  National Committee for Quality
    Assurance, 853
  National Practitioner Data Bank, 101–103
  primary care, 100–105
  provider contract, 1169
  risk management, 878–879
  specialty care physician, 177–178
  Utilization Review Accreditation
    Committee, 864
Credentialing committee, 78
Credentialing verification organization, 100
  certification program, National
    Committee for Quality Assurance,
    857–858
  defined, 1361
  National Committee for Quality
    Assurance, 100–101

Crisis intervention, behavioral health care,
  458
Critical path. *See also* Clinical pathway
  defined, 1361
Cultural bias, 1354
Current Procedural Terminology, 4th
  edition, defined, 1360
Custodial care, defined, 1361
Customer services. *See* Member services

D

Daily hospital log, 592
Data, 579–595
  claims data, 587–588
  confidentiality, 684
  data analysis, member services,
    784–786
  data collection, member services,
    784–786
  elements, 580, 586–590
  encounter-based data, 588
  future of data use, 614–615
  general user needs, 580
  health status questionnaire, 589–590
  measures, 582
  in medical management, 580–583
  medical records-based data, 589
  member survey, 589
  patient satisfaction questionnaire, 589
  prevention, 286, 291
  privacy, 684
  publicly available hospital data, 590
  quality, 582–583
  sample size, 582–583
  security, 684
  sources, 583, 586–590
  time period, 583
  uses, 579
  using system data with other tools,
    580–581
Data warehouse, 590, 669–670
  information system, 679–680
  reporting, 669–670
Date of service, defined, 1361
Days per thousand, defined, 1361
Death spiral, defined, 1361
Decimal dust, defined, 1361
Decision support system, information
  system, 668–669, 682
Deductible, defined, 1361
Deductible carryover, provider excess loss
  coverage, 1009
Deemer clause, 1269
Defined benefit, defined, 1361
Defined contribution, defined, 1361
Delete, defined, 1361
Demand management, 294–298
  return on investment, 296
Demographic cohort, health care
  preferences, 840–841
Demographic shift, home health care, 484
Demonstration project, Federal Employees
  Health Benefits Program, 1056

Denial of coverage
    health maintenance organization, external
        appeals, 1327
    preferred provider organization, external
        appeals, 1327
    state law, external appeals, 1327
Denial of payment, 305–306
    authorization, 336
    member services, 782–783
Dental benefits
    access plan, 1149
    industry, 1148
    referral plan, 1149
Dental health maintenance organization,
    1146–1147
    accreditation, 1152
    compensation, 1150–1151
    credentialing, 1150
    dental delivery system, 1149–1150
    quality improvement, 1151
    recruiting, 1150
    specialty care, 1152
    utilization review, 1151
Dental preferred provider organization,
    1147–1149
    accreditation, 1152
    compensation, 1150–1151
    credentialing, 1150
    dental delivery system, 1149–1150
    quality improvement, 1151
    recruiting, 1150
    specialty care, 1152
    utilization review, 1151
Dental referral plan, 1146
Dependability, 169
Dependent, defined, 1361
Designated admitting physician model,
    utilization management, 321–322
Diagnosis-related group, 188, 603–604
    hospital, 200
Diagnostic and Statistical Manual of Mental
    Disorders, 4th edition, defined, 1362
Diagnostic care group, defined, 1361
Dietition, home health care, 487–488
Differential by day in hospital, 200
Direct access, defined, 1362
Direct contract model
    defined, 1362
    health maintenance organization, 38–39
Direct contracting, defined, 1362
Direct distribution pay plan, 154
Direct mail, advertising, 812
Director of information systems, 77–78
Disability benefits, 157
Disabled, Medicare+Choice, 1097, 1100
Discharge planning
    defined, 1362
    utilization management nurse, 319
Discipline, 631–633
Disclosure, 141–142
    Health Insurance Portability and
        Accountability Act
        group health plans, 1291
        insurers serving small employers, 1291

Discount, 132–133
    outpatient procedures, 204
Discounted fee for service, 178
    subacute care, 500
Disease management, 402–412
    ambulatory visit, 403–404
    ancillary service, 403–404
    barriers, 405
    capabilities, 407
    case management, 399–400
        contrasted, 282
    characteristics specific to, 402–403
    clarification, 402–405
    composing business plan, 405–406
    congestive heart failure, 410, 411
    definition, 402–405
    drivers, 405
    e-commerce, 409–410
    history, 403–405
    linkages, 408–409
    pharmacy benefit management, 444
    prevention, 403
    program elements, 406
    protocol, hospice care, 518–519
    return on investment, 296
    survey of programs, 406–408
Disease management organization, 185
Disenrollment, defined, 1362
Diversion, accounting for, 764–765
Documentation
    Employee Retirement Income Security
        Act, 1257–1259
    provider contract, 1172–1173
Dread disease policy, defined, 1362
Drug formulary
    authorization, 437–438
    decision-making process, 434–435
    defined, 433
    drug access impact, 437–438
    pharmacoeconomics, 435–437
    pharmacy benefit management, 433–438
    selection, 434–435
    state law, 1336
    treatment guidelines, 438
    utilization impact, 437–438
Drug utilization review, 443–444
    pharmacy benefit management,
        443–444
Dual choice, defined, 1362
Dual diagnosis services, behavioral health
    care, 461
Dual option, defined, 1362
Duplicate claims, defined, 1362
Durable medical equipment, defined, 1362

E

E-commerce, 171, 684–687, 688, 689,
    694–709
    brand name, 685–687
    capital markets, 696
    challenges, 707–708
    competition
        differentiators, 695–696

    premium compression, 695–696
    price parity, 695–696
    defined, 694, 1362
    disease management, 409–410
    external impact, 703–705
    functionality, 701–703
    future opportunities, 706–707
    growth, 685
    Health Insurance Portability and
        Accountability Act, Internet-based
        business-to-business growth, 695
    integrated stage, 703
    interactive functionality, 702–703
    internal e-commerce opportunities, 705–
        706
    new distribution channels, 696
    pharmacy benefit management, 421
    semi-integrated functionality, 703
    stages, 688
    static category, 702
    strategy development, 708
    strategy planning, 689
    success factors, 708–709
    technical infrastructure, 709
    technologies, 696–701
    type of information sought by patients,
        685–687, 688
    types, 685, 687
    websites, 685–687
Economic Opportunity Act, 230
Effective date, defined, 1363
Efficiency, 169
    emergency medicine, 357–358
Electronic claims submission, claims and
    benefits administration, 728–729
Electronic commerce. See E-commerce
Electronic communication, member
    services, 779
Electronic connectivity
    contract renewal, 104–105
    credentialing, 104–105
Electronic data interchange, 662–663, 700–
    701
    benefits, 662
    claim scanning, 663
    clearinghouse, 663
    data transmission standards, 662
    defined, 1363
    imaging, 663
    industrywide standards, 662
    pharmacy benefit management, 421
Electronic funds transfer, 699–700
Electronic prescribing, pharmacy benefit
    management, 421–422
Electronic transaction, 171
Eligibility, defined, 1363
Ellwood, Paul, 5–6
Emergency department, defined, 1362
Emergency Medical Treatment and Active
    Labor Act
    defined, 1363
    emergency medicine, 352–355, 358
Emergency medicine, 351–366
    admissions, process, 360–361

areas of conflict, 351
authorization, 352–354
    prudent layperson legislation,
        353–354
clinical pathway, 362
current state, 355–356
definition of emergency, 352
    federal law, 352
efficiency, 357–358
Emergency Medical Treatment and
    Active Labor Act, 352–355, 358
expediting diagnosis and treatment,
    359–360
flexible staffing, 361–362
Health Insurance Portability and
    Accountability Act, 365
improving service, 356–357
Internet, 365
nonurgent (fast track) care, 362–363
opportunities with managed care, 366
patient satisfaction, 356
productivity, 357–358
registration, 358–359
reimbursement, 354–355
state law, 1339
technology impact, 363–365
triage examination, 358
waiting time, 356–357
Employee
    employer-employee relationship, factors
        used in determining, 1252–1253
    rating, 954
    state law, 954
    underwriting, 952–954
        renewal, 953–954
Employee assistance program, 465–466
    defined, 1362
Employee hotline, corporate compliance,
    1319
Employee Retirement Income Security Act,
    1257–1280, 1286, 1302
    administrative services only contract,
        1276
    amendment of plans, 1262–1263
        procedure, 1263
    any willing provider law, 1276–1279
    appeal, 795
    benefit reductions, 1262–1263
    capitated provider contract, 1279–1280
    challenges to benefit denials, 1264–1267
        court action standard of review,
            1266–1267
        jury trial right, 1267
        new disclosure requirements, 1265
        new standards of review, 1265–1266
        new time frames for decision making,
            1265
    civil enforcement, 1267
    claims procedure, 1264–1265
    contract action, 1228–1229
    credentialing, 1272–1273
    defined, 1363
    documentation, 1257–1259
    fiduciary duties, 1263–1264

government reporting requirements,
    1258–1259
liability, 1223, 1224–1225, 1228–1236,
    1337
plan design, 1259–1262
plan document, 1257–1258
plan documentation, discrepancies, 1258
power, 1257
preemption, 1260–1261, 1267–1280
    credentialing, 1272–1273
    deemer clause, 1269
    negligent representations by managed
        care organization to providers, 1273–
        1274
    principles, 1268–1269
    savings clause, 1268–1269
    state insurance regulation, 1275–1280
    utilization review, 1271–1272
    vicarious liability for medical
        malpractice, 1269–1271
remedies, 1267
state law
    distinction between insured and self-
        insured plans, 1260–1261
    plan design, 1260–1261
    preemption, 1260–1261
    preemption limits, 1261
    substantive regulations, 1259–1260
    summary of material modifications, 1258
    summary plan description, 1258
Employer, 817–826
    competition, 817–818
    complementary and alternative medicine,
        247
    consumerism, 818, 824–825, 829–831
    cost
        cost-shifting strategies, 818
        how employers purchase value, 820–
            822
        search for value, 822–824
    employer-employee relationship, factors
        used in determining, 1252–1253
    future trends, 824–825, 826
    Internet, 825
    large group employer, 818–819
    medium group employer, 819
    moderate group employer, 819
    quality, 818
    selection process by size of employer, 819
    small group employer, 820
    technology, 824–825
    trends affecting employers, 817–818
Employer group retiree
    federal preemption, 1073
    Medicare, 1072
    Medicare+Choice, 1072
Employer group underwriting, 983–984
    key data, 984–985
Empowerment, consumerism, 843–844
    delegation of treatment decisions, 843
    demand management, 843
    disease management, 843
    Internet, 843–844
    online self care, 843–844

Encounter, defined, 1363
Encounter-based data, 588
End-of-life care, 508–510
    interdisciplinary approach, 509–510
End-stage renal disease
    Medicare, 1101
    Medicare+Choice, 1101
Enrollee, defined, 1363
Enrollment
    claims and benefits administration, 740
    information system, 659–660
        employer group enrollment, 660
        member enrollment, 660
        provider enrollment, 659–660
    Medicare+Choice
        capacity waiver, 1079
        coordinated open enrollment, 1079,
            1080
        disenrollment, 1079, 1080
        eligibility, 1078
        involuntary disenrollment, 1079
    member services, 783
Enterprise-wide data repository. *See* Data
    warehouse
EO Examination Guidelines Handbook,
    health maintenance organization, 932,
    935–944
Episode of illness, provider profile, 606–
    608, 609
Equity, balance sheet, 917
Equity model, defined, 1363
ERISA. *See* Employee Retirement Income
    Security Act
Ethical issues, hospice care, 513–514
Evidence of coverage, defined, 1363
Evidence of insurability, defined, 1363
Exclusive dealing arrangement, antitrust
    law, 1214
Exclusive provider organization, 32
    defined, 1363
Executive director, 76
Expedited appeals process, 792–793
Experience rating
    defined, 1364
    Federal Employees Health Benefits
        Program, 1046
Experience-rated health maintenance
    organization, 40
Explanation of benefits, defined, 1363
External appeal program
    eligibility decision, 792
    information, 793
    payment, 792
    process, 793
    timeline, 793
Extracontractual benefits, defined, 1364

F

Faculty practice plan
    compensation, 159–160
    contracting situation, 99–100
    defined, 1364

False claims liability, Federal Employees
　Health Benefits Program, 1054–1055
Favored nations discount, defined, 1364
Federal budget surplus, 18
　allocating, 18–19
Federal Employee Health Benefit
　Acquisition Regulations, defined, 1364
Federal Employee Health Benefits Program,
　1043–1058
　appeal, 1051–1054
　application process, 1044
　audit, 1051–1054
　　defending, 1053–1054
　　interest claims, 1054
　　lost investment income, 1054
　　process, 1052–1053
　　settling adverse audit findings,
　　　1053–1054
　benefit design, 1044–1045
　community rating, 1043, 1046–1048
　　adjusted community rating, 1047–1048
　　community rating by class, 1047
　　traditional, 1047
　defined, 1364
　demonstration project, 1056
　enrollment reconciliations with local
　　payroll offices, 1055–1056
　experience rating, 1046
　false claims liability, 1054–1055
　federal preemption of state laws, 1056–
　　1057
　market price, 1044
　Office of Personnel Management,
　　1043, 1054–1055
　　policy on error reporting, 1054–1055
　Patients' Bill of Rights and
　　Responsibilities, 1045
　premium, 1044–1045
　quality assurance, 1057
　rating, 1043, 1045–1051
　　multiple rating region, 1051
　　multiyear contract, 1051
　　similarly sized subscriber group,
　　　1048–1051
　record retention, 1051–1052
　relationship to health maintenance
　　organization, 1043–1058
　state law, state premium taxes, 1057
　tax issues, state premium taxes, 1057
Federal health policy
　forces driving, 17–25
　public opinion shapes, 23–25
Federal qualification
　defined, 1364
　health maintenance organization, 6
Federal Racketeer Influenced and Corrupt
　Organizations Act, 1223
Federal Trade Commission, 1203–1204
Federally qualified health center. See
　Community health center
Fee allowance, 132–133
Fee allowance schedule, 178–180
Fee for service, 178
　defined, 1364
　point of service, 136–137

primary care physician, 129–138
　budgeted fee for service, 136
　categories, 130
　coinsurance, 131–132
　determination of fees, 131
　discount, 132–133
　fee allowance, 132–133
　fee maximum, 132–133
　mandatory reductions in all fees, 136
　negotiated fee schedule, 132–133
　out-of-network fee, 132
　relative value scale, 133–134
　sliding scale individual fee allowances,
　　136
　usual, customary or reasonable, 131
　withhold, 135–136
　resource-based relative value scale, 133–
　　134
Fee maximum, 132–133
Fee revenue, 911
Fee schedule, defined, 1364
Fee schedule analysis, integrated delivery
　system, 972–973
Field marketing, 814
Finance director, 77
Financial administration, 907–922
　background, 907–908
　claims and benefits administration, 740
　failure to reconcile accounts receivable
　　and membership, 898–899
　improper incurred but not reported
　　calculations and accrual methods, 897–
　　898
Financial forecast, budgeting, 919–921
Financial institution, 806–807
Financial management, risk management,
　convergence, 882–883
Financial record, Medicare+Choice, right to
　inspect and evaluate records, 1082
Financial statement
　administrative expenses, 915
　components, 908–915
　medical expenses, 911–915
　operating statement, 908–909
　premium revenue, 909–911
　regulatory reporting considerations, 917–
　　919
Fixed revenue, capitation, 1002
Flat rate, specialty care physician, 188
Flexible benefit plan
　defined, 1364
　Medicare, 1065–1067
Flexible gatekeeper, 93–94
Flexible staffing, 361–362
Flow down clause, provider contract, 1179–
　1180
Formulary, defined, 1364
Foundation, defined, 1364
Foundation model integrated delivery
　system, 57–58
Fraud and abuse, 152–153
　defined, 1364
　Healthcare Integrity and Protection Data
　　Bank, 103–105
　home health care, 492–493

integrated delivery system, 66–67
　preventing, 23, 24
Fraud and abuse, defined, 1364
Full professional risk capitation, 124
　defined, 1364
Full-time equivalent, defined, 1364
Functional independent measure
　home care, 608
　nursing home, 608
　rehabilitation facility, 608

G

GAAP accounting, SAP accounting,
　differences, 918
Gag clause, 88
　defined, 1364
Gainsharing, 159, 160
Gantt chart, clinical pathway, 530, 532
Gatekeeper
　behavioral health care
　　employee assistance program, 465–466
　　mental health/substance abuse case
　　　manager, 466
　defined, 1365
　Medicaid managed care, 1107
　primary care physician, 466
General utilization management, 31
Generally accepted accounting
　principles(GAAP), 908
Generation X, health care preferences,
　840–841
Generation Y, health care preferences,
　840–841
Generic drug
　defined, 1365
　pharmacy benefit management, 438
Geographical area, hospital utilization,
　301–305
Glass-Steagall Act, 1352
Global capitation
　defined, 1365
　integrated delivery system, 62–63
Global fee
　primary care physician, 134–135
　specialty care physician, 188
Governance structure, 73–80
Government purchaser, consumerism,
　831–833
Graduate medical education
　cost, 210
　financing, 14–15
　funding, 210
　Medicare, 210–212
　　Budget Reconciliation Act, 211–212
　　direct medical education payment,
　　　210–211
　　indirect medical education payment,
　　　210–211
Gramm-Leach-Bliley Act, 806, 1352
　defined, 1365
Grievance, 79
　arbitration, 796
　formal grievance procedure, 794–797
　appeal, 795–796

appeal to government agencies, 796
arbitration, 796
filing, 794
investigation, 794–795
health maintenance organization, 1326–1327
lawsuit, 796–797
medical grievance review committee, 79
Medicare+Choice, 1072–1073
member services, 788–789, 794–797
preferred provider organization, 1326–1327
state law, 1326–1327
Group, defined, 1365
Group agreement
coordination of benefits, 758–759
subrogation, 758–759
Group model health maintenance
organization, 35–36
defined, 1365
features, 36
Group practice, defined, 1365
Group practice without walls
defined, 1365
integrated delivery system, 49–50

H

HCFA-1500, defined, 1365
Health and Human Services, defined, 1366
Health and welfare benefits, 157
Health Care Finance Administration
Center for Health Plans and Providers, 1092
complementary and alternative medicine, 250
consumer information, 20
defined, 1365, 1366
Health Insurance Portability and
Accountability Act, industry *vs.* federal
agency interpretations, 1301
Medicare, 1088–1093
physician incentive program, 138–143
Health Care Finance Administration
common procedural coding system, defined, 1365
Health care informatics
features required, 474–475
problems, 473–474
Health care information
confidentiality, 22–23
privacy, 22–23
Health Care Network Accreditation
Program, Joint Commission on
Accreditation of Healthcare
Organizations, 865–866
Health Care Quality Improvement Act, 101, 103
Health care system
chaotic, xxix
complementary and alternative medicine, 258–260
complexity, xxix, 1348
creating strategic portfolio, 1356
defined, 1365

essential nonlinearity, 1348
leadership, 1353–1355
options, 1355–1356
outlook, 25–27
parallel system, 229
payors, 677
sensitivity to initial conditions, 1348–1349
strategy, 1353–1355
uncertainty, 1347
legislative sources of relative
predictability, 1351
legislative sources of relative
unpredictability, 1351–1353
sources of relative predictability, 1350–1351
sources of relative unpredictability, 1351
Health Carrier External Review Model Act, 1327
Health informatics, 297–298
pharmacy benefit management, 418–423
Health insurance
business cycle, 886
history, 4
Health Insurance Association of America, defined, 1366
Health Insurance Portability and
Accountability Act, 22, 980–981, 1285–1304
access, 1287–1293
guaranteed availability for certain
individuals, 1291–1292
standards, 1291
access for small groups, 1303
administration, 1299, 1300
administrative simplication, 1295–1299, 1300
amendments, 1294–1295
applicability, 1287–1288
authorization, 338–339
background, 1286–1287
benefits to individuals, 1301–1303
certificate of coverage, 1301
changing market environment, 1301
confidentiality, 583–586, 663–666, 684
Consolidated Omnibus Budget
Reconciliation Act, 1290
continuation coverage, 1294
crediting prior coverage, 1289–1290
data privacy requirement, 583–586
defined, 1366
disclosure
group health plans, 1291
portability and access standards, 1288
guaranteed availability of coverage to
small employers, 1290–1291
guaranteed renewability of group
coverage, 1290
insurers serving small employers, 1291
limits on preexisting condition
exclusions, 1289
nondiscrimination, 1288
overview, 1286–1287

portability, 1287–1293, 1289–1290
standards, 1291
provisions, 1287–1293
special enrollment periods, 1288–1289
state law, 1287
documenting prior coverage, 1290, 1293
e-commerce, Internet-based business-to-
business growth, 695
effects, 1300–1303
emergency medicine, 365
enforcement, 1299, 1300
federal standards, 1287
group-to-individual portability, 1301–1303
guaranteed renewability of individual
coverage, 1291–1293
Health Care Finance Administration,
industry *vs.* federal agency
interpretations, 1301
health care industry business transactions, 584–585
health insurance tax deduction for self-
employed, 1294
impact on insurers, 1300
medical savings account, 1293
Mental Health Parity Act, 1295
mothers' health, 1294–1295
new access initiatives, 1293
newborn, 1294–1295
privacy, 663–666, 684
referral, 312–313
regulation, industry *vs.* federal agency
interpretations, 1301
releasing job lock, 1303
role of federal government before, 1302
security, 684
state role in implementation, 1329–1330
Women's Health and Cancer Rights Act, 1295
Health maintenance organization, 28–30
access to medical services, 1324
accreditation, 865
complementary and alternative medicine, 247
defined, 1366
denial of coverage, external appeals, 1327
development retarded, 6–7
early, 4–5
enrollment, 3, 35
EO Examination Guidelines Handbook, 932, 935–944
federal qualification, 6
financial examinations, 1329
for-profit, history, 5
grievance, 1326–1327
history, 229
licensure, 1323
models, 33–41
multi-state operations, 1330
National Association of Insurance
Commissioners, 1322–1330
preference changes, 39
preferred provider organization, differences, 8
provider issues, 1324

quality assurance, 1325–1325
removing physicians from network, 107–
  108
reports, 1325
Section 501(c)(3)
  health maintenance organization
    challenge, 931–932
  Internal Revenue Service revocation,
    930–931
site visits, 1329
solvency standards and insolvency
  protections, 1327–1329
state Department of Insurance, minimum
  statutory capital requirements, 918
state law, 1323–1330
state licensure, 6
tax issues
  tax exempt, 926–932
  taxable, 922–926
utilization review, 1325–1325
Utilization Review Accreditation
  Committee, 865
Health Maintenance Organization Model
  Act, 5, 6
  community rating, 6–7
  National Association of Insurance
    Commissioners, 1322
  open enrollment, 6–7
Health Maintenance Organization Research
  Network, 224
Health plan. *See also* Specific type
  defined, 1065
  failures, 887
  market share by type, 10
  selection, sample guidelines, 837
  value-added services, 666–673
Health Plan Employer Data Information Set.
  See HEDIS
Health promotion, member services, 788
Health risk appraisal, 298
  defined, 1365
Health risk-bearing entities
  tax issues, 922–933
  types, 926
Health status, underwriting, 946
Health status questionnaire, data, 589–590
Health telematics, pharmacy benefit
  management, 422–423
Healthcare Integrity and Protection Data
  Bank
  credentialing, 103–105
  fraud and abuse, 103–105
HEDIS, 12, 670–673, 785–786, 802, 850
  characterized, 854
  defined, 859, 1365
  domains of care, 670
  HEDIS Compliance Audit, 860–861
  measures, 671–672, 859
    attributes, 860
  Medicare+Choice, 1074, 1075
  National Committee for Quality
    Assurance, 854–855, 858–861
    consumer survey results, 855
    effectiveness of care, 854

patient satisfaction, 855
performance measurement, 858–861
pharmacy data, 445
HEDIS Compliance Audit, 860–861
Heisenberg Uncertainty Principle, 1349–
  1350
HMO. *See* Health maintenance organization
Hold-harmless clause, provider contract,
  1176
Home health aide, home health care, 488
Home health care, 480–495
  advanced clinical practices, 494–495
  case mix measure, 608
  companion, 488
  cost, 481–472, 483
  decreased availability of informal
    caregivers, 484–485
  defined, 481
  demand indicators and predictors, 482–
    486
  demographic shift, 484
  dietition, 487–488
  disciplines, 486
  financing, 490–492
  fraud and abuse, 492–493
  functional independent measure, 608
  history, 481–482
  home health aide, 488
  homemaker, 488
  infusion service, 486
  legislation, 492–493
  limits of care, 480
  Medicaid
    certification, 489
    Conditions of Participation, 489
  medical equipment and supplies, 486
  Medicare
    certification, 489
    Conditions of Participation, 489
  nursing, 486–487
  occupational therapist, 487
  Operation Restore Trust, 492–493
  Patient Evaluation and Conference
    System, 608
  pharmacist, 487
  physical therapist, 487
  providers, 486, 488
    informal, 484–485
  quality measurement, 493–494
  regulation, 488–490, 492–493
  resource utilization group, 608
  respiratory service, 486
  respiratory therapist, 487
  respiratory therapy, 487
  services, 486
  shrinking hospital system, 484, 485
  social worker, 487
  team, 480
  technology, 486
  utilization management, 326
  volunteer, 488
Homemaker, home health care, 488
Hospice care, 510–519
  agency characteristics, 512–513

care provision, 515
community-based home health agency
  hospice, 516
cost, 517, 518
disease state management protocol, 518–
  519
ethical issues, 513–514
extended care or skilled nursing facility
  affiliation, 516
financing, 511–512
Florida Palliative Home Care Program,
  519
free-standing hospice, 515
future integration and affiliation
  strategies, 519
growth projections, 513, 514
Hospice Care of Rhode Island AIDS Case
  Management Program, 519
hospice in nursing homes, 518
hospital-based hospice, 516
hospital-based hospice home care, 516
industry size, 512–513
legal issues, 514–515
managed care, 512
Medicaid, 511–512
Medicare, 512, 1101–1102
Medicare+Choice, 1101–1102
organization, 511
patient characteristics, 513
pediatric hospice program, 518
philosophy, 510–511
policy issues, 513–515
quality improvement, 514
reimbursement, 511–512
risk management, 514
service models, 515–516
specialty programs, 517–519
staffing, 517, 518
structure, 511
utilization management, 325–326
Zen Hospice Project Residence Program,
  517–518
Hospital
  acquisition, physician practices, 64–65
  bed leasing, 203
  capitation, 197, 201–202
  case rate, 200–201
  cash advance, 203
  complementary and alternative medicine,
    249, 258–260
  contact capitation, 202–203
  diagnosis-related group, 200
  differential by day in hospital, 200
  network development, 191–196
  package pricing, 200–201
  percentage of revenue, 201–202
  performance-based reimbursement, 203–
    204
    penalty, 203–204
    quality incentives, 204
    service incentives, 204
    withhold, 203–204
  periodic interim payment, 203
  provider excess loss coverage, 1005–1010

reimbursement, 196–205
  outpatient procedures, 204–205
  straight charges, 197
  types, 196–205
service-related case rate, 200
sliding scale discount on charges, 198–199
sliding scale per diem, 200
straight discount on charges, 198
straight per diem charge, 199–200
subacute care
  hospital-based skilled nursing facility
    unit, 497–498
  long-term care hospital, 498
  specialty hospital-based subacute
    skilled nursing facility units, 498–499
Hospital contracting, 191–205
  data development, 193
  goal setting, 193–194
  hospital management roles, 195–196
  hospital network development, 191–196
  markets with high managed care
    penetration, 194
  markets with low managed care
    penetration, 193–194
  negotiating strategy, 192–193
  plan management roles, 194–195
  renegotiating existing contracts, 191
  selecting hospital, 192
Hospital report, 592–593
Hospital rounding, utilization management
  nurse, 318
Hospital services, defined, 1017
Hospital utilization
  data, 300–301
  geographical area, 301–305
  variations, 301–305
Hospital-based practitioner, compensation,
  159
Hospital-based specialist, 159
Hospitalist
  defined, 1366
  utilization management, 321–322
Hypertensive management, 649–652

I

Identification card, member services, 783
Imaging, 698–699
  electronic data interchange, 663
Incentive system. *See also* Physician
  incentive program
  nonutilization measures, 166–174
  patient behavior change, 647
  risk management, 882–883
  structures, 974–975
Incurred but not reported, defined, 1366
Indemnification, provider contract, 1177
Indemnity insurance, 30–31
  managed care overlays, 30–31
Independent contractor, integrated delivery
  system, 1251–1255
Independent group model health
  maintenance organization, 36

Independent practice association, 1241
  contracting situation, 97–99
  defined, 1366
  integrated delivery system, 45–47
  removing physicians from network, 107–108
Independent practice association model
  health maintenance organization, 37–38
Individual nongovernment market
  rating, 954
  state law, 954
  underwriting, 952–954
  renewal, 953–954
Information, 828–829
  consumer demand for meaningful
    information, 836–839
  increasing access to, 800–801
  Joint Commission on Accreditation of
    Healthcare Organizations, public
    access, 868
  in medical management, 580–583
  National Committee for Quality
    Assurance, decisions, 855–856
Information dissemination
  Medicare
    coordinated open enrollment, 1078
    plan performance information, 1078
  Medicare+Choice
    coordinated open enrollment, 1078
    plan performance information, 1078
Information economy, 676–677
Information services department, 673–674
  activities, 675
  organizational structure, 673
  purpose, 675
Information sharing, academic health center,
  219–220
Information system, 658–675
  behavioral health care, 473–476
    features required, 474–475
    integration of health care and
      behavioral health care systems, 475–476
  claim payment, 658–659
  confidentiality, 684
  core managed care information system,
    658–662
  data sets, 669–670
  data warehouse, 679–680
  decision support system, 668–669, 682
  enhancers, 669–670
  enrollment, 659–660
    employer group enrollment, 660
    member enrollment, 660
    provider enrollment, 659–660
  enterprise-wide information systems, 680
  information infrastructure, 677
  interconnectivity, 678–679, 680
  knowledge management system, 683–684
  medical management information system,
    668
  pharmacy benefit management, 418–423
  premium billing, 660–661
  privacy, 684

provider reimbursement, 661–662
  security, 684
  value-added services, 666–673
Information technology
  business strategy, 677–678
  capital budgeting, 687–689
  consumerism, 834–835
  managed care organization stakeholders'
    needs, 690
  market need, 677–678
  outsourcing, 691–692
  priorities of health care provider
    organizations, 678
  uses, 680–681
Information technology department
  client relationships, 689–691
  customer teams, 691
  organizational structure, 689–691
  reporting relationships, 689
  service level agreements, 691
Infusion service, home health care, 486
Innovation, 9. *See also* Change
  academic health center, 214–215
  systems inability to manage business,
    901–902
Innovative product, 839
Inpatient care, 579–580
  provider profile, 603–606
    case mix classification systems, 603–606
Institutional utilization management, 313–324
  methods, 314–324
Insurance, provider contract, 1177
Insurance company
  tax issues, 926
  taxable health maintenance organization,
    922–924
Integrated delivery system, 29, 42–71, 803
  accessing marketplace, 69
  accessing revenue, 69
  acquisition, physician practices, 64–66
  actuarial cost modeling, 972
  actuarial services, 971–975
    creating incentive structures, 974–975
    measuring results, 975
  advisory committees, 1245–1246
  antitrust law, 67, 1250–1251
  behavioral health care
    historic structures, 467–468
    importance of planned integrated
      delivery systems, 467
    managed care objectives, 467–469
    move to provider networks, 468–469
    provider structures, 467–469
  change, 71
  charitable benefit, 1247–1248
  committees, 1244–1245
  compensation, 1248–1249
    physicians, 1248–1249
  competition, covenants not to compete,
    1255
  conflict of interest policy, 1246–1247
  consolidated medical group, 50–52

contracting situation, 98–99
core values, 69
critical success factors, 68
defined, 42, 43–44, 1241, 1366
delegated board authority, 1245
evolution, 272
external environment, 69
failures, 887
fee schedule analysis, 972–973
financial administration, 70
foundation model integrated delivery
    system, 57–58
fraud and abuse, 66–67
global capitation, 62–63
goals, 42, 69
governance, 1244
group practice without walls, 49–50
highly integrated delivery systems, 43–44
history, 42
incentives, 71
independent contractor, 1251–1255
independent practice association, 45–47
internal environment, 69
joint venture, 63–64
legal issues, 1241–1256
    pitfalls, 66–68
level of success, 43
licensure, 67–68
management services organization, 56–57
    differences, 1241
managing performance, 70
market characteristics
    heavily penetrated markets, 44
    underpenetrated markets, 44–45
medical group practice, 50–52
medical management, 69
Medicare/Medicaid provider numbers,
    1250
member services, 771–772
models, 1242–1243
nonmedical management, 70
operational integration, 1241–1242
organizational model, 69
performance management, 70
physician ownership model integrated
    delivery system, 59–60
physician practice management
    company independent practice
        association, 47–49
    for-profit, comprehensive physician
        practice management
        company independent practice
        association, 47–48
    specialty physician practice
        management company independent
        practice association, 48–49
physician-hospital organization, 52–56
    closed physician-hospital organization,
        54
    differences, 1241
    open physician-hospital organization,
        53–54
    specialist physician-hospital
        organization, 56

practice acquisition, 1249–1250
private inurement, 66
provider-sponsored organization, 60–62
    licensure, 61
    solvency, 61
    structure, 61
providing insurance function, 63–64
removing physicians from network, 107–
    108
size, 43
staff model integrated delivery system,
    58–59
structural integration, 1242
tax exempt status, 1247–1248
tax issues, 932, 1247–1248
tax-exempt health risk-bearing entity, 932
terminology, 1241
types, 42–43, 45
valuation, 1249–1250
virtual integration, 62
Integrated health care organization, defined,
    1366
Integrated Service Network grant,
    community health center, 236
Integrated services, 799
Integrated Services Delivery Initiative,
    community health center, 236
Intensive care unit, case mix measure, 608
Interactive voice response, 697–698
Interconnectivity, information system, 678–
    679, 680
Interest income, 911
Intermediate care nursing facility, utilization
    management, 324–325
Internal Revenue Service, 922–933
    Revenue Ruling 68-27, 923
    Technical Advice Memorandum 9412002,
        923
    Technical Advice Memorandum 9416001,
        923–924
    Technical Advice Memorandum 9723005,
        925
International Classification of Diseases, 9th
    revision, defined, 1366
Internet, 684–687, 696–697, 801, 843–844
    administration, 844, 845
    brand name, 685–687
    categories of transactions, 701
    consumerism, 834–835
    emergency medicine, 365
    employer, 825
    growth of acceptance, 695
    health plan web site, 666–667
    Medicare+Choice, 1083
    member services, 779
    new distribution channels, 696
    pharmacy benefit management, Internet
        pharmacies, 429–430
    primary care physician, 106–107
        physician interaction with plan, 107
    technology services, 666
    type of information sought by patients,
        685–687, 688
    vs. traditional business rules, 685, 686

Intranet, 697
    member services, 667–668
Inventory control, claims and benefits
    administration, 718–721, 722
Investments, balance sheet, 915

J

Joint Commission on Accreditation of
    Healthcare Organizations, 850, 865–869
    accreditation categories, 868
    cooperative accreditation agreements,
        868–869
    defined, 1367
    document review, 867
    feedback sessions, 867–868
    final on-site survey activities, 868
    function interviews, 867
    Health Care Network Accreditation
        Program, 865–866
    history, 850, 865
    information, public access, 868
    interviews with network leaders, 867
    major initiatives, 868–869
    mission, 850, 865
    opening conference, 867
    ORYX initiative, 869
    scoring compliance against track record
        requirements, 867
    subacute care, defined, 505
    survey
        process, 866–868
        scope, 866
    survey team composition, 867
Joint venture, integrated delivery system,
    63–64

K

Kaiser Permanente/State Compensation
    Insurance Fund of California Alliance
    Project, 1158
Knowledge management
    benefits, 683
    defined, 683
    information system, 683–684

L

Lag study, defined, 1367
Large case management, 31
Large group
    rating, 958–961, 966–967
        degree of community rating, 958–961
        rate structure, 958
    underwriting, 965–966
        eligible enrollees, 957–958
        issue, 955–956
            during plan year, 956–957
        renewal, 957
Lawsuit
    financial penalty, 887
    grievance, 796–797

Leadership, 170
  academic health center, 214–215
  health care, 1353–1355
Learned helplessness, 640, 641
Legal issues
  bad faith action, 1225–1228
  hospice care, 514–515
  integrated delivery system, 1241–1256
    pitfalls, 66–68
  liability, 1221–1239
  medical management activity, 1221–1239
    contract actions related to, 1224–1229
    negligence actions related to, 1229–
      1235
    obligations to conduct, 1222–1223
    recommendations, 1235–1238
  pharmacy benefit management,
    427–428
  provider contract, 1165–1181, 1182–
    1193, 1194
    hospital agreement, 1193–1202
    primary care physician agreement,
      1182–1193
  subrogation, case law, 760–761
Legislation
  consumer protection, 21–22
  financial losses, 887–888
  home health care, 492–493
  managing change, 25–26
  pace of change, 25–26
  physician incentive program, 138–143
  policy decision, 17–27
Length of stay, 84–85
  utilization management, maximum length
    of stay, 316
Letter of intent, provider contract,
  compared, 1166–1167
Liability. *See also* Other party liability
  bad faith action, 1225–1228
  board of directors, 75–76
  claims and benefits administration, 712–
    713
  compensation, civil liability in physician
    compensation programs, 143–144
  Employee Retirement Income Security
    Act, 1223, 1224–1225, 1228–1229,
    1229–1236, 1269–1271, 1337
  legal issues, 1221–1239
  medical management activity
    common law, 1223–1224
    contract actions related to, 1224–1229
    negligence actions related to, 1229–
      1235
    recommendations, 1235–1238
  physician, 84
  state law, 1234–1235
    health plan liability, 1336–1338
Licensure, 61
  health maintenance organization, 1323
  integrated delivery system, 67–68
  preferred provider organization, 1323
  state law, 1323
Lifestyle benefits, consumerism, 839
Line of business, defined, 1367

Loss triangles, 913–914
Low-balling, 891–892

M

Mail, member services, 775
Malpractice, 84
  Employee Retirement Income Security
    Act, 1269–1271
  insurance coverage, 157
Managed Behavioral Healthcare
  Organization, accreditation, 856–857
Managed care
  1985 to present, 9–15
  adolescent years, 5–9
  as big business, 3
  changes in health care organization, 873–
    875
  chaos, 1347–1349
  community health center
    operational responses, 234–237
    strategic responses, 234–237
  continuum, 30
  creating strategic portfolio, 1356
  defined, 1099
  dental benefits, 1146–1153
  enrollment, 29
  feedback, 1349
  future directions, 1346–1356
  future issues, 13–15
  health insurance choices, 82–83
  history, 229
  hospice care, 512
  interplay between public and private
    sectors, 13–14
  market overview, 804
  maturation, 10–12
  myths, 82–88
  overview, 3–15
  pre-1970, 4–5
  predicting federal health program outlays,
    19
  regulatory evolution, 17–27
  restructuring, 12–13
  reversing entropy, 1349–1350
  terminology, 29–30
  variety of organizations, 3
  workers' compensation
    bundling health, disability and workers'
      compensation benefits, 1157–1158
    case studies, 1158, 1160
    changing corporate culture, 1159
    comprehensive medical events
      management, 1159–1160
    employer perspective, 1159
    Kaiser Permanente/State Compensation
      Insurance Fund of California
      Alliance Project, 1158
    product integration, 1158
    success factors, 1157
    toward integration, 1155–1161
    twenty-four hour coverage, 1157–1158
    worker expectations, 1158–1159

Managed care organization
  academic health center
    defining respective roles, 223
    education and training in creating
      value, 223–225
    innovative management techniques,
      224
    long-term benefits, 224
    new role for managed care
      organization, 223–225
    price competition, 224
  basic product, 798–800
  challenges facing, 800–804
  clinical trial, 87
  committees, 78–79
  common problems, 888–903
  components, 799
  consolidation, 803
  consumer strategy development,
    consumerism, 845–846
  consumer/client service function, 814
  defined, 1367
  enrollees' health status, 85
  failure of management to produce or
    understand reports, 899–900
  failure to deal with difficult or
    noncompliant providers, 902–903
  failure to educate and reeducate providers,
    902
  failure to reconcile accounts receivable
    and membership, 898–899
  failure to track correctly medical costs
    and utilization, 900–901
  fee for service problems, 137–138
  growth
    failure to manage reduction in, 894–
      896
    uncontrolled growth, 893–894
  health plan, 814–815
  hubris, 903
  hybrid form, 29
  improper incurred but not reported
    calculations and accrual methods, 897–
    898
  industry profits, 88
  information infrastructure, 677
  key decision makers, 804–807
  key management positions, 76–78
  low-balling, 891–892
  management control structure, 79–80
  overextended management, 899
  ownership of physician practices, 65–66
  physician income, 88
  predatory pricing, 891–892
  process of distribution, 798–816
    alternative distribution, 807
    decision makers, 804–807
    distribution channels, 805–807
    employees, 808
    employers, 807–808
    marketing strategy, 807
    providers, 808
  regulatory reporting considerations, 917–
    919

rural areas, 1133–1144
    Agency for Health Care Policy and
        Research, 1136
    Balanced Budget Act, 1137
    building successful managed care,
        1137–1142
    commitment, 1137–1138
    context, 1135–1137
    critical mass, 1136
    development, 1137
    enrollment, 1134–1135
    financing, 1139
    future directions, 1142–1144
    Heart of America health maintenance
        organization, 1142
    market assessment, 1138
    marketing, 1141–1142
    Marshfield Clinic, 1142
    Medicaid, 1138–1139
    Medicare, 1138, 1142
    Medicare+Choice, 1137
    need for, 1137
    negotiating internally and externally,
        1142
    organization design, 1140
    partnership between local providers and
        commercial insurance entity, 1143
    Physician-Hospital-Community
        Organizations, 1143
    plan design, 1139–1140
    prerequisites for success, 1136–1137
    primary care case management model,
        1135
    provider-sponsored managed care
        plans, 1143
    public policies, 1136
    quality assurance, 1140–1141
    rural provider network, 1143–1144
    status, 1134–1135
    successful, 1134–1135
    unique characteristics, 1133–1134
selection criteria, 830
sensitivity to initial conditions, 1348–
    1349
systems inability to manage business,
    901–902
types, 28–41
underwriting, 977–999
    basic lessons learned, 998–999
    community rating, 986
    failure to use, 896
    historical overview, 977–979
    market factors, 985
    trends, 985
    unrealistic projections, 890–891
Managed Care Plan Network Adequacy
    Model Act, 1324
Managed health care, defined, 1367
Management
    hubris, 903
    management control, 73–80
    overextended management, 899
    systems inability to manage business,
        901–902

Management information system
    claims and benefits administration, 739–
        743
        claims system information, 742
    underwriting, 979–980
Management services organization
    defined, 1369
    integrated delivery system, 56–57
        differences, 1241
    physician-hospital organization,
        differences, 1241
    tax issues, 933
    tax-exempt health risk-bearing entity,
        933
Mandated benefits, defined, 1367
Mandatory external review, defined, 1367
Mandatory outpatient surgery, utilization
    management, 315
Market price, Federal Employees Health
    Benefits Program, 1044
Marketing, 813–814, 1141–1142
    Medicare, 1095
    Medicare+Choice, 1081, 1093, 1095
        description of plan, 1081
        notifications to enrollees, 1081
        prior approval, 1081
        prohibited marketing, 1081
    personnel, 815–816
        compensation, 816
    pharmacy benefit management, 423
    sales, 810
    senior, 1093
Marketing director, 77
Marketing research, 813
Marshfield Clinic, 1142
Master group contract, defined, 1367
Master member index, defined, 1368
Maximum allowable charge, defined, 1367
Maximum out-of-pocket cost, defined, 1367
McCarran-Ferguson Act, 1286
Media, consumerism, 834
Medicaid, 230–231, 1105–1122
    beneficiary growth, 1106
    decrease, 230
    eligibility, 1094–1095
    evolution, 1106–1107
    home health care
        certification, 489
        Conditions of Participation, 489
    hospice care, 511–512
    integrated delivery system, Medicare/
        Medicaid provider numbers, 1250
    Medicaid environment, 1106–1107
    Medicare-Medicaid eligible person,
        1094–1095
    origins, 1106–1107
    reforms, 23
    risk contract, 969–970
        rating, 970
        underwriting, 970
    state health department, 1342
    state social service or welfare department,
        1342
    waiver, community health center, 233

Medicaid managed care, 1107–1122
    access, 1113–1114
    accountability, 1116
    administration
        administrative capacity, 1117
        administrative performance, 1117
        adversarial contracting environment,
            1117–1118
    background, 1107–1108
    choice, 1110–1111
    community health center, 233–234
    compensation, 1112
    contemporary context, 1119–1120
    contractual terms, 1111–1112
    cost, 1114, 1121
    design, 1109–1110
    devolution of authority from federal to
        state governments, 1116
    eligibility, 1110–1111
    enrollment, 1108, 1109, 1110–1111
    future directions, 1120–1122
    gatekeeper program, 1107
    health maintenance organization
        enrollment of beneficiaries, 1107–1108
    implementation, 1109–1110
    models, 1107–1108
    modest savings, 1117
    operational features, 1108–1113
    patient satisfaction
        consumer satisfaction, 1115–1116
        responsiveness, 1115–1116
    planning, 1109–1110
    policy issues, 1120–1122
    political context, 1107, 1120–1121
    primary care case management, 1107
    program models, 1110
    quality of care, 1114–1115
        monitoring, 1112–1113
        oversight, 1112–1113
    rates, 1112
    scarcity of data on outcomes, 1117
    shortfalls, 1116–1119
    special need groups, 1118–1119
    successes, 1113–1116
    sustainable relationships, 1121
Medical advisory committee, 79
Medical charting, 169
Medical consumerism program, 296–297
Medical director, 76–77
    compensation, 158–159
    failure to deal with difficult or
        noncompliant providers, 902–903
    utilization management, responsibilities,
        322–323
Medical education. See also Graduate
    medical education
    academic health center, 206–225
    complementary and alternative medicine,
        248–249
    corporate compliance, 1311
    failure to educate and reeducate providers,
        902
    Medicare, 1096
    Medicare payment, 1069

Medicare+Choice, 1096
physician practice behavior, 620–621
Medical equipment and supplies, home
health care, 486
Medical expenses
financial statement, 911–915
tracking, 900–901
Medical grievance review committee, 79
Medical group, contracting situation, 97
Medical group practice, integrated delivery
system, 50–52
Medical informatics, 297–298
Medical loss ratio
capitation, 1001
defined, 1001, 1367
Medical management
bad faith action, 1225–1228
information system, 668
legal issues, 1221–1239
contract actions related to, 1224–1229
negligence actions related to, 1229–
1235
obligations to conduct, 1222–1223
recommendations, 1235–1238
liability
common law, 1223–1224
contract actions related to, 1224–1229
negligence actions related to, 1229–
1235
recommendations, 1235–1238
policy administration, claims and benefits
administration, 712
practice management, comparison, 283
premium management, comparison, 283
return on investment, 294–295, 296
Medical necessity, 83–84
coverage denial rates, 83–84
decision appeal
eligibility decision, 792
expedited appeals process, 792–793
information, 793
payment, 792–793
Medical policy, defined, 1367
Medical record, 169, 589
computerized medical record, 681–682
consent form, 379
credentialing review, 104
National Committee for Quality
Assurance, 854
Medical savings account, 1063, 1293
defined, 1368
Medicare, 230, 1060–1085
Balanced Budget Act, 1060–1085
choice, 1090–1091
growth, 1090–1091
benefit design, 1095
benefit information form, 1072
capitation, 1067–1072
changing dynamics of delivery system,
1096–1103
competitive bidding, 1092
continuation areas, 1067
cost plan option repeal, 1065
education, 1096

eligibility, 1094–1095
employer group retiree, 1072
end-stage renal disease, 1101
flexible benefits, 1065–1067
government as regulator and competitor,
1091–1092
graduate medical education, 210–212
Budget Reconciliation Act, 211–212
direct medical education payment,
210–211
indirect medical education payment,
210–211
growth, 1089–1090
Health Care Finance Administration,
1088–1093
history, 1060, 1087, 1088–1089
home health care
certification, 489
Conditions of Participation, 489
hospice care, 512, 1101–1102
increasing consumer choices, 19–20
information dissemination
coordinated open enrollment, 1078
plan performance information, 1078
integrated delivery system, Medicare/
Medicaid provider numbers, 1250
marketing, 1095
Medicare-Medicaid eligible person,
1094–1095
member services, 1096
membership geographical distribution,
1094
mid-year benefit change, 1072
minimum enrollment, waiver of
requirement, 1062
part A, 1088
part B, 1089
participation, 1089–1090
payment, 1067–1072
adjusted community rate proposal
requirements, 1070–1071
announcement of rates, 1070
blended rate, 1068–1069
computation of rates, 1070
increases, 1068
limits on charges, 1071
minimum payments, 1068
new entrant bonus, 1069
removal of medical education, 1069
risk adjustment, 1069
supplemental benefits, 1071–1072
user fees, 1069–1071
waiving of charges, 1071–1072
point-of-service plan, 1064–1065
predicting federal health program outlays,
19
preferred provider organization, 1063–
1064
premium support, 19
prescription drugs, 20
pricing, 1095
private fee-for-service plan, 1064
provider-sponsored organizations, 1062–
1063

public policy challenges, 1091
quality of care, 1102–1103
corporate compliance, 1103
quality initiatives, 1103
reforms, 23, 24–25
repeal of 50/50 rule, 1062
retiree, 1094
risk contract, 1087
eligibility, 1061–1062
rating, 968–969
state licensure, 1061–1062
underwriting, 968–969
risk contractors, 11
risk enrollees, 11
sales, 1095
service area, 1065–1067
special groups, 1094–1095
trust fund solvency, 17–19
major areas of development, 21–25
Medicare managed care, TRICARE,
compared, 1131–1132
Medicare supplement, 967–968
rating, 968
underwriting, 968
Medicare+Choice, 626
advance directive, 1072
ancillary provider, 1099–1100
appeal, 1072–1073
Balanced Budget Act, 1086, 1087
benefit design, 1095
benefit information form, 1072
capitation, 1067–1072
care coordinator, 1099–1100
changing dynamics of delivery system,
1096–1103
competitive bidding, 1092
consumer protection, 1076–1077
contacts, 1083
continuation areas, 1067
contract requirements, 1073–1075
contracting process, 1082–1083
modification, 1082–1083
termination, 1082–1083
contractor monitoring, 1081–1082
defined, 1368
disabled, 1097, 1100
education, 1096
employer group retiree, 1072
end-stage renal disease, 1101
enrollment
capacity waiver, 1079
coordinated open enrollment, 1079,
1080
disenrollment, 1079, 1080
eligibility, 1078
involuntary disenrollment, 1079
federal preemption, 1072–1073
federal regulatory requirements, 1092–
1093
financial record, right to inspect and
evaluate records, 1082
future trends, 1083–1085, 1103–1104
government as regulator and competitor,
1091–1092

grievance, 1072–1073
health plan's view, 1086–1104
HEDIS, 1074, 1075
hospice care, 1101–1102
information campaign, 20–21
information dissemination
    coordinated open enrollment, 1078
    plan performance information, 1078
Internet, 1083
marketing, 1081, 1093, 1095
    description of plan, 1081
    notifications to enrollees, 1081
    prior approval, 1081
    prohibited marketing, 1081
member services, 1096
mid-year benefit change, 1072
network design, 1097–1099
payment, 20, 1067–1072, 1087–1088
    adjusted community rate proposal
        requirements, 1070–1071
    announcement of rates, 1070
    average adjusted per capita cost
        payment formula, 20
    blended rate, 1068–1069
    computation of rates, 1070
    increases, 1068
    limits on charges, 1071
    minimum payments, 1068
    new entrant bonus, 1069
    prompt payment to noncontracted
        providers, 1078
    removal of medical education, 1069
    risk adjustment, 1069, 1087
    supplemental benefits, 1071–1072
    user fees, 1069–1071
    variables, 1068
    waiving of charges, 1071–1072
physician incentive plan, 1075–1076
premium tax, 1072–1073
pricing, 1095
provider protections, 1077–1078
public policy challenges, 1091
quality, 1102–1103
    corporate compliance, 1103
    quality initiatives, 1103
quality standards, 1074–1075
    deemed compliance, 1075
    evolving, 1075
    external review, 1075
risk adjustment, 1090
sales, 1095
senior, 1097
    frail elderly, 1100–1101
special populations, 1100
staffing, 1097–1099
state law, preemption, 1072–1073
Medicine, as commodity, 210
Medigap insurance, 1087
    defined, 1368
Member, defined, 1368
Member eligibility, provider excess loss
    coverage, 1031–1032
Member months, defined, 1368

Member rights and responsibilities, 772,
    773–774
    National Committee for Quality
        Assurance, 853–854
Member services, 771–797, 814
    accessing by individual member, 775–779
    appeal, 782–783
        external review of medical necessity
            decisions, 791–794
    claims and benefits administration, 712,
        740, 748
    claims issues, 781–783
        claims problems compared with service
            problems, 790–791
    complaint, 788–789
    contact management, 667–668
    data analysis, 784–786
    data collection, 784–786
    defined, 771
    denial of payment, 782–783
    electronic communication, 779
    enrollment, 783
    functions, 771–772
    grievance, 788–789, 794–797
    health promotion, 788
    hours of availability, 780
    identification card, 783
    integrated delivery system, 771–772
    Internet, 779
    Intranet, 667–668
    mail, 775
    Medicare, 1096
    Medicare+Choice, 1096
    member education program, 786–788
    network access, 783–784
    non-English communication, 780–781
    outreach program, 784
    paper-based communication, 775
    patient satisfaction, 785–786
    primary care physician, selection, 783–
        784
    proactive approaches, 786–788
    provision of general information, 774
    service, 779–780
    service problems, 793–794
    soliciting member suggestions and
        recommendations, 788
    special services and affiliations, 788
    staffing, 774
        automated support, 775
    telephone, 775–779
        automated call distributor, 776
        direct inward dialing, 776
        interactive voice response unit, 776–
            777
        outbound predictive care dialer, 778
        performance standards, 778–779
        toll-free line, 776
        types, 775–778
    training, 772–774
    trends analysis, 786, 787–788
    types of member-specific services, 781–
        784

Member survey, data, 589
Mental Health Parity Act
    behavioral health care, 461
    defined, 1368
    Health Insurance Portability and
        Accountability Act, 1295
Mental health services
    behavioral health care, 460–461
    provider excess loss coverage, 1009
Merger, antitrust law, 1213–1214
Midlevel practitioner
    defined, 1368
    primary care, 95–96
    staffing, 95–96
Mid-year benefit change
    Medicare, 1072
    Medicare+Choice, 1072
Military health system, 1124
    defined, 1368
Mixed model, defined, 1368
Mixed model health maintenance
    organization, 39
Monopolization, Sherman Act, 1215–1219
    attempts to monopolize, 1217–1218
    Health First case, 1218–1219
    monopoly power, 1216
    wrongful conduct, 1216–1217
Monthly summary report, 592
Moral hazard, defined, 1368
Most favored nation clause, antitrust law,
    1214–1215
Multilingual services, 780–781
Multiple employer welfare association,
    defined, 1368
Multiple rating region, 1051
Multispecialty group, defined, 1369
Multiyear contract, 1051

N

National advertising, 814
National Association of Insurance
    Commissioners, 908, 924, 1322
    coordination of benefits, 756
        Order of Benefits Determination, 756,
            757
    health maintenance organization, 1322–
        1330
    Health Maintenance Organization Model
        Act, 1322
    managed care regulation, 1322–1343
    Preferred Provider Arrangement Model
        Act, 1322
    preferred provider organization, 1322–
        1330
National Automated Clearing House
    Association, defined, 1369
National Center for Complementary and
    Alternative Medicine, 249
National Committee for Quality Assurance,
    849, 851–861
    accreditation, 802
        decisions, 855–856

new health plans, 858
review process, 855–858
areas of review, 852
Consumer Assessment of Health Plans
Study 2.0H, 857, 860
consumerism, 833–834
credentialing, 853
credentialing verification organization,
100–101
certification program, 857–858
defined, 1369
HEDIS, 854–855, 858–861
consumer survey results, 855
effectiveness of care, 854
history, 851–852
information, decisions, 855–856
medical record, 854
member rights and responsibilities, 853–
854
performance measurement, 858–861
Physician Organization Certification, 858
preferred provider organization
accreditation program, 857
preventive services, 854
Quality Compass, 861
quality improvement, 852
quality management, 852
reviewers, 852
utilization management, 852–853
National Council for Prescription Drug
Programs, defined, 1369
National Health Services Corps, 232–233
National Institutes of Health
complementary and alternative medicine,
249
Office of Dietary Supplements, 249
National Practitioner Data Bank,
credentialing, 101–103
National Provider Identification, defined,
1369
National Subacute Care Association,
subacute care, defined, 505
Negligence, 1224, 1229–1235
medical management program design,
1229–1230
participating provider
compensation, 1230–1232
selection and supervision, 1230
participating providers, 1230–1234
Negotiated fee schedule, 132–133
Negotiating, hospital contracting, 191–205
Network, capabilities, 799
Network access, member services, 783–784
Network design, Medicare+Choice, 1097–
1099
Network formation, academic health center,
215–216
Network model health maintenance
organization, 36–37
defined, 1369
New entrant bonus, 1069
New Orleans Managed Care Demonstration,
1128

No-balance-billing clause, provider contract,
1176
Noncompliance, physician practice
behavior, 630–633
Non-English communication, member
services, 780–781
Non-health maintenance organization plans,
186–187
Nonparticipating, defined, 1369
Nonphysician practitioner
primary care, 95–96
staffing, 95–96
Nonplan liability claim, 758
Nonurgent (fast track) care, emergency
medicine, 362–363
Notification
provider contract, 1177
provider excess loss coverage, 1030–1031
Nurse advice line, 295
Nursing, home health care, 486–487
Nursing home
case mix measure, 608
functional independent measure, 608
Patient Evaluation and Conference
System, 608
resource utilization group, 608

O

Observation unit, defined, 1369
Obstetrics and gynecology
direct access, 93
primary care, 93
Occupational therapist, home health care,
487
Office of Managed Care, defined, 1370
Office of Personnel Management
appeal, 1051–1054
audit, 1051–1054
defined, 1370
Federal Employees Health Benefits
Program, 1043, 1054–1055
policy on error reporting, 1054–1055
state law, 1342
Office of the Inspector General, defined,
1369
Office staff, orientation, 105, 106
Office-based care, 580
Omnibus Reconciliation Act, defined, 1369
Online self care, 843–844
Online transaction processing system,
pharmacy benefit management, 420
Open access health maintenance
organization, 39–40
authorization, 341–342
Open access plan, report, 593–594, 595
Open enrollment
Health Maintenance Organization Act,
6–7
Medicare+Choice, 1078, 1079
Open enrollment period, defined, 1370
Open panel health maintenance
organization, defined, 1370

Operating statement, financial statement,
908–909
Operation Restore Trust, home health care,
492–493
Operational finance, 907–922
background, 907–908
Operational risk, 875–876
Operations director, 77
Optical character recognition, 698–699
Orientation
office staff, 105, 106
primary care physician, 105
ORYX initiative, Joint Commission on
Accreditation of Healthcare
Organizations, 869
Other party liability, 755–770
accounting for, 763–766
activities, 756
capitation, 766–768
hospitals, 768
physicians, 767–768
characterized, 756
defined, 756
mechanisms, 756
outsourcing, 768–769
policy issues, 766
Outcome
academic health center, 219–220
ambulatory care, 575–578
characterization, 557
comparative risk-adjusted, 570–572
cost reduction, 570–572
criteria for quality assurance, 541–542
outcome measurement, 548, 556–578
behavioral health care, 472–473
comparing risk-adjusted clinical
outcomes, 562–565
data collection, 560–561
data on risk-adjusted costs, 567–570
developing risk-adjustment models,
561–562
development, 559–560
goals, 556–557
measurement domains, 556, 557
measuring comparative risk-adjusted
clinical outcomes, 558–567
performance evaluation, 565–567
risk factors, 559–560
subacute care, 504
using adverse outcome rates to reduce
costs, 570–572
relating clinical outcomes to processes of
care, 572–575
Outdoor advertising, 812
Outlier, defined, 1370
Out-of-area cost per day, provider excess
loss coverage, 1008
Out-of-network cost per day, provider
excess loss coverage, 1008
Out-of-network fee, 132
Out-of-network fee schedule,
provider excess loss coverage,
1012–1013

Outpatient care, 580
  bundled charge, 204
  discounts on charge, 204
  outpatient procedure unit, utilization
    management, 325
  package pricing, 204
  provider excess loss coverage, 1008–1009
    technical services, 1015–1016
  reimbursement, 204–205
  utilization report, 593, 594
  visit, 204–205
Outreach program, member services, 784
Outsourcing
  claims and benefits administration, claims
    processing, 753–754
  other party liability, 768–769
Overpricing, 892–893

P

Package pricing
  defined, 1370
  hospital, 200–201
  outpatient procedures, 204
  specialty care physician, 188
Paper-based communication, member
  services, 775
Par provider, defined, 1370
Patient base maintenance, academic health
  center, 215–218
Patient behavior change, 637–652. *See also*
  Change
  action plans, 646, 648
  coaching, 648–649
  communication, 646, 647
  community systems, 642
  contract, 646
  Humana's CHIP Program, 649–652
  incentive, 647
  models for affecting, 641–646
  patient-provider models, 642–644
  reinforcers, 646–647, 648
  relapse, 644–645
  reminder system, 647
  reward, 647
  social support, 648–649
  stepped model, 644
  system-based models, 641–642
  tools, 646–649
  tracking methods, 646
  worksite models, 645–646
Patient education
  member services, 786–788
  senior, 1096
Patient Evaluation and Conference System
  home care, 608
  nursing home, 608
  rehabilitation facility, 608
Patient Protection Act, 1234
Patient relations, 170, 171–172
Patient satisfaction, 142–143, 171–172
  emergency medicine, 356
  HEDIS, 855

Medicaid managed care
  consumer satisfaction, 1115–1116
  responsiveness, 1115–1116
  member services, 785–786
  new health care consumer defined, 835–
    836
Patient satisfaction questionnaire, 589
  data, 589
Patient satisfaction survey, quality
  management program, 544–546
Patient's rights
  legislation, 871
  Patients' Bill of Rights, 22
  Patients' Bill of Rights and
    Responsibilities, Federal Employees
    Health Benefits Program, 1045
Pattern review, utilization management,
  323–324
Pay and pursue, defined, 1370
Payment. *See also* Reimbursement factor
  ambulatory patient group, 204–205
  ambulatory payment classification, 204–
    205
  ancillary service, 347–349
  emergency medicine, 354–355
  hospice care, 511–512
  hospital, 196–205
    outpatient procedures, 204–205
    straight charges, 197
    types, 196–205
  in-network hospital expenses, 1006
  Medicare, 1067–1072
    adjusted community rate proposal
      requirements, 1070–1071
    announcement of rates, 1070
    blended rate, 1068–1069
    computation of rates, 1070
    increases, 1068
    limits on charges, 1071
    minimum payments, 1068
    new entrant bonus, 1069
    removal of medical education, 1069
    risk adjustment, 1069
    supplemental benefits, 1071–1072
    user fees, 1069–1071
    waiving of charges, 1071–1072
  Medicare+Choice, 20, 1067–1072, 1087–
    1088
    adjusted community rate proposal
      requirements, 1070–1071
    announcement of rates, 1070
    average adjusted per capita cost
      payment formula, 20
    blended rate, 1068–1069
    computation of rates, 1070
    increases, 1068
    limits on charges, 1071
    minimum payments, 1068
    new entrant bonus, 1069
    prompt payment to noncontracted
      providers, 1078
    removal of medical education, 1069
    risk adjustment, 1069, 1087

  supplemental benefits, 1071–1072
  user fees, 1069–1071
  variables, 1068
  waiving of charges, 1071–1072
  outpatient procedures, 204–205
  physician. *See* Physician compensation
  physician-hospital organization, 1175
  provider contract, 1173–1176, 1175
  subacute care, 500–501
  utilization management
    authorization, 305–306
    denial, 305–306
Pediatric hospice program, 518
Peer review, 542, 548
  appropriateness evaluation, 542–543
Peer review organization, defined, 1372
Penalty, 203–204
Pended claims management, claims and
  benefits administration, 721–724
Pended/suspended claim, defined, 1370
Per diem reimbursement
  defined, 1371
  limit, provider excess loss coverage,
    1006, 1007
  subacute care rate, 500, 501, 502
Per employee per month, defined, 1371
Per member per month, 1000
  defined, 1371
  pricing, complementary and alternative
    medicine, 255–256
Per member per year, defined, 1371
Per thousand members per year, defined,
  1372
Percentage of revenue, hospital, 201–202
Performance measurement, 849–870
  academic health center, 219–220
  HEDIS, 858–861
  measurement system, 12
  National Committee for Quality
    Assurance, 858–861
  oversight by type of organization, 850–851
  pharmacy benefit management, 446–447
    budgeting, 446–447
    performance goals, 446–447
    planning, 446–447
Performance-based fee for service, 130,
  136–137, 180
Performance-based reimbursement, hospital,
  203–204
  penalty, 203–204
  quality incentives, 204
  service incentives, 204
  withhold, 203–204
Periodic interim payment
  defined, 1371
  hospital, 203
  specialty care physician, 188–189
Personal attention, consumerism, 842
Personnel
  marketing, 815–816
    compensation, 816
  sales, 815–816
    compensation, 816

Pharmaceutical industry, industry-sponsored clinical research, 208
Pharmaceutical manufacturer discount and rebate contract, pharmacy benefit management, 438–439
Pharmacist, home health care, 487
Pharmacoeconomics, drug formulary, 435–437
Pharmacy
　capitation, 121–122
　cost, 121–122, 804
　services, 344
Pharmacy and therapeutics committee, 79, 433, 434–435
Pharmacy benefit management, 423–426
　authorization, 437–438
　contract, pharmacy provider contract, 431–432
　copayment, 439–444
　　physician response to rising copayments, 441–442
　　relationship to formulary positioning, 442–443
　　tiers, 440, 441, 442
　disease management, 444
　drug formulary, 433–438
　drug utilization review, 443–444
　e-commerce, 421
　electronic data interchange, 421
　electronic prescribing, 421–422
　financial basis, 413–415
　future directions, 447
　generic drug, 438
　genesis, 423–424
　health informatics, 418–423
　health telematics, 422–423
　information system, 418–423
　Internet pharmacies, 429–430
　legal issues, 427–428
　managing supply and demand, 418
　mandatory generic substitution program, 438
　marketing, 423
　medical claims integration, 420
　online transaction processing system, 420
　performance measurement, 446–447
　　budgeting, 446–447
　　performance goals, 446–447
　　planning, 446–447
　pharmaceutical manufacturer discount and rebate contract, 438–439
　pharmacy benefit design, 427
　pharmacy claims adjudication system, 419–420
　pharmacy provider audits, 432–433
　pharmacy provider network, 429–432
　physician dispensing, 430
　physician provider network, 428
　policy and procedure manual, 432
　principles, 415–416
　program components, 426–428
　quality improvement, 444–445
　　HEDIS, 445

retail community pharmacy network, 430–431
　specialized distribution networks, 429–430
Pharmacy benefit management company
　hybrid pharmacy program management using, 425
　rationale, 425
　reintegrating value of pharmacy benefit management services, 425–426
Physical therapist, home health care, 487
Physician. *See also* Specific type
　care management, 272–273
　compensation, 147–165
　　access, 171
　　administrative policies and procedures compliance, 171
　　after-hours call duty, 169
　　attitude, 170
　　authorization requirements, 171
　　benefits, 157
　　closed panel calculation example, 172
　　closed panel evaluation categories, 169–170
　　dependability, 169
　　design alternatives, 153–156
　　direct distribution pay plan, 154
　　distribution of ancillary revenues, 152
　　e-commerce, 171
　　efficiency, 169
　　electronic transaction, 171
　　evaluation categories, 168–172
　　evaluation system problems, 167–168
　　factors considered, 166–167
　　fraud and abuse, 152–153
　　hospital-based specialist, 159
　　information system, 661–662
　　leadership, 170
　　management of outside resources, 170
　　measurement issues, 156
　　medical charting, 169
　　medical knowledge, 169
　　multispecialty group example, 161–162
　　nonutilization-based incentive compensation, 166–174
　　objective criteria, 167–168
　　open panel calculation example, 172–174
　　open panel evaluation categories, 170–172
　　panel size and status, 171
　　participation, 170
　　patient care management, 169–170
　　patient relations, 170, 171–172
　　patient satisfaction, 166, 171–172
　　pay plan design issues, 150–153
　　performance measure development, 162–163
　　plan network use, 171
　　practice profile, 167
　　precertification requirements, 171
　　productivity, 169
　　productivity plan, 153–154

　　quality, 166
　　quality management, 171
　　regulatory considerations, 152
　　relative value unit plan example, 161
　　risk level, 151–152
　　salary plus variable pay plan, 154–156
　　salary-only pay plan, 154–155
　　staff relations, 170
　　Stark regulations, 152
　　structure contexts externally managed, 147
　　by subgroup, 149
　　subjective criteria, 168
　　traditional concepts, 148–150
　　trend in managed care organization, 620
　　utilization, 170
　　weighing factors, 172–174
　complementary and alternative medicine, 248–249
　contracting, 175–178
　　how many of each type, 175–176
　　situation, 97
　income in managed care organization, 88
　liability, 84
　physician-patient interaction, 87–88
　primary *vs.* specialty care designation, 176–177
　provider excess loss coverage, 1010–1016
　requirements per 100,000 population, 176
　restructuring, 817
Physician directory, 106–107
Physician incentive program
　defined, 1371
　Health Care Finance Administration, 138–143
　legislation, 138–143
　Medicare+Choice, 1075–1076
　regulation, 138–143
　　disclosure, 141–142
　　patient satisfaction, 142–143
　　significant financial risk, 139
　　stop loss, 139–141
　state law, 138
Physician Organization Certification, National Committee for Quality Assurance, 858
Physician ownership model integrated delivery system, 59–60
Physician practice, integrated delivery system acquisition, 64–66
Physician practice association, defined, 1371
Physician practice behavior, 618–633
　autonomy, 621–623
　bad habits, 624–625
　change
　　active involvement of managers, 627–628
　　clinical protocol, 629–630
　　discipline, 631–633
　　feedback, 628–629
　　formal continuing medical education, 628

general approaches to changing
  behavior, 626–628
practice guidelines, 629–630
programmatic approaches, 628–630
reward effectiveness, 627
sanctions, 627, 631–633
small group programs, 630
stepwise approach to changing
  behavior, 631
translating goals and objectives, 626–627
control, 621–623
  control of patient care, 622
  control of quality, 622–623
  where care is received, 622
cost, 619
differentiation among competing plans,
  625–626
education, 620–621
environment, 619–620
evolution, 619
importance, 618
noncompliance, 630–633
role conflict, 623
understanding insurance function of plan,
  623–624
understanding of economics, 625
Physician practice management company
  failures, 887
independent practice association, 47–49
integrated delivery system
  for-profit, comprehensive physician
    practice management company, 47–48
  specialty physician practice
    management company, 48–49
Physician profile. See Provider profile
Physician profiling vendor, provider profile
  features, 610, 611
  selection criteria, 610, 611
  services, 610–614
Physician utilization data, 299–300
Physician-hospital organization, 9
defined, 1371
integrated delivery system, 52–56
  closed physician-hospital organization,
    54
  differences, 1241
  open physician-hospital organization,
    53–54
  specialist physician-hospital
    organization, 56
management services organization,
  differences, 1241
payment, 1175
provider contract, 1175
tax issues, 932
tax-exempt health risk-bearing entity, 932
Physician-Hospital-Community
  Organizations, 1143
Physician-owned ancillary service, 345–346
Plan average report, 590–591
PlanID, defined, 1371
Point-of-service, defined, 1371

Point-of-service health maintenance
  organization, 33
Point-of-service plan, 29, 32–33, 127–129
authorization, 334–335
capitation, non-health maintenance
  organization plans, 186–187
fee for service, 136–137
Medicare, 1064–1065
state law, 1330–1331
Policy period, provider excess loss
  coverage, 1009–1010, 1016
Population covered, provider excess loss
  coverage, 1015
Population growth, aging, 509
Powerlessness, 640, 641
Practice guidelines, 552–553, 629–630
risk management, externally imposed, 881
Practice management
  medical management, comparison, 283
  premium management, comparison, 283
Practice management network, community
  health center, 236
Practice profile, 167
Preadmission testing, utilization
  management, 315
Precertification
  defined, 1372
  requirements, 171
  utilization management, 314–315
Predatory pricing, 891–892
Preemption
  employer group retirees, 1073
  Medicare+Choice, 1072–1073
Pre-existing condition, defined, 1372
Preferred Provider Arrangement Model Act,
  National Association of Insurance
  Commissioners, 1322
Preferred provider organization, 28–30, 31–32
access to medical services, 1324
accreditation, 857, 864–865
characteristics, 31–32
defined, 1372
denial of coverage, external appeals, 1327
enrollee information, 1323–1324
enrollment, 3
evolution, 8
fee revenue, 911
financial examinations, 1329
grievance, 1326–1327
health maintenance organization,
  differences, 8
licensure, 1323
Medicare, 1063–1064
multi-state operations, 1330
National Association of Insurance
  Commissioners, 1322–1330
provider issues, 1324
quality assurance, 1325–1325
reports, 1325
site visits, 1329
solvency standards and insolvency
  protections, 1327–1329
state law, 1322–1330

utilization review, 1325–1325
Utilization Review Accreditation
  Committee, 864–865
Premium, Federal Employees Health
  Benefits Program, 1044–1045
Premium billing, information system,
  660–661
Premium management
  medical management, comparison, 283
  practice management, comparison, 283
Premium receivable, balance sheet, 915–916
Premium revenue, 909–911
  financial statement, 909–911
  rating methods, 909
  retroactive billing, 910
  self-billing, 910
Premium source group report, 591–592
Premium support, 19
Premium tax, Medicare+Choice,
  1072–1073
Prenatal care, 87
Prescription drug, Medicare, 20
Prescription drug benefit, 413–447
  cost, 413–415, 416
    cost components, 415–417
Prevention, 283–293
  clinical preventive services, 285
  clinical setting, 287–291
  community programs, 286, 291
  creating prevention systems, 290–291
  data system, 286, 291
  disease management, 403
  environmental preconditions, 290
  evolutionary stage of local health care
    marketplace, 285, 286
  goals, 287
  health data systems, 285–286
  importance, 285
  managed care organization benefits, 285
  National Committee for Quality
    Assurance, 854
  need for, 285
  population-based (member) programs,
    286, 291
  prevention system processes, 289
  preventive care, defined, 1372
  preventive program, 799
  primary vs. secondary prevention, 290
  public policy, 286, 292
  services, 298
  typology, 285–286
Pricing
  claims and benefits administration,
    746–748
  Medicare, 1095
  Medicare+Choice, 1095
Primary care
  academic health center, 216–217
  credentialing, 100–105
  midlevel practitioner, 95–96
  nonphysician practitioner, 95–96
Primary care case management, 11–12
  defined, 1370
  Medicaid managed care, 1107

Primary care physician, 93–108
  capitation, 110, 111, 112–127
    age, 114–115
    benefits reductions, 127
    capitation payment calculation, 114
    capitation pool, 118–121
    carve-out, 116
    chance, 126
    copayment levels, 127
    effect of benefits design on
      reimbursement, 127–129
    financial risk, 116–118
    full professional risk capitation, 124
    gender, 114–115
    inappropriate underutilization, 126
    individual *vs.* pooled risk, 122–124
    institutional services, 118–121
    medical expenses for which primary
      care physician is not at risk, 121
    pharmacy costs, 121–122
    point-of-service plan, 127–129
    problems with, 126–127
    reasons to capitate, 125–126
    referral, 118–121
    reimbursement per visit, 126
    reimbursement variation by product, 129
    reinsurance, 121–122
    risk/bonus arrangement, 118
    scope of covered services, 113–114
    service risk, 116–118
    stop-loss, 121–122
    variation factors, 114–116
    withhold, 117, 118
  compensation, 110–144, 197
    average percentage of contracts
      reimbursed through capitation, 112
    basic models of reimbursement, 111–
      113
    capitation, 111
    capitation geographic variation, 112, 113
    direct contract model health plans, 110
    fee for service, 111
    relative value scale, 111
    salary, 111
  defined, 1370
  fee for service, 129–138
    budgeted fee for service, 136
    categories, 130
    coinsurance, 131–132
    determination of fees, 131
    discount, 132–133
    fee allowance, 132–133
    fee maximum, 132–133
    mandatory reductions in all fees, 136
    negotiated fee schedule, 132–133
    out-of-network fee, 132
    relative value scale, 133–134
    sliding scale individual fee allowances,
      136
    usual, customary or reasonable, 131
    withhold, 135–136
  gatekeeper
    behavioral health care, 466
    flexible gatekeeper, 93–94

global fee, 134–135
Internet, 106–107
  physician interaction with plan, 107
member services, selection, 783–784
network maintenance, 105–106
orientation, 105
primary *vs.* specialty care designation,
  176–177
recruiting, 94–95
  access needs, 94–95
  closed panel access needs, 95
removing physicians from network, 107–
  108
requirements per 100,000 population, 176
resource-based relative value scale, 133–
  134
role, 93
specialty physicians as primary
  physicians, 310–311
in specialty services management, 307–
  309
utilization management, hospital, 319–
  320, 320–321
Primary care preferred provider
  organization, 32–33
Print advertising, 812
Privacy
  data, 684
  health care information, 22–23
  Health Insurance Portability and
    Accountability Act, 663–666, 684
  information system, 684
Private fee-for-service plan, Medicare, 1064
Private inurement
  defined, 1372
  integrated delivery system, 66
Process criteria, quality assurance, 540–541
Product mix, 799
Productivity, 169
  claims and benefits administration, 729–
    731
  emergency medicine, 357–358
Productivity measure, 156, 162
Productivity-based pay plan, 153–154
Professional expense account, 157
Professional services agreement, defined,
  1372
Profit
  stabilization, 886
  volatility, 886
Prospective review
  defined, 1372
  utilization management, 314–315
Protected health information, defined, 1371
Provider. *See also* Specific type
  defined, 1065, 1372
  failure to deal with difficult or
    noncompliant providers, 902–903
  failure to educate and reeducate providers,
    902
  payment, information system, 661–662
Provider contract
  acceptance of enrollee patients, 1172
  annual calendar, 1166

  closing, 1180
  common clauses, 1168–1180
  confidentiality, 1172–1173
  contract structure, 1167–1168
  coordination of benefits, 759–760, 1175–
    1176
  credentialing, 1169
  declarations, 1180
  definitions, 1168–1169
  documentation, 1172–1173
  enrollee complaints, 1172
  flow down clause, 1179–1180
  hold-harmless clause, 1176
  indemnification, 1177
  insurance, 1177
  key factors, 1168–1180
  key objectives, 1166
  legal issues, 1165–1181, 1182–1193,
    1194
    hospital agreement, 1193–1202
    primary care physician agreement,
      1182–1193
  letter of intent, compared, 1166–1167
  names, 1168
  negotiating salary, 1167
  no-balance-billing clause, 1176
  nondiscriminatory requirements, 1171
  notification, 1177
  other-party liability, 1175–1176
  payment, 1173–1176
  physician-hospital organization, 1175
  provider obligations, 1169–1173
  provider qualifications, 1169–1170
  provider services, 1170–1171
  provider subcontracts, 1179–1180
  provisions, 1168–1180
  quality management, 1171–1172
  recitals, 1168
  relationship of parties, 1176
  risk sharing, 1174–1175
  subrogation, 759–760, 1175–1176
  suspension, 1177–1179
  table of contents, 1168
  term, 1177–1178
  termination, 1177–1179
  use of name, 1177
  utilization management, 1171–1172
Provider excess loss, defined, 1370
Provider excess loss coverage, 1000–1039.
  See also Stop-loss coverage
  administration of claims, 1029–1030
  aggregate coverage, 1004
  aggregate excess rate development, 1023–
    1025
  average daily maximum, 1006, 1007
  cancellation, 1029
  carrier expense ratio, 1010, 1016
  catastrophic losses, 1003
  changes to provider agreement, 1029
  claims eligibility, 1009–1010, 1016
  coverage availability, 1032
  deductible carryover, 1009
  effective date, 1016
  eligible service, 1025–1026

experience-specific, 1016–1023
process, 1016–1023
in-network average cost per inpatient day, 1007–1008
in-network definition, 1026–1027
in-network fee schedule, 1011
in-network services, 1011
limitations, 1028–1029
loss reporting guidelines, 1030, 1031
manual hospital-specific rating, 1005–1010
manual physician-specific rating, 1010–1016
member eligibility, 1031–1032
mental health, 1009
notification, 1030–1031
out-of-area cost per day, 1008
out-of-area emergency, 1028
out-of-network, 1028
cost per day, 1008
fee schedule, 1012–1013
outpatient services, 1008–1009
technical services, 1015–1016
paid definition, 1028
per diem limit, 1006, 1007
policy coverage form, 1025–1032
policy period, 1010, 1016
policy provisions, 1029–1030
population covered, 1015
premium change, 1029
proof of loss, 1031, 1032
provider risk contracting, 1003–1004
referral, 1028
reimbursement factor, 1005–1006, 1011
reported definition, 1028
reporting eligibility of claims, 1029–1030
resource-based relative value, 1011–1012, 1013–1014
responsibility matrix, 1025–1028
sample policy language, 1034–1039
specific coverage, 1004
specific excess rate development, 1004–1016
subrogation, 1030
substance abuse, 1009
target loss ratio, 1010, 1016
termination, 1029
totally confined, 1028
types, 1004
of care facilities defined, 1025
of population covered, 1006–1007
variables affecting manual specific rating, 1004–1005
Provider network, 799
antitrust law, 1207–1211
anticompetitive effects, 1209–1210
efficiencies, 1211
exclusive physician networks, 1208
foreclosure, 1210
networks falling outside of safety zones, 1208–1209
nonexclusive physician networks, 1208
per se, 1209–1211
physician union, 1211–1213
recent cases, 1211

risk sharing, 1208
rule of reason, 1209–1211
safety zones, 1207–1208
behavioral health care, 466–467
scope, 466–467, 468–469
selection criteria, 467, 468
size, 466–467, 468–469
Provider profile, 163, 164, 550–551, 580, 595–614
ambulatory payment classification, 602–603, 604
case mix, 600–610
characteristics, 597–600
cost, 600
data elements, 586–587
defined, 580
episode of illness, 606–608, 609
individual physician, 591
inpatient care, 603–606
case mix classification systems, 603–606
limitations, 595
physician profiling vendor
features, 610, 611
selection criteria, 610, 611
services, 610–614
principles, 595–596
provider identification, 597–598
public vs. internal disclosure, 596–597
quality improvement, 595
resource intensity, 601
scientific criteria, 599
severity of illness, 600–610
severity of service, 601
specialty identification, 598–599
statistical technique, 599–600
comparison to norm, 599–600
treatment difficulty, 601
users of, 596
uses, 595
Provider relations, 814
Provider risk contracting, provider excess loss coverage, 1003–1004
Provider services, claims and benefits administration, 712, 740
Provider-sponsored organization, 1243–1244
defined, 1372
integrated delivery system, 60–62
licensure, 61
solvency, 61
structure, 61
state law, 1331–1332
Psychiatric hospitalization, behavioral health care, alternatives, 458
Psychotherapy, behavioral health care, 458
Public perception, consumerism, 834
Public policy, prevention, 286, 292

Q

QISMC, defined, 1372
Quality, 83, 799–800, 801–802
community health center, 242
employer, 818
employer quality measures, 802

Medicaid managed care, 1114–1115
monitoring, 1112–1113
oversight, 1112–1113
Medicare, 1102–1103
corporate compliance, 1103
quality initiatives, 1103
Medicare+Choice, 1102–1103
corporate compliance, 1103
quality initiatives, 1103
role in employer contracting decisions, 14
technology, 678
Quality assurance, 1140–1141
behavioral health care, 469–473
external monitoring, 470–472
inservice training, 472
network providers, 470
provider credentialing, 472
staff qualifications, 472
utilization criteria, 471–472
Federal Employees Health Benefits Program, 1057
health maintenance organization, 1325–1343
outcome criteria, 541–542
peer review, 542
appropriateness evaluation, 542–543
preferred provider organization, 1325–1343
process criteria, 540–541
state law, 1325–1343
structure criteria, 539–540
traditional, 539–543
Quality Compass, 861
Quality improvement
dental health maintenance organization, 1151
dental preferred provider organization, 1151
hospice care, 514
National Committee for Quality Assurance, 852
pharmacy benefit management, 444–445
HEDIS, 445
provider profile, 595
quality improvement system for managed care, defined, 1372
Quality management committee, 78
Quality management program, 171, 539–554, 864
components, 543–544
continuous improvement, 544–554
appropriateness evaluation, 548
benchmarking, 548
comparing results, 550
consumer education, 553–554
defining indicators to measure performance, 549–550
encounter outcome measures, 546–547
establishing performance expectations, 550
feedback, 550–552
identifying processes and outcomes that meet customer need, 546–547
improvement agenda, 554
improvement implementation, 552–554

managing health, 547
monitoring performance, 550
outcomes assessment, 548
peer review, 548
practice guidelines, 552–553
provider profile, 550–551
quality improvement teams, 553
quality management matrix, 549
report card, 551–552
screening, 546
service quality, 547
standards comparison, 547–548
treating disease, 546
National Committee for Quality
 Assurance, 852
process model, 544–554
provider contract, 1171–1172
satisfaction survey, 544–546
Quality measurement
claims and benefits administration, 735–
 737
audit, 735–737
standards, 735
home health care, 493–494
maturation, 12
Quality standards, Medicare+Choice, 1074–
 1075
deemed compliance, 1075
evolving, 1075
external review, 1075
Qui tam sui, defined, 1373

R

Radio, advertising, 812
Rate, defined, 1373
Rating, 947–951, 952
commercial group market, 954–967
common to most markets, 945–954
data sources, 950
employee, 954
Federal Employees Health Benefits
 Program, 1045–1051
multiple rating region, 1051
multiyear contract, 1051
similarly sized subscriber group, 1048–
 1051
formula, 949–950
base rate development, 947–949
conversion of rates from member to
 employee, 950
management report, 951
retention, 950
functions by market, 952–970
individual nongovernment market, 954
large group, 958–961, 966–967
degree of community rating, 958–961
rate structure, 958
Medicaid risk contract, 970
Medicare risk contract, 968–969
Medicare supplement, 968
self-employed individual, 954
small group, 958–961, 964–965
degree of community rating, 958–961

National Association of Insurance
 Commissioners model laws,
 964–965
rate structure, 958
renewal, 965
state regulations, 964–965
Reasonable layperson standard, defined, 1373
Rebundlers, defined, 1373
Record retention
audit, 1051–1052
Federal Employees Health Benefits
 Program, 1051–1052
Recovery, accounting for, 766
Recruiting
dental health maintenance organization,
 1150
dental preferred provider organization,
 1150
primary care physician, 94–95
access needs, 94–95
closed panel access needs, 95
Referral
capitation, 118–121
dental benefits, 1149
Health Insurance Portability and
 Accountability Act, 312–313
prohibition, 311
review of reasons for, 311–313
self-referrals by members, 313
utilization management, 306
Registration, emergency medicine,
 358–359
Regulation
Health Insurance Portability and
 Accountability Act, industry *vs.* federal
 agency interpretations, 1301
home health care, 488–490, 492–493
managed care organization, regulatory
 reporting considerations, 917–919
managing change, 25–26
pace of change, 25–26
physician incentive program, 138–143
disclosure, 141–142
patient satisfaction, 142–143
significant financial risk, 139
stop loss, 139–141
policy decision, 17–27
regulatory pressure, 802–803
underwriting, 980–981
Rehabilitation facility
case mix measure, 608
functional independent measure, 608
Patient Evaluation and Conference
 System, 608
resource utilization group, 608
Reimbursement factor, provider excess loss
 coverage, 1005–1006, 1011
Reinsurance, 1000
capitation, 121–122
defined, 1373
Reinsurance recoverable, 911
Relative risk, by managed care structure,
 875–876
Relative value scale, 178–180
Relative value unit, defined, 1374

Reminder system, patient behavior change,
 647
Report, 579–595. *See also* Specific type
ad hoc reports, 581
application, 586–590
authorization, 341
case management, 382–383
concurrent review reports, 388–392
preadmission reports, 388–392
daily hospital log, 592
failure of management to produce or
 understand reports, 899–900
format, 581
future of data use, 614–615
general user needs, 580
hospital report, 592–593
individual physician, 591
monthly summary report, 592
open access plan, 593–594, 595
outpatient utilization report, 593, 594
plan average report, 590–591
premium source group report, 591–592
routine reports, 581
specialty-focused hospital-based report,
 592–593
types, 590–594
Report card, 551–552
academic health center, 219–220
Reproductive health services, 87
Reserves, defined, 1373
Resource intensity, provider profile, 601
Resource utilization group
home care, 608
nursing home, 608
rehabilitation facility, 608
Resource-based relative value scale, 178–
 180
defined, 1373
fee for service, 133–134
primary care physician, 133–134
provider excess loss coverage, 1011–
 1012, 1013–1014
Respiratory service, home health care, 486
Respiratory therapist, home health care, 487
Respiratory therapy, home health care, 487
Retainer, specialty care physician, 187
Retroactive billing, premium revenue, 910
Retrospective review
defined, 1373
utilization management, 323–324
Return on investment
case management, 296
demand management, 296
disease management, 296
medical management program, 294–295,
 296
Revenue, pressures, 677
Revenue Ruling 68-27, 923
Risk adjustment, Medicare+Choice, 1090
Risk contract, defined, 1373
Risk financing, 883
Risk management, 871–885
California, 871–872
capitation, 882
case law, 879–880

clinical decision making, 879
clinical risk, 878
corporate negligence, 876–879
  direct liability, 876–877
  vicarious liability, 877–878
cost control program, 882–883
credentialing, 878–879
defined, 1373
evolution, 871–872
external environmental assessment, 873, 874
financial management, convergence, 882–883
hospice care, 514
incentive payment system, 882–883
internal environment assessment, 873
key measures of success, 873, 874
multi-site challenges, 881–882
objectives, 872
operational risk, 875–876
practice guidelines, externally imposed, 881
standards of care, externally imposed, 881
utilization management, 879
  reducing utilization management exposure, 880–881
Risk pool deficit allocation, capitation, 1002–1003
Risk pool liability, balance sheet, 916–917
Risk pool profit allocation, capitation, 1002
Risk sharing, 1208
  provider contract, 1174–1175
Risk-adjusted practice profiling tool, 168
Risk-based capital, defined, 1373
Risk/bonus arrangement, 118
Role conflict, physician practice behavior, 623
Rounding physician model, utilization management, 321–322
Rule of small numbers, defined, 1374
Rural areas, managed care organization, 1133–1144
  Agency for Health Care Policy and Research, 1136
  Balanced Budget Act, 1137
  building successful managed care, 1137–1142
  commitment, 1137–1138
  context, 1135–1137
  critical mass, 1136
  development, 1137
  enrollment, 1134–1135
  financing, 1139
  future directions, 1142–1144
  Heart of America health maintenance organization, 1142
  market assessment, 1138
  marketing, 1141–1142
  Marshfield Clinic, 1142
  Medicaid, 1138–1139
  Medicare, 1138, 1142
  Medicare+Choice, 1137
  need for, 1137

negotiating internally and externally, 1142
organization design, 1140
partnership between local providers and commercial insurance entity, 1143
Physician-Hospital-Community Organizations, 1143
plan design, 1139–1140
prerequisites for success, 1136–1137
primary care case management model, 1135
provider-sponsored managed care plans, 1143
public policies, 1136
quality assurance, 1140–1141
rural provider network, 1143–1144
status, 1134–1135
successful, 1134–1135
unique characteristics, 1133–1134

S

Salary plus variable pay plan, 154–156
Salary-only pay plan, 154–155
Sales
  closing, 811
  communications, 814
  consumer sale, 811
  marketing, 810
  Medicare, 1095
  Medicare+Choice, 1095
  needs, 809
  personnel, 815–816
    compensation, 816
  process, 809–812
  proposal, 809–811
  prospecting, 809
  sales function, 813
  target opportunities, 809
  underwriting, collaboration, 979, 984
  underwriting risk, 809
Same-day surgery, utilization management, 315
Sanction, 627, 631–633
SAP accounting, GAAP accounting, differences, 918
Screening, 546
Second opinion, 380–381
  defined, 1374
Section 1115 waiver, defined, 1374
Section 501(c)(3), health maintenance organization
  Internal Revenue Service revocation, 930–931
  organization challenge, 931–932
Section 501(m), tax exempt health maintenance organization, after enactment, 927–930
Security
  data, 684
  Health Insurance Portability and Accountability Act, 684
  information system, 684

Self-billing, premium revenue, 910
Self-care, 296–297
  defined, 1374
Self-efficacy, 639–640
Self-employed individual
  rating, 954
  state law, 954
  underwriting, 952–954
    renewal, 953–954
Self-funded plan
  defined, 1374
  state law, 1333–1334
Self-insured health maintenance organization, 40
Self-insured plan, 819, 820
  defined, 1374
Senior client
  characterized, 1086
  demographics, 1088
  education, 1096
  health care options, 1087–1088
  health care preferences, 841
  marketing, 1093
  Medicare+Choice, 1097
    frail elderly, 1100–1101
Senior executive, hubris, 903
Sentinel effect, defined, 1374
Service area, defined, 1374
Service bureau, defined, 1374
Service plan, defined, 1374
Service-related case rate, hospital, 200
Severity of illness, provider profile, 600–610
Severity of service, provider profile, 601
Shadow pricing, defined, 1374
Shared decision-making program, 297
Sherman Act
  concerted conduct, 1205
    inferring, 1206–1207
  monopolization, 1215–1219
    attempts to monopolize, 1217–1218
    Health First case, 1218–1219
    monopoly power, 1216
    wrongful conduct, 1216–1217
  per se illegality, 1205–1206
  rule of reason, 1206
  Section 1, 1205–1207
  Section 2, 1215–1219
  vertical and horizontal restraints, 1206
Shock claim, defined, 1374
Shoe box effect, defined, 1375
Significant financial risk, defined, 1374
Similarly sized subscriber group, 1048–1051
Single point of entry, defined, 1375
Single specialty management, 185
Skilled nursing facility, subacute care, 498
Sliding scale discount on charges, hospital, 198–199
Sliding scale per diem, hospital, 200
Small group
  rating, 958–961, 964–965
    degree of community rating, 958–961
    National Association of Insurance Commissioners model laws, 964–965

rate structure, 958
renewal, 965
state regulations, 964–965
underwriting, 961–964
eligible enrollees, 957–958
issue, 955–956, 961–964
during plan year, 956–957, 964
renewal, 957, 964
Smoking, 637, 643–644
Social Security, trust fund solvency, 17–19
major areas of development, 21–25
Social support, patient behavior change,
648–649
Social worker, home health care, 487
Southeast Region Preferred Provider
Organization Project, 1129–1130
Specialty care
academic health center, 217–218
access, 86
dental health maintenance organization,
1152
dental preferred provider organization,
1152
utilization management, 306–309
authorization system, 307
definition of specialist services, 306
methods, 307
primary care physician role, 307–309
selection of referral and consulting
providers, 306
Specialty care physician
authorization, 342
bundled case rate, 188
capitation
carve-out, 187
common problems, 186–187
contact capitation, 182–183
disease management organization, 185
financial risk, 187
geographic distribution, 184
management of referral volume, 186
organizational models, 184–186
organized groups, 184
potential to increase utilization, 186
by primary care physician choice, 186
single specialty management, 185
specialty independent practice
association, 184
specialty network manager, 185
subcapitation of specialty care
physician by other specialty care
physician, 183–184
case rate, 188
cash advance, 188–189
compensation, 197
ambulatory patient group, 188
capitating specialty care physician
while paying primary care physician
via fee-for-service, 182
capitation, 187
contact capitation, 182–183
diagnosis-related group, 188
discounted fee-for-service, 178

fee allowance schedule, 178–180
hourly and salary arrangements, 187–
188
models, 178
performance-based fee-for-service, 180
relative value scale, 178–180
resource-based relative value scale,
178–180
risk and reward, 189
straight fee-for-service, 178
subcapitation of specialty care
physician by other specialty care
physician, 183–184
types of reimbursement arrangements,
178–184
credentialing, 177–178
flat rate, 188
global fee, 188
package pricing, 188
periodic interim payment, 188–189
as primary physicians, 177
retainer, 187
specialty physicians as primary
physicians, 310–311
Specialty health maintenance organization,
40–41
Specialty independent practice association,
184
Specialty network manager, defined, 1375
Specialty utilization management, 31
Specialty-focused hospital-based report,
592–593
Speech language pathologists, home health
care, 487
Staff model health maintenance
organization, 34–35
defined, 1375
Staff model integrated delivery system, 58–
59
Staff relations, 170
Staffing
authorization, 337–338
claims and benefits administration, 716–
718
development, 732–734
ratios, 718
coordination of benefits, 761
corporate compliance, 1312–1313
emergency medicine, flexible staffing,
361–362
hospice care, 517, 518
Medicare+Choice, 1097–1099
member services, 774
automated support, 775
midlevel practitioner, 95–96
nonphysician practitioner, 95–96
subrogation, 761
utilization management, 316
Utilization Review Accreditation
Committee, staff qualifications
standards, 863
Stakeholder, complementary and alternative
medicine, 245–251

Standards of care, risk management,
externally imposed, 881
Stark regulations, 152
defined, 1375
State attorney general, 1203–1204
State Department of Insurance, health
maintenance organization, minimum
statutory capital requirements, 918
State health department, 1341
Medicaid, 1342
State insurance department, 1341
State law, 1322–1343
access to medical services, 1324
access to specialty care, 1335–1336
administrative services only, 1334
antitrust law, physician antitrust
exemptions, 1338
any willing provider law, 1334–1335
clinical mandates, 1339–1341
denial of coverage, external appeals, 1327
Department of Defense, 1342
Department of Health and Human
Services, 1341–1342
Department of Labor, 1341
drug formulary, 1336
emergency care, 1339
employee, 954
Employee Retirement Income Security
Act, 1224
distinction between insured and self-
insured plans, 1260–1261
plan design, 1260–1261
preemption, 1260–1261
preemption limits, 1261
enrollee information, 1323–1324
Federal Employees Health Benefits
Program, 1056–1057
state premium taxes, 1057
financial examinations, 1329
grievance, 1326–1327
Health Insurance Portability and
Accountability Act, 1287
health Insurance Portability and
Accountability Act, 1329–1330
health maintenance organization, 1323–
1330
individual nongovernment market, 954
liability, 1234–1235
health plan liability, 1336–1338
licensure, 1323
managed care legislation, 1334–1341
mandated benefits, 1339–1341
Medicaid, mandatory health maintenance
organization enrollment programs,
1108
Medicare+Choice, preemption, 1072–
1073
multi-state operations, 1330
Office of Personnel Management, 1342
physician incentive program, 138
point-of-service plan, 1330–1331
preemption, state insurance regulation,
1275–1280

preferred provider organization, 1322–
1330
provider issues, 1324
provider-sponsored organization, 1331–
1332
quality assurance, 1325–1325
regulation by market segment, 1341–1343
regulation of managed care, 1322–1343
regulatory agencies, 1342–1343
reports, 1325
self-employed individual, 954
self-funded plan, 1333–1334
site visits, 1329
solvency standards and insolvency
protections, 1327–1329
specialty health maintenance
organization, 1332
third-party administrator, 1333
utilization review, 1325–1325
as practice of medicine, 1338–1339
utilization review organization, 1333
State licensure
health maintenance organization, 6
Medicare risk contract, 1061–1062
State of domicile, defined, 1375
State regulation, accounting policy, 907–908
State social service or welfare department,
Medicaid, 1342
State tax, state premium tax, 925
Statistical technique, provider profile, 599–
600
comparison to norm, 599–600
Statutory accounting practices (SAP), 908
Step-down unit, utilization management,
325
Stop-loss coverage, 139–141. *See also*
Provider excess loss coverage
capitation, 121–122
defined, 1375
Straight discount on charges, hospital, 198
Straight fee for service, 130
Straight per diem charge, hospital, 199–200
Strategic sales goals, 802
Structure criteria, quality assurance, 539–
540
Subacute care, 496–507
accreditation, 501–502
capitation, 501
case management, 503–504
categories, 496, 506–507
chronic subacute care, 506–507
clinical staff, 503
continuum of care, 499, 500
defined, 496
discounted fee for service, 500
future sites, 499
general subacute care, 506
hospital
hospital-based skilled nursing facility
unit, 497–498
long-term care hospital, 498
specialty hospital-based subacute
skilled nursing facility units, 498–
499

Joint Commission on Accreditation of
Healthcare Organizations, defined, 505
long-term transitional subacute care, 507
National Subacute Care Association,
defined, 505
outcomes measurement, 504
patients, 496–497
payment, 500–501
per diem rate, 500, 501, 502
programs of care, 502–503
provider selection, 501–504
providers, 497–499
skilled nursing facility, 498
transitional subacute care, 506
Subacute care facility, defined, 1375
Subacute care nursing facility, utilization
management, 324–325
Subauthorization, 336–337
Subrogation, 757
defined, 1375
group agreement, 758–759
legal issues, case law, 760–761
organizational placement, 761
procedure, 763
provider agreement, 759–760
provider excess loss coverage, 1030
staffing, 761
subscriber agreement, 758–759
Subscriber. *See also* Member
defined, 1375
Subscriber agreement
coordination of benefits, 758–759
subrogation, 758–759
Substance abuse
behavioral health care
alternatives to restrictive treatment, 458
services, 459–460
provider excess loss coverage, 1009
Survivor benefits, 157
Suspension, provider contract, 1177–1179
Sutton's law, defined, 1375

T

TAM. *See* Technical Advice Memorandum
Target loss ratio, provider excess loss
coverage, 1010, 1016
Tax Equity and Fiscal Responsibility Act,
defined, 1375
Tax exempt health maintenance
organization, 927–932
Section 501(m), after enactment, 927–930
Tax issues, 922–933
Federal Employees Health Benefits
Program, state premium taxes, 1057
health maintenance organization
tax exempt, 926–932
taxable, 922–926
insurance company, 926
integrated delivery system, 932, 1247–
1248
management service organization, 933
physician-hospital organization, 932
state premium tax, 925

unrelated business income, 933
Tax Reform Act, Section 501(m), 927
Taxable health maintenance organization,
922–926
accrued claim liability, 924–925
status as insurance company, 922–924
withhold arrangement, 925–926
Tax-exempt health maintenance
organization, Internal Revenue Service
guidelines on examinations, 932
Tax-exempt health risk-bearing entity
integrated delivery system, 932
management service organization, 933
physician-hospital organization, 932
unrelated business income, 933
Technical Advice Memorandum 9412002,
923
Technical Advice Memorandum 9416001,
923–924
Technical and Miscellaneous Revenue Act,
928
Technology, 828–829
cost, 678
employer, 824–825
home health care, 486
quality of care, 678
systems inability to manage business,
901–902
Technology assessment, 14
Telephone
member services, 775–779
automated call distributor, 776
dirct inward dialing, 776
interactive voice response unit, 776–
777
outbound predictive care dialer, 778
performance standards, 778–779
toll-free line, 776
types, 775–778
telephone rounding, utilization
management nurse, 317–318
telephone-based case management, 374–
375
Television, advertising, 812
Temporary Assistance to Needy Families,
defined, 1375
Termination, provider contract, 1177–1179
Termination date, defined, 1375
Texas Health Care Liability Act, 1234–1235
Theory of self-efficacy, 639–640
efficacy expectancy, 640
outcome expectancy, 640
Third-party administrator
defined, 1376
state law, 1333
Third-party recovery, 757
contractual support, 758–760
requirements, 758–760
Time loss management, defined, 1375
Training, 472
academic health center, 206–225
claims and benefits administration, 732–
734
member services, 772–774

Treatment difficulty, provider profile, 601
Treatment guidelines, drug formulary, 438
Trends analysis, member services, 786, 787–788
Triage
    defined, 1376
    emergency medicine, 358
TRICARE, 1124–1132
    beneficiary assistance, 1127
    benefits, 1126
    cost sharing, 1127
    defined, 1376
    eligibility, 1126
    future directions, 1132
    history, 1124
    legal authority, 1125
    managed care demonstrations, 1127–1130
    managed care support contracts, 1131
    Medicare managed care, compared, 1131–1132
    military medical benefits program, 1125–1126
    options, 1126
    origins, 1127–1130
    program, 1130–1131
    responsibilities, 1125
Triple option, defined, 1376
Turfing, 168
Turnaround time, claims and benefits administration, 731–732
Twenty-four hour care, defined, 1376
Twenty-four hour coverage program, case management, 399

U

UB-92, defined, 1376
Unbundling, defined, 1376
Undercapitalization, 888–890
Underwriting, 945–947
    ability to pay, 946
    administrative service only underwriting, 997
    benefit plan compatibility, 996
    commercial group market, 954–967
    common to most markets, 945–954
    defined, 1376
    demographic factors, 981
        norms, 996
    economic factors, 981
    effective, 997–999
    employee, 952–954
        renewal, 953–954
    employee eligibility, 995
    employee out-of-pocket cost, 996
    employee participation, 995
    employee-employer relations, 995
    employer group, 983–984
        key data, 984–985
    employer stability, 994–995
    enrollment factors, 981–982
    failure to use, 896
    functions by market, 952–970
    health status, 946

high-risk groups, 995
individual nongovernment market, 952–954
    renewal, 953–954
industry factors, 982
as internal control, 982–983
large group, 965–966
    eligible enrollees, 957–958
    issue, 955–956
    during plan year, 956–957
    renewal, 957
major risk factors, 981–982
managed care organization, 977–999
    basic lessons learned, 998–999
    community rating, 986
    historical overview, 977–979
    market factors, 985
    trends, 985
management information system, 979–980
Medicaid risk contract, 970
Medicare risk contract, 968–969
Medicare supplement, 968
minimum contract size, 996
other coverage, 946
during plan year, 947
premium differential, 995–996
presistency, 946–947
principles, 994–997
probability, 982
provider practices, 982
regulation, 980–981
at renewal, 947
sales, collaboration, 979, 984
selection factors, 982
self-employed individual, 952–954
    renewal, 953–954
small group, 961–964
    eligible enrollees, 957–958
    issue, 955–956, 961–964
    during plan year, 956–957, 964
    renewal, 957, 964
    summary, 996–997
underwriting cycle, 886
Unearned premium, balance sheet, 916
Unfair competition law, enforcement, 1203–1204
Uninsured person, 14–15
    increase, 230
Unrelated business income
    tax issues, 933
    tax-exempt health risk-bearing entity, 933
Upcoding, defined, 1376
U.S. Department of Defense
    managed care programs, 1124–1132
    state law, 1342
U.S. Department of Health and Human Services
    defined, 1366
    Office of Inspector General, corporate compliance, 1306–1320
    state law, 1341–1342
U.S. Department of Justice, Antitrust Division, 1203–1204

U.S. Department of Labor, state law, 1341
Usual, customary or reasonable, 131
    defined, 1376
Utilization
    complementary and alternative medicine, 256–258
    hospital utilization data, 300–301
    measurements, 298–301
    physician utilization data, 299–300
    tracking, 900–901
    variations, 301–305
Utilization management, 294–327, 799. *See also* Utilization review
    alternatives to acute care hospitalization, 324–326
    behavioral health care, 463–464, 469–470
    case management
        concurrent review, 384–388
        concurrent review reports, 388–392
        preadmission review, 384–388
        preadmission review reports, 388–392
    claims and benefits administration, 740
        utilization management-claims clash, 753
    claims review, 323
    concurrent review, 315–323
    designated admitting physician model, 321–322
    e-commerce, 305
    home health care, 326
    hospice care, 325–326
    hospitalist model, 321–322
    institutional utilization management, 313–324
        methods, 314–324
    intermediate care nursing facility, 324–325
    mandatory outpatient surgery, 315
    maximum length of stay, 316
    medical director, responsibilities, 322–323
    National Committee for Quality Assurance, 852–853
    outpatient procedure unit, 325
    pattern review, 323–324
    payment
        authorization, 305–306
        denial, 305–306
    preadmission testing, 315
    precertification, 314–315
    primary care physician, hospital, 319–320, 320–321
    prospective review, 314–315
    provider contract, 1171–1172
    referral, 306
    retrospective review, 323–324
    risk management
        reducing utilization management exposure, 880–881
        risk management, 879
    rounding physician model, 321–322
    same-day surgery, 315
    specialty care, 306–309
        authorization system, 307
        definition of specialist services, 306

methods, 307
primary care physician role, 307–309
selection of referral and consulting
    providers, 306
staffing, 316
step-down unit, 325
subacute care nursing facility, 324–325
workers' compensation, 31
Utilization management nurse, 316–319
discharge planning, 319
follow-up, 319
hospital rounding, 318
information gathering, 317
review against criteria, 318–319
telephone rounding, 317–318
Utilization review, 83–84. *See also*
    Utilization management
coverage denial rates, 83–84
dental health maintenance organization,
    1151
dental preferred provider organization,
    1151
Employee Retirement Income Security
    Act, 1271–1272
health maintenance organization, 1325–
    1325
history, 8
preferred provider organization, 1325–
    1325
state law, 1325–1325
    as practice of medicine, 1338–1339
Utilization Review Accreditation
    Commission, 850
defined, 1376
Utilization Review Accreditation Committee
accessibility, 863
accreditation, 864–865, 865
    member protection, 864
    network management standards, 864
    process, 862
    provider credentialing, 864
    quality management, 864

appeal, 863
confidentiality, 862–863
credentialing, 864
governance, 861–862
health maintenance organization, 865
health utilization management standards,
    862–863
history, 850, 861–862
preferred provider organization, 864–865
program qualifications, 863
staff qualifications standards, 863
Utilization review committee, 79
Utilization review organization
defined, 1376
state law, 1333

V

Valuation, integrated delivery system, 1249–
    1250
Value proposition, care management, 279
Value-added products and services, 799
Vicarious liability, 877–878
Virtual integration, integrated delivery
    system, 62
Virtual merger, antitrust law, 1213–1214
Visit, outpatient procedures, 204–205
Voice response unit, 697–698
Volunteer, home health care, 488

W

Waiting time, emergency medicine, 356–
    357
Wellness program, case management, 398–
    399
Well-woman care, 87
Wickline v. State of California, 879–880

Wilson v. Blue Cross of California, 880
Withhold arrangement, 117, 118, 135–136,
    203–204
taxable health maintenance organization,
    925–926
Women's Health and Cancer Rights Act,
    Health Insurance Portability and
    Accountability Act, 1295
Women's health care, 86–87
cancer, 86–87
Workers' compensation
benefits, 1154–1155
case management, developing protocols,
    1159
cost
    early controls, 1155–1157
    origin of social contract, 1154
defined, 1376
managed care
    bundling health, disability and workers'
        compensation benefits, 1157–1158
    case studies, 1158, 1160
    changing corporate culture, 1159
    comprehensive medical events
        management, 1159–1160
    employer perspective, 1159
    Kaiser Permanente/State Compensation
        Insurance Fund of California
        Alliance Project, 1158
    product integration, 1158
    success factors, 1157
    toward integration, 1155–1161
    twenty-four hour coverage, 1157–1158
    worker expectations, 1158–1159
utilization management, 31
Worksite wellness program, 8–9
Wraparound plan, defined, 1377

Z

Zero down, defined, 1377